Principles and
Practice of
Geriatric Medicine

Principles and Practice of Geriatric Medicine

Edited by

M. S. J. Pathy

Department of Geriatric Medicine
University of Wales College of Medicine

A Wiley Medical Publication

JOHN WILEY & SONS
Chichester · New York · Brisbane · Toronto · Singapore

British Library Cataloguing in Publication Data:

Pathy, M.S.J.
   Principles and practice of geriatric medicine.
   1. Geriatrics
   I. Title
   618.97   RC952

ISBN 0 471 10346 2

Library of Congress Cataloging in Publication Data:
Main entry under title:

Principles and practice of geriatric medicine.

   (A Wiley medical publication)
   Includes index.
   1. Geriatrics—Addresses, essays, lectures. I. Pathy,
M. S. J. II. Series. [DNLM: 1. Geriatrics. WT 100 P957]
RC952.P73 1985   618.97   83–17115
ISBN 0 471 10346 2

Typeset by Input Typesetting Ltd, London SW19 8DR
Printed and bound in Great Britain by the Bath Press Ltd, Bath, Avon

List of Contributors

J. N. Agate CBE MD FRCP

Formerly of the Department of Geriatric Medicine
The Ipswich Hospital
Ipswich, UK.

Sir Ferguson Anderson MD FRCP

Rodal
Moor Road
Strathblane
Glasgow, UK

Joan Andrews MD FRCOG FRCS

Consultant Gynaecologist
St. David's Hospital
Cardiff, UK

K. Andrews MD MRCP

Consultant Geriatrician and Honorary Lecturer in
Geriatric Medicine
University Hospital of South Manchester
Manchester, UK.

A. Azcona MD

Clinical Research
Sandoz Ltd.,
4002 Basle
Switzerland

A. K. Banerjee FRCP

Honorary Lecturer in Geriatric Medicine
University of Manchester and
Consultant Physician
Department of Medicine for the Elderly
Bolton General Hospital
Gt. Manchester, UK.

D. Bellamy DPhil

Professor of Zoology
University College
Cardiff, UK

J. E. Birren PhD

Executive Director
Ethel Percy Andrus Gerontology Center
University of Southern California, USA

Eda T. Bloom PhD

Geriatric Research, Education and Clinical Center
Veteran's Administration,
Los Angeles, California, USA

D. Coakley MD FRCPI

Consultant Physician in Geriatric Medicine
St. James' Hospital
Dublin, Eire

Gillian Cole DPM MD MRCPath

Senior Lecturer in Neuropathology
University of Wales College of Medicine
Cardiff, UK.

P. Courpron MD

Maison de Sante et de Cure Medicale Antoine
Charial
Francheville, France

J. R. Cox MD FRCP MRCGP MRCPsych

Consultant Physician
Department of Medicine
Nether Edge Hospital
Sheffield, UK.

A. C. Crisp BA BPhil MEd ABPsS

Principal Clinical Psychologist
Liverpool Health Authority and
Part-time Lecturer
Department of Psychology
University of Liverpool, UK

D. L. Crosby FRCS

Consultant Surgeon
University Hospital of Wales
Cardiff, UK

Ann D. M. Davies BA PhD Dip Psych FB PaS

Senior Lecturer in Psychology
University of Liverpool, UK

B. H. Davies MB BCh MRCP

Consultant Physician and Director
Asthma Research Unit
Sully Hospital
Penarth, UK.

Ena Davies MCST

Senior Lecturer
Cardiff School of Speech Therapy
South Glamorgan Institute of Higher Education
Cardiff, UK

T. J. Deeley FRCR Director
South Wales Radiotherapy and Oncology Service
Velindre Hospital
Cardiff, UK

M. J. Denham MD FRCP
Consultant Physician in Geriatric Medicine
Northwick Park Hospital and Clinical Research
Centre
Harrow, UK

M. Devas MChir FRCS
Professor of Orthopaedics
University Sains Malaysia
Miden
Penang, Malaysia

M. J. Dew MD MRCP
Senior Registrar in Medicine
Bridgend General Hospital
Bridgend, UK

M. Druguet MD
Maison de Sante et de Cure Medicale Antoine
Charial
Francheville, France

Joyce D. Edwards PhD MSc MCST
Chief Speech Therapist
St. David's Hospital
Cardiff, UK

A. N. Exton-Smith MD FRCP
Barlow Professor of Geriatric Medicine
University College
London, UK

D. J. Farrar MS FRCS
Consultant Urologist
Selly Oak Hospital
Birmingham, UK

T. Gibson MD FRCP
Consultant Physician
Department of Rheumatology
Guy's Hospital
London, UK

P. A. Graham FRCS
Consultant Ophthalmologist
University Hospital of Wales
Cardiff, UK

J. A. Muire Gray MD
Community Physician
Radcliffe Infirmary
Oxford, UK

M. F. Green MA FRCP
Consultant Physician
Department of Geriatric Medicine
Princess Elizabeth and King Edward VII Hospitals
Guernsey

R. A. Griffiths BM FRCP MRCGP
Consultant Physician in Geriatric Medicine
Radcliffe Infirmary
Oxford, UK

M. R. P. Hall MA BM FRCP
Professor of Geriatric Medicine
Southampton General Hospital
Southampton, UK

M. Hildick-Smith MD FRCP
Consultant Physician in Geriatric Medicine
Nunnery Fields Hospital
Canterbury, UK

S. P. Hodgson MB ChB MRCPsych
Consultant Psychogeriatrician
Withington Hospital
Manchester, UK

H. M. Hodkinson MA DM FRCP
Barlow Professor of Geriatric Medicine
University College London and Middlesex Hospital
Joint School of Medicine
St Pancras Hospital
London

B. Isaacs MD FRCP
Charles Hayward Professor of Geriatric Medicine
Selly Oak Hospital
Birmingham, UK

R. A. Jackson MD MRCP
Consultant Physician
Highlands Hospital
London, UK

D. J. Jolley MB BS DPM FRCPsych
Consultant Psychogeriatrician
Withington Hospital
Manchester, UK

A. Kalache MD MSc MCFM
Department of Community Medicine and General
Practice
University of Oxford, UK

B. A. Kottke MD PhD
Professor of Medicine
Mayo Medical School
Rochester, Minnesota, USA

R. W. Lindsay MD

*Professor of Medicine and
Head
Division of Geriatric Medicine
University of Virginia, USA*

B. Livesley MD MRCP

*Department of Clinical Gerontology
St. Francis' Hospital
London, UK*

T. Makinodan PhD

*Director of Geriatric Research
Education and Clinical Center
West Los Angeles VA Medical Center
California, USA*

R. Marks MB BSc FRCP MRCPath

*Professor of Dermatology
University of Wales College of Medicine
Cardiff, UK*

F Meacher MRCPI

*Research Fellow
Department of Clinical Pharmacology
Royal College of Surgeons of Ireland
Dublin, Eire*

R. G. S. Mills FRCS

*Senior Lecturer and
Consultant
University Hospital of Wales
Cardiff, UK*

J. S. Morris MD FRCP

*Consultant Physician and
Gastroenterologist
Bridgend General Hospital
Bridgend, UK*

W. O'Callaghan MD FRCPI

*Department of Clinical Pharmacology
Royal College of Surgeons in Ireland
Dublin, Eire*

J. Ohmura MD

*Visiting Professor
Teikyo University
School of Medicine
Tokyo, Japan*

K. O'Malley MD FRCPI

*Professor of Clinical Pharmacology
Royal College of Surgeons in Ireland
Dublin, Eire*

P. W. Overstall MB MRCP

*Consultant in Geriatric Medicine
The General Hospital
Hereford, UK*

The late **Sir Alan Parks** MD MCh FRCS
MRCP

*Consultant Surgeon
St Marks Hospital and the London Hospital
London, UK*

M. S. J. Pathy FRCP

*Professor of Geriatric Medicine
University of Wales
College of Medicine
Cardiff, UK*

K. Persson

*Research Associate
Texas Research Institute of Mental Sciences
Houston, USA*

W. J. Peterson

*Education and Clinical Center
West Los Angeles VA Medical Center
California, USA*

G. A. D. Rees MB BCh FFARCS

*Consultant Anaesthetist
University Hospital of Wales
Cardiff, UK*

J. Runcie MB ChB FRCP

*University Department of Geriatric Medicine
University of Glasgow, UK*

T. Samorajski PhD

*Chief
Neurobiology Section
Texas Research Institute of Mental Sciences
Houston, USA*

W. A. Shalaby MD MRCP

*Consultant Physician in Geriatric Medicine
Tickhill Road Hospital
Doncaster, UK*

R. J. Shephard MD PhD

*Director
School of Physical and Health Education and
Professor of Applied Physiology
University of Toronto, Canada*

R. Spiegel PhD

*Clinical Research
Sandoz Ltd
Basel, Switzerland*

B. Steen MD PhD

*Professor of Geriatric Medicine
Lund Universty
Malmö, Sweden*

viii

M. Takasugi PhD
Department of Surgery
University of California
Los Angeles, USA

P. S. Timiras MD PhD
Professor of Physiology
University of California
Berkely, USA

D. M. Walker MD FDSRCS MRCPath
Department of Oral Medicine and Oral Pathology
University of Wales College of Medicine
Cardiff, UK

S. G. P. Webster MD MA MRCP
Consultant Physician
Department of Geriatric Medicine
Addenbrooke's Hospital
Cambridge, UK

Ruth B. Weg PhD
Associate Professor of Biology/Gerontology
Ethel Percy Andrus Gerontology Center
University of Southern California
Los Angeles, USA

B. O. Williams MD FRCP
Consultant Geriatrician
Gartnavel General Hospital
Glasgow, UK

J. Williamson MB ChB FRCPE
Professor of Geriatric Medicine
University of Edinburgh, UK

Anita, Woods
Texas Research Institute of Mental Sciences
Houston, USA

P. O. Yates MD FRCPath
Professor of Neuropathology
The University
Manchester, UK

T. T. Yoshikawa MD
Chief
Division of Geriatric Medicine
Veterans Administration
Los Angeles, USA

Contents

Preface

In some parts of the world, notably Europe, North America and Japan, the impact of an expanding elderly population resulting from an era of unprecedented reduction in the diseases of early life has already had a dramatic effect on the epidemiology of disease. Within the foreseeable future no nation will escape a similar increase in the number of its elderly citizens with similar changes in the disease profile of its society. In the developed industrial nations Governments and medical schools, recognizing this phenomenon, are increasingly encouraging teaching and research in the medicine of later life. The objective of this textbook, written by authors of international repute, is to provide in a single volume a comprehensive reference source for all who are involved in the medicine of old age. Some overlap with textbooks of general medicine is inevitable but appropriate emphasis and attention is given to those disorders which are of particular relevance to the elderly.

Whilst this is primarily a clinical textbook, an account is given of the fundamental changes associated with ageing which are so inextricably interlinked with diseases that their study is essential to our understanding and management of elderly sick and disabled people.

Equally important for those treating and caring for the old is an understanding of the influence, for good or ill, of the social environment within which the elderly have to function and its effect on their health.

Knowledge of programmes aimed at the promotion and maintenance of health, early detection of its impending breakdown and the organization and provision of services for health care are additional essential components of a complete account of the medicine of old age.

The early chapters of the book provide a general perspective of old age and the process of ageing. Preventive aspects together with accounts of nutrition and sleep in the elderly and the interpretation of biochemical data in older patients, precede the main clinical section which occupies the greater part of the text. The later chapters cover rehabilitation, the management of the dying patient and aspects of the delivery of health care.

I acknowledge with gratitude the willing help of my colleagues, Dr. Deirdre Hine and Dr. D. Gwyn Seymour who read through much of the text and provided valuable criticisms and suggestions; and to my secretaries Mrs. Lorraine Spriggs who did much of the typing and the arduous task of checking references, and Mrs. Sylvia Bevan. I am indebted to Dr. Ralph Marshall and his team in the Department of Medical Illustration at the University Hospital of Wales for preparing a number of figures and photographs.

1
Introduction

1.1

INTRODUCTION

M. S. J. Pathy

It is now some 20 years since Williamson (1964) and Anderson (1966) reported on the magnitude of unreported illness in old people. Low expectations, a belief that many of the features of illness are the inevitable consequences of age rather than disease, active concealment of illnesses and a high incidence of depression appear to be some of the cardinal determinants influencing the high incidence of unreported disease in old age.

Disease may present insidiously and may be considered as a normal state by many old people, and often no less frequently by their physician. The traditional teaching that symptom-dominated presentations such as pain, cough, breathlessness, vomiting, weight loss, represent the features of medical breakdown, overshadows the significance of problem orientated presentations in diseases of old age.

Osler rightly taught that all signs and symptoms should lead to one diagnosis because he was primarily concerned with the medicine of children and young adults; he brilliantly codified the major presenting features of disease (1898). However, the elimination of the widespread infectious diseases of Osler's era by public health measures, and a greater general prosperity in developed countries and major demographic changes have dramatically changed the population age structure and the pattern of disease. General medical teaching has consistently avoided the emotionally intellectual trauma of overtly accepting that the major illnesses in late 20th. century medicine are predominantly in middle and old age. Teachers of medical practice often continue to preach the medical tenets of an era that no longer exists, and to concentrate on clinical rubrics apposite to unique diseases in the otherwise fit and physiologically elite and to give unbalanced precedence to the curable as against the treatable.

Social breakdown in old age is rarely only social, but often represents an overt marker of medical breakdown. Requests for domiciliary support services or for admission to nursing homes or other forms of residential care are indicators of altered well-being more often than physiological decline. Any old person whose level of functional competence has changed over a definable period of weeks or months is demonstrating the clinical features of medical impairment every bit as much as his younger neighbour who seeks a physician's help for palpitation.

Unless the clinical significance of the problem-orientated presentation of disease is given due emphasis, many old people will have their frailty and impaired competence labelled as the process of ageing, and the opportunity for successful therapeutic intervention will be incontrovertibly lost.

References

Anderson, W. F. (1966). 'The prevention of illness in the elderly: the Rutherglen experiment in medicine of old age'. Proceedings of a conference held at the Royal College of Physicians of London, London. Pitman.

Osler, W. (1898) *Principles and Practice of Medicine*. Young J. Pentland, Edinburgh and London.

Williamson, J., Stokoe, I. H., Gray, S., Fisher, M., Smith, H., McGhee, A. and Stephenson, E. (1964). 'Old people at home: their unreported needs'. *Lancet*, **1**, 1117–1120.

2

An Historical Overview of Geriatric Medicine: Definition and Aims

Principles and Practice of Geriatric Medicine
Edited by M. S. J. Pathy
© 1985 John Wiley & Sons Ltd

2.1

An Historical Overview of Geriatric Medicine: Definition and Aims

Sir Ferguson Anderson

The principle of caring for the elderly is an accepted part of the policy of any civilized nation and their very numbers in many societies encouraged a search for a planned methodology of medical care. Future population projections indicate a massive increase in the numbers of very elderly people throughout the world and this causes concern as many require both medical and social help. While this increase raises problems for the developed countries even greater difficulties lie ahead for the developing countries where the issue is complicated by the rapid urbanization of many agricultural communities, thus splitting up families and changing long-established customs.

The World Health Organization (1963) produced a useful classification of older people dividing them by chronological age into three stages: (a) middle aged persons (45 to 59); (b) the elderly (60 to 74); (c) the aged (75 and over). The point was made that the requirements of the two older groups were different; the elderly should be regarded as a resource and use found for their skills, knowledge, and experience if they desire this. The aged, in contrast, in many instances need assistance of various kinds. In Scotland those people over 85 years of age require in the majority of cases some form of help to enable them to continue to live in their own homes (Akhtar *et al.*, 1973).

GERIATRIC MEDICINE

Geriatric medicine (clinical gerontology) has been defined as the branch of general medicine concerned with the health and the clinical, social, preventive, and remedial aspects of illness in the elderly. Charcot (1881) wrote 'The importance of a special study of diseases of old age would not be contested at the present day' and in 1909 Nascher defined the word 'geriatrics' as the subdivision of medicine which is concerned with old age and its diseases (Freeman, 1979). Dr Marjory Warren was appointed in 1935 to the West Middlesex Hospital when the adjacent Poor Law Infirmary was taken over and she developed in that infirmary a special geriatric unit in which accurate diagnosis and her own outstanding gift of personal rehabilitation were practised (Warren, 1948). The principles of geriatric medicine evolved from these concepts, namely that old age is not a disease, that accurate diagnosis is essential, that many illnesses of elderly people are remediable, and that bedrest without reason is dangerous. Morris (1942) revealed the essential elements of a geriatric service and the British Medical Association (1949) laid excellent guidelines for the speciality of geriatric medicine. Sheldon (1948) published an important survey on the condition of older people living in their own homes and Lord Amulree and Trevor Howell (1974) in 1947 encouraged further progress by founding the Medical Society for the Care of the Elderly which became the British Geriatrics Society. From 1950 onwards, a group of physicians who had learnt the rewarding techniques of Marjory Warren, like Tom Wilson, George Adams, and Taylor Brown, began to take up appointments as physicians specializing in geriatric medicine. At that time (1950) the International Association of Gerontology was founded in Liège to promote gerontological research in the biological, clinical, and social fields and to train highly qualified personnel in the field of ageing. Monroe (1951) described diseases in old age and continued the clinical description of illness in the elderly given by Thewlis (1919), Rolleston (1922), Cowdry (1939), and Steiglitz (1943).

The idea of prevention of illness in older people and of attempting health maintenance was initiated by Anderson and Cowan (1955) and Williamson and coworkers (1964) described the 'iceberg' of unreported illness with the plan of seeking out disease in supposedly healthy elderly people. Day hospital practice started in Cosin's Cowley Road Unit in Oxford in 1958 and subsequent development of this was recorded by Brocklehurst (1973) and Hildick-Smith (1980). Adams and Hurwitz (1963) by describing the mental barriers to the rehabilitation of stroke patients stimulated interest in this distressing illness. Exton-Smith (1955) and Agate (1963) published textbooks which encouraged the academic teaching of this subject.

The establishment of Institutes of Gerontology in Kiev and Baltimore produced the scientific information necessary for the study of 'normal ageing' while the more recently founded Institute of Gerontology in Tokyo, closely associated with a nursing home for the elderly, continues this work.

Roth (1955) provided essential facts about mental disease in old age and this stimulated the appointment of consultant psychiatrists specially interested in psychogeriatrics (Robinson, 1972). The reports of the Royal College of Physicians of Edinburgh (1963, 1970) pointed out deficiences in the care of the elderly in Scotland and suggested solutions, while in 1965 a chair of geriatric medicine was established at the University of Glasgow. The World Health Organization (1974) published a report on the organization of geriatric care and this was followed by another British Medical Association booklet on the same subject (1976).

The development of geriatric care in the Netherlands, Sweden, U.S.S.R., Australia, the United States, and the United Kingdom is described by Brocklehurst (1975). More recently the possibilities of using the Veterans Administration Hospitals in the United States and Canada have further matured by the development of active geriatric units with the prospect of immense expansion.

The concern felt by the nations of the world in regard to the massive projected increase in the numbers of people over 60 years and especially of the very old was expressed at a special meeting of the United Nations on ageing held in Vienna from 24 July to 6 August 1982. Pleas were made for the use of older people as a resource and for the abolition of legislation against the older person, e.g. mandatory age-related retirement. Recommendations were tabled for more data to be collected on a worldwide basis and to be monitored in regard to the well-being of the elderly. In the United Kingdom there are now 14 chairs of geriatric medicine and many young physicians are specializing in the subject, with similar progress being made in psychogeriatrics. Postgraduate courses of training in these specialities have been outlined by the appropriate Royal Colleges.

METHODOLOGY OF GERIATRIC MEDICINE

It has been said with some justification that no two physicians practising geriatric medicine work in the same way. Certain principles guide their activities founded on the belief that there is a sufficient body of scientific knowledge to form a viable speciality. It is generally agreed that older people are happier and healthier in their own homes if they are fit enough to be there and so desire; that they are ill not because of advancing age but due to illness; that they have an altered physiology which may render the presentation of disease atypical; that pathology when it occurs is commonly multiple; and that older people have an immense potential for recovery.

The altered physiology of the elderly is due to a diminished reserve capacity in individual organs and to alterations in sensory input. Apart from the frequently observed impairment of hearing, the sensation of pain may be diminished, postural control may be defective, and autonomic nervous system deterioration may occur. Perception of ambient temperature is lessened and in the individual elevation of temperature is not a reliable guide in diagnosis.

The result of these changes is to alter the presenting symptoms of disease, to make the onset of serious illness insidious, and to increase the difficulty of accurate diagnosis. This is further complicated by the frequent occurrence of many illnesses at the same time.

Medical students should receive specialized instruction in their undergraduate training so that every doctor has a working knowledge of geriatric medicine. The physican practising this subject as a consultant must initially have been well trained in general (internal) medicine and thereafter receive further specialized instruction in geriatric medicine.

In clinical examination the usual history taking may be useless and information must be received from a relative or friend. Much time has to be allocated to this and particular enquiry must be made into the previous illness or operations. It would be helpful if there was an internationally agreed sign which the surgeon would engrave at the lower end of the operation scar indicating the precise character of the operative procedure, as so commonly the old person has forgotten completely what was done and even why the operation was performed. Previous drug therapy should be noted in view of the increased sensitivity of the elderly to drug intolerance. Physical examination often includes formal tests for mental state. This gives information not only about the presence or absence of brain failure but also as to the accuracy of the history and statements made during physical tests.

The methodology of geriatric medicine is concerned with (a) maintenance of health; (b) illness in old people; (c) placement (Fig. 1):

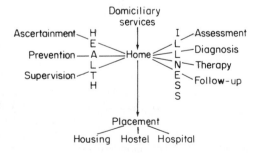

Figure 1

(a) Maintenance of health includes health education of the elderly, identification of early illness, prevention of further disability where possible, and continuing supervision of those found to be at risk.

(b) Illness in old people demands immediate assessment of (1) the total condition of the patient in regard to physical, mental, and social health and of (2) a knowledge of the home conditions, of the presence or absence of caring relatives, and of the possibility of keeping the patient in that particular environment or of return to it following admission and discharge from hospital. This will usually be undertaken by the family doctor or a member of the health care team or on request by the physican practising geriatric medicine. Diagnosis or more commonly a list of diagnoses will be made, correct placement of the elderly patient ensured, appropriate therapy prescribed, and follow-up after recovery arranged.

(c) Placement of the individual becomes important as age advances and guidance may be required as to where to live or, if illness supervenes, the correct place for treatment. The social worker or district nurse may be initially involved, but frequently the general practitioner will be contacted, perhaps through an ascertainment scheme. Knowledge about where the elderly person can go is essential and the element of choice should be introduced with the abiding principle that home is best when this is possible. Information on available services must not only be given to doctors, but to social workers, nurses, home helps, voluntary workers, ministers of religion, the wardens of sheltered housing, and indeed all who come in contact with the elderly and the older people themselves. Facts about the availability of housing for the elderly or specialized housing, e.g. sheltered (warden supervised), should be obtained . The scope of the local authority, the voluntary and the health services should be widely advertised.

The flow of patients from the geriatric unit will depend on the supporting services, e.g. continuing treatment beds, psychogeriatric help, local authority hostel accommodation, and housing facilities. The existence of efficient domiciliary services including a night nursing service is an absolute requirement for the successful care of the elderly. Without these or if there is failure in any one part of the overall plan the concept of a comprehensive geriatric service fails.

The main points of difference between general (internal) medicine and geriatric medicine with the relative interests of physicians practising these specialities can be summarized as shown in Table 1.

Table 1   Differences between general (internal) medicine and geriatric medicine

	General medicine	Geriatric medicine
	Relative interest	
Health Education of the elderly	0	++
Ascertainment of unreported illness	0	++
Knowledge of home conditions	+	++
Atypical presentation of disease	+	++
Multiple pathology	0	++
Physical and mental disease	+	++
Medication problems	+	++
Continuing care	0	++
Comprehensive patient care and teamwork	0	++

Health Education

Health education is required throughout life and Mehigan (1978) showed that 35 per cent. of the beds in a 500 bedded teaching hospital were occupied by patients suffering from the effects of cigarette smoking and a further 25 per cent. were used for the treatment of diseases induced by the abuse of alcohol or drugs, accidents, obesity, faulty dietetic habits. He called these illnesses life style diseases. In the elderly many studies (Fentem and Brassey, 1979) have revealed the importance of physical exercise in the improvement of health in older people. In the mind of the public and of many older people the time of retirement and the onset of old age are regarded as synonymous with the occurrence of ill health, but Akhtar and coworkers (1973) have shown that it is the very old who have the greatest amount of disease. Continuing health education by the media, press, television and radio is necessary not only to encourage appropriate exercise but to provide information about diet, accident pre-

vention, and advice regarding the preservation of mental health. Constructive use of the young old to help the aged and information about the formation of new voluntary services or the correct way to obtain statutory services is constantly necessary. This is a field of intense interest to the physician practising geriatric medicine but not to the general physician or the internist.

Ascertainment of Unreported Illness

The need for some form of health surveillance or ascertainment was demonstrated by Anderson and Cowan (1955) and by Williamson and coworkers (1964). There can be few physicians practising geriatric medicine who have not experienced the feeling of how much more they could have done for their patients if they had had the opportunity of seeing them at an earlier date. By ascertainment in many instances it has been possible to demonstrate certain categories of old people who are especially at risk. The Canadian Task Force, (1979), reporting on periodic health examinations found routine checks generally uneconomic. For most age groups they suggested certain examinations which might be carried out by the physican when the individual reported with a complaint, but in infancy and in old age they recommended calling the presumed healthy person to the doctors' clinic for a series of tests. Some parameters should be measured annually and others at longer intervals and the view was expressed that much of this work could be undertaken by non-medical trained staff. In the United Kingdom many ways of seeking out early illness have been tried either by the family doctor or by a member of the health care team, e.g. the health visitor. People found to require help must, after a satisfactory plan for the future has been organized, be kept under supervision with the aim of maintaining them in their own homes where possible. The physician trained in geriatric medicine should be capable of giving advice and helping when asked in the planning of such a service (Anderson, 1976).

Knowledge of Home Conditions

A knowledge of the home conditions of the older patient is of immense value and is part of the concept of comprehensive patient care. The family doctor is aware of this and many physicians practising geriatric medicine visit their elderly patients before hospital admission. This affords the opportunity to reassure older people that they are not going into hospital to die but to get better and this will greatly help not only the patient but also the physican when planning future home discharge. A word of caution can also be given to relatives, if any, that the patient may be returning home. Appropriate preparation and adaption of the house can be undertaken while the patient is in hospital with saving of time when discharge home is contemplated. A member of the health care team or a social worker may undertake this work; the information obtained is invaluable.

Atypical Presentation of Disease

Old people often find it difficult to state clearly their complaint and cannot be hurried. Time must be found for history taking. Disease presents in altered fashion for many reasons, mainly associated with the changing physiology of the older person. Pain, its intensity, and its site are not reliable guides to the diagnosis of illness in the upper age range. The myocardial infarction without pain has been well documented by Pathy (1967). The occurrence of a fractured femur with no complaint of pain is common knowledge and the painless perforation of a duodenal ulcer is frequently diagnosed as a silent myocardial infarction. The fleeting pains of osteomalacia are sometimes attributed to hysteria and the unusual siting of pain may also be misleading, e.g. the patient with a gastric ulcer who presents with a pain in the neck or upper chest. The defective postural sense of the old may be made worse by almost any illness so that the presenting symptom may be a sudden intensification of episodes of falling; the falls now come in groups and the old person is constantly unsteady. This complaint demands investigation. The acute onset of mental confusion or of urinary incontinence is a cry for help and again complete examination and appropriate tests are indicated. Elevation of temperature will not be found in illness as in younger patients and the pulse rate and respiratory rate are often more reliable indicators of disease. Cardiac failure

may present with tiredness, insomnia, or mental confusion. The bustling man may be noted by his wife to be sitting constantly in his chair and have become very quiet. He may have occasional falls and be suffering from postural hypotension. The unusual presentation of disease is the bait which lures the keen clinician into the speciality of geriatric medicine and is seen less frequently in general medicine.

Multiple Pathology

The atypical presentation of disease tests the physician's diagnostic skill and when this is complicated by the presence of multiple pathology the mind of Sherlock Holmes is required to disentangle the symptoms and signs. In contrast to the younger patient, the simultaneous presentation of many illnesses, often of minor nature in themselves yet having an additive effect on the patient's condition, is an everyday occurrence. An example is the elderly lady who lived alone and was referred to the hospital as a case of senile dementia. After clinical examination she was found to have severe corns on her feet causing her to take to bed, faecal impaction (the result of bed rest and dehydration), and wax in her ears rendering her out of touch with her neighbours. In hospital she was constantly trying to climb out of bed in the endeavour to go to the bathroom and was unable to hear the words of reassurance spoken to her by the nurses. Following the clearing of her ears and her bowels and the attention of the chiropodist she was able to return home 14 days later. The teaching of the search for a single pathology to account for all the symptoms and signs which is usually correct in the young or middle aged is seldom applicable to the elderly.

Physical and Mental Disease

The frequent intertwining of physical and mental illness in the elderly must be appreciated. With advancing age the loss of reserve function in the brain renders the onset of mental confusion (acute brain failure) more likely when, due to physical disease, the cerebral circulation is in any way diminished. Affective illness is also common and depression is frequently found in association with physical disease e.g. following a stroke. Depression in older patients often presents as a somatic symptom like insomnia or constipation without an overt complaint of depression. Diagnosis is difficult and only after a prolonged interview or a repeat consultation will the depression become evident. The specialist in psychogeriatrics can be of immense help in such cases and especially in the differential diagnosis of depression and dementia. These combined problems of physical and mental illness are less frequently encountered by the general physican or internist.

Medication Problems

Old people like drugs and tend to hoard medicines in their cupboards at home. As they often come with many complaints the temptation to the physician to try and alleviate each symptom is great. An order of priority of therapy is required with the most serious illness treated first. When more than three drugs are prescribed the physician must pause and consider if all are essential; only exceptionally will a large number of preparations be required. The more drugs given, the more likely is the occurrence of drug interaction. It is good practice to place a time limit on many drugs and after that period has elapsed to stop the drug and observe the subsequent progress of the patient. Certain questions should always be asked before a drug is given, 'Have you ever received this medicine before and did it upset you?' The patient may frequently not remember, but there may be a record of previous medication. A history of previous drug sensitivity is especially important in regard to antibiotics.

Four main principles emerge for drug therapy:

(a)   The diagnosis should be accurate.
(b)   There must be an indication for the use of a drug.
(c)   The drug must be used in the correct dose for an elderly person.
(d)   The drug should be used initially for a limited period and its effects reviewed.

Continuing Care

When an elderly patient is ill and therapy has been given the physician must continue to supervise the condition of the old person and may undertake this personally or by the use of a member of the health care team. In hospital practice, after a period of initial assessment the elderly patients may be sent home or be referred to a continuing care hospital unit where ideally they will remain under the supervision of the same physician who treated them in the assessment unit. If the patient is discharged to his own home, arrangements should be made for follow-up by the general practitioner or a member of the health care team. In the same way if old people have been ill at home and cared for by their own doctors follow up should be arranged by them. Continuity of care is essential otherwise recurrence of the illness is likely as many of the precipitating factors of the original disease may still be present.

Comprehensive Patient Care and Team Work

The physician practising geriatric medicine must endeavour to treat the physical, mental and social illnesses of his patients. The rehabilitation and resettlement of the patient in its widest sense will be the aim; in particular he will attempt to return the older individual to his own home. Failing this other appropriate accommodation will be necessary with the knowledge and consent of the patient. He will attain these objectives by utilizing the skills and experience of his colleagues, i.e. the physiotherapists, occupational therapists, chiropodists, and orthotists. Many others – social workers, the psychologist, the speech therapist, and the audiometrician – will provide special skills; other consultants in many other fields such as the ophthalmologist, the dermatologist, the surgeon, the gynaecologist, and the dentist will also be essential for advice and assistance. Teamwork is vital in the care of the ill old person.

The skills of the physician practising geriatric medicine have been acquired from the general physician, the psychiatrist, the family doctor, and the members of the health care team such as nurses, physiotherapists, occupational therapists, and chiropodists and his colleagues in social medicine. In summary, the idea of comprehensive patient care is in many ways a return to the old-fashioned physician and in stressing the difference between general (internal) medicine and geriatric medicine no impression should be given that the physician practising geriatric medicine is better than his physician colleagues; he is, however, different.

REFERENCES

Adams, G. F., and Hurwitz, L. J. (1963). 'Mental barriers to recovery from strokes', *Lancet,* **2,** 533–537.

Agate, J. (1963). *The Practice of Geriatrics,* William Heinemann Medical Books Ltd, London.

Akhtar, A. J., Broe, G. A., Crombie, A., McLean, W. M. P., Andrews, G. A., and Caird, F. I. (1973). 'Disability and dependence in the elderly', *Age Ageing,* **2,** 102–110.

Anderson, W. F. (1976). 'The effect of screening on the quality of life after seventy', *J. R. Coll. Physicians Lond.,* **10,** 2, 161–169.

Anderson, W. F., and Cowan, N. R. (1955). 'A consultative health centre for older people', *Lancet,* **2,** 239–240.

British Medical Association (1949). *The Care and Treatment of the Elderly and Infirm,* British Medical Association, London.

British Medical Association (1976). *Services for the Elderly,* British Medical Association, London.

Brocklehurst, J. C. (1973). 'Role of day hospital care', *Br. Med. J.,* **4,** 223–225.

Brocklehurst, J. C. (1975). *Geriatric Care in Advanced Societies,* MTP, Lancaster.

Canadian Task Force (1979). 'The periodic health examination', *Can. Med. Assoc. J.,* **121,** 3–45.

Charcot, J. M. (1881). *Clinical Lectures on Senile Diseases,* The New Sydenham Society, London.

Cowdry, E. V. (1939). *Problems of Ageing: Biological and Medical Aspects,* Williams and Wilkins, Baltimore.

Exton-Smith, A. N. (1955). *Medical Problems in Old Age,* Wright and Sons Ltd, Bristol.

Fentem, P. H., and Brassey, E. J. (1979). *The Case for Exercise,* Sports Council Research Working Papers No. 8, Sports Council, London.

Freeman, J. T. (1979). *Aging,* Human Sciences Press, New York.

Hildick-Smith, M. (1980). 'Geriatric day hospitals: Practice and planning', *Age Ageing,* **9,** 38–46.

Howell, T. (1974). 'Origins of the British Geriatrics Society', *Age Ageing,* **3,** 69–72.

Mehigan, J. A. (1978). 'The doctor's life style', *Ir. Med. J.,* **71,** 174–178.

Monroe, R. T. (1951). *Diseases in Old Age,* Harvard University Press, Cambridge.

Morris, N. (1942). 'De Senectute', *Surgo,* **8,** 28–34.

Pathy, M. S. (1967). 'Clinical presentation of myocardial infarction in the elderly,' *Br. Heart J.,* **29,** 190–199.

Robinson, R. A. (1972). 'The evolution of geriatric psychiatry', *Med. Hist.,* **16,** 184–193.

Rolleston, H. (1922). *Medical Aspects of Old Age,* Macmillan, London.

Roth, M. (1955). 'The natural history of mental disorder in old age', *J. Ment. Sc.,* **101,** 281–301.

Royal College of Physicians of Edinburgh (1963). *The Care of the Elderly in Scotland,* Royal College of Physicians of Edinburgh.

Royal College of Physicians of Edinburgh (1970). *The Care of the Elderly in Scotland: A Follow-up Report,* Royal College of Physicians of Edinburgh.

Sheldon, J. H. (1948). *The Social Medicine of Old Age,* Oxford University Press.

Steiglitz, E. J. (1943). *Geriatric Medicine,* W. B. Saunders, Philadelphia.

Thewlis, M. (1919). *Geriatrics; A Treatise on Senile Conditions; Diseases of Advanced Life and Care of the Aged,* C. W. Mosby, St Louis.

Warren, M. (1948). 'Care of the hemiplegic patient', *Medical Press,* **219,** 396–398.

Williamson, J., Stokoe, I. H., Gray, S., Fisher, M., Smith, A., McGhee, A., and Stephenson, E. (1964). 'Old people at home: Their unreported needs', *Lancet,* **1,** 1117–1120.

World Health Organization (1963). *Report of a Seminar in the Health Protection of the Elderly and Aged and the Prevention of Premature Ageing,* Regional Office in Europe, Copenhagen.

World Health Organization (1974). *Planning and Organization of Geriatric Services: Report of a WHO Expert Committee,* WHO Tech. Rep. Ser. No. 548.

3

Aged and Ageing:
A Perspective

Principles and Practice of Geriatric Medicine
Edited by M. S. J. Pathy
© 1985 John Wiley & Sons Ltd

3.1

Social and Community Aspects of Ageing

J. A. Muir Gray

DEMOGRAPHY OF AGEING

The Greying of Nations

The greying of nations (Butler, 1979) is a metaphor which has been used to describe the demographic changes which have taken place in all industrially developed countries this century. It describes an increase both in the numbers of elderly people and in the proportion of the population which is elderly. Just as the greyness of a head depends not only on the absolute number of white hairs but on their distribution and frequency in relationship to the hairs which are of the original colour, so it is important to consider both the absolute and relative numbers of elderly people in the ageing of a population.

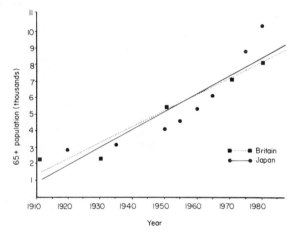

Figure 1   Increase in numbers of elderly people in Japan (over 65 population) and the United Kingdom (men over 65, women over 60). (From Maeda, 1978, and Pearce, 1975)

Absolute Ageing

In all developed countries there has been a rapid growth in the numbers of elderly people; in developing countries there has also been an increase, though not so marked (Chapter 30.4). The increase in the numbers of older people in the United Kingdom and Japan (Fig. 1) is typical of the changes which have taken place in all developed countries.

The size of this phenomenon has led to the increase in the numbers of very elderly people being described as a modern epidemic, but this term is unfortunate for two reasons. Firstly, it is unfortunate because of the connotations of the word epidemic, a term usually used to describe an outbreak of cholera or plague. Old age is not a disease and old people are not an epidemic. Secondly, it is unfortunate because it is etymologically incorrect. An epidemic is an affliction which comes down on the people: 'epi-demos'. The older members of a society have not come down on it, they are part of it – an integral and important part. Furthermore, the numbers of old people in society have not increased suddenly and unexpectedly because it was obvious for many years that the numbers of elderly people would increase as the middle aged grew older.

The Causes of Absolute Ageing

The increase in numbers of older people is not, as is commonly thought, due to the activities of the medical profession 'keeping all these old people alive'. The increase is not primarily due to an increase in expectation of life of elderly people; it is due to the increased expectation of life at younger ages (see Fig. 2). Also, medical science has had little to do with the reduction in mortality and thus the increase in life expectancy which began long before effective medical treatments or services were widely available.

Table 1   Expectancy of life at the age of 1. (From the Royal Commission on the National Health Service, HMSO, 1979

Country	Males	Females
Australia	68.5	75.4
Canada	69.7	77.0
France	69.5	77.1
Norway	71.4	77.7
Sweden	72.0	77.4
United States	68.0	75.6
West Germany	68.6	74.9
England and Wales	69.5	75.6
Scotland	67.7	74.0
Northern Ireland	67.0	73.6

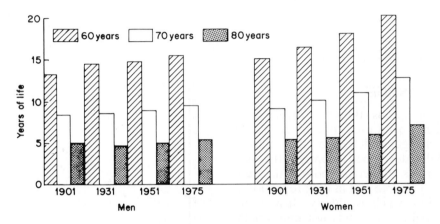

Figure 2   Expectancy of life in Great Britain. (From Wilcock, Gray, and Pritchard, 1982. Reproduced by permission of Oxford University Press)

The number of elderly people in a society depends on the number of births 70 years previously and the subsequent mortality of that cohort over 70 years. The increase in the number of old people in Britain can be explained by analysing the number of births and the infant mortality rate in the last decades of the nineteenth century (Fig. 3) and the mortality experience of the cohorts born at the turn of the century as they grew older. The most important cause of absolute ageing is the increasing size of cohorts surviving to reach old age.

The Male-to-Female Ratio

The ratio of men to women in the older age groups is an aspect of population ageing meriting special mention. The expectation of life at the age of (see Table 1) is about 6 years greater for female infants in Britain than it is

for males, and this gap is of the same magnitude in all developed countries, as is the difference between the life expectancy at the age of 60, which is about 3½ years.

There are biological reasons and social reasons for this difference and thus for the fact that there are more old women than old men. Biologically, the higher mortality of male foetuses and male infants and the inhibitory effect of oestrogens on the development of atherosclerosis both play a part. However, social influences appear to be more important. Earlier this century there were more men than women among the elderly of several developed countries and the reversal of the sex ratio is a relatively recent phenomenon. The change would seem to have been due to the differing life styles of men and women in which the prevalence of cigarette smoking, high alcohol consumption, and exposure to hazards of the work-place have thus far penalized men in comparison to women. A higher death rate of men than women during wars has also affected the ratio while higher rates of mortality from homicide and road traffic accidents contribute their effect during peacetime.

As the life styles of men and women become more alike the gap will probably narrow: changes in female morbidity and mortality associated with increased consumption of alcohol and cigarettes are trends already apparent.

Relative Ageing

The relationship of the number of older to the number of younger people in a society is of importance. Three factors determine the rate of relative ageing: fertility rates, mortality rates, and, at national level, patterns of migration.

As a country develops economically, the first effect is usually a decline in mortality, which increases the numbers of older people, but it is not until fertility declines, usually about 20 years later, that the relative age of the population begins to increase. This has happened in all the developed countries, except those whose age structure has been significantly affected by immigration, e.g. Canada, Australia, and New Zealand.

In all the developed countries about 1 person in 6 is more than 65 years old (Fig. 4), except those in which the effects of migration are still evident. However, as the simple percentage is too crude a measure for long-term planning three other indices are more illuminating:

(a) The index of ageing=

$$\frac{\text{number of people over pensionable age} \times 100}{\text{population under 15}}$$

(b) Demographic dependency ratio:=

$$\frac{\text{number of people over pensionable age}}{\text{and number of children under 15}} \times 100$$

$$\text{number of people 15 to pensionable age}$$

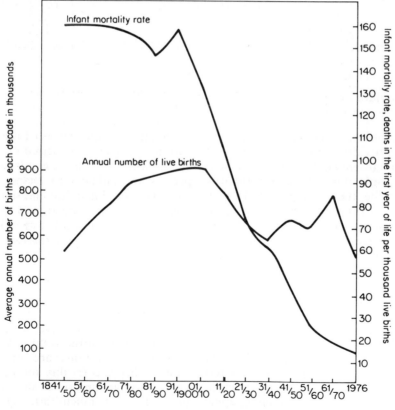

Figure 3   Number of live births and infant mortality rate in Great Britain

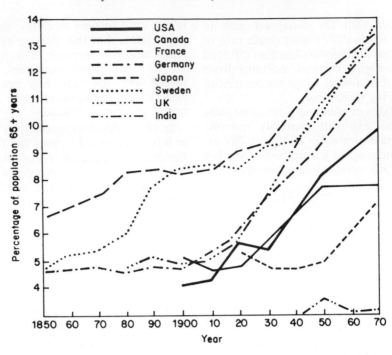

Figure 4   Percentage of the population aged 65 and over. (From Hendricks and Hendricks, 1977)

(c)   Old age dependency ratio:=

$$\frac{\text{number of people over pensionable age} \times 100}{\text{number of people 15 to pensionable age.}}$$

Of these, the index of ageing is of least use in planning or providing services – although of interest to demographers. The old age dependency ratio is useful for both those primarily concerned with the management and planning of staff-intensive caring services and for economists and actuaries trying to forecast the financial consequences of pension policies.

Any forecast of the economic consequences of demographic trends must take into account changes in the birth rate as well as changes in the numbers of elders. Increased expenditure on health care of the elderly will be offset by reductions in expenditure on education if the birth rate falls. For this reason the demographic dependency index is probably the most useful of the three, although even it is too general to be particularly helpful and a more detailed analysis of the effects of demographic trends on economic activity, hospital use, and the use of education services have to be calculated. An example of this approach is given by the graphs prepared by the Office of Population Censuses and Surveys (Fig. 5).

It is important to emphasize that these projections are highly speculative. The trends in the numbers of elderly people can be predicted with a relatively high degree of confidence because mortality rates of middle aged and older people are unlikely to change dramatically. However, the birth rate and the level of economic activity are notoriously difficult to predict, and the indices can all be changed significantly by altering the retirement age.

Retirement Migration

The distribution of old people, and thus their proportion in the population, varies very much from one part of the country to another. The reasons for this range are, in part, variations in mortality and fertility rates. There is, however, another important reason why some regions have a much older population than others – the migration of elderly people.

In America the general trend has been a migration from the north to the south, especially to Florida, Arizona, Nevada, and California. In England there has also been a move to the south, particularly to the south coast (Figs 6 and 7). A detailed study of the phenomenon of retiring to the seaside (Karn, 1977) showed that people moved soon after retirement, often to places they had liked as holiday resorts, and that they moved for a variety of reasons (Table 2).

Table 2   Main reasons for retirement move. (From Karn, 1977)

	Bexhill	Clacton
Sample number	503	487
REASONS FOR MOVING		
Better climate; cleaner air; sea air	33	19
Health reasons	11	18
Flat country	1	1
To get away from town or live in a quiet place	16	10
To live in a bungalow	4	9
Having to leave a tied house	5	5
The expense of living in the previous place	5	9
To have a change	7	9
To join friends or relations	10	15
Other	7	6

Appreciation of this pattern of migration led to public concern and couples contemplating a move were advised of the problems which could result from 'pulling up their roots'. However, the research gave reassuring results and suggested that:

In conclusion, then, it seems that the experience of retirement to the coast had not been one that most retired people had regretted. In addition those people who had regretted their move had done so, not so much because they regretted moving at all, 'pulling up their roots', but because they did not like certain features of the place they had chosen. The dissatisfied in Bexhill often said they thought they would have liked the countryside better and those in Clacton missed the activity and variety of the city. These results fit in with the comments of people who intended to move from the resorts; an unexpectedly large number of them were seeking another retirement resort on the coast or in the country rather than returning to the place from which they came.

For fit elderly people the move was a success. Those who became disabled, however, faced great problems because few resorts had been able to develop health and social services to a sufficient degree to meet the demands generated by populations of whom one quarter or one third were over the age of sixty-five (Karn, 1977).

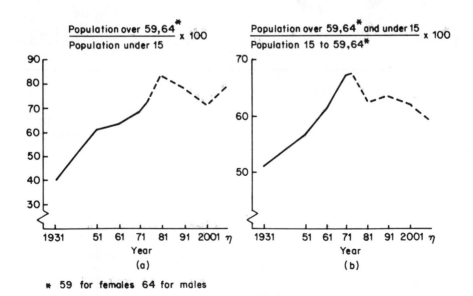

$$\frac{\text{Population over } 59,64^*}{\text{Population under } 15} \times 100$$

$$\frac{\text{Population over } 59,64^* \text{ and under } 15}{\text{Population } 15 \text{ to } 59,64^*} \times 100$$

Year

(a)

(b)

* 59 for females 64 for males

Figure 5 (a) Old age dependency ratio and (b) demographic dependency ratio

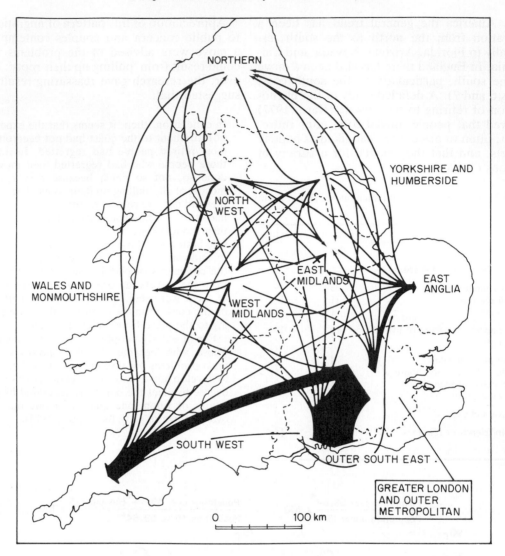

Figure 6   Migration of elderly people

The Changing Family

Before making any statement about the part which the modern family plays in looking after its elders it is essential to take into account some of the changes which have taken place in family size and structure during the era of industrialization and urbanization (Gray and Wilcock, 1981).

The age at which children marry and leave home has decreased (see Table 3). The proportion of marriages which end in divorce has increased (Leate, 1976). Population mobility has increased. The proportion of women who work has increased: in 1921 only 8.7 per cent. of women worked; in 1976 the proportion was 44.3 per cent.

Table 3   Percentage of females married: England and Wales. (From Leate, 1976)

Year	Aged 20–24	Aged 45–49
1931	26	83
1939	34	84
1951	48	85
1961	59	90
1971	59	92
1974	58	93

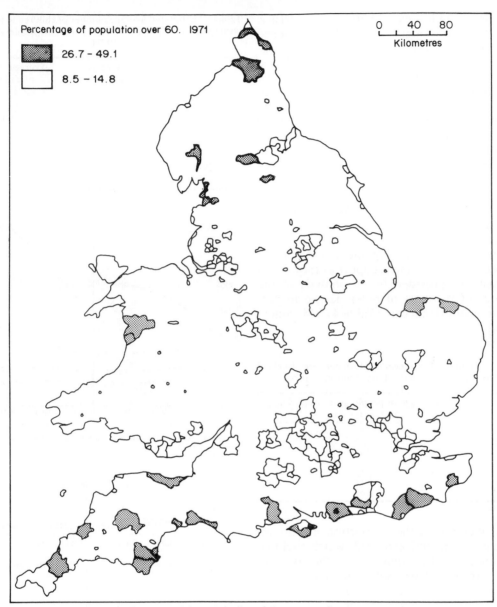

Local authorities in the highest and lowest deciles of the range of percentages of population aged 60 + in 1971

Figure 7　Local authorities in the highest and lowest deciles of the range of percentages of population aged over 60 in 1971

These trends all make it more difficult for people to look after their elderly relatives when they become dependent. Nevertheless, there is no evidence that the modern family in Britain cares less for its elders than did the family in the past.

The belief that families do not care for elderly people is a variant of the more general belief that there was an era before the industrial revolution in which elderly people were loved, respected, and cared for by relatives and neighbours. This belief is a myth and the belief that families cared better in the past is also untrue, although it is has been believed for a long time. The report of the Royal Commission on the Poor Laws and Relief of Distress stated in 1909 that 'there is not the same disposition to assist one another as there was years ago' and the Royal Commissioners, who reported on the Poor Laws in 1832, made the even more uncompromising statement that 'the duty of supporting parents and children in old age is so strongly enforced by our natural feelings that it is well performed, even among savages, and almost always so in a nation deserving the name civilized. We believe that England is the only European country in which it is neglected.'

Data to support the argument that families provide at least as much support as they did in the past are provided by an analysis of the statistics of numbers of older people in permanent institutional care (Table 4), (Moroney, 1976).

Table 4   Trends in long term institutional care: England and Wales 1911–1933. (From Moroney, 1976)

Year	Percentage of people aged over 65 in institutional care
1911	5.17
1921	3.39
1931	2.91
1952	2.10
1961	2.77
1973	2.88

The increase in the proportion institutionalized between 1952 and 1973, which could be attributed to the influence of the Welfare State, can in fact be explained simply by the relative increase in the numbers of very elderly people within the over 65 age group. There has been an increase in the number of people aged over 80 who are in residential care and hospital (Fig. 8) but this is probably due more to the relative decline in the numbers of middle aged children who are available to help than to any decrease in the willingness to care (Table 5) (Grimley Evans, 1976).

Further evidence has been provided by two studies of family support for dependent elderly relatives which did not reveal any widespread refusal to care or any tendency to shift responsibility for care onto the Welfare State, i.e.

Table 5   Estimated average number of children to parents born in different years 1811 to 1921 (From Grimley Evans, 1977)

Year of birth of parent	Average number of children	Average number of children surviving to age 45
1871	4.8	2.7
1881	4.1	2.5
1891	3.3	2.2
1901	2.6	2.0
1911	2.2	1.7
1921	2.0	1.6

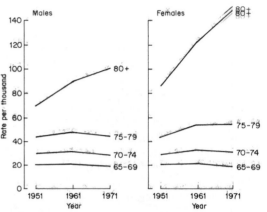

England and Wales census: persons in institutions on census day, age-specific rates per thousand

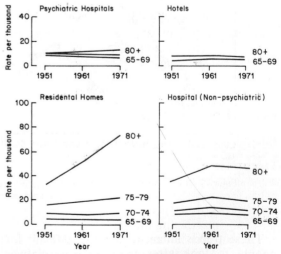

England and Wales census: persons in institutions on census day, age-specific rates per thousand

Figure 8   England and Wales census: persons in institutions on census day, age-specific rates per thousand. (From Grimley Evans, 1977)

statutory services, (Isaacs, 1971, Lowther and Williamson, 1966).

It is true that most professionals who work with elderly people see more cases in which the family's refusal to contribute to the support of an old person precipitates admission to or delays discharge from an institution. There is, however, no evidence that the proportion of families doing this is increasing. The increase simply reflects the increase in the numbers of very frail elderly people. Furthermore, these families who do give up usually do so for good reasons. One common reason is that their relationship with the elderly relative, usually a parent, is not one which fosters the desire to care. Not all old people are nice old people, and some old people have done little to earn the love or gratitude of their children. Indeed, in many cases it is surprising that the children are willing to continue caring for as long as they do for parents who do not appear to have been loving or caring, or for parents who were violent to them in childhood. The second reason why some families refuse to continue caring is that they have been offered too little too late. No matter how loving a family may be, the capacity of the relatives to cope can be eroded by continuous and unremitting demands.

MORTALITY AND MORBIDITY

Before discussing the data which describe the pattern of mortality and morbidity in old age it is important to emphasize certain caveats which must be borne in mind when considering these statistics.

Deficiencies in the Data

Invalidity and Unreliability

The first and most important point to emphasize is that the data from which the statistics are calculated are often inaccurate. Mortality data are particularly suspect because of the common difficulty in assigning the cause of death to one condition. This is due in part to the nature of disease, e.g. the frequent presence of multiple pathology and the fact that atypical presentation is so common. Consider how many deaths are said to be due to 'home accidents' or 'falls' without mention of osteoporosis, ver-

tebrobasilar insufficiency, or any of the other predisposing causes. The inaccuracy of death certification is, however, also due to the attitudes towards death in old age. Many doctors are willing to accept death in old age as being due to 'heart failure' or 'pneumonia'. The older the age group studied the less is the effort made to establish the true cause of death.

A prospective study of 1,152 hospital autopsies in Edinburgh clearly demonstrated the increasing inaccuracy of certification with age (Table 6). This increase in inaccuracy was evident in both the main diagnosis and the other associated conditions recorded on the death certificate. The authors of this article recognized the fact that multiple pathology makes diagnosis more difficult in old age but were of the opinion that it was 'unlikely that it explains entirely the inverse relationship between accuracy of diagnosis and the age of the patient' (Cameron and McGoogan, 1981).

Table 6   Percentage confirmation of clinical diagnoses by age at post-mortem. (From Cameron and McGoogan, 1981)

Age	Percentage confirmation		
	Ia	Ib	II
Under 45 years (50 cases)	78	58	32
45–54 years (115 cases)	73	43	23
55–64 years (300 cases)	68	37	21
65–74 years (392 cases)	61	32	17
More than 75 years (295 cases)	47	26	13

Ia: major underlying cause leading to death.
Ib: conditions resulting from Ia which were ultimately responsible for death.
II: other unrelated conditions which contributed to death.

An important cause of inaccuracy in morbidity data is that they are reported by old people themselves or by their helpers. There is good evidence that the reliability of such data is suspect, whatever the age of the respondent, and this could be a more serious problem with very elderly people whose memory is impaired by the effects of ageing or by dementia. However, the effects of memory impairment may be offset in some people by the fact that their lives are so uneventful that events which might be forgotten by busier people are remembered.

Overprecision

Precision and accuracy have to be clearly distinguished from one another as they can be mutally exclusive and there is new evidence that the desire to become more precise has led to inaccuracy in death certification in old age.

In times past it was common for doctors to state 'senility' as a cause of death, and the Ninth Revision of the International Classification of Disease still has 'old age' as a cause of death. It appears in Section XVI – Symptoms, Signs and Ill-defined Conditions – as category 797 – Senility – without mention of psychosis – old age. However, the proportion of deaths ascribed to old age has fallen progressively and now the great majority of deaths of older people are ascribed to a specific disease. However, the precision is misleading and it now appears that a larger number of people die principally as a result of the ageing process than the number that are classified as doing so.

A review of 200 autopsies of people more than 85 years old demonstrated that 'no acceptable cause of death other than complications of the ageing syndrome, was identified in at least 30% of cases' (Kohn, 1982). The author argued that 'senescence' should be accepted as a cause of death in the United States. The temptations of a precise diagnosis on the death certificate has therefore led to an inaccuracy in the data on causes of death in old age. 'The effects of ageing' may seem to be less precise than 'myocardial infarction' but it is often a more accurate description of the cause of death.

Incompleteness

Although epidemiological and social surveys are deficient because some of the evidence is invalid or unreliable they are at least complete. Other types of data are incomplete, particularly those presenting the incidence or prevalence of problems which ae based on the contacts old people initiate with health or social services. Because older people have, in general, difficulty in contacting help and have low expectations the incidence or prevalence measured by counting the number of events known to the health or social services will give too low an estimate of the true incidence or prevalence. The actual need is often much greater than the demands (Williamson, 1981).

Fortunately this is now widely appreciated and there is increasing evidence about the prevalence and incidence of disease which is based on complete population surveys rather than on the demands made by elderly people. However, data on the utilization of health and social services is still too often taken as an indicator of need.

Deficiencies of Cross-sectional or Prevalence Studies

Much of the data concerning elderly people is collected by prevalence or cross-sectional studies, i.e. they are based on a single examination of a population at one particular time. Such studies usually simply express the results by correlating the findings with chronological age. Implicit in such a simple correlation is the assumption that the groups are directly comparable and therefore that any differences observed are due to the ageing process. However, differences between age groups are often due to factors which were operating at a much earlier stage in the life of the cohort being studied.

Let us consider mortality from tuberculosis as an example. The mortality rate in 1971–75 was noted to be higher in older age groups (Table 7). This gives a fairly depressing picture of old age because it suggests that the incidence of tuberculosis increases with age. If, however, the death rates for successive generations or cohorts are presented (Fig. 9) the picture is transformed and a much more encouraging picture of the resilience of older people and their response to treatment is obtained because mor-

Table 7   Deaths per million population from respiratory tuberculosis: England and Wales, 1971–75. (From Adelstein, 1977).

Age group	35–39	40–44	45–49	50–54	55–59	60–64	65–69	70–74	75–79	80–84	85+
Males	7	14	28	51	71	93	140	195	233	262	258
Females	6	8	18	20	23	21	28	37	44	55	65

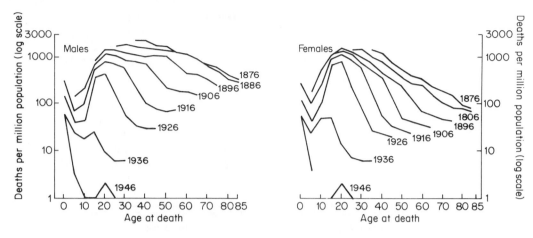

Figure 9   Pulmonary tuberculosis: annual death rates by age in selected cohorts. 1920–1975, England and Wales. (From Adelstein, 1977)

tality from tuberculosis is decreasing even among the oldest members of society.

It is easy to identify factors in which the cohorts of different ages differ from one another in ways which affect mortality and morbidity. Depending on their year of birth, different cohorts may have been exposed to widely differing influences on their health, frequently environmental and social.

People in their eighties differ from younger people not only because they are more affected by the ageing process but also because they suffered more diseases in their childhood. Rheumatic fever, rickets, tuberculosis, poliomyelitis, measles complicated by bronchiectasis, and middle ear infection are diseases of childhood which have permanent sequelae but which are no longer common today.

Other factors, such as the epidemic of encephalitis lethargica during and after World War I, air pollution during the decades in which coal was the principal source of energy, and more recently the increase in cigarette smoking, particularly in men but in the postwar years also in women, all affect in varying degrees and in different ways the health of those who survive into old age.

In addition to the possibility that factors operating in childhood have had pemanent sequelae two other possibilities must always be borne in mind when the incidence of disease is seen to be different in old age:

(a)   differences in diagnosis, e.g. less effort is

put into the establishment of an accurate diagnosis in older age groups;

(b)   older people have been exposed to noxious stimuli for a longer time.

These factors have to be borne in mind when studying statistics relating to older people. Cancer statistics offer a good example of the problems and pitfalls.

Two trends are striking: firstly the incidence of many cancers increases with age, and, secondly, the incidence of some cancers is increasing among older age groups (Table 8). However, the former fact is probably due to the longer exposure of older people to carcinogenic agents, working on the premise that about 90 per cent. of all cancers are environmental in origin (Doll and Peto, 1981) and the latter is probably due to more accurate diagnosis.

Table 8   Trends in age specific registration rates: 1975 registration rates (all sites), expressed as a percentage of 1968 rates. (From Coggan and Acheson, 1981)

Sex	Age (years)					
	25–34	35–44	45–54	55–64	65–74	75+
Male	111	93	108	106	115	128
Female	114	97	110	115	119	132

The fact that cancer appears to be increasing more quickly among older people than in younger age groups has stimulated a number of epidemiological studies, particularly re-

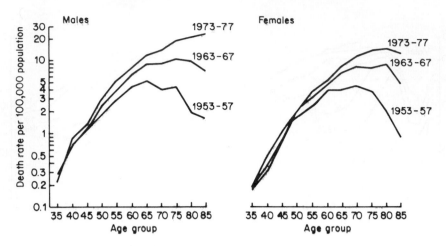

Figure 10   Age and sex-specific death rates for multiple myeloma over 5-year periods during the last 3 decades in England and Wales. (From Velez, Beral, and Cuzick, 1982)

search into those cancers which have shown the most rapid increase in older age groups. Multiple myeloma is one of these and the mortality from this cancer has increased in older people in both Britain and the United States (Fig. 10).

There are two possible explanations for this trend. The first is that there has been a real increase in incidence; in other words the cohort consisting of people who are aged over 70 in 1973–77 is one in which the age-specific incidence of multiple myeloma or cancer is greater than in the cohort of people who were the same age in 1953–57, and an analysis of mortality of both cohorts indeed shows that there has been a change in the age specific mortality from multiple myeloma (Fig. 11).

However, there has also been an improvement in diagnosis and ascertainment during this same period, and this has had an effect on the numbers of people certified as dying from multiple myeloma. There is evidence to suggest that failure to ascertain or record the true cause of death from diseases such as myeloma or leukaemia is more common among older people and that therefore the increase in myeloma mortality may be due to more complete ascertainment and recording of the true cause of death in the older age groups.

The conclusion of epidemiologists is that both real increase in incidence and an apparent increase have occurred in the case of myeloma (Velez *et al.*, 1982).

However, it is not only physical factors which are important; social differences are also important. For example, cross-sectional studies of intelligence are misleading because the intelligence of people aged 80 cannot be simply compared with the intelligence of those in their twenties and thirties. Even more important, however, is the fact that it is now appreciated that the amount of education a person has had

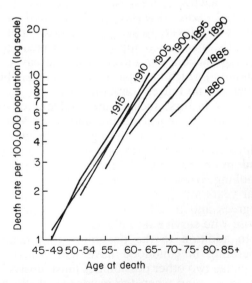

Figure 11   Mortality from multiple myeloma in England and Wales indifferent cohorts born in 5-year periods between 1880 and 1915. (From Velez, Beral, and Cuzick, 1982)

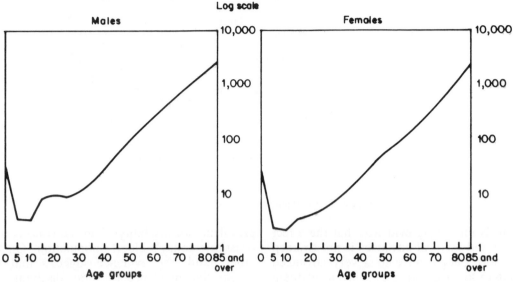

Figure 12   Death rates by age and sex

influences their intelligence as measured by psychological tests. That is to say, the comparison of a cohort of people many of whom left school at 14 with a cohort of people many of whom have had a university education is invalid and gives the impression that the ageing process causes a more serious decline in intellectual ability than it actually does.

An understanding of the health of older people, therefore, has to have a historical perspective and any attempt to plan services for older people has to take into account those factors which affect the health of middle aged and young people.

Table 9   Age-specific death rates showing differences between males and females: (England and Wales, 1973). (From Farmer and Miller, 1977, p. 59)

Age at death	Death rates per million living		Age at death	Death rates per million living	
	Male	Female		Male	Female
Less than 1 year	18,573	14,348	45–54	7,231	4,372
1–4	770	605	55–64	20,422	10,222
5–14	370	236	65–74	51,514	26,848
15–24	957	421	75–84	117,711	76,630
25–34	1,007	579	85+	242,101	195,985
35–44	2,250	1,552	All ages	12,400	11,518

Mortality Statistics

Although the deficiencies in the available data have been emphasized there is no doubt that the age-specific death rate increases steadily with age, increasing by a factor or two in each 10-year age group, and that males have a higher mortality than females at all ages (Table 9), (Fig. 12).

Causes of Death

The common causes of death in old age, as recorded on death certificates, are shown in Fig. 13, although the diagnoses, particularly in the over 75 age group, must be regarded with suspicion.

These data are of interest, provided that one bears in mind the numerous sources of inaccuracy, but are not of much use for service planning. For this purpose the increase in the numbers of old people is of much greater importance. This may not be as alarming as it appears to be at first sight since there is some evidence that the prevalence of disability in those who will be 85 at the turn of the century will not be as great as in the 85 year olds of today.

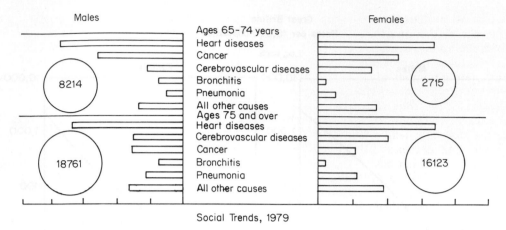

Social Trends, 1979

Figure 13   Common causes of death in old age

There is increasing evidence that the effect of social and medical advances is not to keep many more people alive to a very advanced age but to keep a higher proportion of them alive until they reach the end of the lifespan usual for members of the human species, which may be about 85. This effect is known as the rectangularization of the survival curve (see figs 14 and 15).

Also there is evidence that the effects of geriatric medicine are not simply to postpone the onset of disability to a later age but, in the words of the motto of the World Health Organization, to 'add life to years', and the cohorts who are becoming older appear to reach old age fitter and more active, with a lower prevalence of disability, than the cohorts who constitute today's elderly population. On the other hand, the evidence suggests that the age-specific incidence of some disabling diseases, notably arthritis and dementia, is not decreasing and that the hypothesis of Fries is misleadingly optimistic (Schneido and Brady, 1983).

Predicting the Future

Of central importance to the planning of the health and social services for elderly people is

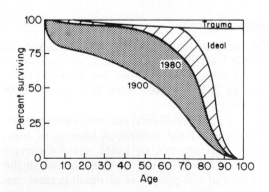

Figure 14   The increasingly rectangular supply curve. About 80 per cent (stippled area) of the difference between the 1900 curve and the ideal curve (stippled area + hatched area) had been eliminated by 1980. Trauma is now the dominant cause of death in early life. (From Fries, 1980)

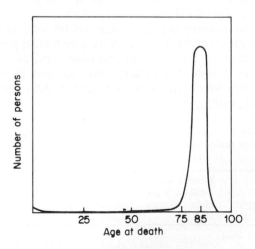

Figure 15   Mortality according to age in the absence of premature death. The morbidity curve is made rectangular and the period of morbidity compressed between the point of the end of adult vigour and the point of natural death. (From Fries, 1980)

the ability to predict their numbers, and this requires the prediction of changes in mortality rates among middle aged and older people.

The mortality rates of old people in future depend upon a number of factors.

Differences in the cohorts. Differences in the experience of the cohorts of people who are becoming older may lead to a decrease in mortality, e.g. the decrease in the incidence of rheumatic fever which has taken place will be reflected by a decrease in the prevalence of chronic rheumatic heart disease. For the same reason there will be a decline in deaths due to tuberculosis. Cohort effects may, however, lead to an increase in mortality, e.g. the increase in the prevalence of smoking among women which has taken place several decades after the increase in the prevalence among men will be reflected in an increase in smoking-related diseases among older women in the future. Differences in the cohorts of people becoming old also affect the prevalence of disease and disability in old age and the attitudes of older people.

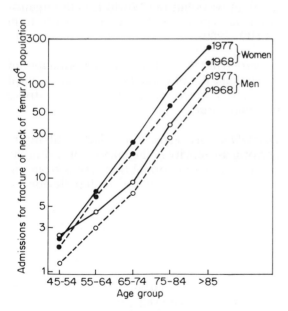

Figure 16 Hospital inpatient admission rates (England and Wales) for men and women in 1968 and 1977 where diagnosis on admission was fracture of neck of femur (Hospital In-Patient Enquiry). Standard errors approximately 10 per cent of rates shown. (From Lewis, 1981)

Improved medical care. Changes in medical care, for example the development of an effective influenza vaccine coupled with a change in the attitudes of doctors to preventive medicine, could lead to a reduction in mortality.

Social Changes

Changes in the life style of those who are old could also be important. If, for example, large numbers of elderly people took up hang-gliding mortality rates would be affected. Ridiculous though this example may seem there is evidence that the age-specific incidence rate of fractured neck of femur is increasing (Fig. 16).

Among the reasons suggested for this are an increase in the consumption of alcohol which may be a cohort effect, i.e. an increase in the number of people becoming old who abuse alcohol rather than a change in the social life of older people, and an increase in the levels of activity of elderly people resulting from changing attitudes of older people themselves and of those who are caring for them.

The Actuarial approach

The actuary has to take these and other factors into account and try to predict changes in mortality rates. One way of doing this is to assume that the mortality rates in a country could fall to the lowest rates for that age group recorded elsewhere, the assumption being that the genetic differences between populations are insignificant. However, the assumptions change from year to year depending upon the evidence available. Consider the difference in the forecasts for improvement in mortality of older men and women made by the Government Actuary in 1973 and 1978 (Table 10).

Table 10 Percentage improvement in mortality expected in the next 40 years. (From *Population Projections*, 1973 and 1978, HMSO)

Age	Males		Females	
	1973 forecast	1978 forecast	1973 forecast	1978 forecast
57	25	6	25	3
67	18	20	24	14
77	7	15	20	17
87	2	13	6	19

Morbidity Statistics

It is essential to define the terms that will be used in this section as there is some difference in the way they are used from one part of the world to another.

Disease and Illness

These terms are often used synonymously but each has been given its own meaning by social scientists.

Diseases are the entities which doctors agree are to be accepted as being diseases, e.g. diabetes or tuberculosis, and they are the same in whatever social class or culture they occur. This may seem self-evident but it is important to remember that many conditions which were once considered diseases no longer exist – soldier's heart and neurasthenia are two obvious examples – and that new diseases are discovered from time to time – normal pressure hydrocephalus is an example of a 'new' disease.

An illness is 'the subjective response of the patient to being unwell; how he, and those around him, perceive the origin and significance of the event; how it affects his behaviour or relationships with other people; and the steps he takes to remedy this situation' (Helman, 1978). Illness varies very much from one social group and culture to another and for older people illness is a different experience than it is for younger people.

Many patients have both disease and illness but some people have diseases without being ill, the person with a symptomless undetected carcinoma for example, and others feel ill without having any disease which can be identified as the cause of their illness (Fig. 17).

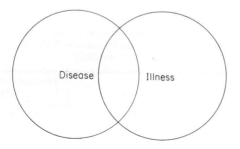

Figure 17   Disease and illness

Some of the people who feel ill without having any detectable disease are relieved when told this and the symptoms may be alleviated simply by being reassured but many older people continue to have symptoms and to feel ill even though no disease can be found to explain their problems.

Disease, Disability, and Handicap (Fig. 18)

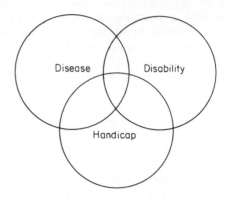

Figure 18   Disease, disability, and illness

Different people often use these terms in different ways but the World Health Organisation has agreed a definition for each term (WHO, 1980).

Impairment. Any loss or abnormality of psychological, physiological, or anatomical structure or function, e.g. the effect of a stroke on brain tissue.

Disability. Any restriction or lack of ability to perform an activity in the manner or within the range considered normal that results from impairment, e.g. limitations in hip flexion or quadriceps strength.

Handicap. A disadvantage for an individual resulting from an impairment or disability that limits or prevents the fulfilment of a role that is normal for someone of that age and sex in their particular social and cultural condition, e.g. difficulties with self-care.

The term 'disablement' is accepted by the WHO as a useful term to describe any experience or impairment, disability, or handicap but the terms 'infirmity', 'invalidity', 'crippled', 'abnormality', 'defect', and 'incapacity' are regarded by the WHO as being too imprecise to be used as technical terms.

The correct use of these terms is as nouns not adjectives, i.e. instead of 'the elderly disabled' or 'the handicapped' it is better to refer to 'elderly people with disabilities'.

Nosological Problems

Epidemiological data about disease will be presented throughout the book and in this section we wish to concentrate on certain nosological problems which complicate epidemiological studies of disease in old age.

Some diseases are relatively simple. Either the neck of a femur is fractured or it is not, although epidemiological studies of fractured neck of femur are complicated by the fact that a small proportion impact and do not present in the same way as the classic, displaced fracture. This, however, is a problem resulting from the difficulty in diagnosing the disease. It is not a true nosological problem and there are many other examples in which diagnosis is difficult because the diagnostic techniques currently available cannot detect minor degrees of the disease.

Nosological problems result from difficulties in defining disease.

The continuous variable. One type of nosological problem is presented by the types of disorder in which the disorder is a matter of degree, that is to say there appears to be no significant qualitative difference between the person with the 'disease' and the person who is considered to be normal.

High blood pressure and osteoporosis are two examples of this type of disorder. All people have 'high' blood pressure; the issue is how high is too high to leave untreated. This is particularly difficult in old age because so little is known about the natural history of the disease. What is the significance of a blood pressure of a 70 year old man which proves to be 194/112 after a series of careful readings? We cannot answer that question for that individual. All that can be done is to deduce the risk he is running from the data which we have on the implications of this level of blood pressure in men of his age, allowing for the presence or absence of other risk factors and the

inadequacies of the available data, and to try to set that against the benefits and risks of instituting treatment, again from inadequate data.

Similarly with osteoporosis; at what bone mass should the prescription of oestrogens be considered? Again the data are limited and costs, risks, and benefits have all to be considered in a cost-effectiveness calculus when making health policy decisions, and in the clinical context when making decisions about an individual patient (Weinstein, 1980).

Disorders of this sort present particular problems for both clinician and policy maker because it is impossible to distinguish normal from abnormal clearly and unequivocally. For the clinican the question is whether or not to intervene; for the policy maker the question is whether or not to devote resources to developing a programme for the treatment of the condition.

Let us consider the costs and benefits of the use of oestrogens as a means of preventing osteoporosis, and therefore fractures, as an example of the type of dilemma faced by the policy maker. The complex calculus of costs and benefits has been most clearly presented by Milton Weinstein who wrote:

> The analytic framework used here is that of cost-effectiveness analysis. This model assumes that health-care resources are limited and that the societal objective is to use those resources to achieve the greatest possible health benefit. Health interventions that provide the greatest benefit per dollar of resources consumed would thus receive the highest priority for those resources. The cost-effectiveness approach requires that all resource costs be measured in the same units and that all health benefits be measured in the same units. It does not require (as does benefit-cost analysis) that benefits be measured in the same (monetary) units as costs. Hence, in this analysis, health-care costs will be measured in dollars, but health benefits will be measured in years of life expectancy. Considerations of the quality of life may be incorporated if, instead of life expectancy, the concept of 'quality-adjusted life expectancy' is used as the unit of benefit.
>
> The objective of the analysis that follows, then, is to assess the components of the following cost-effectiveness ratio:

$$\frac{C}{E} = \frac{\triangle C_{Rx} + \triangle C_{SF} - \triangle C_{Morb}}{\triangle Y - \triangle Y_{SE} + \triangle Y_{Morb} + \triangle Y_{Symp}}$$

The numerator (C), measured in dollars, represents the net increase in health-care costs. The first term $(\triangle C_{Rx})$, is the direct cost of treatment, including drugs, physician visits, and routine tests. The second term $(\triangle C_{SE})$ represents the costs induced by the side effects and complications of treatment – for example, the costs of surgery for uterine bleeding or endometrial cancer. The last term in the numerator $(\triangle C_{Morb})$ represents the savings associated with the prevention of morbid events, notably fractures of the hip and wrist.

The denominator (E), measured in years of life expectancy (or 'quality-adjusted' life expectancy), represents the net health benefit of treatment. The first term $(\triangle Y)$ denotes the net effect on life expectancy, incorporating both the positive and negative effects of treatment on mortality. The present analysis proceeds in two stages: in the first the change in life expectancy $(\triangle Y)$ is the only health effect of concern, and in the second, effects on quality of life may be incorporated according to the subjective values and preferences of the decision maker. For this second stage of analysis, the remaining three terms in the denominator come into play: $\triangle Y_{SE}$ represents the negative quality adjustment associated with the side effects and complications of treatment, $\triangle Y_{Morb}$ represents the positive quality adjustment associated with the prevention of morbid events, and $\triangle Y_{Symp}$ represents the positive quality adjustment associated with the relief from symptoms. The denominator of the ratio is of interest in its own right; it represents a risk-benefit analysis from the perspective of the patient concerned about the net impact of treatment on her life and health but not about resource cost (Weinstein, 1980).

Obviously the equation varies depending upon a number of variables, notably (a) the criteria for treatment (should all women be treated or just those with evidence of osteoporosis and those who have menopausal symptoms?) and (b) the duration of treatment (should treatment be continued for 10 or 15 years?). Precisely the same type of analysis can be made of the same factors relating to the decision of whether or not screening for high blood pressure is cost-effective (Weinstein and Stason, 1976).

Diagnostic difficulties. In high blood pressure and osteoporosis it is possible to measure the relevant variable accurately, it is the interpretation of the significance of the result of that measurement which causes the problems. There are other conditions in which the differential diagnosis is much more difficult, particularly the distinction between disease and normal ageing, and this difficulty can affect assessments of incidence and prevalence.

Consider the problems in attempting to measure the prevalence of degenerative joint disease. What criteria should be used, symptomatic or radiological? What should be regarded as 'normal ageing' and what as 'disease'? What should the disease be called? Some doctors would classify patients who had no symptoms of inflammation as having osteoarthrosis, reserving the term osteoarthritis for those who had symptoms; others would classify all cases as osteoarthrosis; and yet others would classify all as having osteoarthritis. Similar problems occur with many other conditions, notably with attempts to measure the prevalence of mild dementia, and have to be taken into account when considering morbidity data.

Aetiological problems. The collection and presentation of data about disease in old age often show an increase in age-specific incidence which gives a graph that is almost exponential in shape, epitomized by the graph of the age-specific incidence of fractured neck of femur.

However, as we have already emphasized, it is essential to consider the experience of each cohort and other factors which could be a source of bias before assuming that the increased incidence in older age groups is due to the ageing process.

EPIDEMIOLOGY OF DISABILITY AND HANDICAP

There is a large overlap between the 'handicapped' and 'the elderly', as Amelia Harris showed in her classic study of the *Handicapped and Impaired in Great Britain* which was published in 1971. The proportion of people who are impaired and handicapped increases in older age groups (Table 11). More than half of all handicapped men and more than two-thirds of all the women who are handicapped are over the age of 65. Of very severely handicapped people one-half are over the age of 75.

Epidemiology of Disability

The disabling diseases which cause handicap in old age are:

Table 11   Proportion impaired or handicapped. (From Harris, 1971)

Age group	Numbers impaired	Numbers impaired per 1,000	Numbers[a] handicapped	Numbers handicapped per 1,000	Numbers very severely handicapped	Numbers very severely handicapped per 1,000
16–29	89,000	7.5	19,000	1.6	5,000	0.4
30–49	366,000	28.6	97,000	7.6	12,000	0.9
50–64	833,000	85.9	281,000	28.9	26,000	2.7
65–74	915,000	194.6	349,000	74.3	35,000	7.4
Over 75	867,000	333.5	381,000	146.5	80,000	30.7
Total	3,071,000		1,128,000		157,000	

[a]This group includes those who were 'appreciably, severely or very severely handicapped', i.e. those who need 'some support, considerable support and special care', respectively.

(a) Arthritis and osteoarthrosis (see Chapter 25.3)
(b) Stroke (see Ch. 16.9)
(c) Parkinson's disease (see Ch. 16.13)
(d) Blindness (see Ch. 18.1)
(e) Dementia (see Ch. 17.1)

The epidemiology of each of these will be found within the chapter on that disease. This chapter is more concerned with the epidemiology of the common disabilities resulting from the diseases. The data on disabilities which are available are less satisfactory than the data on the incidence and prevalence of the disabling diseases.

The common disabilities are:

(a) Muscle weakness
(b) Joint stiffness
(c) Breathlessness
(d) Inability to control or coordinate movements, e.g. because of tremor or spasticity
(e) Disorders of balance

It is not possible to deduce the prevalence of these disabilities from the prevalence of the common disabling diseases because each of the diseases may cause more than one disability (see Fig. 19).

The prevalence figures quoted in Table 12 are based on the replies given by elderly people to questions asked in the course of a social survey. Objective evidence about the prevalence of these disabilities is scarce and the interpretation of the data is difficult. Data on handicap are more plentiful.

Table 12   Percentage of elderly people suffering from common disabilities. (From Abrams, 1977)

Disability	Age group 65–74	Over 75
Unsteady on feet	22	49
Poor eyesight	32	42
Breathless after any effort	29	35
Giddiness	23	31
Always feel tired	25	29
Arthritis or rheumatism	50	58

The Epidemiology of Handicap

The two common problems are mobility problems and difficulty with self-care and although the two are obviously interrelated they will be discussed separately.

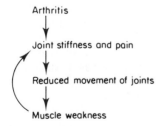

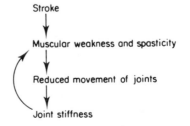

Figure 19   Disabilities caused by diseases

Table 13 Personal mobility. (From Hunt, 1978)

Personal mobility	Men percentages	Women percentages
Bed-fast permanently	0.1	0.4
Bed-fast temporarily, usually house-bound	0.1	0.3
Bed-fast temporarily, usually goes out	0	0.4
House-bound permanently	3.3	4.4
House-bound temporarily, usually goes out	2.1	2.8
Usually goes out with assistance	3.2	10.5
Usually goes out	91.2	81.1
Total	100.0	100.0

Mobility Problems

Ninety per cent. of men and 80 per cent. of women are able to go out and about without assistance (Table 13). The prevalence of mobility problems increases with age (Table 14). The higher average age of women only partly explains the higher prevalence of mobility problems in women, since impaired mobility is more common among women in each age group.

Table 14 Relationship of mobility problems to age. (From Hunt, 1978, p. 68)

Age group	Percentage permanently bed-fast	Percentage permanently house-bound	Percentage requiring assistance
65–69	0	1.1	3.2
70–74	0	2.5	6.6
75–79	0.4	4.9	9.6
80–84	1.0	9.7	12.5
85 and over	1.9	17.7	26.8

The reason why women more frequently have mobility problems than men is probably that arthritis and rheumatism, the most common cause of impaired mobility (Table 15), are more common among women. Even those who are able to get about outside their homes have problems, again most commonly due to arthritis (Table 16).

Elderly people also have problems with mechanized transport. Car ownership and availability is lower among older people and they have greater difficulty in using public transport because of the prevalence of disabling diseases.

Table 15 Cause of loss of mobility or of being bed-fast or house-bound. (From Hunt, 1978)

Bed-fast and house-bound persons, weighted	(174)
(unweighted figure)	(150)
Description of illness or disability[a]	%
Arthritis, rheumatism	36.2
Pulmonary conditions	17.2
Strokes, paralysis	14.9
Blindness, failing sight	14.4
Circulatory conditions	13.8
Cardiac conditions, blood pressure	13.2
Effects of accidents	9.8
Nervous conditions	4.6
Other specific illnesses or conditions	29.9
Old age, other vague descriptions	6.9

(Some people named more than one complaint.)
[a]It should be noted that the word 'disability' here and elsewhere is based on the answers to specific questions which called for a self-diagnosis by the informant or a proxy. We would not therefore be justified in using the terminology 'impairment, disability or handicap' as this would imply greater precision than is warranted.

Table 16 Mobility problems outside the home. (From Age Concern, 1978)

Environmental challenge	Percentage of all elderly people	Percentage of elderly people with arthritis
Hills and ramps	31	68
Traffic and road crossing	23	48
Uneven pavements	16	73
Steps and kerbs	4	59
No problem	40	Not recorded

Difficulties with Self-Care

The survey of *The Elderly At Home* revealed that the tasks which people find difficult most frequently were cutting toe nails and bathing.

It is, however, important to remember that it is not only the major tasks that cause depression and frustration. Many minor household tasks become impossible in old age (Table 18). The failure to perform these tasks and the resultant deterioration and delapidation of home and garden often cause as much distress to the old person who has a disability as does the inability to care for herself.

To solve the problems of a person who has a handicap doctors have to work with other professionals. The teamwork required can best be illustrated in in an algorithum (Fig. 20).

Table 17 Percentage in each age group who are unable to perform each task. (From Hunt, 1978)

	Age-group				
	65–69	70–74	75–79	80–84	85 and over
Elderly persons, weighted	(1,409)	(1,162)	(697)	(392)	(209)
(unweighted figures)	(725)	(629)	(688)	(375)	(205)
Unable to do without help or totally unable to:	%	%	%	%	%
Bath oneself	4.4	11.7	20.2	32.6	51.2
Wash oneself	0.8	1.0	2.3	4.6	7.2
Get to lavatory	0.4	1.3	2.8	5.1	6.2
Get in and out of bed	0.6	1.1	2.7	4.4	4.8
Feed oneself	0.1	0.3	1.3	1.8	2.4
Shave (men); do hair (women)	0.5	0.6	2.5	3.8	4.3
Cut own toenails	12.5	21.3	34.6	42.4	56.9
Get up and down steps, stairs	1.6	3.8	10.1	12.8	18.6
Get around house or flat	0.2	0.8	2.2	4.6	6.2
Go out of doors on own	4.4	9.5	16.5	23.5	48.9
Use public transport	5.3	9.3	15.1	23.8	37.9

GROWING OLD – THE SOCIAL PROCESS

Although the distinction is arbitrary it is useful to try to separate the effects of the physical processes affecting people as they grow older from the effects of the social consequences of attaining an advanced chronological age. There are three of these physical processes – ageing, disease, and the progressive loss of fitness – and these overlap with each other and with the social process which is often called growing old (Fig. 21).

In this chapter we will consider the social problems which occur as a result of growing old.

The Threshold of Old Age

Society imposes many arbitrary rules which depend on the age of an individual. A child in Britain has to have its birth registered by 42 days of age, it must attend school at 5 and remain there till 16, at which age it can leave school, although barred from legally buying an alcoholic drink until 2 years later. Similarly,

Table 18 Percentages unable to perform each task (by sex and age; housewives and those living alone are shown separately). (From Hunt, 1978)

	Total	Age group				
		65–69	70–74	75–79	80–84	85 and over
Elderly persons, weighted	(3,869)	(1,409)	(1,162)	(697)	(392)	(209)
(unweighted figures)	(2,622)	(725)	(629)	(688)	(375)	(205)
Unable to:	%	%	%	%	%	%
Open screw-top bottles[a]	9.7	5.3	8.4	11.5	18.4	24.4
Do little sewing jobs[a]	14.9	9.7	11.8	17.1	27.6	35.4
Jobs involving climbing	43.0	28.0	37.7	57.1	67.3	80.4
Use a frying pan	5.4	2.1	2.8	6.0	13.8	24.9
Make a cup of tea	2.6	0.9	1.4	2.9	6.4	12.9
Cook a main meal	8.8	4.6	6.8	10.0	18.1	26.8
Cut the lawn[b]	47.1	38.4	44.5	55.2	61.0	67.9
Do light jobs in garden[b]	19.3	10.0	15.4	27.0	34.7	49.8
Sweep floors	11.3	5.5	8.0	14.8	23.2	34.4
Wash floors	21.7	10.9	15.9	30.8	42.6	62.2
Make fires, carry fuel[b]	6.0	3.1	4.3	8.6	11.2	17.2
Wash clothes	14.5	6.8	10.8	20.2	29.1	39.7
Clean windows inside	23.6	11.4	17.6	32.3	48.0	65.1
Clean windows outside[b]	52.5	37.2	50.4	64.0	76.3	84.7
Wash paintwork	23.9	11.6	16.3	32.3	50.5	70.8
Minor repairs (e.g. fuses)	49.8	35.3	46.0	62.0	73.2	84.2
Repairs and redecoration inside	60.5	41.4	58.3	77.6	87.5	94.3
Repairs and redecoration outside[b]	49.2	42.0	46.6	53.7	65.6	65.6

[a]Bed-fast informants were asked about these tasks. They are assumed to be unable to do others.
[b]Informants who would not have to perform these tasks (e.g. because they had no garden) are included in the base figures so that the figures given show the percentages of all elderly for whom the tasks present problems. The percentages to whom these do not apply are: lawn 29.7 per cent., garden 22.6 per cent., solid fuel fires 55.8 per cent., windows outside 3.1 per cent., redecorations outside 35.9 per cent.

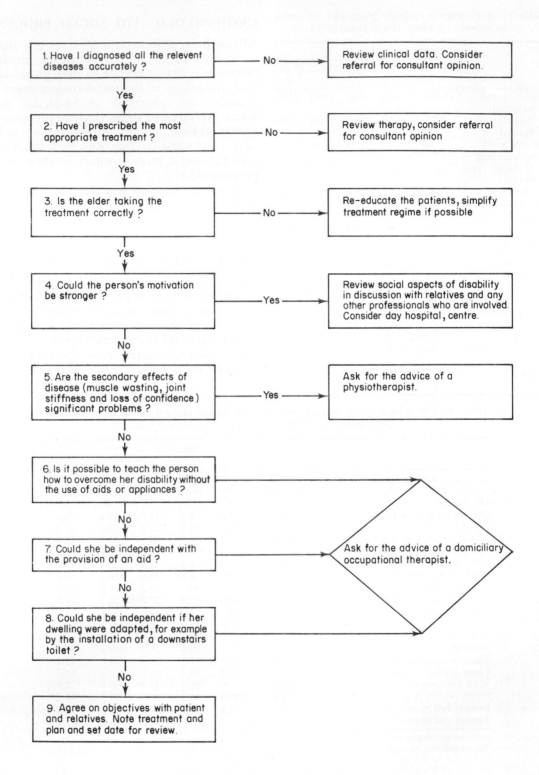

Figure 20   The handicap algorithm

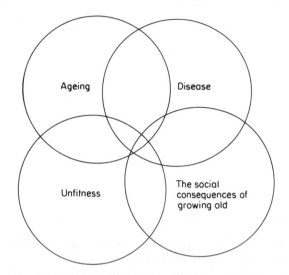

Figure 21   Ageing, disease, unfitness, and the social consequences of growing old

Table 19   The official pension age in 10 European countries. (From Union Bank of Switzerland, *Social Security in Ten Industrial Nations*, 1977)

	Men	Women
Belgium	65	60
Federal Republic of Germany	65	65
Finland	65	65
Canada	65	65
Great Britain	65	60
Netherlands	65	65
Austria	65	60
Sweden	65	65
Switzerland	65	62
United States of America	65	65

people perceive old age as starting at various chronological ages depending on their point of view and, even more important, their own chronological age. For example, a 15 year old may regard someone who is 27 as 'old' whereas a 45 year old man would be alarmed if he thought that someone considered him 'old'. A consultant in geriatric medicine would classify someone who is 74 as 'young' although he would be considered old by most people. In general, however, old age is considered to start at retirement.

Retirement Age

The age at which an individual must retire varies from country to country (Table 19) and from job to job. This age is known as the retirement or 'pension age'. Some jobs have a pension age that is lower than the national or statutory pension age, e.g. in some countries miners can retire at 55 and some jobs allow workers to retire after a certain number of years in employment.

Policemen, for example, can retire at 50 provided that they have completed 30 years' service. Retirement at such an early age usually results in a reduction in the pension that the retired person receives compared with the pension he would receive were he to stay on to the official pension age. For this reason many

people continue to work for a few years after the earliest age at which they could retire but a large number still retire before the statutory pension age.

Choosing a Pension Age

The pension age is chosen to meet political and economic objectives and not because the ages of 60 or 65 have any physical significance, a point that is important to emphasize in pre-retirement lectures.

The history of the pension age in Britain illustrates this fact. The first statutory pension age was 70, which was chosen in preference to 65 because it cost £2 million less. The age dropped to 65 in 1928 partly because this had been desired for many years but also in response to the high rate of unemployment that prevailed at the time. The pension age for women was, however, reduced to 60 in 1940 for good social reasons and not just as a matter of economic expediency. It was appreciated in the 1930s that it had been customary for men to marry women who were a few years younger and as a result many couples experienced hardship because the husband was forced to retire and support his wife on a single pension until she too reached the pension age of 65. The lowering of the female pension age to 60 allowed both to obtain a pension at the same time. Of course, single women benefitted from this innovation but it was primarily introduced to help married couples. Similar political and economic constraints will influence future changes in policy.

The Pension Age in the Future

Although there has been a vigorous campaign against compulsory retirement in several countries, notably in America where it was led by Claude Pepper, a 77 year old Democrat from Florida, the general trend is for lower pension ages. Many factors have contributed to this trend, e.g. the shrinkage of the labour force due to automation with high unemployment among younger age groups, the provision of better pensions making retirement more attractive, and increasing awareness of the fact that work was less important and retirement less damaging to the well-being of the older person than was thought hitherto.

If the pension age were to be reduced politicians would have to choose from a number of options presented to them by economists and actuaries. The British government was presented with the following options in a policy paper on the retirement age.

(a) Lowering the pension age of men to 60. This would cost about £2,000 million at 1980 prices.
(b) Raising the pension age of women to 65. This would not have any economic costs, indeed there would be savings, but would be politically unacceptable and would aggravate unemployment.
(c) Choosing a common pension age of 62.5 years. This would cost £800 million at 1980 prices and would also be politically unacceptable.
(d) Choosing a pension age for men and women which would have no financial costs, namely 64.2 years. This would also be politically unacceptable and would aggravate youth unemployment.

What seems to be the most likely course of events is that the pension age of men will drift gradually downwards, and the cost of this will be largely met by occupational pension funds whose actuaries will take this trend into account when planning the levels of future contributions and pensions. As the funding of pensions is gradually moving towards a 'pay as you go' system, i.e. one in which payments are made not from a fund composed of the past contributions of the pensioners but from the contributions of those who are working, the costs of lowering of the pension age will be paid not by impersonal pension funds but by everyone who is employed. To keep down unemployment we may have to lower the pension age and if we also wish to increase the level of the pension compared with the average wage the burden will fall on those who are of working age and in work.

The Effects of Retirement

Until recently the theory that work plays a valuable part in maintaining health and well-being has influenced our views of the effect of retirement. The theory argued that the worker identified with his work to such a degree that his view of himself and his position in society is dominated by the nature and social status of his work. To support this theory it was pointed out that it was customary to say of someone that 'he is a doctor' or that 'he is a joiner' or that 'she is a teacher' and not that 'he does medicine' or that 'his job is joinery' or that 'she teaches'. Because the person's identity was so closely identified with his work, it was assumed that retirement would lead to an identity crisis, and a very gloomy picture of retirement was held until recent studies showed this theory to be false. The two main effects of retirement are a drop in income and the loss of frequent contact with friends (Cohn, 1979) and it seems that few people are doing jobs that are so enthralling and exciting that they suffer a major existential shock as a result of compulsory retirement.

The widely held belief that retiring predisposes the person to a fatal heart attack has not been demonstrated epidemiologically (Gonzalez, 1980). Indeed, a review of the health consequences of retirement showed that the effect of retirement on health is usually beneficial, (Portnoi, 1981).

In conclusion, then, retirement leads to a change in the social and psychological circumstances of the individual and this may have a deleterious effect on mental health and thus on the physical well-being of an individual, but for most people the social and psychological aspects of life in retirement are more enjoyable and healthier than the social and psychological rewards of work.

For some people the change in physical circumstances that occurs on retirement also has an influence on health and this can be either beneficial or harmful. People who have been in active jobs may become less active and this may lead to unfitness and physical deterioration. For many, however, the change in the physical environment is beneficial to their health either because they leave unsatisfactory working conditions, such as polluted air or conditions in which the risk of injury is high, or because retirement offers the opportunity of a change in life style which is beneficial to health. For example, the person who commutes to and from a sedentary job is able to take more exercise; the natural history of retirement is, for the majority, 'good news'.

Preparation for Retirement

In recent years there has been a growth in preretirement education. Many people do not receive any preretirement education but it has become the practice in many firms to arrange for employees who are approaching retirement to have six or eight sessions to help them prepare for retirement. Although the trend is away from didactic lectures and towards discussions based on the knowledge and experience of the workers themsevles, older people should not be taught like children.
The types of topics which most doctors discuss are:

(a) the benefits of exercise in old age;
(b) basic information on diet and weight control;
(c) advice on stopping smoking;
(d) advice on the benefits of mental activity and engagement with other people;
(e) advice on cervical cytology and blood pressure measurement;
(f) advice on the best way to use health services, including the speaker's views on the benefits of a 'health check-up' at retirement.

In addition, the speaker should emphasize that the retirement age was not chosen because there is any increase in the rate of ageing or the incidence of disease at that age and that retirement is not usually followed by a deterioration in health. Indeed, the speaker should try to emphasize that the opposite is the case and that the health of most people improves after retirement. The Pre-Retirement Association and the Workers' Educational Association are active in this field in the United Kingdom and the Open University is also involved. However, the main need is for both employers and trades unions to accept the importance of preparation for retirement. Many firms offer only 10 or 20 hours of instruction and only a small proportion invite both husbands and wives but to help prepare someone for retirement requires more than a few tutorial sessions in the last month or two of one's working life. What is required is a greater commitment of both employers and unions to the need for preparation for retirement and preretirement programmes that start several years before the day on which the individual has to retire.

Social Problems

When people talk about the social problems of elderly people they are usually referring to certain practical problems that occur more frequently among older people, principally poverty, housing problems, difficulties with heating and isolation.

Aetiology

There are reasons why older people suffer from certain types of social problem more frequently than younger people.

Poverty. Many of the problems of older people are simply due to poverty.

Immobility. The high prevalence of disabling disease combined with the difficulties older people have with public transport, compounded by poverty which restricts their use of cars and taxis, make them less mobile than younger people and immobility is the cause of many social problems. The person who is immobile may be unable to fetch in coal or visit a number of shops to find the best bargain, or to go to the housing department or to the social security office or to see her Member of Parliament, to cite just a few of the ways in which immobility can aggravate social problems.

Communication difficulties. The higher prevalence of visual impairment, hearing loss, aphasia, and dementia among older people increases their social vulnerability and the probability that they will suffer from social difficulties.

Unassertiveness. Because of their upbringing older people are, in general, less assertive than younger people. Because many were brought up in a culture in which the individual had fewer rights than he has today many are less inclined to appeal against official decisions, to seek the help of their elected representative, or to try to overcome bureaucratic inertia than younger people.

Poverty

The word poverty is so commonly used that it may seem unnecessary to define but the word has two meanings which are important to distinguish – absolute poverty and relative poverty – and this distinction is particularly important in a time in which there are rapid fluctuations in prices and wages.

Absolute poverty is defined by comparing a household's income with the level of prices of the basic commodities necessary for life – the subsistence level, sometimes called the 'poverty line' or 'bread line'. Those whose incomes are below the minimum level necessary for subsistence are deemed to be in absolute poverty (Gray and Wilcock, 1981).

The definition of relative poverty is made by comparing a household's income with the average level of incomes in their society. Although an individual's income may be sufficient to provide himself and his dependents with the necessities of life he may find his relative poverty upsetting because it symbolizes his low status; J. K. Galbraith, a famous American economist, has described the condition of relative poverty eloquently: 'People are poverty stricken when their income, even if it is adequate for survival, falls markedly below that of the community. Then they cannot have what the larger community regards as the minimum necessary for decency and they cannot wholly escape, therefore, the judgement of the larger community that they are indecent. They are degraded, for in the literal sense they live outside the grades or categories which the community regards as acceptable.'

In the past, pensions have been set at a level

calculated to be that which will prevent absolute poverty. Central government calculates the level of pensions with respect to the pensioner price index, a modification of the retail price index adjusted to reflect the spending patterns of retired households which differ slightly from those below retirement age, principally by the greater proportionate amount spent on heating by older people.

Relative to the value of average industrial earnings the pension has not increased very markedly. In 1978 the pension was worth twice the amount of money it was worth in 1948 but the increase in relative terms was only from 30 per cent. of the average industrial wage to 37 per cent. In 1978 the Trades Union Congress stated that pensions were to be set at half the average earnings level believing, as do many other people, that the low relative value of pensions reflects and perpetuates the low value society places on elderly people.

In 1975 pensions were index-linked to rise in line with prices or wages, whichever was rising faster. The new pension scheme introduced in 1979 linked the basic pension to prices and the additional pension to earnings so that retired people should not become more impoverished in either absolute or real terms in the future, and all political parties are committed to increasing both the absolute and relative values of the pension if sufficient wealth is available.

The Prevalence of Poverty

The number of elderly people who are in absolute poverty can be estimated from the number who receive a supplementary pension because only those whose income is below the poverty line referred to in the previous section are eligible. In 1978 about 1.7 million people received supplementary pensions and the Department of Health and Social Security estimated that about 600,000 more might be eligible if they were to apply. Other measures of poverty are the numbers of pensioners claiming assistance with rent, nearly 800,000 in 1978, and rates, 1.8 million in 1978. The lowest level of eligibility for assistance with rent and rates, for these allowances are proportional to the pensioner's income, is higher than the level of eligibility of the supplementary pension, but not by very much, so that many of those in receipt of rent and rate rebates will be near the poverty line. (The numbers quoted for rent and rates rebates underestimate the number in this income group because the proportion of eligible people who actually claim – the 'take-up' of the benefits – is not 100 per cent.) Probably about 2 million pensioners live below or near the poverty line.

Compared with households in which the head is employed, pensioner households spend a higher proportion of their income on essentials – food, heating, and housing – and therefore less on goods such as alcohol, tobacco, electrical equipment, and clothes, and less on services such as holidays or eating out. Evidence from the Ministry of Agriculture's National Food Survey in 1974 suggested that old people spend as much on food as younger people and that their purchase of prime foods such as meat, cheese, milk, eggs, vegetables, bread, and fruit was very similar but this survey, like all food surveys, did not give results which were completely reliable; for example, the fact that people are told that they are being included in a government survey influences their pattern of food purchasing. It seems that most pensioners have little money for luxuries but they have enough for the necessities of life, although many find heating costs a problem.

What is hidden by the simple comparison of 'pensioner households' with 'young households', however, is that there is a very wide range of wealth within the group of pensioner households. In general, older people are poorer (Fig. 22).

The wide disparity is not due to a drop in income as people grow older but to the fact that the proportion of people in each age group who have an occupational pension decreases the older the age group considered. This in turn is due to the fact that occupational pensions are a relatively recent innovation and it is therefore only younger retired people, those retiring more recently, who have qualified for them. The difference between the income of different age groups of retired people is accentuated because men die younger than women, on average, so that the older groups consist of relatively more women, many of whom are eligible for neither national insurance or occupational pensions and depend on a supplementary pension which is set at the lowest social security rate. Absolute and relative poverty is most common therefore among elderly women, particularly those who never married.

Prevention and Treatment

Poverty is the cause of many problems of elderly people. It is a major cause of housing and heating problems, it contributes to nutritional problems, and leads to isolation and therefore the sequelae of isolation. Furthermore, it symbolizes and perpetuates the poor image that older people have of themselves.

Obviously governments have the greatest opportunity for the prevention and treatment of poverty but government is not an isolated institution with a will of its own. Governments represent and reflect the electorate and if enough people press for higher pensions they will be introduced. The fault lies not in government but in society.

There is, however, much that every member of society can do to give direct help to any old person they meet. The doctor or nurse who meets elderly people can help in the prevention and treatment of poverty in three ways:

(a) By being aware of the range of benefits that are available including charitable sources of finance, and informing the elderly people they meet about them. There is no need for detailed knowledge but everyone should know what benefits are available and where to apply for each type of benefit.

(b) By helping those elders who have communication problems to make contact with the appropriate authority by offering assistance with form filling or letter writing.

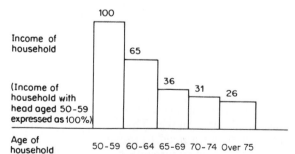

Figure 22   Income of household for various age groups. (From Age Concern, 1977)

(c) By emphasizing that the social security benefits are not charity but are one of the rights of every elderly person and by re-assuring and supporting the person who fears, or feels, humiliation at the hands of officials.

The relationship between doctor and patient often offers a very good opportunity for the prevention and treatment of poverty.

Housing Problems

Environmental Problems

For some older people the cause of their housing problem is not their dwelling but its environment. Many of those who moved into dwellings in the city centres when they were first married have seen the neighbourhood in which they live change and find the change alarming. Some feel that the area has 'gone down', that those who now live there do not have the same standards as they do, and that they are now aliens in a hostile environment in which they once felt at home. The problems of elderly people in city centres and areas of urban deprivation are serious and difficult to remedy because the only remedy is a move to another area in which the person may feel equally alien, although the majority of those who move settle well and happily.

Structural Problems

Often it is the dwelling itself that is the principal cause of the old person's concern. Common problems and their solutions can most easily be presented in a table (Table 20).

The services listed here are not universally available and even where such services exist older people often have difficulty mobilizing them, for the reasons already discussed. Every doctor can help by being aware of the range of services available, suggesting ways in which the dwelling can be improved and by helping the person to contact the appropriate services.

Difficulties Caused by Disability

Sometimes the dwelling itself is suitable until the onset of disability, and the type of problem that most commonly causes a housing problem

Table 20   Solutions to housing problems

Problem	Solution
Lack of toilet, bath, or hot water	The provision of grants and loans to help those who do not have the necessary capital
Difficulties with decorating, minor repairs such as broken windows and major repairs such as rewiring	Help from voluntary services with decorating and minor repairs Provision of grants and loans for major repairs
The cost of rent and rates or property taxes	The provision of financial help with heating costs
Problems caused by disability	Adaptation of the dwelling
Difficulty with heating	Installation of more effective and efficient heating apparatus Improved insulation

is the onset of a disabling disease that affects the old person's ability to climb the stairs, either stairs inside the house leading to the bathroom and toilet or the stairs leading to an apartment. Sometimes the circulation space within the house is too small to allow easy movement from room to room for a person using a wheelchair or walking aid.

The optimum solution to this type of difficulty is adaptation of the dwelling, and the domiciliary occupational therapist is the professional with the skill to do this.

Making a Move

The doctor's opinion about housing decisions is often as highly respected as his opinion about health decisions, particularly on that most difficult decision – 'should I move or stay put?'. Obviously each case is unique but it is possible to list guidelines for decision-making. Tables 21 and 22 give good and bad reasons for moving.

In general, every attempt should be made to solve the housing problem from which the old person feels she has to move away to remove the need for a move. That is not to say that there is never a need to move.

Sheltered or congregate housing is the type of housing which most people think of when new housing for elderly people is mentioned,

Table 21 Bad reasons for moving

1. Because of structural problems; the possibility of solving the structural problem should always be explored first.

2. Because of financial problems; the provision of the full range of financial benefits may solve the problem.

3. Because of disability; the advice of an occupational therapist should be sought.

4. To move away from an area in which the old person feels 'no-one cares'; more people may be assisting than she is prepared to recognize.

Table 22 Good reasons for moving

1. To move nearer a daughter or relative who is willing and able to offer care.

2. To move away from a dwelling that is impossible to repair, improve, or adapt.

3. To move away from an environment that is causing severe depression or anxiety.

4. To move to sheltered housing if there is a need to have someone to call for emergencies.

although many move to independent flats or bungalows. It offers security and reassurance and a well-designed and heated environment to elderly people and thus meets the needs of many frail elderly people, particularly those who are:

(a) nervous of living alone;
(b) anxious that they are not able to call anyone if they should fall ill;
(c) at risk of hypothermia;
(d) isolated, although it should be said that some people feel just as isolated in sheltered housing as in an independent dwelling.

It is not always suitable for the person who has antisocial tendencies or for the very confused person because the warden cannot cope with a large number of dependent people or with very dependent people. The fact that the warden lives on site has many benefits but it also has its drawbacks because she may be called incessantly by a confused person. It may be that the provision of more staff, i.e. the creation of 'very sheltered housing', will overcome some of the problems in sheltered housing, but it is always important to remember that the majority of disabled elderly people live and will continue to live in independent dwellings.

Heating Problems and Hypothermia

The biological and clinical aspects of hypothermia are discussed in Chapter 16.14. In this section the social causes and cures will be discussed (Wicks, 1978).

Social Risk Factors

The following factors increase the risk of hypothermia:

(a) low income;
(b) housing which is difficult to heat;
(c) ineffective or inefficient heating apparatus;
(d) depression;
(e) alcohol abuse;
(f) the old person's reluctance to use heating.

Housing Problems

The type of housing conditions which increase the risk of hypothermia may be summarized in a table (Table 23). It is usually possible to solve these heating problems and rarely necessary for an older person to move to obtain better heating.

Table 23

Housing problem	Solution to be advised to friends and relatives
Draughts round doors and windows	Ask volunteers to help with draught exclusion.
	Ask environmental health officer if help is avilable to replace doors and windows.
Size of house	Concentrate heating on a few rooms but remember that if one part of the house is cold draughts will be common and pipes will freeze
Inadequate loft insulation	Ask environmental health officer for advice about insulation grants.
Thin curtains	Line curtains with any thick material.

Faulty Heating Apparatus

The inverse heating law states that the greater the risk of hypothermia the worse the heating apparatus. The heating apparatus of older people is often ineffective, i.e. unable to produce a sufficient heat for the person's needs, or inefficient, i.e. unable to produce heat at reasonable cost. For example, a small 1-kw radiant electric fire is ineffective whereas a large 3-kw radiant fire may be effective but not efficient. The best solution is to supply a new type of heating apparatus but there are two obstacles – lack of finance and the attitudes of the old person who is at risk.

Many older people are caught in a poverty trap, unable to spend the capital necessary to get better value for money from their weekly income, but it is often possible to raise the necessary capital from statutory and voluntary services.

Even if this is possible, however, the old person may refuse to change her ineffective inefficient source of heat and this should be respected, especially if it is an open fire. Efforts must then be concentrated on the provision of background heat and the promotion of personal central heating and insulation, namely warm food and drink, exercise and activity, and warmer clothes and bedding.

It is important to remind relatives that the gas or electricity boards are willing to advise on the best setting for central heating, for some old people switch off a system that is 'too expensive' solely because the timer and thermostat are wrongly set.

Reluctance to Use Heating

The most difficult problems are often those in which the central issue is the reluctance of the old person to use her heating. This reluctance stems from the beliefs and attitudes of the old person about heating and hypothermia. Fear of debt has already been discussed (see page 000) and is a common cause of reluctance to use the available heating apparatus, but there are other causes and the best way to try to change the old person's attitude is firstly to ask her to explain it and to listen carefully and courteously to her theories before starting to try to influence them (see Table 24).

In the end it may be necessary to give up the attempt to persuade the old person and to resort to 'doctor's orders', simply telling the old person that she has to have more heat. However, the type of old person who is reluctant to use heat is often very difficult to influence

Table 24

Cause of reluctance to use heating	Possible line of argument
'I have never had a warm house, I'm used to it' – failure of the old person to appreciate that her body needs more heat due to the effects of ageing on the thermoregulatory mechanisms.	Explanation of the fact that the ageing process makes people more vulnerable to cold.
'Fresh air's good for you' – many elderly people were brought up in the belief that cold fresh air was an effective preventive and therapeutic measure for respiratory disease; remember the 'treatment' for tuberculosis before antibiotics.	Explanation that it is now known that fresh air is not necessary for good health, that it is acceptable to sleep with the window closed and that it is actually good for one's health to have heating in the bedroom.
'I prefer it this way' – reflecting the fact that some older people equate warmth and comfort with self-indulgence and sensuality.	Very difficult to change this attitude except perhaps by arguing that it is foolish not to have adequate heat when older, if only for the benefit of home helps and nurses who come to help.

no matter how polite or deferential she may be when speaking to her doctor.

Attitudes of Other People

The term 'social problem' is usually used to describe the practical problems faced by many elderly people – the problems of deprivation. However, these practical problems, poverty, bad housing, difficulty with heating, and isolation, arise because of more subtle and less obvious social problems. The reason elderly people so frequently have such practical problems is that there are certain attitudes which constitute the main social problem of elderly people.

Low Esteem

Most societies in the developed countries of the Western world hold elderly people in low esteem. This is symbolized by the low level of income of people who have retired compared with those of working age. This reflects the importance of work in the value system of developed countries and elderly people, like others who are unable to work or who are out of work, e.g. single parents, young disabled people, and the unemployed, are held to be less valuable members of society and less entitled to receive shares of the wealth of that society. It is true that elderly people often receive preferential treatment compared with these other groups, e.g. there are social security regulations that confer benefits on elderly people solely on account of their chronological age, but in the main elderly people are treated like others who do not appear to contribute to our society. Elderly people, of course, do make a contribution to society and many of them have made a very great contribution to society in the past, but past contributions are not considered as being important when assessments of value are being made.

Not only are modern societies those in which work is seen to be important, they are societies in which wealth is also an important determinant of status. The low income of elderly people, therefore, not only symbolizes the low esteem in which they are held, it also perpetuates it. There is a myth about old age in times past and the myth is that there was at one time a 'Golden Age' for elderly people, an age in which it was good to be old and in which elderly people were loved and respected. The myth has become elaborated with time and some people believe that the Golden Age was destroyed by the industrial revolution because the traditional skills of elderly men and women which they passed on to the younger generations by the fireside and in the inglenook were rendered redundant by the speed of change at that time (Fischer, 1977).

Attractive though this myth is there is no substance for it in fact. There never was a Golden Age for elderly people (Laslett, 1968). Rich and powerful elderly people were certainly respected in times past and held on to their position of power and respect for as long as they could. They were not, however, loved as well as respected. In fact, they were often hated by their children because they kept the younger generations in subjugation for so long; the story of King Lear illustrates the tensions between the generations perfectly (Thomas, 1976).

It was only rich elderly people who were in positions of power and respect. Poor elderly people usually finished up in the workhouse

and it is important to remember that in many societies the proportion of elderly people living in institutions was higher in times past than it is today.

Underestimation

The abilities of elderly people are underestimated by many of those who meet them, including, unfortunately, many of those who meet them in a professional capacity. It is assumed that all the problems of old age are due to the ageing process and are therefore untreatable. It is also assumed by people who underestimate the abilities of elderly people that the normal ageing process and dementia are one and the same and it is common to hear elderly people being said to be 'dementing'.

The consequences of this underestimation are considerable and serious. One consequence is that problems are often accepted for too long; relatives and helpers assume that the old person's incontinence or immobility is due to 'her age' whereas it is due to a treatable condition. Even if the treatable condition is diagnosed, the friends and relatives may be reluctant or poorly motivated to help the elderly person take her treatment and follow the advice she has been given because they do not believe that rehabilitation is possible in old age. Regrettably this is still a view held by some professionals, including some doctors. (Gray and Wilcock, 1981).

There are other unfortunate consequences. The tendency to agree with an old person whatever she says is another manifestation of the underestimation of elderly people, it being assumed by some people that all elderly people are dementing and therefore unable to argue or debate or even to make a correction. This can cause or aggravate confusion, for nothing is more confusing than being agreed with if one is making a mistake. It can also cause or aggravate behaviour problems, for nothing makes behaviour problems worse more quickly than allowing the problem behaviour to take place without normal sanctions or expressions of displeasure. Too often this happens with elderly people and once the diagnosis of dementia is made the problem becomes even worse, for friends and relatives too often assume that every problem is due to dementia and overlook correctable factors which are aggravating the elderly person's confusion, e.g. urinary tract infection or the side-effects of medication.

This underestimation is a consistent prejudice called ageism. Ageism, like racism or sexism, is a prejudice and the person who is prejudiced has a set of beliefs and expectations about anyone displaying a certain characteristic. In the case of racism it is a racial characteristic, in the case of sexism it is a person's gender, whereas in ageism it is a person's chronological age. Fortunately there are moves to counter ageism, as there are moves to counter racism and sexism, but one of the most difficult problems in trying to reduce ageist prejudice is that many old people also share the beliefs that form the basis of the ageist prejudice and are not prepared to challenge those who underestimate their abilities or potential.

Guilt and Overprotection

There has never been a better time to be elderly than the present day if one is frail and disabled, particularly if one is poor. Society does care for elderly people and people are concerned about what they can do to help their elders. This caring attitude is very welcome and praiseworthy but there are certain aspects of it which are less laudable. At least some of the protective and caring feelings towards elderly people which prevail in society stem from the underestimation of the ability of elderly people to appreciate their own problems and to find their own solutions. In addition, some people become protective because they feel guilty and their caring attitude stems more from guilt than from love.

Elderly people who are in difficulty or at risk evoke different types of emotional reaction from their friends, neighbours, and relatives. Some evoke a positive caring reaction, one that stimulates the person who is upset to try to help the elderly person constructively. However, it is not uncommon for the reaction to be a guilty reaction and for the person who is upset by the plight of an elderly neighbour to call for the neighbour's removal 'for her own good'. The guilt arises from the fact that the person who feels guilty does not try to take a constructive effort to solve the old person's problem and the reasons for this are that they think that the caring should be provided by the statutory services or that they do not wish to appear nosy or intrusive. Whatever the reason for the inactivity of the friend or neighbour or relative the result is often feelings of guilt and the way in which the individual tries to resolve and allay his guilty feeling is to call for 'something to be done', which usually means putting the old person in a home 'for her own good'.

There are two ways in which these feelings of guilt can be prevented. One is to improve the conditions of elderly people. The second way is to clarify the relationship between friends, neighbours, relatives, and volunteers and those professionals who work, and are very highly paid for their work, in health and social services, because it is the confusion between those who are paid and those who are not paid as to what each expects of the other that inhibits many friends, neighbours, and relatives from stepping in to help and thus creates and perpetuates feelings of guilt.

Therefore it is only by changing the position of elderly people in society and by changing the relationship between voluntary helpers and professional helpers that feelings of guilt can be prevented and elderly people can be put under less pressure to go into a home or to be 'looked after' to allay the anxieties of others.

HEALTH BELIEFS AND ATTITUDES OF OLDER PEOPLE

Individuals make decisions about their health, such as:

(a) is this symptom one which requires treatment?
(b) can I treat it myself or do I need to see my doctor?
(c) how quickly should I see the doctor?
(d) should I follow the doctor's advice?

Decisions are made on the basis of information but information is not simply a collection of isolated facts. The facts are always influenced by the context in which they are transmitted or received. As stated by the doctor, they will be interpreted according to the beliefs of the individual, e.g. whether he believes his symptoms to be due to a disease or to 'old age'. Similarly, a person's interpretation of the facts is influenced by his attitudes towards disease and health services, e.g. the decisions a woman makes following the discovery that she has a lump in her breast are influenced by her degree of anxiety about cancer and the nature of her relationship with her family doctor. Beliefs and attitudes are therefore of vital importance in both preventive and clinical medicine (Gray and Wilcock, 1981)

Ageist Beliefs – 'It's My Age I Expect'

The term 'ageism' was coined after the terms 'racism' and 'sexism' and it is analagous to them. These terms are the names given to prejudices. Each prejudice is towards a group of people who happen to share a certain characteristic. In ageism the characteristic is advanced chronological age. The person who holds ageist views believes that all people over the age of 65 are of declining intelligence, unable to change or learn, rigid, conservative, and dull. He assumes that any physical or mental change is due to the ageing process and is therefore untreatable. He also has a certain set of expectations about the way older people should behave, e.g. that it is not normal for older people to drink to excess, show an interest in members of the opposite sex, or even to argue forcibly with people with whose views they disagree. Many old people hold ageist views and assume that all physical and mental changes are due to 'old age', i.e. the ageing process.

It is only in the last few decades that some doctors have appreciated the difference between the effects of the ageing process and the effects of disease, it is not surprising that many people assume that all the changes they see in old age are due to 'old age'. This assumption seems to have been held for thousands of years and older people grew up in a society in which it was an unchallenged prevailing belief. They acquired it when young and most have carried it into old age.

Effects of Ageist Beliefs

The two main effects are:

Failure to seek help for treatable medical problems – 'what else can you expect at my age?'.

(b) Failure to comply with medical advice –

'it was kind of the doctor to give me tablets but there's no point in taking them, it's just old age that's the problem'.

Practical Implications

It is important to try to correct this mistaken belief at every opportunity.

In talks, lectures, and leaflets given or distributed to groups of older people it is essential to emphasize the difference between ageing and disease. Often people ask how they can tell the difference and it is difficult to answer this question in general terms. However, one useful rule of thumb which many older people find helpful is to be told that if they have noticed that their problem has developed within a period of time that can be defined precisely, it should be assumed to be due to disease. For example, if the symptom has developed 'in the last six weeks', or 'since Christmas', or 'since my daughter last came to see me', or 'in the last six months', it is a symptom which requires medical attention. If, on the other hand, it is a symptom which has come on gradually, 'over years' or 'since I got married', it is probably due to the ageing process, or to a loss of fitness, or to both processes acting together.

Imprecise though this distinction may be most older people find it helpful and useful.

At initial assessment it is possible and important to emphasize the distinction between ageing and disease, thus gently correcting the mistaken beliefs of the elderly person. When a patient is describing her symptoms she can be told that 'they sound like the symptoms of a treatable disease and not just due to your age'. When the diagnosis is made the old person should be told that it is a disease and not just the name given to describe an aspect of the ageing process. When treatment is prescribed it should be emphasized that it is to combat the effects of disease.

At follow-up and review the opportunity should be taken to educate an elderly patient about the difference between ageing and disease and the beneficial effects of the physiotherapy or drug therapy.

When speaking to relatives and friends, who play a major part in forming and modifying health beliefs, it is essential to try to influence their beliefs. They should be given the same message and encouraged to reinforce the old person's belief that her problems are treatable because they are due to a disease and not inevitable sequelae of the ageing process.

Religious Beliefs – 'It's God's Will'

People who are old today were brought up in a culture in which religion played a more important part than it does today.

The Effects of Religious Beliefs

One important effect of a strong religious faith may be a fatalistic approach to life. This is marked among elderly Moslems for whom 'the Will of Allah' is omnipotent and omnipresent but is also found among Christians, particularly among the more fundamentalist Churches. However, the elderly Christian who believes that his suffering is due to 'God's Will' is rarely unwilling to accept help because of this, viewing doctors, nurses, antibiotics, anaesthetics, and all the other wonders of modern medicine as being other manifestations of God's Will and therefore to be accepted joyfully. Occasionally, however, an old person refuses offers of help because of his belief that God has decided that he should suffer.

A more common consequence of a strong religious faith is the interpretation of problems as a punishment for some past sin or transgression. Sickness is described in the *Book of Common Prayer* as a 'fatherly correction', 'God's visitation', and the 'chastisement of the Lord' sent 'to correct and amend you'. Another, slightly more comforting view, also given in the *Book of Common Prayer*, is that 'there should be no greater comfort to Christian persons than to be made to like unto Christ, by suffering patiently adversities, troubles and sicknesses'. Thus, sickness is 'profitable' for the Christian sufferer.

For many people suffering and sickness in old age are seen as profitable, as giving opportunities for looking at, and valuing, life in a fresh light and as opportunities for appreciating the love and friendship of those who are close. For others, however, the development of disease results in suffering either because the person thinks he can identify a cause for his problems – 'I often think it's all due to the unkindness I showed to my daughter all those years ago' – or because he cannot understand why he should suffer – 'It doesn't seem right, I go over and over it in my mind', 'I've helped people all my life. It doesn't seem fair'; 'I can't understand why God has let it happen to me'.

A person who is distressed by this type of thought may become preoccupied or even obsessed by it, raging against the influence and unfairness of her suffering. The clinical consequences of this can be a serious inability to adapt satisfactorily to the demands of a disabling disease, and it is probable that the pain threshold will be lowered by the agitation and that symptoms such as pain, pruritis, or breathlessness will be more distressing and less responsive to drug therapy.

Practical Implications

Firstly, it is essential to think about this aspect of suffering at initial assessment. Many patients suffer a great deal because they cannot find an acceptable answer to the question, 'Why me, why am I suffering?', or even to an adequate opportunity for discussing the question with someone else. There is no easy answer to this question but the opportunity of discussing it often gives considerable relief. A good approach is to open the discussion by saying something like, 'Many older people feel bitter because they are suffering while other people are spared, do feelings like that ever bother you?' The person may simply say, 'It's just bad luck I suppose' or 'There are others worse off than me so I can't complain', and are obviously not bothered by such questions. In the case of the person who is however, such an opportunity will usually be accepted if he respects and trusts his doctor.

The second practical implication is the need to establish close links between the hospital or community health staff and the local ministers of religion. The minister of religion should be an integral member of every team of workers caring for elderly people because he has a valuable contribution to make to comprehensive health care. The spiritual dimension of care should not be ignored.

Pessimistic Attitudes – 'I'm All Right, It Could Be Worse'

Many elderly people have a pessimistic outlook on life and, because of this, do not seek help, follow advice, or participate enthusiastically in a rehabilitation programme.

This pessimism may be due to the mistaken belief that all the problems of old age are due to the age process and therefore untreatable. There are, however, other reasons why many older people have a pessimistic outlook.

Lower Standards

The standard of living of many older people, although lower than it was immediately before retirement, is often higher than it was in the 1920s or 1930s.

> Mr S. was an Old Contemptible and fought through the mud of France. In his middle seventies he lived in a damp council house disabled by bronchitis and a stroke. The district nurse and social worker tried to raise money to buy him a gas fire for his bedroom but without success. They went to break the news to him, a little apprehensive about the effect of the disappointment. They need not have been worried. He was not in the least bothered. 'Don't worry, son', he said to the doctor, 'sixty years ago today I was up to my waist in mud and water'.

Consider how many women in the past often had to struggle to feed both husband and children, while hiding from them the fact that they themselves were not eating enough. No matter how great the deprivation that an woman has to face in old age it may appear slight in comparison with the difficult times she has known in the past.

Lower Expectations

Many older people do not have high expectations and their outlook is summarized in the phrase, 'could be worse'. To understand the reason for this we should consider how often their generation has been disappointed by unkept promises, such as the promise of 'the war to end all wars', or 'homes fit for heroes', or 'peace in our time'. They have grown sceptical and prefer to adopt the 'could be worse' approach to life rather than allow their hopes to be built up by promises of rehousing or financial help or rehabilitation.

Lower Assertiveness

Older people want less and they demand less, not only because their expectations are lower but also because they are less assertive than younger people. This is a reflection of the attitudes in the society in which people who are old today grew up, a society in which one could be evicted or fired with neither notice nor appeal, a society in which the most vigorous and assertive were either killed or debilitated during World War I. As Erich Maria Remarque wrote in his classic *All Quiet on the Western Front*.

> Had we returned home in 1916, out of suffering and the strength of our experiences we might have unleashed a storm. Now if we go back we will be weary, broken, burnt out, rootless and without hope.

The attitudes of those who stayed at home were also irrevocably changed by that war:

> I remember that I was delivering milk on one street and all the women were standing at the door, waiting for telegrams. Then the post came and one after another they all keeled over, the whole street was affected there were so many deaths. It was after that, I believe, that they stopped putting men from the same street or village in the same platoon.

It is important, however, to remember that war has not affected all older people in the same way. Similarly the attitudes of members of any one generation are influenced by national and local cultural characteristics. Old people in America obviously have different attitudes from old people in Britain or France and within the one country there are also marked differences. The attitudes of elderly people who were miners, brought up in a culture in which working people were well organized, are different from the attitudes of retired farm workers in Oxfordshire or Berkshire.

The implications of this are that it is essential to take a biographical approach to work with older people: to learn about their experiences when they were young and the culture in which they grew up and to consider the biography of each patient as important as his description of his symptoms.

Practical Implications

Services for elderly people must be organized and delivered with this pessimism in mind. They will not seek help or demand their rights as readily or vociferously as younger people.

They need not only information about what is available but encouragement to apply. Everyone who meets elderly people has an important part to play and information about health and social services should not be restricted only to professionals but should be given to home helps, priests, voluntary workers, and relatives and friends.

The style in which the help is given is also important. Older patients need help from people who are lively, enthusiastic, and positive; many need to be given hope as the first step in the giving of help.

The objectives of any intervention should be stated explicitly and the initial targets should be those that can be attained without too much difficulty. Nothing succeeds like success in overcoming pessimism and the old person who feels overwhelmed by a host of insuperable health and social problems is more effectively encouraged by the identification and solution of one or two specific problems in the first instance than by a grand plan in which the ultimate objective is presented as the target at which she should aim.

Finally, it is important to remember that it may be unethical to challenge an old person's pessimistic, accepting approach to life or to disturb her tranquillity and equanimity by exhorting her to accept that things could be better if only she would cooperate. Old people, like young people, have a right to opt out.

Fearful Attitudes

Many older people are afraid and it is important to be aware of the common fears for three reasons:

(a) Because fear is a cause of anxiety and depression.
(b) Because the fears may influence the behaviour and the health of the person who is afraid.
(c) Because it is often easy to prevent or allay the fears which occur in old age.

Fear of Isolation

The effects of isolation vary from one person to another depending upon personality, level of education, degree of sensory deprivation, and the speed of onset of the disabling disease. Some people adapt much more easily than

others. However, certain effects are commonly encountered:

(a) Nutritional problems
(b) Intellectual deterioration
(c) Depression
(d) Dependence on those people who remain in contact

Effects of Fear of Isolation

The fear of isolation can reduce the motivation of a disabled person to become independent. Consider the situation of an old person who is severely disabled and who is being rehabilitated. The doctor and therapists plan a programme to help her 'get better' or 'improve' or 'regain independence'. These goals sound attractive in theory but how attractive are they in practice? What 'reward' does the old person face if she takes the drugs, works at her physiotherapy, and struggles to use the aids provided by the occupational therapist in the kitchen and bathroom? The answer is that the consequences would be that the home help and the meals-on-wheels lady would be stopped from coming to help her prepare food and the district nurse would be stopped from coming to help her bathe. She will certainly have 'improved' or 'been successfully rehabilitated' from the medical perspective, but her life may be much less enjoyable for the simple reason that about one-half of her important social engagements have been discontinued.

Practical Implications

This is not an easy fear to overcome, in part because the person is usually unaware of these motives but also because it is rarely possible to tell someone that if she regains her independence in washing or dressing she will be able to go to a day centre due to scarcity of provision. Isolation will reduce this fear but in the short term an approach which may be useful is to tell the old person that the more she does for herself the easier it is for those who are helping her, rather than saying the less will she need them.

Fear of Debt

'If I dropped down dead today there's one thing: I wouldn't owe a penny to anyone.'

Attitudes to debt have changed dramatically this century. In the past debt was feared because the debtor was treated unsympathetically and harshly and because it often led to eviction and institutionalization – 'to the workhouse'. Many older people are proud of the fact that they owe nothing to anyone whereas the professionals who are helping are often deeply in debt with overdrafts and mortgages, which may be a source of worry but are rarely a source of shame.

Effects of Fear of Debt

There are three common problems resulting from this fear. The first is refusal to spend money on clothes or on the upkeep and decoration of the old person's house, with the result that both the old person and his dwelling become tattered and worn. This is sometimes accompanied by a reluctance to wash. The other two problems – refusal to spend money on food or on fuel – are much more serious, with the latter being the more common.

Fear of debt is an uncommon cause of nutritional problems although many older people limit their intake of certain foods, notably meat, because of cost, but reluctance to spend money on fuel is more common and is sometimes a factor in hypothermia cases. Often the person most at risk is not the person without any money but the person who has the money to spend on fuel but who refuses to spend it. The fear of debt is most commonly encountered as a fear of fuel bills for three reasons:

(a) Many older people find it difficult to estimate how much fuel they are using and, thus, do not know how much money they are spending.
(b) They are expected to use fuel before they pay for it, whereas they have always been accustomed to paying for goods and services before using them.
(c) It is common practice to pay fuel bills quarterly whereas many older people have always been accustomed to weekly budgeting.

Practical Implications

It is obviously impossible to alter the basic personality of the old person who is becoming anxious about her income and expenditure. It is, however, often possible to mitigate the effects of the drop in income that occurs on retirement and to reduce the psychological impact of inflation.

The first step is to try to keep every older person in touch with economic reality. The more a person goes to the shops, discusses price rises with others, is told that her pension is being increased in line with prices, and has the opportunity to discuss with other retired people how best to make ends meet, the less likely she is to become obsessed by the cost of living and the fear of debt. With this type of anxiety, as with so many, the opportunity to discuss the source of the worry with others who are similarly affected is often a very effective way of reducing the level of anxiety. It may also be useful for those who are helping the old person to reveal that they are in debt without being forced to go to live in an institution.

In addition to an attempt to influence attitudes it is essential to offer elderly people who are afraid of debt alternative ways of paying for fuel. The best approach is to help the old person to pay for her fuel in small regular instalments, by means of a standing order or the purchase of gas or electricity stamps. Many older people are used to the idea of a thrift club or coal club and only need to be informed about the possibility of this type of arrangement to see its advantages.

Sometimes it is necessary to try to provide heating for an older person which she cannot turn off, e.g. storage heaters. Someone who is fit and alert will obviously be able to turn off a storage heater but if the problem is in part due to the old person's inability to think logically because of dementia, she may not even appreciate that the storage heater is a source of heat and therefore leave it on. It is, of course, a serious step to decide that an old person is incompetent and unable to manage her affairs and it is not one that should be taken lightly.

Fear of Institutionalization

Many older people are afraid of being 'put in' a home or of being 'kept in' if they agreed to go in for what is promised to be a stay of short duration. These fears stem in part from the experiences of being pushed about that many older people had when younger, of being evicted without warning, or fired without notice or redress, and, in particular, of seeing older people being admitted to the workhouse with little or no choice. Secondly, they derive from the fact that many older people feel helpless as a result of their physical disability and their sense of social inferiority.

This fear may be intensified by the pressure applied by relatives who make statements such as 'We'll get the doctor, he'll make you see sense' or 'If you don't agree to go they can have you taken away'.

Effects of Fear of Institutionalization

Two consequences of this type of fear are common: firstly, a reluctance on the part of the older person to admit that she has problems and, secondly, a reluctance to go to hospital for day care or for admission for a limited period of time.

If an old person is suspicious that someone has come to put her in a home or to persuade her to go into a home she may be unwilling to admit that she has problems or may try to play down their severity. If she is lonely she may be reluctant to admit it because she fears that the solution offered will not be more visitors to her at home or the provision of transport to go where she wishes but a place in an old people's home. Similarly if she cannot cope with housework she may fear that an admission of this will lead not to increased domiciliary help but to efforts to force or persuade her to go into a home to be looked after. The safest course for the old person who is suspicious or uncertain of the intentions of the person assessing her is therefore to say, 'I'm all right'.

Reluctance to leave home even for day care is common among people who are afraid that people are conspiring to arrange for them to be put in a home.

Practical Implications

The fact that our policies are devoted to keeping people out of long-stay care is still poorly appreciated by many older people who have an image of doctors and social workers scouring the countryside trying to cajole, persuade, or force people into long-term care. It is there-fore essential to educate the public about the aims and objectives of geriatric medicine.

Secondly, it is important to find out what the person who has referred the problem and the others who are involved expect to happen and what they have told the old person will happen. It is simple to ask, 'What were you hoping for when you asked for my advice?' and 'What have you told the old person about my visit?'. If the relative answers that she is hoping for permanent admission and that she has told the old person that the doctor 'will make her see sense' or 'have her taken away', the attitude of the old person to the consultation can be anticipated.

Thirdly, it is essential to reassure the old person explicitly very early during the consultation, by saying, for example, 'It's my job to help you stay on in your own home if that's what you want to do'.

All these sweeping generalizations require qualification and the most important qualification is to emphasize that this general account of the pessimism of older people, as with all the other attitudes, varies very much from one individual to another (Beauvoir, 1970; Blythe, 1979).

REFERENCES

Abrams, M. (1977). *Three Score Years and Ten*, Age Concern, London.
Adelstein, A. (1977). 'Tuberculosis deaths: A generation effect', *Population Trends*, **8**, 20–23.
Age Concern (1977). *Profiles of the Elderly*, Vol. 1.
Age Concern (1978). *Problems of the Elderly*, Vol. 6, pp. 7–8, Age Concern.
Beauvoir, S. de (1970). *Old Age*, Trans. P. O'Brian. Weidenfeld & Nicholson, André Deutch.
Blythe, R. (1979). *The View in Winter*, Allen Lane.
Butler, R. N. (1979). *The Graying of Nations: Creative Responses*, Age Concern, London.
Cameron, H. M., and McGoogan, E. (1981). *J. Path.*, **133**, 273–283.
Coggan, D., and Acheson, E. D. (1981). 'Trends in cancer morbidity in England and Wales', *Health Trends*, **13**, 89–93.
Cohn, R. M. (1979). 'Age and the satisfaction from work', *J. Gerontol.*, **34**, 264–272.
Doll, R., and Peto, R. (1981). *The Causes of Cancer*, Oxford University Press, Oxford.
Faimer, R. D. T., and Miller, D. L. (1977). *Lecture Notes on Community Medicine*, Blackwell Scientific Pubs., Oxford.

Fischer, D. H. (1977). *Growing Old in America*, Oxford University Press.

Fries, J. F. (1980). N Engl. J. Med., **303**, 130–134.

Gonzalez, E. R. (1980). 'Retiring may predispose to a fatal heart attack', *JAMA*, **243**, 13–14.

Gray, J. A. M., and Wilcock, G. K. (1981). *Our Elders*, Oxford University Press.

Grimley Evans, J. (1977). 'Current issues in the United Kingdom', in *Care of the Elderly* (Eds A. N. Exton Smith and J. Grimley Evans), Academic Press, London.

Harris, A. (1971). *Handicapped and Impaired in Great Britain*, HMSO.

Hunt, A. (1978). *The Elderly at Home*, HMSO.

Hunt, A. (1978). *Problems of the Elderly*, Vol. 6, pp. 7–8, Age Concern, London.

Isaacs, B. (1971). 'Geriatric patients: do their families care?', *Br. Med. J.*, **4**, 282–286.

Hendricks, J., and Hendricks, C. D. (1977). *Ageing in Mass Society: Myths & Realities*, Winthrop, Englewood Cliffs.

Karn, V. (1977). *Retiring to the Seaside*, Routledge and Kegan Paul, London.

Kohn, R. R. (1982). 'Cause of death in very old people', *JAMA*, **247**, 2793–2797.

Laslett, P. (1968). *The World We Have Lost*, Methuen, London.

Leate, R. (1976). 'Marriage and divorce', *Social Trends*, **Spring**, 3–8.

Lewis, A. F. (1981). 'Fracture of neck of femur: changing incidence', *Br. Med. J.*, **283**, 1217–1218.

Lowther, C. P., and Williamson, J. (1966). 'Old people and their relatives', *Lancet*, **2**, 1459–1460.

Maeda, D. (1978). 'Ageing in Eastern society', in *The Social Challenge of Ageing*, (Ed. David Hobman), p. 98, Croom Helm, London.

Moroney, R. M. (1976). *The Family and the State*, Longman, London.

Pearce, D. (1975). 'Births and family formation patterns', *Social Trends*, **1**, 6–8.

Portnoi, V. A. (1981). 'The natural history of retirement', *JAMA*, **245**, 1752–1754.

Shneider, E. L. and Brody, J. A. (1983) Ageing, Natural Death and the Comparison of Morbidity: Another View. *N. Engl. J. Med. 854–855*.

Thomas, K. V. (1976). 'Age and authority in Early Modern England', *Proc. Br. Acad.*, **62**.

Velez, R., Beral, V., and Cuzik, J. (1982). 'Increasing trends of multiple myeloma mortality in England and Wales 1950–79: Are the changes real?', *J.N.C.I.*, **69**, 387–392.

Weinstein, M. C. (1980). 'Estrogen use in post menopausal women—costs, etc., and benefits', *N. Engl. J. Med.*, **1980**, 303–308.

WHO (1980). *International Classification of Impairments, Disabilities, and Handicaps*, World Health Organization.

Wicks, M. (1978). *Old and Cold – Hypothermia and Social Policy*, William Heinemann, London.

Wilcock, G. K., Gray, J. A. M. and Pritchard, P. M. M. (1982). *Geriatric Problems in General Practice*, Oxford University Press.

Williamson, J. (1981). 'Screening, surveillance and case-finding', in *Health Care of the Elderly* (Ed. T. Arie), pp. 194–213, Croom-Helm, London.

3.2

Immunity and Ageing[1]

E. T. Bloom, W. J. Peterson, M. Takasugi, T. Makinodan

INTRODUCTION

That immune functions undergo changes with age has been well documented and is discussed in various reviews (Callard, 1981; Doggett *et al.*, 1981; Leech, 1980; Makinodan and Kay, 1980; Meredith and Walford, 1979;).[2] It is not surprising therefore that increased attention has been given to the role that immune dysfunction plays in diseases of the elderly. Two reasons can be offered. (a) It is becoming apparent that age-induced abnormalities of the immune system contribute to many major acute and chronic diseases of the elderly. (b) Immunorestorative measures could provide an option in addition to the conventional drug therapy for controlling diseases of the elderly.

In this chapter we will address ourselves first to immune functions which are vulnerable to ageing, then to the cellular changes responsible for the functional alterations, and finally to methods for returning immune functions to levels approaching those of younger mature individuals.

IMMUNOLOGICAL FUNCTIONS VULNERABLE TO AGEING

Age-related alteration in normal immunological functions has been observed in humans and in all experimental animals examined, including mice, rats, hamsters, and dogs. The onset and rate of change with age, however, can vary with the species, strains within species, and immunological indices. Most immunological activities show a decline with age, some show an increase, and a few show no significant change.

Cell-Mediated Immunity

It can be seen that in general T-cell-dependent cell-mediated immunological functions decline with age *in situ*. They include a primary delayed type of hypersensitivity skin reactions, resistance to challenge with syngeneic, allogeneic, and xenogeneic tumour cells, resistance to challenge with virus, protozoans, and certain types of bacteria, and primary skin allograft rejection.

There have been conflicting reports in the literature, but only a few. For example, in the case of delayed hypersensitivity skin reaction, no decrease with age in the intensity of reaction or in the frequency of individuals with positive skin reaction has been observed. The failure to detect a decrease could be that the individuals examined may have been subjected to a secondary, rather than a primary, delayed type of hypersensitivity skin reaction, as the test antigens employed were those commonly found in our environment.

Various *in vivo* and *in vitro* T-cell and T-cell-dependent immunological activities have also been shown to decrease with age. They include graft-versus-host reaction, cytolytic T-cell response, mixed lymphocyte reactions, mitogenic response to the plant lectins, phytohaemaglutinin (PHA) and concanavalin A,

[1]This publication was supported in part by V. A. Medical Research Funds, Department of Energy Contract EY-76-S-03–0034, NIH Grant No. CA30187, and NIH Contract NO1-CP43211.

[2]Readers should refer to these reviews for specific references which have been omitted in this chapter to conserve space.

helper T cell activity, T cell growth factor production, and suppressor T cell activity.

Conflicting findings have been reported. The most serious concerns suppressor T cell activity, which has been studied in mice and humans. In mice, it was found that autoimmune disease-resistant long-lived mice show an increase with age, while the autoimmune disease-susceptible, short-lived mice show a decrease, as cited above. The decrease in suppressor cell activity could account for the emergence of autoantibody and autoimmune disease in the older short-lived mice, but the increase in suppressor activity with age cannot account for the increase observed in autoantibody frequency in long-lived mice. Equally perplexing are the results obtained in humans. Thus, an increase in concanavalin-A-stimulated suppressor factor production and an increase in the number of T cells with Fc receptors for immunoglobulin (Ig) G (presumably T suppressor cells) have been observed. The complexity of the suppressor activity phenomenon is reflected by the observation that concanavalin-A-activated suppressor cells from elderly individuals produce less suppressor factors but suppress the mitogenic response of autologous cells to a greater extent than do those of the young. The lack of correlation within an age group between the two suppressor assays indicates that multiple factors influence the overall suppressor influence on responder cells.

It should be noted that in contrast to the age-related decline in activity of cytolytic and graft-versus-host T cells reactive against allogeneic cells, those which are autoreactive increase with age. This is consistent with the observation that resistance to tolerance induction against modified self cells increases with age. Similarly, humoral autoreactivity and resistance against development of autoreactive humoral immunity also increase with age, which will be discussed later.

The influence of age on two other types of cell-mediated immunological activities, which in general do not involve mature T-cells as the responder cells, has been examined recently – namely the natural cell-mediated cytolytic (NCMC) and antibody-dependent cytolytic cell (ADCC) activities. No decline with age could be detected in ADCC activity in mice. NCMC activity does not decline with age in rats, but

does so in mice. The differences between mice and rats may be due to interspecies variability or to differences in the cytotoxicity testing methods. In humans, the results are also contradictory, as both no change and an increase in NCMC and ADCC activities have been observed. The difference in NCMC and ADCC activities observed in humans between investigators could be due to demographic and sampling discrepancies.

Humoral Immunity

The ability to mount a primary but not necessarily a secondary antibody response decreases with age. Moreover, decreases can occur at the time when the thymus begins to involute and when the circulating level of serum thymic hormone factors begins to decrease. This would suggest that ageing may be affecting thymus-derived T cells which regulate the antibody response in addition to possibly the antigen-specific B responder cells. This suspicion has been verified by the subsequent demonstration that the antibody response of B cells to complex natural antigens generally requires the help of T cells. There have been reports showing no decline in primary antibody responses, especially against bacterial and viral vaccines. One explanation is that the individuals have been previously exposed to the antigen and therefore are, in fact, mounting a secondary response.

Associated with the declining capacity to mount a primary antibody response to complex antigens with age, we find a decrease in (a) the circulating levels of isoantibody and heteroantibody starting shortly after the thymus begins to involute, (b) the avidity of murine antibodies, (c) the ability of murine B cells to transform into antibody-secreting cells upon stimulation with gram-negative bacterial lipopolysaccharide (LPS), and (d) the concentration of IgA in the nasal secretion in humans.

We also find that certain other B-cell-dependent immunological indices decrease minimally with age, and they include: (a) the circulating level of IgM in humans, (b) the ability to develop Arthus-type hypersensitivity in mice, and (c) the proliferative capacity of B cells of certain inbred strains of mice in response to LPS stimulation.

B-cell mediated immunological indices

which show an increase with age include: (a) circulating levels of IgG and IgA in humans, (b) the frequency of individuals with monoclonal gammopathies in humans and mice, (c) the frequency of individuals with circulating autoantibodies in humans and mice, (d) murine B cells transforming into autoantibody-forming cells upon stimulation with LPS, and (e) resistance to tolerance induction in mice.

The existence of positive and negative correlations between age and most cell- and antibody-mediated immunological indices underscores the complexity of the mechanisms responsible for the changes of immunological activities with age. The magnitude of the problem is further magnified, as it would appear that age-related changes in immunological activities of the spleen need not correlate with those of the peripheral lymph nodes, which in turn need not correlate with those of gut-associated lymphoid tissues. These age-associated and organ-related differences in immunological activities strongly implicate the involvement of multiple factors in modulating antigen-responsive T and B cells.

It is clinically important that with alteration in immune functions with age, individuals become more vulnerable to infectious, autoimmune and immune complex, and cancerous diseases, as is the case in immunodeficient children and immunosuppressed adults. What is not clear is whether the diseases compromise normal immune functions or whether a decline in normal immune functions to threshold levels predisposes individuals to diseases. We favour the latter explanation because of the following observations: (a) the onset of decline in immune functions under the influence of T cells (lymphocytes that differentiate within the thymus or under thymic influence) can occur as early as sexual maturity when the thymus begins to involute, which is long before immunodeficiency diseases of the elderly are manifested; (b) immunodeficiency, wasting disease, amyloidosis, and autoimmunity in neonatally thymectomized mice and in genetically susceptible mice can be prevented, or at times even reversed, by reconstituting them with young but not old syngeneic thymus or spleen grafts; (c) adult humans subjected to immunosuppressive drug therapy are many times more vulnerable to cancer than are normal adults; (d) patients with primary immu-

nodeficiencies in which the immune systems fail to develop normal activity are vulnerable to autoimmunity, amyloidosis, and certain forms of cancer; and (e) cessation of immunosuppressive therapy following inadvertent transplantation of cancer along with renal transplant leads to the prompt rejection of the tumour and even of widely disseminated cancer.

The intriguing possibility exists that a delay, reversal, or prevention of the decline in normal immune functions could delay the onset and/or minimize the severity of certain diseases of the elderly. However, before any attempt is made to intervene with disease processes, it would seem that an understanding of the basic mechanism(s) responsible for the loss of immunological vigour is both desirable and essential. It is not surprising, therefore, that much of the research in immunosenescence has currently been centered on the basic mechanism responsible for it.

MECHANISMS OF AGE-RELATED ALTERATIONS IN IMMUNOLOGICAL ACTIVITIES

Alterations in immunological activities of ageing mice could result from changes in the immune cells, changes in their milieu, or both. To differentiate between the influence of cells from that of their milieu, the cell transfer method was employed. In this assay, immunocompetent cells from young (Y) and old (O) mice undergo antisheep red blood cell responses in immunologically inert old and young syngeneic recipients, respectively (Y → O) and (O → Y). The results showed that both types of change affect the immune response, but much of the normal age-related alteration can be attributed to changes in the immune (donor) cells, i.e. (Y → Y) > (Y → O) > (O → Y) > (O ⟶ O).

Cellular Milieu

Systemic non-cellular factors were shown to influence the immune response. Spleen cells from young mice were cultured with the test antigen either in the spleen or peritoneal cavity of immunologically inert young (or old) recipients by the cell transfer method and the cell-impermeable diffusion chamber method, respectively. A twofold difference in response was observed between young and old recipients at both sites, indicating that the factor(s) is systemic. The fact that the effect was observed in cells grown in cell-impermeable diffusion chambers further indicates that a noncellular factor is involved. A comparable two-fold difference was observed also when bone marrow stem cells were assessed in the spleens of young and old syngeneic recipients, indicating that the systemic, non-cellular factor(s) influences both lympho- and haematopoietic processes.

The factor(s) could be a deleterious substance of molecular or viral nature, or it could be an essential substance that is deficient in old mice. Unfortunately, we know very little because this area of research has not progressed as rapidly as anticipated.

Cellular Changes (Extrathymic)

Parenchymal versus Stromal Cells

The cells of the immune system can be divided into two classes: (a) parenchymal cells, which include the stem cells (generally referring to all precursor cells), macrophages, B cells, and T cells, and (b) stromal cells which include the fibroblasts, epithelial cells, and smooth muscle cells. In general, the parenchymal cells tend to be more easily dispersed mechanically and are more sensitive to physical and chemical insults. Based on these considerations, it would appear from the cell transfer studies discussed above that both the parenchymal and stromal cells are affected by ageing but that the parenchymal cells are affected more than the stromal cells. Thus, immune cells from young donors performed better in young recipients than in old recipients, and old cells performed better in young recipients than in old recipients but not better than young cells in old recipients.

Relatively little is known about the effect of ageing on stromal cells, since few studies have been performed, with two possible exceptions. One on thymic epithelial tissue will be discussed subsequently.

Parenchymal Cells

Three types of cellular changes could cause a decline in normal immune functions: (a) an absolute decrease in cell number through death, which may be caused by autocytolytic cells; (b) a shift in the proportion of subpopulations of cells (e.g. an increase in the number of suppressor cells and/or decrease in helper cells); and (c) a decrease in functional efficiency caused, perhaps, by somatic mutation. A study on cellular changes in young and old mice showed that all three types of interactions can occur. About 60 per cent of responses of the individual old mice with reduced activity appeared to have been caused by an increase in the number or activity of suppressor cells, about 30 per cent by a shift in the limiting cell types, and about 10 per cent by a decrease in the functional efficiency of effector cells or their progenitors. These results discourage the pooling of tissues from individual old mice, a practice routinely carried out by many for convenience. They also demonstrate the complexity of approaching the age effect of the immune system at the level of tissues.

Stem cells. Any intrinsic alteration in the stem cells can affect the other cells of the immune system. Thus, there has been a continuing search for alteration in the stem cells. The percentage of stem cells with the ability to colonize in the spleen, commonly referred to as spleen colony-forming units (CFU-S), which are found most abundantly in the bone marrow, decreases with age in some, but not all, strains of mice. Because the number of nucleated cells in the bone marrow tends to increase with age, the total number of CFU-S in the bone marrow does not change significantly in those strains showing a decrease in CFU-S concentration.

The transplantation potential of adult stem cells is less than that of young cells, as demonstrated by the simultaneous serial transplantation of marker stem cells from young and adult donor mice. Unlike stem cells passaged *in vivo,* whose self-replicating ability can be exhausted, stem cells can self-replicate *in situ* throughout the natural lifespan of an individual. However, both the ability of stem cells to expand clonally and their rate of division decreases with age, as does their ability to repair X-ray induced damage, their ability to home to the thymus, and their rate of B cell formation.

As to the issue of whether age-related kinetic alterations of stem cells are likely to affect the immune capacity of old individuals, we believe that they are crucial to the old individual in stress. For example, immunologically immature young mice and immunologically inadequate old mice develop autoantibodies to erythrocytes following parainfluenza infection. However, young mice with autoantibodies do not become anaemic, whereas the old mice do. Thus, when stressed, as with infection, old individuals may not be able to maintain homeostasis by increasing cellular production to compensate for increased cellular destruction. The kinetic limitations on stem cell reserve may also account for the clinical observation that elderly individuals with sepsis frequently do not have an elevated white cell count, although they may have a shift to less mature leucocytes in their peripheral blood smears. The significance of young stem cells was also demonstrated in an immunorestorative study, which demonstrated that the grafting into old mice of newborn thymus is effective in elevating their immunological responsiveness for an extended period of time, provided young stem cells are also present.

Macrophages. Early studies on the role that macrophages play in the alteration of immunological activities with age were centered on those residing in the peritoneal cavity because of their accessibility. These studies showed that neither the number of macrophages in the peritoneal cavity nor their handling of antigens during both the primary and secondary immune responses is adversely affected by age. Furthermore, the activity of lysosomal enzymes in splenic and peritoneal macrophages is increased rather than decreased with age. Subsequent studies showed that the capacity of splenic macrophages and other adherent cells to cooperate with T and B cells in the initiation of antibody response *in vitro* was also unaffected by age.

B cells. Although the total number of B cells in humans and mice does not change appreciably with age, the size of certain subpopulations may change as indicated by the increase in circulating levels of IgG and IgA in humans and in benign monoclonal gammopathies in humans and mice.

Qualitative changes in the B cells also appear to be occurring with age. For example, the ability of old B cells to respond to T-cell-dependent antigens, even in the presence of young T cells, is impaired. The alteration may be at the surface membrane level, as indicated by changes in the receptor-mediated signalling mechanism of B cells with age. Alteration in the receptor-mediated signalling mechanism could account for the inability of LPS to transform B cells of old mice into antisheep RBC-secreting cells, although they did proliferate as well as LPS-stimulated B cells from young mice. In this regard, the rate of capping and shedding of crosslinked surface immunoglobulins by B cells was seen to be slower in old rats than in young rats, and this age-related kinetic alteration was associated with a decrease in the density of surface immunoglobulins. Decrease in the density of surface immunoglobulins has also been noted in circulating B cells of ageing humans. At the intracellular level, B cells of old, but not of young, rats were shown to possess altered mitochondria; i.e. mitochondria that are often swollen, containing myelin-like fibres, with reduced numbers of cristae.

T cells. Decrease in the number of T cells has been detected in certain, but not all, strains and hybrid stocks of ageing mice examined; and, furthermore, the pattern and magnitude of change in the number of T cells are dependent upon the tissue and organ; i.e. whether it is in the spleen, lymph nodes, bone marrow, or thymus.

In humans, the number of circulating T cells has been reported either to decrease progressively after adulthood or remain the same. The evidence that the proportion of T cell subpopulations is shifting with age is abundant. For example, an increase has been observed in the proportion of short- to long-lived T cells in the blood, lymph nodes, and spleen with age. Another example is the faster decline with age in the rate of mitogenic response to PHA than to Con A.

T helper cell activity declines with age in long-lived mice which also show an increase in T suppressor cell activity. Of course, a decrease in T suppressor activity has also been observed in a certain strain of mice, but these mice are short-lived. In humans the situation is less clear-cut regarding the T regulatory cells, since both the T helper and suppressor cell activities seem to decline with age, as discussed earlier.

Qualitative changes with age are also evident. At the membrane level, two observations support the view that surface receptors change with age – one indicating loss and the other an emergence of new receptors. The loss is reflected by the decrease in the surface density of Thy 1 antigens with age, as judged by immunofluorescence. Evidence for the emergence of new receptors comes from two observations: (a) young mice can undergo syngeneic graft-versus-host response when injected with syngeneic cells from old but not young donors and (b) young mice can be induced to undergo syngeneic mixed lymphocyte reaction and synthesize cytotoxic antibodies by injecting syngeneic cells into them from old but not young donors. These observations have obvious implications for certain diseases of ageing, particularly neoplasia and auto-immune-immune complex diseases, since it has been shown that continuous graft-versus-host reactions can increase the incidence of lymphoid tumour formation and autoimmunity.

Intracellular changes have also been detected. At the cytoplasmic level, both morphological and functional changes have been observed. Thus, for example, swollen mitochondria containing myelin-like structure with reduced numbers of cristae have been observed electron microscopically in T cells of old, but not young, humans. At the nuclear level, an increase in the loss of chromosomes in T cells has been observed with age, the loss of X and Y chromosomes being the most prevalent.

Other cells. This category of cells comprises those parenchymal cells that are not T cells, B cells, macrophages, or stem cells. They include cells with NCMC and ADCC activities, which were discussed earlier.

Cellular Changes (Thymic)

Since the involution of the thymus, which occurs at about the time of sexual maturity, precedes the age-related decline in T-cell-dependent immune responses, thymic involution has been suspected to be responsible for the decline. Some of the observations in support of this suspicion are as follows:

(a) Peak thymus weight is attained later in life in long-lived mice and they retain a greater thymus-to-body weight ratio later in life than do short-lived mice.

(b) Adult thymectomy of autoimmune-susceptible and autoimmune-resistant mice accelerates the decline in T-cell-dependent humoral and cell-mediated immune responses, increases autoimmunity, and decreases longevity.

(c) Graft of thymus from young mice into syngeneic old mice can offer partial immunological restoration, as does *in vivo* treatment of old mice and humans with thymic hormones.

(d) Dietary restriction, which extends life expectancy in mice, slows the rate of immunological maturation and the subsequent decline in immunological vigour, and these functional alterations are associated with the stunting of thymus growth, specifically of the cortical tissue.

Since thymus involution is associated with atrophic changes in its epithelial tissue that synthesizes thymic hormonal factors, a series of studies were performed to assess the capacity of ageing thymic grafts to generate factors needed for the maturation of precursor stem cells into mature T cells. The results revealed that the ability of thymic grafts to produce factors decreases with age.

In view of these observations, the thymus has been implicated as the ageing 'clock' of T cells. Three possible mechanisms can be proposed to account for ageing of the thymus, which can be triggered by intrinsic or extrinisic factors. One is clonal exhaustion; i.e. thymus cells have a genetically programmed clock mechanism to self-destruct and die after undergoing a fixed number of divisions. The mechanism would be similar to that of the Hayflick phenomenon, which is seen in fibroblasts *in vitro*. It would require that the thymus 'count' the number of migratory thymocytes leaving it or the number of divisions thymocytes undergo, or both. Another possible mechanism is gene deregulation, either intrinsically involving transposons, or through viral infection. The third possible mechanism is a stable molecular alteration at the non-DNA level through subtle error-accumulating mechanisms.

RESTORATION OF IMMUNE FUNCTIONS OF THE AGED

Attempts have been made in experimental rodents to restore immune functions of the aged animals to levels approaching those of younger mature individuals for two reasons: (a) an effective method could be used in geriatric preventive medicine and (b) an effective method could be used as a probe to study cellular and molecular mechanisms of age-related immune dysfunction. Of the attempts made, cell and tissue grafting and chemical treatment have shown significant restorative effects, and therefore they will be discussed.

It should be noted that methods have also been attempted to delay the onset and/or decrease the rate of declining normal immune functions. However, these will not be discussed here, since the effect seems to occur through perturbation of the developmental phase of life. Thus, for example, the most effective method for delaying the onset of immunosenescence has been caloric restriction early in life, a life-extending method first described in rats nearly 50 years ago.

Cell and Tissue Grafting

Since the loss of normal immune functions with age does not begin until after the thymus begins to involute, it is not surprising that attempts have been made experimentally to potentiate immune functions of old mice by implanting into them thymic grafts from genetically compatible young mice. Unfortunately, the results were at best marginal. Subsequent studies revealed that the loss of normal immune functions with age is due to (a) changes in the T cell population, (b) reduced rate at which old stem cells can expand clonally and generate progeny cells, (c) inability of involuted thymus to transform precursor cells into T cells efficiently, and (d) emergence of deleterious factors with age. When this information became available, both young bone marrow stem cells and newborn thymic lobes were grafted into long-lived old mice which had been exposed to a low-dose X-irradiation beforehand. This treatment restored their immune functions to levels approaching those of younger adult mice. The restorative effect was observed for 6 to 11 months after grafting in

mice with an MLS of 28 months (an equivalent of 0.22 to 0.39 of an MLS, or about 16 to 28 human years). No attempt was made to assess the effect of grafting on lifespan.

Studies on susceptibility to infection have also generated encouraging preliminary data. They showed that old mice can be made to resist lethal doses of virulent *Salmonella typhirmurium* by transferring spleen cells from young mice immunized beforehand with a vaccine.

Future studies in this area should resolve what effect, if any, grafting will have on the frequency and severity of diseases of the aged and whether cell and tissue grafting can alter the MLS of short-lived and long-lived mice. The results discussed here of the effects of grafting on immune functions would indicate that three criteria must be met for a graft to be effective in modulating age-related diseases and MLS, if immunity plays a major role:
(a) More than one type of tissue should be included in the graft.
(b) The potentially deleterious cellular environment of the host needs to be minimized to enable the graft to flourish.
(c) The graft must have a long lasting immunopotentiating effect.

Chemical Treatment

Three kinds of chemicals have been tested for their immunorestorative properties on old individuals: (a) thymic factors, (b) multistranded polynucleotides, and (c) antioxidants, including sulphydryl compounds.

Knowing that the contribution of the thymus to the immune system is a source of T cell differentiation-promoting factors, it would seem obvious that thymic factors would be used extensively to restore immunological activities of the aged. Surprisingly, however, they have been used only sparingly. In one study it was found that a thymus humoral factor (THF) can enhance the T-cell-dependent graft-versus-host activity *in vitro* of spleen cells of old, but not of young mice. This would indicate that THF is not acting as a non-specific adjuvant agent, since it would have also enhanced the graft-versus-host activity of young spleen cells. In another study, a substantial restoration of the capacity of old spleen cells to form high-affinity antibody, but not the total antibody-forming capacity, was demonstrated by exposing them to thymopoietin or to thymus tissue. In the third study, it was found that the number of T cells of old individuals can be increased by exposing their white blood cells to thymosin *in vitro*.

Double-stranded polynucleotides are also effective immunorestorative chemicals. Thus, it has been shown that double-stranded poly-adenylic-polyuridylic acid complexes can restore the T-cell-dependent antibody response of middle aged mice to that of young adult mice, and the supernatant of cultures of thymocytes treated with double-stranded polynucleotides is equally effective as an immunorestorative agent. This latter demonstration would suggest that the double-stranded polynucleotide restores immunological vigour of ageing mice by acting on T cells.

The use of antioxidants stems from the hypothesis that ageing is caused by mutation of somatic cells triggered in part by free radicals. Based on this hypothesis, antioxidants have been incorporated into the diet of ageing mice, and the results indicate that free-radical inhibitors can enhance the antibody response of adult and middle aged mice. In a related study, it was found that coenzyme Q_{10}, a non-specific stimulant of mitochondrial electron transport process of respiration, can enhance the level of antibody response of old mice to a level approaching that of adult mice.

Various sulphydryl compounds have been employed in enhancing various non-immunological and immunological cellular activities. One of these that shows some promise is levamisole, an antihelminthic drug, which has been used successfully to restore the declining immune functions of ageing mice. However, its effectiveness is demonstrable only when administered *in vivo* over an extended period, but not *in vitro*. This would suggest that levamisole itself may not be exerting its enhancing effect directly on the immune cells, but rather through either another cell type or a metabolite.

The most commonly used sulphydryl compound by immunologists is 2-mercaptoethanol (2-ME). Studies on its immunorestorative actions on ageing mice show that it enhances the antibody-forming capacity of splenic cells of old mice preferentially over that of young mice (old, 500 per cent; young, 30 per cent). That

2-ME is also an effective immunorestorative agent in intact old mice was demonstrated by restoring the antibody-forming capacity of long-lived old mice to that of young mice by giving 3 weekly injections of 4 μg of 2-ME. These results would suggest that 2-ME and related chemicals may have practical applications. The mode of action of 2-ME is not known. This is not surprising in view of the multitude of possible biochemical effects that sulphydryl compounds can have on cell structure and functions, ranging from SH/SS exchange reactions at the membrane level, to the antioxidant and metal chelating effects.

In summary, cellular and tissue grafting and chemical treatment appear to be promising for serving as probes to understanding the nature and mechanism(s) of age-related immune dysfunction. The former approach should enable one to determine the cell type or types most severely affected functionally and the latter approach the nature of the changes associated with it at the subcellular level. In terms of the practical application, chemical treatment could also serve as an effective method.

CONCLUDING REMARKS

The elucidation of the age-related alterations in immune functions is of great importance in light of the rising susceptibility of the elderly to infections, the likelihood that immunosenescence might also contribute to the age-related rise in cancer, and the role autoantibodies and immune complexes might play in general physical deterioration of ageing individuals through their participation in subclinical chronic tissue damages.

An attempt has been made to summarize our present knowledge on immune functions which are vulnerable to ageing with focus on the functional alterations and on methods for restoring immune functions to levels approaching those of younger mature individuals.

It would appear that alterations of immune functions can begin as early as when an individual reaches sexual maturity. The alterations are due to changes in the parenchymal and stromal immune cells and their milieu. Cell loss, shift in the proportion of subpopulations, and qualitative cellular changes, the three possible types of changes that can cause the decline, have all been detected. The most visible cellular target of ageing appears to be the T cells, and changes in their subpopulations involved in regulation are highly prominent. Since the changes are closely linked with the involution and atrophy of the thymus, an understanding of its changes could be a key to understanding immunosenescence. To compliment current mechanistic studies which are focused on the processes responsible for the disruption of cell-to-cell and intracellular communications, studies on restoration of the ageing immune system are evolving. An effective manipulative method will not only contribute to our understanding of immunosenescence, but will also open new avenues for treating the pathogenesis of ageing and providing geriatric preventive medicine.

Considering that the pathogenesis of ageing appears to be shifting away from the classical extrinsically-caused to intrinsically-caused diseases, current ongoing studies on immunosenescence should have a considerable impact on geriatric medicine.

ACKNOWLEDGEMENT

We wish to thank Mr J. Sproul for capable assembly of the manuscript.

REFERENCES

Callard, R. E. (1981). 'Aging of the immune system', in *Handbook of Immunology in Aging* (Eds M. M. B. Kay and T. Makinodan), pp. 103–122, CRC Press, Boca Raton, Florida.

Doggett, D. L., Chang, M.-P., Makinodan, T., and Strehler, B. L. (1981). 'Cellular and molecular aspects of immune system aging', *Mol. Cell. Biochem.*, **37**, 137–156.

Leech, S. H. (1980). 'Cellular immunosenescence', *Gerontology*, **26**, 330–345.

Makinodan, T., and Kay, M. M. B. (1980). 'Age influence on the immune system', in *Advances in Immunology* Vol. 29, (Eds H. Kunkel and H. Dixon), pp. 287–330, Academic Press, New York.

Meredith, P. J. and Walford, R. L. (1979). 'Autoimmunity, histocompatibility, and aging', *Mech. Ageing Dev.*, **9**, 61–77.

3.3

Biology of Ageing

D. Bellamy

INTRODUCTION

Research into the events leading to a decline in the capacity for adaptation lags far behind studies on the basic mechanisms of growth, maturation, and tissue maintenance. Our understanding of the biology of ageing has not kept pace with the spectacular successes of clinical medicine, so that there is now a great discrepancy between the amount of money spent and knowledge available to keep young people alive and that devoted to maintaining the aged in good physical and mental condition.

Although the impetus to study ageing arises largely from practical problems of human ageing, the field has a much wider scope than geriatric medicine. The area of investigation described as gerontology has lines of study that extend deeply into biology. From this standpoint, the overall aim of the experimental gerontologist is to discover how it comes about that different organisms have characteristic lifespans. The past life-history of the species as well as its present lifespan must be investigated. Within this general area of inquiry, there are two important subsidiary aims: to examine the possible connection between development and ageing and to seek methods of pharmacological, dietary, and environmental regulation in order to improve the quality of human life in the later decades. It is in this very broad sense that gerontology is a unified body of biological knowledge with clear guidelines of principle which have been little explored.

We do need to study the principles of ger-ontology in depth for sound academic and social reasons. At the academic level, ageing may be viewed as an inevitable outcome of life being organized as an interlocking system of unstable chemicals and sequential chemical reactions that tend to drift towards disorder. From this aspect, life is a strategy to overcome ageing. This places the study of chemical deterioration at the centre of biochemistry and molecular biology. Until recently, gerontology has made little impact on biochemical thought but this is simply due to the separate historical development of both subject areas and is not due to any fundamental disharmony in subject matter. In this context, the philosophy of the gerontologist is likely to be of great importance to the future development of biochemistry and molecular biology. It provides additional scope for formulating new concepts and increasing fundamental knowledge of living chemical systems. Also, ageing will never be fully comprehended until we have gained an understanding of the workings of youthful processes and because of this complementary relationship, biochemistry and gerontology will be bound together in their future development.

A need and desire to understand the temporal deterioration of living systems is beginning to arise from many fundamental areas of biochemistry. Since clock-like mechanisms are involved in the manifestation of many biomedical phenomena such as cancerous growth and the failure of reproduction, gerontological investigations are clearly of general academic relevance to the fields of physiology and behaviour.

The two changes just mentioned have important medicosocial implications and are also obviously on the borderline between the academic and practical goals of gerontology. Future practical rewards of research on ageing will be gained from efforts to accommodate successfully the extra years of human life won by medical research over the past century. This work will depend on fundamental knowledge and the results of clinical investigations.

The present low level of support for biological investigations connected with ageing is partly due to the way in which gerontology developed within medicine, from what was the low status field of geriatrics. Ageing, as a well-defined body of knowledge has been omitted from most biological and medical curricula, leaving a large gap in the training of those who should be able to further research. To these historical impediments may be added a current bias against research proposals, arising from ignorance on the part of those in competing fields; the high cost of maintaining stocks of animals of known pedigree into old age; and the difficulties that many specialists encounter in moving into what is essentially an interdisciplinary area of research, where it is hard to separate causes from effects at different levels of organization. There is also a largely unassessed factor arising from the fears of many scientists, who could potentially contribute to gerontology, that the study of ageing might provide a way of prolonging life and so add to our present unsolved social problems.

There are two approaches to restore the present unbalanced accumulation of knowledge, both of which require a deliberate increase in the proportion of our national educational and research budgets that are devoted to gerontology.

An early objective must be to provide new educational resources and research training programmes, backed by appropriate funds for research. More support must be given to research in fields other than biochemistry. While there can be little doubt that ageing will be ultimately explained in molecular terms, it is not easy to integrate the findings of molecular biology into the levels of organization familiar to the physiologist and experimental psychologist. An awareness of this methodological gap is important to the future balanced development of gerontology. Applying the dictum, often attributed to Virchow, 'the study of

things caused must precede the study of the causes of things', biochemical observations only have significance to the extent that they fit the time course of loss of adaptability of the whole organism. There is a strong feeling among gerontologists that molecular biology often receives support on the mistaken assumption that studies at this fundamental level will automatically provide meaningful answers to questions which, of necessity, arise at a higher level.

To gain a better perspective of ageing, we must also pay more attention to the way in which the conditions of early life influence terminal processes. In the biological field, there is also a need to carry out more investigations into ageing in a wider range of organisms— plant, animal, and microbe. More work is needed on ageing in natural populations. This aspect of comparative gerontology is a relatively new growth point, and being closely connected with ecology, provides an area of communication with a number of interdisciplinary fields, such as biochemistry, genetics, endocrinology, and nutrition. While mortality factors in the wild are different from those acting in the laboratory, from current knowledge we cannot yet say that death in these two environments results from the operation of different basic chemical processes.

Evidence is accumulating that the loss of behavioural adaptability may be important in the natural selection of wild populations. This highlights two other important growth points in the ageing field: behavioural gerontology and the associated areas of neurophysiology and endocrinology, where we can expect a future demand for increased temporal information.

Experimental gerontology is much more than the study of terminal processes, and this chapter is an attempt to place research on ageing firmly in a developmental perspective. Increasingly, life is viewed as a continuum in which past physicochemical events and previous environments influence future behaviour at all levels. In this respect gerontology provides a much needed forum where extreme specialist views may be moderated and, as such, will play an important socioscientific role in the future development of biology and medicine.

Only in a prescientific sense is ageing one

phenomenon. A better viewpoint would be to regard it as a symbolic term summarizing a diversity of different and unrelated processes. It is futile to search for one central process of ageing and a single definition and research approach that is all embracing, bearing in mind the great range of organisms and environments. A broad-based biological view of ageing is required at the present time because the physiological basis of ageing is well established and the general molecular principles of ageing are emerging. The next phase will be one of increasing specialism. Future workers will enter ageing research from one level only and will not be aware of the significance of their findings at other levels of complexity. It is the aim of this chapter to present the topic of ageing in the broadest possible perspective. Therefore, each section represents a particular viewpoint of a group of research workers which sees ageing as a particular manifestation of biology.

AGEING AS AN ASPECT OF BIOLOGY

Terminology

The description of every biological system, be it cell, individual, or population, must be qualified by its age and the time of day of observation. Although some processes of physiological function are repeated many times within a lifespan and others only once or twice, it is likely that repeat processes are never identical. Ageing is one of the time scales of life delineating progressive change within a lifespan. Processes of heredity require the passage of a few generations to become clarified while evolution occupies many lifespans.

This kind of grand temporal survey is too wide in scope to be used as a basis for practical research. Nevertheless, it has to be the overriding philosophy of a biologist. In particular, when a living system is studied in a particular phase, the time scale of the problem should never be too narrow so as to block the broad temporal vista. Events during each time interval can only be fully understood in terms of what preceded them and what is to follow. From this viewpoint the choice of the definitions that we use to split life into manageable segments must be made with great care. They are important guidelines for the articulation of research and the gathering of relevant facts, and are also important in the transmission of ideas.

Many terms have been used to describe the various aspects of the life-cycle: 'development', 'differentiation', 'maturation', and 'senescence' have been used by specialists, usually in connection with the study of one particular phase of life. These definitions reflect a restricted viewpoint and have the effect of cutting the life-cycle into arbitrary segments. Some of the apparent divisions may have no biological relevance when a broader perspective is taken. The terminology may actually impede research and communication.

Many protozoa, unicellular algae, malignant cell lines, and the vegetative parts of plants appear to be capable of unlimited cultivation as clones without a general decline in vigour. Lack of ageing also characterizes the germ cell line. In this respect, ageing appears to be the inevitable outcome of a bodily organization where reproductive cells require the support of a relatively large volume of cellular resources not directly concerned with reproduction. Simple metazoan organisms such as hydra and the planarian worms appear to contain a reservoir of non-ageing embryonic-type cells.

For those organisms showing a progressive deterioration of function with time, four landmarks in the life-history are the time of fertilization; the time of sexual maturation; the time when growth ceases; and the time of death. This raises the question, 'Is the period of growth related to the duration of life?' Put more specifically, 'Is ageing a continuation of the same general process constituted by the phenomena of growth?' This is a productive beginning in any discussion of the nature of ageing because growth and ageing are viewed as processes which relate to the pattern of the total life-history. It also makes it possible to ask subsidiary questions concerning the likelihood of control of ageing through the interplay of factors which are known to be important in the regulation of growth.

There are difficulties in defining both 'ageing' and 'development' (Table 1). To many biologists the term 'ageing' is used to describe any time-dependent change with respect to life-history. However, it is necessary to place some restriction on the defintion in order to arrive at a category of changes which is useful in formulating problems open to experiment. For example, definitions of ageing do not include the time-dependent changes of development; development includes the events of differentiation, growth, and maturation which

Table 1 Some definitions of ageing

1. An ageing process is any process occurring in an individual which renders that individual more likely to die in a given time interval as it grows older.
2. Ageing can be defined as that universal attribute of all multicellular organisms which is characterized by time-dependent, reproducible alterations in structure, which may or may not be peculiar to each species or strain.
3. Senescence is that part of the total ageing process which occurs during the last trimester of an adult existence and during which time-related structural and functional changes of a degradative nature predominate in certain organs and tissues, such as to lead ultimately to the diminished capacity of the individual to survive the assaults of both the internal and external surrounding environments.
4. Old age is a major involution of the living organism.
5. All living matter changes with time in both structure and function, and the changes which follow a general trend constitute ageing. Ageing begins with conception and ends only with death.
6. Ageing is a decrease of intracellular water, with maintenance of extracellular water and a varying fat mass.
7. An ageing process is one that occurs in all members of a population, that is progressive and irreversible under usual conditions, and that begins or accelerates at maturity in those systems which undergo growth and development.
8. Ageing is a gradual decline in an organism's adaptation to its normal environment following the onset of reproductive maturity.
9. Ageing is described as a biological process which causes increased susceptibility of an organism to diseases.
10. Ageing is merely the vector sum of a number of morbid processes, most of which take time to develop and often a long time to reach serious climax.
11. Ageing can be defined as an increasing probability for the individual to contract one of the degenerative diseases.
12. Ageing processes may be defined as those which render individuals more susceptible as they grow older to various factors, intrinsic or extrinsic, which may cause death.
13. Ageing stands for the mere increase in years without overtones of increasing deterioration and decay. Senescence means ageing accompanied by that decline of bodily faculties and sensibilities and energies which ageing colloquially entails.
14. Ageing is the process of progressive entropy or the decrease in the information content of the organism until a minimum is reached which is incompatible with life.

aid survival until the individual is a reproductive competent adult, whereas ageing processes lead to a failure to adapt to the environment and ultimately result in death. Points of difficulty arise because many developmental events are the obvious precursors of ageing phenomena and some progressive changes begin before or shortly after birth and continue unabated throughout life. Despite this, many workers would restrict the term 'ageing' and eliminate from consideration any changes which do not render the individual more likely to die in a given time interval as it grows older. Good examples of systems that deteriorate early and which do not show up as an increase in mortality are the regression of the human female reproductive system, loss of scalp hair, and the ageing of the human eye. This particular difficulty of definition has been recognized and another category, 'senescence', introduced which includes only those events which contribute to the decreased resistance to death. However, it is generally accepted that very few ageing phenomena could be proved not to influence mortality. Also, the force of mortality depends very much on the environment. It is of no obvious disadvantage for civilized man not to be able to run a 5-minute mile at the age of 50. Nevertheless, the well-documented decline in human athletic performance from the second or third decade should be included as an early ageing process in a less sophisticated society, where predators had the ability to run faster than human prey. There is also the possibility that delayed secondary responses to early primary changes may increase the chances of death after a considerable lag period. For example, there is a marked decrease in bone density in human females that is partly related to the decline in the female reproductive system. The mean age for menopause is about 50 years whereas the mean age at which half of the bone loss has taken place occurs almost 20 years later. Comparable data for men show that the loss of bone is considerably less and starts at least a decade later. This faster and earlier loss of bone in women is associated with a dramatic rise in fractures of the long bones which has no counterpart in men. In the later years complications, such as pneumonia, arising from fractures are an important cause of death.

Perhaps our difficulties of definition arise

because it is implicit in most current classifications that ageing phenomena have unique causes. It is by no means clear that there is such a compartmentation and the view may be advanced that development and ageing result from the operation of the same basic cellular processes. Further, if the term development is used comprehensively to cover the whole life-cycle, ageing will then appear as a subordinate process. Differences between early and late events of development are that early events lead to perfection of function and late events result in the deterioration of function. From this aspect, gerontology is the scientific study of the irreversible deterioration in those structures and functions which have a definite peak or plateau of development in all members of the species. Although a particular aspect of ageing may appear at an arbitrary age of the subject, the study should not be restricted to the period after the system in question has reached its maximum efficiency because the causes of deterioration may be found in an earlier phase of life.

Although environment is important in the expression of failures in biological organization, ageing is, fundamentally, a loss of precision in the systems specifying form and function. The causes are chemical deterioration, physiological errors, and variability of gene expression which are manifest as a loss of adaptability resulting from a decline in tissue and functional reserves. There may not be an obvious link with the increased probability of death, but a major feature is that the homeostatic systems of the body become less efficient in combating fluctuations in the external world. On this basis, ageing begins before there is a marked increase in mortality. In humans, a steady decline in physiological performance is first noticeable during the third decade of life; the corresponding stage in the white rat (life-span 800 days) occurs at about 100 days; in fruit fly cultures *Drosophila* (lifespan 27 days) ageing of some systems begins at about 10 days. Therefore, it appears that in this context phenomena of ageing may occupy well over half the maximum lifespan in laboratory populations.

The wide temporal range of life that the gerontologist has to cover, together with the fact that ageing is most clearly manifest at the most complex level of organization, yet can only be fully comprehended at the simplest level, means that the biology of ageing has an exceptionally broad intellectual base. This interdisciplinary aspect is illustrated in Table 2 which, starting from the general definition of ageing already given, lists the objects of study and processes of interest to the biologist. Until recent years, this comprehensive viewpoint has not been accepted by most research workers and this has been partly responsible for an unbalanced research strategy and compartmentation of ideas. Ageing is still largely isolated from the mainstream of biological knowledge. Also, there has been much fruitless methodological argument as to whether one should first develop a general testable hypothesis, describe the ageing organism in detail, or enumerate possibilities which are then eliminated one by one. While the decisive approach in science is inevitably an experimental one, all viewpoints are valid and it is apparent that the popular yet extremely biased position of model-making has mitigated against the collection of information on the natural history of ageing.

Table 2 Scope of research on ageing
General definition: gerontology is the scientific study of deterioration in those structures and functions that have a definite peak or plateau of development in all members of the species.

Objects of study	Processes of interest
Molecules	Chemical deterioration
	Enzyme synthesis
Enzymes	Differential expression of genes
	Growth
Organs	Physiological regulation
	Reproduction
Organisms	Behavioural adaptability
	Heredity
Populations	Natural selection

Machine analogies

Many advances in science have come by posing complicated problems in terms of the workings of machines and a number of mechanical analogies have been proposed to define ageing. It is not surprising that ageing has long been viewed as a clock-like process. This has led, in turn, to the view that a biological 'clock' determines the rate at which the organism deteriorates. Further ideas along this line raise the possibility that if the clock could be tampered with, particularly in order to make it run more slowly, the rate at which age deterioration occurs could be slowed down and life thereby prolonged.

As judged by the different times at which various systems reach their peak performance and the different rates at which they deteriorate, it is clear there must be several clocks operating, even in the simplest organisms. Also, since the onset of some characteristic ageing phenomena can be preferentially accelerated or delayed by experimental treatment, some or all of the clocks must function independently of each other. On the whole, the clock concept has not been very useful in defining ageing because the analogy does not match a process that, once it has run down, cannot be restarted.

Another mechanical analogy, based on the continuous playing of a gramophone record, although it highlights the most fundamental characteristic of cellular function, namely the capacity to repeatedly transcribe coded information with decreased fidelity, suffers from the same disadvantage as the clock idea, in that the record of life can only be played once. If it is assumed that life is controlled by the repeated playing of the same record, from what we know about the biochemical transcription process, the music, i.e. the integrated function of the cell, is not quite the same each time the record is played. This is partly because a 'wearing out' of the record of life may occur by repetitive use with cracks appearing due to chemical deterioration with the passage of time, and also because the music of life itself affects the score which is heard on subsequent playing; to begin with, playing improves the score, but, later, playing causes it to deteriorate. Providing that the record player and the record are taken to have these unusual technical properties, the analogy represents development in the broadest sense. It takes account of feedback from the transcribed information governing cellular function, which is able to alter the 'groove pattern' for the next playing. However, as with the clock analogy, it is necessary to postulate the existence in the body of several 'records' with separate 'players' to take account of the multifactorial basis of ageing.

The important evolutionary aspect of ageing is illustrated in the 'space probe analogy'. This likens an individual life to the voyage of a space probe that has been designed and programmed to pass close to a distant planet and transmit its findings back to base. Once the mission is completed the craft will continue to function but increasingly, with the passage of time, various units will begin to break down due to inevitable chemical deterioration of the key components, and, perhaps, frictional wearing. Eventually the probe will 'die' when its main transmitter fails. This model may be taken to represent an organism that is programmed by evolution to have a well-defined lifespan of its non-replaceable parts in relation to the stresses of its surroundings, but once this period has been exceeded, various bodily systems fail to respond appropriately because of changes in the configuration and chemistry of the various components which are no longer appropriate to function. The analogy is particularly useful in highlighting the importance of chemical deterioration in biological ageing. It is also apt in that it takes account of the fact that the lifespan selected by evolution in the wild, i.e. a period comparable to that taken by the space probe to achieve its objective, is the most important biological milestone from which the road to old age begins. The lives of man and his domesticated animals in protected environments continue beyond the lifespan set by evolution because of removal of mortality factors that played a part in the past evolution of the species. On this view, death in old age occurs because the adaptive evolutionary programme is exceeded when a species is in an environment more favourable than the one in which it evolved.

Any imperfection of function which results in a progressive deterioration in the organism could be classed as ageing and from this viewpoint alone it is likely that, as in the space probe, there are many causes and consequently many processes of ageing. The length of the natural life-cycle is the end-point of evolution and the way in which this is established by natural selection need not be identical or even similar in different species. A common physiological cause of ageing in the various organs within an individual is also unlikely on the grounds that they differ so much in both structure and function. In addition the available experimental evidence supports the idea of organ ageing being chemically self-contained and

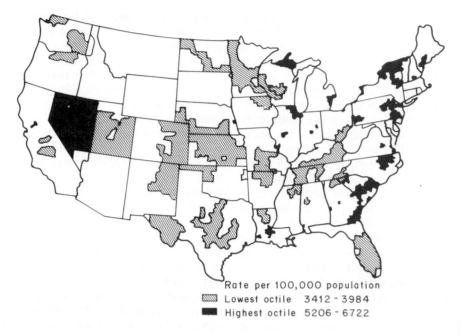

Figure 1   All-causes death rates: white males 65 to 74, 1959–1961. (From Sauer and Donnell, 1970)

not dominated by systemic factors. This multi-factorial theory of ageing is opposed to the less likely unitary hypothesis which states that there is only one process which is responsible for the general loss of adaptability in all organs.

AGEING AS THE CONSEQUENCE OF A PROTECTIVE ENVIRONMENT

The Natural Environment

Consideration of ageing in relation to development takes the discussion of longevity firmly into the realm of evolution, with questions arising on the origins and nature of the wild lifespan compared with the maximum observed lifespan and extended longevity of laboratory animals.

Most life tables and mortality curves have been constructed using laboratory species or domesticated populations. For many species it is known that these tables frequently show maxima of life expectancy which are much higher than the greatest lifespans recorded in the wild. There is a strong possibility that this discrepancy may throw light on the nature of

ageing, but very few accurate comparisons of lifespans have been made for species in different environments. This is because of the great practical difficulties in obtaining reliable life tables from the natural environment.

Life tables are simply constructed by counting the numbers of individuals of different ages in a population. This tends to give a static picture, whereas the wild population is governed by at least five basic numerical changes. An input of individuals occurs through births and immigration; an output occurs through deaths (natural and by predation) and emigration; also over several lifespans, the total population size may change drastically (Fig. 1).

Information about mortality in the wild is collected by methods according to the habits of the species in question. These methods involve knowing, respectively: age at death; numbers of survivors out of an initial definite number; and the age structure of the population at one point in time with mortality rate inferred from the fall in size of the older age classes.

Mortality in wild populations is simple to measure when reproduction and migrations can be ignored and the population examined repeatedly as it decreases in size. However, this is only possible with animals which have an annual life-cycle, a short reproduction period, and a small range of movement. More often than not the death rate in a population is difficult to measure and one must resort to estimating the birth rate in steady state populations or defining age at death by the accumulation of animal remains which are resistant to decay, such as bones in vertebrates, the shells of molluscs, and the cuticle of insects.

The two most commonly used practical methods of assessing age of wild animals are the mark-recapture technique and the evaluation of some feature in captive animals that is known to be affected in a well-defined way by the passage of time. Use of the latter method often requires that the structure in question be calibrated by the mark-recapture method. This method is of limited value. Where it is carried out on a large scale, as in bird-ringing, it provides data on the maximum and minimum lifespans, but the small fraction of the population ringed, together with the very low returns and ring loss from older birds, make it difficult to obtain firm statistical data. There is also the possibility that the stress of capture and marking may shorten the lifespan of the birds after release. Also, birds and other animals that allow themselves to be caught may differ significantly in their physiology from those in the bulk of the population. For terrestrial species the method can only be used to advantage where it is certain that there is no

movement of animals into and out of the experimental sampling area and the sample of animals trapped is a large fraction of the population giving a respresentative cross-section. In this respect, it has been used successfully to measure the lifespan of isolated populations restricted physically to small well-defined geographical areas (Table 3).

So far, little can be said about the age-linked mortality factors in the wild in relation to ageing in the laboratory. This area provides common ground for the gerontologist to collaborate with the ecologist. From what has just been said, it is clear that the study of animal populations is technically difficult to carry out in the wild. This is not the case with many species of higher plants and some of the most detailed analyses of life-cycle strategies have been carried out on plant models.

Demographic botanical studies are clearly in the realm of ecology. Broadly speaking, ecologists attempt to describe how organisms behave in nature and try to explain such fundamental questions as why certain organisms live in a particular place, what regulates their numbers, and what maintains particular species patterns. More specifically, many ecologists are concerned with obtaining information on the sizes of populations in successive developmental stages, so that a life table may be constructed and an attempt made to determine factors that regulate population size in relation to chronological age. The census of

Table 3 Life tables for wild house mice on Skokholm Island. (From Berry and Jakobson, 1971)

Date of birth												
	March–April			May–June			July–August			September–October		
Month	Observ-ed No.	No. of survivors[a]	Life expect-ancy (weeks)	Observ-ed No.	No. of survivors[a]	Life expect-ancy (weeks)	Observ-ed Nos.	No. of survivors[a]	Life expect-ancy (weeks)	Observ-ed Nos.	No. of survivors[a]	Life expect-ancy (weeks)
May–June	276	1,000	13.9									
July–August	–	530.0	13.3	307	1,000	15.5						
Sept.–Oct.	93	283.0	12.5	139	600.0	14.3	1,383	1,000	14.3			
Nov.–Dec.	30	152.3	10.9	114	360.0	12.3	798	600.0	12.3	518	1,000	11.0
Jan.–Feb.	–	68.5	10.2	72	162.0	13.3	–	270.0	13.4	–	400.0	12.4
March–April	12	30.8	15.8	28	72.9	15.7	183	121.5	15.8	71	160.0	15.8
May–June	3	18.5	14.7	11	43.7	14.7	82	72.9	14.7	54	96.0	14.7
July–August	0	11.1	13.0	0	26.2	12.9	–	43.7	13.0	–	57.6	13.0
Sept.–Oct.		6.7	10.0		15.7	9.9	25	26.2	10.1		34.6	10.1
Nov.–Dec.		4.0	5.2		9.4	5.1	0	1.6	4.9		2.1	4.9
Jan.–Feb.		0.4	4.3		0.9	4.3	0	1.6	4.9		2.1	4.9
March–April		0			0	0		0.2	4.3		0.2	4.3
May–June							0				0	

[a]Calculated from mortality rates.

populations and the definition of stages at which mortality factors operate are necessary first steps in estimating ecological productivity. However, generally, neither animal nor plant ecologists pay attention to the determination of specific mortality factors operating in natural populations on an age basis.

If with further study it turns out that the maximum laboratory lifespan of organisms is always greater than that in the wild, it may be that part of the increase in longevity in captivity is due to the experimenter selecting genotypes for good adaptation to laboratory conditions. A more likely explanation, however, is that the major causes of death in wild populations are the physical and biotic insults of a fluctuating environment. From studies on the changes in the mean value of certain characters and their decreased variability it is known that many animals differ characteristically in their order of dying, even when life expectancy does not change very much with age. Therefore it is the natural lifespan in the wild that must be under selection pressure. Nevertheless, there are many natural populations where deaths appear to follow an accident rate curve. Further, in asking the question which processes render the individual more likely to die in a given time interval as it grows older, we are likely to obtain different answers from laboratory strains compared with wild types. This is not to say that age changes leading up to death in wild-type populations have a different fundamental basis.

Pathology and Ageing in Protective Environments

Early workers, in seeking to clarify a chemical change in terms of a fundamental ageing phenomenon, regarded it necessary to rule out pathological processes. Those who entered gerontology from medical fields took great pains to emphasize that every effort should be made to clarify the distinction between the pathological features of ageing from what were termed the fundamental physiological aspects; only the latter aspects should be considered in formulating theories of ageing. From this standpoint, the definition of ageing in the human population is greatly complicated because it is likely that primary biochemical defects may give rise to pathologies in a random way.

Experimental animals also show pathological ageing as evidenced from the onset of latent infectious diseases, some of which, such as pneumonia and ear disease, become clearly developed in advanced old age.

Apart from diseases and pathologies, such as pneumonia, that are well defined as originating in the environment, it is extremely difficult to make a distinction between intrinsic (normal) and extrinsic (abnormal) ageing. One approach is to take the lowest common denominators in the longest lived and shortest lived individuals as being probable primary causes. In this respect, it is worth stressing that, as yet, no case of human old age has been found in which all or several organs and functions show only slight or no changes with ageing. However, the existence of a few human individuals who die in extreme old age, with a relatively small number of degenerative features, indicates that there is a fundamental baseline from which most individuals deviate to different extents.

This whole problem of defining the fundamental features of ageing was well summarized by Korenchevsky, the founder of experimental gerontology. His view was that two differential criteria should be used:

(a) Changes which occur only in the majority of old organisms but not in all old individuals should not be considered as features of pathological ageing, because they are not necessarily present and are apparently avoidable in old age.
(b) Those features in old individuals which are the same or very close to the features in all adult or young persons should be considered as associated with the normal physiological ageing.

The assumptions are that there is one or only a limited number of basic changes and that all individuals age in the same way. Unfortunately, neither of these two assumptions has any experimental basis. A common dilemma is exemplified by the possibly apocryphal autopsy of a male aged 102 which revealed generalized atherosclerosis, thrombosis of the left femoral, popliteal and tibial arteries and of the accompanying veins, terminal bronchopneumonia, a carcinoid tumour of the ilium, enlargement of the thyroid, and chronic emphysema; the cause of death was gangrene of the left foot!

While many pathologies in old age result from the decreased resistance to microbial disease, studies on germ-free mice have shown that infections are not an important fundamental aspect of ageing. Ageing, germ-free mice show the same pattern of non-infectious pathological conditions as do conventionally maintained animals. There is also clear evidence that the introduction of germ-free conditions to a laboratory where rodent strains are already well managed by conventional methods does not increase lifespan; in some experiments germ-free conditions have actually reduced longevity!

The fact that certain diseases show a well-defined age incidence has led to several ideas in which the pathology is seen as the outcome of a developmental process. Gout usually attacks men between the ages of 40 to 50. This disease is marked by painful inflammation of the joints caused by urate deposits and is the major manifestation of hyperuricaemia. Hyperuricaemia may appear in the third decade before there is any discomfort in the joints. This is a hereditary condition with a well-defined genetic mechanism, which suggests that other diseases may arise with secondary complications that are late manifestations of inborn metabolic disorders implying that genetic variation in susceptibility to common primary processes of ageing may account for non-uniform pathological change.

A developmental origin for some pathologies is evident from the fact that they appear to have a highly localized incidence within the body. For example, arteritis occurs frequently in the renal artery of old mice but is seldom seen in the arteries supplying other tissues (Table 4). It is difficult to escape the conclusion, when the basic structure and function of all arteries are very similar, that a subtle programme aspect of phenotypic expression is responsible for the pathology.

Degenerative conditions have a diverse and complex origin and one is immediately struck by the difficulties, not only in defining the cause of death in old organisms but also the nature of disease. Taking the broad view that disease is a malfunction that affects people in a random fashion begs the question, 'Are fatal degenerative conditions, individually described

Table 4 Frequency distribution of major sites of arteritis in ageing RF mice

Artery	Frequency of involvement
Renal	32/64
Aorta	28/64
Coronary	10/64
Ovarian	9/64
Uterine	9/64
Splenic	6/64
Axillary	5/64
Adrenal	3/64
Hepatic	3/64
Gastric	2/64
Cervical/mediastinal	2/64
Pancreatic	1/64
Thymic	1/64
Spermatic	1/64
Superior mesenteric	1/64

as diseases, in fact ageing processes?' The answer to this question depends on whether disease is defined as being due to random events, unrelated to age, or as a progressive deterioration that occurs in only a fraction of the population at a given age. Korenchevsky's dictum is that the only difference between an ageing progress and a disease is that an ageing process occurs in all of the population. To a certain extent, this type of discussion points to the futility of arguing that only those clinical phenomena should be considered within the province of gerontology that are manifest in the bulk of the population, particularly when it is known that for all populations phenotypic variability is widespread. Stating this another way, if we were allowed to live long enough no doubt we would each encounter many disease conditions at different chronological ages dependent upon genotype and environment, all of which could be expressions of a range of deteriorating developmental programmes.

The Protective Environment

When a population of animals is maintained under controlled laboratory conditions, all members have the same environmental history, yet they do not die at the same instant in time. The number of individuals remaining alive at set intervals out of a given number recorded at birth plotted against time results in a curve. There is a great spread in the age at death indicative of variability in resistance to death. The actual shape of the mortality curve denotes the age–frequency distribution of the times of death and is not fundamentally related to the rate or kind of ageing of a given population. The spread in the timing of death could arise because the population was not uniform in genotype. If it was genetically homogeneous, events must have occurred at random which resulted in accidental deaths or different rates of ageing. Measurements of the rate of death at different ages yield age-specific death rates which show for human populations in advanced countries that once the mean lifespan is exceeded, the probability of dying doubles at regular intervals.

The curve of human mortality is at a minimum at around the age of 12. A distinctive feature of the curve is the smoothness that defines the increasing force of mortality in later life. A successful theory of the origin and evolution of senescence must explain the coherence of this curve.

Life tables and the derived mortality curves are useful in making comparisons between ageing in two or more populations which differ with respect to environment, genetics, or the experience of random internal events which may influence the rate of ageing. They show the times of decreasing 'fitness' in terms of the death rate and it is possible by comparing life tables to detect the differential effects of a changed environment upon the life expectancy at different ages, implying that the fitness of individuals varies with age and also with environment.

From this aspect it has been argued that discussion on the nature of ageing should centre on the maximum lifespan rather than on life expectancy. As the latter is a measure of an organism's response to both environmental and intrinsic ageing processes and because it takes into account all possible influences on the population, there can be little doubt that life expectancy is of greater value in evaluating the role of developmental processes in furthering survival. However, when intrinsic ageing processes only are being examined they may be assessed appropriately in terms of maximum lifespan, since this is more a species end-point and is assumed to be a measure of genetic potential attained under the most favourable environmental influence.

A particular difficulty in the use of mortality curves derived from long-lived species is that the terminal deaths of a particular population may refer to individuals that experienced environmental conditions greatly different from those that the younger members of the same species now experience in the same environment. This can usually be overcome with the commonly used laboratory animals bred in constant conditions which have a well-established genotype and for other longer-lived animals by calculating generation life tables each based on the observed mortality of a single generation of births.

Animals tend to have a lifespan which is characteristic of the species implying that ageing is under genetic control. It is this genetic element of longevity which probably accounts for the thousand-fold variation in the maximum lifespan between species in captivity (Table 5). The data refer to studies in which maximum

Table 5 Age distribution of maximum observed lifespans of animals

| Maximum lifespan (yr) | Numbers of species with reliable records | | | | | |
| | Invertebrates | Vertebrates | | | | |
		Fish	Amphibia	Reptiles	Birds	Mammals
0–5	8	3	2	–	4	6
5–10	5	–	–	–	4	4
10–20	3	–	1	–	1	2
20–30	–	–	3	3	8	7
30–40	1	1	–	1	2	1
40–50	1	–	–	1	–	–
50–60	1	2	–	–	1	–
60–70	–	–	–	–	3	–
70–100	–	1	–	3	3	1
Over 100	–	–	–	–	1	1
Totals	19	7	6	8	27	22

lifespan was assessed from the survivors of small initial populations; most of the records came from zoos with good records of animal husbandry, and, in the case of long-lived fish, from maximum scale counts in a large catch. Very few species have been investigated and the species distribution between the various age classes is probably indicative only of the ease with which the species may be studied. The overall range of lifespan from the smallest metazoans, with a maximum lifespan of a few days, to man, with a lifespan of over 100 years, is about 1:3500. This is about the same longevity range found in the higher plants. The existence of these well defined lifespan patterns indicates that the variation in the characteristic lifespans of species depends on the genetic constitution selected in the course of evolution.

With regard to protected human populations, it has been estimated that longevity is about 90 per cent. heritable. However, many geneticists would say that the environmental, non-genetic component is much greater than 10 per cent. Studies on the genetics of human longevity usually take the conventional viewpoint that there is a distinction between, on the one hand, genetic effects of one major mutant gene following a single-factor type of inheritance which causes premature or pathological disturbances and, on the other, a more general genetic influence resulting from the interaction of many genes. The latter, polygenic mode of inheritance is thought to be responsible for a large measure of variability in lifespan in the human population but it is difficult in practice to distinguish polygenic effects from single factor pathological processes.

Data on the heritability of the human lifespan comes classically from studies on identical twins, which have much smaller mean differences in ages at death compared with fraternal twins (Table 6). Longitudinal twin data show that all measurable differences are more pronounced for ageing two-egg twins than for identical twins arising from the same fertilized egg. The relevant parameters included physical features, mental abilities, and pyschological disturbances and social adjustments. This is also borne out by the smaller intrapair lifespan differences of identical twins. Also one-egg twin partners are more than twice as similar in causes of death as two-egg pairs of the same or opposite sex. Additional support for strong genetic influences is that there are marked parental effects, in that ages at death of offspring are related to the parental age at death.

Studies of this type are the best one can get to a genetic analysis of the human factors of longevity. It might be argued that the similarities between ages at death in single-egg twins arise from the tendency of the pairs to seek similar environments but on the whole the similarity in ageing patterns of monozygotic twins occurs even when each member of a pair has experienced a different physical and social environment. Where an identical twin has experienced a vastly different environment from the other it is sometimes possible to see that cosmetic effects of skin ageing depend greatly on environment.

Table 6   Differences in lifespan[a] between one-egg and two-egg human twins. (From Kallmann, 1961)

Year of analysis	Male		Female	
	One-egg twins	Two-egg twins	One-egg twins	Two-egg twins
1948	46.7	89.1	29.4	61.3
1950	48.0	73.8	18.2	41.3
1952	40.7[c]	79.1[c]	30.7[c]	69.5[c]
1954	50.6	68.9	22.9[c]	65.6[c]
1956–57	60.0	64.5	36.9[b]	68.2[b]
1958–59	62.5	65.0	55.4	80.9

[a]Mean intrapair differences in months of same sex senescent twin pairs over the age of 60.
[b]Equals difference between one-egg and two-egg pairs significant at 5 per cent. level.
[c]Equals difference between one-egg and two-egg pairs significant at 1 per cent. level.

Table 7 Mean lifespans of several strains of laboratory mice and rats

Strain	Females		Males	
	Number	Longevity mean (SE)	Number	Longevity mean (SE)
AKR	79	312 (9.4)	79	350 (10.8)
NZB	111	441 (21.1)	110	459 (13.3)
A	68	558 (19.7)	65	512 (21.1)
BALB/c	33	561 (30.3)	35	509 (26.3)
C57BL	29	580 (35.8)	31	645 (34.2)
C57L	26	604 (27.6)	22	473 (30.9)
LACG	40	617 (26.2)	36	536 (38.9)
A2G	51	644 (19.4)	49	640 (21.8)
C57BR/cd	46	660 (22.7)	45	577 (29.8)
LACA	38	664 (29.9)	41	660 (38.5)
129/RrJ	36	666 (23.2)	35	699 (29.8)
C3H	193	676 (9.8)	147	590 (18.6)
DBA/1	39	686 (33.3)	35	487 (35.9)
CE	23	703 (37.3)	20	498 (48.5)
DBA/2	23	719 (35.4)	22	629 (42.1)
NZW	20	733 (42.8)	28	802 (34.0)
WA	22	749 (40.1)	25	645 (29.9)
P	10	782 (51.9)	14	729 (42.9)
CBA	38	825 (32.5)	37	486 (39.0)

The importance of genotype in determining longevity comes out more clearly from studies of inbred experimental animals where environment can be controlled very precisely. For the laboratory mouse, genetic variants can be obtained that differ by a factor of about three in maximum lifespans between strains (Table 7). Hybrids of the F1 generation have been shown to have a mean lifespan that is greater than that of either of the parent inbred lines. Differences in longevity of laboratory populations are associated with differences in the rate of decline in physiological vigour and incidence of pathologies. With respect to the latter point, the frequency distribution and extent of pathological changes of human subjects are clearly genetically conditioned. For example, at the histological level generalized atheroma is considered almost a normal finding in the aortic arch for a person over the age of 60 yet is rarely found in the pulmonary artery of the same person. With respect to genotype, twin studies indicate a greater concordance of cause of death from cancer and tuberculosis in one-egg twins compared with two-egg twins. Also, cause of death in mouse strains is strain specific. Deaths from cancer in the CBA mouse result mainly from hepatomas; in the AKR/J mouse, lymphoid leukaemia is more common and mammary tumours have a high frequency in CBA female mice. Removal of one major cause of death by selection can be expected to unmask another major cause with a high incidence at a greater chronological age.

Statistically, the genetic element in the human lifespan is illustrated by the extra 4 years which are added to the mean lifespan by having all four grandparents surviving to 80 years of age. On the other hand, the environmental influence is indicated statistically by the average life expectancy in cities being 5 years shorter than that in a rural environment.

The dependence of lifespan on environment is a common finding in laboratory animals. Some of the early work was carried out on simple aquatic animals such as rotifers and water fleas which pointed to the importance of temperature, chemical composition of the surrounding environment, and nutritional status. The nutrititional status is of considerable importance, first because the two extremes of over- and undernutrition lead to a decrease in longevity, but also because a moderate reduction in calorie intake which retards growth extends the lifespan of animals at the evolutionary extremes of bodily organization.

The influence of the environment may be explored using mortality survival curves obtained for natural populations. These vary considerably with regard to general shape. Most differ considerably from the rectangular curve characteristic of European and North American human populations and laboratory rodents in that the plateau is either attenuated or absent altogether. It is possible that some of the extreme deviations from the rectangular type represent the operation of mortality factors unrelated to ageing. A useful analogy to indicate random death, independent of age, is that of the accidental breakage of drinking glasses through continuous use. The probability of breakage would have nothing to do with the age of the glasses and if new glasses were continually added in order to keep pace with breakages, the same percentage of those present at the beginning of every time interval would be expected to attain the end-point of breakage during that interval. The age-specific mortality rate would be constant. The percentage of a given number surviving would fall off rapidly at first, then more slowly, because the numbers of individuals dying at each 'age' is in constant proportion to those of that age present. This model may represent the mortality in natural populations, subject to infection with disease or predation, both recurring randomly and with no age discrimination. The mortality curve is similar to that for the decay of a radioactive isotope.

With regard to human populations exposed to severe ecological hazards, a curve with a slight inflection is characteristic of primitive peoples where the life style is dominated by a harsh environment. It may also have been a feature of human populations throughout the formative period of biological evolution. These two ways of looking at the human mortality curve, in terms of historical change and existing geographical differences, indicate that the recent advance in what might be described as environmental control measures – such as improved nutrition, medicine, and public health – has greatly increased the mean lifespan and life expectancy of the human populations in the developed world without affecting the rate of ageing.

There have been reports, usually from remote parts of the world, of individuals reaching ages considerably above 100. It is often difficult or even impossible to check claims beyond the age of 120 years but there can be no doubt from reliable demographic records that some human populations have a much higher proportion of individuals over the age of 80 than is found in Britain and North America. However, the number of these extra 'long-livers' is still only a very small fraction of a given birth cohort. Birth records are particularly suspect in remote areas but it does appear as if the exceptionally long-lived survivors invariably occur in small isolated communities. Often the aged in these communities have a high social status. This, together with the simple diets that characterize these communities opens up possibilities that unique environmental influences (past or present) produced the extended lifespans.

Taking the North American life expectancy as a population mean it would be expected that other populations would be found with a lower proportion of individuals living beyond the eighth decade. This is indeed the case and the risk of dying between the ages of 45 to 65 also varies substantially from country to country and within large countries. For example, between 1962 and 1964, out of 20 countries compared with the United States, 17 had death rates in the age group 45 to 64 that were lower than in the United States. Between the ages of 65 to 74 ten countries had lower rates. The reasons for these differences are not known with any degree of certainty but when generous allowance is made for environmental differences there is still room for genetic explanations.

In a more detailed study on geographical differences of death rates in the United States, the highest rates from all causes occurred predominantly near the East Coast but equally high figures came from states very far removed from this area such as Nevada and Hawaii (Fig. 1). In general the areas with the lowest rates are concentrated in the West Central and mountain areas. These geographical differences in death rate increase with age.

Death rates from cardiovascular and renal diseases are lowest in the West Central areas and it appears that high death rates from these diseases are associated with metropolitan development. This is also true of malignant growths, many of which are now thought to be largely environmental in origin. Deaths from these three causes tend to be correlated in the United States although this is not always true in other countries. At the socioeconomic level, rural farm areas tend to have the lowest death rates from all causes. Here, another causative factor may be low population density. Other correlations that meet the usual standards of statistical significance are for deaths from cardiovascular and renal diseases to be linked with regions of high rainfall and low elevation. High fluctuation in mean January daily temperature is linked with a low death rate from cancers apart from lung cancer. Such correlations, while interesting, are practically meaningless in defining the exact nature of the mortality factors at work. More statistical analysis along these lines is likely to add to our understanding of the role of more environmental factors in human mortality as well as bearing on the mortality in other animal species.

The shift from the 'declining' curve to the 'rectangular' curve in developed human societies does not appear to have resulted from an extension of the maximum lifespan. Indeed, the actuarial interpretation of 'rectangular' curves is based on the assumption that they are derived historically from 'declining' curves mainly by a fall in deaths during infancy and childhood with a smaller contribution from lowered death rates in early middle age. Thus, living conditions improve allowing more of the population to reach a biologically limited mean lifespan.

A differential mortality rate appears to be a sex-linked feature of many animals. In humans, the male death rate is higher than that of the female over the entire lifespan. At birth, the ratio of males to females is 106:100. There is evidence that a differential death rate of males is a feature of interuterine life with estimated primary sex ratios of between 110 and 160 males to every 100 females. In some birds, reptiles, and some insects, the female has the shorter lifespan. However, a frequent feature appears to be that the shorter-lived sex is the one which has the XY chromosome combination. The higher death rate in XY individuals has not been properly explored, but a working hypothesis is that it is related to the action of recessive alleles on the X chromosome for which there are no counteracting alleles in the Y chromosome. Human demographic data have been obtained which indicate that the sex difference in mortality is largely an endocrine phenomenon, being absent in male groups that were castrated before puberty (Table 8). In this respect the sex difference in longevity appears to be in some way connected with different patterns of development.

Table 8   Survival curves of male human subjects castrated at different ages. (From Hamilton and Mestler, 1969

Castrated at	Median lifespan
8–14 years	76.3
15–19 years	72.9
20–29 years	69.6
30–39 years	68.9
Non-castrate	64.7

The fact that species have a characteristic lifespan has prompted correlation analysis of various species characters in an effort to define those which play a dominant role in longevity.

On a comparative basis, within the mammalian class, there is a highly significant relation between lifespan and body weight. This regression accounts for about 60 per cent. of the variance of lifespan of 63 species of placental mammals. A better fit of lifespans is obtained when regressions are calculated on brain weight (which accounts for 76 per cent. of lifespan variance), although the wide scatter in this plot indicates that other factors are also involved in the lifespan variance.

Although generally in large species the brain is relatively smaller than that in related small species, the different parts of the brain show disproportionate evolutionary development. Also, there is a trend in numerous lines for a successive increase in relative brain size as well as a relative larger brain. This implies that a larger brain was a selective advantage, possibly because there is greater central nervous control over bodily functions. It may also be the basis for hybrids frequently having a greater longevity than inbred lines, i.e. it is postulated that hybrids by virtue of possessing two distinct control systems have better stablizing mechanisms compared with inbred types. Because body weight correlates highly with brain weight the view has been taken that evolution of the brain has been a major factor in changing lifespan by allowing the maintenance of an improved physiological regulation nearer to some kind of biochemical ideal. On this idea, brain development has tended to reduce the magnitude of physiological variations and so reduce the probability of irreversible deleterious changes that contribute to ageing. Although this idea is attractive, because mortality seems to be associated proximally with failures in physiological regulation, there is no comparative data on the efficiency of homeostasis within the mammals to substantiate it.

AGEING AS AN EXPRESSION OF REPRODUCTIVE STRATEGY

Plants

Almost all published research on plant demography deals with natural populations, and plants in many respects offer better models for studying the evolution of ageing. There are, however, fundamental differences between the growth form of higher plants and that of higher animals which affect their population behaviour. For example, after germination of a young seedling several structural units accumulate having their own proliferating cell masses, such as leaves, axillary buds and branched root structures. Each higher plant in this sense may be regarded as a subpopulation of cells having growth potential in all its parts. From this viewpoint, a count of the numbers of plants in a given area provides limited information. The two levels of phenotypic expression, the number of plants and the number of growth units per plant, must be examined simultaneously. Births and deaths may occur at either level; death may be of a whole plant or of a part—a leaf, a shoot, a main branch, a root, or a rootlet. Also, the environment may influence birth and death at both demographic levels. In order to clarify this view of the higher plant, the term 'ramet' has been used to describe the subpopulation of discrete functional units within the individual and the term 'genet' has been used to describe the genetic identity of the individual.

Life-cycles and longevity of flowering plants form a continuum separated for convenience into the categories of annual, biennial, and perennial. Annuals range from those that set seed only weeks from germination to species where the growth cycle requires four to six months for completion. Annuals are typically monocarpic, i.e., they die in the year in which they set seed, though in some cases it seems to be the onset of winter or drought that kills rather than any intrinsic annual programme. Among perennials a useful distinction is made between those with and those without an accumulating ageing vegetative body. In general, this division is associated with the competitive advantage of height which can only be gained at the expense of accumulating a perennial ageing structure and dead supporting tissue.

Both reproductive age and reproductive frequency have profound effects on the development of a population of plants and the consequences of various types of fecundity pattern occupy a central role in contemporary ecological theory. Theoretically, a rapid life-cycle might involve a seed that germinates to expose a green photosynthetic flower that rapidly seeds with immediate germination. The flower would stock the new seeds with organic reserves and support a root for the necessary mineral uptake. What is actually seen is a variety of compromises in which precocity of reproduction is balanced against the advantages of growth of a vegetative structure. Some annual species are well fitted to live in an unpredictable environment. If the season turns out to be short, some seed will have been produced although the plant would die before its full reproductive capacity was attained. However, in a long season the full reproductive potential can be fully exploited. Often plants die through frost damage or environmental deterioration while still in the process of producing more flower buds. In other annuals a relatively long period of vegetative growth precedes a rapid onset of reproduction. This change is often seasonal and governed by photoperiod. Death follows the setting of seeds indicating that the act of seed production initiates an ageing process. A complication in this interpretation is that most annual species are rigidly seasonal by virtue of their germination mechanisms. These considerations inevitably open up a discussion of evolutionary strategies and indicate how the biology of ageing impinges on the area of ecology concerned with the evolution of life-cycles.

The most accurate record of age deterioration in reproduction comparable to animal data may be for grasses. For example, the yield of seed per acre of the grass *Bromus marginatus* declines by about 70 per cent. from the second to fifth years after sowing. With regard to trees, after the juvenile period, their seed output tends to increase with age to an optimal age for seed bearing; most trees produce their best seed crop in middle age, which may last from several decades to a century or more. Seed production of trees tends to decline at the same time as a physiological deterioration appears and pathological symptoms become frequent. It is difficult to rule out soil nutrient exhaustion as a factor in these simultaneous changes. The size and age of trees are usually related, but the seed yield of individual trees is more closely linked with size than with age.

A period of great reproductive activity reduces vegetative growth in trees just as in certain long-lived animal species, implying an internal competition for resources. The evidence is an inverse relationship between mast years in oak trees and the appropriate annual wood increment. For example, the annual ring width of beech trees in good mast years, which occurs every 6 or 7 years, may be only half the average ring width in less fertile years and the reduced increments continue for an additional 2 years.

Competition between reproduction and subsequent growth in perennial plants is part of a general negative influence of reproduction on the future reproductive performance of the parent and its subsequent survival. The idea is re-enforced by another generality that species which reproduce only once before death (semelparous) have shorter lifespans than species which reproduce repeatedly during their lifespans (iteroparous).

Animals

Within closely related animal species reproductive effort is larger in semelparous species than in iteroparous species (Table 9). This has been used as the basis of a 'competition hypothesis' which has led to a general theory of natural death (Calow, 1979).

The competition hypothesis was inferred from the following statements:

(a) A fall in growth rate due to loss of materials and energy from the parent into its gametes is thought to reduce the future breeding potential of terrestrial isopods by reducing the size reached by the parent at future breeding seasons. This can occur in any organism where (1) reproduction occurs before growth ceases in the adult, (2) reproductive activity impairs growth, (3) reproduction is positively correlated with size. These conditions are known to hold for some coelenterates, annelids, bivalves, various crustacea, some fishes, amphibia, and reptiles.

(b) Competition between growth and reproduction occurs in perennial plants.

(c) Reserve materials might also be important in supporting the parent through periods of hardship so that failure to accumulate or to maintain reserves as a result of reproduction might contribute to a reduction in adult survival and subsequent fecundity.

(d) By diverting resources from metabolic processes involved in vital functions reproduction can weaken the parent, possibly in an irreversible fashion. For example, during starvation, mated female water-boatmen (*Corixidae*) will use material from flight muscles to maintain egg output and this muscle will not regenerate

Table 9   Estimates of reproductive output in several species of gastropod. (From Calow, 1979)

	Egg biomass, snail biomass	Egg production Total absorbed energy (%)	Proportion of non-respired absorbed energy
Semelparous species			
Lymnaea peregra	3.05	–	–
Physa fontinalis	2.17	–	–
P. Gyrina	2.01	22	–
Planorbis contortus	1.18	20	79
Ancylus fluviatilis	1.89	17.5	51
Ferrissia rivularis	–		45
Iteroparous species			
Lymnaea palustris	0.19	2.3	27
L. stagnalis	0.43	–	–
Bythinia tentaculata	0.21	5	25
Helisoma trivolvis	–	16	33
Malampus bidentatus	0.89	–	80

afterwards. Hence during nutritive disturbance the life expectancy of the female is adversely and irreversibly influenced by reproduction. Virgin females, on the other hand, allow gonads to shrink during starvation and preserve the flight muscles. Under these conditions virgins live longer than the mated females. Similar results have been obtained for other insects.

(e) The use of energy for reproduction in stressed parents may prevent other vital metabolic subsystems from maintaining 'desired states' and may render the parental system as a whole more susceptible to disturbances.

(f) Reproduction may lead to increased metabolic demands not directly associated with gamete loss itself but which nevertheless compete with parental metabolism.

Calow's general theory of natural death attributes senescence to the gradual withdrawal of resources from the soma to support the gonads as the organism matures.

In this connection, growth of an organism is the outcome of resource competition between the various populations of cells comprising its organs. Although there is a high degree of central control of resource utilization through the brain and its neurosecretory system, cells in organs appear to have basic endogenous programmes for self-regulation of size and shape which the endocrine system can only accelerate or retard. At an elementary level of analysis this differential sharing of materials and energy within the body is expressed by the differential growth which occurs between organs. In mammals, the brain has a preferential command of resources during early development when it makes its greatest contribution to body weight. As maturity approaches preference is given to other organ systems. Presumably the shifting pattern of differential growth relates to an evolutionary programming of individual organs to receive the correct allocations of materials and energy concomitant with the continuation of the genotype in evolution.

Although it has not been deeply investigated, it is likely that surveillance and repair in each organ would also come under evolutionary pressures to be kept to a minimum in order to conserve resources for growth and reproduction. These processes might even be reduced at a stage when some imperfections would not be disadvantageous in the short term. Maintaining life as a balanced system of imperfections would be advantageous only within the natural lifespan. In protective environments the continuation of a 'resources withdrawal' programme in any organ system would eventually become non-adaptive and appear as degenerative disease.

The theory of natural death is an attractive biological proposition because it concerns the evolution of systems for getting the most from limited environmental resources by sharing them between different cellular phenotypes within the body according to the survival value of the organs at different stages of life. However, we are still far from applying the theory as an all-embracing biological principle to account for the loss of adaptabilities which we call ageing.

AGEING AS A LOSS OF SYSTEMS PRECISION

As organisms age they show more individuality. Eventually, in people, this variability is manifest as the various causes of death found in the population. Also, as organisms become older they become less adaptable to changes in the environment. Both of these characteristics imply a loss of precision in biochemical, physiological, and behavioural systems. Biochemical failures are the most fundamental features of ageing systems but the biologist cannot handle the biochemistry of the complex multifactorial aspects of whole organism ageing and must resort to simple systems that are amenable to precise description and experiment.

The classification of whole body data and the analysis of blood and urine, both of which are expressions of the working of very complex systems, are of limited value. This is partly because of cohort effects which arise from selective mortality of certain phenotypes at well-defined ages. Longitudinal studies are better than cross-sectional sampling but the practical difficulties of organizing these at the level of both people and experimental animals make it unlikely that data will become available quickly to allow individual rates of ageing to be followed over large fractions of a lifespan.

In any case, we now have sufficient descriptive data enabling us to outline the general features of human ageing, and to take the next step of analysis the gerontologist must work with simpler systems, resorting to the use of various models of human ageing that are taken largely for convenience. Whole animal models only come into their own when behavioural ageing is under investigation.

Homeostasis and Development

When we come to examine the reasons for the increased force of mortality in old organisms, there are two possible levels of function, corresponding to the organ and the cell, where the living system may be considered to fail. For most organs, there appears to be little evidence that malfunctions, either through disproportionate growth, the failure of repair mechanisms, or loss of cells, occur on a scale sufficient to increase the chances of the organism dying. On this plane, however, one is clearly dealing with the deterioration of complex interacting organ systems, comprising sensory detectors, nervous system, endocrine system, and effectors. Taken together, several deviant organ subsystems may result in a failure to produce the correct degree of response in relation to alterations in the external and internal environment. Lack of ability of a subsystem to respond appropriately to a disturbed environment does not appear to be due to the failure of any single component. For example, the endocrine system probably fails to meet demand because of both a fall in the rate of secretion of hormones and the inability of the target tissue to make the appropriate response to the hormones (Bellamy, 1967). Often, structural changes in several components of the effector organs are alone sufficient to limit mechanical aspects of an endocrine response.

Death in the context of organ function involves a series of events which occur over a small fraction of the lifespan, possibly amounting to only a few hours. That is to say, organisms die as the result of internal fluctuations in body chemistry which can no longer be contained through homeostatic regulation; a small shift in metabolism which could be counteracted in youth becomes amplified to the point of preventing a vital function. Thus, death in old organisms may result from minor changes in the environment.

The normal low tolerance and limited capacity for self-regulation of metabolic systems imply that the individual processes concerned in regulation rarely operate under conditions which an engineer might consider optimal. Also, the organs, even at the peak of development, are never quite perfect. As we have seen, tolerance and imperfection appear to be the necessary prerequisites, as well as the consequences, of natural selection, with genetical polymorphism being established through the action of a balance of defects. This is another way of saying that the population carries a genetical load and every individual has some constructional defect resulting from gene sets which will eventually show up as deleterious combinations. At this point gerontology becomes bound up with an analysis of the mechanism that regulates the changing pattern of active genes responsible for development. Development, especially plants and insects, is typically a morphogenetic process leading to death almost immediately after reproduction. The prevention of sexual reproduction, e.g. by the elimination of flowers in monocarpic plants and ovaries in invertebrate animals, can significantly increase the lifespan, but only by modifying the morphogenetic programme. In this context, the morphogenetic programme is selected to favour those intrinsic homeostatic mechanisms that create a reproductively efficient organism within a narrowly defined period after fertilization. This period is determined in relation to the total environmental factors contributing to natural selection which, where they have been measured, are mainly predation and disease. Once removed from the action of these selective forces in the wild environment, the programme would be expected to run on and diverge in a random, senseless way. Selection in the new protective environment would act against the population through age-dependent failures in the various regulatory mechanisms. Most models of ageing are concerned with failures which eventually appear under the controlled environment conditions of the laboratory.

Mathematical Models

A model in gerontology may be defined as a system that is taken as being representative of a major feature of ageing and which opens up the possibility of experimental manipulation.

Models used to investigate loss of precision and adaptability fall into two categories of mathematical models and biological ones. Mathematical models may be further subdivided into those that are used for the prediction of mortality rates and those that indicate a possible mechanism of ageing. An example of a predictive model is the human study made by Keyes dealing with the relationship between the concentration of cholesterol in the blood and the risk of coronary heart disease (Fig. 2).

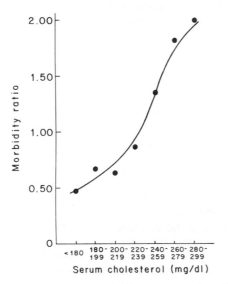

Figure 2 Relationship between coronary heart disease and serum cholesterol. (From Kannel *et.al.*, 1971)

This model starts from descriptive analysis which indicates that in all the large-scale surveys, the risk pattern of mortality from the disease, or of developing myocardial infarction, proves to be much the same. To specify this common pattern, it is assumed that the total risk of future infarction is given by a term denoting the effects of all influences unrelated to serum cholesterol, to which is added a function of predisease cholesterol. These two terms yield mathematical expressions which are simple exponential or logarithmic equations.

These equations were first tested in data from over 6,000 individuals followed from 6 to 15 years, during which time 251 either had infarcts or died from coronary disease. The individuals were grouped according to classes of predisease cholesterol, the group risk was

known in retrospect, and the constants in the equations determined by the method of least squares. Using these constants, the average predicted values for risk correlated highly with the observed risk. This model only deals with the group risk to certain cohorts of the population, and does not throw any light on individual risk. Also, because it was difficult to discriminate between environmental and genetic factors in their distinct contributions to mortality, the fundamental basis is obscure. This highlights a special difficulty in that the genotype may predispose an individual to environmental influences that may or may not be relevant to mortality.

Many mathematical models with a mechanistic basis have been constructed in an effort to explain the fact that for a large number of organisms, a curve of the fraction of population surviving versus time shows a definite S-shape, usually skewed to the left. The logarithmic derivative of this curve can be described by the Gompertz function or some similar expression. All of these curves have essentially two parameters. One is a scale factor converting something like 'speed of living' into units of absolute time. The other parameter is related to the width of the plateau or shoulder of the S-curve and is an expression of stability or precision of the biological system. There are many mathematical models which will result in S-curves of survivors and in each of them the two parameters acquire a distinct, precise meaning. However, between 90 and 10 per cent. survival, the curves are indistinguishable. Therefore, they may be used to analyse only initial and final mortalities based on the characteristics of the first few descendants and the last few survivors. The use of these models allows a very limited insight into the mechanisms of ageing in the bulk of the population between these two extremes.

The first to treat the aetiology of degenerative disease quantitatively were Armitage and Doll who in 1954 showed that mortality curves could be predicted on the basis of a multifactor model (Fig. 3) (See Curtis, 1967.)

If a disease arises through a series of steps each having its own rate constant it can be shown that if the number of cells at risk is large and the probability of occurrence of the steps is low, mortality data will follow a line described by the relationship

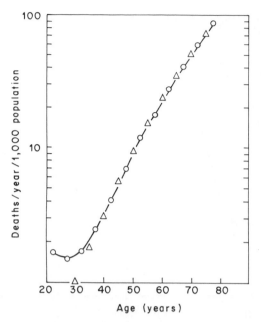

Figure 3   Application of a mathematical model of multistep genesis of disease to human mortality curve ○ United States males, 1960; △ theoretical. (From Curtis, 1967)

$$\frac{dN}{dt} = Kt^{n-1}$$

where N is the percentage of persons contracting the disease, t the time, n the number of steps in the process, and K a constant depending on the probability of each step, the population under study, and the environment. Calculated death rates for all causes best fit with actual data on the assumption that there is on average 6 steps in the reaction sequences. This idea may be presented diagrammatically as the multifactorial theory of ageing (Fig. 4), where each ageing process, in which each has its own probability or rate constant, is postulated to give rise to each of the degenerative diseases.

Burch, Murray, and Jackson (1971) extended this approach to show that the incidence of autoimmune diseases, cardiovascular disease, and phenotypic expressions of ageing such as baldness and loss of teeth fit a multiple factor model. His unified theory of growth and disease contains the assumption that pathogenesis of most age-dependent disorders may be divided into two principal phases termed initiation and development. Initiation occurs

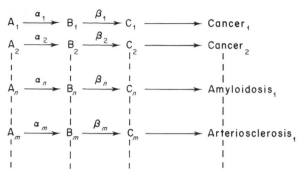

Figure 4   The multifactorial theory of ageing, (from Curtis, 1967)

through random and somatic gene mutation in stem cells that regulate growth and size of target tissues throughout the body. It is postulated that each tissue has a specific central control system and that disease is initiated with a somatic mutation that has occurred at random in a distinctive stem cell. The mathematical model is described by the equation

$$P_t = S(1 - e^{-Kt^r})^n$$

where P_t is the prevalence of the disease at any age;

S is the proportion of the population predisposed to the disease;

K is a constant dependent upon the number of stem cells at risk and the average mutation rate;

t is the age of initiation measured from birth;

r is the number of specific genes that have to mutate.

In Fig. 5 the log of prevalence of greying hair in men is plotted against log age minus a correction factor. The correction factor which is necessary for the points to be fitted to a smooth curve defines the latent period that elapses from the time of initiation to the manifestation of greyness.

Unfortunately, however, these physiological systems are not simple and the complete mathematical expression of models of those systems of interest to gerontologists inevitably contain non-linear terms and equations of a high order, necessitating the use of computer methods to obtain solutions. Also, when an attempt is made to formalize and apply mathematical methods to a particular regulating system, some decision must be made as to how the

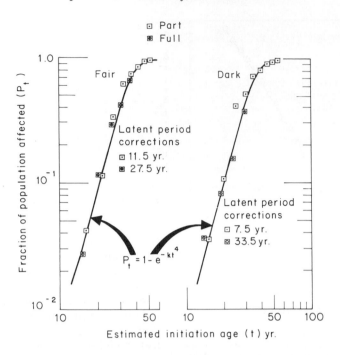

Figure 5 Age-specific prevalence of the greying of hair in men. Data for fair-haired men on left; data for dark-haired men on right. The same theoretical curve, $P_t = 1-e^{-kt^4}$ is plotted in both panels.

system is supposed to work. A model must be specified with regard to the regulation of input in respect of output. Difficulty in interpretation arises because a model that has the known properties of a given biological system may achieve the correct overall end points and yet regulate quite differently from the real system. Even where the biological system is reasonably well known, the application of mathematical analysis has frequently added little to our understanding. Nevertheless, the initial act of model building where the problem is formulated in terms of block diagrams, flow paths, and simple mathmatical equations is useful in that the precise identification and rigorous definition of previously vague concepts is required. This formulation provides insight and clarification obtainable in no other way but may also lead to the construction of elaborate theoretical models based on hypothetical mechanisms. Generalizations may also rise to the status of precisely determined relationships without adequate information to evaluate the validity of the model. Additionally, very few events can be formulated as precise flow dia-

grams or even put into quantitative terms. Generally, the situation can be roughly described by the old saying, namely, that engineers deal with primitive situations in an elegant way, while biologists must tackle elegant situations by primitive means. Only exceptionally is it possible to isolate part of these processes and make this simplified system amenable to quantitative treatment. From this viewpoint, all experiments in gerontology are approximation models based on the axiom that organisms are in many ways regulatory machines. So far, mathematical models of ageing originating from these premises are usually invulnerable to experiments but are useful, in that they often lead to the generation of new data when the model is put to the test.

Biological Models

When using biological models to examine the loss of adaptability, we may feel that we are on firm ground; however, it must always be remembered that a particular biological system is chosen as a model because it is not identical to the phenomenon in which we are really interested. It should be evaluated with scepticism.

Many intact and partly dissected living systems have been used as models in ageing research because they appeared to offer a simplified state with advantageous properties for elucidating a particular aspect of ageing. No doubt, many more such models will become available in the future and it is therefore difficult to deal predictively with the future potential of biological research, particularly as many past models have not been adequately exploited. Therefore what follows is merely an attempt to show the diversity of models available with only in some cases an assessment of their future potential. Only a limited selection of the various biological models that have been used to investigate loss of precision is presented to point out the strengths and weaknesses of the modelling philosophy.

Models for Cellular Ageing.

Microorganisms and cell cultures have been used as biological models mainly because of their mean uniformity when sampled and because their external environment can be defined and controlled. These simple cell models are designed to overcome the experimental difficulties that arise in the study of cells in organs. A disadvantage is that they differ greatly from the integrated organ systems comprising the human body. Microorganisms have the advantage over cell cultures in that they may be subjected to genetic analysis in order to test theories of irreversible genetic damage. Experimental systems used are of two kinds relating to the two kinds of cells which are for convenience recognized by gerontologists in the human body, namely cells capable of reproducing by division and those highly differentiated cells such as muscle that cannot divide.

Bacteria. Resting bacterial spores, if they are not induced to divide for some time, show survival curves that are linear when log survivors are plotted against time. The same is true for non-dividing vegetative cells. This is expressed by

$$N = N_0 \omega^{-1t}$$

where N is the number of survivors alive at time T_0 out of an initial population N_0, and l is constant. On this formula a constant proportion of survivors die per unit time interval; thus the chances of a bacterial cell dying in a given unit of time is independent of the age of the cell. Although proliferating bacteria are far removed from ageing human subjects, a model for the ageing of postmitotic cells has been proposed, using mutant bacteria that require thymine for proliferation. Thus, a suspension may be grown synchronously in a chemically defined medium, harvested, washed, and resuspended in the same growth medium minus thymine. Omission of the vital pyrimidine would prevent DNA synthesis and consequently cell division could not take place. This model would have the advantage of giving unlimited numbers of highly active, growing but not dividing cells. They would all be of approximately the same age, without the complications of intercellular reactions, and the suspensions could be studied to the point of death. Very little work has been carried out on this type of microbial model. The loss of bacteria from the population occurs in the same fashion as the loss of teacups by breakage in a cafeteria. By analogy, death in bacteria may occur because of subjection to a low but constant probability of having an internal chemical accident.

Recent studies on dividing bacteria have shown that clones derived from single cells have a finite lifespan when constrained to reproduce by binary fission. This phenomenon of a finite lifespan of dividing cells was revealed originally with protozoan cultures.

Protozoa. Although cultures of microorganisms cannot be regarded as analogous to cultures of metazoan cells, they have been examined from time to time in an attempt to throw light on cellular ageing. The first work on protozoa was stimulated by predictions that because protozoans were pure germ plasm, they must inevitably be immortal.

When ciliates are cultured on a large scale, the character of a population as measured by the mean properties of all phenotypes present at any time will characteristically go through a series of temporal changes akin to sexual maturation, followed by senescence. Cultures derived from single organisms show a decline or clonal ageing, resembling ageing in multicellular systems. These changes occur while the cells are dividing by binary fission. In the laboratory, a particular clone will eventually die out after its component organisms have passed through the fission cycle a certain number of times. New clones may arise from a clone that is undergoing clonal ageing if sexual reproduction, i.e. conjugation or autogamy, takes place and these processes prevent clonal ageing.

To summarize, this work on experimental cultures of protozoa has shown that once a clone has embarked by binary fission upon its life history, the course of certain events is predictable and is irreversibly set. Genes may modify the phenotype expressed at a particular stage or alter the timing of aspects of the cycle. That is to say, a given character of the population comes to phenotypic expression at a fixed time to be followed by another character arising from the expression of different genetic information, even though a particular stage may last hundreds of fissions. In this way, the cells of a clone transform from one life-cycle stage to the next. This change may be such that a new region of the chromosomes is now susceptible to environmental induction and hence expression (as in the case of a mating-type locus) or the expression may require no inducers. Thus the fission life-cycle results from a programme where successive genetic regions become activated. It appears that all of the cell components may experience characteristic structural changes during the lifespan of a clone; alterations of the cilia and their arrangement, and malformations in the gullet, the micronuclei and the macronuclei are especially striking. New structurally perfect clones arise and new life-cycle is possible only when a macronucleus is produced by the events of fertilization. Hence the renewal of this organelle is indispensable for rejuvenation.

Any clock-like mechanism may trigger many genetic loci, leading to different biological characteristics, but it is not at all clear whether there is a single master clock set in motion at the first division or whether different clocks are activated in sequence.

Protozoan models have characteristics of ageing in the metazoa but what is their value? If it is assumed that all living things are built to a common plan, studies on ageing micro-organisms raise questions which have an important bearing on ageing of higher animals. What are the mechanisms by which cells with a common mitotic lineage, cultivated in a constant environment, develop an orderly sequence of phenotypes? Also, how does nuclear reorganization halt the process of ageing and transform a degenerating cell into a totipotent individual? Other models containing dividing cells relevant to the study of these questions may be found in the de-differentiation of planarians, the conversion of iris epithelial cells to lens cells in vertebrate embryos, and, in plants, the conversion of leaf epidermis cells into meristematic tissue. This list serves to illustrate how problems of ageing impinge upon those of development. Rejuvenation in all of these systems appears to be initiated by virtue of cells finding themselves in a new environment and is mediated by some kind of nuclear reorganization.

Human red cells. The value of the red cell as a model in gerontology may be examined from two different aspects. Firstly, when blood is sedimented the reticulocytes are preferentially distributed at the top of the cell column. As the reticulocyte is a young cell its position is indicative of cells newly formed and released into the circulation. The lower sedimentation rate of reticulocytes is due to their greater water content and consequent lower density. The remaining cells sediment in the column roughly according to age, with the oldest, most dense cells being found at the bottom. One of the ways of separating these cells according to age is to rely on their differences in density (Fig. 6). Centrifugation of a mixture of cells through non-water-miscible mixtures of different specific gravities has been used in order to provide samples for analysis. By means of a brief injection of radioactive iron into donor animals a limited population of cells can be labelled and followed as an identifiable cohort through the entire lifespan. When this approach is combined with sedimentation of samples taken at various times after administration of the isotope, radioactivity first appears in the top layer of cells and then progressively descends the column.

Young cells from the top of a column of sedimented cells are more resistant to osmotic lysis than the older cells at the bottom and if

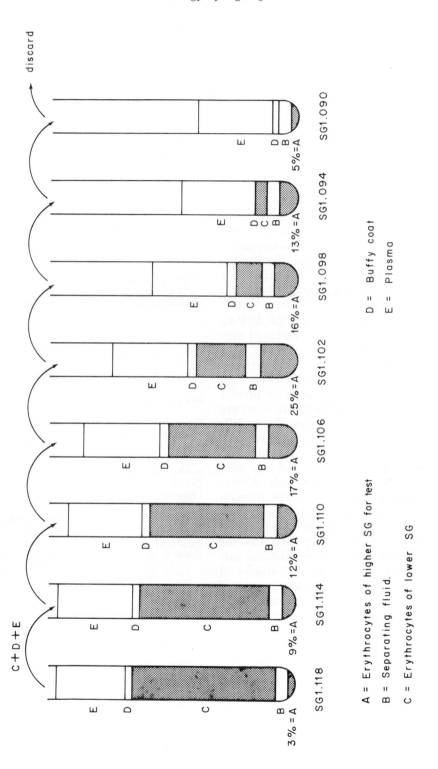

Figure 6   Separation of red cells into age cohorts by differential flotation. (From Yaari, 1969)

cells labelled with radioactive iron are subjected to different hypotonic solutions the amount of radioactive haemoglobin liberated by cell lysis reflects the age of the cells destroyed. Serial studies by this technique indicate that red cells gradually become progressively more susceptible to osmotic lysis during their lifespan.

Age changes in the structure of the red cell are directly related to a decrease in surface area. Chemical analysis indicates less lipid in old cells and structural changes may also be inferred from the different ionic compositions and the behaviour in mechanical fragility tests. There are also well-defined alterations in cell energetics with the rate of glycolysis decreasing progressively with increasing age. There also appears to be a lower level of active transport in older cells with a fall in the steady-state ratio of potassium to sodium.

There is a decrease in the ratio of ATP to ADP which correlates with a decreased survival of ATP in deficient cells as they age, both *in vivo* and *in vitro*. This relationship between age and enzymic activity has been sufficiently developed to enable investigators to predict the mean age of a red cell population on the basis of certain enzyme activities (Table 10). There also appears to be an increased concentration of methaemoglobin in older cells, the increase being appreciable at about fifty days of age, steadily increasing afterwards. Alongside this a number of studies have demonstrated a drop in the ability to reduce methoaemoglobin to haemaglobin is a function of cell age. The same decay curve is found for methaemoglobin reduction as for red cell survival. The fall-off is the reductive capacity of the cell may be explained as one outcome of a generally diminished glucose utilization with a resultant decrease in reduction capacity.

The higher oxygen saturation in older cells (increased affinity) has been described as macromolecular changes within the cell and possibly to alterations in the structure of the haemoglobin molecule that progressed with age. Increased amounts of haemoglobin A3 have been described in older cells. One of the component parts of this haemoglobin contains haemoglobin A with one of two sulphydral groups of each beta chain blocked by a glutathione residue. It is also possible that the increased affinity of haemoglobin for oxygen in

Table 10   Chemical changes in human red cells ageing *in vivo*. (Data taken from Prankard, 1961, and Loehr and Waller, 1961)

Enzyme changes	
Glucose-6-phosphate dehydrogenase	Increased activity in young cells
6–Phosphogluconic dehydrogenase	Increased activity in young cells
Phosphohexose isomerase	Increased activity in young cells
Triosephosphate dehydrogenase	Slight or no increased activity in young cells
Aldolase	Increased activity in young cells
Hexokinase	Increased activity in young cells
Lactic dehydrogenase	Little or no difference in young cells
Methaemoglobin reductase	Increased activity in young cells
Purine nucleoside phosphoyrlase	Little or no difference
Cholinesterase	Increased activity in young cells
Catalase	Increased activity in young cells
Oxalacetic glutamic *transaminase*	Increased activity in young cells
Pyruvate kinase	Increased activity in young cells
Glutathione reductase	No difference between old and young cells
Glyoxalase	No increase in young cells
Metabolic changes	
Glycolysis	Increased in young cells
Oxygen utilization	Decreased in young cells
Nucleoside utilization	Increased in young cells
Constituent changes	
Phosphate esters	Decrease in 2, 3-diphosphoglyceric acid
NAD	Decreased in old cells
Glutathione (reduced)	No difference
Total – SH	Increased in young cells
Lipids	Increased in young cells (but not per unit surface area)
Electrolytes:	
Potassium	Increased in young cells
Sodium	Decreased in young cells
Magnesium (Mg^{2+})	Decreased in old cells
^{42}K exchange	Decreased in young cells
Water	Increased in young cells
Methaemoglobin	Increased in old cells
Oxygen dissociation	Decreased in old cells
Storage changes	
Phosphate esters	Decreased breakdown of ATP and 2, 3-diphosphoglyceric acid in young cells
Electrolytes	Decreased loss of potassium from young cells

older cells in dependent on the intracellular concentration of triosephosphate which decreases as red cells age.

In summary, it appears that largely through changes in the structure of its molecules and consequent loss of metabolic capabilities the human red cell is unable to maintain the necessary reducing capacity to protect haemoglobin deleterious changes. These changes may also be responsible for alterations in the cell membrane that eventually lead to destruction of the cell. Old red cells are more susceptible to haemolysis by immune antibodies. In addition there may be an accumulation of metabolites inhibitory to the metabolic activity of the cell. Although the red cell undergoes the process of ageing and it seems probable that its final destruction is the result of this ageing process there is no direct evidence to establish this as fact. It may well be that the changes noted so far are mechanisms desinged to hold off final destruction as long as possible.

Ageing in vitro. Blood transfusions are given either to restore blood volume or to supply viable red cells, and for both purposes stored blood can, as a rule, effectively replace fresh blood. Cells stored under the best conditions in an acid citrate or dextrose preservative at between 4 and 7 °C undergo morphological and biochemical alterations (Table 11). Cells become more spherical with an associated increase in osmotic and mechanical fragilities. The glycolytic rate drops and organic phosphate compounds decline with the release of inorganic phosphate. There is also a fall in cell potassium and a rise in intracellular sodium. These altered cells when transfused to a recipient are destroyed at a rate dependent upon the duration of storage of the blood. Storage for 3 weeks results in a fall of 15 per cent. in the viability and at 4 weeks there is a 40 per cent. drop in viability. Since the normal human red cell population is destroyed in the body at a rate of about 1 per cent. per day the lowered survival of blood cells after 3 to 4 weeks of storage is consistent with the expected in vivo losses from ageing. This indicates that the ageing of red cells that occurs in the body continues when blood is stored. However, many of the changes in stored red cells are different from those that occur in aged cells in the body.

Table 11 Changes in red cell volume and the concentration of intracellular ions on storage of citrated human blood stored at 4 °C. (From Harris and Maizels, 1952)

Time weeks	0	1	1	4	8
Cells lysed (%)	0	0	0.5	2.0	4.2
Cells:					
pH, 20 °C	7.54	7.36	7.28	7.15	7.00
v^b	100	103	119	131	135
Na meg,/l cells^a	12	53	93	115	131
K meg,/cell^a	102	69	56	47	46
(Na)	17	73	104	114	124
(K)	146	95	63	47	43
(HbO$_2$)	45	33	21	12	5
(Phosphate)	50	47	38	31	24
(Citrate^a)	0	0	7	16	30
Plasma:					
(Na)	189	166	156	152	146
(K)	3	25	38	49	53
(HbO$_2^-$) (by lysis)	0	0	0	0.1	0.2
(Phosphate)	1.0	1.5	1.7	3.3	6.4
(Citrate)	85	85	85	86	70

^{a} Contents corrected for changes in volume by reference to the original cell volume.
^{b} Volume as a percentage of original cell volume.
Brackets indicate concentrations, e.g. (HbO$_2$) = concentration of oxyhaemoglobin anion, meq/l of cell or plasma water.

For example, in stored red cells, ATP diminishes rapidly with time whereas in the body this change occurs very slowly. This discrepancy between the changes occurring in cells on storage and those ageing in the body is not surprising when it is considered that the metabolic conditions on storage are greatly different from those in the body. The low temperature ensures that much less metabolic energy is available so that those processes that depend upon a steady supply of ATP may degenerate irreversibly. So far the techniques of blood preservation have been designed simply from the point of view of obtaining the largest number of surviving cells in relation to the longest possible storage time. In order to study red cell ageing *in vitro* as a continuation of the process in the body it is necessary to duplicate as far as possible the conditions obtained during circulation, i.e. to have a high temperature, a good oxygenation, and a steady supply of blood glucose. So far *in vitro* models have not met these strict criteria.

Changes in the haemopoetic stem cells. Information on the failure of specification in the red cell stem line as the body ages is not so clear cut. At a gross morphological level there are no differences between bulk samples of human red cells from young and old donors with respect to mean corpuscular volume, red cell count, and haemoglobin concentration. However, whole blood viscosity does fall with age, being nearly 35 per cent less comparing mean ages of 21 and 80 years. This is taken to mean that the red cells of old people are more easily deformed. In turn, this must be related to a change in specification of the red cell membrane by the stem line, but there is as yet no detailed evidence to support this view.

Organ Models

At the level of organs, many systems have been examined because they show marked age changes, and several of these changes have led to particular theories of ageing. Organ models suffer from the disadvantage that they are composed of diverse cellular elements that may age in different ways, and they do not lend themselves readily to experimentation, particularly under conditions *in vitro*. From this aspect, virtually no gerontological work has been done with organ perfusion because of the technical problems involved. Despite the poor experimental returns from many organ models, however, there is still much scope for research, particularly using tissues which show marked histological changes with the passage of time and others which may be easily transplanted.

Tissues such as ovary and adrenal cortex, which change with age dramatically at the histological level from the point of view of the random appearance of structural abnormalities, were intensively studied by early gerontologists, and it is encouraging to see work beginning with these tissues into cellular involution at the biochemical level. These models may also be expected to throw light on the failure of endocrine control.

A large proportion of the organ models have the shortcoming that they are not capable of experimental manipulation, and the theories are not vulnerable to experiment.

Ageing of the human lens.

As we age the lens becomes yellower and absorbs more light particularly at the blue end of the spectrum. The gradual increased threshold of vision, which is a consistent feature of human ageing, is partly due to this increased pigmentation. The lens goes on increasing in size by continued division of the anterior layer of epithelial cells through-

out life, resulting in thickness gradually increased by about 7 μn per year; no cells are shed. The epithelium growth process is stable; in particular it is not subject to any form of cancerous transformation. Most of the lens is filled with fibrous material derived from the epithelial cells by a process of differentiation. Experimentally it has been found that this is reversible and the fibrous cells in the centre of the lens can revert to their former undifferentiated state in culture. The lens changes in shape by a gradual bulging of the posterior pole in later life.

Young's modulus of the capsule progressively declines, indicating a threefold decrease in elasticity during an average lifespan. By inducing radial forces on the lens through spinning, it is known that the structure is reversibly deformable although older lenses are more difficult to deform. It is thought that all focusing power is eventually lost through changes in the physical properties of the crystalline lens as it ages. Because of the greater difficulty in deforming the lens substance of older lenses the muscular force must be increased enormously to look at near objects.

At the chemical level there is a gradual decrease in the proportion of soluble protein in the lens, and proteins isolated by electrophoresis from old lenses are less sharply defined as electrical species, suggesting that there is a progressive deterioration of protein molecules postsynthetically. For a specific enzyme, glutathione reductase, there is an increased heat liability. This change occurs around the beginning of the third decade when the proportion of heat labile enzyme increases from about 5 to 25 per cent. with little change thereafter. The shift occurs in the nucleus of the lens. It is likely, therefore, to be a post-translational event. The time at which the biochemical changes occur contrasts with the time of onset of the greatest change in physical properties which occurs at the middle of the fourth decade. At this time there is a rise in the incidence of senile cataract; this may be seen clearly from the statistics of cataract extraction. The number of cataracts extracted increases fortyfold over the next 5 decades. The female incidence of cataract is consistently higher than in men at all ages. There is also strong evidence for geographical differences in the incidence of cataract.

The lens model is important in that, like the red cell model, it indicates the importance of protein deterioration in ageing. It is also the only organ where chemical changes can be directly connected with physiological failure.

Organ transplants. Ovary and skin transplants have been important in establishing the principle of intrinsic multifactorial ageing, and transplant models have scope for furthering research into new theoretical areas of gerontology dealing with the ageing of mitotic clones.

Of various transplant models, normal skin epidermis may be repeatedly propagated to greatly exceed the lifespan of the donor. On the other hand, mammary duct epithelium transplanted in the fat pad shows a progressive age-dependent change, not in dividing capacity but in growth rate. There is no fall with repeated passage in the percentage of 'takes', but the time to reach maximum size increases linearly with clonal age. The clone can outlive the donor, but there is a clock-like mechanism that results in slower growth. This phenomenon appears to be similar to the decline in colony-forming ability of transplanted marrow stem cells, which are otherwise stable as a clone. Thus, transplant models will clearly yield much new information about the modifiability of age changes in differentiated cells with regard to both intrinsic alterations and systemic influences.

Plants

Whole plants and organs. Plant models have so far been little used in gerontology despite the fact that plants grown under laboratory conditions offer more scope for the precise specification of the total environment than most animal cultures. However, the fact that plants are capable of multidirectional growth means that they can grow away from their 'past'. This unique feature, which resides in the general distribution of undifferentiated meristematic tissue that is capable of rapid multiplication presents opportunities for testing ideas on cellular ageing of mitotic cells in plant systems. Useful models in this context may come from those plants that appear to be capable of propagation indefinitely by vegetative methods. The existence of these apparently immor-

tal characteristics of meristems is of the utmost importance in that ageing of dividing cells does not appear to be fundamentally a limited process. A start on investigating these tissues has already been made with the root tip organ system which has yielded information on the short-term changes in cells originating in the root tip which differentiate as they age.

Much work has also been done on leaves which show sequential and multiple senescence. Partial and total senescence of the entire plant appears to be due to the existence of various hormonally directed ageing programmes, all of which are affected by environmental factors and some linked to reproduction. Studies on senescing leaves have pointed to the importance of failures in genetic expression in the senescent process and this view has been supported by experiments on the loss of viability in stored seeds. In this respect plant organ models are useful in relation to animal studies, particularly those on monocarpic species, which closely resemble those animals where programmed death appears to be a major feature of the reproductive process.

Studies of ageing of entire plants are limited in that most botanical experiments have been set up to study the ageing of roots and leaves. Nevertheless, one of the earliest studies on plant ageing was concerned with the loss of vigour of a species where vegetative propagation is a major mode of reproduction. In a constant and favourable environment each frond of the aquatic surface spreading duckweed *Lemna minor* has a finite life and rate of ageing which is characteristic of the clone in its particular environment. The fronds become detached from the mother plant as a normal event in vegetative propagation. Thereafter each one ages, showing a progressive decrease in the size of its daughter fronds. Ageing is not of consequence in the production of daughter fronds, nor is it due to a lack of obvious growth factors in the ageing fronds. Certain environmental factors, such as temperature and nutrient content of the medium, affect the rate of ageing (Table 12) whereas others such as light intensity and length of day do not. The area of daughter fronds appears to be determined by some material in the mother frond which diminishes or is inactivated as the mother frond gets older.

Table 12   Ageing in *Lemna minor* during vegetative reproduction. (From Wangerman and Lacey, 1955)

Amount of nutrient added (mg/l)	Length of life (days)		Relative rate of ageing	
	Mean	SE	Mean	SE
0	78.9	2.29	0.116	0.028
0.05	53.8	1.36	0.156	0.005
0.10	53.5	0.92	0.184	0.009
0.25	50.7	1.40	0.184	0.014
0.50	53.4	1.82	0.188	0.012
2.00	58.2	1.74	0.181	0.010

Seeds. Most observations on seed longevity have been made with artifically, rather than naturally, stored seeds. Two long experimental studies have been made involving the deliberate burial of seed. In 1897 seed of 23 different species was buried in inverted bottles of sand in a field at a depth of 45 cm. Samples have been taken from these containers at 13 intervals, the most recent being 90 years after the start of the experiment. The species include two trees, a biennial, and two perennials, the remainder being all annuals. Some seed of the trees and five of the herbaceous species died out in less than 5 years; three species remained viable after 80 years and only one germinated after 90 years. Radiocarbon techniques have been used to age specimens of seeds of the lotus obtained from soil samples at 1,040 ± 210 years, the seeds being still fertile.

Experimentally, seeds have value as models for studying organ ageing because they have the following unique features:

(a)   No cell division occurs during storage so that if deviant cells arise they are not selected out.

(b)   Cell division may be easily initiated at any time.

(c)   The availability of self-pollinating species makes it easy to obtain homozygous material for genetical studies and so test for mutations arising in storage.

(d)   Species are available with small numbers of large chromosomes so that nuclear changes may be detected at cell division.

(e)   Seeds are easily subjected to different experimental environments during storage.

(f)   Large numbers of seeds are readily obtainable for experiment.

(g)   Conditions of storage may be arranged so that accidental deaths may be avoided.

It is characteristic of all experimental populations investigated that the percentage of viable seeds falls with age, and this is correlated with a gradual rise in phenotypic variability in plants obtained on germination, particularly with regard to the frequency of mutant characters. Indeed, chromosome abnormalities are readily detected by histological methods in the roots of several species of plants grown from old seeds. Although the proportion of abnormalities increases with temperature and moisture content during storage, there is little doubt that the changes are brought about by intrinsic processes in the seeds. The interplay between the intrinsic process and environmental variables makes it possible to alter the rate of the seed ageing and examine the seeds for viability and corresponding changes in the frequency of chromosome aberrations. From such experiments these two parameters are highly correlated.

The evidence is in favour of the basic change, being one involving chromosome breakage occurring during storage which takes place entirely in the interphase state. These nuclear aberrations appear in seeds and also become detectable under the microscope when the cells of the embryo begin to divide on germination. Thus, it may be postulated that death of the embryo is the result of the accumulation of cellular damage associated with chromosome breakage. On this idea, for any given percentage seed survival, the mean frequency of aberrant cells in the survivors would be constant irrespective of how rapidly viability declined and would be independent of the storage conditions. On the whole this is observed except for the most severe environmental conditions, when the chromosome aberrations are less than would be anticipated (Fig. 7).

Although chromosome damage is a reliable index of ageing in seeds it is unlikely to be a causal factor in seed deterioration. This is because cells with damaged chromosomes are eliminated during early growth, for example, of the root tips. This probably takes place because these grossly abnormal cells cannot compete with normal cells. The elimination of aberrant cells in this way throws doubt on the

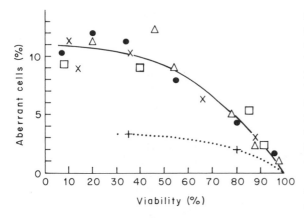

Figure 7   Viability in relation to the frequency of aberrant cells in surviving seeds of the broad bean. The unbroken curve represents the relationship typical of all treatments except the most severe treatment (at 45 °C and 18.0% m.c.), which is represented by a broken line.

general importance of somatic mutations in dividing cells as a cause of ageing. Cytological damage is likely to be an extreme indication of generalized damage to chromosomes. In this respect, quite minor alterations in nucleic acids could lead to complete disorganization of cellular function. Selection pressure does not eliminate minor aberrations of this type which behave as recessive mutants and can be easily detected by breeding experiments in the F2 generation.

The explanation put forward to explain the loss of viability of seeds falls into two classes. Most workers have favoured the idea that storage results in a gradual accumulation of mutagens within the seed. The experimental tests of this hypothesis have involved extracting seeds and testing extracts for mutagenic activity on various dividing systems. Results from this work have not been conclusive, possibly due either to the lack of specificity in the test situation or to the absence of any detectable effect, which by itself cannot be used to eliminate the theory.

The other possibility, which has been used to explain the phenomenon, is usually stated in terms of random molecular accidents. Theoretically, this process, which would involve a constant rate of appearance of chromosome damage with time, may be distinguished from the accumulation of mutagen where the rate of chromosome damage should increase with time. The fact that the number of viable seeds that can be tested for chromosome damage gradually declines because of the operation of the mortality process under investigation introduces a bias into the measuring procedure which becomes greater with time. Thus, it is not possible in practice to ensure the necessary mathematical precision required to distinguish between the two processes where the terminal experimental cohorts represent a small fraction of the phenotypes originally available.

A third possibility, that so far has not received much supporting experimental evidence, postulates that the ageing of seeds occurs through the random occurrence of molecular accidents to embryonic cells with death occurring when a critical number of dead cells has been exceeded. Ageing of the embryonic cells would then be analogous to the ageing of bacteria. Unfortunately, there is at the moment no way of verifying or eliminating this idea in any experimental model.

Programmed ageing of leaves. Plant leaves have long been regarded as suitable models for the study of ageing. In his classical writings on ageing in plants, Molisch suggested in the 1920s that ageing resulted from the loss of organic materials from the leaves as they were transported to the developing seeds. This is now seen as an oversimplified view which has to be modified to take account of shifts in the balance of the various plant hormones that have been discovered. Leaves have lifespans which are often considerably shorter than the whole plant, ranging from a few weeks in short-lived arid zone species to several decades in long-lived trees. The time at which a leaf is shed is under hormone control but the ultimate timing may be governed by environment, by reproductive activity occurring elsewhere in the plant, and by the workings of a genetic programme indigenous to the leaf which produces a gradual decline in the biochemical systems of maintenance. It may be argued that the latter type of system is the most suitable simple model for the ageing of organs that deteriorate long before the death of the organism. Leaf ageing may then be analogous to ageing of the ovary and certain lymphoid system organs in vertebrates.

It has been emphasized by Woolhouse (1972) that the physiology of a particular leaf

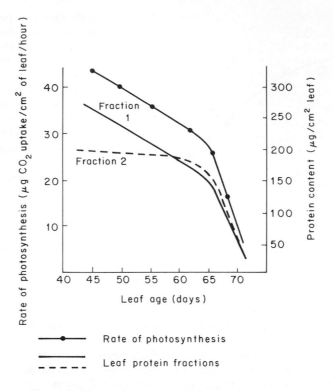

Figure 8   Biochemical and physiological changes in the
third pair of leaves of the plant Perilla fructescens. (From
Woolhouse, 1972)

is likely to be strongly influenced by its position relative to centres of hormone production, such as distance from the growing apex or root. With this in mind, he carried out elegant biochemical studies on the phenomenon of sequential senescence using a plant *(Perilla fructescens)* which enabled him to standardize observations on a particular leaf produced at a well-defined developmental phase of the life-cycle (Fig. 8).

The species chosen normally exhibited an annual life-cycle with death of the plant following flowering induced by a shortening day length. Experimentally the lifespan could be prolonged for several years by inhibiting reproduction through growing in an artificial photoperiod that was longer than that which triggered flowering.

Young plants produce up to eight successive leaf pairs on the main stem. This number appears to be a species character and the lowest pair always becomes moribund by the time the ninth new pair of leaves begins to expand.

Woolhouse confined his studies to the third successive pair of leaves, starting at the time when the first leaf attained its full expansion at about 40 days. Photosynthesis declined steadily up to about 65 days and then more rapidly until the death of the leaf at about 70 days of age. A general feature of the leaves which aged in this way is that there is a general decline in the content of soluble proteins. There is also a parallel decline in the amount of ribonucleic acid present. The causes of these changes is still under discussion. A likely possibility is that the primary event is the cessation of the production of humoral factors within the leaf which are essential for its maintenance. All the known plant hormones appear to be involved in the control of leaf metabolism and the exact changes in hormone balance underlying leaf ageing is likely to be complex.

The central idea that has come from the study of leaf ageing models is that there is a shift in the flow of genetic information. This ultimately leads to the death of the leaf but it also results in changes in the pattern of proteins. Changes in protein pattern are also evident as a major biochemical feature of the ageing of postmitotic organs in animals and it is possible that common mechanisms are involved (Fig. 9).

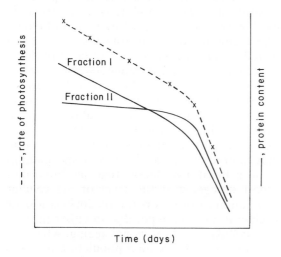

Figure 9 Changes in the protein pattern in ageing leaves. (From Woolhouse, 1967)

Root tips. The mode of meristematic growth by which narrow zones of cells proliferate outwards at the growing points of the vegetative body of plants enables models of cellular ageing to be constructed based on the cytological changes that occur at different distances from the growing point. Distance from a meristem is broadly equivalent to time that has elapsed from the last cell division. Root tips of plants that are easily grown under greenhouse conditions, such as the broad bean and onion, have been widely used in this context. Analysis of the changes has involved histological and biochemical techniques.

For many cells that originate in the meristematic zones, changes occurring after division lead to differentiation into support and conducting tissue. The end-point is death of the cell, suggesting that meristematic growth may be used as a model for studying the origins of cellular death which is a feature of organ involution in animals. Botanical work of this kind is complementary to animal studies of epidermal growth of gut and skin.

Meristems of young plants have a very high

rate of cell division, enabling studies to be mounted to investigate the frequency of occurrence of chromosome abnormalities and the subsequent fate of the cells containing them.

Ageing of Eggs and Sperm

Throughout the living world, it appears that ageing results in a decline in fertility. For laboratory rodents this is a well-defined feature of serial reproduction (Fig. 10) and is due to failures in fertilization, implantations, gestation, and neonatal care. The egg makes a contribution to this phenomenon and in rabbits and hamsters it is concluded that eggs obtained from old mothers have undergone ageing in that very few develop following fertilization and transfer to the uterus of young mothers. In line with this, unfertilized eggs transferred from old rabbits shortly after ovulation and fertilized in young females show a two- to sevenfold increase in cleavage failures. The primary defect in old eggs probably results from the ageing of ova in the ovary. This increases the chances of non-viable eggs being ovulated as the mother ages. It also results in maternal age effects appearing in the phenotype of offspring arising from eggs in that 'bad' but fertile eggs appear frequently in older females. The best known example in the human female is Down's syndrome, or mongolism, which is due to trisomy at chromosome 21. The incidence of mongolism is of the order of 1 in 2,500 mothers under 30, 1 in 1,200 between 30 and 34 years and 1 in 300 at 35 to 39 years. This progressive steady rise in frequency continues until the menopause.

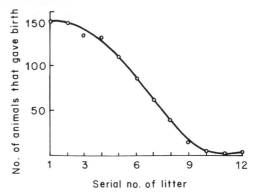

Figure 10 Decline in fertility of female laboratory rats. (From Ingram, Mandl, and Zuckerman, 1958)

Ageing of oocytes takes place in the ovary but may also occur between the time of ovulation and conception, in the reproductive tract. The full complement of eggs is formed in the human ovary during embryonic development so that the eggs released in a middle aged woman have been laying as primordia in the ovary for over 40 years. From what we know about the ageing of seeds, which occurs during storage in a far less chemically reactive environment, it is perhaps surprising that egg ageing is not more dramatic. There is a steady decline in the number of ova in the mammalian ovary. For women, the estimated number at birth is of the order of half a million which steadily decreases to about 85 per cent by middle age (Table 13). Large numbers are progressively lost by a process known as atresia. In a given ovary many more ova develop during each reproductive cycle than will ovulate. Those which do not ovulate degenerate and this degeneration process is described by the term atresia. It is difficult to see the advantages of this apparently wasteful procedure except in terms of a periodic mechanism for selecting the best eggs from a particular batch for fertilization. In this respect the follicular cells which fail to support an atretic follicle and so bring about the degeneration of the egg which it contains may be responding to chemical signs of ageing in that ovum. From this point of view, the system may have evolved as an automatic self-destruct mechanism in order to vet the ova for chemical deterioration and so prevent genetic abnormalities appearing in the offspring. Recent work bearing on this question has been carried out by removing ova from early atretic follicles of sheep and transferring them for fertilization in another ewe. So far it appears that the ova will support full development of young. Therefore the questions concerning the advantages of atresia and of performation of ova at one point in time cannot be answered except that in some respects the ageing of ova may be advantageous.

Ovarian ageing is not just a process of simple functional decline and structural atrophy, but involves the gradual failing of a homeostatic mechanism governing ovarian morphology. The declining number of follicles is correlated with the gradual development of other proliferative cell groups, most frequently composed of tubules, cords, and nodules of cells derived mainly from the germinal epithelium. These proliferative changes are probably due to a decline in the numbers of ova in that depletion of oocytes by irradiation or transplantation may imitate the senile changes. These findings fit a general hypothesis that an important aspect of ageing at the level of the cellular population of organs is the precocious loss or decline in one cell type, due to either postmitotic cellular death or clonal ageing, which results in a loss of a cellular population that was part of the regulatory process that maintained a youthful and adaptive morphology. It is tempting to think of this as resulting from a deficiency in some short distance inhibitor of growth of the supporting cells but as yet there is no direct evidence.

Unlike ovogenesis, spermatogenesis continues from puberty throughout life. However, there is evidence for ageing in the testes at a histological level – e.g. in the increase in its collagen concentration. Also, the stem cell lines and the supporting cells appear to deteriorate in that basic fertility of sperm from domestic lifestock shows a slow decline in fertility of about 1 per cent. per annum after reaching a peak early in maturity (Fig. 11). There is clear evidence for an increase in the number of abnormal sperm in the ejaculate from aged human subjects and recent work on laboratory rats indicates that sperm maturation may be blocked at this stage.

Despite this, it is clear that the mammalian ovary fails completely in terms of ovulation and is often exceeded in function by spermatogenesis. There are several physiological possibilities to account for the cessation of ovarian function. It does not seem to be due to exhaustion of the oocyte store but is more likely to be bound up with the loss of ability to re-

Table 13   Number of follicles in human ovaries at different ages. (From Block, 1952)

Age (years)	Mean no. of follicles	
	Primary	Growing
6–9	484,000	15,400
12–16	382,000	7,300
18–24	155,000	6,800
25–31	59,000	3,500
32–38	74,000	6,200
39–44	8,300	2,600

Only a few hundred of those present at birth will be lost by ovulation. Most will degenerate by the process of atresia.

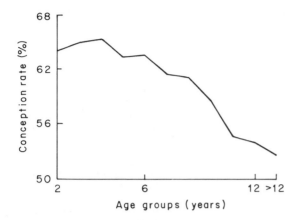

Figure 11 Decline in fertility of bull spermatozoa in relation to donor age. (From Bishop, 1970)

spond to gonadotrophins. In line with this, menopause in women is associated with a marked drop in the plasma oestrogen concentration and a rise in the gonadotrophin level. Despite this clear-cut endocrine change it is not possible to assign ovarian failure directly to a failure of the organ to respond to gonadotrophin. In general, the histological signs of degeneration are the same as in other tissues, indicating that the process of ovarian ageing is a function of diverse cells in an organ system and is not itself unique but proceeds at a faster rate than in other organs.

Ageing of the primary germ cells raises questions as to its importance in reproduction. Evidence for heritable genetic defects comes from well-established experiments which show that certain abnormalities in offspring which appear to be related solely to maternal age are capable of being transmitted to subsequent generations. The classical work was carried out on rotifers and protozoans. Similar studies have been carried out on inbred strains of mice. For example, mice in successive litters show differences in susceptibility to chemically induced fibromas, mainly through the latent period for tumour induction as well as in the characteristics of malignancy defined by survival time and invasiveness. There seems to be an inverse relation between survival time and latent period, although two mechanisms appear to be evident. In the Prunt strain female mice develop tumours earlier in succeeding litters, even though the males do not do so. Female mice show more tumours with the ability to invade into the abdomen than do males. The number of mice with malignant tumours indicating a decline in invasiveness is reduced in mice of both sexes in successive litters. Survival time is also influenced by litter seriation. These experimental results indicate that there are two hereditary mechanisms in susceptibility and malignancy which change during the lifespan in the female mouse and are handed down to her progeny as a result of age changes in the ova.

With regard to ageing of eggs and sperm in the reproductive tract, the lifespan of mammalian eggs after ovulation is very short, although it appears to exceed the period during which fertilization would normally occur. Delay in fertilization beyond the norm leads to polyspermy in mammalian eggs due to a failure of the 'blocking' system that normally prevents the entry of extra sperm after fertilization. With a normal time interval between ovulation and fertilization, polyspermy is usually about 1 to 2 per cent., whereas if mating is delayed, a tenfold increase in frequency is not uncommon. Polyspermic fertilization with only one extra sperm is commonly responsible for abortion in early pregnancy of the triploid embryo.

Sperm after maturation go through a series of changes leading eventually to loss of the ability to fertilize which is followed by death. Motility is retained for a considerable period after the ability to fertilize is lost. These changes in the rabbit with ligated vasa efferentia take about 60 days. Changes in sperm over this period are accompanied by an increase in the frequency of intrauterine mortality and abnormalities of the foetus which go alongside a decreasing fertility. Also, aged sperm are not able to compete with fresh ejaculate despite the fact that they may be successful when used alone. The lifespan of sperm in the female reproductive tract appears to be only about 50 per cent. of that in ligated male ducts. The major failure appears to be at fertilization.

Experiments have been carried out on the ageing of stored sperm from domestic livestock where there is an economic importance in artificial insemination. At −196 °C fertility of bull sperm can be retained for up to 12 months and as the storage temperature is increased the rate of loss of fertility increases, giving survival up to 6 months at −79 °C and 2 days at 4 °C.

As fertility declines on storage there is an increasing embryonic mortality after fertilization which is thought to be due to changes in genetic information carried by the sperm. These changes may be similar to those in seeds but little experimental work has been carried out in this direction.

It appears that the early stages of the ageing of mature sperm in vivo and in vitro have certain features in common. The initial histological change is the swelling of the acrosome with structural abnormalities in the acrosomal and other membranes. Associated with this is a loss of potassium, intracellular nucleotide coenzymes and lipoproteins, and enzymes derived from a range of intracellular organelles. While there does not seem to be a loss of DNA the DNA–protein complex does appear to undergo subtle changes in that nucleic acid–protein extracts prepared from fresh sperm differ antigenically from those from aged specimens. This may be responsible for the decline in fertilization ability which occurs before the cessation of motility and metabolic activity.

Conclusions

Studies of a wide range of organisms and organs have indicated that cellular ageing is expressed as a common set of histological changes (Table 14). So far, the biochemical basis of any of these structural characteristics has not been elucidated and there are many possibilities to be investigated. There is always the temptation to propose a unitary hypothesis to account for all of the phenomenon of ageing (Fig. 12) but the many alternatives of multifactorial origin are very difficult to eliminate.

Similarly, research on the various model systems described has strongly influenced current thinking in the gerontological field, but with so few potentially useful systems investigated perhaps it is unfortunate that some experimental results have been given undue prominence and have too strongly influenced the direction of research. However, this is an inevitable outcome of the way in which experimental biological research must proceed. Care must be taken before a particular model is chosen for study, with regard to its general applicability and manipulative potential. Despite the obvious limitations of application to pressing medical problems which exist in all models,

the experimental gerontologist who searches the entire living world for his material does not justify the derision which all too often he meets when presenting his findings to the geriatric profession. While it is true that medical re-

Table 14 Age changes in nervous tissue of the nucleus – salient features of past work. (From Hasan and Glees, 1973)

Author	Commonly observed changes
Hodge (1894)	1. Failure of nucleoli to stain osmium tetroxide 2. Occurrence of shrunken irregularly shaped nuclei 3. A loss of the capacity of stained nucleu to darken as a result of fatigue
Matzdorff (1948)	1. Diffuse nuclear staining 2. Clumping of the previously finely divided nuclear chromatin 3. Shrinkage of nucleus and cytoplasm
Kuhlenbeck (1954)	1. Shrunken and elongated nuclei 2. Loss of nuclear cytoplasmic contrast in stained specimens 3. Nuclear pycnosis and hyperchromatosis
Buttlar-Brentano (1954)	Occurrence of multiple nuclei and nucleoli associated with advanced age
Andrews (1956)	1. Decreased contrast between nucleus and cytoplasm witha dvancing age 2. A greater degree of basophilia of the 'nuclear sap' in the nucleus of the senile nerve cells 3. Increase in number of lobed and binucleate cells in animals of advanced age

Table 15 Summary of the sequence of age changes and their major governing factors

Sequence of age changes	Major governing factors
Inability to maintain the specification of cellular form and function of early development.	Genetic developmental programme of resource partition.
	Early calorie intake.
Appearance of malformed and malfunctional cells in all organs and organisms.	Random biochemical errors and intrinsic chemical damage.
Slowed organ responses.	Specific environmental risks.
Loss of physiological ability.	
Apperance of degenerative diseases.	
Morbidity and mortality.	

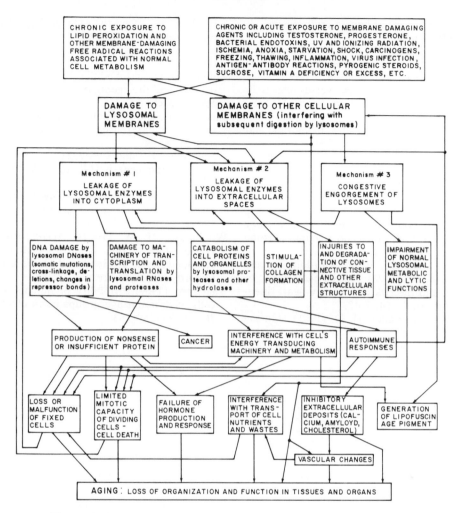

Figure 12   Postulated role of lysosomes in ageing. (From Hochschild, 1970)

search must be initiated with distressing human conditions firmly in mind and the relevant models selected accordingly, the biological basis of ageing will never be elucidated by maintaining a purely geriatric approach.

REFERENCES

Bellamy, D. (1967). 'Hormonal effects in relation to ageing in mammals', *Soc. Exp. Biol. Symp.*, **XXI**, 427–453.

Berry, R. J., and Jakobson, M. E. (1971). 'Life and death in an island population of the house mouse', *Exp. Gerontol.*, **6**, 187–197.

Bishop, M. W. H. (1970). 'Ageing and reproduction in the male', *J. Reprod. Fert.*, Suppl. 12, 65–87.

Block, E. (1952). 'Quantitative morphological investigations of the follicular system in women', *Acta. Anat.*, **14**, 108–123.

Burch, P. R. J., Murray, J. J., and Jackson, D. (1971). 'The age-prevalence of *Arcus senilis*, greying of hair and baldness: Etiological considerations', *J. Gerontol.*, **26**, 364–372

Calow, P. (1979). 'The cost of reproduction – A physiological approach', *Biol. Rev.*, **54**, 23–40.

Curtis, H. J. (1967). 'Radiation and ageing', *Soc. Exp. Biol. Symp.*, **XXI**, 51–63.

Hamilton, J. B. and Mestler, G. E. (1969). 'Mortality and survival: Comparison of eunuchs with intact men and women in a mentally retarded population', *J. Gerontol.*, **24**, 395–411.

Harris, E. J., and Kellermyer, R. W. (1961). *The Red Cell*, Academic Press.

Harris, E. J., and Maizels, M. (1952). 'Distribution

of ions in suspensions of human erythrocytes', *J. Physiol.*, **118**, 40–53.

Hasan, M., and Glees, P. (1973). 'Ultrastructural age changes in hippocampal neurons, synapses and neuroglia', *Exp. Gerontol.*, **8**, 75–83.

Helman, C. G. (1981). 'Disease versus illness in general practice', *J. R. Coll. Gen. Pract.*, **31**, 548–552.

Hochschild, R. (1971). 'Lysosomes, membrane and ageing', *Exp. Gerontol.*, **6**, 153–166.

Ingram, D. L., Mandl, A., and Zuckerman, S. (1958). 'The influence of age on litter-size', *J. Endocr.*, **17**, 280–285.

Kallmann, F. J. (1961). Genetic factors in ageing: Comparative and longitudinal observations on a senescent twin population', in *Psychopathology of Ageing* (Eds P. H. Hoch and J. Zubin', Grune and Stratton, New York.

Kannel, W. N., Castelli, W. P., Gordon, T., and McNamara, P. M. (1971). 'Serum cholesterol, lipoproteins, and the risk of coronary heart disease', *Ann. Int. Med.*, **74**, 1–12.

Loehr, G. W., and Waller, H. D. (1961). 'On the biochemistry of erythrocyte ageing', *Folia Haemat, Leipzig,* **78**, 385–402.

Prankerd, T. A. J. (1961). *The Red Cell*, Blackwell, Oxford.

Roberts, E. H. and Abdulla, F. H. (1967). 'Nuclear damage and the ageing of seeds', *Soc. Exp. Biol. Symp.*, **XXI**.

Sauer, H. I., and Donnell, H. D. (1970). 'Age and geographic differences in death rates', *J. Gerontol.*, **25**, 83–86.

Wangerman, E., and Lacey, H. J. (1955). 'Studies in the morphogenesis of leaves', *New Phytol.*, **54**, 182–198.

Woolhouse, H. W. (1967). 'The nature of senescence in plants', *Soc. Exp. Biol. Symp.*, **XXI**, 179–213.

Woolhouse, H. W. (1972). *Ageing Processes in Higher Plants*, pp. 179–213, Oxford Biology Reader (Eds J. J. Head and O. F. Lowestein), Oxford University Press.

Yaari, A. (1969). 'Mobility of human, red blood cells of different age groups in an electric field', *Blood*, **33**, 159–163.

3.4

Physiology of Ageing: Aspects of Neuroendocrine Regulation

P. S. Timiras

INTRODUCTION

Although the pathology of ageing has received considerable study in terms of combating specific high risk diseases associated with old age, the physiology of ageing, or the study of 'normal' function in the aged has not aroused great interest. This relative neglect is due to the difficulty, partly, of isolating 'normal' from 'abnormal' ageing processes and, partly, of circumscribing their temporal boundaries in physiological terms (Finch and Hayflick, 1977; Kanungo, 1980; Masoro, 1981, Timiras, 1972). The first difficulty is common to all stages of the lifespan; the second is peculiar to the ageing period. In contrast to other periods where the onset is clearly marked by specific physiological events (e.g. menarche as a marker of puberty), ageing has thus far defied all attempts to establish objective landmarks to characterize its onset. Indeed, the demarcation between maturity and old age (or senescence) is arbitrarily fixed by socioeconomic (e.g. age of retirement) rather than biologic factors. Thus, ageing may be defined temporarily as 'that period in the lifespan that begins at some indeterminate period following maturity and, after a progressive decline in functional competence and increase in disease susceptibility, terminates in death'.

In most textbooks of human and animal physiology, adulthood, characterized by great functional stability and competence, serves as the classic reference point for the discussion of both development at one extreme of the lifespan and ageing at the other. In view of the decrement in physiological competence that prevails in old age, physiologists have further defined ageing as 'the sum total of all changes that occur in the living organism and lead to functional impairment and death'. Yet, it must be recognized that functional competence is multifaceted and that optimal performance differs from age to age and from one parameter to another. It would be unsound, if not physiologically incorrect, to assume that a function is maximally efficient only during adulthood and that differences in the earlier and later years necessarily represent immaturity or deterioration, respectively. Rather, physiological competence must be viewed as having several levels of integration, depending on the requirements of the organism and the type and severity of the challenges to which the organism is exposed. With ageing, however, alterations at molecular, cellular, tissular and organismal levels do occur and contribute to the progressively decreasing capacity of the organism to maintain its viability.

It must be emphasized, however, that this decline is not uniform but shows considerable variability among inividuals and species, in both the rate and the magnitude of age-related changes in cells, tissues and organs. Furthermore, deteriorative changes in one such element or structure do not always signal the ageing of the whole organism. In certain functions, the regulation of the organism remains quite efficient well into old age (80 to 90 years in humans). For example, blood sugar levels and acid–base balance represent two functions which possess a number of alternate control mechanisms and their regulation remains relatively stable into old age. Other functions of the body begin to age relatively early in adult life and decline rapidly, as is the case of such sensory functions as vision and hearing which begin to diminish in late adolescence and early adulthood and continue to decline steadily thereafter, culminating at around 50 years of age. Other ageing processes begin very early in life, but because ageing is a continuous, slow process, we observe their effects only when these have progressed sufficiently to induce alterations that can be identified or validated by available testing methods or cause overt pathological manifestations. An example is atherosclerosis, a deteriorative, irreversible alteration of the arterial wall which leads to significant cardiovascular impairment. Although the atherosclerotic lesion often starts in infancy, its consequences (e.g. coronary occlusion, aneurysm, cerebral hemorrhage, gangrene) become manifest in middle and old age (see Chapter 13). Establishing a profile of physiological ageing, 'ageing charts' comparable to growth charts employed for evaluating development during childhood would be extremely valuable; however, the compilation of the necessary data is hampered by the type of variability described above as well as the lack of systematic studies in healthy, aged populations. In humans, most of our current information is not only sporadically acquired but is primarily generated from hospitalized individuals; in animals, maintenance of colonies of aged laboratory animals is quite costly and the study of aged animals in the wild extremely difficult.

In the absence of a complete profile of the ageing organism and cognizant of the temporal variability of ageing changes, physiologists usually have focused on the study of those age-related changes that involve integrative mechanisms. These mechanisms maintain homeostasis, i.e. insure the constancy of the internal environment despite the ever-changing external environment. With ageing, one of the principal expressions of the declining functional competence is the decreasing capacity of the organism to adapt to external demands, especially those involving stress conditions. Thus, ageing may be further defined as 'a de-

creasing ability to survive stress'. For example, the relative stability of blood sugar levels and acid–base balance in old age, mentioned above, is based upon measurements taken under 'basal' or 'resting' conditions; when the same tests are made under increased physiological demand (e.g. sustained muscular exercise, environmental changes), the efficiency of the organism to maintain levels within normal limits or the rapidity with which these levels return to normal demonstrate marked differences between young and old. Indeed, physiologically stressing a system brings to light age differences not otherwise detectable and also clearly demonstrates the declining ability of the ageing organism to withstand or adequately respond to stress. In view of the above considerations, the present chapter will describe in some detail the changes associated with old age in three major integrative systems – nervous, endocrine, and circulatory – but only briefly survey other body systems, particularly as they relate to the maintenance of homeostasis. An attempt will be made to correlate the regulatory role of neural and endocrine signals in the developing organisms with similar signals in the aged. The possibility has been raised by this and other physiologists that, at least in highly complex organisms, ageing may result from failure, that is, desynchronization, of various homeostatic adjustments rather than deterioration of a single organ or tissue. In this view, the various phases of the lifespan are regulated by a 'pacemaker' control system, perhaps situated in the brain, which triggers, by neural and endocrine signals, the passage from one stage of the lifespan to another. Thus, the life-cycle would involve a biological clock in which development and ageing represent a continuum of events along a rigorously regulated timetable between fertilization and death (Timiras, 1978; Timiras, Choy, and Hudson, 1981; Walker and Timiras, 1982).

AGEING OF THE CENTRAL NERVOUS SYSTEM: NEUROTRANSMITTER IMBALANCE

The central nervous system (CNS) undergoes morphological, chemical, and functional changes with ageing that are the subject of numerous investigations directed to identify – and eventually to prevent or to remedy – key changes both in normal (i.e. free of overt neurologic pathology) and pathological (i.e. senile dementia, Alzheimer's disease) states (see Chapter 16.1) (Timiras and Bignami, 1976; Barbagallo-Sangiorgi and Exton-Smith, 1980). In general, while studies in humans have focused on the functional decrements (e.g. memory loss, prolonged reaction time, decreased sensory inputs, sleep disturbances) that afflict a large proportion of the elderly (see Chapters 6 and 16), studies in animals reveal that, in the absence of pathology and under favourable environmental conditions, the CNS undergoes relatively little change and, indeed, retains some capacity for rehabilitation even at advanced ages (Connor, Diamond, and Johnson, 1980a, 1980b; Cotman and Scheff, 1979; Diamond, Johnson, and Gold, 1977).

For example, brain atrophy and neuronal loss were considered originally as inevitable morphological correlates of the aged brain, but current studies show that brain atrophy is restricted primarily to some specific diseases and, under physiological conditions, neuronal loss is essentially an early life event; when it occurs at later ages, it is limited regionally and associated with gliosis, perhaps of a compensatory nature (Bondareff, 1980; Brizzee *et al.*, 1969; Brizzee, Sherwood, and Timiras, 1968).

While the consequences of neuronal loss may not be as catastrophic as hitherto believed, it is undeniable that the CNS undergoes subtle but progressive changes with age which include, among others, intraneuronal and intraglial accumulation of lipofuscin (age pigments) – an indicator of intracellular metabolic

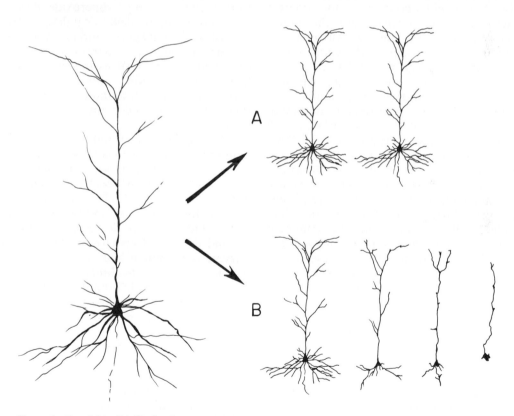

Figure 1   Dendritic distribution in two populations of ageing pyramidal neurons in the cerebral cortex. The fate of two populations of ageing pyramidal neurons: (A) basal dendrites of pyramidal neurons in the occiptal cortex of 3 month old rats living in an enriched environment are similar to the dendritic branching pattern seen in enriched 22 month old animals (Connor, Diamond, and Johnson, 1980a); (B) other populations, e.g. Betz cells incat and man, show progressive loss of the dendritic array, an indication of synaptic impairment 'Scheibel *et al.*, 1975) (Courtesy of Dr M. C. Diamond, University of California, Berkeley, and Dr A. B. Scheibel, Universty of California, Los Angeles)

impairment – and reduction in the number or denudation (i.e. loss of spines) of dendrites – an indicator of synaptic impairment (Scheibel *et al.*, 1975; Schiebel and Tomiyasu, 1978). The latter, necessarily associated with corresponding changes in neurotransmission represents functionally one of the most critical decrements associated with ageing and may be responsible for many of the neurological and psychiatric disturbances of the elderly. The enormous redundancy of the CNS often causes such disturbances to be ascribed to simple or even multifactorial functional imbalances rather than to an absolute loss of a single function, neurotransmitter, or group of cells. Considerable variation occurs in the type and levels of the neurotransmitter most affected (e.g. ageing-related reduction in midbrain noradrenaline (norepinephrine) levels; selective vulnerability of dopaminergic neurons to oxidative damage), in the CNS area where the effects are most marked (e.g. greatest dopamine reduction in substantia nigra with ageing in several animal species and in Parkinson's disease in humans), and in the neurological and mental consequences of neurotransmitter deficits (e.g. impaired cholinergic transmission in hippocampus and cerebral cortex associated with memory disturbances) (Timiras *et al.*, 1983; Timiras, Hudson, and Miller, 1982; Vernadakis and Timiras, 1982; Whitehouse *et al.*, 1982). Thus, in a classical example of neurotransmitter imbalance such as Parkinson's disease – a disease often found in older individuals – the neurotransmitter dopamine is progressively lost allowing the neurotransmitter acetylcholine to dominate. These neurotransmitter changes are associated with specific cell loss (i.e. midbrain catecholaminergic neurons) showing that a focal or selective cellular or chemical loss may result in or contribute to a functional imbalance and attendant clinical deficits (Finch, 1978; McGreer, Yu, and Suzuki, 1977; Wree *et al.*, 1980).

With ageing, one may hypothesize that selective vulnerability or resistance of relatively small populations of neurones possessing critical regulatory functions delineates a pattern of neural and endocrine signals which dictate the functional characteristics of the senescent phenotype. In this sense, major neurotransmitter losses need not be postulated with ageing (and, in fact, do not occur under physiological conditions); rather, selective alterations might be sufficient to desynchronize neurotransmitter balance and thereby disorganize the corresponding neural and endocrine signals which regulate homeostasis and adaptation.

Some current evidence, although still circumstantial, is indicative of a decrease in the number and function of catecholaminergic neurones with age. For example, in contrast to other brainstem nuclei in which total cell counts show no significant loss, a selective reduction of pigmented neurones in the midbrain catecholaminergic nuclei has been reported in aged humans. Such loss may be ascribed to damage inflicted by free radicals (e.g. superoxide anions, hydrogen peroxide, derived hydroxyl radical) in the neurone, also illustrated indirectly by the intracellular presence of protective enzymes (e.g. superoxide dismutase, glutathione peroxidase, catalase) deputed against such damage. Another hypothesis to explain the relative vulnerability of dopaminergic neurones underlines the susceptibility of these cells to hypoxia although no definitive correlation has been found between decreased dopamine levels and cerebral atherosclerotic involvement.

The selective vulnerability of the catecholaminergic systems contrasts with the apparent selective resistance of serotonergic neurones (Calas and Van Den Bosch de Aguilar, 1980; Timiras *et al.*, 1983; Timiras and Hudson, 1980; Timiras, Hudson, and Miller, 1982). Despite some reports of decreased serotonin levels and decreased activity of the synthesizing enzyme (tryptophan hydroxylase) with ageing in one strain of rats (Meek *et al.*, 1977) our own studies in female Long-Evans rats indicate that serotonergic systems do not change significantly with ageing (fig. 2). In addition to the well-known developmental change occurring between birth and weaning (22 days of age in the rat), adult serotonin values are attained by 40 days of age (age of sexual maturation) and remain essentially constant into old age (24 months and beyond) in all brain areas studied; this neurochemical constancy is in agreement with structural studies. Inasmuch as catecholaminergic levels decrease in several of the same areas with ageing, the ratio of serotonin to noradrenaline (norepinephrine) and to dopamine progressively increases. For ex-

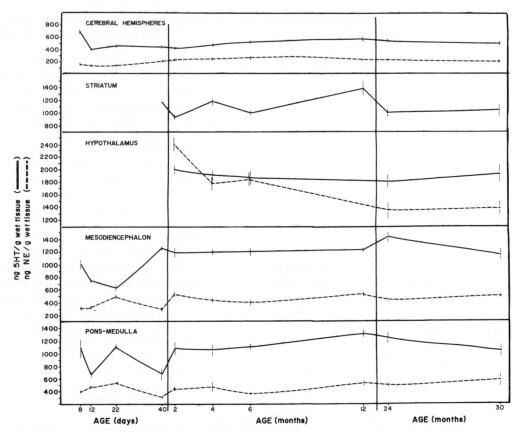

Figure 2 Monoamine levels in specific brain regions of female Long-Evans rats throughout development and ageing. At 8, 12, and 22 days of age, the cerebral hemispheres included the striatum and the mesodiencephalon included the hypothalamus. Note that while both serotonin and norephinephrine undergo early developmental changes, levels remain relatively constant into old age (maximum age, 36 to 40 months), a period of high morbidity and mortality. In the hypothalamus (site of neuroendocrine regulatory mechanisms), the ratio between serotonin and norephinephrine increases with age due to a decline in noradrenaline (norephinephrine) levels. In the striatum, serotonin levels decrease between 12 and 24 months of age and thereafter seem to remain constant. Dopamine levels (not shown here) also decrease progressively with age; as their decline is greater than that of serotonin, the serotonin-to-dopamine ratio increases. (From Timiras *et al.*, 1983; Timiras and Hudson, 1980; Timiras, Hudson, and Miller, 1982)

ample, in the hypothalamus, the ratio of serotonin to noradrenaline (norepinephrine) rises from 0.8 at 2 months to 1.4 at 24 months; in the corpus striatum, the ratio of serotonin to dopamine rises from 0.09 at 2 months to 0.12 at 24 months. Concomitant with the relative stability of steady-state levels, the metabolic enzymes of serotonin do not appear to decline with age. Indeed, a previous report presents evidence for increased serotonin metabolism in the hypothalamus of ageing male rats (Simpkins *et al.*, 1977). Cathecholaminergic and serotonergic signals are known to control or modulate endocrine function through the stimulation or inhibition of hypothalamic neurosecretory products and these, in turn, play a key role in the synthesis and release of pituitary hormones. Hence, an imbalance between these neurotransmitter systems (and eventually other, as yet poorly defined, systems) may trigger those endocrine changes responsible for the passage from one life stage to the other (e.g. puberty/menopause; growth/cessation of growth; adulthood/senescence) (Muller, Nistico, and Scapagnini, 1977; Scapagnini *et al.*, 1980).

In addition to alterations in steady-state concentration and metabolism of neurotransmitters, other changes with ageing may involve neurotransmitter receptors and the interaction between a neurotransmitter and its recognition sites (Makman *et al.*, 1980). Neurotransmitter receptor functions have been examined at various ages by several investigators and in most studies the number of receptors was found to decrease with age, an observation in agreement with the decreased number of dendrites. Whether the reduction in the number of receptors is also associated with a reduced receptor affinity remains to be conclusively demonstrated, the available data being too few and often contradictory to permit a valid conclusion. Nevertheless, the picture that emerges from these studies is one of reduced responsiveness with ageing. For example, serotonin levels and metabolism undergo a characteristic circadian rhythm that has been implicated in the regulation of several cyclic functions such as sleep, locomotor activity, agressive behaviour, sex behaviour, temperature regulation, and regulation of hypophysiotropic hormones. Similarly, catecholamines undergo circadian rhythms in several brain areas, including the hypothalamus and the pineal gland, under normal conditions, and these rhythms may be altered by modifying the light/dark cycle, the diet, or by administration of neurotropic drugs. In human beings (as well as other animals and plants) certain time variations (e.g. daily, weekly, monthly, yearly) are maintained in the absence of any known environmental periodicity. For example, circadian rhythms persist during flight in extraterrestrial space (for the few weeks experienced thus far). It is suggested that the persistence of such rhythms may be due to the presence of an endogenous 'synchronizer' acting through neural and endocrine signals (Halberg, 1982). However, due to disease or environmental changes, some rhythms among the spectrum of biological frequencies best attuned to optimal health may shift; when these shifts do occur, they may lead to deficits in physiologic performance and longevity. Thus, the circadian rhythm of urinary catecholamine in men and women varies with age from 20 to 99 years; in both sexes, circadian amplitude (absolute and averaged) decreases, with most of the decrease occurring after 65 years, but without apparent change in the acrophase (i.e. highest values within a single period). As shown in the next section, hor-

monal rhythms also show some shifts with ageing (Tables 1 and 2). For example, it has been suggested that a peak in the circadian serotonin cycle triggers the surge of luteinizing hormone (LH) preceding ovulation; given the proper hormonal (oestrogen) environment, the actual levels of serotonin are less important for inducing the LH surge than a properly timed peak in the neurotransmitter (Walker, Cooper, and Timiras, 1980). Thus, depression of the peak by the neonatal administration of serotonin inhibitors (e.g. parachlorophenylalanine or testosterone) or displacement of the peak (e.g. by altering the light/dark cycles) will block the LH surge and will alter the timetable of reproduction by accelerating both the onset of sexual maturation and that of sexual senescence (Walker and Timiras, 1980). Similarly, delaying the brain maturation and, presumably, the maturation of serotonergic systems by neonatal hypothyroidism alters the timetable of reproductive function (Walker and Timiras, 1981). While we await the collection of more information, current evidence supports the proposition that CNS ageing is associated with a progressive imbalance in neurotransmission resulting from differential changes in levels, metabolism and/or receptors of neurotransmitters, and/or a desynchronization of their rhythmicity.

AGEING OF THE ENDOCRINE SYSTEM: CHANGES IN HORMONAL SUPPLY, DEMAND, AND BINDING

The study of the changes in endocrine function which occur with old age is confronted by considerable difficulties related to the multitude of existing variables, some of which are peculiar to the endocrines and some of which are shared, to a greater or lesser extent, by all other body systems. Among the first, the most important are the nature of the endocrine function, itself exquisitely responsive to a large variety of environmental (internal and external) stimuli, and the accumulated effects on the endocrines of the stress and diseases to which the individual is exposed throughout the lifespan. For endocrines, as for other tissues, competence at any given age depends on past and present biological and psychological events; the older the individual, the greater the cumulative influence of prior experience. Another factor of practical importance

Table 1   Ageing-related changes in structures and function in pituitary-adrenocortical and pituitary-thyroid axes. Parameters studied and changes recorded

Pituitary-adrenocortical axis	Pituitary-thyroid axis
Adrenal structure	*Histology*
Weight (relative to body weight) unchanged; weight (absolute) increased (Calloway, Foley, and Lagerbloom, 1965) Cortical thickness unchanged (Khelimskii, 1964) Nodular hyperplasia, increased (Dobbie, 1969) Lipofuscin accumulation, connective tissue proliferation, necrosis, lipid loss, capillary dilation (Bourne, 1967)	Flattened follicular epithelium decreased mitosis, increased connective tissue, distended follicles (Cooper, 1925; Dogliotti and Nuzzi, 1935; Mustacchi and Lowenhaupt, 1950; Stoffer *et al.*, 1961) Increased micronodules (Dogliotti and Nuzzi, 1935; Irvine and Hodkinson, 1978) Unchanged follicles in some individuals (Korenchevsky, 1961; Mustacchi and Lowenhaupt, 1950)
Plasma ACTH, basal	Unchanged thyrotrope (Ryan, Kovacs, and Ezrin, 1979)
Unchanged (Blichert-Toft, 1971, 1975)	*Thyroid radioactive iodine uptake*
Pituitary ACTH	Essentially unchanged (Gaffney, Gregerman, and Shock, 1962; Oddie *et al.*, 1968) Decreased (Quimby, Werner, and Schmidt, 1950; Perlmutter and Riggs, 1949)
Unchanged (Jensen and Blichert-Toft, 1971)	
Circadian ACTH periodicity	
Unchanged (Jensen and Blichert-Toft, 1971)	*Protein bound iodine (PBI)*
ACTH response to stress	Unchanged (Braverman, 1966; Ohara *et al.*, 1974; Taylor, Thompson, and Caird, 1974; Wenzel *et al.*, 1974) Decreased (Azizi *et al.*, 1975, Hesch *et al.*, 1976)
Insulin induced Unchanged (Cartlidge *et al.*, 1970; Friedman, Green, and Sharland, 1969) Decreased (Hochstaedt, Schneebaum, and Shadel, 1961) Ether stress, unchanged or decreased (Tang and Phillips, 1978)	*Serum T$_4$*
	Unchanged free T$_4$ (Braverman, Dawber, and Ingbar, 1966; Hansen, Skousted, and Siersback-Lielsen, 1975; Hesch *et al.*, 1976; Ohara *et al.*, 1974; Wenzel *et al.*, 1974)
Steroid-induced suppression of ACTH (measured by corticosteroid response)	Reduced T$_4$ (Bermudez, Sunks, and Oppenheimer, 1975; Herman *et al.*, 1974) Elevated T$_4$ (Burrows *et al.*, 1975)
Decreased (Dilman, Ostroumova, and Tsyslina, 1979) Unchanged (Friedman, Green, and Sharland, 1969; Gittler and Friedfield, 1962)	*Serum T$_3$*
Adrenal response to exogenous ACTH	Unchanged (Braverman, Dawber, and Ingbar, 1966; Olsen, Laurberg, and Weeke, 1978) Reduced T$_3$ (Bermudez, Surks, and Oppenheimer, 1975; Hansen, Skovsted, and Siersback-hielsen, 1975; Herman *et al.*, 1974; Hesch *et al.*, 1976, Rubenstein, Butler, and Werner, 1973) Reduced only in illness (Burrows *et al.*, 1975; Olsen, Laurberg, and Weeke, 1978)
Adrenal androgen excretion (dehydroepiandrosterone) decreased (Antonioni *et al.*, 1968) Cortisol, unchanged (Friedman, Green, and Sharland, 1969; Hochstaedt, Schneebaum, and Shadel, 1961; West *et al.*, 1961) 17-OH-corticosteroids, unchanged (Gitter and Friedfield, 1962)	
Glucocorticoids levels	*T$_4$ secretory rate*
Plasma corticoids, basal unchanged (Blichert-Toft, 1975; Cartlidge *et al.*, 1970; Friedman, Green, and Sharland, 1969; Gherondache, Romanoff, and Pincus, 1967; West *et al.*)	Declined (Gregerman and Solomon, 1967) Can be greatly increased in acute phase of illness in elderly (Gregerman and Solomon, 1967)
Circadian corticosteroid periodicity	*T$_4$ I^{131} deiodination*
Peak, unchanged (Blichert-Toft, 1975; Grad *et al.*, 1971) Peak, delayed (Serio *et al.*, 1970) Higher midnight level (Friedman, Green, and Sharland, 1969)	Greatly decreased *(in vivo)* (Gregerman, Gaffney, and Shock, 1962; Inada *et al.*, 1964; Oddie, 1966; Stern-Nielsen and Friis, 1973) Can be decreased in illness (Gregerman and Solomon, 1967)

Table 1 *Continued*

Pituitary-adrenocortical axis	Pituitary-thyroid axis
Volume of cortisol distribution space Unchanged (West *et al.*, 1961) Decreased (Samuels, 1956) *Cortisol half-life (T 1/2)* Increased (Samuels, 1956, Serio *et al.*, 1969; Tyler *et al.*, 1955; West *et al.*, 1961) *Cortisol secretion rate* Decreased (Romanoff *et al.*, 1961) *17-OH corticosteroid secretion rate* Decreased (Gittler and Friedfield, 1962; Grad *et al.*, 1967; Moncola, Gorney, and Prettel, 1963; Romanoff *et al.*, 1961; West *et al.*, 1961) Unchanged when measured per creatine excreted (Romanoff *et al.*, 1961) *Adrenal androgens* Androsterone, etiocholanolone, dehydroepiandrosterone (DHEA), urinary excretion, decreased (Gherondache, Romanoff, and Pincus, 1967) Decreased plasma DHEA (Migeon *et al.*, 1957; Yamaji and Ibayashi, 1969) *Aldosterone* Decreased (with ageing) (Flood *et al.*, 1967) Renin decreased (Horky *et al.*, 1975; North *et al.*, 1977; Weidmann *et al.*, 1975) *Glucocorticoid receptors (number)* Liver, decreased (Singer, Ito, and Litwack, 1973)	*T_4 I^{131} distribution space* Depends only on weight, not on age (Oddie, Meade, and Fisher, 1966) *Binding of serum T^4 to thyroid binding globulin* Essentially unchanged (Braverman, Dawber, and Inglar, 1966) *T_3 I^{131} metabolic clearance rate (MCR)* Unchanged MCR (Wenzel and Horn, 1975) *Serum TSH, basal* Unchanged (Mayberry *et al.*, 1971) Slightly increased (Cuttelod *et al.*, 1974; Lemarchand-Beraud, and Vanotti, 1969; Ohara *et al.*, 1974) Slightly reduced, (Olsen, Laurberg, and Weeke, 1978) *TSH periodicity* Unchanged (Blichert-Toft, Hummer, and Dige-Petersen, 1975) *TSH response to TRH* Unchanged in females, decreased in males (Azizi *et al.*, 1975; Blichert-Toft, Hummer, and Dige-Petersen, 1975; Snyder and Utiger, 1972) Increased (Ohara *et al.*, 1974) Decreased in women, unchanged in men (Wenzel *et al.*, 1974) *Thyroid hormones output in response to exogenous TSH* Unchanged (Baker *et al.*, 1959; Einhorn, 1958) Reduced (Lederer and Bataille, 1969) *T_4 to T_3 peripheral conversion* Reduced *in vivo* (Wenzel and Horn, 1975) *T_4 I^{131} tissue binding* Unchanged (Holm *et al.*, 1975)

Table 2 Ageing-related changes in structure and function for growth hormone-prolactin and insulin-glucagon. Parameters studied and changes recorded

Growth hormone and prolactin	Insulin and Glucagon
Pituitary, GH Somatotropes, unchanged (Calderon, Ryan, and Kovacs, 1978; Pasteels *et al.*, 1972) GH content, unchanged (Gershberg, 1957)	*Islet histology* Decreased beta/alpha cell ratio (Seifert, 1954) Increased amyloid deposition (Schwartz, Kurucz, and Kuracz, 1965)

Table 2   *Continued*

Growth hormone and prolactin	Insulin and Glucagon

Plasma GH levels

Unchanged (Cartlidge *et al.*, 1970; Dudl *et al.*, 1973; Lazarus and Young, 1966)
Decreased (Danowski *et al.*, 1969; Dilman, 1976; Vidalon *et al.*, 1973)

GH response to stimuli

Insulin-induced hypoglycaemia, unchanged
(Kalk *et al.*, 1973; Sacher, Finkelstein, and Hillman, 1971)
Arginine unchanged (Blichert-Toft, 1975; Dudl *et al.*, 1973; Root and Oski, 1969)
Suppression by glucose load, unchanged (Benjamine *et al.*, 1970; Root and Oski, 1969)
Reduced (Sandberg *et al.*, 1973; Dilman, 1976)
Protein 'Bovril' ingestion reduced (Buckler, 1969)
Anesthesia reduced (Blichert-Toft, 1975)
Exercise reduced (Bazzare *et al.*, 1976)
L-dopa reduced (Bazzare *et al.*, 1976)

Daily GH secretion and sleep-related GH release

Reduced (Bazzare *et al.*, 1976; Carlson *et al.*, 1972; Finkelstein *et al.*, 1972; Thompson *et al.*, 1972)

Tissue response

Unchanged nitrogen retention (Root and Oski, 1969)
Increased free fatty acids, decreased Na$^+$ ('metabolic response') (Rudman *et al.*, 1971)
Reduced hydroxyprolinuria (Root and Oski, 1969)
Reduced inhibition of glucose consumption by red cells *in vitro* (Root and Oski, 1969)
Reduced binding to thymocytes (Talwar, Harjan, and Kidway, 1976)

Metabolic clearance rate

Unchanged (Taylor, Finster, and Mintz, 1969)

Pituitary, prolactin

Mammotropies involuted (Baker and Yu, 1977)
Unchanged
(Kovacs *et al.*, 177; Pasteels *et al.*, 1972)
Increased incidence of prolactin Secreting microadenomas
(Kovacs, Bohns, and Versteeg, 1979)
Prolactin content unchanged
(Yamaji *et al.*, 1976).

Circulating prolactin levels

Males, increased (Vekemans and Robyn, 1975)
Unchanged (Frantz *et al.*, 1972; Yamaji *et al.*, 1976, Frantz *et al.*, 1972)
females, decreased (Vekemans and Robyn, 1975, Vermeulen, 1978)

Prolactin Response to TRH

delayed, prolonged elevation of serum prolactin (Yamaji *et al.*, 1976)

No significant degeneration (Andrew, 1944, Feldman, 1955)
no significant difference in insulin content (Jorpes and Rastgeldi, 1953; Wrenchall, Bogoch, and Ritchie, 1952)

Glucose tolerance

Decreased (Andres, 1971; Davidson, 1979)
Unchanged in non-obese men (Kimmerling *et al.*, 1977)

Fasting serum insulin

Unchanged (Dudl and Ensinck, 1972, 1977)

Insulin response to glucose (in vivo)

Increased after oral glucose (Andres and Tobin, 1977, Davidson, 1979)
Unchanged after oral glucose (Davidson, 1979)
Unchanged after intravenous glucose (Davidson, 1979)
Decreased acute response, delayed peak (Andres and Tobin, 1977; Davidson, 1979)
Reduced (intravenous glucose clamp) (Andres and Tobin, 1977)

Insulin half-life (T 1/2) and metabolic clearance rate (MCR)

Unchanged MCR (Andres and Tobin, 1977; Barbagallo–Sangiori *et al.*, 1970; DeFronzo, 1979; McGuire *et al.*, 1979)
Increased T 1/2 (Orskov and Christensen, 1969)

Plasma pro-insulin after oral glucose

Increased (Duckworth and Kitabchi, 1972, 1976)

Basal (fasting) serum glucagon

Unchanged (Dudl and Ensinck, 1972, 1977)

Glucagon levels after glucose or arginine

Unchanged arginine response (Dudl and Ensinck, 1972; Fedele *et al.*, 1977)
Unchanged glucose response (Dudl and Ensinck, 1977; Nonaka and Tarui, 1977)

Insulin effects on glucose metabolism (in vitro)

Decreased (with maturation) adipocyte response (Gries and Steinke, 1967) contributing to the difficulty of interpreting the functional significance of age-related changes in endocrines is concerned with the methods of measurement, e.g. the type of diagnostic test (secretory activity, hormone levels in blood and urine, free versus conjugated hormones, hormone synthesis and metabolism, intracellular hormone transport, and binding) and the time of testing (time of the day, nutritional state, sleep/wakefulness states). It should be emphasized that useful clinical tests may fail completely to reveal significant age-related physiological and biochemical events. An unaltered hormone level in blood is no indication that the corresponding endocrine function is unaffected by ageing but rather that a number of processes, each influenced by age, have established a new equilibrium. Conversely, standards of normality in clinical tests must take into account the effects of ageing that occur throughout the population. For example, the presence of high blood glucose in a large proportion of the elderly (see below) has resulted in the probable overestimation of the incidence of diabetes – rather than a better understanding of age-related changes in glucose tolerance – and the initiation of unnecessary therapeutic measures. As with neurotransmitters, hormones are secreted in an episodic or cyclical pattern which may show age-related changes in terms of amplitude and frequency. These cycles may be affected differentially by feedback control mechanisms (often situated in the hypothalamus), the responsiveness of which may change with increasing age. Another important aspect of age-related decrements in hormone effectiveness focuses on a changing sensitivity and/or responsiveness of target tissues to the hormones. Such age-related changes may be manifested by a decrease or compensatory increase in the number and affinity of receptors, changes in membrane composition and in membrane-associated transport systems, intracellular binding proteins and other sites, and reactions expressing hormonal effects.

A number of recent reviews are available which cover the ageing of the endocrine glands in detail (Cole, Segall, and Timiras, 1982; Everitt and Burgess, 1976; Greenblatt, 1978; Gregerman and Bierman, 1981). In this chapter, only a short summary of major findings is presented and summarized in Tables 1 and 2. The

ageing of the gonads is discussed further in Chapters 3.5, 21, and 26.1 and therefore will not be reviewed here.

Pituitary–Adrenocortical Axis

Morphological changes are mostly involutional in nature (note the exception, however, of massive hypertrophy and hyperactivity of the adrenal cortex in some species such as the Pacific salmon) and include accumulation of lipofucsin and formation of nodules. In man the plasma levels of the most important glucocorticoid, cortisol, remain unaltered while its circadian rhythm is altered slightly. Secretory rates decrease about 30 per cent. over the entire lifespan although the circulatory levels remain unchanged because of the associated prolongation of corticoid half-life which is suggestive of a reduced peripheral demand and/or a slowing of the metabolic disposition of the steroid.

A decline in the responsiveness of target cells to glucocorticoids is suggested by the reduction in cortisol and corticosterone receptors in several tissues (Roth, 1979a, 1979b). Likewise, the ability of glucocorticoids to induce specific cellular metabolic actions may be impaired with ageing, e.g. the ability of these hormones to inhibit substrate activity in the rat. Glucose oxidation in rat splenic leucocytes and adipocytes declines with age in proportion to the reduction in splenic and adipocyte glucocorticoid receptors (Roth, 1975). In contrast, enzyme induction by glucocorticoids in the liver may be somewhat slowed (Rahman and Peraino, 1973) but ultimately not diminished (Adelman and Freeman, 1972).

Aldosterone, the most important mineralocorticoid, shows reduced secretory rate and plasma levels, apparently secondary to defective renin secretion resulting from a defect of juxtaglomerular beta-adrenergic receptor adenylate cyclase. Adrenal androgen (primarily dehydroepindrosterone) secretions are progressively reduced with ageing and this depression results in decreased plasma levels; the significance of this decrease is not known. In terms of quantity, the adrenal androgens equal or even exceed that of the other adrenal steroids combined; yet the interpretation of the age-related decrease in these androgens awaits a better understanding of their function.

The effect of ageing on the response of the human adrenal to the pituitary adrenocorticotropic hormone (ACTH) is controversial. Under steady-state conditions, pituitary and plasma ACTH levels remain essentially the same into old age. The ACTH response to stress – typically characterized by an increased ACTH secretion from the pituitary and corresponding stimulation of glucocorticoids from the adrenal cortex – also seems to remain unaltered with respect to glucocorticoids although it may be depressed with respect to androgens.

Adrenal Medulla

Under basal adrenal medullary functions, urinary excretion of catecholamines remains unchanged with ageing (Kärki, 1956), or shows a reduction in absolute and averaged circadian amplitude after 65 years of age (Halberg, 1982), or increases (Giorgino *et al.,* 1969), the increase being greater after standing and isometric exercise (Ziegler, Lake, and Kopin, 1976). Urinary elevation, further supported by studies of increased adrenal medullary catecholamines in rats (Kvetnansky *et al.,* 1978), has been interpreted as a compensatory reaction to the apparently increasing refractoriness of target tissues to catecholamines. For example, the ability of dopamine to stimulate adenylate cyclase in the corpus striatum decreases progressively with age (Puri and Volicer, 1977), together with a lowered dopamine binding demonstrated in rats (Roth, 1979a, 1979b), mice (Finch, 1979), and rabbits (Makman *et al.,* 1980). Responsiveness to adenylate cyclase, on the other hand, remains unchanged in adipocytes (Cooper and Gregerman, 1976) or is even increased in hepatocytes (Kalish *et al.,* 1977). This lack of uniformity in pattern may be ascribed to the differential responsiveness of tissues to catecholamines. It may also be influenced by other hormones (e.g. glucocorticoids, thyroid hormones) known to affect catecholamine metabolism and receptors, while these hormones themselves may be undergoing age-related changes. Alterations of membrane structure and function are considered by many to be of critical importance during ageing. Little direct information on age-related changes in membrane function is available except some studies of altered lipid composition of plasma membrane in liver. The changes described in relation to adenylate cyclase activity and its response to various hormones, many of which act on the membrane and/or membrane-associated molecules, point indirectly to an instability of the membrane and altered activity of the membrane-associated enzymes (not only adenylate cyclase but also ATPases are susceptible to hormonal, particularly thyroid, activity) (Valcana and Timiras, 1969).

Pancreas

The endocrine function of the pancreas mediated through the secretion of insulin, glucagon and somatostatin is primarily concerned with glucose metabolism. Most studies, therefore, have utilized various tests of glucose metabolism as indices of age-related pancreatic changes. With ageing, such tests show moderate but progressive alterations. For example, more than 50 per cent. of randomly selected subjects over 60 years of age have significantly impaired glucose tolerance tests when compared with younger controls, blood glucose levels taking longer to return to normal after oral or parenteral glucose administration. These findings have led to considerable controversy as a result of the apparent necessity of labelling, based on this criterion, more than half of the old population as diabetics (Andres, 1971; Andres and Tobin, 1977; Davidson, 1979). This clinical dilemma may be resolved by introducing age-corrected normograms for the glucose-tolerance tests (Andres and Tobin, 1977) or by substituting elevated fasting glucose, rather than decreased glucose tolerance, as the principal criterion for diagnosis. The progressive lowering of glucose tolerance with ageing cannot be denied and a number of factors have been invoked to explain its aetiology: increased insulin resistance perhaps associated with obesity; decreased tissue binding and sensitivity to insulin and glucagon; elevated free fatty acids and glucagon release; increased levels of proinsulin.

While historically the majority of authors have been concerned with the age-associated increased incidence of diabetes, in recent years, the focus is whether ageing may be accelerated in diabetes. Patients with diabetes mellitus display an increased incidence and early onset of several signs commonly associated with ageing: cataracts, microangiopathy, neuropathies, dystrophic skin changes, reduced proliferative capacity of fibroblasts, accelerated rate of collagen ageing, increased incidence of autoimmunity, and accelerated atherosclerosis.

Hormones originating in the gastrointestinal tract participate in glucose homeostasis. One of these hormones, somatostatin, a polypeptide secreted by the pancreas and other tissues (including the hypothalamus), does not seem to be altered by ageing (Raizes *et al.*, 1976). Further studies, however, are necessary to understand the involvement of this and other gastrointestinal hormones in ageing.

Parathyroid

The hormones secreted by this gland do not appear to be consistently altered with ageing. A study of immunoassyable parathyroid hormone shows a decline after 60 years of age in white men but not white women and variable effects depending on the race (Roof *et al.*, 1976), while in other studies the hormone levels increase with ageing (Wiske *et al.*, 1979). In the latter experiments, some of the biologically inactive fragments of the hormone molecule may be responsible for the high immunoassyable levels (Berlyne *et al.*, 1975) but the biological significance of these changes with respect to hormone action remains to be clarified. Similarly, little is known of the changes with ageing in thyrocalcitonin and their impact on the ageing of the organism. A decrease in radioimmunoassayable thyrocalcitonin has been reported in humans, more in men than in women (Deftos *et al.*, 1979). Since thyrocalcitonin decreases bone resorption, its potential usefulness in the therapy of age-related demineralization and osteoporosis has been explored, but without beneficial results (Jowsey *et al.*, 1971).

Pituitary

Of the hormones of the anterior pituitary some are discussed in other chapters (see Chapters 21 to 23) together with the respective target endocrine. This section will consider growth hormone, prolactin, and the hormones of the posterior pituitary.

Pituitary and plasma growth hormone (GH) levels undergo little change with ageing in humans and a number of animal species under resting and stressful conditions. However, the characteristic peak in GH secretion observed during sleep in young and adult subjects is reduced or is absent in the elderly. GH responses to some specific stimuli (e.g. hypoglycaemia, glucose load, arginine administration) do not show clear-cut differences between young and old individuals. As in the case of insulin, obesity (increasing with age) may represent a complicating factor in GH regulation and lead to reduced response of GH to hypoglycaemia. Changes in prolactin levels with ageing are sex and species dependent and probably secondary to changes in circulating estrogens (which decrease in females at monopause) and hypothalamic dopamine (which also decreases with ageing as described in the preceding section).

Regulation of the neurohypophyseal hormones, oxytocin and vasopressin, secreted in the hypothalamus and stored in the posterior pituitary, is impaired with ageing although the mechanism of such impairment remains to be elucidated. Supraoptic and paraventricular nuclei from which the hormones are secreted show striking age-specific cytologic changes (particularly the oxytocin-producing cells) without evidence of cell destruction. Increased sensitivity of vasopressin secretion to inhibitory (e.g. alcohol) and excitatory (e.g. increased plasma osmolality) stimuli has been reported in older subjects. As illustrated by the heightened vasopressin response, this hypersensitivity may serve to compensate for the reduced renal ability to conserve salt and water in the ageing human (Helderman *et al.*, 1978). Some attempts to prevent or slow the physiological decline associated with age-related changes in neurohypophyseal hormones include administration of these hormones, especially oxytocin, to improve health and reduce mortality, and administration of vasopressin to improve memory (Legros *et al.*, 1978; Oliveros *et al.*, 1978). The import of such treatments remains controversial.

Pituitary–Thyroid Axis

The hormones of the thyroid gland, thyroxine (T4) and triidothyronine (T3), have traditionally sparked the interest and imagination of investigators seeking hormonal determinants of senescence. Individuals affected by hypothyroidism develop certain signs of 'precocious senility' including a reduced metabolic rate, hyperlipidemia, and accelerated atherosclerosis, early ageing of skin and hair, slow reflexes, and mental deterioration. Since these patients improve markedly after hormonal replacement therapy, it has been argued that similar symptoms in normally ageing individuals may represent effects secondary to thyroidal involution with age. In view of the well-known action of thyroid hormones in controlling development, it seemed logical to suspect that these hormones might also control the rate or site of ageing. As early as the turn of this century, experimenters optimistically attempted rejuvenation or prolongation of life through hormone administration. While administration of thyroid hormones to some animals (rats) seemed to shorten rather than prolong life, others (fowl) showed an apparent dramatic rejuvenation. However, the ageing process in euthyroid elderly humans was never significantly slowed or altered by the repeated administration of these hormones.

Whether and to what extent the dysthroidal state is associated with ageing remains unanswered. Morphological changes in the thyroid gland of an involutional nature (e.g. fibrosis, cellular infiltration, follicular alterations) do occur in some elderly individuals, often accompanied by a moderate decrease in T4 secretion and in T4 and T3 levels. Intervening illnesses and stress, however, appear to be responsible in great part for this reduction in plasma levels. A potent inhibitor of thyroid hormone binding to serum proteins has been described in extrathyroidal tissues of man (and rat) and its presence has been associated with reduced serum T4 (and T3) in some patients critically ill with non-thyroidal illnesses (Chopra *et al.*, 1982). Although age-related changes of this inhibitor protein remain to be established, it is possible to relate this finding to the hypothesis that in older animals (rats) an inhibitory factor (perhaps a pituitary hormone) is secreted which prevents the binding of thyroid hormones to their receptors and thereby induces a *de facto* condition of hypothyroidism even though hormone levels remain unaffected (Denckla, 1974).

The maintenance of normal serum T4 levels in older humans, despite reduced secretory activity, has been interpreted as reflecting a sharp reduction in peripheral deiodination. Most circulating T4 is deiodinated to either T3 or reverse T3, primarily in the liver and kidney, while a small fraction is directly conjugated to glucoronides and sulphates for disposal through the bile. The progressive reduction in T4 degradation with ageing may, therefore, reflect primarily decreased peripheral monodeiodination. Indeed, T4 and T3 conversion in vitro (Köhrle *et al.*, 1979; Ooka, 1979) and in vivo (Wenzel and Horn, 1975) declines with ageing, although the latter study in the human may not be completely conclusive (Ingbar, 1978).

Conversion of T4 to T3 (i.e. a lesser to a more active catabolic hormone) is generally reduced in conditions where catabolism predominates (e.g. fasting, non-specific illnesses, dexamethasone therapy). This suggests that there is a homeostatic "wisdom" in the arrangement whereby conversion of T4 to T3 is inhibited when catabolism is already overactive (Chopra *et al.*, 1978). From this perspective, the age-related decline in thyroid hormone metabolism would reflect not so much a reduced demand for tissue utilization as an increased demand for 'protection'.

With ageing, a number of experimental animals (rats, mice, rabbits) have lowered T4 levels, associated with higher TSH levels, and progressive increase in TSH polymorphic forms (e.g. high molecular weight, 'big' TSH) (Choy, Klemme, and Timiras, 1982). In rats, not only are TSH levels increased with ageing but the typical circadian cyclicity of the hormone is abolished. The functional significance of TSH rhythmicity is still obscure; however, the loss of specific signals with ageing may be important in view of recent reports of 'down regulation' of TSH receptors. In humans, the majority of studies describe unchanged or slightly increased TSH levels without marked changes in circadian periodicity. For TSH as well as for the thyrotropin-releasing hormone (TRH), current results are in conflict, particularly in relation to sex differences, a decrease in TRH having been reported exclusively in either males or females, depending on the author. Other studies show increased TSH responsiveness to TRH in apparently normal elderly subjects in whom T4 levels are un-changed and basal TSH levels slightly in-creased (Ohara *et al,* 1974).

This brief summary of endocrine ageing dis-closes that one of the striking characteristics of the endocrinology of the elderly is the discrep-ancy between the presence of structural alter-ations and multiple signs and symptoms of hormonal dysfunction with the apparent per-sistance of normal endocrine activity. With the exception of the ovary which exhausts its re-productive and endocrine functions at a spe-cific time during the lifespan (see Chapter 26.1), most endocrine glands continue to syn-thesize and release hormones, albeit at some-what altered levels, until death. Major alterations with ageing may involve peripheral hormone metabolism or the response of per-ipheral tissues to hormonal regulation. Thus, increased insulin resistance and decreased thy-roxine and glucocorticoid metabolic rate may be interpreted as a reduction in peripheral de-mand. The most common explanation offered for this decline in demand is a loss of meta-bolically active tissue mass with ageing. Several factors, however, argue against this interpret-ation: declines begin early in life before any significant cell loss; putative cell loss may not occur at all in healthy individuals as shown in recent studies in humans (Lesser and Markov-sky, 1979) and in rats (Lesser, Deutsch, and Markovsky, 1980); and alterations in potas-sium and creatinine excretion taken as indices of cell loss may, indeed, be the consequence of a primary endocrine alteration. Another ex-planation may lie in some metabolic alterations in target tissues with ageing such as a decline in protein synthesis which, however, begins with the cessation of growth and continues to fall throughout the remaining lifespan. The parallel fall in metabolic rate, whole-body pro-tein synthesis, and thyroid hormone 'utiliza-tion' lends to this hypothesis. Thyroid hormones, necessary for growth and develop-ment when energy requirements are very high, may become detrimental when the only energy needed is for homeostasis. In addition to adverse catabolic effects, they may induce suc-cessive alterations in neuroendocrine pace-makers, leading to a loss of temporal organization of endocrine and metabolic func-tions and consequent degenerative changes (see Walker and Timiras, 1982).

AGEING OF THE CARDIOVASCULAR SYSTEM AT REST AND WITH EXERCISE

The pathophysiology of the circulation in the elderly is further discussed in Chapters 13 and 14. This brief discussion is intended to place the topic within the perspective of age-related changes in control systems which regulate homeostasis. It is generally accepted that age-ing, accompanied by a more sedentary state, restricts the functional capacities of the car-diovascular system. This is manifested by re-duced cardiovascular and pulmonary reserves and decreased strength and endurance of car-diac muscle associated with increased cardiac weight and volume, accumulation of lipofucsin in myocardium, and atherosclerotic lesions in the arterial wall, initiated at early ages and progressive throughout life (Weisfeldt, 1980). Yet some aspects of cardiac function and meta-bolism are not significantly altered under rest-ing conditions. This is true for cardiac action potentials, duration and strength of contrac-tion and relaxation, and nucleotide and phos-phate content (despite some decline in mitochondrial enzymatic activity) (Cantwell and Watt, 1974; Hodgson and Buskirk, 1977; Kaman *et al.,* 1978). When the older individ-ual, however, is exposed to severe (dynamic) exercise, the maximal capacity of the cardiov-ascular system to deliver oxygen to the working muscles is reduced compared to that of younger subjects (Granath, Jonsson, and Strandell, 1970; Niinimaa and Sheppard, 1978; Strandell, 1976). As dynamic exercise (i.e. iso-metric contraction as in swimming, jogging, bicycling, etc.) is being used increasingly as a preventative modality against these very car-diovascular diseases of ageing – atherosclerosis and hypertension – it is important to under-stand the normal responses of the elderly to exercise (see Chapter 4). Despite an abundant literature on this subject, little consistent in-formation is available (Raven and Mitchell, 1980; Skinner, 1973). The lesser ability of the ageing circulatory system to adapt optimally to demands for increased work has been ascribed to several, probably simultaneously acting, fac-tors: metabolic alterations such as decreased metabolic rate, obesity, lack of physical train-ing; impairment of cardiac function such as hypokinesia and reduced output; stiffening and narrowing of arteries due to atherosclerosis;

imbalance of nervous regulation such as decreased sympathetic drive, responsiveness to catecholamines and number of beta receptors. Hormones also interact with the circulatory system: primarily thyroid hormones act synergistically with catecholamines to regulate cardiac rate and contractility and corticosterioids influence the development and activity of metabolic enzymes for catecholamines (in adrenal medulla and other tissues). Possibly some of the age-related changes in the effects of catecholamines on target tissues such as the heart and arterial wall – and, by extrapolation, the deficits in cardiovascular adjustments with ageing – are dependent on alterations in neural and hormonal regulation.

HOMEOSTASIS AND STRESS: AGE-RELATED CHANGES IN NEUROENDOCRINE SIGNALS FOR ADAPTATION AND SURVIVAL

While the range of neural and hormonal changes in the elderly, briefly reviewed above, varies considerably from slight to severe depending on the CNS area and the endocrine gland, the capacity of the organism to adapt to the environment irreversibly declines with advancing age and ultimately fails, resulting in disease and death. In view of the crucial roles of the nervous and endocrine systems in homeostasis and their complex interrelations, the decrement in adaptive capability characteristic of old age may be related to the impairment of neuroendocrine controls rather than to absolute defects in one system or the other. The consequences of such impairment would involve and be mediated through altered circulatory and other visceral and somatic adjustments. In parallel with other events of the lifespan that are regulated by neuroendocrine signals, such as growth, development, and reproduction, ageing may similarly be considered as dependent on neuroendocrine regulation or, alternatively, as consequent to the failure of this regulation.

According to the first view, ageing is the result of a genetically determined, precisely timed process in which clocks or pacemakers provide signals for passage through the life programme. Specific neuronal impulses, transmitted through stimulatory or inhibitory neurotransmitters, modulate the activity of neurosecretory cells of the hypothalamus. Such neurosecretions induce or inhibit release of pituitary hormones which, in turn, would act directly on target cells (e.g. GH, prolactin) or would induce (e.g. TSH, ACTH) other endocrine cells to secrete their hormones. Other hormones (e.g. insulin) are secreted under the influence of nervous and metabolic stimuli. The involvement of the classic monoaminergic and cholinergic neurotransmitters and the more recently considered peptidergic neurotransmitters (e.g. substance P, encephalins, endorphins) in the regulation of many endocrine, visceral, and sensorimotor functions (e.g. sleep

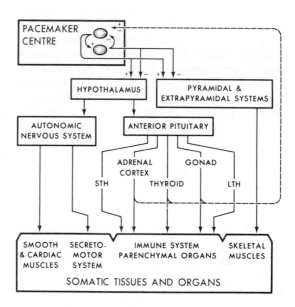

Figure 3 Schema for programmed neuroendoctrine regulation of the lifespan. Timed signals (clocks or pacemakers) direct the passage from one period to another throughout the lifespan. Excitatory (+) or inhibitory (−) neurons, feeding back to each other by direct or indirect neural processes, create stimulatory (+) or repressive (−) influences on brain areas such as the hypothalmus (control of autonomic nervous and neuroendocrine systems) and pyramidal and extrapyramidal nervous systems (control of skeletal muscle tone and movement). These influences then affect structure and function of musculature (smooth, cardiac, and striated), exocrine glands, the immune system, and parenchymal organs. With aging, it is hypothesized that he neuroendocrine signals lead to loss in muscle tone and function, alterations or decline in elaboration of many secretions, cardiovascular impairment, immunologic suppression, parenchymal organs – and therefore homeostatic – performance loss, and many other physiologic deficits associated with senescence. Dashed line represents hypothetical feedback influences of thyroid and steriod hormones on regulatory centres of the brain.

patterns, locomotor activity, reproduction, pain and euphoria, thermoregulation, blood pressure) are well known. As described above, with ageing, qualitative and quantitative changes do occur in the release and metabolism of some of these neurotransmitters as well as of a number of hormones. These changes could trigger such decrements in physiological performance as characterize the 'passage' from adulthood to senescence and signal the terminal period of the lifespan.

An alternative to the hypothesis that ageing is a programmed period of the lifespan is the view that ageing may be the consequence of the cessation of a pacemaker-regulated programme which is exclusively limited to the developmental period. In this context, the lifespan may be divided into two distinct but sequential periods: until adolescence, physiological performance improves progressively according to a genetic programme expressed through neural (e.g. mediated through the neurotransmitter serotonin) and endocrine (e.g. mediated through thyroid hormones) sig-

nals which regulate ontogenetic transformations and selective mechanisms promoting the survival of the individual until reproductive maturity has been attained. In the later period, including late adulthood and senescence, performance is progressively impaired due to failure of optimal integration of homeostatic control systems because at this time they lack any programmed regulation.

Several levels of integration have been proposed where alterations leading to ageing may originate as well as the mechanisms through which they may act. Some of the observations thus far have led to a number of hypotheses which include the following.

The Hypothalamic Disregulation Hypotheses

The hypothalamic disregulation hypotheses suggest that age-related changes in the hypothalamus – in terms of differential ageing of several nuclei, or loss or impairment of feedback sensitivity to hormones, or shifts in hypothalamic secretions – may be responsible for

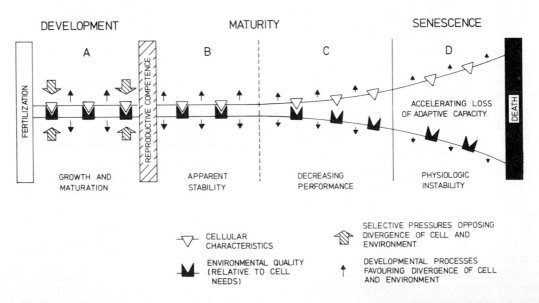

Figure 4 Schema for programmed neuroendocrine regulation of growth and development. Timed signals (clocks or pacemakers) direct the timetable of development until reproductive competence has been achieved. Thereafter, in the absence of a programme, synchrony of neuroendocrine signals is lost, leading to internal disorder, physiologic decline, pathology, and death. Ontogenic, biochemical, and physiological organization, essential to maturational processes, requires coordinated change of cellular internal environmental conditions to ensure survival. Selective pressures favouring survival during development lead to the establishment of mechanisms that integrate cell needs and environmental quality. Integrating forces are absent beyond reproductive maturity, when selective pressures are lost; temporal reorganization, residual from development, continues beyond maturity, leading to internal disorder, physiologic decline, pathology, and death (Walker and Timiras, 1982).

physiological and pathological correlates of ageing (Dilman, 1976; Frolkis and Bezrukov, 1979).

The Neurotransmitter Hypotheses

The neurotransmitter hypotheses implicate neurotransmitter excess or deficit, or imbalance among two or several neurotransmitters in discrete brain areas as directly responsible for specific functional alterations. With the advent of neurotransmitter agonists and antagonists, these hypotheses, by focusing on neurotransmitter alterations, suggest that ageing may be amenable to pharmacological interventions (Ordy, 1979). Indeed, several reports show that administration of certain centrally acting drugs, including some which may act as metabolic precursors, alters various aspects of ageing. On the basis of the selective vulnerability of dopaminergic systems discussed above, the dopamine precursor L-dopa was administered at a young age and retarded growth, reduced overall tumour incidence, delayed the onset of ageing in mice (Cotzias *et al.*, 1974, 1977), and affected favourably the early stages of presenile dementia (Jellinger *et al.*, 1980). Iproniazid, a monoamine oxidase inhibitor, and lergotrile or bromocriptine, alkaloids capable of mimicking the neuroendocrinological effects of dopamine, are capable of reinitiating oestrous cyclicity in old rats, and, at least for the first two, of restoring some aspects of physiological competence as well as extending the lifespan (Clemens and Fuller, 1977; Quadri, Kledzik, and Meites, 1973). Reduction in the levels of brain serotonin, by parachlorophenylalanine (PCPA), an inhibitor of its synthesis, or dietary restriction of tryptophan, its amino acid precursor, seems to retard growth and maturation as well as the onset of ageing of some specific functions (e.g. reproduction, thermoregulation) and possibly prolongs the lifespan (Segall *et al.*, 1978; Segall and Timiras, 1976). With respect to the cholinergic system, while normal individuals show little change in acetylcholine content in old age, in dementia (including Alzheimer's disease) the activity of choline acetyltransferase, the synthesizing enzyme for acetylcholine, is decreased in the cerebral cortex (e.g. hippocampus, nucleus basalis of Meynart) (Whitehouse *et al.*, 1982). In addition, a number of studies in humans and other species have shown that cholinergic dysfunction may be related to the memory impairments of old age and have suggested, at least as an empirical approach, that replacement therapy with choline or lecithin, the natural dietary source, might be beneficial in restoring memory deficits. Although positive effects with dietary or pharmacological replacement therapy have been reported in some elderly subjects and aged animals, the nature of these effects is relatively transient and inconsistent among subjects as well as with respect to the optimal dose (Bartus *et al.*, 1980). An issue of critical importance here, as in the previous cases of monoamine replacement or blockade, is whether choline (or a monoamine or other precursor) manipulations induce alterations in CNS cholinergic (or other neurotransmitter) systems capable of influencing behaviour and function.

The Pituitary Hypotheses

The pituitary hypotheses include some contrasting points of view: according to some investigators, ageing phenomena are the consequence of a deficiency of pituitary hormones (Herman, 1976), while according to others ageing may be due to qualitative (e.g. increased proportion of polymorphic forms with high and low molecular weights) and quantitative (e.g. increased levels of gonadotropins, prolactin, a factor inhibiting thyroid hormone metabolic actions) changes in pituitary secretion (Choy, Klemme, and Timiras, 1982; Denckla, 1974; Everitt, 1980; Timiras, Choy, and Hudson, 1981). Removal of the pituitary (by surgical, pharmacological, or dietary means) prolongs physiological competence and postpones the onset of ageing (Everitt, 1980). A corollary to this theory is the hypothyroid hypothesis which suggests that many signs and symptoms of ageing depend on decrements of thyroid hormone actions (see above and also Walker and Timiras, 1982).

Progeria and Progeroid Syndromes

Progeria and progeroid syndromes emphasize the role of genetic factors in determining the length of the lifespan and of genetic variants in determining accelerations or decelerations of changes in the senescent phenotype. Progeria (premature old age) and progeroid (progeria-like) syndromes resemble but do not quite duplicate all the pathophysiology of ageing, each syndrome representing an acceleration of some of the characteristics associated with normal ageing. The aetiology of these syndromes is obscure, but among the several causes proposed that of neuroendocrinological dysfunction is supported by stunted growth, failure of gonadal maturation, diabetes, and a combination of these conditions.

The Stress Theory of Ageing

The stress theory of ageing applies the cellular hypotheses of 'wear and tear' and autointoxication to the organismic level and amalgamates them with neuroendocrinological theories of ageing involving the hypothalamo-pituitary-adrenocortical axis. Central to this theory, as formulated first by Selye, is the role of the adrenal gland, particularly the cortex, as the endocrine gland indispensable for adaptation and survival (Selye, 1950, 1974). Exposure to environmental or psychological stimuli (stress) both of a detrimental nature and with a positive influence induces a sequence of neural and endocrine events leading first to the activation of defence mechanisms necessary for survival (the so-called alarm reaction), followed by a period of enhanced adaptive capacity (the stage of resistance), and terminating with loss of the capacity to adapt (the stage of exhaustion). The passage from one stage to the other would be dictated by the efficiency of the hypothalamo-adrenocortical axis in synchronizing (a) nervous stimuli from the stress conditions, (b) hormonal secretions from the pituitary and the adrenals, and (c) the sensitivity of peripheral target tissues and cellular functions to the adrenocortical hormone levels and rhythmicity. The composite of these neuroendocrine reactions and their resulting cellular and tissular responses would constitute a 'general adaptation syndrome' which, in its triphasic sequence, seems to resemble the timetable of the individual life: at an early age, adaptive capacity is not completely developed; with adulthood, resistance reaches an optimum; and thereafter declines until death.

Interesting as the stress theory may appear, it is difficult to reconcile it with the apparent adequate adrenocortical function in the elderly reported in the preceding section. Even more controversial is the suggestion that 'diseases of adaptation' may ensue from repeated exposure to stress. Such diseases involving primarily the circulatory (e.g. hypertension, atherosclerosis) and immune (e.g. arthritis, autoimmune diseases) systems are all commonly associated with old age. Indeed, the induction of disease by a variety of stresses in humans may contribute to ageing, as in animals exposure to stress may induce 'precocious ageing', a decrement in one or several functions at an earlier than expected chronological age.

Which of these neuroendocrine hypotheses for ageing is the correct one remains to be verified. In fact, the neuroendocrine theory of ageing itself awaits verification, as do all other theories of ageing discussed throughout this textbook. The concept of pacemaker or 'command' cells situated in specific brain areas and acting through neural and hormonal signals provides a useful model. Identification of the responsible signals may lead to a better understanding of the ageing process and its causes. More importantly, perhaps, the rapid advances in recent years in neuropharmacology and endocrinology make it possible to modify the signals and hence, perhaps, to influence the ageing process. Thus, a defect produced at any level of the functional neuroendocrine pathways may be expected to produce secondary ageing changes which can be appropriately prevented or attenuated by specific interventions.

REFERENCES

Adelman, R. C., and Freeman, C. (1972). 'Age-dependent regulation of the glucokinase and tyrosine aminotransferase activities of rat liver *in vivo* by adrenal, pancreatic and pituitary hormones', *Endocrinology,* **90**, 1551–1160.

Andres, R. (1971). 'Aging and diabetes', *Med. Clin. North Am.,* **55**, 835–845.

Andres, R., and Tobin, J. D. (1977). 'Endocrine systems', in *Handbook of the Biology of Aging* (Eds C. E. Finch and L. Hayflick), pp. 357–378, Van Nostrand Reinhold, New York.

Andrew, W. (1944). 'Senile changes in the pancreas of Wistar Institute rats and of man', *Am. J. Anat.,* **74**, 97–127.

Antonioni, F. M., Porro, A., Serio, M., and Tinti, P. (1968). 'Gas chromatographic analysis of urinary 17-ketosteroids response to gonadotropin and ACTH in young and old persons', *Exp. Gerontol., 3*, 181–192.

Azizi, F., Vagenakis, A. G., Portnoy, G. F., Rapoport, B., Ingbar, S. H., and Braverman, L. E., (1975). 'Pituitary-thyroid responsiveness to intramuscular thyrotropin-releasing hormone based on analyses of serum thyroxine, triiodothyronine, and TSH concentration', *N. Engl. J. Med., 292*, 273–277.

Baker, B. L., and Yu, Y. Y. (1977). 'An immunocytochemical study of human pituitary mammotropes from fetal life to old age', *Am. J. Anat., 148*, 217–249.

Baker, S. P., Gaffney, G. W., Shock, N. W. and Landowne, M. (1959). 'Physiological response of 5 middle-aged and elderly men to repeated administration of TSH', *J. Gerontol., 14*, 37–47.

Barbagallo-Sangiori, G., and Exton-Smith, A. N. (Eds) (1980). *The Aging Brain Neurological and Mental Disturbances,* Plenum Press, New York.

Barbagallo-Sangiori, G., Laudiciana, E., Bompiano, G. D., and Durante, F. (1970). 'The pancreatic beta-cell response to intravenous administration of glucose in elderly subjects', *J. Am. Geriatr. Soc., 18*, 529–538.

Bartus, R. T., Dean, R. L., Goas, J. A., and Lippa, A. S. (1980). 'Age-related changes in passive avoidance retention and modulatin with dietary choline', *Science, 209*, 301–303.

Bazarre, T. L., Johanson, A. J., Huseman, C. A., Varman, M. M., and Blizzard, R. M. (1976). 'Human growth hormone changes with age', in *Growth Hormone and Related Peptides* (Eds A. Pecile and H. Muller), pp. 261–270, Excerpta Medica, 381, Amsterdam.

Benjamin, F., Casper, D. J., Sherman, L., and Kolodny, H. D. (1970). 'Growth hormone, age and the endometrium', *N. Engl. J. Med., 283*, 375.

Berlyne, G. M., Ben-Ari, J., Kushelev, A., Idelman, A., Galinsky, D., Hirsch, M., Shainikin, R., Yagi, I., and Zlotnik, M. (1975). 'The etiology of senile osteoporosis: Secondary hyperparathyroidism due to renal failure', *Q. J. Med., 44*, 505–521.

Bermudez, F., Surks, M. I., and Oppenheimer, J. H. (1975). 'High incidence of decreased serum T$_3$ in patients with non-thyroidal disease', *J. Clin. Endocrinol. Metab., 41*, 27–40.

Blichert-Toft, M. (1971). 'Assessment of serum corticotrophin concentration and its nyctohemeral rhythm in the aged', *Gerontol. Clin., 13*, 215–220.

Blichert-Toft, M. (1975). 'Secretion of corticotrophin and somatotrophin by the senescent adenohypophysis in man', *Acta. Endocrinol., 78* (Suppl. 195), 1–157.

Blichert-Toft, M., Hummer, L., and Dige-Petersen, H. (1975), 'Human TSH level and response to TRH in the aged', *Gerontol. Clin., 17*, 191–203.

Bondareff, W. (1980). 'Synaptic organization as a function of aging', in *Neural Regulatory Mechanisms During Ageing* (Eds R. C. Adelman, J. Roberts, G. T. Baker, III, S. I. Baskin, and V. J. Cristofalo), pp. 143–158, Alan R. Liss, Inc., New York.

Bourne, G. G. (1967). 'Ageing changes in the endocrines', in *Endocrines and Ageing* (Ed. L. Gittman), pp. 66–75, Charles C Thomas, Springfield, Illinois.

Braverman, L. E., Dawber, N. A., and Ingbar, S. H. (1966). 'Observations concerning the binding of thyroid hormones in sera of normal subjects of varying ages', *J. Clin. Invest., 45*, 1273–1279.

Brizzee, K. R., Cancilla, P., Sherwood, N., and Timiras, P. S. (1969). 'The amount and distribution of pigments in neurons and glia of the cerebral cortex. Autofluorescent and ultrastructural studies', *J. Gerontol., 24*, 127–135.

Brizzee, K. R., Sherwood, N., and Timiras, P. S. (1968). 'A comparison of cell populations at various depth levels in cerebral cortex of young adult and aged Long-Evans rats', *J. Gerontol., 23*, 289–298.

Buckler, J. M. (1969). 'The effect of age, sex and exercise on the secretion of growth hormone', *Clin. Sci., 37*, 765–774.

Burrows, A. W., Shakespear, R. A., Hesch, R. D., Cooper, E., Aickin, C. M., and Burker, C. W. (1975). 'Thyroid hormones in the elderly sick: T$_4$ euthyroidism, *Br. Med. J., 4*, 437–439.

Calas, A., and Van Den Bosch de Aguilar, P. (1980). 'Comparative radioautographic study of serotonergic neurons in young and senescent rats', in *The Psychogiology of Aging: Problems and Perspectives* (Ed. D. G. Stein), pp. 59–80, Elsevier North Holland Inc., Amsterdam.

Calderon, L., Ryan, N., and Kovacs, K. (1978). 'Human pituitary growth hormone cells in old age, *Gerontology, 24*, 441–447.

Calloway, N. O., Foley, C. F., and Lagerbloom, P. (1965). 'Uncertainties in geriatric data II. Organ size', *J. Am. Geriatr. Soc., 13*, 20–28.

Cantwell, J. D., and Watt, E. O. (1974). 'Extreme cardiopulmonary fitness in old age', *Chest, 65*, 357–359.

Carlson, H. E., Gillin, J. C., Gordon, P., and Snyder, F. (1972). 'Absence of sleep-related growth hormone peaks in aged normal subjects and acromegaly', *J. Clin. Endocrinol. Metab., 34*, 1102–1105.

Cartlidge, N. E. F., Black, M. M., Hall, M. R., and Hall, R. (1970). 'Pituitary function in the elderly', *Gerontol. Clin., 12*, 65–70.

Chopra, I. J., Solomon, D. H., Chopra, O., Wu, S. Y., Fisher, D. A., and Nakamura, Y. (1978). 'Pathways of metabolism of thyroid hormones', *Recent Prog. Horm. Res., 34*, 521–567.

Chopra, I. J., Solomon D. H., Chua, T., Guadalupe N., and Eisenberg, J. B. (1982). 'An inhibitor of the binding of thyroid hormones to serum proteins is present in extra-thyroidal tissues', *Science*, **215**, 407–409.

Choy, V. J., Klemme, W. R., and Timiras, P. S. (1982). 'Variant forms of immunoreactive thyrotropin in aged rats', *Mech. Ageing Dev.*, **19**, 273–278.

Clemens, J. A., and Fuller, R. W. (1977). 'Chemical manipulation of some aspects of aging', in *Pharmacological Interventions in the Ageing Process, Advances in Experimental Medicine and Biology*, Vol. 97, pp. 187–206, Plenum Press, New York.

Cole, G. M., Segall, P. E., and Timiras, P. S. (1982). 'Hormones during ageing', in *Hormones in Development and Ageing* (Eds A. Vernadakis and P. S. Timiras), pp. 477–550, SP Medical and Scientific Books, New York.

Connor, J. R., Diamond, M. C., and Johnson, R. E. (1980a). 'Occipital cortical morphology of the rat: Alterations with age and environment', *Exp. Neurol.*, **68**, 158–170.

Connor, J. R., Diamond, M. C. and Johnson, R. E. (1980b). 'Ageing and environmental influences on two types of dendritic spines in the rat occipital cortex', *Exp. Neurol.*, **70**, 371–379.

Cooper, B., and Gregerman, R. I. (1976). 'Hormone-sensitive fat cell adenylate cyclase in the rat. Influences of growth, cell size and ageing', *J. Clin. Invest.*, **57**, 161–168.

Cooper, E. R. A. (1925). *The Histology of the More Important Human Endocrine Organs at Various Ages*, Oxford University Press, London.

Cotman, C. W., and Scheff, S. W. (1979). 'Compensatory synapse growth in aged animals after neuronal death', *Mech. Ageing Dev.*, **9**, 103–117.

Cotzias, G. C., Miller, S. T., Nicholson, A. R., Maston, W. M., and Tong, L. C. (1974). 'Prolongation of the lifespan in mice adapted to large amounts of L-Dopa', *Proc. Natl. Acad. Sci.*, **7**, 2466–2469.

Cotzias, G. C., Miller, S. T., Tong, L. C., Papavasiliou, P. S., and Wang, Y. Y. (1977). 'Levodopa, fertility and longevity', *Science*, **196**, 549–551.

Cuttelod, S., Lemarchand-Bergaud, T., Magnenat, P., Perret, C., Poli, S., and Vannotti, A. (1974). 'Effect of age and role of kidneys and liver on TSH turnover in man', *Metabolism*, **23**, 101–113.

Danowski, T. S., Tsai, T., Morgan, C., Sieracki, J., Alley, R., Robbins, T., Sabeh, G., and Sunder, J. H. (1969). 'Serum growth hormone and insulin in females without glocose intolerance', *Metabolism*, **18**, 811–820.

Davidson, M. B. (1979). 'The effect of ageing on carbohydrate metabolism: A review of the English literature and a practical approach to the diagnosis of diabetes mellitus in the elderly', *Metabolism*, **28**, 688–705.

DeFronzo, R. A. (1979). 'Glucose intolerance and ageing. Evidence for tissue insensitivity to insulin', *Diabetes*, **28**, 1095–1101.

Deftos, L. J., Weisman, M. H., Williams, G. H., Karpf, D. B., Frumar, A. M., Davidson, B. H., Parthemore, J. G., and Judd, H. L. (1979). 'Age- and sex-related changes of calcitonin secretion in humans', in *Endocrine Aspects of Ageing* (Ed. S. G. Korenman), Summary of papers presented at a conference jointly sponsored by the National Institute on Ageing and the Endocrine Society, Bethesda, Maryland, 18–20 October.

Denckla, W. D. (1974). 'Role of the pituitary and thyroid glands in the decline of minimal O$_2$ consumption with age', *J. Clin. Invest.*, **53**, 572–581.

Diamond, M. C., Johnson, R. E., and Gold, M. W. (1977). 'Changes in neuron and glia number in the young, adult and ageing rat occipital cortex', *Behav. Biol.*, **20**, 409–418.

Dilman, V. M. (1976). 'The hypothalamic control of ageing and age-associated pathology. The elevation mechanism of ageing,' in *Hypothalamus, Pituitary and Ageing* (Eds A. V. Everitt and J. A. Burgess), pp. 634–667, Charles C. Thomas, Springfield, Illinois.

Dilman, V. M., Ostroumova, M. N., and Tsyrlina, E. V. (1979). 'Hypothalamic mechanisms of ageing and of specific age pathology – II. On the sensitivity threshold of hypothalamo-pituitary complex to homeostatic stimuli in adaptive homeostasis', *Exp. Gerontol.*, **14**, 175–181.

Dobbie, J. W. (1969). 'Adrenocortical nodular hyperplasia: The ageing adrenal', *J. Pathol.*, **99**, 1–18.

Dogliotti, G. C., and Nuzzi, N. G. (1935). 'Thyroid and senescence: Structural transformations of the thyroid in old age and their functional interpretation', *Endocrinology*, **19**, 289–292.

Duckworth, W. C., and Kitabchi, A. E. (1976). 'The effect of age on plasma proinsulin-like material after oral glucose', *J. Lab. Clin. Med.*, **88**, 359–367.

Dudl, R. J., and Ensinck, J. W. (1977). 'Insulin and glucagon relationships during ageing in man', *Metabolism*, **26**, 33–41.

Dudl, R. J., Ensinck, J. W., Palmer, H. E., and Williams, R. H. (1973). 'Effect of age on growth hormone secretion in man', *J. Clin. Endocrinol.*, **37**, 11–16.

Einhorn, J. (1958). 'Studies on the effect of thyrotropic hormone on thyroid function in man', *Acta. Radiol.*, **160**, (Suppl.), 1–107.

Everitt, A. V. (1980). 'The neuroendocrine system and ageing', *Gerontology*, **26**, 108–119.

Everitt, A. V., and Burgess, J. A. (Eds) (1976).

Hypothalamus Pituitary and Ageing, Charles C. Thomas, Publisher, Springfield, Illinois.

Fedele, D., Valerio, A., Molinari, M., and Crepaldi, G. (1977). 'Glucose tolerance, insulin, and glucagon secretions in ageing', *Diabetologia,* **13**, 392.

Feldman, M. (1955). 'The pancreas in the aged: An autopsy study', *Geriatrics,* **10**, 373–374.

Finch, C. E. (1978). 'Age-related changes in brain catecholamines. Synopsis of findings in C57 BL-65 mice and other rodent models', in *Ageing and Neuroendocrine Relationships* (Eds C. E. Finch, D. E. Potter, and A. D. Kenney), pp. 15–39, Plenum Press, New York.

Finch, C. E. (1979). 'Neuroendocrine mechanisms and ageing', *Fed. Proc.,* **38**, 178–183.

Finch, C. E., and Hayflick, L. (Eds) (1977). *Handbook of the Biology of Aging,* Van Nostrand Reinhold, New York.

Finkelstein, J. W., Roffwarg, H. P., Boyar, J. M., Kream, J., and Hellman, L. (1972). 'Age-related changes in the 24-hour spontaneous secretion of growth hormone', *J. Clin. Endocrinol.,* **35**, 665–670.

Flood, C., Gherondache, C., Pincus, G., Tait, J. F., Tait, S. A. S., and Willoughby, S. (1967). 'The metabolism and secretion of aldosterone in elderly subjects', *J. Clin. Invest.,* **46**, 960–966.

Friedman, M., Green, M. F., and Sharland, D. E. (1969). 'Assessment of hypothalamic-pituitary-adrenal function in the geriatric age group', *J. Gerontol.,* **24**, 292–297.

Frolkis, V. V., and Bezrukov, V. V. (1979). *Aging of the Central Nervous System, Interdisciplinary Topics in Gerontology* (Ed. H. P. von Hahn), Vol. 16, Karger, Basel.

Gaffney, G. W., Gregerman, R. I., and Shock, N. W. (1962). 'Serum protein bound iodine concentration in blood of euthyroid men aged 18 to 94 years', *J. Clin. Endocrinol. Metab.,* **22**, 784–794.

Gershberg, H. (1957). 'Growth hormone content and metabolic actions of human pituitary glands', *Endocrinology,* **61**, 160–165.

Gherondache, C. N., Romanoff, L. P., and Pincus, G. (1967). 'Steroid hormones in aging men', in *Endocrines and Aging* (Ed. L. Gitman), pp. 76–101, Charles C. Thomas, Springfield, Illinois.

Giorgino, R., Scardapane, R., Nardelli, G. M., and Tafaro, E. (1969). 'Surrene e senescenza. Aspetti dell'attivita' della midollare', *Folia Endocrinol.,* **22**, 215–224.

Gittler, R. D., and Friedfield, L. (1962). 'Adrenocortical responsiveness in the aged', *J. Am. Geriatr. Soc.,* **10**, 153–159.

Grad, B., Kral, V. A., Payne, R. C., and Berenson, J. (1967). 'Plasma and urinary corticoids in young and old persons', *J. Gerontol.,* **22**, 66–71.

Grad, B., Rosenberg, G. M., Liberman, H., Trach-

tenberg, J., and Kral, V. A. (1971). 'Diurnal variation in serum cortisol level of geriatric subjects', *J. Gerontol.,* **26**, 351–357.

Granath, A. Jonsson, B., and Strandell, T. (1970). 'Circulation in healthy old men studies by right-heart catheterization at rest and during exercise in supine and sitting position', in *Medicine and Sport: Physical Activity and Aging* (Eds D. Brunner and E. Jokl), pp. 48–79, University Park Press, Baltimore.

Greenblatt, R. B. (Ed.) (1978). *Geriatric Endocrinology, Aging,* Vol. 5, Raven Press, New York.

Gregerman, R. I., and Bierman, E. I. (1981). 'Aging and hormones', in *Textbook of Endocrinology* (Ed. R. H. Williams), 6th ed., pp. 1192–1212, Saunders, Philadelphia.

Gregerman, R. I., Gaffney, G. W., and Shock, N. W. (1962). 'Thyroxine turnover in euthyroid man with special reference to change with age', *J. Clin. Invest.,* **41**, 2065–2074.

Gregerman, R. I., and Solomon, N. (1967). 'Acceleration of thyroxine and triiodothyronine turnover during bacterial pulmonary infections and fever: Implications for the functional state of the thyroid during stress and in senescence', *J. Clin. Endocrinol. Metab.,* **27**, 93–105.

Gries, F. A., and Steinke, J. (1967). 'Comparative effects of insulin on adipose tissue segments and isolated fat cells of rat and man', *J. Clin. Invest.,* **46**, 1413–1421.

Halberg, F. (1982). 'Biological rhythms, hormones and aging', in *Hormones in Development and Aging* (Eds A. Vernadakis and P. S. Timiras), pp. 451–476, SP Medical and Scientific Books, New York.

Hansen, J. M., Skovsted, L., and Siersback-Nielsen, K. (1975). 'Age-dependent changes in iodine metabolism and thyroid function', *Acta. Endocrinol.,* **79**, 60–65.

Helderman, J. H., Vestal, R. E., Rowe, J. W., Tobin, J. D., Andres, R., and Robertson, G. L. (1978). 'The response of arginine vasopressin to intravenous ethanol and hypertonic saline in man: The impact of aging', *J. Gerontol.,* **33**, 39–47.

Herman, E. (1976). 'Senile hypophyseal syndromes', in *Hypothalamus, Pituitary and Aging* (Eds A. V. Everitt and J. A. Burgess), pp. 157–170, Charles C. Thomas, Springfield, Illinois.

Herman, J., Rusche, H. J., Kroll, H. J., Hilger, P., and Kruskemper, H. L. (1974). 'Free triiodothyronine (T₃) and thyroxine (T₄) levels in old age', *Hormone Metab. Res.* **6**, 239–240.

Hesch, R. D., Gatz, J., Pope, J., Schmidt, E., and von zur Huhlen, A. (1976). 'Total and free 3′, 5′ triiodothyronine and thyroid hormone binding globulin concentration in elderly human persons', *Eur. J. Clin. Invest.,* **6**, 139–145.

Hochstaedt, B. B., Schneebaum, M., and Shadel,

M. (1961). 'Adrenocortical responsibility in old age', *Gerontol. Clin.*, **3**, 239–246.

Hodgson, J. L., and Buskirk, E. R. (1977). 'Physical fitness and age, with emphasis on cardiovascular function in the elderly', *J. Am. Geriatr. Soc.*, **25**, 385–402.

Holm, A. C., Lemarchand-Beraud, T., Scazziga, B. R., and Cuttelod, S. (1975). 'Human lymphocyte binding and deiodination of thyroid hormones in relation to thyroid function', *Acta Endocrinol.*, **80**, 642–656.

Horky, K., Manek, J., Kopecka, J., and Gregorova, A. (1975). 'Influence of age on orthostatic changes in plasma renin activity and urinary catecholamines in man', *Physiol. Bohemoslov.*, **24**(6), 481–488.

Inada, M., Koshiyame, K., Torizuka, K. A., Kagi, H., and Miyake, T. (1964). 'Clinical studies of the metabolism of ^{131}I-thyroxine', *J. Clin. Endocrinol. Metab.*, **24**, 775–784.

Ingbar, S. H. (1978). 'The influence of age on the human thyroid hormone economy', in *Geriatric Endocrinology*, (Ed. R. B. Greenblatt), *Aging* Vol. 5, pp. 13–31, Raven Press, New York.

Irvine, R. E., and Hodkinson, H. M. (1978). 'Thyroid disease in old age', in *Textbook of Geriatric Medicine and Gerontology* (Ed. J. C. Brocklehurst), 2nd ed., pp. 451–494, Churchill Livingston, Edinburgh.

Jellinger, K., Flament, H., Riederer, P. Schmid, H., and Ambrozi, L. (1980). 'Levodpa in the treatment of (pre) senile dementia', *Mech. Ageing Dev.*, **14**, 253–264.

Jensen, H. K., and Blichert-Toft, M. (1971). 'Serum corticotrophin, plasma cortisol and urinary excretion of 17-ketogenic steroids in the elderly (age group: 66–94)', *Acta. Endocrinol.*, **74**, 511–523.

Jorpes, E., and Rastgeldi, S. (1953). 'Insulin content of human pancreas', *Acta Physiol. Scand.*, **29**, 163–169.

Jowsey, J., Riggs, B. L., *et al.* (1971). 'Effects of prolonged administration of porcine calcitonin in postmenopausal osteoporosis', *J. Clin. Endocrinol.*, **33**, 752–758.

Kalish, M. I., Katz, M. S., Pineyro, M. A., and Gregerman, R. I. (1977). 'Epinephrine- and glucagon-sensitive adenylate cyclases of rat liver during aging: Evidence for membrane instability associated with increased enzymatic activity', *Bio-Chim. Biophys. Acta.*, **483**, 452–466.

Kalk, J., Vinik, A. I., Pimstone, B. L., and Jackson, W. P. U. (1973). 'Growth hormone response to insulin hypoglycemia in the elderly', *J. Gerontol.*, **28**, 431–433.

Kaman, R. L., Raven, P. B., Carlisle, C., and Ayres, J. (1978). 'Age related changes in cardiac enzymes as a result of jogging exercise in man', *Med. Sci. Sports*, **10**, 46–47.

Kanungo, M. S. (1980). *Biochemistry of Ageing*, Academic Press, New York.

Kärki, N. T. (1956). 'The urinary excretion of noradrenaline and adrenaline in different age groups, its diurnal variation and the effect of muscular work on it', *Acta. Physiol. Scand.*, **39** (Suppl. 132), 7–96.

Khelimskii, A. M. (1964). 'Age changes in dimensions of adrenal cortex', *Fed. Proc.* **23**, (Translation Suppl.), T1250-T1252.

Kimmerling, G., Javorski, C., and Reaven, G. M. (1977). 'Aging and insulin resistance in a group of nonobese male volunteers', *J. Am. Geriatr. Soc.*, **25**, 349–353.

Köhrle, J., Ködding, R., Wong, C. C., and Hesch, R. D. (1979). 'Age-dependent changes of thyroxine-deiodination in rat liver', *Acta Endocrinol.*, Suppl 225, 20.

Korenchevsky, V. (1961). 'Thyroid gland', in *Physiological and Pathological Ageing* (Ed. G. H. Bourne), pp. 311–332, Hafner Publishing Co., Inc., New York.

Kovacs, G. L., Bohus, B., and Versteeg, D. H. G. (1979). 'The effects of vasopressin on memory processes: The role of noradrenergic neurotransmitter', *Neuroscience*, **4**, 1529–1537.

Kovacs, K., Ryan, N., Horvath, E., Penz, G., and Ezrin, C. (1977). 'Prolactin cells of the human pituitary gland in old age', *J. Gerontol.*, **32**, 534–540.

Kvetnansky, R., Jahnova, E., Torda, T., Strbak, V., Balaz, V., and Macho, L. (1978). 'Changes of adrenal catecholamines and their synthesizing enzymes during ontogenesis and aging in rats', *Mech. Ageing Dev.*, **7**, 206–216.

Lazarus, L., and Young, J. D. (1966). 'Radioimmunoassay of human growth hormone in serum using ion-exchange resin', *J. Clin. Endocrinol. Metab.*, **26**, 213–218.

Lederer, J., and Bataille, J. P. (1969). 'Senescence et fonction thyroidienne', *Ann. Endocrinol.*, **30**, 598–603.

Legros, J. J., Gilot, P., Seron, X., Claessens, J., Adams, A., Moeglen, J. M., Audibert, A., and Berchier, P. (1978). 'Influence of vasopressin on learning and memory', *Lancet*, **1**, 41–42.

Lemarchand-Beraud, T., and Vanotti, A. (1969). 'Relationship between blood thyrotropin level, protein bound iodine and free thyroxine in man under normal physiological conditions', *Acta. Endocrinol.*, **60**, 315–326.

Lesser, G. T., Deutsch, S., and Markovsky, J. (1980). 'Fat-free mass, total body water, and intracellular water in the aged rat', *Am. J. Physiol.*, **238**, R82-R90.

Lesser, G. T., and Markovsky, J. (1979). 'Body water compartments with human aging using fat-free mass as the reference standard', *Am. J. Physiol.,* **238**, R215-R220.

McGeer, P. L., Yu, B. P., and Suzuki, J. S. (1977). 'Aging and extrapyramidal function', *Arch. Neurol.,* **34**, 33–35.

McGuire, E. A., Tovin, J. D., Berman, M., and Andres, R. (1979). 'Kinetics of native insulin in diabetic, obese, and aged men', *Diabetes,* **28**, 110–120.

Makman, M. H., Gardner, E. L., Thal, L. J., Hirschhorn, I. D., Seeger, T. F., and Bhargava, G. (1980). 'Central monoamine receptor systems: Influence of aging, lesion and drug treatment', in *Neural Regulatory Mechanisms During Aging* (Eds R. C. Adelman, J. Roberts, G. T. Baker, III, S. I. Baskin, and V. J. Cristofalo), pp. 91–127, Alan R. Liss, Inc., New York.

Masoro, E. J. (1981). *CRC Series Handbook of Physiology in Aging,* CRC Press, Inc., Boca Raton, Florida.

Mayberry, W. E., Gharil, H., Bilshel, J. M., and Sizmore, G. W. (1971). 'Radioimmunoassay for human thyrotrophin, clinical value in patients with normal and abnormal thyroid function', *Ann. Int. Med.,* **74**, 471–480.

Meek, J. L., Bertilsson, L. Cheney, D. L., Zsilla, C., and Costa, E. (1977). 'Aging-induced changes in acetylcholine and serotonin content of discrete brain nuclei', *J. Gerontol.,* **32**, 129–131.

Migeon, C. J., Keller, A. R., Lawrence, B., and Shepard, T. H. (1957). 'Dehydroepiadrosterone and androsterone levels in human plasma. Effect of age and sex; day to day and diurnal variations', *J. Clin. Endocrinol. Metab.,* **17**, 1051–1062.

Moncloa, F., Gomez, R., and Prettel, E. (1963). 'Response to corticotrophin and correlation between the clearance of creatinine and urinary sterioids in aging', *Steroids,* **1**, 437–444.

Muller, E. E., Nistico, G., and Scapagnini, U. (Eds.) (1977). *Neurotransmitters and Anterior Pituitary Function,* Academic Press, New York.

Mustacchi, P. O., and Lowenhaupt, E. (1950). 'Senile changes in the histologic structure of the thyroid gland', *Geriatrics,* **5**, 268–273.

Niinimaa, V., and Shephard, R. J. (1978). 'Training and oxygen conductance in the elderly. II. The cardiovascular system', *J. Gerontol.,* **33**, 362–367.

Nonaka, K., and Tarui, S. (1977). 'Aging and endocrine pancreas', *Folia Endocrinol. Jap.,* **53** (12), 1321–1327.

North, R. H., Lassman, N., Tan, S. Y., Fernandez-Cruz, A., and Mulrow, P. J. (1966). 'Age and the related renin–aldosterone system', *Arch. Intern. Med.,* **137**, 1414–1417.

Oddie, T. H., Meade, J. H., and Fisher, D. A. (1966). 'An analysis of published data on thyroxine turnover in human subjects', *J. Clin. Endocrinol. Metab.,* **26**, 425–436.

Oddie, T. H., Myhill, J., Pirnique, F. G., and Fisher, D. A. (1968). 'Effect of age and sex on the radioactive iodide uptake in euthyroid subjects', *J. Clin. Endocrinol. Metab.,* **28**, 776–782.

Ohara, H., Kobayashi, T., Shiraishi, M., and Wada, T. (1974). 'Thyroid function of the aged as viewed from the pituitary-thyroid system', *Endocrinol. Jap.,* **21**, 377–386.

Oliveros, J. C., Jandali, M. K., Jinsit-Berthier, M., Remy, R., Benghezal, A., Audibert, A., and Moeglen, J. M. (1978). 'Vasopressin in amnesia', *Lancet,* **1**, 42.

Olsen, T., Laurberg, P., and Weeke, J. (1978). 'Low serum triiodothyronine and high serum reverse triiodothyronine in old age: An affect of disease not age', *J. Clin. Endocrinol. Metab.,* **47**, 1111–1115.

Ooka, H. (1979). 'Changes in extrathyroidal conversion of thyroxine (T_4) to 3, 3′, 5′-triiodothyronine (T_3) *in vitro* during development and aging of the rat', *Mech. Ageing Dev.,* **105**, 151–156.

Ordy, J. M. (1979). 'Geriatric psychopharmacology: Drug modification of memory and emotionality in relation to aging in human and non-human primate brain', in *Brain Function in Old Age* (Eds F. Hoffmeister and C. Muller), pp. 435–455, Springer-Verlag, Berlin.

Orskov, H., and Christensen, N. J. (1969). 'Plasma disappearance rate of injected human insulin in juvenile diabetic, maturity onset diabetic and non-diabetic subjects', *Diabetes,* **18**, 653–659.

Pasteels, J. L., Gausset, P., Danguay, A., Ecotros, F., Nicoll, C. S., and Varavudhi, P. (1972). 'Morphology of the lactotropes and somatotropes of man and rhesus monkeys', *J. Clin. Endocrinol. Metab.,* **34**, 959–967.

Perlmutter, M., and Riggs, D. S. (1949). 'Thyroid collection of radioactive iodide and serum protein-bound iodine concentration in senescence, in hypothyroidism, and hypopituitarism', *J. Clin. Endocrinol. Metab.,* **9**, 430–439.

Puri, S. K., and Volicer, L. (1977). 'Effect of aging on cyclic AMP levels and adenylate cyclase and phosphodiesterase activities in the rat corpus striatum', *Mech. Ageing Dev.,* **6**, 53–58.

Quadri, S. K., Kledzik, G. S., and Meites, J. (1973). 'Reinitiation of estrous cycles in old, constant estrous rats by centrally acting drugs', *Neuroendocrinology,* **11**, 248–255.

Quimby, E. H., Werner, S. C., and Schmidt, C. (1950). 'Influence of age, sex, and season upon radioactive iodide uptake by the human thyroid', *Proc. Soc. Exp. Biol. Med.,* **75**, 537–540.

Rahman, Y. E., and Peraino, C. (1973). 'Effects of age on enzyme adaptation in male and female rats', *Exp. Gerontol.,* **8**, 93–100.

Raizes, G. S., Elahi, D., *et al.* (1976). 'Effect of aging on the gastrointestinal mediation of insulin response: The role of gastric inhibitory polypeptide', *29th Annual Scientific Meeting of the Gerontological Society*, p. 50 (abstract).

Raven, P. B., and Mitchell, J. (1980). 'The effect of aging on the cardiovascular response to dynamic and static exercise', in *The Aging Heart* (Ed. M. L. Weisfeldt), *Aging*, Vol. 12, pp. 269–296, Raven Press, New York.

Romanoff, L. P., Morris, C. W., Welch, P., Rodriquez, R. M., and Pincus, G. (1961). 'The metabolism of cortisol-4-^{14}C in young and elderly men. I. Secretion rate of cortisol and daily excretion of tetrahydrocortisol, allotetrahydrocortisol, tetrahydrocortisone and cortolone (20α and 20β)', *J. Clin. Endocrinol.*, **21**, 1413–1435.

Roof, B. S., Piel, C. F., Hansen, J., and Fudenberg, H. H. (1976). 'Serum parathyroid hormone levels and serum calcium levels from birth to senescence', *Mech. Ageing Dev.*, **5**, 289–304.

Root, A. W., and Oski, F. A. (1969). 'Effects of human growth hormone in elderly males', *J. Gerontol.*, **24**, 97–105.

Roth, G. S. (1975). 'Age-related changes in glucocorticoid binding by rat splenic leukocytes – possible cause of altered adaptive responsiveness', *Fed. Proc.*, **34**, 83–85.

Roth, G. S. (1979a). 'Hormone action during aging: Alterations and mechanisms', *Mech. Ageing Dev.*, **9**, 497–514.

Roth, G. S. (1979b). 'Hormone receptor changes during adulthood and senescence: Significance for ageing research', *Fed. Proc.*, **38**, 1910–1914.

Rubenstein, H. A., Butler, V. P., and Werner, S. C. (1973). 'Progressive decrease in serum T$_3$ with human aging: RIA following extraction of serum', *J. Clin Endocrinol. Metab.*, **37**, 347–353.

Rudman, D., Chyatte, S., Patterson, J., Gerron, G., O'Beime, I., Barlow, J., Ahmann, P., Jordan, A., and Mosteller, R. (1971). 'Observations on the responsiveness of human subjects to human growth hormone', *J. Clin. Invest.*, **50**, 1941–1949.

Ryan, N., Kovacs, K., and Ezrin, C. (1979). 'Thyrotrophs in old age. An immunocytologic study of human pituitary glands', *Endokrinologie*, **73** (2), 191–198.

Sachar, E. J., Finkelstein, J., and Hellman, L. (1971). 'Growth hormone responses in depressive illness', *Arch. Gen. Psych.*, **25**, 263–269.

Samuels, L. T. (1956). 'Effects of aging on steriod metabolism', in *Hormones and the Aging Process* (Eds E. T. Engle and G. Pincus), pp. 21–33, Academic Press, New York.

Sandberg, H., Yoshime, N., Maeda, S., Symonds, D., and Zavodnick, J. (1973). 'Effects of an oral glucose load on serum immunoreactive insulin, free fatty acid, growth hormone and blood sugar

levels in young and elderly subjects', *J. Am. Geriatr. Soc.*, **21**, 433–439.

Scapagnini, U., Canonico, P. L., Drago, F., Amico-Roxas, M., Toffano, G., Valeri, P., and Angelucci, L. (1980). 'Neuroendorinology and aging of the brain', in *The Aging Brain – Neurological and Mental Disturbances* (Eds G. Barbagallo-Sangiorgi and A. N. Exton-Smith), pp. 33–49, Plenum Press, New York.

Scheibel, M. E., Lindsay, R. D., Tomiyasu, U., and Scheibel, A. B. (1975). 'Progressive dendritic changes in aging human cortex', *Exp. Neurol.*, **47**, 392–403.

Schiebel, A. B., and Tomiyasu, U. (1978). 'Dendritic sprouting in Alzheimer presenile dementia', *Exp. Neurol.*, **60**, 1–8.

Schwartz, P., Kurucz, J., and Kurucz, A. J. (1965). 'Fluorescence microscopy demonstration of cerebrovascular and pancreatic insular amyloid in presenile and senile states', *J. Am. Geriatr. Soc.*, **13**, 199–205.

Segall, P. E., Ooka, H., Rose, K., and Timiras, P. S. (1978). 'Neural and endocrine development after chronic tryptophan deficiency in rats, I. Brain monoamine and pituitary responses', *Mech. Ageing Dev.*, **7**, 1–17.

Segall, P. E., and Timiras, P. S. (1976). 'Pathophysiologic findings after chronic tryptophan deficiency in rats: A model for delayed growth and aging', *Mech. Ageing Dev.*, **5**, 109–124.

Seifert, G. (1954). 'Zur Orthologie und Pathologie des qualitativen Inselzellbilder (nach Bensley-Terbruggen)', *Virchows Arch.*, **325**, 379–396.

Selye, H. (1950). *Stress—The Physiology and Pathology of Exposure to Stress*, Acta Inc. Medical Publishers, Montreal, Quebec.

Selye, H. (1974). *Stress without Distress*, J. B. Lippincott Co., Philadelphia.

Serio, M., Piolanti, P., Capelli, G., DeMagistris, L., Ricci, F., Anzalone, M., and Giusti, G. (1969). 'The miscible pool and turnover rate of cortisol in the aged and variations in relation to time of day', *Exp. Gerontol.*, **4**, 95–101.

Serio, M., Piolanti, P., Romano, S., DeMagistris, L., and Guisti, G. (1970). 'The circadian rhythm of plasma cortisol in subjects over 70 years of age', *J. Gerontol.*, **4**, 95–97.

Simpkins, J. W., Mueller, G. P., Huang, H. H., and Meites, J. (1977). 'Evidence for depressed catecholamine and enhanced serotonin metabolism in aging male rats: Possible relation to gonadotropin secretion', *Endocrinology*, **100**, 1672–1678.

Singer, S., Ito, H., and Litwack, G. (1973). '^{3}(H) cortisol binding by young and old human liver cytosol proteins in vivo', *Int. J. Biochem*, **4**, 569–573.

Skinner, J. S. (1973). 'Age and performance', in

Limiting Factors of Physical Performance (Ed. J. Keul), pp. 271–282, Thieme, Stuttgart.

Snyder, P. J., and Utiger, R. D. (1972). 'Response to thyrotropin releasing hormone in normal men', *J. Clin. Endocrinol. Metab.*, **34**, 1096–1098.

Stern-Nielsen, L. K., and Friis, T. (1973). 'Age dependence of thyroxine metabolism in euthyroid patients', *Ugeskr. Laeg.*, **135**, 640–644.

Stoffer, R. P., Hellwig, C. A., Welch, J. W., and McCusker, E. N. (1961). 'The thyroid gland after age 50', *Geriatrics*, **16**, 435–443.

Strandell, T. (1976). 'Cardiac output in old age', in *Cardiology in Old Age* (Eds F. T. Caird, J. L. C. Doll, and R. D. Kennedy), pp. 81–99, Plenum Press, New York.

Talwar, G. P., Hanjan, S. N., and Kidway, Z. (1976). 'Growth hormone action on thymus and lymphoid cells', in *Growth Hormone and Related Peptides* (Eds A. Pecile and E. E. Muller), Vol. 381, pp. 104–115, Exerpta Medica, Amsterdam.

Tang, F., and Phillips, J. G. (1978). 'Some age-related changes in pituitary-adrenal function in the male laboratory rat', *J. Gerontol.*, **33**, 377–382.

Taylor, A. L., Finster, J. L., and Mintz, D. H. (1969). 'Further studies of thyroid function tests in the elderly at home', *Age Ageing*, **3**, 122–125.

Taylor, B. B., Thompson, J. A., and Caird, F. I. (1974). 'Further studies of thyroid function tests in the elderly at home', *Age Ageing*, **3**, 122–125.

Thompson, R. G., Rodriguez, A., Kowarski, A., and Blizzard, R. M. (1972). 'Growth hormone: Metabolic clearance rates, integrated concentrations, and production rates in normal adults and the effect of prednisone', *J. Clin. Invest.*, **51**, 3193–3199.

Timiras, P. S. (1972). *Developmental Physiology and Aging*, Macmillan, New York.

Timiras, P. S. (1978). 'Biological perspectives on aging: In search of a master-plan', *Am. Sci.*, **66**, 605–613.

Timiras, P. S., and Bignami, A. (1976). 'A pathophysiology of the aging brain', in *Special Review of Experimental Aging Research, Progress in Biology* (Eds M. F. Elias, B. E. Eleftheriou, and P. K. Elias), pp. 351–378, EAR Inc., Bar Harbor, Massachusetts.

Timiras, P. S., Choy, V. J., and Hudson, D. B. (1981). 'Neuroendocrine pacemaker for growth, development and ageing', *Age Ageing*, **11**, 73–88.

Timiras, P. S., Cole, G., Croteau, M., Hudson, D. B., Miller, C., and Segall, P. E. (1983). 'Changes in brain serotonin with aging and modification through precursor availability' in *Aging Brain and Ergot Alkaloids* (Eds. A. Agnoli, G. Crepaldi, P. F. Spano, and M. Trabucchi), pp. 23–35, Raven Press, New York.

Timiras, P. S., and Hudson, D. B. (1980). 'Changes

in neurohumoral transmission during aging of the central nervous system', in *Neural Regulatory Mechanisms During Aging* (Eds R. C. Adelman, J. Roberts, G. T. Baker, III, S. I. Baskin, and V. J. Cristofalo), pp. 25–51, Alan R. Liss, Inc., New York.

Timiras, P. S., Hudson, D. B., and Miller, C. (1982). 'Developing and aging brain serotonergic systems', in *Molecular and Cellular Mechanisms of Aging in the Central Nervous System* (Eds G. Filogamo, E. Giacobini, G. Giacobini, and A. Vernadakis), pp. 173–184, Raven Press, New York.

Tyler F. H., Eik-Nes, K., Sandberg, A. A., Florentin, A. A., and Samuels, L. T. (1955). 'Adrenocortical capacity and the metabolism of cortisol in elderly patients', *J. Am. Geriatr. Soc.*, **3**, 79–84.

Valcana, T., and Timiras, P. S. (1969). 'Effects of hypothyroidism on ionic metabolism and Na^+K^+ activated ATP phosphohydrolase in the developing rat brain', *J. Neurochem.*, **16**, 935–943.

Vekemans, M., and Robyn, C. (1975). 'Influence of age on serum prolactin levels in women and men', *Br. Med. J.*, **4**, 738–739.

Vermeulen, A. (1978). 'Sex hormone levels in post-menopausal women: Influence of number of years since the menopause, age and weight', *J. Endocrinol.*, **77**, 2p.

Vernadakis, A., and Timiras, P. S. (Eds) (1982). *Hormones in Development and Aging*, SP Medical and Scientific Books, New York.

Vidalon, C., Khurana, R. C., Chae, S., Gigick, C. G., Stephan, T., Nolan, S., and Danowski, T. S. (1973). 'Age-related changes in growth hormone in non-diabetic women', *J. Am. Geriat. Soc.*, **21**, 253–255.

Walker, R. F., Cooper, R. L., and Timiras, P. S. (1980). 'Constant estrus: Role of rostral hypothalamic monoamines in development of reproductive dysfunction in ageing rats', *Endocrinology*, **107**, 249–255.

Walker, R. F., and Timiras, P. S. (1980). 'Loss of serotonin circadian rhythms in the pineal gland of androgenized female rats', *Neuroendocrinology*, **31**, 265–269.

Walker, R. F., and Timiras, P. S. (1981). 'Serotonin in development of cyclic reproductive function', in *Serotonin: Current Aspects of Neurochemistry and Function, Advances in Experimental Biology and Medicine*, (Eds B. Haber, S. Gabay, M. R. Issidorides, and S. G. A. Alivisatos), Vol. 133, pp. 515–539, Plenum Press, New York.

Walker, R. F., and Timiras, P. S. (1982). 'Pacemaker insufficiency and the onset of aging', in *Cellular Pacemakers* (Ed. P. Carpenter), pp. 396–425, Wiley Interscience, New York.

Weidmann, P., Myttenaere-Burisztein, S., Maxwell, M. H., and Lima, J. (1975). 'Effect of aging on plasma renin and aldosterone in normal man', *Kidney Int.* **8**, 325–333.

Weisfeldt, M. L. (Ed.) (1980). *The Aging Heart. Its Function and Response to Stress, Aging,* Vol. 12, Raven Press, New York.

Wenzel, K. W., and Horn, W. R. (1975). 'Triidothyronine (T_3) and thyroxine (T_4) kinetics in aged men', *7th International Thyroid Conference*, Abstract, Boston, Excerpta Medica, International Congress Series 361, p. 89.

Wenzel, K. W., Meinhold, H., Herpich, M., Adlkofer, F., and Schleusner, H. (1974). 'TRH-Stimulation Test mite alters-und geschlechtsabhaengigem TSG-Ansteig bei normal Personen', *Klin. Wschr.,* **52**, 721–727.

West, C. D., Brown, H., Simons, E. L., Carter, D. B., Kumagai, L. I., and Englert, E., Jr (1961). 'Adrenocortical function and cortisol metabolism in old age', *J. Clin. Endocrinol. Metab.,* **21**, 1197–1207.

Whitehouse, P. J., Price D. L., Struble, R. G., Clark, A. W., Coyle, J. T., and DeLong, M. (1982). 'Alzheimer's disease and senile dementia: Loss of neurons in the basal forebrain', *Science,* **215**, 1237–1239.

Wiske, P. S., Epstein, S., *et al.* (1979). 'Increases in immunoreactive parathyroid hormone with age', *N. Engl. J. Med.,* **25**, 1419–1421.

Wree, A., Braak, H., Schleicher, A., and Zilles, K. (1980). 'Biomathematical analysis of the neuronal loss in the aging human brain of both sexes, demonstrated in pigment preparations of the pars cerebellaris loci coerulei', *Anat. Embryol.,* **161**, 105–119.

Wrenchall, G. A., Bogoch, A. and Ritchie, R. C. (1952). 'Extractable insulin of the pancreas', *Diabetes,* **1**, 87–107.

Yamaji, T., and Ibayashi, H. (1969). 'Plasma dehydroepiandrosterone sulfate in normal and pathological conditions', *J. Clin. Endocrinol. Metab.,* **29**, 273–278.

Yamaji, T., Shimamoto, K., Ishibashi, M., Kosaka, K., and Orimo, H. (1976). 'Effect of age and sex on circulating and pituitary prolactin levels in human', *Acta. Endocriol.,* **83**, 711–719.

Ziegler, M. G., Lake, C. R., and Kopin, I. J. (1976). 'Plasma noradrenaline increases with age', *Nature,* **261**, 333–335.

Principles and Practice of Geriatric Medicine
Edited by M. S. J. Pathy
© 1985 John Wiley & Sons Ltd

3.5

Sexuality in Ageing

Ruth B. Weg

One of the glories of society is to have created woman where nature had made only a female; to have created a continuity of desire where nature thought only of perpetuating the species; and in fine, to have invented love.

Honoré de Balzac
French novelist (1799–1850)

INTRODUCTION

Balzac did not suggest that a society created only a young woman; he saw beyond reproduction and extolled the creation of a continuity of desire, and therefore potentially all life long – he put no age constraints on love. Yet the evolution of cultural values over the years has brought with it the burden of ageism. This abhorrence and fear of aging has not only assigned the wrinkled, grey elders to hidden, useless roles, not only removed them from full view and full participation in the present and future of society, but has conspired to deprive them of a part of their humanity – their sensual and sexual natures.

To be socialized from childhood forward that becoming old also means becoming sexless, unlovable, and unloving is to believe – to dread the middle and later years – and often to fulfil the predicted prophecy. With that as a beginning either older persons do not acknowledge desire and capacity or if they do, guilt may be a not so silent accompaniment. The emotional and psychological pleasures of intimacy, the delights of caress and touch, of physical closeness, and the ecstasies of inter-

course or orgasm have been reserved only for the fulsome bodies of youth and earlier adult years. Such images and assumptions continue to persist despite research to the contrary, and in face of developing recognition of elders as persons replete with acknowledged needs, desires, and capacities.

Few systematic, well controlled human sexuality studies exist and fewer still have explored sensuality/sexuality and the later years. But those inquiries that have included some old indicate that the 'sexless older person' is a myth (DeNicola and Peruzza, 1974; Friedeman, 1979; Kinsey, Pomeroy, and Martin, 1948; Kinsey *et al.*, 1953; Masters and Johnson, 1966, 1970; and Pfeiffer and Davis, 1972). Nevertheless, the more than 26.8 million people over 65 in America (Weg, 1984) remain classified essentially in the twilight zone of 'neuter' – little or no desire, capacity, or activity. This erroneous stereotype has also contaminated the thinking of a great many health professionals whose formal and informal learning have taken place within a largely Victorian context.

Change in societal attitudes and practices is, nevertheless, inevitable. Its rate and direction will be moulded by reality factors: the rapid ageing of world populations, the application of new information regarding both sexuality and ageing, and ongoing research designed by competent gerontologists and geriatricians. Old age is no longer a rare happening and is perceived as a predicted, expected stage in the last half of life. The over 65 has become the fastest growing segment of the population with every indication for a similar rate into the twenty-first century. Not only are there more than 8 per cent. more people over 65 than in early 1900s in America, but the average lifespan is approximately 27 years longer and women outnumber men (by 148 to 100). Such numbers can no longer be labelled 'special problem', and would appear to create a formidable pressure group for significant attitudinal and behavioural changes concerning the sensuality and sexuality of age.

MYTHOLOGY OF THE SEXLESS OLD

It is no accident that contemporary Western societies have not yet conferred full sexual citizenship on the old. It would appear that it was 'natural' for man and woman (as with other animals) to have sexual intercourse, as part of physical activity. With the growth of the human family through the centuries came the acceptance of marital, procreative sexuality over all other sexual activities, thus enabling the relegation of the later, barren years to asexuality. The development of Christianity is marked by the increasing idealization of celibacy and the declaration of sex as evil (Bullough, 1976; Tannahill, 1980). However, the Renaissance and the Protestant Reformation held that sex was not sinful, and there was little virtue, per se, in chastity and celibacy. Women were still largely for child bearing and the satisfaction of men's sexual desires. But the Victorian era was yet to come – the imprint of its sexual repression is still recognizable.

Victorianism – a long era of reserve, prudery, and modesty (especially among women)—began about the 1840s with remnants still vital well into the twentieth century. It was a period of apparent contradictions. The first antipornography law was passed, yet prostitution was legal. Masturbation was disapproved and identified as the culprit for a range of illnesses, including insanity (Bullough and Bullough, 1977; Tannahill, 1980). Women continued to be described as less than man, physically and cognitively, persons of little or no libido or capacity for sexual response (Haller and Haller, 1977; Masters, Johnson, and Kolodny, 1982). Moreover, virginity was expected of the female (even virgin prostitutes were in demand) and sexual athletics of the male.

Sexuality has been perceived alternately as: natural, evil; pleasurable, procreative; health and/or illness; power, weakness. . . . In recent years, other important human dimensions have been integrated with sexuality to include intimacy, love, friendship and play, caring, and it is now considered increasingly an area of personal concern and choice (Datan and Rodeheaver, 1983; Gagnon and Henderson, 1975; Gagnon and Simon, 1973). It is clear that sensual, sexual behavior is learned and that the stereotype of asexual elders is also learned. Education and other therapeutic interventions are available for unlearning and new learning (Guarino and Knowlton, 1980).

No period in human history has escaped the drive to maintain and enhance sexual capacities with alchemy, sorcery, magic, and the scores of elixirs and potions. Since the common measures of youth and immortality potential were sexual capacity and performance (Trimmer, 1970), vigour and long life have frequently been equated with sexual activity and potency. It is, therefore, understandable that society continues a multiple search that may be as old as humankind – the search for the extension of sexual potency, youth, and finally immortality. Today the magic of ginseng and gerovital has captured (for some) the imagination and hopes for the energy and passion of youth. Ageing and old are then outside of the sexual realm, perceived as the enemy – to be banished and denied.

Yet human sensuality/sexuality is more than biology of genitalia, more than procreation, intercourse, hormones, or orgasm and is a function of all that contributes to the whole man or woman at any age. It is the whole person/personality that participates in a relationship with another – not the genitalia. The whole person experiences, remembers, and desires the pleasures and pain of a relationship in which sexual expression may or may not play a major role. Indeed, the whole person, alone into the later years, still remains a sexual human being with the frustrations and hunger for affection and loving which may no longer be readily at hand. Sexual expression and the power given to it by society is, for most, young or old, a connection with vigour and life, a relationship – and a symbol of reaffirmation of self (Weg, 1980, 1981b, 1983).

It is with a sense of how and why the cruel

stereotypes of ageing and sexuality came to be that we can look at the research and the changing reality with some perspective.

RESEARCH: THE SCIENTIFIC ERA

Important legitimatization of human sexuality as an area of research and the first documentation of American sexual behaviour were the works of Kinsey and coworkers (Kinsey, Pomeroy, and Martin, 1948; Kinsey *etal*., 1953). Their massive survey produced findings which recognized – for the first time – the variation and range of human sexual behaviour among men and women. There is little doubt that this major work was crucial in the identification of normative standards of American sexual behaviour (Leiblum and Pervin, 1980; Masters, Johnson, and Kolodny, 1982). In the attempt to be dispassionate and traditionally scientific, Kinsey and coworkers chose a quantifiable entity – the number of encounters and/or orgasms consequent to a spectrum of sexual activities – self-stimulation; fellatio or cunnilingus; intercourse; homosexual, heterosexual, and/or bisexual interactions. The lack of attention to the quality and meaning of human relationships beyond the physical has continued to have negative effects on the perception of sexual older persons, their relationships and needs.

The scientific perspective was extended in the 1960s and 1970s by the pioneering inquiry of Masters and Johnson into the physiology of sexual arousal and response (Masters and Johnson, 1966, 1970). This laboratory investigation using a range of stimuli – 'masturbation, coitus with a partner, artificial coition, and stimulation of the breasts alone' (Crooks and Baur, 1980, p. 25) – was a first. A signal contribution of Masters' and Johnson's study was the unequivocal documentation of the identical, physiological nature of clitoral and vaginal female orgasms. In so doing they freed millions of women from the Freudian dogma which labelled them as childlike and/or inadequate if they failed to experience a so-called vaginal orgasm during intercourse (Leiblum and Pervin, 1980). Despite the foregoing investigations the diminished sexual image of old persists.

The best available sources related to the sexuality of later life are the longitudinal studies that document the assessment of change in mental and physical parameters over time – sexual activity included. The Duke Center for the Study of Aging and Human Development began their study in 1954, and the findings attested to the persistent social and sexual interest and capacity into the ninth decade of those elders in moderately good physical and psychological health (Pfeiffer and Davis, 1972). In addition to earlier issues of frequency of encounter and/or orgasm, longitudinal studies included questions of interest and enjoyment now and in the past. There were enquiries about intimate others or spouses – a sense of persons, their relationships and desires. For both men and women, interest, frequency, and enjoyment of sexual expression in the earlier years were good predictors of interest and activity in the later years, a finding also reported earlier by Kinsey for women in their postmenopausal years). The availability of an interested marriage partner proved to be a critical factor for older women, and health status a major variable for men. Generally, the Duke study found that women attributed cessation to their male mates (lack of libido, illness), confirmed by the men. While it is true that interest and activity decline with age – the lack of any sexual activity was generally consistent with illness of one or both of the partners, or death of a partner. A variable picture of individual male sexual activity over time was more complex than the simple decrease in sexual activity with age implies: 58 per cent. of their sample reported diminished activity or none, and 42 per cent. indicated a continuation or an increase. Among the oldest males, 78 and older, 20 per cent. still reported an increase in sexual activity (Verwoerdt, Pfeiffer, and Wang, 1969). Older women, on the other hand, were characterized by little or no sexual activity – 74 per cent.; any sustained activity and decreased activity measured 10 per cent. each, and 6 per cent. showed an increase. By 72 to 77 years of age, no women reported sustained or increasing activity and 10 per cent. showed decreasing levels (Verwoerdt, Pfeiffer, and Wang, 1969).

Although only 4.5 per cent. of the total study population were over 65, Masters' and Johnson's work unequivocally supported the earlier findings of Kinsey and coworkers, (1948, 1953) and Pfeiffer and Davis (1972). 'There is no time limit drawn by the advancing years of female sexuality', and in supportive physical and emotional situations, the male maintains 'a capacity for sexual performance that frequently may extend to and beyond the 80 year-old age level' (Masters and Johnson, 1966).

The Baltimore Longitudinal Study on Ageing (Martin, 1975) has presented data on sexual behaviour of white, married, well-educated, and urban men between the ages of 25 and 85. Although they also report a decrease in the incidence of sexual activity – 62 per cent. of men in their seventies reported coital activity and 23 per cent. between 70 and 79 years indicated masturbatory behaviour.

Data from other countries suggest that cohort similarities exist. An inquiry into the sex lives of Italian men and women between 62 and 81 years (free of disease) found 85 per cent. of males still coitally active with the expected decrease in frequency. It is encouraging that most experienced sexual satisfaction after age 60 similar to or greater than in the younger years (DeNicola and Peruzza, 1974). The older women reported less coital activity (53 per cent.), but with little difference in frequency between active men and women.

In Denmark, Hegeler (1976) found a series of steep drops in coital incidence in males from 75 to 78 per cent. in their sixties to 24 per cent. among those between 76 and 80, and continuing sharp decreases beyond 80. Masturbatory activity also diminished, but more gradually – from 60 per cent. among 51 to 55 year olds to a plateau at 21 to 23 per cent. among 80 to 95 year olds. Fewer studies have included women, but those that have also report decreases in orgasmic response and frequency of coitus. More importantly, there is repeated reference to the fact that a proportion of the decreased activity is a function of either male desire and/or illness, or the unavailability of a suitable partner (Christenson and Gagnon, 1965; Kinsey *et al.*, 1953; Masters and Johnson, 1966). The Duke study reported similar patterns – an analysis of data from all 4 interviews of 39 persons (20 male, 19 female) during a 10 year span demonstrated a decrease of sexual activity from 70 to 25 per cent. in the males and a more variable picture for females, with an increase from 16 to 21 to 25 per cent. and then a drop to 15 per cent. (Pfeiffer *et al.*, 1969).

It would appear from a number of studies (Christenson and Gagnon, 1965; Christenson and Johnson, 1973; Pfeiffer and Davis, 1972) that marital status is a significant variable in sexual activity among older women reported as highest in the married, followed by the divorced, widowed, and never married. However, women's interest in sexuality is unaffected by marriage (Verwoerdt, Pfeiffer, and Wang, 1969). On the other hand, neither sexual behaviour or interest among men are affected by marital status (Pfeiffer and Davis, 1972).

A recent survey in the United States of 800 adults between 60 and 91, living in communities in all major regions of the country, found that a majority of respondents had a strong, continuing interest in sexual expression, a belief that sexual activity is supportive to physical and mental well-being, show little embarrassment or anxiety about sexuality, and for a large number of both men and women 'sex' is better in the later years. The respondents in an earlier pilot study demonstrated by their answers (and questions) that they are not only aware of today's changing sexual behaviour but they are more comfortable with oral sex, and with sexual intimacies without the sanctity of marriage than one would have expected (Starr and Weiner, 1981).

Bretschnaider and McCoy (1983) reported data from a study of 202 men and women aged 80 to 102 years living in retirement communities in the northern California region. This, too, was a survey – using a questionnaire, self-administered and anonymous. They also found interest, continuity with past activity, and statements that the sexuality of their lives was still important.

Institutionalization does not eliminate desire and need but expression is often frustrated by embarrassed, ignorant staff and/or mechanical, inhuman rules of 'appropriate' institutional behaviour (Kassell, 1983). One attending physician reported, after 12 years among nursing home elders, that sexual desire and physical love existed in a significant number of the elderly as 'an important integral part of their lives' (West, 1975). A more recent exploration of sexuality among institutionalized aged (in 15 nursing homes in two Texas counties) confirms earlier findings and looks more specifically at the variables of sexual history, interest, attitudes, and knowledge and their relationship to sexual activity of elders in institutions (White, 1982).

Mainstream research in sexuality and age suggests the 'continuum' nature of sexual expression throughout the lifespan. Therefore, an examination of the climacteric may illuminate the sequence of changes through the middle and into the later life stages.

THE CLIMACTERIC AND BEYOND

Climacteric, for a long time, was assumed to be a 'feminine' experience, equating it with menopause, but new information has enlarged its meaning and usefulness. Climacteric is now described as a period that generally begins between 40 and 50 years with a probable duration of 5 to 10 years, and is characterized by a host of changes applicable to men and women: hormonal, circulatory, neuronal, emotional, and psychological symptoms.

The Female

The climacteric includes a gradual sequence of phases, differing in time, degree, and extent in one individual, and among women: reduced fertility, irregular menses, final cessation of menses or menopause, blood vessel instability, atrophy in genital and other systemic tissues, and hormonal changes. Body contours are generally less round and firm, muscle tone and skin elasticity diminish, affecting the appearance of limbs and abdomen.

A number of subjective symptoms are often attributed to all women, but in fact investigations suggest that the perimenopausal and menopausal experience is a highly individual one. Some women recognize minor or no changes during this period, whereas others report one or more of the following: hot flush, headache, sweating, dizziness, high blood pressure, palpitation, anxiety, nervousness, depression, appetite loss, and insomnia (Bates, 1981; Weg, 1981b). It is apparent that a number of these could have various other aetiologies unrelated to menopause, since some of the symptoms are found equally as often in younger women (McKinlay and McKinlay, 1973).

Recent research has given renewed credence to the biological base – oestrogen depletion –

of depression, anxiety, and headaches, since all were found to be hormone responsive (Dennerstein *et al.*, 1978; Durst and Maoz, 1978; Greenblatt *et al.*, 1979; Lauritzen, 1973; Durst and Maoz, 1978). There are those who maintain that these essentially emotional and psychological complaints are a response to the destructive psychosocial situation for many women in contemporary cultures (Alington-Mackinnon and Troll, 1981; Bart, 1976; Detre, Hayashi, and Archer, 1978; Neugarten and Datan, 1976; Utian, 1975; Weg, 1978). Findings from crosscultural investigations are also suggestive. In societies that reward women who reach the end of fertility, women report a very low level of symptoms (Flint, 1976). However, in societies that punish women who have outlived their youth and productivity, women describe more severe symptoms (Van Keep, 1976). Those women who have not identified totally with wife, mother, and housekeeper roles and have established additional, purposive roles (such as work) report minimal or no symptoms (Bart, 1976; Neugarten and Datan, 1976).

The Male

There is finally increasing professional acceptance of the reality of a climacteric among men. This syndrome, as with climacteric women, is not measurably expressed in all men nor is it experienced similarly by those men who describe some discomfort or troublesome changes (Albeaux-Fernet, Bohler, and Karpas, 1978; Greenblatt *et al.*, 1979; Vermuelen, Rubens and Verdonck, 1972). The group of symptoms that have been documented are variable: feelings of weakness, fatiguability, increased irritability; diminished libido, frequent loss of potency; listlessness, poor appetite, weight loss; difficulty with concentration (Henker, 1977; Kolodny, Masters, and Johnson, 1979; Weg, 1983). These are, as with menopausal associated complaints, also attributable to other causes such as anaemia, malignancy, or depression. Therefore, to isolate the male climacteric as a primary causative factor, Kolodny, Masters, and Johnson (1979) suggest diagnostic clues such as a subnormal plasma testosterone level (below 325 ng per 100 ml) and remission of the foregoing symptoms after 2 months of testosterone replacement therapy.

The hot flush, considered so characteristic of female menopause (in some women), may be absent from the male climacteric because oestrogen is maintained at a constant level, contributing to vasomotor stability (Greenblatt *et al.*, 1979).

AGEING, SEXUAL PARTNERS: PHYSIOLOGY/BEHAVIOUR

The double standard of ageing (Sontag, 1972) still exists, and sexual ageing is no exception (Weg, 1980, 1983). Middle aged and older men retain an aura of sexually attractive maturity and distinction, often into their seventies, despite flab, paunch, and greying. Many men confront their own ageing and mortality, possibly for the first time, and any small change in sexual capacity appears to bring them closer to old age and death. They may panic at the occasional episode of erectile failure or ejaculatory retardation and assume that the end of sexual vigour is close (Masters and Johnson, 1970; Weg, 1978, 1981b). Some attempt to recapture lost youth by seeking younger partners for confirmation of vitality while others accept without hope, by withdrawing from sexual activity. Other contributing factors in problematic sexual behaviour include work-a-holic behaviour, excessive drinking and eating, plus boredom with a long-time mate.

Menopausal, postmenopausal, and older women whose fertility and reproduction have come to an end are largely perceived as no longer attractive, sexy young things (Butler and Lewis, 1976). Rather, they are most frequently viewed as wrinkled, greying, neutered – lost to society as the decoration they once were. In this climate, the traditional woman, socialized for family and hearth, may find herself wanting – unlovable and unloving (Weg, 1977).

Kaplan (1974) has found that male sexuality is at a maximum at 18 to 20 years and generally declines steadily with the years. Under American socialization, female sexual responsiveness is at a low, possibly non-existent, level in the teens. Her activity peaks in her late thirties and forties and is maintained at that level into the sixth decade and beyond, depending upon opportunity and social supports. Unlike the prevailing stereotype, menopausal and postmenopausal women report heightened libido and interest, possibly as a function of unopposed testosterone in face of lowered oestrogen levels (Kaplan, 1974). Strong sexual drive of middle aged and older women persists with or without a partner. Interest in sexual expression and sexual activity of the ageing female would appear to be out of phase with those of the ageing male, creating frustrations and unmet expectations.

Physiological and affective changes with significance for sexual activity begin in the middle years and are measurable in the late years. Gradual reduction in sex hormones, alteration in anatomy and function of genital tissues and organs, and declining efficiency in the circulatory and nervous systems all contribute to changes in function with added years. There are departures from earlier patterns of responsiveness in the 4 phases of intercourse (as suggested by Masters and Johnson, 1966). Time required for lubrication, erection, and excitement is longer, and the intensity of physiological response in both men and women is diminished. Significant individual differences in the sexual system and its responses do exist (as in other organ systems).

THE OLDER WOMAN

Major anatomical and functional changes in older women result from hormonal depletion (oestrogen) and diminution of neuronal responsivity and circulatory effectiveness. A decrease in fat and glandular tissue and a reduction in elasticity and muscle tone leave breasts less full and firm and other body dimensions more angular, but do not interfere directly with sexual function. The loss of vulval tissue, reduction in the cervix, body of uterus and ovaries, and a slight decrease in size of the clitoris also have a minimal, if any, effect on responsiveness. The most significant effects on the physical and emotional well-being and sexual behaviour are those tissue and hormonal reductions that take place in the vagina and related soft tissues.

Age-related differences in the vaginal canal that are centrally involved include: length and circumference are reduced, the rugal pattern gradually smooths out, the mucosa thins, and the elasticity is decreased. Oestrogen-deficient vaginitis and reduced lubrication (both the wall 'sweating' phenomenon as well as Bartholin gland activity) are common complaints with age. Thinning, dry vaginal walls may make intromission difficult, painful (dyspareunia), and result in bleeding. Urethra and bladder undergo modest atrophy, but may complicate genital symptoms. Intercourse may stimulate burning and frequent urination in already irritated, inflamed atrophic bladder and urethra. Uterine contractions during orgasm may be spasmodic and painful rather than rhythmic and pleasurable. Therefore, coitus may be uncomfortable enough for some women to lose interest or find little satisfaction in sexual expression. However, even with hormonal replacement therapy which helps to slow the loss in elasticity and tissue and to improve lubrication, there are still normal age changes in responsivity identifiable in each of the four phases – excitement, plateau, orgasm, and resolution (Masters and Johnson, 1966, 1970; Weg, 1981b, 1983).

Time for lubrication is increased from 15 to 40 seconds to as much as 5 minutes, but is comparable to the delay in the ageing male. Vascongestion of the genital tissues is diminished. The clitoral response remains fairly intact and includes the elevation and flattening on the anterior border of the symphysis. Duration of orgasm is measurably reduced between 50 to 70 years. The spread of contractions may be similar to that of younger women, but may be spastic rather than rhythmic, and reduced from 3 to 5 to 1 or 2. Freudian wisdom contended that there were two kinds of female climax labelled the vaginal orgasm, in 'mature' women only, and the clitoral orgasm, a sign of narcissism and sexual inadequacy (Freud, 1960). As this myth prevailed, convinced that orgasm through coition (indirect stimulation of clitoris) was the only mature behaviour, most women suffered silently. However, as mentioned earlier, the Masters and Johnson (1966, 1970) research has exposed the myth. They found little or no difference in the response of the pelvic viscera to effective stimulation of the breast, clitoris, or via coition. Nevertheless, many women prefer coition because of multiple, psychological reasons. Rapid resolution, as with older men, is characteristic of female sex steroid imbalance.

Masters and Johnson (1970) found that there is 'no objective evidence to date to suggest any appreciable loss in sensate focus', largely due to the relatively intact clitoris. Although the skewed sex ratio among older men and women finds women without available opposite sex partners, the older woman remains physiologically advantaged. There is no diminution of earlier multiorgasmic capacity (Kinsey *et al.*, 1953; Martin and Johnson, 1970; Roszak, 1969). Many postmenopausal women report a heightened desire, arousability, interest, and intact activity after hysterectomy – reasonable, since fertility is separable from libido and capacity (Post, 1967).

In view of a fairly intact, sexual system and physiological competence for the physical pleasures of sexuality, why do older women experience difficulty in remaining sexual, human beings? Large numbers of average women (single or married) in their sixties or seventies may have the kind of sexual feelings for which there is no outlet – and frustration, guilt, or shame grow. It is not uncommon for presenting symptoms to include physical and psychological symptoms: headaches, back problems, bowel and vaginal concerns, insomnia, anxiety, depression, or phobias. If she is over 60 now, her psychosociosexual heritage most likely has been the 'no no's' related to the touching and enjoyment of sexual pleasures by oneself and/or with partners. Her sexuality has been appropriate only in procreation – not pleasure. She has had to live through reeducation and resocialization to put early repression behind her. Her opportunities for social intercourse and affectionate relationships with men of her own or near cohorts have diminished with the years.

If single, she is likely to outnumber the single men in her cohort (at times as high as 10 to 1) in the social situations in the community at large, at centres or nursing homes. Older widowers remarry quickly, and generally to younger women, whereas most older women who outlive men by 8 years end up alone (5.3 times as many widows as widowers). Most older men are married – 77 per cent. as compared to 38 per cent. for older women (Weg, 1981a).

If she is still married but her mate has withdrawn from sexual activity, or has become involved with other, generally younger women, or he is ill, she may be in great need. On the other hand, many an older wife may be grateful for this avoidance because she feels her wrinkled, sagging body is unlovable – she is

embarrassed, sad, and rejects physical closeness. In either circumstance she may be in starvation – for affection, touching, and release.
Masturbation, a self pleasuring and physical
outlet available to all men and women, has
become increasingly common in the older
woman, but may still be very difficult for some
to accept (Catania and White, 1982).

THE OLDER MALE

There is a fundamental difference in reproductive ageing of the older male since there is no
total cessation of fertility – spermatogenesis
may continue into the ninth decade (MacLeod
and Gold, 1953). As with the female, tissue
and hormonal changes contribute to gradual
functional changes. Muscles lose tone and
strength – sag is more evident; testes become
smaller, more flaccid; fewer viable sperm are
produced in the narrowing testicular tubules;
the prostate gland enlarges, hardens, and its
contractions grow weaker; the volume and viscosity of seminal fluid is diminished; and the
force of ejaculation decreases. Some studies
describe a gradual reduction in testosterone
levels, beginning about 10 years later than the
oestrogen fall in women; others maintain that
testosterone concentration is the same in older
men, possibly greater (Harmon and Tsitouras,
1980; Rutherford, 1956; Stearns *et al.*, 1974;
Vermeulen, Rubins, and Verdonck, 1972;
Witherington, 1974).

There is less frequent intercourse, and decrease in the intensity of sensation, speed of
reaching an erection, and the force of ejaculation. The ability to maintain an erection
longer, based on the reduction in ejaculatory
demand, fits well with the longer time needed
for the older woman to reach an appropriate
excitation level, and increases the potential for
arousal and orgasm in both. There are, however, normal age changes in each of the phases
which can be expected (Masters and Johnson,
1970; Weg, 1981b, 1983).

Excitement builds slowly and generally requires longer, direct stimulation to the penis.
Erection takes longer to attain, and the middle
aged and older male often needs more caressing and stroking, direct penile stimulation, orally or manually, to assist in reaching
engorgement and erection. Penile circumference increases during the plateau, but is

marked by the reduction or absence of pre-
ejaculatory fluid emission common in the
younger years. Orgasm is of shorter duration,
and generally there is a reduced or absent first
stage or ejaculatory demand. The second
stage, the expulsion of the seminal fluid bolus
through the penis, is completed within one or
two contractions in the older male, contrasted
with the four or more of the younger male.
The loss of erection and return of the penis to
a flaccid state may take only a few seconds
compared to the minutes or hour of the
younger male. The subsequent refractory
period may be extended from the 2 minutes of
the younger male to 12 to 24 hours.

The longer refractory period of the older
male (Masters and Johnson, 1970) is not comparable to any change in the older female and
may be particularly threatening. However,
with appropriate information, there is little
reason to view this as a deterrant to the intimacy and love making which may grow even
more meaningful as other of life's activities
decrease.

Though he is perceived in a more positive
light, he too suffers the consequences of early
socialization and ageism. If he has retired, the
worker role, a primary source of male identity
and ego support in Western societies, is generally no longer there. Sexual and emotional
difficulties appear to be frequently psychogenic
in origin rather than a function of hormonal or
other physiological changes (Notman, 1980).
As he grows older, the male continues to be
afraid of ageing, his waning attractiveness, and
the gradual changes in sexual responsiveness;
he blames boredom in a long-term relationship
for disinterest and apparent reduction in activity. Though the quality of sexual response does
change, the pattern of behaviour tends to be
part of a continuum of desire, frequency, and
enjoyment with the earlier years.

If he has been a father, parenting has also
decreased in its significance since most of the
children are out on their own. He, too, may
have experienced a difficult emotional and/or
physical time during the climacteric; nevertheless, his sexual capacities and function actually
change very little. If he is single and in his
seventies, his adult children or other relatives
may view any evidence of his sexual needs as
abnormal. For those older men who reach out
to younger women and are rebuffed, even rid-

iculed (albeit subtly), confirmation of his fears may result in depression and inadequacy in many aspects of daily living.

BARRIERS TO SEXUAL EXPRESSION

As documented earlier, normal ageing of the sexual system does leave older persons interested and able to remain effective sexual partners, but chronic disease, surgery, alcohol, and other drug abuse have been implicated in sexual difficulties. Current sophistication in medicine concerning their effects on sexual behaviour assists the practitioner in working towards prevention or modification of negative consequences.

With the years both susceptibility to and incidence of chronic disease (coronary, cerebrovascular, diabetes, pelvic, arthritis) increase. Frequently, the palliative treatment has included techniques and drugs which play havoc with libido and the capacity for erection, lubrication, and orgasm. The responsible practitioners keep this in mind and plan (with the patient) the kind of treatment that will, if possible, leave sexual potential intact.

Alcohol, marijuana, and tranquillizers all weaken erection and delay ejaculation so that their abuse adds to an already slowed sexual response – unabated use may lead to long-term impotency. Antihypertensive medication may cause erectile failure (the major side-effect), decrease in libido, and retardation in ejaculation. In addition, many hypertensive patients are convinced that in view of the illness, sexual activity may be dangerous. Beta-adrenergic blockers have also been involved with increased impotence (Kayne, 1976; Weg, 1978).

In an inquiry of 100 female diabetics, Ellenberg (1977) observed that 82 maintained normal sexual drive and orgastic capacity. Despite continued libido, sexual dysfunction can occur: in women, vaginal lubrication decreases; in men, erectile failure is the single most frequent effect, but retrograde and premature ejaculation are also found. Numerous investigators have found that 50 per cent. of the diabetic males cannot stimulate erection by masturbation or any other method (Kolodny *et al.*, 1974). Neuropathy and disturbed circulation are typical in diabetes of long duration, both intimately involved with engorgement and erection of the penis (Faerman *et al.*, 1974; Mel-

man and Henry, 1979; Weiss, 1972). Surgical techniques – implantation of penile prosthesis – in selected patients with organic impotence have been helpful in improving 'psychological and sexual status' (Finney, 1977; Schiavi, 1979; Small, 1976).

Coronary disease has resulted in frequent termination of sexuality, particularly following a myocardial infarction. For the sake of an estimated 0.6 to 0.8 per cent. of sudden coronary death during intercourse, the benefits of human warmth and sexuality are lost to many (Butler and Lewis, 1976; Hellerstein and Friedman, 1970). The therapeutic objective relates to a restoration of the pre-illness level of activity. It is important as well to educate and assure the spouse, especially to explain that the physiological cost of sexual activity is low, and thus attempt to prevent overprotection and invalidism. Generally, when the patient has recovered so that he is able to climb 1 or 2 flights of stairs or walk several blocks briskly, sexual activity can be resumed safely. At times, prophylatic nitroglycerine is recommended to avoid angina during intercourse (Wagner and Sivarajan, 1979). Recommendations to a coronary patient usually relate to cessation of smoking, reduced cholesterol and lipid intake, weight reduction, and regular, mild exercise, but rarely to sexual matters. This leaves the patient to act on hearsay, myths, and fears unless he or the clinician raise the issue. Such a lack will often result in minimization of activity or abstinence which can lead not only to frustration and a sense of invalidism, but also to marital unhappiness – none of which is good rehabilitative therapy. Women also have cardiac problems though to a significantly lesser degree. Much of the research and author commentary have been largely oriented to the male patient so that counselling for her will be fashioned (as it should be with men) on an individual case basis. Derogatis and King (1981), evaluating the concept of coital coronary and the empiric evidence that has accumulated, conclude that the evidence to date is grossly deficient. Without further research, information and advice to elders and practitioners are leavened with hearsay and impressions.

Pelvic surgery has, often without direct cause, meant an end to effective sexual activity for large numbers of older men and women. Although clinical data suggest that prostatectomies and hysterectomies appear to depress desire and orgasmic capacity, there is no indication that these are inevitable consequences of surgery (Weg, 1978, 1983). With the improvement in surgical procedures for prostate removal, blood and nerve supply are only rarely affected.

Preoperative explanation and postoperative follow-up counselling have reduced the numbers of patients who failed to return to sexual activity (Finkle and Prian, 1966) and minimized the psychological impact.

Colostomies, ileostomies, and mastectomies can also become barriers to the resumption of sexual activity. Sensitive, patient, and understanding partners and health practitioners are essential in the rehabilitation to full function. The core of the problem is body image – loss, mutilation, shame, and embarrassment. People with these surgeries consider their less than whole bodies as deformed and unlovable, and find it difficult to feel sexy and loving (Rollin, 1976). It is essential, therefore, to keep communication open to give the patient and spouse (or other family members) permission to voice their fears, concerns, and anger so that a close relationship can be reestablished. As most practitioners know, it is at such periods of major loss and depressed self-esteem that tender, loving care and open admission of fear and/or loathing are most required. Because these surgeries are usually cancer dependent, the fear of recurrence and death persists for long periods.

It has been suggested that masturbation may help preserve potency in older men and vaginal lubrication in older women. Moreover, it stimulates sexual appetite, is contributory to general well-being, and releases tensions (Masters and Johnson, 1970; Weg, 1983). Most older men have few inhibitions or barriers regarding masturbation since early socialization was likely to find this acceptable sexual behaviour. Realistically, the imbalance in the sex ratio, the preponderance of widows over widowers, and fewer social outlets suggest that for many older women masturbation may be the only means for sexual pleasure and release. Discussion of sexual feelings, and the variety of sexual behaviours that do exist for most older persons, may lead more easily to inquiry about how she perceives masturbation. Permission and encouragement may be needed, but any description of masturbation as 'must' for a healthy, sexual system is as oppressive as the negative socialization in childhood.

ALTERNATIVE SEXUAL BEHAVIOUR

Most of this discussion has concentrated on heterosexuality – the mainstream of sexual behaviour of the human family. Yet, the range of human sexual behaviour has and does include bisexuality and homosexuality. Homophobia and ignorance of homosexuality have led to well-known stereotypes, which are slowly being moderated with facts. Increasingly, health professionals perceive homosexual men and women as similar and as different from each other as are the heterosexuals (Bell and Weinberg, 1978).

Recent studies of particular homosexual communities suggest that older 'gays' and 'lesbians' fare better than earlier thought. In a study of ageing male homosexuals in Los Angeles, Kelly (1977) found that, contrary to the frequent 'youth-oriented' label, older 'gays' preferred contact with men of their own cohort and 50 per cent. reported 'satisfactory sexual lives'. Middle class older 'gays' and those who spend time in gay bars tend to be youth focused whereas working class and younger gay men are more interested in older or same-age partners (Harry and DeVall, 1978).

'Lesbians' appear to have fewer problems than 'gays' because of long-term commitment to an interpersonal relationship – they are more often involved in a longer semipermanent to permanent one (Bell, 1971). Older 'lesbians' may have a larger pool of eligible partners than older heterosexual women (Laner, 1979) in view of the skewed ratio of 100 men to 148 women in those over 65. Victorian socialization and current attitudes may continue to mimimize the possibilities for 'lesbian' and/or affectional relationships among older women and thus obviate the warmth, friendship, and support that these women can find in each other.

THE HEALTH PROFESSIONAL: CHALLENGES, OPPORTUNITIES

Factors other than those already detailed, also have their impact on the sexual system: the mental health status of self and a sexual partner, living arrangements (e.g. privacy), economics, transportation, community (people, social agencies, and physical conveniences). The clinician who wishes to be helpful would have to be aware of how all of these variables interact with each other and affect the person's sexuality. This may be especially true with patients in their later years who are frequently at risk in any number of these areas.

The health professional is in a unique position to: offer necessary sex education so that age-related normative changes in sexuality are understood, give supportive non-judgemental counsel if the situation requires it, suggest chemical or psychological therapy, and, when appropriate, supply authoritative permission for the sexual feelings that many elders have and may or may not suppress.

A good doctor–patient relationship will permit and encourage the use of preventive, educational and therapeutic approaches as needed, before and at the time men and women begin to experience any troublesome changes in the peri- or postclimacteric years. Some who have worked with older patients assign failures in sexual activity to the earlier years but 'perpetuated by defects in communication' (Glover, 1977).

The older person/patient will rarely open the visit to the office or clinic with a sexual problem. Clues to sexual concerns and/or problems may often be found in vague presenting problems and remarks, apparently unrelated to sexuality, or in rather direct, specific complaints or questions, e.g. prostate discomfort or vaginitis. The attentive listener can pursue the conversation for further information to enable appropriate assessment.

When careful physical and chemical examination yield very little in an older woman patient, the practitioner would do well to wonder if 'deliberate control, denial and repression of sexual feelings' have not produced most of the symptoms (Reenshaw, 1982).

There is every reason to enquire of such an older woman, as part of a conversation about any complaints, how comfortable or satisfying she finds the affectional/sexual part of her life. When lack of motivation, weariness, irritability, and non-specific pain continue in the older man and cannot be explained by physical and biochemical facts, he too deserves the clinician's enquiry into sexual matters. He may feel less 'manly' to have to share the facts of his problem.

Common symptoms among elders such as fatigue, apathy, headache, backache, also diminish libido and responsivity. Rather than assume they are age dependent, it seems prudent to check out physical disorders – anaemia, internal bleeding, infection, liver or kidney dysfunction. Successful treatment of any disease or illness will raise the wellness level, and the potential for sexual interest and activity. Wellness is dependent on acceptance and harmony of body, mind, and spirit. Love and loving are special mortar for the integration of these human dimensions, and kindle hope and commitment to life today and tomorrow.

Symptomology can be misread (with insufficient sexual history) and the individual may be unnecessarily medicated and/or institutionalized. Prior prerequisites for a positive patient–clinician relationship are the professional's knowledge base in human sexuality and the lifespan, comfort with his or her own sexuality, and the commitment to caring for the whole person rather than the disease alone. Those helping professionals who are unaware of gerontological research results cannot incorporate this new information into practice, and continue to deny or ignore the sexuality of the later years (Sander, 1976). Open communication with the older patient is primary and necessary to any meaningful exchange on any topic, but especially sexuality. A number of specific patient and clinician interchanges has been useful in supplying workable frameworks (Charatan, 1978; Glover, 1978; Shearer and Shearer, 1977; Wise, 1977). Collectively, they cover important considerations.

Encouragement of Discussion

The physician or other helping professional (a nurse or physician's assistant) to whom the patient comes for general health care, preventive counselling, disease treatment, or rehabilitation may have to exercise initiative in beginning a relaxed, informal discussion. If at all possible, a baseline of sexual behaviour developed before the person is old would be helpful. Whether professional or patient takes the first step, sympathetic, non-judgemental listening is in order.

History Taking

Attention to good history taking should not only provide complete past and current medical, physical, and drug status, but also psychosocial and sexual histories.

If frank pathology exists known to have particular negative consequences for sexuality, such as diabetes, hypertension, cardiac dysfunction, and various surgical procedures (colostomy, ileostomy, mastectomy, hysterectomy, prostatectomy), both emotional and physiological concerns will undoubtedly be present. Good history taking may uncover the origin of erectile failure in the male or dyspareunia in the woman – in physical, drug, psychogenic factors or a combination of age-related normal changes and pathology.

Plan: Advice, Counsel, and Action

The treatment approach will, of course, develop from the nature of the problem and person. Older persons are individuals and differ from each other as they age in sexuality as in other aspects. Only in stereotypic thinking are all aged alike – invalid, incompetent, and sexless. The real older person that you see will have a separate sexual history that calls for individual considerations. Sexual activity in the later years (as in the younger) has significance for mental and physical health status, only recently recognized among health professionals. The health professional is in a position to provide understanding management of any related problems (Masters and Johnson, 1981).

Ageism has set the stage in the last 50 years for the widespread disinterest and reluctance in treating elders for any sexual difficulty or dysfunction. Masters (1974) has called this a major disservice by the medical and behavioural professionals. At their clinic, Masters and Johnson (1966, 1970) report a 50 per cent. success rate with older couples in the restoration of satisfying sexual activity. If the general practitioner, family physician, or geriatrician is unable to help, then referral to a therapist who specializes in sexual problems is appropriate. The objective for the clinician and the older person is to maximize remaining sexual capacities and desires physiologically, psychologically, and socially.

Effectiveness and pleasure as a sexual partner among ageing men and women are at risk if there are extended periods of coital continence (whether voluntary or involuntary); continued masturbatory activity does not appear to correct for the consequences of prolonged lack of activity (Masters and Johnson, 1981). Men and women could profit from professional help in regaining potency in the male and vaginal competence in the female.

In instances where libido is depressed, where vaginal lubrication is low, and the lack of full erections are disturbing, serious consideration could be given to hormone replacement therapy for women and men. There have been disagreements about the value of testosterone therapy, yet more recent clinical studies report fair to excellent results in about 66 per cent. of patients using injectable testosterone or subcutaneously implanted pellets (Witherington, 1974). A low testosterone level (and libidinal, erectile problems) could reasonably be treated in this way. More recent studies suggest that health status rather than lowered testosterone may be the problem (Harmon and Tsitsouras, 1980; Sparrow, Bosse, and Rowe, 1980). Hormone replacement (oestrogen and progesterone) is now the more acceptable therapy for peri- and post menopausal women and would seem to have largely replaced oestrogen therapy. This treatment is effective in enhancing comfort and ability to function sexually; it reduces vasomotor instability, vaginitis, and inadequate lubrication with no excess of endometrial cancer over the incidence among those with no hormone therapy (Greenblatt, 1977; Jern, 1973; Nachtigall, 1976). This procedure has thus far not been implicated in increased risk for endometrial cancer, phlebitis, or suggested liver damage that were indicated for oestrogen use alone.

Further clinical and biochemical analyses may be called for to identify any medical condition such as prostate disorder, urinary inflammation or infection, maturity-onset diabetes, or polypharmacy (details are discussed elsewhere in this volume) which could be involved. A detailed review of postinfarct or post-surgical sexual behaviour – what is safe, what can be expected – may be desirable or necessary.

In some instances, education on normal age changes will dispel inappropriate fears of inadequacy or 'performance anxiety'. At times, just the assurance that a satisfying sexual relationship does not require a fully erect penis or an intact uterus will make the difference. Careful discussion of the particular age changes in the physiology of sexual response will correct false expectations and prevent frustration and fear when the time for responsivity grows longer and duration of orgasm shorter. There is, in fact, no diminution in the quality of sensual pleasure – and there is 'hope' in the reminder that since sexual behaviour is learned, relearning and new learning are possible at any age.

SUMMARY

Clearly, the facts document that the gradual anatomical and physiological changes in the ageing sexual system (and related systems) are insufficient to account for society's neuter stereotype or the self-imposed withdrawal from sexual activity by older persons.

The clinical and social research suggest that the most destructive, limiting barrier to sexual activity in the later years is not the real but gradual decrease in physiological capacities and behaviour but the negative, societal feedback concerning sexuality in the last half of life.

Self-esteem and confidence, attributes that nurture love of self and others, are already at risk since investment in work, parenting, and community roles diminish (or are effectively eliminated). Any additional assault heightens the sense of loss and inadequacy. Because of shrinking life's experiences, there may be even greater need for enhancement of caring, loving relationships (Weg, 1978, 1980, 1983).

Research in the first half of this century established sexuality as an area of scientific enquiry, with major emphasis on the physical dimensions of orgasm, intercourse, and masturbation. These have been the important, reportable behaviours among old and young and have served to minimize the affectional, sensual, and relationship qualities that endow human sexual expression with meaning beyond release. This genital emphasis continues, exacerbated by many current therapy programmes and countless 'how to' illustrated pamphlets and manuals, largely technique-focused, and directed to the eradication of physical, sexual dysfunction and the insurance of orgasm.

What has been generally ignored or minimally discussed are the nature and significance of interpersonal relationships in the later years. Little attention has been given to the differences in the meaning of friendship with time, in changing love patterns. The importance of affection and intimacy in the same sex and different sex relationships among elders is only now beginning to appear in the literature (Kelly, 1977; Marmor, 1980; Money, 1980; Parron and Troll, 1978; Reedy, 1978; Saflios-Rothschild, 1977; Weiss, 1983).

What has been considered too minor or too difficult to study are the qualities of interactions among older persons – the companionable, supportive, and happy liaisons with or without intercourse. Unnoticed are gentle, but often lifegiving, connections – the holding and touching, hand in hand, arm in arm, and the caring for one another (Butler and Lewis, 1976). Overlooked are the continuing 'sexual dreams, hopes and fantasies' of older men and women (Reenshaw, 1982). What of the emotional and physical starvation of many lonely older women, who in keeping with their early Victorian socialization, confront the present and the future alone and abstinent, without hope of contact or warmth?

For persons old today, there is another limiting factor that sex education for the middle and later years could easily eliminate – ignorance – which breeds dysfunction, anxiety, despair, and withdrawal. This ignorance extends into many areas: the individuality and diversity of sexual interest and behaviour among older persons, the importance of sensitivity to one's partner's needs and comfort with one's own needs, those changes that do take place, possible adaptations for satisfactory sexual activity in the face of disease, ways to revitalize longtime relationships, and how to love again.

Older persons are also frustrated in their sexual behaviour by anxious middle aged offspring and unknowing health professionals who deny that sexuality is lifelong, and see active, interested elders as abnormal. Removing this imposed barrier entails a widespread change in perspective and specific attitudes concerning human sexuality and especially the sexuality of the later years.

And, finally, limitations can be mollified by

the concern and guidance of the primary health care professional who has discarded the stereotypes of age and the sexless old, who is prepared to relate to the whole person and his/her sexuality as part of that wholeness, and who is prepared to be non-judgemental and accepting of diverse needs and behaviours. There is a caution to be exercised so that society and health professionals avoid a new stereotype which establishes the 'older sexual athlete' as the model elder, recognized by the same drives, passions, and behaviours of the earlier years. This mythology would be equally confining, damaging, and inhibiting, removing the options for sexual behaviour, the birthright of every person.

It is inescapable that, for most elders, sexuality in the later years is not the same as in youth, but few realities are. Impressive is the realization that most people are interested and able to remain sexual human beings into the ninth and tenth decades. Butler (1975) suggests that as with other aspects of ageing, sexuality has a developmental potential: 'new insights and new levels of feeling during a lifetime of lovemaking' are or can be acquired. He discussed two languages of sex: one is more direct and explosive and is the orgasmic communication that has been counted, measured, and specified; the other is an experential language and involves caressing, touching, and tenderness. Both languages may be learned and practised early in life, yet the first language is more typical of youth and the second associated with later life. Freedom from the mythology and power that have been identified with sexuality would support the use of both languages for lifespan sexual expression.

There are thousands of ways to love and be loved – there must be one or more that fits best with each person/personality at every stage of life. Heightened awareness and commitment of health care professionals, changing media images of age, and improving self-esteem among elders themselves are welcome signs in the breakdown of ageism, and the creation of a positive social environment in which people will want to love, growing old and alive.

'If you would be loved, love and be lovable.'
Benjamin Franklin (1706–1790)

REFERENCES

Albeaux-Fernet, M., Bohler, C. S. S., and Karpas, A. E. (1978). 'Testicular function in aging male', in *Geriatric Endocrinology Aging*, Vol. 5, p. 201 (Ed. R. B. Greenblatt), Raven Press, New York.

Alington-Mackinnon, D., and Troll, L. E. (1981). 'The adaptive function of the menopause: A devil's advocate position', *J. Am. Geriatrics Soc.*, **XXIX**(8), 349–353.

Bart, P. (1976). 'Depression in middle aged women', in *Female Psychology: The Emerging Self* (Ed. S. Cox), Science Research Associates Inc., Chicago, Illinois.

Bates, G. (1981). 'On the nature of the hot flash', *Clin. Obst. Gynecology*, **24**(1), 231–241.

Bell, A. P., and Weinberg, M. S. (1978). *Homosexualities: A Study of Diversity Among Men and Women*, Simon and Shuster, New York.

Bell, R. R. (1971). *Social Deviance*, Dorsey Press, Homewood, Illinois.

Bretschaider, J., and McCoy, N. (1983). *Sexual Attitudes and Behavior among Healthy 80–102 Year Olds*, Paper presented at Sixth World Congress of Sexology, Washington, DC., 22–27 May 1983.

Bullough, V. L. (1976). *Sexual Variance in Society and History*, Wiley, New York.

Bullough, V., and Bullough, B. (1977). *Sin, Sickness, and Sanity*. New American Library, New York.

Butler, R. N. (1975). 'Sex after 65', in *Quality of Life: The Later Years* (Eds L. E. Brown and E. O. Lewis), The American Medical Association, Publishing Sciences Group, Inc., Action, Maryland.

Butler, R. N.. and Lewis, M. I. (1976). *Sex After Sixty*. Harper and Row Publishers, New York.

Catania, J. A., and White, C. B. (1982). 'Sexuality in an aged sample: Cognitive determinants of masturbation,' *Arch. Sexual Behaviour* **11**, 237–245.

Charatan, F. B. (1978). 'Sexual function in old age', *Med. Aspects of Human Sexuality*, **12**(9), 150–164.

Christenson, C. V., and Gagnon, J. H. (1965). 'Sexual behavior in a group of older women', *J. Gerontol*, **20**, 351–356.

Christenson, C. V., and Johnson, A. B. (1973). 'Sexual patterns in a group of older never-married women', *J. Geriatric Psychiatry*, **6**, 80–98.

Crooks, R., and Baur, K. (1980). *Our Sexuality*, p. 433, The Benjamin-Cummings Publishing Co., Inc., Menlo Park, California.

Datan, N., and Rodeheaver, D. (1983). 'Beyond generativity: Toward a sensuality of later life', in *Sexuality in the Later Years: Roles and Behavior* (Ed. R. B. Weg), pp. 279–288, Academic Press, New York.

DeNicola, P., and Peruzza, M. (1974). 'Sex in the aged', *J. Am. Geriatrics Soc.*, **XXII**,380–382.

Dennerstein, L., Laby, B., Burrows, G. D., and Hyman, G. T. (1978). 'Headaches and sex hormone therapy', *Headache*, **18**, 146.

Derogatis, L. R., and King, K. M. (1981). 'The coital coronary: A reassessment of the concept', *Arch. Sexual Behaviour*, **10**, 325–335.

Detre, T., Hayashi, T., and Archer, D. F. (1978). 'Management of the menopause', *Ann. Intern. Med.*, **88**, 373.

Durst, N., and Maoz, B. (1978). *The Effect of Estrogen Therapy on the Psychic State and Social Adaptation of Post Menopausal Women*, Paper read at the Second International Congress of Menopause, Jerusalem, June 1978.

Ellenberg, M. (1977). 'Sexual aspects of female diabetic', *Mt. Sinai J. Med. N.Y.*, **44**, 495–500.

Faerman, I., Glocer, L., Fox, D., Jadzinksy, M. (1974). N., and Rappaport, M. 'Impotence and diabetes. Histological studies of the autonomic nervous fiber of the corpora cavernosa in impotent, diabetic males', *Diabetes*, **23**, 971–976.

Finkle, A., and Prian, D. V. (1966). 'Sexual potency of elderly men before and after prostatectomy', *JAMA.*, **196**, 139–143.

Finney, R. P. (1977). 'New hinged silicone penile implant', *J. Urol.*, **118**, 585–587.

Flint, M. (1976). 'Cross-cultural factors that affect age of menopause', in *Consensus on Menopause Research* (Eds. P. A. Van Keep, R. B. Greenblatt, and M. Albeaux-Fernet), University Park Press, Baltimore, Maryland.

Freud, S. (1960). *The Letters of Sigmund Freud* (Ed. E. L. Freud), Basic Books, New York; originally published 1935.

Friedeman, J. S. (1979). 'Sexuality in older persons', *Nursing Forum*, **XVIII**,(1), 92–101.

Gagnon, J. H., and Henderson, B. (1975). *Human Sexuality: An Age of Ambiguity*, Social Issues Series No. 1, Educational Associates, division of Little, Brown and Co., Boston, Massachusetts.

Gagnon, J., and Simon, W. (1973). *Sexual Conduct: The Social Sources of Human Sexuality*, Aldine, Chicago, Illinois.

Glover, B. H. (1977). 'Disorders of sexuality and communication in the elderly', *Comprehensive Therapy*, **3**(6), 21–25.

Glover, B. H. (1978). 'Sex counseling', in *The Geriatric Patient* (Ed. W. Reichel), pp. 125–133, HP Publishing Co., Inc., New York.

Greenblatt, R. B. (1977). 'Estrogens in cancer change the way you treat post menopausal patients', *Mod. Med*, Mar. **1977**, 47.

Greenblatt, R. B., Nezhat, C., Roesel, R. A., and Natrajan, P. K. (1979). 'Update on the male and female climacteric', *J. Am. Geriatrics Soc.*, **XXVII**(11), 481.

Guarino, S. C., and Knowlton, C. N. (1980). 'Planning and implementing a group health program on sexuality for the elderly', *J. Gerontol. Nursing*, **6**, 600–603.

Haller, J. S., and Haller, R. M. (1977). *The Physician and Sexuality in Victorian America*, Norton, New York.

Harmon, S. M., and Tsitouras, P. D. (1980). 'Reproductive hormones in aging men', *J. Clin. Endocrinol. Metab.*, **51**(1), 35–40.

Harry, J., and DeVall, W. (1978). 'Age and sexual culture among homosexually oriented males', *Arch. Sex Behav.* **7**, 199.

Hegeler, S. (1976). *Sexual Behavior in Elderly Danish Males*, Paper presented at International Symposium on Sex Education and Therapy, Stockholm, Sweden.

Hellerstein, H. K., and Friedman, E. H. (1970). 'Sexual activity in the post-coronary patient', *Arch. Intern. Med.*, **125**, 987–999.

Henker, F. O., III. (1977). 'A male climacteric syndrome: Sexual, psychic, and physical complaints in 50 middle aged men', *Psychosomatics*, **18**(5), 23.

Jern, H. Z. (1973). *Hormone Therapy of Menopause and Aging*, Charles C. Thomas, Springfield, Illinois.

Kaplan, H. S. (1974). *The New Sex Therapy*, Brunner-Mazel, New York.

Kassel, V. (1983). 'Long term care institutions', in *Sexuality in the Later Years: Roles and Behavior*, (Ed. R. B. Weg), pp. 167–184, Academic Press, New York, 1983.

Kayne, R. C. (1976). 'Drugs and the aged', in *Nursing and the Aged* (Ed. J. M. Burnside), pp. 436–451, McGraw-Hill.

Kelly, J. (1977). 'The aging male homosexual: Myth and reality', *Gerontologist*, **17**, 328–443.

Kinsey, A. C., Pomeroy, W. B., and Martin, C. I. (1948). *Sexual Behavior in the Human Male*, W. B. Saunders, Philadelphia, Pennsylvania.

Kinsey, A. C., Pomeroy, W. B., Martin, C. I., and Gebhard, P. H. (1953). *Sexual Behavior in the Human Female*, W. B. Saunders, Philadelphia, Pennsyvania.

Kolodny, R. C., Kahn, C. B., Goldstein, H. H., and Barnett, D. M. (1974). 'Sexual dysfunction in diabetic men', *Diabetes*, **23**, 306–309.

Kolodny, R. C., Masters, W. H., and Johnson, V. E. (1979). *Textbook of Sexual Medicine*, Little, Brown and Co., Boston, Massachusetts.

Laner, M. R. (1979). 'Growing older female: Heterosexual and homosexual', *J. Homosexuality*, **4**(3), 267.

Lauritzen, C. (1973). 'The management of the pre-menopausal and post-menopausal patient', *Frontiers Hormone Research*, **2**, 2.

Leiblum, S. R., and Pervin, L. (1980). *Principles*

and Practice of Sex Therapy, Guildford Press, New York.

MacLeod, J., and Gold, R. Z. (1953). 'The male factor in fertility and infertility: VII. Semen quality in relation to age and sexual activity', *Fertility and Sterility*, **4**, 194–209.

McKinlay, S., and McKinlay, J. (1973). 'Selected studies on the menopause.' *J. Biosocial Sci.*, **5**, 533–555.

Marmor, J. (Ed.) (1980). *Homosexual Behavior*, Basic Books, New York.

Martin, C. E. (1975). 'Marital and sexual factors in relation to age, disease and longevity', in *Life History Research in Psychopathology* (Eds R. D. Wirt, G. Winokur, and M. Roff), Vol. 4, pp. 326–347, University of Minnesota Press, Minneapolis, Minnesota.

Masters, W. H. (1974). 'From remarks at a meeting', Reported in *Los Angeles Times,* 4 May, 1974.

Masters, W. H., and Johnson, V. (1966). *Human Sexual Response*, p. 223, Little, Brown and Co., Boston, Massachusetts.

Masters, W. H., and Johnson, V. (1970). *Human Sexual Inadequacy*, p. 337, Little, Brown and Co., Boston, Massachusetts.

Masters, W. H., and Johnson, V. E. (1981). 'Sex and the aging process', *J. Am. Geriatrics Soc.*, **XXIX**(9), 385–390.

Masters, W. H., Johnson, V. E., and Kolodny, R. C. (1982). *Human Sexuality*, p. 337, Little, Brown and Co., Boston, Massachusetts.

Melman, A., and Henry, D. (1979). 'The possible role of the catecholamines of the corpora in penile erection', *J. Urol.*, **121**, 419–421.

Money, J. (1980). *Love and Love Sickness*, The John Hopkins University Press, Baltimore, Maryland.

Nachtigall, L. (1976). 'Behind the estrogen-cancer headline' *Medical World News*, **17**, 39.

Neugarten, B., and Datan, N. (1976). 'The middle years', *J. Geriatr. Psychiat.*, **9**(1), 45.

Notman, M. (1980). 'Adult life cycles', in *The Psychobiology of Sex Differences and Sex Roles* (Ed. J. Parsons), Hemisphere Publishing Co., Washington, DC.

Parron, E. M., and Troll, L. E. (1978). 'Golden wedding couples: Effects of retirement on intimacy in long standing marriages', *Alternative Lifestyles*, **1**(4), 447–464.

Pfeiffer, E., and Davis, G. C. (1972). 'Determinants of sexual behaviour in middle and old age', *J. Am. Geriatrics Soc.*, **20**, 151.

Pfeiffer, E., Verwoerdt, A., and Wang, H. S. (1970). 'Sexual behavior in aged men and women', in *Normal Aging* (Ed E. Palmore), pp. 229–303, Duke University Press, Durham.

Post, F. (1967). 'Sex and its problems', *Practitioner*, **199**, 377.

Reedy, M. N. (1978). 'What happens to love? Love, sexuality and aging', in *Sexuality and Aging* (Ed. R. Solnick), rev. ed., p. 184, Andrus Gerontology Center, University of Southern California Press, Los Angeles, California.

Reenshaw, D. C. (1982). 'Sex and older women', *Med. Aspects of Human Sexuality*, **16**(1), 132–139.

Rollin, B. (1976). *First, You Cry*, J. B. Lippincott, Philadephia, Pennsyvania.

Roszak, B. (1969). 'The human continuum', in *Masculine/Feminine* (Eds. B. Roszak and T. Roszak), p. 305, Harper and Row, New York.

Rutherford, R. N. (1956). 'The male and female climacteric', *Postgraduate Med.*, **50**, 125.

Saflios-Rothschild, C. (1977). *Love, Sex and Sex Roles*, Prentice-Hall, Englewood Cliffs, New Jersey.

Sander, F. (1976). 'Aspects of sexual counseling with the aged', *Social Casework*, **57**(8), 504–510.

Schiavi, R. C. (1979). 'Sexuality and medical illness, specific reference to diabetes', in *Human Sexuality: A Health Practitioner's Text* (Ed. R. Green), pp. 203–212, Williams and Wilkins Co., Baltimore, Maryland.

Shearer, M. R., and Shearer, M. L. (1977). 'Sexuality and sexual counseling in the elderly', *Clin. Obst. Gyn.*, **20**(1), 197–208.

Small, M. P. (1976). 'Small-carrion penile prosthesis', *Mayo Clin. Proc.*, **51**, 336–338.

Sontag, S. (1972). 'The double standard of aging', *Sat. Rev.*, **55**, 29–38.

Sparrow, D., Bosse, R., and Rowe, J. W. (1980). 'The influence of age, alcohol consumption and body build on gondal function in man', *J. Clin. Endocrinol. Metab.,* **51**, 508–512.

Starr, B. D., and Weiner, M. B. (1981). *The Starr-Weiner Report on Sex and Sexuality in the Mature Years*, McGraw-Hill, New York.

Stearns, E. L., MacDonnell, J. A., Kaufman, B. J., Padua, R., Lucman, T. S., Winter, J. S. D., and Faiman, C. (1974). 'Declining testicular function with age: hormonal and clinical correlates', *Am. J. Med.* **57**, 761–766.

Tannahill, R. (1980). *Sex in History*, Stein and Day, New York.

Trimmer, E. J. (1970). *Rejuvenation, The History of An Idea*. A. S. Barnes and Co., Inc., Cranberry, New Jersey.

Utian, W. H. (1975). 'Definitive symptoms of post menopause incorporating use of vaginal parabasal cell index', *Front. Horm. Res.*, **3**, 74.

Van Keep, P. A. (1976). 'Psychosocial aspects of the climacteric', in *Consensus on Menopause Research* (Eds. P. A. Van Keep, R. B. Greenblatt, and M. Albeaux-Fernet), p. 6, University Park Press, Baltimore, Maryland.

Vermuelen, A., Rubens, R., and Verdonck, L. (1969). 'Testosterone secretion and metabolism in male senescence.' *J. Clin. Endocrinol. Metab.* **34**:730–735, 1972.

Verwoerdt, A., Pfeiffer, E., and Wang, H. S. (1969). 'Sexual behavior in senescence. II. Patterns of sexual activity and interest', *Geriatrics*, **24**, 137–154.

Wagner, N. N., and Sivarajan, E. S. (1979). 'Sexual activity and the cardiac patient', in *Human Sexuality* (Ed. R. Green), pp. 193–200, Williams and Wilkins Co., Baltimore, Maryland.

Weg, R. B. (1977). 'More than wrinkles', in *Looking Ahead: A Woman's Guide to the Problems and Joys of Growing Older* (Eds. L. E. Troll, J. Israel, and K. Israel), p. 22, Prentice-Hall, Inc., Englewood Cliffs, New Jersey.

Weg, R. B. (1978). 'Drug interaction with the changing physiology of the aged: Practice and potential', in *Drugs and the Elderly* (Ed. R. C. Kayne), pp. 103–142, Andrus Gerontology Center, University of Southern California Press, Los Angeles, California.

Weg, R. B. (1980). 'The physiology of sexuality in aging', in *Sexuality and Aging* (Ed. R. Solnick), pp. 48–65, University of Southern California Press, Los Angeles, California.

Weg, R. B. (1981a). *The Aged: Who, Where, How Well*, Gerontology Center, Leonard Davis School of Gerontology, Los Angeles, California.

Weg, R. B. (1981b). 'Normal aging changes in the reproductive system', in *Nursing and the Aged* (Ed. J. M. Burnside), pp. 362–373, McGraw-Hill, New York.

Weg, R. B. (1983). 'The physiological perspective', in *Sexuality in the Later Years: Roles and Behavior* (Ed. R. B. Weg), pp. 40–80, Academic Press, New York.

Weg, R. B. (1984). 'Selective characteristics of the aging in the United States', in *Retirement Preparation* (Ed. H. Dennis), pp. 7–28, Lexington Books, Lexington, Maryland.

Weiss, H. D. (1972). 'The physiology of human penile erection', *Ann. Intern. Med.*, **76**, 793–799.

Weiss, L. (1983). 'Intimacy and adaptation', in *Sexuality in the Later Years: Roles and Behavior* (Ed. R. B. Weg), pp. 147–166, Academic Press, New York.

West, N. D. (1975). 'Sex in geriatrics: Myth or miracle?', *J. Am. Geriatrics Soc.*, **XXIII**(12), 551.

White, C. B. (1982). 'Sexual interest, attitudes, knowledge and sexual history in relation to sexual behavior in the institutionalized aged', *Arch. Sexual Behavior*, **11**, 11–21.

Wise, T. N. (1977). 'Sexuality in chronic illness', *Primary Care*, **4**(1), 199–208.

Witherington, R. (1974). 'The controversial male climacteric', in *Clinician: Male and Female: An Endocrine Update* (Ed. L. Mastroiana), Medcom Press, New York.

4

Preventive Aspects
of Geriatric Medicine

4.1

Preventive Aspects of Geriatric Medicine

J. Williamson

The dramatic triumphs of preventive medicine in the late nineteenth and early twentieth centuries arguably represent the greatest boon that medicine will ever make to mankind. The public health measures of that epoch were directly responsible for the control of pandemic and epidemic communicable diseases and thus have been directly responsible for the 'geriatric problem' of today through ensuring that a large majority were able to live out their normal life span.

Despite this record of remarkable achievement, preventive medicine today is a neglected topic and often little more than lip service is paid to it in undergraduate and specialist training. An obvious example is the contrast between the money and resources (including some of the most highly trained doctors) which are spent upon investigation and treatment of ischaemic heart disease and the relative neglect and lack of interest in its prevention. There is evidence recently that this imbalance is being noted and voices are now raised in proclaiming the importance of preventive medicine (Department of Health and Social Security, 1976).

Prevention in old age suffers the extra disadvantage that it is widely assumed that physical, mental, and social deterioration are inescapable and hence nothing can be (or even should be) done about them. Nothing could be further from the truth and it becomes clearer year by year that in this field rests the best hope of containing, in a humane and economical way, the rising demands from ageing populations.

Any effective modern geriatric service therefore must possess a firm commitment to prevention in the widest sense. This implies not merely prevention of disease but also the prevention and limitation of disability and the promotion of better health. This enables old people to age with greater independence, satisfaction, and happiness. Nor is this effort to be confined to the individual old person but it must be extended to include the whole family. This involves the spouse where the patient is married and in all cases the supporting daughter or daughter-in-law. A well supported family, sensibly informed of the nature of the elderly patient's condition and assured of appropriate and timely help in meeting his or her needs, will continue to function much more effectively and for a longer time than a family denied such support.

This approach, of course, necessitates close collaboration with other services, especially primary medical care and social services. Indeed, the effective collaboration of services by itself possesses a powerful preventive potential.

CLASSIFICATION OF PREVENTION

Prevention may be divided into primary, secondary, and tertiary stages (Morris, 1975).

Primary Prevention

In its purest form, this means 'true' prevention, i.e. the eradication of disease as by ensuring proper diet as a means of elimination of malnutrition or by isolation of infectious cases and immunisation of populations in the control of such conditions as poliomyelitis and smallpox.

The Place of Immunization in the Elderly

As has been pointed out elsewhere in this volume (see Chapter 3.2), immune competence declines in old age and old patients are thus more prone to infection. Their infections also tend to be more severe, more likely to be fatal, to lead to delay in recovery, or to a permanent reduction in the level of functioning. The value of immunization must thus be considered.

The infection which regularly afflicts communities and may have serious consequences is influenza and effective immunization is now available. Should this be used more widely among the elderly? Most people argue that there is a case for influenza immunization in some institutional populations because of the high risk of epidemics within such closed communities. The indication for immunization would be an approaching epidemic. For it to be effective the strain of influenza virus should be known, the appropriate vaccine must be available, and the immunization must be given several weeks before exposure to allow the required level of humoral immunity to develop. Polyvalent pneumococcal vaccines may also be of use in limiting the spread of infection in an institution (Craig and Shang, 1981; Fiumara and Waterman, 1979).

Immunization of the staff of institutions caring for older people is equally, if not more, important. While there may be debate about the advisability of keeping the 'old man's friend' at bay in old people whose lives are nearing their end and for whom there is little but unhappiness left, there can be no doubt that reducing staffing levels (especially nursing staff) in these institutions through illness can only lead to considerable increase in misery for the residents.

In the field of chronic disease, primary prevention is a complex problem involving many factors. There may be a genetic predisposition, as in some cancers, ischaemic heart disease, and even in some forms of dementia. Environmental factors are important as in the case of atmospheric pollution and dust as a cause of chronic respiratory disease and behavioural factors can be a principal cause, as in cigarette smoking and other forms of unhealthy life style.

Thus, some of the main disabling conditions in old age may have their origins in much earlier life and primary prevention must be focused upon younger groups in the population. Unhealthy dietary habits in old age are often a continuation of similar habits in youth so that mothers should be told that by encouraging proper diet in their children they will contribute to the better health of future generations of old people.

Healthy exercise is no less important to the older person than it is for the young and middle aged and studies have shown that the body composition of those elderly who have continued to exercise regularly conforms much more closely to the 'ideal' than that of those who do not exercise (Tanner, 1964). It is, of course, difficult to prove conclusively that the better physique of those who continue to exercise regularly into old age is due entirely to such exercise since these individuals tend to be much more health conscious in other respects and hence less likely to smoke or drink to excess (Shephard, 1977).

What is, however, now beyond dispute is that, even in old age, it is possible to improve fitness and exercise tolerance by careful training regimes (see Chapter 28). A recent Swedish study showed that after a 12-week course of thrice-weekly physical training, 70 year old healthy men showed significant improvements in fitness compared to matched controls. They showed a 26 per cent increase in maximum oxygen uptake, lower heart rates on submaximal exercise, and marked increase in muscle strength. In addition, needle biopsy of thigh muscle before and after the training showed a significant increase in the proportion of type one muscle fibres (Aniansson *et al.* 1980).

Further encouragement comes from experiments which have shown that similar measurable improvements may be induced in mental and social function. Tests of cognitive function were carried out before and after training in 'figural relations' among elderly subjects. Test subjects showed significant improvements in function compared to controls and this lasted for at least 4 months (Plemons, Willis, and Baltes, 1978). Similar results in the improvement of memory were claimed by Langer and

Rodin (1976) after attempts to secure mental arousal among elderly nursing home residents. The same research showed that when elderly residents were offered more choice over their life styles and more control of their environments, they became more active, interested, and involved (Langer *et al.*, 1979).

There is a strong inference that some of the losses in physical, mental, and social function which are commonly observed in old age are not the result of ageing or disease but simply of disuse. The disuse is related to the prevalent negative and defeatist stereotype of old age. Further research is clearly needed to confirm these findings and to indicate how these experiments may best be translated into improved management of the elderly.

Screening for Precursors of Disease (Risk Factors)

Within the scope of primary prevention is the search for precursors of disease (or screening for risk factors) in asymptomatic individuals. Commonly sought precursors of disease are hypertension, hypercholesterolaemia, raised intraocular tension, and cervical metaplasia (by taking cervical smears). Once screening of this sort was introduced a number of centres were set up where 'multiphasic screening' could be carried out. Healthy people were encouraged to go to these centres (and their employers to send them) for electrocardiograms, chest X-rays, and a wide range of investigations including blood and urine testing for a variety of components. Few studies have been done to assess the value of multiphasic screening but one of the best designed trials failed to show benefits in morbidity or mortality in screened subjects as compared to controls. There was no reduction in use of health or social services as a result of screening (South-East London Screening Study Group, 1977). Largely as a result of this study multiphasic screening within the National Health Service in the United Kingdom has not been encouraged. The South-East London investigation involved middle aged subjects (45 to 64 years) and it may be assumed that similar procedures in an older group would be unlikely to prove any more rewarding – the probability is that they would be much less useful.

Despite these negative findings pleas continue to be made for the detection of risk factors among the elderly, especially in relation to hypertension which has been shown in younger groups to be closely related to ischaemic heart disease and stroke. The Framingham Study has shown that the adverse results of raised systolic or diastolic pressure appeared to be continued in the age group 64 to 75 and so a strong plea has been made for the discovery of hypertension and its effective treatment even in older patients (Kannel, McGee, and Gordon, 1976). The force of this argument has recently been blunted by the article by Oliver (1982). He cautions using drugs to 'correct' a risk factor since only a minority with such characteristics will develop the feared consequence, whether it be myocardial infarction or stroke. The risks of use of such drug treatment on a wide scale are considerable and for the majority of those with risk factors who will not develop the 'consequence', these drug risks are unwarranted and therefore may be unacceptable. It is also stated that 'aggressiveness in the use of these drugs should be inversely proportional to age' and it is certain that those involved in the clinical medicine of old age will endorse this statement. Two recent prospective studies from the United Kingdom have failed to show a significant relationship between raised blood pressure and morbidity or mortality from stroke or heart disease in older subjects (Evans, Prudham, and Wandless, 1980; Milne, 1981).

The present situation as regards drug treatment for hypertension in the elderly (without symptoms directly related to raised blood pressure) accords with the sound Scots legal verdict of 'not proven'. The alert physician will continue to weigh up the advantages and disadvantages for individual patients, including the considerable risks of postural hypotension and even the precipitation of stroke through overzealous reduction of raised blood pressure in individuals whose autoregulatory control of cerebral perfusion is impaired (Wollner *et al.*, 1979).

Secondary Prevention

This implies the earlier detection of disease thus affording a better chance of curing or at least halting its progression. In this way the prevalence of disease and its severity in the community may be reduced. Early diagnosis is the basis of good clinical medicine and it is highly relevant to the problems of ageing societies. The indentification of early features of disease requires better education in gerontology and geriatric medicine for medical students and postgraduates, especially for those who plan to become general practitioners. All doctors must be able to recognize both the manifestations of normal ageing and of the presentation of disease in old age so that the two are not confused. The frequency of multiple pathology and atypical presentation must be realized.

Likewise, doctors and nurses should be alive to the frequency with which social stress may present in old age with somatic symptoms which may vary from headaches, insomnia, and anorexia to complaints of giddiness and dysponea. Failure to suspect the psychosomatic basis of these conditions may mean that the doctor will prescribe a medication (often a psychotropic drug). The patient cannot possibly benefit from such irrational therapy and is at risk rom adverse reactions. In addition, if the underlying psychosocial factor is not detected, there will be scant chance of alleviating it.

Tertiary Prevention

This is the detection of established disease and disability in patients who are not receiving appropriate treatment and support. This may reduce the risk or speed of deterioration, of relapse, and of complication: overall disability in a community may also be reduced, leading to a corresponding reduction in dependency among the elderly.

In the elderly in whom chronic and multiple diseases are the rule, there is less sharp distinction between secondary and tertiary prevention. Both become a matter of effective case finding with a view to the earlier detection of conditions which have progressed to disability, or may do so.

In younger patients there are forces which influence the patient to report his or her health problems, and thus to obtain investigation and treatment. The man may feel that his earning capacity will be threatened and the woman fears that her role as mother and family manager (plus, increasingly, her earning capacity) is endangered. These forces are weaker in old age since there is now no job for the man and the elderly widow has lost her previous roles as mother, wife, and manager. Very old people also may have formulated their ideas of appropriate use of health services prior to the provision of a comprehensive 'free' Health Service and they simply do not understand the need to report disabling conditions to their doctors. Whatever are the reasons, it is well known that elderly people tend to be slow to report their disabilities and it is still quite common to find old people with well-established conditions who have made no effort to see their doctor. The fact that some doctors may be rather ignorant of their problems and dismiss their symptoms with remarks such as 'What can you expect at your age?' does not encourage these reluctant old people to come forward. They may also fear that if they divulge their problems they will be under threat of loss of independence or of being 'put away'. They rightly value their independence and have great fear of loss of control over their lives and that others may 'take over'. It must be admitted that the past record of insensitive handling of old peoples' problems with the provision of inappropriate remedies by the medical profession makes it easy to understand this reluctance.

Studies of non-reporting of disabling conditions in old age have shown that some conditions are more likely than others to go unnoticed (Williamson *et al.*, 1964).

Conditions relating to the locomotor system (including foot troubles), the urinary system, and to mental disturbance are especially likely to go unreported (Fig. 1). These are, however, conditions of the greatest importance, because of their direct effects in causing pain and discomfort and also because they readily lead to secondary consequences. Thus a locomotor disability which reduces mobility may lead to restriction of social life, reduction in the capacity for self-care, and hence to social deterioration. Problems with bladder function such as frequency and precipitancy of micturition, exhausting nocturia, and any degree of incontinence are also liable seriously to restrict social intercourse and life satisfaction. Deterioration in cognitive function due to a dementing condition rapidly impairs the ability to cope with the day-to-day demands of life. This may often be exaggerated by the characteristic lack of

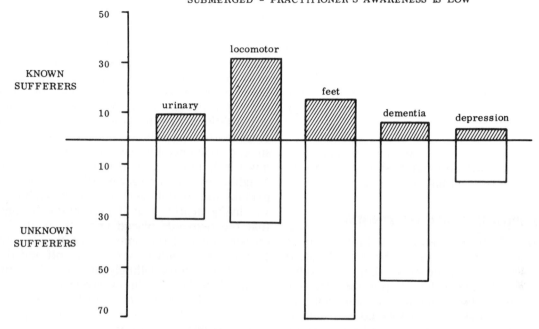

Figure 1   Unknown disabilities in older persons. Disabilities in which most of the iceberg is submerged – practitioner's awareness is low. 'Reproduced from J. Williamson, in *Essays in Health Care of the Elderly*, Ed. T. Arie, p. 197, Croom Helm Ltd, London)

insight associated with dementia so that the patient remains largely unaware of the deterioration which is occurring. The importance of an undiagnosed depression in an old person is clear. What all these commonly non-reported conditions share is the tendency to reduce social competence and to erode morale and self-esteem, both vitally important in enabling the elderly to cope with usual problems of ageing including reduced income, reduced family and social life, and the losses of bereavement which crowd in on them.

High-Risk Groups of Old People

It would be impractical to suggest that all old people should be subjected to a repeated process of case finding and it is certain that many cope very successfully throughout their long lives and do not need this service. However, an indication of some high-risk categories of old people for whom some form of case finding

is justified may be helpful. These include the following:

(a)   The very old, i.e. those aged 85 or more. It has been shown (Akhtar *et al.* 1973) that 4 out of 5 persons aged over 85 are unable to cope with all the demands of daily living and require some degree of help.

(b)   The socially isolated, i.e. those who have become separated from their families.

(c)   The bereaved. The commonest bereavement is the old lady who loses her husband, but it must also be remembered that the loss of a son or daughter in old age is just as significant – the old lady may readily harbour feelings of guilt as she asks herself 'Why could it not have been me?'

(d)   Those already in receipt of help such as social security, home help, district nurse, etc.

(e) Those recently discharged from hospital. Have all the necessary supporting services been ordered and have they arrived?

(f) Those recently rehoused (or otherwise relocated). Old people take badly to having their roots pulled up and may require much help to put new ones down.

(g) Those living in areas of multiple deprivation in inner city areas where they may live in fear of vandalism, robbery, or violence.

These are a few of the more common danger groups but each community should attempt to form its own local high-risk lists.

THE PROCESS OF CASE FINDING

At present there is no precise information as to how case finding should be carried out. It is, however, very probable that a workable pattern will emerge based upon the detection of functional loss. This would mean that persons in high-risk categories would be visited by a 'case finder'. This person would most appropriately be a health visitor, although any well-motivated trained general nurse could readily be taught to carry out the process (Milne *et al.*, 1972). Detailed enquiry would be conducted into mobility, ability to cope with the essentials of daily living, visual acuity, and hearing capacity. A survey would be made of the breadth and depth of family and social contacts and cognitive mental function and mood assessed.

The important problems of old people may in this way be detected by a non-medically trained person. Many of such problems may then be resolved by direct action by the visiting nurse/case finder, e.g. if shortage of money or problems in paying heating bills have been detected, social services may be invoked; if loneliness is detected, the family may be contacted and further visiting and support stimulated. An important area for enquiry is medication and a full review of current medication should be undertaken.

An advantage of this functional approach is that it leads readily to the inclusion of family and other carers in the case-finding procedure. Thus the old lady who is quietly dementing but still managing in her own home with regular help from her daughter may appear herself to have few unmet needs, but it is essential to find out what is the emotional cost of this arrangement to her family and neighbours. Her daughter may be under considerable stress as she struggles to cope with her own job, her home, family, and husband. It is plain that the early detection of stress in the daughter is of the greatest importance since if she once becomes too stressed or is taken beyond 'the end of her tether', then her ability to continue will cease and 'rejection' occurs. All experience suggests that once this has occurred, the breakdown in family support is usually irreversible. Neighbours must be seen in the same way as persons who readily give help to an aged person living nearby, but if they gradually find that the demands placed upon them are increasing beyond the limits which they regard as reasonable then they will back off and the support previously willingly given may be withdrawn. It is therefore in everyone's best interest to include carers in the case-finding process in order that family and community support may be continued at optimal levels.

As already stated, there is as yet no certainty as to the scope and content of the optimum case-finding procedure. Published studies have tended to concentrate upon the detection of disease (Currie *et al.*, 1974; Williams, 1974). This has inevitably led to an unnecessarily narrow approach with relative neglect of functional loss. Case finding aimed at the detection of pathology is in the aged difficult to achieve with scientific precision because of the great variability in the effects of pathological changes in this age group. Thus the results of pure tone audiometry may yield a poor idea of functional hearing since an identical decibel loss in two individuals may be accompanied by marked differences in hearing capacity if one patient has significant dementia and the other has not. Similar X-ray changes of osteoarthrosis of knees may be associated with widely differing degrees of functional impairment (Chamberlain, 1973). This has tended to discourage those who have tried to do research in case finding and it is therefore important to concentrate efforts upon detection of loss of function which avoids these constraints to a large extent.

Suggested Checklist for Case Finding in Old Age

The enquiry may be envisaged as being conducted on two levels: level I is the detection of functional loss for which the nurse herself will seek a remedy and level II is the detection of functional disturbance which will necessitate referral to the general practitioner.

EVALUATION OF CASE FINDING

The question will be posed as to the effectiveness of these case-finding proposals. This is

Level I	*Action*
Loneliness	Advice, referral to voluntary agencies, family stimulation, installation of electronic alarm system
Widowhood	Counselling patient and family.
Effects of rehousing (or other relocation)	Counselling. Arrange contact with appropriate local agencies
Family dispersal	Counselling patient and family. Help with installation and cost of telephone
Family apathy	Counselling family, invoking voluntary agencies
Signs of family stress or exhaustion	Counselling, prompt offer of day care, respite admission to appropriate level of care. Continued support for family
Fear and uncertainty (e.g. fear of falling and being unable to get up)	Electronic alarm. Search for hazards in the house. Instruction on how to rise from floor
Heating in home. Checking ambient temperature in living room, bedroom and bathroom	Advice on better heating, home insulation and clothing, electric blanket, etc. Advice on how to obtain special heating allowances
Medication. Inspection of medication in patient's home	Check that patient understands the reasons for medication and the dosage regime
Vision. Simple test of functional vision. Inspection of spectacles in use	Refer to optician
Hearing. Simple hearing assessment	Refer to hearing aid centre

Level II	*Action*
Elicitation of cardiorespiratory problems, dyspnoea, cyanosis, cough, sputum, wheeze, leg oedema	Refer to general practitioner
Locomotor. Examine gait, ask about pain and stiffness, examine principal joints and feet. Inspect footwear	Refer to general practitioner or chiropodist
EXCRETORY PROBLEMS	
Bladder Frequency, nocturia, dysuria, prostatism, incontinence	Refer to general practitioner

Bowel
  Constipation
    Alteration in bowel habit. Use of laxatives
	Refer to general practitioner
	Advice on diet

POSTURAL CONTROL	
Assess gait and postural stability. Elicit history of falls, blackouts Examine environment for hazards	Refer to general practitioner Make environment safer
COGNITIVE FUNCTION AND MOOD	
Apply tests of memory, orientation, and mood.	Refer to general practitioner

extremely difficult to determine. Lowther, McLeod, and Williamson, (1970) reported on 300 patients who had been involved in a case-finding scheme in Edinburgh. At follow-up 18 to 30 months after the case finding, 29 per cent were judged to be still enjoying some benefits. Williams (1974) reviewed a group of 200 patients 1 year after initial assessment and concluded that 27 per cent were still showing benefits from their involvement. These evaluation attempts were uncontrolled and hence their exact meaning is not completely certain. Tulloch and More (1979) conducted an investigation of a scheme of 'screening and surveillance' in patients aged 70 and over in one general practice. The patients in the scheme were compared over a 2-year period with matched controls. There were no startling differences in the two groups although the study group had significantly lower mean duration of hospital inpatient care. This study failed to indicate the scope and nature of the case-finding process and perhaps its main lesson is the great difficulty of evaluation of these services.

An encouraging feature of these studies has been the very high levels of cooperation among the elderly subjects with acceptance rates as high as 95 per cent.

The main need now seems to be for a clear statement on the content and scope of case finding for elderly subjects.

A bonus to be expected from the institution of case finding is that it encourages doctors, nurses, and others to think in terms of prevention and may make work with the elderly more interesting and rewarding, thus helping to destroy the negative stereotype of old age which has been held by so many health professionals.

SERVICES FOR THE ELDERLY – THEIR PREVENTIVE ROLE

It will be apparent from the foregoing that most or all of available community services fulfil some preventive function. Housing, for example, contributes to primary prevention insofar as grouped or sheltered housing helps old people to avoid or reduce loneliness. Housing for disabled elderly fulfils a tertiary preventive role by making it possible for elderly disabled persons to function more effectively and independently in their home environment. It is satisfactory to note, therefore, the considerable improvements which have taken place in housing, especially the increased provision of sheltered housing. Even the installation of an electronic alarm system may have a powerful preventive effect by reducing the level of anxiety felt by the old person who may be haunted by the fear of 'something happening' and being unable to summon help.

The extensive network of voluntary agencies has considerable preventive value not only by providing services and support for the less-fit elderly but also through offering to the fit elderly a range of opportunities for positive roles and satisfying work in their organizations.

These and other services will be described more fully elsewhere.

REFERENCES

Akhtar, A. J., Broe, A., Crombie, A., McLean, W. M. R., Andrews, G. R., and Caird, F. I. (1973). 'Disability and dependence in the elderly at home', *Age Ageing,* **2**, 102–110.

Aniansson, A., Grinby, G., Rundgren, A., Svanborg, A., and Orlander, J. (1980). 'Physical training in old men', *Age Ageing,* **9**, 186–187.

Chamberlain, J. O. P. (1973). 'Screening elderly people', *Proc. R. Soc. Med.,* **66**, 38–39.

Craig, T. B., and Shang, P. L. (1981). 'Mortality among elderly psychiatric patients basis for preventive intervention', *J. Am. Geriatr. Soc.,* **29**, 181–185.

Currie, G., MacNeill, R. M., Walker, J. G., Barrie, E., and Mudie, E. (1974). 'Medical and social screening of patients aged 70 to 72 by an Urban General Practice Health Team', *Br. Med. J.,* **2**, 108.

Department of Health and Social Security (1976). *Prevention and Health: Everybody's Business,* HMSO, London.

Evans, J. G., Prudham, D., and Wandless, I. (1980). 'Risk factors for stroke in the elderly', *The Ageing Brain* (Eds G. Barbagallo-San Giorgio and A. N. Exton-Smith), pp. 113–126, Plenum Press, London.

Fiumara, N. J., and Waterman, G. E. (1979). 'State wide geriatric immunization program with polyvalent pneumococcal vaccine (pneumovax r)', *Curr. Ther. Res.,* **25**, 185.

Kannel, W. B., McGee, D., and Gordon, T. (1976). 'A general cardiovascular risk profile: The Framingham Study', *Am. J. Cardiol.,* **38**, 46–51.

Langer, E. J., and Rodin, J. (1976). 'The effects of choice and enhanced personal responsibility for the aged: A field experiment in an institutional setting', *J. Pers. Soc. Psychol.,* **34**, 191–198.

Langer, E. J., Rodin, J., Beck, P., Weinman, C., and Spitzer, L. (1979). 'Environmental determinants of memory improvement in late adulthood', *J. Pers. Soc. Psychol.,* **37**, 2003–2013.

Lowther, C. P., McLeod, R. D. M., and Williamson, J. (1970). 'Evaluation of early diagnostic services for the elderly', *Br. Med. J.,* **3**, 275–277.

Milne, J. S. (1981). 'A longitudinal study of blood pressure and stroke in older people', *J. Clin. Exp. Gerontol.,* **3**, 135–159.

Milne, J. S., Maule, M. M., Cormack, S., and Williamson, J. (1972). 'The design and testing of a questionnaire and examination to assess physical and mental health in older people using a staff nurse as the observer', *J. Chronic. Dis.,* **25**, 385–404.

Morris, J. N. (1975). *The Uses of Epidemiology*, Churchill Livingstone, Edinburgh.

Oliver, M. F. (1982). 'Risks of correcting the risks of coronary disease and stroke with drugs', *N. Engl. J. Med.,* **306**, 297–298.

Plemons, J. K., Willis, S. L., and Baltes, P. B. (1978). 'Modifiability of fluid intelligence in aging: A short-term longitudinal training approach', *J. Gerontol.,* **33**, 224–231.

Shephard, R. J. (1977). 'Physical Activity and Aging'. Croom Helm, London.

South-East London Screening Study Group (1977). 'Controlled trial of multiphasic screening in middle age: Results of the South East London Screening Study', *Int. J. Epidemiol.,* **6**, 357–363.

Tanner, J. M. (1964). *The Physique of the Olympic Athlete*, Allen and Unwin, London.

Tulloch, A. J., and Moore, V. (1979). 'A randomized controlled trial of geriatric screening and surveillance in general practice', *J. R. Coll. Gen. Pract.,* **29**, 733–742.

Williams, I. (1974). 'A follow-up of geriatric patients after sociomedical assessment', *J. R. Coll. Gen. Pract.,* **24**, 341–346.

Williamson, J., Stokoe, I. H., Gray, S., Fisher, M., Smith, A., McGhee, A., and Stephenson, E. (1964). 'Old people at home. Their unreported needs', *Lancet,* **1**, 1117–1120.

Wollner, L., McCarthy, S. T., Soper, N. D. W., and Macy, D. J. (1979). 'Failure of cerebral autoregulation as a cause of brain dysfunction in the elderly', *Br. Med. J.,* **1**, 1117–1118.

5

Physical Fitness:
Exercise and Ageing

Principles and Practice of Geriatric Medicine
Edited by M. S. J. Pathy
© 1985 John Wiley & Sons Ltd

5.1

Physical Fitness: Exercise and Ageing

R. J. Shephard

INTRODUCTION

The typical medical curriculum provides little or no instruction in the area of physical fitness. Anatomy, physiology, and biochemistry are reviewed in the context of a hypothetical 'basal state', and clinical teaching pays little heed to the principles of fitness assessment and exercise prescription. In a young patient, the margin of exercise tolerance is usually broad, so that inappropriate advice from the physician may do little harm. Ageing narrows the range of adaptability (Rowlatt and Franks, 1973), and in geriatric medicine there is much less scope for error. Inappropriate exercise prescription in the elderly person may prove ineffective, while a relatively small increase in the prescribed activity may be sufficient to cause serious injury or even death. A clear understanding of physical fitness, exercise, and ageing is thus of particular importance to the physician.

The present chapter looks briefly at the nature of physical fitness and, in the context of the elderly patient, discusses methods of assessment, norms of fitness, implications of declining fitness, principles of exercise prescription, and potential gains from a training programme. Detailed discussion of the biology of physical activity and ageing is given by Shephard (1978a).

THE NATURE OF PHYSICAL FITNESS

The World Health Organisation (Anderson *et al.*, 1971) described physical fitness very simply as 'the ability to perform muscular work satis-factorily'. Shephard has discussed the nature of physical fitness (1977) and the physiological determinants of working capacity (1978b, 1982a) in detail. In a young individual, fitness is task-specific – the sprinter needs an abundance of fast-twitch muscle fibres, well-charged with anaerobic metabolites, while the distance runner requires well-developed slow-twitch muscle fibres with a capacity to burn fat rather than glycogen.

The occasional elderly person also has specific needs associated with participation in age-class 'masters' sports competitions (Kavanagh and Shephard, 1977). In general the motivated elderly may engage in activities aimed at developing fitness in order to widen their range of independent living and pleasurable activities while maintaining and developing positive health.

The prime requirements to meet these important but less ambitious goals are:

(a) a good state of nutrition and general health;

(b) maintenance of an adequate system to transport oxygen from the atmosphere to the working muscles (the 'maximum oxygen intake'; (see Shephard *et al.*, 1968; Taylor, Buskirk, and Henschel, 1955);

(c) slowing of the normal tendency to loss of lean tissue and bone minerals;

(d) avoidance of an excessive build-up of body fat,

(e) preservation of flexibility;

(f) avoidance of an intensity of activity inducing abnormal electrocardiographic responses.

NORMS OF FITNESS FOR THE ELDERLY

Few reliable figures are available to indicate the 'normal' fitness anticipated of an elderly person. It is difficult to obtain exercise test volunteers from among the elderly population, and those who volunteer for examination inevitably tend to be the more active members of the community. Moreover, it is far from clear whether functional loss is an inevitable consequence of ageing, or whether it reflects merely a diminution of habitual physical activity.

In support of a true ageing process, the rate of loss of aerobic power is much the same for 'masters' athletes and for sedentary older individuals (Kavanagh and Shephard, 1977; Shephard, 1978a, 1978b, 1980); the functional deterioration amounts to about 5 per cent. per decade from the age of 25 to 65 years, with some possible acceleration of loss thereafter. The main difference between the continuing athletes and sedentary subjects is that the ageing line for the athletes is set at a higher level (an advantage of some 10 ml/kg min of oxygen transport at all ages). The usual finding for a 65 year old subject, irrespective of sex, is a maximum oxygen intake of 25 to 30 ml/kg min; however, this can often be increased to 35 to 40 ml/kg min through several years of rigorous training.

Muscle strength apparently remains at the young adult level until 40 to 45 years of age, but thereafter there is an increasingly rapid deterioration of performance. If strength is assessed in terms of handgrip force, typical values for a 65 year old man and woman are 45 kg (450 N) and 29 kg (290 N), respectively. The lean tissue loss at 65 years can be as large as 5 kg, 20 per cent. of the total lean mass found in a young adult. The lean tissue per centimetre of stature thus diminishes from the young adult values of 300 to 340 g/cm (men) and 270 to 310 g/cm (women) to 240 to 275 g/cm (men) and 210 to 250 g/cm (women). The effects of overall muscle wasting are exacerbated by local changes at sites of injury or arthritis. Regional differences can be evaluated by tape measurements of limb circumference with appropriate allowance for overlying body fat or by appropriately sited soft-tissue radiographs. The local musculature varies widely from one individual to another, and it is advisable to use the opposite limb as a control, though this may also have undergone some wasting if the patient's general activity has been restricted.

The thickness of subcutaneous fat is commonly several millimetres greater than the average found in young adults of ideal body mass (10 to 11 mm in male, 13 to 14 mm in female). There is no evidence that such fat accumulation is necessary or even a desirable accompaniment of ageing (Sidney, Shephard, and Harrison, 1977).

Many patients aged 65 years and older show an 'abnormal' ECG response to physical activity (see Table 6). Fortunately, not all such records are due to ischaemia; in women particularly, a substantial proportion are benign (Cumming, Dufresne, and Samm, 1973; Sidney and Shephard, 1977b). Prognostic warnings based upon a supposed abnormality of the ECG should be given in guarded terms. The ceiling of heart rate at the age of 65 averages at least 170 beats/min in men and 160 beats/min in women (Lester *et al.*, 1968, Sidney and Shephard, 1977a), with a limiting systolic blood pressure of 180 to 200 mmHg (24 to 27 kPa). If diet is adequate, haemoglobin levels should be much as in a normal young adult (14.5 to 15 g/dl in men, 13 to 13.5 g/dl in women (Elwood, 1971). However, the cardiac stroke volume is less well sustained than in a young person, particularly at high work rates (Niinimaa and Shephard, 1978).

THE ASSESSMENT OF PHYSICAL FITNESS

General Health

A general medical examination is an important component of physical fitness assessment in the elderly. Chronic disorders may limit the inherent physical fitness of the individual (Brown and Shephard, 1967).

Physical restrictions upon movement often occur in the elderly, though progressive disengagement from normal society (Cumming and Henry, 1961) may be the main cause of inactivity. Joint mobility may be reduced by rheumatoid or osteoarthritis. Corns, calluses and other podiatric problems may make walking painful. Confidence may be weakened by instability of the knee joints. A variety of neuromuscular disorders can affect both balance and muscle function. Loss of vision is a severe handicap to a person who previously had normal sight. Some degree of emphysema or chronic bronchitis is common and this leads to unpleasant breathlessness if vigorous activity is attempted. Angina or intermittent claudication may reduce physical activity. Varicose veins reduce central blood volume, the maximum cardiac output, and thus physical performance (Carlsten, 1972).

Nutrition is important in terms of (a) the control of obesity, (b) optimization of the serum lipid profile, and (c) maintenance of a normal haemoglobin concentration. Oxygen transport, and thus the ability to perform sustained work, depends heavily upon the oxygen capacity of the blood. Effort tolerance is limited in patients with low haemoglobin levels and estimation of the haemoglobin concentration is an important aspect of fitness assessment.

Maximum Oxygen Intake

The direct measurement or the prediction of maximum oxygen intake is a vital component of fitness assessment at all ages (Shephard, 1977, 1978a, 1978b). Anaerobic energy processes are unable to sustain muscle activity for more than about a minute. Common everyday activities such as walking are dependent on the ability of the heart and lungs to transport oxygen to the working tissues, the variable reported as the 'maximum oxygen intake'.

Treadmill walking to exhaustion can be used to determine the maximum oxygen intake of healthy individuals in the seventh, eighth, and ninth decades of life (Sidney and Shephard, 1977a). Ideally such measurements include an 'on-line' indication of oxygen consumption, continuous electrocardiographic monitoring, electronic averaging of the ECG waveform, and blood pressure recording at 30 second intervals. The 'maximum' can then be demonstrated as a plateau of oxygen consumption (increase less than 2 ml/kg min in response to a further increase of treadmill speed or slope). At least three-quarters of subjects reach a plateau at their first test, and about a half of the remainder do so with repetition of the procedure (Shephard, 1978a, 1978b). Subsidiary criteria of a maximum effort include heart rate and blood lactate (Table 1). The maximum heart rate of a 65 year old person is usually higher than the 155 beats per minute that was once suggested (Åstrand, 1960). Sidney and Shephard (1977a) observed average readings of 172 beats/min in men and 161 beats/min in women who had a good maximum effort, while Lester and coworkers (1968) reported values as high as 177 beats/min for sedentary 65 year old men. Limiting blood lactate readings (11

Table 1. Characteristics of good maximum effort in elderly subjects studied by Sidney and Shephard (1977a)

Variable	Percentage of sample showing characteristic	
	Men	Women
	(*n* = 19)	(*n* = 20)
Oxygen consumption plateau ≤ 2 ml/kg min	79	75
Heart rate plateau ≤ 5 beats/min	63	75
Heart rate ≥ 160 beats/min	84	60
Respiratory gas exchange ratio ≥ 1.00	100	80
≥ 1.15	37	20
Arterial blood lactate ≥ 8.8 mmol/l	78	50
Systolic blood pressure ≥ 200 mmHg (26.7 kPa)	58	35

mmol/l) are less than in a young person (Sidney and Shephard, 1977a) but are likewise higher than was once believed.

The day-to-day coefficient of variation for a well-performed direct measurement of maximum oxygen intake is extremely small (2.2 to 2.5 per cent., see Shephard, 1978a). If a treadmill is available without ancillary equipment, it is possible to determine the time to exhaustion (see Table 2), using a protocol of speeds and slopes set by Bruce (Bruce, Kusumi, and Hosmer, 1973; see also, Cumming, 1978). Such times are moderately well correlated with the directly measured maximum oxygen intake, although in extending the protocol to the elderly it should be stressed that stiff joints and poor coordination may increase the oxygen cost of walking. A given endurance time implies a higher maximum oxygen intake than would be the case in a young person.

Predictions of maximum oxygen intake from submaximum data almost all exploit the supposed linear relationship between heart rate and oxygen intake or the equivalent rate of working (Åstrand, 1960). Unfortunately, the errors inherent in such predictions are exaggerated in an older person. Not only is there disagreement on the maximum heart rate to be used in calculations, but there is a considerable interindividual variation of this maximum rate (SD ± 12 beats/min; Shephard, 1978a). Moreover, older patients have difficulty in sustaining cardiac stroke volume at high workloads (Niinimaa and Shephard, 1978), thereby threatening the required linearity of the heart rate to oxygen intake relationship. If oxygen consumption is predicted from the work performed on a staircase or a cycle ergometer, due account must be taken of the low mechanical efficiency of effort (e.g. the net mechanical efficiency of cycling in a 65 year old is 21.5 per cent. rather than the 23.0 per cent. value found in a young adult, Shephard, 1978a). The cumulative consequence of these various difficulties is a prediction so liable to error that it cannot be used to advise the individual on fitness status. Sidney and Shephard (1977a) reported the mean and SD of the discrepancy between direct treadmill measurements and cycle ergometer predictions as -25 ± 15 per cent in elderly men and -5 ± 16 per cent in elderly women.

Cooper (1968) found that the distances a person can run in 12 minutes was a simple test of aerobic fitness. The procedure can work well in young and highly motivated subjects, but 12 minutes of all-out activity from an elderly person who is in poor physical condition is hazardous. Even in better-trained older persons problems of interpretation arise from a low mechanical efficiency of running. Sidney and Shephard (1977a) suggested using the following equations to estimate the maximum oxygen intake ($V_{O_2}(max)$) of subjects aged 65 years and older:

Men:
$$V_{O_2} (max) = 12.4 \ (S, km) + 21.5 \ ml/kg \ min$$
(10% c.v.)

Women
$$V_{O_2} (max) = 11.4 \ (S, km) + 11.9 \ ml/kg \ min$$
(16% c.v.)

Table 2.　Prediction of maximum oxygen intake from endurance time during progressive exhausting exercise

Duration (min)	Speed (km/h)	Slope (%)	Approximate oxygen cost	
			Middleaged men (Bruce, Kusumi, and Hosmer, 1973)	Elderly men (22% loss of efficiency) (Shephard, 1978*)
3	2.72	10	17.4	21.2
4	4.00	12	19.8	24.2
5	4.00	12	22.3	27.2
6	4.00	12	24.8	30.3
7	5.44	14	27.9	34.0
8	5.44	14	31.1	37.9
9	5.44	14	34.3	41.8
10	6.72	16	37.4	45.6
11	6.72	16	40.6	49.5
12	6.72	16	43.8	53.4

Canadian Home Fitness Test

In this test the subject climbs a double 8-inch (20.3 cm) step to a rhythm established by a long-playing gramophone record (Bailey, Shephard, and Mirwald,1976). The heart rate is counted immediately following a 3-minute bout of stepping, and on the basis of this subjects are allocated to an age and sex specific fitness category (Table 3). A multiple regression formula also allows the prediction of the maximum oxygen intake value from the duration of stepping, body weight, heart rate, and age (Jetté *et al.*, 1976).

The maximum oxygen intake score is generally expressed relative to body weight. This penalizes the obese person, although many authors regard this as legitimate, since the body weight must be displaced during most types of physical activity. There have been few measurements beyond the seventh decade of life, but one may anticipate a deterioration of a score at least as rapid as that seen in earlier decades (about 5 ml/kg min for every 10 years of adult life). The absolute maximum oxygen intake (1/min) is the statistic relevant to weight-supported activities (e.g. propulsion of a wheelchair).

Lean Tissue

Measurements of lean tissue mass and bone mass can be undertaken in specialized centres, using such techniques as nitrogen activation, calcium activation, and determinations of the naturally occurring isotope $^{40}K^+$. When applying these methods in the elderly there are some uncertainties of data interpretation, since neither the water nor the potassium content of the tissues reach the levels established through studies of normal young adults. Lean tissue mass may be determined more simply by subtracting fat mass from total body mass. In a young person, lean tissue ranges from 270 to 340 g/cm of stature, depending on sex and body build. However, the ratio falls as muscle protein is lost from the body with ageing.

Measurement of the Maximum Isometric Force of One or More Muscle Groups

Clarke (1966) has argued that there is a correlation of about 0.8 between handgrip force and the general muscularity of an individual. His conclusion seems reasonably well-established for a young person, unless there is an unusual occupational or athletic development of the wrist muscles. However, there remains a need to validate this approach in the assessment of individuals older than 60 to 65 years (see, for example, Fisher and Birren, 1947).

Body Fat

The physician has traditionally relied upon actuarial tables of 'ideal weights' to assess the extent of obesity (Society of Actuaries, 1959). Such figures (Table 4) are currently undergoing substantial revision, and in any event can be misleading in the elderly, since additional body mass due to an accumulation of body fat can be masked by a loss of muscle and a decrease of bone density (Shephard, 1977).

Measurement of the thickness of a double fold of skin and subcutaneous fat, using standardized calipers (Harpenden or Cambridge),

Table 3.   Canadian Home Fitness Test Scores for male subjects aged 60–69 years.*

Fitness category	Stepping rate	Duration of exercise	Ten second recovery pulse count
	(per min)	(min)	
Undesirable	66	3	≥ 24
Minimum	84	6	≥ 23
Recommended	84	6	≤ 22

* Subjects are required to climb a 40.6 cm double step at a rhythm set by a long-playing record (obtainable from Fitness and Amateur Sport Directorate, Health and Welfare, Canada, Journal Building, Kent, at Laurier Ave., Ottawa).

The maximal oxygen consumption can be predicted by the equation $\dot{V}_{O_2} = 42.5 - 16.6\ (E) - 0.12\ (M) - 0.12\ (f_h) - 0.24\ (A)$, where $\dot{V}_{O_2}$ is the oxygen cost of stepping (1/min), M is the body mass (kg), f_h is the recovery heart rate, and A is the age (years).

The recommended time (T, min) to walk or jog 1.6 km is then given by $T = 44.7 - 0.27\ (\dot{V}_{O_2}) - 12.3\ H + 0.015\ M$, where $\dot{V}_{O_2}$ is the maximum oxygen intake as predicted from the Canadian Home Fitness Test, H is the subjects height and M is the body mass (kg).

Table 4. 'Ideal' body weights, based on the data of the Society of Actuaries (1959) for subjects of average body build; in elderly subjects who have lost much lean tissue, the body mass may be up to 5 kg lower than shown, unless there is a compensatory increase of body fat

Height (no shoes, cm)	Ideal weight (indoor clothing, kg)	
	Men	Women
157.5	57.6	54.2
160.0	58.9	55.8
162.6	60.3	57.8
165.1	61.9	60.0
167.6	63.7	61.7
170.2	65.7	63.5
172.7	67.6	65.3
175.3	69.4	66.8
177.8	71.4	68.5
180.3	73.5	—
182.9	75.5	—

is a simple line of approach. Skinfold readings may be interpreted in their own right, relative to data for a young and healthy individual of ideal body mass (Table 5), or they may be converted to body density and thus percentage body fat, using equations such as those of Durnin and Womersley (1974) and Siri (1956). The latter approach has come under heavy criticism in recent years (Lohman, 1981; Shephard, 1978b; Shephard Hatcher, and Rode, 1973). There are a wide variety of possible prediction formulae giving more than twofold variation in estimates of body fat (Shephard, 1978b). Unfortunately, search for a 'better' formula is likely to prove fruitless. There can never be any guarantee that the relative proportions of subcutaneous and internal fat will be similar in different individuals, and there is little basis

Table 5. Skinfold thicknesses in a young subject with 'ideal' body weight (based on data of Shephard, 1978a)

Skinfold	Thickness of double fold of skin and fat (mm)	
	Men	Women
Chin	6	7
Triceps	8	16
Chest	12	9
Subscapular	12	11
Suprailiac	13	15
Waist	14	15
Suprapubic	11	21
Knee (medial)	9	12
Average (all 8 folds)	10	14

for the supposition that lean tissue has a constant density such as 1.10 in all subjects.

Interindividual variations of lean tissue density are equally a source of criticism when body fat is determined by hydrostatic weighing. The heaviest component of lean tissue is bone and loss of calcium from bones is particularly likely to invalidate hydrostatic estimates in older subjects.

Bidimensional measurements of fat, muscle, and bone shadows can be made in soft-tissue radiographs (Tanner, 1965). This method of studying body composition is not very popular among younger subjects because of the X-irradiation. A second disadvantage is that only one region of the body is sampled. However, there is less objection to soft-tissue radiography on an older person, and information obtained in this manner may be particularly helpful in assessing the local regeneration of muscle following a limb injury (Fried and Shephard, 1969).

Flexibility

Flexibility comprises both static and dynamic components. Dynamic flexibility is important to an athlete, but in the average older person the key factor is the range of motion that can be developed at a given joint, assuming that a reasonable time is allowed for completion of the movement. For precise data, a goniometer may be attached to the body part, taking care to make its axis of rotation coincident with that of the joint. Specific movements can be evaluated by simpler pieces of apparatus; for instance, the Dillion 'sit and reach' test examines forward flexion of the back in terms of the maximum forward movement of the palms when the feet are resting against a vertical board.

Electrocardiogram

The two main danger signs in the exercise electrocardiogram are ST segmental depression and premature ventricular contractions. The ST segmental change is regarded as indicative of myocardial oxygen lack if it assumes a horizontal or downsloping form, or is upsloping with a residual depression of more than 1 mm (0.1 mV) at the commencement of the T wave. Subjects can safely continue an exercise test until a depression of at least 0.2 mV is seen. If it is necessary to halt a test for either ST depression or symptoms such as anginal pain, it is useful to record the corresponding heart rate–systolic blood pressure product as a measure of the cardiac workload that the subject can tolerate.

Occasional premature ventricular contractions are a normal response to physical activity. However, testing should be stopped if the frequency of 'extra beats' reaches 3 in 10 seconds or if there is a coupling of the abnormal contractions. Other adverse aspects of premature ventricular contractions are a multifocal origin and occurrence at an early point in the cardiac cycle. As with ST depression, such changes usually reflect underlying ischaemic heart disease.

The diagnostic sensitivity of the ECG is improved by the use of multiple chest leads, examination of both exercise and recovery tracings, and by exercising close to maximum effort (Shephard, 1980). During exercise there is some loss of specificity, with an increase in the number of false positive results. This is a particular problem in older individuals, a high proportion of whom show some abnormality of the exercise electrocardiogram (Table 6); not all of these abnormalities are attributable to ischaemic heart disease. Much can be learnt using a single (CM_5) lead (Shephard, 1977) and a portable electrocardiogram. Analysis is facilitated by electronic averaging tools that will superimpose 16 or 32 tracings, exclude abnormal waveforms, and calculate statistics such as ST depression and ST slope.

Table 6   Reported frequency of 'abnormal' electrocardiograms in elderly subjects. (For details of references, see Shephard, 1978a; information reproduced by permission of Croom Helm Publishers)

Author	Percentage of abnormal records	
	Men	Women
Åstrand (1969)	35	55
Brown and Shephard (1967)	—	36
Cumming *et al.* (1972/3)	37	33
Doan *et al.* (1965)	46	—
Kasser & Bruce (1969)	25	—
Kavanagh and Shephard (1977)	17[a]	—
Profant *et al.* (1972)	—	100
Riley *et al.* (1970)	32	21
Sidney and Shephard (1977)	29	36

[a]Masters' class athletes.

Special Assessments

In some elderly patients, lower limb disability will require assessment by special test equipment such as arm ergometers or treadmills modified to accommodate wheelchairs (Kelsey *et al.*, 1982). The principles of maximum oxygen intake assessment remain much as when using the legs, although on interpreting the results it must be remembered that the available power is needed to propel not only the patient but also a wheelchair. Moreover, the mechanical efficiency of most wheelchairs is quite low, so that a substantial oxygen transport is needed to accomplish even a modest amount of external work.

Conclusion

Given some patience and ingenuity, a remarkable proportion of the elderly population can undertake a standard fitness assessment of the type discussed above. However, there are plainly some groups (particularly in extended care institutions) who are too frail or too sick to tolerate normal methods of testing. Little formal consideration has yet been given to the fitness testing of such individuals, but the safest and most promising approach is probably to examine the metabolic activity of each patient in the context of his or her daily routine. Key concepts include (a) the voluntarily chosen rate of a movement such as walking (typically 35 to 40 per cent. of maximum oxygen intake; Hughes and Goldman, 1970), (b) the type of large muscle activity that makes the person too breathless to talk (usually the anaerobic threshold, 60 to 70 per cent. of maximum oxygen intake), and (c) the corresponding heart rates and ECG waveforms (as recorded by telemetry or portable tape-recorder).

IMPLICATIONS OF DECLINING FITNESS

Several arguments can be advanced for an increase rather than a decrease of physical activity as a person becomes older. A policy of increased physical activity seems likely to prolong independence, improve general life style, induce favourable psychological effects, and lessen the risk of developing several serious types of medical disorder.

Prolongation of Independence

A combination of ageing and disease or injury may lead to progressive dependency. Training gives a larger margin of oxygen transport over basal metabolism, reversing this trend. Once retirement has occurred the elderly are in general unlikely to undertake sufficient voluntary activity to induce the 10 ml/kg min advantage of aerobic power seen in an athlete. A more realistic training response of 3 to 4 ml/kg min would suffice to maintain independence for a further 6 or 7 years.

General Lifestyle

An increase of habitual activity encourages an adequate dietary intake and tends to discourage smoking. The elderly can ill afford the acute doubling of the work of breathing induced by smoking (Rode and Shephard, 1971). Dieting becomes more effective in reducing body fat if it is accompanied by an increase of physical activity.

Psychological Advantages

Following retirement, many workers undergo a progressive disengagement from society (Cumming and Henry, 1961) until they have few residual interests. Physical activity does much to counter this trend. It takes the individual into new situations, encourages the making of new friends, and provides new topics for conversation. The act of moving has an immediate arousing effect upon the brain, and increased personal strength gives a renewed self-confidence. There may finally be more subtle links between memory and the learning process, of the type discussed by Piaget (1956) and the French school of education psychologists. Based on this last concept, there is currently much interest in the 'université de la troisième âge', a form of university extension class that provides both mental and physical stimulation to the elderly.

Medical Prophylaxis

The value of enhanced activity is well established in obesity and maturity-onset diabetes. In other disorders such as hypertension and bone demineralization, a regular exercise programme induces a significant change, but the improvement of status is too small to have much therapeutic usefulness. In a third group of maladies, such as ischaemic heart disease and chronic obstructive lung disease, regular training brings about a substantial subjective improvement, but it has yet to be shown that morbidity or mortality is reduced.

PRINCIPLES OF EXERCISE PRESCRIPTION

General Conditions

The pattern of exercise that is prescribed for an older person inevitably depends upon its purpose. If the main goal is to escape from loneliness, a group recreational programme will be accepted with greater enthusiasm than a regimen of solitary jogging. If the intention is to reduce excess body fat, a moderate intensity of walking for increasing periods of the day will prove more effective than attempts at vigorous jogging. In some instances there will be a need to strengthen specific muscles or to increase mobility about particular joints, and a skilled occupational therapist may be of great value in adapting an interesting hobby to this purpose.

Any programme that is proposed must be readily accessible to an elderly person. Many older people no longer have a car or the funds to make an extensive journey by private or public transport. Where possible, programmes for institutionalized patients should be arranged 'on-site'; frequent reminders and encouragement are necessary to ensure participation.

The availability of equipment and specific facilities along with the interests and aptitudes of the individual patient are relevant to prescribing exercise.

Warm-Up and Warm-Down

The general principles of warm-up and warm-down are particularly important in an older person. A preliminary gentle stretching of the muscles to be exercised is helpful in reducing the risk of musculoskeletal injuries (de Vries, 1980), while a gradual progression from moderate to more vigorous activity over a period of 5 to 10 minutes reduces the likelihood of provoking a cardiac dysrhythmia (Barnard *et al.*, 1973).

Circulatory adaptations during the recovery period are less effective than in a younger individual. There is thus a greater risk of loss of consciousness from postural hypotension and an increased chance that an abnormal cardiac rhythm may develop (McDonough and Bruce, 1969). The warm-down should allow at least 5 minutes of activity at a steadily diminishing tempo. A subsequent excessively hot shower or exposure to a hot and humid changing environment should be avoided.

Aerobic Activity

The main segment of an exercise class should provide a period of moderate aerobic activity. Ideally, there would be some 30 minutes of activity at 60 per cent. of maximum oxygen intake, performed 5 times per week while the condition of the patient was being improved, and 3 times per week for maintenance of fitness (Pollock, Ward, and Foster, 1979; Shephard, 1975, 1977). However, many elderly patients are in such poor physical condition that they need to approach this target gradually. The exercise that is prescribed should not leave a participant feeling more than pleasantly

tired the following day. It may be necessary to commence training at 50 rather than 60 per cent. of maximum oxygen intake, splitting the required activity into two 10–15 minute sessions rather than a single bout of 30 minutes.

Any large muscle exercise such as vigorous walking, swimming, cycling, or cross-country skiing (see Table 7) will theoretically develop aerobic fitness (Cooper, 1968; Shephard 1977). However, because of degenerative changes in joints and limited support from surrounding muscles, the incidence of injuries can be alarming; some overenthusiastic jogging programmes have found that more than 50 per cent. of participants were quickly incapacitated by orthopaedic problems (Kilbom *et al.*, 1969; Mann *et al.*, 1969). In older patients, it is possible to develop just as large an oxygen consumption by fast walking as by jogging. Moreover, the stress on the knee joints and weight-supporting bones is only about one-third as great during walking as during jogging. The approximate relationship between walking and oxygen consumption is shown in Table 8.

Table 8 Approximate oxygen cost of walking at various speeds

Speed (km/h)	Oxygen cost (ml/kg min)	
	Middle age	Elderly[a]
1.6	5.0	6.1
3.2	9.0	11.0
4.8	12.5	15.3
6.4	16.0	19.5
7.2	20.0	24.4
8.0	24.0	29.3

[a]Assuming a 22% decrease in the efficiency of effort.

Swimming is a good method of beginning the conditioning process, particularly for an obese or a disabled patient; however, there is need for closer supervision than in a walking programme. An obese person can float with relatively little expenditure of energy; an appropriately graduated schedule of swimming speeds and distances should thus be established for each patient. If a well-heated pool is available, calisthenics against the resistance of the water (aquabics; see Lawrence, 1981) can provide a useful type of group activity, particularly for patients with joint disorders. Cycling has the disadvantage that a major part of the effort is sustained by the quadriceps. It provokes a

Table 7 Approximate oxygen cost of selected recreational activities. Note that data are obtained on young adults and values are probably higher for elderly subjects. (Based on data collected by the Public Health Committee, Ontario Medical Association)

Activity	Oxygen cost (ml/kg min)
Shuffleboard	9
Fishing	9
Billiards	10
Bowling	10
Horseshoe pitching	10
Golf (power cart)	10
Sailing	12
Archery	12
Table tennis	14
Golf (no cart)	14
Waltzing	14
Cross-country skiing (level)	18
Fishing (wading)	21
Hiking	21
Hunting	21
Snow-shoeing	21
Square dancing	21
Dancing (rhumba)	21
Tennis	28

greater rise of blood pressure than would the development of an equivalent oxygen consumption by fast walking or swimming. Gentle cross-country skiing on level, well-groomed trails is an excellent large muscle activity. However, impaired coordination and decalcification of bones increase the risk of injury.

The gentle playing of competitive sports such as tennis, golf, and curling can add interest to the activity of a fit older person. However, partners and opponents should be chosen to ensure an appropriate tempo of play. Determination to beat a better preserved opponent can have fatal consequences for a patient with incipient myocardial ischaemia (Shephard, 1974). The risk of such an occurrence depends greatly upon the personality of the individual. Some people need an element of competition to sustain their interest in physical activity, but it is often these same people who are unwilling to accept defeat philosophically. If vision is poor, there are increased risks of injury from the ball, the opponent's racket, and collision with obstacles. Moreover, sudden twisting movements can exacerbate a previous back or knee injury.

Rhythmic calisthenics can provide the basis for a useful warm-up while increasing the range of motion at the joints that are exercised. However, the movements that are prescribed should be gentle and smooth to avoid causing injuries. Routines that involve the support of body weight (such as repeated 'push-ups') are best avoided, since they induce an excessive rise of blood pressure and thus cardiac workload.

The exercise potential of normal daily living both in the garden and in the home should be exploited. Within the home, many simple domestic chores have an appropriate intensity for an older person (Table 9). However, activities such as fixing high shelves and painting ceilings cause an undesirable rise of blood pressure (Åstrand, Gahary, and Wahren, 1968).

Among institutionalized patients, thought should be directed to maximizing daily activity. The stairways provide a valuable resource.

Muscle Strengthening

'Muscle building' programmes have been regarded as undesirable on at least three counts: (a) sustained isometric contractions cause a

Table 9 Approximate oxygen cost of household activities. Note: data are obtained on young adults, and values are probably higher for elderly subjects. (Based on data collected by the Public Health Committee, Ontario Medical Association)

Activity	Oxygen cost (ml/kg min)
Standing	5
Writing at desk	5
Typing	9
Working on car	9
Housework (scrubbing, waxing)	10
Cutting wood (power saw)	10
Stocking shelves	12
Painting	14
Paper hanging	14
Carrying trays and dishes	14
Mowing lawn (power mower)	14
Carpentry	18
Gardening	18
Carrying 15 to 25 kg	18
Mowing lawn (hand mower)	18
Chopping wood (axe or saw)	21
Shovelling light earth (10 spades/min)	21
Carrying 35 to 45 kg	28

rise of blood pressure, increasing the cardiac workload, (b) skeletal muscle is developed without a corresponding augmentation of cardiac muscle, and (c) the patient may believe that a bout of isometric training is all that is required to sustain personal fitness.

In a young person, aerobic exercise is usually sufficient to sustain an adequate muscle mass. However, this is not necessarily true for an older individual. The strengthening of appropriate muscle groups by a regimen of isometric contractions can do much to stabilize knee joints and minimize lower back problems. Development of the lower abdominal muscles may help to reduce the risk of herniae. Local exercises may also be necessary if a body part has been immobilized following bone injury.

An excessive rise of blood pressure can be avoided if contractions are held for 10 seconds or less, and fortunately this duration of stimulus seems adequate to induce muscle hypertrophy (Hettinger, 1961). The other problems of isometric training can be minimized if the need for aerobic activity is also impressed upon the patient.

Reduction of Body Fat

The most effective regimen for the reduction of body fat involves creation of a slight negative energy balance through a combination of increased physical activity and some restriction of diet. Each 29 kJ (7 kcal) of energy is equivalent to 1 g of fat. A 1,000 kJ energy deficit (500 kJ reduction of food intake, 500 kJ of brisk walking) burns 34 g of fat per day or 1 kg per month.

A steady loss of this type has several advantages over more drastic 'spot' reducing programmes. In particular, (a) the muscle wasting and hyperkalaemia of overvigorous dieting are avoided, (b) the exercise component helps to arouse the patient, avoiding the depression of rigorous dieting alone, (c) physical activity may cause an increase of blood sugar, thereby reducing appetite, (d) the prescription includes some pleasant positive elements as well as prohibitions, and (e) the gradual approach to weight loss helps in the creation of an improved lifestyle, with a reduced risk of recidivism.

A very heavy person may not be capable of increasing daily energy expenditure by 500 kJ immediately. However, the required energy expenditure can be attained by a persistent and progressive approach. If the feet and knee joints are sound, the patient should be encouraged to walk a little further every day, until a distance of at least 2 km can be tolerated twice a day. The speed of movement must also be increased in easy stages. The initial velocity may be as low as 1.5 to 2.0 km/h, but this should be boosted every few days until a rate of 5 to 6 km/h is well-accepted.

There has been much discussion on the value of moderate exercise in correcting an abnormal lipid profile (Kavanagh *et al.*, 1982; (Shephard *et al.*, 1980). A modest increase of physical activity is often associated with a small increase of HDL cholesterol and/or a decrease of LDL cholesterol. However, the changes in serum lipids seem due to an associated alteration of lifestyle – cessation of smoking, reduction of alcohol intake, selection of a low fat diet, and weight loss rather than exercise per se. The volume of exercise (15 to 20 km per week) needed to change the lipid profile in its own right is beyond the tolerance of many elderly individuals.

Flexibility

A wide range of vigorous normal activities does much to maintain flexibility. Joints that have been restricted by arthritis, injury, or prolonged immobilization require particular attention. The static range of movement must be extended a little each day by gentle passive stretching, while the dynamic range must be broadened by devising interesting forms of occupational therapy. Various forms of heat treatment help in the mobilization process.

Adapted Exercise Prescription

A substantial proportion of elderly persons have some type of medical abnormality that necessitates a more cautious approach to exercise prescription.

At least 20 per cent. of those over the age of 60 years show exercise-induced ST segmental depression suggestive of ischaemic heart disease. A variety of abnormal ECG rhythms and waveforms are also observed, both at rest and during exercise. Some of these findings would be considered as absolute contraindications to exercise in a younger person. However, the elderly may decide to enjoy life at some risk rather than hope to extend existence by a few months of cloistered inactivity.

If there is a history of exercise-induced angina, the best response is to a modified interval pattern of training: 1 to 1½ min bursts of vigorous movement are interspersed with equal periods of slow walking to allow oxidation of anaerobic metabolites (Kavanagh and Shephard, 1975). If inhalation of cold air precipitates angina, the patient may arrange to exercise indoors or can wear a jogging mask (Kavanagh, 1970). Severe cases may take a trinitrin tablet or similar medication prior to exercising. The threshold of angina is set by cardiac workload, proportional to the product of heart rate and systolic blood pressure. As fitness improves, the heart rate associated with a given external work rate decreases, and heavier work can be undertaken before angina appears.

Sustained isometric contractions should be avoided if there is evidence of hypertension. Nevertheless, the overall effect of an increase of habitual activity seems (a) a decrease of resting systemic pressure and (b) an ability to sustain cardiac stroke volume against a higher load after exercise.

Vascular disease of the limbs may give rise to intermittent claudication. The appropriate pattern of training is then an intermittent exercise schedule. There have been several reports that regular, progressive activity extends the function of affected individuals, possibly by opening up alternative vascular pathways to the ischaemic muscles (Hedlund and Porjé, 1964; Larsen and Lassen, 1966).

A varying degree of chronic obstructive lung disease is common in the elderly population. Undue dyspnoea from vigorous exercise impairs motivation. A prescription that keeps the work rate below the anaerobic threshold, usually 60 to 70 per cent. of the maximum oxygen intake, is one therapeutic measure. Bronchospasm precipitated by inhalation of very cold or very dry air should be avoided. A jogging mask or even a scarf over the mouth can be a helpful protection against the cold. For indoor exercise a humidifier may be necessary.

Patients requiring adapted exercise programmes include those with orthopaedic problems, limb disabilities such as hemiplegia and paraplegia, impaired balance, and deterioration of the special senses.

Motivation

At all ages, motivation is a key component of a successful exercise programme. Gains of fitness disappear over a few weeks of inactivity or bed-rest, and participants must thus be encouraged to lifelong activity.

If a patient is to persist with a prescribed exercise, it must be perceived as safe, convenient, and appropriate relative to his or her age. The person supervising group activities must have empathy for the needs, desires, and potential of an older person. An overly athletic instructor can have a discouraging, negative impact upon both body image and motivation (Sidney and Shephard, 1977c). Classes grouped by age and disability are helpful to both real and perceived safety, overcoming some of the self-consciousness and embarrassment that older people find in the early stages of renewed activity.

The rewards expected from the activity programmes should be explored through 'open-ended' questions, and the 'feedback' of information should be adjusted accordingly. Some older people will be seeking companionship, social interchange, and fun, but in most cases the prime motivation will be to improve health and fitness. Consultations and evaluations should thus stress the gains of health and fitness that have been realized through the programme. It is initially easy to demonstrate an improved score, whether this be a gain of aerobic power registered by a simple procedure such as the Canadian Home Fitness Test (Table 3), or an improvement in body composition (a decrease of skinfold thickness without necessarily any change of body mass). The extent of weekly gains diminishes progressively as an individual approaches the standard for a fit person of his age. There are then two alternatives: (a) the programme can be explained as a campaign of maintenance, in the face of advancing age, or (b) attention can be drawn to items of performance which are still improving (e.g. the distance walked without fatigue). A helpful technique in emphasizing the extent of physiological gains is to relate scores to the anticipated rate of ageing.

Supervision

Controversy continues on the extent of supervision that is necessary for exercise testing and exercise programmes. The risk of a cardiac emergency in any given hour of activity is quite low, even for elderly patients.

Vigorous physical activity probably increases the risk of a cardiac episode by a factor of 4 to 5 during the time that the patient is exercising (Shephard, 1974). However, it is less clear whether a vigorous life style increases or decreases the risk measured over the next year of life. Exercise should thus be commended as the basis of a happier life rather than as a guarantor of longevity.

The role of the physician should probably be restricted to the preparation of exercise guidelines, encouragement of appropriate exercise in the elderly, and the identification of subgroups in whom exercise is either contraindicated or requires close supervision. Both injuries and emergencies will be reduced if a few simple rules are followed, including:

(a) avoidance of outdoor exercise in extreme heat or cold (Shephard, 1976);

(b) avoidance of outdoor exercise on ice-covered surfaces;

(c), a gentle progression of the exercise prescription;

(d) a restriction of activity to a total dose of exercise that leaves the patient pleasantly tired the next day;

(e) a temporary halting of activity if symptoms suggest angina, premature ventricular contractions, or excessive breathlessness;

(f) an adequate warm-up and warm-down;

(g) avoidance of sudden twisting and jerking movements;

(h) avoidance of forms of exercise that tax sight or balance; and

(i) avoidance of vigorous activity during intercurrent infections.

The specific problem of cardiac emergencies can be best tackled by encouraging exercise in pairs, and by educating the general public in techniques of cardiac resuscitation (Cobb *et al.*, 1975).

GAINS FROM A TRAINING REGIMEN

There has been much discussion as to whether the elderly are less trainable than younger individuals. The training process involves both regulatory and morphological adaptations to vigorous exercise (Holmgren, 1967). The ability of the body to adapt to exogenous stress diminishes with age, so that an impaired regulatory response might be anticipated in an elderly individual. Equally, the morphological response to training requires the synthesis of new tissue in heart and skeletal muscle – a process that is likely to be more difficult to initiate with advancing age.

The physiological response to training has been interpreted in several different ways. An important variable is the individual's initial fitness, and some authors have classified such baseline data without reference to age (Grimby and Saltin, 1971). This is unsatisfactory, although we lack a good alternative basis for an initial objective categorization of elderly subjects. The most appropriate method of expressing gains in performance is contentious. If improvements of test score are presented in absolute terms, the training response usually decreases with age, but if improvements are expressed as a percentage of the initial value, the response of the elderly may exceed that of younger individuals. Adequacy of testing in

frail individuals requires experience. If the initial measurement is 'symptom-limited', premature halting of the test due to fear on the part of the patient or the examining physician will result in underscoring. If the examination is repeated after the confidence of both parties has been increased by a period of vigorous activity, the test may be pushed closer to a true physiological limit, with a large apparent gain of fitness.

Perhaps more important than physiological gains are the psychological rewards of training. The patient feels more cheerful, is more alert, and is better able to care for him- or herself. Psychological gains can sometimes be demonstrated by paper and pencil psychological tests such as the Profile of Mood States (Morgan, 1979), the Minnesota Multiphasic Personality Inventory (Kavanagh *et al.*, 1977), and the Taylor Manifest Anxiety Scale (Sidney and Shephard, 1977c), but failing eyesight and lack of patience with complex forms militate against a clear statistical result when such procedures are applied to elderly populations. The physician must thus be content to observe the improvement in his patients and accept their self-reports.

In the words of Henry Blackburn (1974): 'Moderate activity is a part of balanced, satisfying living, and it is the safe and hygienic prescription of the thoughtful physician for his patients, the high risk and the healthy alike.'

References

Andersen, K. L., Shephard, R. J., Denolin, H., Varnauskas, E., and Masironi, R. (1971). *Fundamentals of Exercise Testing*, WHO, Geneva.

Åstrand, I. (1960). 'Aerobic work capacity in men and women with special reference to age', *Acta. Physiol. Scand..*, **49** (Suppl. 169), 1–92.

Åstrand, I., Gahary, A., and Wahren, J. (1968). 'Circulatory responses to arm exercise with different arm positions', *J. Appl. Physiol.*, **25**, 528–532.

Bailey, D. A., Shephard, R. J., and Mirwald, R. L. (1976). 'Validation of a self-administered home-test of cardio-respiratory fitness', *Can. J. Appl. Sport Sci.*, **1**, 67–78.

Barnard, R. J., MacAlpin, R. N., Kattus, A. A., and Buckberg, G. D. (1973). 'Ischemic response to sudden strenous exercise in healthy men', *Circulation*, **48**, 936–942.

Blackburn, H. (1974). 'Disadvantages of intensive exercise therapy after myocardial infarction', in

Controversy in Internal Medicine (Ed. F. Ingelfinger), p. 162, W. B. Saunders, Philadelphia, Pennsylvania.

Brown, J. R., and Shephard, R. J. (1967). 'Some measurements of fitness in older female employees of a Toronto department store', *Can. Med. Assoc. J.*, **97**, 1028–1213.

Bruce, R. A., Kusumi, F., and Hosmer, D. (1973). 'Maximal oxygen intake and nomographic assessment of functional aerobic impairment in cardiovascular disease', *Am. Heart J.*, **85**, 546–562.

Carlsten, A. (1972). 'Influence of leg varicosities on the physical work performance', in *Environmental Effects on Work Performances* (Eds G. R. Cumming, A. W. Taylor, and D. Snidal), Can. Assoc. of Sports Sciences, Ottawa.

Clarke, H. H. (1966). *Muscular Strength and Endurance in Man*, Prentice-Hall, Englewood Cliffs, New Jersey.

Cobb, L., Baum, R. S., Alvarez, H., and Schaffer, W. A. (1975). 'Resuscitation from out of hospital ventricular fibrillation: 4 year follow-up', *Circulation*, **52** (Suppl. 3), 223–235.

Cooper, K. H. (1968). *Aerobics*, Evans, New York.

Cumming, E., and Henry, W. E. (1961). *Growing Old: The Process of Disengagement*, Basic Books, New York.

Cumming, G. R. (1978). 'Body size and the assessment of physical performance', in *Physical Fitness Assessment, Principles, Practice and Application* (Eds R. J. Shephard and H. Lavallée), pp. 18–31, C. C. Thomas, Springfield, Illinois.

Cumming, G. R., Dufresne, C., and Samm, J. (1973). 'Exercise e.c.g. changes in normal women', *Can. Med. Assoc. J.*, **109**, 108–111.

de Vries, H. (1980). *Physiology of Exercise for Physical Education and Athletics*, 3rd ed., Dubuque, Iowa.

Durnin, J. V. G. A., and Womerlsey, J. (1974). 'The relationship of total body fat, "fat-free mass" and total body weight in male and female human populations of varying ages', *J. Physiol. (Lond.)*, **213**, 33.

Elwood, P. C. (1971). 'Epidemiological aspects of iron deficiency in the elderly', *Gerontol. Clin. (Basel)*, **13**, 2–11.

Fisher, M. B., and Birren, J. E. (1947). 'Age and strength', *J. Appl. Psychol.*, **31**, 490–497.

Fried, T., and Shephard, R. J. (1969). 'Deterioration and restoration of physical fitness after training', *Can. Med. Assoc. J.*, **100**, 831–837.

Grimby, G., and Saltin, B. (1971). 'Physiological effects of physical conditioning', *Scand. J. Rehabil. Med.*, **3**, 6–14.

Hedlund, S., and Porjé, J. B. (1964). 'Cirkulationstörnigar hos äldre. Synpunkter på fysiologi och fysik träning som terapiform', *Svenska Läk – Tidn.*, **61**, 2970–2985.

Hettinger, T. (1961). *Physiology of Strength*, C. C. Thomas, Springfield, Illinois.

Holmgren, A. (1967). 'Commentary', in Proc. Int. Symp. on Physical Activity and Cardiovascular Health, *Can. Med. Assoc. J.*, **96**, 794.

Hughes, A. L., and Goldman, R. F. (1970). 'Energy cost of hard work', *J. Appl. Physiol.*, **29**, 570–572.

Jetté M., Campbell, J., Mongeon, J., and Routhier, R. (1976). 'The Canadian Home Fitness Test as a prediction of aerobic capacity', *Can. Med. Assoc. J.*, **114**, 680–682.

Kavanagh, T. (1970). 'A cold weather jogging mask for angina patients', *Can. Med. Assoc. J.*, **103**, 1290–1291.

Kavanagh, T., and Shephard, R. J. (1975). 'Conditioning of postcoronary patients: comparison of continuous and interval training', *Arch. Phys. Med. Rehabil.*, **56**, 72–76.

Kavanagh, T., and Shephard, R. J. (1977). 'The effects of continued training on the ageing process', *Ann. N. Y. Acad. Sci.*, **301**, 656–670.

Kavanagh, T., and Shephard, R. J. (1982). 'Influence of exercise and lifestyle variables upon HDL cholesterol following myocardial infarction. *Arteriosclerosis* **3**, 249–259.

Kavanagh, T., Shephard, R. J., Tuck, J. A., and Qureshi, S. (1977). 'Depression following myocardial infarction: the effects of distance running', *Ann. N.Y. Acad. Sci.*, **301**, 1029–1038.

Kelsey, J. C., Davis, G. M., Kofsky, P. R., and Shephard, R. J. (1981). Cardiorespiratory fitness and muscular strength in the lower-limb disabled. *Canad. Med. Assoc. J.*, **125**, 1317–1323.

Kilbom, Å., Hartley, L. H., Saltin, B., Bjure, J., Grimby, G., and Åstrand, I. (1969). 'Physical training in sedentary middle-aged and older men. I. Medical evaluation', *Scand. J. Clin. Lab. Invest.*, **24**, 315–322.

Larsen, O. A., and Lassen, N. A. (1966). 'Effect of daily muscular exercise in patients with intermittent claudication', *Lancet* ii, 1093–1096.

Lawrence, G. (1981). *Aquafitness for Women*, Wiley/Everest, Toronto.

Lester, F. M., Sheffield, L. T., Trammell, P., and Reeves, T. J. (1968). 'The effect of age and athletic training on maximal heart rate during muscular exercise', *Amer. Heart J.*, **76**, 370–376.

Lohman, T. G. (1981). 'Skinfolds and body density and their relation to body fatness: A review', *Hum. Biol.*, **53**, 181–226.

McDonough, J., and Bruce, R. A. (1969). 'Maximal exercise testing in assessing cardiovascular function', *J. S.C. Med. Assoc.*, **65** (Suppl. 1), 26–33.

Mann, G. V., Garrett, L. H., Farlie, A., Murray,

H., and Billings, F. T. (1969). 'Exercise to prevent coronary heart disease', *Am. J. Med., **46**,* 12–27.

Morgan, W. P. (1979). 'Psychologic aspects of heart disease', in *Heart Disease and Rehabilitation* (Eds M. L. Pollock and D. H. Schmidt), pp. 105–119, Houghton Mifflin, Boston, Massachusetts.

Niinimaa, V., and Shephard, R. J. (1978). 'Training and oxygen conductance in the elderly. I. The respiratory system. II. The cardiovascular system', *J. Gerontol.* 35, 351–367.

Piaget, J. (1956). 'Motricité, Perception et Intelligence,' Enfance, 9, 9–14. March/April 1956.

Pollock, M. L., Ward, A., and Foster, C. (1979). 'Exercise prescription for rehabilitation of the cardiac patient', in *Heart Disease and Rehabilitation* (Eds. M. L. Pollock and D. H. Schmidt), pp. 413–445, Houghton Mifflin, Boston, Massachusetts.

Rode, A., and Shephard, R. J. (1971). 'The influence of cigarette smoking upon the work of breathing in near maximal exercise', *Med. Sci. Sports Exerc.*, 3, 51–55.

Rowlatt, C., and Franks, L. M. (1973). *Aging in Tissues and Cells*, Churchill-Livingstone, Edinburgh.

Shephard, R. J. (1974). 'Sudden death – a significant hazard of exercise?', *Br. J. Sports Med.*, 8, 101–110.

Shephard, R. J. (1975). 'Future research on the quantifying of endurance training', *J. Human Ergol. (Tokyo)*, 3, 163–181.

Shephard, R. J. (1976). 'Environment and sports medicine', in *Sports Medicine* (Eds J. Williams and P. Sperryn), 2nd ed., Arnold, London.

Shephard, R. J. (1977). *Endurance Fitness*, University of Toronto Press, Toronto.

Shephard, R. J. (1978a). *Physical Activity and Aging*, Croom Helm, London.

Shephard, R. J. (1978b). *Human Physiological Working Capacity*, Cambridge University Press, London.

Shephard, R. J. (1980). *Ischaemic Heart Disease and Exercise*, Croom Helm, London.

Shephard, R. J. (1982a). *Physiology and Biochemistry of Exercise*, Praeger, New York.

Shephard, R. J. (1982b). *The Risks of Passive Smoking*, Croom Helm, London.

Shephard, R. J., Allen, C., Benade, A. J. S., Davies, C. T. M., di Prampero, P. E., Hedman, R., Merriman, J. E., Myhre, K., and Simmons, R. (1968). 'The maximum oxygen intake – an international reference standard of cardio-respiratory fitness', *Bull. WHO,* 38, 757–764.

Shephard, R. J., Hatcher, J., and Rode, A. (1973). 'On the body composition of the Eskimo', *Eur. J. Appl. Physiol.*, 30, 1–13.

Shephard, R. J., Youldon, P. E., Cox, M., and West, C. (1980). 'Effects of a six month industrial fitness programme on serum lipid concentrations', *Atherosclerosis*, 35, 277–285.

Sidney, K. H., and Shephard, R. J. (1977a). 'Maximum and submaximum exercise tests in men and women in the seventh, eighth and ninth decades of life', *J. Appl. Physiol.*, 43, 280–287.

Sidney, K. H., and Shephard, R. J. (1977b). 'Training and e.c.g. abnormalities in the elderly', *Br. Heart J.*, 39, 1114–1120.

Sidney, K. H., and Shephard, R. J. (1977c). 'Attitudes towards health and physical activity in the elderly. Effects of physical training programme', *Med. Sci. Sports Exerc.*, 8, 246–252.

Sidney, K. H., Shephard, R. J., and Harrison, J. (1977). 'Endurance training and body composition of the elderly', *Am. J. Clin. Nutr.*, 30, 326–333.

Siri, W. E. (1956). In *Advances in Biological and Medical Physics* (Eds J. H. Laurence and C. A. Tobias), Academic Press, London.

Society of Actuaries (1959). *Build and Blood Pressure Study*, Society of Actuaries, Chicago, Illinois.

Tanner, J. M. (1965). 'Radiographic studies of body composition in children and adults', in *Human Body Composition. Approaches and Applications* (Ed. J. Brozek), pp. 211–235, Pergamon, Oxford.

Taylor, H. L., Buskirk, E. R., and Henschel, A. (1955). 'Maximal oxygen intake as an objective measure of cardio-respiratory performance', *J. Appl. Physiol.*, 8, 73–80.

6

The Pharmacology of
Ageing

Principles and Practice of Geriatric Medicine
Edited by M. S. J. Pathy
© 1985 John Wiley & Sons Ltd

6.1

The Pharmacology of Ageing

K. O'Malley, F. Meagher, W. O'Callaghan

Pharmacology is the science that deals with the action of drugs in the body. Pharmacology embraces diverse aspects of drug knowledge. In this chapter we are concerned with the main aspects of drugs as they relate to the elderly. The first of these is the epidemiology of drug prescribing, and various other aspects of drug consumption. Secondly, we consider what happens to drugs in the body after they are administered – pharmacokinetics. There are important changes in pharmacokinetics with ageing and depending on which drug one is concerned with they may be of sufficient magnitude to affect the response observed. Finally, there are some examples of altered responsiveness to drugs in the elderly; for a given amount of drug at the site of action there is an altered magnitude or duration of response.

Clearly the end result of the doctor writing a prescription is determined by many factors – some physiological, others psychological, and yet others sociological. We start by considering drug prescribing and drug consumption in the elderly.

DRUG PRESCRIBING

The increasing size of the geriatric population (arbitrarily defined as over 65 years of age) in developed countries in recent years is well documented. At present 14 per cent. of the population of the United Kingdom and 10 per cent. of that of the United States are aged 65 years and over (OPCS Monitor, 1981; U.S. Bureau of the Census, 1979). With the continuing so-cioeconomic improvement and advances in medical technology, this trend is expected to continue. Increased life expectancy is associated with an increase in age-related disabilities.

Treatment of the elderly patient presents the physician with a great challenge. Multisystem disease becomes more prevalent and the non-specific presentation of disease in the elderly is well recognized. Their response to illness may be changed by the alterations in physiological function. Compensatory mechanisms and functional reserves are impaired. For example, cardiac output declines approximately 1 per cent. per year from the age of 19 to 86. The capacity to metabolize some drugs in the liver and to eliminate other drugs via the kidney is reduced in the elderly (Crooks, O'Malley, and Stevenson, 1976), and altered tissue sensitivity with ageing may result in a variable response (Castleden *et al.*, 1977; Shepherd *et al.*, 1977). An awareness and clear understanding of the implications of these changes is essential to the prescriber if the value of drug treatment in this age group is to be maximized.

In view of the multiple pathology associated with ageing, it is perhaps to be expected that the elderly are prescribed a greater number of drugs than the younger population. Polypharmacy appears to be the rule rather than the exception. This has been confirmed by many studies to be the case, both in hospital patients (Christopher *et al.*, 1978) and patients in the community (Law and Chalmers, 1976). Dunnell and Cartwright (1972) showed that people in Great Britain take on average 2.2 drugs and that the elderly take twice as much. The problem is confounded further by factors such as poor eye sight, impaired intellect, confusion, and reduced manual dexterity.

The striking increase in the number and potency of available drugs in the last 20 years is pertinent. Clinicians are faced with the problem of keeping their knowledge of drugs in step with recent developments. They have somehow to familiarize themselves with this growing repertoire and above all to ensure the drugs are used to the patients' advantage. The information that is available to the clinician concerning the expected effect of the new drug on the elderly patient is, sadly, often scanty. Extra care when prescribing to this group is therefore mandatory. The volume of prescribing among the elderly has been studied by different groups of workers. In Britain those aged over 65 comprise 15 per cent. of the population but account for 33 per cent. of the national expenditure on drugs (Judge and Caird, 1978). Law and Chalmers (1976) found that in one general practice 87 per cent. of those over 75 years received regular drug treatment, 34 per cent. taking three or more different drugs each day. Skegg, Doll, and Perry (1977) showed a positive correlation between the volume of prescribing and increasing age. They also found that psychotropic drugs were the main group prescribed. Similar results have been found in Sweden where Boethius (1977) demonstrated changes in the prescribing of drugs by therapeutic groups and age. The elderly received the greatest number of prescriptions per person and there was an increase in the prescribing of psychotropics, hypoglycaemics, analgesics, and cardiovascular drugs with increasing age.

The number of consultations occurring as a percentage of the total number of patients in a given age range rises with age and the incidence of non-prescribing consultations is lower in the older age groups (Whitfield, 1973). Similar high prescribing rates are found among elderly hospitalized patients. In a multicentre study involving 42 geriatric medicine departments in Britain (Williamson, 1979) it was found that, of nearly 2,000 patients aged 65 and over, 81.3 per cent. were receiving drugs at the time of admission with 55.4 per cent. receiving one to three drugs and 25.9 per cent. receiving four to six drugs. The most frequently prescribed groups of drugs were diuretics, analgesics, and antipyretics and psychotropic drugs (Table 1). In a cross-sectional one-day survey of 873 elderly people in Dundee hospitals, Christopher and coworkers (1978) found the average number of drugs prescribed per patient was 3.6. The most widely used group of drugs in this study were hypnotics.

Table 1 Most commonly prescribed drugs. (From Williamson, 1979)

	Male (%)	Female (%)	Total (%)
Diuretics	35.9	38.2	37.4
Analgesics and antipyretics	23.2	29.6	27.4
Antidepressants, tranquillizers, and psychomimetics	21.3	24.9	23.7
Hypnotics, sedatives, and anticonvulsants	22.6	22.0	22.2
Digitalis	18.3	21.0	21.1
Salts (potassium)	15.1	16.0	15.7

The practice of 'repeat' prescriptions exposes the elderly to unnecessary risk. Dunnell and Cartwright (1972) estimated that 75 per cent. of prescriptions given to elderly patients are repeat prescriptions. Walker (1971) has also clearly shown the extent to which repeat prescribing is age related. These prescriptions are often for psychotropic drugs and patients may have been taking these for many years with inadequate supervision. In a survey of psychotropic drug prescribing in general practice, Dennis (1979) found that repeat prescriptions are often given without the patient seeing the doctor. His analysis showed that the longer the repeat prescribing had taken place, the older the patient was likely to be and the less closely were they monitored by their general practitioner. Reliance on self-referral by the elderly is unsafe and this makes this area all the more problematic (Shaw and Opit, 1976).

Prescribing habits of doctors are affected by many factors. It is generally acknowledged that the topic of geriatric pharmacology is neglected at the undergraduate level. Joyce, Last, and Weatherall (1967) found that the possession of higher qualifications was associated with lower prescribing rates among general practitioners. In a study on sources of drug information used by general practitioners, Eaton and Parish

(1976) found the Monthly Index of Medical Specialities (MIMS) was the most popular, being used by 77 per cent. to select an appropriate drug for treatment and by 96 per cent. to check on dose and/or tablet strength. It was also rated by a large proportion (76 per cent.) of doctors as a source of information used to check on adverse drug effects and contraindications. It is clear, however, that MIMS is a far from adequate source of such information in relation to the treatment of most patients, but particularly to that of the elderly. It does not in fact list adverse effects and there is no modification of drug dosage and administration for the elderly. The British National Formulary has a special section on geriatric prescribing. However, it is clear that the ever increasing number and potency of drugs combined with a relative dearth of information on their use in the elderly mitigates against good prescribing in this population.

Adverse Drug Reactions

An adverse drug reaction has been defined by the WHO (1970) as any response to a drug 'that is noxious and unintended and which occurs at doses used in man for prophylaxis, diagnosis or treatment'. This definition is regarded as inadequate by many. For instance, it does not include suicide which is an obvious adverse reaction, albeit intentional. Nor does it include accidental drug poisoning. It has been suggested that the definition should include therapeutic failures. Karch and Lasagna (1975) put forward the following addition to the WHO definition: '. . . including failure to accomplish the intended purpose'. The lack of agreement among workers as to their understanding of the term 'adverse drug reaction' is clearly undesirable.

Further confusion arises from the classification of adverse drug reactions as 'probable', 'possible', 'unlikely', etc. A reaction that one investigator judges to be 'possible' may be considered 'probable' by another. In addition,

these descriptive terms are often not defined in reports. The lack of standardization renders the comparison of results of different studies of doubtful value. Recently attempts to improve precision in the diagnosis of adverse drug reactions have been made (Karch and Lasagna, 1977; Kramer et al., 1979; Naranjo et al., 1981). These consist of algorithms that provide detailed operational criteria for ranking the probability of causation when an adverse drug reaction is suspected.

Incidence and Causes of Adverse Drug Reactions

In spite of the problem of lack of standardization, there is evidence that adverse drug reactions occur more commonly in the elderly. Adverse drug reactions in hospitalized patients have been estimated to occur at a frequency of between 10 and 13.6 per cent. (Schimmel, 1964; Seidl et al., 1966., Smith, Seidl, and Cluff, 1966). Levy and coworkers, (1980) and Hurwitz (1969) (Table 2) have clearly shown increasing age to be associated with adverse drug reactions. It has also been shown (Caranosos, Stewart, and Cluff, 1974; Hurwitz and Wade, 1969) that drug-induced illness leading to hospitalization occurs more frequently among elderly patients (Table 3). A direct relationship has been suggested between the number of drugs a patient receives and the probability of acquiring an adverse reaction (Cluff, Thornton, and Seidl, 1964). The increased incidence of adverse drug reactions among elderly patients is probably due, in part, to the greater number of drugs taken by this group. Caranosos, Stewart, and Cluff (1974), in their series of 6,063 consecutive admissions found that one-third of the drug reactions were produced by eight drugs (Table 4). The first four of this group are among those drugs commonly prescribed to the elderly. Toxic effects of some drugs occur more often in the elderly. For a given amount of administered digoxin higher blood levels are observed in older in-

Table 2 Age and drug reactions. (From Hurwitz, 1969)

Age of patients (years)	Number of given drugs	Number with reactions	Rate (%)
< 60	667	42	6.3
60 +	493	76	15.4

Table 3 Adverse drug reactions and admissions by age group. (From Caranosos, Stewart, and Cluff, 1974)

Age range (years)	All admissions number (%)	Adverse drug reaction number (%)
11–20	294 (6.5)	11 (6.2)
21–30	782 (12.9)	19 (10.7)
31–40	746 (12.3)	20 (11.3)
41–50	1,006 (16.6)	21 (11.9)
51–60	1,225 (20.2)	33 (18.6)
61–70	1,213 (20.0)	44 (24.9)
71–80	546 (9.0)	26 (14.7)
81–90	139 (2.3)	3 (1.7)
91–100	12 (0.2)	0 (0.0)
Total	6,063 (100.0)	177 (100.0)

Table 4 Drugs implicated in adverse drug reactions. (Caranosos, Stewart, and Cluff, 1974

Drugs	Number of times cited
Aspirin	25
Digoxin	24
Warfarin	12
Sodium hydrochlorthiazide	11
Prednisone	8
Vincristine Sulphate	6
Norethindrone	6
Frusemide	5
7 Drugs	4
15 Drugs	3
31 Drugs	2
48 Drugs	1

Total number of drugs cited 109
Total number of times all drugs cited 280

dividuals (Ewy *et al.*, 1969), due mainly to the reduced clearance of the drug. Reduced drug elmination contributes to the increased incidence of adverse reactions among old people.

Patients' sex has been shown to be another risk factor in the development of adverse drug reactions – women being more susceptible (Seidl *et al.*, 1966; Stewart and Cluff, 1971),

both in absolute terms and in proportion to their numbers. The greater number of drugs taken by women (Stewart and Cluff, 1971) contributes to this finding.

Smith, Seidl, and Cluff (1966) have shown that the overall rate of adverse reactions is increased in patients with decreased renal function (Table 5), a finding particularly pertinent to the elderly population.

There have been conflicting reports on the effect of adverse drug reactions on the duration of patients' hospital stay. Hurwitz (1969) failed to find a significant prolongation of hospitalization. This, however, is contrary to the findings of other workers (Ogilvie and Ruedy, 1967; Seidl *et al.*, 1966). Unfortunately, none of these studies relate the prolongation of hospital stay to age, but it is tempting to suggest that this is greater among the elderly. It has been suggested that patients who have had an adverse reaction in the past are predisposed to having a further one while hospitalized (Hurwitz, 1969).

Compliance

Ineffective treatment due to poor patient compliance has been increasingly recognized over the past 10 years as another major pharmacotherapeutic problem. Compliance has been defined as the extent to which the patients' behaviour coincides with the clinical prescription (Haynes, 1979). The elderly are not alone in showing a less than perfect relationship between drugs that are prescribed for them and those they take. Poor compliance is often the result of extraneous factors – intellectual impairment, poor vision, reduced manual dexterity, etc. The difficulty encountered when trying to separate these unintentional non-compliers from the deliberate non-compliers is obvious. Inadequacy in quantifying compliance

Table 5 Rates or adverse drug reactions: effect of renal function. (From Smith, Seidl, and Cluff, 1966.)

	Patients	Patients with reactions	Rate (%)
BUN* 20 or less	753	68	9.0
BUN 21–40	114	21	18.4
BUN 41 or greater	33	8	24.2
Total	900	97	10.8

* BUN = Blood urea nitrogen.

renders an accurate estimate of its frequency difficult. There are many different studies showing a great disparity in the incidence of non-compliance. Haynes (1976) reviewed 37 of these and only in 7 did he find an association between decreasing compliance and increasing age. Parkin and coworkers (1976) found that among patients who deviated from prescribed drug treatment after discharge from hospital, non-comprehension accounted for the majority. The responsibility of ensuring maximum compliance with therapy lies with the physician. It is he who initiates therapy and he who must provide appropriate follow-up. He must identify those elderly patients who are likely to be 'unintentional' non-compliers and take the necessary steps to overcome this problem. Although the ultimate outcome of non-compliance is the same whatever the cause, the methods of dealing with the problem are different (O'Hanrahan and O'Malley, 1981). Above all, the regimen for the elderly patient must be simple. Gibson and O'Hare (1968) found that three drugs was the maximum number alert elderly patients could manage. This finding has been confirmed by Dass, Maddock, and Whittingham (1977). The fact that an elderly patient does not question any instructions should not be taken to mean that the patient understands them. Comprehension and recall of prescription directions are necessary for correct drug taking.

Errors in drug taking are directly related to the degree of mental impairment. Those patients who err are likely to make multiple mistakes. Schwartz (1962) found that the average number of errors per error-making patient was 2.6. The most frequent error was of omission, followed by errors in drug dose, timing, and sequence. These findings serve to emphasize the importance of clear written instructions. The labelling of medicines 'to be taken as directed' is clearly inappropriate for many elderly patients. Poor compliance could be further minimized in the elderly by the use of appropriate drug packaging. Drugs should be packaged in clear glass containers to allow the elderly to recognize their tablets. These containers should also open without undue difficulty.

Active teaching of elderly patients to take their drugs correctly is another method of improving compliance (Wandless and Davie, 1977). This must be done prior to discharge from hospital. Atkinson, Gibson, and Andrews (1978) suggest that occupational therapists could successfully incorporate this item into their activities of daily living programme.

There is no simple answer to the problem of non-compliance but the physician must always have a high index of suspicion as the primary problem is the identification of the defaulter. The various methods of improving compliance described above, in conjunction with judicious prescribing, can then be implemented.

Improving Prescribing

Improvement in the quality of geriatric prescribing could be brought about in many ways. Initially an accurate diagnosis is vital. A careful history from the patient and/or relatives, mindful of the non-specific presentation of disease in the elderly must be obtained. An awareness of the pharmacology of each drug prescribed and its altered handling by these patients is also essential. In the interests of good compliance, the general principle of prescribing as few drugs as possible and at the lowest effective dose should be adhered to. Having initiated therapy, the doctor has an obligation to assess the efficacy and to regularly review the need for continued treatment. Dall (1970) reviewed a group of 80 elderly patients receiving digoxin on a maintenance basis and found that in almost 75 per cent. of the group, digoxin could be stopped, without ill effect. Elderly patients must be encouraged to bring all their drugs to each consultation so that these can be closely scrutinized and careful records kept of those that required to be 'repeated'. Enquiries about adverse reactions must be made at each visit, the doctor being mindful of the tolerance of the elderly and their consequent failure to report symptoms of drug toxicity.

RESPONSIVENESS TO DRUGS

Responsiveness to drugs refers to the readiness with which the organism responds and to what extent and duration. As will be outlined in the pharmacokinetic section, age alters the way in which the body handles drugs and such changes have been shown or may reasonably be expected to affect the patient's response. This results from the fact that the magnitude and duration of drug effect is proportional to the amount of free drug in the vicinity of the site of drug action. In discussing responsiveness to drugs we must take into account not only the amount of drug present at the site of action but in addition relate this to the pharmacological effect. If the effect is greater or less for a given amount of drug we say that the responsiveness is increased or decreased.

Change at different levels of organization may account for alterations in responsiveness. Drug receptor numbers or affinity may be affected or there may be changes in membrane structure and function in old age. Diminution in effectiveness in homeostatic mechanisms is a hallmark of ageing and as drugs act by perturbing biochemical and physiological systems the older patient may not have the capacity of restoring function to the status quo. An example is blood pressure control where the decrease in baroreflex sensitivity seen in the elderly (McGarry *et al.*, 1983) puts them at particular risk of postural hypotension with some blood pressure lowering drugs.

It is not possible to measure the amount of free drug at the site of action though we can extrapolate from the amount of drug in the plasma, particularly the concentration of free drug. There are relatively few studies where responsiveness has been measured in this way. Perhaps the best example is that of Vestal and coworkers (1979b) who examined heart rate response to isoprenaline and propranolol as a function of age. They showed that responsiveness to both drugs was diminished in the older subjects. Using a model system, the human lymphocyte, Dillion and coworkers (1980) showed that responsiveness to isoprenaline was lower in cells from old people.

Many unwanted effects of drugs affect the central nervous system. Castleden and George (1979) examined the responsiveness of the elderly and young to the benzodiazepine hypnotic nitrazepam and showed that there was no difference in pharmacokinetics in young and old but that the magnitude and duration of CNS depression was greater in the elderly. This may reflect greater access of nitrazepam to the site of action in the older brain or possibly there are changes in the relevant receptors with ageing. Reidenberg and coworkers (1978) showed that the elderly are more sensitive to the CNS depressant effects of another benzodiazepine,

diazepam. They studied the use of diazepam as an intravenous premedication in young and elderly. There is also evidence that there is an increased responsiveness in the elderly to a third benzodiazepine, temazepam (Salem, 1981).

The anticoagulant effect of warfarin is also increased (O'Malley *et al.*, 1977). In the absence of alterations in steady-state plasma levels the degree of anticoagulation increases with ageing (Shepherd *et al.*, 1977).

From the foregoing it can be seen that we cannot generalize with regard to responsiveness to drugs in the elderly. In some cases responsiveness is increased while in others it is decreased. We are quite ignorant of the mechanisms involved in these changes and clearly further study into this important aspect of pharmacology is required.

PHARMACOKINETICS

The ageing process is associated with anatomical, physiological, and pathological changes which may significantly alter various aspects of pharmacokinetics in the elderly. Such age-related changes may contribute to altered drug effects in the elderly both therapeutic and toxic. The large interindividual variation in some pharmacokinetic parameters seen in the elderly may reflect the difference between chronological and biological ageing. This limits to some extent the application of general principles to individual cases.

Drug Absorption

The rate and extent of absorption are independent parameters (Greenblatt and Koch-Weser, 1975). Rapid absorption is required for prompt therapeutic effect while the extent of absorption determines steady-state drug concentration and therefore the pharmacological effect with chronic dosage.

After administration a medication disintegrates. The drug then dissolves and is absorbed. Disintegration and dissolution can be affected by both the formulation of the medication and various factors within the gut. The ability to absorb chemicals is a characteristic of the membranes of the gastrointestinal tract. In most cases drug absorption is achieved by passive diffusion across membranes but the absorption of some sugars and other nutrients is by active transport mechanisms.

Despite many age-related changes in the gastrointestinal tract which would in theory affect drug absorption (Bender, 1968), there are only minor alterations in drug absorption in the elderly (Stevenson *et al.*, 1981). There have not been many examples of a clinically significant diminution in drug absorption in man. Many drugs have been studied and the data are summarized in the review of Stevenson and coworkers (1981).

Drug Distribution

The pattern of drug distribution depends upon the physiochemical properties of the drug in question and the body composition of the subject. Fat-soluble drugs cross membranes easily and spread widely throughout the body. In contrast, polar drugs cross membranes less easily and largely remain in lean body tissue. Additional factors determining drug distribution include binding to plasma proteins and red cells as well as the blood flow to particular organs and tissues. This change in body composition, plasma protein concentration, or regional blood flow may affect the distribution of individual drugs.

In general the elderly tend to be smaller than younger patients. Total body water is reduced both in absolute terms (Shock *et al.*, 1963) and as a percentage of body weight (Edelman and Liebman, 1959; Vestal *et al.*, 1975), declining by 10 to 15 per cent. between the second and eight decades. At the same time body fat increases (Novak, 1972). The net effect of these changes is a reduction in lean body mass per unit of total body weight (Forbes and Reina, 1970), largely due to the increased fat content. Therefore it may be expected that drugs which are largely distributed in body water or lean body mass achieve higher blood levels in the elderly.

Volume of Distribution

The apparent volume of distribution of a drug is a proportionality factor which related the mass of a drug in the body to its plasma concentration in an effort to describe the extent of drug distribution in a mathematical fashion. As expected, the apparent volume of distri-

bution of fat-soluble drugs such as chlordiazepoxide (Shader *et al.*, 1977), chlormethiazole (Nation *et al.*, 1976), diazepam (Klotz *et al.*, 1975), and lignocaine (Nation, Triggs, and Selig, 1977) increases with age, whereas that of polar drugs such as propicillin (Simon *et al.*, 1972) and ethanol (Vestal *et al.*, 1977) is reduced.

Protein Binding

Free drug concentration also determines drug distribution and elimination. It is dependent on the degree of drug binding to plasma proteins and red cells. Serum albumin concentration is reduced in old age but this reduction may be related to disease and immobility rather than to age per se (Woodford-Williams *et al.*, 1964). In addition, the normal metabolic response to a reduced albumin pool appears to be impaired in elderly subjects (Misera, Loundon, and Staddon, 1975). This reduction in serum albumin is associated with a decrease in the maximum binding capacity of warfarin (Hayes, Langman, and Short, 1975a), phenytoin (Hayes, Langman, and Short, 1975b), and carbenoxolone (Hayes, Sprackling, and Langman, 1977). However, at therapeutic concentrations there is no age-related change in protein binding of warfarin (Shepherd *et al.*, 1977) or phenytoin (Bender *et al.*, 1975).

Therefore the capacity for binding to albumin may be smaller in older subjects, but this may be of little significance at therapeutic concentrations of single drugs, where the capacity is not exceeded. When elderly patients are taking many drugs, the reduced albumin binding capacity may be more significant and result in a displacement of bound drugs with consequent increases in free drug concentrations. Indeed, the free drug concentrations of phenylbutazone, salicylate, and sulphadiazine have been noted to be greater in elderly patients on multiple-drug therapy compared to those of similar age on one drug only (Wallace, Whiting, and Runcie, 1976).

A small reduction in protein binding by highly bound drugs such as warfarin or phenytoin results in a large percentage increase in plasma free drug concentration. More free drug is therefore available for distribution and elimination. A new equilibrium is reached and free drug concentration returns to its original level while total plasma drug concentration is reduced. This results in a larger volume of distribution for total drug but no change in that for free drug (Klotz, 1976). It follows that the net effect is not of great significance for long-term steady-state levels.

The binding of drugs to red blood cells is decreased with advancing age. Pethidine (Chan *et al.*, 1975) and chlormethiazole (Nation, Triggs, and Selig, 1977) display less binding to erythrocytes in the elderly than in younger subjects, with a resultant increase in free drug concentration, at least in the acute situation.

Regional Distribution

Whereas the apparent volume of distribution is a useful measurement of the extent of uptake of a drug in the tissues it provides no indication of drug concentration at the site of action. Drug distribution to and within individual tissues and organs depends on factors such as organ blood flow and vascularity, tissue lipid content and local pH. The measurement of drug distribution to different organs in man is difficult and little data are available on this aspect of pharmacokinetics. This point is illustrated by diazepam, the volume of distribution of which is increased in the elderly (Klotz *et al.*, 1975). Thus one would expect that plasma concentrations would be lower and thus that an equieffective sedatory dose would be higher in the elderly than in younger subjects. However, as nothing is known of the effect of age on brain uptake of diazepam, a prediction based on the volume of distribution alone is not valid. Indeed, the effective sedatory dose of diazepam is reduced in the elderly compared to younger subjects (Reidenberg *et al.*, 1978). Therefore, predictions regarding the clinical efficacy of drugs cannot be based on indices of distribution characteristics alone.

Drug Metabolism

Though conventional biochemical indices of hepatic function show no age-related decline (Kampmann, Sniding, and Moller-Jorgensen, 1975) certain physiological and anatomical changes occur which may influence hepatic drug metabolism.

Hepatic blood flow, which is particuarly im-portant for the clearance of drugs with high hepatic extraction ratios such as propranolol and lignocaine, declines with age (Wood *et al.*, 1979). Estimations of this decline range from 0.3 to 1.5 per cent. per year. In addition, autopsy studies show that liver mass, relative to body weight, declines after middle age (Geokas and Haverback, 1969).

Hepatic clearance of metabolized drugs depends on two factors, hepatic blood flow and the activity of drug metabolizing enzymes – intrinsic hepatic clearance. Elimination of most drugs such as antipyrine, diazepam, and phenylbutazone is dependent mainly on intrinsic hepatic clearance, because these drugs have a small hepatic extraction ratio. Systemic elimination of other drugs with a moderate to large extraction ratio, such as propranolol, lignocaine, and chlormethiazole, is intermediate, depending on both intrinsic clearance and hepatic blood flow. Drugs with a moderate or high hepatic extraction ratio undergo extensive first-pass metabolism in the liver after oral administration and thus their bioavailability is low. The bioavailability of chlormethiazole (Nation *et al.*, 1976), propranolol (Castleden and George, 1979), and labetalol (Kelly *et al.*, 1982) is greater in the elderly, indicating that presystemic hepatic extraction declines with age (Fig. 1).

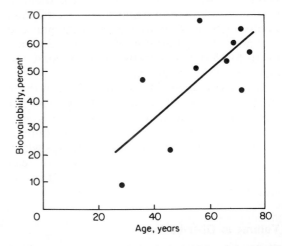

Figure 1   Increasing bioavailability of labetalol with age reflects diminishing first pass metabolism (Kelly *et al.*, 1982)

In man the drug most widely used to assess hepatic metabolism is antipyrine. It is a model drug for the estimation of intrinsic hepatic metabolizing capacity because it is well absorbed after oral administration, has minimal binding to plasma proteins, and is almost completely metabolized in the liver. Since it has a low hepatic extraction ratio its clearance is independent of hepatic blood flow; rather, metabolism is determined by the activity of hepatic microsomal enzymes.

Plasma elimination half-life of antipyrine is prolonged and its clearance is reduced in the elderly (O'Malley *et al.*, 1971; Liddell, Williams, and Briant, 1975). Initially it was thought that this change was related to age alone. However, it has become clear that environmental factors, particularly cigarette smoking, are more important than age (Wood *et al.*, 1979; Vestal *et al.*, 1975).

The intrinsic hepatic clearance of propanolol and the total systemic clearance of antipyrine, both of which reflect hepatic drug metabolizing capacity, declines with age in smokers but not in non-smokers. The systemic clearance of propranolol, which depends on both hepatic blood flow and intrinsic hepatic clearance, is inversely related to age in smokers only. The clearance of indocyanine green, which is an index of hepatic blood flow, declines with age irrespective of smoking. Therefore, smoking it seems is associated with a higher rate of intrinsic drug metabolism in the young. Hepatic blood flow declines with age and is not related to smoking.

In addition to cigarette smoking poor nutrition and vitamin deficiencies could contribute to the decline in antipyrine elimination observed in the aged (Smithard and Langman, 1971). Elderly hospitalized non-smokers showed no difference in antipyrine elimination when compared to a younger group. However, non-hospitalized non-smoking elderly patients, who may have a poorer nutritional status than hospitalized patients, showed a reduction in antipyrine elimination (Swift, Homeida, and Roberts, 1978). On the other hand, it is possible that the enhanced antipyrine elimination in the hospitalized group is related to enzyme induction by unidentified agents.

Age-related changes have also been noted in the rate of metabolism of other metabolized drugs. The clearance of chlordiazopoxide (Roberts *et al.*, 1978), chlormethiazole (Nation *et al.*, 1976), desmethyldiazepam (Klotz and

Muller-Scydlitz, 1979), and quinine (Salem and Stevenson, 1977) is lower in the elderly. The clearance of acetanilide (Playfer *et al.*, 1978), diazepam (Klotz *et al.*, 1975), lignocaine (Nation, Triggs, and Selig, 1977), lorazepam (Kraus *et al.*, 1978), and warfarin (Shepherd *et al.*, 1977) is unchanged with age.

In advancing age there is also a variable change in the elimination of drugs which are not oxidized. The clearance of carbenoxolone (Shepherd *et al.*, 1977) and paracetamol (Fulton, James, and Rawlins, 1979) declines with advancing age while that of aspirin (Salem and Stevenson, 1977) is unaltered. Clearances of nitrazepam, which is reduced in the liver, is unchanged (Kangas *et al.*, 1979). The plasma half-life of isoniazid which is acetylated is unchanged in the elderly (Farah *et al.*, 1977). However, in some of the above studies (Fulton, James, and Rawlins, 1979; Kangas *et al.*, 1979; Roberts *et al.*, 1978) clearance values were not corrected for body weight. As elderly patients are generally smaller than the young, a lower absolute clearance value may reflect lower body weight and not reduced drug metabolizing capacity.

Few data are available on the effects of ageing on hepatic enzyme induction potential in man. The elimination of antipyrine and quinine was observed to increase in the young but not in the elderly (Salem *et al.*, 1978) following treatment with the inducing agent, dichloralphenazone. However, the mean baseline clearance of antipyrine was high in the elderly group, being similar to the mean postinduction clearance in the young group, suggesting for some reason that metabolism in the elderly group in this study was maximally stimulated at the outset. Theophylline metabolism appears to be at least partially inducible in the elderly (Cusack *et al.*, 1980).

In summary, hepatic blood flow declines with age which increases the bioavailability of drugs such as propranolol which have a high first pass metabolism. The decline in blood flow does not seem to affect the metabolism of drugs with small hepatic extraction ratios. Intrinsic hepatic drug metabolizing capacity is little altered by age per se but is altered by environmental factors such as cigarette smoking. Some alterations in the elimination of non-oxidized drugs have been described but these may relate to alterations in other pharmacokinetic parameters rather than to changes in metabolism alone.

RENAL EXCRETION OF DRUGS

Many physiological and pathological changes occur in the ageing kidney. In humans, kidney weight declines by about 20 per cent. between the fourth and eighth decades (McLachlan, 1978). The major amount of weight loss occurs in the cortex. These changes are related to a reduction in renal blood flow per unit mass of renal tissue (Hollenberg *et al.*, 1974).

Renal function declines steadily with age. Glomerular filtration rate and renal plasma flow are reduced (Davies and Shock, 1950), their decline becoming apparent from the age of 40 years onwards. Therefore, a 70 year old person would be expected to have a glomerular filtration rate 35 per cent. less than that of a young adult. As well as this, there is a parallel decline in renal tubular function. The maximum reabsorptive capacity for glucose falls with age (Muller, McDonald, and Shock, 1952), as does urine concentrating ability (Rowe, Shock, and Defromzo, 1976). These observations were made in healthy subjects with no evidence of renal disease and so are likely to reflect the influence of age per se.

The decline in creatinine clearance is not accompanied by an elevation of serum creatinine in elderly persons, because creatinine production is also reduced in old age in proportion to a decline in lean body mass. Therefore, a normal serum creatinine in elderly patients should not be equated with normal renal function.

Drug elimination by the kidneys is invariably reduced in old age. The excretion of many important drugs is reduced including digoxin (Ewy *et al.*, 1969), dihydrostreptomycin (Vartia and Lakola, 1960), gentamycin (Lumholtz *et al.*, 1974), kanamycin (Kristensen *et al.*, 1974), penicillin G (Kampmann *et al.*, 1972; Kampmann and Molholm-Hansen, 1979), and tetracycline (Kramer *et al.*, 1978). A proportional relationship has been observed between creatinine clearance and renal clearance of digoxin (Ewy *et al.*, 1969), quinidine (Ochs *et al.*, 1978) and sulphmetiazole (Triggs *et al.*, 1975). Therefore, calculation of creatinine clearance provides a simple means of predicting drug plasma clearance, and therefore daily requirements.

Unlike hepatic drug elimination, which has some age-dependent trends and also has marked interindividual variation, drug elimination by the kidney appears to predictably decline with age (see Chapter 26.2).

REFERENCES

Atkinson, L., Gibson, I., and Andrews, J. (1978). 'An investigation into the ability of elderly patients to take prescribed drugs after discharge from hospital and recommendations concerning improving the situation', *Gerontology*, **24**, 225–234.

Bender, A. D. (1968). 'Effect of age on intestinal absorption: Implications for drug absorption in the elderly', *J. Am. Geriat. Soc.*, **16**, 1331–1339.

Bender, A. D., Post, A., Meuer, J. P., Higson, J. E., and Reichard, G. (1975). 'Plasma protein binding of drugs as a function of age in adult human subjects', *J. Pharm. Sci.*, **64**, 1711–1713.

Boethius, G. (1977). 'Prescription of drugs 1970–1975 in the County of Jamtland, Sweden', PhD Thesis, Ostersund and Karolinska Institutet Huddinge, University Hospital, Huddinge, Sweden, 1977.

Caranosos, G. J., Stewart, R. B., and Cluff, L. E. (1974). 'Drug-induced illness leading to hospitalization', *JAMA*, **228**, 713–717.

Castleden, C. M., and George, C. F. (1979). 'The effects of ageing on the hepatic clearance of propranolol', *Br. J. Clin. Pharmacol.*, **7**, 49–54.

Castleden, C. M., George, C. F., Marcer, D., and Hallett, C. (1977). 'Increased sensitivity to nitrazepam in old age', *Br. Med. J.*, **1**, 110–112.

Chan, K., Kendall, M. J., Mitchard, M., and Wells, W. D. E. (1975). 'The effect of ageing on plasma pethidine concentration', *Br. J. Clin. Pharmacol.*, **2**, 297–302.

Christopher, L. J., Ballinger, B. R., Shepherd, A. M. M., Ramsay, A., and Crooks, G. (1978). 'Drug prescribing patterns in elderly. A cross-sectional study of in-patients', *Age & Ageing*, **7**, 74–82.

Cluff, L. E., Thornton, C. F., and Seidl, L. G. (1964). 'Studies on the epidemiology of adverse drug reactions. I. Methods of surveillance', *JAMA*, **188**, 976–983.

Crooks, J., O'Malley, K., and Stevenson, I. H. (1976). 'Clinical pharmacokinetics in the elderly', *Clin. Pharmacokin.*, **1**, 280–296.

Cusack, B., Kelly, J. G., Lavan, J., Noel, J., and O'Malley, K. (1980). 'Theophylline kinetics in relation to age: The importance of smoking', *Br. J. Clin. Pharmac.*, **10**, 109–114.

Dall, J. L. C. (1970). 'Maintenance digoxin in elderly patients', *Br. Med. J.*, **2**, 705–706.

Dass, B. C., Maddock, S. G., and Whittingham, G. C. (1977). 'Special problems of medication in a survey of 114 elderly people at home, in welfare homes and in hospital', *Mod. Geriat.*, **7**, 22–25.

Davies, D. F., and Shock, N. W. (1950). 'Age changes in glomerular filtration rate effective renal plasma flow and tubular excretory capacity in adult males', *J. Clin. Invest.*, **29**, 496–507.

Dennis, P. J. (1979). 'Monitoring of psychotrope prescribing in general practice', *Br. Med. J.*, **2**, 1115–16.

Dillon, N., Chung, S., Kelly, J. G., and O'Malley, K. (1980). 'Age and beta adrenoceptor-medicated function', *Clin. Pharmacol. Ther.*, **27**, 769–772.

Dunnell, K., and Cartwright, A. (1972). *Medicine Takers, Prescribers and Hoarders*, Routledge and Kegan Paul, London.

Eaton, G., and Parish, P. A. (1976). 'Sources of drug information used by general practitioners', *J. Roy. Coll. Gen. Practit.* **26** (Suppl. 1), 58–64.

Edelman, I. S., and Liebman, J. (1959). 'Anatomy of body water and electrolytes', *Am. J. Med.*, **27**, 256–277.

Ewy, G. A., Kapadia, G. C., Yao, L., Lullin, M., and Marcus, F. I. (1969). 'Digoxin metabolism in the elderly', *Circulation,* **39**, 449–453.

Farah, F., Taylor, W., Rawlins, M. D., and James, O. (1977). 'Hepatic drug acetylation and oxidation: Effects of ageing in man', *Br. Med. J.*, **2**, 155–156.

Forbes, G. B., and Reina, J. C. (1970). 'Adult lean body mass declines with age: Some longitudinal observations', *Metabolism,* **19**, 653–663.

Fulton, B., James, O., and Rawlins, M. D. (1979). 'The influence of age on the pharmacokinetics of paracetamol', *Br. J. Clin. Pharmacol.*, **7**, 418p.

Geokas, M. C., and Haverback, B. J. (1969). 'The ageing gastrointestinal tract', *Am. J. Surg.*, **117**, 881–892.

Gibson, I. J. M., and O'Hare, M. M. (1968). 'Prescription of drugs for old people at home', *Geront. Clin.*, **10**, 271–280.

Greenblatt, D. J., and Koch-Weser, J. (1975). 'Clinical pharmacokinetics', *New Eng. J. Med.*, **293**, 702–705 and 964–969.

Hayes, M. J., Langman, M. J. S., and Short, A. H. (1975a). 'Changes in drug metabolism with increasing age. 1: Warfarin binding and plasma proteins', *Brit. J. Clin. Pharmacol.*, **2**, 69–71.

Hayes, M. J., Langman, M. J. S., and Short, A. H. (1975b). 'Changes in drug metabolism with increasing age. 2: Phenytoin clearance and protein binding', *Br. J. Clin. Pharmacol.*, **2**, 73–79.

Hayes, M. J., Sprackling, M., and Langman, M. J. S. (1977). 'Changes in plasma clearance and protein binding of carbenoxolone with age, and their possible relationship with adverse drug effects', *GUT,* **18**, 1054–1058.

Haynes, R. B. (1976). 'A critical review of the "determinants" of patient compliance with therapeutic regimes', in *Compliance with Therapeutic Regimes* (Eds D. L. Sackett and R. B. Haynes), pp. 26–39, The Johns Hopkins University Press, Baltimore.

Haynes, R. B. (1979). In *Compliance in Health Care* (Eds R. B. Haynes, D. W. Taylor, and D. L. Sackett), pp. 1–7, The Johns Hopkins University Press, Baltimore and London.

Hollenberg, N. K., Adams, D. F., Solomon, H. F., Rashid, A., Abrams, H. L., and Merrell, J. P. (1974). 'Senescence and the renal vasculature in normal man', *Circ. Res.*, **34**, 309–316.

Hurwitz, N. (1969). 'Predisposing factors in adverse reactions to drugs', *Br. Med. J.*, **1**, 536–539.

Hurwitz, N., and Wade, O. L. (1969). 'Intensive hospital monitoring of adverse reaction to drugs', *Br. Med. J.,* **1**, 531–536.

Joyce, C. R. B., Last, J. M., and Weatherall, M. (1967). 'Personal factors as a cause of differences in prescribing by general practitioners', *Br. J. Prev. Soc. Med.*, **21**, 170–177.

Judge, T. G., and Caird, F. E. (1978). *Drug Treatment of the Elderly Patient*, Pitman Medical, London.

Kampmann, J. P., and Molholm-Hansen, J. E. (1979). 'Renal excretion of drugs', in *Drugs and the Elderly* (Eds J. Crooks and I. H. Stevenson), pp. 77–87, Macmillan, London.

Kampmann, J., Molholm-Hansen, J., Siersback-Nielsen, K., and Laursen, H. (1972). 'Effect of some drugs on penicillin half-life in blood', *Clin. Pharmacol. Ther.*, **13**, 516–519.

Kampmann, J. P., Sniding, J., and Moller-Jorgensen, I. (1975). 'Effect of age on liver function', *Geriatrics,* **30**, 91–95.

Kangas, L., Iisalo, E., Kanto, J., Lehtinen, V., Pynnonen, S., Ruikka, I., Salminen, J., Sillapaa, M., and Syvalahti, E. (1979). 'Human pharmacokinetics of nitrazepam: Effect of age and diseases', *Europ. J. Clin. Pharmacol.*, **15**, 163–170.

Karch, F. E., and Lasagna, L. (1975). 'Adverse drug reactions – a critical review', *JAMA,* **234**, 1236–1241.

Karch, F. E., and Lasagna, L. (1977). 'Towards the operational identification of adverse drug reactions', *Clin. Pharmacol. Ther.*, **21**, 247–254.

Kelly, J. G., McGarry, K., O'Brien, E. T., and O'Malley, K. 'Bioavailability of labetalol increases with age', *Br. J. Clin. Pharmacol.*, **14**, 304–305.

Klotz, U. (1976). 'Pathophysiological and disease-induced changes in drug distribution volume: Pharmacokinetic implications', *Clin. Pharmacokin.*, **1**, 204–218.

Klotz, U., Avant, G. R., Hoyumpa, A., Schenker, S., and Wilkinson, G. R. (1975). 'The effects of age and liver disease on the disposition and elimination of diazepam in adult man', *J. Clin. Invest.*, **55**, 347–359.

Klotz, U., and Muller-Scydlitz, P. (1979). 'Altered elimination of desmethyldiazepam in the elderly' (letter), *Br. J. Clin. Pharmacol.*, **7**, 119–120.

Kramer, M. S., Leventhal, J. M., Hutchinson, T. A., and Feinstein, A. R. (1979). 'An alogrithm for the operational assessment of adverse drug reactions. 1. Background, description and instructions for use', *JAMA*, **242**, 623–632.

Kraus, J. W., Desmond, P. V., Marshall, J. P., Johnson, R. F., Spenker, S., and Wilkinson, G. R. (1978). 'Effects of ageing and liver disease on disposition of lorazepam', *Clin. Pharmacol. Ther.*, **24**, 411–419.

Kristensen, M., Hølholm-Hansen, J., Kampmann, J., Lymholtz, B., and Siersback-Nielsen, K. (1974). 'Drug elimination and renal function', *J. Clin. Pharmacol.*, **14**, 307–308.

Law, R., and Chalmers, C. (1976). 'Medicines and elderly people: A general practice survey', *Brit. Med. J.*, **1**, 565–568.

Levy, M., Kewitz, H., Altwein, W., Hillebrand, J., and Eliakim, M. (1980). 'Hospital admissions due to adverse drug reactions: A comparative study from Jerusalem and Berlin', *Europ. Clin. Pharmacol.*, **17**, 25–31.

Liddell, D. E., Williams, F. M., and Briant, R. H. (1975). 'Phenazone (antipyrine) metabolism and distribution in young and elderly adults', *Clin. Exp. Pharmacol. Physiol.*, **2**, 481–487.

Lumholtz, B., Kampmann, J., Siersback-Nielsen, K., and Mølholm-Hansen, J. (1974). 'Dose regimen of kanamycin and gentamycin', *Acta Med. Scand.*, **190**, 521–524.

McGarry, K., Laher, M., Fitzgerald, D., Horgan, J., O'Brien, E., and O'Malley, K. (1983). 'Baroreflex function in elderly hypertensive patients', *Hypertension*, **5**, 763–766.

McLachlan, M. S. F. (1978). 'The ageing kidney', *Lancet*, **2**, 143–146.

Misera, D. P., Loundon, J. M., and Staddon, G. E. (1975). 'Albumin metabolism in elderly patients', *J. Gerontol.*, **30**, 304–306.

Muller, J. H., McDonald, R. K., and Shock, N. W. (1952). 'Age changes in the maximal rate of renal tubular reabsorption of glucose', *J. Gerontol.*, **7**, 196–200.

Naranjo, C. A., Busto, U., Sellers, E. M., Sandor, P., Ruiz, I., Roberts, E. A., Janecek, E., Domecq, C., and Greenblatt, D. J. (1981). 'A method for estimating the probability of adverse drug reactions', *Clin. Pharmacol. Ther.*, **30**, 239–245.

Nation, R. L., Learoyd, B., Barber, J., and Triggs, E. J. (1976). 'The pharmacokinetics of chlormethiazole following intravenous administration in the aged', *Europ. J. Clin. Pharmacol.*, **10**, 407–415.

Nation, R. L., Triggs, E. J., and Selig, M. (1977). 'Lignocaine kinetics in cardiac patients and aged subjects', *Br. J. Clin. Pharmacol.*, **4**, 439–448.

Novak, L. P. (1972). 'Ageing, total body potassium, fat-free mass and cell mass in males and females between 18 and 85 years', *J. Gerontol.*, **27**, 438–444.

Ochs, H. R., Greenblatt, D. J., Woo, E., and Smith, T. W. (1978). 'Reduced quinidine clearance in elderly subjects', *Am. J. Cardiol.*, **42**, 481–485.

Office of Population Censuses and Surveys Monitor (1981). Ref. PPI 81/5, Office of Population Censuses and Surveys, London.

Ogilvie, R. E., and Ruedy, J. (1967). 'Adverse drug reactions during hospitalization', *Canad. Med. Assoc. J.*, **97**, 1450–1457.

O'Hanrahan, M., and O'Malley, K. (1981). 'Compliance with drug treatment', *Br. Med. J.*, **283**, 298–330.

O'Malley, K., Crooks, J., Duke, E., and Stevenson, I. H. (1971). 'Effect of age and sex on human drug metabolism', *Br. Med. J.*, **3**, 607–609.

O'Malley, K., Stevenson, I. H., Ward, C., Wood, A. J. J., and Crooks, I. (1977). 'Determinants of anticoagulant control in patients receiving warfarin', *Br. J. Clin. Pharmacol.*, **4**, 309–314.

Parkin, D. M., Henney, C. R., Quirk, J., and Crooks, J. (1976). 'Deviation from prescribed drug treatment after discharge from hospital', *Br. Med. J.*, **2**, 686–688.

Playfer, J. R., Baty, J. D., Lamb, J., Powell, C., and Price-Evans, D. A. (1978). 'Age related differences in the disposition of acetanilide', *Br. J. Clin. Pharmacol.*, **6**, 529–535.

Reidenberg, M. M., Levy, M., Warner, H., Coutinho, C. B., Swaritz, M. A., Yu, G., and Chempko, J. (1978). 'Relationship between diazepam dose, plasma level, age and central nervous system depression', *Clin. Pharmacol. Ther.*, **23**, 371–376.

Roberts, R. K., Wilkinson, G. R., Branch, R. A., and Shenker, S. (1978). 'Effect of age and parenchymal liver disease on the disposition and elimination of chlordiazepoxide (Librium)', *Gastroenterology*, **75**, 479–485.

Rowe, J. W., Shock, N. W., and Defromzo, R. A. (1976). 'The influence of age on renal response to water deprivation in man', *Nephron.*, **17**, 270–278.

Salem, S. A. M. (1981). 'Studies of the psychomotor effects of drugs in man', PhD Thesis, The Queen's University of Belfast, N. Ireland.

Salem, S. A. M., Rijjayabun, P., Shepherd, A. M. M., and Stevenson, I. H. (1978). 'Reduced induction of drug metabolism in the elderly', *Age*

Ageing, 7, 68–73.

Salem, S. A. M., and Stevenson, I. H. (1977). 'Absorption kinetics of aspirin and quinidine in elderly subjects', *Br. J. Clin. Pharmacol., 4*, 397pp.

Schimmel, E. M. (1964). 'The hazards of hospitalization', *Ann. Intern. Med., 60*, 100–110.

Schwartz, D. (1962). 'Medication errors made by elderly chronically ill patients', *Am. J. Pub. Health., 52*, 2018–2029.

Seidl, L. G., Thornton, G. F., Smith, J. W., and Cluff, L. E. (1966). 'Studies on the epidemiology of adverse drug reactions. III. Reactions in patients on a general medical service', *Bull. Johns Hopkins Hosp., 119*, 299–315.

Shader, R. I., Greenblatt, D. J., Harmatz, J. S., Frank, R. I., and Koch-Weser, J. (1977). 'Absorption and disposition of chlordiazepoxide in young and elderly male volunteers', *J. Clin. Pharmacol., 17*, 709.

Shaw, S. M., and Opit, L. J. (1976). 'Need for supervision in the elderly receiving long-term prescribed medication', *Br. Med. J., 1*, 505–507.

Shepherd, A. M. M., Hewick, D. S., Moreland, T. A., and Stevenson, I. H. (1977). 'Age as a determinant of sensitivity to warfarin', *Br. J. Clin. Pharmacol., 4*, 315–320.

Shock, N. W., Watkin, D. M. Yiengst, B. S., Norms, A. H., Gaffney, G. W., Gregerman, R. I., and Falzone, J. A. (1963). 'Age differences in the water content of the body as related to basal oxygen consumption in males', *J. Gerontol., 18*, 1–8.

Simon, C., Malerczy, K. V., Muller, U., and Muller, G. (1972). 'Zur Pharmakokinetik von Propicillin bei geriatrischen Patienten im Vergleich zu jungeren Erwachsenen', *Dtsch. Med. Wochenschr., 97*, 1999.

Skegg, D. C. G., Doll, R., and Perry, J. (1977). 'Use of medicines in general practice', *Br. Med. J., 1*, 1561–1563.

Smith, J. W., Seidl, L. G., and Cluff, L. E. (1966). 'Studies on the epidemiology of adverse drug reactions. V. Clinical factors influencing susceptibility', *Ann. Intern. Med., 65*, 629–640.

Smithard, D. J., and Langman, M. J. S. (1971). 'Drug metabolism in the elderly', *Br. Med. J., 3*, 520–521.

Stevenson, I. H., Salem, S. A. M., O'Malley, K., Cusack, B., and Kelly, J. G. (1981). 'Age and drug absorption', in *Drug Absorption* (Eds L. F. Prescott and W. S. Nimmo), pp. 253–261, ADIS Press, Sydney.

Stewart, R. B., and Cluff, L. E. (1971). 'Studies on the epidemiology of adverse drug reactions: VI. Utilization and interactions of prescription and non-prescription drugs in outpatients', *Johns Hopkins Med. J., 129*, 319–331.

Swift, C. G., Homeida, M., and Roberts, C. J. C.

(1978). 'Antipyrine disposition and liver size in the elderly', *Europ. J. Clin. Pharmacol., 14*, 149–152.

Triggs, E. J., Nation, R. L., Long, A., and Ashley, J. J. (1975). 'Pharmacokinetics in the elderly', *Eur. J. Clin. Pharmacol., 8*, 55.

U.S. Bureau of the Census, (1979). *Statistical Abstract of the United States: 1979*, 100th ed, Washington, D.C.

Vartia, K. O., and Lalola, E. (1960). 'Serum levels of antibiotics in young and old subjects following administration of dihydrostreptomycin and tetracycline', *J. Gerontol., 15*, 392–394.

Vestal, R. E., McGuire, E. A., Tobin, J. D., Andres, R., Norris, A. H., and Mezey, E. (1977). 'Ageing and ethanol metabolism', *Clin. Pharmacol. Ther., 21*, 343–354.

Vestal, R. E., Norris, A. H., Tobin, J. D., Cohen, B. H., Shock, N. W., and Andres, R. (1975). 'Antipyrine metabolism in man: Influence of age, alcohol, caffeine and smoking', *Clin. Pharmacol. Ther., 18*, 425–432.

Vestal, R. E., Wood, A. J. J., Branch, R. A. Shand, D. G., and Wilkinson, G. R. (1979a). 'Effect of age and cigarette smoking on propranolol disposition', *Clin. Pharmacol. Ther., 26*, 8–15.

Vestal, R. E., Wood, A. J. J., and Shand, D. G. (1979b). 'Reduced β-adrenoceptor sensitivity in the elderly', *Clin. Pharmacol. Ther., 26*, 181–186.

Walker, K. (1971). 'Repeat prescription recording in general practice', *J. Roy. Coll. Gen. Practit., 21*, 748–751.

Wallace, S., Whiting, B., and Runcie, J. (1976). 'Factors affecting drug binding in plasma of elderly patients', *Br. J. Clin. Pharmacol., 3*, 327–330.

Wandless, I., and Davie, J. W. (1977). 'Can drug compliance in the elderly be improved?', *Br. Med. J., 1*, 359–361.

Whitfield, M. J. (1973). 'A study of prescribing in general practice, 1969–1970', *J. Roy. Coll. Gen. Practit., 23*, 168–182.

Williamson, J. (1979). 'Adverse reactions to prescribed drugs in the elderly', in *Drugs and the Elderly* (Eds J. Crooks and I. H. Stevenson), Macmillan Press, London.

Wood, A. J. J., Vestal, R. E., Wilkinson, G. R., Branch, R. A., and Shand, D. G. (1979). 'Effect of ageing and cigarette smoking on antipyrine and indocyanine green elimination', *Clin. Pharmacol. Ther., 26*, 16–20.

Woodford-Williams, E., Alvarez, A. S., Webster, D., Landless, B., and Dixon, M. P. (1964). 'Serum protein patterns in "normal" and pathological ageing', *Gerontologica, 10*, 86–99.

World Health Organization (1970). 'International drug monitoring – the role of the hospital', *Drug Intelligence Clin. Pharmacol., 4*, 101.

7

Sleep and Its Disorders

Principles and Practice of Geriatric Medicine
Edited by M. S. J. Pathy
© 1985 John Wiley & Sons Ltd

7.1

Sleep and Its Disorders

R. Spiegel, A. Azcona

As people grow older their sleep changes in subjective and objective quality and sleep disorders become more frequent. Many ageing persons notice that their sleep is less deep, suffers more interruptions, and is less refreshing than in younger years. These changes lead many of them to seek medical assistance. Reversal of day and night rhythms of wakefulness and sleep is a phenomenon mainly occurring in severely deteriorated old people and its disturbing consequences almost regularly lead to drug therapy.

Thus, physicians in hospital and private practice are often confronted with sleep disorders in the elderly and have to decide if and when prescribing a sleep-inducing drug is appropriate. They will also ask themselves which other medical and social measures should be taken in this situation. This chapter attempts to give answers to the following questions:

(a) How common are sleep disorders in advanced age and how can they be clinically defined?
(b) What has modern sleep research contributed to an understanding of these disorders?
(c) What therapeutic possibilities are there?

EPIDEMIOLOGY OF SLEEP DISORDERS IN OLD AGE

About 10 per cent. of all young adults complain frequently, or continuously, of insomnia.

The incidence of subjective disturbance of sleep increases with age and reaches 25 per cent. and more in people over 60 years. All subjective disorders of sleep – difficulties with sleep onset, frequent interruptions of sleep during the night, early waking – are 3 to 4 times more common in elderly than in young people (Miles and Dement, 1980; Spiegel, 1981). Almost all studies show that sleep disorders are more common in elderly women than in elderly men. In accordance with the increased frequency of sleep disorders, there is a tendency towards increased ingestion of sleep-inducing drugs in old age (Fig. 1), in spite of the fact that these drugs produce frequent, and sometimes severe, untoward effects in the elderly (Greenblatt and Allen, 1978; Greenblatt, Allen, and Shader, 1977).

Sleep disorders can be classified according to several criteria. The most simple and descriptive classification differentiates between delayed sleep onset, interrupted sleep, and early awakening. A more aetiologically oriented approach distinguishes between primary and secondary sleep disorders: primary insomnia is not caused by other medical or psychiatric diseases; secondary insomnia is caused by or is part of another disease. A recent classification of wake and sleep disorders (ASDC, 1979) is quite complex in that descriptive, aetiological and electrophysiological aspects are combined to provide 4 categories of disturbances, each containing 8 to 18 different syndromes. As the disorders of initiating and maintaining sleep (DIMS) are by far the

197

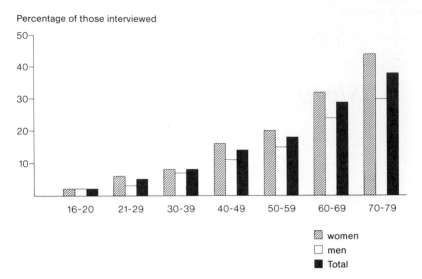

Figure 1   Age and consumption of sleep medication. Data from a representative investigation carried out in West Germany (see Spiegel, 1981, p. 12). The subjects were asked whether they 'sometimes' took sleep medication. The increase in consumption with age is steady and progressive

most common, this chapter will concentrate on this category.

In practice, sleep disorders appear in the form of subjective complaints from either the patients themselves or through their relatives or surroundings. At any event, the physician is confronted with a subjective symptom whose aetiology and objective correlates he at first does not know. Furthermore, neither he nor the patient know for sure how much sleep is normal and necessary; both are influenced by presumptions and social norms. For this reason, the treatment of sleep disorders is frequently subject to emotional and arbitrary decisions. It is therefore of interest to review the empirical knowledge gathered about sleep in the elderly and to examine how this knowledge could be put to practical use.

PHYSIOLOGY OF SLEEP: CHANGES IN OLD AGE

Polygraphic sleep recordings comprise the simultaneous registration of the EEG, electromyogram, and electrooculogram plus other physiological indicators during the whole night. This non-invasive technique permits a continuous registration of sleep, its course, and so-called stages during the night without essen-

tially disturbing the sleeper. Polygraphic sleep recordings are usually made in specialized sleep laboratories, but telemetric techniques also permit sleep to be recorded in more natural surroundings. According to polygraphic criteria, sleep may be divided into several stages (see Rechtschaffen and Kales, 1968): stages 1 to 4 correspond approximately to sleep depth, as established by wake experiments. REM (rapid eye movement) sleep is the time when most dreams appear (see overview by Webb and Cartwright, 1978).

During the night an adult person goes through 3 to 5 so-called NREM–REM cycles (Fig. 2), i.e. sections of about 80 to 120 minutes' duration, consisting of the longer NREM (non-REM) and a shorter REM sleep part. Slow wave sleep (SWS) indicates a sleep stage with very high and slow EEG waves; it is a deep form of sleep that requires intense stimuli in order to wake a person up. SWS appears mainly during the first 2 NREM–REM cycles, and it is in this period that most growth hormone secretion peaks occur. After sleep deprivation or bodily exertion, SWS increases and this is presumably correlated with an intensive recuperation phase of the body. Very little is known about the other sleep stages and their relation to biological and psychological par-

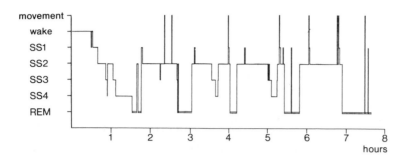

Figure 2   The NREM–REM cycle of sleep. This 'hypnogram' of a 25 year old healthy subject illustrates the chronological sequence of polygraphic sleep stages (SS) in a single night. In reality, the transition from 'lighter' to 'deeper' sleep stages, e.g. from 1 to 2, does not occur in the form of steps, but smoothly. Upwards 'shifts', however, are generally abrupt, as a result of body movements or brief awakenings

ameters; there are, nevertheless, many hypotheses or speculations (see Fishbein, 1981; Meddis, 1975).

Sleep parameters alter with increasing age (Fig. 3): SWS decreases after adolescence and REM sleep is reduced in people over 60 years. With increasing age, sleep is interrupted more frequently by awakenings, and elderly people have a lower sleep efficiency, i.e. they must spend a longer period in bed in order to obtain the same net sleeping time. Sleep changes typical of old age are more pronounced in men, many elderly women showing almost no alterations in their sleep patterns in relation to youth (Webb, 1982).

It can be asked whether such changes, occurring in healthy elderly persons, are physiological concomitants of ageing or if they are related to pathological, although subclinical, states. This question is difficult to answer as there are, during the ageing process, functional changes in most systems and the distinc-

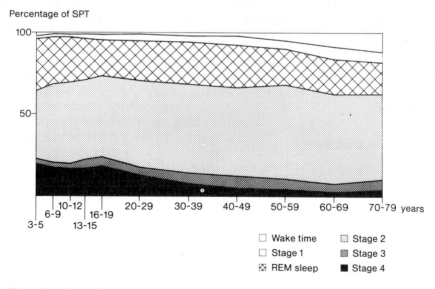

Figure 3   Age and percentages of sleep stages (females). The duration of stage 4, expressed as a percentage of SPT (sleep period time, i.e. the time from sleep onset until final awakening in the morning), decreases sharply once adulthood is reached. The percentage of stage 1 increases slightly with age. Awakenings during the sleep period increase considerably with age. The percentual share of REM sleep falls slightly in advanced age (see Spiegel, 1981, p. 92)

tion between normal and pathological states is less clear than in youth.

The decrease of SWS, particularly pronounced in elderly men, is probably age-related, as is the reduction of REM sleep. The mechanisms which cause these changes are unknown. On the other hand, many of the frequent sleep interruptions in the elderly might be partly related or even due to respiratory disorders (see below). The relation between the duration of REM sleep and the intellectual status of elderly people (Prinz, 1980; Spiegel, 1982) is disputed.

There is some overall agreement between polygraphic data and the subjective descriptions of sleep in the elderly: both indicate that sleep becomes less deep, shows more interruptions, and is, at least for many elderly, less refreshing. On the other hand, complaints of disturbed sleep are more frequent in elderly women while, according to polygraphic criteria, it is the elderly men who show more evidence of deteriorated sleep. This discrepancy indicates that sleep disorders and objective sleep alterations are not identical and that the experience of sleep is very much dependent on factors within the individual. Furthermore, although correlations between subjective and objective sleep assessments are generally positive, elderly men without complaint of disturbed sleep tend to overestimate their sleeping time, while insomniac men have a tendency to underestimate it. In contrast, women – both good and poor sleepers – have repeatedly been shown to be accurate estimators of sleep times.

PATHOGENESIS OF INSOMNIA

There are many causes and conditions which may induce sleep disorders. Most often it is the concurrence of several factors which leads to a sleep disorder, and especially in old age it is necessary to consider a multifactorial aetiology (Dement, Miles, and Carskadon, 1982). In this sense, the factors enumerated below are not meant to be mutually exclusive, although they are relevant as far as therapy is concerned. We distinguish between:

(a) 'situative' factors,
(b) psychological and psychiatric factors,
(c) iatrogenic factors and drug abuse,

(d) sleep disorder as a symptom of cerebrovascular disease,
(e) sleep disorder as a consequence of other organic diseases,
(f) sleep apnœa syndrome,
(g) primary insomnia.

'Situative' Factors of Insomnia

Traffic noise and other kinds of disturbing noises from the surroundings can prevent sleep, especially in elderly people whose wake threshold is lower. Noisy surroundings delay sleep onset, and wake periods during the night may become much extended. Falling asleep will be particularly difficult if the patient feels annoyed or hurt by inconsiderate or supposedly malevolent neighbours. Sleeping with closed windows, cotton wool in the ears, and similar measures may be helpful. Changing the bedroom over to a quieter part of the house is to be considered, but this may not be possible for various reasons. If the patient feels very cold, falling asleep may be difficult. Some patients go to bed early only because they are alone and want to get warm. They wake up in the early hours of the morning and cannot fall asleep again.

Few of these factors can be influenced by purely medical measures. Thus it is more important to work together with district nurses, social workers, and local organizations who will assist the patient in a practical way. If this can be done it will also give the patient the feeling that someone is caring for him.

A typical state of situative insomnia is one which occurs after a patient is referred to a home for the elderly or to a hospital. In these cases the temporary use of sleeping tablets may be helpful. Morbid brooding during the night and the fear of being alone will be suppressed, and the patient will find it easier to acclimatize to the new situation.

Psychological and Psychiatric Factors

Mourning and sorrow after the loss of a spouse, friend, one's home, or professional situation are normal reactions to the frequent losses so typical of old age. More attention, practical advice, and help and understanding from the family and other members of the community will support the elderly person; the physician should be ready to listen to the patient and to give practical help as far as is desired by the patient. Even in such situations the temporary use of a sleeping pill can be indicated.

Acute depressive reactions after severe losses cannot always be distinguished from prolonged depressive phases occurring as a consequence of repeated, cumulative losses. Both reactive and endogenous major depressive episodes (APA, 1980) are accompanied by sleep disorders. The kind of sleep disorder, be it difficulty in falling asleep or interruptions of sleep, does not distinguish between endogenous and reactive depression since the continuity of sleep is disturbed in old age anyhow. Very frequently insomnia is the first symptom of a depressive phase, and insomnia commonly remains as the last symptom once the depression has cleared up. However, even severe insomnia alone is not sufficient for a diagnosis of depression (Reynolds *et al.*, 1983). More important are depressive mood, hopelessness, fear of the future, loss of interest, self-reproaches, and vital symptoms such as loss of appetite and energy. Sleep disorders as a symptom of depression are usually treated with sedative antidepressants (see the next section).

Iatrogenic Insomnia and Drug Abuse

Some drugs which are commonly prescribed in old age may disturb sleep, e.g. alpha-methyldopa and reserpine-like antihypertensive drugs. These compounds influence biogenic amines in the brain and may produce insomnia. Diuretics indirectly exert a disturbing effect on sleep if they are administered in the evening because they produce nycturia. Patients with Parkinson's disease who are receiving L-dopa may experience sleep disturbances. Beta-blockers sometimes produce nightmares and lively dreams. If a patient receiving such drugs complains of disturbed sleep, the physician should not primarily prescribe a sleep-inducing drug but consider a change in the medication causing disturbed sleep.

Caffeine is a central nervous system stimulant, and coffee and tea may disturb sleep. Sensitivity to the arousing action of caffeine varies greatly among individuals and also within the same individual. Therefore, patients who complain of sleeplessness should be routinely questioned regarding coffee and tea ingestion, and consumption should be reduced in the evening. This also applies to persons who are not aware of any stimulant effect of these beverages or who claim that they need a good cup of coffee in order to be able to sleep.

Such habits are generally easy to change, but alcoholics – who often have a severe sleep problem – are difficult to convince of the need to give up drinking. While a glass of red wine or beer can facilitate sleep, larger quantities of alcohol disturb sleep: the initial sedating effect is usually followed in the early morning hours by rebound sleeplessness. Besides, large amounts of beer produce a need to micturate and thereby interrupt sleep. Alcoholism is especially a problem of men, although sleeplessness is only a part – and usually not the most important one – of the alcoholic syndrome.

Dependency on hypnotics is particularly relevant in the present context. Since sleeping pills do not eliminate the causes of disturbed sleep, insomnia will reappear once treatment with hypnotics is discontinued if its causes have not been treated in the meantime. Insomnia after drug withdrawal may be even worse than before drug treatment. Although the mechanism of this phenomenon is not well understood, there is empirical evidence that hypnotics with a short biological half-life will produce withdrawal insomnia within 1 to 3 nights, while compounds with longer half-lifes produce a similar picture several days later (Breimer and Jochenson, 1983; Kales *et al.*, 1983). The phenomenon of rebound insomnia should be known to practising physicians, and the patient should also be aware of what may happen when the regular intake of hypnotics is discontinued. Rebound insomnia is a transient phenomenon but may ultimately lead to drug dependence.

Sleeplessness as a Symptom of Cerebrovascular Disease

Disturbed sleep, accompanied by other subjective complaints, frequently appears in initial stages of cerebrovascular disease. Typical is the triad of headaches, dizziness, and tiredness during the day (cf. Chapter 16.8), together with sleep inversion in more advanced cases.

These symptoms, however, are not specific enough to permit a positive diagnosis. As cerebral infarction is only rarely the initial manifestation of cerebrovascular disease, the differentiation from signs of 'normal' ageing, symptoms of depression, or degenerative types of dementia may be difficult. Correct diagnosis is established using the following methods: inspection of the fundus oculi, neurological status including Doppler sonography, EEG, and computer tomography. Positron emission tomography (PET) and nuclear magnetic resonance (NMR) techniques may also be helpful in the future.

Hypnotic drugs are basically indicated but may produce paradoxical reactions, including excitation and confusion, in some patients with cerebrovascular disease. Whether treating the underlying disease with vasodilating substances (vincamine, naftidrofuryl, dihydroergotoxine, etc.) is useful has been put into doubt (Cook and James, 1981); management of insomnia is often achieved by using sedative neuroleptics such as thioridazine, laevomepromazine, and similar drugs.

Disturbed Sleep Related to Other Medical Diseases

Sleeplessness very often accompanies the course of other diseases. Three physiopathological mechanisms are of interest here. Because of the sudden impairment of vital functions like respiration and circulation, sleep may be disrupted in certain conditions such as pulmonary œdema following left ventricular insufficiency and acute cor pulmonale after lung embolism. In these cases, the patient may awake suddenly during the night with extreme anxiety and tachypnoea and will not be able to fall asleep again. These syndromes need to be carefully distinguished from sleep disorders related to anxiety and affective disorders. Their treatment is purely medical and use of sleep-inducing drugs is clearly contraindicated.

A second mechanism which disturbs sleep during the course of medical disease is fear, anxiety, and despair, often related to both acute and chronic illnesses. In these cases, talking to the patient and reassurance are indicated. Sleep-inducing drugs can also be used as an adjuvant to these measures.

Disruption of sleep may be due to pain, for example, from duodenal ulcer, angina pectoris, rheumatoid arthritis, or osteoarthrosis. In some instances, such as duodenal ulcer, the pain is typically exacerbated during the night, and the patient wakes up without being able to fall asleep again. The superimposed anxiety makes things more difficult. Specific treatment directed towards the underlying cause of the pain will prove far more helpful than hypnotics.

The Problem of Sleep Apnœa

Changes in sleep with ageing are not limited to subjective quality and EEG characteristics but also involve vital functions such as respiration. Apnœic episodes, i.e. cessation of air flow for 10 seconds and more, have received special attention in recent years. They seem to occur in a high percentage (more than 30 per cent.) of healthy people over 60 years (Ancoli-Israel *et al.*, 1981; Carskadon and Dement, 1981) and may be even more pronounced in patients with complaints of disturbed sleep (Coleman *et al.*, 1981; Reynolds *et al.*, 1980). Even though the samples investigated in these studies are not necessarily representative of the total population (Coleman *et al.*, 1982) sleep apnœa appears to be a medical problem in many elderly, unknown until recently. Patients suffering from sleep apnœa typically complain of sleepiness during the day (Parkes, 1981) but also frequently of disturbed sleep at night. As a rule, they are unaware of the severe disruption of respiration which occurs every night with a frequency of up to 150 times and which may damage their health. Adequate diagnosis of this otherwise hidden syndrome and appropriate therapy are therefore important.

As it is impossible to perform routine polygraphic sleep recordings of all persons aged over 60 years, clinical characteristics of individuals at risk should be emphasized. It has been found that sleep apnœa is associated with male sex, overweight, a history of throat operations, loud snoring during the night, restlessness during sleep, hypertension with cor pulmonale, heart failure. Of these, high blood pressure, right ventricular failure (cor pulmonale), and heart failure are clinically relevant. Thus, patients suffering from one of these diseases and complaining of disturbed sleep should not be treated with sleeping pills, as even benzodiazepines produce a small but potentially dangerous suppression of respiration. Obstructive sleep apnœa is surgically treated by tonsillectomy, thyroidectomy, and, in severe cases, tracheostomy (see Weitzman, 1981).

Primary Insomnia

Diagnosis of primary insomnia may be made after other underlying causes of sleeplessness have been excluded. The incidence of primary insomnia is difficult to estimate, as different studies used different criteria for the exclusion of causative factors of insomnia, and some authors even deny the existence of primary insomnia. Younger patients with primary insomnia frequently show depressive traits, although a major depressive disorder cannot be diagnosed. However, in older age psychopathological factors of insomnia probably play a minor role (Miles and Dement, 1980; Roers *et al.*, 1983).

Primary insomnia in old age is frequently treated with sleep-inducing drugs. In severe cases sedative neuroleptics are preferred, and patients who show clear-cut depressive symptoms may be treated with sedating antidepressants.

THERAPY OF SLEEPLESSNESS

The following remarks refer to insomnia which persists after underlying and accompanying diseases have been appropriately treated. Although a distinction is made between pharmacological and non-pharmacological therapies, the division is less sharp in practice in that the two approaches can and should be combined in many cases.

Pharmacological Therapy of Insomnia

Almost all publications on hypnotics begin or end with cautionary remarks and emphasize that even recently introduced preparations should be prescribed with great circumspection in the elderly. Caution was justified with some of the older sleep-inducing drugs which have a small safety margin (bromides, barbiturates) or produce dependency and addiction (barbiturates, methyprylone, methaqualone). Even the most recent and frequently taken hypnotics (benzodiazepines) are not completely free of negative aspects. Although their toxicity and addiction potential are low, they do present risks which can be summarized under the headings of long duration of action, risk of cumulation, and dependency potential. Neuroleptics and antidepressants, if taken as sleeping aids, have their limitations, too. (Table 1).

Benzodiazepines

The commonly used benzodiazepine hypnotics are nitrazepam, flurazepam, flunitrazepam, oxazepam, temazepam, and triazolam. They differ mostly with regard to potency and duration of action: nitrazepam, flurazepam, and flunitrazepam show relatively long-lasting effects, temazepam and oxazepam intermediate effects, and triazolam shorter-lasting ones. Hypnotics with shorter duration of action are generally preferred, particularly because potential after-effects on the following day such as sleepiness, amnesia, confusion, and muscle weakness are most undesirable in the elderly. However, compounds with very short duration of action like midazolam and triazolam have been reported to induce early morning insomnia after regular use for 1 to 2 weeks (Kales *et al.*, 1983). Consequently, the drugs of first choice for geriatric use are temazepam, oxazepam, and, if taken late in the night, triazolam. Nevertheless, side-effects may also occur with these compounds as individual susceptibility differs markedly. Benzodiazepines interfere little with other drugs during metabolic catabolism.

Pharmacokinetic characteristics of some of the benzodiazepines are quite complicated (see Breimer, 1979): nitrazepam has a half-life of about 30 hours and therefore, if administered repeatedly, tends to cumulate. Flurazepam has been reported to have a short plasma half-life, but its main metabolite, *N*-desalkyl-flurazepam, is pharmacologically active and has a plasma half-life of between 37 and 289 (!) hours. Untoward after-effects and cumulation are therefore likely and have indeed been reported (Oswald *et al.*, 1979). Temazepam and triazolam are, in regard to their pharmacokinetic properties, better drugs as they have short half-lives (4 to 10 hours for temazepam, 5 to 10 hours for triazolam) and produce no or only small quantities of pharmacologically active metabolites. Flunitrazepam is similar to the longer-acting preparations such as nitra-zepam and flurazepam.

There have been doubts, however, whether plasma levels of benzodiazepines correspond to concentrations at relevant central nervous system sites. Furthermore, pharmacokinetic differences between various compounds are not necessarily reflected in untoward after-effects and/or the risks of drug accumulation (Johnson and Chernik, 1982).

Although long-acting drugs ought to be avoided due to their after-effects and risk of cumulation, there have been claims that such compounds offer some advantage if chronically administered (Kales *et al.*, 1983). Rebound insomnia after drug withdrawal is delayed as slowly eliminated metabolites are still active in the organism, and it is assumed that patients will not make a connection between drug with-drawal and insomnia recurring with a few nights' delay. Therefore, cessation of drug treatment should be easier if long-acting drugs are utilized. However, one must doubt whether this is a real advantage, since severe overshoot insomnia was reported after discon-tinuation of flurazepam with a delay of 5 to 7 nights (Greenblatt *et al.*, 1981). The presence of centrally active metabolites in the organism of elderly patients in whom quick medical in-terventions may become necessary is certainly unwarranted. Interestingly, it is mainly elderly men who show delayed metabolism of some benzodiazepines (see Chapter 5), whereas in women age differences are much less pronounced.

Other Hypnotics

Some of the older sleep-inducing drugs, like chloral hydrate and related substances, are effective, produce only slight after-effects on the following day, and are generally well tol-erated. Repeated use may lead to partial loss of effect, although results on this topic are equivocal. The gastrointestinal tolerance of chloral hydrate has been improved with new galenical preparations and is satisfactory if the drugs are taken with or after meals. Chloral hydrate and its derivatives are inexpensive and still widely used for treating elderly insom-niacs, especially in homes and hospitals.

Although barbiturates enjoy a dubious repu-tation and their use has been discouraged by the British National Formulary, they are still prescribed as hypnotics. According to their duration of action they are classified as short-, intermediate-, and long-acting derivatives. Short-acting barbiturates like hexobarbital are preferred in patients with sleep difficulties in the first few hours of the night, while patients who tend to wake up towards the end of the night are often prescribed intermediate-lasting compounds such as cyclobarbital. The long-acting barbiturates like phenobarbital tend to cumulate and to produce severe hangover effects and should not be prescribed in the elderly. The advantage of the barbiturates is their high efficacy in inducing sleep; their dis-advantages include the possibility of drug add-iction, cumulation, and high toxicity in overdose, as well as their interference with the metabolism of other drugs. Affective changes and psychotic developments have been de-scribed after prolonged and high-dose therapy. For these reasons, barbiturates should only be used as a last resort.

We shall not deal with drugs like glute-thimide, methyprylon, and methaqualone be-cause the disadvantages of these hypnotics overweigh their possible advantages. Also not recommended for the elderly are anticholi-nergics and antihistaminics, although their sed-ative effect is well documented.

Neuroleptics and Antidepressants

Disturbed sleep appearing as a part of schizo-phrenic psychosis or mania is routinely treated with neuroleptic drugs (Chapter 17). Depres-sive patients with sleeplessness are usually pre-scribed antidepressants, especially sedative ones like trimipramine, doxepin, or amitrip-tyline. However, antidepressants should not be used for treating insomnia in patients who are not depressed, since their anticholinergic ac-tion may lead to unnecessary complications in the elderly.

If disturbed sleep and day–night reversal oc-cur in the context of organic brain syndromes, paradoxical reactions to barbiturates and also benzodiazepines are occasionally observed, or the doses needed for inducing sleep are so high that motor and cognitive disturbances must be feared. In these instances the use of sedative neuroleptics like thioridazine, laevomepro-mazine, and floropipamid are recommended, although cardiovascular and extrapyramidal actions of these compounds must be kept in mind. In hospitalized and particularly in bed-ridden patients these drugs are usually preferred to benzodiazepines because they do not cause ataxia or amnesic syndromes.

RECOMMENDATIONS

For light and moderate sleep disturbances, especially in ambulatory patients:

Valeriana preparations; hop preparations (rarely prescribed in the United Kingdom)
Intermediate to short-acting benzodiazepines such as:

Temazepam	10–20 mg	Beware of muscle relaxation,
Oxazepam	10–20 mg	ataxia, amnesia, paradoxical
Triazolam	0.125–0.25 mg	reactions, and habituation

For severe sleep disorders, especially in hospitalized patients:

Dichloralphenazone	1.3–1.95g	Beware of
Chloral hydrate	500 mg	habituation and
Triclofos	750 mg	addiction

Sedative neuroleptics such as:

Thioridazine	10–25 mg	Beware of
Laevomepromazine	6–25 mg	cardiovascular
Floropipamid	40 mg	effects, especially hypotension and extrapyramidal symptoms
Short-acting barbiturates (last resort, no chronic use)		Beware of toxicity, addiction, etc.; not recommended by the BNF

Table 1

Treatment of Insomnia without Drugs

There are numerous recommended ways of inducing sleep without resorting to drugs, although many of these supposedly effective methods contradict one another: cold showers, warm showers, intensive activity or little activity before going to bed, a warm bedroom, a cool bedroom, etc., are suggested by various authors, but obviously few of these measures have been put to adequate test. Unfortunately, this is also the case with several psychotherapeutic and relaxation techniques whose efficacy, particularly in elderly insomniacs, has not been established in properly designed studies.

There are some recommendations which seem to be supported by knowledge about insomnia and by common sense. In sleeplessness which is mainly a problem within the patient rather than his surroundings, treatment should be directed towards correcting false expectations concerning 'normal sleep' and reducing the tensions which prevent sleep onset. A first point to emphasize to the patient is that the need to sleep and the duration of sleep vary greatly among and within individuals. There is neither a physiological nor a statistical law according to which healthy individuals must sleep 7 or 8 hours per night. Many people are doing fine on 4 or 5 hours of sleep per night, others need 10 and more hours in order to feel recovered in the morning.

Another point to be made is that, according to present knowledge, one or even several nights without sleep or poor sleep will not harm the body or health in any way: 'The organism gets as much sleep as it needs.' To support this the physician might refer to experiments with total sleep deprivation which lasted 10 days and had to be given up, not because the subjects were exhausted but because the experimenters became too tired. Emphasis should also be put on the fact that sleep undergoes physiological changes with ageing (see above). It is, therefore, by no means alarming if an elderly person notices subjective sleep changes and from time to time feels like taking a nap during the day (Prinz *et al.*, 1982). Counselling by the physician should attempt to counteract the belief in the importance of immediately falling asleep in the evening, and of quickly going back to sleep after waking up during the night – situations which are experienced by many insomniacs as an examination of great importance. Patients should be given an opportunity to describe the real or supposed consequences of not sleeping properly. Although many of them will not be able to describe objectively the sequelae of insomnia, the physician must realize that for many elderly people time spent alone in the dark means lonesomeness, brooding, and despair. Even if no formal psychotherapy is within the reach of the practising physician, to be listened to with sympathy may be reassuring for many patients.

CONCLUDING REMARKS

The division between pharmacological and non-pharmacological therapy of insomnia in old age is less distinct than may appear from many critical publications. Even physicians with psychotherapeutic orientation and who are primarily interested in the problems which lead to sleeplessness will find that sometimes the use of drugs is necessary and gives the patient assistance when he most needs it. On the other hand, no patient should be prescribed hypnotic drugs without being informed about their desired and possible undesired effects. This will include a precise information (not a warning!) about the consequences of prolonged drug intake, i.e. habituation and possible withdrawal insomnia. All the sleep-inducing drugs used nowadays produce some degree of dependency if administered chronically, and insomnia will sooner or later reappear if its reasons are not eliminated otherwise. Thus patients should be aware that they will possibly suffer from worse sleeplessness for several nights after cessation of drug treatment, but this does not mean that their sleep mechanism has been damaged in any way. Rebound insomnia is the result of a physiological adaptation which occurs in similar ways after many kinds of drug. It can be avoided if sleep-inducing drugs are not taken for longer than 3 to 5 consecutive nights, i.e. if the patient is willing to discontinue the drug during weekends or holidays, when even a couple of slightly disturbed nights would not be of great importance.

REFERENCES

American Psychiatric Association (1980). DSM-III. *Diagnostic and Statistical Manual of Mental Disorders*, 3rd. ed., APA, Washington, D.C.

Ancoli-Israel, S., Kripke D. F., Mason, W., and Messin, S. (1981). 'Sleep apnea and nocturnal myoclonus in a senior population', *Sleep,* **4**, 349–358.

ASDC (1979). 'Association of Sleep Disorders Centers: Diagnostic classification of sleep and arousal disorders', *Sleep*, **2**, 1–137.

Breimer, D. D. (1979). 'Pharmacokinetics and metabolism of various benzodiazepines used as hypnotics', *Br. J. Clin. Pharmac.*, **8**, 7S-13S.

Breimer, D. D., and Jochemson, R. (1983). 'Pharmacokinetics of hypnotic benzodiazepines in man', *Sleep 1982. Sixth Eur. Congr. Sleep Res., Zürich 1982*, pp. 89–109, Karger, Basel.

Carskadon, M. A., and Dement, W. (1981). 'Respiration during sleep in the aged human', *J. Gerontol.*, **4**, 420–423.

Coleman, R. M., Miles, L. E., Guilleminault, Ch. C., Zarcone, V. P., van den Hoed, J., and Dement, W. C. (1981). 'Sleep–wake disorders in the elderly: A polysomnographic analysis', *J. Am. Geriatr. Soc.*, **7**, 289–296.

Coleman, R. M., Roffwarg, H. P., Kennedy, S. J., *et al.* (1982). 'Sleep–Wake disorders based on a polysomnographic diagnosis', *JAMA*, **247**, 997–1003.

Cook, P., and James, I. (1981). 'Cerebral vasodilators', *New Engl. J. Med.*, **305**, 1508–1512 and 1560–1564.

Dement, W. C., Miles, L. E., and Carskadon, M. A. (1982). 'White Paper on Sleep and Ageing', *J. Am. Ger. Soc.*, **30**, 25–50.

Fishbein, W. (Ed.) (1981). *Sleep, Dreams and Memory. Advances in Sleep Research*, Vol. 6, MTP Press, Lancaster.

Greenblatt, D. J., and Allen, M. A. (1978). 'Toxicity of nitrazepam in the elderly: A report from the Boston collaborative drug surveillance program', *Br. J. Clin. Pharmac.*, **5**, 407–413.

Greenblatt, D. J., Allen, M. D., and Shader, R. I. (1977). 'Toxicity of high-dose flurazepam in the elderly: A report from the Boston collaborative drug surveillance program', *Clin. Pharmacol. Ther.*, **21**, 355–361.

Greenblatt, D. J., Divoll, M., Harmatz, J. S., MacLaughlin, D. S., and Shader, R. I. (1981). 'Kinetics and clinical effects of flurazepam in young and elderly noninsomniacs', *Clin. Pharmacol. Ther.* **30**, 475–486.

Johnson, L. C., and Chernik, D. A. (1982). 'Sedative-hypnotics and human performance', *Psychopharmacology*, **76**, 101–113.

Kales, A., Soldatos, C. R., Bixler, E. O., and Kales, J. D. (1976). 'Early morning insomnia with rapidly eliminated benzodiazepines', *Science*, **220**, 95–97.

Kales, A., Soldatos, C. R., Bixler, E. O., Kales, J. D. (1983). 'Rebound insomnia and rebound anxiety: A review', *Pharmacology*, **26**, 121–137.

Meddis, R. (1975). 'On the function of sleep'. *Anim. Behav.*, **23**, 676–691.

Miles, L. E., and Dement, W. C. (1980). 'Sleep and ageing', *Sleep.*, **2**, 119–220.

Oswald, I., Adam, K., Borrow, S., and Idzikowski, C. (1979). 'The effects of two hypnotics on sleep, subjective feelings and skilled performance', in *Pharmacology of the States of Alertness* (Eds P. Passouant and I. Oswald), pp. 51–63, Pergamon, Oxford.

Parkes, J. D. (1981). 'Day-time drowsiness', *Lancet*, **2**, 1213–1218.

Prinz, P. N. (1980). 'Sleep changes with ageing', in *Psychopharmacology of Ageing*, (Eds C. Eisdorfer and W. E. Fann), pp. 1–12, Spectrum, New York.

Prinz, P. N., Peskind, E. R., Vitaliano, P. P., Raskund, M. A., Eisdorfer, C., Zemcuznikov, N., and Gerber, C. J. (1982). 'Changes in the sleep and waking EEGs of nondemented and demented elderly subjects', *J. Am. Ger. Soc.*, **30**, 86–93.

Rechtschaffen, A., and Kales, A. (Eds) (1968). *A Manual of Standardized Terminology, Techniques and Scoring System for Sleep Stages of Human Subjects*, Public Health Service, U.S. Government Printing Office, Washington, D.C.

Reynolds, Ch. F., Coble, P. A., Black, R. S., Holzer, B., Carroll, R., and Kupfer, D. J. (1980). 'Sleep disturbances in a series of elderly patients: Polysomnographic findings', *J. Am. Geriatr. Soc.*, **28**, 164–170.

Reynolds, Ch. F., Spiker, D. G., Hahin, I., and Kupfer, D. J. (1983). 'Electroencephalic sleep, ageing, and psychopathology: New data and state of the art', *Biol. Psychiat.*, **18**, 139–155.

Roers, T., Zorick, F., Sicklesteel, J., Wittig, R. and Roth, T. (1983). 'Age-related sleep–wake disorders at a sleep disorder center', *J. Am. Ger. Soc.*, **31**, 364–370.

Spiegel, R. (1981). '*Sleep and sleeplessness in advanced age*', *Advances in Sleep Research* (Series Ed. E. D. Weitzman), Vol. 5, Spectrum, New York.

Spiegel, R. (1982). 'Aspects of sleep, daytime vigilance, mental performance and psychotropic drug treatment in the elderly', *Gerontology*, **28**, (Suppl. 1), 68–82.

Webb, W. B. (1982). 'Sleep in older persons: sleep structures of 50- to 60-year-old men and women', *J. Gerontol.*, **37**, S81–S86.

Webb, W. B., and Cartwright, R. D. (1978). 'Sleep and dreams', *Ann. Rev. Psychol.*, **29**, 223–252.

Weitzman, E. D. (1981). 'Sleep and its disorders', *Annu. Rev. Neurosci.*, **4**, 381–417.

8

Interpretation of
Biochemical Data

Principles and Practice of Geriatric Medicine
Edited by M. S. J. Pathy
© 1985 John Wiley & Sons Ltd

8.1

Interpretation of Biochemical Data

H. M. Hodkinson

Few would now deny that adequate investigation of the elderly patient is an essential basis for effective treatment. However, biochemical investigation of the elderly was very much neglected in the past. Happily, the situation has greatly changed over the past 15 years. This has been due in part to the increasing recognition of geriatric medicine but has also been greatly helped by the widespread introduction of laboratory automation so that a comprehensive battery or 'profile' of biochemical tests is now readily available in practically every hospital. In consequence, there has been a striking growth in our understanding of biochemical investigation in old age over the past decade which has been shown to have many special difficulties. Despite the advances in our understanding there are still many challenges.

REFERENCE RANGES IN OLD AGE

Improvements in the availability of biochemical tests quickly led to the realization that there was an almost total lack of appropriate reference ranges for the elderly. Earlier studies of the effects of age on ranges, for example that of Roberts (1967), were most often based on healthy blood donors but stopped short at the maximum permitted age of 65. However, a number of studies of healthy elderly subjects were begun in the early 1970s and reference ranges are now available for all the commonly used tests. These have been summarized by Caird (1973) and Hodkinson

(1977). Table 1 shows some of the more important reference ranges; many of these are not very different to those appropriate to younger adults. Even where ranges are significantly different in the statistical sense, the changes are not of such a magnitude as to be of practical importance. One of the more marked changes is the fall in serum albumin with age, but even this only amounts to a reduction of 2 or 3 grams per litre on the young adult level and is far less striking than the falls which may result from the general effect of illness in the age group. The only range which is markedly different in old age is that of serum phosphate which falls considerably in old men so that the appropriate range is considerably lower than for young men and indeed than for old women.

Changes in reference ranges in old age are thus generally small in extent and should not give rise to major problems in interpretation of biochemical investigations in elderly patients.

INVESTIGATION OF ILL OLD PEOPLE

If age itself has relatively minor effects on biochemical test results, this is not so in the case of a number of effects which relate to the special characteristics of ill old people. The elderly are often gravely ill, commonly have some degree of renal impairment, usually have multiple pathology, and are frequently on many different drugs as treatment. All these characteristics have important effects on bio-

Table 1 Reference ranges for biochemical tests in healthy old people

Test	Reference range	Author
Serum albumin	33–49 g/l	Leask, Andrews, and Caird (1973)
Serum globulin	20–41 g/l	Leask, Andrews, and Caird (1973)
Sodium	135–146 mmol/l	Leask, Andrews, and Caird (1973)
Potassium	3.6–5.2 mmol/l	Leask, Andrews, and Caird (1973)
Bicarbonate	20–31 mmol/l	Leask, Andrews, and Caird (1973)
Urea	3.9–9.9 mmol/l	Leask, Andrews, and Caird (1973)
Creatinine	52.159 μmol/l	Leask, Andrews, and Caird (1973)
Uric acid	148–461 μmol/l	Leask, Andrews, and Caird (1973)
Calcium (women)	2.19–2.68 mmol/l	Leask, Andrews, and Caird (1973)
Calcium (men)	2.19–2.59 mmol/l	Leask, Andrews, and Caird (1973)
Phosphate (women)	0.85–1.33 mmol/l	Hodkinson (1977)
Phosphate (men)	0.65–1.23 mmol/l	Hodkinson (1977)
Alkaline phosphatase	3.6–14.5 KAU	Hodkinson and McPherson (1973)
SGOT	11–33 IU/l	Hodkinson (1977)
Bilirubin (women)	3.12 μmol/l	Reed *et al.* (1972)
Bilirubin (men)	2.17 μmol/l	Reed *et al.* (1972)
Random blood glucose	3.4–9.3 mmol/l	Denham (1972)

chemical test results. Furthermore, many diseases may present in a non-specific or atypical way in old age. If we are not to miss important and eminently treatable diseases such as osteomalacia, hypothyroidism, or thyrotoxicosis we are obliged to use profile tests as screening tests rather than employ them in the more usual diagnostic manner. This leads to special interpretational difficulties. Let us examine these special difficulties in more detail.

Effects of Illness

Illness in elderly patients is often severe. For example, 37 per cent of patients admitted to a department of geriatric medicine were judged to have clinical evidence of constitutional upset (Hodkinson and Hodkinson, 1980a). Homeostasis is far more vulnerable in old age (Mukherjee, Coni, and Davison, 1973), and severe illness may often result in some degree of hyponatraemia. The reference range of 135 to 146 mmol/l for sodium in healthy old people may thus be contrasted with a range of 128 to 147 mmol/l found in an unselected series of patients admitted to a geriatric department (Hodkinson, 1975). Approximately 20 per cent of the patients have sodium values below the lower limit of the reference range and, while some of this hyponatraemia can be ascribed to drugs, it appears to be mainly a consequence of illness itself and to represent the syndrome of inappropriate secretion of anti-diuretic-hormone of greater or lesser degree. Similar disturbance of serum potassium also occurs with

ranges of 3.6 to 5.2 mmol/l in well old people but 2.9 to 5.2 mmol/l in patients admitted to the geriatric department. Again only a proportion of the hypokalaemia found in the elderly patients can be attributed to drug effects and it more often appears to be a consequence of illness itself.

Even more striking than these effects of illness on sodium and potassium, however, are the powerful effects on a variety of serum proteins. Hypoalbuminaemia is very commonly found and similar changes appear to affect other carrier proteins such as thyroxine-binding globulin and iron-binding protein (Hodkinson, 1975). These changes appear to reflect the severity of constitutional upset and are thus quite powerful prognostic indicators (Hodkinson, 1981). The magnitude of such changes quite outweighs the effects of age itself for while albumin is 2 or 3 g/l lower in the healthy elderly than in young adults, it is 8 grams lower again in elderly patients admitted to hospital (Hodkinson, 1977). The practical consequences of such protein changes on biochemical test interpretation are that we must not fail to recognize that low values of substances which are substantially protein-bound are more likely to be due to low carrier proteins than to any specific alteration in the metabolism of the substance carried. Hypoalbuminaemia is the commonest cause of hypocalcaemia and lowered thyroxine-binding globulin accounts for most low serum T4 values in ill old people. We need to correct for these changes by, for example, correcting calcium for protein concentrations and using FTI to assess thyroid status when we are dealing with ill patients, if we are not to be misled. We may be equally misled where serum proteins are spuriously elevated by dehydration, and clinically obvious dehydration was found in 1 in 7 patients admitted to a geriatric department (Hodkinson and Hodkinson, 1980a).

Consequences of Renal Impairment

There is a physiological decline in renal function with age which is reflected by the somewhat higher reference range for urea in old age of 3.9 to 9.9 mmol/l (Leask, Andrews, and Caird, 1973), compared with that of 3.5 to 7.2 mmol/l in middle life (Roberts, 1967). The elevation of serum creatinine is, however, partly annulled by the generally lower muscle mass of elderly subjects, particularly women, and this is of sufficient magnitude in elderly patients for correction of creatinine for body weight to be advisable (Denham, Hodkinson, and Fisher, 1975). Creatinine is generally considered to be a better guide to the glomerular filtration rate than urea, but in the elderly it is urea that is marginally superior even when creatinine has been corrected for body weight (Denham, Hodkinson, and Fisher, 1975). Urea and creatinine in combination give a marginally improved prediction of the glomerular filtration rate, but the increased precision probably does not repay the practical inconvenience of calculation or the use of a nomogram (Hodkinson, 1977). Interpretation of these tests is in other respects no different than in younger age groups.

The relatively minor physiological changes associated with ageing are totally overshadowed by those produced by clinical renal impairment in elderly patients. The reference range of 3.9 to 9.9 mmol/l for urea in well old people can be compared with a range of 3.1 to 20.6 mmol/l in elderly patients (Hodkinson, 1977). Impairment is most commonly associated with dehydration though intrinsic renal disease and postrenal pathology may also be responsible or causation may be multifactorial. This high frequency of renal impairment has major consequences in connection with a number of tests which are not performed as indices of renal function but are nonetheless dependent upon it. Thus, for example, phosphate results are markedly skewed towards higher values in elderly patients so that the test is of very little value in the recognition of osteomalacia or in the differential diagnosis of hypercalcaemia when there is any degree of renal impairment. Similarly uric acid results are skewed upwards in ill old people and interpretation becomes difficult.

Effects of Multiple Pathology

Multiple disease may often complicate test interpretation. We may wish to use alkaline phosphatase as a screening test for osteomalacia in elderly patients, but unfortunately there are many other conditions which also raise alkaline phosphatase. In one reported series of elderly patients only 14 per cent of raised alkaline phosphatase results in women proved to be due to osteomalacia and none in men (Hodkinson and MacPherson, 1973). A raised alkaline phosphatase result is thus of no great value in the diagnosis of osteomalacia in an ill elderly person unless we are able to exlude other causes of elevation such as liver disease, fractures, Paget's disease, or rheumatoid arthritis, all of which have a higher prevalence.

Disturbances Due to Drugs

Elderly patients are often on multiple drugs. Clinicians tend to be largely unaware of the multitude of potential disturbances of biochemical test results which may be a consequence of drug administration. Even a decade ago the literature describing such drug effects ran to more than 9,000 references (Young *et al.*, 1972).

The effects may be *in vivo* ones and clinicians are generally more familiar with these, e.g. hypokalaemia and hyponatraemia from diuretics or hyperglycaemia or hyperuricaemia from thiazides. Test disturbances due to the hepatotoxic or nephrotoxic effects of drugs are also familiar. Other *in vivo* effects are less well known however. A common and important example in geriatric practice is the transient but often quite striking elevation in serum T4 which may follow L-dopa administration and which may lead to an erroneous diagnosis of thyrotoxicosis if the clinican is ignorant of the connection. Another common cause of major test abnormalities is the administration of the sex and anabolic steroids. All of these may produce a marked fall in serum phosphate and a lesser fall in serum calcium so as to mimic the biochemical findings in osteomalacia. Major changes in levels of thyroxine-binding globulin also result, oestrogens giving elevation and androgens and anabolics a decrease. In consequence, there are marked changes in T4 and T3 levels because of altered binding though free levels or FTI are unaffected. Further examples of possible *in vivo* disturbances of test results are lowering of 25-hydroxy vitamin D levels from enzyme induction due to antiepileptic drugs and thyroid hormone disturbances due to displacement from thyroxine-binding globulin by competitive binding of such drugs as phenylbutazone or phenytoin. Elevation of bilirubin may be caused by competition for biliary excretion by radiological contrast media and lowering of uric acid from enhanced renal excretion due to drugs such as aspirin or phenylbutazone.

There are a considerable number of ways in which test results may be affected by in vitro mechanisms. There may be simple contamination as by a wide variety of iodine compounds in the case of protein-bound iodine which used to be widely used as a measure of circulating thyroid hormone levels before specific assays were generally available. Drugs may inhibit reactions used to measure enzymes; e.g. nitrofurantoin and ethionamide may lower the measured values of alkaline phosphatase and LDH in this way. Crossreactions with reagents used in colorimetric analyses may give spuriously high values; e.g. L-dopa may elevate creatinine measured by the Jaffé reaction. Other drugs may similarly give higher readings in fluorimetric analyses as spironolactone or fucidin may in the case of cortisol. Drugs which are oxidizing or reducing substances may affect oxidation–reduction reactions; e.g. other reducing substances may be measured as glucose when reduction methods are employed. Drug binding to albumin may interfere with analysis when a dye-binding estimation is used, salicylates may lead to a falsely low albumin in this way.

These are just some of the many possible drug effects on biochemical test results and such disturbances are probably far more common than is realized. In particular we have very little idea what may happen with multiple drug therapy. The clinician needs to be constantly on his guard if he is not to be misled by such occurrences. He cannot expect to keep abreast of all possible pitfalls and should make full use of the advice and experience of his laboratory colleagues when unexpected test results suggest the possibility of drug effects.

DISCRIMINATORY POWER OF TESTS IN THE ELDERLY PATIENT

As we have seen, test results in ill old people are likely to be subjected to a number of disturbing influences, whether from constitutional upset, renal impairment, the presence of multiple pathology, or drug therapy. The consequence of these phenomena is that the discriminatory power of tests is considerably reduced in the elderly patient. Improved knowledge and understanding may minimize but cannot avoid this blunting of biochemical diagnostic tools. To compensate for this inescapable weakening of the power of tests one must endeavour to squeeze the maximum information from test results by employing the optimal strategy in their interpretation.

The Basics of Test Interpretation

To help see the issues clearly it is worth looking at a simplified hypothetical situation. Consider a test which can only take two values, positive or negative, and which is known to be positive in 95 per cent of cases of certain disease but positive in only 5 per cent of healthy subjects. We now wish to apply the test to a patient we think may well have the disease. Let us be rather precise and say that we judge the patient's chances of having the disease to be 50 per cent. This clinical estimate has been made before the test and is therefore termed a prior probability.

Given these conditions the resulting probabilities can be assessed. Our model is that we are drawing a sample test from a hypothetical population of test results, half of which are derived from subjects without the disease and half from those with the disease. The half without disease will contribute $0.5 \times 0.05 = 0.025$ positive tests and the half with disease $0.5 \times 0.95 = 0.475$. There is a total proportion of 0.5 of positive tests in the population, therefore

(0.025 + 0.475). It follows that if we draw a positive test result it has a probability of 0.475/0.5 = 0.95 of having come from a subject with the disease. Thus a positive test in this situation leads to a revised probability (termed the posterior probability) of 95 per cent for disease.

Now let us compare this finding with what happens using the same test but with a different prior probability of 5 per cent. The 95 per cent without disease will contribute $0.95 \times 0.05 = 0.0475$ positive results and the 5 per cent with disease $0.05 \times 0.95 = 0.0475$ positive results. In this case a positive result leads to a posterior probability of only 50 per cent $(0.0475/(0.0475 + 0.0475) = 0.5)$ compared with the previous result of 95 per cent.

This simple example clearly shows that the power of a positive test to predict disease is very much dependent on prior probability and falls as the prior probability decreases. This is true of any test but a weaker test becomes very weak indeed when prior probabilities are low.

Most biochemical tests, of course, give continuous results rather than a simple positive or negative value. It is tempting to simplify interpretation by converting them to two values by using the reference range (or as it is often rather dangerously called the 'normal range'). We can call the test negative if it is in the range and positive if it is outside it. Misleadingly, however, the term normal range often leads to the categories being referred to as 'normal' and 'abnormal', with much resulting confusion for, by definition, 5 per cent of healthy subjects will have results out of the range but these are clearly not 'abnormal'. Indeed, if we perform a number of independent tests on a healthy subject we expect only the proportion of 0.95^n of such sets of n tests to have all the results within the range. Beyond 13 tests this proportion falls below half $(0.95^{14} = 0.49)$!

A crude normal range approach may serve adequately in more straightforward situations. If we strongly suspect a disease and the relevant test is out of the range in the appropriate direction we can reason that only 2½ per cent of results of healthy people would be thus and can take it as powerful support for the diagnosis. Our hypothetical example has shown us that this is likely to be so. The danger of this unsophisticated approach is when prior probability is low. We know that the test will be far weaker in this situation. It is also intuitively obvious that a more extreme result must favour disease more than one just outside the reference limit and that we are throwing away valuable information when we convert our continuous test values into two broad categories.

The 'Normal Range' Approach to Test Interpretation

We need a better strategy. Our simple example of a test taking only positive and negative values has shown us that the essential requirements for optimal test interpretation are:

(a) an estimate of the prior probability of disease;
(b) knowledge of the distribution of test results in health (i.e. the reference range);
(c) knowledge of the distribution of test results in the presence of the disease.

It is an unfortunate fact that while we can estimate prior probability from our clinical knowledge and experience and while reference ranges are available, the literature rarely provides adequate information as to the distribution of test results in disease, though this is equally important. However, where this has been determined, it is usual to find that the distributions in health and disease are similar in type (both normal or both log-normal), have similar spreads as measured by their standard deviations and, though having different means, usually considerably overlap each other as shown in the hypothetical example of Fig. 1.

In Fig. 1 the test value scale on the horizontal axis is in standard deviation units, while the vertical axis corresponds to the relative prob-

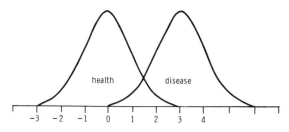

Figure 1   Diagnostic test situation when prior probability of disease is 50 per cent.

ability density, i.e. heights under the curves are proportional to the chances of that value occurring in health or disease respectively. The actual size of the two populations corresponds to the area under each curve and so Fig. 1, where the curves are of the same size, represents a situation where the prior probability for disease is assessed at 50 per cent. As the height under a curve is a measure of the relative probability density it follows that if we wish to determine the posterior probability of disease, given any test value, we have simply to look at the heights under the curves at that point and can then determine the posterior probability simply by taking the ratio of the height under the disease curve divided by the combined heights under the two curves. We can see that in this example a test value exactly at the upper normal limit (+ 1.96 S.D.) would strongly favour the diagnosis of disease. However, the upper normal limit has no special significance; the really important value is that given by the intersection of the two curves (+ 1.5 S.D. in this example), for at this value, the 'critical limit' (Murphy and Abbey, 1967), health and disease are equally likely, while above this value the probability of disease progressively rises above the 50 per cent value.

Test Interpretation in the Screening Situation

We have already commented that it is often of considerable relevance in the elderly to search for a number of diseases which are eminently treatable, but which may often present atypically, or be clinically inapparent, yet have prevalences which are low enough to make test interpretation difficult but high enough to warrant a serious search for the condition. For example, osteomalacia has an incidence of approximately 3 per cent in elderly women and is often clinically inapparent. Hyperthyroidism with an incidence of a little over 2 per cent is also often atypical in its presentation so that only a proportion of cases can be recognized without the help of screening tests (Bahemuka and Hodkinson, 1975). Figure 2 models a situation of this kind. The curves are identical to those in Fig. 1, save that their relative sizes have changed to represent a prior probability of only 5 per cent. It will be seen that the critical limit has now moved from + 1.5 to + 2.5 S.D. and it is only beyond + 3.5 S.D. that

higher probabilities of disease are indicated. This can be compared to the previous model illustrated in Fig. 1 and it can then be clearly seen that far more extreme test values are needed to achieve the same diagnostic significance. While the test was diagnostic in most of the disease population in the 50 per cent prior probability situation, a substantial proportion of the disease population now falls in the uncertain area of overlap of distributions, showing that the test has a very much reduced discriminatory power in this screening situation. We can see from these two simple examples that we can apply the same principles that were possible with a simple test giving only positive and negative values to our continuous test results.

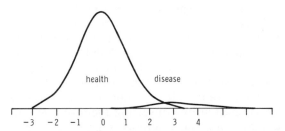

Figure 2 Diagnostic test situation when prior probability of disease is 5 per cent.

We are now not discarding any useful information given by the actual value of the test. If the distributions of the test in health and disease are accurately known, an actual posterior probability can readily be calculated using quite simple calculations which can easily be performed on a pocket calculator (Hodkinson, 1977). However, even if we were not in a position to make accurate calculations of this sort, we can learn from this approach and, in particular, it shows us that we must be extremely cautious in interpretation of test results when prior probabilities are low. The commonest clinical error is to think that screening tests are far more powerful than they really are and to overdiagnose rather than underdiagnose the disease.

Using Tests in Combination

We are often in a situation where there are several tests which can help in the diagnosis of a disease. For example, in the case of osteomalacia we would commonly wish to make use of serum calcium, serum phosphate, and the alkaline phosphatase results. If we use the crude normal range approach we can only interpret the tests by using some sort of pattern recognition strategy. In other words, we would pay more attention to test abnormalities which involved all three tests being disturbed in the appropriate direction. Fortunately we can do better than this for there is an efficient way to combine the information from several tests and use the resulting information in the way we have just described. The statistical method used is that of discriminant function analysis, though this has as yet been rather little used despite its great potential value. Examples of its application are to the diagnosis of osteomalacia (Hodkinson and Hodkinson, 1980b) and to the differential diagnosis of hypercalcaemia in elderly patients (Grero and Hodkinson, 1977). The essence of discriminant function analysis is to find the linear combination of values of a number of tests which achieve the widest separation between two or more defined groups. The principle can perhaps be most readily grasped in visual terms by looking at the situation where two tests are being applied to two groups. This is shown in an idealized way in Fig. 3, the two circles representing the distribution of the individual observations in the two groups of the two tests x and y. Viewing these results from either the x or the y axis shows that there is considerable overlap for each of the tests between the two groups. However, if the distributions are viewed from a new axis, z, we can see that there is virtually complete separation of the test results of the two groups. Discriminant function analysis finds this best axis, combining the test values as a new variable, the discriminant function, which takes the form $z = ax + by$, where a and b are coefficients found by the analysis of the previous cases. The function can then be calculated for subsequent cases and can then be interpreted exactly as though it were a single test value.

REFERENCES

Bahemuka, M., and Hodkinson, H. M. (1975). 'Screening for hypothyroidism in the elderly inpatient', *Br. Med. J.* **2**, 601–603.

Caird, F. I., (1973). 'Problems of interpretation of laboratory findings in the old', *Br. Med. J.*, **4**, 348–351.

Denham, M. J. (1972). 'The value of random blood glucose determinations in a screening method for detecting diabetes mellitus in the elderly patient', *Age Ageing*, **1**, 55–59.

Denham, M. J., Hodkinson, H. M., and Fisher, M. (1975). 'Glomerular filtration rate in sick elderly inpatients', *Age Ageing,* **4**, 32–35.

Grero, P. S., and Hodkinson, H. M., (1977). 'Hypercalcaemia in elderly hospital inpatients: Value of discriminant analysis in differential diagnosis', *Age Ageing,* **6**, 14–19.

Hodkinson, H. M., and MacPherson, C. K. (1973). 'Alkaline phosphatase in a geriatric inpatient population', *Age Ageing*, **2**, 28–33.

Hodkinson, H. M. (1975). 'Diagnostic and prognostic aspects of routing laboratory screening of the geriatric inpatient', D. M. Thesis, University of Oxford.

Hodkinson, H. M. (1977). *Biochemical Diagnosis of the Elderly*, Chapman and Hall, London.

Hodkinson, H. M., and Hodkinson, I. (1980a). 'Death and discharge from a geriatric department', *Age Ageing,* **9**, 220–228.

Hodkinson, H. M., and Hodkinson, I. (1980b). 'A discriminant function for the biochemical diagnosis of osteomalacia in elderly subjects and its relevance to interpretation of borderline bone histological findings', *J. Clin. Exp. Gerontol.,* **2**, 123–131.

Hodkinson, H. M. (1981). 'Value of admission profile tests for prognosis in elderly patients', *J. Am. Ger. Soc.,* **29**, 206–210.

Leask, R. G. S., Andrews, G. R., and Caird, F. I. (1973). 'Normal values of sixteen blood constituents in the elderly', *Age Ageing*, **2**, 14–23.

Mukherjee, A. P., Coni, N. K., and Davison, W. (1973). 'Osmoreceptor function among the elderly', *Gerontol. Clin.,* **15**, 227–233.

Murphy, E. A., and Abbey, H. (1967). 'The normal range – a common misuse', *J. Chronic. Dis.,* **20**, 79–88.

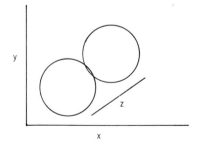

Figure 3 Diagnostic two-way plot of results of two tests (x and y) in two diagnostic groups, showing how a discriminant function (shown as the z axis) improves discrimination.

Reed, A. H., Cannon, D. C., Winkelman, J. W., Bhasin, Y. P., Henry, R. J., and Pileggi, V. J. (1972). 'Estimation of normal ranges from a controlled sample survey: I, Sex and age related influence on SMA 12/60 screening group of tests', *Clin. Chem.*, **18** 57–66.

Roberts, L. B. (1967). 'The normal ranges, with statistical analysis for seventeen blood constituents', *Clin. Chim. Acta.,* **16**, 69–78.

Young, D. S., Thomas, D. W., Friedman, R. B., and Pestaner, L. C. (1972). 'Effects of drugs on clinical laboratory tests', *Clin. Chem.,* **18**, 1041–1303.

9

Ageing and Infectious Diseases

9.1

Ageing and Infectious Diseases

T. Yoshikawa

Until the practice of antisepsis, the availability of antimicrobial chemotherapy, and the institution of vaccination entered modern society, infections were the most important cause of death in humans. Thus, infectious diseases played a major role in the shortened life expectancy observed prior to the mid-twentieth century. A comparison between 1935 and 1968 of reported deaths for select infections in the United States illustrates the impact infections have had on survival of mankind. Whereas such diseases as pertussis, measles, diphtheria, scarlet fever, tetanus, acute poliomyelitis, tuberculosis, and syphilis caused significant number of deaths in 1935, they contributed insignificantly to mortality in 1968 (U.S. Department of Commerce, 1937; U.S. Department of Health, Education and Welfare, 1970). However, despite the eradication of many infectious diseases affecting the general population, infections ostensibly have a major impact on morbidity and mortality in geriatric patients (Yoshikawa, 1983). From the perspective of practising clinicians, empirically it appears that the elderly are more prone to acquire infectious diseases and to suffer greater complications. If, however, a careful analysis is made of objective data from *limited* clinical studies and observations, the conclusion that the aged are generally more susceptible to *all* infections is not substantiated. Recently available information suggests that *select* infections may attack the old in higher numbers or cause greater morbidity and mortality.

HOST RESPONSE TO INFECTION WITH INCREASING AGE

Microbe–Host Interaction

For microorganisms to produce infections, they must be pathogenic or virulent to the host. In fact, the great majority of bacteria that humans encounter are non-pathogenic and therefore harmless. Microbial virulence is dependent on several factors: (a) the ability of the microbe to gain access to the host (e.g., penetrating the skin or mucous membrane); (b) the ability of the microbe to replicate or multiply in the host; (c) inhibition or avoidance of host defence mechanisms by the microbe; and (d) production of damage or injury to the host (McCloskey, 1979). Another perspective is to view infection as a host–parasite relationship. Development of infection is directly dependent on the number of microbes to which the host is exposed and microbial virulence, and is inversely related to the functional integrity of the host's defence mechanism against microbial invasion. This can be described by a simple formula as:

$$\text{Infection} = \frac{\text{quantity of organism} \times \text{virulence}}{\text{host defence mechanisms}}$$

Thus, the probability of infection occurring will be high if the inoculum is high, the microbe is highly virulent, or host defence mechanisms are diminished. Certain bacteria such as *Pseu-*

domonas aeruginosa and *Staphylococcus aureus* are highly virulent and require a smaller inoculum to cause infection compared to less virulent organisms such as *S. epidermidis*. Alternatively, relatively avirulent microbes can become pathogens if the quantity of organisms exposed to the host is large or if the defence mechanism of the host is compromised.

Risk Factors for Infection in the Elderly

With the above principles and concepts, several factors can be identified which might be contributing to the apparent propensity of the elderly for acquiring certain infections. These risk factors are environmental exposure, physiological changes with ageing, diseases that increase susceptibility to infection, and aberrations of host defence mechanisms (Gardner, 1980).

Environmental Exposure

The greater the exposure to microbes, the greater the risk for infection. The life span for men and women has increased. Associated with this longevity is increasing affliction with chronic illnesses, which require more hospitalization. The elderly are hospitalized in acute care facilities, on the average, twice as long as those persons under 65 years (U.S. Bureau of Census, 1978). Additionally, the average age of patients in nursing homes is approximately 84 years. Once hospitalized, any patient has a significant risk (nearly 5 per cent.) of acquiring a hospital-acquired infection. More significantly, this risk increases with age, especially over the age of 60 years, for nosocomial urinary tract infection, pneumonia, bactaeremia, and surgical wound infections (Haley *et al.*, 1981). It has been estimated that the elderly have a threefold higher risk for nosocomial infection than the average population (Freeman and Gowan, 1978). The most common pathogens causing nosocomial infections are gram-negative bacilli (Riley, 1977). Hence, the hospitalized geriatric patient has a high incidence of gram-negative bacillary infections. Another observation that in part explains this phenomenon is that the aged who are hospitalized or placed in nursing homes have a high incidence of pharyngeal colonization with gram-negative bacilli (Valenti, Trudell and Bentley, 1978). Whether this colonization is strictly age-related or influenced equally or to a lesser degree by other factors (e.g. antibiotics, underlying disease) has not been clearly defined.

Physiological Changes with Ageing

With advancing age, there is a decremental change of structure in most organs and tissues. These age-related abnormalities are reviewed in other sections of this text and have been extensively discussed by others (Goldman, 1979). The organ changes may involve not only its structure but also physiology. These alterations may ultimately impact on the host's defence mechanisms against microorganisms, and contribute to the increased risk of infection in the elderly.

Diseases of the Aged that Increase Susceptibility to Infection

Certain diseases that are associated with higher frequency of infection appear to have a significant predilection for the elderly. Select malignancies such as those arising from the stomach, pancreas, breast, lung, and prostate as well as multiple myeloma and chronic lymphocytic leukaemia attack the old more frequently. Diabetes mellitus and prostatic hypertrophy are other examples. All of these diseases have a high association with various infectious diseases (Bodey, 1975; Edwards *et al.*, 1979; Serpick, 1978; Twomey, 1973).

Aberrations of Host Defence Mechanisms

Of all the risk factors contributing to the infections in the elderly, the integrity of the host's defence mechanisms against microbial invasion may be the most important. Although it is unlikely that current research has identified every important host defence mechanism against microbial invasion, there are several mechanisms that appear to play a significant role in preventing and eradicating infectious pathogens from man: mechanical factors, phagocytosis, immune processes, and complement activity.

Mechanical Factors

The intact skin is a formidable mechanical barrier for preventing invasion by microorganisms, since very few have the innate ability to penetrate this tissue. Only by a physical disruption of the skin (e.g. trauma, burn, insect bite, surgery, etc.) can microbes gain access to the host through the skin. The skin's milieu or environment is also effective in inhibiting or minimizing microbial replication. The relative dryness of the skin, the mild acid state, and the normal skin flora create an unsuitable environment for most pathogenic microorganisms (Tramont, 1979). Additionally, fatty acids and other secretory products from various skin glands may have microbicidal activity. In the elderly, many of the age-related physiological changes of the skin may affect its antimicrobial defence mechanisms; thinning of the epidermis and decreased glandular secretions are examples of such changes. Increased trauma and injuries in the old compromise the skin's mechanical barrier. Pressure sores in the aged disrupt the integrity of the epidermal structure and function. Mucous membranes act also as mechanical obstacles against microorganisms. Both cilia and mucus secreted by glands in the respiratory tract act to trap invading microbes, which can then be removed by coughing. Peristalsis may be a mechanism of the intestinal tract to remove harmful pathogens. Whether anatomical changes of the mucous membranes occur normally with age has not been well studied. Such age-associated changes or disorders as atrophic gastritis, diverticulosis, or colonic cancer also alter mucosal surfaces and indirectly may contribute to a greater risk to intra-abdominal infection.

Phagocytosis

Phagocytosis of microorganisms can be accomplished by granulocytes (neutrophils, eosinophils, and basophils), monocytes, and macrophages. Of these cells, the characteristics and kinetics of neutrophil phagocytosis are best known. Phagocytosis by neutrophils is a complex series of events culminating in microbial death. The functional integrity of neutrophil phagocytosis depends on cell movement (chemokinesis or chemotaxis), microbial attachment and engulfment, metabolic activity or respiratory burst (conversion of oxygen to active bactericidal metabolites), degranulation, and microbicidal activity. Studies that compared intracellular killing of *Staphylococcus aureus* by neutrophils from old versus young healthy

volunteers showed no significant difference (Palmblad and Haak, 1978; Phair *et al.*, 1978a). Similar studies performed in hospitalized patients demonstrated abnormal neutrophil function in all age groups but no difference between young and old (Phair *et al.*, 1978b). One investigation has shown significantly lower neutrophil chemiluminescence responses in individuals over 70 years (Van Epps, Goodwin, and Murphy, 1978). However, concurrent microbicidal studies were not performed.

Little is known about the integrity of phagocytosis of tissue macrophages in humans with advancing age. Limited data in animals suggest that ageing does not significantly influence the phagocytosis capacity of macrophages (Perkins, 1971).

Immune Processes

In Chapter 2 the immunological changes that occur with ageing are described and will not be discussed here. However, it should be mentioned that certain infectious pathogens are most frequently associated with defects in either cell-mediated immunity or humoral immunity. This is not to say that an overlap or dependency between the two arms of the immune system does not occur with these infections. Moreover, with greater understanding and newer immunological techniques, it is clear that previously held concepts of immunity to certain microorganisms are much more complex. For example, certain infections that previously were thought to be defended by the host through humoral mechanisms only are now shown to be modulated by certain T lymphocytes (helper or suppressor cells).

With disturbances in the humoral immune system, there is a significant incidence of infections with encapsulated bacteria and, to a lesser extent, gram-negative bacteria. These organisms include *Streptococcus pneumoniae, Haemophilus influenzae, Neisseria meningitidis,* and *Pseudomonas aeruginosa* (Pitchon and Sorrell, 1980). Other infections that appear to occur with greater frequency in patients with hypogammaglobulinaemia or dysgammaglobulinaemia are pneumonia caused by *Pneumocystis carinii* and *gastrointestinal giardiasis.*

Cell-mediated immunity plays an important role in host defences against microbial invasion from several perspectives: its own intrinsic microbicidal mechanisms (e.g. cytotoxicity), its interaction with macrophages (e.g. attraction, activation, memory), and its regulatory role in humoral-mediated immunity. As a very broad, general rule, cell-mediated immunity is important against intracellular bacterial infections, many viral infections, mycobacterioses, most fungal infections, and select protozoa and helminthic infections (Pitchon and Sorrell, 1980). Table 1 lists common pathogens that are isolated in patients with defects primarily in cell-mediated immunity.

Table 1 Pathogens associated with defects in cell-mediated immunity

Class of microorganism	Pathogen
Bacteria	*Listeria monocytogenes*
	Salmonella sp.
Viruses	Rubella
	Varicella-zoster
	Vaccinia
	Cytomegalovirus
Mycobacteria	*Mycobacterium tuberculosis*
	Non-tuberculous mycobacteria
Fungi	*Candida albicans*
	Coccidiodes immitis
	Cryptococcus neoformans
Protozoa	*Toxoplasma gondii*
	Pneumocystis carinii
Helminthic	*Strongyloides stercoralis*

Complement Activity

Both the classical and alternate pathways of complement play important roles in host defence against infection. The multiplicity of physiological effects of the complement system that affect microbial invasion include vascular permeability, leucocyte function, and microbial lysis. The complement system interacts with the affector and effector pathways of the humoral immune system, and facilitates phagocytosis by neutrophils and macrophages. Thus aberrations or deficiencies of individual or several components of complement do result in a higher frequency of infection, i.e., *Neisseria* organisms, encapsulated bacteria, and *Salmonella* (Root, 1979). Investigations of the complement system with increasing age have been few in number. In such limited studies, select complement components appear not to diminish in activity in the elderly population (Palmblad and Haak, 1978; Phair *et al.*, 1978a).

Clinical Features of Infection in the Elderly

It is beyond the scope of this chapter to enumerate all the symptoms and signs of every major infection encountered by the aged population. However, a few general comments should be made. Careful, controlled comparative studies have yet to be done in terms of clinical responses to infection in the old versus the young. Thus, much of our statements, recommendations, and teaching is based on empirical observations and day-to-day clinical experiences.

A hallmark or diagnostic feature of infection is the presence of fever. It appears that advancing age may blunt the ability of an individual to mount a febrile response to an infection. Some clinicians have encountered elderly patients who have had documented infections but no demonstrable hyperpyrexia (Gleckman and Hibert, 1982). Whether this lack of fever response is related to ageing, underlying disease, severity of infection, or level of patient debility is not known.

Besides the possible absence of fever, another perplexing diagnostic problem in the elderly is the non-specific nature of symptoms (or no symptoms) in the presence of active infection. For examples, old patients with bacteriuria frequently are asymptomatic (Wolfson *et al.*, 1965) or the elderly with a urinary tract infection may present to the clinician with confusion, loss of cognition, weakness, and anorexia rather than complaining of dysuria, frequency, fever, and chills. Thus, it should be remembered that any relatively acute change in the well-being of an otherwise stable or well geriatric patient could be due to an active infectious disease process.

Another difficulty for clinicians in diagnosing infections in the aged is the concomitant presence of several chronic diseases, which not infrequently may mask or confuse the clinical presentation of an infection. For example, chest pain in the old may be ascribed to a myocardial infarction or angina rather than pneumonia; confusion and nuchal rigidity may lead the physician to a diagnosis of a stroke and cervical osteoarthritis instead of meningitis; or anorexia and weight loss may lead to a cancer evaluation where tuberculosis is the underlying disease. Such diversity of diseases commonly found in the geriatric patient, therefore, taxes the clinical skills and acumen of physicians when an infectious process is suspected.

IMPORTANT INFECTIONS IN THE ELDERLY

Based on current available data, those infectious diseases that appear to occur more frequently or cause greater morbidity and mortality in the geriatric population are shown in Table 2 (Yoshikawa 1981). Pulmonary infections, genitourinary infections, and herpes zoster infections are discussed in other sections of this textbook.

Table 2 Important infectious diseases of the elderly

Pneumonia (including influenza)
Tuberculosis
Urinary tract infection
Intra-abdominal infections
Gram-negative sepsis
Skin and soft tissue infections
Infective endocarditis
Meningitis
Bacterial arthritis
Herpes zoster infection

Intra-abdominal Sepsis

Biliary Tract Infection

Epidemiology. Gallstones reportedly occur in 15 to 20 million persons in the United States (Smith & Wiener, 1980). Because the complications of cholelithiasis (cholangitis, gangrene, perforation, and common duct stones) are more common in the old, the morbidity and mortality are higher than for young or middle-aged persons. Infected bile occurs with the greatest frequency in patients over 70 years (54 to 72 per cent.) (Chetlin and Elliot, 1971; Keighley *et al.*, 1975). Mortality following biliary tract surgery in the elderly is nearly 7 per cent, compared to less than 2 per cent. for the general population (Morrow, Thompson and Wilson, 1978) (see Chapter 27).

Pathophysiological changes. The gallbladder may be simply inflamed (acute cholecystitis) or become infected and rapidly progress to acute purulent cholecystitis, empyema, gangrene, perforation, or suppurative cholangitis. Hepatic, subhepatic and subphrenic abscesses; peritonitis; and bacteraemia with or without hypotension are serious extrabiliary tract extensions of this infection.

Clinical features. Abdominal pain is a constant symptom with both acute and chronic cholecystitis. Pain is frequently located within the epigastric or right upper quadrant, although some patients experience pain substernally or in the left upper quadrant (generally chronic cholecystitis). Pain may radiate, generally posteriorly to the back; referred pain to the right shoulder is not uncommon. Nausea, vomiting, dyspepsia, or flatulence usually accompany or precede abdominal pain. Jaundice and peritoneal signs are evidence of more severe and extensive infection. Mental confusion, disorientation, and disregard for food may be early signs of sepsis in the aged. Although fever is an important sign of infection, only three-quarters of the elderly with acute cholecystitis may show a temperature rise (Morrow, Thompson, and Wilson, *et al.* 1978). The gallbladder may be palpable in 30 per cent. of cases, but right upper quadrant tenderness may be absent in one-third of elderly patients (Smith and Wiener, 1980).

Diagnostic procedures. Plain X-ray films of the abdomen may occasionally show gallstones (10 per cent. of cases). Abdominal ultrasonography is rapid, safe, and valuable in detecting stones and abscesses, and should be performed on suspected cases of biliary tract disease or infection. If this test is negative, cholecystography (oral or intravenous) should be performed to confirm or deny the presence of cholecystitis. Use of computed tomography for diagnosis of biliary tract disease has been limited.

As with all cases of suspected infection, obtaining blood cultures is essential. A complete blood count and liver function tests are important. At surgery, bile should be cultured aerobically and anaerobically. The most common pathogens isolated from patients with bactobilia are, in descending order of frequency, *Escherichia coli*, *Klebsiella* sp., *Enterobacter* sp., *Streptococcus* sp. (enterococcus), anaerobic streptococci, and *Bacteroides fragilis*.

With emphysematous cholecystitis, *Clostridium perfringens* may be recovered from bile.

Treatment. General supportive care including intravenous fluids, nasogastric suction, and analgesics should be started. Antispasmodics may be hazardous in the elderly because of potential glaucoma, obstructive uropathy, and cardiac tachyarrhythmia. After stabilization of the patient, surgical intervention should be prompt. Cholecystectomy is the treatment of choice. Because of the high frequency of bactobilia in patients over 70 years, preoperative antibiotics are recommended by some clinicians (see Chapter 27).

Antibiotic therapy for septic patients (or preoperative prophylaxis) should include drugs that will be effective against most of the previously mentioned pathogens (primarily the gram-negative bacilli). Combinations of an aminoglycoside and ampicillin or a cephalosporin has been the most popular regimen recommended by infectious disease specialists and surgeons. Second-generation cephalosporins such as cefoxitin or cefamandole have been useful for biliary tract infections in limited studies. Whether the newer, third generation cephalosporins or broad-spectrum penicillins will be effective for gallbladder infections remains to be seen.

Postoperatively, pneumonia, hepatic failure, intra-abdominal abscesses, biliary fistula, pancreatitis, cardiopulmonary failure, and renal dysfunction may occur as complications of biliary tract surgery.

Appendicitis

Epidemiology

Appendicitis in the elderly may constitute 4 to 7 per cent. of all cases (Owens and Hamit, 1978). This disorder afflicts 1 out of every 15 persons after the age of 50 years. The risk of appendicitis is 1:35 for women and 1:50 for men (Peltokallio and Jauhiainen, 1970). The mortality and complications of appendicitis in geriatric patients are exceedingly high compared to younger counterparts. Mortality rates in the elderly of 7, 11.7, and 16 times higher than young patients have been reported (Peltokallio and Jauhiainen, 1970; Williams and Hale, 1963; Yusuf and Dunn, 1979). As many

as 20 per cent. of patients over 60 years and 24 per cent. over 75 years may suffer death as a complication of acute appendicitis (Albano, Zielinski, and Organ, 1975; Owens and Hamit, 1978). Delay in diagnosis (resulting in gangrene and perforation), the presence of other concomitant diseases, and postoperative complications are the major reasons for such high death rates. Wound infection, intra-abdominal sepsis, postoperative pneumonia, and cardiopulmonary dysfunction are responsible for the postoperative complication rate of 35 to 68 per cent. in the aged with appendicitis (see Chapter 27).

Pathophysiological Changes

Gangrene and perforation are common pathological findings at surgery, occurring in as many as 30 to 60 per cent of elderly patients with appendicitis (Goldenberg, 1955; Peltokallio and Jauhiainen, 1970; Thorbjarnarson and Loehr, 1967; Williams and Hale, 1963). Anatomical changes of the appendix in the older person include narrowing and obliteration of the lumen of the appendix, thinning of the mucosa, and arteriosclerosis (Thorbjarnarson and Loehr, 1967). Under such conditions, it is not surprising that minimal obstruction of the appendix results in vascular thrombosis, gangrene, rapid inflammation, and perforation.

Clinical Features

Acute appendicitis in the old may present with classical clinical findings: abdominal pain, later locating to the right lower quadrant; anorexia, nausea, and/or vomiting; fever; and palpable abdominal tenderness, localized rebound and rectal tenderness (Owens and Hamit, 1978; Peltokallio and Jauhiainen, 1970; Yusuf and Dunn, 1979). However, such typical findings may be absent or symptoms may be atypical (Albano, Zielinski, and Organ, 1975). The average duration of symptoms of appendicitis before patients seek medical attention is longer in elderly patients than in the young. This delay combined with a greater frequency of incorrect diagnosis of appendicitis in the old by physicians contribute to the higher morbidity and mortality in this age group (Albano, Zielinski, and Organ, 1975; Owens and Hamit, 1978; Yusuf and Dunn, 1979).

Diagnostic Procedures

Plain X-rays of the abdomen may show localized ileus in one-third of patients (Yusuf and Dunn, 1979). White blood cell counts above 10,000/mm^3 occur in nearly 80 per cent. of patients (Williams and Hale, 1963; Yusuf and Dunn, 1979); conversely, 20 per cent. may not show leucocytosis. Blood cultures are recommended because of the high incidence of gangrene and perforation; however, its diagnostic value in this condition has not been clearly elucidated.

Treatment

The treatment of choice is appendectomy. Preoperative antibiotic therapy is most likely warranted, although controlled trials in the elderly with appendicitis are lacking. The microflora of perforated and/or gangrenous appendices is a mixture of anaerobic and aerobic bacteria, similar to the colonic faecal flora (Lorber and Swenson, 1975; Stone, Kolb, and Geheber, 1975). Therefore, antimicrobial regimens should include drugs effective against aerobic gram-negative bacilli (*E. coli* primarily) and anaerobic organisms including *Bacteroides fragilis*.

Diverticulitis

Epidemiology

Diverticulosis increases in frequency with advancing age. From barium enema studies of unselected patients or studies from autopsy examinations, the incidence of diverticular disease is at least 40 per cent. over the age of 70 years (Debray *et al.*, 1961; Parks, 1975). The most common complication of diverticulosis is acute diverticulitis (Boles and Jordan, 1958). The exact incidence of inflammatory complications of diverticular disease is unclear since diagnosis is made by autopsy, clinical features, or radiological findings – the latter two methods being frequently imprecise. It appears that the risk for development of diverticulitis increases with the passage of time with the incidence varying from 10 to 40 per cent. after a period of 5 to 20 years (Parks, 1975). Mortality from acute diverticulitis depends on several variables including the presence of other dis-

eases (e.g. cardiovascular, renal), severity of diverticular disease (i.e. peritonitis, obstruction, large abscess), and/or development of bactaeremia. The mortality rate from inflammatory diverticular disease may be as high as 12 per cent. (Kyle, 1968).

Pathophysiological Changes

Colonic diverticula develop most frequently in the left colon, particularly the descending and sigmoid colon. Diverticulitis is not simply an infectious, inflammatory process of the lumen of the diverticulum. It is a perforation of the diverticulum, the majority of which are microperforations and thus are subclinical (Cello, 1981). Adjacent local peritonitis with adhesion of mesentery prevents extension of the inflammatory process. This pattern of diverticulitis has been termed pericolitis (Cello, 1981) or acute phlegmonous (non-perforated) diverticulitis (Hughes, 1975). Other variants (more severe forms) of diverticulitis include pericolic abscess with or without intestinal obstruction; perforated diverticulitis with peritoneal cavity communications; and mesocolic gangrenous diverticulitis (Hughes, 1975).

Clinical Features

The signs and symptoms of diverticulitis may vary, depending on the extent of the disease, and at times, in the elderly, the clinical findings may be atypical, non-specific, or absent. However, most commonly, patients complain of lower abdominal pain, usually in the left lower quadrant, constipation (occasionally diarrhoea with narrowed but not obstructed colon), fever, and chills. Examination often reveals a palpable, tender, sausage-shaped mass in the left lower quadrant, localized left lower abdominal tenderness and guarding, diminished bowel sounds, and/or rectal tenderness. With perforation and generalized peritonitis, clinical findings of sepsis, adynamic ileus, generalized abdominal guarding, and percussion, evidence of free air may be present.

Diagnosis

The differential diagnosis of diverticulitis in the elderly is primarily carcinoma of the colon. Other diseases to be considered include inflammatory bowel disease (Crohn's disease), ischaemic colitis, and appendicitis. Plain upright abdominal X-rays are generally unremarkable unless ileus, obstruction, free intraperitoneal air, or large mass are present. Careful and gentle sigmoidoscopy should be performed (providing the patient is not severely ill) to exclude mass lesions. A colon contrast study, only after several days of hospitalization, using water-soluble agents such as Hypaque is recommended (Cello, 1981). Bowel preparation or air sufflation should be avoided. Both endoscopy and contrast study in patients with acute diverticulitis may result in perforation of the colon. Gallium scan and abdominal computed tomography may be helpful in localizing pericolic abscesses. Blood cultures should be obtained in septic patients.

Treatment

Most patients with diverticulitis may be managed medically (Larson, Masters, and Spiro, 1976). Mild cases (without evidence of sepsis, peritonitis, large abscesses or obstruction) may be treated with bowel rest. The role of antibiotics in such mild cases is unclear (Cello, 1981). Oral tetracycline has been most commonly prescribed for mild uncomplicated cases of diverticulitis. With more severe cases, but not requiring surgery, intravenous antibiotics are recommended. Since the microorganisms involved in diverticulitis are the faecal flora, antibiotics must be effective against aerobic gram-negative bacilli and anaerobic bacteria including *B. fragilis* (Lorber and Swenson, 1975; Stone, Kolb, and Geheber, 1975). In such severely ill patients a combination of an aminoglycoside and clindamycin or metronidazole would be an effective chemotherapeutic regimen. Surgical intervention should be reserved for (a) patients treated medically who fail to clinically respond; (b) evidence of a pericolic abscess that fails to resolve on medical

management; (c) colonic perforation; (d) fistula formation; (e) bowel obstruction; (f) generalized peritonitis; (g) gangrenous diverticulitis; and (h) suspected colonic carcinoma.

Hepatic Abscesses

Epidemiology

Hepatic abscesses may account for 13 per cent. of all cases of intra-abdominal abscesses (Altemeier *et al.*, 1973). Several series reporting on liver abscesses show that the elderly are particularly susceptible to this infection and the mortality is exceedingly high (Butler and McCarthy, 1969; Lazarchick *et al.*, 1973; Rubin, Swartz, and Malt, 1974). Table 3 summarizes these data. The primary source of infection in the aged with hepatic abscesses are the intra-abdominal infections previously described: biliary tract infection, diverticulitis, and appendicitis. Bowel carcinoma with perforation may also be a primary cause in the aged. In all age groups, the primary source may be cryptogenic in approximately 20 to 40 per cent. of cases (Butler and McCarthy, 1969; Lazarchick *et al.*, 1973).

Pathophysiological Changes

Liver abscesses occur primarily by microorganisms travelling from the biliary tract or portal venous system, or spread of a contiguous infection to the liver. Haematogenous or bacteraemic spread to the liver may also occur. Hepatic abscess may be microscopic, macroscopic, solitary or multiple. Most solitary abscesses are located in the right side of the liver (Butler and McCarthy, 1969; Lazarchick *et al.*, 1973); abscesses associated with biliary tract disease are most frequently multiple in number.

Table 3　Incidence and mortality of hepatic abscesses in the elderly

References	Total number of cases	No. of cases over 60 years (%)	No. died over 60 years (%)
Butler and McCarthy (1969)	31	16 (52)	9 (57)
Lazarchick *et al.* (1973)	75	29 (37)	—[a]
Rubin, Swartz, and Malt (1974)	53	30 (57)	23 (77)

[a] Not stated by age groups.

Clinical Features

Fever is the most constant complaint; in fact, many cases may present as fever of undetermined origin (Butler and McCarthy, 1969). Malaise, fatigue, anorexia, and weight loss are common non-specific symptoms. In elderly patients, the occurrence of confusion and dementia may lead the clinician away from the diagnosis of an abdominal infection. Palpable liver enlargement is found in half the patients and tenderness in the right upper quadrant occurs in 40 per cent. of cases.

Diagnosis

Anaemia may be seen in 50 to 100 per cent. of patients with hepatic abscesses (Butler and McCarthy, 1969; Rubin, Swartz, and Malt, 1974). Leucocytosis (leucocyte count over 10,000/mm^3) occurs in one-half to two-thirds of cases. Liver function tests that are variably abnormal include the serum bilirubin, serum alkaline phosphatase, prothrombin time, and serum albumin. A standard chest X-ray not infrequently may demonstrate elevation of the right hemidiaphragm with or without a pleural effusion. Abdominal ultrasonography will rapidly detect large abscesses but a negative test does not exclude liver abscesses that might be microscopic. Isotopic liver scan is an excellent test for diagnosing hepatic abscesses. Computed tomography and gallium scan are also useful diagnostic tests.

Blood cultures are important to obtain since over 40 per cent. of patients may show bacteraemia (Lazarchick *et al.*, 1973), particularly those with multiple abscesses (61 per cent.). Moreover, with good anaerobic techniques, 54 per cent. of patients with anaerobic liver abscesses may show bacteraemia (Sabbaj, Sutter, and Finegold, 1972). The organisms most commonly isolated from pyogenic liver abscesses are the enteric gram-negative bacilli, particularly *E. coli,* and anaerobic organisms including streptococci, *Bacteroides*, and *Fusobacterium* (Kreger *et al.*, 1980; Rubin,Swartz, and Malt, 1974).

Treatment

Surgical drainage is the cornerstone of successful treatment of liver abscesses. At the time of surgery, abscess fluid must be carefully examined by Gram stain and then cultured for aerobic and anaerobic organisms. Prior to culture data, antibiotic therapy should include drugs that are active against organisms previously mentioned. Penicillin G, clindamycin, chloramphenicol, erythromycin, aminoglycoside, and cephalosporins have been administered in different combinations for treatment of liver abscess. Duration of therapy is controversial and has been dependent on whether the abscess is solitary, multiple, microscopic or macroscopic, drained, or excised. Therapy varying in duration from 3 weeks to 4 months has been advocated (Rubin, Swartz, and Malt, 1974; Sabbaj, Sutter, and Finegold, 1972). As a general guideline, multiple, macroscopic, and drained lesions require longer therapy.

Gram-Negative Sepsis

Epidemiology

Bacteraemia or sepsis caused by aerobic or facultative anaerobic gram-negative bacilli occurs in approximately one out of every 100 patients admitted to the hospital (Kreger *et al.*, 1980). Gram-negative bacilli are the most frequent cause of bacteraemia in the United States (McCabe, 1973) and are the aetiological agents for the majority of nosocomial infections (Riley, 1977). Recent data suggests that the age-specific attack rate for gram-negative bacillaemia is highest in patients over 60 years and increases further in individuals over 80 years (Kreger *et al.*, 1980). Hypotension or shock occurs most frequently in the elderly (Hodgkin and Sanford, 1965; Weil, Shubin, and Biddle, 1964). Mortality rate for the aged with gram-negative bacteraemia is 70 per cent. or greater (Weil, Shubin, and Biddle, 1964), primarily because of hypotension and poor cardiovascular reserve. For both community- and hospital-acquired gram-negative bacillaemia in the old, urinary tract infection and intra-abdominal sepsis are the most common primary sources of infection (Esposito *et al.*, 1980; Kreger *et al.*, 1980).

Pathophysiological Changes

The pathological and physiological events in gram-negative bacillaemia appear to be initiated by endotoxin, the complex lipopolysaccharide found in the cell wall of gram-negative organisms (Yoshikawa, 1980). Endotoxin activates the complement, coagulation, fibrinolytic and kallikrein–kinin systems (Young, 1979). Components of complement regulate inflammation, influence chemotaxis of neutrophils, increase vascular permeability, and affect microbial killing. Bradykinin increases vascular permeability and causes vasodilation. Coagulation and fibrinolytic systems induce disseminated intravascular coagulation. Histopathological changes following gram-negative sepsis include microthrombi in blood vessels, hemorrhage, and necrosis of tissues.

Clinical Features

The classical clinical pattern of gram-negative bacillary sepsis is the abrupt onset of shaking chills, followed by fever and hypoperfusion of organ structures. However, in elderly or debilitated patients, mental confusion, hypothermia, respiratory alkalosis, or unexplained hypotension may be the presenting clinical findings (Yoshikawa, 1980). Early in sepsis, peripheral vasodilation ('warm shock') may be observed. However, with prolonged hypotension, tachycardia and vasoconstriction rapidly ensue. Patients appear cold and clammy, and are peripherally cyanotic. In severe cases of septic shock, disseminated intravascular coagulation (hemorrhage), renal cortical necrosis (oliguria), hepatic failure (jaundice), and/or adult respiratory distress syndrome (respiratory failure) may dominate the clinical findings.

Diagnosis

Blood cultures yielding gram-negative bacilli confirm the diagnosis. Such cultures are positive in nearly 70 per cent. of the patients (Young, 1979). Conversely, a negative blood culture does not exclude this diagnosis. All potential sites (i.e., urinary tract, lungs, soft tissue, wounds, cerebrospinal fluid, intraabdominal structures) of primary infection should be actively investigated and specimens obtained for staining and culture. Peripheral leucocytosis occurs frequently although leucopenia or a normal leucocyte count is not uncommon. Such coagulation studies as platelet count, prothrombin time, factor V and VIII activity, fibrinogen levels, and the presence of fibrin split products should be serially tested in severely ill patients or patients with evidence of haemorrhage.

Treatment

First and foremost is correction of the shock and hypotension, if present. In the elderly patient, fluid replacement with saline, plasma, or lactated Ringers' solution should be carefully administered under haemodynamic monitoring by way of a pulmonary artery or central venous pressure catheter. The risk of precipitating cardiac failure or pulmonary congestion is very high in elderly patients with septic shock. Use of vasoactive drugs such as dopamine may be helpful in managing hypotension after intravascular volume depletion is corrected. The value or non-value of corticosteroids in managing septic shock is still hotly debated. Although one prospective, double-blind study of patients with gram-negative bacteraemic shock showed significant benefit of pharmacologic doses of corticosteroids (Schumin, 1976), another large study (uncontrolled) failed to show clinical improvement with these agents regardless of the severity of the underlying disease (Kreger, Craven, and McCabe, 1980).

Antibiotic therapy should be selected on the basis of the primary source of infection (e.g. urinary tract infection). However, if the aetiology of sepsis is unclear, the antibiotic regimen should include at least an aminoglycoside (i.e., gentamicin, tobramycin, or amikacin). This antibiotic then can be combined with a cephalosporin, a broad-spectrum penicillin, clindamycin, chloramphenicol, or a semisynthetic antistaphylococcal penicillin.

Careful monitoring of serum aminoglycoside concentrations, renal function, acid–base and electrolyte balance, arterial oxygenation, cardiac function, and liver functions are essential during therapy.

Soft Tissue Infection

Epidemiology

The major causes of skin and soft tissue infection are related to trauma, postoperative wounds, diabetic peripheral vascular disease, and decubitus or pressure ulcers. Trauma and injury to lower extremities are frequently consequences of instability in standing and ambulation in the old. Postoperative wound infection is significantly higher in the elderly as a result of greater morbidity (and mortality) from intra-abdominal sepsis (see previous section).

Infected diabetic foot ulcers are common occurrences in the geriatric population (Louie *et al.*, 1976). Decubitus ulcer is a problem of old age, since the elderly more frequently suffer diseases that result in chronic immobility and bed rest (e.g. cerebral vascular accidents).

Pathophysiological Changes

The underlying pathological changes will depend on the primary disease process. However, when infection ensues, cellulitis, necrosis or gangrene may develop in the skin. Extension to underlying muscle can result in myositis; bacteraemia with sepsis occurs commonly in elderly patients.

Clinical Features

Cellulitis, regardless of the initiating cause, will be the earliest sign of skin infection. The skin is red, tender, and often indurated. Depending on the organism and the cause of the cellulitis, the infection can be severe enough to show tissue necrosis or gangrene (usually in postoperative abdominal wound infections). Purulence, drainage of serosanguinous fluid and gas in tissue may be present. Foul-smelling drainage or tissue indicates the presence of anaerobic bacteria.

Diagnosis

The diagnosis is made clinically. Blood cultures are essential, especially in patients with infected decubitus ulcers. Bacteraemia from decubitus ulcers in the elderly has a high mortality rate (Galpin *et al.*, 1976). Needle aspiration of tissue fluid or pus should be performed and examined immediately by Gram stain. Aerobic and anaerobic cultures are important diagnostic tests in these infections. Abdominal wounds, diabetic foot ulcers, and decubitus ulcers are commonly invaded by both aerobic and anaerobic bacteria. If tissue gas is suspected, plain X-rays may confirm this diagnosis.

Treatment

Antibiotic therapy is the mainstay of therapy for most soft tissue infections. If tissue necrosis, gangrene, or localized purulence is present or the extent of infection is unclear, surgical intervention is indicated. Depending on the process, incision, excision, or drainage may be performed.

Antibiotic selection should be determined ultimately by results of microbiological studies. In the absence of such data, trauma-related soft tissue infection should be initially treated with an antistaphylococcal drug such as oxacillin, nafcillin, methicillin, or a cephalosporin. Abdominal wound infections, infected decubitus ulcers, and infected diabetic foot ulcers require antibiotics effective against anaerobic and aerobic (gram-negative bacilli and staphylococci) bacteria.

Infective Endocarditis

Epidemiology

During the antibiotic era, there has been a change in age distribution of infective endocarditis (Cantrell and Yoshikawa, 1983). As examples, the average ages for patients with infective endocarditis from two large medical centres were 55 and 56 years, respectively (Garvey and Neu, 1978; Von Reign *et al.*, 1981). Those patients over the age of 60 years may account for 30 per cent. or more of all cases of infective endocarditis (Hartman and Myers, 1959; Weinstein and Rubin, 1973). Males dominate over females despite the greater number of women over the age of 65 years. The mortality associated with infective endocarditis increases with age (Pearce and Guze, 1961) and may exceed 70 per cent. (see Table 4).

Pathophysiological Changes

Elderly patients stricken with infective endocarditis generally have some anatomical abnormality of their valves. Most common findings at autopsy are rheumatic disease, de-

Table 4 Infective endocarditis in patients over the age of 60 years

References	Total number of cases	M:F[a]	Underlying valve disease (%)	Murmur present (%)	Strep.[b] or staph. (%)	Mortality (%)
Wallach *et al.* (1955)	18	14:4	100	—[c]	44	—[d]
Gleckler (1958)	10	6:4	100	100	100	40
Hartman and Myers (1959)	7	3:4	100	100	100	28
Cummings, Furman, and Dunst (1960)	12	7:5	—[c]	75	42[e]	67
Applefeld and Hornick (1974)	29	—[c]	52	66	66	72
Thell, Martin, and Edwards (1975)	42	29:13	63	68	57	—[d]

[a] Male to female ratio.
[b] Streptococcus or staphylococcus.
[c] Not reported or incompletely reported.
[d] Autopsy study.
[e] Total of 6 patients with no blood cultures performed or negative blood cultures.

generative or atherosclerotic changes, and congenital abnormalities (Thell, Martin, and Edwards, 1975; Wallach *et al.*, 1955). Presumably, the abnormal valve serves as a focus for thrombus formation followed by bacteraemia, multiplication of microorganisms on the valve, and development of a vegetation (Wallach *et al.*, 1955). However, in some studies of infective endocarditis in the aged, no underlying valvular pathology could be identified in 32 to 48 per cent. of cases (Applefeld and Hornick, 1974; Thell, Martin, and Edwards, 1975).

Clinical Features

The clinical findings in old patients with infective endocarditis can be quite variable. It is not uncommon that the diagnosis is not considered antemortem in the majority of elderly patients (60 per cent.) (Thell, Martin, and Edwards, 1975). Fever is present in most patients (Thell, Martin, and Edwards, 1975), but nearly 20 per cent. may not demonstrate a temperature of 100°F or greater (Applefeld and Hornick, 1974). Heart murmurs are found in 66 to 100 per cent. of elderly patients, depending on the reported series (see Table 4). Peripheral manifestations of infective endocarditis (splinter hemorrhage, Osler's nodes, Janeway's lesions, splenomegaly) occur in less than half of the cases or may even be absent. More importantly, in the elderly with valve infection, many patients present with symptoms unassociated directly with the heart: confusion, delirium, agitation, depression, weight loss, anorexia, weakness, or uraemia may be the presenting complaints (Gleckler, 1958). In one report,

over one-third of the patients presented to the hospital with neurological signs, most commonly coma or acute hemiplegia (Applefeld and Hornick, 1974). Additionally, old patients have other associated diseases that may predispose to bacteraemia or obscure the diagnosis of endocarditis (e.g. infected decubitus ulcer, genitourinary infection).

Diagnosis

Definitive diagnosis of infective endocarditis can only be made by demonstration on histology or by microbiology of valve infection from surgical or autopsy specimens. Clinical diagnosis of infective endocarditis is valid if blood cultures are repeatedly positive in a patient with (a) a murmur or predisposing heart disease and peripheral findings of endocarditis, or (b) blood culture are negative or intermittently positive in a patient with fever, new regurgitant murmurs, and peripheral manifestations of endocarditis (Von Reyn *et al.*, 1981). Other criteria for diagnosing infective endocarditis would include multiple positive cultures with echocardiographic evidence of valvular vegetations.

It is recommended that three sets of blood cultures be obtained, preferably several hours apart. Anaemia and leucocytosis are constant findings. Urinalysis and renal function tests are recommended to detect haematuria, proteinuria or azotaemia – signs of renal involvement from infective endocarditis. Echocardiography, either single (M) mode or two-dimensional mode, is a useful instrument to detect valvular vegetations.

Treatment

High doses of bactericidal antibiotics administered intravenously is the therapy of choice for infective endocarditis. Generally, antibiotics could be withheld until specific identification of the aetiological agent from the blood is made. However, under certain conditions, empiric antibiotic therapy (before microbiological data are available) is warranted. These conditions include the presence of (a) haemodynamic instability (congestive heart failure); (b) aortic valve involvement; (c) emboli to major organs (brain, lung, kidneys); and (d) myocardial involvement. Since streptococci and staphylococci are most frequently isolated from elderly patients with valve infections (Applefield and Hornick, 1974; Gleckler, 1958; Hartman and Myers, 1959; Thell, Martin, and Edwards, 1975; Wallach *et al.*, 1955), antibiotics effective against these bacteria should be administered for empiric therapy. A combination of ampicillin and a penicillinase-resistant semisynthetic penicillin is an appropriate regimen. Aqueous penicillin G could be substituted for ampicillin for streptococcal therapy. However, an aminoglycoside should be added in order to effectively manage group D enterococci *(S. faecalis)*. Cephalosporins may be used for staphylococcal infection. In penicillin-allergic patients, a drug such as vancomycin is optimal since it is bactericidal for most streptococci and staphylococci. Antibiotic therapy should be continued for 4 to 6 weeks. Serum bactericidal titre should be monitored at least on a weekly basis; a titre exceeding 1:8 is desirable.

Surgical intervention should be reserved for infective endocarditis cases with the following complications: (a) progressive congestive heart failure; (b) prosthetic valve infection failing on medical management or a valve with dehiscence; (c) fungal valve infection; and (d) repetitive emboli on therapy.

Meningitis

Epidemiology

Meningitis is an infectious disease primarily of the paediatric age group. However, in the adult population, the elderly seem to have an inordinately high predilection for certain types of bacterial meningitis. The elderly are particularly susceptible to meningitis caused by *S. pneumoniae* (pneumococcus) and unusual pathogens such as gram-negative bacteria and *Listeria monocytogenes* (Cherubin *et al.*, 1981; Finland and Barnes, 1977; Fraser, Henke, and Feldman, 1973; Massanari, 1977; Weiss *et al.*, 1967). More importantly, bacterial meningitis in the old results in an exceedingly high mortality rate (Yoshikawa and Norman, 1981). In patients over 70 years, pneumococcal meningitis may cause a mortality rate of over 80 per cent. (Finland and Barnes, 1977). Aged patients with meningitis caused by *L. monocytogenes, E. coli,* or *Klebsiella* sp. may experience death rates of 83, 96, and 100 per cent. respectively (Cherubin *et al.*, 1981).

Pathophysiological Changes

Pneumococcal meningitis develops by contiguous spread of *S. pneumoniae* infection or bacteraemia from an extrameningeal infection. Otitis media, mastoiditis, sinusitus, head trauma, and pneumonia are common infections or disorders predisposing to pneumococcal meningitis (Finland and Barnes, 1977; Weiss *et al.*, 1967). Gram-negative bacillary meningitis develops following trauma, surgery of the head, or bacteraemia from an extrameningeal focus of infection (Crane and Lerner, 1979; Mangi, Quintilliani, and Andriole, 1975). The pathogenic mechanism for *Listeria* meningitis has not been clearly defined, although meningeal infection following bacteraemia is suspected.

Clinical Features

Most elderly patients with bacterial meningitis will demonstrate fever, mental confusion, and nuchal rigidity (Massanari, 1977). Headache, visual disturbances, or complaints resulting from intracranial hypertension may be experienced. However, in the aged patient, altered mental function, stupor, or coma may be interpreted as a stroke or dementia. Additionally, the common occurrence of degenerative cervical osteoarthritis in the elderly may make the finding of nuchal rigidity difficult to interpret.

Diagnosis

The single most important test to confirm the diagnosis of bacterial meningitis is examination of the cerebrospinal fluid (Yoshikawa, 1980). The cerebrospinal fluid should be immediately examined by Gram stain – a properly performed stain will reveal an organism in 75 per cent. of proven cases of bacterial meningitis. The fluid should then be sent immediately for total and differential cell count, protein, glucose, and culture. Bacterial meningitis typically will show in the cerebrospinal fluid a total cell count exceeding 500 cells/mm^3, 90 per cent. or greater neutrophils, elevated protein concentration, and depressed glucose content (Yoshikawa, 1980).

Blood cultures should be obtained on all patients. A diagnostic evaluation should be pursued for pericranial and extrameningeal sites of infection with microbiological and radiological studies.

Treatment

Pneumococcal meningitis should be treated with high-dose, intravenous penicillin G (20 million units a day) or ampicillin (12 grams a day). In patients allergic to penicillin, chloramphenicol is an excellent alternative drug for this infection. Gram-negative bacillary meningitis therapy requires intravenous aminoglycoside antibiotics supplemented with intrathecal doses, since these drugs penetrate into the cerebrospinal fluid poorly. Ideally, the cerebrospinal fluid concentration of aminoglycoside should be 5 to 10 times the minimum inhibitory concentration of the drug against the pathogen (Yoshikawa, 1981). Careful monitoring of renal function and auditory changes is extremely important when administering aminoglycosides, especially in the elderly. Frequent measurements of serum concentration of aminoglycosides are recommended. For susceptible pathogens, gram-negative bacillary meningitis is effectively treated with such newer third-generation cephalosporins as moxalactam or cefotaxime (Landesman, Cherubin, and Corrado, 1982). *Listeria monocytogenes* meningitis is best treated with ampicillin or penicillin G (Cherubin *et al.*, 1981); the addition of an aminoglycoside is advocated by some clinicians.

Therapy for at least 2 weeks may be necessary, especially for gram-negative bacillary meningitis. Repeat lumbar punctures to re-examine the cerebrospinal fluid should be performed within 48 hours following initiation of antibiotic therapy and as needed thereafter.

Bacterial Arthritis

Epidemiology

Excluding disseminated gonococcal disease (dermatitis–arthritis syndrome), the elderly especially appear to be vulnerable to joint infection caused by bacteria (Argen, Wilson, and Wood, 1966; Norman and Yoshikawa, 1983; Phair, 1979). The presence of some type of underlying disease (e.g., diabetes mellitus, malignancy) and/or previous joint disease (trauma, osteoarthritis, gout, pseudogout, rheumatoid arthritis) are important factors in predisposing the elderly to bacterial arthritis (Goldenberg *et al.*, 1974; Goldenberg and Cohen, 1976). *Staphylococcus aureus* is the most frequent pathogen isolated (Goldenberg and Cohen, 1976), although gram-negative bacilli are also important causes of bacterial arthritis in the aged (Goldenberg *et al.*, 1974).

Pathophysiological Changes

Presumably, most infections of the joint in the aged occur as a result of bacteraemia (most often transient), with bacteria entering the joint. However, iatrogenically induced bacterial arthritis can develop following arthrocentesis. A neutrophilic inflammatory response develops (often exceeding 100,000 cells/mm^3) in the synovial fluid following bacteria multiplication. Joint damage and contiguous osteomyelitis may complicate bacterial arthritis.

Clinical Features

In the elderly, the knee joint is most commonly infected (followed by hips, shoulders, and wrists) (Newman, 1976). The afflicted joint is typically painful, tender, swollen, hot, and red (Argen, Wilson, and Wood, 1966; Goldenberg and Cohen, 1976). The range of motion is limited. Fever is commonly present but may be absent. Evidence of extra-articular infection (e.g. pneumonia, skin infection, urinary tract infection) may be found with careful examination (Argen, Wilson, and Wood, 1966).

Diagnosis

Septic arthritis is confirmed by isolation of the pathogen from synovial fluid. Therefore, performance of arthrocentesis is essential for diagnosis. The fluid should be gram-stained and analysed for leucocyte count and differential, mucin clot formation, and glucose content. Poor mucin clot, depressed glucose content, and leucocyte elevation with neutrophil predominance is characteristic for most bacterial arthritides.

Joint X-ray for evidence of damage and osteomyelitis are important for evaluation of the severity of the disease. Blood cultures should be obtained on all patients.

Treatment

Therapy should be focused on three aspects: antibiotics, drainage, and immobilization. Antibiotics should be administered for a minimum of 2 weeks and as long as 4 to 6 weeks, depending on clinical and microbiological response. Generally, intra-articular injection of antibiotics are unnecessary. Drugs should be administered parenterally until significant resolution of the infection has occurred. Closed drainage of the joint by needle aspiration should be frequently performed as needed in order to (a) relieve joint pressure, (b) remove autolytic enzymes and necrotic tissue, and (c) examine fluid for culture and cellular changes (Argen, Wilson, and Wood, 1966). Larger joints such as the hips may require open surgical drainage (Goldenberg and Cohen, 1976). Afflicted joints should be immobilized by splints but given passive range of motion at least once or twice a day in order to prevent ankylosis or flexion contracture. Despite appropriate treatment, patients with gram-negative bacillary arthritis frequently have poor outcomes and mortality is as high as 25 per cent. (Goldenberg *et al.*, 1974).

REFERENCES

Albano, W. A., Zielinski, C. M., and Organ, C. H. (1975). 'Is appendicitis in the aged really different?' *Geriatrics*, **30**, 80–88.

Altemeier, W. A., Culbertson, W. R., Fullen, W. D., Shook, C. D. (1973). 'Intra-abdominal abscesses', *Am. J. Surg.*, **125**, 70–79.

Applefeld, M. M., and Hornick, R. B. (1974). 'Infective endocarditis in patients over 60', *Am. Heart J.*, **88**, 90–94.

Argen, R. J., Wilson, C. H., Jr, and Wood, P. (1966). 'Suppurative arthritis. Clinical features of 42 cases', *Arch. Intern. Med.*, **117**, 661–666.

Bodey, G. P. (1975). 'Infections in cancer patients', *Cancer Treat. Rev.*, **2**, 89–128.

Boles, R. S., and Jordan, S. M. (1958). 'The clinical significance of diverticulosis', *Gastroenterology*, **35**, 579–582.

Butler, T. J., and McCarthy, C. F. (1969). 'Pyogenic liver abscess', *Gut*, **10**, 389–399.

Cantrell, M., and Yoshikawa, T. T. (1983). 'Aging and infective endocarditis', *J. Am. Geriat. Soc.*, **31**, 216–222.

Cello, J. P. (1981). 'Diverticular disease of the colon', *West J. Med.*, **134**, 515–523.

Cherubin, C. E., Marr, J. S., Sierra, M. F., Becker, S. (1981). 'Listeria and gram-negative bacillary meningitis in New York City, 1972–1979. Frequent causes of meningitis in adults', *Am. J. Med.*, **71**, 199–209.

Chetlin, S. H., and Elliot, D. W. (1971). 'Biliary bacteremia'. *Arch. Surg.*, **102**, 303–307.

Crane, L., and Lerner, M. (1979). 'Non-traumatic gram-negative bacillary meningitis in the Detroit Medical Center, 1964–1974 (with special mention of cases due to *Escherichia coli*)', *Medicine (Balt.)*, **57**, 197–209.

Cummings, V., Furman, S., Dunst, M. (1960). 'Subacute bacterial endocarditis in the older age groups', *JAMA*, **172**, 137–141.

Debray, C., Hardouin, J. P., Bescancon, F., Raimbault, J. (1961). 'Frequence de la diverticulose colique selon l'âge etude statisque â partin de 500 lavements barytes', *Semaine des Hôpitaux de Paris*, **37**, 1743–1745.

Edwards, J. E., Jr, Tillman, D. B., Miller, M. E., Pitchon, H. E. (1979). 'Infection and diabetes mellitus', *West J. Med.*, **130**, 515–521.

Esposito, A. L., Gleckman, R. A., Cram, S., Crowley, M., McCabe, F., Drapkin, M. S. (1980). 'Community-acquired bacteraemia in the elderly: analysis of one hundred consecutive episodes', *J. Am. Geriat. Soc.*, **28**, 315–319.

Finland, M., and Barnes, M. W. (1977). 'Acute bacterial meningitis at Boston City Hospital during 12 selected years, 1935–1972', *J. Infect. Dis.*, **136**, 400–415.

Fraser, D. W., Henke, C. E., and Feldman, R. A. (1973). 'Changing patterns of bacterial meningitis in Olmsted County, Minnesota, 1935–1970', *J. Infect. Dis.*, **128**, 300–307.

Freeman, J., and McGowan, J. E., Jr (1978). 'Risk

factors for nosocomial infection,' *J. Infect. Dis.*, **138**, 811–819.

Galpin, J. E., Chow, A. W., Bayer, A. S. Guze, L. B. (1976). 'Sepsis associated with decubitus ulcers', *Am. J. Med.*, **61**, 346–350.

Gardner, I. D. (1980). 'The effect of aging on susceptibility to infection', *Rev. Infect. Dis.*, **2**, 801–810.

Garvey, G. J., and Neu, H. C. (1978). 'Infective endocarditis – an evolving disease. A review of endocarditis at the Columbia-Presbyterian Medical Center, 1968–1973', *Medicine (Balt.)*, **57**, 105–127.

Gleckler, W. J. (1958). 'Diagnostic aspects of subacute bacterial endocarditis in the elderly', *Arch. Intern. Med.*, **102**, 761–765.

Gleckman, R., and Hibert, D. (1982). 'Afebrile bacteremia: A phenomenon in geriatric patients', *JAMA*. **248**, 1478–1480.

Goldenberg, D. L., Brandt, K. D., Cathcart, E. S., Cohen, A. S. (1974). 'Acute arthritis caused by gram-negative bacilli: a clinical characterization', *Medicine (Balt.)*, **53**, 197–209.

Goldenberg, D. L., and Cohen, A. S. (1976). 'Acute infectious arthritis. A review of patients with nongonococcal joint infections (with emphasis on therapy and prognosis)', *Am. J. Med.*, **60**, 369–377.

Goldenberg, I. S. (1955). 'Acute appendicitis in the aged', *Geriatrics*, **10**, 324–327.

Goldman, R. (1979). 'Decline in organ function with aging', in *Clinical Geriatrics* (Ed. I. Rossman), 2nd ed., pp. 23–59, J. B. Lippincott, Philadelphia.

Haley, R. W., Hooton, T. M., Culver, D. H., Stanley, R. C., Emori, T. G., Hardison, C. D. Quade, D., Shachtman, R. H., Schaberg, D. R., Shah, B. V., Schatz, G. D., (1981). 'Nosocomial infections in U.S. hospitals, 1975–1976. Estimated frequency of selected characteristics of patients', *Am. J. Med.*, **70**, 947–959.

Hartman, T. I., and Myers, W. K. (1959). 'Occurrence of bacterial endocarditis in older individuals', *Geriatrics*, **14**, 374–380.

Hodgin, U. G., and Sanford, J. P. (1965). 'Gram-negative bacteraemia. An analysis of 100 patients', *Am. J. Med.*, **39**, 952–960.

Hughes, L. E. (1975). 'Complications of diverticular disease: inflammation, obstruction and bleeding', *Clin. Gastroenterol.*, **4**, 147–170.

Keighley, M. R. B., Drysdale, R. B., Burdon, D. W., Alexander-Williams, J. (1975). 'Antibiotic treatment of biliary sepsis', *Surg. Clin. North Am.*, **55**, 1379–1390.

Kreger, B. E., Craven, D. E., Carling, P. C., McCabe, W. R. (1980). 'Gram-negative bacteraemia. III. Reassessment of etiology, epidemiology and ecology in 612 patients', *Am. J. Med.*,

68, 332–343.

Kyle, J. (1968). 'Prognosis in diverticulitis', *J. Royal Coll. Surg. Edinburgh*, **13**, 136–141.

Landesman, S. H., Cherubin, C. E., and Corrado, M. L.(1982). 'Gram-negative bacillary meningitis. New therapy and changing concepts', *Arch. Intern. Med.*, **142**, 939–940.

Larson, D. M., Masters, S. S., and Spiro H. M. (1976). 'Medical and surgical therapy in diverticular disease. A comparative study', *Gastroenterology*, **71**, 734–737.

Lazarchick J., deSouza Silva, N. A., Nichols, D. R., Washington J. A. (1973). 'Pyogenic liver abscess', *Mayo Clin. Proc.*, **48**, 349–355.

Lorber, B., and Swenson, R. M. (1975). 'The bacteriology of intra-abdominal infections', *Surg. Clin. North Am.*, **55**, 1349–1354.

Louie, T. J., Barlett, J. G., Tally, F. B., Sherwood, L., Gorbach, M. D. (1976). 'Aerobic and anaerobic bacteria in diabetic foot ulcers', *Ann. Intern. Med.*, **85**, 461–463.

McCabe, W. R. (1973). 'Gram-negative bactaeremia', *Disease-a-Month*, December **1973**, 1–38.

McCloskey, R. V. (1979). 'Microbial virulence factors', in *Principles and Practice of Infectious Diseases* (Eds G. L. Mandell, G. R. Douglas Jr, and J. E. Bennett), Chap. 1, pp. 3–11, John Wiley, New York.

Mangi, R., Quintilliani, R., and Andriole V. (1975). 'Gram-negative meningitis', *Am. J. Med.*, **59**, 829–835.

Massanari, R. M. (1977). 'Purulent meningitis in the elderly: when to suspect an unusual pathogen', *Geriatrics*, **32**, 55–59.

Morrow, D. J., Thompson, J., and Wilson, S. E. (1981). 'Acute cholecystitis in the elderly. A surgical emergency', *Arch Surg.*, **113**, 1149–1152.

Newman, J. H. (1976). 'Review of septic arthritis throughout the antibiotic era', *Ann. Rheum. Dis.*, **35**, 198–205.

Norman, D. C., and Yoshikawa, T. T. (1983). 'Responding to septic arthritis', *Geriatrics*, **38**, 83–86.

Owens, B. J., and Hamit H. F. (1978). 'Appendicitis in the elderly', *Ann. Surg.*, **187**, 392–396.

Palmblad, J., and Haak, A. (1978). 'Ageing does not change blood granulocyte bactericidal capacity and levels of complement factors 3 and 4', *Gerontology*, **24**, 381–385.

Parks, T. G. (1975). 'Natural history of diverticular disease of the colon', *Clin. Gastroenterol.*, **4**, 53–69.

Pearce, M. L., and Guze, L. B. (1961). 'Some factors affecting prognosis in bacterial endocarditis', *Ann. Intern. Med.* **55**, 270–282.

Peltokallio, P., and Jauhiainen, K. (1970). 'Acute appendicitis in the aged patient. Study of 300 cases after the age of 60', *Arch. Surg.*, **100**, 140–143.

Perkins, E. H. (1971). 'Phagocytic activity of aged mice', *J. Reticuloendothel. Soc., 9*, 642–643.

Phair, J. P. (1979). 'Aging and infection: a review', *J. Chron. Dis., 32*, 535–540.

Phair, J. P., Kauffman, C. A., Bjornson, A., Gallagher, J., Adams, L., Hes, E. V. (1978a). 'Host defenses in the aged: evaluation of components of the inflammatory and immune responses', *J. Infect. Dis., 138*, 67–73.

Phair, J. P., Kauffman, C. A., Bjornson, A., (1978b). 'Investigation of host defense mechanisms in the aged as determinants of nosocomial colonization and pneumonia', *J. Reticuloendothel. Soc., 23*, 397–405.

Pitchon, H. E., and Sorrell, T. C. (1980). 'Infection in the immunocompromised host', in *Infectious Diseases. Diagnosis and Management* (Eds T. T. Yoshikawa, A. W. Chow, and L. B. Guze), Chap. 27, pp. 253–261, Houghton Mifflin, Boston.

Riley, H. D., Jr (1977). 'Hospital-acquired infection', *South Med. J., 70*, 1265–1266.

Root, R. K. (1979). 'Humoral immunity and complement', in *Principles and Practice of Infectious Disease* (eds G. L. Mandell, R. G. Douglas, Jr, and J. E. Bennett), Chap. 3, pp. 21–63, John Wiley, New York.

Rubin, R. H., Swartz, M. N., and Malt, R. (1974). 'Hepatic abscess: changes in clinical, bacteriological and therapeutic aspects', *Am. J. Med., 57*, 601–610.

Sabbaj, J., Sutter, V. L., and Finegold, S. M. (1972). 'Anaerobic pyogenic liver abscess', *Ann. Intern. Med. 77*, 627–638.

Schumin, W. (1976). 'Steroids in the treatment of clinical septic shock', *Ann. Surg., 184*, 333–341.

Serpick, A. A. (1978). 'Cancer in the elderly', in *The Geriatric Patient* (Ed. W. Reichel), pp. 109–117, HP Publishing.

Smith, J. K., and Wiener, S. P. (1980). 'Life-threatening infections in the elderly. Abdominal and pelvic infections', *Drug Ther., 6*, 23–32.

Stone, H. H., Kolb, L. D., and Geheber C. E. (1975). 'Incidence and significance of intraperitoneal anaerobic bacteria', *Ann. Surg., 181*, 705–715.

Thell, R., Martin, F. H., and Edwards, J. E. (1975). 'Bacterial endocarditis in subjects 60 years of age and older', *Circulation, 51*, 174–182.

Thorbjarnarson, B., and Loehr, W. J. (1967). 'Appendicitis in patients over the age of 60', *Surg. Gynec. Obstet., 125*, 1271–1281.

Tramont, E. D. (1979). 'General or nonspecific host defense mechanism', in *Principles and Practice of Infectious Diseases* (Ed. G. L. mandell, G. R. Douglas, Jr, and J. E. Bennett), Chap. 2, pp. 13–21, John Wiley, New York.

Twomey, J. J. (1973). 'Infections complicating multiple myeloma and chronic lymphocytic leukemia', *Arch. Intern. Med., 132*, 562–565.

United States Bureau of Census (1978). *Statistical Abstract of the United States, 1978*, Government Printing Office, Washington, D.C.

United States Department of Commerce, Bureau of Census (1937). *Mortality Statistics, 1935*, Government Printing Office, Washington, D.C.

United States Department of Health, Education and Welfare, Public Health Service (1970). *Vital Statistics of the United States, 1968*, Vol. II, *Mortality*, Government Printing Office, Washington, D.C.

Valenti, W. M., Trudell, R. G., and Bentley, D. W. (1978). 'Factors predisposing to oropharyngeal colonization with gram-negative bacilli in the aged', *New Engl. J. Med., 298*, 1108–1111.

Van Epps, D. E., Goodwin, J. S., and Murphy, S. (1978). 'Age-dependent variations in polymorphonuclear leukocyte chemiluminescence', *Infect. Immun., 22*, 57–61.

Von Reyn, C. F., Levy, B. S., Arbeit, R. D., Friedland, G., Crumpacker, C. S. (1981). 'Infective endocarditis: an analysis based on strict case definitions', *Ann. Intern. Med., 94* (part 1), 505–518.

Wallach, J. B., Glass, M., Lukash, L. Angrist, A. A. (1955). 'Bacterial endocarditis in the aged', *Ann. Intern. Med., 42*, 1206–1213.

Weil, M. H., Shubin, H., and Biddle, M. (1964). 'Shock caused by gram-negative microorganisms. Analysis of 169 cases', *Ann. Intern. Med., 60*, 384–399.

Weinstein, L., and Rubin, R. H. (1973). 'Infective endocarditis – 1973', *Prog. Cardiovasc. Dis., 26*, 239–274.

Weiss, W., Figueroa, W., Shapiro, W. H. Flippin, H. F. (1967). 'Prognostic factors in pneumococcal meningitis', *Arch. Intern. Med., 120*, 517–524.

Williams, J. S., and Hale, H. W., Jr (1964). 'Acute appendicitis in the elderly. Review of 83 cases', *Ann. Surg., 162*, 208–212.

Wolfson, S. A., Kalmanson, G. M., Rubini, M. E., Guze, L. B. (1965). 'Epidemiology of bacteriuria in a predominantly geriatric male population', *Am. J. Med. Sci., 250*, 168–173.

Yoshikawa, T. T. (1980). 'Meningitis and encephalitis', in *Infectious Diseases. Diagnosis and Management* (Eds T. T. Yoshikawa, A. W. Chow, and L. B. Guze), Chap. 5, pp. 45–56, Houghton Mifflin, Boston.

Yoshikawa, T. T. (1980). 'Septic shock', in *Infectious diseases. Diagnosis and Management* (Eds T. T. Yoshikawa, A. W. Chow, and L. B. Guze), Chap. 25, pp. 233–242, Houghton Mifflin, Boston.

Yoshikawa, T. T. (1981). 'Important infections in elderly persons', *West J. Med., 135*, 441–445.

Yoshikawa, T. T. (1983). 'Geriatric infections diseases: an emerging problem', *J. Am. Geriat. Soc.*, **31**, 34–39.

Yoshikawa, T. T., and Norman, D. C. (1981). 'Meningitis. A disease of young and old', *Consultant,* **21**, 175–192.

Young, L. S. (1979). 'Gram-negative sepsis', in *Principles and Practice of Infectious Diseases* (Eds G. L. Mandell, G. Douglas Jr, and J. E. Bennett), Chap. 47, pp. 571–608, John Wiley, New York.

Yusuf, M. F., and Dunn, E. (1979). 'Appendicitis in the elderly: learn to discern the untypical picture', *Geriatrics*, **34**, 73–79.

10
Nutrition

10.1

Nutrition

Bertil Steen

INTRODUCTION

As it has been said in a pertinent remark 'in the field of medicine, it has become more and more recognized that a proper diet during a disease is a prerequisite if the specific therapy is going to have an optimal effect' (Isaksson, 1975). This statement is obviously valid in the highest age groups since the prevalence of disease rapidly increases with age.

The absolute as well as the relative number of elderly increases in most countries, although at very different levels. In some countries in western Europe the proportion of people aged 65 and over is approaching 20 per cent.

The elderly are a heterogeneous group of individuals in many important aspects of nutrition. This is true in relation to degree of health and disease, degree of physical activity, psychological and sociomedical characteristics and not the least age per se – with a range of more than 40 years. Some authors, therefore, divide these age groups into 'young elderly' (aged 65 to 75) and 'old elderly' (over 75 years of age). However, the latest edition of the American Recommended Dietary Allowances (Food and Nutrition Board, 1980) groups individuals aged 51 and over together into one age group.

In a country like Sweden where institutional living is relatively common among the elderly, only a few per cent. of people up to the age of 75 live outside their own homes. In the age group 80 to 89 years more than three-quarters live in their own homes and only 14 and 9 per cent. live in homes for the elderly and hospitals/nursing homes, respectively. Even at the age of 90 and over it is as common to live in one's own home as in a home for the elderly in Sweden.

Many earlier studies – mainly based on cross-sectional techniques – have shown ageing to be accompanied by a linear decrease of function in many organ systems from a maximum at the age of 20 to 30. However, longitudinal studies have shown that many functions might be relatively unaltered during a major part of adult life. Relatively small but significant changes in nutrition during a healthy adult life up to the age of 70 can be exemplified by some body composition parameters (Bruce *et al.*, 1980; Steen *et al.*, 1977) and many psychological characteristics (Berg, 1980). However, variation around average values is great at advanced ages – also in groups of healthy individuals.

Changes in the consumption of many food items during this century in Western societies are unfavourable to low energy consumers like many elderly people. For example, during this period of time the Swedish per capita consumption of bread/other flour products and potatoes/other starches has decreased very markedly. At the same time the fat proportion of energy intake has increased from about 20 per cent. in the year of 1900 to almost 40 per cent. currently, and the sugar proportion of energy intake from about 5 to about 15 per cent. The situation today in a country like Sweden is that approximately one third of the energy intake is derived from sucrose and fat for cooking and/or spreading – i.e. from food items of no or low nutrient density.

The relation between food restriction and longevity in laboratory animals, first shown by McCay, Crowell, and Maynard (1935), has been extensively studied and the original results confirmed (e.g. Nolen, 1972; Ross and Bras, 1971). This highly significant inverse relationship between the quantity of food consumed and the duration of life in rats is illustrated in Fig. 1 (Ross, 1976a). Rats on a restricted food regimen during their first year of life live considerably longer than rats on an *ad libitum* food regimen. The mechanisms behind this phenomenon are not fully elucidated, although Sacher (1977) pointed out that food restriction acts by decreasing the ageing rate. Furthermore, food restriction seems to influence the incidence of chronic diseases (Coleman *et al.*, 1977; Masoro, 1976; Ross, 1976b; Ross and Bras, 1974, 1975).

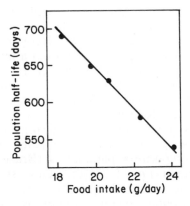

Figure 1   Example of the relationship between the quantity of food consumed by male rats, given freedom of dietary choice and length of life. (From Ross, 1976a, p.51. Reproduced by permission of John Wiley & Sons, Inc., New York)

There are many reasons why altered needs for energy and nutrients for elderly individuals require discussion: physical activity, metabolism of cells and organs, and degree of health and disease are all subjected to alterations in old age.

An altered cell metabolism has been shown in some respects. Thus, Chen, Warshaw, and Sanadi (1972) reported signs of lower respiratory activity in isolated mitochondria from hearts of old rats. However, other studies have

failed to find any reduction in oxygen uptake of tissue slides, homogenates or isolated mitochondria from rat heart, liver or kidney (Barrows, 1966). Preliminary experiments by Sugarman and Munro (1980) suggest that the ageing cell may have less capacity to transport some nutrients into the cytoplasm. If this is the case, this may be compensated for by higher blood concentrations of nutrients in the blood perfusing different organs. Indeed some nutrient fractions in blood such as glucose have a higher concentration in old age than earlier in life.

Changes in the enzyme patterns have been demonstrated (Wilson, 1973), e.g. a decrease of mitochondria and an increase of lysozymes corresponding to the reduction of respiratory and an increase of hydrolytic enzymes.

Ageing also reduces the capacity to regulate metabolism (Munro, 1980). The time taken to induce enzymes with hormones becomes longer with increasing age (Adelman, 1970, 1971; Roth, 1975). The reduced enzymatic adaptability and inducibility is, thus, a striking feature of old cells (Wilson, 1973).

REQUIREMENTS

There exist numerous nutritional standards and 'recommendations' to help in judging the adequacy of diets of individuals or groups of individuals. Most standards are based upon results from younger age groups – in some instances remodelled for the use in elderly people. Minimal requirements which would with a definable degree of certainty 'keep an average person free from frank nutritional disease' (Judge, 1974) should be distinguished from optimal requirements which 'will promote an optimal state of health' (Darke, 1972). Hegsted (1972, 1975) has reviewed different kinds of nutritional standards and their proper use.

For the purpose of this chapter it is practical to adhere to the kind of recommendations represented by the American Recommended Dietary Allowances (Food and Nutrition Board, 1980), the ninth edition of which will be referred to in the text as RDA 1980. They are 'designed for the maintenance of good nutrition of practically all healthy people in the USA', and they are 'intended to provide for individual variations among most normal per-

Table 1 Recommended daily dietary allowances designed for the maintenance of good nutrition of practically all healthy people in the United States. (Reproduced from *Recommended Dietary Allowances*, 9th ed., National Academy Press, Washington, D.C.)

	Males		Females	
	Age 23–50	Age 51+	Age 23–50	Age 51+
Weight (kg)	70	70	55	55
Height (cm)	178	178	163	163
Protein (g)	56	56	44	44
Vitamin A (μg retinol equivalents)	1,000	1,000	800	800
Vitamin D (μg)	5	5	5	5
Vitamin E (μg α-tocopherol equivalents)	10	10	8	8
Vitamin C (mg)	60	60	60	60
Thiamin (mg)	1.4	1.2	1.0	1.0
Riboflavin (mg)	1.6	1.4	1.2	1.2
Niacin (mg niacin equivalents)	18	16	13	13
Vitamin B-6 (mg)	2.2	2.2	2.0	2.0
Folacin (μg)	400	400	400	400
Vitamin B-12 (μg)	3.0	3.0	3.0	3.0
Calcium (mg)	800	800	800	800
Phosphorus (mg)	800	800	800	800
Magnesium (mg)	350	350	300	300
Iron (mg)	10	10	18	10
Zinc (mg)	15	15	15	15
Iodine (μg)	150	150	150	150

sons as they live in the United States under usual environmental stresses' (Table 1). Another standard gives different levels for high intake, acceptable intake and low/minimum intake, respectively (Eeg-Larsen *et al.*, 1971).

Energy

The major explanation for the reduction of energy metabolism with age is probably the decreasing number of cells in the organs, loss of metabolizing tissue, and reduced physical activity (Shock, 1972), although some intracellular age induced changes on the enzyme level might also be responsible.

Energy expenditure and energy intake are, thus, lower in old age than earlier in life. This seems to be related more to a decrease of physical activity than to a decrease of basal metabolic rate. In the Baltimore longitudinal study the external energy expenditure and the basal metabolic rate (BMR) were 1,175 kcal/4.9 MJ and 1,636 kcal/6.9 MJ, respectively, in 30 year old males, and 640 kcal/2.7 MJ and 1,324 kcal/5.6 MJ, respectively, in 80 year old males (McGandy *et al.*, 1966). Total energy expenditure in that study, thus, amounted to 2,811 kcal/11.8 MJ and 1,924 kcal/8.2 MJ, respectively, in the two age groups (Fig. 2). The proportion of the decrease of energy expenditure related to a reduced physical activity might of course differ very much between different populations due to differences in habits.

It is an especially difficult task to give recommendations for energy intake in a group of individuals which is so heterogenous as the elderly in regard to the degree of health and physical activity. Energy intake, however, is of great importance to many elderly for two reasons. On the one hand ordinary food in most Western countries has a low nutrient density because of a high proportion of fat and refined sugar. Small portions of the same kind of food as in early adult life might, therefore, give too little essential nutrients. On the other hand, energy intake is of utmost importance to nitrogen balance in individuals with low intakes of energy and protein. This will be dealt with later on.

RDA 1980 gives as energy values for the age group 51 years and over 2,400 kcal/10.1 MJ and 1,800 kcal/7.6 MJ for males and females, respectively. The age group 51 years and over is a very heterogeneous one. The differences between the body weights of different aged populations and the reference person in the oldest (51+) RDA 1980 group (70 and 55 kg for males and females, respectively) can be marked which might obviously be of considerable importance in the requirements of both

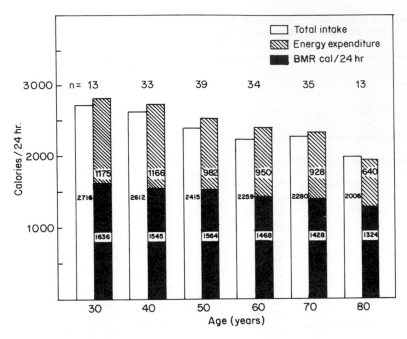

Figure 2 Average daily energy balance in normal males aged 30 to 80 years. (From McGandy *et al.*, 1966)

energy and some nutrients. As an example, the body weights at the ages of 70, 75, and 79 in a Swedish population were 73, 70, and 69 kg for males and 67, 65, and 63 kg for females, respectively (Steen, Isaksson, and Svanborg, 1981), which for females is much higher than the RDA 1980 reference woman.

Protein

Even for younger age groups there is no uniform opinion regarding the minimal requirements of protein and this is even more so for the higher age groups. Scrimshaw (1976) reviewed past and present allowances of protein and suggested that the 'safe allowance of protein' (0.57 and 0.52 g/kg for males and females, respectively) of FAO/WHO (1973) is too low.

Earlier studies – e.g. Kountz, Hofstatter, and Ackermann (1951) – suggested that elderly people have an increased protein requirement. Albanese and coworkers (1957) found that a positive nitrogen balance was obtained with an average daily intake of 0.9 g/kg. Recent balance studies have shown that some elderly individuals require more dietary protein to maintain equilibrium (Munro and Young, 1978; Uyau, Scrimshaw, and Young 1978). The

average needs for maintaining a positive nitrogen balance may not deviate in healthy elderly compared to younger individuals (Cheng *et al.*, 1978; Zanni, Calloway, and Zezulka 1979).

The level of serum albumin is frequently lower in healthy elderly individuals than in younger subjects (Yan and Franks, 1968). Although it has been reported in the literature that elderly people with low protein intake have lower albumin levels (Acheson and Jessop, 1962), most authors deny a consistent relationship between protein intake and albumin levels (Anderson *et al.*, 1972). Some age-dependent factor in albumin synthesis might be a more likely explanation than malnutrition (Exton-Smith, 1978; Munro, 1981; Watkin, 1978).

Werner and Hambraeus (1972) found the elderly to have a reduced tolerance to high protein loads; in their studies a daily protein intake of 100 g or more often resulted in higher faecal nitrogen loss than in younger persons. Even if this normally is of minor importance, the elderly should avoid large meals and have smaller meals more evenly distributed throughout the day.

The requirements of the essential amino acids methionine and lysine have been reported to be high in the elderly (Tuttle *et al.*, 1965). Ackerman and Kheim (1964) found that the concentrations of six essential amino acids, valine, methionine, leucine, isoleucine, phenylalanine, and lysine, were lower in elderly than in younger adults. On the other hand, Wehr and Lewis (1966) reported a significantly higher concentration of ornithine in the elderly. Young (1976) gave data suggesting that leucine, isoleucine, and valine metabolism was similar in young and elderly subjects. Data on essential amino acid requirements in old age are scarce and somewhat contradictory, and further studies are needed in this field.

There seems to be no need for different allowances of protein in healthy elderly individuals. However, the dietary protein requirement in disease states is often increased (Isaksson, 1973). An adequate protein intake is essential for many elderly because of the high prevalence of, for instance, infections, leg ulcers, and other more or less chronic diseases. For example, in an unselected population of 70 year old people in western Sweden, chronic bronchitis (based on WHO criteria) was prevalent in 18 per cent. of males and 9 per cent of females, and 9 per cent. of the women had bacteriuria (Svanborg, 1977).

Isaksson (1973) performed nitrogen balance studies on hospital patients with a variety of diseases (Fig. 3). Out of 23 studies where the protein intake was as high as 0.9 to 1.5 g/kg body weight, 12 showed a negative nitrogen balance and 3 out of 22 studies showed a negative balance even at levels of protein intake of 1.6 g/kg or more.

RDA 1980 recommends 0.8 g/kg in the 51 + age group. This corresponds to 56 g for the reference male and 46 g for the reference female, and is regarded as an 'acceptable' intake by Eeg-Larsen and coworkers (1971).

There are good reasons to believe that for the whole group of elderly – healthy as well as diseased – this figure is a minimum one.

The protein status has to be viewed in the light of the energy situation in the elderly and chronically diseased. Individuals with a low protein intake may have an increased need for energy to maintain nitrogen balance (Garza, Scrimshaw, and Young, 1976). Furthermore, energy intake seems to have a greater effect on nitrogen balance than has protein intake in persons with marginal intakes of protein and energy (Calloway, 1975).

The problem for the majority of healthy elderly people living at home in developed countries is to lower energy intake while maintaining the quality of food. For many chronically diseased, very old, and frail institutionalized patients the dietary problem is largely a quantitative one, with an urgent need to consume enough energy. Malnutrition in hospitalized patients has been reported from many countries such as Denmark (Hessov, 1977), Sweden (Steen, 1980), the United Kingdom (Hackett, Young, and Hill 1979), and the United States (Steffee, 1980).

Nursing home patients may have many reasons for a decreased energy intake. Restricted physical activity, bad appetite, motor or psychic impairment and sometimes poor dental state or oral hygiene. In one study (Steen, 1980) protein intake calculated from urinary analyses of nitrogen in geriatric nursing home patients was lower than 0.8 g/kg body weight in more than one third of the patients.

Maintenance of energy and nutrient intake at an acceptable level is an important task in geriatric medicine. Energy intake may sometimes be lower than normal basal metabolism, suggesting that adaptation to low energy intake must have taken place. The distribution of meals throughout the day is therefore important. It is essential to have a good quality and quantity of the breakfast meal, to separate lunch and dinner, and to distribute the meals over larger parts of the day than is often the case in hospitals and nursing homes.

Other Nutrients and Food Constituents

As can be seen from Table 1 the recommended daily allowances according to RDA 1980 do not differ between the 'elderly' age group and

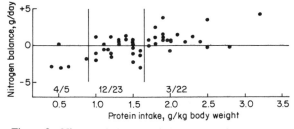

Figure 3   Nitrogen balance in 23 patients at different levels of protein intake. (From Isaksson, 1973. Reproduced by permission of S. Karger AG, Basel)

other adult age groups in most respects. Therefore, only a sample of nutrients and food constituents of special importance or possible gerontological or geriatric importance will be discussed in this context. These are vitamin D, thiamin, ascorbic acid, calcium, iron, and potassium.

Vitamin D

The eighth edition of RDA (Food and Nutrition Board, 1974) did not recommend any daily intake of vitamin D for the normal healthy adult, since the requirement 'seems to be satisfied by nondietary sources'. However, in the ninth edition (RDA 1980) an allowance of 5 micrograms is included.

The importance of a satisfactory dietary intake of vitamin D, especially in house-bound elderly with no access to sunlight, has been increasingly recognized. For many years it has been repeatedly claimed that osteomalacia due to such dietary insufficiency might play a role in the genesis of skeletal rarefaction in elderly people (Exton-Smith, Hodkinson, and Stanton, 1966). Gallagher and coworkers (1979) have reported on age-dependent differences of serum concentrations of 1–25-dihydroxycholecalciferol – differences which might be caused by an impaired renal metabolism of 25-hydroxy-vitamin D.

Thiamin

The recommendation of the RDA 1980 is 0.5 mg per 1,000 kcal/4.2 MJ. However, since there are early reports of an impaired utilization of thiamin in higher age groups (Horwitt *et al.*, 1948, Oldham, 1962) the RDA 1980 also suggests an allowance of 1 mg per day in individuals with an energy intake of less than 2,000 kcal/8.4 MJ.

Ascorbic Acid

The RDA 1980 value of the allowance of ascorbic acid is 45 mg – not corrected for losses during storage and preparation. Such losses are often in the order of magnitude of 50 per cent., and may be very variable due, among other things, to different cooking techniques.

Low ascorbic acid levels in the elderly have been reported by many authors (e.g. Andrews

and Brook, 1966; Loh and Wilson, 1971), especially in males, in residents in homes for the elderly, and during the winter (Andrews, Brook, and Allen, 1966; Kataria, Rao and Curtis, 1965) Supplementation studies (Andrews, Letcher, and Brook, 1969; Burr, Hurley, and Sweetnam, 1975) have shown that 40 to 80 mg taken daily increases leucocyte levels, but the clinical importance of such supplementation needs to be further elucidated.

Calcium

The recommended daily allowance of calcium is 800 mg per day (RDA 1980). However, it seems that some adults remain in calcium balance despite lower calcium intakes. The 'practical allowance' for adults has even been suggested to be between 400 and 500 mg per day (FAO/WHO, 1962).

The aetiology of osteoporosis is still under debate (see Chapter 25.2). It is clearly not a simple deficiency disease. However, supplementation of calcium has been reported to induce calcium retention and relieve bone pain (Avioli, 1977; Nordin, 1962). The efficiency of calcium absorption seems to decrease with advancing age (Avioli, McDonald, and Lee, 1965; Bullamore *et al.*, 1970). At least to some extent, this is probably due to vitamin D deficiency, and the low absorption might be reversible on vitamin D treatment (Nordin, 1971).

Physical activity may alter calcium balance, and house-bound immobile elderly may suffer from calcium losses for that reason. Furthermore, physiological imbalance may lead to a negative calcium balance (Malm, 1958). During the last decade some evidence has been put forward that borderline or low calcium intakes – less than 500 mg per day – might infer risk for losses of calcium (Johnson, Alcantara, and Linkswiler, 1970; Linkswiler, Joyce, and Arnaud, 1974).

Iron

RDA 1980 gives the recommended iron value of 10 mg for both sexes in these age groups. There seems to be evidence that the absorption of iron in old age is not different from that in younger age groups (Brünschke, Mehls, and Zschenderlein, 1967; Frieman, Tauber, and

Tulsky, 1963). Marx (1979) studied with a double-isotope technique and total-body scanning the absorption and uptake of iron in different body compartments. He found no age differences regarding mucosal uptake, transfer, and retention of iron. However, the erythrocyte uptake after 2 weeks was lower than in a younger control group.

Of practical importance in elderly people is the common occurrence of iron loss from the gastrointestinal tract, which gives rise to a higher demand for nutritional iron (see Chapter 11.3). The most common sources of such bleeding is an atrophic gastric mucosa, especially in elderly on aspirin treatment, and a diverticular colon.

Potassium

In the common recommendations of dietary intakes, potassium is seldom explicitly mentioned. RDA 1980 states that healthy adults need about 2.5 g per day of potassium (about 65 mmol). Judge and Cowan (1971) claim that the minimal satisfactory dietary intake of potassium per day is 60 mmol.

Dermal and faecal losses of potassium are in the order of magnitude of 15 mmol (Isaksson and Sjögren, 1967), and since normal kidneys are able to retain all but 10 to 15 mmol, these recommendations may be too high in healthy individuals. However, the kidneys react more sluggishly to potassium deficiency than to sodium depletion, and potassium may be lost in significant amounts during the first 2 weeks of severely insufficient dietary intake. Inadequate dietary intake is one of many causes of potassium deficiency and gastrointestinal and renal conditions are also causes of major significance (Steen, 1981).

In elderly patients potassium deficiency is often not the result of a single aetiological factor, but rather due to a combination of conditions, such as insufficient dietary intake of potassium, diuretic treatment, and one or more conditions with secondary aldosteronism, such as liver cirrhosis and chronic heart disease.

Dietary Fibre

This relatively new concept is usually defined as the sum of the indigestible carbohydrate and carbohydrate-like components of food, including cellulose, lignin, hemicellusoses, pentosans, gums, and pectins. It is, thus, a broader term than crude fibre, which comprises only a portion of the cellulose and lignin.

The practical importance of dietary fibre lies in its relation to many conditions common in higher age groups, such as constipation, colonic cancer, and diabetes (for a review, see Burkitt and Trowell, 1975; Roth and Mehlman, 1978).

The RDA 1980 does not recommend a specific level of fibre intake. The absorption of minerals might be impaired by very high intakes of dietary fibre (Reinhold *et al.*, 1976). However, most elderly populations in developed countries should be recommended to moderately increase the consumption of fibre-rich food items such as vegetables and wholegrain cereal products.

Water

Needless to say water is essential to all biological functions in the body. For a discussion of the total, extracellular, and intracellular body water, see the body composition section of this chapter.

Water is lost from the body by kidneys, intestines, lungs, and skin. These losses might increase in conditions such as diarrhoea, febrile states, and renal diseases, which are common in older age groups (reviewed by Massler, 1979).

The sensation of thirst diminishes with age, especially in the very old. Many elderly are, therefore, at risk of developing a negative water balance, particularly in the presence of infection with fever, and severe symptoms, such as confusional states and circulatory collapse, may result.

DIETARY SURVEYS

Methods

The nutritional status of a population cannot be classified by dietary surveys alone. Collection of social, psychological, and medical data are necessary – especially in surveys in developing regions of the world – together with the assessment of clinical signs of malnutrition, anthropology, biochemical analyses, and biophysical tests (Jeliffe, 1966). However, surveys of dietary intake of energy and nutrients and meal habits give basic data for judging the nutritional state of any population. Methodology varies markedly in different studies, and since the validity of the methods is also different, attention to the methods chosen in different studies is of special importance.

Weighing methods, record methods, and interview methods are used to evaluate dietary intake (Roine and Pekkarinen, 1968). Record and interview methods are based upon the use of food tables. Individual dietary surveys (for reviews, see Marr, 1971; Steen, 1977a) using interview techniques are usually performed either according to the 24-hour recall method (Wiehl, 1942) or the dietary history method originally described by Burke (1947). The 24-hour recall method means that the probands are interviewed about their food consumption during the last 24 hours, while the dietary history interview method illustrates the ordinary food habits of the probands.

Isaksson (1980) drew attention to the necessity of performing validity tests in dietary surveys, e.g. with comparisons of nitrogen analyses of 24-hour urine samples and the calculated dietary intake of protein. Steen, Isaksson, and Svanborg, (1977) compared the 24-hour recall and the dietary history methods using validity tests. They showed that in a population of 70 year olds the urinary nitrogen method of calculating protein intake gave results not significantly different from the dietary history data, but significantly higher than the 24-hour recall values. They concluded that the dietary history method was the more valid of the two interview techniques.

Another major methodological question in nutrition surveys is to what extent the sample investigated is representative for the population under discussion. In many published studies it is not possible to judge the degree of representativeness of the examined probands. This can be revealed only by a thorough analysis of the non-responders. This might be easier in countries with access to register data (Steen, Isaksson, and Svanborg, 1977).

Results from Elderly Populations

There are several surveys of dietary habits in elderly populations, especially on intakes of energy and nutrients. Knowledge in this field is inadequate for many regions of the world and discussion will be largely based on surveys from Sweden and the United Kingdom, namely the gerontological and geriatric population study in Göteborg, Sweden (Lundgren, Steen, and Isaksson, 1984; Rinder et al., 1975; Steen, Isaksson, and Svanborg, 1977), the studies by the U.K. Department of Health and Social Security from six areas in the United Kingdom in 1967–68 (Panel on Nutrition of the Elderly, 1972) and 1972–73 (Committee on Medical Aspects of Food Policy, 1979), and the survey by McLeod, Judge, and Caird (1974a, 1974b, 1975) in Glasgow.

In the Swedish study a representative sample of 182 males and 188 females aged 70 were examined in 1971–72 with the dietary history method. In 1976–77, 129 males and 140 females were reexamined at the age of 75 (73 per cent.), together with a new group of 70 year olds – 101 males and 99 females. In the United Kingdom studies 365 people aged 65 years and over were examined in 1967–68 and reexamined 5 years later in 1972–73. The original sample from 1967–68 comprised 879 elderly people from four areas in England and two in Scotland. The Glasgow study comprised 45 males and 95 females aged 67 to 74, and 92 females aged 75 and over.

The United Kingdom and Glasgow studies were based mainly on the 7-day record method, while the Swedish study used the 24-hour recall and the dietary history method. For reasons explained above the dietary history method was considered the more valid in the Swedish study and the results referred to below are based upon this method.

The first United Kingdom study showed an average daily intake of energy of 9.8 and 8.8 MJ for the age groups 65 to 74 and 75 years of age and over, respectively. This corresponds closely to the Glasgow study of 65 year olds and older with an energy intake of 9.7 MJ and 7.3 MJ for males and females, respectively. The Swedish study of 70 year olds revealed energy intakes of 9.8 MJ for males and 8.1 MJ for females, corresponding well to the British studies (Table 2).

Lonergan, Milne, and Williamson (1973), who studied the energy expenditure of elderly people according to principles of Durnin and Passmore (1967), reported very similar calcu-

Table 2 Intake of energy and nutrients in 70 year olds, calculated using the dietary history method. M: mean value, SD: standard deviation, 1st: 1st decentile, m: median value, 9th: 9th decentile. (From Steen, Isaksson, and Svanborg, 1977. Reproduced by permission of *Acta. Medica Scandinavica* and the authors)

	Males					Females				
	M	SD	1st	m	9th	M	SD	1st	m	9th
Energy (kcal)	2,344[a]	574.3	1,728	2,292	2,951	1,928[a]	545.3	1,262	1,888	2,578
(MJ)	9.8[a]	2.4	7.3	9.6	12.4	8.1	2.3	5.3	7.9	10.8
Protein (g)	74[a]	18.7	51	72	97	63	16.5	45	61	85
Fat (g)	96[a]	32.3	63	91	130	80	30.1	47	77	117
Carbohydrates (g)	279[a]	73.4	201	274	366	227	73.8	141	221	315
Calcium (mg)	1,033[a]	414.0	514	1,021	1,632	927	368.0	514	885	1,384
Iron (mg)	16.5[a]	4.17	11.7	16.0	21.4	14.0	4.37	9.0	13.3	19.6
Potassium (mmol)	79[a]	22.2	52	78	109	68	25.1	46	65	97
Vitamin A (µg retinol)	15.5[a]	801.5	678	1,281	2,881	1,357	684.2	555	1,242	2,287
Thiamin (mg)	1.4[a]	0.35	1.0	1.4	1.9	1.2	0.43	0.8	1.2	1.7
Riboflavin (mg)	1.8[a]	0.61	1.0	1.8	2.6	1.6	0.54	1.0	1.5	2.3
Ascorbic acid (mg)	82[a]	41.7	38	76	129	87	53.7	34	74	162

[a] Further daily intake of energy from wine and liquor was reported by about 10 per cent. of males and 1–2 per cent. of females.

lated energy expenditure figures for males (9.8 MJ), and energy intake calculated with a 2-day record method was 10.1 MJ. For females their average calculated energy expenditure of 8.2 MJ was similar to the figure in the Swedish study of 70 year olds. On the other hand, the calculated energy intake of the females in the Lonergan study was a little lower, namely 7.3 MJ.

The variation of the average values was great in all studies, with standard deviations being in the order of 25 per cent. Regional variation in energy intake was not large in the United Kingdom studies, although in males energy intake was reported below the average in the two northern urban areas.

The proportions of energy intake derived from protein, carbohydrates, and fat were not significantly different in these studies and it seems that these groups of elderly people eat a food of similar composition as people of other age groups, but in smaller quantities. This statement is supported by the findings of the three groups of studies regarding most nutrients.

Protein

The protein intakes were on average high in all the studies, but as was the case with other nutrients as well, the variation was fairly large.

Thus, in the Swedish study not less than 18 per cent. of the subjects showed values below 0.7 g/kg body weight. Animal protein constituted the main part of the protein ingested in these countries, the main food items in this respect being fish, meat, eggs, cheese, and milk. In the British studies at least, milk seems to be of more importance to women than to men.

Vitamin A

The average vitamin A intake was high in the British studies except for women above 75 years of age.

Nicotinic Acid

The two British studies showed lower than recommended average values and about 5 per cent. of the subjects were shown to have in-

takes less than the 'minimum safe level' of 4.4 mg per 1,000 kcal per day (FAO/WHO, 1967).

Riboflavin

Riboflavin intake in the lower decentile groups of both sexes in the Swedish study was below the minimum recommendation value of 0.4 mg per 1,000 kcal per day, and in the British studies not less than one-third of men and one-fifth of women showed intake values below that level.

Ascorbic Acid

The average ascorbic acid status seems to be much better in Sweden than in the United Kingdom. In the British studies mean ascorbic acid intakes were only just above the recommended level of 30 mg per day. About 5 per cent. of the subjects had less than 10 mg of ascorbic acid daily. However, the regional variation was considerable.

Vitamin D

The average vitamin D intakes – not estimated in the Swedish study – were well below recommended levels in the British women and at these levels in men, with a considerable variation.

Calcium

Calcium intakes were on average high in all studies, but the British studies showed some regional variation depending on differences in milk consumption.

Iron

Iron intake was on average above 10 mg per day in the Swedish study and in the British men. However, the British women showed lower average values, and the lower decentile value in the Swedish women fell just below that level.

Summary

Taking all studied nutrients together it may be generally concluded that a substantial proportion of subjects showed intakes below recommended standards although the average intake values were rather high.

Obvious undernutrition seems to be uncommon in the elderly in Europe. For example, in the first United Kingdom study in 1967–68, 3 per cent. of the probands aged 65 and over were judged to be malnourished. Six weeks later the incidence in the same probands of this longitudinal study had increased to 7 per cent. and was twice as large among subjects aged 80 years or more compared with those under 80 years of age. In all except perhaps one subject, malnutrition, however, was associated with non-nutritional disease.

If undernutrition is uncommon, overnutrition is a problem in large areas of Europe. Overnutrition may be combined with undernutrition of essential nutrients such as protein, minerals, and vitamins. The risk is especially obvious in low-energy consumers. Inadequate dietary habits, when they exist, seem to depend more on cultural and traditional factors and culinary preferences than on economic reasons.

The Swedish study suggested that the average 70 year old person should increase his consumption of green vegetables and potatoes or other starches. It is recommended that those at risk – about 10 per cent. of the 70 year old subjects – should attempt to increase the daily number of good meals and to increase the consumption of foods rich in protein, thiamin, and riboflavin.

Nutritional support to this group of elderly is advisable since an improved nutritional status might be one of many factors enabling the elderly to live independently in their own homes. Higher education and higher income seemed to be related to more adequate dietary intakes of a couple of nutrients in the Swedish study.

In the British studies house-bound subjects had smaller mean intakes than those subjects not confined to their homes. Social factors associated with undernutrition were living alone (for men only), bereavement, having no regular cooked meals, being in social classes IV and V, and being in receipt of supplementary benefit. The authors concluded that the provision of more money alone to the individual concerned would not, however, necessarily have been the most effective means of improving nutritional status.

RELATION BETWEEN ORAL HEALTH AND DIETARY INTAKE

Among many factors, such as social factors, physical disease, and psychological impairment, the dental state may be expected to have a relation to dietary intake, (see Chapter 11.1). In the study of the relation between the dental state and dietary habits it is necessary to take these confounding factors into consideration in the statistical analyses (Heath, 1972).

Odontological surveys of elderly populations inside (for a review see Mäkilä, 1977) and outside (for a review see Österberg, Hedegård, and Säter, 1984) institutions have often revealed an unsatisfactory oral health situation in these age groups. This is often in contrast to the relatively good general health situation, at least in the 'younger elderly'.

For example, in a large representative group of 70 year old Swedes, half of the subjects were edentulous in both jaws and one-fifth in one jaw. Half of the endentulous subjects had worn their dentures for more than 10 years and only 14 per cent. had satisfactorily functioning dentures and acceptable occlusion. Furthermore, a clinically healthy oral mucosa was seen in only 25 per cent. of that population and was more frequently seen in the floor of the oral cavity. Denture-related lesions were most common (denture stomatitis in 42 per cent. and 'irritation denture hyperplasia' in 38 per cent.). Leucoplakia was recorded in 21 per cent. and was more common in the edentulous subjects and the male smokers than in others. Although there was a highly significant correlation between subjective dryness of the mouth and the number of drugs consumed and diseases, there was no correlation between the stimulated secretion and the intake of diuretic drugs (Österberg and Carlsson, 1979; Österberg *et al.*, 1983a, 1983b, 1983c.)

Oral health in elderly populations shows marked cohort effects in short intervals of time. Seventy year old people in Sweden in 1976–77 showed a significantly lower prevalence of edentia, a lower degree of oral invalidity and, consequently, a better oral health than 70 year olds five years earlier in 1971–72 (Österberg, Hedegård, and Säter, 1984).

Literature data regarding the influence of dental state upon the dietary intake are contradictory and somewhat confusing. Berry

(1972) showed that individuals over the age of 75 with an impaired masticatory efficiency had a lower energy intake and meat consumption than a control group with satisfactory masticatory efficiency. The condition of dentures influences the dietary habits of denture wearers, as shown by Neill (1973) and Söremark and Nilsson (1972). Edentulous persons with dentures have been shown to have higher blood levels of ascorbic acid and pantothenic acid than those without dentures (Mäkilä, 1968, 1970). Also, other authors have shown a relation between different nutritional data, such as intake of some nutrients, including protein, and body weight (Davidson *et al.*, Ruikka, Sourander, and Kasanen, 1967) and dental state.

However, Bates, Elwood, and Foster (1971) could not find any support for the hypothesis that a natural dentition is necessary for the elderly to maintain a satisfactory nutritional state, and similar conclusions were drawn by Neill (1973) and Hartsook (1974).

As was pointed out by Heath (1972), it is necessary to make a distinction between intake of energy and nutrients, on the one hand, and dietary selection of different food items, on the other.

Many authors have found that elderly people with a poor dental state experienced difficulty in ingesting items such as meat and hard foods (Bates and Murphy, 1968; Bender and Davies, 1968; Heath, 1972; Mäkilä, 1968). Few, however, have found a similar relationship between dental state and the intake of nutrients.

Österberg and Steen (1982) studied the relation between the dental state, expressed by Eichner classes and subgroups (Eichner, 1955) on one hand, and the intake of food items, energy, and nutrients on the other. A relation was observed regarding single food items, so that the intakes of, for example, chicken and vegetables were higher and the intake of sausages lower in men with a better dental state. No significant relation between dental state and intake of energy and single nutrients was found. When the analysis was extended to subjects with low intakes of one or more nutrients, this group was overrepresented in the lower Eichner subgroups. These correlations remained unchanged in men, and also when socio-economic factors were kept constant in the statistical analyses.

BODY COMPOSITION

The composition of the human body is of the utmost interest from both a gerontological and geriatric point of view. It reflects genetic and environmental factors, such as physical activity, nutrition, and disease, as well as ageing processes per se. Changes in cardiac and renal function that might influence the amount of body water are common in later life, even in individuals without obvious symptoms of cardiac and renal disease. Knowledge of geriatric clinical pharmacology and clinical chemistry has to be enhanced by data of body composition because of changes of drug distribution volumes with age. The amount of body fat and of body cell mass are important parameters when judging the net effect of energy intake and expenditure, and the body cell mass is a better reference point than body weight or body surface area when studying, for example, energy exchange and work performance.

Concepts and Methods

The concepts of body composition and the nomenclature of the body compartments are somewhat confusing (Fig. 4). A very common concept is the lean body mass (LBM), which is body weight minus neutral fat, i.e. a mass similar to – but not identical with – a fat-free body.

However, although lean body mass has a relatively constant specific weight in healthy individuals, it is from a biological point of view a heterogenic body compartment. Lean body mass thus comprises body cell mass, fat-free extracellular solids, and extracellular water.

Several years ago Moore and coworkers (1963) proposed that the concept of lean body mass should be avoided. They suggested that the concept of body cell mass should be used as a better estimate of the metabolically active tissue, and therefore be used as a reference when, for example, studying oxygen consumption and requirements of energy and nutrients.

As is shown in Fig. 4, many laboratories now prefer to divide body weight into body cell mass, extracellular water (ECW), body fat, and fat-free extracellular solids (FFECS). The fat-free extracellular solids are present primarily in the skeleton and in the connective tissue.

Over the years many techniques have been

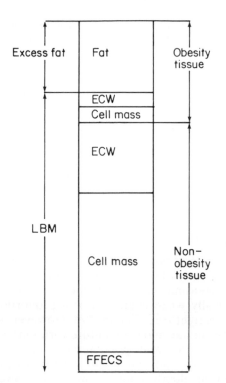

Figure 4   Anatomical definitions of the concepts of non-obesity and obesity tissue and of lean body mass (LBM) and excess fat. ECW: extracellular water, FFECS: fat-free extra cellular solids

have been discussed by Berg and Isaksson (1970) and Steen and coworkers (1977).

Body compartments are calculated from the determination of body weight, body height, total body potassium and total body water (Fig. 5). Total body potassium is determined with a high-sensitivity whole-body counter with plastic scintillators (Sköldborn, Arvidsson, and Andersson, 1972) to measure the gamma radiation from the naturally occurring radionuclide ^{40}K, which constitutes a constant fraction of all body potassium in the body. Total body water is determined with a tritiated water dilution technique (Berg and Isaksson, 1970; Lindholm, 1967; Steen *et al.*, 1977). Since most body potassium is located intracellularly and the potassium can be considered to be in constant relation with the cell mass, and since the intracellular water can also be considered to be constant, this technique allows the estimation of the different body compartments from the measured parameters mentioned.

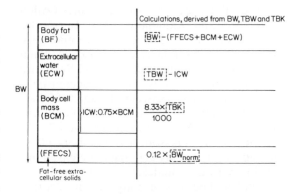

Figure 5   Four-compartment model of body composition as derived from measurements of body weight (BW), total body water (TBW), and total body potassium (TBK), ICW is the intracellular water, and BW norm is the 'normal' body weight for height. (From Bruce *et al.*, 1980. Reproduced by permission of The Scandinavian Journal of Clinical and Laboratory Investigation)

used to get an impression of the body composition in man (for reviews see Moore *et al.*, 1963; Steen, 1977a; Steinkamp *et al.*, 1965). These methods range from cadaver analyses (Forbes, Cooper, and Mitchell, 1953), anthropological measurements (Barter and Forbes, 1963), absorption of fat-soluble gases (Hytten, Taylor, and Taggart, 1966), isotope dilution methods to calculate the total body water (Lindholm, 1967) and body cell mass (Moore *et al.*, 1963), whole-body potassium counting (Sköldborn, Arvidsson, and Andersson, 1972), and measurements of subcutaneous fat thickness with radiography (Garn, 1957) and with calipers (Pascale *et al.*, 1955). There is an advantage in using combined measurements in this respect.

The isotope methods for determining body composition which have been used for two decades at the Department of Clinical Nutrition, University of Göteborg, Sweden (Berg and Isaksson, 1970; Lindholm, 1967), are described below. The errors inherent in such methods

Simple methods are necessary in practical clinical work, using for instance weight-to-height ratios of different kinds and skinfold and girth measurements. The validity of such methods has been investigated in several papers. Such validity studies have to be performed for different age groups, since the relations between somatometric measurements and body compartments need not be the same for all ages. In a representative population of 70 year olds Steen and coworkers (1977) showed that it was possible from body weight and subscapular skinfold thickness in males and thigh and triceps skinfolds in females to obtain a proportion of explained variance of body fat of 58 and 76 per cent., respectively. In the subjects studied there was a good correlation between body fat and the difference between body weight and an 'ideal' body weight in common use in Scandinavia.

Body Cell Mass

The decreasing number of cells in the organs and the increasing disuse of skeletal muscle tissue with age result in a decreasing body cell mass. At the age of 70 skeletal muscle has been shown to have lost 40 per cent. of its maximal weight in early adult life as compared to 18 per cent. for the liver, 9 per cent. for the kidneys, and 11 per cent. for the lungs (Korenchevsky, 1961). The decrease with age of body cell mass has been illustrated by several studies (Allen, Anderson, and Langham, 1960; Burmeister and Bingert, 1967; Forbes and Reina, 1970; Novak, 1972; Shukla *et al.*, 1973). A longitudinal study (Steen, Isaksson, and Svanborg, 1979) showed that body cell mass decreased by approximately 1 kg between the ages of 70 and 75 years (Table 3). In a further longitudinal study of these males and females aged 70, 75, and 79, Steen, Isaksson, and Svanborg (1981) showed that the body cell mass decreased during this period in males, but not significantly in females. The loss of body weight occurring in both sexes corresponded more to loss of body cell mass in males than in females, while the weight loss corresponded more to loss of body fat in females than in males.

A comparison between people aged 54 and 70, respectively, showed that body cell mass was similar in these two age groups in females, but showed a lower value in 70 year old females than in 54 year old males (Steen *et al.*, 1977). It was suggested that retired males at the age of 70 have a lower physical activity than in active middle life and, therefore, a smaller amount of muscular tissue, while the physical activity in females might be similar in the two age groups. These sex differences are in accordance with the results from other investigators (Munro, 1981).

Table 3   Average values of body weight (BW), body cell mass (BCM), extracellular water (ECW), and body fat (BF) at the ages of 70 and 75. NS.: $p > 0.05$, x: $p < 0.05$, xx: $p < 0.01$. (Reprinted from Steen, Isaksson, and Svanborg, 1979, pp. 185–200, by courtesy of Marcel Dekker, Inc.)

	Males			Females		
	70 yr	75 yr	S	70 yr	75 yr	S
BW	76.1	73.2	x	66.2	64.5	x
BCM	28.6	27.6	xx	20.3	19.7	x
ECW	22.5	20.2	xx	16.9	15.3	xx
BF	17.8	18.0	x	22.5	23.1	NS

Body Fat

The study of body fat is of obvious importance in the study of obesity. Most data have shown an increasing amount of body fat with age, especially when expressed as a proportion of body weight (see Chapter 22). However, since energy intake and expenditure varies markedly between different populations, the average amount of body fat might vary between the different elderly populations. In the Swedish longitudinal study (Steen, Isaksson, and Svanborg, 1979, 1981) the amount of body fat did not change in any noteworthy way between the ages of 70 and 75, but decreased by 2 kg between 75 and 79 in females. As indicated above the loss of body weight occurring in both sexes between the ages of 70 and 79 seemed to correspond more to loss of body cell mass in males than in females, and to a decrease of body fat in females.

Skerlj, Brozek, and Hunt (1953) found that subcutaneous fat was deposited more on the trunk than on the extremities in old compared to young women. Another type of age-dependent redistribution of fat was described by Durnin and Womersley (1974), who found that there was an increase of deep adipose tissue relative to subcutaneous fat with age.

Body Water

Body water decreases with advancing age in most studies (Shock *et al.*, 1963). However, this trend might be less significant in the highest age groups, as shown by Bruce and coworkers (1980); in their studies the age dependence was not great. A possible explanation for this might be that the trend of a decreasing amount of total body water might be counteracted by the fact that a change in cardiac and renal function might increase the amount of body water in individuals without obvious signs of heart or kidney disease. The relative amount of extracellular water, furthermore, might increase with age since the ratio between extracellular and intracellular water which is around 1 in younger age groups, and lower for males, seems to be higher at the age of 70 and about the same for the sexes (Steen *et al.*, 1977).

SOCIAL, PSYCHOLOGICAL, AND PUBLIC HEALTH ASPECTS

Domiciliary Support

There seems to be an overall agreement in most countries, regardless of the kind of health care system, that elderly people should be helped to lead independent lives in their own homes for as long as possible. Indeed, most elderly people live in their own homes and in many countries enhanced social services might further increase this proportion; home-help services are of particular importance (International Federation on Ageing, 1975a). In many countries social services tend to show greater regional differences than the health services. For a review on public health aspects of nutrition of the elderly, see Steen (1977b).

Voluntary Agencies

Voluntary bodies (International Federation on Ageing, 1975b) are often engaged in domiciliary services. However, the organization and extent of such services vary from country to country. For example, voluntary bodies play a relatively small role in the Scandinavian countries.

Voluntary activities may be directed towards the delivery of meals-on-wheels, the provision of social and/or luncheon clubs, and home visits to the elderly. One major advantage is that such activities often provide not only the recipients but also the volunteers themselves with important social contact.

Access to good kitchen facilities such as a refridgerator and a deepfreeze unit may help considerably in food planning and, therefore, result in savings, including the avoidance of food wastage.

In some countries the elderly, especially those with a physical handicap, are actively encouraged to keep an emergency store of food for one or two days in case of temporary illness or bad weather. Such an emergency store may contain certain food items such as dried milk, tins of soup, meat, fish and vegetables, instant potatoes, crispbread, and coffee/tea.

Meals-on-wheels are an important complement to other public health activities regarding nutrition in the elderly. They must, however, be considered only 'second best' to activities where elderly come together for meals and meet others in, for example, luncheon clubs, local cafés, and day centres. Some elderly might be dependent on meals-on-wheels in the winter but manage to come to a day centre in the summer.

Education

The crucial importance of education of the elderly in dietary matters should be borne in mind. It may be provided through, for example, leaflets, radio and television programmes, and lectures.

Leaflets should be easy to read, in large print type, spaciously and attractively laid out. Television and radio are probably the best media to reach many elderly, especially the housebound.

The dietary educational problems of the elderly cannot be treated altogether separately from educational activities aimed at the population as a whole. The ultimate goal is to improve general dietary habits. Members of society other than the elderly (especially cooks, health instructors, and home-helps) should also be made aware of the ageing process and basic gerontological and geriatric nutritional problems.

Alcohol

The relations between dietary habits and the use and misuse of alcohol are at least twofold. Alcohol abusers have an increased risk of acquiring bad food habits and alcohol intake increases energy intake without improving the intake of essential nutrients. Alcohol thus lowers the nutrient density of the food. Alcohol abuse is not uncommon in the elderly (Mellström, Rundgren, and Svanborg, 1981).

Smoking

Smoking habits are also related to the nutritional state of individuals and groups of individuals. A comparison of the dietary habits between non-smokers and smokers in a Swedish 70 year old male population (Mellström *et al.*, 1981) revealed no differences regarding intake of energy and nutrients. However, body weight, subscapular and triceps skinfold, and waist girth were significantly lower in the smokers. Thus, there was a difference of 5.5 kg in body weight between smokers and non-smokers.

Summary

A meal ought to be a social event, and limitations of the psychological and social quality of the meal situation might seriously predispose to inadequate dietary habits. This seems to be a common factor to many of the risk groups which different studies have revealed, such as men living alone (Steen, Isaksson, and Svanborg, 1977), widows (Lundgren, Steen, and Isaksson, 1984), elderly with a physical handicap, and those having few cooked meals (Caird, Judge, and MacLeod, 1975). These considerations are also applicable to elderly patients in institutional care, where every effort should be made to improve the social qualities of the meal situation.

REFERENCES

Acheson, R. M., and Jessop, W. J. (1962). 'Serum proteins in a population sample of males 65–85 years. A study by paper electrophoresis', *Gerontologia*, **6**, 193–205.

Ackerman, P. G., and Kheim, T. (1964). 'Plasma amino acids in young and older adult human subjects', *Clin. Chem.*, **10**, 32–40.

Adelman, R. C. (1970). 'Impaired hormonal regulation of enzyme activity during ageing', *Fed. Proc.*, **34**, 179–182.

Adelman, R. C. (1971). 'Age-depending effects in enzyme induction – a biochemical expression of ageing', *Exp. Gerontol.*, **6**, 75–87.

Albanese, A. A., Higgons, R. A., Orto, L. A., and Zavattaro, D. N. (1957). 'Protein and amino acids

needs of the aged in health and convalescence', *Geriatrics*, **12**, 465–475.

Allen, T. H., Anderson, E. C., and Langham, W. H. (1960). 'Total body potassium and gross body composition in relation to age', *J. Gerontol.*, **15**, 348–357.

Anderson, W. F., Cohen, C., Hyams, D. E., Millard, P. H., Plowright, N. M., Woodford-Williams, E., and Berry, W. T. C. (1972). 'Clinical and subclinical malnutrition in old age', in *Nutrition in Old Age* (Ed. L. A. Carlsson), pp. 140–146, Almqvist and Wiksell, Uppsala.

Andrews, J., and Brook, M. (1966). 'Leucocyte-vitamin C content and clinical signs in the elderly', *Lancet*, **1**, 1350–1351.

Andrews, J., Brook, M., and Allen, M. A. (1966). 'Influence of abode and season on the vitamin C status of the elderly', *Geront. Clin.*, **8**, 257–266.

Andrews, J., Letcher, M., and Brook, M. (1969). 'Vitamin C supplementation in the elderly: A 17-month trial in an old person's home'. *Br. Med. J.*, **2**, 416–418.

Avioli, L. V. (1977). 'Osteoporosis. Pathogenesis and therapy'. In *Metabolic Bone Disease* (Eds L. V. Avioli and S. M. Krane), Vol. 1, pp. 307–385, Academic Press, New York.

Avioli, L. V., McDonald, J. E., and Lee, S. W. (1965). 'The influence of age on the intestinal absorption of 47 Ca in women and its relation to 47 Ca absorption in post-menopausal osteoporosis', *J. Clin. Invest.*, **44**, 1960–1967.

Barrows, C. H. (1966). 'Enzymes in the study of biological ageing', in *Perspectives in Experimental Gerontology* (Ed. N. W. Shock), pp. 169–181, C. C. Thomas, Springfield, Illinois.

Barter, J., and Forbes, G. B. (1963). 'Correlation of potassium-40 data with anthropometric measurements', *Ann. N. Y. Acad. Sci.*, **110**, 264–270.

Bates, J. F., Elwood, P. C., and Foster, W. (1971). 'Studies relating mastication and nutrition in the elderly', *Geront. Clin.*, **13**, 227–232.

Bates, J. F., and Murphy, W. M. (1968). 'A survey of an edentulous population', *Br. Dent. J.*, **124**, 116–121.

Bender, A. E., and Davies, L. (1968). 'Milk consumption in the elderly', *Br. J. Geriatr. Pract.*, **5**, 331–335.

Berg, K., and Isaksson, B. (1970). 'Body composition and nutrition of school children with cerebral palsy', *Acta. Paediatr. Scand. (Suppl.)*, **204**, 41–52.

Berg, S. (1980). 'Psychological functioning in 70- and 75-year-old people. A study in an industrialized city', *Acta. Psychiatr. Scand. (Suppl.)* **288**.

Berry, W. T. C. (1972). 'Mastication, food and nutrition', *Dent. Practr. Dent. Rec.*, **22**, 249–255.

Bruce, Å., Anderson, M., Arvidsson, B., and Isaksson, B. (1980). 'Body composition. Prediction of normal body potassium, body water and body fat in adults on the basis of body height, body weight and age', *Scand. J. Clin. Lab. Invest.*, **40**, 461–473.

Brüschke, G., Mehls, E., and Zschenderlein, B. (1967). 'Die Eisenresorption in hohen Lebensalter', *Deutsch. Gesundh.*, **22**, 1639–1640.

Bullamore, J. R., Gallagher, J. C. Wilkinson, R., Nordin, B. E. C., and Marshall, D. H. (1970). 'The effect of age on calcium absorption', *Lancet*, **2**, 535–537.

Burke, B. S. (1947). 'The dietary history as a tool in research', *J. Am. Diet. Assoc.*, **23**, 1041–1046.

Burkitt, D. P., and Trowell, H. H. (1975). *Refined Carbohydrate Foods and Disease*, Academic Press, New York.

Burmeister, W., and Bingert, A. (1967). 'Die quantitativen Veranderungen der menschlichen Zellmasse zwischen dem 8. und 90. Lebensjahr', *Klin. Wochenschr.*, **45**, 409–416.

Burr, M. L., Hurley, R. J., and Sweetnam, P. M. (1975). 'Vitamin C supplementation of old people with low blood levels', *Geront. Clin.*, **17**, 236–241.

Caird, F. I., Judge, T. G., and MacLeod, C. (1975). 'Pointers to possible malnutrition in the elderly at home', *Geront. Clin.*, **17**, 47–54.

Calloway, D. H. (1975). 'Nitrogen balance of men with marginal intakes of protein and energy', *J. Nutr.*, **105**, 914–923.

Chen, J. C., Warshaw, J. B., and Sanadi, D. R. (1972). 'Regulation of mitochondrial respiration in senescence', *J. Cell. Physiol.*, **80**, 141–148.

Cheng, A. H. R., Gomez, A., Bergan, J. G., Lee, T. C., Monckeberg, F., and Chichester, C. O. (1978). 'Comparative nitrogen balance study between young and aged adults using three levels of protein intake from a combination wheat-soymilk mixture', *Am. J. Clin. Nutr.*, **31**, 12–22.

Coleman, G. L., Barthold, S. W., Osbaldiston, G. W., Foster, S. J., and Jonas, A. M. (1977). 'Pathological changes during aging in barrierreared Fischer 344 male rats', *J. Gerontol.*, **32**, 258–278.

Committee on Medical Aspects of Food Policy. (1979). *Nutrition and Health in Old Age*, Department of Health and Social Security, Reports on Health and Social Subjects No. 16, HMSO, London.

Darke, S. (1972). 'Requirement for vitamins in old age', in *Nutrition in Old Age* (Ed. L. A. Carlsson), pp. 107–117, Symposia of the Swedish Nutrition Foundation X.

Davidson, C., Livermore, J., Anderson, P., and Kaufman, S. (1962). 'The nutrition of a group of apparently healthy ageing persons', *Am. J. Clin. Nutr.*, **18**, 181–199.

Durnin, J. V. G. A. and Passmore, R. (1967). *Energy, Work and Leisure*, Heinemann, London.

Durnin, J. V. G. A., and Womersley, J. (1974). 'Body fat assessed from total body density and its estimation from skinfold thickness: Measurements on 481 men and women aged from 16 to 72 years', *Br. J. Nutr.*, **32**, 77–97.

Eeg-Larsen, N., Isaksson, B., Nicolaysen, R., and Wretlind, A. (1971). 'Veiledning til vurdering og planlegging av kosthold', Landforeningen for kosthold og helse, Universitetsforlaget, Oslo.

Eichner, K. (1955). 'Über eine Gruppeneinteilung des Lückengebisses für die Prothetik', *Dtsch. Zahnaerztl. Z.*, **18**, 1831–1834.

Exton-Smith, A. N. (1978). 'Nutrition in the elderly', in *Nutrition in the Clinical Management of Disease* (Eds J. W. T. Dickerson and H. A. Lee), pp. 72–104, Edward Arnold, London.

Exton-Smith, A. N., Hodkinson, H. M., and Stanton, B. R. (1966). 'Nutrition and metabolic bone disease in old age', *Lancet*, **2**, 999–1001.

FAO/WHO (1962). 'Calcium requirements', Report of an FAO/WHO Expert Committee on Calcium requirements, *WHO Tech. Rep. Ser.*, **230**, FAO, Rome.

FAO/WHO. (1967), 'Requirements of vitamin A, thiamine, riboflavine, and niacin', *WHO Tech. Rep. Ser.*, **301**, Geneva.

FAO/WHO (1973). 'Energy and protein requirements', *WHO Tech. Rep. Ser.*, **522** Geneva.

Food and Nutrition Board. (1974) *Recommended Dietary Allowances*, 8th ed., Nat. Acad. Sci., Washington, D.C.

Food and Nutrition Board (1980). *Recommended Dietary Allowances*, 9th ed., Nat. Acad. Sci., Washington, D.C.

Forbes, R. M., Cooper, A. R., and Mitchell, H. H. (1953). 'The composition of the adult human body as determined by chemical analysis', *J. Biol. Chem.*, **203**, 359–366.

Forbes, R. M., and Reina, J. C. (1970). 'Adult lean body mass declines with age: Some longitudinal observations', *Metabolism*, **19**, 653–663.

Freiman, H. D., Tauber, S. A., and Tulsky, E. G. (1963). 'Iron absorption in the healthy aged', *Geriatrics*, **18**, 716–720.

Gallagher, J. C., Riggs, B. L., Eisman, J., Hamstra, A., Arnaud, S. B., DeLuca, H. F. (1979). 'Intestinal calcium absorption and serum vitamin D metabolites in normal subjects and osteoporotic patients. Effect of age and dietary calcium', *J. Clin. Invest.*, **64**, 729–736.

Garn, S. M. (1957). 'Roentgenogrammetric determinations of body composition', *Human Biol.*, **29**, 337–353.

Garn, S. M., Rothmann, C. G., and Wagner, B. (1967). 'Bone loss as a general phenomenon in man', *Fed. Proc.*, **26**, 1729–1736.

Garza, C., Scrimshaw, N. S., Young, V. R. (1976).

'Human protein requirements: The effect of variations in energy intake within the maintenance range', *Am. J. Clin. Nutr.*, **29**, 280–287.

Hackett, A. F., Yeung, C. K., Hill, G. L. (1979). 'Eating patterns in patients recovering from major surgery – a study of voluntary food intake and energy balance', *Br. J. Surg.*, **66**, 415–418.

Hartsook, E. I. (1974). 'Food selection, dietary adequacy and related dental problems of patients with dental prosthesis', *J. Prosthet. Dent.*, **32**, 32–40.

Heath, M. R. (1972). 'Dietary selection by elderly persons, related to dental state', *Br. Dent. J.*, **132**, 145–148.

Hegsted, D. M. (1972). 'Problems in the use and interpretation of the Recommended Dietary Allowances', *Ecology of Food and Nutrition*, **1**, 255–265.

Hegsted, D. M. (1975). 'Dietary standards', *J. Am. Diet. Assoc.*, **66**, 13–21.

Hessov, I. (1977). 'Energy and protein intake in elderly patients in an orthopedic surgical ward', *Acta. Chir. Scand.*, **143**, 145–149.

Horwitt, M. K., Liebert, E., Kreisler, O., and Wittman, P. (1948). *Investigations of Human Requirements for B-Complex Vitamins*' NRC Bull. no. 116, Nat. Acad. Sci., Washington, D.C.

Hytten, F. E., Taylor, K., and Taggart, N. (1966). 'Measurement of total body fat in man by absorption of ^{85}Kr', *Clin. Sci.*, **31**, 111–119.

International Federation on Ageing (1975a). *Home-help Services for the Ageing around the World*, Washington, D.C.

International Federation on Ageing (1975b). *The Voluntary Agency as an Instrument of Social Change*, Washington, D.C.

Isaksson, B. (1973). 'Clinical nutrition. Requirements of energy and nutrients in diseases', *Bibl. 'Nutr. Diet'.*, **19**, 1–10 (Karger, Basel).

Isaksson, B. (1975). 'Future trends in clinical nutrition', *Bibl. 'Nutr. Diet'.*, **21**, 163–176 (Karger, Basel).

Isaksson, B. (1980). 'Urinary nitrogen output as a validity test in dietary surveys', *Am. J. Clin. Nutr.*, **33**, 4–12.

Isaksson, B., and Sjögren, B. (1967). 'A critical evaluation of the mineral and nitrogen balances in men', *Proc. Nutr. Soc.*, **26**, 106–116.

Jeliffe, D. B. (1966). *The Assessment of the Nutritional Status of the Community (with special reference to field surveys in developing regions of the world)*, WHO, Geneva.

Johnson, N. E., Alcantara, E. N., and Linkswiler, H. M. (1970). 'Effect of protein intake on urinary and fecal calcium and calcium retention of young adult males', *J. Nutr.*, **100**, 1425–1430.

Judge, T. G. (1974). 'Nutrition in the elderly', in *Geriatric Medicine* (Eds W. F. Anderson and T.

G. Judge), pp. 231–245, Academic Press, London and New York.

Judge, T. G., and Cowan, N. R. (1971). 'Dietary potassium intake and grip strength in older people', *Geront. Clin.*, **13**, 221–226.

Kataria, M. S., Rao, D. B., and Curtis, R. C. (1965). 'Vitamin C levels in the elderly', *Geront. Clin.*, **7**, 180–189.

Korenchevsky, V. (1961). In *Physiological and Pathological Ageing* (Ed. G. H. Bourne), Karger, Basel.

Kountz, W. B., Hofstatter, L., and Ackermann, P. (1951). 'Nitrogen balance studies in four elderly men', *J. Gerontol.*, **6**, 20–33.

Lindholm, B. (1967). 'Changes in body composition during long-term treatment with cortisone and anabolic steroids in asthmatic subjects', *Acta. Allerg. (Kobenhavn)*, **22**, 261–288.

Linkswiler, H. M., Joyce, C. L., and Arnaud, C. R. (1974). 'Calcium retention of young adult males as affected by level of protein and of calcium intake', *Trans. NY Acad. Sci.*, **36**, 333–340.

Loh, H. S., and Wilson, C. W. M. (1971). 'Relationship between leucocyte ascorbic acid and haemoglobin levels at different ages', *Int. J. Vitam. Nutr. Res.*, **41**, 259–267.

Lonergan, M. E., Milne, J. S., and Williamson, J. (1973). 'Physical activity and energy expenditure of elderly men and women in Edinburgh, Scotland', *Geront. Clin.*, **15**, 113–123.

Lundgren, B. K., Steen, B., and Isaksson, B. (1984). 'Dietary habits in 70- and 75-year-old males and females. Longitudinal and cohort data from a population study', In preparation.

McCay, C. M., Crowell, M. F., and Maynard, L. A. (1935). 'The effect of retarded growth upon the length of life span and upon the ultimate body size', *J. Nutr.*, **10**, 63–79.

McGandy, R. B., Barrows, C. H., Jr, Spanias, A., Meredith, A., Stone, J. L., and Norris, A. H. (1966). 'Nutrient intakes and energy expenditure in men of different ages', *J. Gerontol.*, **21**, 581–587.

McLeod, C. C., Judge, T. G., and Caird, F. I. (1974a). 'Nutrition of the elderly at home. I. Intakes of energy, protein, carbohydrates and fat', *Age Ageing*, **3**, 158–167.

McLeod, C. C., Judge, T. G., and Caird, F. I. (1974b). 'Nutrition of the elderly at home. II. Intakes of vitamins', *Age Ageing*. **3**, 209–220.

McLeod, C. C., Judge, T. G., and Caird, F. I. (1975). 'Nutrition of the elderly at home. III. Intakes of minerals', *Age Ageing*, **4**, 49–57.

Mäkilä, E. (1968). 'Effect of complete dentures on the dietary habits and serum thiamin, riboflavine and ascorbic acid levels in edentulous persons', *Suom. Hammaslääk. Toim.*, **64**, 107–111.

Mäkilä, E. (1970). 'Serum values of some mineral

elements in edentulous persons', *Suom. Hammaslääk. Toim.*, **66**, 196–199.

Mäkilä, E. (1977). 'Oral health among the inmates of old people's home. 1. Description of material. Dental state' *Proc. Finn. Dent. Soc.*, **73**, 53–63.

Malm, O. J. (1958). 'Calcium requirement and adaptation in adult men', *Scand. J. Clin. Lab. Invest.*, **10**, 1–289.

Marr, J. W. (1971). 'Individual dietary surveys. Purposes and methods', *World Rev. Nutr. Diet.*, **13**, 105–164 (Karger, Basel).

Marx, J. J. M. (1979). 'Normal iron absorption and decreased red-cell iron uptake in the aged', *Blood*, **53**, 204–211.

Masoro, E. J. (1976). 'Physiologic changes with ageing', *Curr. Concepts Nutr.*, **4**, 61–76.

Massler, M. (1979). 'Geriatric nutrition 11: Dehydration in the elderly', *J. Prosthet. Dent.*, **42**, 489–491.

Masoro, E. J. (1976). 'Physiologic changes with aging'. *Curr. Concepts Nutr.*, **4**, 61–76.

Mellström, D., Rundgren, Å., Jagenburg, R., Steen, B., and Svanborg, A. (1981). 'Tobacco smoking, ageing and health among the elderly. A longitudinal population study of 70-year-old men and an age cohort comparison', *Age Ageing*, **11**, 45–58.

Mellström, D., Rundgren, Å., and Svanborg, A. (1981). 'Previous alcohol consumption and its consequences for ageing, morbidity and mortality in men aged 70–75', *Age Ageing*, **10**, 277–286.

Moore, F. D., Olesen, K. H., McMurrey, J. D., Parker, H. V., Ball, M. R., and Boyden, C. M. (1963). *The Body Cell Mass and Its Supporting Environment*, Saunders, Philadelphia and London.

Munro, H. N. (1980). 'The status of the elderly. Major gaps in nutrient allowances', *J. Am. Diet. Assoc.*, **76**, 137–141.

Munro, H. N. (1981). 'Nutrition and ageing', *Br. Med. Bull.*, **37**, 83–88.

Munro, H. N., and Young, V. R. (1978). 'Protein metabolism in the elderly', *Postgrad. Med.*, **63**, 143–148.

Neill, D. J. (1973). 'The relationship between masticatory performance and diet', *Proc. Roy. Soc. Med.*, **66**, 598–599.

Nolen, G. A. (1972). 'Effect of restricted dietary regimens on the growth, health and longevity of albino rats', *J. Nutr.*, **102**, 1477–1494.

Nordin, B. E. C. (1962). 'Calcium balance and calcium requirements in spinal osteoporosis', *Am. J. Clin. Nutr.*, **10**, 384–390.

Nordin, B. E. C. (1971). 'Clinical significance and pathogenesis of osteoporosis', *Br. Med. J.*, **1**, 571–576.

Novak, L. P. (1972). 'Aging, total body potassium, fat-free mass and cell mass in males and females between ages 18 and 85 years', *J. Gerontol.*, **27**, 438–443.

Oldham, H. G. (1962). 'Thiamine requirements of women', *Ann. NY Acad. Sci.*, **98**, 542–549.

Österberg, T., Hedegård, B., and Säter, G. (1984). 'Variation in dental health in 70-year-old men and women in Gothenburg, Sweden. A cross-sectional epidemiological study including longitudinal and cohort effects', *Swed. Dent. J.*, In press.

Österberg, T., and Steen, B. (1982). 'Relation between dental state and dietary intake in 70-year-old men and women in Göteborg, Sweden. A population study', *J. Oral Rehabil.*, **9**, 509–521.

Panel on Nutrition of the Elderly (1972). *A Nutrition Survey of the Elderly*,. Department of Health and Social Security, Reports on Health and Social Subjects No. 3, HMSO, London.

Pascale, L. R., Grossman, M. I., Sloane, H. S., and Frankel, T. (1955). 'Correlations between thickness of skin folds and body density in 88 soldiers', *Hub. Biol.*, **27**, 165–176.

Reinhold, J. G., Faradji, B., Abadi, P., and Ismail-Bligi, F.(1976). 'Decreased absorption of calcium, magnesium, zinc and phosphorus by humans due to increased fiber and phosphorus consumption as wheat bread', *J. Nutr.*, **106**, 493–503.

Rinder, L., Roupe, S., Steen, B., and Svanborg, A. (1975). '70-year-old people in Gothenburg. A population study in an industrialized Swedish city. I. General presentation of the study', *Acta. Med. Scand.*, **198**, 397–407.

Roine, P., and Pekkarinen, M. (1968). 'Methodology of dietary studies', in *Richtlinien gesunder Ernährung. Inter Z. Vit. forsch.* (Ed. G. Ritzel), Vol. 31, Beiheft 11.

Ross, M. H. (1976a). 'Nutrition and longevity in experimental animals', in *Nutrition and Ageing* (Ed. M. Winick), pp. 43–57, John Wiley and Sons, New York, London, Sydney, Toronto.

Ross, M. H. (1976b). 'Nutrition and longevity in experimental animals', *Curr. Concepts Nutr.*, **4**, 43–57.

Ross, M. H., and Bras, G. (1971). 'Lasting influence of early caloric restriction on prevalence of neoplasms in the rat', *J. Nat. Cancer Inst.*, **47**, 1095–1113.

Ross, M. H., and Bras, G. (1974). 'Dietary preference and diseases of age', *Nature*, **250**, 263–264.

Ross, M. H., and Bras, G. (1975). 'Food preference and length of life', *Science*, **190**, 165–167.

Roth, G. S. (1975). 'Age-related changes in glucocorticoid binding by rat splenic leucocytes: Possible cause of altered adaptive responsiveness', *Fed. Proc.*, **34**, 183–185.

Roth, H. P., and Mehlman, M. A. (Eds) (1978). 'Symposium on role of dietary fiber in health', and *Am. J. Clin. Nutr.*, **31**, 1–291.

Ruikka, I., Sourander, L. B., and Kasanen, A.

(1967). 'The dentition of the aged in Turku in the light of a sampling study', *Suom. Hammaslääk. Toim.*, **63**, 3–10.

Sacher, G. A. (1977). 'Life table modification and life prolongation', in *Handbook of the Biology of Ageing* (Eds C. E. Finch and L. Hayflick), pp. 582–628, Van Nostrand, New York.

Scrimshaw, N. S. (1976). 'Strengths and weaknesses of the committee approach – an analysis of past and present recommended dietary allowances for protein in health and disease', *New Engl. J. Med.*, **294**, 136–142 and 198–203.

Shock, N. W. (1972). 'Energy metabolism, caloric intake and physical activity of the ageing', in *Nutrition in Old Age* (Ed. L. A. Carlsson), pp. 12–21, Symposia of the Swedish Nutrition Foundation X, Almqvist and Wiksell, Uppsala.

Shock, N. W., Watkin, D. M., Yiengst, M. J., Norris, A. H., Gaffney, G. W., Gregerman, R. I., and Falzone, J. A. (1963). 'Age differences in the water content of the body as related to basal oxygen consumption in males', *J. Gerontol.*, **18**, 1–9.

Shukla, K. K., Ellis, K. J., Dombrowski, C. S., and Cohn, S. H. (1973). 'Physiological variation of total-body potassium in man', *Am. J. Physiol.*, **224**, 271–274.

Skerlj, B., Brozek, J., and Hunt, E. E. (1953). 'Subcutaneous fat and age changes in body built and body form in women', *Am. J. Phys. Anthropol.*, **11**, 577–600.

Sköldborn, H., Arvidsson, B., and Andersson, M. (1972). 'A new whole body monitoring laboratory', *Acta. Radiol. (Suppl.)*, **313**, 233–241.

Söremark, R., and Nilsson, B. (1972). 'Dental status and nutrition in old age', in *Nutrition in Old Age* (Ed. L. A. Carlsson), pp. 147–164, Symposia of Swedish Nutrition Foundation X.

Steen, B. (1977a). 'Nutrition in 70-year-olds. Dietary habits and body composition. A report from the population study 70-year-old people in Gothenburg, Sweden', *Näringsforskning*, **21**, 201–223.

Steen, B. (1977b). 'Public health aspects in nutrition of the elderly', WHO, Copenhagen.

Steen, B. (1980). 'Intake of protein in geriatric long-term care patients', *Aktuel. Gerontol.*, **10**, 515–517.

Steen, B. (1981). 'Hypokalemia – Clinical spectrum and etiology', *Acta. Med. Scand. (Suppl.)*, **647**, 61–66.

Steen, B., Bruce, Å., Isaksson, B., Lewin, T., and Svanborg, A. (1977). 'Body composition in 70-year-old males and females in Gothenburg, Sweden. A population study', *Acta. Med. Scand. (Suppl.)*, **611**, 87–112.

Steen, B., Isaksson, B., and Svanborg, A. (1977). 'Intake of energy and nutrients and meal habits in 70-year-old males and females in Gothenburg, Sweden. A population study', *Acta. Med. Scand. (Suppl.)*, **611**, 39–86.

Steen, B., Isaksson, B., and Svanborg, A. (1979). 'Body composition at 70 and 75 years of age. A longitudinal population study', *J. Clin. Exper. Gerontol.*, **1**, 185–200 (Marcel Dekker, New York).

Steen, B., Isaksson, B., and Svanborg, A. (1981). 'Body composition at 70, 75, and 79 years of age. A longitudinal population study', *Proceedings from Twelfth International Congress of Nutrition*, San Diego, p. 102.

Steffee, W. P. (1980). 'Malnutrition in hospitalized patients', *JAMA*, **244**, 2630–2635.

Steinkamp, R. C., Cohen, N. L., Siri, W. E., Sargent, T. W., and Walsh, H. E. (1965). 'Measures of body fat and related factors in normal adults. 1. Introduction and methodology', *J. Chronic. Dis.*, **18**, 1279–1307.

Sugarman, B., and Munro, H. N. (1980). 'Altered accumulation of zinc by aging human fibroblasts in culture', *Life Sci.*, **26**, 915–920.

Svanborg, A. (1977). 'Seventy-year-old people in Gothenburg. A population study in an industrialized Swedish city. II. General presentation of social and medical conditions', *Acta. Med. Scand. (Suppl.)*, **611**, 5–37.

Tuttle, S. G., Bassett, S. H., Griffith, W. H., Mulcare, D. B., and Swendseid, M. E. (1965). 'Further observations on the amino acid requirements of older men', *Am. J. Clin. Nutr.*, **16**, 229–232.

Uyau, R., Scrimshaw, R. S., and Young, V. R. (1978). 'Human protein requirements. N-balance response to graded intakes of egg protein in elderly men and women', *Am. J. Clin. Nutr.*, **31**, 779–785.

Watkin, D. M. (1978). 'Nutrition for the ageing and the aged', in *Modern Nutrition in Health and Disease*, (Eds R. S. Goodhart and M. E. Shills), 6th ed., pp. 781–813, Lea and Febiger, Philadelphia, Pennsylvania.

Wehr, R. F., and Lewis, G. T. (1966). 'Amino acids in blood plasma of young and aged adults', *Proc. Soc. Exp. Biol. Med.*, **121**, 349–351.

Werner, I., and Hambraeus, L. (1972). 'The digestive capacity of elderly people', in *Nutrition in Old Age* (Ed. L. A. Carlsson), pp. 55–59, Almqvist and Wiksell, Uppsala.

Wiehl, D. G. (1942). 'Diets of a group of aircraft workers in southern California', *Milbank Mem. Fund. Q.*, **20**, 329–366.

Wilson, P. D. (1973). 'Enzyme changes in ageing mammals', *Gerontologia*, **19**, 79–125.

Yan, S. H. Y., and Franks, J. J. (1968). 'Albumin metabolism in elderly men and women', *J. Lab. Clin. Med.*, **72**, 449–454.

Young, V. R. (1976). 'Protein metabolism and needs in elderly people', in *Nutrition, Longevity and Ageing* (Eds M. Rockstein and M. L. Sussman), pp. 67–102, Academic Press Inc., New York.

Zanni, E., Calloway, D. H., and Zezulka, A. Y. (1979). 'Protein requirements of elderly men', *J. Nutr.*, **109**, 513–524.

11
Gastrointestinal Disease

11.1

Oral Disease

D. M. Walker

INTRODUCTION

Doctors rather than dentists have the opportunity of regularly examining the mouths of their elderly patients. For this a better source of light than that of the average battery pencil torch is recommended (that of a dental unit is ideal). A pair of dental hand mirrors serves both to illuminate the oral cavity (by reflected light) and retract the cheeks and lips. Subtle changes in the oral mucosa are better examined by drying the altered surface with a gauze square.

A systematic examination of the lips, cheeks, sulci, teeth, gingivae, floor of the mouth, the ventral and dorsal surfaces of the tongue, palate, and oropharynx in turn will ensure that early lesions are not missed. A note should be made of the fit, stability, and cleanliness of any dentures. The dentures should then be removed to disclose any inflammation of the supporting mucosa or of hyperplastic tissue at the denture periphery.

TEETH

Age Changes

A progressive yellow-brown discoloration of the teeth results from staining by extrinsic pigments from beverages, particularly tea, from tobacco, and probably from oral bacteria. Due to the deposition of secondary (posteruptive) dentine the pulp recedes from the crown and the root canal becomes narrow and thread-like. Starting at their periphery the dentinal

tubules become progressively obliterated by deposition of calcified peritubular dentine by the odontoblast processes. The roots of the teeth become increasingly translucent and brittle and tend to fracture easily during extractions.

The odontoblast layer lining the pulp chamber becomes irregular and discontinuous. The pulp tissue undergoes a patchy fibrosis and fine calcific deposits are laid down throughout the pulp or rounded pulp stones, composed of dentine, may form.

Attrition

The incisal edges and cusps, and to a lesser extent the approximal surfaces, of the teeth are worn away during chewing. On the usual soft Western diet the loss of tooth tissue is not rapid, unless the teeth are habitually ground together or clenched, often during sleep (nocturnal bruxism).

Abrasion

Misdirected and overenthusiastic horizontal toothbrushing produces substantial grooves at the necks of the teeth. Dentine exposed by this abrasion is often sensitive, toothbrushing may be inhibited, and a plaque–caries sequence initiated.

Erosion

In excess, grapefruit, lemon juice, or other soft drinks of low pH may demineralize the surface of the enamel and the underlying dentine. Eventually shallow concavities appear on the labial surfaces and incisal edges of the maxillary incisors and the characteristically imbricated enamel surface becomes smooth and thin.

By contrast, oral regurgitation of gastric acid in reflux oesophagitis will progressively dissolve the palatal surfaces of the teeth. Fillings stand proud from the eroded surface.

Dental Caries

Although new carious lesions of fissures and approximal surfaces are uncommon in the elderly, a gradual loss of interest in dental hygiene or loss of the dexterity needed for toothbrushing may lead to plaque accumulation and caries at the necks of the teeth (Baum, 1981) or tooth surfaces contacting dentures. Regular attention from a dental hygienist can have surprisingly good results in preventing or arresting caries in this situation. A 0.2% chlorhexidine mouthwash is an effective topical antibacterial agent which is a useful adjunct to mechanical measures in prevention of the accumulation of dental plaque.

GINGIVAE AND PERIODONTAL MEMBRANE

Age Changes

In most elderly people the gingivae (gums) have receded and the roots of the teeth become partially exposed. The epithelial attachment (junctional epithelium) which forms a cuff around the tooth surface below the gingival sulcus migrates apically onto the cementum during this gingival recession. Although Gottlieb (1946) considered that gingival recession was part of a physiological ageing process, it may in fact be a feature of the almost universal low-grade chronic periodontitis caused by plaque. For example, recession of the gums with age does not occur in germ free animals (Amstad-Jossi and Schroeder, 1978).

Localized Gingival Swelling (Epulis)

Partly because they usually arise in relation to standing teeth, solitary swellings of the gum or epulides are less frequent in the elderly. The fibrous epulis, a localized chronic inflammatory hyperplasia of the gingiva, is the commonest, and occurs interdentally. It is a response to an irritant such as plaque, calculus or a cavity margin. The treatment will include excision of the hyperplastic swelling and removal of the cause.

Generalized Gingival Enlargement

Generalized enlargement of the gingivae usually represents a chronic inflammatory hyperplasia induced by dental plaque, but is uncommon in the seventh or later decades.

The excessive collagen deposition in the gingival overgrowth seen in patients taking Phenytoin seems to be another type of reaction to plaque, but modified by the anticonvulsant.

Leukaemia

Leukaemic infiltration of the gingivae results in a dramatic enlargement in a matter of weeks, in contrast with the insidious increase in other types of enlargement. This clinical feature of leukaemia is more characteristic of the acute monocytic or myeloid varieties.

There are gingival haemorrhages which are spontaneous, free, and generalized, unlike the localized and limited bleeding typical of chronic gingivitis which occurs only after eating or toothbrushing. In leukaemia, mucosal purpura and ecchymoses are also commonly found, as is ulceration of the interdental gingival papillae resembling a Vincent's infection.

Scurvy

The haemorrhagic and erythematous gingivae in scurvy (Fig. 1) are probably also a form of inflammatory hyperplasia induced by plaque, conditioned by ascorbic acid deficiency. Although the body stores of vitamin C as assessed by leucocyte ascorbic acid levels are commonly diminished in the elderly (Exton-Smith and Caird, 1980), frank scorbutic gingivitis is rare, partly no doubt because most old people are edentulous.

Chronic Gingivitis and Periodontitis

After the age of 40, chronic periodontal disease is the major cause of tooth loss (Allen,

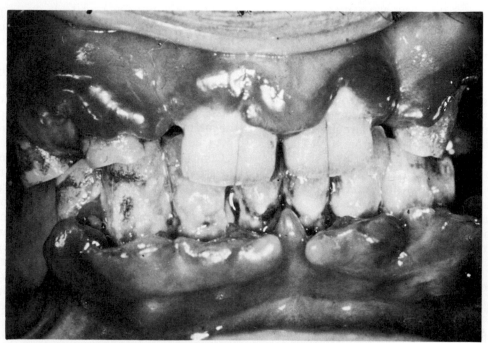

Figure 1   Gingival enlargement in scurvy. (By courtesy of Professor B. E. D. Cooke)

1944). This commences as a gingivitis initiated by the accumulation of dental plaque at the necks of the teeth. The gingivae which are normally pink and stippled and firmly applied to the teeth become darkened, oedematous, and glazed, and bleed easily. The normal shallow groove or sulcus formed by the gum at its junction with the tooth becomes pathologically deepened to form a pocket from which an inflammatory exudate slowly seeps, giving the bad taste, halitosis, and bleeding which are the characteristic and trivial symptoms of early periodontal disease. Gradually the collagen fibres of the periodontal membrane and the alveolar supporting bone may be destroyed by this inflammatory reaction to plaque until eventually the teeth may become grossly mobile, interfering with mastication. Less commonly an acute periodontal abscess may supervene.

After a detailed clinical and radiographic assessment, a long-term treatment plan can be proposed. In some older patients with gingivitis or limited degree of periodontitis, there is a good response to instruction in toothbrushing to remove plaque and a course of scaling and polishing of the teeth. Loose, painful useless teeth should be extracted. Where the retention of teeth with deep residual periodontal pockets is planned, regular scaling combined with root planing under local anaesthesia is usually preferable in the elderly to surgical elimination of the pockets by gingivectomies. Discomfort from exposed root dentine is an indication for application of an autopolymerizing resin by a dental surgeon, or home use of a toothpaste containing strontium chloride (Sensodyne).

ORAL MUCOSA

Age Changes

Epithelium

There are few studies of the age changes in the oral epithelium and the results conflict (Holm-Pedersen, 1978; Miles, 1972). Quantitative analysis does suggest that the palatal oral epithelium and its stratum corneum becomes thicker in old age despite earlier reports to the contrary (Richman and Abarbanel, 1943). Wearing dentures tends to reduce this effect. Oral epithelium may differ in its behaviour at different sites within the mouth, and the gingival epithelial cell population was found not to vary with age (Löe and Karring, 1971).

Studies of the epithelial cell kinetics of the rodent oral mucosa have concluded that epithelial turnover slows down in the elderly, with a lengthening of the mitotic cycle (Barakat, Toto, and Choukas, 1969; Karring and Löe, 1973).

Deficiencies of iron and B complex vitamins are more common in older people and are also associated with epithelial atrophy (Frantzell, Tornquist, and Waldenstrom, 1945; Miles, 1972).

Like the sense of smell, the sensitivity of taste becomes less acute in the elderly (Harris and Kalmus, 1949), for example, to sweet, sour, and bitter substances, but not to salt. This can be partly related to the reduced number of taste buds in the tongue (Jenkins, 1978).

Connective Tissue

With age, the corium of the oral mucosa becomes less cellular (Squier, Johnson, and Hackemann, 1975). The collagen of the oral mucosa is probably subject to the progressive intra- and intermolecular crosslinking which is a feature of ageing skin (Jackson, 1965) and becomes less soluble (Sams and Smith, 1965; Troy, 1968) and less elastic (Elden, 1970). If the age-associated loss of dermal collagen of the skin (Shuster and Bottoms, 1963) also affects the oral mucosa, it might explain why mastication is painful for some elderly denture wearers. The mucosal collagen undergoes degeneration, fragmentation, and hyalinization with basophilia in the elderly subjects. The ectopic sebaceous glands become larger and more numerous in the lips and cheeks of old people (Miles, 1958, 1963, 1972).

Many dilated veins resembling caviar on the ventral surface of the tongue are also common.

The foliate papillae representing leaf-like folds of the mucosa covering accumulations of lymphoid tissue (the 'lingual tonsil') on the posterolateral margins of the tongue (Simpson, 1964) are a further normal feature noticed by elderly men and women, particularly against a background of cancerophobia. Sometimes these structures enlarge during an upper respiratory tract infection, particularly in the edentulous subject, and become subsequently traumatized by ill-fitting lower dentures.

With senescence there is also an irregular atrophy of the adipose tissue of the cheeks and lips. As a result the minor labial salivary glands become more obvious and may present as 'nodules' in the lips of elderly ladies with cancerophobia.

To summarize, the histological changes in the epithelium or corium of the oral mucosa are relatively minor, and insufficient to account for the dry, burning sensation of the lips and tongue to which many elderly women are subject (see page 279).

Clinically significant degenerative changes in the skin of elderly people are only apparent in regions exposed to sunlight. The vermilion border of the lower lip is subject to solar irradiation and may become irregularly mottled as a result, due to alternating atrophy and hyperkeratosis. There is solar 'elastotic' degeneration of the collagen and the lamina propria. Crusted nodules representing solar keratoses or early invasive squamous cell carcinomas may subsequently develop and require excision, and in continuity with it the whole of the unstable vermilion border, in a 'lip-shave' operation.

INFECTIONS

Infections of the Oral Mucosa

In practice, candidosis in its various forms is the only common infection in patients aged 70 or more, in contrast to the wider range of infectious disorders in children and young adults.

Systemic Factors

The systemic factors which predispose to candidal infection have been listed by Winner and Hurley (1964), and the most important in patients over 70 years are:

(a) Dehydration
(b) Diabetes mellitus
(c) Drugs – steroids
            antibiotics
            immunosuppressive
(d) Malignant disease
(e) Anaemias, iron deficiency, neutropoenia
(f) Postoperative states

Local Factors

Local factors seem to interact importantly with these systemic influences in promoting candidal infection of the mouth (Walker *et al.*, 1981b). The wearing of complete dentures, particularly continuously, boosts oral candidal populations (Arendorf and Walker, 1979).

Smoking significantly increases the candidal carrier rate (Arendorf and Walker, 1980) and most patients with chronic hyperplastic candidosis have had a history of cigarette smoking, (see page 275) usually with a high tobacco consumption.

Salivary flow is a further local factor which influences candidal populations. Patients with xerostomia due to Sjogren's syndrome have high oral candidal populations (Tapper-Jones, Aldred, and Walker, 1980) and are susceptible to thrush (Chisholm and Mason, 1975a).

The interaction of systemic and local factors is apparent in diabetes mellitus when only patients wearing dentures, particularly continuously, had evidence of oral candidosis (Tapper-Jones, Aldred, and Walker, 1981). Surprisingly the mode of therapy, degree of diabetic control, duration of the disease, or age of onset did not affect yeast populations.

Oral candidoses may be classified as follows.

Thrush (acute pseudomembranous candidosis). The creamy white plaques, resembling milk curds, on the oral mucosa with an inflammatory surround are familiar in geriatric practice. The pseudomembrane can be easily wiped off.

Denture stomatitis (chronic atrophic candidosis). Denture stomatitis is a symptomless inflammation confined to the denture-bearing area of the palatal mucosa. It is the response to an overgrowth of *Candida albicans* in the microbial plaque colonizing the fitting surface of the maxillary prosthesis (Davenport, 1970) which is usually worn day and night (Arendorf and Walker, 1979). The yeast is transported in the saliva to the commissures where it may also initiate an angular stomatitis. The patient should not wear the dentures overnight but should instead immerse the dentures in a proprietary denture cleaner, e.g. Dentural (Walker *et al.*, 1981a).

Antibiotic sore mouth (acute atrophic candidosis). Similarly, patients developing an acute 'antibiotic sore mouth' (Lehner, 1966) after broad-spectrum antibiotic therapy are usually denture wearers. The tongue becomes sore, red, and the filiform papillae are lost, whereas the remaining fungiform papillae become prominent. In contrast, when healthy dentate volunteers are given tetracycline experimentally, there is only a brief and modest rise in oral candidal populations and candidal infection does not supervene.

Chronic hyperplastic candidosis (candidal leukoplakia) (See page 275).

Angular cheilitis. The skin lateral to the commissures is erythematous, fissured, or eroded (Fig. 2). This is most commonly due to candidal infection (MacFarlane and Helnarska, 1976) from organisms derived from the fitting surface of the upper denture (Arendorf and Walker, 1979) passing in the saliva to this site. The palatal denture-bearing mucosa is erythematous and may exhibit a nodular hyperplasia (denture stomatitis). Allergy to the acrylic resin material of the denture base, is by contrast, an extremely rare cause of maxillary denture stomatitis.

The patient should be instructed in the cleaning of the dentures and asked to remove them at night since continuous wearing favours candidal colonization of the prosthesis (Arendorf and Walker, 1979).

Old dentures in which the vertical height has been substantially reduced due to excessive wear of the teeth may contribute to angular cheilitis and a dental opinion is then advisable. Angular cheilitis may be a feature of iron deficiency anaemia in which case papillary atrophy of the tongue, particularly its lateral margins, is usually also present. Although angular stomatitis is said to be a feature of vitamin B complex or folic acid deficiency (Rose, 1971), confirmed cases are rarely encountered, although chronic folate deficiency is not uncommon in a geriatric population (DHSS, 1972).

Median rhomboid glossitis. A rhomboidal depapillated area of mucosa often irregularly keratinized develops in the midline of the dorsum of the tongue, in its middle or posterior third. It may cause intermittent soreness or more commonly is an incidental finding. It appears to be an acquired chronic oral candidosis (Cooke, 1975b) rather than, as was previously supposed, a developmental anomaly. Ampho-

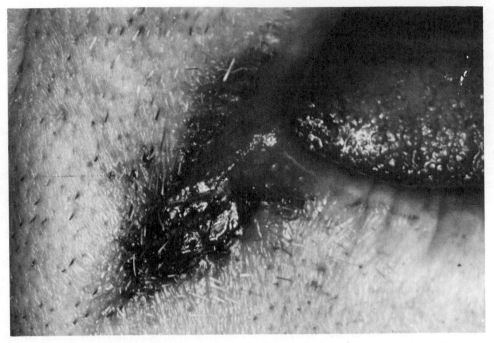

Figure 2   Angular cheilitis due to candidal infection from organisms passing in the saliva from the fitting surface of the upper denture

tericin lozenges (10 mg) dissolved orally t.d.s. will relieve any symptoms but the condition is otherwise harmless.

BLACK HAIRY TONGUE

This represents an elongation of the filiform papillae distributed about the midline of the posterior third of the tongue. The papillae become discoloured by pigment-forming bacteria and possibly by dietary constituents. The long papillae may prove nauseating or cause alarm by their unsightliness. The cause is unknown but reassurance as to the absence of any serious infection is important. The patient can remove the papillae mechanically by simply scraping with a stiff toothbrush or spoon.

ULCERATIVE AND BULLOUS LESIONS OF THE ORAL MUCOSA

The range of ulcerative and erosive conditions of late onset to affect the mouth is relatively narrow (see Table 1). Thus, acute primary herpes simplex infections for practical pur-

poses do not occur, and the common aphthous ulceration has often spontaneously remitted by the sixth decade (Cooke, 1977). Failure to recognize erosive lichen planus or mucous membrane pemphigoid presenting as recurrent 'mouth ulcers' often leads to delays in instituting the appropriate treatment.

Other bullous disorders of the elderly such as bullous pemphigoid only rarely or insignificantly affect the mouth but in the case of pemphigus vulgaris, (see Chapter 20.1) patients may present with oral "ulcers". The mouth ulcers of Behcet's syndrome first occur in the second and third decades.

Recurrent Oral Ulceration

Traumatic Ulcers

Traumatic ulcers are the most frequent. They arise in the sulci at the periphery of ill-fitting dentures or in the buccal mucosa as a result of cheek biting. The ulcers are typically shallow and shelving with an irregular or linear outline and once the local cause is eliminated, healing is swift.

Lichen Planus (see Chapter 20.1)

In oral lichen planus the basic lesions are white papules or striae forming a reticular or annular pattern on the buccal mucosa or lateral margins of the tongue, often with a bilaterally symmetrical distribution.

Other appearances, such as cotton wool patches or confluent white plaques have been described on the tongue (Cooke, 1954). The desquamative gingivitis affects the attached gingiva on its buccal or labial aspects, rather than lingual or palatal surfaces in areas where there are standing teeth. A bullous form of lichen planus is a rare variant.

In the erosive form, lichen planus may present as recurrent oral ulceration. In a series of 50 patients with oral lichen planus, only 5 had skin lesions, and most patients were women in the fifth and sixth decade of life (Cooke, 1954), whereas in 85 per cent of patients presenting with skin lesions the condition has remitted spontaneously after 18 months (Samman, 1968), men being affected more often than women. Lichen planus confined to the mouth has a different natural history. The erosive form is relatively frequent and the disorder may have a protracted course, sometimes taking 10 years to involute.

Table 1   Ulcerative and bullous conditions of the oral mucosa in the elderly

---

Recurrent oral ulceration
   Traumatic ulceration
   Lichen planus
   Drug-induced ulceration

Persistent oral ulcer
   Squamous cell carcinoma

Bullous disorders
   Mucous membrane (cicatrizing) pemphigoid
   Herpes zoster
   Pemphigus vulgaris and pemphigus vegetans
   Subepithelial haemorrhagic bullae

Occasionally the lesions heal as a white mucosal plaque (Cooke, 1975a) or as localized areas of depapillation of the tongue. It is in the erosive lichen planus in elderly women that a squamous cell carcinoma may eventually supervene, although others have questioned whether oral lichen planus does carry an increased risk of malignancy (Krutchkoff, Cu-

tler, and Laskowski, 1978). The keratinized white margins of the erosions usually serve to distinguish lichen planus from those due to mucous membrane pemphigoid. A biopsy of the intact keratinized margin will clinch the diagnosis.

In most cases no cause can be isolated, although stress, particularly a bereavement, may be followed by exacerbation (Samman, 1968). In a small minority, drugs seem to induce lichen planus. The arsenicals, gold and barbiturates, have been implicated and more recently antihypertensives such as alpha-methyl-dopa or beta-adrenergic blocking agents such as labetalol (Gange and Wilson Jones, 1978) or propanolol (Hank, 1980). Rifampicin, a more recent antituberculous drug, has been associated with the eruption, as were PAS and INAH in the past.

Reassurance that the condition is harmless is frequently all that is needed. A 2% aureomycin mouthwash for 3 days will relieve symptoms due to secondary bacterial infection in the erosive form. Topical corticosteroids may relieve the burning sensation or soreness of the involved mucosa, such as beta-methasone 17-valerate (Betnovate) in 0.1 mg pellets, dissolved orally q.d.s., or 0.1% triamcinolone in an adhesive paste (adcortyl in Orabase), or 0.05% fluocinonide in Orabase (Pimlott and Walker, 1983).

In severe forms where eating and swallowing become intolerable to the point of weight loss and the patient's life has become miserable, a limited course of systemic corticosteroids is justified, e.g. prednisone, 5 mg q.d.s. for 1 month, reducing gradually to a maintenance dose of 5 to 10 mg daily. Usually the systemic therapy can be tailed off and discontinued within 12 months.

Drug-Induced Ulceration

Ulceration confined to the lateral margins and ventral surface of the tongue, floor of mouth, and lower half of the buccal mucosa is characteristic of the erosions produced by emepronium bromide (Cetiprin) used to treat urinary incontinence and frequency (Strouthidis, Mankikar, and Irvine, 1972) in elderly, senile, or psychiatric patients who instead of swallowing the tablets allow them to dissolve in the floor of the mouth (Fig. 3). Aspirin held

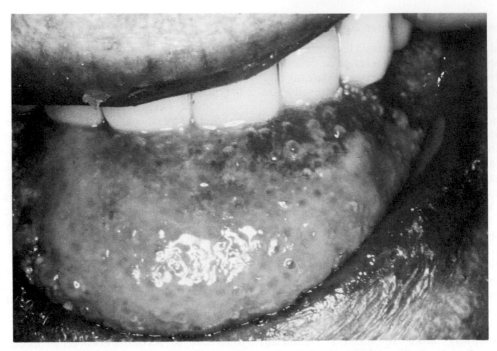

Figure 3   Ulceration of tongue induced by emepronium bromide (Cetiprin) in senile female patient

in the cheek to relieve an aching tooth also causes an erosion covered by necrotic epithelium.

Persistent Oral Ulcer

A solitary enlarging oral ulcer in the elderly persisting for more than 3 weeks despite treatment should be regarded as a squamous cell carcinoma until proved otherwise and a biopsy is mandatory.

Bullous Lesions

Mucous Membrane Pemphigoid (*Cicatricial Pemphigoid*) (see Chapter 20.1)

This is the commonest mucosal blistering disorder in the elderly. The oral mucosa is almost invariably affected and also the nasal mucosa and conjunctiva in most cases, but skin lesions affect only half the patients (Lever, 1953). Subepithelial bullae arise on the maxillary gingivae, hard and soft palate, and buccal mucosa (Fig. 4). The bullae are generally clear, tense, a few millimetres to a centimetre in diameter, and take some hours to rupture, leaving painful erosions (Cooke, 1960). Desquamative gingivitis associated with standing teeth may also be present, but the keratinizing lesions of lichen planus are absent. In severe forms, dysphagia indicates lesions of the pharynx and oesophagus and hoarseness, laryngeal involvement. An association with rheumatoid arthritis has been reported. The buccal and labial sulci become reduced in depth, particularly in the lower jaw, due to scarring resulting from the subepithelial bullae, just as the synechiae tend to obliterate the conjunctival fornix in the eye. As a consequence dentures become unstable and need frequent adjustment.

The experienced clinician can usually make the diagnosis on the clinical features but a biopsy of an intact bulla will confirm it to be subepithelial with a chronic inflammatory infiltrate in the subjacent corium. Deposits of IgG, IgA, and C3 are detectable in the basement membrane zone by direct immunofluorescent examination (Griffith *et al.*, 1974). Serum antibodies to basement membrane are generally absent (Holubar, Honigsmann, and Wolff, 1973). The treatment consists of the occasional use of a 2% aureomycin mouthwash to combat secondary infection, together with topical or systemic corticosteroids, according to the indications and regimes described for erosive lichen planus (see page 271). It is important to seek an early ophthalmic opinion in the event of ocular involvement.

Herpes Zoster

This infection due to the varicella zoster virus affects middle aged and elderly patients in particular. The sensory ganglion of the trigeminal nerve is quite often involved. After a prodromal phase of severe facial pain and cutaneous hyperaesthesia, the characteristic unilateral grouped mucocutaneous vesicles appear. The eruption develops on the skin of the cheek, lower eyelid, and lip in maxillary nerve lesions; intraorally erosions spread on the ipsilateral mucosa of the upper lip and palate as far as the midline. In mandibular division involvement, the rash is commonly situated on the skin of the chin in the distribution of the mental nerve, and intraorally on the buccal mucosa and ipsilateral half of the dorsum of the tongue. Loss of taste signals involvement of the chorda tympani and facial paralysis indicates that the geniculate ganglion is affected (the Ramsay–Hunt syndrome).

High-dose steroids, e.g. 15 mg of prednisone q.d.s. for 5 days at the outset, are effective in alleviating the pain and severity of the lesions and reducing the incidence of the severe postherpetic neuralgia or paraesthesia that afflict the elderly patient. Topical application of Herpid-S to the skin vesicles speeds healing and the pain due to secondary infection of the mouth erosions is relieved by Mysteclin syrup (10 ml) used as a mouthwash t.d.s. for 4 days or by 0.1% aqueous idoxuridine (the ophthalmic preparation) BP (10 ml) used as a mouthwash 5 times daily for 4 days. Intravenous acyclovir therapy also appears promising.

Pemphigus Vulgaris and Pemphigus Vegetans

The serious, even life threatening bullous eruption often appears in the mouth before the skin is affected. Its onset is commonly in middle age, but the geriatrician will meet patients in whom the bullae have persisted into later life. It is important to distinguish pemphigus vulgaris from other bullous or ulcerative conditions of the oral mucosa. Direct immunofluorescent examination of frozen sections of

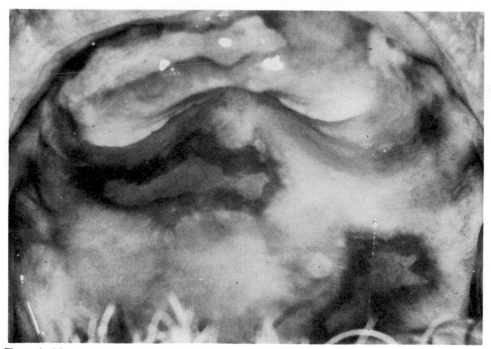

Figure 4 Mucous membrane pemphigoid (cicatricial pemphigoid) presenting as erosions of palate and gingivae

a biopsy of an intact bulla reveals IgG deposits with an intercellular distribution in the prickle cell layer. This auto antibody of the IgG class directed against the intercellular glycoprotein of normal prickle cells is also detectable in the patient's serum. Diagnosis at this stage is important in that the condition is easier to manage if corticosteroids or immunosuppressive therapy are given at an early stage. Pemphigus vegetans differs from pemphigus vulgaris in that vegetations are formed and the mucosa heals with an irregular granular surface, men are more frequently affected, and the clinical course is generally milder.

Subepithelial Haemorrhagic Bullae

Young or middle aged women are principally affected. During or shortly after eating, a haemorrhagic bulla forms rapidly in the subepithelial region of the mucosa of the soft palate or cheeks. Occasionally the palatal swellings may enlarge to the point where the patient may fear asphyxiation, but he or she soon learns to rupture the bullae with a fingernail. Without any interference, the extravasated blood soon bursts through the oral epithelium, forming a painful erosion. Mysteclin syrup (10 ml) held in the mouth for 5 minutes t.d.s. relieves soreness from secondary bacterial infection. No haemostatic defect has been identified.

DENTURE-INDUCED HYPERPLASIA

This is a benign mucosal hyperplasia induced by the irritant effect of the periphery of a denture. Leaf-like folds of hyperplastic mucosa arise, particularly in the lower labial sulcus, in relation to the margin of an overextended or unstable lower denture.

WHITE LESIONS

One third of oral keratoses arise in patients aged 60 or more (Waldron and Shafer, 1975). A keratosis (leukoplakia) may be defined as 'a white patch which cannot be characterized clinically and pathologically as any other disease' (WHO, 1978).

The white lesions of thrush, lichen planus, and aspirin burns are thus excluded by this definition.

The keratoses may be classified as follows:
(a)   Tobacco smoker's keratosis
(b)   Frictional keratosis
(c)   Tertiary syphilis
(d)   Chronic hyperplastic candidosis
(e)   Idiopathic
(f)   Sublingual keratosis

Smoker's Keratosis

Most patients presenting with oral keratoses are pipe or cigarette smokers. In a pipe smoker's keratosis umbilicated white papules stud the palate. The palatal mucosa protected by the upper denture remains unchanged. Histologically there is a keratosis of the palatal epithelium surrounding the orifices of minor salivary glands. There is no epithelial dysplasia and this is not a premalignant lesion (Pindborg, 1980). If the patient stops smoking, the mucosa generally returns to normal within a year (Roed-Petersen and Pindborg, 1980).

In cigarette smokers, the buccal mucosa is principally affected and has a diffuse white sheen, except where protected by the teeth.

Frictional Keratosis

A frictional keratosis is a linear white lesion in the occlusal plane in the cheeks and lips or lateral margins of the tongue. There may be an obvious occlusal error in a denture or a jagged natural tooth. Smoking often seems to be a co-irritant. If the sources of trauma is dealt with, the mucosa returns to normal. Histologically there is a parakeratosis or hyperkeratosis confined to the superficial layers of the epithelium, without epithelial dysplasia (Rushton, Cooke, and Duckworth, 1972).

Tertiary Syphilis

A syphilitic glossitis is one of the oral manifestations of tertiary syphilis. The tongue is blunt and fibrosed and feels like a 'bladder of lard'. The normal papillae of the anterior dorsum are characteristically replaced by areas of keratosis and atrophy. This field change of the mucosa is followed in up to 19 per cent of cases (Nielsen, 1942) by squamous cell carcinomas which are often multiple.

Although penicillin injections are often hopefully administered, there is no evidence that this alters the natural history of the tertiary oral lesions.

Chronic Hyperplastic Candidosis (Candidal Leukoplakia)

Cawson (1966, 1969) showed that a high proportion of leukoplakias with histological evidence of candidal infiltration underwent carcinomatous change. Clinically these appear as speckled white plaques at the commissures of the tongue or palate which are firmer than, and often slightly depressed below, the surrounding mucosa (Fig. 5). In addition to the candidal hyphae in the superficial epithelial layers, there is acanthosis and epithelial dysplasia of the stratum spinosum and a chronic inflammatory infiltrate in the corium. The treatment is excision or cryotherapy and anticandidal therapy.

Idiopathic

White plaques without an obvious cause such as tobacco smoking more frequently undergo malignant transformation.

Sublingual Keratoses

These are supple, wrinkled, white plaques on the ventral surface of the tongue or the floor of the mouth, often symmetrically distributed about the midline. Kramer, El-Labban, and Lee (1978) observed that these lesions which are usually banal histologically have an unexpectedly high rate of malignant transformation.

ERYTHROPLAKIA

This bright red velvety mucosal plaque is an uncommon but sinister lesion which is disproportionately frequent in older patients. It is often asymptomatic and detected during a routine examination of the mouth. Squamous cell cancer can be a complication in as many as 50 per cent of cases (Shafer, 1975; Shafer and Waldron, 1975).

SUMMARY

The management of the individual elderly patient presenting with an oral keratosis requires

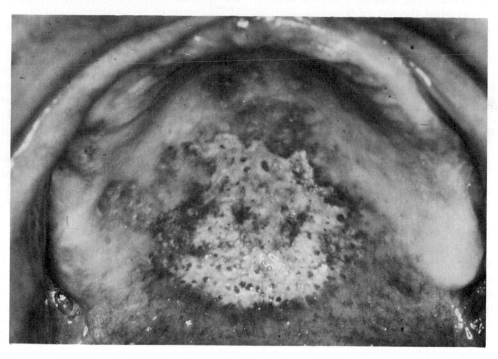

Figure 5   Fenestrated appearance of chronic hyperplastic candidosis (candidal leukoplakia) in a diabetic woman who was a cigarette smoker and wore dentures

some thought. In large-scale studies, 2 to 6 per cent progress to a cancer over 10 years (Banoczy, 1977; Einhorn and Wersall, 1967; Silverman *et al.*, 1976). However, a carcinoma occurred in 7.5 per cent of patients aged 70 to 89 years, whereas in patients under 50 years of age the corresponding value was 1 per cent. Speckled leukoplakias, sublingual keratoses, and white plaques on the tongue are more sinister. A biopsy should be performed since the presence and severity of epithelial dysplasia does have some value in predicting the risk of an oral cancer with the exception of sublingual keratoses. Any dysplastic lesions and all sublingual keratoses should be excised or removed by cryotherapy.

ORAL CANCER

Incidence

Although oral cancer accounts for only 2 per cent of malignant tumours registered in the United Kingdom, approximately half of the patients registered died from the disease (Binnie *et al.*, 1972). The incidence of oral cancer rises steeply after the age of 50 years, and 70 per cent of patients presenting with cancer of the tongue are over 65 years. The relationship between the log rate and log age is linear. Males are affected more often than females but the difference in incidence between the sexes has become less pronounced in recent years, due to a more marked downward trend in men than women.

Aetiology

Tobacco, alcohol, syphilis, and possibly iron deficiency may be aetiological factors in oral cancer. Wynder and Stellman (1977) demonstrated a relationship between the tobacco consumption of cigar and pipe smokers and the risk of oral cancer. Although Doll and Hill (1964a, 1964b) found that cigarette smokers developed cancer of the mouth more frequently than non-smokers, they pointed out that the mortality from oral cancer fell by 36 per cent between 1942 and 1962, a period in which tobacco consumption rose, and deaths from lung cancer increased by 325 per cent.

Heavy alcohol consumption is associated with a tenfold increase in the incidence of oral carcinoma (Graham, *et al*, 1977; Wynder, Bross, and Feldman, 1957); and alcohol and tobacco consumption seem to combine to accelerate the onset of the tumour (Bross and Coombs, 1976; Feldman *et al.*, 1975; Fortier, 1975). That the association between alcohol and oral cancer may be indirect is suggested by the recent decline in frequency in oral cancer at a time when alcoholism is becoming more prevalent.

Syphilis seems to be an aetiological factor in a minority of oral cancers, particularly of the tongue (Fry, 1929; Levin, Kress, and Goldstein, 1942; Wynder, Bross, and Feldman, 1957), although the number of patients with cancer of the mouth who have positive serological reactions is low in contemporary practice.

Iron Deficiency

Although the Patterson–Kelly (Plummer–Vinson) syndrome does carry a material risk of a postcricoid carcinoma, the reported association between iron deficiency and cancer of the mouth (Ahlbohm, 1936; Wynder *et al.*, 1957) seems to be weaker.

Clinical Appearances of Oral Cancer

On the lower lip, a persistent crusted lesion of the vermilion border, often superimposed on a diffuse solar cheilosis, should be regarded as a squamous cell carcinoma until proved otherwise, and the diagnosis established histologically.

Within the mouth, most carcinomas arise in a horseshoe area comprising the lateral margins of the tongue (Saxena, 1970), floor of mouth, mandibular alveolus, and lower buccal sulcus. The tumour may appear as a raised nodule (Fig. 6), an ulcer with indurated margins, or an indurated or fissured white plaque. It should be stressed that limitation of tongue movements, severe pain, trismus, and lymph node involvement are all late signs.

A biopsy should be performed if there is any doubt as to the nature of the lesion. Unrecognized oral cancers are still treated with topical medicaments or antibiotics for long periods with distressing consequences. The patient's fear of the treatment is one reason why they

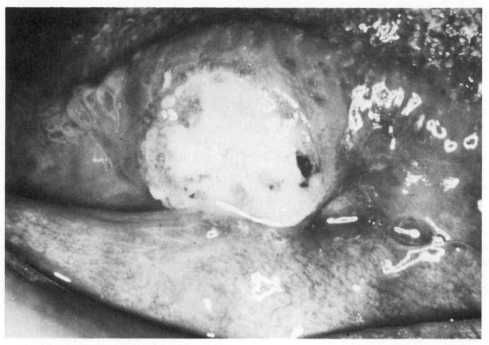

Figure 6 Squamous cell carcinoma presenting as an ulcerated swelling of the lateral margin of the tongue

delay consulting their doctor or dentist, often until the tumour is advanced or inoperable (Williams, 1973). Most patients are edentulous and elderly and have long ceased to attend a dentist regularly (Pogrel, 1974). Long delays before elderly patients presenting with oral cancer were referred to hospital by their medical and dental practitioners have been documented by Cooke and Tapper-Jones (1977).

The prognosis for oral cancer depends largely upon the stage (i.e. size of tumour and evidence of metastases) at presentation and its site (Binnie *et al.*, 1972).

Spread to the submental submandibular and subsequently to the jugular or other cervical lymph nodes takes place relatively late in the natural history of oral cancer and has an adverse effect on survival (Blady, 1971; Kalnins *et al.*, 1977; Spiro *et al.*, 1974). Distant metastases, e.g. to the lung, do occur but are less common (Castigliano and Rominger, 1954).

The site of the cancer is the other important prognostic factor in oral malignancy. Whereas most elderly patients with lip cancer are cured of their disease, cancer of the tongue is fatal in 8 out of 10 cases (Binnie *et al.*, 1972). Whereas most lip tumours are diagnosed at an early stage, presumably due to their conspicuousness, most intraoral cancers in the elderly are advanced (Williams, 1981) and the prospects for survival correspondingly worsened. Other prognostic factors such as the sex of the patient, histological grading, and method of treatment are less important.

Treatment

Oral cancer is treated by surgery or radiotherapy or a combination, with additionally in some cases chemotherapy using bleomycin or *cis*-diaminedicholorplatinum (*cis*-DDP).

Elderly patients with oral cancer fare appreciably worse in terms of survival from the disease compared with younger patients with TNM matched tumours. That potentially curative surgery or radiotherapy may sometimes be refused by the older patient or withheld in view of the patient's age might be a reason for this poorer prognosis.

THE JAWS

Age Changes

The structure and size of the alveolar processes of the jaws are dependent upon the presence of the teeth which they support. The alveolar bone forms as the teeth develop and erupt and is resorbed after extractions. If the periodontal tissues remain healthy, the alveolar bone loss with age is minimal. Conversely, progressive periodontal disease results in loss of the alveolar bone supporting the teeth (Boyle, Via, and McFall, 1973). As in other bones, the jaws of the elderly participate in any generalized osteoporosis (Atkinson and Woodhead, 1968; Manson and Lucas, 1962; Von Wowern and Stoltze, 1980) and the resorption of alveolar bone in an individual will reflect the net effect of both local and systemic factors.

Swellings of the Jaws

Due to Irregular Alveolar Resorption after Extractions

Uneven resorption after extractions results in an irregular contour of the edentulous alveolus. Patients may misinterpret the resulting prominences as being due to neoplasms, retained roots, or unerupted teeth. Particularly in the mandible, this loss of alveolar bone can result in instability of dentures. Surgical procedures such as grafting bone from the iliac crest or rib cartilage, or deepening the sulci with skin grafts, do improve the stability of prostheses but preprosthetic surgery in patients aged over 70 years is not to be undertaken lightly.

Unerupted Teeth, Roots, and Cysts

There is usually a dental cause, e.g. a dental abscess or a cyst, for swellings of the jaws, whatever the time of life. In the elderly edentulous subject presenting with a swelling of the alveolus causing a loss of fit of dentures, a radiograph will often reveal a residual dental cyst or an unerupted tooth, sometimes with an associated dentigerous cyst. Unerupted teeth tend to become more superficial due to the gradual resorption of the overlying denture-bearing alveolar bone. Secondary bacterial infection of the surrounding soft tissues ensues when communication of the tooth with the mouth is established. Frequent mouthbaths with a 0.2% chlorhexidine mouthwash (Corsodyl), a course of penicillin V (250 mg q.d.s. for 5 days), and a simple analgesic such as paracetamol should be prescribed and the patient instructed not to wear their denture meanwhile. After at least 2 weeks, the tooth should be removed.

Retained roots may become exposed and require removal, but asymptomatic roots buried deeply in the jaws are common incidental radiographic findings (Ritchie, 1973) and can be left, unless there is evidence of cyst formation.

Ameloblastoma

This locally invasive tumour of odontogenic epithelium arises centrally in the jaws, particularly in the third molar region or angle of the mandible. It may present as a swelling or cause a loss of fit of a denture. A multilocular radiolucency is the characteristic X-ray appearance although some tumours are monolocular. The ameloblastoma typically presents at the age of 40 years, but older patients can be affected. Since recurrences after removal take up to 10 years to develop, the removal of ameloblastomas in elderly patients can be more conservative than the wide resection of the jaws which is usual for younger subjects.

Paget's Disease

This osteodystrophy is present in approximately 1 per cent of the population aged 61 years or more (Monroe, 1951). It involves the facial skeleton in a minority of cases and the maxilla is more often affected than the mandible in both the polyostotic and also the rare monostotic forms of the disease (Stafne and Austin, 1938). The calvarium of the skull is a frequent site for the lesions of Paget's disease and the enlargement imparts an inverted triangle shape to the head (Cooke, 1956).

In the jaws, pain and facial deformity are the usual presenting features. The maxilla is usually diffusely enlarged with a tendency to obliteration of the vault of the palate, palatal tilting of the teeth, or loss of fit of dentures. The covering gingivae may be hyperaemic.

In the resorptive phase, the lesion is radio-lucent (e.g the osteoporosis circumscripta of the calvarium) (Rushton, 1948) but the cotton wool patches representing subsequent sclerosis are a commoner radiographic finding. The lamina dura around the teeth may be lost (Cahn, 1951). The usual trabecular structure of the bone is replaced by a coarse fibrillar pattern (Cooke, 1956).

A craggy hypercementosis of the teeth in regions of the jaws affected by long standing Paget's disease may make extractions difficult (Fox, 1933).

Severe infection of the sockets may follow extractions in sclerotic areas in elderly patients, whereas postextraction haemorrhage is a feature in the vascular osteoporotic phase in younger subjects.

Calcitonin injections give some relief of pain in Paget's disease. Diphosphonates such as sodium etidronate have become the standard treatment.

Sarcoma is an extremely rare complication of jaw lesions (Barry, 1969). Cardiac failure is only seen in the polyostotic type of Paget's disease.

SALIVARY GLAND DISORDERS

Age Changes in Salivary Function

Studying autopsy material, Waterhouse and coworkers (1973) demonstrated that a mean 25 per cent of the secretory parenchyma of major salivary gland tissue is replaced by fat and fibrous tissue in old people. Some of the epithelial cells become enlarged and their cytoplasm becomes granular and eosinophilic. Such cells have been termed oncocytes (Batsakis, 1979).

Clinical measurements of salivary secretion have generally shown a corresponding decline in salivary secretion with age (Bertram, 1967; Meyer and Necheles, 1940), although Chisholm and Mason (1975a,b) found that this only applied to female subjects.

The wide range of salivary flow rates in the general population makes it difficult to demonstrate reduced salivary function in individual patients complaining of a dry mouth unless the xerostomia is virtually complete.

The Dry Mouth

Idiopathic

A dry burning sensation of the lips or mouth is a common and distressing complaint in elderly people. The salivary flow rates usually prove to be normal and the oral mucosa is clinically healthy.

Cooke (1972) suggested that this dry burning sensation resulted from atrophy of the oral mucosa but no supporting histological evidence is available.

Although this complaint is most common in the postmenopausal female, a recent study by Ferguson and coworkers. (1981) suggests that hormonal factors are not in fact involved. Women who had had bilateral oophorectomy were treated with oestrogen or placebo. Symptoms of dryness or burning of the mouth did not respond to the hormonal replacement. The presence or absence of these symptoms was instead found to correlate with the degree of neurosis. The complaint of a dry mouth seems to be a symptom of the anxiety and depression common in advanced age rather than of a reduced production of saliva.

Dehydration

Dryness of the mouth is a feature of undiagnosed diabetes mellitus but more often marks the terminal stages of senility when patients cease to take adequate amounts of fluid, sometimes from apathy or to loss of the neuromuscular coordination required for drinking and swallowing. A feeding cup may be helpful but sometimes the decision has to be taken as to whether the patient should be admitted to hospital and intravenous fluid replacement instituted.

Smoking

Some of the patients referred with a xerostomia are heavy smokers. The roughened texture of the oral mucosa exhibiting a smoker's keratosis of the epithelium (see above) may be responsible for the sensation of a dry mouth but there is no evidence that smoking directly affects salivary flow in the long term.

In the majority of patients who can be persuaded to stop smoking, the keratosis is reversible and the mucosa returns to normal after 1 year (Roed-Petersen and Pindborg, 1980). The patient whose smoking habit has persisted into old age is more resistant to advice to stop smoking.

Drug-Induced Xerostomia

Antidepressants, antihypertensives, or antihistamines are the three common causes of drug-induced xerostomia. Of the antidepressants, tricyclic preparations such as chlorpromazine can inhibit salivation although this drug has largely been superseded in contemporary psychiatric practice.

Alpha-methyldopa (Aldomet), although useful in the treatment of hypertension, has the disadvantage of causing xerostomia. Beta-adrenergic blocking drugs such as practolol used to treat hypertension and angina may occasionally inhibit salivary secretion. Besides the xerostomia, a further adverse effect of practolol was a serious keratoconjunctivitis sicca, leading to corneal perforation and blindness, and less frequently retroperitoneal fibrosis and pleural fibrosis (Wright, 1975). There are reports of occasional similar oculomucocutaneous reactions to other Beta-blocking agents such as oxprenolol (Holt and Waddington, 1975) and propanolol (Cubey and Taylor, 1975).

Antihistamine drugs such as chlorpheniramine (Piriton) can also cause some dryness of the mouth.

Few objective studies of the effect of drugs on salivary flow have been reported but the subjective reaction of patients to the same drug seems to be very individual. Secondly, with time, patients become largely acclimatized to the xerostomia. The effect on salivary flow is dose-dependent and only a few patients experience troublesome dryness of the mouth with the above drugs at the lower end of the therapeutic range, but at a high dose virtually all patients complain of the xerostomia.

Sjögren's Syndrome

Sjögren's syndrome (Sjögren, 1933) is a triad of keratoconjunctivitis sicca, xerostomia, and in most cases rheumatoid arthritis or another connective tissue disorder. Two out of the three major components are considered sufficient for the diagnosis (Bloch *et al.*, 1965). The term 'sicca syndrome' (primary sicca syndrome) is reserved for cases with only dryness of the eyes and mouth. The aetiology of Sjögren's syndrome is not understood, but studies of the HLA phenotype of patients indicate that genetic factors are involved (Moutsopoulos *et al.*, 1979).

Although a few cases of Sjögren's syndrome present over the age of 70 years (Bloch *et al.*, 1965), most elderly patients with this disorder have had symptoms since middle age.

As in any severe xerostomia, the patient complains of difficulty in swallowing solids, in speaking, aberrations in taste, and the sheer discomfort of the parchment-like mucosa.

A bilateral angular cheilitis is a common finding. The dorsum of the tongue is atrophic and subdivided by fissures giving a cobblestone appearance (Hadden, 1888). The usual pool of saliva in the floor of the mouth is absent, and the mucosa of the cheeks is smooth and glazed and readily adheres to instruments. Isolated beads of mucus may stand out on the mucosa of the soft palate. There is widespread caries, affecting the cervical margins of the teeth or at unusual sites such as incisal edges (Fig. 7). Candidal infections of the mouth are frequent (MacFarlane and Mason, 1974; Tapper-Jones, Aldred, and Walker, 1980). Dentures become unstable. The major salivary glands, most noticeably the parotid glands, may be persistently enlarged in approximately half the patients (Bloch *et al.*, 1965). Typically the swelling is firm, diffuse, and bilateral.

Alternatively, some patients experience intermittent painful swellings of the parotid gland which subside spontaneously within a few days. These acute swellings often represent ascending bacterial infections of the secretory ducts.

Measurement of the stimulated parotid flow rate appears to be the most sensitive method for detection of salivary hyposecretion in Sjögren's syndrome (Chisholm and Mason, 1973). A labial salivary gland biopsy will show replacement of secretory acini by a lymphocytic and plasma cell infiltrate (Chisholm and Mason, 1968) and sialography is also useful diagnostically (Bloch *et al.*, 1965).

Rarely the inflammatory infiltrate of the salivary glands is generalized to involve regional and other lymph nodes, lung, kidneys, spleen,

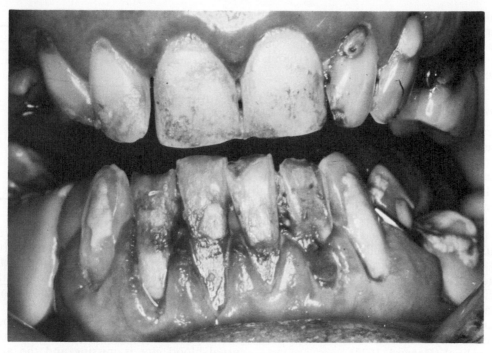

Figure 7   Caries in Sjögren's syndrome. Increased susceptibility to caries in a patient with Sjögren's syndrome affecting cervical margins of teeth

bone marrow, muscle, or liver (Anderson and Talal, 1971). The term 'pseudo-lymphoma' has been applied to this extraglandular lymphoproliferation. Malignant lymphomas have also been described (Anderson and Talal, 1971; Azzopardi and Evans, 1971; Batsakis *et al.*, 1975).

The ophthalmic diagnosis is made on a subnormal Schirmer test result (Schirmer, 1903), rose bengal staining of the conjunctiva (Duke-Elder, 1965), and slit lamp examination to detect punctate or filamentary keratitis, the most satisfactory test (Buchanan *et al.*, 1976).

The serum autoantibodies to salivary gland duct epithelium found in some patients with Sjögren's syndrome (Bertram and Halberg, 1964; Halberg *et al.*, 1965; MacSween *et al.*, 1967) are not specific for that disease. A wide array of other autoantibodies has been detected (Buchanan *et al.*, 1976; Bunim *et al.*, 1964; Whaley *et al.*, 1973).

Associated connective tissue disorders. Instead of rheumatoid arthritis, systemic lupus erythematosus (Morgan, 1954), systemic sclerosis (Schaposnik, Bergna, and Conti, 1956), po-

lyarteritis nodosa, and dermatomyositis (Bloch *et al.*, 1965) may be present in Sjögren's syndrome.

The wide-ranging other features occasionally found in Sjögren's syndrome are reviewed by Shearn (1971).

Management of Sjögren's syndrome. Hypromellose (1%) eye drops alleviate the xerophthalmia of Sjögren's syndrome. The problem of replacing the normal 1500 ml daily salivary secretion for a patient with severe xerostomia has not yet been solved. Artificial substitutes for saliva have not been very successful. A simple preparation combining a sialogogue with a lubricant which helps a few patients is as follows:

Citric acid, 4.5 g
Lemon essence, 1 ml
Saccharin solution, 0.5 ml
Carboxymethylcellulose '5000', 1% to 100 ml

but many patients revert to taking frequent sips of water. Lemon sweets stimulate any residual salivary secretion.

Topical fluoride applications to the teeth and regular scaling, polishing and instruction in effective toothbrushing are important in combating the severe caries in profound xerostomia.

Postirradiation Xerostomia

Salivary glands involved by radiotherapy for malignant disease of the head and neck may undergo atrophy and fibrosis of the secretory parenchyma and a temporary xerostomia results. If a patient is still dentate, an unusual form of dental caries may occur, the decay characteristically encircling the necks of the teeth (Frank, Herdly, and Philippe, 1965). Careful toothbrushing and stannous fluoride gel (0.4%) applied topically can prevent this postirradiation caries in cooperative patients.

Radiation can also impair healing of the jaws, especially the mandible, and extractions or even mild trauma from a denture may be complicated by osteoradionecrosis (radiation osteomyelitis) (Regaud, 1922).

'Excessive Saliva'

Middleaged and elderly patients may complain that they are producing excessive amounts of saliva. Hypersalivation may occur as a response to wearing dentures for the first time but is usually short lived. Prolonged ptyalism may be an adverse reaction in iodism or after parasympathominetic or other drugs, or in poisoning by mercury (and mercurial diuretics) or other heavy metals (see the review by Chisholm and Mason, 1975b).

In most patients complaining of 'excessive saliva', the salivary flow rates are within normal limits. The affected individual seems to have become overaware of what is in fact a normal volume of saliva but does not swallow it as usual. This seems to be an obsessional trait and explanations and reassurances as to the mechanism are usually unavailing.

FACIAL PAIN

Dental Causes

As in younger subjects, a carious tooth is the commonest cause of facial pain (Table 2). Ex-

Table 2 Facial Pain

1. Dental causes
     Dental caries and periodontal disease
     Infected sockets
     Retained roots, unerupted teeth
     Jaw cysts
2. Temporomandibular joint pain
3. Trigeminal neuralgia
4. Postherpetic neuralgia
5. Periodic migrainous neuralgia
6. Giant cell arteritis
7. Myocardial ischaemia
8. Ocular causes
9. Atypical (psychogenic) facial pain
10. Trotter's syndrome

acerbation of the pulpitis by hot or cold drinks is characteristic. A transient hypersensitivity to thermal or osmotic stimuli (e.g. sweet substances) can be due to dentine exposed at the necks of the teeth by toothbrush abrasion or periodontal disease.

The pain of an infected socket may be very severe and continuous. On examination the usual blood clot is missing and the alveolar bone lining the socket is exposed. Unerupted teeth, jaw cysts, and retained roots are painful only when secondary bacterial infection has supervened due to communication with the mouth becoming established.

Temporomandibular Joint Pain

Pain from the temporomandibular joint is a frequent symptom in old people according to Agerberg and Osterberg (1974). These workers found radiographic evidence of erosion, flattening, lipping, and other degenerative changes and features of osteoarthrosis of this joint. Toller (1974) delineated two groups of patients complaining of pain from the temporomandibular joint in a clinical, radiographic, and histological study. Mandibular condyles with the microscopic and radiological features of osteoarthrosis were encountered more often over the age of 40 years (Ogus and Toller, 1981) whereas in young women with similar pain and spasm of the masseter and pterygoid muscles, there were no abnormal histological or positive X-ray findings and the condition is known as the pain–dysfunction syndrome. In this younger group, the study of Feinmann and Harris (1984) showed a positive response to antidepressants, but not to wearing a simple splint over the teeth. This suggests that much of the pain is psychogenic. A study by Fine (1971) showing that the same group were more neurotic than were control subjects is consistent with this hypothesis.

Occlusal factors may play a part in some cases of temporomandibular joint pain. Some patients lack posterior teeth or have old dentures with a reduced vertical dimension. The provision of satisfactory full or partial dentures to restore the occlusion is still a wise measure. A simple explanation, a soft diet, and some jaw exercises are often sufficient. For a few middle aged or elderly patients fulfilling the criteria for osteoarthrosis of the temporomandibular joint who do not respond to the conservative measures, condylectomy on the affected side brings relief. Two-thirds of the patients suffering from rheumatoid arthritis have evidence of temporomandibular joint involvement but presentation with pain and crepitus from this site are usually due to secondary degenerative changes arising after many years of the disease (Ogus and Toller, 1981). Erosion of the anterior and superior articular surface with subarticular pseudo-cysts is the characteristic radiographic change (Ogus, 1975).

Trigeminal Neuralgia (see page 657)

The patient is usually over 50 years of age at presentation (Harris, 1952). The diagnosis is made on the history in the absence of any physical signs. More females are affected than males. The patient complains of a paroxysmal pain of frightening intensity, arresting any activity. The pain is usually brief (less than 2 minutes) and confined to one or more divisions of the trigeminal nerve, most commonly both the maxillary and mandibular divisions (Penman, 1968). It is almost invariably unilateral, particularly affecting the right side of the face. The pain may be provoked by washing or towelling the skin of the face or eating (Harris, 1940). It may occur several times daily for weeks or months and then remit spontaneously only to recur with greater severity with increasingly brief remissions. Carbamazepine (Tegretol) or phenytoin form the treatment of choice. Occasionally patients cannot tolerate these drugs or develop a blood dyscrasia. For these and for a minority for whom the pain becomes uncontrollable, even at high doses of drugs,

surgical management by alcohol injection, avulsion, or cryotherapy of the peripheral nerve affords relief in most cases and only rarely is injection of the Gasserian ganglion or injection or division of its sensory root required nowadays in the author's experience. Selective radiofrequency electrocoagulation appears promising.

Usually some years after onset of the disease, 3 to 4 per cent. of patients with multiple sclerosis will develop trigeminal neuralgia. Compression of the trigeminal nerve will produce facial pain, e.g. by trigeminal neurinoma, acoustic neurinoma, basilar and other arterial malformations, or cerebellopontine angle tumours in general, but the pain rarely resembles true trigeminal neuralgia (Graham, 1976).

In unusual cases, the bone changes of Paget's disease may give rise to pain simulating trigeminal neuralgia.

Postherpetic Neuralgia

This is particularly distressing to the elderly who may become depressed to the point of contemplating suicide. It is a common sequel to herpes zoster infection of the ophthalmic division of the trigeminal nerve. On examination there may be atrophic scars from the eruption with a segmental distribution. The skin is hyperaesthetic or dysaesthetic. Application of vibrators or freezing sprays may help some patients. Reassurance that the prognosis is good and prescription of adequate analgesics is sufficient for most. Prednisone or amantidine therapy combined with local application of topical idoxuridine to the vesicles in the first 4 days of the eruption help to prevent or reduce the incidence and pain of postherpetic neuralgia.

Periodic Migrainous Neuralgia (Cluster Headache)

There may be an ipsilateral lacrimation and conjunctival injection and nasal stuffiness. The pain is usually felt in or around the orbit. Young males are predominantly affected. The pain lasts for up to 2 hours. It tends to occur late at night or in the early hours of the morning, in a regular manner, daily for several weeks or months, and then remits for months, only to recur (Harris, 1926). This clustering of attacks in time is a useful diagnostic feature.

Giant Cell Arteritis

Middle aged or elderly patients are affected (see Chapter 25.1). They usually present with a headache but alternatively pain confined to the face may be a symptom of involvement of the temporal or facial branches of the external carotid artery. The pulses are typically absent and tender nodular thickenings may be palpable along the course of the vessel. Alternatively, the lumen of the affected artery may be merely narrowed and pain during mastication results from the ischaemia of masseter and temporalis muscles. The patient looks ill and there may be an associated weight loss and anorexia. The ESR is usually significantly elevated. There is a good response to systemic prednisone therapy. Sudden blindness which is sometimes bilateral can follow ophthalmic artery involvement and an early ophthalmic opinion is advisable in all cases of giant cell arteritis.

Myocardial Ischaemia

Although pain of cardiac origin may radiate to the mandible, it is very rare for the pain to be confined to the jaw.

Ocular Causes

In acute glaucoma, the pain is felt in the globe of the eye itself and visual disturbances, photophobia, and lacrimation are usual. The eye is characteristically red, hard, and tender to palpation.

Atypical Facial Pain

The patients are usually middle aged or elderly women. The complaint is of a continuous diffuse pain affecting both jaws, spreading across the midline (unlike toothache), and is not confined to the territory of any of the branches of the trigeminal nerve. The pain, however, does not usually keep the patient awake or interfere with daily activities and can be described by the patient with a composed or even cheerful facial expression. Often previous dental treatment such as extractions is blamed. Mastication or taking cold or hot sweet foods have no effect on the pain in contrast to that from pulpitis. Clinically and radiographically there are no abnormalities in the mouth, teeth, or jaws. Often the patient has had a clearance because of the pain. In many patients there are features of anxiety and depression (Lascelles, 1966) or of an obsessional trait (Harris, 1974). Treatment with a psychotropic drug, particularly antidepressants, e.g. prothiaden (Feinmann and Harris, 1984) or amitryptiline, is beneficial but the relapse rate is high (Rudge, 1979). Requests for the extraction of sound teeth should be resisted.

Trotter's Syndrome

Pain from a nasopharyngeal carcinoma may be referred to the mandibular or maxillary divisions of the trigeminal nerve. An ipsilateral conductive deafness and immobility of the soft palate and an enlarged cervical lymph node are characteristic of the syndrome.

DENTAL CARE OF THE ELDERLY

General Considerations

Most British people aged 65 or more are edentulous (Beal and Dowell, 1977; Grey *et al.*, 1970) and complaints referable to the mouth often originate from the patients' dentures. These prostheses are erroneously regarded by their wearers as being permanent fixtures designed to last the rest of the patient's life. Once rendered edentulous, the habit of regular dental attendance is usually lost and thus many oral lesions in old people are unfortunately advanced and early detection of oral cancer in this age group is the exception (Williams, 1981).

Since mastication with dentures is considerably less efficient than with natural teeth, complete denture wearers may choose a diet rich in carbohydrate which requires a minimum of mastication (Neill, 1961, 1965). However, Bates, Elwood, and Foster (1971) did not find that an unsatisfactory dentition in the elderly was associated with any nutritional deficiencies.

The dental treatment of old people poses particular problems (Lawental and Meisel, 1983). Brittle, broken-down teeth, often with gross abrasion and attrition, are more difficult to restore satisfactorily, the more so because few elderly patients can tolerate lengthy sessions in the dental chair. A significant proportion have difficulty in visiting a dentist because of transport problems or because they are bedridden or confined to a wheelchair and cannot manage the stairs or steps of a dentist's premises. Many dentists will provide treatment on a domiciliary basis, however. The cost of dental treatment is another reason why some old people may not seek dental care (Council on Dental Health and Health Planning, Osborne *et al.*, 1979). Others are simply afraid of dental treatment (Fløystrand *et al.*, 1982).

Until recently, only the exceptional patient has attended regularly for dental treatment into old age and hopelessly neglected dentitions with carious exposure of the pulp and mobile teeth encrusted with calculus and plaque in the final stages of periodontal disease are only too common (Fig. 8). Such dental remnants are often surprisingly painless and the enthusiastic eradication of all dental disease is usually inappropriate. A dental clearance is both taxing and unpleasant for the older patient. There is also anxiety that the present

trend to retaining some natural teeth until later life (Beal and Dowell, 1977) will carry aged patients beyond the point where the new muscle skills required to wear dentures can be learnt (Brill, Tryde, and Schübeler, 1960).

Medical Disorders and Drug Interactions

The medical disorders which commonly affect old people will influence their dental treatment. Cardiovascular diseases, cerebrovascular disease, asthma, and obstructive airways disease are common and local anaesthesia for dental treatment is preferable to general anaesthesia where possible. Local anaesthetics containing the vasoconstrictor felypressin have no adverse effects and are as effective as those with noradrenaline or adrenaline which carry at least a theoretical risk for these patients. Adequate sedation, with, for example, oral diazepam, is important before dental treatment for the anxious cardiac patient. For patients with a history of rheumatic fever, congenital heart disease, or cardiac surgery, an oral dose of 3 g of amoxycillin is recommended as a prophylaxis against infective endocarditis to be administered 1 hour before procedures

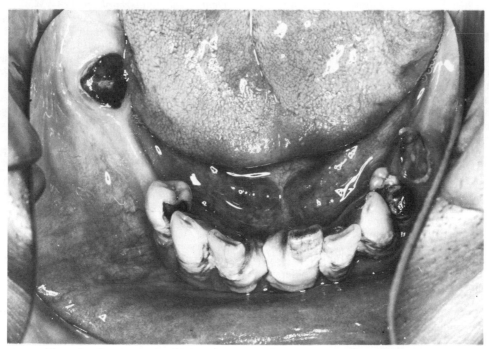

Figure 8   Gross caries, calculus deposits, and gingival recession in an elderly patient

likely to cause a bacteraemia, e.g. scaling, extractions, or root canal treatment (Oakley and Darrell, 1981).

Dental treatment is also complicated by the drug therapy of the elderly patient.

Those who have taken corticosteroids over the previous 2 years may have adrenocortical suppression and a booster intravenous injection of hydrocortisone immediately prior to dental treatment is advisable, even in patients on low doses of steroids.

Elderly patients taking cytotoxic or immunosuppressive therapy are at increased risk from infections following surgical procedures in the mouth. A full blood count and platelet count should be performed immediately prior to any oral surgery to exclude a drug-induced anaemia, neutropoenia, or thrombocytopaenia and most dental surgeons prescribe antibiotics prior to extractions or other surgical procedure in the immunocompromised. In patients taking anticoagulants who need extractions, the dose of anticoagulants will have to be reduced until the prothrombin time (BCR) is sufficiently reduced to avoid a postextraction haemorrhage. Close liaison between physician and dental surgeon is essential.

REFERENCES

Agerberg, G., and Osterberg, T. (1974). 'Maximal mandibular movements and symptoms of mandibular dysfunction in 70 year old men and women', *Svensk Tandlakare-Tidskr.*, **67**, 147–164.

Ahlbohm, H. E. (1936). 'Simple achlorhydric anaemia, Plummer–Vinson syndrome and carcinoma of the mouth, pharynx and oesophagus in women', *Br. Med. J.*, **2**, 331–333.

Allen, E. F. (1944). 'Statistical study of primary causes of extractions', *J. Dent. Res.*, **23**, 453–458.

Amstad-Jossi, M., and Schroeder, H. E. (1978). 'Age-related alterations of periodontal structures around the cemento-enamel junction of the gingival connective tissue composition in germ-free-rats', *J. Periodont. Res.*, **13**, 76–90.

Anderson, L. G., and Talal, N. (1971). 'The spectrum of benign to malignant lymphoproliferation in Sjögren's syndrome', *Clin. Exp. Immunol.*, **9**, 199–221.

Arendorf, T. M., and Walker, D. M. (1979). 'Oral candidal populations in health and disease', *Br. Dent. J.*, **147**, 267–272.

Arendorf, T. M., and Walker, D. M. (1980). 'The prevalence and intra-oral distribution of *Candida albicans* in man', *Arch. Oral. Biol.*, **25**, 1–10.

Atkinson, P. J., and Woodhead, C. (1968). 'Changes in human mandibular structure with age', *Arch. Oral. Biol.*, **13**, 1453–1463.

Azzopardi, J. G., and Evans, D. J. (1971). 'Malignant lymphoma of parotid associated with Mikulicz disease (benign lymphoepithelial lesion)', *J. Clin. Pathol.*, **24**, 744–752.

Banoczy, J. (1977). 'Follow up studies in oral leukoplakia', *J. Maxillofac. Surg.*, **5**, 69–75.

Barakat, N. J., Toto, P. D., and Choukas, N. C. (1969). 'Ageing and cell renewal of oral epithelium', *J. Periodontol.*, **40**, 599–602.

Barry, H. C. (1969). *Paget's Disease of Bone*, E. & S. Livingstone Limited, Edinburgh and London.

Bates, J. F., Elwood, P. C., and Foster, W. (1971). 'Studies relating mastication and nutrition in elderly', *Gerontologia Clinica*, **13**, 227–232.

Batsakis, J. G. (1979). (Clinical and pathological considerations', in Tumours of the Head and Neck, pp. 57–58, Williams and Wilkins Company, Baltimore.

Batsakis, J. G., Bernacki, E. G., Rice, D. H., and Stebler, M. E. (1975). 'Malignancy and the benign lympho-epithelial lesion', *Laryngoscope*, **85** (2), 389–399.

Baum, B.J. (1981). 'Characteristics of participants in the oral physiology component of the Baltimore longitudinal study of aging', *Community. Dent. Oral. Epidermiol.*, **9**, 128–134.

Beal, J. F., and Dowell, T. B. (1977). 'Edentulous and attendance patterns in England and Wales 1968–1977', *Br. Dent. J.*, **143**, 203–207.

Bertram, U. (1967). 'Xerostomia. Clinical aspects, pathology and pathogenesis', *Acta. Odontol. Scand.*, **25**, Suppl. 49, 1–126.

Bertram, U., and Halberg, P. (1964). 'A specific antibody against the epithelium of the salivary ducts in sera from patients with Sjögren's syndrome', *Acta. allerg.*, *(Kbh)*, **19**, 458–466.

Binnie, W. H., Cawson, R. A., Hill, G. B., and Soaper, A. (1972). *Oral Cancer in England and Wales. A National Study of Morbidity, Mortality, Curability and Related Factors*, Office of Population Censuses and Surveys, HMSO, London.

Blady, J. V. (1971). 'The present status of treatment of cervical metastases from carcinoma arising in the head and neck region', *Am. J. Surg.*, **111**, 56–59.

Bloch, K. J., Buchanan, W. W., Wohl, M. J., and Bunim, J. J. (1965). 'Sjögren's syndrome. A clinical, pathological and serological study of sixty-two cases', *Medicine*, **44**, 187–230.

Boyle, W. D., Via, W. F., and McFall, W. T. (1973). 'Radiographic analysis of alveolar crest height and age', *J. Periodontol.*, **44**, 236–243.

Brill, N., Tryde, G., and Schübeler, S. (1960). 'The role of learning in denture retention', *J. Prosthet. Dent.*, **10**, 468–475.

Bross, I. D. J., and Coombs, J. (1976). 'Early onset of oral cancer among women who drink and smoke', *Oncology*, **33**, 136–139.

Buchanan, W. W., Whaley, K., MacSween, R. N. M., Williamson, J., and Ferguson, M. M. (1976). 'Sjögren's syndrome and liver disease in rheumatoid arthritis', in *Non-articular Forms of Rheumatoid Arthritis*, Proceedings of the Fourth ISRA Symposium, Stafleu's Scientific Publishing Company, The Netherlands.

Bunim, J. J., Buchanan, W. W., Wertlake, P. T., Sokoloff, L., Bloch, K. J., Beck, J. S., and Alepa, F. P. (1964). 'Clinical, pathologic and serologic studies in Sjögren's syndrome. Staff Conference at the National Institute of Health', *Ann. Intern. Med.*, **61**, 509.

Cahn, L. R. (1951). "The jaws in generalised skeletal disease', *Ann. R. Coll. Surg.*, **8**, 115–140.

Castigliano, S. G., and Rominger, C. (1954). 'Distant metastases from carcinoma of the oral cavity', *Am. J. Roentgenol., Rad. Ther. Nucl. Med.*, **71**, 997–1006.

Cawson, R. A. (1966). 'Chronic oral candidiasis and leukoplakia', *Oral Surg.*, **22**, 582–591.

Cawson, R. A. (1969). 'Leukoplakia and oral cancer', *Proc. R. Soc. Med.*, **62**, 610–615.

Chisholm, D. M., and Mason, D. K. (1968). 'Labial salivary gland biopsy in Sjögren's disease' *J. Clin. Pathol.*, **21**, 656–660.

Chisholm, D. M., and Mason, D. K. (1973). 'Salivary gland function in Sjögren's syndrome. A review', *Br. Dent. J.*, **135**, 393–399.

Chisholm, D. M., and Mason, D. K. (1975a). In *Salivary Glands in Health and Disease*', Saunders, London.

Chisholm, D. M., and Mason, D. K. (1975b). 'Disturbance of salivary gland secretion: Sjögren's syndrome', in *Oral Mucosa in Health and Disease* (Ed A. E. Dolby), pp. 447–466, Blackwell, Oxford.

Cooke, B. E. D. (1954). 'The oral manifestations of lichen planus', *Br. Dent. J.*, **106**, 1–9.

Cooke, B. E. D. (1956). 'Paget's disease of the jaws: Fifteen cases', *Ann. R. Coll. Surg.*, **19**, 223–240.

Cooke, B. E. D. (1960). 'The diagnosis of bullous lesions affecting the oral mucosa', *Br. Dent. J.*, **109**, 131–138.

Cooke, B. E. D. (1972). 'The atrophic oral mucosa: The dry burning feeling', *Scott. Med. J.*, **17**, 39–49.

Cooke, B. E. D. (1975a). 'Leukoplakia buccalis: An enigma', *Proc. R. Soc. Med.*, **68**, 337–341.

Cooke, B. E. D. (1975b). 'Median rhomboid glos-

sitis: Candidiasis and not a developmental anomaly', *Br. J. Dermatol.*, **93**, 399–405.

Cooke, B. E. D. (1977). 'Recurrent oral ulceration', *Proc. R. Soc. Med.*, **70**, 354–357.

Cooke, B. E. D., and Tapper-Jones, L. M. (1977). 'Recognition of oral cancer: Causes of delay', *Br. Dent. J.*, **142**, 96–98.

Council on Dental Health and Health Planning, bureau of Economic and Behavioral Research (1983). 'Oral health status of Vermontnursing home residents', *J. Am. Dent. Assoc.*, **104**, 68–69.

Cubey, R. B., and Taylor, S. H. (1975). 'Ocular reaction to propanolol and resolution on continued treatment with a different beta-blocking drug', *Br. Med. J.*, **4**, 327–328.

Davenport, J. C. (1970). 'The oral distribution of *Candida* in denture stomatitis', *Br. Dent. J.*, **129**, 151–156.

Department of Health and Social Services (1972). *A Nutrition Survey of the Elderly*. Report on Public Health and Medical Subjects', No. 3, HMSO, London.

Doll, R., and Hill, A. B. (1964a). 'Mortality in relation to smoking: Ten years' observations of British doctors', *Br. Med. J.*, **i**, 1399–1410.

Doll, R., and Hill, A. B. (1964b). 'Mortality in relation to smoking: Ten years' observations of British doctors', *Br. Med. J.*, **i**, 1460–1467.

Duke-Elder, S. (1965). In *System of Ophthalmology*, Vol. III, Part I, p. 129, and Part II, p. 648, Henry Kimpton, London,

Einhorn, J., and Wersall, J. (1967). 'Incidence of oral carcinoma in patients with leukoplakia of the oral mucosa', *Cancer*, **20**, 2189–2193.

Elden, H. R. (1970), 'Biophysical properties of ageing skin', in *Advances in Biology of Skin* Eds W. Montagna, J.P. Bentley, and R.L. Dobson, Vol. X, pp. 321–252, Appleton-Century-Crofts, New York.

Exton-Smith, A. N., and Caird, F. I. (1980). *Metabolic and Nutritional Disorders in the Elderly*, p. 33, John Wright, Bristol.

Feinmann, C. and Harris, M (1984). *Br. Dent. J.* **156**, 165–168 and 205–208.

Feldman, J. G., Hazan, M., and Nagarajan, M., *et al.* (1975). 'A case control investigation of alcohol, tobacco and diet in head and neck cancer', *Prev. Med.*, **4**, 444–463.

Ferguson, M. M., Carter, Julie, Boyle, P., McHart, D., and Lindsay, R. (1981). 'Oral complaints related to climacteric symptoms in oöphorectomized women', *J. R. Soc. Med.*, **74**, 492–498.

Fine, E. W. (1971). 'Psychological factors associated with non-organic temporomandibular joint pain dysfunction syndrome', *Br. Dent. J.*, **131**, 402–404.

Fløystrand, F., Ambjørnsen, E., Valderhaug, J.,

and Norheim, P.W. (1982). 'Oral status and acceptance of dental services among some eldrly persons in Oslo', *Acta. Odont. Scand.*, **40**, 1–8.

Fortier, R. A. (1975). 'Étude sur les facteurs etiologiques des cancers buccauxpharyngés dans la province de Québec', *J. Can. Dent. Assoc.*, **41**, 235–241.

Fox, L. (1933). 'Paget's disease (osteitis deformans) and its effects on maxillary bones and teeth', *J. Am. Dent. Assoc.*, **20**, 1823–1829.

Frank, R. M., Herdly, J., and Philippe, E. (1965). 'Acquired dental defects and salivary gland lesions after irradiation for carcinomas', *J. Am. Dent. Assoc.*, **70**, 868–883.

Frantzell, A., Tornquist, R., and Waldenstrom, J. (1945). 'Examination of the tongue: A clinical and photographic study', *Acta. Med. Scand.*, **122**, 207–237.

Fry, H. J. B. (1929). 'Syphilis and malignant disease; serological study', *J.Hygiene*, **29**, 313–322.

Gange, R. W., and Wilson Jones, E. (1978). 'Bullous lichen planus caused by labetalol', *Br. Med. J.*, **1**, 816–817.

Gottlieb, B. (1946). 'The new concept of periodontoclasia', *J. Periodontol.*, **17**, 7–23.

Graham, J. G. (1976). 'Facial pain', in *Twelth Symposium on Advanced Medicine*, D.K. Peters, Ed, pp. 149–162, Pitman Medical Books, London.

Graham, S., Dayal, H., Rohrer, T., *et al.* (1977). 'Dentition, diet, tobacco and alcohol in the epidemiology of oral cancer', *J. Natl. Cancer. Inst.* **59**, 1611–1618.

Gray, P. G., Todd, J. E., Slack, G. L., and Bulman, J. S. (1970). *Adult Dental Health in England and Wales in 1968*, HMSO London.

Griffith, M. R., Fukuyama, K., Tuffanielli, D., and Silverman, S. (1974). 'Immunofluorescent studies in mucous membrane pemphigoid', *Arch. Dermatol.*, **109**, 195–200.

Hadden, W. B. (1888). 'On "dry mouth" or suppression of the salivary and buccal secretions', *Trans. Clin. Soc. London*, **21**, 176–179.

Halberg, P., Bertram, U., Söberg, M., and Nerup, J. (1965). 'Organ antibodies in disseminated lupus erythematosus', *Acta.med.Scand.*, **178**, 291–295.

Hank, J. L. (1980). 'Lichenoid drug eruption induced by propanolol', *Clin. Exp. Dermatol.*, **5**, 93–96.

Harris, H., and Kalmus, H. (1949). 'The measurement of taste sensitivity to phenylthiourea (PTC)', *Ann.Eugen.*, **15**, 24–31.

Harris, M. (1974). 'Psychogenic aspects of facial pain', *Br. Dent. J.*, **136**, 199–202.

Harris, W. (1926). In *Neuritis and Neuralgia*, Oxford University Press, Oxford.

Harris, W. (1940). 'Analysis of 1,433 cases of paroxysmal trigeminal neuralgia (trigeminal-tic) and end-results of gasserian alcohol injection', *Brain*, **63**, 209–224.

Harris, W. (1952). 'Fifth and seventh cranial nerves in relation to nervous mechanism of taste sensation; new approach', *Br. Dent. J.*, **1**, 831–836.

Holm-Pedersen, P. (1978). *Aging in Oral Tissues*, Department of Periodontology, The Royal Dental College, Aarhus, Denmark.

Holt, P. J. A., and Waddington, E. (1975). 'Oculocutaneous reaction to oxprenolol', *Br. Med. J.*, **2**, 539–540.

Holubar, K., Honigsmann, H., and Wolff, K. (1973). 'Cicatricial pemphigoid', *Arch. Dermatol.*, **108**, 50–52.

Jackson, D. (1965). 'The mortality of permanent teeth', *Br. Dent. J.*, **118**, 158–162.

Jenkins, G. N. (1978). *The Physiology and Biochemistry of the Mouth*, 4th ed., pp. 553–554, Blackwell Scientific Publications, Oxford.

Kalnins, I. K., Leonard, A. G., Sako, K., Razack, M. S., and Shedd, D. P. (1977). 'Correlation between prognosis and degree of lymph node involvement in carcinoma of the oral cavity', *Am. J. Surg.*, **134**, 450–454.

Karring, T., and Löe, H. (1973). 'The effect of age on mitotic activity in rat oral epithelium', *J. Periodontol. Res.*, **7**, 271–282.

Kramer, I. R. H., El-Labban, N., and Lee, K. W. (1978). 'The clinical features and risk of malignant transformation in sublingual keratosis', *Br. Dent. J.*, **144**, 171–180.

Krutchoff, D. J., Cutler, L., and Laskowski, S. (1978). 'Oral lichen planus. The evidence regarding malignant transformation', *J. Oral. Pathol.*, **7**, 1–7.

Lascelles, R. G. (1966). 'Atypical facial pain and depression', *Br. J. Psychiatry.*, **112**, 651–659.

Lehner, T. (1966). 'Classification and clinico-pathological features of candidal infections in the mouth', in *Symposium on Candida infections*, (Eds H.I. Winner, and R. Hurley, pp. 119–137, Churchill Livingstone, Edinburgh.

Lever, W. F. (1953). 'Pemphigus', *Medicine (Baltimore)*, **32**, 1–123.

Levin, M. L., Kress, L. C., and Goldstein, H. (1942). 'Syphilis and cancer; reported syphilis prevalence among 7,761 cancer patients', *N Y State. J. Med.*, **42**, (ii), 1737–1745.

Löe, H., and Karring, T. (1971). 'The three-dimensional morphology of the epithelium-connective tissue interface of the gingiva, as related to age and sex', *Scand. J. Dent. Res..*, **79**, 315–326.

Howental, U., and Mersel, A. (1983). 'The elderly patient', *Oral Surg.*, **55**, 142–144.

MacFarlane, T. W., and Helnarska, S. J. (1976). 'The microbiology of angular cheilitis', *Br. Dent. J.*, **140**, 403–406.

MacFarlane, T. W., and Mason, D. K. (1974).

'Changes in the oral flora in Sjögren's syndrome', *J. Clin. Pathol.*, **27**, 416–419.

MacSween, R. N. M., Goudie, R. B., Anderson, J. R., Armstrong, E., Murray, M. A., Mason, D. K., Jasani, M. K., Boyle, J. A., Buchanan, W. W., and Williamson, J. (1967). 'Occurrence of antibody to salivary duct epithelium in Sjögren's disease, rheumatoid arthritis and other arthritides. A clinical and laboratory study', *Ann. Rheum. Dis.*, **26**, 402–411.

Manson, J. D., and Lucas, R. B. (1962). 'A microradiographic study of age changes in the human mandible', *Arch. Oral. Biol.*, **7**, 761–769.

Meyer, J., and Necheles, H. (1940). 'Studies in old age. IV. The clinical significance of salivary, gastric and pancreatic secretion in the aged', *JAMA*, **115**, 2050–2055.

Miles, A. E. W. (1958). 'Sebaceous glands in the lip and cheek mucosa of man', *Br. Dent. J.*, **105**, 235–248.

Miles, A. E. W. (1963). 'Sebaceous glands in oral and lip mucosa', in *Advances in Biology of Skin*, (Eds W. Montagna, R. A. Ellis, and A. F. Silver, Vol IV, pp. 1–32, Pergamon Press, Oxford.

Miles, A. E. W. (1972). ' "Sans teeth". Changes in the oral tissues with advancing age', *J. R. Soc. Med.*, **65**, 801–806.

Monroe, R. T. (1951). *Diseases of Old Age*, p. 304, Harvard University Press, Cambridge Massachusetts.

Morgan, W. S. (1954). 'Probable systemic nature of Mikulicz's disease and its relation to Sjögren's syndrome', *N. Engl. J. Med.*, **251**, 5–10.

Moutsopoulos, H. M., Mann, D. L., Johnson, A. H., and Chused, T. M. (1979). 'Genetic differences between primary and secondary sicca syndrome', *N. Engl. J. Med.*, **301** (4), 761–763.

Neill, D. J. (1961). *Aetiology and Treatment of Angular Cheilitis*, Proceedings of the British Society of Prosthetic Dentistry.

Neill, D. J. (1965). 'Symposium on denture sore mouth. I. An aetiological review', *Dent. Pract.*, **16**, 135–138.

Nielsen, J. (1942). 'Om cancer i de øvre luft- og spiseveje', *Tandlaegebladet*, **46**, 1–23.

Oakley, C. M., and Darrell, J. H. (1981). 'Prophylaxis against streptococcal endocarditis', *Br. Dent. J.*, **150**, 178–179.

Ogus, H. D. (1975). 'Rheumatoid arthritis of the temporomandibular joint', *Br. J. Oral. Surg.*, **12**, 275.

Ogus, H. D., and Toller, P. A. (1981). *Common Disorders of the Temporomandibular Joint*, p. 20, John Wright and Sons, Bristol.

Osborne, J., Maddick, I., Gould, A., and Ward, D. (1979). 'Dental demands of old people in Hampshire', *Br. Dent. J.*, **146**, 351–355.

Penman, J. (1968). *Handbook of Clinical Neurology*, Volume 5. (Ed. P. J. Vinken and G. W. Bruyn), Vol. 5, pp. 296 and 323, North Holland Publishing Co.

Pimlott, S. J., and Walker D. M. (1983). A random double blind clinical trial of the efficancy of fluocinonide in the treatment of recurrent aphthous ulceration', *Br. Dent. J.*, **154**, 174–177.

Pindborg, J. J. (1980). *Oral Cancer and Precancer*, p. 82, John Wright and Sons, Bristol.

Pogrel, M. A. (1974). 'The dentist and oral cancer in the North-East of Scotland', *Br. Dent. J.*, **137**, 15–20.

Regaud, C. (1922). 'Sur la sensibilite du tissue osseux normal vis a vis des radiations X et Y et sur le micoxience de l'osteo-radio-necrose', *C. R. Soc. Biol. (Paris)*, **87**, 629–632.

Richman, M. J., and Abarbanel, A. R. (1943). 'Effect of estradiol and diethylstilbestrol upon the atrophic human buccal mucosa with a preliminary report on the use of estrogens in the management of senile gingivitis', *J. Clin. Endocrinol.*, **3**, 224–226.

Ritchie, G. M. (1973). 'A report of dental findings in a survey of geriatric patients', *J. Dent.*, **1**, 106–112.

Roed-Petersen, B., and Pindborg, J. J. (1980). 'Unpublished observations', cited in *Oral Cancer and Pre-cancer* by J. J. Pindborg, John Wright and Sons, Bristol.

Rose, J. A. (1971). *The Aetiology of Angular Cheilitis: A Clinical, Mycological and Serological Study*, M. Phil. Thesis. University of London.

Rudge, G. H. A. (1979). *A Study of Atypical Facial Pain and its Association with Depressive Illness*, M.Sc.D.Thesis, (University of Wales).

Rushton, M. A. (1948). 'Osteitis deformans affecting the upper jaw and osteoporosis circumspecta of the skull', *Br. Dent. J.*, **84**, 189–192.

Rushton, M. A., Cooke, B. E. D., and Duckworth, R. (1972). *Oral Histopathology*, p. 165, E. S. A. Livingstone, Edinburgh.

Samman, P. D. (1968). In *Textbook of Dermatology*, (Eds. A. Rook, D. S. Wilkinson, and F. J. G. Ebling), p. 1197, Blackwell, Oxford.

Sams, W. M., and Smith, J. G. (1965). 'Alterations in human dermal fibrous connective tissue with age and chronic sun damage', in *Advances in Biology of Skin* (Ed. W. Montagna), Pergamon Press, Oxford.

Saxena, V. S. (1970). 'Cancer of the tongue: local control of the primary', *Cancer*, **26**, 788–794.

Schaposnik, F., Bergna, L. J., and Conti, A. (1956). 'Sindrome de Sjögren y lupus eritematoso diseminado', *Rev. Clin. Espan.*, **59**, 102–105.

Schirmer, O. (1903). 'Studien zur Physiologie und Pathologie der Tränenabsonderung und Tränenabfuhr', *Graefe Arch. Opthal.*, **56**, 197.

Shafer, W. G. (1975). 'Oral carcinoma in situ', *Oral Surg.*, **39**, 227–238.

Shafer, W. G., and Waldron, C. A. (1975). 'Erythroplakia of the oral cavity', *Cancer*, **36**, 1021–1028.

Shearn, M. A. (1971). *Sjögren's Syndrome*, Vol. II. in the series, *Major Problems in Internal Medicine*, W. B. Saunders Co., Philadelphia.

Shklar, G., Meyer, I., and Zacarian, S. A. (1969). 'Oral lesions in bullous pemphigoid', *Arch. Dermatol.*, **99**, 663–670.

Shuster, S., and Bottoms, E. (1963). 'Senile degeneration of skin collagen', *Clin. Sci.*, **25**, 487–491.

Silverman, S., Bhargava, K., Mani, N., *et al.* (1976). 'Malignant transformation and natural history of oral leukoplakia in 57,518 industrial workers of Gujarat, India', *Cancer*, **38**, 1790–1795.

Simpson, H. E. (1964). 'Lymphoid hyperplasia in foliate papillitis', *J. Oral. Surg.*, **22**, 209–214.

Sjögren, H. (1933). 'Zür Kenntnis der Keratoconjunctivitis sicca (keratisis filiformis bei hypofunktion der Tränendrüsen)', *Acta. Ophth. Suppl.*, **2**, 1–151.

Spiro, R. H., Alfonso, A. E., Farr, H. W., and Strong, E. W. (1974). 'Cervical lymph node metasis from epidermoid carcinoma of the oral cavity and oropharnyx. A critical assessment of current staging', *Am. J. Surg.*, **128**, 562–567.

Squier, C., Johnson, N. W., and Hackemann, M. (1975). 'Structure and function of normal human oral mucosa', in *Oral Mucosa in Health and Disease*, (Ed A. E. Dolby), pp. 1–112, Blackwell, Oxford.

Stafne, E. C., and Austin, L. T. (1938). 'Study of dental roentgenograms in cases of Paget's disease (osteitis deformans), osteitis fibrosa cystica and osteoma', *J. Am. Dent. Assoc.*, **25**, 1202.

Strouthidis, T. M., Mankikar, G. D., and Irvine, R. E. (1972). 'Ulceration of mouth due to emepronium bromide', *Lancet*, **i**, 72–73.

Tapper-Jones, L., Aldred, M., and Walker, D. M. (1980). 'Prevalence and intra-oral distribution of Candida albicans in Sjögren's syndrome', *J. Clin. Pathol.*, **33**, 282–287.

Tapper-Jones, L. M., Aldred, M. J., and Walker, D. M. (1981). 'Candidal infections and populations of *Candida albicans* in the mouths of diabetics', *J. Clin. Pathol.*, **34**, 706–711.

Toller, P. A. (1974) 'Temporomandibular arthropathy', *Proc. R. Soc. Med.*, **67**, 153.

Troy, W. R. (1968). 'Changes in human skin in the light of current theories of ageing', *J. Soc. Cosmetic. Chem.*, **19**, 829–840.

Von Wowern, N., and Stoltze, K. (1980). 'The pattern of age-related bone lost in mandiblis', *Scand. J. Dent. Res.*, **88**, 134–146.

Waldron, C. A., and Shafer, W. G. (1975). 'Leoplakia revisted. A clinicopathological study of 3,256 oral leukoplakias', *Cancer*, **36**, 1386–1392.

Walker, D. M., Stafford, G. D., Huggett, R., and Newcombe, R. G. (1981a). 'Evaluation of two agents for the treatment of denture stomatitis', *Br. Dent. J.*, **151**, 416–419.

Walker, D. M., Tapper-Jones, L. M., Arendorf, T. M., and Aldred, M. J. (1981b). 'The interaction of local and systemic factors in oral candidal colonisation and infection', *Acta. Stomatologica Internationalia*, **151**, 416–419.

Waterhouse, J. P., Chisholm, D. M., Winter, R. B., Patel, M., and Yale, R. S. (1973). 'Replacement of functional parenchymal cells by fat and connective tissue in human submandibular salivary glands; an age-related change', *J. Oral. Pathol.*, **2**, 16–27.

Whaley, K., Webb, J., McAvoy, B. A., Hughes, G. R. V., Lee, P., MacSween, R. N. M., and Buchanan, W. W. (1973). 'Sjögren's syndrome. 2. Clinical associations and immunological phenomena', *Quart .J. Med.*, **42**, 513–548.

Williams, R. G. (1973). 'The management of mouth cancer', *Ann. R. Coll. Surg.*, **52**, 49–52.

Williams, R. G. (1981). 'The early diagnosis of carcinoma of the mouth', *Ann. R. Coll. Surg.*, **63**, 423–425.

Winner, H. I., and Hurley, R. (1964). In *Candida albicans*, p. 64, J. & A. Churchill Limited, London.

World Health Organization, Collaborating Reference Centre for Oral Precancerous Lesions (1978). 'Definition of leukoplakia and related lesions: An aid to studies on oral precancer', *Oral. Surg.*, **46**, 517–539.

Wright, P. (1975). 'Untoward effects associated with practolol administration: Oculomuco-cutaneous syndrome', *Br. Med. J.*, **1**, 595–598.

Wynder, E. L., Bross, I. J., and Feldman, R. M. (1957). 'A study of the etiological factors in cancer of the mouth', *Cancer*, **10**, 1300–1323.

Wynder, E. L., Hultberg, S., Jacobsson, F., and Bross, I. J. (1957). 'Environmental factors in cancer of the upper alimentary tract. A Swedish study with special reference to Plummer–Vinson (Paterson–Kelly) syndrome', *Cancer*, **10**, 470.

Wynder, E. L., and Stellman, S. D. (1977). 'Comparative epidemiology of tobacco-related cancers', *Cancer Res.*, **37**, 4608–4622.

Principles and Practice of Geriatric Medicine
Edited by M. S. J. Pathy
© 1985 John Wiley & Sons Ltd

11.2

Absorption of Nutrients in Old Age

S. G. P. Webster

INTRODUCTION

In the times before scientific medicine was evolved, physicians were well aware of the associations between eating and ageing. Dietary advice was provided to ensure a long and vigorous life. Once achieved, old age, was recognized as a period requiring special attention to eating habits.

Unfortunately the scientific revolution has overlooked these associations. However, we do have evidence of the effect of calorific intake on longevity and there is some evidence of age changes in the digestive tracts of both animals and man.

Since McCay's work over 40 years ago (McCay *et at.*, 1935, 1939, 1941) there has been a steady accumulation of evidence that a dietary reduction of 30 to 50 per cent. in some animal models will prolong life by 50 to 100 per cent. The earlier the restrictions begin the more successful is the subsequent retardation of growth and prolongation of life. Such changes have been demonstrated in a variety of experimental species. It will always remain unthinkable to perform such rigid and restrictive experiments in man. However, encouragement to limit calorific intake is easily justified. Not only is life prolonged but the frequency of a variety of pathological changes has been found to be reduced in experimental animals on restricted diets (Berg and Simms, 1960; Ross, 1972; Ross and Bras, 1973).

EXPERIMENTAL STUDIES IN ANIMALS

Animal work concerning the effect of age on the gut is confined mainly to studies carried out on rodents – and in many instances the observations are not pursued into the terminal stages of the animal's life. Many investigators have limited their studies to comparisons between very young and mature animals. In the majority absorption seems to be most effective in the period before weaning. There tends to follow a decline in efficiency leading to a period of functional and structural stability. Further changes in both structure and function appear to take place in old age, although the results from different workers are sometimes conflicting.

The small bowel of the rat shortens with age (Penzes and Skala, 1977), but increases in weight in mice (Moog, 1977). The latter may be due to a generalized thickening secondary to increases in fibrous tissue (Andrew and Andrew, 1957) or the deposition of amyloid, (Moog, 1977).

There is conflicting evidence about the number of mucosal villi present in the small gut of aged animals. Penzes and Skala (1977) claim that the number remains static in rats throughout adult life, but Hohn, Gabbert, and Wagner (1978) and Clarke (1977) report both villous atrophy and an associated reduction in enzyme levels in the proximal small bowel. In mice a reduction in the number of villi has been claimed.

The technique of autoradiography with titrated thymidine (Lesher, Fry, and Kohn, 1961; Lesher and Sacher, 1968) has been used to demonstrate a prolonged generation time of crypt cells in the elderly duodenum and prolonged transit times for the cells to pass from the crypts to the villous tips.

Animal work concerning the function of the ageing gut is sparse and the results are variable. There have, however, been reports of reduced monosaccharide absorption (Phillips and Gilder, 1940) and impairment of calcium handling (Hansard, Comar, and Dairs, 1954; Hansard and Crowder, 1957; Henry and Kon, 1953; Schachter, Dowdle, and Schenker, 1960), reduced iron absorption (Yeh, Soltz, and Chow, 1965), thiamidine (Draper, 1958), and cadmium (Kello and Kostial, 1977).

Both jejunal surface area and passive permiability to fatty acids and glucose have been shown to be reduced in aged rabbits (Thomson, 1979, 1980).

POSSIBLE AGE-RELATED CHANGES IN MAN

Available information on age changes in the small intestine in man is limited. Small bowel biopsies in the elderly are difficult to justify, but where this has been possible changes have been demonstrated.

Dissecting microscopic examination of specimens obtained from the first part of the jejunum by the double-tube technique has revealed a reduction in finger-like villi with a corresponding increase in broader villous forms – even to the extent of long ridges and convolutions being seen in patients without gastrointestinal symptoms (Webster and Leeming, 1975b). The villi are significantly shorter than those found in young controls, but mucosal thickness remains unchanged. Estimates of mucosal surface area have also been made on specimens removed from subjects over a wide age range and the specimens from the elderly have shown a significant reduction in surface area (Warren, Pepperman, and Montgomery, 1978).

CLINICAL ASPECTS

Functional efficiency declines in most systems with increasing age and it would be surprising if the gut did not follow this general trend.

Increasing general frailty and weight loss may occur in the old without evidence of any specific underlying cause. Weight reduction will occur in the presence of a well-maintained appetite and a known adequate and balanced diet. Fifty subjects observed during a 3 to 5 year period in an American institution (Pelz, Gottfried, and Soos, 1968) of 330 residents lost on average 11 lb (5 kg) (a fifth of them lost over 27 lb (12.3 kg) each). Half of these subjects showed evidence of malabsorption on simple testing, but none had significant bowel symptoms. These results suggest that at least 7 per cent. of residents in old people's homes are likely to have impaired absorptive ability.

A Birmingham study (Montgomery *et al.*, 1978) of the ageing gut found that 12 per cent of asymptomatic hospital patients had laboratory evidence of malabsorption. Not all malabsorption in old people is silent and non-specific. It should be possible to identify the underlying pathology in just over half of the cases who present with bowel complaints or disorders secondary to nutrient deficiencies.

The elderly are not immune from diseases normally associated with youth. For example, coeliac disease has been diagnosed for the first time in very old age, and about 5 per cent. of cases with coeliac disease are diagnosed in patients over 65 years of age (Badenoch, 1960). However, when cases of steatorrhoea in the elderly are studied, twice as many (50 per cent.) as in younger age groups are found to be due to pancreatic disease and 25 per cent. to coeliac disease (Price, Gazzard, and Dawson, 1977).

Small bowel contamination by abnormal bacteria accounts for the majority of remaining cases to which a specific diagnosis can be applied. The underlying structural abnormality is most likely to be a previous partial gastrectomy with a blind loop or small bowel diverticular disease, but stasis secondary to any constriction may be responsible.

Postgastrectomy malabsorption accounts for about 10 per cent. of diagnosable cases of malabsorption and small bowel diverticular disease for about twice as many. The latter is a very common condition in the elderly, affecting about 10 per cent., but only 2 to 3 per cent. of these with diverticulae are likely to show evidence of malabsorption (Pearce, 1980).

Many generalized conditions affecting the elderly may have some detrimental effect on absorption. Skin conditions (Marks and Shuster, 1970) such as psoriasis (Barry *et al.*, 1971), dermatitis herpetiformis, and scleroderma are good examples. Conditions associated with an arteritis, such as rheumatoid arthritis (Pettersson, Wegelius, and Skrifuars, 1970), may, on occasion, lead to malabsorption and deficiency states.

Xylose absorption has traditionally been used as the indicator of small bowel function. Early work with xylose revealed a marked reduction in absorption in the elderly, but the work was discounted later as it was realized that the effect of renal impairment could have distorted the results. The introduction of combined oral and intravenous xylose tests circumvented the renal complications (Kendal and Nutter, 1970). Using this technique, Webster and Leeming (1975a) demonstrated significant impairment of xylose absorption in 26 per cent. of a series of geriatric inpatients.

Studies with calcium probably present us with our best available evidence of a gradual reduction of absorption with increasing age. However, this may be due to a deficiency of 1:25-$(OH)_2D$, a metabolite of vitamin D which normally promotes calcium absorption through the gut. The gut may therefore be an innocent bystander in this reduction in absorption (Gallagher *et al.*, 1979).

There is conflicting evidence concerning the absorption of iron by the elderly (Jacobs and Owen, 1969; Marx, 1979). Where workers have shown an age-related reduction it may be a consequence of maldigestion rather than malabsorption. There is undoubtedly an increase in gastric atrophy and a reduction in acid secretion with increasing age (Baron, 1963). This may well be the reason why reduced iron appears to be absorbed normally by all ages, but other forms present the elderly with difficulties.

Gastric deficiencies due to atrophy are also likely to be responsible for impaired absorption of vitamin B_{12} (Hyams, 1964). Defects at the terminal ileum are rare and usually found only in the presence of a specific pathology, such as Crohn's disease.

Similar explanations, i.e. maldigestion, may account for changes reported in fat absorption in old age. Several studies have noted that the addition of pancreatic extract to the test meals given to elderly subjects has reduced any age difference. Delay in gastric emptying may, in some instances, be at least partially responsible for the reported reduced blood levels of fat derivatives in older persons (Webster *et al.*, 1977).

FOLATE DEFICIENCY, THE AGEING GUT AND NUTRITION

The frequency of low folate levels in the elderly is high – up to 24 per cent. of various groups of old people who have been studied (Webster and Leeming, 1979). The deficiency is usually ascribed to dietary inadequacy but it is hard to accept this explanation. The true dietary requirement is uncertain – estimates as high as 200 micrograms have been proposed, but 50 micrograms per day (Herbert, 1962) seems a more accurate amount. The value of the greater part of dietary folate, i.e. the polyglutamate forms, has never been seriously considered and their degree of availability to us is not accurately known. There are also difficulties in making allowances for the amount of folate lost in food during its cooking and storage – although information for cooked food is now becoming available (Hurdle, Barton, and Searles, 1968). Clearly there are difficulties in assessing dietary folate but inadequate diets are probably less common than previously thought – probably less than 10 per cent. of elderly subjects (Webster, 1973).

Ill-health

Ill-health has also been suggested as a cause of the increased frequency of folate deficiency in the aged, but the study of groups of differing health status does not support this argument. Webster (1973) studied a group of 44 subjects to assess the role of folate depletion in old age. The results of the study suggest that the critical level of dietary folate is between 50 and 95 micrograms daily. If the intake is in this range then only subjects with normal absorption will be able to maintain a normal red cell folate level. However, if surplus free folate is available, i.e. 150 micrograms, then the degree of malabsorption found in elderly patients is rarely sufficient to cause a deficiency state.

However, the bulk (75 per cent.) of our dietary folate is in polyglutamate form and there is evidence that this is not as readily available to the old as to the young (Baker, Jaslow, and Frank, 1978). Changes in the jejunal mucosa may prevent the absorption of the complicated forms of folate. These changes may be a reduction in the number of cells (as would occur with shorter, broader villi as described previously) or a normal number of cells but with a reduced enzyme content.

These studies with folate demonstrate the vulnerability of many elderly patients. A minor reduction in absorptive ability in the presence of a reduced or borderline folate intake may precipitate a deficiency state.

In conclusion, about one-quarter of elderly patients have evidence of impaired small bowel function. This is possibly due to a reduced small bowel surface area as a consequence of broader and shorter villi. Almost half of these elderly people take only just enough free folate to maintain normal folate levels, providing absorptive ability is not impaired. This combination of factors is a likely reason why almost one-quarter of elderly patients show evidence of low red cell folate levels. The same mechanism may also explain the frequency of other deficiency states found in old age.

SMALL BOWEL DISEASE

Small bowel disease should be suspected when there is evidence of nutritional deficiency and malnutrition and maldigestion have been excluded. Symptoms of small bowel disease are usually vague or absent and the patient's history is therefore of little assistance in making a diagnosis. There may be complaints of vague abdominal discomfort, weight loss, and tiredness but overt steatorrhoea or any other recognizable alteration in bowel habit is rare.

Disorders of small bowel function and structure which require investigation in elderly patients are: coeliac disease, mesenteric ischaemia, small bowel diverticular disease lymphomatous infiltration of the small bowel, and tuberculosis.

Coeliac Disease

The diagnosis of coeliac disease in the elderly relies on the same diagnostic criteria as in younger subjects. Malabsorption of xylose and fat should be demonstrated, together with deficiencies of folate and possibly iron. Obtaining such information in frail elderly subjects can be very difficult and special care and patience is required. A small bowel biopsy is essential for confirmation of the diagnosis. Preferably a repeat biopsy should also be taken after a glu-

ten free diet has been prescribed. Only if the atrophic changes seen on the first biopsy are shown to have responded to diet can the diagnosis be upheld. Adherence to a strict gluten-free diet is difficult, tedious, and expensive and can be justified in the elderly only if it is essential for the control of troublesome symptoms. Nutritional deficiencies can usually be more easily corrected by the addition of large dietary supplements of pure forms – e.g. folic acid, calcium, and vitamin D.

Mesenteric Ischaemia

Chronic small bowel ischaemia may lead to weight loss and malabsorption in association with abdominal pain after eating and the finding of a central abdominal bruit. The pain (abdominal angina), however, may be difficult to differentiate from that of peptic ulceration and gall bladder and large bowel disease. The demonstration of widespread vascular disease is usually possible – e.g. ischaemic heart disease, previous cerebrovascular accidents, and peripheral vascular disease. There is also evidence of aortic disease – dilation and calcification – in most instances. The definitive investigation is arteriography in order to show mesenteric vessel narrowing. However, it is rarely possible to justify this procedure in the elderly as the widespread nature of the vascular pathology will be a contraindication to surgical correction. Dick and coworkers, (1967) found only 5 positive cases in 100 aortograms and only 2 of these were suitable for surgery. All five positive cases were patients over 59 years of age. Unfortunately the management of most cases will be restricted to advice about taking small frequent nutritious meals, in order that pain can be avoided or minimized. Any deficiency states which may have arisen should be corrected.

Small Bowel Diverticular Disease

Elderly patients with evidence of malabsorption, plus vague abdominal discomfort, and sometimes diarrhoea, should undergo small bowel barium study to exclude small gut diverticular disease. When such lesions are found by chance during barium investigations for other conditions they are usually innocent; they are liable to colonization with bacteria and may then be responsible for malabsorption. The deficiencies will be mainly of fat soluble vitamins as their absorption becomes impaired as the bacteria deconjugate the bile salts and make them ineffective. B12 deficiency may also occur due to consumption of the vitamin by the bacteria. However, folate levels can become high as the same organisms may produce extra amounts of folate which will be available for absorption. The combination of nutritional deficiency with high or normal folate levels is sometimes an important clue that small bowel diverticular disease is responsible.

Additional, valuable, tests are those which indicate abnormal and prolific bacterial contamination of the small bowel. Examples are urinary indican estimations, the radioactive carbon glycocholate breath test, and blood estimates of volatile fatty acids.

Treatment in most cases will consist of nutrient replacement and sterilization of the diverticulae with a broad spectrum antibiotic, such as tetracycline. If the responsible pouches are very numerous, then surgical removal can be justified.

Lymphomatous Disease

Lymphomatous changes may occur in the small bowel due to previously unrecognized and untreated coeliac disease. It may also be part of a generalized lymphoma, in which case evidence of other system involvement may be apparent.

The diagnosis is difficult to make – histological evidence may be obtained from small bowel biopsies, but lymphangiograms or laparotomy may be the only successful method of confirming the diagnosis. Treatment will depend on the nature of the lesions and should be under the guidance of an oncologist.

Intestinal Tuberculosis

Tuberculosis may affect the terminal ileum and caecum. The diagnosis may be suggested by the presence of TB elsewhere and suggestive changes on a small bowel barium meal. Confirmation can only be obtained by removal of tissue at laparotomy. Although rare, this condition needs to be considered because of the increasing predilection of tuberculosis for the elderly.

REFERENCES

Andrew, W., and Andrew, N. W. (1957). 'An age involution in the small intestine of the mouse', *J. Gerontol.*, **12**, 136–149.

Badenoch, J. (1960). 'Steatorrhoea in the adult', *Br. Med. J.*, **2**, 879–887.

Baker, H., Jaslow, S. P., and Frank, O. (1978). 'Severe impairment of dietary folate utilization in the elderly', *J. Am. Geriatr. Soc.*, **26**, 218–221.

Baron, J. H. (1963). 'Studies of basal and peak acid output with an augmented histamine test', *Gut*, **4**, 136–144.

Barry, R. E., Salmon, R. R., Read, A. E., and Warin, R. P. (1971). 'Mucosal architecture of the small bowel in cases of psoriasis', *Gut*, **12**, 873–877.

Berg, B. N., and Simms, H. S. (1960). 'Nutrition and longevity in the rat. II. Longevity and onset of disease with different levels of food intake', *J. Nutr.*, **71**, 255–263.

Clarke, R. M. (1977). 'The effects of age on mucosal morphology and epithelial cell production in rat small intestine', *J. Anat.*, **123**, 805–811.

Dick, A. P., Graff, R., Grieg, D., McG Peters, N., and Sarner, M. (1967). 'An arteriographic study of mesenteric arterial disease. 1. Large vessel changes', *Gut*, **8**, 206–220.

Draper, H. H. (1958). 'Physiological aspects of ageing. I. Efficiency of absorption and phosphorylation of radiothiamine', *Proc. Soc. Exp. Biol. Med.*, **97**, 121–124.

Gallagher, J. C., Riggs, L., Eisman, J., Hamstr, A., Arnaud, S. B., and Deluca, H. F. (1979). 'Intestinal calcium absorption and serum vitamin D metabolites in normal subjects and osteoporotic patients', *Amer. Soc. Clin. Invest.*, **64**, 729–736.

Hansard, S. L., Comar, L. L., and Davis, G. K. (1954). 'Effects of age upon the physiological behaviour of calcium in cattle', *Am. J. Physiol.*, **177**, 383–389.

Hansard, S. L., and Crowder, M. H. (1957). 'The physiological behaviour of calcium in the rat'. *J. Nutr.*, **62**, 325–339.

Henry, K. M., and Kon, S. K. (1953). 'The relationship between calcium retention and body stores of calcium in the rat. Effect of age and vit. D', *Br. J. Nutr.*, **7**, 147–159.

Herbert, V. (1962). 'Minimal daily adult folate requirement', *Arch. Intern. Med.*, **110**, 649–652.

Hohn, P., Gabbert, H., and Wagner, R. (1978). 'Differentiation and ageing of the rat intestinal mucosa. II. Morphological, enzyme histochemical and disc electrophoretic aspects of aging of the small intestinal mucosa', *Mech. Ageing Dev.*, **7**, 217–226.

Hurdle, A. D., Barton, D., and Searles, I. H.

(1968). 'A method for measuring folate in food and its application to a hospital diet', *Am. J. Clin. Nutr.*, **21**, 1202–1207.

Hyams, D. E. (1964). 'The absorption of vitamin B₁₂ in the elderly', *Geront. Clin.*, **6**, 193–206.

Jacobs, A. M., and Owen, G. M. (1969). 'The effect of age on iron absorption', *J. Gerontol.*, **24**, 95–96.

Kello, D., and Kostial, K. (1977). 'Influence of age and milk diet on cadmium absorption from the gut', *Toxicol. Appl. Pharmacol.*, **40**, 277–282.

Kendal, M. J., and Nutter, S. (1970). 'The influence of sex, body weight and renal function on the xylose test', *Gut*, **11**, 1020–1023.

Lesher, S., Fry, R. J. N., and Kohn, H. A. (1961). 'Influence of age on transit time of cells of mouse intestinal epithelium', *Lab. Invest.*, **10**, 291–300.

Lesher, S., and Sacher, G. A. (1968). 'Effects of age on cell proliferation in mouse duodenal crypts', *Exp. Geront.*, **3**, 211–217.

McCay, C. M., Crowell, M. F., and Maynard, L. A. (1935). 'The effect of retarded growth upon the length of life span and upon the ultimate body size', *J. Nutr.*, **10**, 63–79.

McCay, C. M., Maynard, L. A., Sperling, G., and Barnes, L. (1939). 'Retarded growth life span, ultimate body size and age changes in the albino rat after feeding diets restricted in calories', *J. Nutr.*, **18**, 1–13.

McCay, C. M., Maynard, L. A., Sperling, G., and Osgood, H. S. (1941). 'Nutritional requirements during the latter half of life', *J. Nutr.*, **21**, 45–60.

Marks, T., and Shuster, S. (1970). 'Small intestinal mucosal abnormalities in various skin diseases – fact or fancy?', *Gut*, **11**, 281–291.

Marx, J. J. M. (1979). 'Normal iron absorption and decreased red cell iron uptake in the aged', *Blood*, **53**, 204–211.

Montgomery, R. D., Haeney, M. R., Ross, I. N., Sammons, H. G., Barford, A. V., Balakrishnan, S., Mayer, P., Culank, L. S., Field, J., and Gosling, P. (1978). 'The ageing gut: A study of intestinal absorption in relation to nutrition in the elderly', *Quart. J. Med.*, **47**, 197–211.

Moog, F. (1977). 'The small intestine in old mice. Growth, alkaline phosphatase and disacchridase activities and deposition of amyloid', *Exp. Gerontol.*, **12**, 223–235.

Pearce, V. R. (1980). 'The importance of duodenal diverticula in the elderly', *Postgrad. Med. J.*, **56**, 777–780.

Pelz, K. S., Gottfried, S. P., and Soos, E. (1968). 'Intestinal absorption studies in the aged', *Geriatrics*, **23**, 149–153.

Penzes, L., and Skala, I. (1977). 'Changes in the mucosal surface area of the small gut of rats of different ages', *J. Anat.*, **124**, 217–222.

Pettersson, T., Wegelius, O., and Skrifuars, B. (1970). 'Gastrointestinal disturbances in patients with severe rheumatoid arthritis', *Acta. Med. Scand.*, **188**, 139–144.

Phillips, R. A., and Gilder, H. (1940). 'The relation of age nutrition and hypophysectomy on the absorption of dextrose from the gastro-intestinal tract', *Endocrinology*, **27**, 601–604.

Price, H. L., Gazzard, B. G., and Dawson, A. M. (1977). 'Steatorrhoea in the elderly', *Br. Med. J.*, **1**, 1582–1584.

Ross, M. H. (1972). 'Length of life and calorie intake', *Am. J. Clin. Nutr.*, **25**, 834–838.

Ross, M. H., and Bras, G. (1973). 'The influence of protein under and over nutrition on spontaneous tumour prevalence in the rat', *J. Nutr.*, **103**, 944–963.

Schachter, D., Dowdle, E. B., and Schenker, H. (1960). 'Active transport of calcium by the small intestine of the rat', *Am. J. Physiol.*, **198**, 263–274.

Thomson, A. B. R. (1979). 'Unstirred water layer and age-dependent changes in rabbit jejunal D glucose transport', *Am. J. Physiol.*, **236** (6), E 685–691.

Thomson, A. B. R. (1980). 'Effect of age on uptake of homologous series of saturated fatty acids into rabbit jejunum', *Am. J. Physiol.*, **239** (2), G 363–371.

Warren, P. M., Pepperman, M. A., and Montgomery, R. D. (1978). 'Age changes in small intestinal mucosa', *Lancet*, **2**, 849–850.

Webster, S. G. P. (1973). 'Changes in proximal small bowel function and structure in the elderly and their relevance to folate status', MD Thesis. University of London.

Webster, S. G. P., and Leeming, J. T. (1975a). 'Assessment of small bowel function in the elderly using a modified xylose tolerance test', *Gut*, **16**, 109–113.

Webster, S. G. P., and Leeming, J. T. (1975b). 'The appearance of the small bowel mucosa in old age', *Age Ageing*, **4**, 168–174.

Webster, S. G. P., and Leeming, J. T. (1979). 'Erythrocyte folate levels in young and old', *J. Am. Geriatr. Soc.*, **27**, 451–454.

Webster, S. G. P., Wilkinson, E. M., and Gowland, E. (1977). 'A comparison of fat absorption in young and old subjects', *Age Ageing*, **6**, 113–117.

Yeh, D. J., Soltz., W., and Chow, B. F. (1965). 'The effect of age on iron absorption in rats', *J. Gerontol.*, **20**, 177–180.

11.3

Age and Gastrointestinal Disease

J. S. Morris, M. J. Dew

There are no age specific disorders of gastrointestinal function and although cellular changes occur and structural support is altered throughout the gastrointestinal tract with increasing age as elsewhere in the body, function is maintained above requirements, in the absence of localized disease. Disorders and diseases, however, become more common with advancing age, including impaired oesophageal motility, gastric atrophy, gallstones, and gastrointestinal malignancy at all sites. The study of gastrointestinal disease in the elderly is therefore an extension of existing gastroenterology into an area which, although recognized clinically, has little supportive scientific data, partly because of the difficulty in obtaining such information in elderly subjects.

THE OESOPHAGUS

The oesophagus has long ceased to be regarded as a convenient passage for ingested food into the stomach, and much research in the last two decades has drawn attention to its physiology and, in particular, to the lower oesophageal sphincter.

Anatomically the oesophagus is, under resting conditions, a hollow tube closed at the top by the sphincter-like arrangement of the striated muscle fibres of the cricopharyngeous and at the lower end by the lower oesophageal sphincter which is a physiological sphincter with no anatomic counterpart (Fyke, Code, and Schlegel, 1956; Pope, 1967). The oesophagus has two muscle coats: an outer longitudinal layer and an inner circular one. In the upper two thirds the muscle is striated blending with smooth muscle and consists entirely of smooth muscle in the lower third. It is lined by non-keratinized stratified squamous epithelium which meets the gastric mucosa approximately 40 cm from the teeth. The vascular supply derives from the inferior thyroid artery and branches of the descending thoracic aorta with a portion at the lower end supplied from the left gastric artery. The venous drainage is to the superior vena cava and the azygos vein in its upper parts, while the lower part drains to the portal venous system. The lymphatic vessels enter the cervical nodes, the mediastinal nodes, and also the coeliac and gastric lymph nodes. The lymphatic communications are rich and allow the rapid spread of oesophageal tumours.

The Nerve Supply

The nerve supply is important for the fibres subserve the afferent and efferent pathways of the swallowing reflex. The swallowing centre is found in the medulla and afferent impulses arrive at the centre through the superior branch of the vagus and the glossopharyngeal nerve. Efferent impulses leave the centre by means of the V, VII, X, and XII cranial nerves from the nucleus ambiguus. The vagus nerve also supplies the body and lower oesophagus and the fibres synapse in Auerbach's plexus with short postganglionic fibres supplying groups of muscle cells. Nerve fibres probably contribute little to the resting lower oesophagus sphincter tone and vagal impulses probably relax rather than contract the sphincter (Weisbrodt, 1976).

The Act of Swallowing

The act of swallowing is mainly reflex and is stimulated by food coming into contact with the fauces, hypopharynx, and upper part of the oesophagus. Peristaltic waves carry the food bolus down the oesophagus and when they arrive at the lower oesophageal sphincter relaxation of the sphincter occurs. The competence of the sphincter depends on both vagal and humoral influences.

Age and Motility (Presbyoesophagus; see Soergel, Zboralske, and Amberg, 1964)

This abnormality of oesophageal motility is the one most commonly associated with age. Manometric and cine-radiographic studies show that a large number of swallows are followed, not by peristaltic waves, but by non-peristaltic tertiary waves. Failure of the lower oesophageal sphincter to relax may result. Original studies of presbyoesophagus were influenced by the coexistence of other disorders such as senile dementia, diabetes, and peripheral neuropathy, and lead to difficulty in relating the presence of tertiary contractions to definitive symptoms.

It has been suggested, however, that most tertiary contractions relate to the presence of oesophagitis, and its clinical counterpart heartburn. In patients with tertiary contractions alone, spasm and dysphagia do not occur.

The predominant clinical presentation of an oesophageal motility disorder is dysphagia. Dysphagia is a sensation of food sticking during the act of swallowing and should be distinguished from a similar sensation in hysterical patients unassociated with the swallowing act (globus hystericus). The clinical history in dysphagia is of great diagnostic help and the cause may be deduced in 80 per cent on clinical grounds alone.

In motility disturbances, dysphagia for both solids and liquids, particularly if they are hot or cold, occurs from the outset. Pharyngeal causes of dysphagia give rise to a choking sensation and oronasal regurgitation of food and liquids just taken. Of itself dysphagia is not painful although pain may occur in diffuse oesophageal spasm and in achalasia (Cohen, 1979).

Recent reviews have drawn attention to the syndrome of 'angina-like' pain in patients with angiographically proven normal coronary arteries (Rosenthal and Cooper, 1979). Oesophageal studies in some of these patients have shown reflux oesophagitis or oesophageal spasm (Brand, Ilves, and Pope, 1980), sometimes provoked by the intravenous administration of ergometrine (Dart *et al.*, 1980).

Nitrites may be useful in oesophageal pain leading to even greater confusion with pain of cardiac origin (Swammy, 1977).

In routine clinical practice the cornerstone of investigation of oesophageal motility is the barium swallow examination with cine-radiography. Manometric studies have done much to help in the understanding of motility abnormalities but are seldom of use in the clinical situation.

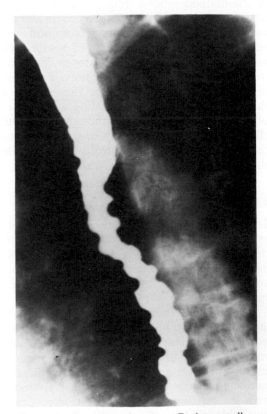

Figure 1 Oesophageal spasm. Barium swallow showing typical "corkscrew" appearance

Diffuse Oesophageal Spasm (Fig. 1)

This was first recognized as a radiographic abnormality by Schatzki (1933). Creamer, Donohue, and Code, (1958) provided the definitive description; 'Immediately following the act of swallowing, barium fills and distends the oesophagus as in health, but as the primary peristaltic wave reaches the arch of the aorta, the lower half of the oesophagus suddenly becomes distorted and puckered into a series of pockets giving it a beaded appearance.' Descriptions such as functional diverticula, pseudo-diverticulosis, segmental spasms, non-sphincter spasm, knuckleduster and corking or corkscrew oesophagus have been applied (Creamer, Donohue, and Code, 1958). A minority of patients have symptoms which include dysphagia, particularly for solid foods, and pain. Overall the proportion of patients presenting with dysphagia who prove to have oesophageal spasm is small. Confusion with angina is possible and such motor abnormalities are common in patients with normal corronary arteriograms (Brand, Martin, and Pope, 1977; Svensson *et al.*, 1978).

Pseudo-Bulbar Palsy

This is the commonest neuromuscular disorder causing dysphagia in the elderly (Fischer *et al.*, 1965). It results from bilateral cortical cerebrovascular events. Usually bilateral pyramidal tract signs coexist – the uvula is fixed and the gag reflex is absent. The disorder is mainly due to incoordinate activity of spastic pharyngeal muscles. In addition manometric studies have revealed a variety of abnormalities including diffuse oesophageal spasm, decreased peristaltic activity and abnormalities in the lower oesophageal sphincter (Fischer *et al.*, 1965), so that the dysphagia may not result entirely from the bulbar nuclei denervation of the pharynx and upper oesophageal sphincter.

Clinically regurgitation of foods, and particularly liquids, occurs and fits of coughing and choking are common. Pneumonia may result from oesophageal overspill. Treatment of the condition is directed to maintaining the patient's nutrition over the initial 2 to 3 weeks to allow any spontaneous recovery to occur. Gastrostomy has been largely superceded by the placement of a fine bore polythene tube –

perhaps with the help of endoscopy—and is often life saving. Division of the cricopharyngeus may be helpful, particularly in those with adequate tongue movement, to push the food back into the pharynx (Mills, 1975).

Motility Disturbances in Other Diseases

Diabetes

Motility disturbances have been observed in patients with autonomic or peripheral diabetic neuropathy (Mandelstam *et al.*, 1969). Dysphagia may result although it is uncommon. The motility disturbance results in disordered peristalsis with delay in oesophageal emptying. Tertiary contractions are common.

Parkinson's Disease

Cine-radiographic studies have revealed motility disturbances in the majority of patients with Parkinson's disease. Symptoms of dysphagia are unusual. The motility disturbances increase difficulty in the initiation of swallowing with motor disturbances in the pharynx, and diminished or absent oesophageal perisalsis (Fischer *et al.*, 1965; Logemann, Blonsky, and Boshes, 1975; Pallis and Lewis, 1974). It is difficult to be sure that some changes are not purely those of ageing.

Alcohol Ingestion

Autonomic alcohol neuropathy leads to reduction of peristaltic activity and oesophageal sphincter tone (Winship *et al.*, 1968). Again symptoms are unusual.

Achalasia

In this condition the oesophageal smooth muscle atrophies consequent upon disease of the dorsal motor nuclei of the vagus nerve and Wallerian degeneration of Auerbach plexuses. Propulsive peristalsis is affected and the lower oesophagus sphincter is unable to relax.

The disease presents mainly in those under 50 years of age. Patients presenting older than this possibly do so as a result from a progression of diffuse oesophageal spasm (Vantrappen, Janssens, and Hellemans, 1979). It may occur in later life as a non-metastatic complication of malignancy, particularly of pancreatic, gastric, or bronchial origin (Davis *et al.*, 1975).

Scleroderma

Oesophageal disease may present in the absence of typical skin manifestations of scleroderma (Atkinson and Summerling, 1966; Rodnan and Fennell, 1962). Deteriorating oesophageal function sometimes coincides with improvement of the cutaneous manifestations of the disease (Garrett *et al.*, 1971). Atrophy of the oesophageal smooth muscle occurs, resulting in the development of an atonic, non-peristaltic tube (Atkinson and Summerling, 1966). Motor activity is retained in the upper oesophageal striated muscle. Dysphagia results and is more marked when the patient is supine. Radiographic investigation of the patient with scleroderma is not complete without observations of swallowing while lying.

Associated gastrooesophageal reflux is common and results from atrophy of the oesophageal sphincter. The diminished peristaltic activity prevents acid clearance and can lead to peptic strictures (Atkinson and Summerling, 1966).

Rheumatoid Arthritis

Laryngeal arthritis and disorders of the cricoarytenoid joints are common in rheumatoid disease (Montgomery, 1963; Montgomery and Goodman, 1980).

Reduced oesophageal peristalsis and lowered oesophageal sphincter pressure are seen in rheumatoid patients and seems to bear no relation to the extent or duration of the disease or to other evidence of peripheral neuropathy (Sun *et al.*, 1974). Drugs used to control the disease may be responsible for some of the oesophageal abnormalities. Symptoms of dysphagia and heartburn occur in approximately a quarter of patients.

Polymyositis and Dermatomyositis

These diseases, which are associated with malignancy in older patients, lead to focal degenerative changes in groups of striated muscle cells and a pharyngeal type of dysphagia (see Ch. 25.1). Derangement of oesophageal motility and lower oesophageal sphincter pressure also occur (Atkinson, 1976).

Gastrooesophageal Reflux

Gastrooesophageal reflux occurs normally after meals and does not usually give rise to symptoms (Dent *et al.*, 1980). The gastric contents are rapidly cleared by primary and secondary oesophageal contractions (Wallin and Madsen, 1979). The amount of reflux is controlled mainly by the lower oesophageal sphincter. The sphincter mechanism is affected by various physiological and pharmacological agents and is often disturbed by the patient's habits. Thus smoking and drinking alcohol lower the oesophageal sphincter pressure as does the ingestion of fat, but not protein. Glucagon secretion and cholecystokinin have also been shown to reduce the pressure. Oesophageal sphincter pressure is also lowered in ascites and obesity. The sphincter pressure is increased by gastrin, antacids, and by intravenous metolopromide. Oesophageal clearance of refluxed gastric contents is dependent on motility and ultimately the integrity of the autonomic nerve supply. The diminished motility of the ageing oesophagus lessens the organ's ability to clear acid and refluxed bile and promotes oesophageal symptoms (Hollis and Castell, 1974; Soergel, Zboralske, and Amberg, 1964). In addition those conditions which affect oesophageal motility (see above) also lessen the ability to clear refluxed acid leading to oesophagitis. The situation is complicated by the observation that oesophagitis of itself induces changes in oesophageal motor function and lowers the sphincter pressure (Eastwood, Castell, and Higgs 1975). Cimetidine has been shown to improve sphincter pressure in patients with symptomatic reflux while it has no effect in normal individuals (Freeland, Higgs, and Castell, 1977; Goodhall and Temple, 1980).

The predominant clinical feature of oesophageal reflux is a retrosternal burning discomfort originating in the epigastrium and radiating into the chest. The symptom is made worse by bending and may awake the patient from sleep. Fluid is often regurgitated into the mouth.

The assessment of oesophagitis is difficult.

Barium swallow and endoscopic appearances even with oesophageal biopsy do not correlate well with clinical symptoms. Manometric studies are useful in research laboratories, but have little part to play in routine clinical situations. Acid perfusion studies are useful in assessing the contribution of oesophageal disease to symptoms (Bernstein and Baker, 1958).

Hiatus Hernia

Herniation of the stomach into the thoracic cavity is increasingly frequent with age and can be demonstrated in over 70 per cent of patients over 70 years of age (Stilson *et al.*, 1969). In clinical terms these hernias are often of dubious significance, particularly since the lower oesophageal sphincter pressure is unaffected (Atkinson, 1962). Similarly the endoscopic presence of oesophagitis occurs equally in those with or without a hiatus hernia. Further the existence of a hiatus hernia does not compromise sphincter function if the intra-abdominal pressure is raised (Wernly *et al.*, 1980). A hiatus hernia, however, does delay gastric emptying which tends to promote reflux (Donovan *et al.*, 1977).

A hiatus hernia may cause problems in the elderly if it becomes incarcerated in the chest when it is associated with pain, dysphagia, anaemia, and respiratory problems (Fig. 2).

Barret's Oesophagus

This is probably best regarded as a consequence of reflux oesophagitis although early descriptions suggested that it arose from congenital ectopic islands of gastric mucosal cells (Mossberg, 1966). Gastric-type mucosa within the oesophagus secretes both acid and pepsinogen perpetuating the underlying oesophagitis and sometimes causes an oesophageal peptic ulcer and possibly stricture formation. Adenocarcinoma of the oesophagus is a further possible complication (Haggitt *et al.*, 1978). Barret's oesophagus is best detected by endoscopy, the gastric-type mucosa appearing as orange/yellow patches contrasting against the glistening pink normal oesophageal mucosa (Gibbs, 1976).

Increased gastrooesophageal reflux occurs after partial gastrectomy (Cox, 1961; McKeown, 1958). Vagotomy itself does not reduce lower oesophageal sphincter tone (Temple *et al.*, 1981) and the increased reflux is possibly explained by associated gastric stasis (Alexander-Williams and Cox, 1969). However, patients with duodenal ulcers also have increased gastrooesophageal reflux and reduced lower oesophageal sphincter pressures (Wallin, 1980).

Management of Reflux Oesophagitis

The aims of management are to diminish acid attack, to improve oesophageal acid clearance, and perhaps to modify the sensitivity of the oesophageal mucosa.

The treatment of obesity is associated with the improvement of reflux symptoms, presumably because obesity increases intra-abdominal pressure leading to increased gastrooesophageal reflux. Reflux is also worsened by posture, and the patient should avoid bending at the waist and sleep with the head of the bed propped to diminish reflux at night. Many patients when told to alter their sleeping position do so by increasing the number of pillows, which is not useful as it serves to increase intra-abdominal pressure and promote reflux. Smoking and alcohol ingestion each lower oesophageal sphincter pressure and should be avoided. Antacids often provide immediate relief of symptoms presumably by neutralizing gastric acid but also possibly by reflexly increasing the secretion of gastrin by raising gastric pH. Gastrin increases sphincter pressure. Cimetidine has been used in the treatment of reflux oesophagitis but the clinical improvement it provides is not as dramatic as is the symptom relief when the drug is used in peptic ulcer. Metoclopamide improves sphincter pressure and has been used in some patients. The drug is potentially hazardous in elderly patients because of the possibility of inducing extrapyramidal manifestations.

Improvement in oesophageal clearing of acid may be expected by improving posture and weight reduction, but the effects of individual manoeuvres are difficult to assess. Improvement in mucosal sensitivity may theoretically derive from the use of carbenoxolone but the value of this drug alone remains to be proved. The combination of carbenoxolone with alginic

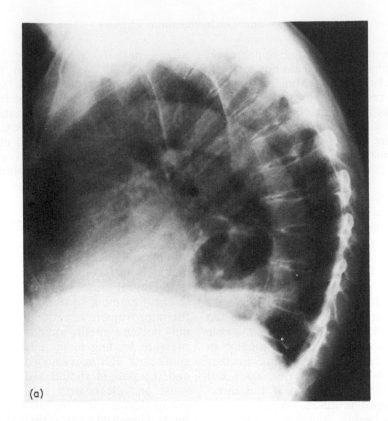

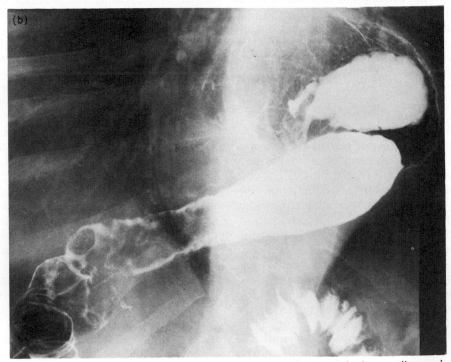

Figure 2 a&b, Lateral chest X-ray showing a fixed hiatal hernia. A barium swallow and meal reveals an intrathoracic stomach

acid is less useful in elderly patients because of its association with water retention, raised blood pressure, and hypokalaemia. The combination of a local anaesthetic agent such as oxethazaine with antacids is favoured by some clinicians in the treatment of reflux oesophagitis, although the evidence that it is useful is not available. Physical barriers protecting the oesophageal mucosa are provided by alginic acid/sodium alginate preparations which, in the presence of hydrochloric acid, produce a foaming gel and by mixtures containing polymethyl silexane.

Failure to control reflux symptoms medically leads to the consideration of surgery. Various forms of antireflux surgery are performed but the most popular is probably the Nissen fundoplication (Nissen, 1961). Physiological assessment of this operation has shown a definitive increase in the lower oesophageal sphincter pressure postoperatively (Demeester *et al*, 1974).

Structural Abnormalities of the Oesophagus

Postcricoid Webs (Fig. 3)

These occur within 1 to 2 cm of the pharyngo-oesophageal junction either in the hypopharynx or cervical oesophagus. The webs arise anteriorly, extend laterally and are occasionally circumferential. In 10 per cent of patients the webs are multiple (Chisholm *et al.*, 1971a). The webs are covered by normal oesophageal stratified squamous epithelium with supporting subepithelial connective tissue. Histologically there is no evidence of chronic inflammation.

Postcricoid webs are associated with dysphagia but many are asymptomatic and discovered at routine barium examination (Nosher, Campbell, and Seaman, 1975). The webs occur more commonly in patients with iron deficiency anaemia, and are found mainly in females. The majority of webs arise in patients over the age of 50 years (Chisholm *et al.*, 1971a, 1971b).

The association of iron deficiency manifest as glossitis and koilonychia, with postcricoid webs was pointed out early in the present century (Kelly 1919; Paterson, 1919; Vinson, 1922). Further work tends to confirm the as-

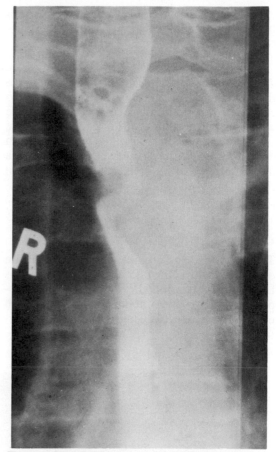

Figure 3 Postcricoid web in a patient with iron deficiency, anaemia and dysphagia

sociation but the pathogenesis of the web and its relationship to iron deficiency remains obscure. Anaemic patients with postcricoid webs are usually iron deficient because of gastrointestinal bleeding or excessive menstrual blood loss; nutritional causes of iron deficiency are unusual (Chisholm *et al.*, 1971a). The situation is complicated by the occurrence of dysphagia and iron deficiency in the absence of a post cricoid web (Elwood *et al*, 1964; Jones, 1961).

The most striking complication of a postcricoid web is the development, in up to 10 per cent. of patients, of postcricoid or high oesophageal malignancy (Chisholm, 1974). The malignancy may present at any time after the diagnosis of the postcricoid web. The effect of iron replacement in preventing the development of a carcinoma is unknown.

The diagnosis of postcricoid webs depends on barium swallow and particularly cineradiography.

Treatment. Iron replacement often improves the dysphagia whilst there may be a little or no change in the radiological appearance of the web. Further episodes of iron deficiency in the same patient may be associated with the return of the dysphagia. Dysphagia associated with a large web or stricture is unaffected by iron therapy and may necessitate repeated oesophageal dilatations.

Lower Oesophageal Webs

These are rare and are not associated with iron deficiency. Dysphagia, when it occurs, is treated by dilatation through a flexible oesophagoscope or by nibbling at the web with endoscopic biopsy forceps (Tedesco and Morton, 1975).

Oesophageal Rings (Fig. 4)

Ring-like constrictions at the lower end of the oesophagus are seen commonly during barium swallow examinations. The rings are eponymously termed Schatzki rings (Schatzki and Gary, 1953). Histologically the mucosal rings are of two types (Goyal, Bauer, and Spiro, 1971). In the first type the ring is found at the gastrooesophageal junction and consists of connective tissues and fibres of the muscularis mucosa but do not contain muscle coat fibres. The second type of ring occurs 2 to 3 cm above the gastrooesophageal junction, perhaps at the site of the physiological lower oesophageal sphincter, and contains muscle fibres. They are seldom the cause of symptoms although they may be the site of a bolus obstruction and cause intermittent dysphagia.

Pharyngeal Pouch

A pharyngeal pouch (Zenker's diverticulum) occurs as the result of protrusion of the phar-

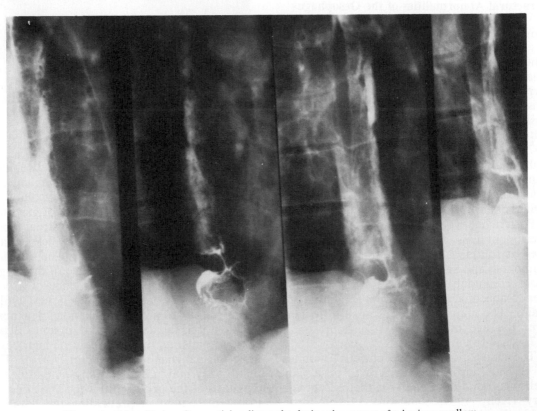

Figure 4   Schatzki ring. Sequential radiographs during the course of a barium swallow

yngeal mucosa posteriorly between the oblique fibres of the inferior pharyngeal constrictor and the transverse muscle fibres of the cricopharyngeus. It is commoner in elderly patients (Ellis *et al.*, 1969; Holinger and Jensik, 1973). With the passage of time the pouch may enlarge. Manometric and radiological studies suggest that the primary physiological defect is incoordinate action of the cricopharyngeal muscle, so that the upper sphincter works prematurely leading to the development of high pressures in the pharynx during swallowing (Ardran and Kemp, 1961; Ellis *et al.*, 1969).

The pouch fills with food during eating and may become sufficiently large to cause dysphagia or even compress the trachea. As well as dysphagia the patient complains of effortless regurgitation of recently ingested food and may notice a swelling in the neck. Regurgitation and overspill from the pouch at night results in respiratory complications.

The diagnosis may be made by a lateral chest X-ray when an air/fluid level is seen posterior to the larynx. The appearances during barium swallow are unequivocal.

Treatment Treatment is surgical. A cricopharyngeal myotomy is a rapid procedure which can be performed endoscopically (Dohlman and Mattsson, 1960). Resection of the pouch is not always necessary (Holinger and Jensik, 1973).

Midoesophageal Diverticula

Midoesophageal diverticula are regarded wrongly as being due to traction of the oesophagus by fibrous tissue arising from tubercular lymph nodes. It is now thought that they arise mainly as a result of oesophageal motor dysfunction and the consequent development of high pressure areas giving a 'blow out' effect (Kaye, 1974). Indeed midoesophageal diverticula may not be constant and a case has been recorded where a diverticulum has occurred above a bolus obstruction only to disappear when the obstruction was relieved (Pope, 1978). The condition is usually asymptomatic and dysphagia is more likely to result from the underlying motor abnormality. Surgical removal is not necessary.

Epiphrenic Diverticula

Epiphrenic diverticula are found rarely and occur principally in elderly men in the terminal 3 or 4 cm of the thoracic oesophagus (Hurwitz, Way, and Haddad, 1975). Radiologically the diverticula appear globular and measure up to 4 cm in diameter. Pathologically herniation of the oesophageal mucosa through the muscle coat is seen. The likely cause is a motility disturbance and the majority of patients have high-pressure peristaltic waves in the lower oesophagus associated with poor relaxation of the lower oesophageal sphincter. They are associated frequently with other oesophageal disorders such as oesophagitis and oesophageal carcinoma. Some patients complain of dysphagia but it is difficult to be certain that the dysphagia is the result of the diverticulum or the underlying motor dysfunction. Surgical removal of the diverticulum appears hazardous and if surgery is thought necessary oesophageal myotomy is preferable (Allan and Clagett, 1965).

Benign Oesophageal Strictures

Benign oesophageal strictures arise as the result of various insults on the oesophageal mucosa which result in fibrosis and scarring. The most common cause is reflux oesophagitis. In the elderly a long history of dysphagia is not inevitable, and this is important when considering whether the stricture is malignant or not. Strictures are particularly likely to occur when the oesophagitis is associated with gastric epithelialization of the oesophagus (Barret's oesophagus). Drug ingestion, particularly slow release potassium preparations, cause strictures as do nasogastric tubes left in place for long periods. Ingestion of corrosive liquids with suicide attempt may result in stricture formation. Most oesophageal strictures are found in the lower and middle regions of the oesophagus but may be found at any level (Williamson, 1975).

Investigation (of benign strictures). The preliminary examination of the patient with dysphagia is a barium swallow. A benign stricture appears as a smooth tapered abnormality with the overlying mucosa intact throughout its length. Malignant strictures appear irregular with ulceration and possibly evidence of extension of the tumour into the mediastinum (Fig. 5). Direct inspection is mandatory and histological and cytological specimens should be obtained. Endoscopy of an elderly patient is not without hazard and perforation may occur if the endoscopist is too adventurous.

Management of a benign stricture. Prevention of strictures associated with reflux oesophagitis is theoretically possible with the introduction of H_2 blockers such as cimetidine and the results of long-term studies are awaited with interest. The use of slow-release potassium preparations should be avoided in patients with existing oesophageal disease (Collins *et al.*, 1979). The prompt treatment of oesophageal corrosive injury by lavage and perhaps the careful placement of a wide-bore nasogastric tube with supportive therapy may help prevent stricture formation.

In the patient with an established stricture assessment of nutrition is of primary importance in deciding its management. The patient who is not losing weight and whose life style is not too disrupted can be advised to chew their food carefully and to avoid tough foods which are likely to stick in the oesophagus. If reflux oesophagitis is present, antireflux measures should be suggested (page 300), and these may lead to clinical and radiological evidence of improvement of the stricture. In patients with nutritional problems early oesophageal dilatation is necessary. Techniques of dilatation have changed over recent years, and the one now most often employed by the skilled endoscopist was described by Puestow (1955) and modified by Price, Stanciu, and Bennett (1974). Under light sedation a flexible oesophagoscope is introduced and a flexible guide wire is passed through the biopsy channel of the endoscope into the stomach under radiological control. The endoscope is then withdrawn and a dilator is passed over the guide wire. The stricture is progressively dilated using olives of increasing diameter. The guide wire, dilating olives, and introducer are recovered together to prevent knotting of the wire which may cause oesophageal perforation (Sanderson and Trotter, 1980). Following the dilatation the stricture site should be reinspected endoscopically and the patient should remain on clear fluids for 24 hours. This procedure is rapid and is particularly well tolerated by elderly patients (Olgilvie, Fergusson, and Atkinson, 1980). The incidence of oesophageal perforation is under 0.1 per cent. which compares favourably with other methods such as the use of a rigid oesophagoscope and blind bougienage (Eastman and Sali, 1980). If oesophageal perforation occurs following endoscopic dilatation, a nasogastric tube should be introduced and antibiotics administered. The necessity of early surgery is uncertain (Skinner, Little and DeMeester, 1980).

The procedure may be repeated but in about 40 per cent. of patients only one dilatation is necessary (Olgilvie, Fergusson, and Atkinson, 1980). Following dilatation medical means of reducing oesophageal reflux and postural and dietary advice should be given to the patient. In a controlled trial of patients with a stricture associated with reflux oesophagitis, cimetidine did not influence the frequency or number of endoscopic dilatations (Ferguson, Dronfield, and Atkinson, 1979).

Surgical resection of strictures carries a high mortality, but if repeated dilatations are difficult or unsuccessful, antireflux surgery should be considered (Larrain, Csendes, and Pope, 1975).

Benign Oesophageal Tumours

Benign oesophageal tumours are unusual. The commonest is the leiomyoma which seldom achieves a size large enough to cause symptoms and is found incidentally during the course of barium swallow investigations or at autopsy.

Malignant Oesophageal Disease (Fig. 5)

Approximately 7,500 cases of oesophageal cancer occur in the United States each year, and there is a marked male predominance (Wynder *et al.*, 1976). The disease occurs more commonly in the elderly and in most reported series the average age of the patients is over 60 years (Langman, 1971; Miller, 1962).

There is speculation as to the cause of oesophageal cancer and various studies have shown a marked geographic variation in disease incidence, suggesting that environmental or dietary factors are important. (Editorial, 1974). Alcohol ingestion is associated with the

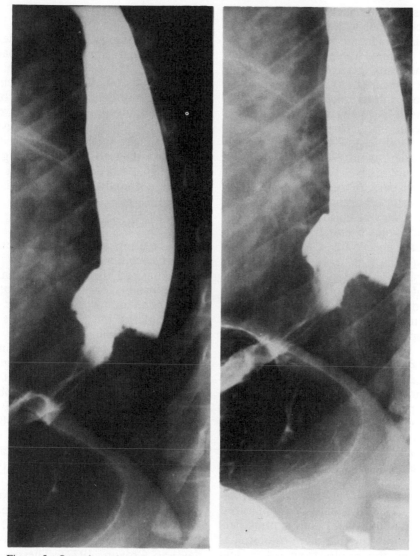

Figure 5 Oesophageal carcinoma. Proximal dilatation of the oesophagus above a stricture with shouldering giving rise to an "apple core" appearance. A soft tissue mass is evidence of an extensive lesion

development of oesophageal cancer particularly, in users of tobacco. The evidence that tobacco alone induces oesophageal cancer is less convincing (Wynder *et al.*, 1976). Other dietary factors appear to be a diet deficient in protein and vitamins A and C (Joint Iran–International Agency, 1977). Genetic factors are less obvious although tylosis and oesophageal cancer have occurred together in some families (Harper, Harper, and Howel Evans, 1970).

Oesophageal cancer complicates the Patterson–Kelly syndrome (Chisholm *et al.*, 1971a) and is also seen in association with a benign peptic stricture and hiatus hernia (Olgilvie, Fergusson, and Atkinson, 1980).

Oesophageal cancers are mainly squamous in type. Adenocarcinomas may develop in an oesophagus which is the site of Barret's change and fundal gastric adenocarcinoma can extend into the oesphagus and present with dysphagia.

Rapid local spread of these tumours occurs because of rich lymphatic drainage and at presentation subdiaphragmatic lymph node deposits are found in up to 10 per cent. of cancers of the cervical oesophagus, up to 30 per cent. of cancers of the middle third, and up to 50 per cent. of lower third cancers (Rubin, 1974). Distant metastases involving the lung, liver, and bones occur in approximately a third of cases.

Patients present with dysphagia which is often rapidly progressive. Weight loss and dehydration occur early in the course of the disease. Deep boring mid-sternal pain occurs in some and there may be episodes of acute pain associated with bolus obstruction.

Oesophageal cancers are readily diagnosed radiologically in most patients. Indirect laryngoscopy may be valuable in high oesophageal or pharyngeal tumours. Fibre-optic endoscopy is a useful adjunct to radiology and provides further information with histological and cytological samples.

Treatment of oesophageal cancer Radical oesophageal surgery is disappointing and in the best hands only up to 30 per cent. survive 5 years. The perioperative mortality is high (Gunnlaugsson *et al.*, 1970). Elderly patients fare even less well and attempts at radical surgery are probably not justified. Radiotherapy provides a realistic alternative and gives 5-year survival rates comparable to those of surgery, particularly for tumours higher in the oesophagus (Pearson, 1975). It should be emphasized that the figures quoted are from centres particularly involved in the treatment of oesophageal cancer and the results from other, less specialized, centres may be even more gloomy.

In many instances the only treatment that can be offered the patient is palliative by the insertion of a Mousseau-Barbin, Souttar, or Celestin tube. The recent introduction of a method of inserting such tubes by fibre-optic endoscopy has provided a valuable advance for the medical profession, and, hopefully, their patients. Complications such as perforation of the oesophagus occurs in up to 15 per cent. of patients. The maximal survival time following insertion of the tube is 2 to 3 years. One of the main advantages of the tube is to allow the patient's nutrition to be improved and perhaps enable subsequent radiotherapy.

Extrinsic Oesophageal Problems

Mediastinal tumours, lymph nodes, and even left atrial enlargement may encroach upon the oesophagus and cause dysphagia. Congenital abnormalities usually present in childhood but extrinsic compression by afferent blood vessels may occur in later life (Lincoln *et al.*, 1969; Pope, 1978). Dysphagia lusoria results from an aberrant right subclavian artery arising from the descending aorta and passing behind the oesophagus. Aortic aneurysms of the thoracic aorta occasionally cause dysphagia.

Drugs and the Oesophagus

The increasing availability of new drugs and different compilations of new therapeutic agents has led to the recognition of drug-induced oesophageal disease. At present drugs account for only a small number of oesophageal problems, but this number is expected to increase with time.

An important recent study has indicated that drugs may remain in the oesophagus for longer than 5 minutes without the patient being aware of their presence (Evans and Roberts, 1976). The presence of motility disturbances, common in the elderly, or organic obstructive lesions will increase the time in which drugs remain in contact with the oesophageal mucosa and enhance the drug's ability to cause damage.

The drugs commonly reported as causing oesophageal disease are slow-release preparations of potassium (McCall, 1975; Pemberton, 1970; Sumithran, Tim, and Chiam, 1979; Whitney and Croxon, 1972). The oesophageal effects of the drug are severe and include ulceration, stricture formation, perforation, and haemorrhage. The damage has sometimes a fatal outcome. Many of the recorded patients have rheumatic heart disease and left atrial enlargement causing narrowing of the oesophagus. Other drugs reported as causing oesophageal damage include Emepronium bromide used as a urinary antiseptic (Barrison, Trewly, and Kane, 1980; Collins *et al.*, 1979), tetracyclines (Crowson, Head, and Ferrante, 1976; Schneider, 1977), clindamycin, quinidine, aspirin containing analgesics and indomethacin (Agdal, 1979; Carlsborg, Cumlien, and Olsson, 1978; Froese, 1979; Teplick *et al.*,

1980). An important though unusual cause of oesophageal drug-induced injury is the mistaken ingestion of 'Clinitest' urine testing tablets.

Effects of Oesophageal Disease

Dysphagia is an uncomfortable and unpleasant symptom which leads to reduced and altered nutritional intake, particularly in the elderly. Foodstuffs such as meat and bread which form boluses are excluded from their diet and in their place fluids or semifluid foods are taken – often only tea! The increased time required to eat a meal usually results in reduced intake. Anorexia may be a prominent feature particularly in mitotic lesions. Painful bolus obstruction may occur with carcinomas and result in the patient being afraid to eat.

Malnutrition and weight loss are common features of oesophageal disease and dehydration soon follows oesophageal obstruction. Anaemia may occur from blood loss from oesophagitis or the oesophageal stricture itself, if malignant. It may result from malnutrition.

Pulmonary complications result from oesophageal obstruction and retention of food stuffs with overflow into the bronchial tree, particularly at night. These include recurrent bronchitis, aspiration pneumonia, bronchiectasis, and pulmonary fibrosis.

Infections of the Oesophagus (Fig. 6)

Oesophageal Candidiasis

Candida albicans is a mycelia forming yeast producing oropharyngeal (thrush) and oesophageal infection (Monilial oesophagitis). These infections usually occur in debilitated patients with conditions such as carcinoma and lymphoma and in patients with diabetes or after antibiotics. Infection is characterized by small white plaques on the buccal mucosa extending into the pharynx, and sometimes for variable distinces down the oesophagus. Occasionally the infection is localized to the oesophagus.

Patients complain of a burning soreness in the mouth and throat with particular sensitivity to hot and cold liquids. With oesophageal involvement dysphagia is a prominent symptom and may be severe (Buckle and Nichol, 1964).

Diagnosis. The diagnosis can usually be easily made by inspection of the oropharyngeal region and by swabbing the affected areas. When infection is confined to the oesophagus abnormalities are seen on barium swallow examination. Multiple small irregularities of the oesophageal wall occur which are sometimes mistaken for varices (Fig. 6) and endoscopically appear similar to the oropharyngeal lesions. Brush cytology confirms the diagnosis (Kodsi *et al*, 1976).

Treatment. Most infections are controlled by local nystatin or miconazole therapy. Persistent, severe, or systemic infection can be treated with intravenous miconazole (Rutgeerts and Verhagen, 1977).

Herpetic Oesophageal Infection

Patients with immunodeficiency often due to malignant disease are susceptible to herpetic infection which occasionally affects the oesophagus. Multiple small ulcers 1 to 3 mm in diameter are found at the affected site, often with secondary monilial infection. Occasionally the infection may extend into the respiratory passages. Endoscopic biopsy shows inclusion bodies typical of herpes simplex (Howiler and Goldberg, 1976). There is no treatment of proven value. Improvement occurs if the patient's underlying condition responds to therapy (Lightdale *et al.*, 1977). Cytosine arabinoside may be helpful.

THE STOMACH AND DUODENUM

The stomach functions as a reservoir and because of its acid environment helps to sterilize food. Controlled amounts of food pass from the stomach to the small intestine for absorption. By its churning movements the stomach breaks down ingested food; the gastric enzyme pepsin is not an important digestive enzyme.

The stomach has three muscle coats, an outer longitudinal layer and an inner circular layer which is expanded at its distal end to form the pylorus. A series of oblique muscle fibres placed submucosally makes up the third layer. The stomach is lined by glandular mucosa capable of secreting acid, mucus, and intrinsic factor necessary for the absorption of vitamin B_{12}.

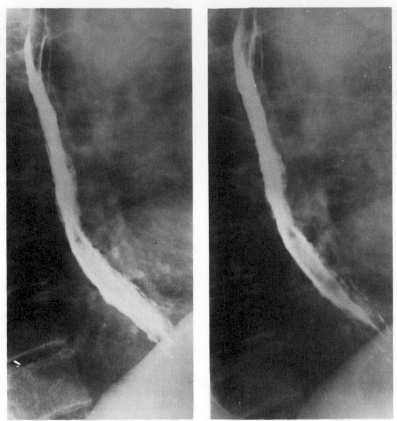

Figure 6   Oesophageal moniliasis. This appearance may be confused with oeso-
pageal varices

The arterial blood supply is derived from the coeliac axis. The right and left gastric arteries supply the lesser curvature of the stomach and the right and left gastroepiploic arteries supply the greater curve. The short gastric arteries provide blood to the fundus and the superior aspect of the greater curve.

Gastric innervation is provided by the vagus nerve, the two major trunks of which pass through the oesophageal hiatus to lie anteriorly and posteriorly to the lesser curve. Sympathetic fibres, both afferent and efferent, accompany the arterial blood supply and originate in the coeliac plexus.

Lymphatic drainage from the stomach is to the suprapancreatic and supramesenteric nodes which communicate with the nodes around the oesophagus. There is no communication of the lymphatics with those from the duodenum which explains the spread of gastric carcinoma caudally.

Hydrochloric acid is produced by the parietal or oxyntic cells of the gastric mucosa in response to gastrin or vagal stimulation. Gastric acid output is greatest in teenage and declines steadily with age (Bloomfield and Keefer, 1928). Direct estimation of stimulated or non-stimulated gastric acid secretion is therefore of little relevance in the elderly. Pepsinogen is also secreted by gastric parietal cells and rapidly converted to pepsin in the acid gastric environment. Small quantities of gastric pepsinogen 'spill' over into the bloodstream and serum pepsinogen levels reflect not only pepsinogen secretions but also acid secretion (Samloff, Secrist, and Passaro, 1975). Nothing is known of the effect of age on this system.

The intrinsic factor is a glycoprotein produced by the body and fundus of the stomach which binds to ingested vitamin B_{12}. The intrinsic factor bound vitamin B_{12} is actively absorbed in the terminal small intestine.

Atrophic gastritis, a condition associated with ageing, is associated with diminished production of intrinsic factor.

Gastric mucus produced by gastric mucosal cells plays a major role in protecting the mucosa from acid/pepsin attack and breakdown of mucus production may play a role in ulcer production (Rhodes, 1972).

Gastric Motility

During eating the stomach dilates to accommodate the volume of ingested food without significant increases in pressure. Muscular contractions propel food distally and at the same time exert a churning effect which mixes food and acid in the antrum. Gastric emptying is complex and the rate of emptying is strongly influenced by the amount of fat ingested. The stomach is able to empty itself of different foodstuffs at different rates. Liquids leave the stomach quickly, the pylorus tending to retain solid foods (Kelly, 1980). Digestible solids are also emptied from the stomach more rapidly than non-digestible solids (Hinder and Kelly, 1977).

Diseases of the Stomach – Gastritis

The incidence of gastritis rises with age so that evidence of it is found in 50 per cent. of patients over the age of 60 years. It is difficult to correlate the inflammatory and pathological changes of gastritis with dyspeptic symptoms (Edwards and Coghill, 1966).

Acute Gastritis

This condition is seen frequently in acutely ill patients commonly as a result of major intracranial haemorrhage, hepatic failure, and severe trauma. Aspirin and alcohol ingestion are also associated with its occurrence. Recent studies of gastrointestinal haemorrhage suggest that acute gastritis is responsible for up to 20 per cent. of hospital admissions (Allan and Dykes, 1976). The haemorrhage is usually minor but may be torrential necessitating radical gastrectomy.

Endoscopic examination reveals a congested haemorrhagic mucosa with multiple small ulcers affecting principally the fundus and body of the stomach.

The changes are thought to occur as a result of disruption of the protective mucosal barrier, perhaps as the result of mucosal ischaemia, as a consequence of hypotension, or to a direct toxic effect of drugs or alcohol. Disruption of the barrier allows luminal hydrogen ions to diffuse into mucosal cells causing damage.

Management of acute gastritis involves replacing blood loss where this occurs and the use of antacids or histamine blockers such as ranitidine or cimetidine to neutralize or reduce gastric acid secretion. These agents are also recommended for prophylactic use in seriously ill patients likely to develop acute gastritis.

In patients who survive, the gastric mucosa returns to normal within 48 hours.

Chronic Gastritis

Two categories of chronic gastritis are recognized which have been arbitrarily designated Type A and type B (Strickland and Mackay, 1973). Type A gastritis affects the glands of the body of the stomach sparing the antral secreting glands. Reduced acid secretion with high levels of serum gastrin occur and parietal cell antibodies are formed. The end stage of the process is atrophic gastritis (Fig. 7) with consequent failure of intrinsic factor production, malabsorption of vitamin B_{12}, and megaloblastic anaemia. The progress of the condition is slow and may occur over 20 years. Histologically there is a mucosal infiltrate and loss of gastric mucosal glands. Intestinal metaplasia may occur, and groups of cells organized into villi with absorptive function are described.

Type B gastritis is a less distinct entity the effects of which are seen mainly in the antrum with loss of mucosa and glands. There is no evidence of autoimmune disease, progression to chronic gastritis is unusual, and intrinsic factor production is maintained.

These changes occur most likely as the result of gastric irritants such as alcohol, aspirin, tobacco, or the ingestion of hot liquids. Histologically the changes of type B are similar to those seen in type A.

Bile Reflux Gastritis

Bile is probably toxic to the gastric mucosa and is associated with gastritis in both animals and

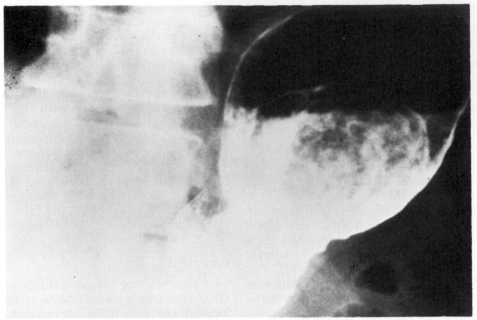

Figure 7   Atrophic gastric mucosa with an intra-gastric bezoar

man, and may play a role in the development of gastric ulcer (Delaney, 1975; Flint and Grech, 1970; Rhodes, 1972). The constituents of bile which are potential toxins include bile acids, lysolecithin, and pancreatic enzymes. As in aspirin injury the main effect of these toxins is on the gastric mucosal barrier, allowing back diffusion of hydrogen ions.

Postoperative Gastritis

Following partial gastrectomy a distal gastritis is common and the subsequent development of an atrophic gastritis is frequent (Johnston, 1966). Bile acids and pancreatic enzymes are postulated toxins, with reduced gastric acid allowing bacterial overgrowth.

Severe changes produce dyspepsia and vomiting and occult bleeding may lead to anaemia. Where the clinical effects and macroscopic changes are severe various biliary diversion procedures have been advocated. The incidence of gastric carcinoma following gastrectomy is increased (Domellöf, 1979).

Peptic Ulcer

The term peptic ulcer is used to describe those ulcers which occur as a result of acid or pepsin attack on the gastrointestinal mucosa. Peptic ulcers occur not only in the stomach or duodenum but also in the lower oesophagus (Barret's ulcer) and in relationship to a Meckel's diverticulum in the ileum.

Epidemiology

Peptic ulcers are common in Western society and evidence is accruing of their incidence in developing countries, particularly India and Africa (Malhotra, 1967; Gatumbi and Roy, 1970; Tovey and Tunstall, 1975).

In both the United States and the United Kingdom, hospital admission rates of patients with peptic ulcers have fallen sharply in recent years (Brown, Longman, and Lambert, 1976; Elashoff and Grossman, 1980). Although this may reflect an altered approach to treatment or the availability of ulcer-healing agents, the concomitant decrease in mortality rates suggests that peptic ulcer disease is less prevalent. The incidence of ulcer perforation which possibly reflects the incidence of ulcer disease has fallen in the United Kingdom but remained static in the United States. (Brown, Longman, and Lambert, 1976; Elashoff and Grossman, 1980).

Elderly patients tend to predominate among

those admitted to hospital for peptic ulcer disease and patients over 60 years of age account for nearly 50 per cent. of those with gastric ulcer and for 40 per cent. of those with duodenal ulcer. In elderly patients the major mortality occurs and age is the largest risk factor in patients with peptic ulcer disease. Considering peptic ulcer as a whole, 15 to 20 per cent. of patients are over the age of 60 years, and about half of these patients develop their first ulcer symptoms at this age (Cutler, 1958; Leverat *et al.*, 1966; Narayanan and Steinheber, 1976). McKeown (1965), reviewing a personal series, suggested that peptic ulcer was the principal cause of death in 4.2 per cent. of autopsies performed on elderly patients.

Both gastric and duodenal ulcer are more common in patients from lower social classes at all ages (Litton and Murdoch, 1963; Registrar General, 1971). The disease occurs with increasing frequency in hepatic cirrhosis and chronic renal failure whilst in diabetes it is less common possibly as a result of vagal neuropathy (Dotevall, 1959; Hosking *et al.*, 1975).

Drugs may be important in the development of peptic ulcer. Since World War II a rising incidence of gastric ulcer has occurred in Australia (Billington, 1965). Further work has incriminated the increasing use of high dose aspirin therapy over a prolonged period (Chapman and Duggan, 1969; Levy, 1974). Positive evidence relating peptic ulcer to drug ingestion, however, particularly the non-steroidal anti-inflammatory agents, is lacking (Cooke, 1978; Zentler-Munro and Northfield, 1979). In patients taking anti-inflammatory drugs dyspeptic symptoms are common. Steroids drugs are often incriminated as a cause of peptic ulcer, but a major review of the world literature has failed to confirm this suggestion (Conn and Blitzer, 1976).

Blood group O is associated with a twofold increase in the incidence of duodenal and pre-pyloric ulcers (McConnell, 1966). There is probably no association with peptic ulceration and the HLA system (Baron, Longman, and Wastell, 1980).

Giant Peptic Ulcer

In patients over the age of 60 years 'giant' ulcers over 3 cm in diameter may be seen (Strange, 1959). These occur along the lesser curve and are often reported radiologically as malignant ulcers. Giant ulcers in the duodenum occur less commonly. Haemorrhage is a frequent complication but such ulcers rarely perforate, healing is slow and erratic, and recurrences are common. Surgery of these ulcers is associated with a high mortality.

Symptoms of Peptic Ulcer Disease in the Elderly

Classical symptoms of peptic ulcer disease occur in the elderly and, as in other age groups, it is not possible on clinical grounds alone to distinguish between gastric and duodenal ulcer (Edwards and Coghill, 1968). In the elderly, however, vague symptoms such as generalized ill-health, anorexia, weight loss, vomiting, or even diarrhoea may be the only clinical associate of radiologically proven peptic ulcers. As in younger age groups, perforation may occur with no preceding history of peptic ulcer symptoms. In elderly patients the classical evidence of perforated peptic ulcer such as sudden abdominal pain and rigidity may not occur (Coleman and Denham, 1980).

Duodenal Ulcer (Fig. 8)

Acid Secretion

Increased acid secretion is a feature of duodenal ulcer disease (Baron, 1963; Fordtran and Walsh, 1973). The number of parietal cells is increased, perhaps because of a genetic predisposition or as a result of increased stimulation (Cox, 1952). Patients with a duodenal ulcer produce more acid as a result of stimulation with pentagastrin or histamine than do control non-ulcer subjects (Isenberg *et al.*, 1975, McLoy, Girvan, and Baron 1978). Vagal overactivity has also been demonstrated (Dragstedt, 1956; Gedde-Dahl, 1975). Acid production is inhibited in normal subjects by a low intragastric pH but in duodenal ulcer subjects this inhibition fails (Walsh, Richardson, and Fordtran, 1975). Little work relating duodenal ulcer to acid secretion in the elderly is available, and it is perhaps surprising that duodenal ulcer occurs in this group as gastric acid production falls with age; clearly local duodenal factors may be more important than acid secretion.

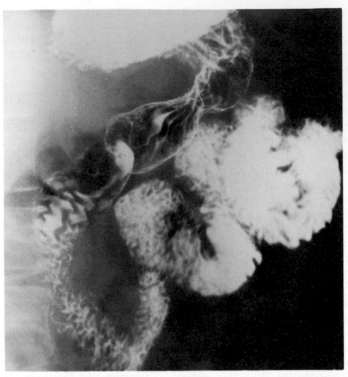

Figure 8   Duodenal ulcer

Local Duodenal Factors and the Development of Duodenal Ulcer

Angiographic studies of the duodenal cap have shown areas of ischaemia which may account for the localization of ulcers (Piasecki, 1974). Duodenitis is often seen preceding the development of a duodenal ulcer and may be associated with gastritis.

Diagnosis

Duodenal ulcers are demonstrated radiologically in 80 to 90 per cent. of subjects by double contrast barium meals (Herlinger, Glanville, and Kreel, 1977; Rogers *et al.*, 1976). Endoscopy improves the diagnostic rate but its use is probably best restricted to those patients with X-ray negative dyspepsia or in whom the presence of chronic duodenal disease radiologically casts doubt on the presence of an active ulcer. Endoscopy is usually safe in elderly patients and well tolerated, but is associated with a degree of morbidity and mortality which is not the case with radiological investigations (Colin-Jones *et al.*, 1978). Premedica-

tion with valium may cause respiratory depression and occasional death and the elderly patient is at particular risk. Aspiration pneumonia may occur both as the result of valium and manoeuvres aimed at anaesthetizing the throat.

Medical Treatment of Duodenal Ulcer

Major advances in the management of duodenal ulcer have occurred in the past decade. Formerly advocated treatment including small frequent meals, high milk diets, milk drips, bland diets, and small-dose antacids are now largely redundant. Although none of these treatments have been shown to heal ulcers, ulcers did heal and the consideration of any ulcer healing agent must allow for a high placebo response rate and the natural tendency for ulcers to heal with time.

H₂ Blocking Drugs

The first of the H_2 blocking agents was metiamide which, because of bone marrow toxicity, was replaced by cimetidine. The drug was developed as the result of a theoretical concept that a histamine receptor occurred on the parietal cell which was not blocked by conventional antihistamines. The drug has proved highly effective and blocks acid secretion in response to gastrin and vagal stimulation in a dose-dependent reversible manner. Ulcer healing rates of between 70 and 90 per cent. have been achieved in multicentre trials (Bodemar and Walan, 1976; Burland and Simplins, 1977; Venables *et al.*, 1978). and in all studies the improved healing rate compared with placebo is significant (Binder *et al.*, 1978). Those ulcers which fail to heal may respond to larger doses of the drug (Bardhan, 1981).

A major problem of cimetidine treatment is the ulcer recurrence rate when treatment is stopped. Perhaps as many as 80 per cent. of ulcers recur endoscopically within a year, which contrasts with a figure of 65 per cent. recurrence at a year in those treated with placebo (Burland *et al.*, 1978). Ulcer recurrence may, however, be lessened by continuing the nightly dose of cimetidine over a prolonged period (Blackwood, Mandgai, and Northfield, 1978). In younger patients the long-term safety of cimetidine and hypoacidity is questioned, although this argument should not apply to elderly patients in whom long-term ulcer healing and the avoidance of surgery are the main aims of treatment. Although ulcer recurrence occurs when H_2 receptor blockade is stopped there is no evidence that this is because of rebound hyperacidity.

Few side-effects have been reported from the use of cimetidine. Worries with respect to bone marrow suppression and liver toxicity have not be substantiated. Gynaecomastia occurs, but is rare, and the development of galactorrhoea following the stimulation of prolactin by cimetidine is unusual. Elderly patients and those with poor renal function have high blood levels of cimetidine following an oral dose (Redolfi, Borgogelli, and Lodola, 1979; Schentag *et al.*, 1981). In elderly patients cimetidine has been reported to cause confusion (Basavaraju *et al.*, 1980). Reduced doses of cimetidine would seem sensible in elderly patients and patients with renal insufficiency although side-effects in these groups are not common.

A few patients have been described who developed gastric carcinoma while on treatment with cimetidine (Elder, Ganguli, and Gillespie, 1979; Hawker, Museroft, and Keighley, 1980; Reed, Cassell, and Walters, 1979). A cause-and-effect relationship has yet to be established and the possible carcinogenicity of cimetidine should be disregarded in the elderly. Theoretically the cancer risk of cimetidine is related either to anacidity allowing the conversion of ingested nitrates to carcinogens or to the metabolites of cimetidine which might possibly be carcinogenic (Muscroft *et al.*, 1981; Reed *et al.*, 1981; Ruddell *et al.*, 1978).

An alternative to cimetidine, ranitidine, has recently been introduced. It has a longer duration of action than cimetidine and does not induce hyperprolactinaemia, thus avoiding the possibility of galactorrhoea (Woodings *et al.*, 1980).

High-dose antacid therapy. The administration of large volumes of antacid, about 300 ml each day, have been shown to induce ulcer healing (Peterson *et al.*, 1977). The ingestion of such large volumes of antacid, however, is difficult for they are unpalatable and their high sodium, aluminium, and phosphate levels have the potential of serious side effects.

Mucosal protective agents. Carbenoxolone reinforces the mucosal barrier. It is probably less useful in the case of duodenal ulcer than in gastric ulcer, but there is evidence that healing of duodenal ulcer occurs compared with placebo (Brown *et al.*, 1972; Davies and Reed, 1977). Unfortunately the drug has a mineralo-corticoid effect inducing fluid retention, hypertension and hypokalaemia so that its use is not recommended in the elderly.

Tripotassium dicitrate bismithate (de-nol). Several trials have demonstrated a beneficial effect of this compound on the healing of duodenal ulcer (Connon, 1977; Coughlin, Kupa, and Alp, 1977). Side-effects are not recorded and its only disadvantage is a rather unpleasant taste. Combinations of De-Nol and cimetidine may be useful in healing ulcers in the elderly, avoiding the necessity for surgery.

Smoking and Peptic Ulcer

Healing rates of duodenal ulcer are probably adversely affected by continued cigarette smoking and the incidence of ulcers is higher in those who smoke, (Friedman, Siegelaub, and Seltzec, 1974; Jedrychowski and Popiela, 1974; Sonnenberg *et al.*, 1980). With the advent of cimetidine smoking has less effect on ulcer healing than previously.

Surgical Management of Duodenal Ulcer

The morbidity following duodenal ulcer surgery is high and some operations gave an appreciable mortality, particularly in the elderly. Proximal gastric vagotomy may avoid some of these problems but ulcer recurrence is high (Kronborg and Madsen, 1975; Storey *et al.*, 1981). Following definitive surgical management of an ulcer, recurrence may be treated medically with cimetidine or De-Nol (Festen *et al.*, 1979; Gugler *et al.*, 1979).

Gastric Ulcer (Fig. 9)

The symptoms of gastric ulcer are ill-defined particularly in the elderly. It may present with anaemia, weight loss or general malaise, and dyspeptic symptoms can be absent.

Acid Secretion

Acid studies in gastric ulcer are variable and suggest changes in acid secretion depending on the site of the ulcer. Ulcers along the lesser curve (type I) are seen particularly in the elderly and are associated with low acid secretion. Gastric ulcers in association with a duodenal ulcer (type 2) and prepyloric ulcers (type 3) are associated with normal or increased acid production (Wormsley and Grossman, 1965).

The Gastric Mucosal Barrier

The gastric mucosa is protected from acid and pepsin digestion by a thin lining layer of mucus. This protective layer is breached by several agents allowing back diffusion of hydrogen ions into the mucosa. Bile disrupts the mucosal barrier and studies have shown that bile reflux is increased in patients with gastric ulcer.

Diagnosis of Gastric Ulcer

Double-contrast barium studies are successful in demonstrating the majority of gastric ulcers but radiology cannot always provide evidence

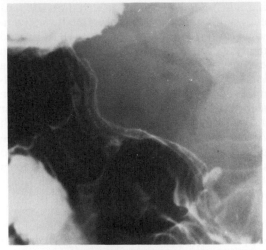
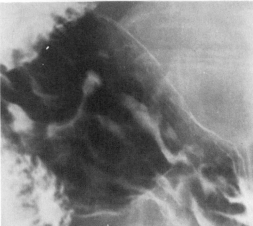

Figure 9   Lesser gastric ulcer. The ulcer shows evidence of bleeding with a "flow" of barium

of malignancy. Some 5 per cent. of apparently benign ulcers, radiologically, prove on subsequent endoscopy to be malignant. It is good practice to endoscope all patients with gastric ulcer in order to obtain histological and cytological material. Failing this, repeat radiological examination after 12 weeks medical treatment is important, when over 90 per cent. of ulcers should be healed (Ashton *et al.*, 1982).

Medical Management of Gastric Ulcer

H₂ blockers. Benign gastric ulcers are associated with a normal or reduced acid output, but do not occur in the absence of acid. The reduction of acid output with cimetidine encourages ulcer healing although the effects are not as dramatic as in the case of duodenal ulcer (Ciditira *et al.*, 1977; Colin-Jones, Cockel, and Schiller, 1978; Frost *et al.*, 1977). Full-dose treatment over a longer period than that used for duodenal ulcer is advised. Gastric ulcers, however, often recur after H_2 blockade is stopped and long-term maintenance therapy may be necessary (Bodemar and Walan, 1978). It is important to appreciate that some histologically malignant gastric ulcers have healed under the influence of cimetidine (Taylor *et al.*, 1978).

Carbenoxolone. Difficulties with carbenoxolone have already been noted (see page 315) and while it is a potent healing agent its use cannot be advocated in the elderly.

De-nol. De-Nol also speeds the healing of gastric ulcer and the absence of side-effects makes it a useful agent (Brogden *et al.*, 1976).

Surgery for Gastric Ulcer

Morbidity and mortality of gastric ulcer surgery is high and surgery is best avoided in the elderly. The morbidity has been lessened by replacing the former operation of partial gastrectomy by vagotomy and a drainage operation combined with ulcer excision (Clarke, Lincoln-Lewis, and Williams, 1972; Kennedy, Kelly, and George, 1972).

Over the last decade the use of surgery in the management of both duodenal and gastric ulcer has declined, reflecting perhaps the falling incidence of duodenal ulcer and the availability of ulcer healing agents (Brown, Langman, and Lambert, 1976; Elashoff and Grossman, 1980; Penn, 1980). The effect that ulcer healing agents, particularly H_2 blockers, have on the natural history of ulcers is unknown and studies of the eventual outcome of peptic ulcers treated with such drugs, particularly in the elderly, are awaited with interest.

Gastrointestinal Bleeding

Gastrointestinal bleeding in the elderly provides a challenge for both the physician and the surgeon. Despite advances in management over the last half century, the mortality rate has changed little, and remains at around 10 per cent. in most published series. One of the reasons for the unchanged mortality rate is the greater representation of elderly patients among those with gastrointestinal bleeding. In 1927 only 2 per cent. of patients were over 60 years of age (Bulmer, 1927) whereas in recent series about 40 to 50 per cent. of patients were over 60 years of age (Fig. 10). Analysis of published series suggests that the risk of gastrointestinal bleeding is three times greater in the over 60 age group that in those under 30 years of age. A further factor contributing to the unchanged mortality from gastrointestinal bleeding is that about half the deaths are judged inevitable, occurring in patients with gastric carcinoma or patients with bleeding associated with terminal liver disease.

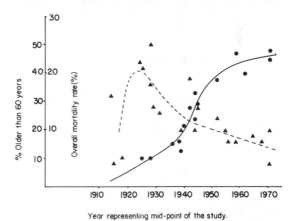

Year representing mid-point of the study.

Figure 10   Percentage of patients over 60 years of age (●) and mortality rate (▲) for gastrointestinal bleeding in major European series.
(Allan and Dykes, 1976, *Quart. J. Med.* **45**, 533–550)
Reproduced by kind permission of the editor

Causes of Gastrointestinal Bleeding (Table 1)

Peptic ulceration is the principal cause of gastrointestinal bleeding in all age groups. Males and females with gastric ulcers over the age of 60 are more likely to bleed than younger patients, a similar increased risk applies to the elderly man with a duodenal ulcer. Bleeding from an erosive gastritis accounts for about one fifth of all causes of gastrointestinal bleeding but is rarely severe. Mallory-Weiss tears at the oesophago-gastric junction account for an increasing number of episodes of bleeding and the classical history of severe vomiting preced-ing the bleeding is not always obtained. Bleed-ing from gastric carcinoma is rarely severe.

Cirrhosis of the liver is being diagnosed more frequently in elderly patients and bleed-ing varices occur in this age group – providing particularly difficult problems in management. Bleeding from smooth muscle tumours in the gastrointestinal tract is a rare cause of gastro-intestinal bleeding and tends to occur more often in younger people. Melaena from lesions on the right side of the colon can occur from a solitary diverticulum or rarely from a segment of angiodysplasia (Boley *et al.*, 1977; Editorial, 1981; Tarin *et al.*, 1978). Angiodysplasia is an acquired lesion occurring with increasing fre-quency with age and being found in the right colon or small bowel. Examination of resected specimens reveal distension of the veins of the bowel wall which penetrate the mucosa so that uncovered vessels impinge on the bowel lu-men. Not surprisingly the diagnosis is often delayed and colonoscopy and arteriography may be apparently normal.

Table 1 Causes of gastrointestinal bleeding. (Adapted from Allan and Dykes, 1976. Reproduced by kind per-mission of Drs Allan and Dykes)

Cause	Male	Female	Total
Duodenal ulcer	26	4	30
Gastric ulcer	9	10	19
Gastric erosions	12	5	17
Mallory–Weiss syndrome	2	0	2
Gastric cancer	4	1	5
Varices	0.5	1	1.5
Miscellaneous	8.5	8	16.5
Not established	6	3	9
	68%	32%	100%

Severity of Gastrointestinal Haemorrhage

Retrospectively the severity of a bleed can be assessed by the transfusion requirement. At the outset vital signs such as pulse rate and blood pressure are important and indicate a need for transfusion. Following a bleed a drop in central venous pressure is an early sign of rebleeding and often precedes changes in pulse and blood pressure. On admission about a third of patients do not require transfusion and a further third require only a 2 to 4 unit trans-fusion. In the remainder bleeding is heavy and recurrent and it is in this group that surgical

intervention is indicated. Not surprisingly this latter group provides the highest number of deaths. Rebleeding is particularly common in the elderly with a gastric ulcer.

Investigation of Gastrointestinal Bleeding

Endoscopy, when performed within 24 hours of admission, provides a definitive diagnosis of the source of the bleeding in over 90 per cent. of patients. The success rate diminishes pro-gressively with a delay between admission and endoscopy (Bown *et al.*, 1981). Radiology de-monstrates a potential source of bleeding in approximately 80 per cent. of patients pro-vided the technique is adequate (Fraser, 1978; Thoeni and Cello, 1980). The superior diag-nostic efficiency of endoscopy does not appear to translate into more successful clinical man-agement particularly in avoiding deaths (Allan and Dykes, 1976; Morris *et al.*, 1975; Sandlow *et al.*, 1974). The universal adoption of early endoscopy in the diagnosis of gastro-intestinal bleeding is debatable and many clinicians re-serve emergency endoscopy for those in whom surgery appears inevitable. In this instance en-doscopy is performed in the anaesthetic room and can provide the surgeon with vital infor-mation as to the source of the bleeding.

Medical Management of Gastrointestinal Bleeding

Assessment of individual medical measures has not demonstrated a useful effect on the out-come of gastrointestinal bleeding. The use of cimetidine is disappointing with only a small benefit being recorded in patients bleeding from gastric ulcer (Hoare *et al.*, 1979) and a major beneficial effect being restricted to those with liver disease who have bled or threaten to bleed (MacDougall and Williams, 1978). Tra-nexamic acid, an oral fibrinolytic agent, is also ineffective (Biggs, Hugh, and Dodds, 1976). High-dose antacid therapy is apparently useful in preventing bleeding in high risk patients such as those with head injury or major burns (Hastings *et al.*, 1978; Priebe *et al.*, 1980). It is rare for patients who have gastrointestinal bleeding to have concurrent abnormalities of coagulation, but where these occur they should be reversed.

Bleeding from oesophageal varices provides

a particular challenge (Fig. 11). Any form of portocaval shunt is contraindicated in the elderly because of the high operative mortality and incidence of portosystemic encephalopathy postoperatively. Indeed, the use of portocaval shunting in younger patients with oesophageal varices due to chronic liver disease is increasingly questioned. The initial treatment of bleeding varices is adequate blood transfusion and correction of clotting abnormalities. Attempts should be made to clear blood from the gut so that protein absorption is diminished and hepatic encephalopathy avoided. Sterilization of the gut with neomycin, gentle purgation with lactulose, or even magnesium sulphate enemata are of value. Bleeding often stops spontaneously. In those patients who continue to bleed intravenous vasopressin is considered although this is not without hazard in elderly patients. Vasopressin is a potent vasoconstrictor which may constrict coronary arteries in vulnerable age groups. Since it is designed to constrict splanchnic blood vessels hepatic arterial inflow may be further embarrassed and liver function deteriorates. Continued bleeding can be controlled by balloon tamponade using a Sengstaken tube. This technique is hazardous and demands high standards of nursing and medical care. A four channel tube is used with one tube in the oesophagus above the oesophageal balloon which is constantly aspirated to prevent overspill of upper gastrointestinal secretions into the lungs. The oesophageal balloon should be deflated for 1 to 2 hours every 12 to 24 hours to prevent necrosis of the oesophageal wall.

A direct surgical attack on varices is preferred by many without the use of balloon tamponade. Oesophageal transection, done early, is useful and controls bleeding. This latter operation is being replaced by the use of a stapling gun which allows an abdominal approach and is technically easier.

Once initial bleeding is controlled long-term management of the varices is contemplated. Sclerotherapy of oesophageal varices was introduced over 40 years ago (Crafoord and Frenckner, 1939) but has only recently with the advent of fibre-optic endoscopy, become popular. To ensure obliteration of vessels endoscopic injection is repeated at monthly intervals until the varices disappear. Complications occur in about 5 to 10 per cent.

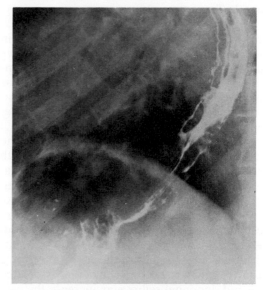

Figure 11   Oesophageal varices

of patients and include dysphagia due to stricture formation and oesophageal perforation with mediastinal abscess, but recent figures indicate that the survival rate has improved with technical advances (MacDougall *et al.*, 1982).

Transhepatic embolization of the portal vein has been used to effect long-term control of variceal bleeding but the technique is difficult and few centres see enough patients to develop expertise (Sherlock, Smith-Laing, and Dick, 1981).

Surgical Management of Gastrointestinal bleeding

About one-fifth of patients admitted with gastrointestinal bleeding require surgical intervention. The timing of surgery is difficult and there are few useful guidelines. Clearly planned surgery by experienced personnel is preferable to emergency surgery and the operation performed should be the least necessary to control haemorrhage. Surgery in the elderly is controversial and some have claimed that surgical intervention in this group contributes significantly to mortality (Schiller, Truelowe, and Williams, 1970).

Laser therapy with the laser beam being directed through the endoscope is a recently introduced means of controlling intestinal bleeding and its use, particularly in the elderly, remains to be explored (Laurence *et al.*, 1980).

Gastric Tumours

The incidence of gastric cancer has fallen in the last few decades both in Western countries and Japan. The reasons for this fall are unknown. Massive screening programmes such as those available in Japan are unlikely to account for the falling incidence which was already declining before their introduction.

Premalignant conditions occur in the stomach. An increased risk is associated with chronic atrophic gastritis, pernicious anaemia, and previous partial gastrectomy. The postulated cause of this risk is anacidity where a rise in the gastric pH allows the conversion of ingested nitrites to potential carcinogens (Ruddell *et al.*, 1976, 1978). In the case of patients with partial gastrectomy the association of a distal gastritis is common and the associated bile and duodenal reflux may increase the cancer risk.

The role of nitrites in the development of gastric cancer is much discussed. High dietary levels of nitrites are associated with a high incidence of gastric cancer in areas such as Chile and Japan (Marquardt, Rufino, and Weisburger, 1977; Zaldiver, 1970). As well as environmental factors genetic factors are important. Expatriate Japanese in the United States continued to experience an increased cancer risk (Stemmermann, 1977) and a further study has suggested a high incidence in those who are 'genetically' Welsh (Ashley, 1969). In addition an increased risk of gastric cancer is associated with possession of blood group A, perhaps because pernicious anaemia is also associated with this blood group (Callender *et al.*, 1971).

Gastric Polyps

Adenomatous gastric polyps are as much of a risk for gastric carcinoma as are colonic polyps for colonic cancer. Multiple gastric polyps are not associated with a similar risk (Owen, 1979).

Superficial Gastric Cancer

This is an unusual gastric tumour but it is important to recognize for the 5-year survival rates following surgery approach 90 per cent. The cancer is confined to the mucosa. A shallow ulcer is seen endoscopically, the base of which is benign histologically whereas the edges are histologically malignant. The lesions occur in the antrum and are occasionally multicentric. Patients with superficial cancer present, on average, 5 years younger than do patients with other forms of gastric cancer. The clinical expression of the disease is ill defined, leading to difficulties in diagnosis. Dyspepsia or other symptoms of peptic ulceration are unusual and gastrointestinal bleeding is rare. Rarely this lesion is discovered incidentally at laparotomy.

Gastric Cancer (Fig. 12)

Gastric cancer presents with a variety of symptoms including anorexia, nausea and vomiting, weight loss, abdominal pain, and anaemia. Gastric cancer may present in the elderly with symptoms which are not typical of upper gastrointestinal disease.

Presentation of gastric cancer occurs at any age although the majority of patients are over the age of 50 years. The diagnosis is seldom in doubt when standard techniques such as double-contrast barium meal and endoscopy are used.

No effective treatment exists for gastric cancer and the majority of patients are dead within 5 years of presentation. Surgery offers the best chance of a 'cure' but often the disease has

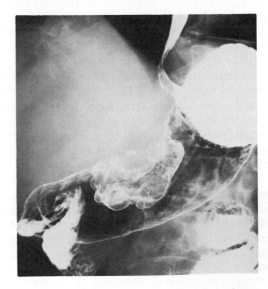

Figure 12   Advanced gastric cancer on the lesser curve

spread beyond the stomach at laparotomy. Palliative surgery is often the most that can be offered. Chemotherapy and radiotherapy make little contribution.

Smooth Muscle Tumours (Fig. 13)

These tumours are unusual and present either with gastrointestinal bleeding or abdominal pain. Radiological investigation is valuable when a submucosal tumour with ulceration is seen. Endoscopy is less helpful since biopsy of a submucosal tumour is not possible. Malignant smooth muscle tumours are difficult to distinguish from gastric ulcers but may be more amenable to surgery. They do not spread to lymph nodes.

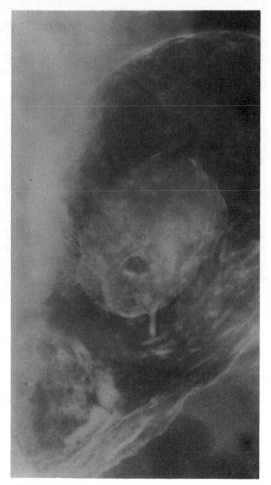

Figure 13 Smooth muscle tumour of the stomach. Central ulceration and a fimbrimated outline are characteristic

Gastric Lymphomas

These tumours are clinically and radiologically indistinguishable from gastric cancer but the distinction should be attempted as the response to surgery is much better than for gastric carcinoma.

Gastric Motility

Impaired gastric motility is an unusual clinical problem. It occurs principally in two conditions, diabetes mellitus and following vagotomy. In the diabetic patient it is a part of a more generalized autonomic neuropathy and there is often marked peripheral neuropathy. Gastroparesis also occurs in diabetic ketoacidosis in a reversible way, perhaps related to 'vagal paralysis' as a result of hyperglycaemia, and the presence of acetone and ketone bodies with altered potassium balance (Taub, Moriani, and Birkin, 1979).

Reduced gastric emptying has been noted in other gastric disorders such as gastric ulcer (Garrett, Summerskill, and Code, 1966).

Drug Therapy

Metaclopramide and bethanechol can be shown by electrophysiological techniques to improve gastric motor activity on both postoperative and diabetic stomach (Malagelada *et al.*, 1980). Unfortunately the clinical effect is less certain.

THE COLON AND RECTUM

The colon is lined by columnar epithelium comprising mainly of secretory mucus cells. There are two muscle coats, the inner coat of circularly arranged fibres which contract to produce the saculations or haustra and three outer bands of longitudinal muscle, the taenia coli. Contraction of the longitudinal muscle provides a propelling force for the onward movement of colonic contents.

The colon is not a digestive organ but acts rather as a reservoir. It is important in conserving intestinal fluid for while 1 to 2 l of fluid enter the colon each day the faecal mass contains less than 0.5 l.

The arterial supply of the colon is derived from the superior mesenteric artery which supplies the right side and the inferior mesenteric artery which supplies the left side. The splenic flexure is supplied from anastomosing vessels from both arteries and it is this part of the colon which is most vulnerable to ischaemic colitis. The rectum is supplied by branches from the internal iliac arteries. The venous drainage of the colon is to the portal vein whereas veins from the rectum drain into the inferior vena cava. This provides a site of potential portocaval shunting in chronic liver disease although varices seldom seem to develop.

The colon is richly supplied by lymphatics which accompany blood vessels and drain into the para-aortic nodes. Innervation of the colon occurs both through the sympathetic and parasympathetic system. The sympathetic nerve supply is from the coeliac and splenic nodes derived from the fifth thoracic and second lumbar nerve roots. The parasympathetic nerve supply occurs through the terminal branches of the vagus. Parasympathetic stimulation increases colonic motility and helps to propel the faecal mass. Sympathetic stimulation has an opposite effect.

Colonic Motility

The control mechanisms of various forms of colonic motility are ill understood. The entry of food into the upper small intestine leads to the passage of material from the terminal ileum into the caecum – the so-called gastroileal reflex. This reflex is possibly mediated by the hormone gastrin. The gastroileal reflex also seems to stimulate colonic activity which results in the movements of faecal mass along the colon. Further movement within the colon serves to mix and perhaps prevent colonic contents from entering the rectum. Eventually faeces enter the upper rectum and stimulate the defaecation reflex. The centre of the defaecation reflex is found in the sacral spinal cord and is served by efferent fibres travelling in sympathetic nerves which relax the upper anal sphincter. The lower anal sphincter is under voluntary control (see Chapter 11.4).

Normal Bowel Habit

Over 90 per cent. of a normal adult population have a bowel action which varies from three times daily to three times a week (Connell *et al.*, 1965). Bowel habits outside this range should be considered as abnormal, but the most important consideration of bowel habit is to note a recent change. In the elderly, bowel habit alters with changes in mobility, preventing access to lavatory facilities and the effect that exercise has on defaecation being important. Diet and drugs each play a particular role in causing changes in bowel habit in the elderly.

Abnormal Colonic Motility

Irritable Colon Syndrome

The irritable colon syndrome is a common disorder in the young and middle aged but is diagnosed only reluctantly in the elderly. Patients present with a wide range of abdominal symptoms of which pain is prominent and either constipation or diarrhoea occurs. Barium enema and sigmoidoscopy are normal.

Electrophysiological measurements demonstrate increased colonic contractions in response to stimulants such as emotion, eating, and hormones such as cholecystokinin (Harvey and Read, 1973; Ritchie, 1977). There are no good studies relating age to colonic motility and symptoms, which in the young are of the irritable colon syndrome, are ascribed to diverticular disease in the elderly. Abnormal colonic motility is associated with diverticular disease and it is tempting to suggest that diverticular disease is the result in the elderly of earlier irritable colon.

Diverticulosis

Diverticulosis is unknown in African communities, but is seen in up to 60 per cent. of elderly patients from Western countries on barium enema or at autopsy (Painter and Burkitt, 1971). Diverticula occur as the colonic mucosa herniates through the inner muscle coats consequent upon increased tone and hypertrophy. In the absence of inflammation it is unlikely that these blind-ended sacs cause symptoms of themselves. Any symptoms that do occur are probably the result of colonic spasm.

With respect to diet, lack of roughage is

currently suspected as being important in the genesis of both the irritable colon and diverticular disease (Painter, 1969; Painter and Burkitt, 1971). The addition of bulk to the diet in the form of bran tends to improve the symptoms of irritable bowel (Brodribb, 1977; Manning *et al.*, 1977), although this experience is questioned by others (Ornstein *et al.*, 1981; Soltoft *et al.*, 1976). Other preparations including peppermint oil capsules (Rees, Evans, and Rhodes, 1979) and an antispasmodic such as mebeverine may be helpful.

Diverticulitis

Diverticulitis (see Chapter 9) occurs as the result of inflammation of a colonic diverticulum. Diverticula may contain faecal material and if the pressure within the colon rises the diverticulum is excluded from the colonic lumen and an abscess may develop which can extend into the paracolic area. Inflammation and infection may result in the development of a stricture a stricture or vesico-colic fistula can occur. A palpable mass is present in 30 per cent. of individuals. Bleeding does occur but is unusual, and its presence should alert the clinician to the possibility of colonic neoplasia, polyps, and angiodysplasia.

Cathartic Colon

Thirty or forty years ago public hoardings were urging people to take care of their bowels and persuading them of the merits of various commerical purgative preparations. Ritual weekly purgation was commonplace at all levels of society. It was against this background that our present elderly population grew up. It is therefore not surprising that bowels assaulted by various purgatives in youth continue to be assaulted in old age.

Chronic purgative ingestion makes the bowel less and less responsive to the effects of the purgative despite increasing its dosage, producing eventually a cathartic colon. The patient has chronic constipation. Radiologically the haustral pattern of the colon is lost and large areas of the colon become featureless and redundant. Pseudo-strictures may occur. Pathological examination shows the colon to be thin walled with neuronal degeneration affecting the intrinsic network and axons.

Black pigmentation may be seen sigmoidoscopically as the so called melanosis coli (Cooke, 1977).

Treatment is difficult. Clearly purgatives must be stopped and a high fibre diet, bulking agents, and an osmotic laxative such as lactulose given. Recovery is uncertain and in some colectomy provides the only solution.

Diarrhoea in the Elderly

Diarrhoea when it occurs is a major problem in the elderly. Deprived social circumstances and poor sanitary facilities make its management difficult. A common cause of elderly diarrhoea is faecal impaction with overflow of faecal contents, sometimes amounting to incontinence. Diarrhoea is occasionally iatrogenic and is a recognized complication of methyl dopa, bethanidine, mefenamic acid, and antibiotic therapy. Infections are less common in the elderly but may occur causing great distress and disruption of fluid and electrolyte balance.

Inflammatory Bowel Disease

The cause of inflammatory bowel disease is unknown. The possibility that it is infective has been examined but is as yet not proven (Philpotts *et al.*, 1980). Two organisms are recognized as causing an acute colitic illness – *Campylobacter* and *Clostridium difficile*—but their involvement in chronic disease is unlikely. There is some familial expression for both Crohn's disease and ulcerative colitis (Binder *et al.*, 1966; Lewkonia and McConnell, 1976). Inflammatory bowel disease is not associated with a particular tissue type (Asquith *et al.*, 1974; Lewkonia *et al.*, 1974).

Presentation of Inflammatory Bowel Disease and Age

Inflammatory bowel disease has a bimodal age incidence peaking at 25 to 44 years old and in the 60 to 80 age group (Evans and Acheson, 1965; Garland *et al.*, 1981). The bimodal age presentation occurs both for ulcerative colitis and Crohn's disease. The improved management of middle aged patients with inflammatory bowel disease leads to the survival of patients into old age and further problems of management for the physician responsible for the care of the elderly.

Acute Fulminating Ulcerative Colitis

This condition presents at any age. The initial presentation may cause difficulties in distinguishing it from an infective diarrhoea. The patient complains of profuse diarrhoea with blood and pus in the stools. Systemic effects are common and the patient may be malnourished, have fever and tachycardia, and disturbances of acid/base balance occur. Stool cultures are mandatory with particular emphasis being laid on the presence of *Campylobacter* or *Clostridium difficile*. Proctoscopy and limited sigmoidoscopy without biopsy suggest the diagnosis of ulcerative colitis. Barium enema examination should never be performed in the acute situation for fear of perforating the colon.

The great danger is the development of acute toxic dilatation of the colon. The danger is greatest in those who have fulminating colitis with fever, tachycardia, a high ESR, a high white cell count, and disturbances of acid/base balance. Patients presenting with acute colitis should have such indices measured daily together with plain X-rays of the abdomen. Such X-rays are of twofold importance. Firstly, it is unlikely, though not impossible, that areas of colon which contain faeces are the site of acute colitis. Secondly, the plain X-rays of the colon allow the assessment of the degree of colonic distension. If the transverse diameter of the colon exceeds 10 cm the danger of perforation is imminent (Fig. 14).

The management of acute colitis is urgent and large doses of corticosteroids (the equivalent of 60 mg of Prednisolone a day) intravenously are required. Oral feeding is

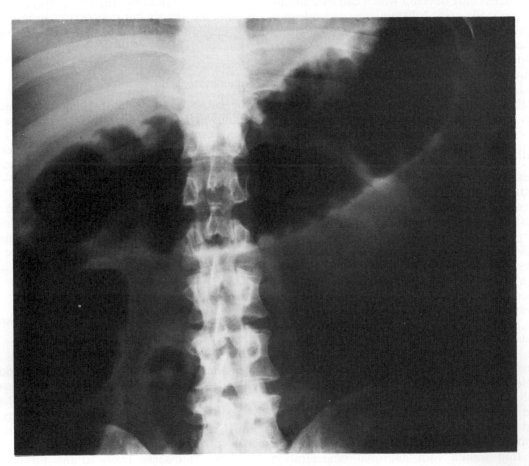

Figure 14   Toxic dilatation of the colon in acute colitis

discontinued and fluid and electrolytic balance is maintained by intravenous infusion. Because of the profuse diarrhoea, special attention to potassium levels is paid. The contribution of antibiotic agents to the patient with acute fulminating colitis is controversial although it is fair to state that most clinicians feel that agents such as metronidazole and gentamycin have a role. Where acute symptoms do not settle or where radiological evidence of toxic dilatation occurs, surgery must be considered sooner rather than later as a life-saving measure, even in the elderly (Goligher, Hoffman, and De Dombal, 1970).

Ulcerative Colitis and Proctitis

Ulcerative colitis does not always involve the whole colon. Disease limited to the rectum, proctitis, is common and seldom does this progress. Commonly the patient presents with blood-stained diarrhoea and gross systemic effects are unusual. The diagnosis is supported by sigmoidoscopy where the rectal mucosa is granular and bleeding and the rectal lumen contains blood and mucus. Rectal biopsy shows the inflammation is limited to the mucosa with loss of goblet cells and a chronic inflammatory infiltrate. It is an important practical point to suggest that barium enema examination should not be performed for 7 days following rectal biopsy, for it is during this time that the danger of colonic perforation as a consequence of radiological examination is greatest. Eventual barium enema reveals the extent of the colitis which is characterized by loss of haustral pattern and pseudo-polypformation in long-standing disease (Figs 15 and 16).

The initial treatment of an acute attack of proctitis or limited colitis is again corticosteroids which may be administered by enema or by mouth. It is unlikely that steroid administration by the rectal route reaches much further than the splenic flexure (Matts and Gaskell, 1961).

Following the successful management of an acute attack of colitis relapse is prevented by Sulphasalazine (Misievicz *et al.*, 1965; Svartz, 1942). The prevention of relapse has now been shown to persist for some years (Dissanayake and Truelove, 1973). In addition to its prophylactic effect in preventing relapse Sulphasalazine is useful in treating acute colitis (Baron *et*

al., 1962). Unfortunately a third of colitic patients may be unable to tolerate long-term Sulphasalazine because of gastrointestinal side-effects which may be avoided by using the drug other than in tablet form. Pharmacologically the drug contains sulphapyridine and 5-aminosalicylic acid which is probably the active constituent (Azad-Kahn, Piris, and Truelove, 1977; Campieri *et al.*, 1981; Van Hees, Bakker, and Van Tongeren, 1980). Developments in providing a rectally administered form of Sulpasalazine or of its active constituent are current and the results of their wider application awaited with interest.

Azathioprine has been used in ulcerative colitis without apparent advantage (Jewell and Truelove, 1974; Rosenberg *et al.*, 1975). Gastroenterologists were excited by the suggestion that disodium chromoglycate was useful in proctitis and localized colitis but its early promise is unconfirmed by subsequent experience (Buckell *et al.*, 1978; Dronfield and Langman, 1978); Heatley *et al.*, 1975; Mani *et al*, 1976; Willoughby *et al*, 1979)

Crohn's Disease

Crohn's disease affects the whole gastrointestinal tract although the commonest site of involvement is in the terminal ileum. All age groups are affected.

Crohn's Colitis

The whole colon may be involved although segmental or skip lesions, where portions of the colon are spared, are also seen. Rectal sparing is usual in patients with otherwise extensive colitis and this serves as a useful distinction from ulcerative colitis. Perianal disease with discoloration of the perianal region, abscesses, and fistulae may be the sole expression of the illness or appear in combination with either colonic or small intestinal involvement. Perianal disease is unusual in ulcerative colitis and also serves as a useful distinguishing feature of Crohn's disease.

The diagnosis is suggested by the use of sigmoidoscopy and rectal biopsy with barium enema examination and occasionally colonoscopy. Sigmoidoscopic examination may reveal an inflamed, bleeding rectal mucosa which is impossible to distinguish from ulcerative coli-

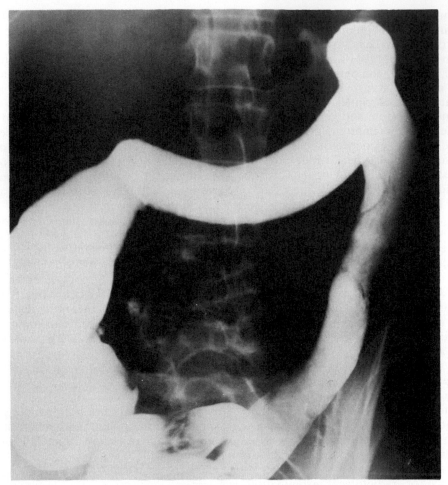

Figure 15 Total ulcerative colitis. The mucosa is ulcerated and the haustral pattern is lost

tis. Occasionally multiple aphthoid-type ulcers are seen which are typical of Crohn's disease. Rectal biopsy reveals inflammation extending into the submucosa. Non-caseating granulomata are characteristic and occasionally seen on rectal biopsy. Rectal biopsy of a macroscopically normal rectum may provide histological evidence of disease where disease occurs at other sites in the intestinal tract.

Barium enema examinations indicate the site and extent of disease. Changes confined to one or two segments of the colon with deep penetrating ulcers – the so-called 'rose thorn ulcers'—are characteristic (Fig. 17). Where the radiological changes are diffuse, the distinction from ulcerative colitis may be impossible. Ileal involvement occurs more commonly in Crohn's disease although changes in the ileum may be seen in severe ulcerative colitis—'backwash ileitis'.

The association radiologically of Crohn's disease of the colon with diverticular disease presents a difficult clinical problem. Both conditions occur in the elderly and sometimes occur together. The combination is increasingly recognized in those over 40 years of age with a mean age of about 60 years. Patients present with typical colitic symptoms and the coexistence of the two conditions may not be recognized until the pathologist's report on a surgically removed segment of colon is available (Marshak, Janowitz, and Present ,1970; Ritchie and Lennard-Jones, 1976; Schmidt *et al.*, 1968).

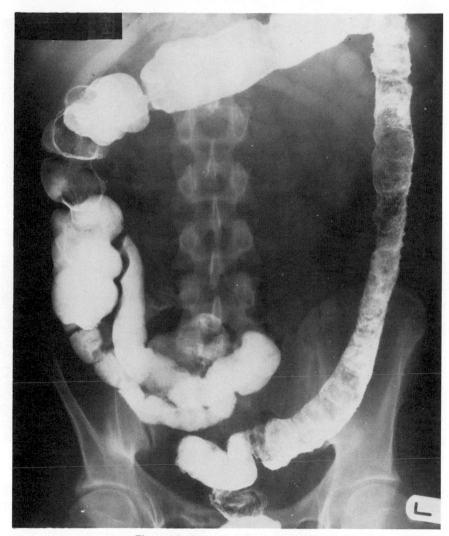

Figure 16   Left sided ulcerative colitis

The treatment of Crohn's colitis is that of ulcerative colitis. The results of treatment of Crohn's colitis are not as impressive as those for ulcerative colitis and surgery is more frequent (Allan *et al.*, 1977). Rectal sparing often allows an ileorectal anastomosis rather than the more mutilating ileostomy to be performed.

Ischaemic Colitis

Ischaemic colitis occurs predominantly in elderly patients. A history of previous cardiovascular disease such as myocardial infarction, intermittent claudication, or hypertension is common. The splenic flexure area of the colon is most often affected but other sites of the colon, including the rectum, are involved (Marston, 1977).

The recognition of ischaemic colitis is recent and has resulted from experimental evidence in dogs and clinical observations in humans (De Villiers, 1966; Marston *et al.*, 1969). Ischaemic colitis sometimes occurs following reconstructive aortic surgery or rectal excision of carcinoma resulting in interference with the inferior mesenteric artery (Goligher, 1954; Gonzalez and Jaffe, 1966).

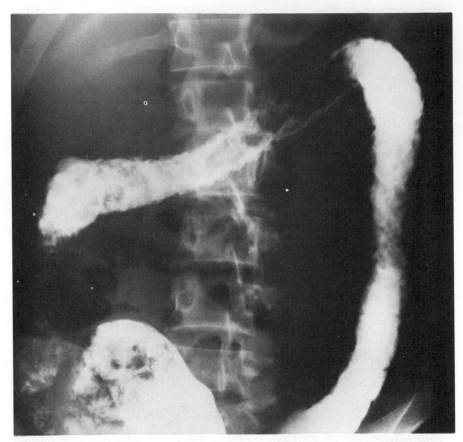

Figure 17   Crohn's colitis, with deep ulcers and a "cobbelstone" mucosa

Arteriography of the colonic vasculature may fail to reveal localized arterial obstruction since the clinical picture is also caused by small vessel thrombosis, venous thrombosis, transient hypotension following myocardial infarction, and hyperviscosity states.

The clinical presentation of ischaemic colitis is sudden. The patient complains of abdominal pain and blood-stained diarrhoea. The symptoms may settle within hours or persist for some weeks. Occasionally the patient becomes acutely unwell with fever, tachycardia, and signs of an intra-abdominal catastrophe leading to exploratory laparotomy.

In patients who do not come to immediate laparotomy the diagnosis of ischaemic colitis is made at subsequent barium enema examination. In the early stages radiological examination reveals the characteristic thumbprinting sign due to mucosal oedema. Later a smooth tapering stricture may appear (De Dombal, Fletcher, and Harris, 1969) (Fig. 18). In fortunate patients the clinical symptoms and radiological signs disappear.

Vascular radiographic procedures are best avoided for they carry the risk of extension of the vascular insufficiency. Colonoscopy is useful in that it helps to distinguish vascular lesions from other causes of a segmental colitis, but should not be performed in the acute situation.

Treatment of the condition is largely conservative. Corticosteroids and Sulphasalazine are of no value.

Infective Colitis

Of two recent pathogens associated with colitic illness *Campylobacter* is the most common. The diarrhoea induced by *Campylobacter* results from inflammatory change in the rectal mucosa which may be indistinguishable from

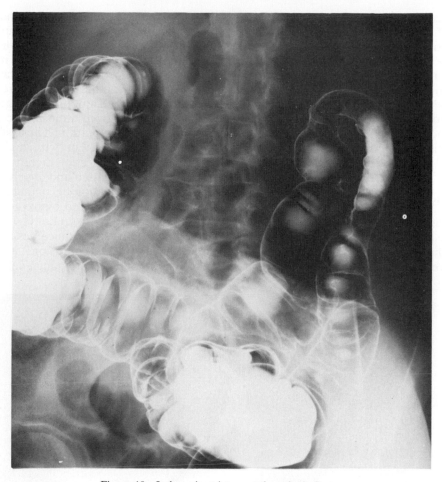

Figure 18   Ischaemic stricture at the splenic flexure

an acute idiopathic proctitis (Price, Jecokes, and Sanderson, Willoughby, Piris, and True-love, 1979). The organism has been isolated from the stools of domestic pets and chickens and these form an important reservoir for human infection. In the majority of cases the illness is acute and non-recurring, but the symptoms and signs may persist for as long as 6 months. The diagnosis may only be made by bacterial examination of the faeces. In most the disease is self-limiting but in severe infection erythromycin may prove useful.

Diarrhoea following antibiotics is common. It occurs particularly in the elderly and can occur with any antibiotic although that associated with lincomycin or clindamycin is best described. In severe cases there is gross structural change in the colon. Classically islands of normal mucosa occur between areas of severe ulceration presenting the appearance of a pseudo-membrane. Barium enema examination reveals an extensive colitis with rectal involvement; the small bowel is affected only rarely and toxic megacolon is unusual.

The organism responsible for antibiotic-induced diarrhoea is *Clostridium difficile (George et al,* 1978; Larson *et al,* 1978). This organism is not usually present in stool cultures but the administration of antibiotics suppresses the growth of normally found colonic bacteria allowing *Clostridium difficile* to overgrow. The organism forms a toxin which is cytopathic and probably induces the mucosal damage (Chang, Lauermann, and Batlett, 1979).

A history of recent antibiotic ingestion should be sought of all patients who present an acute colitis. Sigmoidoscopy reveals the presence of a pseudo-membrane in most cases. Bacterial confirmation of the offending organism may be obtained by careful stool culture.

The recommended treatment is with vancomycin or oral metronidazole. The diarrhoea does not always respond, particularly in the elderly, and recurrences are common. Parenteral nutrition may be necessary in the severely ill. The initial mortality rate is high and ranges between 10 and 20 per cent.

Pneumatosis Cystoides Intestinalis

This is a rare condition presenting principally in later life. It is debatable whether it is commoner in the colon or the small intestine. The disorder presents usually as an incidental find-

ing on barium examination of rounded multiple filling defects in the colonic lumen (Fig. 19). The aetiology remains unknown but there is a definite association with both respiratory disease and pyloroduodenal ulceration. The gas-filled cysts contain a high percentage of nitrogen and a small amount of oxygen and are probably derived from atmospheric air rather than bacterial fermentation. The cysts may disappear during treatment with high pressure oxygen therapy, suggesting there is an equilibrium between formation and absorption of the gas contents, absorption becoming more rapid if the nitrogen is replaced by oxygen.

The disorder is essentially benign and asymptomatic. Its importance lies in its recognition which prevents confusion with other diseases such as polyps, carcinoma, and ischaemic

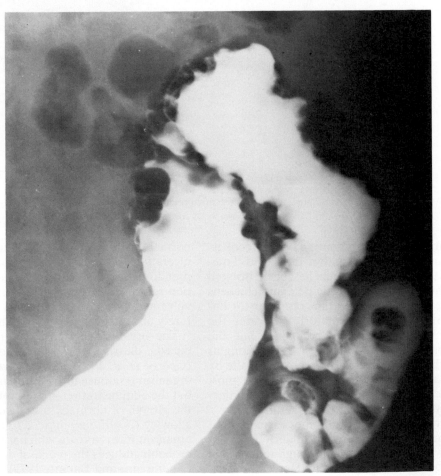

Figure 19   Pneumatosis cystoides intestinalis. A barium enema showing smooth round
filling defects at the splenic flexure

colitis and avoids unnecessary laparotomy. Left-sided disease of the colon leads to abdominal pain and even rectal bleeding.

Colorectal Polyps and Carcinoma

Three groups of polyps occur in the colon: adenomas, villous adenoma or papilloma, and an intermediate histological group. With all groups there is a risk of malignant change which is related mainly to size. Polyps which have a diameter greater than 2 cm have a malignant change rate of up to 50 per cent. The risk of malignant change is greater for villous adenoma than for other polyps (Panish, 1979).

The suggestion has been made that all colonic carcinoma derive from polyps (Morson, 1962). The postulated mechanism is that malignant change occurs in the tip of the polyp and invasion of the submucosa occurs through the stalk. The actual sequence has been observed in some patients while in others it is not uncommon to find remnants of an adenomatous polyp in relation to a resected carcinoma.

Most polyps are, unfortunately, asymptomatic. They may present with rectal bleeding but often are discovered during the course of barium enema examinations when it is difficult to believe that they produced the symptoms which led to the radiological examination. Villous papilloma occasionally presents with hypokalaemia as the result of the profound watery diarrhoea.

Because of the risk of malignant change all colonic polyps must be removed either through the sigmoidoscope or the colonoscope. Histological examination of the base of the polyp is mandatory and any doubt with respect to malignancy should lead to colonic resection.

Colorectal Cancer

There are wide geographical variations in the incidence of colorectal cancer. The incidence is apparently highest in Westernized society and low in the Third World countries. Dietary factors have been discussed in the aetiology of colonic cancer and recently the lack of dietary fibre has been implicated as a major factor. Stool examination of unaffected individuals from high and low risk areas have revealed high bile acid concentrations in stool specimens from the areas of higher risk (Hill, 1974; Hill

et al., 1975). The reason for the high bile acid content of such stools is thought to be the coexisting high concentration of bacteria which are capable of metabolizing bile acids into potential carcinogens. The theory is completed by the suggestion that diets rich in fibre promote the excretion of bacteria by decreasing whole bowel time and also that dietary fibre adsorbs potential carcinogens and leads to their quicker expulsion.

Several conditions are associated with a higher than expected risk of colorectal cancer. Familial polyposis is inherited as an autosomal dominant and in such patients polyps develop through the colon by the age of 20 years. Total colectomy is indicated in the mid-twenties in order to avoid the complication of carcinoma which occurs before 50 years of age; this problem is seldom one which taxes physicians involved in the care of the elderly. Ulcerative colitis is a recognized premalignant condition. The risk is associated with the extent of colonic involvement and rises in patients who have had the disease for longer than 10 years. The role of prophylactic colectomy in such patients, particularly in the elderly age group, is difficult. Our personal view is that the problems of major surgery and an ileostomy in an elderly patient far outweighs the dangers of colonic cancer and is not justified. Constant vigilance for the development of cancer is vital, for these tumours have up to a 50 per cent 5-year survival rate (Ritchie, Hawley, and Lennard-Jones, 1981). There is also an increased risk of colonic cancer in Crohn's colitis (Gyde *et al.*, 1980).

Colorectal cancer presents in all age groups but the risk is highest in those over the age of 60 years (Goligher, 1980). The principal complaint is that of an altered bowel habit, tenesmus, rectal bleeding, and contamination of the stool with slime. Constipation with abdominal pain occurs in those with an obstructing lesion. Occasional patients present with secondary deposits. Iron deficiency anaemia is a common presentation in the elderly.

Over 50 per cent of the tumours are left sided in the lower sigmoid colon and rectum. Left-sided lesions present early with obstructing symptoms whereas right-sided lesions present late because they have little effect on bowel habit.

The diagnosis is made by rectal examination,

sigmoidoscopy, and barium enema (Fig. 20).

Surgical resection in the best hands leads to a 20 to 50 per cent 5-year survival rate (Franklin and McSwain, 1970; Slaney, Waterhouse and Powell, 1968), and these rates can be achieved in the elderly (Adam, Calabrese, and Volk, 1972). Several factors affect survival, not the least of which is adequate colonic resection and antibiotic cleansing before surgery. Tumours confined histologically to the bowel wall have a 90 per cent 5-year survival rate.

LIVER, BILIARY TRACT, AND PANCREAS

The liver is a lobular organ whose structure depends greatly on its vascular supply and drainage and its relationship with the biliary system. The liver lobule may be regarded as a filter which connects portal venous inflow to hepatic venous outflow. The basic structural support to the liver is the portal tract which in health contains only a small amount of fibrous tissue. Within the portal tract are the radicles of the portal vein which is formed by the junction of the splenic and superior mesenteric vein and carries nutrients and products of bacterial metabolism from the gut. Arterial blood is supplied by the hepatic artery which arises from the coeliac plexus. The portal tract also contains bile ductules which originate at the level of the bile canaliculus which is simply the corrugated surface of a liver cell. The bile ductules join to form the right and left hepatic ducts and these in turn form the common bile duct which enters the second part of the duodenum. Within the portal tract are sympathetic nerves which synapse in the coeliac plexus, with the right and left vagus and the right phrenic nerve. Lymph vessels found in the portal tract drain to nodes at the porta hepatis.

The portal tract is separated from the hepatic lobule by a distinct layer of liver cells called the limiting plate. The hepatic lobule is composed of hepatocytes arranged in columns radiating from the hepatic veins. Each hepatocyte is in communication with an adjoining hepatocyte and has a biliary canaliculus and a surface facing the hepatic sinusoid and space of Disse. Sinusoids contain tissue fluid and are lined by endothelial and Kupfer cells which play a part in the immunological system. The space of Disse is the potential space between the liver cell and the sinusoid.

Hepatic veins originate in the centre of the liver lobule, one from the left lobe and two from the right lobe of the liver, which drain to the inferior vena cava. Smaller venous channels drain directly from the caudate lobe into the inferior vena cava.

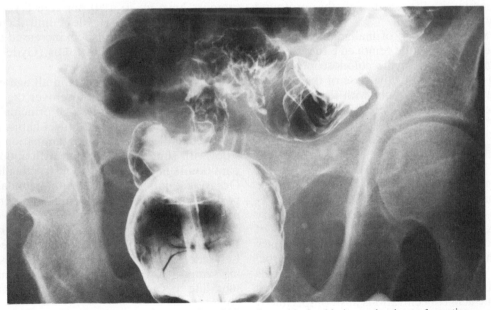

Figure 20   Carcinoma at the recto-sigmoid junction, with shouldering and stricture formation

Bilirubin Metabolism

The breakdown of haemoglobin, myoglobin and respiratory enzymes occurs mainly in the reticuloendothelial system of the liver and spleen and results in the formation of bilirubin. About one fifth of the circulating bilirubin is produced by immature erythropoeitic cells in the bone marrow and the spleen, or formed in the liver from the breakdown of haem, cytochromes, and other sources.

Unconjugated bilirubin thus formed is very sparingly soluble in water and is carried in the plasma reversibly bound to albumin. Uptake of unconjugated bilirubin into the hepatocyte is preceded by the dissociation of the bilirubin/albumin complex. This probably occurs at the level of the sinusoidal/plasma membrane. The bilirubin is transported within the liver cell, bound to proteins such as ligandin, to the endoplasmic reticulum. Within the endoplasmic reticulum, the water-insoluble bilirubin is conjugated under the influence of an enzyme, bilirubin UDP glucuronyl transferase, to a water-soluble bilirubin glucuronide in which form it is excreted with the bile. An active transport mechanism occurs at canalicular level for the hepatic excretion of bilirubin diglucuronide. Within the colon bacterial hydrolysis of the conjugated bilirubin occurs and urobilinogens are formed. Little is known of the effect of age on bilirubin metabolism.

Disorders of Bilirubin Metabolism

Increased production of bilirubin occurs in haemolytic states and leads to modest elevations of the serum unconjugated bilirubin. Other evidence of haemolysis such as anaemia or reticulocytosis is evident but biochemical indicators of liver disease such as serum transaminases and alkaline phosphatase are not affected.

Familial Unconjugated Hyperbilirubinaemia (Gilbert's Syndrome)

Population studies have revealed that almost 10 per cent of otherwise normal individuals have unconjugated hyperbilirubinaemia (Owens and Evans, 1975). Unconjugated hyperbilirubinaemia is more commonly found in men. The principal biochemical abnormality appears to be reduction in the hepatic levels of UDP glucuronyl transferase leading to failure of production of bilirubin glucuronides. In some individuals evidence of mild haemolysis or dyshaemopoeisis is apparent although such abnormalities are not sufficient to account for the hyperbilirubinaemia. There are no convincing clinical symptoms and serum transaminase and alkaline phosphatase levels are normal. Hepatic histology is never abnormal although it is seldom necessary to resort to liver biopsy to establish the diagnosis. The importance of the condition lies in its recognition for it frequently appears in elderly patients who have had a heart attack or developed a stroke and whose calorie intake is subsequently decreased. Fasting leads to diminution of intrahepatic levels of UDP glucuronyl transferase, explaining why unconjugated hyperbilirubinaemia may be noticed for the first time in such patients. Restriction of calorie intake has been used to diagnose the abnormality (Owens and Sherlock, 1973) and the administration of phenobarbitone, by inducing the hepatic glucoronating system, reduces the levels of serum bilirubin (Black and Sherlock, 1970).

Other unconjugated hyperbilirubinaemias including the Crigier–Najjer, the Dubin–Johnson, and the Rotor types present in young people and are never a problem in the elderly.

Bile Acid Metabolism

Bile acids are produced within the liver from cholesterol and form the major excretory pathway for cholesterol from the body. The liver produces two primary bile acids, cholic and chenodeoxycholic acid, and these are excreted into the bile as glycine and taurine salts. Within the intestine bile salts undergo bacterial dehydroxylation and two secondary bile salts are produced: deoxycholic acid from cholic acid and lithocholic acid from chenodeoxycholic acid.

Bile salts are not only an important pathway of cholesterol metabolism but are vital for the solubilization of cholesterol within the bile. Additionally bile acids promote bile flow and the dihydroxy bile acids cause a net secretion of fluid into the colon if they occur there in excess and consequently stimulate colonic motility. Whether bile acids promote colonic function in normal circumstances is uncertain.

Bile acids promote the absorption of fats and fat-soluble vitamins by their ability to form micelles. The bile acid molecule has two sides one of which has an affinity for fat and the other for water. In conjunction with lecithin bile salts arrange themselves into spheres so that the hydrophobic (fat soluble) part of the molecule face the inside and the hydrophilic (water soluble) part of the molecule face the outside. Fat and fat-soluble vitamins are therefore carried within the centre of the micelle while the water-soluble part of the molecule face the aqueous conditions of the small intestine and thus are carried to their absorptive sites. As well as being involved in the intestinal solubilization of fat, bile acids probably influence the function and secretion of pancreatic enzymes and are also important in the intramucosal resynthesis of triglycerides. The detergent properties of bile acids help in fat emulsification which precedes lipolysis although the mechanical churning action of the gastrointestinal tract is probably more important in breaking up fat globules.

The enterohepatic circulation of bile acids is an efficient method of conserving these substances in the body. In health the majority of secreted bile acid is actively reabsorbed from the terminal ileum and recycled through the liver so that less than 5 per cent of the total bile acid pool is lost from the body in each 24 hours.

Bile Acid Metabolism and Age

Little is known of the effect of age on the bile acid composition of the bile. Age, however, does lead to increased saturation of the bile with cholesterol but whether this is due to increase in cholesterol concentration, diminution in total bile acid production, and/or phospholipid concentration, or even to a lowered water phase, is not certain. The net result of increased bile cholesterol saturation is to lead to the development of gallstones.

Bile Acids and Liver Disease

In cholestatic liver disease total concentrations of serum bile acids are raised and this may be the cause of the associated pruritis. Depletion of the total bile acid pool by the anionic exchange resin cholestyramine relieves itching in many patients. There are no specific changes in the serum levels of individual bile acids associated with liver disease but the total serum level of bile acid, particularly after a meal, is high in patients with chronic hepatocellular disease and may be a sensitive laboratory test (Kaplowitz, Kok, and Javitt, 1973). Biliary bile acid levels are lowered in chronic liver disease reflecting hepatocellular function and possible cholestasis. Fat solubilization may be affected and steatorrhoea result.

Bile Acids in Disease of the Terminal Ileum

Loss of the terminal ileum either as the result of disease or following surgical resection leads to a constant drain of the bile acid pool for which the liver is eventually unable to compensate. Loss of bile acid leads to saturation of the bile with cholesterol, and hence the formation of cholesterol gallstones, and to the defective absorption of fat and fat-soluble vitamins. Overspill of the unabsorbed bile acid into the colon causes profound diarrhoea as the result of 'cathartic' action of bile salts. The diarrhoea is often controlled with cholestyramine which protects the mucosa although further bile acid loss results. In steatorrhoea associated with bile acid deficiency an alternative mechanism of diarrhoea exists. The unabsorbed fats enter the colon as long-chain fatty acids where they are acted upon by intestinal bacteria to form hydroxy-fatty acids. These substances again exert a cathartic effect. The removal of long-chain triglyceride from the diet and its substitution with medium chain fat as a calorie source relieves the diarrhoea.

Structural Liver Damage

Hepatitis

Several forms of viral hepatitis are now recognized. Short-incubation hepatitis (virus A) is a disease of young people and is unlikely to occur in the elderly. The recent introduction, however, of a serological marker for hepatitis A disease may reveal sporadic cases in the elderly. The disease is mild and progression to cirrhosis unlikely. More is known of the epidemiology of long-incubation hepatitis because of the discovery of the hepatitis B surface antigen. It is commoner in younger people but the effects of infection may continue into old age. Hepatitis B infection occurs through exposure to blood or blood products, by homosexual contact, tattooing, and occasionally by insect bites. Persistent damage to the liver may occur and appear as a so-called 'cryptogenic' cirrhosis in the elderly. The development of an aggressive hepatitis occurs in younger people ('active chronic hepatitis') and is associated with early morbidity so that it is unlikely to present in old age. Persistence of HB_sAg may occur in the elderly although is probably rare because the passage of time allows the patient to clear the antigen. Nevertheless, if the carrier state is discovered in the elderly contact with the patient's blood and secretions should be avoided.

In addition to the two forms of hepatitis discussed a further group has recently been studied. The virus responsible is not yet identified and, for convenience, the disease has been termed non-A–non-B hepatitis. The incubation period for this infection is midway between short-incubation and long-incubation hepatitis and non-A–non-B virus is the dominant cause of post-transfusion hepatitis. The disease is usually mild but persisting abnormalities of liver function and even progression to cirrhosis occur. The mildness of the disease may lead to a failure to recognize it in the elderly.

Besides the established virus A, virus B, and non-A–non-B infections other viruses also cause hepatitis. In the elderly the most important is probably infection with the virus herpes simplex which occurs particularly in immunosuppressed individuals. The liver picture, however, seldom predominates and disorders of blood coagulation with involvement of the brain or heart provide the usual clinical manifestations.

Other Hepatic Infections

Pyogenic Liver Abscess

The majority of patients with pyogenic liver abscess are over 60 years of age. Although concomitant diseases such as diabetes and other immunological disorders are common, the condition is often spontaneous. Within the liver the abscess may be single or multiple and the majority occur within the right lobe of the liver. The patient presents with evidence of infection and may complain of abdominal tenderness associated with hepatomegaly. There is usually more than one infecting organism and aerobic and anaerobic bacteria are found. Diagnosis of liver abscess has become easier with radioisotope scanning which reveals a space-occupying lesion within the liver. Ultrasonography is a useful investigation showing the lesion is not solid. Treatment is surgical with the placement of a wide drainage tube in the abscess cavity. Wide-spectrum antimicrobial therapy is essential and should cover *Escherichia coli*, *Anaerobes*, and *Staphylococcus aureus*, even if these organisms are not grown in the laboratory. Follow-up of the treated patient with ultrasonography is essential for such abscesses may recur. The prognosis is poor, often reflecting a failure to consider the diagnosis (Verlenden and Frey, 1980).

Amoebic Liver Abscess

Amoebic liver abscess occurs at all ages and may occur in those patients who have not travelled to areas of the world where amoebiasis is considered endemic. The physical signs and changes on radioisotope and ultrasound examination are as those for pyogenic liver abscess. The abscess is sometimes seen on a straight X-ray of the abdomen or in a right lateral of the chest, and a small posterior effusion may also be noted. The diagnosis may be confirmed by amoebic complement fixation studies. The abscess responds to high dose therapy with metronidazole, obviating the need for surgery in younger people. Since amoebic liver abscess is associated with a high mortality early surgical intervention may be necessary for diagnostic purposes.

Hydatid Liver Disease

This condition seldom produces acute problems in the elderly but is often found in an elderly patient incidentally as hepatic calcification in areas where the disease is common (Fig. 21). If a large cyst is present the approach is surgical although this is probably best per-

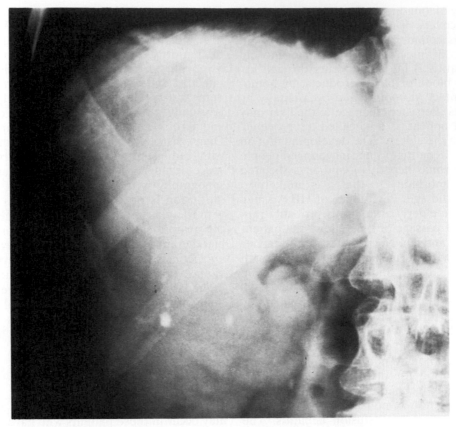

Figure 21   Multiple calcified flecks in the liver due to hydatid disease

formed in centres where there is special expertise for the disease. A cyst can be confidently diagnosed by a hydatid complement fixation test and the Casoni test is now redundant. The antihelmintic agent mebendazole has recently been introduced for the treatment of hydatid disease and the results of its use are awaited with interest.

Chronic Liver Disease

Chronic liver disease is due either to hepatocellular problems or cholestatic disease each of which has classical clinical features.

Chronic Hepatocellular Disease

The patient presents with general symptoms or with complications of chronic hepatocellular disease such as portal hypertension, ascites, and, less frequently, portosystemic encephalopathy. Clinical examination reveals vascular spiders distributed in the drainage area of the superior vena cava, paper-money skin, gynaecomastia, testicular atrophy, pallor, clinical jaundice, pigmentation, and possibly hepatosplenomegaly. The jaundice is not usually intense. In terms of standard liver function tests the serum transaminases are high and the alkaline phosphatase normal or only slightly elevated. These factors have previously been considered as being those of cirrhosis of the liver but they should be considered as problems of chronic hepatocellular failure of which there are many causes.

Causes of Chronic Hepatocellular Disease

Active chronic hepatitis (Syn. juvenile hepatitis, lupoid hepatitis). Although this condition is primarily a disease of young people, elderly individuals are affected. Symptoms and signs of hepatocellular disease occur. Biochemically the serum transaminases are elevated and there is a marked elevation of serum gamma globulin. Smooth muscle antibodies are positive in approximately 60 per cent of patients and the mitochondrial antibody is not found. Liver biopsy provides confirmatory, but not diagnostic, evidence of disease. The portal tracts are inflamed and have a cellular infiltrate of plasma cells and lymphocytes. The limiting cell plates are disturbed and fibrous tissue encroaches on the hepatic lobule capturing groups of liver cells forming 'rosettes'. This histological process is referred to as 'piecemeal' necrosis or 'aggressive' hepatitis. Cirrhosis may or may not be present at initial histological examination. Clearly the diagnosis does not depend on isolated clinical, biochemical, or histological characteristics but on compatible combinations of liver abnormalities. The diagnosis, once made, demands treatment with corticosteroids initially at a high dose which, as the biochemical features improve, can be reduced to a maintenance level of 10 mg daily. Treatment should be continued for 2 years after return to biochemical normality and with the patient carefully followed. If appropriate, the dose of corticosteroid can be lowered by using it in combination with azothioprine, but azothioprine alone is of little use.

Alcoholic liver disease The easy availability of alcohol, its increasing social use, and its comparative low cost makes alcohol the main cause of chronic liver disease in all age groups. A history of excessive alcohol use is often forthcoming from patients or their relatives. Clinically there are symptoms and signs of chronic liver disease and enlargement of the parotid gland and Dupuytren's contracture of the palms are frequent. Biochemically the serum transaminase and gamma glutamyl transpeptidase levels are raised and examination of the peripheral blood film reveals macrocytosis. This latter abnormality reflects a direct toxic effect of alcohol on the bone marrow and not on nutritional deficiencies of folic acid or vitamin B_{12}. Liver biopsy reveals histological features varying from fatty infiltration, piecemeal necrosis, to a developed micronodular cirrhosis. The only treatment is withdrawal of alcohol. The prognosis depends on the clinical

presentation—the more severe the symptoms and signs initially the graver the prognosis.

Other causes of chronic hepatoceullular disease Wilson's disease (hepatolenticular degeneration) does not cause problems in the elderly. Alpha-l-antitrypsin deficiency is associated with chronic liver disease sometimes presenting as an aggressive hepatitis or as cirrhosis. Previous infection with HB_sAg or nonA–nonB virus may present as cirrhosis for the first time in the elderly although there is no available data to estimate their frequency. Drugs causing chronic hepatocellular disease are discussed on page 340.

Chronic Cholestatic Disease

The clinical picture of chronic cholestatic disease differs from that of hepatocellular disease in that signs of hepatocellular failure, e.g. spider naevi, liver palms, and ascites appear at a late stage. The patient complains of malaise and pruritis, particularly at night, is common. Jaundice is usually present and the stools are pale and the urine dark. Considerable hepatomegaly is usual. Progression of the cholestasis leads to difficulty in fat and fatsoluble vitamin absorption so malnutrition is inevitable. Tests of liver function show hyperbilirubinaemia and a raised alkaline phosphatase. Serum transaminases may be slightly elevated.

Primary Biliary Cirrhosis

This condition occurs in middle aged females although it may appear for the first time in the elderly. Many patients these days are diagnosed as the result of finding antimitochondrial antibodies done as a screen or as the result of pruritis with no other symptomatic suggestion of liver disease. On examination the patient may be covered with scratch marks and cholesterol deposits occur in the eyelids and extensor surfaces of the body. As in all cholestatic syndromes the liver is large and the spleen may be palpable as the result of portal hypertension. The antimitochondrial antibody is found in the serum in over 90 per cent of patients and liver biopsy reveals a cellular infiltrate in the portal tract with bile duct damage and possible granuloma in relation to the bile ducts. It is unusual to find classical histological abnormalities in percutaneous needle biopsy and the histological features so described are found, more usually, on an operative biopsy. The diagnosis is further supported by the exclusion of large bile duct obstruction. The first investigation is grey scale ultrasonography of the liver which in obstructive jaundice shows dilated bile ducts above the level of obstruction. Thin-needle percutaneous transhepatic cholangiography is also of use in confirming large bile duct obstruction and more clearly defining the upper level of any obstructive lesion. Retrograde endoscopic cholangiography is a useful adjunct to investigation and delineates the lower level of any obstructive lesion which might be useful to the surgeon. Percutaneous needle biopsy of the liver is best delayed until these diagnostic methods have excluded large bile duct obstruction.

Treatment of primary biliary cirrhosis is mainly supportive. If nutrition is poor calorie intake should be supplemented by medium-chain triglyceride preparations which are more easily absorbed where bile salt concentrations are diminished. Fat-soluble vitamins given intramuscularly help to delay bone disease consequent upon calcium malabsorption, and reverse coagulation defects. Corticosteroid drugs are contraindicated for, not only do they have no effect on the natural history of the disease, they have the disadvantage of promoting bone disease. Whether azothioprine is useful remains to be settled. Recent studies of *D*-penicillamine have suggested its use in late-stage disease.

Bile Duct Carcinoma (Cholangio Carcinoma)

This condition again occurs in the elderly and approximately 25 per cent of cases occur after the age of 65 (Whelton *et al.*, 1969). The patient presents with features of cholestasis and large duct obstruction is confirmed by ultrasound examination and transhepatic cholangiography. The tumour is commonly found at the junction of the right and left hepatic ducts and may spread into the liver. It is important to diagnose the tumour for survival after surgery may be long. Treatment is surgical with a plastic prosthesis being introduced through the tumour into the liver. Recent attempts, which may be particularly valuable for the elderly, to save laparotomy, have included the

introduction of a prosthesis over a guide wire by a percutaneous transhepatic route. (Burcharth, Jensen, and Olesen, 1979).

Bile Duct Stricture

Prolonged biliary stricture produces clinical features of cholestasis with its attendant nutritional problems. The majority of cases follow cholecystectomy although trauma, perforation of a peptic ulcer, chronic pancreatitis, and sclerosing cholangitis are potential causes. The treatment is surgical in most cases.

Differential Diagnosis of Jaundice in the Elderly

A scheme for the diagnosis of jaundice is laid out in Table 2. Despite the fact that conditions such as alcoholic cirrhosis and previous primary biliary cirrhosis occur in the elderly, they are rare and in elderly patients with jaundice a surgical cause is seen in over 80 per cent. (Hueto-Armijo and Exton-Smith, 1962).

Table 2 Differential diagnosis of jaundice

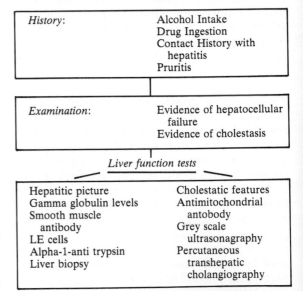

Consequences of Chronic Liver Disease

Ascites

Ascites is a distressing complication of chronic liver disease. It results primarily from fluid retention, the cause of which is uncertain, and is localized within the abdomen because of portal hypertension with hepatic lymphatic obstruction playing a minor role. Chronic liver disease is an important cause of ascites in the elderly but obstruction to hepatic venous outflow and malignancy must be considered. The usual step in the management of ascites is to obtain a small sample of fluid by aspiration for bacteriological culture, protein estimation, and cytology. Bacteriological culture is extremely important, for up to 20% of the patients with chronic liver disease have infected ascites and its prompt treatment improves the patient's condition. Measurement of protein levels helps to distinguish exudates from transudates and cytological examination sometimes provides evidence of malignancy.

The treatment of hepatic ascites should be 'gentle' and rapid losses of fluid should be avoided. Strict bed-rest often leads to a useful diuresis and its effect should always be assessed before recourse to strong diuretic agents. Of the diuretic agents available a naturetic agent such as frusemide and an aldosterone antagonist such as spironolactone are the most popular. Aldosterone antagonists can be used alone but are also useful when used with a loop diuretic. Hypokalaemia should be avoided for it may induce hepatic failure. The treatment of ascites is best controlled by daily patient weighing, aiming for a weight loss of between 0.5 and 1.0 kg each day. Diuretic agents are continued in the long term and patients are advised to reduce the dosage in very hot weather. It is safer to maintain the patient on a dose of diuretic which does not completely relieve fluid retention thus ensuring that the patient does not receive excessive amounts. The potency of modern diuretic agents probably makes fluid restriction redundant.

Hepato-Renal Failure

This condition is a later complication of chronic liver cell disease and often precipitated by overenthusiastic diuresis. The kidneys are histologically normal and the precise nature of the syndrome is unknown. It is thought, however, that diversion of renal cortical blood flow leading to a reduced glomerular filtration rate is important. Disturbances in prostaglandin synthesis are described and may lead to abnormalities of renal blood flow.

Portal Hypertension

The hallmark of portal hypertension is the development of oesophageal varices. Portal pressure rises as a consequence of extrahepatic portal vein obstruction which occurs in the elderly mainly as a result of thrombosis consequent on extrinsic pressure from enlarged lymph nodes in the porta hepatis. Rare cases also present as a late complication of mesenteric vascular occlusions. The main cause of portal hypertension is cirrhosis of the liver. Obstruction to hepatic venous outflow as a result of obstruction to the hepatic veins, or even cardiac failure, also leads to an increased portal pressure but such conditions are seldom associated with oesophageal varices. Portocaval shunting is never justifiable in the elderly patient but repeated endoscopic sclerotherapy promises to be a useful method of controlling variceal bleeding.

Portosystemic Encephalopathy

Although a rare condition, occasionally patients survive into old age having undergone porto-caval anastomosis for the control of portal hypertension. The condition presents with cerebellar and basal ganglion signs. Dementia is common. The cause of the complication is ill understood but absorbed nitrogenous substances which bypass the liver are implicated. Factors which precipitate portosystemic encephalopathy include intercurrent infection, the use of sedative drugs, hypokalaemia, and even severe constipation. Management is difficult and any obvious precipitating factor should be removed. Withdrawal of dietary protein is important and produces some improvement. The amount of protein which the patient should eat is that amount which he can tolerate. Purgation with lactulose is useful in preventing absorption of nitrogenous products. Neomycin, useful in acute hepatic failure, is not indicated in the patient with chronic portosystemic encephalopathy because of ototoxicity. Bromocryptine may be of some use (Morgan *et al.*, 1980).

Drugs and the Liver

Two aspects of the relationship between drugs and the liver are important in the elderly.

Firstly, with increasing age the necessity for drug therapy becomes greater and the potential for toxicity increases. Secondly, it is possible that the ageing liver is less able to metabolize and detoxify drugs so that toxic levels may accumulate in the blood. Information regarding this aspect of the relationship between the liver and drugs is scant.

Drug Hepatotoxicity

In structural terms drugs may produce cholestatic syndromes or induce hepatocellular disease. Additionally drugs may induce hepatic enzymes affecting the metabolism of other drugs and some drugs compete with bilirubin for carrier proteins or acceptor sites in the liver cell affecting the disposal of bilirubin itself.

It is usually drug metabolites that are responsible for hepatic injury rather than the administered drug. The classical example of this kind of injury is that caused by paracetamol. Metabolites of paracetamol are usually conjugated in the liver cell with glutathione and glucoronide making them water soluble and disposable. The amount of glutathione available, however, is limited and saturation of the conjugating system leads to a build-up of paracetamol metabolites which bind to liver cells and cause necrosis. The early administration of glutathione precursors prevents liver damage.

Hepatocellular dysfunction and structural damage may also occur as the result of individual idiosyncrasy to a drug. It is postulated that the drug acts as a hapten by combining with liver antigens and stimulating an immune response. The best example of such a drug is halothane which gives rise to an acute hepatitis in some individuals after repeated exposure. Hepatotoxicity due to methyl dopa is probably also a hypersensitivity reaction.

Cholestatic jaundice as a result of drug toxicity occurs classically following chlorpromazine therapy. The mechanism is uncertain although several features such as an eosinophilia, the low incidence of cholestasis in those who take the drug, and the fact that the reaction is not dose related suggests it is allergic. As well as cholestatic syndromes, however, there is additional undisputed evidence that chlorpromazine induces hepatocellular damage. Cholestatic syndromes which are predictable, i.e. are dose related, result from the administration of some hormones.

The development of a liver abnormality in someone taking a drug should immediately suggest a cause-and-effect relationship. The type of drug reaction is classified by means of standard liver function studies which suggest hepatic or cholestatic disease (see pages 336 and 337).

The Liver in Systemic Disease

Cardiac Failure

Chronic liver disease resulting from cardiac failure is less common since the introduction of modern diuretic therapy. Venous congestion is common, however, and the serum bilirubin may be raised with elevation of serum transaminases to high levels sometimes in excess of 1,000 IU (AST).

Diabetes

Hepatic enlargement is a common consequence of uncontrolled insulin-dependent or maturity onset diabetes. Histologically hepatocytes are filled with vacuoles indicating fatty change. Chronic liver disease does not occur although the combination of diabetes with hepatomegaly should always arouse the suspicion of haemachromatosis.

Amyloid Disease

Hepatic enlargement is a prominent feature of both primary and secondary amyloid disease and often liver biopsy provides the diagnosis. Amyloid may be deposited in the portal tracts and in the Disse space in the hepatic lobules. Amyloid disease is an occasional cause of portal hypertension.

Collagen Disorders

Significant liver disease is rare in collagen disorders although occasionally liver biopsy shows arteritic changes. Portal hypertension does occur in rheumatoid arthritis associated with gross splenomegaly (Felty's syndrome) where the portal blood flow is increased. Histologically fibrosis in the portal tract and of the intrahepatic portal vein radicles may occur as a result of portal hypertension. Scleroderma has been associated with portal hypertension. Most usually there is underlying liver disease such as primary biliary cirrhosis but sometimes no structural liver problem is detected.

Chronic Inflammatory Bowel Disease

Minor reactive and fatty changes are seen in most patients with inflammatory bowel disease. A minority of patients develop an aggressive cirrhosis and chronic biliary disease such as pericholangitis, primary sclerosing cholangitis, and bile duct carcinoma.

Diseases of the Gall-Bladder

Several autopsy surveys have recorded a rise in the prevalence of gallstones with increasing age so that they are found in approximately 30 to 40 per cent of people over the age of 60 (Torvik and Høivik, 1960). An important study in Bristol, however, revealed that the peak ages at which patients present with gallstone symptoms requiring definitive treatment is between 40 and 60 years (Holland and Heaton, 1972). The reason for this is not clear but one inference is that gallstones are less likely to cause symptoms in the elderly. Certainly the cholecystectomy rate in the elderly appears low.

Discussion on the lithogenicity of bile is discussed on page 333. The use of clofibrate as a cholestrol lowering agent, hormone replacement therapy, and other oestrogen preparations are associated with an increased incidence of gallstones.

The presentation of gallstones in the elderly is similar to that in younger people. Painless jaundice, however, occurs and concurrent cholagitis may lead to elevations of liver enzymes which confuse the diagnosis.

The management of the elderly patient with gallstones is difficult. Surgery is attended by a high mortality and morbidity and postoperative chest infections, in particular, are common. Where surgery appears contraindicated the use of chenodeoxycholic acid or ursodeoxycholic acid in patients with non-calcified gallstones who have a functioning gall-bladder should be considered.

Tumours of the Gall-Bladder

Benign tumours of the gall-bladder occur but seldom cause a diagnostic problem. Among benign tumours, polyps, adenomas, and heterotopic tissue deriving from the stomach and intestines are recorded.

Carcinoma of the Gall-Bladder

This is a tumour of people over the age of 60 years. In the majority of patients gallstones are found, suggesting an aetiological relationship, and perhaps a further reason for the removal of gallstones which do not give rise to symptoms in younger people.

Clinically there is a long preceding history of attacks of biliary pain, jaundice, or cholagitis. The diagnosis is often made for the first time at laparotomy. Early tumours may occur as a filling defect on the cholecystogram but often the gall-bladder is non-functioning. Calcification of the gall-bladder occurs in 25 per cent of tumours.

THE PANCREAS

The pancreas is an important digestive organ responsible for the secretion of digestive enzymes including amylase, lipase, and the proteases trypsin and chymotrypsin. The pancreas also secretes fluid isoosmotic with plasma up to rates of 5 litres per minute. The main cations are sodium and potassium at concentrations found in the plasma. Smaller quantities of calcium are found. The main anions are chloride and bicarbonate.

Arterial blood reaches the pancreas from the coeliac and superior mesenteric arteries and venous drainage is to the portal venous system. The lymphatic drainage accompanies the arterial blood supply. Innervation of the pancreas occurs through the vagal nerves. The contribution of neural influence on pancreatic secretion is uncertain and the main stimulus is hormonal.

Inflammatory Disorders of the Pancreas

Acute Pancreatitis

Acute idiopathic pancreatitis is unusual in the elderly but pancreatic inflammation associated with alcoholism and biliary tract disease is common, and indeed the incidence of acute pancreatitis associated with such conditions appears to increase with age. Pancreatitis may also occur in the elderly as a result of diuretic and corticosteroid drugs, and occurs frequently as a complication of hypothermia. Hypercalcaemia, hyperlipidaemia, and oestrogen therapy are also associated with the condition.

The predominant symptom is abdominal pain quickly followed by vomiting. Respiratory difficulties occur and the patient is cyanosed and may even develop a left-sided pleurisy or pleural effusion. On examination the patient is ill with evidence of peripheral circulatory failure and rarely the bluish discoloration of the flanks and around the umbilicus caused by acute haemorrhagic pancreatitis is seen. Evidence of localized or generalized ileus is frequent.

The diagnostic biochemical abnormality is the elevation of the serum amylase. The discriminative value of the amylase-to-creatinine clearance ratios is disputed. Ultrasound examination may reveal pancreatic swelling and is a useful non-invasive method of excluding gallstones.

The treatment of acute pancreatitis is unsatisfactory. General supportive measures such as plasma expansion and oxygen therapy are important. The pancreas is rested by stopping oral intake and nasogastric suction and fluids are infused intravenously. Glucagon inhibits pancreatic exocrine secretion and has been used as a means of resting the pancreas, although the results of controlled trials are inconclusive. Attempts to inactivate released pancreases with Aprotinin (Trasylol) which has a powerful antitryptic effect has been disappointing. Hypocalcaemia, if it occurs, should be corrected; hyperglycaemia should be sought.

The mortality of acute pancreatitis increases with age and with the severity of the disease. Pancreatic abscess and a pancreatic pseudocyst occur and their appearance may be delayed for some weeks following the acute attack.

Chronic Pancreatitis

Chronic pancreatitis is a difficult condition to diagnose and treat; little is known of its cause although alcoholism and malnutrition are each implicated. Calcification of the pancreatic gland occurs (Fig. 22) but this is possibly more common in tropical cases of chronic pancreatitis.

Clinically the predominant complaint is pain and this is associated with manifestations of chronic pancreatic insufficiency such as weight loss and mild diabetes. Jaundice is rare.

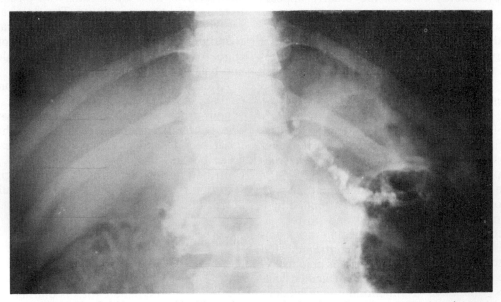

Figure 22   Calcific pancreatitis. The main pancreatic duct is outlined by calcium deposits

Establishing the diagnosis is difficult. Steatorrhoea is often present and levels of faecal fat are often higher than those seen in other forms of malabsorption. Serum levels of amylase or lipase seldom provide useful information.

A useful screening test for chronic pancreatic insufficiency has recently become available. The PABA excretion index is based on the ability of pancreatic chromotrypsin to cleave orally administered *N*-benzoyl-*L*-tyrosolpara aminobenzoic acid. The released paraaminobenzoic acid is easily measured in the urine (Mitchell *et al.*, 1979). Provided hepatic and intestinal function is normal a low PABA excretion index suggests chronic pancreatic insufficiency. Further evidence of exocrine insufficiency may be provided by the analysis of pancreatic enzymes and bicarbonate following a standard test meal. The chemical analysis is, however, difficult and much experience is needed by the individual laboratory before the results are valid. Ultrasonography is useful for assessing pancreatic size but does not completely exclude pancreatic carcinoma. Outlining pancreatic ducts by endoscopic retrograde pancreatography is useful in demonstrating duct abnormalities but is not without risk.

The management of chronic pancreatitis is directed towards pain relief and in this respect surgery, either duct drainage or pancreatectomy, may have a role. Otherwise nutrition is maintained and steatorrhoea relieved by replacing long-chain triglyceride by medium-chain fat in the diet. Enzyme replacements are given with each meal in quantities sufficient to relieve the diarrhoea. Recently H_2 blockers such as cimetidine and ranitidine have been advocated to raise the intragastric pH and prevent acid destruction of pancreatic enzyme.

Pancreatic Cancer

The incidence of pancreatic cancer is increased in patients with chronic pancreatitis and diabetes but apart from these epidemiological observations little is known of the cause of the disease.

Patients present with pain, often severe and radiating through to the back, jaundice, and weight loss. The diagnosis is most often made during the course of the investigation of jaundice and percutaneous transhepatic cholangiography is especially helpful. Pancreatic ultrasonography is useful.

The treatment is surgical. Attempts at radical resection are never justified in the elderly and a simple bypass procedure should be performed which relieves the jaundice. Even in younger people the survival following radical resection and palliative bypass is similar and there is much discussion as to the role of excisional surgery. Chemotherapy combined with high energy radiotherapy may in time become an increasingly important form of treatment.

REFERENCES

Adam, Y. G., Calabrese, C., and Volk, H. (1972). 'Colorectal cancer in patients over 80 years of age', *Surg. Clin. North Am.*, **52** (4), 883–889.

Agdal, N. (1979). 'Medicininiducerede esophagusskader', *Ugeskr. Laeger*, **141**, 3019–3021.

Alexander-Williams, J., and Cox, A. J. (1969). '*After Vagotomy*', Butterworth, London.

Allan, R., and Dykes, P. W. (1976). 'A study of the factors influencing mortality rates from gastrointestinal haemorrhage', *Quart. J. Med.*, **45**, 533–550.

Allan, R. N., Steinberg, D. M., Alexander-Williams, J., and Cooke, W. T. (1977). 'Crohn's disease of the colon: An audit of clinical management', *Gastroenterology*, **73**, 723–732.

Allan, T. H., and Clagett, O. T. (1965). 'Changing concepts in the surgical treatment of pulsion diverticula of the lower oesophagus', *J. Thorac. Cardiovasc. Surg.*, **50**, 455–462.

Ardran, G. M., and Kemp, F. H. (1961). 'The radiography of the lower lateral food channels', *J. Laryngol. Otol.*, **75**, 358–370.

Ashley, D. J. B. (1969). 'Gastric cancer in Wales', *J. Med. Genet.*, **6**, 76–79.

Ashton, M. G., Holdsworth, C. D., Moore, M., Ryan, F. P. (1982). 'Healing of gastric ulcers after one, two and three months of ranitidine', *Br. Med. J.*, **284**, 467–468.

Asquith, P., Mackintosh, P., Stokes, P. L., Holmes, G. K. T., and Cooke, W. T. (1974). 'Histocompatibility antigens in patients with inflammatory bowel disease', *Lancet*, **1**, 113–115.

Atkinson, M. (1962). 'Mechanisms protecting against gastro-oesophageal reflux'. A review, *Gut*, **3**, 1–15.

Atkinson, M. (1976). 'Oesophageal motor changes in systemic disease', *Clin. Gastroenterol.*, **5:1**, 132.

Atkinson, M., and Summerling, M. D. (1966). 'Oesophageal changes in systemic sclerosis', *Gut*, **7**, 402–408.

Azad-Kahn, A. K., Piris, J., and Truelove, S. C. (1977). 'An experiment to determine the active therapeutic moiety of sulphasalazine', *Lancet*, **2**, 892–895.

Bardhan, K. D. (1981). 'What happens to duodenal ulcers that do not respond quickly to cimetidine?', *Gut*, **22**, A880.

Baron, J. H. (1963). 'The relationship between basal and maximum acid output in normal subjects and patients with duodenal ulcer', *Clin. Sci.*, **24**, 357–370.

Baron, J. H., Connell, A. M., Lennard-Jones, J. E., and Jones, F. A. (1962). 'Sulphasalazine and salicylazosulphadimidine in ulcerative colitis', *Lancet*, **1**, 1094–1096.

Baron, J. H., Langman, M. J. S., and Wastell, C. (1980). In *Recent Advances in Gastroenterology* (Ed. I. A. D. Bouchier), Vol. 4, p. 30, Churchill Livingstone, London.

Barrison, I. G., Trewly, P. N., and Kane, S. P. (1980). 'Oesophageal ulceration due to emepronium bromide', *Endoscopy*, **12**, 197–199.

Basavaraju, N. G., Wolf-Klein, G., Silverstone, F. A., and Libow, L. S. (1980). 'Cimetidine-induced mental confusion in elderly', *NY State J. Med.*, **80**, 1287–1288.

Berstein, L. M., and Baker, L. A. (1958). 'A clinical test for oesophagitis', *Gastroenterology*, **34**, 760–781.

Biggs, C., Hugh, T. B., and Dodds, A. J. (1976). 'Transexamic acid and upper gastrointestinal haemorrhage – a double blind trial', *Gut*, **17**, 729–734.

Billington, B. P. (1965). 'Observations from New South Wales on the changing incidence of gastric ulcer in Australia', *Gut*, **6**, 121–133.

Binder, H. J., Cocco, A., Crossley, R. J., Finkelstein, W., Font, R., Friedman, G., Croarke, J., Hughes, W., Johnson, A. F., McGuigan, J. E., Summers, R., Vlahcerce, R., Wilson, E. C., and Winship, D. M. (1978). 'Cimetidine in the treatment of duodenal ulcer', *Gastroenterology*, **74**, 380–388.

Binder, V., Weeke, E., Olsen, J. M., Anthonisen, P., and Riis, P. (1966). 'A genetic study of ulcerative colitis', *Scand. J. Gastroenterol.*, **1**, 49–56.

Black, M., and Sherlock, S. (1970). 'Treatment of Gilbert's syndrome with phenobarbitone', *Lancet*, **1**, 1359–1361.

Blackwood, W. S., Maudgai, D. P., and Northfield, T. C. (1978). 'Prevention by bedtime cimetidine of duodenal ulcer relapse', *Lancet*, **1**, 626–627.

Bloomfield, A. L., and Keefer, C. S. (1928) 'Gastric acidity: Relation to various factors such as age and physical fitness', *J. Clin. Invest.*, **5**, 285–194.

Bodemar, G., and Walan, A. (1976). 'Cimetidine in the treatment of active duodenal and prepyloric ulcers', *Lancet*, **2**, 161–164.

Bodemar, G., and Walan, A. (1978). 'Maintenance treatment of recurrent peptic ulcer by cimetidine', *Lancet*, **1**, 403–407.

Boley, S. J., Sammartano, R., Adams, A., Dibiase, A., Kleinhaus, S., and Sprayregen, S. (1977). 'On the nature and aetiology of vascular ectasia of the colon. Degenerative lesion of ageing', *Gastroenterology*, **72**, 650–660.

Bown, S. G., Salman, P. R., Brown, P., and Read, A. E. (1981). 'Upper gastro-intestinal haemorrhage', *J. R. Coll. Physicians, Lond.*, **4**, 265–268.

Brand, D. L., Ilves, R., Pope, C. E. II (1980). 'Evaluation of oesophageal function in patients with central chest pain', *Acta Med. Scand. Suppl.*, **644**, 53–56.

Brand, D. L., Martin, D., Pope, C. E. II (1977). 'Oesophageal manometrics in patients with angina-like chest pain', *Dig. Dis. Sci.*, **22**, 300–304.

Brodribb, A. J. M. (1977). 'Treatment of symptomatic diverticular disease with a high fibre diet', *Lancet*, **1**, 664–666.

Brogden, R. N., Pinder, R. M., Sawyer, P. R., Speight, T. M., and Avery, G. S. (1976). 'Tripostassium di-citrato bismuthate: A report of its pharmacological properties and therapeutic efficiency in peptic ulcer', *Drugs*, **12**, 401–411.

Brown, P., Salmon, P. R., Htut, T., and Read, A. E. (1972). 'Double blind trial of carbenoxolone sodium capsules in duodenal ulcer therapy, based on endoscopy diagnosis and follow-up', *Br. Med. J.*, **3**, 661–664.

Brown, R. C., Langman, M. J. S., and Lambert, P. M. (1976). 'Hospital admissions for peptic ulcer during 1958–72', *Br. Med. J.*, **1**, 35–37.

Buckell, N. A., Gould, S. R., Day, D. W., Lennard-Jones, J. E., and Edwards, A. M. (1978). 'Controlled trial of disodium cromoglycate in chronic persistent ulcerative colitis', *Gut*, **19**, 1140–1143.

Buckle, R. M., and Nichol, W. D. (1964). 'Painful dysphagia due to monilial oesophagitis', *Br. Med. J.*, **1**, 821–822.

Bulmer, E. (1927). 'The mortality from haematemesis: an analysis of 526 cases', *Lancet*, **2**, 168–171.

Burcharth, F., Jensen, Ll., and Olesen, K. (1979). 'Endoprosthesis for internal drainage of the bilary tract', *Gastroenterology*, **77**, 133–137.

Burland, W. L., Hawkins, B. W., Horton, R. J., and Beresford, J. (1978). 'The longer term treatment of duodenal ulcer with cimetidine', in *Cimetidine, The Westminster Hospital Symposium* (Eds C. Wastell and P Lance), Churchill Livingston, London.

Burland, W. L., and Simplins, M. A. (Eds) (1977). 'Multicenter double blind trial. The effect of cimetidine on duodenal ulceration', in *Cimetidine—*

Proceedings of the Second International Symposium on Histamine H₂ Receptor Antagonists, Excerpta Medica.

Callender, S., Langman, M. J. S., Macleod, I. N., Mosbech, J., and Nielson, K. R. (1971). 'ABO blood group in patients with gastric carcinoma associated with pernicious anaemia', *Gut*, **12**, 465–467.

Campieri, M., Lanfranchi, G. A., Bazzocchi, G., Brignola, C., Sarti, F., Franzin, G., Battocchia, A., Labo, G., and Dal Monte, P. R. (1981). 'Treatment of ulcerative colitis with high dose 5-amino-salicylic acid enemas', *Lancet*, **2**, 270–271.

Carlborg, B., Cumlien, A., and Olsson, H. (1978). 'Medikamentalle esofagusstrikturer', *Lakartidningen*, **75**, 4609–4611.

Chang, T. W., Lauermann, M., and Bartlett, J. G. (1979). 'Cytotoxicity assay in antibiotic associated colitis', *J. Infect. Dis.*, **140**, 765–770.

Chapman, B. L., and Duggan, J. M. (1969). 'Aspirin and uncomplicated peptic ulcer', *Gut*, **10**, 443–450.

Chisholm, M. (1974). 'The association between webs, iron and post-cricoid carcinoma', *Postgrad. Med. J.*, **50**, 215–219.

Chisholm, M., Ardran, G. M., Callender, S. T., and Wright, R. (1971a). 'A follow-up study of patients with post-cricoid webs', *Quart. J. Med.*, **40**, 409–420.

Chisholm, M., Ardran, G. M., Callender, S. T., and Wright, R. (1971b). 'Iron deficiency and autoimmunity in post-cricoid webs', *Quart. J. Med.*, **40**, 421–433.

Ciditira, P. J., Machell, R. J., Farthing, M. J. G., Dick, A. P., and Hunter, J. O. (1977). 'Double blind controlled trial of cimetidine in the healing of gastric ulcer', *Gut*, **20**, 730–734.

Clarke, R. J., Lincoln-Lewis, D., and Williams, J. A. (1972). 'Vagotomy and pyloroplasty for gastric ulcer', *Br. Med. J.*, **2**, 369–371.

Cohen, S. (1979). 'Medical progress: Motor disorders of the oesophagus', *New Engl. J. Med.*, **301**, 184–192.

Coleman, J. A., and Denham, M. J. (1980). 'Perforation of peptic ulceration in the elderly', *Age Ageing*, **9**, 257–261.

Colin-Jones, D. G., Cockel, R., and Schiller, K. F. R. (1978). In *Clinics in Gastroenterology* (Ed. K. F. R. Schiller), Vol. 7:8, p. 782, Saunders, London.

Colin-Jones, D. G., Misiewicz, J. J., Milton-Thompson, G. J., Hunt, R. H., and Golding, P. I. (1978). 'Cimetidine and carbenoxolone in gastric ulcer', in *Cimetidine, The Westminster Hospital Symposium* (Eds C. Wastell, and P. Lance), Churchill Livingstone, London.

Collins, F. J., Mathews, H. R., Baker, S. E., and

Strakova, J. M. (1979). 'Drug induced oesophageal injury', *Br. Med. J.*, **1**, 1673–1676.

Conn, H. O., and Blitzer, B. L. (1976). 'Non-association of adrenocorticosteroid therapy and peptic ulcer', *New Engl. J. Med.*, **294**, 473–479.

Connell, A. M., Hilton, C., Irvine, G., Lennard-Jones, J. E., and Misiewicz, J. J. (1965). 'Variation of bowel habit in two population samples', *Br. Med. J.*, **2**, 1095–1099.

Connon, J. J. (1977). 'Denol, an effective drug in the therapy of duodenal ulceration', *Ir. Med. J.*, **70**, 206–207.

Cooke, A. R. (1978). In *Gastrointestinal Disease*, (Eds M. H. Sleisenger and J. S. Fordtran), Saunders, Philadelphia.

Cooke, W. T. (1977). 'Laxative abuse', in *Clinics in Gastroenterology*, Vol. 6, pp. 659–673, Saunders, London.

Coughlin, C. P., Kupa, A., and Alp, M. H. (1977). 'The effect of tri-potassium di-citrato bismuthate (De-nol) on the healing of chronic duodenal ulcers', *Med. J. Aust.*, **1**, 294–298.

Cox, A. J. (1952). 'Stomach size and its relation to chronic peptic ulcer', *Arch. Pathol.*, **54**, 407–422.

Cox, K. R. (1961). 'Oesophageal stricture after partial gastrectomy', *Br. J. Surg.*, **49**, 307–313.

Crafoord, C., and Frenckner, P. (1939). 'New surgical treatment of varicose veins of the oesophagus', *Acta. Otolaryngol. (Stockh.)*, **27**, 422–429.

Creamer, B., Donohue, F. E., and Code, C. F. (1958). 'Patterns of oesophageal motility in diffuse spasm', *Gastroenterology*, **34**, 782–796.

Crowson, T. D., Head, L. M. and Ferrante, W. A. (1976). 'Oesophageal ulcers associated with tetracycline therapy', *JAMA*, **235**, 2747–2748.

Cutler, C. W. (1958). 'Clinical patterns of peptic ulcer after sixty', *Surg. Gynecol. Obstet.*, **107**, 23–30.

Dart, A. M., Alban Davies, M., Lowndes, R. M., Dalal, J., Rutley, M., and Henderson, A. H. (1980). 'Oesophageal spasm and angina: Diagnostic value of ergometrine (ergonovine) provocation', *Eur. Heart J.*, **1**, 91–95.

Davies, W. A., and Reed, P. I. (1977). 'Controlled trial of duogastrone in duodenal ulcer', *Gut*, **18**, 78–83.

Davis, J. A., Kantrowitz, P. A., Chandler, H. L., and Schatzki, S. (1975). 'Reversible achalasia due to reticulum-cell sarcoma', *New Engl. J. Med.*, **293**, 130–132.

De Dombal, F. T., Fletcher, D. M., and Harris, R. S. (1969). 'Early diagnosis of ischaemic colitis', *Gut*, **10**, 131–134.

Delaney, J. P. (1975). 'Pyloric reflux gastritis; the offending agent', *Surgery*, **77**, 764–772.

Demeester, T. R., Johnson, L. F., and Kent, A. H. (1974). 'Evaluation of current operations for the precention of gastro-oesophageal reflux', *Ann. Surg.*, **180**, 511–525.

Dent, J., Dodds, W. J., Friedman, R. H., Sekiguchi, T., Hogan, W. J., Arndorfer, R. C., and Petrie, D. (1980). 'Mechanism of gastro-oesophageal reflux in recumbent asymptomatic human subjects', *J. Clin. Invest.*, **65**, 256–267.

De Villiers, D. R. (1966) 'Ischaemia of the colon; an experimental study', *Br. J. Surg.*, **53**, 497–503.

Dissanayake, A. S., and Truelove, S. C. (1973). 'A controlled therapeutic trial of long term maintenance treatment of ulcerative colitis with sulphasalazine (Salazopyrin)', *Gut*, **14**, 923–926.

Dohlman, G., and Mattsson, O. (1960). 'The endoscopic operation for hypopharyngeal diverticula: A roetgencinematographic study', *Arch. Otolaryngol.*, **71**, 744–752.

Domellöf, L. (1979). 'Gastric carcinoma promoted by alkaline reflux gastritis with special reference to bile and other surfactants as promotor of postoperative gastric cancer', *Med. Hypotheses*, **5**, 463–470.

Donovan, I. A. M., Harding, L. K., Keighley, M. R. B., Griffin, D. W., and Collis, J. L. (1977). 'Abnormalities of gastric emptying and pyloric reflux in uncomplicated hiatus hernia', *Br. J. Surg.*, **64**, 847–848.

Dotevall, G. (1959). 'Incidence of peptic ulcer in diabetes mellitus', *Acta. Med. Scand.*, **164**, 463–477.

Dragstedt, L. R. (1956). 'A concept of the aetiology of gastric and duodenal ulcer', *Am. J. Roentgenol.*, **75**, 219–229.

Dronfield, M. W., and Langman, M. J. S. (1978). 'Comparative trial of sulphasalazine and oral sodium cromoglycate in the maintenance of remission in ulcerative colitis', *Gut*, **19**, 1136–1139.

Eastman, M. C., and Sali, A. (1980). 'Modern treatment of oesophageal strictures', *Med. J. Aust.*, **1**, 129–130.

Eastwood, G. L., Castell, D. O., and Higgs, R. M. (1975). 'Experimental oesophagitis in cats impairs lower oesophageal sphincter pressure', *Gastroenterology*, **69**, 146–153.

Editorial (1974). 'Leads in oesophageal cancer', *Lancet*, **2**, 504.

Editorial (1981). 'Angiodysplasia', *Lancet*, **2**, 1086–1087.

Edwards, F. C., and Coghill, N. F. (1966). 'Aetiological factors in chronic atrophic gastritis', *Br. Med. J.*, **2**, 1409–1415.

Edwards, F. C., and Coghill, N. F. (1968). 'Clinical manifestations in patients with chronic atrophic gastritis, gastric ulcer, and duodenal ulcer', *Quart. J. Med.*, **37**, 336–360.

Elashoff, J. D., and Grossman, M. I. (1980). 'Trends in hospital admissions and death rates for peptic ulcer in the United States from 1970–78', *Gastroenterology*, **78**, 280–285.

Elder, J. B., Ganguli, P. C., and Gillespie, I. E. (1979). 'Cimetidine and gastric cancer', *Lancet*, **1**, 1005–1006.

Ellis, F. H. Jr., Schlegel, J. F., Lynch, V. P., and Payne, W. S. (1969). 'Cricopharyngeal myotomy for pharyngo-oesophageal diverticulum', *Ann. Surg.*, **170**, 340–349.

Elwood, P. C., Jacobs, A., Pitman, R. G., and Entwistle, C. C. (1964). 'Epidemiology of the Paterson–Kelly syndrome', *Lancet*, **2**, 716–720.

Evans, J. G., and Acheson, E. D. (1965). 'An epidemiological study of ulcerative colitis and regional enteritis in the Oxford area', *Gut*, **6**, 311–324.

Evans, K. T., and Roberts, G. M. (1976). 'Where do all the tablets go?', *Lancet*, **ii**, 1237–1239.

Ferguson, R., Dronfield, M. W., and Atkinson, M. (1979). 'Cimetidine in the treatment of reflux oesophagitis with peptic stricture', *Br. Med. J.*, **2**, 472–474.

Festen, H. P. M., Camers, C. B. H., Driessen, W. M. M., and Van Tongeren, J. H. M. (1979). 'Cimetidine in anastomotic ulceration after partial gastrectomy', *Gastroenterology*, **77**, 83–85.

Fischer, R. A., Ellison, G. W., Thayer, W. R., Spiro, H. M., and Glaser, G. H. (1965). 'Oesophageal motility in neuromuscular disorders', *Ann. Intern. Med.*, **63**, 229–248.

Flint, F. J., and Grech, P. (1970). 'Pyloric regurgitation and gastric ulcer', *Gut*, **11**, 735–737.

Fordtran, J. S., and Walsh, J. H. (1973). 'Gastric acid secretion rate and buffer content of the stomach after eating', *J. Clin. Invest.*, **52**, 645–657.

Franklin, R., and McSwain, B. (1970). 'Carcinoma of the colon, rectum and anus', *Ann. Surg.*, **171**, 811–818.

Fraser, G. M. (1978). 'The double contrast barium meal in patients with acute upper gastro-intestinal bleeding', *Clin. Radiol.*, **29**, 625–634.

Freeland, G. R., Higgs, R. H., and Castell, D. O. (1977). 'Lower oesophageal sphincter response to oral administration of cimetidine in normal subjects', *Gastroenterology*, **72**, 28–30.

Friedman, G. D., Siegelaub, A. B., and Seltzer, C. C. (1974). 'Cigarettes, alcohol and peptic ulcer', *New Engl. J. Med.*, **290**, 469–473.

Froese, E. M. (1979). 'Oesophagitis with clindamycin', *South Afr. Med. J.*, **56**, 826.

Frost, F., Rahbek, I., Rune, S. J., Jensen, K. B., Hoyer, E. G., Krag, E., Madsen, J. R., Wulff, H. R., Garbol, J., Jensen, K. G., Hoylund, M., and Nissen, V. R. (1977). 'Cimetidine in patients with gastric ulcer: A multicentre controlled trial', *Br. Med. J.*, **2**, 795–799.

Fyke, F. E., Code, C. F., and Schlegel, J. F. (1956).

'The gastro-oesophageal sphincter in healthy human beings', *Gastroenterologica*, **86**, 135–150.

Garland, C. F., Lilienfeld, A. M., Mendeloff, A. I., Markowitz, J. A., Terrell, K. B., and Garland, F. C. (1981). 'Incidence rates of ulcerative colitis and Crohn's disease in fifteen areas of the United States', *Gastroenterology*, **81**, 1115–1124.

Garrett, J. M., Summerskill, W. H. J., and Code, C. F. (1966). 'Antral motility in patients with gastric ulcer', *Am. J. Dig. Dis.*, **11**, 780–789.

Garrett, J. M., Winkelmann, R. K., Schlegel, J. F., and Code, C. F. (1971). 'Oesophageal deterioration in scleroderma', *Mayo Clin. Proc.*, **46**, 92–96.

Gatumbi, I., and Roy, A. D. (1970). 'The prevalence of peptic ulcer dyspepsia in a rural community in Kenya', *East Afr. Med. J.*, **47**, 627–633.

Gedde-Dahl, D. (1975). 'Serum gastrin response to food stimulation and gastric acid secretion in male patients with duodenal ulcer', *Scand. J. Gastroenterol.*, **10**, 187–191.

George, R. H., Symonds, J. M., Dimock, F., Brown, J. D., Arabi, Y., Skinagawa, M., Keighley, M. R. B., Alexander-Williams, J., and Burdon, D. W. (1978). 'Identification of *Clostridium difficile* as a cause of pseudomembranous colitis', *Br. Med. J.*, **1**, 695.

Gibbs, D. (1976). 'Endoscopy in the assessment of reflux oesophagitis', in *Clinics in Gastroenterology* (Ed. M. Atkinson), Vol. 5, No. 1, pp. 135–142, Saunders, London.

Goligher, J. C. (1954). 'The adequacy of the marginal blood supply to the left colon after high ligation of the inferior mesenteric artery during excision of rectum', *Br. J. Surg.*, **41**, 351–358.

Goligher, J. C. (1980). In *Surgery of the Anus, Rectum and Colon*, 4th ed., Balliere Tindall, London.

Goligher, J. C., Hoffman, D. C., and De Dombal, F. T. (1970). 'Surgical treatment of severe attacks of ulcerative colitis, with special reference to the advantages of early operation', *Br. Med. J.*, **4**, 703–706.

Gonzalez, L. L., and Jaffe, M. S. (1966). 'Mesenteric arterial insufficiency following abdominal aorta resection', *Arch. Surg.*, **93**, 10–20.

Goodhall, R. J. R., and Temple, J. G. (1980). 'Effect of cimetidine on lower oesophageal sphincter pressure in oesophagitis', *Br. Med. J.*, **1**, 611–612.

Goyal, R. L., Bauer, J. L., and Spiro, H. M. (1971). 'The nature and location of lower oesophageal ring', *New Engl. J. Med.*, **284**, 1175–1180.

Gugler, R., Lindstaedt, H., Miederer, S., Möckel, W., Rohner, H. G., Schmitz, H., and Szekessy, T. (1979). 'Cimetidine for anastomotic ulcers after partial gastrectomy', *New Engl. J. Med.*, **301**, 1077–1080.

Gunnlaugsson, G. M., Wychulis, A. R., Roland, C., and Ellis, F. H. Jr. (1970). 'Analysis of the records of 1657 patients with carcinoma of the oesophagus and cardia of the stomach', *Surg. Gynecol. Obstet.*, **130**, 997–1005.

Gyde, S. H., Prior, P., MacCartney, J. C., Thompson, H., Waterhouse, J. A. H., and Allan, R. N. (1980). 'Malignancy in Crohn's disease', *Gut*, **21**, 1024–1029.

Haggitt, R. C., Tryzelaar, J., Ellis, H., and Colcher, M. (1978). 'Adenocarcinoma complicating columnar epithelium-lined (Barrett's) oesophagus', *Am. J. Clin. Path.*, **70**, 1–5.

Harper, P. S., Harper, R. M. J., and Howel Evans, A. W. (1970). 'Carcinoma of the oesophagus with tylosis', *Quart. J. Med.*, **39**, 317–333.

Harvey, R. F. and Read, A. E. (1973). 'Effects of cholecystokinin on colonic motility and symptoms in patients with irritable bowel syndrome', *Lancet*, **1**, 1–3.

Hastings, P. R., Skillman, J. J., Bushnell, L. S. and Silen, W. (1978). 'Antacid titration in the prevention of acute gastro-intestinal bleeding; a controlled randomized trial in 100 critically ill patients', *New Engl. J. Med.*, **298**, 1041–1045.

Hawker, P. C., Muscroft, T. J., and Keighley, M. R. B. (1980). 'Gastric cancer after cimetidine in patient with two negative pre-treatment biopsies', *Lancet*, **1**, 709–710.

Heatley, R. V., Calcraft, B. J., Rhodes, J., Owen, E., and Evans, B. K. (1975). 'Disodium cromoglycate in the treatment of chronic proctitis', *Gut*, **16**, 559–563.

Herlinger, H., Glanville, J. N., and Kreel, L. (1977). 'An evaluation of the double contrast barium meal (DCBM) against endoscopy', *Clin. Radiol.*, **28**, 307–314.

Hill, M. J. (1974). 'Bacteria and the aetiology of colonic cancer', *Cancer*, **34**, 815–818.

Hill, M. J., Drasar, B. S., Williams, R. E. O., Meade, T. W., Cox, A. G., Simpson, J. E. P., and Morson, B. C. (1975). 'Faecal bile-acids and clostridia in patients with cancer of the large bowel', *Lancet*, **1**, 535–538.

Hinder, R. A., and Kelly, K. A. (1977). 'Canine gastric emptying of solids and liquids', *Am. J. Physiol.*, **233**, E335–340.

Hoare, A. M., Bradby, G. V. H., Hawkins, C. F., Kang, J. Y., and Dykes, P. W. (1979). 'Cimetidine in bleeding peptic ulcer', *Lancet*, **2**, 671–673.

Holinger, P. H., and Jensik, R. J. (1973). 'Halting the progress of Zenker's diverticula', *Geriatrics*, **28**, 133–137.

Holland, C., and Heaton, K. W. (1972). 'Increasing frequency of gall bladder operations in the Bristol clinical area', *Br. Med. J.*, **3**, 672–675.

Hollis, J. B., and Castell, D. O. (1974). 'Oesophageal function in elderly men. A new look at

"Presby oesophagus"', *Ann. Intern. Med.*, **80**, 371–374.

Hosking, D. J., Moody, F., Stewart, I. M., and Atkinson, M. (1975). 'Vagal impairment of gastric secretion in diabetic autonomic neuropathy', *Br. Med. J.*, **2**, 588–590.

Howiler, W., and Goldberg, M. I. (1976). 'Gastro-oesophageal involvement in herpes simplex', *Gastroenterology*, **70**, 775–778.

Heuto-Armijo, A., and Exton-Smith, A. N. (1962). 'Causes and diagnosis of jaundice in the elderly', *Br. Med. J.*, **1**, 1113–1114.

Hurwitz, A. L., Way, L. W., and Haddad, J. K. (1975). 'Epiphrenic diverticulum in association with an unusual motility disturbance: Report of surgical correction', *Gastroenterology*, **68**, 795–798.

Isenberg, J. I., Grossman, M. I., Maxwell, V., and Walsh, J. M. (1975). 'Increased sensitivity to stimulation of acid secretion by pentagastrin in duodenal ulcer', *J. Clin. Invest.*, **55**, 330–337.

Jedrychowski, W., and Popiela, T. (1974). 'Association between the occurrence of peptic ulcers and tobacco smoking', *Public Health*, **88**, 195–200.

Jewell, D. P., and Truelove, S. C. (1974). 'Azathiaprine in ulcerative colitis: Final report on controlled therapeutic trial', *Br. Med. J.*, **4**, 627–630.

Johnston, D. H. (1966). 'A biopsy study of the gastric mucosa in post operative patients with and without marginal ulcer', *Am. J. Gastroenterol.*, **46**, 103–118.

Joint Iran–International Agency (1977). 'Oesophageal cancer studies in the Caspian Littoral of Iran: Results of population studies – a prodrome', *J. Natl. Cancer Inst.*, **59**, 1127–1128.

Jones, R. F. McN. (1961). 'The Paterson–Brown–Kelly syndrome. Its relationship to iron deficiency and post-cricoid carcinoma', *J. Laryngol. Otol.*, **75**, 529–543.

Kaplowitz, N., Kok, E., and Javitt, N. B. (1973). 'Post-prandial serum bile acid for the detection of hepato biliary disease', *JAMA*, **225**, 292–293.

Kaye, M. D. (1974). 'Oesophageal motor dysfunction in patients with diverticula of the mid-thoracic oesophagus', *Thorax*, **29**, 666–672.

Kelly, A. B. (1919). 'Spasm at the entrance to the oesophagus', *J. Laryngol. Rhin. Otol.*, **34**, 285–289.

Kelly, K. A. (1980). 'Gastric emptying of liquids and solids: Roles of proximal and distal stomach', *Am. J. Physiol.*, **239**, G71–76.

Kennedy, T., Kelly, M. J., and George, J. D. (1972). 'Vagotomy for gastric ulcer', *Br. Med. J.*, **2**, 371–373.

Kodsi, B. E., Wickremesinghe, P. C., Kozinn, P. J., Iswasa, K., and Goldberg, P. K. (1976). 'Candida oesophagitis; a prospective study of 27 cases', *Gastroenterology*, **71**, 715–719.

Kronborg, O., and Madsen, P. (1975). 'A controlled randomised trial of highly selective vagotomy vs. selective vagotomy and pyloroplasty in the treatment of duodenal ulcer', *Gut*, **16**, 268–271.

Langman, M. J. S. (1971). 'Epidemiology of cancer of the oesophagus and stomach', *Br. J. Surg.*, **58**, 792–793.

Larrain, A., Csendes, A., and Pope, C. E. II (1975). 'Surgical correction of reflux: An effective therapy for oesophageal strictures', *Gastroenterology*, **69**, 578–583.

Larson, H. E., Price, A. B., Honour, P., and Borriello, S. P. (1978). '*Clostridium difficile* and the aetiology of pseudomembraneous colitis', *Lancet*, **1**, 1063–1066.

Laurence, B. M., Vallon, A. G., Cotton, P. B., Miro, J. R. A., Oses, J. C. S., LeBodic, L., Sudry, P., Frühmorgen, P., and Bodem, F. (1980). 'Endoscopic laser photocoagulation for bleeding peptic ulcers', *Lancet*, **1**, 124–125.

Leverat, M., Pasquier, J., Lambert, R., and Tissot, A. (1966). 'Peptic ulcer in patients over 60; experience in 287 cases', *A. J. Dig. Dis.*, **11**, 279–285.

Levy, M. (1974). 'Aspirin use in patients with major upper gastro-intestinal bleeding and peptic ulcer disease', *New Engl. J. Med.*, **290**, 1158–1162.

Lewkonia, R. M., and McConnell, R. B. (1976). 'Progress report: Familial inflammatory bowel disease – hereditary or environment?', *Gut*, **17**, 235–243.

Lewkonia, R. M., Woodrow, J. C., McConnell, R. B., and Evans, D. A. P. (1974). 'HL-A antigens in inflammatory bowel disease', *Lancet*, **1**, 574–575.

Lightdale, C. J., Wolf, D. J., Marcucci, R. A., and Salyer, W. R. (1977). 'Herpetic oesophagitis in patients with cancer: Ante-mortem diagnosis by brush cytology', *Cancer*, **39**, 223–226.

Lincoln, J. C. R., Deverall, P. B., Stark, J., Aberdeen, E., and Waterston, D. J. (1969). 'Vascular anomalies compressing the oesophagus and trachea', *Thorax*, **24**, 295–306.

Litton, A., and Murdoch, W. R. (1963). 'Peptic ulcer in South West Scotland', *Gut*, **4**, 360–366.

Logemann, J. A., Blonsky, E. R., and Boshes, B. (1975). 'Dysphagia in Parkinsonism', *JAMA*, **231**, 69–70.

McCall, A. J. (1975). 'Slow K ulceration of oesophagus with aneurysmal left atrium', *Br. Med. J.*, **3**, 230–231.

McConnell, R. B. (1966). The Genetics of Gastrointestinal Disorders, pp. 76–111, Oxford University Press, London.

MacDougall, B. R. D., and Williams, R. (1978). 'The role of cimetidine in the management of bleeding in liver disease', in *Cimetidine*, The *Westminster Hospital Symposium* (Eds C. Wastell and P. Lance), Churchill Livingstone, London.

MacDougall, B. R. D., Westaby, D., Theodossi, A., Dawson, J. L., and Williams, R. (1982). 'Increased long-term survival in variceal haemorrhage using injection sclerotherapy', *Lancet*, **1**, 124–127.

McKeown, F. (1965). *Pathology of the Aged*, pp. 219–220. Butterworths, London.

McKeown, K. C. (1958). 'Oesophageal stenosis after partial gastrectomy', *Br. Med. J.*, **2**, 819–823.

McLoy, R. F., Girvan, D. P., and Baron, J. H. (1978). 'Twenty four hour gastric acidity after vagotomy', *Gut*, **19**, 664–668.

Malagelada, J. R., Rees, W. D. W., Mazzotta, J., and Go, V. L. W. (1980). 'Gastric motor abnormalities in diabetic and post-vagotomy gastroparesis: Effect of metoclopramide and bethanechol', *Gastroenterology*, **78**, 286–293.

Malhotra, S. L. (1967). 'Epidemiological study of peptic ulcer in the South of India', *Gut*, **8**, 180–188.

Mandelstam, P., Siegel, C. I., Lieber, A., and Siegel, M. (1969). 'The swallowing disorder in patients with diabetic neuropathy–gastroenteropathy', *Gastroenterology*, **56**, 1–12.

Mani, V., Lloyd, G., Green, F. H. Y., Fox, H., and Turnberg, L. A. (1976). 'Treatment of ulcerative colitis with oral disodium cromoglycate: A double blind controlled trial', *Lancet*, **1**, 439–441.

Manning, A. P., Heaton, K. W., Harvey, R. F., and Uglow, P. (1977). 'Wheat fibre and irritable bowel syndrome: A controlled trial', *Lancet*, **2**, 417–418.

Marquardt, M., Rufino, F., and Weisburger, J. H. (1977). 'Mutagenic activity of nitrite: Human stomach cancer may be related to dietary factors', *Science*, **196**, 1000–1001.

Marshak, R. H., Janowitz, H. D., and Present, D. H. (1970). 'Granulomatous colitis in association with diverticula', *New Engl. J. Med.*, **283**, 1080–1084.

Marston, A. (1977). *Intestinal Ischaemia*, Edward Arnold, London.

Marston, A., Marcuson, R. W., Chapman, M., and Arthur, J. F. (1969). 'Experimental study of devascularization of the colon', *Gut*, **10**, 121–130.

Matts, S. G. F., and Gaskell, K. H. (1961). 'Retrograde colonic spread of enemata in ulcerative colitis', *Br. Med. J.*, **2**, 614.

Miller, C. (1962). 'Carcinoma of thoracic oesophagus and cardia: A review of 405 cases', *Br. J. Surg.*, **49**, 507–522.

Mills, P. C. (1975). 'Cricopharyngeal sphincterotomy and bilateral division of the chorda tympani in bulbar palsy', *Proc. R. Soc. Med.*, **68**, 644–646.

Misiewicz, J. J., Lennard-Jones, J. E., Connell, A. M., Baron, J. H., and Avery-Jones, F. (1965). 'Controlled trial of sulphasalazine in maintenance

therapy of ulcerative colitis', *Lancet*, **1**, 185–188.

Mitchell, C. J., Humphrey, C. S., Bullen, A. W., Kelleher, J., and Losowsky, M. S. (1979). 'Improved diagnostic accuracy of a modified oral pancreatic function test', *Scand. J. Gastroenterol.*, **14**, 737–741.

Montgomery, W. W. (1963). 'Cricoarytenoid arthritis', *Laryngoscope*, **73**, 801–836.

Montgomery, W. W., and Goodman, M. L. (1980). 'Rheumatoid cricoarytenoid arthritis complicated by upper oesophageal ulceration', *Ann. Otol. Rhinol. Laryngol.*, **89**, 6–8.

Morgan, M. Y., Jakobovits, A. M., James, I. M., and Sherlock, S. (1980). 'Successful use of bromocryptine in the treatment of chronic hepatic encephalopathy', *Gastroenterology*, **78**, 663–670.

Morris, D. W., Levine, G. M., Soloway, R. D., Miller, W. T., and Moran, G. A. (1975). 'Prospective, randomized study of diagnosis and outcome in acute upper gastro-intestinal bleeding: Endoscopy versus conventional radiography', *Am. J. Dig. Dis.*, **20**, 1103–1109.

Morson, B. C. (1962). 'Precancerous lesions of the colon and rectum', *JAMA*, **179**, 316–321.

Mossberg, S. M. (1966). 'The columnar lined oesophagus (Barrett's syndrome): An acquired condition', *Gastroenterology*, **50**, 671–676.

Muscroft, T. J., Youngs, D. J., Burdon, D. W., and Keighley, M. R. B. (1981). 'Cimetidine is unlikely to increase formation of intragastric *N*-nitroso-compounds in patients taking a normal diet', *Lancet*, **1**, 408–410.

Narayanan, M.. and Steinheber, F. U. (1976). 'The changing face of peptic ulcer in the elderly', *Med. Clin. North Am.*, **60**, 1159–1172.

Nissen, R. (1961). 'Gastropexy and fundoplication in surgical treatment of hiatal hernia', *Am. J. Dig. Dis.*, **6**, 954–961.

Nosher, J. L., Campbell, W. L., and Seaman, W. B. (1975). 'The clinical significance of cervical oesophageal and hypopharyngeal webs', *Radiology*, **117**, 45–47.

Olgilvie, A. L., Fergusson, R., and Atkinson, M. (1980). 'Outlook with conservative treatment of peptic oesophageal stricture', *Gut*, **21**, 23–25.

Ornstein, M. H., Littlewood, E. R., Baerd, I. M., Fowler, J., North, W. R. S., and Cox, A. G. (1981). 'Are fibre supplements really necessary in diverticular disease of the colon? A controlled clinical trial', *Br. Med. J.*, **282**, 1353–1356.

Owen, D. A. (1979). 'The diagnosis and significance of gastritis', *Pathol. Ann.*, **14**, 247–271.

Owens, D., and Evans, J. (1975). 'Population studies in Gilbert's syndrome', *J. Med. Genet.*, **12**, 152–156.

Owens, D., and Sherlock, S. (1973). 'Diagnosis of Gilbert's syndrome: Role of reduced calorie intake test', *Br. Med. J.*, **3**, 559–563.

Painter, N. S. (1969). 'Diverticular disease of the colon. The disease of the century', *Lancet*, **2**, 586–588.

Painter, N. S., and Burkitt, D. P. (1971). 'Diverticular disease of the colon. A deficiency disease of Western civilisation', *Br. Med. J.*, **2**, 450–454.

Pallis, C. A., and Lewis, P. D. (1974). *The Neurology of the Gastro-intestinal Tract*, Saunders, London.

Panish, J. F. (1979). State of the art. Management of patients with polypoid lesions of the colon. Current concepts and controversies', *Am. J. Gastroenterol.*, **71**, 315–324.

Paterson, D. R. (1919). 'A clinical type of dysphagia', *J. Laryng. Rhin. Otol.*, **34**, 289–291.

Pearson, J. G. (1975). 'Value of radiation therapy: Current concepts in cancer. 42-II Oesophagus treatment – localised and advanced', *JAMA*, **227**, 181–183.

Pemberton, J. (1970). 'Oesophageal obstruction and ulceration caused by oral potassium therapy', *Br. Heart J.*, **32**, 267–268.

Penn, I. (Editorial) (1980). 'The declining role of the surgeon in the treatment of acid-peptic disease', *Arch. Surg.*, **115**, 134–135.

Peterson, W. L., Sturdevant, R. A. L., Frankl, H. D., Richardson, C. T., Isenberg, J. I., Elashoff, J. D., Sones, J. Q., Gross, R. A., McCallum, R. W., and Fordtran, J. S. (1977). 'Healing of duodenal ulcer with an antacid regimen', *New Engl. J. Med.*, **297**, 341–345.

Philpotts, R. J., Herman-Taylor, J., Teich, N. M., and Brooke, B. N. (1980). 'A search for persistent virus infection in Crohn's disease', *Gut*, **21**, 202–207.

Piasecki, C. (1974). 'Blood supply to the human gastro-duodenal mucosa with special reference to the ulcer bearing areas', *J. Anat.*, **118**, 295–335.

Pope, C. E. II (1967). 'A dynamic test of sphincter strength. Its application to the lower oesophageal sphincter', *Gastroenterology*, **52**, 779–786.

Pope, C. E. II (1978). 'The oesophagus'. in *Gastrointestinal Disease* (Eds M. H. Sleisenger and F. S. Fortran), 2nd ed., pp. 502–604, Saunders, London.

Price, A. B., Jewkes, J., and Sanderson, P. J. (1979). 'Acute diarrhoea: Campylobacter colitis and the role of rectal biopsy', *J. Clin. Pathol.*, **32**, 990–997.

Price, J. D., Stanciu, C., and Bennett, J. R. (1974). 'A safer method of dilating oesophageal strictures', *Lancet*, **1**, 1141–1143.

Priebe, H. J., Skillman, J. J., Bushnell, L. S., Long, P. C., and Silen, W. (1980). 'Antacid versus cimetidine in preventing acute gastro-intestinal bleeding. A randomized trial in 75 critically ill patients', *New Engl. J. Med.*, **302**, 426–430.

Puestow, K. L. (1955). 'Conservative treatment of stenosing disease of the oesophagus', *Postgrad. Med. J.*, **18**, 6–14.

Redolfi, A., Borgogelli, E., and Lodola, E. (1979). 'Blood level of cimetidine in relation to age', *Eur. J. Clin. Pharmacol.*, **15**, 257–261.

Reed, P. I., Cassell, P. G., and Walters, C. L. (1979). 'Gastric cancer in patients who have taken cimetidine', *Lancet*, **1**, 1234–1235.

Reed, P. I., and Davies, W. A. (1978). 'Controlled trial of a new dosage form of carbenoxolone (pyrogastrone) in the treatment of reflux oesophagitis', *Am. J. Dig. Dis.*, **23**, 161–165.

Reed, P. I., Smith, P. L. R., Haines, K., House, F. R., and Walter, C. L. (1981). 'Effect of cimetidine on gastric juice N-nitrosamine concentration', *Lancet*, **2**, 553–556.

Rees, W. D., Evans, B. K., and Rhodes, J. (1979). 'Treating irritable bowel syndrome with peppermint oil', *Br. Med. J.*, **2**, 835.

Registrar General (1971). *Decennial Supplements, Occupational Mortality Tables for 1959–69*, HMSO, London.

Rhodes, J. (1972). 'Aetiology of gastric ulcer', *Gastroenterology*, **63**, 171–182.

Ritchie, J. (1977). 'The irritable bowel syndrome. Part II: Manometric and cineradiographic studies', *Clin. Gastroenterol.*, **6** (3), 622–631.

Ritchie, J. K., Hawley, P. R., and Lennard-Jones, J. E. (1981). 'Prognosis of carcinoma in ulcerative colitis', *Gut*, **22**, 752–755.

Ritchie, J. K., and Lennard-Jones, J. E. (1976). 'Crohn's disease of the distal large bowel', *Scand. J. Gastroenterol.*, **11**, 433–436.

Rodnan, G. P., and Fennell, R. H. Jr. (1962). 'Progressive systemic sclerosis sine scleroderma', *JAMA*, **180**, 665–670.

Rogers, I. M., Sokhi, G. S., Moule, B., Joffe, S. M., and Blumgart, L. H. (1976). 'Endoscopy and routine and double-contrast barium meal in diagnosis of gastric and duodenal disorders', *Lancet*, **1**, 901–902.

Rosenberg, J. L., Wall, A. J., Levin, B., Binder, H. J., and Kirsner, J. B. (1975). 'A controlled trial of azathioprine in the management of chronic ulcerative colitis', *Gastroenterology*, **69**, 96–99.

Rosenthal, H. M., and Cooper, J. H. (1979). 'The oesophagus and chest pain with normal coronary arteries', *Am. Heart J.*, **97**, 266–267.

Rubin, P. (1974). 'Cancer of the gastrointestinal tract. Current concepts in cancer 42-II. Oesophagus: Treatment – localised and advanced', *JAMA*, **227**, 175–185.

Ruddell, W. S. J., Bones, E. S., Hill, M. J., Blendis, L. M., and Walters, C. L. (1976). 'Gastric juice nitrite. A risk factor for cancer in the hypochlorhydric stomach?', *Lancet*, **2**, 1037–1039.

Ruddell, W. S. J., Bones, E. S., Hill, M. J. and Walters, C. L. (1978). 'Pathogenesis of gastric cancer in pernicious anaemia', *Lancet*, **1**, 521–523.

Rutgeerts, L., and Verhagen, H. (1977). 'Intravenous miconazole in the treatment of chronic oesophageal candidiasis', *Gastroenterology*, **72**, 316–318.

Samloff, I. M., Secrist, D. M., and Passaro, E. Jr. (1975). 'A study of the relationship between serum Group 1 pepsinogen levels and gastric acid secretion', *Gastroenterology*, **69**, 1196–1200.

Sanderson, C. J., and Trotter, G. A. (1980). 'Eder Puestow oesophageal dilation a new hazard', *Br. J. Surg.*, **67**, 300–301.

Sandlow, L. J., Becker, G. H., Spellberg, M. A., Allen, H. A., Berg, M., Berry, L. H., and Newman, E. A. (1974). 'A prospective randomized study of the management of upper gastrointestinal haemorrhage', *Am. J. Gastroenterol.*, **61**, 282–289.

Schatzki, R. (1933). 'Reliefstudien on der normalen und kronkhaft veranderten speiserohre', *Acta. Radiol. Suppl.*, **18**, 1.

Schatzki, R., and Gary, J. E. (1953). 'Dysphasia due to a diaphragm-like localised narrowing in the lower oesophagus ("lower oesphageal ring")', *Am. J. Roentgenol.*, **70**, 911–922.

Schentag, J. J., Cerra, F. B., Calleri, G. M., Leising, M. E., French, M. A., and Bernhard, H. (1981). 'Age, disease and cometidine disposition in healthy subjects and chronically ill patients', *Clin. Pharmacol*, **29**, 737–743.

Schiller, K. F. R., Truelove, S. C., and Williams, D. G. (1970). 'Haematemesis and melaena with special reference to factors influencing outcome', *Br. Med. J.*, **2**, 7–14.

Schmidt, G. T., Lennard-Jones, J. E., Morson, B. C., and Young, A. C. (1968). 'Crohn's disease of the colon and its distinction from diverticulitis', *Gut*, **9**, 7–16.

Schneider, R. (1977). 'Doxycycline oesophageal ulcers', *Dig. Dis. Sci.*, **22**, 805–807.

Sherlock, S., Smith-Laing, G., and Dick, R. (1981). 'The therapy of bleeding oesophageal varices', *Liver*, **1**, 3–6.

Skinner, D. B., Little, A. G., and DeMeester, T. R. (1980). 'Management of oesophageal perforation', *Am. J. Surg.*, **139**, 760–764.

Slaney, G., Waterhouse, J. A., and Powell, J. (1968). 'Cancer of the colon and rectum and its response to treatment', *Gut*, **9**, 730.

Soergel, K. M., Zboralske, F., and Amberg, J. R. (1964). 'Presbyoesophagus: Oesophageal motility in nonagenarians', *J. Clin. Invest.*, **43**, 1472–1479.

Soltoft, J., Gudmand-Hoyer, E., Krag, B., Kristensen, E., and Wulf, H. R. (1976). 'A double blind trial of the effect of wheat bran on symptoms of irritable bowel syndrome', *Lancet*, **1**, 270–272.

Sonnenberg, A., Schmid, P., Muller-Lissner, S. A.,

Vogel, E., and Blum, A. L. (1980). 'What makes duodenal ulcer heal and relapse', *Gastroenterology*, **78**, 1266.

Stemmermann, G. N. (1977). 'Gastric cancer in the Hawaii Japanese', *Gan.*, **68**, 525–535.

Stilson, W. L., Saunders, I., Gardiner, G. A., Gorman, H. C., and Lodge, D. F. (1969). 'Hiatal hernia and gastro-oesophageal reflux', *Radiology*, **93**, 1323–1328.

Storey, D. W., Boulos, P. B., Ward, M. W. N., and Clark, C. G. (1981). 'Proximal gastric vagotomy after five years', *Gut*, **22**, 702–704.

Strange, S. L. (1959). 'Giant innocent gastric ulcer. Its behaviour and treatment', *Br. Med. J.*, **1**, 476–480.

Strickland, R. G., and Mackay, I. R. (1973). 'A reappraisal of the nature and significance of chronic atrophic gastritis', *Am. J. Dig. Dis.*, **18**, 426–440.

Sumithran, E., Lim, K. H., and Chiam, H. L. (1979). 'Atrio-oesophageal fistula complicating mitral valve disease', *Br. Med. J.*, **2**, 1552–1553.

Sun, D. C. H., Roth, S. M., Mitchell, C. S., and England, D. W. (1974). 'Upper gastrointestinal disease in rheumatoid arthritis', *Am. J. Dig. Dis.*, **19**, 405–410.

Svartz, N. (1942). 'Salazopyrin, a new sulphonilamide preparation. (a) Therapeutic results in rheumatic polyarthritis. (b) Therapeutic results in ulcerative colitis. (c) Toxic manifestations with sulphonilamide preparations', *Acta. Med. Scand.*, **110**, 577–598.

Svensson, O., Stenport, G., Tibling, L., and Wranne, B. (1978). 'Oesophageal function and coronary angiogram in patients with disabling chest pain', *Acta. Med. Scand.*, **204**, 173–178.

Swammy, N. (1977). 'Oesophageal spasm: Clinical and manometric response to nitroglycerine and long acting nitrites', *Gastroenterology*, **72**, 23–27.

Tarin, D., Allison, D. J., Modlin, I. M., and Neale, G. (1978). 'Diagnosis and management of obscure gastrointestinal bleeding', *Br. Med. J.*, **2**, 751–754.

Taub, S., Moriani, A., and Birkin, J. S. (1979). 'Gastro-intestinal manifestations of diabetes mellitus', *Diabetes Care*, **2**, 437–447.

Taylor, R. H., Menzies-Gow, M., Lovell, D., La Brooy, S. J., and Misiewicz, J. J. (1978). 'Misleading response of malignant gastric ulcers to cimetidine', *Lancet*, **1**, 686–688.

Tedesco, F. J., and Morton, W. J. (1975). 'Lower oesophageal webs', *Am. J. Dig. Dis.*, **20**, 381–383.

Temple, J. G., Goodhall, R. J. R., Hay, D. J., and Miller, D. (1981). 'Effects of highly selective vagotomy upon the lower oesophageal sphincter', *Gut*, **22**, 368–370.

Teplick, J. G., Teplick, S. K., Ominsky, S. H. and

Haskin, M. E. (1980). 'Oesophagitis caused by oral medication', *Radiology*, **134**, 23–25.

Thoeni, R. F., and Cello, J. P. (1980). 'A critical look at the accuracy of endoscopy and double contrast radiography of the upper gastrointestinal tract in patients with substantial U.G.I. haemorrhage', *Radiology*, **135**, 305–308.

Torvik, A., and Høivik, B. (1960). 'Gallstones in autopsy series. Incidence, complications and correlations with carcinoma of the gallbladder', *Acta. Chir. Scand.*, **120**, 168–174.

Tovey, F. I., and Tunstall, M. (1975). 'Duodenal ulcer in black populations in Africa south of the Sahara', *Gut*, **16**, 564–576.

Van Hees, P. A. M., Bakker, J. H., and Van Tongeren, J. H. M. (1980). 'Effects of sulphapyridine, 5 amino-salicylic acid and placebo in patients with idiopathic proctitis: A study to determine the active moiety of sulphasalazine', *Gut*, **21**, 623–635.

Vantrappen, G., Janssens, H., and Hellemans, J. (1979). 'Achalasia, diffuse oesophageal spasm, and related motility disorders', *Gastroenterology*, **76**, 450–457.

Venables, C. W., Stephen, J. G., Blair, E. L., Reed, J. D., and Saunders, J. D. (1978). In *Cimetidine. The Westminster Hospital Symposium* (Eds C. Wastell and P. Lance), Churchill Livingstone, London.

Verlenden, W. L., and Frey, C. F. (1980). 'Management of liver abscess', *Am. J. Surg.*, **140**, 53–59.

Vinson, P. P. (1922). 'Hysterical dysphagia', *Minn. Med.*, **5**, 107–108.

Wallin, L. (1980). 'Gastro-oesophageal function in duodenal ulcer patients', *Scan. J. Gastroenterol.*, **15**, 145–150.

Wallin, L., and Madsen, T. (1979). '12-hour simultaneous registration of acid reflux and peristaltic activity in the oesophagus. A study in normal subjects', *Scand. J. Gastroenterol.*, **14**, 561–566.

Walsh, J. H., Richardson, C. T., and Fordtran, J. S. (1975). 'pH dependence of acid secretion and gastrin release in normal and ulcer subjects', *J. Clin. Invest.*, **55**, 462–468.

Weisbrodt, N. W. (1976). 'Neuromuscular organisation of oesophageal and pharyngeal motility', *Arch. Intern. Med.*, **136**, 524–531.

Wernly, J. A., DeMeester, T. R., Bryant, G. H., Wang, C. I., Smith, R. B., and Skinner, D. B. (1980). 'Intra-abdominal pressure and manometric data of the distal oesophageal sphincter', *Arch. Surg.*, **115**, 534–539.

Whelton, M. J., Petrelli, M., George, P., Young, W. B., and Sherlock, S. (1969). 'Carcinoma at the junction of the main hepatic ducts', *Quert. J. Med.*, **38**, 211–230.

Whitney, B., and Croxon, R. (1972). 'Dysphagia caused by cardiac enlargement', *Clin. Radiol.*, **23**, 147–152.

Williamson, R. C. N. (1975). 'The management of peptic oesophageal stricture', *Br. J. Surg.*, **62**, 448–454.

Willoughby, C. P., Heyworth, M. F., Piris, J., and Truelove, S. C. (1979). 'Comparison of disodium cromoglycate and sulphasalazine as maintenance therapy for ulcerative colitis', *Lancet*, **1**, 119–122.

Willoughby, C. P., Piris, J., and Truelove, S. C. (1979). 'Campylobacter colitis', *J. Clin. Pathol.*, **32**, 986–989.

Winship, D. H., Caflisch, C. R., Zboralske, F. F., and Hogan, W. J. (1968). 'Deterioration of oesophageal peristalsis in patients with alcoholic neuropathy', *Gastroenterology*, **55**, 173–178.

Woodings, E. P., Dixon, G. T., Harrison, C., Carey, P., and Richards, D. A. (1980). 'Ranitidine – a new H_2 receptor antagonist', *Gut*, **21**, 187–191.

Wormsley, K. G., and Grossman, M. I. (1965) 'Maximal histolog test in control subjects and patients with peptic ulcer', *Gut*, **6**, 427–435.

Wynder, E. L., Reddy, B. S., McCory, G. D., Weisburger, J. H., and Williams, G. M. (1976). 'Diet and gastro-intestinal cancer', in *Clinics in Gastroenterology*, Vol. 5:3, pp. 485–487, Saunders, London.

Zaldiver, R. (1970). 'Geographical pathology of oral oesophageal, gastric and intestinal cancer in Chile', *Z. Krebsforsch.*, **75**, 1–13.

Zentler-Munro, P. L., and Northfield, T. C. (1979). 'Drug induced gastro-intestinal disease', *Br. Med. J.*, **1**, 1263–1265.

Principles and Practice of Geriatric Medicine
Edited by M. S. J. Pathy
© 1985 John Wiley & Sons Ltd

11.4

The Physiology and Pathophysiology of the Pelvic Floor Musculature

Sir Alan Parks

It is essential to give a brief description of the normal physiology of the anorectal region prior to a consideration of the pathophysiological changes which are found together with their accompanying clinical manifestations.

ANATOMY

Developmentally, the anorectal region is composite in nature, consisting of the termination of the alimentary viscus and the skeletal muscle and fascial tissue which surrounds it. The arrangement may be likened to two tubes, one within the other. The inner consists of the termination of the alimentary viscus (the visceral component), containing only smooth muscle innervated by the autonomic system (Fig. 1). The outer tube, which can be called the somatic or skeletal muscle component, is made up of the external anal sphincter ring together with the puborectalis muscle. Being composed of skeletal muscle, it is subject to conscious activation but is mainly under reflex control. The upper part of the pelvic floor fans out to

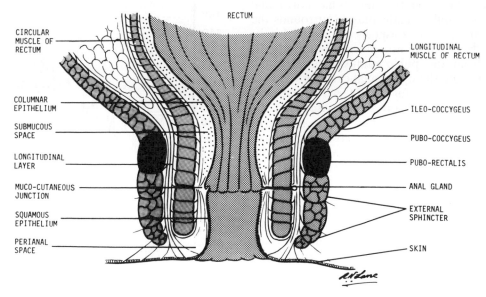

Figure 1   A diagrammatic coronal section through the pelvic floor. The visceral and somatic components can be seen

form a barrier which closes the pelvic hiatus; it has no sphincteric action.

The visceral component contains the usual constituents of a viscus, i.e. a longitudinal layer of muscle on the outside, a circular layer (the internal sphincter), submucosa, and mucosa. The circular layer which forms the internal sphincter is a large muscle mass capable of exerting considerable pressure upon the anal canal. The upper half of the canal is lined by columnar, mucus-secreting epithelium, such as is found in the rectum and colon. The lower half of the canal is lined by squamous epithelium which has, as it were, migrated from the skin in the course of embryological development. This migration confers several advantages; the squamous mucosa is dry and does not secrete mucus. It is also richly innervated with nerve endings and plays an important part in the mechanism of continence (Duthie and Gairns, 1960). In order that the mucosa shall not prolapse, there is a zone of fibromuscular tissue in the midanal canal which anchors the mucocutaneous junction to the underlying internal sphincter.

The somatic or skeletal muscle component of the pelvic floor is made up of the external sphincters together with the puborectalis, the pubococcygeus, and ileococcygeus muscles. The external sphincter which surrounds the lower three-quarters of the anal canal derives its innervation from the inferior haemorrhoidal nerve. The puborectalis muscle surrounds the lateral and posterior aspects of the canal in its upper third but is not present anteriorly. It arises from the pubic ramus anteriorly and passes behind the upper anal canal as a muscle sling. It is a powerful muscle, whose action is partially sphincteric on all the viscera of the pelvic hiatus. An important action is that of maintaining the angulation between the lower rectum and the anal canal, upon which continence is largely dependent. The pelvic floor muscles above the puborectalis, known collectively as the levator ani muscles, have an antigravity function, preventing herniation of abdominal contents through the pelvis. The nerve supply of the levator ani muscles and also the puborectalis muscle is derived from branches of S3 and S4 which descend as the levator nerve on the anterior surface of the muscles. The junction of the two components of the pelvic floor is an embryonic plane of

fusion. Few vascular or nervous structures cross it. Because of this it is an important plane of dissection used for certain operative procedures (Parks, 1975).

PHYSIOLOGY

The Visceral Component

The action of the internal sphincter is markedly different from that of the circular muscle of the rectum above it. It is in a state of continuous tone, which maintains closure of the anal canal and is responsible for the basal pressure recorded in the canal. A pressure profile of the action of the sphincter is shown in Fig. 2. A small pressure probe drawn down from the rectum through the anal canal usually reveals a peak of pressure about half-way along, which is in the region of 60 to 80 cm of water. The length of the canal as detected by pressure measurement is about 3.5 cm; it is greater in men than women and is unaffected by age or parity. Pressures are higher in men but diminish with increase in age in both sexes (Read *et al.*, 1979). Distention of the rectum produces transient relaxation of the internal sphincter (Denny-Brown and Robertson, 1935; Gaston, 1948; Schuster, Hendrix, and Mendeoff, 1963).

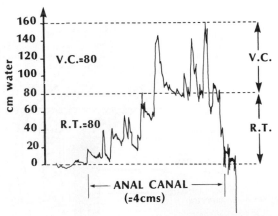

Figure 2   A pressure profile of the anal canal, recordings being taken at 1 cm intervals. Resting tone (RT) due to external sphincter activity is 80 cm water. Voluntary contraction (VC) causes a rise of another 80 cm

Partial recovery occurs and further relaxation takes place with increased filling of the rectum (Fig. 3). With each increment the baseline falls until finally the sphincter relaxes completely. This effect is seen even in patients with complete cauda equina lesions and after a transection of the spinal cord (Frenckner, 1975; Melzak and Porter, 1964). It is absent in patients with Hirschsprung's disease; the myenteric plexus of the rectum is abnormal in this condition, suggesting that the normal reflex response is dependent upon the intrinsic neural plexus of the gut (Aaronson and Nixon, 1972).

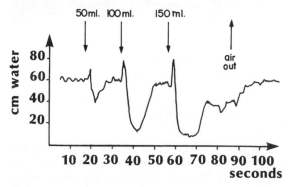

Figure 3 Internal sphincter pressure is recorded.The balloon is distended within the rectum. The internal sphincter tone decreases with each increment

The Somatic Component

The skeletal muscles of the pelvic floor serve two functions, both equally important. The first is to combat the force of intra-abdominal pressure which is considerable in man due to the erect posture. The external sphincter group and puborectalis muscle maintain normal faecal continence. It is essential that these activities be automatically carried out. Muscles which responded only to voluntary or even synergistic stimuli would be unable to make the necessary adjustments in pelvic floor tone which are essential to cope with the many and varied stresses placed upon it. Most skeletal muscles in the body are completely at rest when not in action; an electromyographic needle inserted in such a muscle will show no electrical activity at all. However, voluntary or synergistic contraction produces a burst of electrical potentials (Fig. 4). The situation of the pelvic floor muscles is quite different; they contract constantly at rest, even during sleep (Floyd and Walls, 1953). In order to respond to the differing stresses upon the pelvic floor there are a variety of reflex changes which oc-

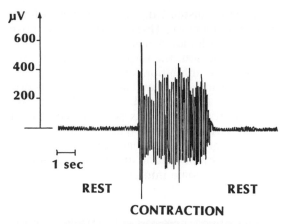

Figure 4 An electromyogram of the extensor muscles of the forearm. There is no activity at rest; when the muscles are tensed, activity commences

cur, resulting in contraction or relaxation, as is appropriate (Parks, Porter, and Melzak, 1962). For instance, when intra-abdominal pressure rises as a result of coughing (Kerrimens, 1969; Parks, Porter, and Melzak, 1962; Phillips and Edwards, 1965), lifting, walking, or for any other reason, there is a marked reinforcement of the tonic activity of the pelvic floor muscles, which will resist this pressure (Fig. 5). Conscious, willed contraction of these muscles is only capable of being sustained for a limited period of time (Phillips and Edwards, 1965).

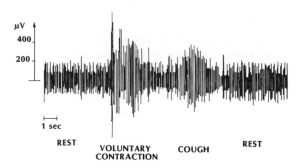

Figure 5 An electromyogram of the pelvic floor muscles shows constant activity at rest. Coughing causes a reflex increase in activity

If the rectum is distended by the action of a balloon placed in it, there is a reflex increase in activity of the external sphincters. This automatic reaction will protect the patient from involuntary defaecation. As the balloon is increasingly distended, so the activity of the sphincters increases (Fig. 6). However, above a certain volume, which varies greatly from person to person, the response changes to one of complete inhibition of sphincter activity. The anal canal gapes and all sphincteric action disappears (Melzak and Porter, 1964). This physiological response is seldom seen under normal circumstances. When, however, the rectum is grossly distended, such as occurs in a patient with impaction of faeces, then it does undoubtedly come into play.

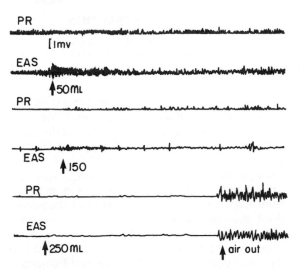

Figure 6   Distention of the rectum causes a reflex increase in external sphincter activity at first. After 250 ml inhibition occurs

An attempt to evacuate the rectum by abdominal straining inhibits the tonic activity of the pelvic floor (Kerrimans, 1969; Parks, Porter, and Melzak, 1962) and allows a stool to be passed without difficulty (Fig. 7). However, there are some who indulge in excessive defaecation straining over many years and, in so doing, may cause permanent damage to the pelvic floor. In this situation the pelvic floor muscles stop contracting and yet are being subjected to the full force of abdominal pressure. Descent of the perineum with passive stretching of the pelvic floor occurs. Provided the episode is of a temporary nature, recovery is usually complete. If the faulty bowel habit persists for years, the pelvic floor may well become permanently stretched (Parks, Porter, and Hardcastle, 1966). Not only will the mus-

cles lengthen and become less efficient but the nerves supplying them are also stretched (Beersiek, Parks, and Swash, 1979; Parks, Swash, and Urich, 1977).

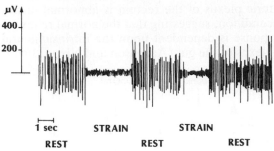

Figure 7   The effect of defaecation straining on the tone in the anal sphincters; inhibition occurs

As has already been mentioned, the tonic contraction of the puborectalis muscle maintains the right-angled relationship between the lower rectum and anal canal. A mechanical valve effect is produced in this way which closes the upper part of the anal canal; the anterior wall of the lower rectum impinges upon the closed anal canal and obstructs it (Parks, 1975). An increase in abdominal pressure alone automatically forces the lower rectal wall even more firmly upon the closed canal, provided the tonic traction of the anal sphincters is present (Fig. 8). Increase in abdominal pressure due to coughing, walking, etc., will automatically seal the upper anal canal and prevent stress incontinence. Ideally, the flap valve should be overcome by the propulsion of rectal content towards the upper anal canal as a result of contraction of the intrinsic musculature of the rectum; it will be automatically lifted off the anal canal in this way.

Sensation

Distention of the rectum in the normal person produces a sensation of fullness in the perineum associated with a feeling of impending evacuation. It has always been believed that this effect was due to stimulation of receptors in the rectal wall itself. Recently, however, it has been shown that this sensation is still present even when the rectum itself has been completely removed and alimentary continuity

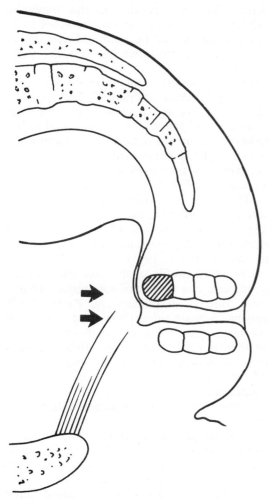

Figure 8   Diagram to show the flap valve produced by the angulation of the lower rectum and anal canal. The anterior wall of the lower rectum impinges upon the closed anal canal

restored by anastomosis of the colon to the anal canal (Lane and Parks, 1977). The receptors for this sensation must therefore lie outside the rectum itself and in all probability are situated in the levator ani muscles (which are known to contain muscle spindles); these cradle the rectal ampulla.

FAECAL INCONTINENCE

As has been shown, the maintenance of normal control is a complex matter at the best of times. Should any abnormality occur, either in the activity of the intestine itself or in the muscles of the pelvic floor, then the mechanism may break down. A person with normal sphincters may find control impossible during an attack of severe diarrhoea. In the elderly patient, who has lost some part of the sphincter muscle mass, merely as the result of ageing, diarrhoea presents a much more difficult problem. Certain neurological conditions affect the pelvic floor muscles, and these may be so severe that even with a normal stool continence is not attained. Finally, there may be organic deficiencies in the muscle ring due to trauma of one variety or another.

Severe Diarrhoea

Even a normal person may be incontinent if afflicted with a sudden episode of diarrhoea. If in addition the person has any defect of the pelvic floor, whether this be due to injury, neurological disease, or even the process of ageing, then they will be much more susceptible to such a situation. Inflammatory disease of the colon, for instance diverticulitis, is a common cause of this state of affairs. Any lesion which secretes mucus can have the same effect, such as a villous papilloma or a carcinoma. Such possibilities must always be borne in mind in the case of a patient who is partially or totally incontinent. Provided that no organic disease is present, and even if a mild degree of sphincter weakness exists, a patient can often be relieved by making the stool more solid in consistency. This can be achieved by an alteration in diet or by the use of one of the drugs which have a delaying effect on intestinal propulsion. A warning note must be sounded about the use of such medication in the elderly. It is very easy to change a state of chronic diarrhoea to one of impaction of faeces. From the patient's point of view, the result is the same; incontinence results.

Impaction of Faeces

The effect of rectal distention on the anal sphincters has already been noted. In certain circumstances the rectum becomes overloaded and lacks adequate power of peristaltic contraction to empty. This may or may not be accompanied by discomfort. The patient's complaint is nearly always that of diarrhoea with complete incontinence. Liquid stool is passed round the impacted mass and is expelled through temporarily inactive and ineffectual anal sphincters. This temporary pathophysiological state is a very important one as, if unrecognized, it can lead to persistent misery for the patient quite unnecessarily. It may occur in young people who have somewhat atonic colons and is often triggered off by an operation, accident, or enforced bed rest. In the young it is often attributed to psychological factors but this is seldom the case and the condition nearly always responds to corrective physical measures. In the elderly it is often considered to be due to senility alone. Lack of physical activity and inattentiveness to bowel function may indeed contribute to the development of impaction but it usually responds to treatment despite advanced years. It is particularly tragic when this condition exists at either end of the age spectrum. The child is condemned to a stigma by his family and schoolmates; the elderly patient is labelled as dirty and may be rejected by the family. Unfortunately, such cases are often left undiagnosed and untreated for many years. This is especially unfortunate, as the treatment is simple; firstly, the impacted mass of stool must be removed, which often requires a general anaesthetic. The chronically distended colon will need time to recover its tone. It will need to be stimulated into activity by daily enemas for 1 to 2 weeks and thereafter an evacuant suppository regime each morning will usually suffice. The latter may be needed for several months.

Neurological Disease

Neuromuscular control of the pelvic floor is centred in the cauda equina; transection above this point seldom causes severe impairment of function once the phase of spinal shock has passed. The rectum empties reflexly and the patient will learn how to induce reflex contraction by stimulation of the anal canal. During the phase of spinal shock, evacuation with the aid of enemata may be needed.

In complete lesions of the cauda equina there is neither muscle activity in the pelvic floor nor is there sensation, and such patients are usually totally incontinent. In an effort to avoid soiling they endeavour to become constipated but this is frequently followed by impaction. The best routine in this inevitably unsatisfactory situation is for the stool to be kept firm and defaecation induced with the aid of glycerine suppositories or even disposable enemata.

There is a variety of incontinence which was previously labelled 'idiopathic'. The sphincter muscles are lax and patulous on clinical examination and there is an absent anal reflex. However, cutaneous sensation is present which implicates the efferent neuron as being defective. There is no contraction in the external sphincter itself but the puborectalis muscle usually responds to voluntary effort. Even so there is loss of tone in the puborectalis muscle, which results in the loss of normal anorectal angulation and impairment of the flap valve mechanism (Parks, 1975).

A pressure profile of the anal canal in this condition shows only minimal pressure change or no tone at all (Henry and Parks, 1980). Pressure increase caused by voluntary contraction varies greatly but is usually considerably less than normal (Read *et al.*, 1979). Routine electromyography may not be grossly abnormal but single-fibre electromyography shows grouping of muscle cells supplied by one axon, indicative of a neuropathic degeneration in the muscle (Fig. 9). Biopsy of the muscles of the pelvic floor has shown a grouping of histochemical types of muscle cells, again indicative of neuropathic change (Beersiek, Parks, and Swash, 1979; Parks, Swash, and Urich, 1977). Similar findings are seen in the carpal tunnel syndrome at the wrist. These changes are believed to be due to stretching of the nerve supplying the pelvic floor either by the excessive defaecation efforts practised over many years or by the result of difficult childbirth.

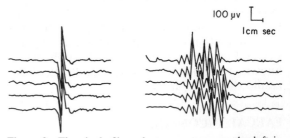

Figure 9 The single-fibre electromyogram on the left is normal, showing only single spikes. On the right the multiple-action potentials denote innervation of many muscle cells by one axon; this is a sign of partial denervation

The external sphincter is always the most severely affected of the pelvic floor muscles. Neuropathic changes diminish the higher up the muscle is in the levator ani group. Because of the deficient tone in the puborectalis muscle, the anorectal angulation upon which the flap valve mechanism depends is impaired (Parks, Porter, and Hardcastle, 1966).

As has already been mentioned, there is a diminution in the muscle mass with advancing years. If the pelvic floor sphincters were already partially weakened by changes such as have been described, then there comes a point when the ageing process tips the balance and incontinence ensues. In the younger patient a neuropathic pelvic floor can be restored to near normality by a reconstruction carried out behind the rectum and anal canal. This results in the reconstruction of the anorectal angle and restores the flap valve mechanism (Parks, 1975). Even in the eighth decade such a procedure can be very effective, provided that there is some residual function present and that the patient is able to cooperate in any postoperative regime.

Injury to the Sphincter Muscle Ring

Complete division of the muscle ring may be caused by childbirth injury, the surgery of anal fistula, or direct trauma, such as that associated with automobile accidents. The female pelvic floor is particularly susceptible to injury incontinence following a degree of damage which would not necessarily cause symptoms in the male. Despite the poor results which followed reconstructive surgery in the past, a satisfactory functional repair can now almost always be achieved, no matter how bizarre the injury. It is necessary to mobilize the ends of the divided muscle, freeing it from scar tissue which binds it down to the fascia in the ischio-rectal fossa. An overlapping repair of the muscle ends is performed and it is wise to protect this with a temporary colostomy (Parks and McPartlin, 1971).

SPECIAL CONSIDERATIONS RELATING TO THE GERIATRIC SITUATION

As has already been mentioned, the elderly patient is more vulnerable to intermittent or persistent diarrhoea due to the progressive weakening of the pelvic floor with age. It is essential that organic causes of diarrhoea are looked for before symptomatic measures are instituted. Impaction of faeces commonly occurs and is inevitably overlooked unless a thorough pelvic examination is performed. However old the patient may be, the treatment is effective; the rectum must be evacuated, if necessary under anaesthesia, followed by the measures previously described. There is one advantage attached to the large, atonic colon so commonly seen in this age group. It has an enormous storage capacity, which can be put to good use by the attending physician. Laxatives administered by mouth frequently result in diarrhoea or irregular bowel action, which is uncontrollable. It is far better to induce colonic evacuation by a stimulus applied rectally. The simplest measure is of course a glycerine suppository; more potent is a suppository containing a contact laxative. In the case of a patient with a large capacity colon which may not empty under normal conditions more than once a week, an enema regime is the most satisfactory. A disposable enema administered every 2 to 3 days may well keep such a person in a state of complete continence, even though the sphincters are weak. By such measures, either singly or in combination, many patients can be freed from the stigma of incontinence, however old they may be. There is little excuse for accepting this state of affairs under the misapprehension that it is inevitable in old people.

With the increased understanding of the physiology and pathophysiology of the pelvic floor in recent years, most of the causes of incontinence are now reasonably well understood. By one means or another it is usually possible to overcome this very severe social disability. Of equal importance is the need to prevent the causes of the condition—causes which may be active during youth but only result in symptoms in later years. Faulty dietary habits over the last hundred years have caused many to suffer from severe constipation with the need to indulge in excessive defaecation straining. Such efforts undoubtedly cause the neuropathic changes described. Health education as to sensible dietary habits is necessary to establish a normal pattern of defaecation, thereby avoiding the muscle changes which can cause such disability in the later years of life. Evidence at present suggests, but is not conclusive, that local neurological damage can be caused by prolonged and difficult labour. It is hoped that a knowledge of the late results which can occur following difficult childbirth will result in measures being taken to prevent this occurring. How much better to prevent such changes than to treat them when they begin to cause symptoms, which may not be until the geriatric age group has been reached.

REFERENCES

Aaronson, I., and Nixon, H. H. (1972). 'A clinical evaluation of anorectal pressure studies in the diagnosis of Hirschprung's disease', *Gut*, **13**, 138–146.

Beersiek, F., Parks, A. G., and Swash, M. (1979). 'Pathogenesis of anorectal incontinence: A histometric study of the anal sphincter musculature', *J. Neurol. Sci.*, **42**, 111–127.

Denny-Brown, D., and Robertson, E. G. (1935). 'An investigation of the nervous control of defaecation', *Brain*, **58**, 256–310.

Duthie, H. L., and Gairns, F. W. (1960). 'Sensory nerve endings and sensation in the anal region of man', *Br. J. Surg.*, **47**, 585–595.

Floyd, W. F., and Walls, E. W. (1953). 'Electromyography of the sphincter ani externus in man', *J. Physiol. (Lond.)*, **122**, 599–609.

Frenckner, B. (1975). 'Function of the anal sphincters in spinal man', *Gut*, **16**, 638–644.

Gaston, E. A. (1948). 'The physiology of faecal continence', *Surg. Gynececol. Obstet.*, **87**, 280–290.

Henry, M. M., and Parks, A. G. (1980). 'The investigation of anorectal function', Hospital Update (January).

Kerrimans, R. (1969). *Morphological and Physiological Aspects of Anal Continence and Defaecation*, Editions Arscia, Brussels.

Lane, R. H. S., and Parks, A. G. (1977). 'Function of the anal sphincters following colo-anal anastomosis', *Br. J. Surg.*, **64**, 596–599.

Melzack, J., and Porter, N. H. (1964). 'Studies of the reflex activity of the external sphincter ani in spinal man', *Paraplegia*, **1**, 277–296.

Parks, A. G. (1975). 'Anorectal incontinence', *Proc. R. Soc. Med.*, **68**, 681–690.

Parks, A. G., and McPartlin, J. F. (1971). 'Late repair of injuries of the anal sphincter', *Proc. R. Soc. Med.*, **64**, 1187–1189.

Parks, A. G., Porter, N. H., and Hardcastle, J. D. (1966). 'Syndrome of the descending perineum', *Proc. R. Soc. Med.*, **59**, 477–482.

Parks, A. G., Porter, N. H., and Melzak, J. (1962). 'Experimental study of the reflex mechanism controlling the muscles of the pelvic floor', *Dis. Colon Rectum.*, **5**, 407–414.

Parks, A. G., Swash, M., and Urich, H. (1977). 'Sphincter denervation in anorectal incontinence and rectal prolapse', *Gut*, **18**, 656–665.

Phillips, S. F., and Edwards, D. A. W. (1965). 'Some aspects of anal continence and defaecation', *Gut*, **6**, 396–406.

Read, N. W., Harford, W. V., Schmulen, A. C., Read, M. G., Santa Ana, C., and Fordran, J. S. (1979). 'A clinical study of patients with faecal incontinence and diarrhoea', *Gastroenterology*, **76**, 747–756.

Schuster, M. M., Hendrix, T. R., and Mendeoff, A. I. (1963). 'The internal anal sphincter response: Manometric studies on its normal physiology, neural pathways and alteration in bowel disorders', *J. Clin. Invest.*, **42**, 196–207.

12
The Haemopoietic System

Principles and Practice of Geriatric Medicine
Edited by M. S. J. Pathy
© 1985 John Wiley & Sons Ltd

12.1

The Haemopoietic System

A. K. Banerjee

INTRODUCTION

A considerable body of knowledge on the age-related changes in the haemopoietic system has accumulated in recent years. Although the clinical presentation of blood disorders may be significantly modified by ageing and diagnosis may require more critical evaluation, basic pathology is largely unchanged and requires similar therapeutic intervention (Banerjee, 1976).

Old age is not particularly immune to any specific blood disorder. This chapter will, however, deal with those haematologic conditions which are more likely to be encountered in later life.

THE BLOOD IN OLD AGE

Red Cell

The quantity and the quality of red cells do not change significantly with advancing age. The mean red cell diameter and the mean corpuscular volume increase slightly from the fifth decade onwards (Olbrich, 1947; Spriggs and Sladden, 1958). A recent Canadian study (Munan *et al.*, 1978) has confirmed this earlier finding; total red cell count and packed cell volume tend to decrease with age in both sexes while the mean corpuscular volume shows some increase.

Red cell osmotic fragility increases slightly (Detraglia *et al.*, 1974). The red cell lifespan has been reported to remain normal (Hurdle and Rosin, 1962; Woodford-Williams *et al.*, 1962). A progressive reduction in red cell mass and total blood volume has also been noted in apparently normal healthy old individuals.

The red cell kinetics are probably the same in the elderly as they are in the young. Active marrow distribution may be reduced with increased presence of fat. Subsequent to an age-related decrease in transferrin level, it is probable that the iron utilization is slightly diminished in old age (Weeke and Krasilnikoff, 1972). However, in routine clinical practice, an adequate marrow erythropoietic response to appropriate haematinic should be expected.

The enzyme content of red cells and its metabolic activities have been studied but the results are inconclusive and conflicting. Brain and Card (1972) have suggested that the red cell adenosine triphosphate (ATP) and diphosphoglyceric acid (DPG) levels decrease with age. The shape and flexibility of red cells depend on their ATP content and ATP-deficient red cells usually become more spherical and less flexible (Lessin, Klug, and Jenson, 1976). Similarly, decrease in DPG level increases the haemoglobin affinity for oxygen with subsequent reduction of oxygen release in the tissues. The ability of red cells to maintain glutathione in its reduced form is diminished, but the total erythrocyte glutathione level increases in older subjects (Bertolini, 1969). The level of red cell sodium has been found to increase only in elderly women (Naylor, 1970).

Although the red cell deformability may increase, the blood viscosity does not show any significant age-related difference in healthy individuals (Roath, 1980).

Lymphocytes

There is a sharp drop in the absolute lymphocyte count during the first two decades of life, after which it remains constant during middle life. Numerous studies have failed to demonstrate a significant change in the absolute lymphocyte count in the later years of life (Bourne and Wilson, 1961; Zacharski, Elveback, and Linman, 1971). MacKinney (1978), in his study of individuals of all ages, has demonstrated an accelerated decline of the total lymphocyte population from the sixth decade onwards. This finding does not prove that the lymphoid cell mass decreases with age and any absolute reduction of lymphocyte count in the very elderly is probably due to a decline in one subpopulation of lymphocytes. Cell culture studies show an age-related loss of one or more chromosomes (hypodiploidy) in the human peripheral lymphocytes and this is probably more evident in females (Martin, Kellet, and Kahn, 1980).

Broadly speaking, the lymphocytes functionally differentiate along two major pathways. The thymus-processed lymphocytes are called T-lymphocytes and are mainly involved in the maintenance of cell-mediated immunity. The other group of lymphocytes are mainly concerned with humoral immunity and are called B-lymphocytes in view of their original association with the Bursa of Fabricius, a cloacal lymphoid organ in the chicken. Although morphologically indistinguishable, T and B cells can be recognized by their differences in membrane structure. T cells bear receptors which react with sheep red cells and such formation of E-rosettes is normally used to identify them. B cells, on the other hand, are demonstrated by fluorescent antibody technique, since they carry immunoglobulins on their membranes. As regards proportional distribution, it has been estimated that in normal adult blood 30 to 75 per cent of the lymphocytes belong to the T type and 10 to 35 per cent are of the B type. T cells and immunity mechanisms are discussed in Chapter 3.2.

Monocytes

The median monocyte count is higher in males of all ages. However, there is evidence of a gentle decline in monocytes from the fifth decade onwards in males but not in females (Munan and Kelly, 1979).

Granulocytes

The number of granulocytes in the peripheral blood does not change with age. In a study of 500 healthy old people without any acute illness, a slight reduction of total leucocytes has been observed (Caird, Andrews, and Gallie, 1972); however, a reduction in lymphocyte levels is more obvious than that of granulocytes. Increased nuclear segmentation and cytoplasmic granulation occurs in the granulocytes of older people.

A greater proportion of neutrophils with higher than four lobes in the nuclei have been noted in the elderly (Bruschke, Thiele, and Schulz, 1960). This minor morphological anomaly of the neutrophils are likely to be due to undetected occult illness rather than an age-associated deviation. In this connection, it is pertinent to note that the presence of an increased proportion of hypersegmented neutrophils is a valuable indicator of a megaloblastic marrow, particularly in the elderly (Adam *et al.*, 1973).

A probable diminution of cell lysosome contents is implicated in the reduction in granules within the cell cytoplasm: the granules are now thought to be lysosomes (Clein, 1972).

Limited kinetic studies of granulocyte formation have been carried out in old age. It is probable that granulocyte mobilization decreases with age (Roath, 1980). Whether granulocyte adherence is increased in the elderly remains doubtful.

Alteration in certain enzymes has also been noted. Granulocyte alkaline phosphatase decreases with age, sometimes to a marked degree (Ray and Pinkerton, 1969). Transketolase activity may decrease whereas peptidase and pyruvate kinase increase with advancing age (Rubinson *et al.*, 1976).

The age-associated changes in platelets, coagulation factors, etc., will be discussed in other appropriate sections of this chapter.

Erythrocyte Sedimentation Rate

Erythrocte sedimentation rate (ESR) is a measure of the suspension stability of red cells in blood. The technique of measuring the ESR is simple but proper standardization is essential. Various methods have been devised and the Westergren technique is now universally accepted.

The rate of sedimentation is influenced by a number of factors. Primarily it depends on the difference in specific gravity between red cells and plasma, but it is also greatly influenced by the extent to which red cells themselves behave. There are external factors such as the environmental temperature, the anticoagulant used, and the time interval between the venepuncture and the performance of the test. The level of fibrinogen or of fibrinmonomer (Lipinsky *et al.*, 1969) and perhaps the amounts of alpha-2 and gammaglobulins in plasma are important influencing factors. Fibrinogen, being an acute phase reactant protein, may alter in various minor illnesses, which may be reflected in the corresponding increase in the ESR. The presence of specific plasma protein 'agglomerin' has been suggested by some workers (Ruhenstroth-Bauer, 1961) as a contributing agent to the ESR activity. The plasma levels of various lipids appear to have an influencing role. The ESR in normal adults under standardized conditions should not exceed 15 mm/h in men and 25 mm/h in women (Lewis, 1974). However, these 'normal' figures may not be applicable to the elderly. It has been suggested that ESR increases with advancing age and this is entirely physiological (Bottiger and Svedberg, 1967; Hayes and Stinson, 1976; Milne and Williamson, 1972).

The range of normal values of ESR in the healthy elderly is controversial. Perhaps the single most important reason for this is the difficulty of identifying an unequivocably healthy elderly population.

ESR is a measure of the presence and severity of a variety of inflammatory and other active disease processes. Unfortunately, the variables are many. Interpretation of a moderate rise in ESR, therefore, cannot be conclusive. On the other hand, a normal ESR does not exclude organic disease.

Anaemia of any kind may result in an increase of ESR and it is therefore necessary to calculate a 'corrected' ESR in patients with anaemia.

Pincherle and Shanks (1967) argue against the suggestion that ESR increase is normal in healthy old age. In a recent study of age and sex matched sample of 200 subjects aged 60–89, Griffiths *et al.*, (1984) have found that on ESR exceeding 19mm/h in men and 22mm/h in women warrants futher investigation. An unexplained increase in ESR is sometimes a feature of occult malignancy, but detailed studies in a group of elderly patients with autopsy follow-up have not supported this (Rai, 1979).

A grossly elevated ESR level of 100 mm/h or more is commonly associated with giant cell arteritis and polymyalgia rheumatica but the correlation is never absolute.

Very low ESRs are found in polycythaemia, in some cases of congestive cardiac failure, and in defibrination syndromes.

Serial measurements of ESR might help in diagnosis and in the assessment of the progress of a disorder, where the initial ESR was very high. For example, a dramatic fall in the ESR following corticosteroid administration in cases of giant cell arteritis may be of great value in the assessment of the patient's overall response to therapy.

Plasma Viscosity

Estimation of plasma viscosity is sometimes considered to be a more useful test than the measurement of the ESR (Eastham, 1973). Viscosity can be a better marker of serum fibrinogen and globulin levels and certainly in disorders like macroglobulinaemia with hyperviscosity syndrome this is of better value than ESR. Similarly, viscosity shows an excellent correlation with haematocrit values and a reduction of the latter corresponds with a fall in the former. Nearly all kinds of vascular and hypertensive disease elevate the blood viscosity and as these disorders are frequent in old age, measurement of viscosity may have a special relevance (Rai, 1981). The normal range for the elderly has not yet been firmly determined and, like ESR, the problems of interpretation remain.

PREVALENCE AND INCIDENCE OF ANAEMIA

Definition

Anaemia is defined as a condition where the level of haemoglobin is lower than it should be for the individual's age and sex. This definition is usually widened to include other variables, but it probably offers the maximum degree of latitude. The question then arises as to what should be the normal range of haemoglobin in the elderly of either sex. The World Health Organisation (1968) suggests a figure of 13 g/dl for males and 12 g/dl for females (see Table 1), as the lower ranges of normal haemoglobin levels. The figures recorded for the 'normal' haemoglobin value in old age has varied in the many surveys from 15.4 g/dl in the males to 12.1 g/dl in the females (Hyams, 1978).

Table 1　Diagnostic criteria of anaemia (WHO, 1968)

	Hb (g/dl)	RBC (10^{12}/l)	PCV	MCH (g/dl)
Male	13	4.7	0.42	34
Female	12	4.0	0.35	34

The reported incidence of anaemia in studies in both the community and among hospital patients (Banerjee, 1975; Bird, Hall, and Schade, 1977; DHSS, 1972; Hill, 1976; MacLennan et al., 1973), has been influenced by the adoption of different diagnostic criteria. The following general conclusions can be made:

(a) Anaemia is not 'physiological' or 'normal' in old age; however, the haemoglobin level in males is probably higher than that in females.

(b) Elderly women are more prone to develop anaemia.

(c) The WHO guidelines (Table 1) should be accepted for the diagnosis of anaemia in the elderly.

With the same diagnostic criteria, widely different 'incidence' figures emerge, varying from as high as 41 per cent. (Morgan, 1967) to as low as 5 per cent. (Elwood, 1971). Nearly all the surveys confirm that the prevalence of anaemia increases with age and is a genuine increase in its occurrence among elderly women.

Mortality and Morbidity

Mortality due to anaemia also increases considerably after 60 years of age (WHO, 1969). Surveys on hospital inpatients in general reveal a much higher incidence among the older patients, which suggests that a considerable morbidity associated with anaemia is seen in hospitals (DHSS, 1970; Powell, Thomas, and Mills, 1968). It may also be true that anaemia when present in the elderly is often the manifestation of a chronic underlying disease (Matzner et al., 1979).

Anaemia should always be taken seriously, a correct diagnosis to establish its nature must be made, and, whenever possible, any underlying pathology must be identified. The treatment of anaemia is relatively simple and the therapeutic response can be remarkably encouraging.

Clinical Features of Anaemia

When a patient presents with severe pallor, gross lassitude and weakness, and readily induced exhaustion, even on mild accustomed activity, the clinical diagnosis is simple and straightforward. In the elderly, associated infirmity and other coexistent pathologies can overshadow the clinical diagnosis of mild to moderate anaemia. In addition, in this age group, anaemia can present in many 'atypical' ways. Such features may be broadly classified in the following groups.

Cardiovascular

Palpitation, breathlessness, and typical retrosternal anginal pains are common. Incipient or frank features of cardiac failure may occur. Associated cardiomegaly with haemic murmurs are frequently reversible on appropriate therapy. Symptoms of peripheral vascular disease, intermittent claudication, can also become obvious. In severe cases, elderly patients may present as acute cardiovascular emergencies.

Psychiatric

Irritability, apathy, forgetfulness, and sleeplessness are fairly common. Acute confusional states and severe depression with or without agitation can also be the presenting feature. Acute psychotic behaviour with paranoia, delusion, and hallucination can occur in some cases. Needless to say, elderly mentally infirm subjects with existing psychomotor problems are more vulnerable.

Neurolocomotor

Dizziness with faints and falls, immobility, increase in postural sway, loss of balance, paraesthesiae, and visual disturbances are significant presenting complaints. Sphincter disturbances, with incontinence, are not uncommon and the possibility of anaemia as a precipitating or a contributory factor should be considered.

Alimentary

Painful glossitis, stomatitis, distorted taste inside the mouth, and intermittent dysphagia, especially on tiredness, are some of the common features. Classic pharyngeal web with sideropenic dysphagia (Plummer–Vinson syndrome) can occur in severe iron-deficiency states, especially in elderly women. Rarely leucoplakia of the buccal mucosa can be present. Loss of appetite, indigestion, constipation, and diarrhoea may either be the result of anaemia or may indeed be the features of the associated disorders causing the anaemia.

Other features

Pallor of the exposed skin is not a very reliable sign as many house-bound elderly may have skin pallor irrespective of anaemia because of inadequate exposure to sunshine. Pallor of the tongue or buccal mucosa is more diagnostic. Generalized pruritus or pruritus vulvae can occur. Changes in nails are not very helpful in the very elderly. However, classical koilonychia, if present, may suggest severe iron deficiency.

Patients with pernicious anaemia may, in addition, present with mild jaundice or with purpura and bleeding due to thrombocytopenia. Signs of advanced subacute combined degeneration of the spinal cord are fairly well recognized. Early peripheral neuropathy with loss of deep reflexes in the ankle and/or lack of vibration sense may not be readily interpreted, as peripheral loss of deep reflex and posterior column sensation is not uncommon in the elderly without obvious pathology. A low grade fever and minimal splenomegaly may be associated with pernicious anaemia.

Social deprivation, self-neglect, isolation, and poverty are commonly associated with anaemia and in many such elderly patients evidence of other forms of malnutrition is also present.

The absolute clinical diagnosis of anaemia in the very elderly, therefore, can be difficult. Accordingly, a routine simple examination of blood is probably justified on every elderly patient irrespective of their appearance or symptoms.

Iron-Deficiency Anaemia

Iron deficiency is the most common single cause of anaemia in the elderly as in other age groups. Anaemia is one of the important manifestations of iron deficiency but iron deficiency may be present in the absence of anaemia. It is, therefore, important to understand the nature of iron metabolism and the various factors which may influence the iron status of the body.

Iron Intake and Absorption

The iron content of an average daily diet is approximately 13.5 mg, of which about 5 to 10 per cent. is usually absorbed. The daily dietary iron requirements for adults of both sexes has been suggested as 10 mg by the Department of Health and Social Security (1972) (see Chapter 10). However, a large number of factors, e.g. reduction in gastric acidity in old age, etc., may influence this and there is evidence that iron intake tends to fall with age (Hallberg and Hogdahl, 1971). A large number of studies have been carried out on iron requirements, dietary deficiency of iron intake, and its causal relationship with the development of iron deficiency and subsequent anaemia in the elderly. Most of the nutritional surveys in this field have shown that the average daily iron intake in the elderly is between 8.5 and 12.8 mg (DHSS, 1972; MacLeod, Judge, and Caird, 1975), that there is no definite relationship between haemoglobin level and dietary iron intake (Davis, Jacobs, and Rivlin, 1967), and that elderly individuals with definite iron deficiency do not necessarily take less dietary iron than others (MacLennan *et al.*, 1973). Nutritional iron inadequacy is a rather uncertain cause of iron deficiency in old age.

Absorption. The state of gastric mucosa and its functional ability are of considerable importance in iron absorption. The role of gastric juice, with adequate hydrochloric acid content, in physiological iron absorption has been firmly established (Jacobs, Bothwell, and Charlton, 1964). With advancing age, the gastric mucosa may suffer atrophic changes with gross reduction of chief and parietal cells; varying degrees of lymphocytic infiltration may give rise to a picture of chronic atrophic gastritis with a considerable reduction in the secretion of acid, pepsin, gastrin, and intrinsic factor (Henderson, Shearman, and Ganguli, 1971). Iron deficiency is a common result of these changes. Prolonged severe iron deficiency can, by itself, give rise to gastric mucosal changes (Jacobs *et al.*, 1966); these changes are usually reversible by iron therapy, but only in younger subjects (Delamore and Shearman, 1965; Shearman, Delamore, and Gardner, 1966). The gastric changes are usually irreversible and progressive in older people and are frequently associated with circulating parietal cell antibodies. It is probable that this form of atrophic gastritis is genetically determined but the situation is far from clear (Delamore, 1972; Jacobs and Worwood, 1974). In addition to the expected malabsorption of iron, there may be increased iron loss in this condition due to high cell turnover and loss of free iron from the gastric mucosa. All these factors may be responsible for the iron deficiency which develops later. High intake of dietary fibre and cereals inhibits iron absorption. Hypochlorhydria induced by hydrogen-receptor antagonists, e.g. Cimetidine, has also been implicated in the poor absorption of iron (Esposito, 1977). Iron absorption depends on body iron stores and may be influenced by other factors. Kinetic analysis has shown that the iron uptake by the human duodenal mucosal 'carrier-enterocyte' is considerably higher in iron deficient patients than in controls (Cox and Peters, 1978). Simultaneous ingestion of ascorbic acid has also been shown to be beneficial (McCurdy and Dern, 1968).

Iron-binding proteins have been identified either within or on the cell surface of certain lymphocytes and macrophages. The macrophages have receptors for lactoferrin and synthesize ferritin. Activated lymphocytes have transferrin receptors and T cells contain transferrin. The overall significance of these factors is not clear but iron may influence lymphoid cell traffic. It has been shown that in both animals and humans, lymphocyte circulation in the gut runs parallel with iron absorption,

being highest in the jejunum and duodenum and lowest in the ileum; in iron deficiency, this pattern is lost (De Sousa, 1981).

Transport, utilization and storage. Iron status can be assessed from the study of the following major iron-containing compartments:
(a) Serum and transport iron, e.g. transferrin
(b) Storage iron, e.g. ferritin and haemosiderin
(c) Iron in haemoglobin
(d) Tissue iron enzymes

These factors are all depleted in a state of advanced iron deficiency.

Serum iron. Serum iron tends to fall with age (Powell, Thomas, and Mills, 1968) but, taken in isolation, this is not necessarily diagnostic of true iron deficiency. A persistently low serum iron can be found in chronic disorders and in malignancy. A fall in serum iron following ingestion of 'All-Bran' (Persson *et al.*, 1975) is probably due to its phytin content. As bran is widely consumed by the elderly, this factor should be borne in mind.

Transferrin. The beta-globulin, transferrin, to which iron is bound to be transported in the plasma, has for many years been used as one of the most useful assessors of true iron status in the body. However, the transferrin level can be influenced by various factors. This can diminish in infections, in cases of protein malnutrition and can be elevated in patients on oestrogen therapy (Banerjee, 1976). To obviate this, the levels of transferrin saturation is a better index of iron deficient erythropoiesis:

$$\text{Transferrin sat.} = \frac{\text{plasma iron } (\mu g/dl) \times}{\text{TIBC } (\mu g/dl)} \, 100$$

A level of 16 per cent. or less is acceptable as diagnostic of iron-deficient erythropoiesis (Bainton and Finch, 1964).

Serum ferritin Over the recent years, radio-immunoassay measurement of serum ferritin has largely superseded serum transferrin estimation. In general, serum ferritin estimation has been found to be more reliable, reproducible, and comparable without the drawbacks of the interpretation of the transferrin levels (*Lancet*,

1979a). Serial measurements of serum ferritin level can be valuable in monitoring the therapeutic progress of patients with iron overload disorders and chronic renal failure (Jacobs and Worwood, 1975). Beck and coworkers (1979) have suggested that serum ferritin and MCV together can predict the accurate iron stores in the bone marrow in at least 70 per cent of patients. A serum ferritin level of below 15 μg/dl is usually accepted as an indicator of diminished iron reserve. In patients with inflammatory disease, however, this level increases considerably because of excessive production of ferritin-protein; under such circumstances, a ferritin level of 55 μg/dl will be a more appropriate lower limit of normality (Blake, Waterworth, and Bacon, 1981). Tests for iron-containing enzymes, e.g. cytochrome oxidase, although sensitive, is beyond the reach of ordinary laboratories. The marrow iron content may be assessed by detailed bone marrow examination but comparative interpretation of marrow examination can be quite difficult (Jacobs and Worwood, 1974).

Diagnosis

Although anaemia of any type and origin can affect the general functioning of the body, iron-deficiency anaemia is particularly relevant.

In young people, the effects of iron-deficiency anaemia have been found to have a direct influence on work productivity and general daily activity patterns, all of which are reversible by appropriate iron therapy (Edgerton *et al.*, 1979). In the frail elderly, the overall clinical effects of iron deficiency are likely to be even more pronounced. The other haematologic and tissue changes attributable to iron deficiency are well recognized (Dallman, 1974). In elderly patients with multiple pathologies, the possibility of a coexistent different variety of anaemia should be borne in mind. Peripheral red cell microcytosis with hypochromia is the classical picture of severe iron deficiency anaemia. Changes in the red cell shape and the presence of target cells are common. A low MCH is a better and more reliable index of hypochromia than the MCHC. A well-stained peripheral film along with the measurements of MCV, MCH, and serum ferritin will probably clinch the correct diagnosis in the majority of patients. Further estimation of serum iron, TIBC, transferrin saturation, and marrow iron content may be useful in doubtful cases (Beck *et al.*, 1979).

Table 2 Common causes of iron deficiency

I. Chronic blood loss	1. Peptic ulcer
	2. Hiatus hernia
	3. Diverticular disease, neoplasms
	4. Haemorrhoids
	5. Ingestion of analgesics, e.g. phenylbutazone, indomethacin, salicytates
	6. Chronic gastritis
	7. Low-grade haematuria
II. Dietary inadequacy	
III. Impaired absorption	1. Gastritis
	2. Following surgery
	3. Ingestion of bran, H_2-receptor antagonist

The classic picture of hypochromic anaemia may be seen in conditions other than iron deficiency and an iron-deficiency state may be present in the absence of anaemia.

Treatment

Following the confirmation of an iron-deficiency anaemia, the causative factor must be identified (see Table 2) and if possible the source of anaemia must be eliminated.

Oral iron. The depleted iron stores should be adequately replenished; in the majority of cases this can be done quite simply by oral iron therapy for several months.

Over 40 oral iron preparations are currently available on prescription in Britain and preparations such as ferrous sulphate, ferrous succinate, ferrous gluconate, and ferrous fumarate are equally useful and are adequately absorbed (*Drugs and Therapeutic Bulletin*, 1979). One 200 mg tablet of ferrous sulphate containing 60 mg of elemental iron, twice daily with or immediately after food, is cheap, effective, and tolerated by most patients.

Gastroenteric side-effects, e.g. nausea, vomiting, constipation, and diarrhoea, may occur at times and are often due to wrong timing, excessive dosage, or to psychological factors. In cases of genuine oral iron intolerance, a different preparation does not usually alleviate the problem. A sustained-release preparation of ferrous sulphate with 105 mg of elemental iron once a day can also be useful; however, like other similar sustained-release tablets, the non-absorbable 'shell' may very rarely accumulate inside the small intestine and cause obstruction. Multiple haematinic therapy must always be avoided without a specific indication. Addition of other vitamin preparations, with the possible exception of ascorbic acid, is unnecessary. Ascorbic acid facilitates iron absorption and as ascorbic acid deficiency is quite common in old age, simultaneous administration of ascorbic acid may be justified (Exton-Smith, 1971). In a number of conditions especially frequent in the elderly, e.g. chronic peptic ulcer, prolonged alcohol and salicylate intake, postgastroenteric surgery etc., both iron and ascorbic acid deficiencies may arise; combined iron and ascorbic acid therapy is indicated under these circumstances.

As regards the duration of therapy, no rigid recommendation equally applicable to each patient can be made. In the absence of adverse factors (e.g. undetected neoplasm), the normal response to adequate oral iron therapy is a haemoglobin rise of 100 to 200 mg/dl per day: most patients would obtain a normal haemoglobin level within 6 to 8 weeks. Following this, oral iron therapy should continue for 3 to 6 months to replenish the body iron stores. Periodic follow-up and haemoglobin estimation should be carried out to detect possible recurrences. In cases of chronic slow blood loss, which cannot be successfully treated, oral iron therapy should continue indefinitely.

Parenteral iron. Parenteral iron therapy should generally be avoided in the elderly. However, in some cases of genuine oral iron intolerance or poor drug takers, iron has to be administered parenterally. Iron–dextran complex is used for the total dose infusion.

Originally introduced into obstetric practice (Basu, 1963), it has since been found to be an effective way of giving parenteral iron in the elderly with safety and simplicity (Andrews, Fairley, and Barker, 1967; Wright, 1967). In many patients, overnight stay in hospital is not required and this procedure can be easily undertaken at a well-organized day hospital. Iron–dextran complex (Imferon) contains 50 mg of elemental iron per mililitre in the form of ferric hydroxide combined with a low molecular weight dextran. Iron–dextran is not bound to transferrin and is stored in the RE system. The iron is utilized fully from the storage sites and is, therefore, effective even in cases of chronic and recurrent deficiency (Kernoff, Dommisse, and Du Toit, 1975).

The total iron (TI) requirement (mg) for an individual is calculated as:

$$\text{TI} = 15 \text{ haemoglobin (g/dl)} \times \text{body weight (kg)} \times 3$$

The calculated quantity of iron–dextran complex is mixed with 100 ml of normal saline to make a 5% solution V/V and the infusion is commenced immediately. The flow should be slow initially at 10 to 15 drops/min for about 15 to 20 min and then be increased to 40 to 50 drops/min, to complete the infusion within 8 hours.

In patients with poor cardiopulmonary state and failure, a diuretic should be administered concomitantly. Anaphylactic reactions are extremely rare.

Prevention of Iron-Deficiency Anaemia

In certain countries of the world, iron-deficiency anaemia is of endemic proportions from a large number of factors, e.g. hookworm disease, malnutrition, and general poverty. A large-scale national iron prophylaxis may prove to be beneficial and cost-effective in that situation (*Lancet*, 1980a).

Although the elderly population in this country are susceptible to iron deficiency, routine 'prophylaxis' with either medicated iron preparations or dietary fortification cannot be justified. Overprescribing iron tablets in the elderly can be dangerous and may conceal serious gastrointestinal pathology by masking the clinically diagnostic anaemia (Reizenstein *et al.*, 1979). Iron therapy should only be given after a full examination and investigation and the patient must be reviewed periodically in an attempt to avoid recurrence.

Anaemia of Chronic Disorder

Although the terminology 'anaemia of chronic disorder' is a relatively recent one, this condition has been recognized for many years under a variety of other names, e.g. anaemia of infection, toxic anaemia, anaemia of neoplasia, simple chronic anaemia, etc. Haematological changes were first noted to occur in infections more than a century ago and it was observed that a reduction in total red cell mass took place in infections (Andral and Gavarett, 1842).

A wider knowledge of haematological disorders in general and the availability of more sophisticated investigatory techniques has generated considerable information on this subject. The anaemia is commonly mild, normocytic, normochromic, and refractory to usual haematinic agents; in severe cases it may be microcytic and hypochromic (Smith, 1974). The conditions under which this type of anaemia can develop are summarized in Table 3.

Table 3   Causes of anaemia of chronic disorder

Chronic infection	Tuberculosis
	Infective endocarditis
	Bronchiectasis
	Lung abscess
	Urinary tract infection
	Osteomyelitis
	Certain fungal infections
	Infection with decubitus sores
Malignant diseases	Metastatic carcinoma
	Renal carcinoma
	Lymphoma
Connective tissue disorders	Rheumatoid arthritis
	Giant cell arteritis and polymyalgia rheumatica
	Polyarteritis nodosa

The genesis of anaemia in these conditions is usually multifactorial and complex and any, or all, of the following mechanisms may be involved (McMurdoch and Smith, 1972; Smith and McMurdoch, 1976):

(a) Defective utilization of the marrow iron at a cellular level affecting haemoglobin synthesis
(b) Mild degree of haemolysis
(c) Depression of marrow function and maturation arrest of erythropoiesis

The levels of both serum iron and transferrin can diminish in acute infections from the first day; however, they become normal when the infection is brought under control. With persistent and chronic infections, these levels remain low and oral iron therapy becomes ineffective. In addition, loss of appetite, which is not uncommon with chronic infection, reduces the intake and the absorption of iron from the gut is impaired. Whatever iron is absorbed is rapidly cleared from the plasma and is deposited at various storage sites in liver, spleen, and bone marrow with a resultant increase in the amount of depot iron and marrow haemosiderin. There is no evidence that the excretion of iron is increased. The utilization of depot iron is reduced and its rate of incorporation in haemoglobin synthesis is impaired. The persistence of a low serum iron level in chronic infections is due to a number of intricate pathological events: decreased intake, poor absorption, increased diversion to storage sites, and inability of the reticuloendothelial cells to release iron from degraded haemoglobin of effete red cells into the plasma. The transferrin level, which remains low in chronic infections, rises gradually when the infection is controlled (Bainton and Finch, 1964; McMurdoch and Smith, 1972; Smith, 1974). The reduced level of transferrin is due to a lack of production or adherence of transferrin to iron-loaded RE cells or to foci of infections (Cartwright and Lee, 1971).

The role of iron and transferrin in the potentiation of or resistance to infection has recently received attention (*Lancet*, 1974). It has been suggested that availability of iron may potentiate infection, while lack of iron may contribute to resistance. It is probable that the ability of microorganisms to compete successfully with the host for iron is a feature of pathogenicity while the ability of the host to limit availability of iron to the pathogen is associated with resistance to infection. Whether iron interferes with specific immune mechanisms, however, remains unclear. It is known that transferrin can act together with antibody and complement to interfere with bacterial RNA synthesis (Smith and McMurdoch, 1976).

The erythrocyte protoporphyrin is increased in anaemia of chronic disorders along with a high amount of free coproporphyrin in urine. Abnormalities of globin synthesis and of red cell stroma may also occur. Although low-grade haemolysis, as evidenced by shortened red cell survival time (Cartwright and Lee, 1971), is not unusual in chronic infection, acute haemolytic episodes can also occur in a number of bacterial, viral, and protozoal infections. Depression of marrow function and erythropoietic maturation arrest can happen and there may be decreased availability of erythropoietin. Ferrokinetic studies show an increased erythrocytic response to anaemia; the marrow proliferative response to anaemia is limited by the availability of iron.

The mechanism of anaemia in connective tissue disorder and some malignant diseases are almost identical to those described in connection with chronic infections.

Among significant factors are chronic blood loss, mild episodic haemolysis, deficiency of folate, and haemodilution due to enlarged spleen. An excessive quantity of ferritin can be detected in the synovial fluid of patients with active rheumatoid arthritis. This ferritin is probably derived from the synovial endothelial cells and has a close association with synovial immune complexes. It is likely that some unspecified factor blocks the release of this storage iron for normal and adequate haemoglobin synthesis (Blake and Bacon, 1981).

A true iron deficiency may arise at times giving rise to a microcytic and hypochromic picture. Table 4 gives the important biochemical distinguishing features of anaemia of chronic disorder, true iron deficiency, and sideroblastic anaemia.

Hume, Dagg, and Goldberg (1973) reported a group of 9 elderly patients who had moderate to severe hypochromic anaemia with complaints of marked tiredness and weakness. Nearly half of them had severe musculoskeletal aches around the shoulder and pelvic girdles. The serum iron and TIBC were low, thereby maintaining adequate transferrin saturation. The ESR was grossly elevated and alpha-2 globulins were increased. The haematological picture was similar to the anaemia of chronic disorder. Although the clinical features were highly suggestive of polymyalgia rheumatica, no associated histological giant cell arteritis was found. However, comparable anaemic states have been described in cases of biopsy-confirmed giant cell arteritis (Paulley and Hughes, 1960) and an 'anaemic giant-cell arteritis' without classical clinical features of the disease has been described recently (Strachan, How, and Bewster, 1980).

Treatment

There is no specific treatment for anaemia of chronic disorder and every attempt should be made to correct the underlying disorder. Conventional haematinics are only useful in cases of proven specific deficiency. Folate supplements may be required in rheumatoid diseases and with chronic haemolytic states. Care should be taken to avoid iron therapy in cases of hypochromic anaemia without iron deficiency. In rheumatoid disease, oral corticosteroids mobilize storage iron in the marrow and sequestered iron in the joints, for haemoglobin synthesis. Under the influence of steroids, the RE system tends to shrink in size with a reduction in activity including that of the phagocytic iron-storing cells of the synovial membrane (Mowat, 1972). Anaemia in polymyalgia rheumatica responds well to oral corticosteroids, which need to be maintained at a low dosage for at least one year (*Lancet*, 1979b). In refractory cases, a regime of periodic blood transfusions with adequate diet is to be recommended.

Table 4   Distinguishing features of anaemia of chronic disorder

	Normal	Chronic disorder	Iron deficiency	Sideroblastic anaemia
Serum iron (μg/dl)	70–150	Low	Low	Normal/increased
TIBC (μg/dl)	300–400	Reduced	Increased	Low
Transferrin sat. (%)	25–40	Usually normal	Reduced	Increased
Sideroblast (%)	20–40	Reduced	Absent	Increased
Reticuloendothelial iron	Adequate	Increased	Absent	Increased
Plasma copper (μg/dl)	81–147	Increased	Increased	Normal
Free RBC Protoporphyrin (μg/dl)	14–79	Markedly increased	Increased	Normal

Sideroblastic Anaemias

Defective globin synthesis from abnormal haemoglobin diseases gives rise to a hypochromic picture but these disorders are not commonly seen in the elderly. A fault in porphyrin synthesis is quite common in old age and gives rise to defective iron utilization and results in a marrow containing a large number of abnormal normoblasts with abundant granules of haemosiderin, commonly called sideroblasts. These iron granules lie in the mitochondrial matrix of developing normoblasts and are arranged around the nucleus like a 'ring' or 'collar'.

Aetiology

The sideroblastic anaemias can be classified as shown in Table 5.

Table 5   Causes of sideroblastic anaemia

I. Hereditary	
II. Acquired	1. Primary and idiopathic
	2. Secondary
	(a) Drugs and chemicals: anti-TB (isoniazide, pyrazinamide, cycloserine) chloramphenicol, phenacetin, cytotoxic agents, ethyl alcohol, lead
	(b) Blood disorders – myeloproliferative conditions, leukaemias, lymphomas
	(c) Deficiency states – malabsorption, partial gastrectomy, folate deficiency
	(d) Miscellaneous – myxoedema, connective tissue disorders

The secondary acquired variety is not uncommon in the elderly (Simpson, 1974). The picture is one of chronic refractory hypochromic microcytic anaemia; occasionally the anaemia may be normocytic or even macrocytic. The serum iron level is usually raised with a high saturation of transferrin. The marrow picture with abundant ring sideroblasts is diagnostic. Ferrokinetic studies show a reduced clearance of iron and an overall depression of iron utilization.

The genesis of alcohol-induced sideroblastic anaemia remains unclear. Well-nourished alcoholics do not develop such a complication; however, alcohol byproduct acetaldehyde does have a toxic effect on the red cell pyridoxine metabolism and this may be a contributory factor. On the other hand, alcohol and acetaldehyde do exert direct depressive effect on the marrow colony-forming units and influence the colony stimulating factors for both erythroid and myeloid series (Meagher, Sieber, and Spivak, 1982). Whether the alcohol-induced changes are caused through the haem-synthetic pathway or through the direct effect on the marrow cell colonies or both is still a matter of conjecture.

In rare instances, no precipitating or associated condition can be detected and the disorder is labelled as 'primary' or 'idiopathic'.

Treatment

When the sideroblastic anaemia is secondary to some other remediable disease, the proper management of the latter may correct the anaemia. Withdrawal of an offending drug or alcohol may be beneficial (Eichner and Hillman, 1971). Folate therapy is indicated in cases with myeloproliferative disorders (Bateman and Beard, 1976) and in chronic alcoholics (Hines and Grasso, 1970). Iron therapy is to be avoided and blood transfusions should be kept to an absolute minimum to avoid iron overload; however, when essential, chelating agents should be administered at the same time. The relationship of pyridoxine with this condition is not very clear. Pyridoxine is a factor necessary for normal haem synthesis and pyridoxine deficient experimental animals have been shown to produce atypical sideroblasts in their marrow. Patients on pyridoxine antagonist drug therapy (e.g. Isoniazide) have been known to develop sideroblastic anaemia. It is, therefore, logical to surmise that pyridoxine deficiency is an important cause of sideroblastic anaemia and that pyridoxine therapy will correct such anaemia. However, apart from occasional instances, pyridoxine has not been found to be of great therapeutic value in this disorder (Crowther and Bateman, 1972). Serum pyridoxal falls with age (Anderson, Peart, and Fulford-Jones, 1970) and therefore pyridoxine therapy may be useful in the elderly with primary acquired sideroblastic anaemia.

In primary sideroblastic anaemia, the intraerythrocytic conversion of pyridoxine to its main active form pyridoxal-5-phosphate is defective (Hines and Grasso, 1970). In occasional patients with primary acquired sidero-blastic anaemia, parenteral pyridoxal-5-phosphate has been found to be beneficial (Mason and Emerson, 1973). However, these claims have not been substantiated (Datta, 1975; Trump *et al.*, 1975). Oral pyridoxine at a dosage of 150 to 200 mg/day should be thera-peutically tried in elderly patients with primary acquired sideroblastic anaemia for 10 to 12 weeks (Banerjee, 1976).

Iron Overload

It is recognized that the overall iron storage in the body steadily increases during the whole of adult life in men and during the postmenopau-sal years in women (Cook, Morgan, and Hoff-brand, 1974). Serum ferritin increases from a median level of 25 μg/l in women in the 18 to 45 age group to about 89 μg/l among postmen-opausal women. From a general epidemiolog-ical point, increased incidence of cardiovascular disease has been correlated with higher amounts of body iron stores (Sullivan, 1981).

Pathological iron overload can be encoun-tered in elderly patients and it can arise from chronic alcoholism, advanced calcific pan-creatic disease, and multiple transfusions. In Hodgkin's disease, T-lymphocytes have been shown to have ferritin on their surface. Increased amounts of abnormal ferritin can also be produced from liver secondaries and in primary bronchial malignancy (Li and Batey, 1977) and they can cause excess deposition of iron in other tissues and organs.

Idiopathic Haemochromatosis

The most important condition where iron overload is preponderant is the genetically determined condition of idiopathic haemo-chromatosis. As the peak incidence of this dis-order is between the fifth and sixth decades, a short discussion of this condition is relevant.

The basic pathology is an unabated and inappropriate absorption of iron. It has been shown that this is due to increased carrier affinity for iron in the enterocyte (Cox and Peters, 1978). The disease is usually familial and a statistically significant association with HLA-A3 and HLA-B14 antigens has been found.

Clinical features. In frank cases, the clinical features are fairly obvious. The patient is usually a middle aged or elderly male with generalized pigmentation, hepatomegaly, and diabetes which can be difficult to control. Approximately half of the patients develop cirrhosis of the liver. Arthritis is a feature of haemochromatosis. This is more common in elderly patients who have had the disease for some time. Involvement of the small joints in the fingers is usual although larger joints may be affected. Characterized by loss of joint space, cysts, and destruction of articular surface, it can simulate other forms of arthritis. Chondrocalcinosis or calcification of cartilages are also common, especially involving the wrists and knee joints (Hamilton *et al.*, 1981).

Investigations. Biochemical investigations show a high saturation of serum transferrin. While an increased concentration of serum fer-ritin is found in more advanced cases of hae-mochromatosis, it is not useful in detecting the disease early – an important distinction from other states of iron overload (*BMJ*, 1977b).

Needle biopsy of liver is probably the most satisfactory way of confirming the diagnosis.

Treatment. In fully developed disease, regular venesection usually improves the overall clini-cal picture and its metabolic effects. As 500 ml of blood removes about 250 mg of iron, there-fore, to reach the normal iron status, removal of 5 to 8 litres of blood may be required over 10 to 12 months. Venesection does not influence the natural history of chondrocalci-nosis or arthritis. In some cases, liver cell car-cinoma can develop as a complication. The first-degree relatives and particularly the male siblings should be screened for iron overload.

Macrocytic Anaemias

Macrocytosis is essentially a descriptive diag-nosis meaning the presence of a large number of red cells of more than normal size in the peripheral blood. The normal upper limit of mean corpuscular volume varies with different laboratories but is usually 100 femto litres and is the best index of red cell size. In alcoholics, this is a useful finding and suggests the toxic effect of alcohol on the developing erythro-cytes (Whitehead, Clarke, and Whitfield, 1978;

Wu, Chanarin, and Levi, 1974). An isolated elevation in the MCV does not necessarily signify any serious underlying disease or anaemia. Persistent macrocytosis requires adequate investigation.

Polychromatic macrocytes may be seen in the peripheral film in patients with increased erythrocyte regeneration but these are not true macrocytes and the MCV remains normal. Red cell size may slightly increase with age (Munan *et al.*, 1978; Okuno, 1972) but the value of MCV remains within the accepted upper normal limit and, as an isolated finding, is of no clinical relevance.

Anaemia associated with macrocytosis and raised MCV always signifies definite pathology, and the various causes are given in Table 6.

Table 6   Causes of macrocytic anaemia

1. With megaloblastic marrow	Vitamin B12 deficiency
	Folate deficiency
2. With normoblastic marrow	Hypothyroidism
	Neoplastic disease
	Sideroblastic anaemia
	Haemolytic anaemia
	Alcoholism
	Cytotoxic drug therapy

Megaloblastic Anaemias

They arise as the direct result of either vitamin B12 or folate deficiency or both. This type of anaemia is well recognized in the elderly and responds extremely well to appropriate therapy.

Precise diagnosis is essential before therapy is instituted. The metabolic pathways of vitamin B12 and folate are interlinked and deficiency of either makes the red cell precursors incapable of adequate DNA production; this leads to a megaloblastic change in the marrow and, among other things, a peripheral macrocytosis and anaemia.

Vitamin B12 was isolated more than 30 years ago and, like folates, was found to be able to reverse severe megaloblastic marrows. The efficacy of B12 and its active coenzymes was established in two main areas: (a) in the synthesis of methionine from homocysteine and (b) in the conversion of methyl malonic acid to succinic acid towards the synthesis of haem. Later, it was also suggested that the B12 coenzymes were necessary for the conversion of 5-methyl tetrahydrofolate to more active tetrahydrofolate (THF) within the folate metabolic path and that in B12 deficiency folate remained 'trapped' as inactive 5-methyl THF (Herbert and Zalusky, 1962). This view has recently been challenged by Chanarin and co-workers (1980), who suggest that failure of methionine synthesis subsequent to B12 deficiency leads to a lack of formate and in turn to inadequate formylation to THF. Formyl THF is the required substrate for the synthesis of active folate polyglutamates (Chanarin *et al.*, 1980).

The various aspects of vitamin B12 and folate status and metabolism in old age have been extensively studied and the main conclusions are summarized below.

Vitamin B12

The level of serum vitamin B12. Serum vitamin B12 level gradually falls with age (Cape and Shinton, 1961; Elsborg, Lund, and Bastrup-Madseu, 1976; Gaffney *et al.*, 1957) but taken in isolation, its aetiology and significance is uncertain. Despite considerable improvement and standardization of assay techniques, this still remains a rather confusing area (England and Linnell, 1980). In man, virtually all cobalamins are attached to an apparently functionless binder, transcobalamin I; accordingly, a low serum B12 (cobalamin) level is a poor predictor of a true deficiency. On the other hand, the metabolically active serum binder, transcobalamin II is a more accurate predictor and the deficiency of this protein causes a severe megaloblastic anaemia even though the conventional serum B12 level is normal. Some conditions, where the B12 assay may be insensitive or non-specific are listed below:

(a) Serum B12 is normal, yet the patient is truly deficient:
  (1) 10 to 20 per cent. of true B12 deficiency, e.g. PA, postgastrectomy, malabsorption, dietary deficiency;
  (2) chronic myeloid leukaemia;
  (3) nitrous oxide inhalation;
  (4) transcobalamin II deficiency.

(b) Serum B12 is low, but the patient is not deficient:
  (1) 30 per cent. cases of megaloblastic anaemia due to folate deficiency;

(2)   75 per cent. of strict vegetarians;

(3)   transcobalamin I deficiency.

As all the above factors may be prevalent in old age, a low serum B12 level must be interpreted critically. A number of antibiotics and antimetabolites and probably chlorpromazine may influence the microbiological assay technique of the vitamin and produce artificially low serum levels.

Vitamin B12 absorption. The approximate daily requirement of 1 μg vitamin B12 is obtained entirely from dietary source. As bacteria only can synthesize B12, a strict vegetarian diet can hardly provide any B12; accordingly, an adequate and proper dietary intake is essential. The stomach plays an important role in B12 absorption by secreting the carrier-glycoprotein, intrinsic factor. The B12–intrinsic factor complex is then absorbed from the last 2 to 3 m of ileum, an area also required for absorption of bile salts. It is now known that bile enhances the absorption of B12 (Teo *et al.*, 1980). The distal ileal enterocytes and the specific B12–intrinsic factor receptors help absorb the 'complex', separate the B12 from the intrinsic factor, and let it bind to the specific carrier protein, transcobalamin II, before it enters the circulation. Whether the normal B12 absorption is impaired with age is doubtful; some workers suggest that this occurs and is probably due to lack of gastric intrinsic factor (Chernish *et al.*, 1957), while others have found no alteration in B12 absorption in the elderly (Hyams, 1964; Tauber *et al.*, 1957).

Reserve vitamin B12. The liver contains 0.5 to 1.2 μg/g and holds most of the reserve vitamin B12, which is normally 1,000 to 2,000 μg. There is no reason to believe there is a natural drop in tissue stores of vitamin B12 in old age.

Impairment of B12 absorption. 4. Vitamin B12 absorption may be impaired in patients with chronic atrophic gastritis, severe chronic pancreatic disorders, and taking certain drugs, e.g. anticonvulsants, para-aminosalicylic acid, neomycin, and potassium chloride, all of which may be particularly relevant in the elderly. Hydrogen-receptor antagonists, which are widely used for peptic ulcer disease, have also been shown (Fielding *et al.*, 1978) to reduce IF output in both basal and augmented conditions and accordingly, after prolonged use, may adversely affect the absorption of B12.

Although the absorption of aqueous cobalamin is not affected by age, Dawson *et al.*, (1984), have recently shown that the overall absorption of protein-bound cobalamin i.e. the dietary B12 is diminished in the elderly. And this is more pronounced in elderly subjects with previous gastric surgery, chronic iron deficiency and prolonged alcoholic indulgence with folate deficiency. Lack of gastric acidity may play a causative role here. Malabsorption of Vitamin B12 from protein-bound sources which is not detected by other conventional tests may give rise to a subnormal serum B12 level with a picture of clinical deficiency.

Folic Acid

Intake of folates. The normal daily intake of free folates should be at least 200 μg (see Chapter 10).

Lack of folates. An absolute dietary lack of folate is reflected by a drop in the serum folate level within a matter of weeks and an overt megaloblastic anaemia develops within 5 months as the total body store of folate is exhausted (Herbert, 1962). As serum folate is subject to constant fluctuations from temporary dietary inadequacies and trivial illnesses, measurement of red cell folate level is much more useful and informative. The latter takes much longer to show any alteration and is a more accurate marker of the true tissue stores.

Blood level. Patients with a serum folate level below 3 μg/litre and an RBC folate below 150 μg/l should be regarded as folate deficient. Using these figures, the DHSS survey (1972) suggests that an approximate 15 per cent. of the elderly living in the community are likely to be deficient.

Similar observations have been made among the more disabled, infirm, and chronically ill elderly subjects residing in institutions (Girdwood, Thomson, and Williamson, 1967). As most of these elderly individuals are not manifestly anaemic, the clinical relevance of this 'low' folate level is uncertain. Thomas and Powell (1971) suggest that the so-called 'normal' range acceptable for the young individuals is probably not applicable to the elderly and that a much lower figure, e.g. a serum level of less than 1 μg/l, should only be regarded as pathologically and clinically significant in the very elderly.

Absorption. Folate is mostly absorbed from the upper small bowel and an adequately functional jejunal mucosa is therefore essential (see Chapter 11.2). Lesher and Sacher (1968) have demonstrated some alteration in small bowel function with age in experimental animals. In a group of non-anaemic elderly patients with low serum folate, definite flattening and broadening of proximal jejunal villi have been identified (Webster and Leeming, 1975). Whether this bowel change is the effect or cause of folate deficiency is uncertain (Webster, 1979). It would be an interesting hypothesis if some physioanatomic age-related change were responsible for a low-grade malabsorption of folate in the elderly.

Diet and Vitamins B12 and Folate

A clinically relevant vitamin B12 deficiency due to dietary inadequacy alone is uncommon at all ages in Western communities. The average mixed and balanced daily diet contains up to 30 μg of vitamin B12 and this amount is reduced to about 0.5 μg in strict vegans. Despite this, a strict vegan does not become B12 deficient, presumably due to maintenance of an intact enterohepatic circulation conserving B12. However, occasionally neurological complications can develop without megaloblastic anaemia (Wokes, Badernoch, and Sinclair, 1955).

A normal mixed Western diet contains about 600 to 700 μg of folate and approximately one-third of this is available for absorption. Folates are easily destroyed by high-temperature cooking with large quantities of water, by ultraviolet light, and by various oxidizing agents. Pasteurization of milk, too, reduces the folate content by reducing the ascorbic acid.

A causal relationship with associated ascorbic acid deficiency cannot be definitely established (Bates *et al.*, 1980).

Anticonvulsant drugs, e.g. phenytoin and barbiturates, can impair folate absorption by interfering with conjugase production at mucosal level; similar problems may also arise with biguanides.

A large number of elderly mentally infirm live in a relatively neglected state of dietary and social deprivation and a general state of subnourishment can be expected in them. Many of these patients have multiple systemic disease, bacterial infections, or tuberculosis, which can affect the absorption of folate (Cook, Morgan, and Hoffbrand, 1974). A low serum folate level is common among patients with dementia (Batata *et al.*, 1967) but whether this low folate status is causally related to their mental state still remains uncertain. Similar reduction in serum folate has also been found in epileptics and in other psychiatric patients. In a recent study, Shorvon and coworkers (1980) have clearly demonstrated a high incidence of affective disorders and depression among female patients with significant folate deficiency. They feel that folate deficiency and mental changes may be causally related, as occasional improvement in the neuropsychiatric state has been observed following supplementation (Botez and Reynolds, 1979).

In the interpretation of a low blood folate level in an elderly patient, influencing clinical, psychiatric, dietary, and environmental factors must be taken into consideration.

Pernicious Anaemia

No routine description of this well recognized condition will be given. However, certain points deserve special emphasis.

Incidence. This is a disease of later life affecting females more often than the males. The gradual age incidence from a large-scale Danish survey can be seen in Table 8.

Table 8 Incidence of pernicious anaemia in various age groups:
cases per 100,000 in each age group. (From Pederson and Mosbech, 1969)

Age group	Males	Females
20–39	3	8
40–59	160	210
60–79	770	1,510
80+	900	2,440

Regional variation has been observed, the disease being more common in northern Scandinavian countries and Scotland compared to the southern parts of England (Hoffbrand, 1974). The peak age at diagnosis is around 60 and the general overall frequency of about 0.1 to 0.2 per cent. increases to around 10 per cent. in the seventh or eighth decades.

Pathogenesis. An immunological basis for the changes in the gastric mucosa is well established. An increased incidence of immunological thyroid deficiency has been observed in patients with overt or latent pernicious anaemia (PA).

Thyroid antibodies can be detected in approximately 5 per cent. of elderly females (Tunbridge *et al.*, 1981). Similarly, antibodies against gastric parietal cells can be found in a sizeable proportion of the normal elderly population (Hooper *et al.*, 1972). It is also recognized that 10 per cent. of patients suffering from primary myxoedema also have pernicious anaemia with positive parietal cell and intrinsic factor antibodies. Thyroid antibodies can be detected in about half of the patients with PA and their relatives also have an increased presence of antibodies (Doniach, Roitt, and Taylor, 1965; Ungar, Whittingham, and Francis, 1977).

More recently a relationship between histocompatability antigens (HLA) and atrophic gastritis with or without PA has been established. In patients without any other endocrine disease, PA is associated with HLA-B7 and B12 whereas those with coexistent endocrine disease are found to have HLA-B8, B15, and B17 (Ungar, Whittingham, and Francis, 1977).

The pattern of HLA-DR antigens has also been closely studied (Ungar *et al.*, 1981) in 66 patients with PA, which included 18 patients with associated endocrine disease, e.g. myxoedema, thyrotoxicosis, diabetes, etc., and 48 patients with no associated endocrine disease. Compared with a control group, all 66 patients showed an increase in HLA-DR2 and DR4 and a decrease in DR3. Significant differences were also found between the 'endocrine' and the 'non-endocrine' subgroups. The authors concluded that the interactive effect related to HLA-DR2/4 and DR4/5 may predispose to PA without endocrine disease whereas the effects related to DR3/4 may predispose to PA in association with endocrine disease.

The neuropsychiatry of B12 deficiency. The detailed neuropsychiatry of vitamin B12 deficiency has not been adequately studied and compared with that due to folate deficiency. Recently Shorvon and coworkers (1980) found abnormalities of the nervous system in about 65 per cent of the patients with frank B12 deficiency.

Peripheral neuropathy is the commonest neurological change followed by organic mental change, depressive illness, and subacute combined degeneration of the spinal cord. Neuropsychiatric changes can be clinically manifest without any significant haematologic alteration.

Diagnosis. In addition to the classic peripheral blood picture with increased hypersegmented polymorph and megaloblastic marrow films, a reduction in total leucocyte count and platelets is common with severe anaemia. The levels of serum unconjugated bilirubin and lactic dehydrogenase (mainly the fast-moving isoenzymes LDH1 and 2) are increased. The serum B12 level, whether assayed microbiologically or by the radioisotope dilution method, is grossly diminished and the level is usually below 100 μg/l (normal is 160 to 900 μg/l). The microbiological assay results correlate well with the clinical severity of the anaemia, but this is influenced by the presence of antbiotics, a point worth remembering while interpreting the findings. In some patients, a definite demonstration of intrinsic factor (IF) deficiency may be necessary. Direct assay of IF in gastric juice is usually beyond the scope of routine laboratories. Lack of free acid in gastric juice following pentagastrin stimulation is a simple test in older people.

The 'Diagnex blue' test can be a useful screening test. The resin is taken by mouth and free acid, if present in the gastric juice, will make it release the azure-A which can be detected in the urine.

Both fasting and postprandial levels of serum gastrin are grossly elevated in patients with pernicious anaemia (Hansky, 1981), and measurement of serum gastrin can be helpful.The fasting level quite often exceeds 600 ng/l as against the normal value of less than 100 ng/l.

The presence of various gastric autoantibodies against intrinsic factor (IFA) is diagnostically more specific than the parietal cell antibodies. In nearly all patients with positive IFA the antibodies are active against the intrinsic factor receptors for B12, and hence such antibodies are called blocking antibodies; however, in approximately two-thirds of the IFA positive cases, a second variety of antibodies which bind to the IF–B12 complex can also be detected. These are known as binding antibodies.

Demonstration of impaired absorption of B12 by the radioisotopic method (Schilling, 1953) has considerable diagnostic value. The classic Schilling test has been superseded by the more recent 'Dicopac' test (Bell, Bridges, and Nelson, 1965), a double isotope urinary excretion test using ^{57}Co and ^{58}Co. The latter test has been found to be of value even if the patient had prior B12 therapy or in cases of megaloblastic anaemia with low levels of both B12 and folate. An extremely low excretion of each isotope has been described as a useful parameter of intestinal malabsorption with normal renal function (Pathy, Pippen, and Kirkman, 1972). An upper limit of the normal range for the urinary ^{57}Co/^{58}Co ratio is usually 1.3 with a lower limit for PA of 2.0. This sharp borderline distinguishing PA from other causes of low serum vitamin B12 is not consistent in the elderly and the overlap in excretion ratios may create difficulty in the interpretation of the result (Pathy, Kirkman, and Molloy, 1979).

Some workers (England and Linnell, 1980) prefer the classic Schilling test, which is helpful in detecting transcobalamin II deficiency, to the Dicopac test.

England and Linnell (1980) suggest the following approach to establish a definite diagnosis of B12 deficiency:

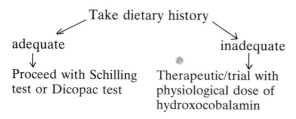

Take dietary history

adequate   inadequate

Proceed with Schilling test or Dicopac test   Therapeutic/trial with physiological dose of hydroxocobalamin

(a) If B12 malabsorption is suggested, use a therapeutic dosage of hydroxocobalamin.
(b) If the Schilling test is normal or the Dicopac test suggests malabsorption, exclude folate deficiency.

Treatment. Before venturing on a lifelong therapy with B12 for suspected PA, the importance of a correct and firm diagnosis is emphasized. Although B12 is not particularly harmful and is well excreted by the kidneys, there is no evidence to suggest that it is useful as a general tonic. The popular practice of treating elderly anaemic patients with multiple haematinic therapy creates great difficulty in establishing the correct diagnosis. Macrocytic anaemias must be adequately investigated before any therapy is commenced.

Five or six daily intramuscular injections of 1000 μg of hydroxocobalamin initially will replenish the deficiency in most cases of pernicious anaemia. A maximum reticulocyte response usually occurs on the fifth to seventh day. Once haematological response is achieved, the uncomplicated patient with PA can be satisfactorily maintained on 250 to 500 μg of hydroxocobalamin once every 1 or 2 months. Hypokalaemia may arise during the initial period of therapy and adequate potassium supplements should be given to an elderly patient during the early phase, especially if she is already depleted of potassium from previous diuretic therapy (Lawson, Murray, and Parker, 1972). Oral iron supplementation should also be given during the first few months as iron deficiency frequently develops during the early treatment phase of classical PA. Blood transfusion should be avoided if possible; otherwise slow transfusion of packed cells under adequate diuretic cover should only be used. In cases with neurologic complications, B12 should be given at a much higher dosage of 1,000 μg once every week or fortnight for at least 6 months.

Gastric carcinoma is five times more common in patients with PA and its pathogenesis has remained unclear. It has recently been shown that the mean nitrite concentration in gastric juice from patients with PA is nearly fifty times greater than that of age matched controls (Ruddell *et al.*, 1978). The intragastric production of carcinogenic *N*-nitroso compounds may be an important aetiological factor for the high incidence of gastric cancer in PA.

Folate Deficiency

The main causes of folate deficiency in the elderly are considered in Table 9.

Table 9 Cause of folate deficiency

I. Inadequate intake	Confusion
	Apathy and immobility
	Poor dietary advice
	Alcoholism
II. Impaired absorption	Small bowel resection
	Mesenteric vascular insufficiency
	Idiopathic steatorrhoea
	Regional enteritis
III. Increased consumption	Neoplasms
	Leukaemias
	Rheumatoid arthritis
IV Drugs	Folic acid antagonists
	Anticonvulsants
	Trimethoprim
V. Excessive loss	Skin diseases – psoriasis, exfoliative dermatitis
	Long-term dialysis

Incidence. Frank megaloblastic anaemia solely due to folate deficiency is relatively uncommon in the elderly (Batata *et al.*, 1967; MacLennan *et al.*, 1973). On the other hand, folate deficiency may be associated with other nutritional deficiencies among generally mal- or subnourished individuals.

Clinical features. As mentioned earlier, mental symptoms can be obvious. Depressive illness and affective disorders have been frequently noted. Peripheral neuropathy and rarely myelopathy resembling subacute combined degeneration of the spinal cord may occur and may respond satisfactorily to folate therapy (Manzoor and Runcie, 1976).

Diagnosis. In florid and severe cases, the bone marrow is frankly megaloblastic and anaemia is obvious with peripheral macrocytosis and an increase in hypersegmented neutrophils. The serum and RBC folate levels drop significantly in such cases. However, in milder cases, the picture may not be so clear. The general significance of serum and RBC folate level measurements has been discussed earlier. Increased urinary excretion of FIGLU after an oral dose of histidine has not been found to be a useful diagnostic test. Various tests for folate absorption and clearance by radioisotope methods have been described but they are not very commonly practised in routine clinical situations.

Treatment. Folic acid is administered orally at a daily dosage of 10 to 20 mg. Folic acid should not be given to patients with inadequately diagnosed megaloblastic macrocytic anaemias as it may precipitate serious neurological complications if given alone in pernicious anaemia. A physiological dosage of 200 μg daily may be used as a diagnostic method for an optimal response.

Non-Megaloblastic Macrocytic Anaemias

Macrocytic anaemia may arise from factors other than vitamin B12 and/or folate deficiency. The marrow is normoblastic, the red cells are enlarged with increased MCV, and the anaemia is usually of a moderate degree which does not respond to either B12 or folate therapy. Table 10 shows the different kinds of macrocytic anaemias.

Table 10 Distinction between macrocytic anaemias of megaloblastic and normoblastic origins

	Megaloblastic	Normoblastic
1. RBC size and shape	Macrocytosis ++++ Poikolocytes ++ Oval macrocytes – common	Macrocytosis ++ Poikilocytes + Oval macrocytes – rare
2. WBC	Macropolycytosis – common	Macropolycytosis – absent
3. Response to B12/folate	Very good	Nil

The availability of more detailed investigations has resulted in more macrocytic anaemias of non-megaloblastic origin being detected in elderly patients (Bahemuka, Denham, and Hodkinson, 1973).

Banerjee (1975) found that 40 per cent. of 282 consecutive acutely ill elderly patients had haemoglobin concentrations of less than 11.4 g/dl. Of the 37 cases with an MCV of more than 105 fl, 90 per cent. had a non-megaloblastic macrocytosis. This study suggests that normoblastic macrocytic anaemia is fairly common in elderly patients. The pathogenesis of such anaemia is not clear.

True enlargement of red cells can occur with increased erythropoietic activity, which is a well recognized feature in alcoholism, chronic liver disorder, renal insufficiency, rheumatoid disease, and hypothyroid states.

The elucidation of non-megaloblastic macrocytosis in the elderly often requires skilful clinical and laboratory orientation.

POLYCYTHAEMIC SYNDROMES

The number of circulating red cells can increase in several conditions. Erythrocytosis as a secondary event to underlying disease must be differentiated from polycythaemia rubra vera, a primary myeloproliferative disorder.

Secondary Erythrocytosis

In the absence of dehydration, a haemoglobin of 17 g/dl or above, a PCV of more than 0.52, and a red cell count of 5×10^{12} per litre or higher suggests erythrocytosis. Secondary erythrocytosis is associated with an increase in red cells only without any increase in leucocytes or platelets. This may arise from a large number of clinical conditions (see Table 11). In these conditions, erythrocytosis is mediated by increased production of erythropoietin.

Table 11   Causes of secondary erythrocytosis

1. Neoplastic disorders	Kidney
	Liver
	Uterus
	Cerebellum
2. Hypoxic respiratory disorders	Chronic obstructive bronchitis
	Pulmonary fibrosis
3. Cardiac disorders	Any condition causing central cyanosis
4. Renal abnormalities	Hydronephrosis
	Cystic disease
5. Others	Chronic alcoholism

Chronic respiratory disorder is probably the most common cause of secondary erythrocytosis in the elderly. The demonstration of a low arterial oxygen tension is diagnostic of pulmonary erythrocytosis. However, the severity of red cell response is variable and, on occasion, marked erythrocytosis occurs with only slight depression of arterial oxygen tension. It has been suggested that intermittent hypoxia at night, especially during REM sleep, may be the major stimulus for increased erythropoietin production and subsequent increase in red cell mass. Erythrocytosis in chronic hypoxic lung disease should be regarded as compensatory,

and the treatment of the basic disorder is all that is usually required. In cases with associated vascular complications, intermittent isovolaemic venesection should be undertaken.

As listed above, certain tumours may produce inappropriate amounts of erythropoietin. Removal of the tumour is the preferred approach. Where surgery is contraindicated, regular venesection will improve the clinical state.

Compensatory Erythrocytosis Due to Abnormalities of Oxygen Transport

Over the last few years, a number of elderly patients have been diagnosed as suffering from erythrocytosis due to the presence of 'high-affinity' haemoglobin in the blood (Charache, Weatherall, and Clegg, 1966; Weatherall *et al.*, 1977). Normally, when haemoglobin takes up or releases oxygen it undergoes changes in its structure. This affects the shape of each polypeptide chain as well as the whole tetramer. However, sometimes substitution of a single amino acid occurs in a particular region of the globin chain which alters the deformability of the whole molecule in such a way that oxygen is less readily released to the tissues. The first such 'high-affinity' haemoglobin was described in an 81 year old male and the 'abnormal' haemoglobin isolated was called haemoglobin-Chesapeake (Charache, Weatherall, and Clegg, 1966). On a detailed predigree study, many members of that patient's family, over three generations, were found to have erythrocytosis. Such 'high-affinity' haemoglobins do not release oxygen easily and as a result the oxygen–disassociation curve is shifted to the left and its shape is altered from a sigmoid to a hyperbolic form. The clinical effect of poor oxygen release is relative anoxia and compensatory erythrocytosis.

To date, a large number of high-affinity haemoglobins have been identified and although their amino acid structures vary from each other, the clinical and haematological effects are very much the same. The diagnosis depends on family history and demonstration of an abnormal haemoglobin by various chemical and electrophoretic techniques. Many elderly patients, who had been diagnosed previously as atypical cases of polycythaemia vera and had not responded to treatment, are now being reviewed and more and more cases of high-affinity haemoglobinopathies are being identified.

Treatment

The treatment in these cases is regular vene-section, usually on a lifelong basis (*BMJ*, 1977a).

Relative Erythrocytosis

Most patients with a mild elevation of red cell values in association with vascular disease do not have a significant elevation of red cell mass. In some, the red cell values are significantly raised because of contraction of the plasma volume. This may be inferred accurately by direct measurement of plasma volume using direct labelled isotopic albumin. The red cell mass does not exceed 32 ml/kg in relative erythrocytosis.

This condition is sometimes seen in heavy smokers due to a chronic low-grade increase in carboxyhaemoglobin in their blood. The increase in red cell values may result in increased blood viscosity and may contribute to ischaemic problems of the carotid, coronary, or peripheral arterial system.

Cerebral Blood Flow in Polycythaemic Disorders

It has been recognized for some years that patients with true polycythaemia are more prone to cerebrovascular disorders. There is also some evidence that a raised PCV, not necessarily accompanied by an increase in red cell mass, as seen in secondary polycythaemia, may also be significant in vascular disease (Burge, Johnson, and Prankerd, 1975). The relationship between cerebral blood flow and high PCV has been studied and it has been shown that a reduction of haematocrit in patients with existing higher values increases the cerebral blood flow considerably. This improvement is due largely to the subsequent reduction of blood viscosity. Whether the cerebral blood flow (CBF) decreases with normal ageing remains controversial (Arnold, 1981), but it is probable that in the severely mentally infirm elderly the CBF is reduced (Melamed *et al.*, 1979; Marshall, 1982), although here, too,

there is some disagreement (McAlpine *et al.*, 1981). Polycythaemic disorders with increased haematocrit value and blood viscosity may be of considerable clinical significance in relation to higher cerebral function in old age. Changes in behaviour and impaired alertness have also been noticed in elderly subjects with increased red cell values. A similar alteration in higher cerebral functions is also seen in patients with hypoxic lung disease with secondary polycythaemia (Wade *et al.*, 1981).

Treatment

Reduction of the haematocrit by regular venesection has been found to be helpful in relieving the various symptoms of vascular disease secondary to polycythaemic disorders.

Venesection reduces the viscosity and improves the cerebral blood flow (Humphrey *et al.*, 1979) with significant improvement in overall higher functions and alertness (Thomas and Willison, 1981). In patients with relative erythrocytosis with a low plasma volume, normovolaemic haemodilution has been recommended (Yates *et al.*, 1979). Even with normal plasma volume, in patients with poor cardiac or renal states and in those where the risks of thromboembolic complications are high, haemodilution without any total volume depletion is much safer (Gottstein, 1981). Venesection with a removal of 200 to 300 ml of blood at a time should be performed with simultaneous slow infusion of an equal amount of low-molecular weight dextran or 6% dextran 70 in normal saline to replenish the lost blood volume.

The therapy is usually repeated at weekly intervals until the haematocrit level recedes to approximately 35 per cent., a goal usually reached within 4 to 8 weeks. Reinfusion of patient's own plasma following venesection has also been found to be useful in some centres.

Polycythaemia Rubra Vera

This primary myeloproliferative disorder is seen mainly in people above 60. Males are more frequently affected. The symptoms are mainly due to increased blood viscosity. Frontal or occipital headache especially on lying down or on awakening in the morning, dizziness, syncope, forgetfulness, depression and

Table 12 Distinguishing features of different polycythaemic states

	Red cell mass	Plasma volume	Enlarged spleen	High WCC and platelets
Primary PRV	Very high	Normal	Present	Present
Secondary	High	Normal	Absent	Absent
Relative and compensatory	Normal	Low	Absent	Absent

irritability can be a few of the presenting features. Redness of eyes and transient motor weakness of a limb tend to be more serious diagnostic markers. Vascular thrombosis, haemorrhage, peptic ulceration, and gout are some of the complicating features. The spleen is palpable in the majority of patients and may progress to a massive enlargement in late-stage myelofibrosis. Generalized pruritus is fairly common and is usually aggravated by exposure to heat or cold; it is characteristically manifest after a bath. Laboratory diagnosis is made by measurement of the red cell mass by the use of an isotopic label, usually ^{51}Cr or ^{32}P. A figure of more than 35ml/kg in men and 32ml/kg in women clearly excludes other forms of compensatory disorders (Table 12).

Total white cell count and platelet count are elevated in the majority of patients. In contradistinction to chronic myeloid leukaemia, another myeloproliferative disease, neutrophil alkaline phosphatase, is raised in more than 70 per cent. of cases. Bone marrow aspirates reveal hypercellularity with proliferation of all types of cells. An increase in reticulin may indicate a transition to myelofibrosis. Leukaemic transformation may occasionally arise. Combined ferrokinetic and erythrokinetic studies show a rapid iron accumulation in bones followed by complete release, increased plasma iron turnover, a normal red cell lifespan, and normal ^{59}Fe surface counting patterns with no evidence of extramedullary erythropoiesis (Lewis, 1976).

Treatment of Primary Polycythaemia

Venesection with removal of 500 ml of blood at a time is mandatory in acutely ill patients with severe polycythaemia. This is particularly important to avoid impending vascular catastrophe. Once the PCV is brought under control, some form of myelosuppressive therapy is desirable. The most effective agent is radioactive phosphorus. The isotope is administered by a single i.v. injection and the usual dose is 3 to 5 mCi. No suppressive effect can be seen within 3 to 4 weeks and the full therapeutic benefit is unlikely to be obtained within 3 months. A second dose may occasionally be required. Cytostatic drugs such as busulphan at a dose of 2 to 4 mg daily or chlorambucil at 4 to 6 mg daily has also been found to be effective. Occasionally, patients may become iron deficient because of chronic haemorrhagic blood loss; oral iron therapy may be warranted in such cases. Iron therapy may also be of value in patients with severe pruritis (Salem *et al.*, 1982).

MYELOFIBROSIS

Pathology

Bone marrow fibrosis can be histologically divided into two grades. Reticulin fibrosis, which is sometimes thought to be an exaggeration of the normal pattern, is found in a wide variety of blood disorders, both benign and malignant. However, such fibrosis may be the precursor of collagen fibrosis which is restricted to a much smaller group of conditions. Here, the whole marrow sinusoidal architecture is disrupted and obliterated with widespread scarring. Probably the best recognized type of collagen fibrosis occurs in idiopathic myelofibrosis. A variety of terms have been used to describe this enigmatic condition and it is now generally regarded as one of the chronic myeloproliferative disorders. Other conditions, e.g. primary polycythaemia rubra vera, chronic myeloid leukaemia, etc., are usually included in this group.

In myelofibrosis, the normal bone marrow becomes grossly fibrosed and, as a result, haemopoietic activity is taken over in various extra-medullary sites, such as the liver and spleen. Isotope studies show a shortened red cell lifespan with evidence of sequestration of cells inside the spleen. Erythropoiesis becomes ineffective and evidence of extramedullary haemopoiesis is markedly evident. The basic aetiology of this condition is not definitely known. Various suggestions, such as autonomous proliferation, exposure to irradiation or chemicals, and viral infection, have been made. It is possible that this is a response of normal stromal cells to abnormal haemopoietic cells or their environment. Its relationship with other disorders such as polycythaemia vera and chronic myeloid leukaemia remains inadequately explained.

Clinical Features

This disorder is primarily a condition of the aged and is clinically characterized by anaemia, a leucoerythroblastic blood picture, massive splenomegaly, and sometimes hepatomegaly. The patients suffer from marked lassitude, loss of weight, and night sweats. Like primary polycythaemia, haemorrhagic manifestation is not uncommon. This is a chronic condition and many patients, if not grossly decompensated, may carry on normally.

Treatment

Drug therapy is unsatisfactory. Cytotoxic drugs should be considered in patients with severe leucocytosis or massive splenomegaly. Splenectomy should only be reserved for patients with adequate marrow function and is not usually recommended in the very elderly (*BMJ*, 1979). Haematinic agents such as folic acid and pyridoxine may be used in selected patients.

REFRACTORY ANAEMIAS

The term 'refractory anaemia' has been in vogue for nearly 40 years and is used to describe a group of anaemias of uncertain aetiology characterized by failure to respond favourably to the conventional haematinic agents. With better understanding of blood disease and with improved diagnostic facilities, few conditions are now included under this heading. Myelofibrosis, diserythropoietic anaemias and classical hypoplastic anaemia are perhaps the better known ones.

Apart from these conditions, over recent years, the syndrome of 'primary refractory anaemia' has been recognized. This is characterized by a qualitative disturbance of erythropoiesis with morphologically and functionally abnormal erythroid cells; some disturbance in leucopoiesis is also seen. Two varieties of such chronic refractory disorder have been identified and they are sometimes collectively described as 'myelodysplastic syndromes' suggesting disturbances in both erythroid and myeloid precursors (Gordon-Smith, 1969). These conditions are common in the elderly.

Pathogenesis

The pathogenesis of this group of anaemias is unclear. Detailed cell culture studies have thrown some light on this condition. Soft agar colony-forming unit assays of the bone marrow show three distinctive growth patterns (Valera and Good, 1980):

(a) Colony formation is slow but is not suppressed by normal cells suggesting a defect intrinsic to the haemopoietic stem cell.

(b) Colony formation is normal with no evidence of suppressor activity, indicating that the defect is due to an abnormality in the stem cell microenvironment.

(c) Colony formation is decreased with obvious suppressor activity, suggesting that the defect results from suppressor cell action. This is the classical situation in primary hypoplastic anaemia.

It is, therefore, probable that the classical hypoplastic anaemia and the other myelodysplastic refractory anaemias are part of a spectrum of pancytopenic disorders with a common pathogenesis.

Myelodysplastic Anaemias

Two clinical varieties have been described. Presentation with clinical symptoms of pancytopenia, e.g. anaemia, recurrent infections, and haemorrhage. The bone marrow is not hypoplastic. It is of normal or of increased cellularity with a gross increase in myeloid precursors and blasts. This may need to be distinguished from smouldering leukaemia, a condition which is also prevalent in the elderly. Some patients do indeed terminate in acute leukaemia; however, the majority remain stable for many years. Bone marrow culture studies is the only way to identify the true nature of the disease.

The second type of refractory anaemia is characterized by proliferative dysplasia. Here, the patient presents with pancytopenia and grossly decreased number of reticulocytes. The bone marrow is normocellular and there is no increase in the proportion of myeloblasts. However, there is associated marked dyserythropoiesis with an increased amount of reticulin. This type of refractory anaemia simulates myelofibrosis but ferrokinnetic studies show an aplastic pattern without any evidence of extramedullary haemopoiesis. Leukaemic transformation does not occur.

Hypoplastic Anaemia

Idiopathic primary hypoplastic anaemia is not uncommon in old age. Peripheral pancytopenia can occur with a number of conditions (Table 13) and a proper examination of the bone marrow along with other relevant clinical features usually point to the correct diagnosis.

Table 13 Common causes of Pancytopenia

Pernicious anaemia
Severe folate deficiency
Severe protein deficiency
Myelofibrosis
Metastatic infiltration of bone marrow
Connective tissue disease, e.g. DLE
Miliary tuberculosis
Acute leukaemia (on rare occasions)
Advanced renal disease
Hypoplastic and refractory anaemia

In the elderly, marrow hypoplasia is commonly secondary to other causes (Table 14).

Table 14 Causes of marrow hypoplasia

1. Exposure to radiation or cytotoxic drugs
2. Idiosyncrasy to certain drugs and chemicals:
(a) Drugs, e.g. phenylbutazone, gold salts, chloramphenicol, sulphonamides
(b) Chemicals, e.g. benzene
3. Marrow depression following:
(a) Certain minor viral infections, e.g. influenza
(b) Bacterial infections, e.g. Legionnaire's disease, etc.
(c) Hepatitis (usually of non-A, non-B type)

The marrow damage is usually transient with the majority of viral infections; however the posthepatitis hypoplasia has a very poor prognosis (Camitta, Storb, and Thomas, 1982).

The clinical presentation is commonly with frank haemorrhage or purpura. However, anaemia of slow onset and/or recurrent infections can also be important presenting features. Physical signs are usually absent. Diagnosis is usually reached by careful clinical history, especially that of drug ingestion. Peripheral counts reveal pancytopenia but it is not unusual to see patients with reduction of only one formed element of the blood. Trephine marrow biopsy is essential to distinguish the disorder from other pathologies. The marrow reticulin is normal or reduced. Ferrokinetic study shows a marked reduction in the utilization of ^{59}Fe.

Treatment

A gross reduction in peripheral neutrophils, platelets, and reticulocytes are indicative of poor prognosis. Supportive treatment with regular transfusion is essential in all cases.

Neutropenia and/or thrombocytopenia require immediate attention in order to avoid any serious clinical crisis. Regular infusions of granulocyte and platelet concentrates may be necessary. Prophylactic use of non-absorbable antibiotics is also justified. Chronic anaemia is not a life threatening disorder and patients usually cope with it quite well.

Androgens and anabolic steroids have been used to stimulate erythropoiesis, but their overall efficacy in severe cases remains doubtful. The drug commonly used is oxymetholone. This drug stimulates erythropoiesis and diminishes the requirement of packed red cell transfusions, but unfortunately does not stimulate the production of the white cells or platelets. A fairly high dosage of 2.5 to 5.0 mg/kg per day is required and the effects are not seen for 12 to 16 weeks. Corticosteroids are sometimes used as a short-term measure to treat thrombocytopenic haemorrhage.

Agents to stimulate the proliferation of stem cells have been tried over the last few years. Preparations of lithium have been particularly studied and occasional benefits have been obtained (Blum, 1979). Lithium inhibits the action of adenyl cyclase and reduces the intracellular levels of cAMP. It enhances the production of colony-stimulating activity which

considered to be a possible modulator of granulopoiesis in vivo (Malloy, Zanber, and Chervenick, 1978). In general, oral lithium
carbonate is relatively non-toxic and should,
perhaps, be used as a possible method of treatment to stimulate granulopoiesis in marrow
hypoplastic disorders (*Lancet*, 1980b).

Therapy with antilymphocyte globulin or
bone marrow transplantation are not likely to
be undertaken in routine geriatric medical
practice.

Although the initial mortality from refractory anaemias is significant, patients who survive one year or more usually have a
reasonable outcome. In patients with a relatively stable marrow, overall prognosis is excellent and they usually die of some unrelated
illness.

HAEMOLYTIC ANAEMIAS

Anaemia due to red cell haemolysis is a complex area of haematology. Frank haemolysis
due to intrinsic defects of red cell and/or its
membrane is not common in geriatric practice,
although occasional patients who have grown
old with intrinsic red cell defect such as thal-
assaemia or hereditary spherocytosis since
childhood may be encountered. Detailed discussions of such conditions are irrelevant to
this chapter. Haemolytic diseases can broadly
be classified as shown in Table 15.

Haemolysis, usually of low grade, is not infrequent in cases of pernicious anaemia and in
some other symptomatic and refractory anaemias. This is important as it may have some
relevance to the clinical features and progress
of the disease; response to conventional therapy may also be influenced. Confirmation of
haemolysis may only be achieved by isotopic
estimation of the red cell lifespan, which is
markedly shortened.

Haemolysis, when present in the elderly, is
usually secondary to some external agent or
due to the presence of autoantibodies to red
cells. Sometimes, autoantibodies are detected
in secondary haemolytic disorders.

Autoimmune Haemolytic Anaemias

Antibodies to red cells are divided into 'warm'
and 'cold' types. Warm antibodies are active
at 37 °C and the cold antibodies are active at

Table 15   Classification of haemolytic anaemias

I. Intrinsic defects	1. Inherited
	Abnormal haemoglobin disease
	Hereditary spherocytosis
	Lack of enzymes, e.g. G6PD, PK, etc.
	2. Acquired
	Dyshaemopoietic anaemias: Vitamin B12 deficiences, leukaemias, hypoplastic anaemias
II. Extrinsic defects	1. Autoimmune
	Idiopathic acquired
	Secondary autoimmune
	Cold haemagglutinin disease (CHAD)
	2.) Secondary to drugs and chemicals, infection, trauma

4 °C. Immunologically, the 'warm' antibodies
are of the IgG subclass and the 'cold' of the
IgM subclass. Not infrequently, such antibodies are associated with other disease processes, but when no associated disorders are
present the autoimmune haemolytic process
can be labelled as idiopathic.

Idiopathic autoimmune haemolytic anaemias associated with 'warm' IgG-type antibodies are uncommon in old age. However,
the subacute or chronic haemolytic state due
to an IgM-type 'cold' antibody is not
infrequent.

Cold Haemagglutinin Disease

Acute transient haemolysis due to cold antibodies may occur following infectious mono-
nucleosis or mycoplasma infections but these
conditions are not common in old age. On the
other hand, chronic haemolytic process due to
IgM antibodies is not unusual. Such primary
cold haemagglutinin disease (CHAD) usually
presents as a mild to moderate haemolytic
anaemia of gradual onset. Raynaud's phenomenon is common and occasional haemoglo-
binuria can occur. The anaemia becomes worse
in cold weather and the direct antiglobulin test
(Coomb's) remains persistently positive.

These antibodies are almost always of the
IgM subclass and monoclonal (Cooper,

Chavin, and Franklin, 1970). They may be associated with the light chains of kappa type. The antibody specificity is usually anti-I with paraprotein IgM(K), but anti-i, anti-p, and other antibodies can also be detected.

In most patients, symptoms become obvious at an average paraprotein level of only 4 g/l. The disease usually runs a chronic course and a gradual monoclonal increase of IgM takes place progressively over several years. Cold antibodies are also seen with malignant lymphoreticular disorders but here the antibodies are more commonly polyclonal.

Treatment

The treatment of CHAD is primarily environmental. The patient should keep warm and avoid unnecessary exposure to cold. Where these measures fail to alleviate symptoms, specific cytotoxic therapy with chlorambucil or penicillamine can be undertaken, but symptoms usually improve only in one third of cases. Plasma exchange, on similar lines as macroglobulinaemia (see later), can be tried but is not of permanent benefit. Corticosteroids, which are of great therapeutic value in warm-antibody infused haemolysis, are of little or no benefit to these patients.

Secondary Autoimmune Haemolytic Anaemias

In general, these are more frequent than the primary idiopathic type. Lymphoma, chronic lymphatic leukaemia, ulcerative colitis, systemic lupus erythematosus, and some ovarian tumours may be associated with IgG type warm antibodies and manifest haemolytic anaemia. The haemolysis may be acute with a sudden fall in haemoglobin or may be slow and progressive. Usual features of haemolysis are clinically apparent; mild jaundice and splenomegaly are common. Laboratory examination reveals reticulocytosis. The reticulocyte level should be corrected in the presence of anaemia, and the following calculation may be used:

$$\text{Corrected \% retic.} = \text{reported \% retic.} \frac{\text{patient's PCV}}{\text{normal PCV}}$$

Bone marrow shows marked erythroid hyperplasia and a corresponding reduction of the myeloid-erythroid cell ratio. Levels of haemoglobin-binding protein haptoglobin are diminished. However, since haptoglobin is an active-phase protein, its level may remain normal or even be higher with associated infections. A rise in serum lactate dehydrogenase isoenzymes may occur but this is usually non-specific. The most confirmatory sign of haemolysis is, however, a reduction of the circulating red cell lifespan. Autologous red cells are incubated with radioisotopic sodium chromate ($^{51}CrO_4$) and are reinjected into the circulation. The gradual loss of red cell radioactivity is then measured over a period of time. By this method, the normal half-life of red cells is between 25 to 32 days. In haemolytic states the half life is grossly reduced. Examination of the peripheral blood film may be informative. The presence of an increased number of atypical and abnormal red cells, e.g. spherocytes, elliptocytes, fragmented red cells, Burr cells, etc., may be seen. A simple, readily available test for immune haemolysis is Coomb's antiglobulin test. It is usually performed using the 'broad-spectrum' reagent and a positive result is followed by specific anti-IgG and anticomplemet testing to detect either warm or cold antibodies. The direct Coomb's test detects the antibodies attached to red cells; the indirect test identifies free circulating antibodies. A few patients with immune haemolysis may not produce a positive result because of insufficient density of the antibody. Unfortunately, lack of sensitivity does not relate the gross differences in the amounts of 'coating' antibodies (Wiley, 1980).

Drugs are well-known inducers of haemolysis and they may also involve immune mechanism.

Treatment

Oral corticosteroids is the treatment of choice. An initial dosage of 40 to 60 mg/day may be required and the response is usually dramatic. Transfusion of carefully crossmatched blood may be necessary at an early stage but the decision of transfusing patients with an active haemolytic process should be made with great care. Appropriate treatment of the underlying disorder is mandatory.

Oxidative Haemolysis

Rarely, patients may have intrinsic deficiency of red cell enzymes, best known of which is lack of glucose-6-phosphate dehydrogenase (G6PD). Although extremely uncommon in this country and certainly in the elderly, it is mainly seen in people of Oriental, Mediterranean, West Indian, and African origin. Accordingly, sporadic cases may be seen in elderly first-generation immigrants. Haemolysis is usually episodic and acute and is very frequently precipitated by ingestion of oxidative drugs, e.g. sulphonamides, nitrofurantoin, antimalarial primaquine, and aspirin. Infective conditions, such as pneumonia, as well as severe diabetic keto acidosis can also precipitate haemolysis in deficient individuals. The appropriate fluorescent spot test supported by G6PD assay will clinch the diagnosis.

THE LEUKAEMIAS

Incidence

Although the incidence and distribution of acute leukaemias have always shown a bimodal picture, recent surveys indicate an absolute increase of this disease in the elderly. Reports from Sweden (Brandt, Nilsson, and Mitelman, 1979), Denmark (Clemmeson, 1974), north and south central regions of the United States (Blair, Fraumeni, and Mason, 1980), Scotland (Kemp, Stein, and Heasman, 1980), and north-western England (Geary, Benn, and Leck, 1979) suggest a genuine increase in acute myeloid leukaemia, especially among the older male population. This rate of increase in the elderly has roughly paralleled the corresponding increase in lung cancer mortality. An increase in coverage of all types of cancer registration and a general improvement in the application of diagnostic techniques in the elderly might suggest that the high diagnostic rates of leukaemia is an artefact. However, increased environmental exposure to various exogenous leukaemogens by elderly individuals with constitutional, hormonal, and perhaps genetic vulnerability is probably the more important basic factor (*Lancet*, 1980c).

Analyses of the age/sex specific registration rates per million population per year for acute myeloid leukaemia, in Scotland, show the rates for males were 65.8 for the 65 to 79 age group and 149.8 for the 80+ age group during the 5 year period 1973–77, as compared to 51.6 and 87.0 for the immediate previous 5 year period 1968–72 (Kemp, Stein, and Heasman, 1980).

Classification

The conventional classification of leukaemia is as follows:
I.   Acute
     (a) Non-lymphoid or myelogenous
     (b) Lymphoid
     (c) Blast crisis of chronic leukaemias
II. Smouldering leukaemia or pre-leukaemia
III. Chronic
     (a) Myeloid
     (b) Lymphatic:
          including hairy cell leukaemia
          prolymphocytic leukaemia

Acute Myelogenous Leukaemias

This form of leukaemia can be subdivided into the following groups (Gralnick *et al.*, 1977; Whittaker *et al.*, 1979) on conventional morphology and special staining methods:
(a) Myeloblastic leukaemia without maturation (M1)
(b) Myeloblastic leukaemia with features of maturation (M2)
(c) Promyelocytic leukaemia with hypergranular cells and abundant Auer rods (M3)
(d) Myelomonocytic leukaemia (M4)
(e) Monocytic leukaemia (M5)
(f) Erythroleukaemia (M6)
(g) ? Megakaryocytic (M7)

The non-myelogenous lymphoid leukaemias are usually classified by immunologic cell marking methods into various B, T, and non-B, non-T lymphocytic varieties.

The correct diagnosis of leukaemias can only be made by appropriate laboratory cytochemical and immunological techniques supported if necessary by more detailed studies of chromosome changes and cell growth patterns. The clinician has to depend on laboratory expertise for a correct diagnosis which is essential before the appropriate management programme can be contemplated.

Clinical Manifestations

The clinical features of frank and florid cases include fever, enlargement of peripheral lymph nodes, purpura and haemorrhage, arthralgia, and rapidly progressive anaemia.

Atypical presentation is not unusual in elderly subjects and may create diagnostic problems. For example, hypoplastic acute leukaemia can present with marrow failure and without evidence of tissue infiltration (Beard *et al.*, 1975), or patients with acute promyelocytic leukaemia (M3) can present with disseminated intravascular coagulation and uncontrollable bleeding.

Acute Leukaemic Blast Crisis on a Chronic Leukaemic State

Terminal blast crisis or metamorphosis is a serious complication of chronic myeloid leukaemia and is extremely resistant to cytostatic chemotherapy. Some cases of chronic myeloid leukaemia can give rise to acute lymphoid blast crisis with a positive Ph chromosome. The haematological picture is usually that of an acute or subacute lymphoblastic leukaemia. A careful diagnosis is essential as many of these cases respond well to conventional chemotherapy for acute lymphoblastic leukaemia (*BMJ*, 1977c; Rosenthal *et al.*, 1977).

Acute myelogenous leukaemia may occur in patients receiving various cytotoxic drugs for treatment of other malignancies (Davis *et al.*, 1973). Melphalan therapy for myeloma (Kyle, Pierre, and Bayrd, 1970) and busulphan for carcinoma of bronchus (Stott *et al.*, 1977) have given rise to various forms of acute non-lymphoid leukaemia after long-term therapy.

'Preleukaemia' or 'Smouldering Leukaemia'

This is an interesting group of leukaemias which may be included under either 'acute' or 'chronic', depending on the stage and management of the disease. The patient presents with a refractory anaemia or a low platelet count or monocytosis. Abnormal development of one or more cell lines may be evident with dyserythropoesis and ring sideroblasts in the marrow or agranular neutrophils with abnormal lysosome development and giant platelets in peripheral blood. The proportion of blast cells in the marrow may be low, around 10 per cent. (pre-leukaemia), or may be higher, around 30 per cent. (smouldering leukaemia). These conditions may follow a subacute or chronic course for several months without requiring therapeutic intervention.

Evidence for a definite leukaemic process can be established by chromosomal studies and cell growth techniques. The sequence may be: preleukaemia → Ph-negative chronic myeloid leukaemia → subacute myelogenous leukaemia → acute myelogenous leukaemia. (Beard and Whitehouse, 1977). In the terminal phase, the picture is similar to the acute disease requiring the same kind of therapeutic intervention, but the prognosis is much worse.

Management of Acute Leukaemia

Treatment has become so complex that it is being increasingly undertaken in special centres of oncology.

The decision of whether to deploy an aggressive chemotherapeutic regime on an elderly patient has to be made with care and compassion. Cognizance of the medical and environmental factors of the individual is essential and the degree to which various supportive resources, e.g. blood, platelet concentrates, and proper nursing care, including effective barrier nursing, are locally available must be considered.

The age per se of the patient used to be considered a major prognostic factor (Crosby, 1968; Rosner *et al.*, 1976), but recent trials of intensive treatment have not supported this belief (Gale and Cline, 1977; Peterson and Bloomfield, 1977). Nevertheless, mortality is much higher in the elderly from haemorrhage and infection, and meticulous care is necessary before selecting the appropriate regime and the dosage schedule.

The following combination chemotherapy is likely to induce a remission in 85 per cent. of cases of acute myelogenous leukaemia (Rees *et al.*, 1977):

Doxorubicin 50 mg/m^2 i.v., day 1
Cytosine arabinoside 100 mg/m^2 i.v., day 1–5
6-Thioguanine 100 mg/m^2 orally b.d., day 1–5

Courses of 5 days' duration are repeated with a 7 to 14 day interval in between until remission is achieved. Such intensive regimes are reasonably tolerated by aged patients and the overall therapeutic efficacy of aggressive chemotherapy remains identical in all ages (Foon *et al.*, 1981).

If adequate supportive care is unobtainable, a less aggressive, oral cytotoxic schedule may be used (Stuart, 1980):

6 Thioguanine 100 mg/m^2 per day ⎫
Cyclophosphamide 100 mg/m^2 per ⎬ Days 1–5
day ⎭

This gives a 2 to 3 day interval between the first two courses with 7 to 10 day intervals between subsequent courses as required. If there is no initial response, drug administration may be increased to 12 hourly with an intravenous dosage of Doxorubicin of 50 mg/m^2 on day 1.

After the initial successful remission, a 4 to 6 weekly maintenance 'pulse' therapy should be continued.

Very recently, attempts are being made to treat some cases of hypoplastic acute myeloid leukaemias with low-dosage cytosine arabinoside. Subcutaneous cytarabine at a dosage of 10 mg/m^2 twice a day for two to three weeks has been found to be particularly useful and tolerated by the elderly patients (Housset *et al.*, 1982; Manoharan, 1983). However, the overall efficacy and precise indications and nature of such regime still need to be adequately evaluated (Desforges, 1983).

Supportive Care and Therapy

Infection. Neutropenia and leucopenia with infection is a major hazard. The patient should be isolated and barrier-nursed in a single cubicle.

Despite this, the endogenous infections may cause problems. Oral chemoprophylaxis with either a combination of framycetin, colistin and nystatin (FRACON) or with cotrimoxazole alone can be useful. It may be difficult to establish a firm diagnosis of an infection. Estimation of serum acute-phase C-reactive protein has been found to be useful. Although a modest rise in C-RP level can be expected in acute leukaemia per se, a grossly elevated level of more than 100 mg/l is highly suggestive of significant bacterial infection (Stuart, 1980).

A combination of intravenous broad-spectrum antibiotics, e.g. gentamicin, flucloxacil-

lin, and carbenicillin, is likely to be successful in the majority of these patients. Granulocyte transfusions can be beneficial. Anaerobic infections should be treated with metronidazole. Superficial candidal infection responds to local nystatin; severe systemic fungal infection may need parenteral amphotericin B, although the newer antifungal ketoconazole may be equally effective. Lung infection with protozoan pneumocystis is relatively rare in the elderly and responds well to a high dosage of oral cotrimoxazole. Until recently, viral infections in these patients were difficult to control, but the newly available antiviral agent Acyclovir is proving to be useful here.

Haemorrhage. Thrombocytopenic bleeding can be a fatal complication. Regular administration of platelet concentrate is life-saving and can be used even on a prophylactic basis.

Acute disseminated intravascular coagulation (DIC) may cause thrombocytopenia and bleeding in this situation. DIC is particularly associated with acute promyelocytic leukaemia (M3) where prophylactic low-dose heparin is occasionally recommended (Drapkin *et al.*, 1978).

Hyperuricaemia. This is a fairly common occurrence during the cytotoxic therapy. Oral allopurinol is effective, although its concurrent use with purine antagonists, e.g. 6-mercaptopurine, may warrant dose reduction of the latter agent; thioguanine does not require such a reduction of dosage.

Acute Lymphatic (Non-Myelogenous) Leukaemia

This condition will not be discussed here as it is relatively uncommon in the elderly. In the event, the natural history, manifestations and the lines of management are the same as they are in younger adults.

Chronic Leukaemias

Chronic Lymphatic Leukaemia (CLL)

This is the most commonly seen form of leukaemia in the elderly. The diagnosis is often reached as a chance finding and most patients with this disorder do not require therapeutic intervention. The detailed indications of therapy depend on the haematologic clinical manifestations which are mentioned later. It is now recognized that chronic lymphatic leukaemia can be the manifestation of a widespread lymphoproliferative disorder. Immunologic cell marker techniques have thrown considerable light on the identification and distinction of several lymphoproliferative disorders (*BMJ*, 1979). A few of these conditions deserve special mention.

T Cell-Chronic Lymphatic Leukaemia

Although the classic CLL is of B-cell variety and manifests the presence of surface immunoglobulin, in a few patients with CLL the lymphocytes form E-rosettes and there are no surface immunoglobulins. These patients are usually elderly and present with considerable splenomegaly with absent or minimal peripheral lymphadenopathy. Skin infiltration is commoner than in B-CLL. The lymphocyte morphology is variable but often there is a folded nucleus and abundant cytoplasm containing azurophilic granules (Reinherz *et al.*, 1979).

Prolymphocytic Leukaemia

This variant was first described by Galton and coworkers (1974), occurring predominently in elderly males. Characterized by massive splenomegaly with minimal lymph node enlargement, the patient presents with general lassitude, loss of weight, and fever. The lymphocytes are mainly of the B-cell type.

Hairy Cell Leukaemia

This B-cell chronic steadily progressive lymphoproliferative disorder is seen mainly among elderly men. The clinical features include massive splenomegaly without marked peripheral lymphadenopathy and a relatively low lymphocyte count in blood. A general neutropenia and/or thrombocytopenia is common and the patient may present with infection or haemorrhage. The cells show numerous short villi around the membrane and have abundant cytoplasm, and homogeneous chromatin with a fine fibrillary pattern. Despite this appearance as histiocytes, they behave as lymphocytes with some phagocytic potential (Catovsky *et al.*, 1974a, 1974b).

Chronic Lymphatic Leukaemia

Management

The management depends on the nature of the disease. Classical B-cell chronic lymphatic leukaemia is staged as follows (Rai *et al.*, 1975):

Stage O: Peripheral lymphocyte >15 × 10^9/litre
Marrow lymphocytes >40% of all nucleated cells
Hb >11 g/dl
Platelets 100 × 10^9/litre
No hepatosplenomegaly or lymphadenopathy

Stage I: As O, but with enlarged lymph nodes

Stage II: As O, but with enlarged spleen or liver or both; lymph nodes may or may not be enlarged

Stage III: As O, I, or II, but Hb conc. <11 g/dl

Stage IV: As O, I, II, or III, but platelet count <100 × 10^9/litre

The medium survival times depend on the staging, which is usually more than 150 months for stage 0 to around 19 months for stages III and IV. More recently Galton (1982) has obtained better prognostic discrimination by the three following clinicopathologic groupings of chronic lymphatic leukaemia arrived at by multivariate analysis:

Group A: (Good prognosis) Hb > 10 g/dl, platelet count > 100 × 10^9/l, fewer than three sites of palpable organ enlargement

Group C: (Bad prognosis) Hb < 10 g/dl or platelets < 100 × 10^9/l

Group B: (Intermediate prognosis) Hb and platelets as in group A but with more than three sites of palpable organ enlargement, the latter meaning enlarged spleen, liver, or localized lymphadenopathy in various parts of the body

Estimation of beta₂-microglobulin, a low molecular weight protein of nucleated cell membrane origin, may be helpful in the staging of this disease. Although the normal concentration of beta₂-microglobulin increases with age, it seldom exceeds 3 mg/l. This level increases progressively to a level of around 17 mg/l in advanced stages of CLL (Späti *et al.*, 1980).

Patients in stages O, I, and II or belonging to group A are probably best managed without any cytotoxic therapy, whereas the conventional oral drug chlorambucil, with or without corticosteroids, is the drug of choice for the more advanced stages. Prolonged therapy is usually required and chlorambucil can be administered either intermittently or continuously at a lower dosage. The usual daily dosage ranges from 2 to 8 mg/m² depending on the therapy schedule.

An important associated feature of untreated CLL, especially in the elderly, is immunodeficiency. The patient suffers from repeated infections, attacks of herpes, etc.

The rarer variants, e.g. prolymphocytic and the hairy cell leukaemias, are refractory to conventional chemotherapeutic regimes. The total lymphocyte cell mass can be reduced by repeated leucapheresis. Splenic irradiation can be attempted in cases of prolymphocytic leukaemia. The course of hairy cell leukaemia can be prolonged and the disease can occasionally achieve a spontaneous remission. In some selected cases, with adequate marrow reserve, splenectomy may be therapeutically justified.

Chronic Myelomonocytic Leukaemia

The classical chronic myeloid leukaemia (CML) is in no way different in the elderly than it is in any other middle aged adult. However, the only variant of CML which deserves a special mention in relation to the very elderly is chronic myelomonocytic leukaemia. This disorder is characterized by splenomegaly and the peripheral blood shows an increase in granulocytes, monocytes, and a population of cells between granulocytes and monocytes. The marrow blast cells are increased but the Ph chromosome, which is present in the classical CML, is lacking. The disease usually runs a prolonged course and is refractory to chemo-

therapy. A terminal blast cell crisis resembling acute myelogenous leukaemia is common.

The management of leukaemic disorders may involve many disciplines—immunology, bacteriology, biochemistry—and the handling of multiple cytotoxic agents requires special skills and facilities. The above discussion is intended as a brief introduction to the subject.

MALIGNANT LYMPHOMA

Non-leukaemic lymphoproliferative malignancies are not uncommon in old age. Characterized by localized or general lymphadenopathy, hepatosplenomegaly, and various systemic symptoms, e.g. fever, weight loss, anaemia, etc., these disorders may pose diagnostic problems. When the disease is at an early stage and is localized, diagnosis is by histological examination of a biopsied lymph node. The two main groups of Hodgkin's and non-Hodgkin's lymphomata are further classified into more detailed histopathological types and require intricate clinical staging. Management depends on the nature and extent of the disease and is usually carried out by a team of oncologists and radiotherapists. Detailed discussion of such conditions is beyond the scope of this chapter.

PARAPROTEIN DISORDERS

Changes of serum globulins may occur in a number of clinical conditions in patients of all ages. The immunological role of globulins has been long appreciated and the term 'immunoglobulin' was introduced to refer to that kind of protein in which specific antibody activity can be detected (Heremans, 1959). Immunoglobulins (Ig) are a heterogeneous collection of serum proteins migrating in the slowest region of electrophoresis and include at least five different types: IgG, IgA, IgM, IgD, IgE, in decreasing order of concentrations. All immunoglobulins have a common basic biochemical structure. Each molecule contains a pair of light chains, Kappa (K) and lambda (L), only one type per molecule, and a pair of heavy chains, gamma, alpha, and so forth. Only one class of heavy chain can link to itself and only one class of light chain can link to a heavy chain in a given immunoglobulin or in a given plasma cell synthesizing the immunoglobulin. The serum Ig levels vary considerably, depending on the general immunological status of the body.

A large number of specific and non-specific disorders give rise to significant alterations; the type and nature of such alteration depends on the basic antigenic stimuli. When only one subclass increases out of a single clone of cells, it is called monoclonal. In other cases the increase in Ig may arise out of two or more cell clones causing a 'di- or polyclonal' gammopathy. Minor protein alteration occurs in 1 per cent. of the general population but the incidence increases with age and abnormal immunoglobulins have been reported in a significant proportion of very old people (Radl *et al.*, 1975).

Some workers have attached considerable importance to the various Ig levels in old age and have equated this with survival (Buckley and Roseman, 1976). In routine practice, significant variation of Ig levels does not occur, even in very old and chronically sick patients (Banerjee, Brocklehurst, and Swindell, 1981).

Myelomatosis, amyloidosis, chronic infections, and lymphoreticular malignancies are associated with an abnormal increase in immunoglobulin levels (Conklin and Alexanian, 1975). Many of these disorders arise out of B-cell dyscrasias involving the haemopoietic system and by far the commonest is myelomatosis.

Myelomatosis

This disease mainly affects older people and is caused by malignant proliferation of a monoclonal population of B-lymphocytes, commonly labelled as malignant plasma cells or 'myeloma' cells. The main features responsible for the major harmful effects are the replacement of the bone marrow by abnormal mitotic cells and excessive production of abnormal proteins.

Clinical Features

Although in some patients myeloma is a chance finding, the majority of cases present with well-recognized symptomatology. These can be grouped as follows: (a) skeletal, (b) neurologic, (c) renal, and (d) metabolic.

Skeletal. Bone pain is the commonest presenting feature and typically occurs in the axial skeleton; it is made worse by movement. Pathological fractures of vertebrae are common, as are the localized swellings, especially in the skull. Occasionally, the patient presents with skeletal deformities of the spine, pelvis, etc., as a result. Radiological manifestation may vary from a single vertebral collapse or an isolated punched-out lesion in the skull to multiple lytic shadows all over the skeletal system. Fractures may be detected. Diffuse rarefaction of bones is seen in occasional patients.

Neurologic. Compression of the spinal cord or nerve roots subsequent to vertebral collapse may present as para- or quadriparesis. Girdle pains, sciatica, and sphincter disturbances can occur. Peripheral neuropathy, carpal tunnel syndrome, etc., may arise as a result of associated amyloidosis.

Renal. Chronic or acute renal insufficiency may be a serious manifestation. Renal infections, tubular damage, hypercalcaemia, etc., are the contributory factors.

Metabolic. Generalized bone involvement may cause severe hypercalcaemia characterized by constipation, dehydration, anorexia, nausea, excessive thirst, etc. Serum uric acid may rise as a result of increased marrow turnover. Severe increase in paraproteins may give rise to hyperviscosity manifestations.

Associated immune-paresis may cause frequent infections. Generalized purpura and bleeding may occur as a result of thrombocytopenia and paraprotein disorder. Rarely, amyloid cardiomyopathy with failure, macroglossia, erythema annulare, hypertrichosis, and yellow discoloration of skin and hair may be some of the atypical presenting features.

The associated protein disturbances have aroused considerable interest. Myeloma is characteristically a malignant proliferation of a single clone of cells secreting one homogeneous paraprotein, i.e. a 'monoclonal' disorder, but a quarter of the patients with this condition exhibit the presence of more than one clone and the tribes of clones increase in frequency after prolonged cytotoxic therapy (Hobbs, 1974). A small number of myeloma sufferers have no paraprotein in their serum.

Typically, the disease is associated with an increase in IgG or IgA levels. Incomplete, low molecular weight light-chain fragments of immunoglobulins may also be synthesized and excreted as Bence–Jones protein (BJP) in the urine.

Immunoelectrophoretically, myelomatosis is of IgG type in 48 per cent., IgA in 22 per cent. and Bence–Jones type in about 22 per cent. Light chains K and L do not coexist; the majority of patients show kappa and a small proportion lambda chains (Hobbs, 1980). A few cases of myeloma with separate increases in IgG, IgD, and IgM levels have also been reported. Clinical manifestation and response to therapy do not usually depend on the nature of the Ig pattern.

Out of the common varieties, IgG lambda-type myelomatosis may have a poorer prognosis than the IgG kappa variety; however, such a relationship is not invariable and definite in all cases (Banerjee, 1977). Similarly, multiband myeloma does not necessarily have any worse prognosis than myeloma associated with a single paraprotein (*BMJ*, 1980).

In the elderly, the diagnosis of myeloma may be unduly delayed. Bone pains and backaches may be attributed to osteoarthritis and age-related osteoporosis, symptoms and signs of renal insufficiency to lack of fluid intake and/or diuretic therapy, and anaemia to dietary inadequacy. Loss of sphincter control due to cord compression, pathological fractures, and extraosseous tumour formation, too, may remain undiagnosed for a long time. A raised serum calcium level does not always produce serious symptoms and the modern multiparameter biochemical reporting often provides the first clue which initiates the full investigative process.

These practical diagnostic difficulties may have considerable influence on the overall prognosis of this disorder (Clinch and Banerjee, 1982).

Management

The prognosis of myeloma depends on a number of factors.

A high serum paraprotein concentration is not necessarily suggestive of a poor prognosis. Severe anaemia, high serum urea, low serum albumin and the presence of excessive urinary Bence–Jones protein and albumin usually indicate a grave prognosis (Hobbs, 1980). In a recent survey of 870 patients attending the Mayo Clinic (Kyle, 1983) the only two significant initial features influencing the duration of survival have been found to be the (a) age and (b) level of urea or creatinine.

A combination of melphalan, (10 mg/m^2) and prednisolone (60 mg/m^2) for 4 consecutive days every 6 weeks has been found to be reasonably tolerated; once the induction of remission is achieved, corticosteroids can be discontinued, especially in the very elderly, to spare their bones from further osteoporosis. Either a 'pulse' therapy with high-dose melphalan or a maintenance with melphalan at a lower dose of around 2 mg/day continuously have both been found to retain excellent remission. It is not unusual for elderly patients to survive such remissions for several years without any problem.

The overall response to therapy is undoubtedly a major factor in inducing a favourable long-term prognosis. The more aggressive M2 regime (cyclophosphamide, melphalan, vincristine, prednisolone, and carmistine [BCNU]) is now considered to be a more effective alternative (Lee, Lake-Lewin, and Myers, 1982).

During the initial stage of therapy, a few important factors should be remembered:

(a) Local lesions, spinal compressions, etc., must be treated with irradiation.

(b) The patient should be adequately hydrated and radiological investigations of kidneys, e.g. IVP, should be avoided if possible.

(c) Severe hypercalcaemia should be corrected and severe anaemia should be treated with transfusions as necessary.

(d) Patients with Bence–Jones proteinurea should be given adequate amounts of oral bicarbonate.

(e) Bone pain should be adequately treated with analgesics.

(f) Hyperviscosity syndrome, if present, may require plasma pheresis.

Benign Monoclonal Gammopathy (BMG)

A monoclonal increase of immunoglobulin is a characteristic feature of myeloma. However, a persistent elevation of a single-band paraprotein may be detected in some apparently normal elderly subjects. It has been suggested that about 1 in 5 of those with monoclonal gammopathy belong to this group called benign monoclonal gammopathy (BMG).

Table 16   Criteria distinguishing BMG and malignant paraprotein disease

	Benign (% incidence)	malignant (% incidence)
1. Ig fragments	0	84
2. Suppression of normal Ig's	10	98
3. Serum paraprotein level > 10 g/l	15	92
4. Progressive rise in paraprotein level	1	99

The transition from a benign state to malignancy is uncommon, but occasional findings indicative of malignancy justify follow-up and cytotoxic treatment (Ritzmann, Daniels, and Levin, 1975).

The genuine BMG may occasionally give rise to hyperviscosity syndrome, amyloidosis, renal tubular problems, thromboembolic complications, etc.

Apart from symptomatic measures, no specific therapy is indicated, but each patient must be followed up and kept under close surveillance. A monoclonal increase in immunoglobulin may occur in patients with chronic liver and intestinal disease and in chronic infections. It is possible that the increased frequency of BMG in the elderly is related to their harbouring more chronic inflammatory disorders compared to patients of younger age groups.

Macroglobulinaemia

A monoclonal increase in high molecular weight IgM or macroglobulin may occur in a variety of conditions, e.g. lymphomas, chronic lymphatic leukaemias, rheumatoid arthritis, cold haemagglutinin disease, various carcinomas, and, indeed, in myelomatosis. These conditions are common in the elderly. Although frequently associated with malignancy, in a significant proportion of cases no underlying mitotic disorder can be found.

The most common cause of a monoclonal rise in IgM is primary macroglobulinaemia (Waldenström, 1944). This is mainly a disease of the elderly and males are more often affected. Pathologically, this condition is graded as a primary malignant disorder of the lymphoreticular system but it is certainly more 'benign' than myeloma. The marrow is infiltrated with a large number of pleomorphic malignant cells with basophilic cytoplasm, resembling lymphocytes and plasma cells, some with PAS positive cytoplasmic inclusions. Because of an excess of paraproteins, there is usually a heavy background staining of the films and marked rouleaux formation of the peripheral red cells. The histology of lymph nodes is commonly preserved although the follicular pattern may be largely lost. Diffuse infiltration with abnormal malignant B-cell clones is the usual feature. IgM-containing cells, mostly of a single light-chain type, may be demonstrated in lymph nodes, bone marrow, and peripheral blood by fluorescent antibody technique. Lymphoid cells from macroglobulinaemic patients can carry both IgM and IgD, the latter being noted primarily on the more immature cells. This is consistent with the hypothesis that the maturation of lymphocytes is associated with a changeover from delta-chain to mu-chain synthesis (Rowe *et al.*, 1973).

Clinical Features

(a) Incipient infiltration of the marrow and associated RE system by malignant cells gives rise to anaemia, infections due to leucopenia, and haemorrhagic manifestation due to thrombocytopenia. Liver, spleen, and lymph nodes may be enlarged.

(b) The presence of excess protein of high molecular weight produces manifestations of hyperviscosity. These include mental changes, headache, lethargy, cerebral and peripheral vascular disease, coma, epistaxis and pulmonary hypertension.

Clinical evidence of hyperviscosity may manifest as dilatation of retinal veins (Fig. 1). However, this is uncommon at a serum IgM level of below 30 g/dl. In more advanced cases the retinal veins become tortuous and eventually their interrupted dilatations may give rise to the classical 'string of sausages' appearance. This is associated with congestion of optic discs; linear and flame-shaped perivenous haemorrhages may occasionally lead to

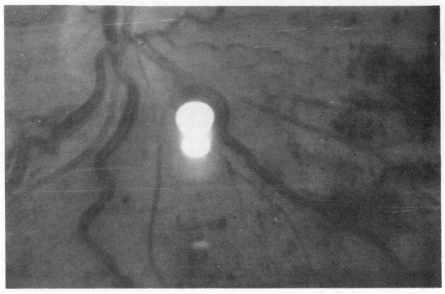

Figure 1   Fundi in Macroglobulanaemia. (By courtesy of Dr P. J. D. Snow)

blindness. Sometimes, associated diffuse amyloidosis causes cardiomyopathy and heart failure.

Unlike myeloma, osteolytic lesions are not seen. However, Bence–Jones nephropathy and renal failure can occasionally occur.

Treatment

(a) The malignant cell proliferation can be suppressed adequately by cytostatic agents. Chlorambucil is the drug of choice although melphalan and cyclophosphamide are effective. Low-dose continuous therapy for an indefinite period is likely to be better tolerated and achieve better results than high-dose intermittent 'pulse' therapy.

(b) Symptoms due to hyperviscosity may warrant urgent relief. Plasma pheresis with a 4L plasma exchange can reduce the serum paraprotein to 5 to 10 per cent. of its initial level. This is followed by regular monthly exchange which usually keeps the patient free of severe symptoms. Rapid and aggressive procedures can precipitate severe hypotension and collapse in an ill elderly patient. The IBM cell separator may play a very useful role here. When fre-

quent plasma pheresis proves ineffective, the oral administration of a thiol-reducing agent penicillamine can cause a substantial decrease in serum macroglobulins and reduce the plasma viscosity.

Amyloidosis

Amyloidosis has been recognized for more than a century as a definite histological and clinical entity, especially in association with long standing inflammatory diseases. The modern concept is that it is an immunological process and occurs in an inadequately controlled immune system. This may explain its high frequency in the very elderly (Walford, 1969). Amyloid is a compound consisting of carbohydrate and protein fractions of immunoglobulin with light- and heavy-chain fragments. The amyloid substance is characterized by its fibrillary ultrastructure and specific staining properties. Broadly, amyloidosis can be classified as primary or secondary. In primary and myeloma-associated amyloidosis immunoglobulin abnormality is obvious. However, in the secondary variety, which is usually associated with chronic inflammatory disease or rheumatoid arthritis, the major component of the amyloid-associated protein has been shown to be unrelated to immunoglobulin (Benditt and Eriksen, 1972). Only primary amyloidosis, therefore, can be counted as a plasma cell or B-cell dyscrasia.

Clinical Features

The clinical manifestations of amyloidosis may include haemorrhagic diathesis, purpura, lymphadenopathy, macroglossia, carpal tunnel syndrome, cardiomyopathy, malabsorptive state, and nephrotic syndrome. Bence–Jones proteinuria can occur. In patients with primary amyloidosis, some form of associated malignancy is not uncommon and a high incidence of renal carcinoma has been noted. The relationship of amyloid and myeloma has been more definitely established. It has been suggested that idiopathic primary amyloidosis and myelomatosis are probably clinical expressions of the same B-cell disorders.

Bence–Jones kappa-type globulin has been identified in urine, serum, and in the synovial fluid of patients with amyloid arthropathy. This may be due to the fact that the amino acid sequence of amyloid protein fragments is homologous with a part of the kappa-type light chain.

Treatment

The primary type of the disease is best treated with cytotoxic drugs effective against other plasma cell disorders, e.g. myeloma. Unfortunately, treatment is not very satisfactory; drugs of the nitrosourea groups, e.g. BCNU, have been found to be beneficial in some cases (Delamore *et al.*, 1975). In patients with chronic inflammatory and/or other disorders, colchicine has been found to be effective in the prevention of secondary amyloid deposits.

Heavy-Chain Disease

These are rare conditions with an excessive synthesis of alpha, gamma, or mu heavy chains with no associated light chains. Alpha heavy-chain paraproteinaemia is the commonest form but is not seen in the elderly. Gamma heavy-chain disease resembles a lymphoma-like condition with a waxing and waning clinical picture. Peripheral pancytopenia with eosinophilia is common. Mu heavy-chain disease strongly resembles chronic lymphatic leukaemia; the diagnosis is clinched by immunoelectrophoresis. This is the rarest variety of all.

Monoclonal Cryoglobulinaemia

Paraproteins can occasionally form crystals or precipitates on exposure to cold and hence the name cryoglobulin. Some cryoproteins are detectable only at low temperatures (16 °C) but others can be demonstrated at a slightly lower (25 to 35 °C) than normal body temperature. The monoclonal cryoglobulins (type I) are mainly associated with lymphoreticular malignancies, whereas the mixed cryoglobulins (types II and III) are often detected in chronic infections, connective tissue and benign lymphoproliferative disorders, and in a variety of liver diseases (Levo, 1980). Trace amounts of mixed IgM–IgG-type cryoproteins are often found in normal individuals (Grey and Kohler, 1973). The protein aggregates can block the skin vessels and, accordingly, the dependent areas of legs, feet, and buttocks are commonly affected. Clinical hypothermia in the elderly can be a common inducer of cryoglobulin activity. The patient should be advised to keep warm and to wear adequate warm clothes. In severe cases, plasma exchange can be helpful.

Polyclonal Increase in Immunoglobulin

A polyclonal increase can sometimes occur in elderly patients. This is usually associated with chronic infections, liver disease, and various other disorders affecting lung, kidneys, and gastrointestinal tract. However, this may not be a regular and universal finding (Hobbs, 1974). Transient paraprotein increase may also be seen after multiple blood transfusions. The appearance of a transient paraprotein is probably a weak manifestation of an antigen–antibody reaction.

PLATELETS AND PURPURA

For proper haemostasis, an adequate number of platelets of good quality is essential. The importance of the functional efficacy of platelets in the blood coagulation process has been appreciated relatively recently. The major difficulties here have always been the complex and rather difficult technical and laboratory procedures necessary to evaluate the platelet function properly. The platelet behaviour also varies considerably between the in vivo and in vitro studies (ten Cate, 1972). Information on the physiology of platelet function in the aged and their general responsiveness in older individuals is somewhat inconsistent and conflicting. Platelet adhesiveness to glass beads has been reported to be increased in the elderly (Bentegeat *et al.*, 1975). Aggregation response to ADP has been found to be more active with age (Grolle *et al.*, 1968; Reading and Rosie, 1980) whereas response to collagen has been reported to decrease (Bankowski, Niewiarowski, and Galasinski, 1967). In a study of 14 healthy subjects with an average age of 80, the glass bead adhesiveness and the aggregation response to ADP was found to be impaired when compared with 27 normal young individuals with an average age of 36 (Banerjee and Etherington, 1974a).

These findings do not necessarily imply that all old people have a basic haemostatic platelet defect which can be manifest clinically, but this may be important and significant in the light of other pathological factors which may have adverse effects on the overall efficiency of platelets.

Irrespective of age, platelet function may be subject to alteration in a number of conditions, e.g. uraemia, macroglobulinaemia, myeloproliferative disorders, and scurvy. Several commonly used drugs such as analgesics and antirheumatics may also do likewise. As these are common factors among elderly patients, the risk of further reduction in their platelet quality with possible haemorrhagic complications must be considered.

Two conditions are particularly relevant in the elderly, scurvy and senile purpura.

Scurvy

Clinical and subclinical scurvy associated with low leucocyte ascorbic acid level is fairly common among the elderly population. Reduction in ascorbic acid level alone is not necessarily associated with clinical scurvy and it is sometimes difficult to assess its overall significance (Banerjee, Lane, and Meichen, 1978). From a haematological point of view, the purpura and bleeding diatheses are due to a generalized defect of collagen synthesis in the capillary wall

endothelium. However, a relationship has been established between defective platelet behaviour and scurvy. It is now known (Born and Wright, 1967; Wilson, McNicol, and Douglas, 1967) that platelet adhesiveness to glass beads and platelet aggregability in general are both reduced in clinical scurvy.

Banerjee and Etherington (1974b) studied the platelet functions in a group of elderly individuals with clinical scurvy and confirmed significant reduction in platelet adhesiveness to glass beads, diminution of platelet aggregability to ADP and collagen, and prolongation of Stypven coagulation time compared with those in young normals. However, when these results were compared with those from normal elderly, the difference was insignificant. This was probably due to the usual reduction in platelet function in old age.

Senile Purpura

Bright red fairly localized purpuric lesions are commonly seen on the exposed skin surface, usually on the dorsum of the hand, in the very elderly. Localized wear and tear and minor trauma to degenerated vessel walls are the suggested aetiologic factors. Skin collagen alters with age and this may be the reason for the vessel wall weakness. The apparent brightness of the lesion and the lack of colour change is probably due to the absence of normal phagocytic response to the extravasated blood (Shuster and Scarborough, 1961).

Not all types of dermal collagen necessarily diminish with age. Although the amount of true elastin is reduced, there is also a qualitative alteration in collagen (Hall, Reed, and Vince, 1974).

The incidence of such 'vascular' purpura is age-related and hence the terminology senile purpura is scientifically correct (Roberts, Andrews, and Caird, 1975; Tattersall and Seville, 1950).

The condition is found to be commoner in males and the overall incidence in both sexes is around 14 per cent. A minor reduction in platelet aggregation to extrinsic collagen has been found (Banerjee and Etherington, 1973).

In summary, senile purpura is primarily due to shearing strain to a thin skin with altered collagen architecture.

Non-thrombocytopenic purpura from allergic vasculitis may result from bacterial sensitiv-ity reaction and drug therapy. Cases of Henoch–Schonlein purpura, primarily a pae-diatric disorder, can also be seen in very old age. However, the clinical features may vary a little and the course may be different.

The relation between drugs and purpura is important. A large variety of drugs can cause purpura either by vascular damage or by caus-ing a reduction in the number of platelets.

Idiopathic Thrombocytopenic Purpura

Whether acute or chronic, this condition is usually seen in younger people. However, this condition can occur at any age (Pitney, 1973). Cases of ITP have been reported in the seventh and eighth decades of life (Weiss, Kock, and Richardson, 1975). In fact, some reports sug-gest that the incidence of ITP in the elderly can be as high as 30 per cent. of the total incidence covering all age groups (Aster and Keene, 1969; Shashaty and Rath, 1978). The natural history of this condition is probably the same as in younger patients but with certain minor differences. Unlike the young, there is no female preponderance. Serious complica-tions are usually rare. Corticosteroid therapy seems to be equally effective but response to splenectomy, in certain cases, is not as satis-factory as in the young (Hyams, 1978).

Other Bleeding Disorders

Acquired Haemophilia

The level of factor VIII does not alter with age. In one detailed study of 80 normal indi-viduals carefully matched for sex and increas-ing age groups, a fairly constant level of factor VIII activity has been demonstrated (Dodds *et al.*, 1975). The same study has shown a sig-nificant increase in the levels of factor VII, IX, and plasminogen.

Classical hereditary haemophilia is not likely to be a diagnostic problem in old age. How-ever, over the last decade or so, a condition resulting from the development of factor VIII-neutralizing antibodies with clinical fea-tures of spontaneous deep tissue haemorrhage has been described. The typical patient is eld-erly and female (*Lancet*, 1981a). Although the majority of patients do not have any concur-rent disorder, there is an association with dis-

orders having an autoimmune or allergic basis. These include rheumatoid arthritis, various forms of carcinoma, different connective tissue disorders, ulcerative colitis, and pemphigus. Occasionally it may be a side-effect of penicil-lin therapy. History of previous blood trans-fusions is usually absent. The diagnosis of acquired haemophilia depends on clinical ob-servation of a bleeding diathesis in a patient with no such bleeding history. Bleeding is spontaneous and usually serious, occurring in deep tissues and joints. Prolonged bleeding af-ter routine surgery or even minor trauma is characteristic. The whole blood clotting time and activated partial thromboplastin time are prolonged whereas the bleeding time and pro-thrombin time are normal. Factor VIII activity in plasma is abnormally low or undetectable. Specific IgG antibodies against factor VIII are present in high titres. The levels of anti-VIII antibodies usually correlate well with severity of haemorrhagic manifestation. Accordingly, spontaneous remission is not uncommon.

Treatment. Any procedure likely to provoke haemorrhage should be avoided. Injections, overenthusiastic mobilization, and aggressive physiotherapy may all cause serious bleeding. Invasive investigations and surgery of doubtful value are contraindicated. Steroids with cyclo-phosphamide seem to be the most effective medical therapy (Green, Schuette, and Wal-lace, 1980). Acute bleeding episodes are un-likely to be corrected by fresh frozen plasma or cryoprecipitates, as they are prone to be rapidly neutralized by the antibodies. Infusion of polyelectrolyte fractionated porcine factor VIII concentrate is the only useful and effec-tive agent. Apart from its prohibitive cost and general non-availability severe thrombocyto-penia can be precipitated in frail old patients. Therefore, the best line of management would be to adopt strict prophylactic measures against iatrogenic haemorrhage (*Lancet*, 1981a).

Fibrinolysis and Associated Disorders

Physiologically, in vivo coagulation activity and fibrinolytic activity exist concurrently. A delicate balance needs to be maintained be-tween these two opposing processes for keep-ing the vascular tree patent.

The plasminogen–plasmin enzyme system is the main fibrinolytic system in the blood. Plasminogen is probably synthesized in the liver and is present at a constant plasma level of 1 to 2 umol/l. Plasminogen is activated to plasmin by a number of plasma and vessel wall activators.

Activated plasmin then dissolves the organized fibrin thrombus into various degradation products. Inhibiting factors are also present and within the plasminogen-plasmin conversion process itself, the relative influence of activators and inhibitors may be of crucial significance (Fig. 2).

With advancing age the fibrinolytic activity diminishes a little (Robertson, Pandolfi, and Nilsson, 1972; Rosing *et al.*, 1973). In a detailed study of elderly subjects with advanced atheromatous vascular disease, increased concentration of prothrombin was detected in the lipid and fibrin-rich plaques. The ratios of plasmin inhibitors to prothrombin was considerably lower than that in normal intima (Smith and Staples, 1981). It is, therefore, likely that once fibrin has accumulated within the intima of vessels, sequestration of such deposits along with other clotting factors continue to happen as a self-generating system. Various studies of vessel wall fibrinolytic activity have been carried out in the elderly. Some workers have suggested that such activity is significantly impaired in leg vessels in old age (Robertson, Pandolfi, and Nilsson, 1972). This observation

may or may not have clinical significance in the increased incidence of thrombotic disease in the lower limbs of elderly patients. Fibrinolytic activity is abnormally low in many thrombotic disorders, e.g. coronary artery disease, peripheral arterial and venous disorders, and cutaneous vasculitis (Kernoff and McNicol, 1977). In postoperative patients with deep vein thrombosis, a fibrinolytic 'shutdown' is preceded by overactivity.

Drugs which enhance fibrinolysis, e.g. phenformin, ethyloestrenol, and stanozolol have all been used with success in the treatment of venous thrombosis (Fearnley *et al.*, 1967), Raynaud's phenomenon (Jarrett, Morland, and Browse, 1978), and various postphlebitic disorders (Burnand *et al.*, 1980).

Onion and garlic can increase blood fibrinolytic activity and reduce the levels of blood lipids and fibrinogen (Sharma, Sharma, and Arora, 1978).

If vascular intima is a major source of fibrinolytic activators, mechanical stimulation and compression of blood vessels might enhance fibrinolysis.

Pneumatic intermittent compression of limbs has been reported to be of value in reducing the incidence of postoperative thrombosis (*Lancet*, 1981b). Whether the benefit is entirely due to activated fibrinolysis or purely mechanical due to an increase in blood flow is open to question. Application of intermittent pneumatic calf compression does not alter the

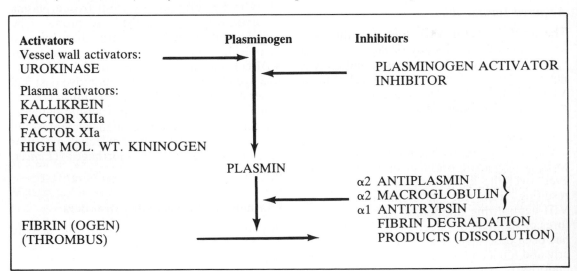

Figure 2   Fibrinolytic system

incidence of post-stroke deep vein thrombosis (Prasad, Banerjee, and Howard, 1982).

Disseminated Intravascular Coagulation (DIC)

In its acute form, this is a serious complication which may arise in patients with multiple trauma and with fulminant stephylococcal and meningococcal septicaemias. Severe hypothermia can also be an important precipitating factor. A more subacute form of DIC can be seen in various forms of malignancy. Prostatic carcinoma with metastases, and malignant tumours of the lung, stomach, colon, breast, and ovary are some of the common causes. Acute promyelocytic leukaemia and some cases of subacute or chronic myelomonocytic and lymphatic leukaemias may give rise to serious haemorrhagic problems (Donati, Poggi, and Semeraro, 1981).

Clinical Features

In severe cases, haemorrhage is the most common and obvious feature. This occurs in the skin in the form of generalized purpura and ecchymoses. Serious gastrointestinal and other mucosal bleeding may be life-threatening. Prolonged oozing from a venepuncture site may be an early warning sign. In a small but significant number of affected patients, clinical thromboembolic disorder may be apparent. Peripheral gangrene or cyanosis, thrombophlebitis, etc., may occur, although major arterial or venous thrombosis is uncommon. The other general and systemic features of DIC include jaundice, uraemia with metabolic acidosis, and cardiorespiratory failure, all of which carry an extremely grave prognosis. On the contrary, in many cases, the process is mild and is detectable only by laboratory investigations. Similarly, when the DIC process is subacute or chronic, the clinical picture may be less obvious. Gram-negative septicaemias are often responsible for low-grade DIC without any frank haemorrhage.

The common trigger appears to be the liberation of the procoagulant thromboplastin in the blood and the term 'consumption coagulopathy' characterizes the decrease in platelets and various clotting factors. The prothrombin time is markedly prolonged, fibrinogen drops below 1g/l and the platelet count is less than 100×10^9 per litre. This, together with fibri-nolysis as shown by increased levels of FDP, explains the bleeding defect.

In addition to the increased coagulative process and fibrinolysis, a decrease in the levels of naturally occurring anticoagulant factors in the blood also becomes obvious. The principal ones in this category are antithrombin and protein C. Antithrombin is a strong inhibitor of thrombin in the plasma as a physiological entity and its level diminishes with age (Odegard, Fagerhal, and Lie, 1976). During any active process of DIC, the concentration of antithrombin falls even further to a very low level (Abildgaard, 1981). Protein C is a vitamin K dependent plasma protein with the property of inhibiting the coagulation cascade. So far, there is no evidence that, like antithrombin, the blood level of protein C alters with age. However, in all types of DIC, whether active or well compensated, the level of protein C also falls to a very low or unmeasurable level (Mannucci and Vigano, 1982).

Treatment of DIC

Needless to say, the associated conditions must be adequately treated. Patients with fulminant infections and septicaemias will require appropriate antibiotics, usually multiple and in high dosage. Patients with leukaemias need to be treated with proper antileukaemic chemotherapy. If the fibrinogen is less than 0.5 g/l, an immediate infusion of fibrinogen can be life-saving. However, the effect will be only transient. Similarly, infusion of platelet concentrates for severe thrombocytopenia or fresh frozen plasma to correct factors V and VIII deficiencies may be required. As the basic process being increased is microcoagulation, heparin therapy has been used with beneficial results. An initial dose of 50 to 100 units/kg with 10 to 15 units/kg per hour thereafter by a slow i.v. infusion is generally enough. As this may create adverse complications in severe thrombocytopenic and in postoperative cases, the decision of instituting heparin therapy in mild to moderate cases of DIC should be made with great caution, and in the majority of patients it should be avoided. Because of a significant drop in the anti-thrombin level in blood, administration of antithrombin by continuous infusion has recently met with success (Abildgaard, 1981).

BLOOD DISORDERS IN MALIGNANCY

Every type of haematologic change may arise in patients with malignant disease. Various treatments of malignancy, e.g. cytotoxic agents, surgery, and irradiation, may have haematological sequelae.

Anaemia is undoubtedly the commonest haematologic manifestation of mitotic disease (Table 17). Changes in white cells, platelets, and the coagulation system can also occur, but these are relatively uncommon and are usually associated with widespread dissemination.

Table 17 Causes of anaemia in malignancy

1. Loss of blood	Haemorrhage
2. Lack of haematinics and nutrients	Iron, folate, vitamin B12, proteins, etc.
3. Lack of adequate iron utilization and erythropoiesis	Anaemia of chronic disorder, sideroblastic anaemia.
4. Increased breakdown of RBC	Haemolysis
5. Suppression and infiltration of marrow	

Iron-deficiency anaemia in malignancy is almost always due to chronic blood loss. Dietary inadequacy or malabsorption of iron may occur but they are not common. Mild iron-deficiency anaemia may be difficult to distinguish from anaemia of chronic disorder.

Demand for folate may increase with accelerated cell turnover in fast-growing tumours. Concurrent infections also increase folate requirement. These factors, associated with dietary inadequacy, can sometimes precipitate severe and acute folate deficiency (Ibbotson, Colvin, and Colvin, 1975). Cytotoxic antifolate drugs and antimicrobial cotrimoxazole may also cause similar problems.

Total gastrectomy or extensive small bowel surgery involving the terminal ileum may give rise to vitamin B12 deficiency. As a rule, B12 deficiency is not common in malignancy, but in some cases of liver cell cancer, especially of the fibrolamellar variety (Paradinas *et al.*, 1982) and in myeloproliferative disorders, a marked increase in serum B12 levels may be observed. Such elevation of serum B12 level is due to an associated increase in the B12-binding protein, transcobalamin (Waxman and Gilbert, 1974).

Low-grade haemolysis is fairly frequent in malignancy and the aetiology is usually autoimmune. Carcinomas of ovary, cervix, breast, stomach, colon, and bronchus may all cause autoimmune haemolysis. The lymphoreticular disorders may cause frank haemolysis. Warm-antibody induced haemolysis is frequently associated with disseminated lymphomata and chronic lymphatic leukaemia.

Leucoerythroblastic Anaemia

Leucoerythroblastic anaemia characterized by the presence of immature red and white cells in the peripheral blood may occur with any form of malignancy and usually signifies the infiltration of bone marrow with foreign mitotic cells. The commoner primary sites are prostate, lungs, and breast. Occasionally, the primary cannot be detected and the marrow infiltration is the only feature of malignancy (Bateman and Beard, 1976).

Many patients with carcinomas and lymphoma have an expanded plasma volume (Price and Greenfield, 1960) and this may contribute to the overall blood picture. Marked splenomegaly, if present, may have a causal role. Inappropriate excessive production of antidiuretic hormone can occur in malignancies of bronchus, pancreas, etc., and in lymphomas and can cause increased retention of water. This can alter the degree of anaemia and haematocrit levels considerably.

Polycythaemia

Rarely, polycythaemia with increased red cell mass can be seen in certain malignant disorders. The pathogenesis of such a change is usually attributed to the increased and perhaps inappropriate production of erythropoietin. The malignant tumours of those organs which tend to cause increased production of erythropoietin are kidney, liver, uterus, and cerebellum (Hammond and Winnick, 1974). Complete surgical removal of these tumours usually corrects the polycythaemia.

Changes in Leucocytes

A marked increase in total leucocyte count along with the appearance of a large number of immature white cells in the peripheral blood can, sometimes, be a feature of advanced malignant disease. However, concurrent fulminant infections or septicaemias may also be responsible for such 'leukaemoid' reaction.

Isolated elevation of only one type of white cell is probably more common. Table 18 gives a list of a few such associations. The exact mechanism of such leukaemoid reaction in malignancy remains uncertain; primary haematologic malignancies and leukaemias must be excluded.

Table 18 Selective leucocyte change in malignancy

1. Lymphocytosis	Malignancies of breast, gastrointestinal tract, bronchus
2. Eosinophilia	Malignancies of bronchus, thyroid, and cervix
3. Neutrophilia	Disseminated malignancy of any kind

Changes in Platelets

An increase in platelet count may be a 'physiological' response to bleeding from a malignant tumour. However, uncommonly an unexplained thrombocytosis may be a marker of an occult malignant lesion (Davis and Ross, 1973). Carcinomas of bronchus, breast, pancreas, kidney, intestines, and ovary are known to cause an increase in the peripheral platelet count. Disseminated malignancies with widespread intravascular coagulation can, on the other hand, result in a dramatic reduction in the number of circulating platelets.

A number of abnormalities of platelet functions has also been described. Defects in platelet aggregation response to various stimuli, in platelet coagulation activities, and in platelet prostaglandin synthetic pathway may be found in various malignant disorders, and they can give rise to clinical haemorrhagic complications (Donati, Poggi, and Semeraro, 1981). Some deficiency in platelet lipoxygenase activity has recently been observed in myeloproliferative disorders (Schafer, 1982).

Coagulation Abnormalities

An increased frequency of vascular thrombosis is a well-recognized feature of malignant disease. There is most commonly seen with mucous-producing adenocarcinomas. Pancreas, colon, stomach, ovary, and lungs are the usual sites. Both venous and arterial thrombosis can occur; non-bacterial thrombotic endocarditis may cause arterial embolization (Rosen and Armstrong, 1973). Apart from spontaneous thromboembolism and thrombosis migrans, patients with malignancy are prone to thrombosis when exposed to haemostatic stimuli. The incidence of postoperative thromboembolic complications rises sharply in patients with cancer.

A generalized bleeding tendency, with or without thrombosis, is sometimes seen in patients with solid tumours. Although this may arise with carcinoma of bronchus, stomach, colon, or breast, the commonest lesion to cause this is carcinoma of prostate (Sun *et al.*, 1979), an extremely common condition in the elderly.

Various haemostatic abnormalities have been observed in patients with malignant disease but these are not necessarily associated with clinical haemorrhage and/or thrombosis. The prothrombin time, the whole blood clotting time, and the partial thromboplastin time may all be shortened, whereas there may be elevation of one or more coagulation factors, fibrinogen and fibrin degradation products with the presence of circulating fibrin monomers. The antithrombin level may be reduced (Sun *et al.*, 1979).

Platelet and/or fibrinogen turnover is increased; this is commonly seen in the absence of other coagulation disturbance and may relate to a specific type of tumour (Lyman *et al.*, 1978). Human malignant tissues and experimental tumours harbour a procoagulant activity (O'Meara, 1958).

Malignant cells have some non-specific 'thromboplastic' activity and this is probably different from that present in the apparently normal tissues, in both quality and quantity. Cancer cells can directly activate the coagulation factor X and this process is entirely distinct from the intrinsic or extrinsic pathways of the blood clotting system (Gordon and Lewis, 1978). The extrinsic pathway can be triggered separately by some malignant tissue factors subsequent to the activation of factor VII in the presence of calcium ions. Platelets can be influenced in malignancy and may become increasingly procoagulant.

Many tumour tissues are known to activate the fibrinolytic process and this is precipitated by a release of a plasminogen-activating substance from the cancer cells. The procoagulant and fibrinolytic activities quite often exist together and it is the relationship between these two processes that is ultimately responsible for the overall clinical effects.

DRUG-INDUCED BLOOD DISORDERS

Approximately 8 out of every 10 old people consume an average of 2.3 prescribed medications at any time. The overall incidence of drug complication among the total elderly population is around 12 per cent. (Williamson and Chopin, 1980).

Drug-related haematologic disorders and side-effects are not frequent in elderly patients. Drugs, by virtue of their direct effects on the haemopoietic system, the marrow and the peripheral blood, can give rise to 'primary' haematologic problems; on the other hand, 'secondary' changes in blood may arise from the effects of drugs on other organs of the body. Perhaps the most relevant and important of these 'secondary' manifestations is iron deficiency anaemia due to chronic blood loss from the gastrointestinal tract.

Anaemia Due to Chronic Blood Loss

Salicylates have been well recognized as gastrointestinal irritants capable of causing dyspepsia and indigestion. Occult bleeding has also been a well-known side-effect. The blood loss is commonly 5 ml/day or less and anaemia rarely occurs (Wood, Harvey-Smith, and Dixon, 1962) except when iron reserve is inadequate. However, higher daily blood loss may produce overt anaemia. Such blood loss with aspirin is dose-related and is dependent on the frequency of administration (Levy, 1974). Simultaneous intake of antacids and hydrogen-receptor antagonists decrease such occult blood loss whereas alcohol increases it. Patients with already existing peptic ulceration, oesophageal varices, and other bleeding diathesis are naturally more prone to iatrogenic gastroduodenal haemorrhage and every attempt should be made to avoid salicylate preparations in these patients.

Non-steroidal anti-inflammatory drugs such as indomethacin and phenylbutazone can cause microbleeding from the upper gastrointestinal tract (Trewby, 1980) and result in iron-deficiency anaemia after long-term therapy. Various statistical figures are frequently used to claim one analgesic's superiority over others, but in any elderly patient (Clinch *et al.*, 1982, 1983), the causal relationship between prolonged analgesic intake and an overt iron-deficiency anaemia must be critically reviewed.

Although on the basis of clinical impression and anecdotal experience, corticosteroid therapy has been implicated with an increased incidence of peptic ulcer, in general, corticosteroids in a low maintenance dosage have not show any correlation with upper gastrointestinal side-effects (Boston Collaborative Drug Surveillance Programme, 1972). When given in conjunction with other irritant analgesic agents, there may be an additive effect and chronic blood loss may be clinically apparent. Enteric coated steroid preparations are usually not safer; for essential use, perhaps the lowest therapeutic dose given less frequently along with antacids and hydrogen-blockers is the best alternative.

No firm statement can be made to the effect that corticosteroids should not be used in the presence of known peptic ulcer disease (Douglas and Bateman, 1981). Very recently, a large-scale study from the United States has strongly suggested that corticosteroids, by themselves, do increase the risk of peptic ulcers and gastrointenstinal haemorrhage (Messer *et al.*, 1983).

Among other commonly used drugs in the elderly, the diuretic, ethacrynic acid (Jick and Porter, 1978), slow K, and potassium chloride (Collins *et al.*, 1979) have been known to cause chronic blood loss from the upper gastrointenstinal tract. Oesophageal ulceration and slow haemorrhage can occur with emepronium bromide (Cetiprin), an agent frequently used to treat urinary incontinence. Alcohol ingestion may render the stomach more susceptible to drug induced haemorrhage.

Anticoagulants will naturally have an additive effect to all these gastroenteric irritants.

Megaloblastic Anaemia

This is probably the least common of the reported major drug-induced haematologic problems and may arise by three major pathogenetic mechanisms (Table 19).

Table 19 Mechanisms of drug-induced megaloblastic anaemia

I. Disturbance of folate metabolism	Anticonvulsants e.g. phenytoin, primidone, barbiturates Antituberculous, e.g. cycloserine Folate antagonists, e.g. trimethoprim and cotrimoxazole, triamterene, aminopterin Miscellaneous, e.g. salazopyrine
II. Malabsorption of vitamin B12	Metformin, neomycin, paramino-salicylic acid, slow K
III. Nucleic acid synthesis inhibitors	Various cytotoxic agents, e.g. azathioprine, thioguanine, cytosine arabinoside

Not infrequently, the clinical and haematological picture become quite severe. As may be expected, people with inadequate body stores of folate or B12 are more likely to be affected.

Hypoplastic Anaemia

Total or selective suppression of bone marrow is a fairly well-known and a relatively common adverse effect of certain drugs. Some commonly used drugs which are most frequently incriminated in marrow hypoplasia are mentioned in Table 20.

Table 20 List of drugs associated with marrow hypoplasia

Antimicrobials	Chloramphenicol
	Sulphonamides
Antirheumatics	Phenybutazone
	Oxyphenbutazone
	Indomethacin
	Gold preparations
Tranquillizers	Chlorpromazine
Anticonvulsants	Phenytoin
Antidiabetics	Chlorpropamide

The mechanisms by which drugs may induce marrow damage can be divided into three broad groups:
(a) Dose-dependent: affecting mainly the formation of cells in the marrow; changes usually reversible.
(b) Conditional or sensitivity effect: defect probably genetically determined; either the target cells or the drug metabolism is abnormal; usually fatal.
(c) Immunological: dose and time relationships are erratic.

However, there may be considerable overlap between these mechanisms and one agent may act through different channels at the same time. From the clinical point of view, the properties of individual drugs and the frequency and dose of their usage are extremely important. Chloramphenicol, for example, is reasonably safe if prescribed for a short while at a lower dosage, whereas with a high dose there is likely to be a dose related erythroid depression or even a reversible panhypoplasia, presumably due to its inhibition of protein synthesis in the cell mitochondria (Yunis, 1973).

It has been suggested that some drugs cause irreversible hypoplasia by not only damaging the pluripotential haematopoietic stem cell but also by a total inhibition of the 'transit' compartment through which the various maturation processes advance. Again, the detailed mechanisms of all aplasias cannot be satisfactorily explained with this hypothesis alone (Geary, 1979).

Gold compounds probably produce marrow damage by a different mechanism. In some cases, the damage seems to be predictable and dose-related, while in others the blood picture may change with dramatic suddenness. Marrow damage with chlorpromazine is usually dose-dependent yet unpredictable. This is probably due to a constitutional defect in marrow cells and the transit compartment only is damaged rather than the stem cells. The changes are usually rapidly reversible (Pisciotta, 1971).

Cytotoxic agents, as a group, are extremely likely to induce marrow aplasia. Both phase-specific (e.g. Ara-C) and cycle-active (e.g. alkylating agents) groups of drugs broadly leave the resting stem cells unharmed; accordingly, despite temporary setbacks, ultimate recovery of marrow is usual. However, the situation may be different in cases of repeated doses, a point especially important in elderly patients.

Haemolytic Anaemia

The mechanisms of drug-induced haemolysis can be classified as follows:

(a) Immune   mechanisms   with   positive
    Coomb's test:

Antimicrobials	Penicillin
	Sulphonamide
	Cephalothin
	Rifampicin
	Isoniazid
Antihypertensive	Methyldopa
Antirheumatics	Mefenamic acid
	Amidopyrine
Tranquillizer	Chlorpormazine
Others	Chlorpropamide
	Quinine
	Quinidine
	Hydralazine
	Procainamide
	Levodopa.

(b) Direct haemolysis:
    Sulphones, phenacetin, acetanilide.

(c) Oxidative haemolysis due to intrinsic red-
    cell defects, enzyme deficiences, etc.:
    Aspirin, primaquine, sulphonamides, sul-
    phones, nitrofurantoin, chloroquine.

Oxidative haemolysis is extremely rare
in routine geriatric practice. Rapid and direct destruction of red cells due to drugs
and chemicals like lead, arsenic, and na-
phthalene are also quite rare these days
and, in general, such interactions are
uncommon.

The various immune haemolysis mechanisms
are seen from time to time but, despite a positive Coomb's test, the detailed mechanisms
are not always adequately understood. Two
different types of immunologically mediated
haemolysis are recognized (Worlledge, 1969):
(a) Immune haemolysis in which the anti-
    bodies are directed against the offending
    drug and cannot be demonstrated unless
    the drug is also present.
(b) Autoimmune haemolysis in which the
    antibodies are directed against the red
    cell antigens and can be detected all the
    time. Drugs like methyldopa, mefenamic
    acid and L-dopa fall into this category.
       About 20 per cent. of patients on meth-
    yldopa, at a relatively high dosage for a
    long time, develop a positive Coomb's
    test of IgG type but fortunately only 0.15
    to 0.3 per cent. of them actually manifest
    clinical haemolysis.

Penicillin, in massive intravenous dosage,
can give rise to immune haemolysis and the
antibodies are attached to red cell membrane.
Hydralazine, on the other hand, can cause a
lupus erythematosus-like clinical picture and in
addition to a positive Coomb's test, a large
number of LE cells can be detected.

Depending on the individual mechanism, the
clinical picture may vary. The haemolysis can
be very rapid and can occur within a few days
of drug exposure in the 'immune' type whereas
in the 'autoimmune' variety (as with methyldopa) it is usually very slow and is only occasionally clinically overt. Withdrawal of the
causative drug is mandatory but in patients on
multiple drug therapy this may be difficult.
Supportive transfusions and corticosteroids
therapy may be required in severe cases.

Thrombocytopenia

This is probably the commonest form of drug
related blood disorder at all ages and is particularly common in the elderly (Bottiger and
Westerholm, 1972). In every case of thrombocytopenia without an obvious cause a drug
must be considered as a possible aetiological
factor and in every case of apparent idiopathic
thrombocytopenia, especially in the elderly, a
drug association must be seriously explored
even if the drug has been consumed some time
ago.

A reduction in platelet count may be a feature of an overall marrow hypoplasia, but
drugs may frequently cause a selective platelet
deficiency. There are two principal mechanisms by which drug-induced selective thrombocytopenia may occur:
(a) immunological with increased destruction
    of platelets in the peripheral blood;
(b) selective depression of megakaryocytes in
    the bone marrow.

In addition, there may be a third mechanism
where there is a dose-related non-immune action of a drug on the platelets, but this is extremely uncommon (De Gruchy, 1975).

The exact pathogenesis of drug-associated immune thrombocytopenia remains unclear and
it is sometimes suggested that in some cases
the metabolite of the causative drug acts as a
hapten in the immunological reaction, rather
than the drug itself.

It is impossible to provide a complete list of

all the drugs which can cause thrombocytopenia. Such cases of thrombocytopenia are being reported constantly.

However, among the commonly prescribed drugs among the elderly in this country, antirheumatic phenylbutazone and antimicrobial cotrimoxazole are probably the most frequent offenders. Table 21 lists some frequently used drugs which are known to cause thrombocytopenia.

Table 21   Drugs which may cause thrombocytopenia

Anti-rheumatics	Phenylbutazone, indomethacin, gold compounds, aspirin, paracetamol.
Anti-microbials	Cotrimoxazole, sulphonamides, chloramphenicol, ristocetin, rifampicin, ampicillin, tetracycline.
Diuretics	Thiazides, frusemide, acetazolamide, spironolactone
Antidiabetics	Chlorpropamide, tolbutamide
Psychotropics	Amitriptyline, imipramine, thioridazine, meprobamate, diazepam.
Cinchona alkaloids	Quinine, quinidine
Others	Carbamazepine, oestrogens, heparin, digitoxin, trinitrin

Many non-ethical products which do not require a doctor's prescription may contain offending ingredients. Various tonics and cramp pills have varying amounts of quinine and are frequently consumed by old people.

The clinical manifestations may vary. Although, classically dramatic, occurring shortly after the ingestion of the last dose, sometimes the onset is slow, and the cessation of bleeding and return of the platelet count to normal do not always happen immediately following drug withdrawal. Generalized purpura and mucous membrane bleeding from the mouth and gastrointestinal tract are fairly typical. The mortality in this complication is around 20 per cent. and the death is most often due to cerebral haemorrhage. The offending drug or drugs must be withdrawn immediately and supportive therapy with platelet concentrates, fresh blood, and corticosteroids should be followed. The patient must also be advised to avoid the suspected drug or drugs and be given an appropriate warning card for future medical attendance.

All prostaglandin-inhibiting drugs can affect the quality of platelets and may indeed precipitate haemorrhagic complications.

Neutropenia and Agranulocytosis

Granulocytes are vulnerable to various commonly used drugs. Drug-induced agranulocytosis is not uncommon among the elderly. Many such offensive drugs, e.g. amidopyrine and its byproducts, are no longer prescribed in the United Kingdom.

Table 22   Drugs associated with granulocytopenia

Antithyroid	Carbimazole methimazole
Antirheumatics	Phenylbutazone oxyphenbutazone
Antimicrobials	Sulphonamides chloramphenicol
Antidiabetics	Sulphonylureas
Tranquillizers and psychotropics	Phenothiazines, meprobamate, amitriptyline, imipramine
Others	Acetazolamide, antazoline, phenytoin, penicillamine

Cytotoxic drugs can also cause reduction in white cells and platelets. Selective neutropenia may occur by two pathogenetic ways:

(a)   Immune sensitivity reaction where a sensitive donor's plasma causes leucocyte agglutination in normal subjects. This is not dose related and a small amount of the drug can precipitate an abrupt crisis.

(b)   Direct toxic effect on the leucocyte nucleic acid synthesis and the mitochondria. This is a dose-dependent response and the drug does not render the patient prone to similar effects on renewed exposure. The neutropenic victims are naturally more susceptible to infections.

The neutrophil count may sometimes drop below 200 per cubic millimetre and the patient requires careful barrier-nursing, antibiotics, etc., until recovery occurs.

Effects of Radiation

An increasing number of elderly patients are receiving exposure to radiation for a variety of therapeutic reasons.

The various haematologic changes following irradiation can be divided into the exposure phase, the delay time, the prodromal phase, the latent phase, the secondary phase of frank hypoplasia, and the convalescent phase (Thoma and Wald, 1959). The rapidity of these reactions naturally depends on the acuteness and severity of the radiation exposure, and frank marrow aplasia may develop within 3 to 6 weeks in an acute radiation sickness.

Of the peripheral-formed elements, lymphocytes are the most radiosensitive. A dose of as low as 25 rad may cause an almost immediately detectable lymphopenia. However, this is also associated with a transient increase in neutrophils which disappears shortly afterwards. A steady and progressive lymphopenia continues to develop for about 15 days. An increased number of multinucleated lymphocytes appear in the peripheral blood. Reduction of lymphocytes is the most persistent index of radiation exposure and may persist for a long time following a large dose. Low-level chronic exposure is not usually associated with a lymphocyte change (Donati and Gantner, 1973). Changes in red cells, haemoglobin, and haematocrit are not frequent and marginal reductions are observed only after 7 to 10 days. Severe thrombocytopenia causing clinical haemorrhage occurs only after acute and large-dose radiation exposure. In other cases, minor thrombocytopenia may occur but this is usually a delayed change and is not of great clinical relevance. The bone marrow may show some early changes in the erythrocyte precursors and this is followed by changes in the white cell and megakaryocyte series.

REFERENCES

Abildgaard, U. (1981). 'Antithrombin and related inhibitors of coagulation', in *Recent Advances in Blood Coagulation* (Ed. L. Poller), Vol. 3, pp. 151–173, Churchill Livingstone, Edinburgh.

Adam, H. M., Dawson, A. A., Wigzell, F. W., and Roy, S. K. (1973). 'Polymorph hypersegmentation in the elderly', *Age Ageing*, 2, 183–188.

Anderson, B. B., Peart, M. B., and Fulford-Jones, C. E. (1970). 'The measurement of serum pyridoxal by a microbiological assay using lactobacillus casei', *J. Clin. Pathol.*, 23, 232–242.

Andral, G., and Gavarret, J. (1842). 'Recherches sur les modifications de proportion de quelques principes de sang, fibrine, globules, materiaux solides du serum et eau dans les maladies'. Cited by F. Nilsson (1948) in *Acta. Med. Scand.*, 130, Suppl. 210.

Andrews, J., Fairley, A., and Barker, R. (1967). 'Total dose infusion of iron-dextran in the elderly', *Scott. Med. J.*, 12, 208–215.

Arnold, K. G. (1981) 'Cerebral blood flow in geriatrics'. *Age Ageing*, 10, 5–9.

Aster, R. H., and Keene, W. R. (1969). 'Sites of platelet destruction in idiopathic thrombocytopenic purpura', *Br. J. Haematol.*, 16, 61–73.

Bahemuka, M., Denham, M. J., and Hodkinson, H. M. (1973) 'Macrocytosis', *Mod. Geriatr.*, 3, 421–422.

Bainton, D. F., and Finch, C. A. (1964). 'The diagnosis of iron-deficiency anaemia', *A. J. Med.*, 37, 62–70.

Banerjee, A. K. (1975). 'Macrocytic anaemia in the elderly' *Mod. Geriatr.*, 5, 12–16.

Banerjee, A. K. (1976). 'Geriatric medicine', in *Haematological Aspects of Systemic Disease* (Eds M. C. G. Israels and I. W. Delamore), 1st ed., pp. 409–439, Holt Saunders, London.

Banerjee, A. K. (1977). 'What protein disorders mean in old age', *Mod. Geriatr.*, 7, 28–33.

Banerjee, A. K., Lane, P. J., and Meichen, F. W. (1978). 'Vitamin C and osteoporosis in old age', *Age Ageing*, 1, 16–18.

Banerjee, A. K., Brocklehurst, J. C., and Swindell, R. (1981). 'Protein status in long-stay geriatric in-patients', *Gerontology*, 27, 161–166.

Banerjee, A. K., and Etherington, M. (1973). 'Senile purpura and platelets', *Gerontol. Clin. (Basel)*, 15, 213–220.

Banerjee, A. K., and Etherington, M. (1974a). 'Platelet function in old age', *Age Ageing*, 3, 29–35.

Banerjee, A. K., and Etherington, M. (1974b). 'Platelet function in elderly scorbutics', *Age Ageing*, 3, 97–105.

Banerjee, A. K., Lane, P. J., and Meichen, F. W. (1978). 'Vitamin C and osteoporosis in old age', *Age Ageing*, 1, 16–18.

Bankowski, E., Niewiarowski, S., and Galasinski, W. (1967). 'Platelet aggregation by human collagen in relation to its age', *Gerontologia*, 13, 219–226.

Basu, S. K. (1963). 'Rapid administration of iron-dextran in late pregnancy', *Lancet*, 1, 1430.

Batata, M., Spray, G. H., Bolton, F. G., Higgins, G., and Wollner, L. (1967). 'Blood and bone marrow changes in elderly patients with special reference to folic acid, vitamin B12 and ascorbic acid', *Br. Med. J.*, 2, 667–669.

Bateman, C. J. T., and Beard, M. E. J. (1976). 'Malignant disease', in *Haematological Aspects of Systemic Disease* (Eds M. C. G. Israels and I. W. Delamore), 1st ed., pp. 131–161, Holt Saunders, London.

Bates, C. J., Fleming, M., Paul, A. A., Black, A.

E., and Mandal, A. R. (1980). 'Folate status and its relation to vitamin C in healthy elderly men and women', *Age Ageing*, **9**, 241–248.

Beard, M. E. J., Bateman, C. J. T., Crowther, D., Wrigley, P. F. M., Whitehouse, J. M. A., Hamilton-Fairley, G., and Bodley Scott, R. (1975). 'Hypoplastic acute myelogenous leukaemia', *Br. J. Haematol.*, **31**, 167–176.

Beard, M. E. J., and Whitehouse, J. M. A. (1977). 'Adult acute leukaemias', in *Recent Advances in Haematology* (Eds A. V. Hoffbrand *et als*), Vol. 2, pp. 175–200, Churchill Livingstone, Edinburgh.

Beck, J. R., Meier, F. A., French, E. E., Brink-Johnson, T., and Cornwell III, G. G. (1979). 'Serum ferritin', *Lancet*, **1**, 1080.

Bell, T. K., Bridges, J. M., and Nelson, M. G. (1965). 'Simultaneous free and bound radioactive vitamin B12 urinary excretion test', *J. Clin. Pathol.*, **18**, 611–613.

Benditt, E. P., and Eriksen, N. (1972). 'Chemical similarity among amyloid substances associated with long standing inflammation', *Lab. Invest.*, **26**, 615–526.

Bentegeat, Pr, Darmendrail, Mlle, Moras, Mille, de Cacqueray-Joiguy, Mme, Choussat, Pr, Galley, Pr, Blein, Cavel, and Dartenuc (1975). 'About the platelet adhesiveness and aggregability on old-aged people', *Abstracts of Tenth Int. Cong. Gerontol., Jerusalem*, **2**, 49.

Bertolini, A. M. (1969). In *Gerontologic Metabolism*, C. C. Thomas, Springfield, Illinois.

Bird, T., Hall, M. R. P., and Schade, R. O. K. (1977). 'Gastric histology and its relation to anaemia in the elderly', *Gerontology*, **23**, 309–321.

Blair, A., Fraumeni, J. F., and Mason, T. J. (1980). 'Geographic patterns of leukaemia in the United States', *J. Chronic Dis.*, **33**, 251–260.

Blake, D. R., and Bacon, P. A. (1981). 'Synovial fluid ferritin in rheumatoid arthritis: An index or cause of inflammation?', *Br. Med. J.*, **282**, 189.

Blake, D. R., Waterworth, R. F., and Bacon, P. A. (1981). 'Assessment of iron stores in inflammation by assay of serum ferritin concentration', *Br. Med. J.*, **283**, 1147–1148.

Blum, S. P. (1979) 'Lithium therapy of aplastic anaemia', *New Engl. J. Med.*, **302**, 713–719.

Born, G. V. R., and Wright, H. P. (1967). 'Platelet adhesiveness in experimental scurvy', *Lancet*, **1**, 477–478.

Boston Collaborative Drug Surveillance Programme (1972). 'Acute adverse reactions to prednisone in relation to dosage', *Clin. Pharmacol. Ther.*, **13**, 694–698.

Botez, M. I., and Reynolds, E. H. (1979). *Folic Acid in Neurology, Psychiatry and Internal Medicine,* Raven Press, New York.

Bottiger, L. E., and Svedberg, C. A. (1967). 'Nor-

mal erythrocyte sedimentation rate and age', *Br. Med. J.*, **2**, 85–87.

Bottiger, L. E., and Westerholm, B. (1972). 'Thrombocytopenia: I. Incidence and etiology', *Acta. Med. Scand.*, **191**, 535–540.

Bourne, G. H., and Wilson, E. M. H. (1961). *Structural Changes of Ageing*, Pitman, London.

Brain, M. C., and Card, R. T. (1972). 'Effect of inorganic phosphate on red-cell metabolism: In vitro and in vivo studies', in *Haemoglobin and Red-Cell Structure and Function* (Ed. G. J. Brewer), *Adv. Exp. Med. Biol.*, Vol. 28, pp. 145–154, Plenum Press, New York.

Brandt, L., Nilsson, P. G., and Mitelman, F. (1979). 'Trends in incidence of acute leukaemia', *Lancet*, **2**, 1069.

British Medical Journal (1977a). 'High affinity haemoglobins', *Br. Med. J.*, **2**, 1040–1041.

British Medical Journal (1977b). 'Idiopathic haemochromatosis', *Br. Med. J.*, **2**, 1242.

British Medical Journal (1977c). 'Lymphoid blast crisis in chronic myeloid leukaemia', *Br. Med. J.*, **2**, 1303–4.

British Medical Journal (1979). 'Cell surface markers in chronic lymphatic leukaemia', *Br. Med. J.*, **2**, 886–887.

British Medical Journal (1980). 'Paraproteinaemia', *Br. Med. J.*, **280**, 273–274.

Bruschke, G., Thiele, W., and Schulz, F. H. (1960). 'Die Abhangiegkeit der Retraktion des Fibringerinnsels van Alter', *Z. Alternsofrsch*, **15**, 185–190.

Buckley, C. E. III, and Roseman, J. M. (1976). 'Immunity and survival', *J. Am. Geriatr. Soc.*, **24**, 241–248.

Burge, P. S., Johnson, W. S. and Prankerd, T. A. J. (1975). 'Morbidity and mortality in pseudopolycythaemia'. *Lancet*, **1**, 1266–1269.

Burnand, K., Clemenson, G., Morland, M., Jarrett, P. E. M., and Browse, N. L. (1980). 'Venous lipodermatosclerosis: Treatment by fibrinolytic enhancement and elastic compression', *Br. Med. J.*, **280**, 7–11.

Caird, F. I., Andrews, G. R., and Gallie, T. B. (1972). 'The leucocyte count in old age', *Age Ageing*, **1**, 239–244.

Camitta, B. M., Storb, R., and Thomas, E. D. (1982). 'Aplastic anaemia: Pathogenesis, diagnosis, treatment and prognosis', *New Eng. J. Med.*, **306**, 645–562.

Cape, R. D. T., and Shinton, N. K. (1961). 'Serum B12 concentration in the elderly', *Geront. Clin.*, **3**, 163–172.

Cartwright, G. E., and Lee, G. R. (1971). 'Annotation. The anaemia of chronic disorders', *Br. J. Haematol.*, **21**, 147–152.

Catovsky, D., Pettit, J. E., Galitto, J., Okos, A., and Galton, D. A. G. (1974a). 'The B-lymphocyte nature of the hairy cell of leukaemic reticu-loendotheliosis', *Br. J. Haematol.*, **26**, 29–37.

Catovsky, D., Pettit, J. E., Galton, D. A. G., Spiers, A. S. D., and Harrison, C. V. (1974b). 'Leukaemic reticuloendotheliosis (? hairy cell leukaemia): A distinct clinicopathological entity', *Br. J. Haematol.*, **26**, 9–27.

Chanarin, I., Deacon, R., Lumb, M., and Perry, J. (1980). 'Vitamin B12 regulates folate metabolism by the supply of formate', *Lancet*, **2**, 505–508.

Charache, S., Weatherall, D. J., and Clegg, J. B. (1966). 'Polycythaemia associated with haemoglobinopathy', *J. Clin. Invest.*, **45**, 813–821.

Chernish, S. M., Helmer, O. M., Fouts, P. J., and Kohlstaedt, K. G. (1957). 'The effect of intrinsic factor on the absorption of vitamin B12 in older people', *Am. J. Clin. Nutr.*, **5**, 561–658.

Clein, G. P. (1972). 'The neutrophil granulocyte', *Br. J. Hosp. Med.*, **7**, 83–88.

Clemmeson, J. (1974). 'On the epidemiology of leukaemia', in *Advances in Acute Leukaemia*. (Eds F. J. Cleton *et al.*), pp. 1–50, North Holland, Amsterdam.

Clinch, D., and Banerjee, A. K. (1982). 'The varied presentations of multiple myeloma', *Geriatric Med.*' **12**, 45–49.

Clinch, D., Banerjee, A. K., Ostick, G. and Levy, D. W. (1982). 'Non-steroidal anti-inflammatory drugs – do they cause gastro-intestinal pathology in the elderly?', (Paper presented at the British Geriatrics Society Meeting at RCP London, November, 1982.

Clinch, D. and Banerjee, A. K., Ostick, G., and Levy, D. W. (1983). 'Non-steroidal anti-inflammatory drugs and adverse gastro-intestinal effects', *J. Royal Coll. Phys.* **7**, 228–230.

Collins, F. J., Mathews, H. R., Baker, S. E., and Strakova, J. M. (1979). 'Drug induced oesophageal injury', *Br. Med. J.*, **1**, 1673–1676.

Conklin, R., and Alexanian, R. (1975). 'Clinical classification of plasma-cell myeloma', *Arch. Intern. Med.*, **135**, 139–143.

Cook, G. C., Morgan, J. O., and Hoffbrand, A. V. (1974). 'Impairment of folate absorption by systemic bacterial infections', *Lancet*, **2**, 1416–1417.

Cooper, A. G., Chavin, S. I., and Franklin, E. C. (1970). 'Predominance of a single μ-chain subclass in cold agglutinin heavy chains', *Immunochemistry*, **7**, 479–483.

Cox, T. M., and Peters, T. J. (1978). 'Uptake of iron by duodenal biopsy specimens from patients with iron deficiency anaemia and primary haemachromatosis', *Lancet*, **1**, 123–124.

Crosby, W. H. (1968). 'To treat or not to treat acute granulocytic leukaemia', *Arch. Intern. Med.*, **122**, 79–80.

Crowther, D., and Bateman, C. J. T. (1972). 'Malignant disease', *Clin. Haematol.*, **1**, 447–473.

Dallman, P. (1974). 'Tissue effects of iron deficiency', in *Iron Biochemistry and Medicine* (Eds A. Jacobs and M. Worwood), pp. 437–475, Academic Press, London.

Datta, S. B. (1975). Letter to the editor, *Mod. Geriatr.*, **5**, 3.

Davis, H. L. Jr, Prout, M. N., McKenna, P. J., *et al.* (1973). 'Acute leukaemia complicating metastic breast cancer', *Cancer*, **31**, 543–546.

Davis, R. H., Jacobs, A. and Rivlin, R. S. (1967). 'Dietary iron and haematological status in normal subjects'. *Br. Med. J.*, **3**, 711–712.

Davis, W. M., and Ross, A. O. M. (1973). 'Thrombocytosis and thrombocythaemia. The laboratory and clinical significance of an elevated platelet count', *Am. J. Clin. Pathol.*, **59**, 243–247.

Dawson, D. W., Sawers, A. H. and Sharma, R. K. (1984) Malabsorption of protein-bound Vitamin B12. *Br. Med. J.* **288**, 675–678.

De Gruchy, G. C. (1975). 'Thrombocytopenia', in *Drug Induced Blood Disorders*, pp. 118–155, Blackwell, Oxford.

Delamore, I. W. (1972). 'Gastro-intestinal disease', *Clin. Haematol.*, **1**, 507–531.

Delamore, I.W., Mallick, N. P., Azam, L., Dosa, S., Williams, G., and McFarlane, H. (1975). 'Monoclonal light chain paraproteinaemia presenting with renal disease and treated with quadruple cytotoxic chemotherapy', *Proc. Int. Soc. Haematol.*, European and African Division, London.

Delamore, I. W., and Shearman, D. J. C. (1965). 'Chronic iron deficiency anaemia and atrophic gastritis', *Lancet*, **1**, 889–891.

Department of Health and Social Security (1970). 'First report by the Panel on Nutrition of the Elderly', Report on Public Health and Medical Subjects No. 123, HMSO, London.

Department of Health and Social Security (1972). 'A nutritional survey of the elderly', Report on Health and Social Subjects No. 3, HMSO, London.

Desforges, J. F. (1983). 'Cytarabine, low-dose, high-dose, no-dose?', *New Eng. J. Med.*, **309**, 26, 1637–1638.

De Sousa, M. (1981). 'A circulation of lymphocytes: Reflections of the questions of how and why', in *Lymphocyte Circulation, Experimental and Clinical aspects*, pp. 197–217, John Wiley, Chichester.

Detraglia, M., Cook, F. B., Stasiw, D. M., and Cerny, L. C. (1974). 'Erythrocyte fragility in ageing', *Biochim. Biophys. Acta.*, **345**, 213–219.

Dodds, W. J., Moynihan, A. C., Benson, R. E., and Hall, C. A. (1975). 'The value of age and sex matched controls for coagulation studies', *Br. J. Haematol.*, **29**, 305–317.

Donati, M. B., Poggi, A., and Semeraro, N. (1981). 'Coagulation and malignancy', in *Recent Ad-*

vances in Blood Coagulation, (Ed. L. Poller), Vol.3, pp. 227–259, Churchill Livingstone, Edinburgh.

Donati, R. M., and Gantner, G. E. (1973). 'Haematological aspects of radiation exposure', in *Blood Disorders Due to Drugs and Other Agents* (Ed. R. H. Girdwood), pp. 241–264, Excerpta Medica, Amsterdam.

Doniach, D., Roitt, I. M., and Taylor, K. B. (1965). 'Autoimmunity in pernicious anaemia and thyroiditis: A family study', *Ann. N.Y. Acad. Sci.*, 12A, 605–625.

Douglas, A. P., and Bateman, D. N. (1981). 'Gastro-intestinal disorders', in *Textbook of Adverse Drug Reactions* (Ed. D. M. Davies), 2nd ed., pp. 202–215, Oxford University Press, Oxford.

Drapkin, R. L., Gee, T. S., Dowling, M. D., Arlin, Z., McKenzie, S., Kempin, S., and Clarkson, B. (1978). 'Prophylactic heparin therapy in acute pro-myelocytic leukaemia', *Cancer*, 41, 2484–2490.

Drugs and Therapeutic Bulletin (1979). 'How many oran iron preparations does a prescriber need?', *Drugs Ther. Bull.*, 17, 33.

Eastham, R. D. (1973). 'ESR vs. plasma viscosity readings in the old', *Br. Med. J.*, 4, 612–613.

Edgerton, V. R., Gardner, G. W., Ohira, Y., Gunawaredena, K. A., and Senewiratne, B. (1979). 'Iron deficiency anaemia and its effect on worker productivity and activity patterns', *Br. Med. J.*, 2, 1546–1549.

Eichner, E. R., and Hillman, R. S., (1971). 'The evolution of anaemia in alcoholic patients', *Am. J. Med.*, 50, 218–232.

Elsborg, L., Lund, V., and Bastrup-Madseu, P. (1976). 'Serum B12 levels in the aged', *Acta. Med. Scand.*, 200, 309–314.

Elwood, P. C. (1971). 'Epidemiological aspects of iron deficiency in the elderly', *Gerontol. Clin. (Basel)*, 13, 2–11.

England, J. M., and Linnell, J. C. (1980). 'Problems with the serum B12 assay', *Lancet*, 2, 1072–1074.

Esposito, R. (1977). 'Cimetidine and iron deficiency anaemia', *Lancet*, 2, 1132.

Exton-Smith, A. N. (1971). 'Nutrition of the elderly', *Br. J. Hosp. Med.*, 5, 639–646.

Fearnley, G. R., Chakravarti, R., Hocking, E. D., and Evans, J. F. (1967). 'Fibrinolytic effects of diguanides plus elthyloestrenol in occlusive vascular disease', *Lancet*, 2, 1008–1011.

Fielding, L. P., Chalmers, D. M., Chanarin, I., and Levi, A. J. (1978). 'Inhibition of intrinsic factor secretion by cimetidine', *Br. Med. J.*, 1, 818–819.

Foon, K. A., Zighelboim, J., Yale, C., and Gale, R. P. (1981). 'Intensive chemotherapy is the treatment of choice for elderly patients with acute myelogenous leukaemia', *Blood*, 58, 467–470.

Gaffney, G. W., Horonick, A., Okuda, K., Meier, P., Chow, B. F., and Shock, N. W. (1957). 'Vitamin B12 serum concentrations in 528 apparently healthy subjects of ages 12–94', *J. Gerontol.*, 12, 32–38.

Gale, R. P., and Cline, M. J. (1977). 'High remission induction rate in acute myeloid leukaemia', *Lancet*, 1, 497–499.

Galton, D. A. G. (1982). 'The chronic leukaemias', in *Recent Advances in Haematology* (Ed. A. V. Hoffbrand), Vol. 3, pp. 183–206, Churchill Livingstone, Edinburgh.

Galton, D. A. G., Goldman, J. M., Wilshaw, E., Catovsky, D., Henry, K., and Goldberg, G. J. (1974). 'Prolymphocytic leukaemia', *Br. J. Haematol.*, 27, 7–23.

Geary, C. G. (1979). 'The pathogeneisis of aplastic anaemia', *Br. J. Hosp. Med.*, 21, 392–402.

Geary, C. G., Benn, R. T., and Leck, I. (1979). 'Incidence of myeloid leukaemia in Lancashire', *Lancet*, 2, 549–551.

Girdwood, R. H., Thomson, A. D., and Williamson, J. (1967). 'Folate status in the elderly', *Br. Med. J.*, 1, 670–671.

Gordon, S. G., and Lewis, B. J. (1978). 'Comparison of pro-coagulant activity in tissue culture medium form normal and transferred fibroblasts', *Cancer Res.*, 38, 2467–2472.

Gordon-Smith, E. C. (1969). 'Bone marrow failure: Diagnosis and treatment', *Br. J. Haematol.*, 16, 167–175.

Gottstein, U. (1981). 'Normovolaemic and hypervolaemic haemodilution in cerebro-vascular ischaemia', *Bibliotheca Haematologica*, 47, 127–138.

Gralnick, H. R., Galton, D. A. G., Catovsky, D., Sultan, C., and Bennett, J. M. (1977). 'Classification of acute leukaemia', *Ann. Intern. Med.*, 87, 740–753.

Green, D., Schuette, P. T., and Wallace, W. H. (1980). 'Factor VIII antibodies in rheumatoid arthritis. Effect of cyclophosphamide', *Arch. Intern. Med.*, 140, 1232–1235.

Grey, H. M., and Kohler, P. F. (1973). 'Cryoimmunoglobulins', *Semin. Haematol.*, 10, 87–112.

Griffiths, R. A., Good, W. R., Watson, N. P., O'Donnell, H. F., Fell, P. J. and Shakespeare, J. M. (1984). Normal erythrocyte sedimentation rate in the elderly. *Br. Med. J.* 289, 724–725.

Grolle, G., Arturi, F., Cercutti, G., and Delijuiano, G. C. (1968). 'Platelet agglutination in young and elderly normal subjects and in arteriosclerotic patients', *J. Gerontol.*, 16, 89–96.

Hall, D. A., Reed, F. B., and Vince, J. D. (1974) 'The relative effects of age and corticosteroid therapy on the collagen profiles of dermis from subjects with rheumatoid arthritis', *Age Ageing*, 3, 15–22.

Hallberg, L., and Hogdahl, A. M. (1971). 'Anaemia and old age – observations in a population sample of women in Goteberg', *Gerontol. Clin. (Basel)*, **13**, 31–43.

Hamilton, E. B. D., Bomford, A. B., Laws, J. W., and Williams, R. (1981). 'The natural history of arthritis in idiopathic haemochromatosis: Progression of the clinical and radiological features over ten years', *Quart. J. Med.*, **199**, 321–329.

Hammond, D., and Winnick, S. (1974). 'Paraneoplastic erythrocytosis and ectopic erythropoietin', *Ann. N.Y. Acad. Sci.*, **230**, 219–227.

Hansky, J. (1981). 'Gut hormones', *Med. International*, **1**, 546–549.

Hayes, G. S., and Stinson, I. N. (1976). 'Erythrocyte sedimentation rate and age', *Arch. Ophthalmol.*, **94**, 939–940.

Henderson, J. T., Shearman, D. J., and Ganguli, P. C. (1971). 'Plasma gastrin concentration and antral gastritis in achlorohydria', *Scott. Med. J.*, **16**, 532.

Herbert, V. (1962). 'Experimental nutritional folate deficiency in man', *Trans. Assoc. Am. Physicians*, **75**, 320.

Herbert, V., and Zalusky, R. (1962). 'Inter-relation of vitamin B12 and folic acid metabolism: Folic acid clearance studies', *J. Clin. Invest.*, **41**, 1263–1276.

Heremans, J. F. (1959). 'Immunochemical studies on protein pathology. The immunoglobulin concept', *Clin. Chim. Acta.*, **4**, 639–646.

Hill, R. D. (1976). 'The prevalence of anaemia in the over-65s in a rural practice', *Practitioner*, **217**, 963–967.

Hines, J. D., and Grasso, J. A. (1970). 'The sideroblastic anaemias', *Semin. Haematol.*, **7**, 86–106.

Hobbs, J. R. (1974). 'Paraproteins', in *Blood and Its Disorders* (Eds R. M. Hardisty and D. J. Weatherall), pp. 1343–1373, Blackwell, Oxford.

Hobbs, J. R. (1980). 'Myeloma', *Medicine* (3rd series), **29**, 1507–1512.

Hoffbrand, A. V. (1974). 'Vitamin B12 and golate metabolism: The megaloblastic anaemias and related disorders', in *Blood and Its Disorders* (Eds R. M. Hardisty and D. J. Weatherall), 1st ed., pp. 392–472, Blackwell, Oxford.

Hooper, B., Whittingham, S., Mathews, J. D., MacKay, I. R., and Curnow, D. H. (1972). 'Autoimmunity in a rural community', *Clin. Exp. Immunol.*, **12**, 79–87.

Housset, M., Daniel, M. T., and Degos, L. (1982). 'Small doses of ARA–C in the treatment of acute myeloid leukaemia: differentation of myeloid leukaemia cells?, *B. J. Haematol.*, **51**, 125–9.

Hume, R., Dagg, J. H., and Goldberg, A. (1973). 'Refractory anaemia with dysproteinaemia. Long term therapy with low dose corticosteroids', *Blood*, **41**, 27–35.

Humphrey, P. R. D., Marshall, J., Ross-Russell, R. W., Wetherley-Mein, G., Du-Boulay, G. H., Pearson, T. C., Symon, L., and Silkha, E. (1979). 'Cerebral blood flow and viscosity in relative polycythaemia'. *Lancet*, **2**, 873–877.

Hurdle, A. D. F., and Rosin, A. J. (1962). 'Red cell volume and red cell survival in normal aged people', *J. Clin. Pathol.*, **15**, 343–345.

Hyams, D. E. (1964). 'The absorption of vitamin B12 in the elderly',. *Gerontol. Clin. (Basel)*, **6**, 193–206.

Hyams, D. E. (1978). 'The blood', in *Textbook of Geriatric Medicine and Gerontology* (Ed. J. C. Brocklehurst), pp. 560–625, Churchill Livingstone, London.

Ibbotson, R. M., Colvin, B. T., and Colvin, M. P. (1975). 'Folic acid deficiency during intensive therapy', *Br. Med. J.*, **4**, 145–147.

Jacobs, A., Lawrie, J. H., Entwistle, C. C. and Campbell, H. (1966). 'Gastric acid secretion in chronic iron deficiency anaemia', *Lancet*, **2**, 190–192.

Jacobs, A., and Worwood, M. (1974). 'Iron metabolism, iron deficiency and iron overload' in *Blood and Its Disorders* (Eds R. M. Hardisty and D. J. Weatherall), 1st ed., pp. 332–391, Blackwell, Oxford.

Jacobs, A., and Worwood, M. (1975). 'The clinical use of serum ferritin estimation', *Br. J. Haematol.*, **31**, 1–3.

Jacobs, P., Bothwell, T., and Charlton, R. W. (1964). 'Role of hydrochloric acid on iron absorption', *J. Appl. Physiol.*, **19**, 187.

Jarrett, P. E. M., Morland, M., and Browse, N. L. (1978). 'Treatment of Raynaud's phenomenon by fibrinolytic enhancement', *Br. Med. J.*, **2**, 523–525.

Jick, H., and Porter, J. (1978). 'Drug induced gastro-intestinal bleeding', *Lancet*, **2**, 87–89.

Kemp, I. W., Stein, G. J., and Heasman, M. A. (1980). 'Myeloid leukaemia in Scotland', *Lancet*, **2**, 732–734.

Kernoff, L. M., Dommisse, J., and Du Toit, E. D. (1975). 'Utilization of iron dextran in recurrent iron deficiency anaemia', *Br. J. Haematol.*, **30**, 419–424.

Kernoff, P. B. A., and McNicol, G. P. (1977). 'Normal and abnormal fibrinolysis', *Br. Med. Bull.*, **33**, 239–243.

Kyle, R. A. (1983). 'Long-term survival in multiple myeloma', *New Eng. J. Med.*, **308**, 314–316.

Kyle, R. A., Pierre, R. V., and Bayrd, E. D. (1970). 'Multiple myeloma and acute myelo-monocytic leukaemia', *New Engl. J. Med.*, **283**, 1121–1125.

Lancet, (1974). 'Iron and resistance to infection', **2**, 325–326.

Lancet, (1979a). 'Serum ferritin', *Lancet*, **1**, 533–

534.

Lancet, (1979b). 'Steroids in polymyalgia rheumatica', *Lancet*, **2**, 341.

Lancet, (1980a). 'Preventing iron deficiency', *Lancet*, **1**, 1117–1118.

Lancet, (1980b). 'Lithium in haematology', *Lancet*, **2**, 626–627.

Lancet, (1980c). 'Epidemiology of leukaemia', *Lancet*, **2**, 727–728.

Lancet, (1981a). Acquired haemophilia', *Lancet*, **1**, 255.

Lancet, (1981b). 'Natural fibrinolysis and its stimulation', *Lancet*, **1**, 1401–1402.

Lawson, D. H., Murray, R. M., and Parker, J. L. W. (1972). 'Early mortality in the megaloblastic anaemias', *Quart. J. Med.*, **41**, 1–14.

Lee, B. J., Lake-Lewin, D., and Myers, J. E. (1982). 'Improved survival times and response rates in multiple myeloma with the use of combination chemotherapy', *Controversies in Oncology*, (Ed. P. H. Wiernick), John Wiley, New York.

Lesher, S., and Sacher, G. A. (1968). 'Effects of age on cell proliferation in mouse duodenal crypts', *Exp. Gerontol.*, **3**, 211–217.

Lessin, L. S., Klug, P. P., and Jenson, W. N. (1976) 'Clinical implications of red cell shape', *Adv. Intern. Med.*, **21**, 451–500.

Levo, Y. (1980). 'Nature of cryoglobulinaemia', *Lancet*, **1**, 285–286.

Levy, M. (1974). 'Aspirin use in patients with major upper gastro-intestinal bleeding and peptic ulcer disease', *New Engl. J. Med.*, **290**, 1158–1162.

Lewis, S. M. (1974). 'The constituents of normal blood', in *Blood and Its Disorders*, (Eds R. M. Hardisty and D. J. Weatherall), 1st ed., pp. 3–67, Blackwell, Oxford.

Lewis, S. M. (1976). 'Polycythaemia vera', *Br. J. Hosp. Med.*, **16**, 125–132.

Li, A. K. C., and Batey, R. G. (1977). 'A tumour inducing iron overload', *Br. Med. J.*, **2**, 1327–1328.

Lipinski, B., Worowski, K., Mysliweic, M., and Farbiszewski, R. (1969). 'Erythrocyte sedimentation and soluble fibrin monomer complexes', *Thromb. Diath. Haemorrh.*, **21**, 196–202.

Lyman, G. H., Bettigole, R. E., Robsob, E., Ambrus, J. L., and Urban, H. (1978). 'Fibrinogen kinetics in patients with neoplastic disease', *Cancer*, **41**, 1113–1122.

McAlpine, C. J., Rowan, J. O., Matheson, M. S., and Patterson, J. (1981). 'Cerebral blood flow and intelligence rating in persons over 90 years old', *Age Ageing*, **10**, 247–253.

McCurdy, P. R., and Dern, R. J. (1968). 'Some therapeutic implications of ferrous sulphate – ascorbic acid mixtures', *Am. J. Clin. Nutrition*, **21**, 284–288.

MacKinney, S. A. (1978). 'Effects of aging on the peripheral blood lymphocyte count', *J. Gerontol.*, **33**, 213–216.

MacLennan, W. J., Andrews, G. R., MacLeod, C., and Caird, F. I. (1973). 'Anaemia in the elderly', *Quart. J. Med.*, **42**, 1–13.

MacLeod, C. C., Judge, T. G., and Caird, F. I. (1975). 'Nutrition of the elderly at home. III. Intake of minerals', *Age Ageing*, **4**, 49–57.

McMurdoch, J., and Smith, C. C. (1972). 'Infection', *Clin. Haematol.*, **1**, 619–644.

Manoharan, A. (1983). 'Low dose cytarabine therapy in hypoplastic acute leukaemia', *New Eng. J. Med.*, **309**, 26, 1652–1653.

Malloy, M. L., Zanber, N. P., and Chervenick, P. A. (1978). 'The effect of lithium on blood and marrow neutrophils'. *Blood*, **52** (Suppl. 1), 228 (abstr.)

Mannucci, P. M., and Vigano, S. (1982). 'Deficiencies of protein C; an inhibitor of blood coagulation', *Lancet*, **2**, 463–467.

Manzoor, M., and Runcie, J. (1976). 'Folate responsive neuropathy: Report of ten cases', *Br. Med. J.*, **1**, 1176–1178.

Marshall,J. (1982). 'Cerebral blood flow', in *Neurological Disorders in the Elderly* (Ed. F. I. Caird', pp. 25–31, Wright PSG, Bristol.

Martin, J. M., Kellet, J. M., and Kahn, J. (1980) 'Aneuploidy in cultured human lymphocytes: I. Age and sex difference', *Age Ageing*, **9**, 147–153.

Mason, D. Y., and Emerson, P. M. (1973). 'Primary acquired sideroblastic anaemia: Response to treatment with pyridoxal-5-phosphate', *Br. Med. J.*, **1**, 389–390.

Matzner, Y., Levy, S., Crossowicz, N., Izak, G., and Hershko, C. (1979). 'Prevalence and causes of anaemia in elderly hospitalised patients', *Gerontology*, **25**, 113–119.

Meagher, R. C., Sieber, F., and Spivak, J. L. (1982). 'Suppression of haematopoietic progenitor-cell proliferation by ethanol and acetaldehyde', *New Eng. J. Med.*, **307**, 845–849.

Melamed, E., Lavy, S., Siew, F., Bentin, S., and Cooper, G. (1979). 'Reduction of rCBF in dementia: Correlation with age matched normal controls and computarized tomography'. *Acta. Neurol. Scand.*, **60** (Suppl. 72), 544–545.

Messer, J. Reitman, D., Sacks, H. S., Smith, H., Jr., and Chalmers, T. C. (1983). 'Association of adrenocorticosteroid therapy and peptic-ulcer disease', *New Engl. J. Med.*, **309**, 21–24.

Milne, J. S., and Williamson, J. (1972). 'The ESR in older people', *Gerontol. Clin.*, **14**, 36–42.

Morgan, R. H. (1967). 'Anaemia in elderly housebound patients', *Br. Med. J.*, **4**, 171.

Mowat, A. G. (1972). 'Connective tissue diseases', *Clin. Haematol.*, **3**, 573–594.

Munan, L., and Kelly, A. (1979). 'Age dependent

changes in blood monocyte populations in man', *Clin. Exp. Immunol.*, **35**, 161–162.

Munan, L., Kelly, A., Petticlere, C., and Dillon, C. (1978). 'Atlas of blood data', University of Sherbrooke, Ontario.

Naylor, G. J. (1970). 'The relationship between age and sodium metabolism in human erythrocyte', *Gerontologia*, **16**, 217–222.

Odegard, O. R., Fagerhal, M. K., and Lie, M. (1976). 'Heparin co-factor activity and antithrombin III concentration in plasma related to age and sex', *Scand. J. Haematol.*, **17**, 258–267.

Okuno, T. (1972). 'Red cell size and age', *Br. Med. J.*, **1**, 569–570.

Olbrich, O. (1947). 'Blood changes in the aged', *Edin. Med. J.*, **54**, 306–321.

O'Meara, R. A. Q. (1958). 'Coagulative properties of cancer', *Irish J. Med. Sci.*, **394**, 474–479.

Paradinas, F. J., Melia, W. M., Wilkinson, M. L., Portmann, B., Johnson, P. J., Murray-Lyon, I. M., and Williams, R. (1982). 'High serum vitamin B12 binding capacity as a marker of the fibrolamellar variant of hepatocellular carcinoma', *Br. Med. J.*, **285**, 840–842.

Pathy, M. S., Kirkman, S., and Molloy, M. J. (1979). 'An evaluation of simultaneously administered free and intrinsic factor bound radioactive cyanocobalamin in the diagnosis of pernicious anaemia in the elderly', *J. Clin. Pathol.*, **32**, 244–250.

Pathy, M. S., Pippen, C. A. R., and Kirkman, S. (1972). 'Free and I.F. bound radioactive cynocobalamin. Simultaneous administration to assess the significance of low serum B12 levels', *Age Ageing*, **1**, 111–119.

Paulley, J. W., and Hughes, J. P. (1960). 'Giant cell arteritis or arteritis of the aged'. *Br. Med. J.*, **2**, 1562–1567.

Pederson, A. B., and Mosbech, J. (1969). 'Morbidity of pernicious anaemia. Incidence, prevalence and treatment in a Danish county', *Acta. Med. Scand.*, **185**, 449–452.

Persson, I., Raby, K. N., Fonns-Bech, P., and Jensen, E. (1975). 'Bran and blood lipids', *Lancet*, **2**, 1208.

Peterson, B. A., and Bloomfield, C. D. (1977). 'Treatment of acute non-lymphocytic leukaemia in elderly patients', *Cancer*, **40**, 647–652.

Pincherle, G., and Shanks, J. (1967). 'Value of the erythrocyte sedimentation rate as a screening test', *Br. J. Prev. Soc. Med.*, **21**, 133–136.

Pisciotta, A. V. (1971). 'Drug induced leucopenia and aplastic anaemia', *Clin. Pharmacol. Ther.*, **12**, 13–18.

Pitney, W. R. (1973). 'The purpuras', in *Blood and Its Disorders* (Eds R. M. Hardisty and D. J. Weatherall), pp. 995–1035, Blackwell: Oxford.

Powell, D. E. B., Thomas, J. H., and Mills, P. (1968). 'Serum iron in elderly hospital patients', *Geront. Clin.*, **10**, 21–29.

Prasad, B. K., Banerjee, A. K., and Howard, H. (1982). 'Incidence of deep vein thrombosis and the effect of pneumatic compression of the calf in elderly hemiplegics', *Age Ageing*, **11**, 42–44.

Price, V. E., and Greenfield, R. E. (1960). 'Anaemia in cancer', *Adv. in Canc. Res.*, **5**, 199–284.

Radl, J., Sepers, J. M., Skvaril, F., Morell, A., and Hijmans, W. (1975). 'Immunoglobulin patterns in humans over 95 years of age', *Clin. Exp. Immunol.*, **22**, 84–90.

Rai, G. S. (1979). 'Erythrocyte sedimentation rate and disease in the elderly', *J. Am. Geriatr. Soc.*, **27**, 382–383.

Rai, G. S. (1981). 'Viscosity, vascular disease and the elderly', *Age Ageing*, **10**, 221–224.

Rai, K. R., Sawitsky, A., Cronkitc, E. P., Chanana, A. D., Levy, R. N., and Pasternack, B. S. (1975). 'Clinical staging of chronic lymphocytic leukaemia', *Blood*, **46**, 219–234.

Ray, P. K., and Pinkerton, P. H. (1969). 'Leucocyte alkaline phosphatase, the effect of age and sex', *Acta. Haematol. (Basel)*, **42**, 18–22.

Reading, H. W., and Rosie, R. A. (1980). 'Age and sex differences related to platelet aggregation', *Biochem. Soc. Trans.*, **8**, 180–181.

Rees, J. K. H., Sandler, R. M., Challener, J., Hayhoe, F. G. J. (1977). 'Treatment of acute myeloid leukaemia with a triple cytotoxic regime: D.A.T.', *Br. J. Cancer*, **36**, 1066–1075.

Reinherz, E. L., Nadler, L. M., Rosenthal, D. S., Moloney, W. C., and Scholssman, S. F. (1979). 'T-cell subset characterisation of human T-C.L.L.', *Blood*, **53**, 1066–1075.

Reizenstein, P., Ljunggren, G., Smedby, B., Agenas, I., and Penchansky, M. (1979). 'Overprescribing iron tablets to elderly people in Sweden', *Br. Med. J.*, **2**, 962–963.

Ritzmann, S. E., Daniels, J. C., and Levin, W. C. (1975). 'Idiopathic (asymptomatic) monoclonal gammopathies', *Arch. Int. Med.*, **135**, 95–106.

Roath, S. (1980). 'Blood disorders and ageing', *Geriatric Med.*, **10**, 73–79.

Roberts, M. A., Andrews, G. R., and Caird, F. I. (1975). 'Skinfold thickness on the dorsum of the hand in the elderly', *Age Ageing*, **4**, 8–15.

Robertson, B. R., Pandolfi, M., and Nilsson, I. M. (1972). 'Fibrinolytic capacity in healthy volunteers at different ages as studied by standardised venous occlusion of arms and legs', *Acta. Med. Scand.*, **191**, 199–202.

Rosen, P., and Armstrong, D. (1973) 'Nonbacterial thrombotic endocarditis in patients with malignant neoplastic diseases', *Am. J. Med.*, **54**, 23–29.

Rosenthal, S., Canellos, G. P., Devitta, V. T., Jr., *et al.* (1977). 'Characteristics of blast crisis in chronic granulocytic leukaemia', *Blood*, **49**, 705–714.

Rosing, D. R., Redwood, D. R., Brakman, P., Astrup, T., and Epstein, S. E. (1973). 'Impairment of the diurual fibrinolytic response in man: Effects of ageing, type IV hyperlipoproteinaemia and coronary artery disease', *Cir. Res.*, **32**, 752–758.

Rosner, F., Sawitsky, A., Grunwald, H. W., and Rai, K. R. (1976). 'Acute granulocytic leukaemia in the elderly', *Arch. Int. Med.*, **136**, 120.

Rowe, D. S., Hug, K., Form, L., and Pernis, B. (1973). 'Immunoglobulin D as lymphocyte receptor', *J. Exp. Med.*, **138**, 965–972.

Rubinson, H., Kahn, A., Boivin, P., Schapira, R., Gregori, C., and Dreyfus, J. C. (1976). 'Aging and accuracy of protein synthesis in man: Search for inactive enzymatic cross-reacting material in granulocytes of aged people', *Gerontology*, **22**, 438–448.

Ruddell, W. S. J., Bone, E. S., Hill, M. J., and Walters, C. L. (1978). 'Pathogeneisis of gastric cancer in pernicious anaemia', *Lancet*, **1**, 521–523.

Ruhenstroth-Bauer, G. (1961). 'Mechanism and significance of erythrocyte sedimentation rate', *Br. Med. J.*, **1**, 1804.

Salem, H. H., Van der Weyden, M. B., Young, I. F., and Wiley, J. S. (1982). 'Pruritus and severe iron deficiency in polycythaemia vera', *Br. Med. J.*, **285**, 91–92.

Schafer, A. J. (1982). 'Deficiency of the platelet lipoxygenase activity in meloproliferative disorders', *New Eng. J. Med.*, **306**, 381–386.

Schilling, R. F. (1953). 'Effects of gastric juice on urinary excretion of radioactive vitamin B12', *J. Lab. Clin. Med.*, **42**, 860–866.

Sharma, K. K., Sharma, S. P., and Arora, S. C. (1978). 'Some observations on the mechanism of fibrinolytic enhancing effect of garlic during alimentary lipaemia in man.' *J. Postgrad. Med.*, **24**, 98–102.

Shashaty, G. G., and Rath, C. E. (1978). 'Idiopathic thrombocytopenia purpura in the elderly', *Am. J. Med. Sci.*, **276**, 263–267.

Shearman, D. J. C., Delamore, I. W., and Gardner, D. (1966). 'Gastric function and structure in iron deficiency', *Lancet*, **2**, 845–848.

Shorvon, S. D., Carney, M. W. P., Chanarin, I., and Reynolds, E. H. (1980). 'The neuropsychiatry of megaloblastic anaemias', *Br. Med. J.*, **281**, 1036–1038.

Shuster, S., and Scarborough, H. (1961). 'Senile purpura', *Quart. J. Med.*, **30**, 33–40.

Simpson, R. G. (1974). 'Disease patterns in elderly', *Br. J. Hosp. Med.*, **12**, 660–667.

Smith, C. C. (1974). 'Toxic anaemia', *Br. Med. J.*, **2**, 606–607.

Smith, C. C., and McMurdoch, J. (1976). 'Infection'. in *Haematological Aspects of Systemic Diseases* (Eds M. C. G. Israels and I. W. Delamore), 1st ed., pp. 342–370, Holt-Saunders, London.

Smith, E., and Staples, E. (1981). 'Haemostatic factors in human aortic intima', *Lancet*, **1**, 1171–1174.

Späti, B., Child, J. A., Kerruish, S. M., and Cooper, E. M. (1980). 'Behaviour of serum β_2-microglobulin and acute phase reactants protein in chronic lymphocytic leukaemia. A multicentre study', *Acta. Haematol. (Basel)*, **64**, 79–86.

Spriggs, A. I., and Sladden, R. A. (1958). 'The influence of age on red cell diameter', *J. Clin. Pathol.*, **11**, 53–55.

Stott, H., Fox, W., Girling, D. J., Stephens, R. J., and Galton, D. A. G. (1977). 'Acute leukaemia after busulphan', *Br. Med. J.*, **2**, 1513–1517.

Strachan, R. W., How, J., and Bewster, P. D. (1980). 'Masked giant cell arteritis', *Lancet*, **1**, 194–197.

Stuart, J. (1980). 'Chemotherapy of the myeloid leukaemias', *J. Roy. Coll. Physicians Lond.*, **14**, 36–41.

Sullivan, J. L. (1981). 'Iron and sex difference in heart disease risk', *Lancet*, **1**, 1293–1294.

Sun, N. C. J., McAfee, W. M., Hum, G. J., and Weiner, J. M. (1979). 'Haemostatic abnormalities in malignancy, a prospective study of one hundred and eight patients. Pt. 1. Coagulation studies', *Am. J. Clin. Pathol.*, **71**, 10–16.

Tattersall, R. N., and Seville, R. (1950). 'Senile purpura', *Quart. J. Med.*, **19**, 151–159.

Tauber, S. A., Goodhart, R. S., Shu, J. M., Blumberg, N., Kassab, J. and Chou, B. F., (1957). 'Vitamin B12 deficiency in the aged', *Geriatrics*, **12**, 368–374.

ten Cate, J. W. (1972). 'Platelet function tests', *Clin. Haematol.*, **1**, 283–294.

Teo, N. H., Scott, J. M., Neale, G., and Weir, D. G. (1980). 'Effect of bile on vitamin B12 absorption', *Br. Med. J.*, **2**, 831–833.

Thoma, G. E., and Wald, N. (1959). 'The diagnosis and management of accidental radiation injury', *J. Occup. Med.*, **1**, 421–438.

Thomas, D. J., and Willison, J. R. (1981). 'Effect of phlebotomy on cerebral blood flow and function', *Bibliotheca Haematologica*, **47**, 139–144.

Thomas, J. H., and Powell, D. E. B. (1971). *Blood Disorders in the Elderly*', 1st. ed., pp. 78, John Wright, Bristol.

Trewby, P. N. (1980). 'Drug induced peptic ulcer and upper gastrointestinal bleeding', *Br. J. Hosp. Med.*, **23**, 185–190.

Trump, B. F., Barrett, L. A., Valigorsky, J. M., and Jiji, R. M. (1975). 'Ultrastructural studies of sideroblastic anaemias', in *Iron Metabolism and Its Disorders* (Ed. H. Kief), pp. 251–253, Excerpta Medica, Amsterdam.

Tunbridge, W. M. G., Brewis, M., French, J. M., Appleton, D., Bird, T., Clark, F., Evered, D., Grimley-Evans, J., Hall, R., Smith, P., Stephenson, J., and Young, E. (1981). 'Natural history of auto-immune thyroiditis', *Br. Med. J.*, **282**, 258–262.

Ungar, B., Mathews, J. D., Tait, B. D., and Cowling, D. C. (1981). 'HLA-DR patterns in pernicious anaemia', *Br. Med. J.*, **282**, 768–770.

Ungar, B., Whittingham, S., and Francis, C. M. (1977). 'Pernicious anaemia: Incidence and significance of circulating antibodies to intrinsic factor and to parietal cells', *Aust. Ann. Med.*, **16**, 226–229.

Valera, E., and Good, R. A. (1980). 'Studies on the pathogenesis of refractory anaemia', *Am. J. Med.*, **68**, 381–385.

Wade, J. P. H., Pearson, T. C., Ross Russell, R. W., and Wetherley-Mein, G. (1981). 'Cerebral blood flow and blood viscosity in patients with polycythaemia secondary to hypoxic lung disease', *Br. Med. J.*, **283**, 689–692.

Waldenström, J. (1944). 'Incipient myelomatosis or essential hyperglobulinaemia with fibrinogenopenia, a new syndrome?', *Acta. Med. Scand.*, **117**, 216.

Walford, R. L. (1969). *The Immunological Theory of Ageing*', Munksgaard, Copenhagen.

Waxman, S., and Gilbert, H. S. (1974). 'Characteristics of a novel serum vitamin B12–binding protein associated with hepatocellular carcinoma', *Br. J. Haematol.*, **27**, 229–239.

Weatherall, D. J., Clegg, J. B., Callender, S. T., Wells, R. M. G., Gale, R. E., Huehns, E. R., Perulz, M. F., Viggiano, G., and Ho, C. (1977). 'Haemoglobin radcliffe: A high oxygen affinity variant causing familial polycythaemia', *Br. J. Haematol.*, **35**, 177–191.

Webster, S. G. P. (1979). 'Is poor dietary intake the cause of folate deficiency?', *Mod. Geriatr.*, **9**, 81–82.

Webster, S. G. P., and Leeming, J. T. (1975). 'The appearance of the small bowel mucosa in old age', *Age Ageing*, **4**, 168–174.

Weeke, B., and Krasilnikoff, P. A. (1972). 'The concentration of 21 serum proteins in normal children and adults', *Acta. Med. Scand.*, **192**, 149–155.

Weiss, G. B., Kock, J. C., and Richardson, H. B. (1975). 'Idiopathic thrombocytopenic purpura in the elderly', *Lancet*, **1**, 411–412.

Whitehead, T. P., Clarke, C. A., and Whitfield, A. G. W. (1978). 'Biochemical and haematological markers of alcohol intake', *Lancet*, **1**, 987–981.

Whittaker, J. A., Withey, J., Powell, D. E. B., Parry, T. E., and Khurshid, M. (1979). 'Leukaemia classification: A study of the accuracy of diagnosis in 456 patients', *Br. J. Haematol.*, **41**, 177–184.

Wiley, J. S. (1980). 'Haemolysis', *Medicine/3rd series*, **28**, 1468–1473.

Williamson, J., and Chopin, J. M. (1980). 'Adverse reactions to prescribed drugs in the elderly', *Age Ageing*, **9**, 73–80.

Wilson, P. A., McNicol, G. P., and Douglas, A. S. (1967). 'Platelet abnormality in human scurvy', *Lancet*, **1**, 975–978.

Wokes, F., Badenoch, J., and Sinclair, H. M. (1955). 'Human dietary deficiency of vitamin B12', *Am. J. Clin. Nutr.*, **15**, 77.

Wood, P. H. N., Harvey-Smith, E. A., and Dixon, A. St J. (1962). 'Salicylates and gastrointestinal bleeding, acetylsalicytic acid and aspirin derivatives', *Br. Med. J.*, **1**, 669–675.

Woodford-Williams, E., Webster, D., Dixon, M. P., and MacKenzie, W. (1962). 'Red cell longevity in old age', *Geront. Clin.*, **4**, 183–193.

World Health Organisation (1968). 'Nutritional anaemias'. Report of a WHO Scientific group. WHO Tech. Rep. Series. No. 405, Geneva.

World Health Organisation (1969). 'Anaemias 1922–1966. Mortality statistics', *WHO Stat. Rep.*, **22**, 409–427.

Worlledge, S. M. (1969). 'Immune drug-induced haemolytic anaemias', *Semin. Haematol.*, **6**, 181–200.

Wright, W. B. (1967). 'Iron deficiency anaemia in the elderly treated by total-dose infusion', *Gerontol. Clinica.*, **9**, 107–115.

Wu, A., Chanarin, I., and Levi, A. J. (1974). 'Macrocytosis of chronic alcoholics', *Lancet*, **1**, 829–830.

Yates, C. J. P., Andrews, V., Berent, A., and Dormandy, J. A. (1979). 'Increase in leg blood flow by normovolaemic haemodilution in intermittent claudication', *Lancet*, **2**, 166–168.

Yunis, A. A. (1973). 'Chloramphenicol toxicity', in *Blood Disorders Due to Drugs and Other Agents* (Ed. R. H. Girdwood), pp. 107–126, Excerpta Medica, Amsterdam.

Zacharski, L. R., Elveback, L. R., and Linman, J. W. (1971). 'Leucocyte counts in healthy adults', *Am. J. Clin. Pathol.*, **54**, 148–150.

13

Disorders of the
Blood Vessels

13.1

Disorders of the Blood Vessels

B. A. Kottke

INTRODUCTION

In attempting to understand the pathophysiology of diseases of the peripheral vasculature, it is useful to understand the normal cell biology of the major cells of the arteries, veins, and lymphatics. Most vascular diseases are associated with an alteration of the biochemistry and physiology of these cells. In the past, much emphasis has been placed on the innervation and vasoconstrictive activity of vessels. Such factors play little role in the pathogenesis of disease except in systemic hypertension and in orthostatic hypotension. Otherwise, their major role is in the haemodynamic control of the circulation, especially in cardiac disease. Only rarely is failure of these neurogenic and vasomotor controls specifically involved in the disease process of peripheral vascular diseases. The basic cell types which comprise the peripheral vessels include: endothelial cells, smooth muscle cells, and fibroblasts. Cells in the circulating blood which commonly interact with these cells include: platelets, macrophages, and lymphocytes.

Endothelial Cells

Endothelial cells are formed during angiogenesis. Characteristically they grow in true monolayers and demonstrate contact inhibition of growth. That is, when the cells reach a confluent stage where they are in contact with each other, their growth ceases. They represent a major histologic cell type (2 kg/70 kg human)

and form the luminal surface of the entire cardiovascular and lymphatic systems (Levine and Mueller, 1979). They play a role in the regulation of vascular permeability and provide a surface which inhibits blood coagulation. It is thought that the latter property is, in part, due to their ability to secrete prostacyclin (PGI_2) from endoperoxides produced by the cyclo-oxygenase pathway of arachidonic acid metabolism (Weksler, Mancus, and Jaffe, 1977). Their identifying characteristics include the presence of factor VIII antigen (Jaffe et al., 1973) and Weibel–Palade bodies (Weibel and Palade, 1964). Normally, in blood vessels the cells are oriented longitudinally in the direction of blood flow. In addition to mechanical and haemodynamic trauma, agents known to be injurious to endothelium include antigen–antibody complexes (Angles-Cano, Sultan, and Clauvel, 1979), and smoking (Fuster et al., 1981; Hladover, 1978).

Fibroblasts

Fibroblasts are a primitive, multipotential type of mesenchymal cell. They do not have any contractile mechanism, but migrate readily. In tissue culture they grow in concentric whorls, have multiple layers, and are easier to culture than most other cell types. They have many of the functional characteristics of more differentiated smooth muscle cells and have been used extensively for the study of genetic disorders of metabolism including studies of lipid and lipoprotein metabolism (Goldstein and Brown, 1977).

Smooth Muscle Cells

The smooth muscle cell is the major cell of the arterial wall. In addition to their contractile properties, these cells are capable of synthesizing collagen (Ross and Klebanoff, 1971), elastin (Ross, 1971), and glycosaminoglycans (Wight and Ross, 1975). They can be differentiated from fibroblasts by: the presence of myofilaments; their growth in a 'hill and valley' configuration in tissue culture; the presence of a basement membrane on electronmicroscopy; and immunological markers. These markers include smooth muscle actin, tropomyosin, and a 55,000 dalton protein of 100 Å filaments (Chamley-Campbell, Campbell, and Ross, 1979). They retain essentially the same metabolic pathways as fibroblasts for the regulation of lipid metabolism and, under appropriate conditions, can accumulate large numbers of lipid droplets (Goldstein *et al.*, 1977). Their growth and proliferation, as well as their ability to migrate, can be stimulated by the platelet-derived growth factor (Ross *et al.*, 1974 and Thorgeirsson, Robertson, and Cowan, 1979).

Platelets

In addition to the cells of the arterial wall, several cells of the circulating blood also play critical roles in the pathophysiology of peripheral vascular disease. Of these, the roles of platelets and of macrophages are best understood. Mammalian platelets (White, 1971) are non-nucleated cells derived from bone marrow megakaryocytes. Their normal life span is about 10 days. Structurally they are usually discoid in shape and contain a prominent and complex microtubular system which is in direct contact with the plasma membrane.

Platelets have two types of membrane-bound granules. One type is the alpha granule which contains platelet factor-4, β-thromboglobulin, fibrinogen, and platelet-derived growth factor (Kaplan *et al.*, 1979 and Witte *et al.*, 1978). One or more of these factors are absent in the platelets of patients with storage pool disease (Weis *et al.*, 1979). Release of alpha granule components occurs with exposure to thrombin or collagen (Kaplan *et al.*, 1979). The other types of platelet granules, the dense granule, contain primarily 5-hydroxytryptamine and adenosine diphosphate (ADP).

Stimulation of platelets with ADP or epinephrine causes secretion of dense granules (Mills, Robb, and Roberts, 1968). Recent studies suggest that the release of these granules is inhibited by aspirin, indomethacin, and other cyclooxygenase inhibitors which prevent the conversion of arachidonic acid to prostaglandins (Linder *et al.*, 1979). Platelet factor-4 (Deuel *et al.*, 1977), the platelet-derived growth factor (Heldin, Westermark, and Wasteson, 1979), and β-thromboglobulin (Moore and Pepper, 1976) have been isolated and chemically characterized.

Circulating platelets undergo a number of well-defined physiological actions. They have the unique property of adhering to areas of endothelial injury or loss. In part, this action is mediated by contact with exposed subendothelial collagen (MacIntyre, 1976) and requires the presence of factor VIII antigen (Fuster *et al.*, 1978). After adherence to endothelium, the platelets undergo the release reaction which involves the secretion of the contents of their alpha and/or dense granules, depending on the nature of the stimulus for the reaction. This reaction is calcium dependent and requires ADP. The release of ADP induces the adherence of platelets to each other, a process that is called aggregation. Such a process further promotes the development of a platelet thrombus. If the sheer stress of flow is sufficiently high, the platelet thrombus or clump may become detached, be carried downstream, and be broken up. Alternatively, the platelet may trigger the coagulation system resulting in the deposition of fibrin and the formation of a red thrombus which causes complete occlusion.

Thus, whether or not a true thrombus is formed depends on the balance between the forces of platelet adherence, platelet aggregation, and stimulation of the coagulation system versus the haemodynamic sheer stresses. The low sheer stress in veins creates a situation where lower forces of adhesion and aggregation are required to form a thrombus than is the case in arteries where the forces capable of dislodging the platelet thrombus or clump are more prominent and thus tend to inhibit arterial thrombus formation. This concept may also partially explain why anticoagulants (which primarily prevent fibrin formation) are more effective in venous disease where reduced flow rather than platelet adherence and aggregation are primary aetiological factors. In contrast, in arterial diseases, where platelet adherence and aggregation and their role in stimulating proliferation of smooth muscle cells are the critical factors, antiplatelet agents are generally more effective. In the case of normal endothelium, the continual production of PGI_2 (a potent inhibitor of platelet aggregation) prevents the initial platelet adherence (Moncada and Vane, 1979).

Investigators in the field have divided the platelet release reaction into two phases. Release I refers to the secretion of the contents of the dense body and is induced by ADP, adrenalin, and low concentrations of collagen. This reaction is abolished by aspirin, although high concentrations of collagen or thrombus can overcome the aspirin effect (MacIntyre, 1976). Release II refers to the release of alpha granule constituents. This release does not appear to be dependent on prostaglandins. It is known that agents (such as dipyridamole), which elevate intracellular cAMP, inhibit the platelet release reaction (Mills and Smith, 1971).

Macrophages

The macrophage is a large phagocytic cell descended from the circulating blood monocyte. Macrophages are non-dividing cells which do not replicate in tissue culture (Edelson and Cohn, 1976). They have an outstanding ability to adhere to glass or plastic in the presence of plasma. When cultured for sufficient periods of time, they also can form large, multinucleated giant cells (Chang and Yao, 1979). In addition to their ability to phagocytose india ink and other particles, the presence of Fc receptors is another characteristic marker for these cells. Other known surface receptors of the cells include those for α-macroglobulin–trypsin complexes (Kaplan and Nielsen, 1979), acetylated LDL (Goldstein *et al.*, 1979), and for the C3b component of complement (Roelants, 1977).

Monocytes appear to be attracted to sites of endothelial injury (Gerrity, 1981). They are capable of producing a growth factor that stimulates proliferation of fibroblasts and smooth muscle cells (Liebovich and Ross, 1976). Macrophages are also a critical compo-

nent of the immune system. With the receptors for the Fc fragment of IgG and complement, they are thought to play a key role in the initial processing of antigen prior to the mounting of a T lymphocyte and/or B lymphocyte immune response by the organism (Roelants, 1977). They also have the capacity to maintain antigen memory by storing antigen and releasing it over an extended period of time (Roelants, 1977). Antigen–antibody immune complexes are thought to play a role in the pathogenesis of many forms of vasculitis. The deposition of these complexes may be associated with the presence of the C3b component of complement (Bellanti, 1978).

THE PATHOGENESIS OF ATHEROSCLEROSIS

Atherosclerosis has been defined as 'a variable combination of the changes of the intima of arteries (as distinguished from arterioles) consisting of the focal accumulation of lipids, complex carbohydrates, blood and blood products, fibrous tissue, and calcium deposits and associated with medial changes' (Study Group, 1958). In terms of current cell biology, the development of an atherosclerotic plaque involves two major interrelated processes which proceed concurrently. The first involves platelet–endothelial interaction and its consequences while the second involves the incorporation and accumulation of intracellular and extracellular lipids.

Endothelial Changes

Most current evidence suggests that endothelial loss or injury is the initial step in the pathogenesis of atherosclerosis. In animal models, increased endothelial permeability has been demonstrated in arterial locations where atherosclerotic plaques preferentially develop (Bjorkerud and Bondjers, 1972; Caplan and Schwartz, 1973). Examination of the endothelial surfaces of arteries from pigs, rabbits, mice, and young humans who died suddenly have shown clumps of formed elements, mainly platelets and leucocytes, at those sites where atherosclerosis characteristically develops (Jørgensen *et al.*, 1972). The cause of this endothelial damage has not been determined. Possibilities include antigen–antibody complex deposition (Angles-Cano, Sultan, and Clauvel, 1979), haemodynamic sheer stresses, and, in humans, smoking (Fuster *et al.*, 1981; Hladover, 1978). To explain the variable susceptibility to atherosclerosis of different individuals, haemodynamic stress must be coupled with some other factors, such as an increased susceptibility to endothelial injury. Since haemodynamic stresses in similar locations are reasonably comparable between different adult individuals, they are probably more important in determining the sites of lesions within a single individual rather than being a cause for differences in susceptibility between individuals.

Once endothelial damage has occurred, platelets adhere to the injured endothelium and undergo the release reaction and degranulation. One of the products released from the granules is platelet-derived growth factor (PDGF) (Heldin, Westermark, and Wasteson, 1979). PDGF is a very potent growth hormone for smooth muscle cells and fibroblasts (Ross *et al.*, 1974). In addition, it also stimulates the migration of smooth muscle cells (Grotendorst *et al.*, 1981; Thorgeirsson, Robertson, and Cowan, 1979). Fibroblasts, glial cells, and smooth muscle cells, but not endothelial cells,

have receptors for PDGF (Heldin, Westermark, and Wasteson, 1981). Thus, the release of PDGF at the sites of endothelial injury and platelet adherence results in the stimulation of nearby smooth muscle cells in the media to re-enter the cell cycle and undergo proliferation. This change causes them to lose their contractile properties (Chamley-Campbell, Campbell, and Ross, 1979), migrate from the media to the subendothelial space via fenestrations in the elastic lamella (Thorgeirsson, Robertson, and Cowan, 1979), and undergo proliferation (Ross *et al.*, 1974). As part of the proliferative process, they secrete elastin and collagen (Ross, 1971; Ross and Klebanoff, 1971) as well as glycosaminoglycans (Wight and Ross, 1975), thus providing the fibroproliferative components of the plaque.

Lipids

In order to understand the second major process involved in atherogenesis, the cellular uptake of lipid, it is necessary to have some understanding of lipid and lipoprotein metabolism. The lipids include free cholesterol, cholesteryl esters, triglycerides, phospholipids, and fatty acids. The salts of fatty acids are soluble

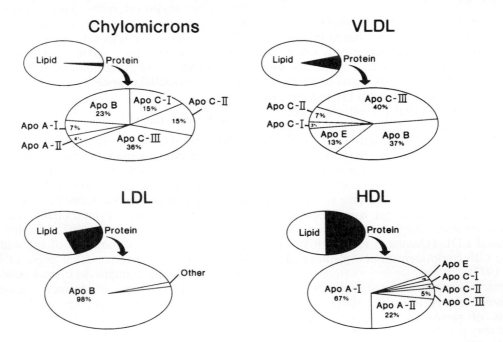

Figure 1   The appropriate composition of the major lipoprotein particles found in plasma. (Reproduced by permission of Mayo Clinic and Mayo Foundation)

and the phospholipids are amphoteric and tend to be located at lipid–water interfaces. The other lipids are all insoluble in water and must be transported in the blood as macromolecular complexes called lipoproteins. Of these lipids, only fatty acids and free cholesterol have the capability of moving freely through cellular membranes. In addition, it must be recalled that the sterol ring cannot be oxidized in animal tissues.

Lipoproteins

For operational convenience, the plasma lipoproteins can be divided into four major classes. These include: chylomicrons (exogenous particles) which are triglyceride rich and are formed by the intestine during fat absorption; very low density lipoproteins (VLDL) (endogenous particles) which are also triglyceride-rich and are secreted by the liver following absorption and during the mobilization of fat stores; low density lipoproteins (LDL) which are cholesterol-rich and are formed in the liver by the degradation of VLDL; and high density lipoproteins (HDL) which are also cholesterol-rich and are formed by both the liver and the intestine. These classes are separated by electrophoresis which is based on differences in electrical charge and by ultracentrifugation which detects differences in density. The protein portion of the lipoprotein particles is made up of apolipoproteins. Figure 1 shows the relative lipid and protein composition of each class of particles as well as their apolipoprotein compositions In addition to their role as carriers of plasma lipid, these apoproteins also have specific roles in the regulation of the enzymes lipoprotein

lipase (LPL) and lecithin-cholesterol acyltransferase (L-CAT) which are critical in the metabolism of lipoproteins as well as in the regulation of the interaction of particles with specific cellular receptors. These specific functions are listed in Table 1.

The assembly of lipoprotein particles involves synthesis in the liver and/or intestine as well as exchange of apoproteins between lipoprotein particles in the plasma. This process, as currently understood, is diagrammed in Fig. 2. As shown there, HDL is secreted by the liver as a bilayer disk containing phospholipids and primarily apolipoprotein E. On entering the plasma the HDL acquires apolipoproteins A-I and A-II from chylomicrons, and phospholipids (Wilson, Ellsworth, and Jackson, 1980), cholesterol, and cholesteryl esters from other lipoproteins and from tissues. The transfer of phospholipids and of cholesteryl esters

HDL AND CHYLOMICRON FORMATION

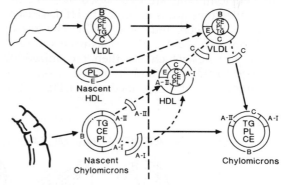

Figure 2   The role of the interchange of apolipoproteins between lipoprotein particles in the formation of circulating plasma lipoproteins. (Reproduced by permission of Mayo Clinic and Mayo Foundation)

Table 1   Human plasma apolipoproteins

Apoprotein	Site of synthesis	Function	Consequences of deficiency
ApoA-I	Intestine, liver	L-CAT activation	Severe atherosclerosis
ApoA-II	Intestine, liver	Lipid binding	Unknown
Apo B	Intestine, liver	Fat transport Receptor recognition	Absorption and neurological disorders
ApoC-I	Liver	LPL activator	Unknown
ApoC-II	Liver	LPL activator	Inhibition of liver remnant
ApoC-III	Liver	LPL inhibition	uptake
Apo D	Liver	Cholesteryl ester transfer	Unknown
Apo E	Liver	Receptor recognition Liver remnant uptake	Unknown

from other lipoproteins is facilitated by the action of specific transfer proteins (Fielding and Fielding, 1980; Hopkins and Barter, 1980; Pattnaik *et al.*, 1980). The C apoproteins of HDL are acquired from VLDL. VLDL is secreted by the liver and, after degradation to remnant particles in peripheral tissues, it is removed by the liver, degraded further, and secreted as LDL (see Fig. 3). Nascent chylomicrons from the lymph provide apolipoproteins A-I and A-II to HDL and then are degraded to remnants in peripheral tissues, followed by further degradation in the liver to LDL (similar to the degradation of VLDL) (Fielding, 1978).

The metabolism of remnant particles is further detailed in Fig. 3. The enzyme lipoprotein lipase (LPL) plays a major role in this process. This enzyme is synthesized and secreted by adipocytes from which it is transferred to the surface of endothelial cells where it acts on circulating lipoprotein particles (Spooner *et al.*, 1979a, 1979b). As the triglycerides of VLDL and chylomicrons are hydrolysed by LPL, the C apoproteins are transferred to HDL (Eisenberg, Bilheimer, and Levy, 1972). The loss of C apoproteins and triglycerides results in remnant particles which are then recognized by hepatic receptors and removed from the circulation and degraded to LDL. The recognition of these particles by the hepatic receptors is dependent on the absence of C apoproteins. Ordinarily these apoproteins inhibit the uptake of intact VLDL and chylomicrons (Shelburne *et al.*, 1980; Windler, Chao, and Havel, 1980). During fat ingestion, the C apoproteins are transferred back to chylomicrons and VLDL (Eisenberg, Bilheimer, and Levy, 1972).

The liver has an immense capacity to remove remnant particles. Hence, they are rarely seen in large quantities in the circulation (Sherrill and Dietschy, 1978). Following hepatic uptake, the remnant particles are rapidly degraded to LDL and secreted by the liver into the peripheral blood.

Defects in LDL removal are responsible for most problems associated with hypercholesterolemia. The removal of LDL from the circulating plasma occurs by an LDL receptor mediated route and by a receptor-independent route (Thompson *et al.*, 1981). In homozygous familial hypercholesterolemia, the LDL receptor route does not function. A similar situation is present in hypothyroidism, but this effect is reversible with thyroid replacement therapy. In heterozygotes the receptor route can be stimulated by treatment with colestipol (a bile acid sequestral resin) or with the experimental

PERIPHERAL METABOLISM OF LIPOPROTEINS

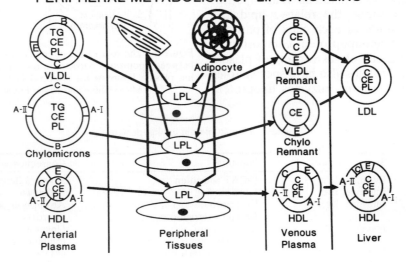

Figure 3   The role of lipoprotein lipase (LPL) in the metabolism of lipoproteins by cells of the peripheral tissues. (Reproduced by permission of Mayo Clinic and Mayo Foundation)

drug mevinolin (Kovanen *et al.*, 1981). Both hepatic LDL receptors (or B-E receptors) and extrahepatic LDL receptors play a role in the receptor dependent route of LDL catabolism (Brown, Kovanen, and Goldstein, 1981).

The LDL receptor-independent route of LDL removal is not well understood. A portion of this route may depend on a proposed scavenger pathway. This proposed pathway is based on the fact that, while macrophages (of all types) do not have LDL receptors, they do have receptors for modified LDL (acetylated LDL). The activity of these acetylated LDL receptors is not regulated, hence, they can pick up enormous quantities of LDL and become classic foam cells (Goldstein *et al.*, 1979). It is proposed that in vivo the delayed catabolism of LDL results in a modification of the LDL-apo B protein which results in its being recognized by this macrophage receptor.

At present it is unclear whether macrophages or smooth muscle cells are the major sources of foam cells in atherosclerotic lesions. It should be noted that the LDL receptor also recognizes apolipoprotein E of remnant particles. This recognition may result in the uptake of remnants in areas of endothelial damage and also may play a role in the uptake of remnants by the liver (Brown, Kovanen, and Goldstein, 1981). There also appears to be a remnant receptor which recognizes normal apolipoprotein E (Sherrill, Innerarity, and Mahley, 1980). Recently the group at the Gladstone Foundation (Hui, Innerarity, and Mahley, 1981; Mahley *et al.*, 1981) have shown that this receptor does not recognize apo B or LDL. It has been called the apo E receptor and is distinct from the LDL or B-E receptor. The Gladstone group showed that the hepatic membranes of young animals contain both E and B-E receptors, while in the liver membranes of adult animals, the hepatic B-E receptors are strikingly reduced in number. The apo E receptor does not recognize the abnormal apo E (apoE-II isomeric form) found in patients with familial dyslipoproteinaemia (Havel *et al.*, 1980). Because of this, patients with this disorder accumulate large quantities of remnants in the circulating plasma. Recently it has been shown that abnormal remnant particles present in cholesterol-fed dogs can be recognized by a receptor present in macrophages (Mahley *et al.*, 1980).

Mechanisms Considered Responsible for Accumulation of Cholesteryl Esters in Atherosclerotic Plaques

This pathway is outlined in Fig. 4. Whether or not accumulation of cholesteryl esters occurs depends on the balance between the uptake of lipoproteins and intracellular cholesterol synthesis versus the removal of intracellular cholesteryl esters. The major cell types of the arterial wall that are involved in this process are smooth muscle cells and macrophages. The relative importance of each of these cell types is still quite controversial.

Lipoprotein Uptake

The best-known uptake process is the LDL receptor pathway described by Goldstein and Brown (Brown, Kovanen, and Goldstein, 1981; Goldstein and Brown, 1977). These authors have demonstrated that normal human fibroblasts and smooth muscle cells have membrane surface, high affinity receptors for LDL. After the binding of LDL to these receptors, it is internalized by endocytosis and transported to lysosomes where the apolipoprotein (apo B) is degraded by lysosomal proteases, while the lipids are hydrolysed by an acidic lysosomal lipase. This results in the subsequent stimulation of the enzyme acylcholesterol acyltransferase (A-CAT) which results in the re-synthesis of cholesteryl esters (especially cholesterol oleate) and an inhibition of the controlling enzyme of cholesterol biosynthesis, HMG-CoA reductase. In cells from patients with familial hypercholesterolaemia, these authors have demonstrated absent, deficient, or defective LDL receptors and, in two families, a defect in the internalization of receptor-bound LDL (Brown and Goldstein, 1976; Goldstein, Kottke, and Brown, 1982). Cells from patients with cholesteryl ester storage disease or Wolman's disease have a deficiency of the lysosomal acidic lipase, and thus accumulate cholesteryl esters (especially cholesterol linoleate) in the lysosomes of the cells (Goldstein *et al.*, 1975).

Specialized high affinity receptors for the uptake of lipoproteins have also been described in macrophages. The best characterized one is a surface receptor that recognizes a modified LDL called acetylated LDL (Gold-

REMOVAL OF CELLULAR CHOLESTEROL

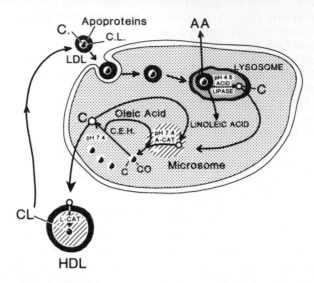

Figure 4   The intracellular metabolism of cholesteryl esters. (Reproduced by
permission of Mayo Clinic and Mayo Foundation)

stein *et al.*, 1979), β-VLDL (Mahley *et al.*,
1980), a lipoprotein that is present in the
plasma of cholesterol-fed animals, or LDL that
has previously been exposed to cultured endothelial cells (Henriksen, Mahoney, and
Steinberg, 1981). It is very likely that in the
future other receptors for specific lipoproteins
will be described in these and other major cells
of the arterial wall.

Sterol Removal
Besides regulation of lipoprotein uptake, cholesteryl ester accumulation is also regulated by
the rate of intracellular sterol removal. As
shown in Fig. 4, this process consists of three
major steps. First, since cholesteryl esters are
very hydrophobic and cannot cross cell membranes, the stored esters (primarily cholesterol
oleate) must be hydroliysed to free cholesterol.
This is accomplished by a neutral enzyme in
the cytoplasm called cholesteryl ester hydrolase (CEH). The second step of removal is the
transfer of free cholesterol through the membrane. The details of this process are not well
understood although it is known that cholesterol can 'flip flop' between the membrane's
inner and outer leaflets (Blau and Bittman,
1978). It can also play a role in regulating the

fluidity of membranes (Kawato, Kinosita, and
Ikegami, 1978; Shepherd and Büldt, 1979).
   The third step involved in cholesterol removal is the uptake of cholesterol from the
outer site of the membrane by an acceptor protein. Most evidence suggests that HDL is the
physiologic acceptor protein and that apolipoprotein A-I and phosphatidylcholine are the
essential components of HDL responsible for
this activity (Stein *et al*, 1975; Stein, Fainaru,
and Stein, 1979).

Drugs and Lipid Metabolism

Recent studies by Brown, Ho, and Goldstein,
(1980) have shown that in macrophages,
stored, intracellular cholesteryl esters are continuously undergoing hydrolysis by the enzyme
cholesteryl ester hydrolase (CEH) and that, in
addition, cholesteryl esters are continuously
being reformed by A-CAT (acylcholesterol
acyltransferase). Thus, A-CAT activity can
regulate the availability of free cholesterol for
transfer across the cell membrane. These authors also showed that exposure of cells that
have been previously loaded with cholesteryl
esters to HDL results in a nearly complete
inhibition of A-CAT with no change in the

rate of cholesteryl ester hydrolysis (Brown, Ho, and Goldstein, 1980). Studies from our laboratory have shown that A-CAT activity can be inhibited by many commonly used pharmacologic agents (Alley *et al.*, 1982; Cornicelli *et al.*, 1981). A recent report indicates that one of these agents, propranolol, also significantly reduces the mortality of patients with previous myocardial infarctions (Kolata, 1981). Thus, several pharmacologic agents in current use may potentially benefit atherosclerosis by promoting excretion of intracellular cholesterol. Further studies of this potential approach to therapy appears warranted. In the case of macrophages, the unregulated uptake of massive quantities of cholesteryl esters may result in cell death and rupture with the accumulation of large quantities of extracellular lipid. In an extracellular location, enzymes for the hydrolysis and removal of this lipid may not be available.

Whether or not smooth muscle cells can differentiate and acquire the characteristics of macrophages remains a very controversial question. While morphologic studies suggest that such a possibility may exist (Geer, 1965), this change has not been reproduced in tissue culture.

In summary, the major cellular processes involved in atherogenesis include: endothelial damage; stimulation of smooth muscle proliferation by the platelet-derived growth factor with a production of large quantities of connective tissue proteins; uptake of specific lipoproteins by specific cell surface receptors; and removal of intracellular lipids by HDL. Alteration of any of these functions can lead to accumulation of lipid in atherosclerotic lesions. Also, it is obvious that there are multiple potential points for possible therapeutic intervention. In advanced atherosclerosis the additional processes of calcification and atheromatosis embolization further extend the pathological process.

EXAMINATION OF PATIENTS WITH PERIPHERAL VASCULAR DISEASE

Taking a History

The first important step in the examination of a patient is the elucidation of an accurate and meaningful history. This is particularly import-

ant in the case of the patient with peripheral vascular disease. The most frequent presenting symptom is pain in an extremity which may either be persistent or intermittent in nature. Types of persistent pain include the following.

Pretrophic or Rest Pain

This form of severe pain is present in gangrenous ulcers and pregangrenous ischaemic tissue. The pain is constant and severe. It is aggravated by elevation. Frequently, patients will hang an extremity over the edge of the bed to obtain relief. Narcotics are usually required for relief.

Pain of Acute Occlusion

This pain is characterized by a sudden onset. It may be excruciating in some instances. In other cases it is primarily described as a continuous numbness and/or tingling.

Pain of Neuropathy

Characteristically, this pain is described as sharp, shooting, and jabbing and occurs as paroxysms.

Pain of Inflammation

This is a relatively mild aching pain associated with inflamed tissue such as seen in thrombophlebitis and more rarely in lymphangitis and arteritis. It is usually relieved with aspirin or similar analgesics.

Intermittent Claudication

Intermittent pain is of particular importance in the evaluation of arterial disease. The most diagnostic and important form of pain is intermittent claudication. It is described as a numbness or aching in the extremity that is always induced by exercise of muscles and ceases promptly when the exercise is stopped. Induction of the pain usually requires a constant amount of exercise. Most importantly, the distress is not brought on by weight-bearing and does not require shifting the weight from the extremity to obtain relief. This pain is diagnostic of muscle ischaemia, usually due to arterial insufficiency. It is one of the most specific symptoms in medicine. In the lower extremities, the location of the distress can frequently provide a clue as to the level of the major arterial obstruction. Claudication in the calf muscles suggests that the obstruction is at or proximal to the level of the popliteal artery. Thigh claudication suggests that the obstruction is at or proximal to the origin of the common femoral artery, while hip, buttock, or back claudication suggests aortic or aorto-iliac obstruction.

The pain of several other common conditions is frequently confused with intermittent claudication. Pain that is induced by weight-bearing and promptly relieved by shifting weight to the other foot or sitting down is usually indicative of osteoarthritis of the hips, knees, or spine. If this type of pain occurs in the feet, it may indicate the presence of plantar neuromas, plantar fasciitis, or osteoporosis.

Very rarely, pain from compression of the cauda equina by hypertrophic ridging or a protruding lumbar disk can at least superficially mimic intermittent claudication. On careful questioning, however, the patient will indicate that the pain is also brought on by bending, lifting, or other movements of the spine and the pain may be associated with numbness, incoordination, or clumsiness. This syndrome has been called 'pseudoclaudication' (Kavanaugh, Svien, and Holnar, 1968). It should be emphasized that it is a rare syndrome. Besides being confused with intermittent claudication, the pseudoclaudication syndrome is most commonly confused with muscle attachment pain of the trochanter of the hip (pseudo-pseudo-claudication). Localized tenderness in this location can be associated with intermittent pain on walking, standing, or lying on the involved side at night. Symptoms may be present for months before the patient is seen. The diagnosis is confirmed with the finding of tenderness over the trochanter of the hip and a normal hip X-ray or rarely the presence of calcification in the area of tenderness. This condition should always be carefully excluded prior to subjecting patients to myelography for suspected pseudoclaudication since it is quickly remedied with the local injection of corticosteroids combined with physical therapy. It is one of the most commonly missed diagnoses in patients with suspected peripheral vascular disease.

Pain of Erythromelalgia

A second type of intermittent pain seen in peripheral vascular disease practice is the pain of erythromelalgia. In this extremely rare condition, the patient notes an intense burning sensation of the soles of the feet. It comes on when the skin temperature reaches a critical level. Patients obtain relief by cooling the feet with a fan or a pan of cold water. As long as the skin remains cool, there is no pain.

Physical Examination of Patients with Peripheral Vascular Disease

Arterial Pulsations, Lower Extremity

The most important part of the examination of a patient with peripheral vascular disease is the evaluation of the arterial pulsations. With practice and experience, it can be done quite accurately. It is useful to use a shorthand system to grade the pulses so that they can be compared from one examination to the next. At our Institution, they are graded from 0 to 4 with 0 denoting an absence of pulsation and 4 indicating a normal pulse; 2 denotes a pulsation that is definitely present but definitely reduced; 3 indicates a slight impairment of the pulse; and 1 denotes a barely palpable pulse. In the large vessels, the presence or absence of bruits should also be noted.

Pedal pulses are best examined with the patient sitting on the examining table with the feet in a dependent position. The dorsalis pedis pulse can be felt on the dorsum of the foot, usually in its midportion between the first and third metatarsals just distal to the ankle. This location can be variable, however, and it must be recalled that bilateral absence of the dorsalis pedis pulse occurs in 10 per cent. of normal individuals. The posterior tibial pulse is best felt posterior and just distal to the medial malleolus. Bilateral absence of this pulse occurs in about 2 per cent. of normal individuals. Hence, absence of both a palpable dorsalis pedis and a posterior tibial pulse is extremely rare in normal individuals.

Examination of the popliteal pulse is best done with the patient supine. The fingers of both hands are placed over the popliteal fossa and the knee is lefted and slightly flexed. The pulse may not be immediately apparent but if one waits a few seconds, it becomes evident. Often one must search over the entire popliteal fossa to locate this pulse. In searching for popliteal aneurysms, it is particularly important to search the upper portion of the popliteal fossa between the insertions of the medial and lateral flexor muscles. While initially, evaluation of the popliteal pulse is difficult, this difficulty is readily overcome by persistent practice. This is best accomplished by initially examining patients with aneurysms. Evaluation of the femoral artery at the groin usually presents no problem. In many individuals, the abdominal aorta can easily be palpated in a relaxed, supine position. Initially, this skill can be developed by routinely feeling the aorta of individuals and/or cautiously evaluating the size of aneurysms of the abdominal aorta. The true width of the aorta can be evaluated by subtracting the apparent thickness of the abdominal wall (felt by pinching it between two fingers) from the apparent thickness of the aorta as determined by palpation. Evaluation of the size of aneurysm by this method is quite accurate when compared to ultrasound measurements. The normal aorta is 2 to 3 cm in diameter. A word of caution, however, is appropriate regarding this examination. A horseshoe kidney can have the same expansile pulsation as an abdominal aortic aneurysm on examination. Hence, one must be certain to rule this possibility out before making a definitive diagnosis of aortic aneurysm.

Arterial Pulsations, Upper Extremity

Examination of the circulation of the upper extremity can be accomplished by evaluating the radial and ulnar pulses at the wrist, the brachial pulse at the upper arm, and the subclavian pulses. Rarely, the radial pulse may be located on the extensor side of the radius rather than on its volar surface. If a question arises as to whether or not the ulnar pulse is present, this can be readily checked by performing the Allen test (Allen, 1929). To perform the test, the examiner compresses the radial artery with his thumb, taking care not to tighten the skin over the ulnar aspect of the wrist. The patient is then instructed to clench his hand in order to squeeze blood out of the hands. Following this, the patient opens his hands partially, *avoiding full extension*. The return of blood to the hand via the ulnar artery can then be observed by the return of the red colour to the skin. The brachial pulse is best felt in the midportion of the upper arm by pressure of the medial surface of the arm so as to compress the artery against the humerus. The subclavian pulses are most easily felt by standing behind the patient who is in a sitting position and searching for the pulses just behind the midportion of the clavicle.

Doppler Ultrasound, Arteries

In recent years, ultrasonic techniques based on the Doppler principle have been developed for the detection of blood flow in arteries. Such instruments are very sensitive and at times can detect flow when a pulse is not palpable. From a practical standpoint, however, the detection of such minimal flows is of limited significance. Since these instruments do not measure flow quantitatively, their practical use is limited to unusual situations. In most cases, the experienced examiner can get all the essential information he needs by examination of the arterial pulses.

Cutaneous Circulation

The second important part of the examination of the patient with arterial disease is the evaluation of cutaneous ischaemia. In the presence of occlusions of the major arteries, the absence or presence of cutaneous ischemia is dependent on the degree of collateral flow.

To evaluate cutaneous ischaemia, the patient is placed supine on the examining table while the examiner elevates the legs and the patient flexes and extends the toes. The relative pallor of the soles of the feet can then be compared. Following the elevation, the patient is asked to sit up quickly with the feet in a dependent position and the time required for the return of colour (normal = 5 seconds) and the filling of superficial veins (normal = 15 to 20 seconds) is determined. Prolongation of colour return and venous filling to 1 minute or more indicates a severe degree of cutaneous ischemia and often is associated with gangrenous ulcers or pregangrenous colour changes in the skin.

Examination of Venous Disorders

In the examination of the patient with suspected venous disease, the examiner should attempt to determine whether or not deep vein obstruction is present and the nature of any swelling that is present. Frequently, when deep vein obstruction is present (especially obstruction of the inferior vena cava), the extremity takes on a violaceous colour when the patient stands for a few minutes. While prominent varicose veins are usually present in patients with deep venous obstruction, they are also often present on a congenital basis and thus are not a useful diagnostic finding. The presence of 'stasis pigmentation', a light brown to nearly black discolouration below the knees and especially over the medial malleolus, is a fairly reliable sign of long-standing deep vein obstruction.

In the evaluation of venous disease, the differential diagnosis of swelling of the lower legs is of critical importance. Ankle oedema characterized by a dependent distribution (i.e. more prominent at the ankle than at the leg above) may be due to cardiac disease and is also frequently related to chronic venous obstruction. It always pits with pressure. This dependent swelling is not characteristic of early, acute thrombophlebitis. If the area of swelling does not pit, it is probably due to lipoedema (accumulation of subcutaneous fat). Also, lipoedema almost never involves the feet. In lymphoedema (lymphatic obstruction) the swelling usually is not dependent but has a cylindrical type of distribution and usually involves the entire leg below the knee and often the entire leg up to the level of the groin.

In sural popliteal phlebitis, the earliest swelling occurs in the calf. This can best be appreciated with the patient supine and the knee flexed at a 90° angle. Standing at the foot of the bed and looking at the medial edge of the tibia, one can readily appreciate a concavity of the calf muscles as they fall away from the midportion of the medial edge of the tibia in normal individuals. In the earliest stages of phlebitis, this concavity of the musculature disappears and the muscles appear as a convex bulge protruding from behind the medial tibial edge. I have found this sign to be much more reliable than attempts to measure calf circumference. It is difficult to make such measurements accurately and small amounts of asymmetry due to atrophy or hypertrophy of calf muscles may cause such measurements to be misleading. The differentiation of acute phlebitis is also aided by the presence of mild aching in the calf, localized tenderness, and increased temperature of the extremity.

Ultransonic Examination, Veins

Ultransonic examination can be very helpful in the detection of venous obstruction of the iliac, superficial femoral, and popliteal veins (Yao and Berger, 1974). Normally, phasic flow sounds can be heard over these veins. These sounds decrease in intensity with inspiration due to increased abdominal pressure and increase in intensity with expiration. They disappear with the increased abdominal pressure of a Valsalva's manoeuver and can be increased by squeezing the muscles of the calf. In the presence of venous obstruction proximally, the sounds are markedly decreased in intensity or absent, and changes with respiration as well as augmentation by compression of the calf muscles is lost. Unless large collaterals have formed, these findings are a reasonably good indication of acute or chronic venous obstruction.

ARTERIOSCLEROSIS

Arteriosclerosis Obliterans

Arteriosclerosis obliterans (ASO) of the lower extremities is primarily a disease of elderly men. A large series reports a relative incidence of only 10 per cent. in women (Bloor, 1961). The disease is virtually a disease of cigarette smokers. In a series of over 400 men, only 2.5 per cent. were non-smokers (Juergens, Barker, and Hines, 1960). This relationship has been confirmed by autopsy studies (Strong and Richards, 1976) and it has been shown that patients with ASO who stop smoking have a much lower incidence of amputation than patients who continue to smoke. As indicated in the earlier section on the pathogenesis of atherosclerosis, smoking probably produces its effects by causing endothelial damage to the arteries (Fuster *et al.*, 1981; Hladover, 1978). Diabetes mellitus is another important aetiologic factor in this disease. It occurs in 15 to 20 per cent. of patients with ASO (Bartels and Rullo, 1958; Schadt *et al.*, 1961). Since 97.5 per cent. of the patients with ASO are smokers, it is apparent that both diabetes and smoking are important etiological factors in many patients. Other factors of lesser importance are hyperlipoproteinaemia and possibly hypertension. The incidence of hyperlipoproteinaemia depends to a large extent on the definition of normal lipid levels, but, even so, levels of blood lipids that are clearly well within the usual norms are common in this disease. Unfortunately, few formal studies have been done as compared to the plethora of such studies of lipids in coronary heart disease.

The pathogenesis of atherosclerosis was discussed in the previous section. As shown in the diagrams in Fig. 5, after the initial endothelial damage, there is a migration of smooth muscle cells from the media into the subendothelial space. These platelet-derived growth-factor-stimulated cells then accumulate lipid until this uptake produces cell necrosis and spilling of lipid and other debris into the extracellular space. The fibroblasts form a fibrous cap resulting in the classical pearly plaque. Subsequent rupture of this plaque then results in distal embolization of atheromatous debris into smaller arterial branches, thus aggravating the distal ischemia.

Clinical Features

Except for the incidental finding of asymmetric subclavian bruits or a decreased blood pressure in one arm, arteriosclerosis of the extremities is confined almost exclusively to the lower extremities. In the elderly, its clinical presentation occurs in one or more of three forms: acute arterial occlusion, intermittent claudication, or severe cutaneous ischaemia with or without gangrene. Acute arterial occlusion will be discussed in a subsequent section.

Intermittent claudication is the most common presenting symptom of ASO. In elderly patients, who are relatively physically inactive, this symptom may occur only after the disease is moderately far advanced. In general, the distance at which symptoms occur when walking at a normal pace on level ground is a fairly good indicator of overall severity. Except for situations resulting from unusual trauma to the skin, cutaneous ischaemia is rarely seen in in-

dividuals whose claudication distance is greater than one block, (approx. 300 metres). The major clinical problem is the diagnosis of ASO in patients with symptoms of one of the other forms of intermittent pain of the lower extremity. When the pain is clearly related to walking and does not occur with weight-bearing, bending, or lifting, one can be quite certain of the diagnosis. In cases where the patient is a poor observer, strolling down the hallway with the patient will often make the diagnosis quite evident. As indicated in the section on vascular examination, the most common sources of confusion are osteoarthritis of the hips and knees (which can be ruled out with examination of the joint motions and appropriate X-rays) and muscle attachment pain of the hip (evidence by tenderness over the hip trochanter and usually negative hip X-rays). If the distress is limited to the feet and ankles, plantar neuromas should be sought. The clinical reduction or absence of pulses is diagnostic. ASO may commonly occur in association with other disorders in elderly individuals and the clinician must carefully sort out the symptoms related to each of the different aetiologies in order to treat the patient effectively. Only rarely is it necessary to conduct ultrasound Doppler studies. While these can readily rule out ASO as an aetiology, in the more common situation where ASO is present in association with an orthopaedic problem, symptoms due to ASO must be clearly identified from those due to orthopaedic causes before considering therapeutic possibilities.

Symptoms of cutaneous ischaemia present the clinician with an urgent, challenging problem. These patients have severe, constant pain in the feet and/or toes which often keeps them awake at night. Often the foot and ankle will be swollen from attempts to obtain relief by sleeping with the foot in a dependent position. The skin frequently has a deep rubor or bluish black colour. Ulcers, when present, are usually located on the toes or heels. When in other locations, they have usually been precipitated by trauma. In areas where their surface is not covered by necrotic debris or infectious exudate, the ulcers have a pale pink base of granulomatous tissue. At times the patient may also have symptoms of ischaemic neuropathy. Often they have associated muscle atrophy, osteoporosis, and contractures.

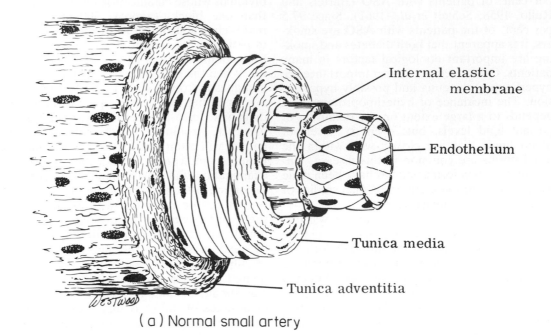

(a) Normal small artery

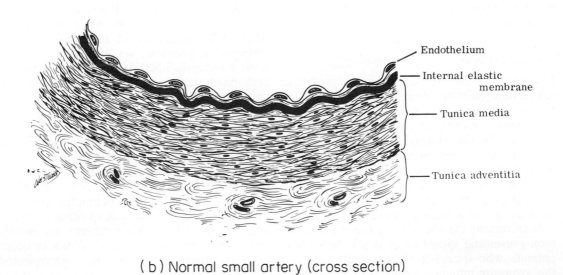

(b) Normal small artery (cross section)

Figure 5   Sequential stages in the pathogenesis of antherosclerosis. (Reproduced by permission of Mayo Clinic and Mayo Foundation)

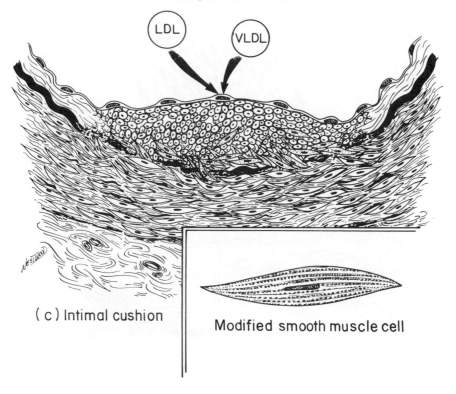

(c) Intimal cushion

Modified smooth muscle cell

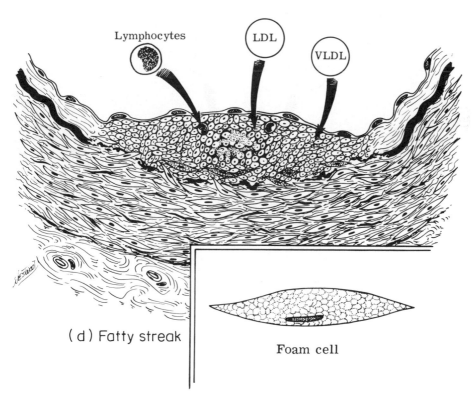

(d) Fatty streak

Foam cell

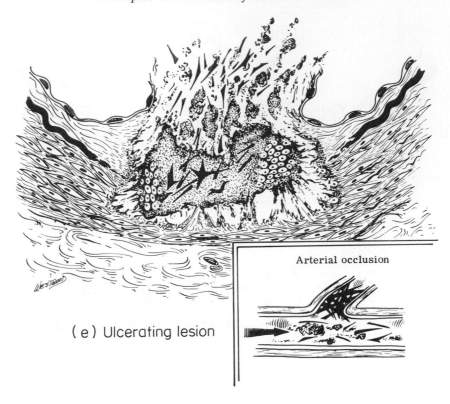

(e) Ulcerating lesion

Arterial occlusion

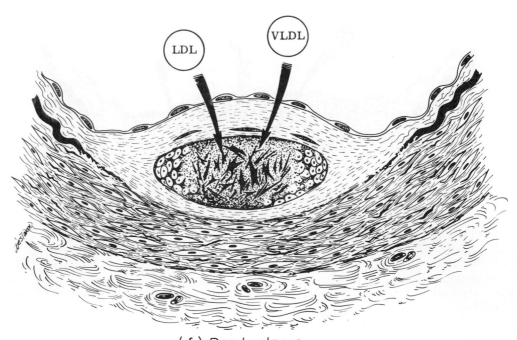

LDL

VLDL

(f) Pearly plaque

On physical examination distal pulses are absent with or without the absence of proximal arterial pulses as well as postural signs of cutaneous ischaemia. When ulcers are present, they are often infected and have copious exudate. It is important to differentiate ulcers due to cutaneous ischaemia from those due to repetitive trauma to areas with absent or diminished sensation. These latter ulcers are characteristically located over pressure points. Their management requires the treatment of secondary infection and the use of pads and special shoes to relieve pressure over the ulcer area. These ulcers have been called neurotrophic ulcers.

Investigations

The initial laboratory investigation of the patient with ASO should include assessment of blood lipids and plasma glucose. In patients with severe cutaneous ischaemia and/or ulcers, X-rays of the feet to rule out osteomyelitis should be obtained. Unless there are clear contraindications, nearly all patients with cutaneous ischaemia should be considered for aortography with visualization of the distal runoff. To obtain adequate visualization of the vessels, with minimum risk, it is important that aortography be done by a radiologist with considerable experience with this technique and with availability of equipment specifically designed for complete visualization of the entire length of the peripheral vessels. In general, the usual equipment used for coronary angiography is not adequate for obtaining the multiple long films required for adequate assessment of the peripheral arteries.

Medical Treatment

The medical treatment of patients with arteriosclerosis is largely supportive and should include modification of the risk factors. The cornerstone of this approach is to convince the patient to completely stop all forms of smoking. To successfully accomplish this, it is important for the clinician to discuss with the patient the history of his smoking, including an evaluation of whether or not he really craves cigarettes and/or just uses them to allay his chronic anxiety. Particular attention should be paid to the reasons why previous attempts to stop smoking have failed (i.e. withdrawal symptoms, a spouse continuing to smoke, social pressures, etc.). Based on these factors, the clinician's approach should be based on a sympathetic and understanding attitude. Frequently, where withdrawal symptoms are the reason for previous failures, the use of mild tranquilizers such as chlordiazepoxide (Librium) 10 mg t.i.d. for a limited period of time may be quite helpful. In other situations, individually tailored approaches should be used. Just admonishing the patient to stop smoking is rarely successful. It is important to point out to the patient that the more popular recommendations regarding control of diabetes and of hyperlipoproteinemia will have little effect in the patient who continues to smoke.

All patients with ASO should receive very specific instructions regarding routine foot care, i.e.: (a) strict avoidance of the use of any form of external heat as a means of warming a cold extremity (i.e. hot soaks, heating pads, hot water bottles, etc.); (b) avoidance of cold injury; (c) avoidance of mechanical injury from trimming corns and callouses, ill fitting shoes, and ingrown toenails; (d) wearing socks at night to prevent the heels from rubbing on the sheets; and (e) the regular use of a lanolin-based cream to lubricate the skin of the feet, thus avoiding the development of skin fissures.

The major principles involved in the treatment of gangrenous ulcers include: removal of necrotic debris, avoidance of chemical trauma from local ointments, systemic treatment of infection, adequate pain relief, bed rest, and exploration of means for improving the blood supply.

Except with very large ulcers, initial debridement should be non-surgical and should include soaking the involved extremity in clear, tepid water, 0.9% saline, or a saturated solution of boric acid for 15 to 20 minutes 3 or 4 times daily with dry dressings between the soaks. When ulcers are present between the toes, the use of dental rolls to separate the toes and thus provide adequate drainage of the lesions may be helpful. If available, the use of a whirlpool to replace one or more of the soaks is also beneficial. Solutions should never be warmer than 32 °C (90 °F). Occasionally enzymatic debridement with Varidase or a similar preparation may be useful. However, it must be used very cautiously for short periods of time (15 to 20 minutes) and be followed by soaks to remove the residual enzyme. When such preparations are used, the ulcer must be inspected daily and treatment discontinued at the first indication of any irritation of the normal tissue. The use of a whirlpool is clearly superior to this enzymatic approach.

Except for this enzymatic debridement, the use of any chemical antiseptics or any ointments on the lesions must be scrupulously avoided. All of these carry the hazard of inducing sensitization and delaying the healing process. All draining ulcers should be cultured and appropriate antibiotic therapy given systemically. The treatment of ischaemic ulcers requires that the patient have adequate relief from pain. Without this, other measures become impossible to implement. Levo-Dromoran (2 to 4 mg every 3 or 4 hours) is very effective and the potential for addiction is extremely low, even with prolonged use. Demerol (Pethidine) or other similar agents with a high incidence of addiction should be avoided in the treatment of these patients. In the treatment of patients with foot ulcers, it is important that the patient wear a thick stocking or a bulky dressing over the entire foot to protect it from rubbing the sheets and producing a new heel ulcer. Also, the knee and ankle joints should be passively or actively extended fully several times a day to prevent contractures.

While vasodilating agents are frequently recommended for the treatment of ischaemic ulcers, there is no good evidence that they are helpful. Also, the pathogenesis of the disease does not suggest that arterial spasm is a critical factor. This lack of effectiveness is also evident from clinical experience.

Surgical Treatment

Decisions regarding the elective surgical treatment of patients with intermittent claudication without significant cutaneous ischaemia depends on a number of important variables. Follow-up studies have shown that, of patients with intermittent claudication as their only symptom of ASO, only 3 per cent required subsequent amputation in a 5-year follow-up period (Juergens, Barker, and Hines, 1960). The amputation rate in diabetic patients is 4 times that of non-diabetic patients (Schadt *et al.*, 1961), and in diabetics, bilateral amputation is frequently required (Silbert, 1952). Another consideration is that many of these patients also have significant associated atherosclerosis of the coronary and cerebral arteries. It was found that 20 per cent. of patients with ASO have coronary artery disease at the time of diagnosis of their ASO (Singer and Rob, 1960). The 5-year survival rates of non-diabetics with femoral artery disease was 76 per cent. versus 93 per cent. in a normal age-matched population, while for diabetics this figure was 54 per cent. (Schadt *et al.*, 1961). Similar survival figures have also been reported in patients with aortic iliac ASO. Thus, one can conclude that the prevention of gangrene and subsequent amputation by themselves are not a reasonable indication for the surgical treatment of patients with intermittent claudication who do not have ischaemic rest pain since it is unlikely that the small risk of limb loss will be altered in these individuals.

Because of the high incidence of associated coronary and cerebrovascular disease in this group of patients, enthusiasm for elective surgery for relief of claudication symptoms must be tempered. Before considering elective surgery, one must be certain that the patient's symptoms are not due to osteoarthritis or muscle attachment pain of the hip which are extremely common in this age group. Usually the pain from these disorders is more troublesome to the individual than intermittent claudication even when both are present. Since symptoms of intermittent claudication without cutaneous ischaemia are the most frequent forms in which the disease occurs, it is apparent that surgical treatment is best reserved for a selected minority of elderly patients with ASO.

Another important factor when considering surgical therapy is the location of the major occlusion. In patients with primarily aortic-iliac disease with little femoral popliteal disease, surgical results are very good in 94 per cent. of cases (Gomes, Bernatz, and Jurgens, *et al*, 1967). While long-term patency depends on many factors, the results with a variety of techniques using synthetic grafts have been excellent. Surgical techniques and synthetic materials used in this area are quite well standardized.

The surgical treatment of femoral-popliteal disease has taken much longer to develop. The initial experience using synthetic material resulted in low, long-term patency rates (Szilagyi *et al.*, 1965; Vollmar, Tiede, and Lauback, 1969). In recent years, with improvements of techniques and the use of reversed saphenous vein grafts, patency rates after long-term follow-up have increased to 70 to 90 per cent. (Vollmar *et al.*, 1969; DeWiese *et al.*, 1966; Darling, Linton, and Razzuk, 1967; Barner *et al.*, 1968). When suitable saphenous veins are not available, newer synthetic materials are being used with fairly good success (Florian *et al.*, 1976).

Recently, encouraging data on the use of dipyridamole and aspirin prior to, during, and after operation in patients undergoing coronary saphenous vein bypass grafts, where the problems of graft occlusion are quite similar to those encountered in femoral-popliteal artery surgery, suggest that the application of this approach to peripheral artery surgery may result in considerable further improvement in graft patency rates (Chesebro *et al.*, 1982). The current dosage schedule of dipyridomole being used at our Institution in patients undergoing coronary saphenous vein bypass surgery is 100 mg 4 times daily for 2 days before surgery; 100 mg twice prior to surgery on the day of surgery; and 75 mg with 325 mg of aspirin 3 times daily beginning 7 hours after surgery.

Since the major cause for early vein graft occlusion is platelet thrombosis, and late occlusions are due to platelet-derived growth-factor-induced intimal smooth muscle cell proliferation, this antiplatelet drug approach is based on sound physiologic and biochemical principles (Unni *et al.*, 1974). Although so far these data are based on grafts in the coronary position, it seems likely that the same situation probably holds true in the femoral-popliteal system as well. The importance of the platelet and its products in vein graft occlusion is also supported by evidence that continued smoking following surgery has a very deleterious effect on the long-term surgical results (Gomes, Bernatz, and Jurgens, 1967).

In the patients with signs of cutaneous ischaemia and/or gangrenous ulcers, there is little question regarding the need for vascular surgery if it is feasible. While occasionally small, and rarely large, gangrenous ulcers may heal with conservative medical measures, this is frequently not the case. Even in situations where healing occurs, the process takes many weeks and usually months of bed-rest or at least very limited activity.

Unfortunately, patients with cutaneous ischaemia also present the greatest difficulties for the vascular surgeon. They are often poor surgical risks and have extensive disease. However, since the alternative is usually evential amputation, an aggressive, carefully planned surgical approach is indicated. This approach must be based on a thorough evaluation of the clinical situation, including high-quality arteriograms. Decisions must be individualized in each case and the patient must be fully cognizant of the seriousness of his disease, the results that can be reasonably expected, and the risks involved. Several principles are especially important in this evaluation. The patient must be prepared to contribute his share by stopping smoking and following the measures of foot care.

In considering femoral-popliteal surgery, the surgeon should be certain that there is no significant proximal disease. If proximal disease is present, this should be treated before or, if feasible, with the distal disease. Failure to appreciate the importance of this point is a major reason for failed femoral-popliteal grafts. The vascular surgeon must have the experience and skills to adapt a variety of techniques to the solution of the individual patient's problems. Rigid adherence to technical detail is essential for success. While reoperation can be considered in cases of graft failures, the success rate of such procedures, even in the hands of experts, is far lower than that of primary grafts.

In the past few years, considerable enthusiasm has developed for the treatment of isolated arterial stenosis and occlusions using percutaneous balloon dilatation (Grüntzig, 1977; Katzen, Chang, and Knox, 1979). Dilatation in the physiological sense is rarely accomplished. Pathological studies show that the intima and media of the arteries are fractured by this technique (Castenedo-Zuniga *et al.*, 1980). Thus, at least theoretically, there are risks of potentially causing aneurysm formation and distal embolization of atherosclerotic debris to small branch arteries. Also, one is left with a section of artery which is devoid of endothelium. A number of investigators have used antiplatelet agents in combination with the procedure to prevent reocclusion. Long-term studies of the potential for aneurysm formation or of the consequences of distal embolization occluding multiple branch vessels have not been reported.

To date, there is no evidence that the results of this procedure equal the excellent results of surgical repair of aortic-iliac lesions or even the results obtained in femoral-popliteal surgery, especially when the results of the addition of pre-, intra-, and postoperative antiplatelet therapy to the surgical procedures are considered. Although the simplicity of the procedure is attractive, the possibility for potentiating distal ischaemia and late complications has not been evaluated. At the present time, I consider this procedure experimental and do not feel it is a reasonable alternative to surgery or that it should be a part of routine vascular practice even in highly selected individuals since these selected cases are also known to have excellent results with conventional surgical approaches.

In the past, surgical sympathectomy has been utilized in the management of patients with ASO and severe cutaneous ischaemia. In general, there is little data concerning its effectiveness. This author has not been impressed with its usefulness in this group, although in young patients with thromboangiitis obliterans (Buerger's disease), I have seen dramatic improvement in a few patients. Occasionally, it may be helpful in patients with primarily femoral-popliteal disease when used in conjunction with arterial surgery.

Unfortunately, too many patients with cutaneous ischaemia come to amputation because of extensive gangrene or intractable, severe pain in a situation where no vascular surgery is possible. While digital amputation can be considered when gangrene is limited to a single digit, such amputations are rarely successful and usually result in an open wound that fails to heal. The only reliable means for judging the appropriate level of leg amputation (above versus below the knee) is for the surgeon to begin the amputation below the knee without a tourniquet and then observe the degree of bleeding from the small arteries and capillaries. If the tissue appears ischaemic and there is little bleeding, then the below knee site should be abandoned and the procedure done above the knee. Because of the debilitated condition of most patients undergoing amputation for arterial occlusive disease, the hospital mortality for this procedure may be high. The patients require expert postoperative care and management of their associated medical conditions.

Acute Arterial Occlusion

Because collateral vessels have not had an opportunity to develop, acute occlusions of major arteries to the extremities present a serious limb- and often life-threatening situation. The occlusion may be of embolic origin or may result from acute thrombosis of a diseased artery. Most emboli arise from a cardiac source (especially left atrial thrombi). Other possible sources include: thrombi or atherosclerotic debris from proximal arterial aneurysms, cardiac tumours, cardiovascular invasive procedures, and prosthetic valves (Green, De Weese, and Rob, 1975).

Thrombotic occlusions are usually associated with arteriosclerosis obliterans or atherosclerotic aneurysms. Rarely, they occur in hypercoagulable states related to lupus erythematous and other forms of collagen disease as well as ulcerative colitis. These are thought to represent primarily disorders of platelet function. Various forms of muscle entrapment of arteries are another rare cause of arterial occlusions.

The severity of symptoms is usually related to the size of the occluded artery. Often, symptoms will improve to some extent after the initial event. This is probably related to clot lysis and fragmentation rather than to spasm. Also, the dislodgement of platelet thrombi in branch vessels may play an important role in this improvement.

The clinical diagnosis of acute arterial occlusion is usually quite clear. The presenting symptom is pain in about 50 per cent. of cases. Other patients present with paraesthesiase and coolness of the extremity. In severe cases, there may be major loss of motor function. The symptoms may come on over several hours or several days. Often, the initial symptoms will partially resolve over several days but, except in mild cases, complete resolution is rare. The most important physical finding is the absence of arterial pulsations distal to the site of occlusion. Postural signs of cutaneous ischaemia also are uniformly present. Frequently, a reduction of distal skin temperature is evident on examination. In cases of severe ischaemia, there is a loss of the ability to wiggle the toes and, in very severe cases, ankle motion is also lost. Careful evaluation of these changes will usually differentiate the disorder from thrombophlebitis.

The medical management of acute arterial occlusion includes: prompt initiation of intermittent heparin therapy (5,000 USP units every 4 hours), protection of the extremity from trauma, and the avoidance of application of heat to the extremity. Hot water bottles, heating pads, and heat cradles can cause serious irreversible damage. Using intermittent heparin rather than continuous heparin infusion greatly facilitates the reversal of heparin therapy with protamine in preparation for surgery.

The advent of the use of the Fogarty balloon catheter has resulted in a major improvement in the management of patients (Fogarty *et al.*, 1963). If necessary, this technique can be accomplished under regional anesthesia in the severely ill patients who frequently develop these occlusions. Unless the acute occlusion is minor or there is prompt relief and full return of limb function, nearly all of these patients should be considered for prompt embolectomy using the Fogarty catheter technique. Even in cases where the aetiology is acute thrombosis in the presence of superimposed occlusive arterial disease, this procedure may tide a patient over until definitive arterial bypass surgery can be done. If it is suspected that the artery was significantly diseased prior to the acute occlusion (as in the case of thrombotic lesions), preoperation arteriography should be obtained. Although in some cases the limb might survive without surgical intervention, embolectomy almost uniformly results in additional preservation of function. This procedure has significantly reduced mortality and improved limb salvage and function in patients with acute arterial occlusions (Green, DeWeese, and Rob, 1975). In general, patients should be maintained on anticoagulants postoperatively to prevent reocclusion. In situations where oedema of the extremity develops as a result of the ischaemia, fasciotomies to prevent compartmental compression and subsequent muscle necrosis should be considered at the time of operation.

Mesenteric Artery Occlusive Disease

Atherosclerosis of the abdominal visceral arteries is a common occurrence which typically involves the proximal portion of the major arteries or alternatively it may occur as a result of impingement of aortic atheromas on the artery orifice. Rare causes of mesenteric artery obstruction include: fibromuscular dysplasia; dissecting haematoma, ergot ingestion, and various types of arteritis. Studies of unselected patients at autopsy have revealed partial obstruction of the coeliac artery in 44 per cent. and of the superior mesenteric artery in 37 per cent of cases (Derrick, Pollard, and Moore, 1959). In spite of this high frequency, only a small proportion of these patients develop clinical symptoms. This probably relates to the excellent collateral blood supply of the intestines. They are supplied by three major vessels, the coeliac, superior mesenteric, and inferior mesenteric arteries plus their branches. The superior mesenteric is connected to the coeliac system by the gastroduodenal and left gastroepiploic branches and to the inferior mesenteric system by the marginal and midcolic branches. Thus, it is not surprising that a patient with symptoms of mesenteric artery obstruction not only has obstruction of the mesenteric artery but this obstruction is often accompanied by severe stenosis or occlusions of either the coeliac or inferior mesenteric artery systems as well.

This clinical syndrome occurs in older patients who often have atherosclerotic disease of other vessels. The usual presenting symptom is one of periumbilical pain occurring immediately or 30 minutes after meals. The severity of the pain may be related to the size of the meal. Moderate to severe weight loss is frequently present (Bircher *et al.*, 1966). In half of the patients, the abdominal pain is atypical. While bowel function is frequently altered in these patients, only a few develop steatorrhoea from villus atrophy. Abdominal bruits may be present but are not specific since such bruits are commonly seen in patients with aortic atherosclerosis.

Since the symptoms of this disorder are very non-specific, most patients will need gastrointestinal diagnostic studies to rule out more common disorders. However, in the usual patient with obscure abdominal pain, the diagnosis of mesenteric artery insufficiency should be considered and selective arteriography done. This procedure can also be useful in identifying other possible causes of obscure abdominal pain. Since occlusions typically involve the origin and first portion of the artery, it is critically important that the lateral views be obtained so that the first portion of the artery is adequately visualized. The only effective treatment is surgical revascularization. This may involve endarterectomy (especially for orifice lesions), arterial bypass, or reimplantation of the mesenteric artery, depending on the specific arteriographic characteristics of the lesion. Since the splenic artery is often an important source of collateral flow, transplants of this artery to the distal mesenteric vessel is rarely a procedure of choice.

Acute mesenteric artery occlusions present an urgent problem. About 40 per cent. are embolic and 40 per cent. involve thrombosis of previously stenotic atherosclerotic lesions. In about 20 per cent., decreased perfusion without an obstructing, organic arterial lesion occurs. This latter situation occurs in patients with vascular collapse due to severe cardiac failure or hypotension. They have a grave prognosis (Laufnur, Lora, and Mittlepunkt, 1964).

In the initial stages of embolus or acute thrombosis, the presenting symptom is unrelenting abdominal pain frequently with vomiting, diarrhoea, and blood loss. Leucocytosis is usually present but abdominal findings on physical examination are minimal or absent. At this stage, there is spasm of the intestinal wall and mucosal infarction. While diagnosis is difficult, the problem can be identified by mesenteric arteriography and the results of surgery are reasonably good. In later stages there is infarction of the full thickness of the intestinal wall, peritonitis, peripheral vascular collapse due to the absorption of toxic substances, and bleeding. At this stage, the diagnosis is obvious but few patients survive regardless of treatment. Thus, early diagnosis and early consideration of arteriography are critical in the management of this disorder. In all cases of acute occlusion, sources of emboli should be sought, and any material removed should be examined for the possibility of embolic cardiac tumours.

ARTERIAL ANEURYSMS

Arterial aneurysms are a common manifestation of atherosclerosis in the elderly. They develop as a result of destruction of the elastic tissue by the atherosclerotic process. The exact mechanism of this destruction is not known. There is evidence that it may be related to the binding of lipoproteins to the elastic tissue once the atherosclerotic process has invaded the arterial media. The most common location for atherosclerotic aneurysms in approximately decreasing frequencies are abdominal aorta, popliteal artery, femoral artery, thoracic aorta, and splenic and renal arteries.

In years past, syphilitic aortitis was a frequent aetiology for aneurysms, especially those in the thoracic aorta. These have become exceedingly rare in recent years. Currently, the vast majority are due to atherosclerosis. Trauma related to rapid acceleration or deacceleration has been the second most common aetiology and appears to be increasing. Many visceral artery aneurysms are thought to be of congenital origin. Nearly all atherosclerotic aneurysms occur after the age of 60 and are approximately 10 times more frequent in males than in females.

Abdominal Aortic Aneurysms

These aneurysms represent a fairly common geriatric problem in men. Often they are asymptomatic and are discovered on physical examination or by the presence of calcification in an abdominal or spine X-ray. Except in obese individuals, these can be detected as an expansile mass greater than 4 cm in diameter. Palpation of the abdominal aorta and determination of its width should be a routine part of any physical examination of a patient over 60 years of age. If this is done, most aneurysms can be identified before they become symptomatic and, when indicated, relatively safe elective rather than more risky emergency surgery can be done. Confirmation of the diagnosis is most readily accomplished by ultrasound scanning with an accuracy of greater than 95 per cent. (Lee *et al.*, 1975). Since these aneurysms are nearly always filled with laminated thrombus, aortography is of little help except when done to assess the distal circulation. In many cases, the thrombus may result in the appearance of a normal aortogram.

When a patient with an aneurysm develops abdominal or back pain, the clinician should strongly suspect that leakage or partial rupture of the aneurysm has occurred or is imminent.

Studies of the prognosis of untreated abdominal aortic aneurysms in 141 cases have shown a 3-year survival rate of 52.5 per cent. and a 5-year survival rate of 36 per cent. (Schatz, Fairbairn, and Jungens, 1962). In earlier studies, when the aneurysms were probably large at the time of diagnosis, the prognosis was even worse (Estes, 1950). In most cases, death occurred from rupture into the retroperitoneal space, rarely from rupture into the gastrointestinal tract, producing an aortoenteric fistula, or occasionally into the vena cava to produce an aortocaval fistula. A frequent complication of the aneurysms is distal ischaemia due to atheromatous embolization to the kidneys and, less commonly, to the skin and muscles of the extremities (Florey, 1945). The only effective treatment for aneurysms is surgical replacement with a synthetic graft. In many large series of patients, the operative risk of elective surgery is less than 5 per cent. In contrast, in a case where rupture has already occurred, requiring emergency surgery, a mortality of 58 per cent. has been reported (Ottinger, 1975). Follow-up studies have shown that successful surgery increases the survival rate to twice that of untreated aneurysms.

Thus, in summary, the presence of an abdominal aortic aneurysm of significant size is a strong indication for prompt elective surgical replacement, especially if the patient is a reasonably good surgical risk.

The late complications of abdominal aortic grafts include: the development of a false aneurysm, particularly at the proximal suture line; graft infection; and, extremely rarely, aortoenteric fistula. Improved surgical techniques in recent years have reduced these complications to very low levels.

Popliteal Artery Aneurysms

Usually these are identified on physical examination as a mass with expansile pulsations. Examination of the popliteal artery for aneurysm should be part of the routine of all physical examinations of patients over 50 years of age. Occasionally, these aneurysms are first noted as curvilinear calcifications on X-ray. Ultrasound scanning has proven to be a valuable tool in confirming the diagnosis of these aneurysms (Carpenter *et al.*, 1976). Arteriography may be needed to define the status of the distal vessels and to aid in planning for surgical resection. In a series of 152 patients, these lesions were bilateral in 59 per cent. and were associated with aneurysms of other arteries (mainly abdominal aorta and femoral arteries) in 45 per cent. of cases (Wychulis, Spittell, and Wallace, 1970). Follow-up studies in 87 patients who were not treated surgically showed that 31 per cent. developed complications in 1 to 8 years and 3.5 per cent. eventually came to amputation. The major serious complication is distal embolization of atheromatous material. Frequently, ischaemia is accelerated by an acute thrombosis or, less commonly, by rupture of the aneurysm. In this area, potential collaterals are often compressed which further accelerates the ischaemia. Surgical treatment is the only satisfactory treatment. Preferably, it should be done early before complications and at a point when vascular continuity with distal vessels can be established. In such cases, the results of surgical treatment are excellent.

Aneurysms of the Thoracic Aorta

At the present time, atherosclerosis is the principle aetiology for these aneurysms with approximately 5 per cent. being related to trauma (Joyce *et al.*, 1964). Although syphilis was formerly a common cause of aneurysms in this area, few such cases have been seen in recent years. Most of these aneurysms are asymptomatic unless they become quite large and compress adjacent organs. They are usually initially discovered on chest X-ray but require fluoroscopy and/or aortography for differentiation from other mediastinal tumours. The overall prognosis for patients with untreated thoracic aortic aneurysms has been reported as a 68% 3-year, 50% 5-year, and 30% 10-year survival. This was not influenced by the location of the aneurysm, but survivorship was further reduced in older patients and in patients with hypertension (Joyce *et al.*, 1964). Thus, the outlook is somewhat better than that of untreated aneurysms of the abdominal aorta, but the lesions still carry a poor prognosis which justifies consideration of surgical treatment if the patient is in good health and no other contraindications are present. This is especially true if there is evidence of significant enlargement over time. The only definitive treatment is surgical excision with replacement by a prosthetic graft. The risk of surgery depends on the location of the aneurysm and the length of the aorta involved. Lesions of the ascending aorta, even with associated replacement of the aortic valve, carry a risk of 10 per cent. when surgery is done by experienced surgical teams (Kidd *et al.*, 1976). Aneurysms of the transverse aortic arch with involvement of the origins of the brachial-cephalic vessels present a formidable challenge and require the use of extracorporeal whole body perfusion, often with perfusion of individual branch vessels. Experience is limited and mortality has been reported as 25 per cent. (Greipp *et al.*, 1975). Aneurysms in the descending thoracic aorta usually occur just distal to the origin of the left subclavian artery. Most are due to atherosclerosis, but this is a common location for traumatic aneurysms. Resection of these aneurysms has a mortality risk of 10 to 12 per cent. An additional risk in the resection of these aneurysms is the risk of spinal cord ischaemia. Several techniques to reduce this risk have been developed (Crawford and Rubio, 1973).

Visceral Artery Aneurysms

The splenic artery is the most common site for aneurysms of the visceral arteries. Most are of atherosclerotic origin. These are usually discovered as calcifications on X-ray. They are asymptomatic in most cases. The diagnosis should be confirmed by selective aortography. Ruptures are uncommon except in females in the third trimester of pregnancy (Spittell *et al.*, 1961). In most instances, elective resection seems reasonable if the patient is in good health and especially if the aneurysm is larger than 1 cm in diameter. Aneurysms of the renal artery are less common but carry the added potential of causing renal-vascular hypertension. They rarely rupture. In cases with significant hypertension, surgical resection appears justified (Vaughan *et al.*, 1971).

Dissecting Aortic Aneurysms

This condition represents one of the most catastrophic diseases of the vascular system. It is usually characterized by an abrupt onset and often by extensive aortic involvement. Little is really known about the aetiology of this disease although there has been much speculation based on gross descriptions of the lesions and its association with hypertension and the Marfan syndrome. Histologic studies using sophisticated techniques and studies of the fine structure of the artery wall in this disease have rarely been reported. While haemodynamic factors and hypertension probably do increase the risk of rupture of these aneurysms and may instigate the acute onset of dissection, it is doubtful that they have any real influence on the basic aetiology. The lesion of aortic dissection has been reproduced in animal models. Lathyrism in rats has been shown to be due to β-aminopropionitrile and aminoacetonitrile (Ponseti and Baird, 1952). These compounds have been shown to poison the enzyme responsible for the cross-linking of elastin between its leucine and desmoleucine residues (Siegel, Pinnell, and Martin, 1970). The copper-deficient pig is another animal model (Shields *et al.*, 1962). It develops dissection because copper is an essential cofactor for the cross-linking of elastin by the enzyme which is poisoned in lathyrism. The blotchy mouse has a genetic deficiency of lysyloxidase activity and has a high incidence of dissecting aneurysms (Rowe *et al.*, 1977). These studies strongly suggest that failure of the biochemical cross-linking of elastin may be a major aetiologic factor in this disease.

Clinical Features

Clinically, aortic dissection predominates in men with a male to female ratio of about 2 or 3:1 and occurs between 40 and 70 years of age. The most common initial symptom is the acute onset of a severe ripping or tearing pain in the thorax (either anterior or posterior). This may present with loss of pulses in extremities and signs of pericarditis. Hypertension is present in 70 per cent. of the cases and may either precede the onset of symptoms or be secondary to involvement of the renal arteries by the dissection itself. Besides the absence of proximal extremity pulses, physical examination may reveal a pericardial friction rub, a tender, wide abdominal aorta on palpation, and, occasionally, bruits along the course of the spine. The picture is often confusing and may be mistaken for an acute myocardial infarction, acute arterial occlusion, or a cerebral vascular accident. In some patients, the pain may be surprisingly minimal. The finding of a new murmur of aortic insufficiency or of a widened mediatinum on chest X-ray should heighten the clinician's suspicion of a dissection, although in some cases the chest X-ray may be normal or show only cardiac enlargement (Earnest, Muhm, and Sheedy, 1979). In some cases, echocardiography may also be helpful (Brown, Popp, and Klastei, 1975; Mintz *et al.*, 1979) (see Chapter 14).

When a dissecting aneurysm is suspected, prompt aortography to confirm the diagnosis, to localize the site of the primary tear, and to determine the extent of the aneurysm should be done. In some difficult diagnostic cases, studies with computer assisted tomography scanning may be helpful.

Management

Untreated, these patients have a very poor prognosis. Reported studies show that 70 per cent. of patients died within 2 weeks of the onset of symptoms and that 50 per cent. of those surviving the acute phase died within a year. The prognosis is worse when the primary tear is in the ascending aorta or arch and when hypertension is present (McCloy, Spittell, and McGoon, 1965).

Wheat (1973) has proposed a detailed protocol of medical treatment for acute dissection. It involves the use of the antihypertensive agents intravenous trimethaphan, reserpine, propranolol, and guanethidine. The selection of these agents was based on the speculation that decreasing the force of ventricular contraction was a critical factor in preventing rupture. The most important factor, however, is the prompt, effective reduction of systolic blood pressure to levels below 120 mmHg, thus maintaining the patient's blood pressure at below normal levels. Many of Wheat's patients were maintained at pressures between 80 and 100 mmHg systolic. When using guanethidine, it should be recalled that the orthostatic hypotensive effect of the agent can be obtained by elevating the head of the bed.

Currently, sodium nitroprusside would seem to be the initial drug of choice, since development of drug tolerance over a few days is not a problem as is the case with trimethaphan. Control is much smoother with nitroprusside and the dose can gradually be reduced as the effects of oral agents such as guanethidine and Inderal are added. The patient should be maintained in an intensive care unit during the treatment programme. The major emphasis should be that of maintaining the blood pressure as low as possible (80 to 120 mmHg systolic) consistent with the maintenance of a reasonably urine output.

If on aortography the aneurysm involves the entire or ascending portion of the aorta, prompt surgical treatment is indicated. If the lesion is limited to the segment distal to the left subclavian artery, surgery may be delayed for 2 to 3 weeks until the patient is stable and periaortic edema has subsided. If pain is not relieved or if pain recurs, prompt surgery is indicated.

The goals of surgery (Appelbaum, Karp, and Kirklin, 1976) are to reduce the potential for external rupture, prevent further dissection, correct any aortic incompetence, and restore potency to occluded vessels. These are accomplished by resecting the area of the primary tear, closing the false channels proximally and distally if they have not been resected, and replacing an incompetent aortic valve with a prosthesis. Occasionally, it is necessary to graft occluded branches as well. Early mortality in surgically treated dissections involving the ascending aorta is approximately 20 per cent. while the operative mortality for lesions involving only the descending aorta is approximately 10 per cent. (Appelbaum, Karp, and Kirklin, 1976; Reul *et al.*, 1975).

VASCULITIS AND RELATED DISORDERS

Vasculitis is a very general term that refers to a large group of diseases which have the presence of inflammation and proliferative changes in the small arteries and arterioles as their major pathologic characteristic. The list includes: periarteritis nodosa, the arteritis of rhematoid arthritis, Goodpasture's syndrome, Wegener's granulomatosis, Cogan's syndrome, Behcet's syndrome, cranial arteritis, Takayashu's disease, systemic lupus erythematous, and scleroderma. Cranial arteritis is the most common of these disorders seen in geriatric practice and is discussed in Chapter 25.1. Since lupus erythematous, Takayashu's disease, and Cogan's syndrome occur primarily in younger individuals, they will not be discussed further (see Chapter 25.3. Most of these diseases are thought to be related to abnormalities in the immune system but the precise mechanisms responsible for the various specific syndromes are not known.

Periarteritis nodosa is a classic example of this group of diseases. It can occur at all ages, but is most frequent in the fifth and sixth decades. Males are affected twice as often as females (Frohnert and Sheps, 1967). The disease is defined by characteristic pathological changes in the arterial wall. Initially, there is endothelial desquamation and fibrinoid degeneration of the media. The media and adventitia are then infiltrated with polymorphonuclear neutrophils, eosinophils, and plasma cells. The vessels then become thrombosed and/or develop small aneurysms. Resultant vascular ischaemia then leads to multiple small infarcts of the involved organs (Arkin, 1930). The disease involves the entire thickenss of the vascular wall and has been called panarteritis. Typically, individual lesions at multiple stages of development can be seen in the same biopsy specimen.

The organs involved in descending order are: kidneys and testes, heart, lung, liver, gastrointestinal tract, pancreas, muscles, and peripheral and central nervous systems (Moskowitz, Baggenstoss, and Slocomb, 1963). Similar lesions can be produced in rabbits by injection of bovine serum albumin to produce serum sickness. Prior depletion of complement or of polymorphonuclear neutrophils prevents development of these experimental lesions (Rich, 1947). Limited studies demonstrating the deposition of immune globulin and complement as detected by immunofluorescence have been done on arteries obtained from patients with this disease. This is obviously an area where much more investigation needs to be undertaken. Gocke and associates (1970) have demonstrated immune complexes of hepatitis B antigen in the lesions and one group (Trepo *et al.*, 1974) has found these complexes in as many as 55 per cent. of patients with polyarteritis nodosa.

The most likely scenario for the pathogenesis of this disease appears to be the stimulation of the immune system to produce large quantities of immune globulins that then deposit on endothelium and cause damage to the endothelial cells. This permits the attraction of platelets and lymphocytes to perpetuate the response and to activate the complement system. This results in an infiltration with polymorphonuclear cells which liberate lysosomal enzymes to produce vascular damage. Thus, potential points of therapeutic intervention could include: avoidance or removal of the unknown factor triggering the immune reaction, prevention of immune complex deposition, and inhibition of the destructive process instigated by the neutrophils.

Clinical Features

Periarteritis nodosa is a widely disseminated disease that can involve multiple body systems. This multisystem involvement is its most characteristic clinical feature. It may have a sudden or an insidious onset and often presents the picture of chronic infection, toxaemia, and cachexia. Low grade fever and leucocytosis are common and, in some cases, eosinophilia is a prominent feature. Involvement of the joints, nervous system, and skin occurs in 50 per cent of the patients. About 50 per cent have classical mononeuritis multiplex. This is a situation in which multiple major nerve trunks are involved, usually in an asymmetric distribution. Skin involvement usually takes the form of infarctive skin ulcers of irregular shape surrounded by normal skin.

Laboratory studies will nearly always show elevation of the erythrocyte sedimentation rate (often over 100 mm/hh) when the disease is active. Evidence of renal involvement with microhaematuria, casts, elevated serum creatine, and hypertension are frequently present. In many cases, the additional finding of evidence of hepatic involvement is an important clue to the consideration of a multisystemic disease such as periarteritis nodosa. Elevated titres of rheumatoid factor and low serum complement are often noted. Only limited studies of the frequency of elevated levels of circulating immune complexes have been done. Selected arteriography of visceral arteries may reveal multiple intraparenchymal aneurysms which may be quite helpful diagnostically (Fleming and Stein, 1965). Occasionally, these aneurysms can cause unilateral or bilateral massive perirenal haematomas (Gamble, DeWeerd, and Dockerty, 1968). Pulmonary involvement with transient or solid exudate and occasionally with cavitation have also been noted (Divertie, 1964). With the possible exception of the patient with classical mononeuritis multiplex and other classical findings, the diagnosis can only be established by positive findings in a biopsy specimen of involved accessible tissue (nerve, skin, muscle, or testicle). Electromyography may be helpful in localizing the site for a nerve or muscle biopsy. Blind muscle biopsies and blind renal or liver biopsies are rarely helpful.

Treatment

Steroids

The prognosis in periarteritis nodosa has been reported as a 12.7% 5-year survival without steroids and a 48% 5-year and 42% 10-year survival rate in patients treated intensively with steroids (Frohnert and Sheps, 1967). In 1950, Schick and associates first reported encouraging results in the treatment of this disease with steroids (Shick *et al.*, 1950). There is no doubt, from subsequent experience, that steroids are beneficial in the management of periarteritis nodosa. One of the major problems has been that 50 per cent. of the surviving patients were still on steroids 10 years after initiation of therapy, presumably because of continuing recurrences (Frohnert and Sheps, 1967). The generally recommended initial starting dose of treatment with steroids is 1 to 1.5 mg of prednisone or its equivalent per kilogram body weight per day until the acute symptoms subside and the sedimentation rate begins to fall. The dose should then be reduced to 0.6 mg/kg to maintain immunosuppression for 4 to 6 weeks. Following this, the dose should be reduced by about 10 per cent. each week until treatment can be discontinued. When a dose of 20 mg/day is reached, it may be beneficial to give the cortisone as a single dose on alternate days to reduce side-effects. While on ster-

oids, the dietary sodium should be restricted, potassium supplements given, and a liberal antacid programme initiated. The use of prophylactic isoniazid (300 mg daily) should be considered, especially if the chest X-ray shows a Ghon complex (Sheps and McDuffie, 1980).

The most difficult aspect of this recommended programme is the period of steroid reduction. It is critically important that the physician see the patient regularly during this period and that the dosage reduction schedule be rigidly adhered to. The patient and physician must be firm and not fall into the trap of attributing every minor ache, pain, or increase in arthralgia as evidence of recurrence which requires an increase of steroid dosage or discontinuation of the programme of steroid withdrawal. These symptoms as well as a transient rise in the sedimentation rate occur in virtually all patients when steroids are reduced. While true reactivation of this disease occurs, this is quite rare. The diagnosis of reactivation should be based only on the occurrence of new skin, nerve, or pulmonary lesions or clear evidence of reduced renal function. Arthralgias are not evidence of reactivity and should be treated with salicylates and other anti-inflammatory agents and not with an increased dosage of steroids. If these principles are followed, it should be possible to eventually discontinue steroids in nearly all patients. This programme of steroid withdrawal and the normal expected symptoms of steroid withdrawal should be thoroughly discussed with the patient and his family prior to initiation of therapy. If this reduction is not accomplished, the patient is committed to a lifetime disability as a steroid cripple with all of its serious consequences of osteoporotic fractures, gastrointestinal bleeding, etc.

Immunosuppressive Drugs

While there has been considerable controversy raised in recent years over the possible use of azathioprine and cyclophosphamide in the management of this disease, there have been no controlled, direct comparison studies. Thus, at the present time, their usefulness is not known. The fairly extensive experience in the use of these drugs in combination with small doses of prednisone in the management of transplant rejection should provide a sound basis for the planning of such comparative studies. In the patient who is extremely toxic, and when high levels of circulating immune complexes can be detected, consideration should be given to the use of plasmapheresis combined with lymphophoresis (Hamblin and Oscier, 1978; Wallace *et al.*, 1979). This approach has had dramatic success in the management of another form of vasculitis, Goodpasture's syndrome, characterized by massive pulmonary hemorrhage and necrotizing proliferative glomerulonephritis (Rosenblatt *et al.*, 1979).

Other Forms of Vasculitis

There are other forms of vasculitis that are difficult to differentiate from periarteritis nodosa and probably are also due to a defect in the immune system. In Wegener's granulomatosis, focal necrotizing lesions develop in the lungs, eyes, and ears, and spread to all organs of the body. Generally, cytotoxic immunosuppression agents have been more effective than steroids in its treatment. Occasionally arteritis is seen in patients with long-standing chronic rheumatoid arthritis. Whether or not these different clinical syndromes are related to differences in the types of circulating immune complexes or to different defects in other aspects of the immune system is not known.

SCLERODERMA

Scleroderma is another multisystem disease with primarily skin and blood vessel involvement. A high frequency of Raynaud's phenomenon is characteristic of the disease. It occurs 3 to 4 times more frequently in women than in men and its onset usually occurs between the third and seventh decade with most cases occurring in the fifth decade (Campbell and LeRoy, 1975). Pathologically, the skin has an increased amount of swollen collagneous connective tissue and fragmentation of the elastic fibres. Small arteries show concentric, subendothelial mucoid proliferation (D'angelo *et al.*, 1969). Cultured skin fibroblasts of these patients have an increased ability to synthesize procollagen (Uitto, Bauer, and Eisen, 1979).

Clinical Features

Raynaud's phenomenon is usually the initial symptom in this disease. Skin changes occur in nearly all cases. The skin becomes tight and atrophic usually over the forearm, hands, neck, and face. Telangiectasia is common in about one-third of the cases demonstrating subcutaneous calcification especially around the joints and fingertips. Feeble esophageal contractions of the lower portion of the esophagus as detected by manometric motility studies is one of the most useful diagnostic procedures for this disease (Mukhopadhyay and Graham, 1976). Pulmonary function studies often reveal a decreased carbon monoxide diffusing capacity. As the disease progresses, pulmonary fibrosis, pericarditis, and myocardopathy develop. The development of advanced renal involvement is the most common cause of death. The term 'mixed connective tissue disease' has been used to describe cases where features of scleroderma overlap those of lupus erythematous and polymyositis.

The prognosis of scleroderma is extremely variable and unpredictable. In general, visceral organ involvement and, especially, renal involvement suggest a poor prognosis. In many cases, the disease may stabilize and remain inactive for many years. Because of the variability, mean survival figures are of little help in predicting the course of a patient's disease. There is no effective treatment for scleroderma other than palliative, supportive care. Steroids, immunosuppressive agents, and numerous other agents have been tried without success.

DISEASES OF THE VEINS

The Pathophysiology of Thromboembolism

The diagnosis and management of patients with thromboembolism has been an area of great controversy for many years. The development of tests with a high sensitivity but questionable specificity and the use of anticoagulant therapy have all contributed to this confusion. To gain a balanced perspective, there is considerable value in reviewing the older studies which were done prior to the use of anticoagulants and the institution of measures for preventing venous stasis. The extensive studies of

Barker and coworkers are of particular value in this regard (Barker *et al.*, 1940, 1941). The critical findings of these studies were: (a) the incidence of fatal pulmonary embolism did not depend on the site of the clinically detected thrombophlebitis; (b) the risks of fatal pulmonary embolism in patients with deep vein thrombophlebitis was 6.5 per cent.; (c) a patient with a pulmonary embolism has a 44 per cent. risk of developing a second pulmonary embolism and an 18 per cent. chance of developing a fatal pulmonary embolism during the same period of hospitalization; (d) the primary factors related to thromboembolism were venous stasis and tissue injury; and (e) pulmonary embolism is extremely rare in patients with thrombophlebitis limited to the 'superficial veins'. (see also p. 492, chapter 14)

In spite of many more sophisticated studies since the 1940s, these concepts remain important guidelines for understanding this disease. It is useful to think of thrombophlebitis and pulmonary embolism as symptoms of a disease whose basic defect is a hypercoagulable state. This concept is supported by the fact that the risk of pulmonary embolism does not depend on the site of clinical thrombophlebitis as would be the case if propagation of the thrombus was the critical event. It suggests that embolism occurs early before the thrombus has been fixed to the wall of the vein secondary to the induction of inflammation.

It is likely that there is a very high incidence of small platelet emboli even in normal individuals but, because of small size, they produce little clinical effect. However, in the face of venous stasis, they may grow to a considerably larger size before becoming detached and thus result in clinical symptoms. This would also explain why the sensitive isotopic scanning techniques detect thromboembolism that cannot be confirmed by venography. It would also be consistent with the findings of a 26.9 per cent. incidence of venous thrombosis in the thigh veins of an unselected series of consecutive autopsies. Of those with thrombi in the thigh veins, 60 per cent. had pulmonary emboli, whereas of those patients without thigh vein thrombosis only a 1.9 per cent. incidence of pulmonary embolism was found (Beckering and Titus, 1969).

Barker's studies (Barker *et al.*, 1941) also point out that once the embolism occurs, the chances of its recurring are very high and the risk of a large, fatal pulmonary embolism becomes nearly 20 per cent. Again, the critical factor is the size of the thrombus prior to its detachment from its origin in the vessel wall versus the process of inflammation which results in a firm attachment and thus prevents dislodgement and embolism. This process of inflammation, however, requires a longer period of time than the development of small platelet thrombi. It is obvious from this point of view that interruption of the veins at any point distal to the inferior vena cava will be totally ineffective. This has been well shown by experience in years past. The studies of Sevitt (1969) have demonstrated the relatively high incidence of venous thrombosis in patients with hip trauma and/or surgery. While venous stasis and the suspected increased platelet–endothelial interaction associated with stasis and tissue injury are the basis for the vast majority of cases of thromboembolism, there are unusual situations in which the basic aetiology is probably quite different.

Diseases associated with certain immunological disorders are occasionally associated with an increased incidence of venous thromboembolism, presumably related to the endothelial damage produced by antigen–antibody complexes. These syndromes include patients with systemic lupus erythematous, certain patients with ulcerative colitis, and patients with thromboangiitis obliterans (Buerger's disease). In some of these instances (especially those associated with ulcerative colitis), the patient's thromboembolism may not be inhibited with the usual levels of anticoagulation.

Certain malignancies are also associated with a high incidence of thromboembolism (see Chapter 12.1, p. 403). In malignancy of the lung, prostate, and ovary it may be the first presenting symptom, while in pancreatic malignancies, it is more likely to occur after metastatic lesions have developed. Again, in many instances, this hyperthromboembolism is not controlled by the usual levels of anticoagulation.

Finally, there is a small group of patients who develop recurrent thromboembolism without any history of injury or immobilization and without any of the aetiologies mentioned above. The majority of these patients are males and, in some but not all instances, a familial aggregation of cases has been noted. Presumably, these patients have some chronic defect in the coagulation mechanism. A familial antithrombin-III deficiency has been reported in some (Filip, Eckstein, and Veltkarp, 1976) and others may have shortened platelet survival time (Steele, Ellis, and Genton, 1978).

Clinical Presentation and Diagnosis of Thrombophlebitis

Except in the unusual circumstances outlined above, thrombophlebitis characteristically occurs in a situation where the patient has been restricted in his activities, particularly when this is related to recent surgery. With current practices of early postoperative ambulation, orthopaedic surgery, with its long periods of required immobilization, is associated with the highest incidence of postoperative thromboembolism. In one of the more common operations in current geriatric practice, hip surgery, the use of prophylactic anticoagulants during the postoperative period has been of considerable value (Coventry, Nolan and Beckenbaugh, 1973). An important advantage in the use of oral prophylactic anticoagulants is that it avoids the use of heparin which is mainly responsible for bleeding into the surgical wound. In contrast, the major risk of bleeding with short-term oral anticoagulants is gastric bleeding.

Some authors have suggested the use of low-dose heparin therapy as originally proposed by Wessler (1975). While this prophylactic approach does reduce the incidence of thrombophlebitis in patients undergoing abdominal and thoracic surgery, it is not as effective as prophylactic oral anticoagulants in preventing thromboembolism following orthopaedic procedures, especially hip surgery.

The Diagnosis of Thrombophlebitis

In patients who are immobilized for extended periods and especially in a postoperative setting, the clinician should always have a high suspicion of thrombophlebitis. Regular examination of the extremities should be routine practice in the follow-up of these patients, especially when a low grade fever is noted.

Details regarding the examination of the extremity have been outlined in the section on the vascular examination. The typical calf swelling, localized tenderness, and increased temperature of the extremity are the most helpful signs. Homans' sign (pain on dorsiflexion of the ankle) is not a reliable sign for phlebitis and should not be used for this purpose. Instead, the calf and Scarpa's triangle should be carefully palpated for localized areas of tenderness and occasionally will reveal a palpable cord. Superficial thrombophlebitis is readily apparent on inspection and palpation of a superficial, tender thrombotic varix or superficial vein. It may be noted as a chemical phlebitis at the site of an intravenous injection.

Many procedures have been developed as possible aids in the diagnosis of thrombophlebitis. These include: ^{125}I fibrinogen leg scanning, impedance plethysmography, radionuclide venography, Doppler flow velocity detection, and contrast venography. All of these have problems which limit their usefulness. Contrast venography is the most useful, but it requires considerable experience for interpretation, especially regarding involvement of the calf veins. If the patient has had a previous episode of phlebitis, one cannot always distinguish between acute changes and those associated with chronic venous insufficiency. The Doppler flow velocity technique in experienced hands can be a useful bedside technique for confirmation of iliofemoral or popliteal venous occlusion. Details of this technique were discussed in the vascular examination section.

The Diagnosis of Pulmonary Embolism

Pulmonary embolism presents in two patterns: the small embolism producing a small pulmonary infarct and a relatively large pulmonary embolism producing at least a lobar sized infarct with corpulmonale and shock.

The small embolism presents well-localized pleuritic pain as its primary symptom. It is often associated with low grade fever and tachycardia. A high fever with a temperature over 101 °F is very rare. Often sticky inspiratory rales, sometimes called an inspiratory friction rub, are heard directly over the area of pleuritic pain during the first 24 hours. Hemoptysis with small quantities of fresh blood or occasional old blood clots is fairly common.

Early examination of the patient affords the best opportunity to make the diagnosis. The chest X-ray is usually negative and an ECG is rarely of value unless pericarditis is suspected.

In the case of the less common larger pulmonary embolism, the pleuritic pain may be diffuse or may even be absent. Dyspnea is quite prominent. Frequently, there is dullness to percussion at one or both lung bases or over the distribution of the middle or, less commonly, the upper lung lobes. The chest X-ray is often positive and the ECG may show a right ventricular strain pattern. In very large, massive emboli, especially when they are multiple, shock and cardiovascular collapse develop rapidly.

The development of techniques for isotope scanning of the lungs has been an important aid to diagnosis (Wagner *et al.*, 1964). The technique is sensitive, but lacks specificity unless the scan is carefully compared with the chest X-ray and ideally with ventilation scanning using radioactive xenon (Wagner and Strauss, 1975). Arterial blood gases, though not always abnormal, can be very helpful. A PO_2 of 80 mmHg or lower while breathing room air should raise a very high suspicion of pulmonary embolism unless some other clear aetiology is present. Blood enzyme levels are of limited value in the differential diagnosis of pulmonary embolism.

The signs and symptoms of pulmonary embolism, except for residual lung scarring, clear within a week. Liquefaction of the infarct and development of a lung abscess is extremely rare. Pulmonary angiography can definitively demonstrate the lesions if it is done within 48 hours. Fibrinolysis of lesions has been documented after longer periods of time (Simon and Sasahara, 1965).

Treatment of Thromboembolism

The first and most important phase of treatment of thrombophlebitis and pulmonary embolism is the prompt initiation of anticoagulant therapy. This is most readily initiated with heparin, 5,000 units every 4 hours. Unless contraindicated, oral anticoagulants should also be initiated promptly. Regular prothrombin times should be obtained on blood samples obtained between 3 and 4 hours after the previous dose of heparin. When the prothrombin time is between 1½ and 2 times the control value in seconds, the heparin can be discontinued. The patient should be at bed-rest and moist heat should be applied to the extremities involved with thrombophlebitis. In the case of thrombophlebitis, acute symptoms will usually clear in 7 to 10 days.

Patients with pulmonary embolism should receive oxygen if they are dyspnoeic. In those with massive emboli, if the systolic blood pressure cannot be maintained above 90 mmHg systolic and the PO_2 cannot be maintained at more than 60 mmHg after 1 hour of intensive medical therapy, and if the pulmonary arteriogram shows greater than 50 per cent. of the total cross-sectional area of pulmonary arteries to be compromised, emergency pulmonary embolectomy should be considered. Such situations, however, are extremely rare (Sasahara and Baramian, 1973). Most patients with fatal pulmonary emboli die within the first hour after the onset of symptoms (Gifford and Graves, 1969).

Fibrinolytic treatment with urokinase or streptokinase has been proposed as an ancillary form of treatment for pulmonary embolism (Bell, 1974). While it hastens the resolution of symptoms, this is accompanied by significant bleeding in one-third of the cases and there is no convincing evidence of long-term benefits. The best way of avoiding long-term lung damage is to recognize thrombophlebitis and the initial small pulmonary emboli. Prompt treatment of these can avoid most of the subsequent massive emboli.

There is controversy as to how long patients should be maintained on anticoagulants following an episode of acute thromboembolism. Everyone agrees that they should be continued until the patient is fully ambulatory. Once the patient has been ambulatory for several weeks, there is no good rationale for further continuation of long-term anticoagulants unless the patient has one of the unusual hypercoagulable states discussed above (i.e. lupus erythematous, malignancy, or idiopathic recurrent thromboembolism) rather than the usual postoperative aetiology. Patients who suffer a postoperative thromboembolic event should be considered for prophylactic anticoagulants following any future significant surgery since they do have a high incidence of recurrence under such circumstances. Prior to ambulation, all patients with thrombophlebitis should be furnished with effective elastic support from the instep to below the knee to prevent the development of chronic venous insufficiency. This may be in the form of an elastic bandage or a custom-fit elastic stocking. Ordinary non-custom fitted elastic stockings are not adequate for this purpose.

Chronic Venous Insufficiency

Chronic venous insufficiency is a condition characterized by chronic venous stasis and increased venous pressure. It is seen in adults of all ages. Most cases of chronic venous insufficiency develop after an episode of thrombophlebitis. Frequently, this may take many years to develop. Rarely it develops as a result of venous compression by tumours or increased venous pressure from an arterial venous fistula. This leads to chronic ankle, foot, and lower leg swelling and brownish and purplish stasis pigmentation. The area surrounding the medial malleolus is usually the most severely involved. Dermatitis may be present and, commonly, skin ulcers occur. At times, these ulcers can become very large. Generally, they are not as painful as ischaemic ulcers.

Treatment

Stasis ulcers usually do not heal but remain chronic as long as the patient is ambulatory. Applications of cream, salves, antibiotic ointments, etc., only compound the problem. With bed rest, elevation of the extremities, and the use of continuous wet compresses (0.25% aqueous solution of aluminous subacetate, 0.9% sodium chloride, or tap water), most of these ulcers will heal quite rapidly. If healing is slow, arterial occlusive disease should be suspected. With very large ulcers, split thickness skin grafting may speed the healing once the ulcer is clean. Following healing of the ulcer and in all other cases of chronic venous insufficiency, the only effective therapy for preventing the development of ulcers or their recurrence is adequate elastic support. In patients without recent ulcers, this can best be done using a custom measured elastic stocking as described in the section on lymphoedema. In the case of recently healed ulcers, the use of a foam rubber pad with an elastic bandage may be helpful.

Lymphoedema

Lymphoedema refers to enlargement of an extremity by oedema secondary to obstructed lymph flow. In aged patients, the most common aetiology is malignancy. Less frequent radiation therapy, lymph node surgery, or episodes of recurrent lymphangitis may be the underlying cause. Most commonly, the condition is unilateral and is usually painless. Stasis pigmentation is absent and the swelling has a cylindrical appearance. Occasionally, squaring of the toes is characteristic.

Localization of the level of obstruction of the lymphatics can be determined by lymphangiography (Kinmonth, Taylor, and Harper, 1955) or computed tomography. The treatment of this disorder is elastic support. Diuretics, in small doses, may be helpful but will not control the swelling without elastic support. The patient should be at bed-rest with the extremity continuously elevated at an angle of at least 45° until all swelling has subsided. Once this has been accomplished, measurements can then be made for a custom-fit elastic stocking. The patient should then wear the stocking whenever the leg is in a dependent position. It must be emphasized that this disease cannot be treated successfully without the use of good and effective elastic support. Many surgical procedures for the treatment of lymphoedema have been proposed. None of these have proven to be particularly effective except for rare instances in which compression by a tumour is the cause of the lymphoedema.

REFERENCES

Allen, E. V. (1929). 'Thromboangiitis obliterans: Methods of diagnosis of chronic occlusive arterial lesions distal to the wrist with illustrative cases', *Am. J. Med. Sci.*, **178**, 237–244.

Alley, M. C., Dempsey, M. E., Bale, L., Dinh, D., and Kottke, B. A. (1982). 'Inhibition of cholesterol esterification in cultured human fibroblats by cardiac glycoside and local anesthetic agents', *Fed. Proc.*, **41**, 1428 (6766).

Angles-Cano, E., Sultan, Y., and Clauvel, J. P. (1979). 'Predisposing factors to thrombosis in systemic lupus erythematous', *J. Lab. Clin. Med.*, **94**, 312–323.

Appelbaum, A., Karp, R. B., and Kirklin, J. W. (1976). 'Ascending versus descending aortic dissections', *Ann. Surg.*, **183**, 296–300.

Arkin, A. (1930). 'A clinical and pathologic study of periarteritis nodosa: A report of 5 cases, one histologically healed', *Am. J. Pathol.*, **6**, 401–426.

Barker, N. W., Nygaard, K. K., Walters, W., and Priestly, J. T. (1940). 'A statistical study of postoperative versus thrombosis and pulmonary embolism. I. Incidences in various types of operations', *Proc. Staff Meeting Mayo Clin.*, **15**, 769–773.

Barker, N. W., Nygaard, K. K., Walters, W. and Priestly, J. T. (1941). 'A statistical study of postoperative versus thrombosis and pulmonary embolism. II. Predisposing factors', *Proc. Staff Meeting Mayo Clin.*, **16**, 1–5.

Barner, H. B., Judd, D. R., Kaiser, G. C., Willman, V. L., and Hanlon, C. R. (1968). 'Blood flow in femoral-popliteal bypass vein grafts', *Arch. Surg.*, **96**, 619–627.

Bartels, C. C., and Rullo, F. R. (1958). 'Unsuspected diabetes mellitus in peripheral vascular disease', *New Engl. J. Med.*, **259**, 633–635.

Beckering, R. E., Jr., and Titus, J. L. (1969). 'Femoral-popliteal venous thrombosis and pulmonary emboli', *Am. J. Clin. Pathol.*, **52**, 530–537.

Bell, W. (1974). 'Urokinase-streptokinase embolism trial: Phase 2 results – A cooperative study', *J. Am. Med. Assn.*, **229**, 1606–1613.

Bellanti, J. A. (1978). 'Immunologically mediated diseases', in *Immunology II* (Ed. J. A. Bellanti), pp. 471–643, Saunders, Philadelphia.

Bircher, J., Bartholomew, L. G., Cain, J. C., and Adson, M. A. (1966). 'Syndrome of intestinal arterial insufficiency and abdominal angina', *Arch. Intern. Med.*, **117**, 632–638.

Bjorkerud, S., and Bondjers, G. (1972). 'Endothelial integrity and viability in the aorta of the normal rabbit and rat as evaluated with dye exclusion tests and interference contrast microscopy', *Atherosclerosis*, **15**, 285–300.

Blau, L., and Bittman, R. (1978). 'Cholesterol distribution between the two halves of the lipid bilayer of human erythrocyte ghost membranes', *J. Biol. Chem.*, **253**, 8366–8368.

Bloor, K. (1961). 'Natural history of arteriosclerosis of the lower extremities', *Ann. R. Coll. Surg. Engl.*, **28**, 36–52.

Brown, M. S., and Goldstein, J. L. (1976). 'Analysis of a mutant strain of human fibroblasts with a defect in the internalization of receptor-bound low density lipoprotein', *Cell*, 663–674.

Brown, M. S., Ho, Y. K., and Goldstein, J. L. (1980). 'The cholesteryl ester cycle in macrophage foam cells', *J. Biol. Chem.*, **255**, 9344–9352.

Brown, M. S., Kovanen, P. T., and Goldstein, J.

L. (1981). 'Regulation of plasma cholesterol by lipoprotein receptors', *Science*, **212**, 628–635.

Brown, O. R., Popp, R. L., and Klaster, F. E. (1975). 'Echocardiographic criteria for aortic root dissection', *Am. J. Cardiol.*, **36**, 17–20.

Campbell, P. M., and LeRoy, E. C. (1975). 'Pathogenesis of systemic sclerosis: A vascular hypothesis', *Semin. Arthritis Rheum.*, **4**, 351–368.

Caplan, B. A., and Schwartz, C. J. (1973). 'Increased endothelial cell turnover in areas of in vivo Evans Blue uptake in the pig aorta', *Atherosclerosis*, **17**, 401–417.

Carpenter, J. R., Hattery, R. R., Hunder, G. G., Bryan, R. S., and McLeod, R. A. (1976). 'Ultrasound evaluation of the popliteal space – Comparison with arthrography and physical examination', *Mayo Clin. Proc.*, **51**, 498–503.

Castenedo-Zuniga, W. R., Fornanek, A., Tadiavarthy, M., Vlodaver, Z., Edwards, J. E., Zollikofer, C., and Amplatz, K. (1980). 'The mechanism of balloon angioplasty', *Diagn. Radiol.*, **135**, 565–571.

Chamley-Campbell, J., Campbell, G. R., and Ross, R. (1979). 'The smooth muscle cell in culture', *Physiol. Rev.*, **59**, 1–61.

Chang, Y. H., and Yao, C. S. (1979). 'Investigation of the human macrophage. I. Collection and in vitro cultivation', *Eur. J. Immunol.*, **9**, 517–520.

Chesebro, J. H., Clements, I. P., Fuster, V., Elveback, L. R., Smith, H. C., Bardsley, W. T., Frye, R. L., Hokmes, D. R. Jr., Vlietstra, R. E., Pluth, J. R., Wallace, R. B., Puga, F. J., Orszulak, T. A., Piehler, J. M., Schaff, H. V., and Danielson, G. K. (1982). 'A platelet inhibitor-drug trial in coronary-artery bypass-operations. Benefit of perioperative dipyridamole and aspirin therapy on early postoperative vein-graft potency', *New Engl. J. Med.*, **307**, 73–78.

Cornicelli, J. A., Gilman, S. R., Krom, B. A., and Kottke, B. A. (1981). 'Cannabinoids impair the formation of cholesteryl ester in cultured human cells', *Arteriosclerosis*, **1**, 449–454.

Coventry, M. B., Nolan, D. R., and Beckenbaugh, R. D. (1973). '"Delayed" prophylactic anticoagulation: A study of results and complications in 2,012 total hip arthroplasties', *J. Bone Joint Surg.*, **55**, 1487–1492.

Crawford, E. S., and Rubio, P. A. (1973). 'Reappraisal of adjuncts to avoid ischaemia in the treatment of aneurysms of descending thoracic aorta', *J. Thorac. Cardiovasc. Surg.*, **66**, 693–703.

D'angelo, W. A., Fries, J. F., Masi, A. T., and Shulman, L. E. (1969). 'Pathologic observations in systemic sclerosis (scleroderma). A study of fifty-eight autopsy cases and fifty-eight matched controls', *Am. J. Med.*, **46**, 428–440.

Darling, R. C., Linton, R. R., and Razzuk, M. A. (1967). 'Saphenous vein bypass grafts for femoral-popliteal occlusive disease: A reappraisal', *Surgery*, **61**, 31–38.

Derrick, J. R., Pollard, H. S., and Moore, R. M. (1959). 'The pattern of arteriosclerotic narrowing of the celiac and superior mesenteric arteries', *Ann. Surg.*, **149**, 684–689.

Deuel, T. F., Keim, P. S., Faineru, M., and Heinrikson, R. L. (1977). 'Amino acid sequence of human platelet factor-4', *Proc. Natl. Acad. Sci., USA*, **74**, 2256–2258.

DeWiese, J. A., Tering, R., Barner, H. B., and Rob, C. G. (1966). 'Autogenic venous femoral-popliteal bypass grafts', *Surgery*, **59**, 28–38.

Divertie, M. B. (1964). 'Lung involvement in connective tissue disorders', *Med. Clin. North Am.*, **48**, 1015–1030.

Earnest, F. IV, Muhm, J. R., and Sheedy, P. F. II (1979). 'Roentgenographic findings in thoracic aortic dissection', *Mayo Clin. Proc.*, **54**, 43–50.

Edelson, P. J., and Cohn, Z. A. (1976). 'Purification and cultivation of monocytes and macrophages', in *Vitro Methods in Cell-Mediated and Tumor Immunity* (Eds B. R. Bloom and J. R. David), pp. 333–340, Academic Press, New York.

Eisenberg, S., Bilheimer, D. W., and Levy, R. I. (1972). 'The metabolism of very low density lipoprotein proteins. II. Studies on the transfer of apoproteins between plasma lipoproteins', *Biochim. Biophys. Acta*, **280**, 94–104.

Estes, J. E. Jr. (1950). 'Abdominal aortic aneurysm: A study of one-hundred and two cases', *Circulation*, **2**, 258–264.

Fielding, C. J. (1978). 'Origin and properties of remnant lipoproteins', in *Disturbance in Lipid and Lipoprotein Metabolism* (Eds J. M. Dietschy, A. M. Gotto, and J. A. Ortko), pp. 83–98, Williams and Wilkins Co., Baltimore.

Fielding, P. E., and Fielding, C. J. (1980). 'A cholesteryl ester transfer complex in human plasma', *Proc. Natl. Acad. Sci. USA*, **77**, 3327–3330.

Filip, D. J., Eckstein, J. D., and Veltkarp, J. J. (1976). 'Hereditary antithrombin III deficiency and thromboembolic disease', *Am. J. Hematol.*, **1**, 343–349.

Fleming, R. J., and Stein, L. Z. (1965). 'Multiple intraparenchymal renal aneurysms in polyarteritis nodosa', *Radiology*, **84**, 100–103.

Florey, C. M. (1945). 'Arterial occlusions produced by emboli from eroded aortic atheromatous plaques', *Am. J. Pathol.*, **21**, 549–565.

Florian, A., Cohn, L. H., Dammin, G. J., and Collins, M. J. Jr. (1976). 'Small vessel replacement with gore-tex (expanded polytetrafluoroethylene)', *Arch. Surg.*, **111**, 267–270.

Fogarty, T. J., Cranley, J. J., Krause, R. J., Strasser, E., and Hafner, C. D. (1963). 'A method for extraction of arterial emboli and thrombi', *Surg. Gynecol. Obstet.*, **116**, 241–244.

Frohnert, P. P., and Sheps, S. G. (1967). 'Long-term follow-up study of periarteritis nodosa', *Am. J. Med.*, **43**, 8–14.

Fuster, V., Bowie, E. J. W., Lewis, J. C., Fass, D. N., Owen, C. A. Jr., and Brown, A. L. (1978). 'Resistance to arteriosclerosis in pigs with von Willebrand's disease', *J. Clin. Invest.*, **61**, 722–730.

Fuster, V., Chesebro, J. H., Frye, R. L., and Elveback, L. R. (1981). 'Platelet survival and the development of coronary artery disease in the young adult: Effects of cigarette smoking, strong family history and medical therapy', *Circulation*, **63**, 546–551.

Gamble, E. E., DeWeerd, J. H., and Dockerty, M. B. (1968). 'Periarteritis nodosa complicated with bilateral spontaneous massive perirenal hemorrhage', *Minn. Med.*, **51**, 767–769.

Geer, J. C. (1965). 'Fine structure of human aortic intimal thickening and fatty streaks', *Lab. Invest.*, **14**, 1764–1783.

Gerrity, R. G. (1981). 'Transition of blood-bovine monocytes into foam cells in fatty lesions', *Am. J. Pathol.*, **103**, 181–190.

Gifford, R. W. Jr., and Graves, L. K. (1969). 'Limitation in the feasibility of pulmonary embolectomy: A clinical pathological study of 101 cases of massive pulmonary embolism', *Circulation*, **39**, 523–530.

Gocke, D. J., Hsu, K., Morgan, C., Bombardieri, S., Lockshin, M., and Christian, C. L. (1970). 'Association between polyarteritis and Australia antigen', *Lancet*, **2**, 1149–1153.

Goldstein, J. L., Anderson, R. G. W., Buja, L. M., Basu, S. K., and Brown, M. S. (1977). 'Overloading human aortic smooth muscle cells with low density lipoprotein-cholesterol esters reproduces features of atherosclerosis in vitro', *J. Clin. Invest.*, **59**, 1196–1202.

Goldstein, J. L., and Brown, M. S. (1977). 'The low-density lipoprotein pathway and its relation to atherosclerosis', *Ann. Rev. Biochem.*, **46**, 897–930.

Goldstein, J. L., Dana, S. E., Faust, J. R., Beaudet, A. L., and Brown, M. S. (1975). 'Role of lysosomal acid lipase in the metabolism of plasma low density lipoprotein – Observations in cultured fibroblasts from a patient with cholesteryl ester storage disease', *J. Biol. Chem.*, **250**, 8487–8495.

Goldstein, J. L., Ho, Y. K., Basu, S. K., and Brown, M. S. (1979). 'Binding site on macrophages that mediates uptake and degradation of acetylated low density lipoprotein, producing massive cholesterol deposition', *Proc. Natl. Acad. Sci. USA*, **76**, 333–337.

Goldstein, J. L., Kottke, B. A., and Brown, M. S. (1982). 'Biochemical genetics of LDL receptor mutations in familial hypercholesterolemia', in

Human Genetics. Part B: Medical Aspects, pp. 161–176, Alan R. Liss Inc., New York.

Gomes, M. R., Bernatz, P. E., and Juergens, J. L. (1967). 'Aortic ilium surgery. Influence of clinical factors on results', *Arch. Surg.*, **95**, 387–393.

Green, R. M., DeWeese, J. P., and Rob, C. G. (1975). 'Arterial embolectomy before and after the Fogarty catheter', *Surgery*, **77**, 24–33.

Greipp, R. B., Stinson, E. B., Hollingsworth, J. F., and Buehler, D. (1975). 'Prosthetic replacement of the aortic arch', *J. Thorac. Cardiovasc. Surg.*, **70**, 1051–1063.

Grotendorst, G. R., Seppa, H. E. J., Kleinman, H. K., and Martin, G. R. (1981). 'Attachment of smooth muscle cells to collagen and their migration toward platelet-derived growth factor', *Proc. Natl. Acad. Sci. USA*, **78**, 3669–3672.

Grüntzig, A. (1977). 'Die perkutane transluminale rekanalisation chronischer arterienverschulusse mit einer neuen dilatationstecknik', Verlog Gerhard Witztroch, Baden-Baden.

Hamblin, T., and Oscier, D. (1978). 'Polyarteritis presenting in thrombocytosis and palliated by plasma exchange', *Postgrad. Med. J.*, **54**, 615–617.

Havel, R. J., Chao, Y.-S., Windler, E. E., Kotite, L., and Guo, L. S. S. (1980). 'Isoprotein specificity in the hepatic uptake of apolipoprotein E and the pathogenesis of familial dysbetalipoproteinemia', *Proc. Natl. Acad. Sci. USA*, **77**, 4349–4353.

Heldin, C.-H., Westermark, B., and Wasteson, A. (1979). 'Platelet-derived growth factor: Purification and partial characterization', *Proc. Natl. Acad. Sci. USA*, **76**, 3722–3726.

Heldin, C.-H., Westermark, B., and Wasteson, A. (1981). 'Specific receptors for platelet-derived growth factor on cells derived from connective tissue and glia', *Proc. Natl. Acad. Sci. USA*, **78**, 3664–3668.

Henriksen, T., Mahoney, E. M., and Steinberg, D. (1981). 'Enhanced macrophage degradation of low density lipoprotein previously incubated with cultured endothelial cells – Recognition by receptors for acetylated low density lipoproteins', *Proc. Natl. Acad. Sci. USA*, **78**, 6499–6503.

Hladover, J. (1978). 'Endothelial injury by nicotine and its prevention', *Experientia*, **34**, 1585.

Hopkins, G. J., and Barter, P. J. (1980). 'Transfers of esterified cholesterol and triglyceride between high density and very low density lipoproteins: In vitro studies of rabbits and humans', *Metabolism*, **29**, 546–550.

Hui, D., Innerarity, T. L., and Mahley, R. W. (1981). 'Lipoprotein binding to canine hepatic membranes – Metabolically distinct apo E and apo B-E receptors', *J. Biol. Chem.*, **256**, 5646–5655.

Jaffe, E. A., Nachman, R. L., Becker, C. G., and Minick, C. R. (1973). 'Culture of human endothelial cells derived from umbilical veins. Identification by morphologic and immunologic criteria', *J. Clin. Invest.*, **52**, 2745–2756.

Jørgensen, L., Packham, M. A., Rowsell, H. C., and Mustard, J. F. (1972). 'Deposition of formed elements of blood on the intima and signs of intimal injury in the aorta of rabbit, pig, and man', *Lab. Invest.*, **27**, 341–350.

Joyce, J. W., Fairbairn, J. F. II, Kincaid, O. W., and Juergens, J. L. (1964). 'Aneurysms of the thoracic aorta. A clinical study with special reference to prognosis', *Circulation*, **29**, 176–181.

Juergens, J. L., Barker, N. W., and Hines, E. A. Jr. (1960). 'Arteriosclerosis obliterans: Review of 520 cases with special reference to pathogenic and prognostic factors', *Circulation*, **21**, 188–195.

Kaplan, J., and Nielsen, M. L. (1979). 'Analysis of macrophage surface receptors. II. Internalization of α-macroglobulin trypsin complexes by rabbit alveolar macrophages', *J. Biol. Chem.*, **254**, 7329–7335.

Kaplan, K. L., Broekman, M. J., Chernoff, A., Lesznik, G. R., and Drillings, M. (1979). 'Platelet α-granule proteins: Studies on release and subcellular localization', *Blood*, **53**, 604–618.

Katzen, B. T., Chang, J., and Knox, W. G. (1979). 'Percutaneous transluminal angioplasty with the Grüntzig balloon catheter', *Arch. Surg.*, **114**, 1389–1399.

Kavanaugh, G. J., Svien, H. J., and Holnar, C. B. (1968). '"Pseudoclaudication" syndrome produced by compression of the cauda equina', *JAMA*, **206**, 2477–2481.

Kawato, S., Kinosita, K. Jr., and Ikegami, A. (1978). 'Effect of cholesterol on the molecular motion in the hydrocarbon region of lecithin bilayers studied by nanosecond fluorescence techniques', *Biochemistry*, **17**, 5026–5031.

Kidd, J. N., Reul, G. J. Jr., Cooley, D. A., Sandiford, F. M., Kyger, E. R. III, and Wukasch, D. C. (1976). 'Surgical treatment of aneurysms of the ascending aorta', *Circulation*, **54**, Suppl. 3, 118–122.

Kinmonth, J. B., Taylor, G. W., and Harper, R. K. (1955). 'Lymphangiography: A technique for its use in the lower limb', *Br. Med. J.*, **1**, 940–942.

Kolata, G. B. (1981). 'Drug found to help heart attack survivors', *Science*, **214**, 774–775.

Kovanen, P. T., Bilheimer, D. W., Goldstein, J. L., Jaramillo, J. J., and Brown, M. S. (1981). 'Regulatory role for hepatic low density lipoprotein receptors in vivo in the dog', *Proc. Natl. Acad. Sci. USA*, **78**, 1194–1198.

Laufnur, H., Nora, P. F., and Mittlepunkt, A. I. (1964). 'Mesenteric blood vessels: Advances in surgery and physiology', *Arch. Surg.*, **88**, 1021–1044.

Lee, K. R., Walls, W. J., Martin, N. L., and Templeton, A. W. (1975). 'A practical approach to the diagnosis of abdominal aortic aneurysms', *Surgery*, **78**, 195–201.

Levine, E. M., and Mueller, S. N. (1979). 'Cultured vascular endothelial cells as a model system for the study of cellular senescence', *Int. Rev. Cytol., Suppl.*, **10**, 67–76.

Liebovich, S. J., and Ross, R. (1976). 'A macrophage dependent growth factor that stimulates the proliferation of fibroblasts in vitro', *Am. J. Pathol.*, **84**, 501–513.

Linder, B. L., Chernoff, A., Kaplan, K. L., and Goodman, D. S. (1979). 'Release of platelet-derived growth factor from human platelets by arachidonic acid', *Proc. Natl. Acad. Sci. USA*, **76**, 4107–4111.

McCloy, R. M., Spittell, J. A. Jr., and McGoon, D. C. (1965). 'The prognosis in aortic dissection (dissecting aortic hematoma or aneurysm)', *Circulation*, **31**, 665–669.

MacIntyre, D. E. (1976). 'The platelet release reaction: Association with adhesion and aggregation, and comparison with secreting response in other cells', in *Platelets in Biology and Pathology* (Ed. J. L. Gordon), pp. 61–83, Elsevier/North Holland Biomedical Press, Amsterdam.

Mahley, R. W., Hui, D. Y., Innerarity, T. L., and Weisgraber, K. H. (1981). 'Two independent lipoprotein receptors on hepatic membranes of dog, swine and man-apo B, E and apo E receptors', *J. Clin. Invest.*, **68**, 1197–1206.

Mahley, R. W., Innerarity, T. L., Brown, M. S., Ho, Y. K., and Goldstein, J. L. (1980). 'Cholesteryl ester synthesis in macrophages: Stimulation by β-very low density lipoproteins from cholesterol-fed animals of several species', *J. Lipid Res.*, **21**, 970–980.

Mills, D. C. B., Robb, I. A., and Roberts, G. C. K. (1968). 'The release of nucleotide, 5-hydroxytryptamine and enzymes from human platelets during aggregation', *J. Physiol.*, **195**, 715–730.

Mills, D. C. B., and Smith, J. B. (1971). 'The influence of platelet aggregation of drugs that affect the accumulation of adenosine 3':5' cyclic monophosphate in platelets', *Biochem. J.*, **121**, 185–196.

Mintz, G. S., Kotler, M. N., Segal, B. L., and Parry, W. R. (1979). 'Two dimensional echocardiographic recognition of the descending thoracic aorta', *Am. J. Cardiol.*, **44**, 232–238.

Moncada, S., and Vane, J. R. (1979). 'Arachidonic acid metabolites and the interactions between platelets and blood-vessel walls', *New Engl. J. Med.*, **300**, 1142–1147.

Moore, S., and Pepper, D. S. (1976). 'Identification and characterization of a platelet specific release product: β-thromboglobulin', in *Platelets in Biology and Pathology* (Ed. J. L. Gordon), pp. 293–311, Elsevier/North Holland Biomedical Press, Amsterdam.

Moskowitz, R. W., Baggenstoss, A. H. and Slocomb, C. H. (1963). 'Histopathologic classification of periarteritis nodosa: A study of 56 cases confirmed at necropsy', *Proc. Staff Meeting Mayo Clin.*, **38**, 345–357.

Mukhopadhyay, A. K., and Graham, D. Y. (1976). 'Esophageal motor dysfunction in systemic diseases', *Arch. Intern. Med.*, **136**, 583–588.

Ottinger, L. W. (1975). 'Ruptured arteriosclerotic aneurysm of the abdominal aorta: Reducing mortality', *JAMA*, **233**, 147–150.

Pattnaik, N. M., Montes, A., Hughes, L. B., and Zilversmit, D. B. (1978). 'Cholesteryl ester exchange protein in human plasma – Isolation and characterization', *Biochim. Biophys. Acta*, **530**, 428–438.

Ponseti, I. V., and Baird, W. D. (1952). 'Scoliosis and dissecting aneurysm of the aorta in rats fed with "lathyrus odoratus" seeds', *Am. J. Pathol.*, **28**, 1059–1077.

Reul, G. J. Jr., Cooley, D. A., Hallman, G. L., Reddy, S. B., Kyger, E. R. III, and Wukasch, D. C. (1975). 'Dissecting aneurysm of the descending aorta – Improved surgical results in 91 patients', *Arch. Surg.*, **110**, 632–640.

Rich, A. R. (1947). 'Hypersensitivity in disease with special reference to periarteritis nodosa, rheumatic fever, disseminated lupus erythematous, and rheumatoid arthritis', *Harvey Lect.*, **42**, 106–147.

Roelants, G. E. (1977). 'The regulatory role of macrophages in immune recognition', in *B and T Cells in Immune Recognition* (Eds F. Loor and G. E. Roelants), pp. 103–121, John Wiley, London.

Rosenblatt, S. G., Knight, W., Bannayan, G. A., Wilson, C. B., and Stein, J. H. (1979). 'Treatment of Goodpasture's syndrome with plasmapheresis – A case report and review of the literature', *Am. J. Med.*, **66**, 689–696.

Ross, R. (1971). 'The smooth muscle cell. II. Growth of smooth muscle in culture and formation of elastic fibers', *J. Cell Biol.*, **50**, 172–186.

Ross, R., Glomset, J., Kariya, B., and Harker, L. (1974). 'A platelet-dependent serum factor that stimulates the proliferation of arterial smooth muscle cells in vitro', *Proc. Natl. Acad. Sci. USA*, **71**, 1207–1210.

Ross, R., Klebanoff, S. J. (1971). 'The smooth muscle cell. I. In vivo synthesis of connective tissue proteins', *J. Cell Biol.*, **50**, 159–171.

Rowe, D. W., McGoodwin, E. B., Martin, G. R., and Grahm, D. (1977). 'Decreased lysyloxidase activity in the aneurysm prone-nottled mouse', *J. Biol. Chem.*, **252**, 939–942.

Sasahara, A. A., and Baramian, E. M. (1973). 'Another look at pulmonary embolectomy', *Ann. Thorac. Surg.*, **16**, 317–320.

Schadt, D. C., Hines, E. A. Jr., Juergens, J. I., and Barker, N. W. (1961). 'Chronic atherosclerotic occlusion of the femoral artery', *JAMA*, **175**, 937–940.

Schatz, I. J., Fairbairn, J. F. II, and Juergens, J. L. (1962). 'Abdominal aortic aneurysms: A reappraisal', *Circulation*, **26**, 200–205.

Sevitt, S. (1969). 'Venous thrombosis in injured patients (with some observations on pathogenesis)', in *Thrombosis* (Eds S. Sherry, K. M. Brickhous, E. Genton, *et al.*), pp. 29–49, National Academy of Sciences, Washington, D.C.

Shelburne, F., Hanks, J., Meyers, W., and Quarfordt, S. (1980). 'Effect of apoproteins on hepatic uptake of triglyceride emulsions in the rat', *J. Clin. Invest.*, **65**, 652–658.

Shepherd, J. C. W., and Büldt, G. (1979). 'The influence of cholesterol on head group mobility in phospholipid membranes', *Biochim. Biophys. Acta*, **558**, 41–47.

Sheps, S. G., and McDuffie, F. C. (1980). 'Vasculitis', in *Peripheral Vascular Disease* (Eds J. L. Juergens, J. A. Spittell, and J. F. Fairbairn II), pp. 493–553, Saunders, Philadelphia.

Sherrill, B. C., and Dietschy, J. M. (1978). 'Characterization of the sinusoidal transport process responsible for uptake of chylomicrons by the liver', *J. Biol. Chem.*, **253**, 1859–1867.

Sherrill, B. C., Innerarity, T. L., and Mahley, R. W. (1980). 'Rapid hepatic clearance of the canine lipoproteins containing only the E apoprotein by a high affinity receptor', *J. Biol. Chem.*, **255**, 1804–1807.

Shick, R. M., Baggenstoss, A. H., Fuller, B. F., and Polley, H. F. (1950). 'Effects of cortisone and ACTH on periarteritis nodosa and cranial arteritis', *Proc. Staff Meeting Mayo Clin.*, **25**, 492–494.

Shields, G. S., Coalson, W. F., Kimball, D. A., Carnes, W. H., Cartwright, G. E., and Wintrope, M. M. (1962). 'Studies on copper metabolism. 32. Cardiovascular lesions in copper-deficient swine', *Am. J. Pathol.*, **41**, 603–621.

Siegel, R. C., Pinnell, S. R., and Martin, G. R. (1970). 'Cross-linking of collagen and elastin. Properties of lysyloxidase', *Biochemistry*, **9**, 4486–4492.

Silbert, S. (1952). 'Amputation of the lower extremity in diabetes mellitus: A follow-up study of 294 cases', *Diabetes*, **1**, 297–299.

Simon, M., and Sasahara, A. A. (1965). 'Observations on the angiographic changes in pulmonary thromboembolism', in *Pulmonary Embolic Disease* (Eds A. A. Sasahara and M. Stein), pp. 214–224, Grune and Stratton, New York.

Singer, A., and Rob, C. (1960). 'The fate of the claudicator', *Br. Med. J.*, **2**, 633–636.

Spittell, J. A. Jr., Fairbairn, J. F. II, Kincaid, O. W., and ReMine, W. H. (1961). 'Aneurysm of the splenic artery', *JAMA*, **175**, 452–456.

Spooner, P. M., Chernick, S. S., Garrison, M. M., and Scow, R. O. (1979a). 'Development of lipoprotein lipase activity and accumulation of triacylglycerol in differentiating 3T3-L1 adipocytes', *J. Biol. Chem.*, **254**, 1305–1311.

Spooner, P. M., Chernick, S. S., Garrison, M. M., and Scow, R. O. (1979b). 'Insulin regulation of lipoprotein lipase activity and release in 3T3-1L adipocytes', *J. Biol. Chem.*, **254**, 10021–10029.

Steele, P., Ellis, J. Jr., and Genton, E. (1978). 'Effects of platelet supernatant, anticoagulant and fibrinolytic therapy in patients with recurrent venous thromboembolism', *Am. J. Med.*, **64**, 441–445.

Stein, O., Fainaru, M., and Stein, Y. (1979). 'The role of lysophosphatidylcholine and apolipoprotein A₁ in the cholesterol-removing capacity of lipoprotein-deficient serum in tissue culture', *Biochim. Biophys. Acta*, **574**, 495–504.

Stein, Y., Glangeaud, M. C., Fainaru, M., and Stein, O. (1975). 'The removal of cholesterol from aortic smooth muscle cells in culture and landschutz ascites cells by fractions of human high-density apolipoproteins', *Biochim. Biophys. Acta*, **380**, 106–118.

Strong, J. P., and Richards, M. L. (1976). 'Cigarette smoking and arteriosclerosis in autopsied men', *Atherosclerosis*, **23**, 451–475.

Study Group (1958). 'Classification of atherosclerotic lesions', *W.H.O. Tech. Rep. Ser.*, **143**, 1–20.

Szilagyi, D. E., Smith, R. F., Elmquist, J. G., Gonzalez, A., and Elliott, J. P. (1965). 'Angioplasty in the treatment of peripheral occlusive arteriopathy: A surgery of 12 years experience', *Arch. Surg.*, **90**, 617–628.

Thompson, G. R., Soutar, A. K., Spengel, F. A., Jadhav, A., Gavigan, S. J. P., and Myant, N. B. (1981). 'Defects of receptor-mediated low density lipoprotein catabolism in homozygous familial hypercholesterolemia and hypothyroidism in vivo', *Proc. Natl. Acad. Sci. USA*, **78**, 2591–2595.

Thorgeirsson, G., Robertson, A. L. Jr., and Cowan, D. H. (1979). 'Migration of human vascular endothelial and smooth muscle cells', *Lab. Invest.*, **41**, 51–62.

Trepo, C. G., Zuckerman, A. J., Bird, R. C., and Prince, A. M. (1974). 'The role of circulating hepatitis B antigen/antibody immune complexes in the pathogenesis of vascular and hepatic manifestations in polyarteritis nodosa', *J. Clin. Pathol.*, **27**, 863–868.

Uitto, J., Bauer, E. A., and Eisen, A. Z. (1979). 'Scleroderma-increased biosynthesis of triple-helical type I and type II procollagens associated with unaltered expression of collagenase by skin fibroblasts in culture', *J. Clin. Invest.*, **64**, 921–930.

Unni, K. K., Kottke, B. A., Titus, J. L., Frye, R. L., Wallace, R. B., and Brown, A. L. (1974). 'Pathologic changes in aortocoronary saphenous vein grafts', *Am. J. Cardiol.*, **34**, 526–532.

Vaughan, T. J., Barry, W. F. Jr., Jeffords, D. L., and Johnsrude, I. S. (1971). 'Renal artery aneurysms and hypertension', *Radiology*, **99**, 287–293.

Vollmar, J., Tiede, M., and Lauback, K. (1969). 'Procedures for chronic femoral-popliteal occlusions: A report of 546 operations', *J. Cardiovasc. Surg.*, **9**, 297–301.

Wagner, H. N. Jr., Sabiston, D. C. Jr., Iio, M., McAfee, J. G., Meger, J. K., and Langan, J. K. (1964). 'Regional pulmonary blood flow in man by radioisotope scanning', *JAMA*, **187**, 601–603.

Wagner, H. N. Jr., and Strauss, H. W. (1975). 'Radioactive tracers in the differential diagnosis of pulmonary embolism', *Prog. Cardiovasc. Dis.*, **17**, 271–282.

Wallace, D. J., Goldfinger, D., Gatti, R., Lowe, C., Fan, P., Bluestone, R., and Klinenberg, J. R. (1979). 'Plasmapheresis and lymphoplasmapheresis in the management of rheumatoid arthritis', *Arthritis Rheum.*, **22**, 703–710.

Weibel, E. R., and Palade, G. E. (1964). 'New cytoplasmic components in arterial endothelium', *J. Cell Biol.*, **23**, 101–112.

Weis, H. J., Witte, L. D., Kaplan, K. L., Lages, B. A., Chernoff, A., Nossel, H. L., Goodman, B. S., and Baumgartner, H. R. (1979). 'Heterogeneity in storage pool deficiency: Studies on granule-bound substances in 18 patients including varieties deficient in α-granules, platelet factor-4, β-thromboglobulin, and platelet-derived growth factor', *Blood*, **54**, 1296–1319.

Weksler, B. B., Marcus, A. J., and Jaffe, E. A. (1977). 'Synthesis of prostaglandin I₂ (prostacyclin) by cultured human and bovine endothelial cells', *Proc. Natl. Acad. Sci. USA*, **74**, 3922–3926.

Wessler, S. (1975). 'Small doses of heparin and a new concept of hyper-coagulability', *Thromb. Diath. Haemorrh.*, **33**, 81–86.

Wheat, M. W. Jr. (1973). 'Treatment of dissecting aneurysms of the aorta: Current status', *Prog. Cardiovasc. Dis.*, **16**, 87–101.

White, J. G. (1971). 'Platelet morphology', in *The Circulating Platelet* (Ed. S. A. Johnson), pp. 45–121, Academic Press, New York.

Wight, T. N., and Ross, R. (1975). 'Proteoglycans in primate arteries. II. Synthesis and secretion of glycosaminoglycans by arterial smooth muscle cells in culture', *J. Cell Biol.*, **67**, 675–686.

Wilson, D. B., Ellsworth, J. L., and Jackson, R. L. (1980). 'Net transfer of phosphatidylcholine from plasma low density lipoproteins to sphingomyelin-apolipoprotein A-II complexes by bovine liver and human plasma phospholipid exchange proteins', *Biochim. Biophys. Acta*, **620**, 550–561.

Windler, E., Chao, Y.-S., and Havel, R. J. (1980). 'Determinants of hepatic uptake of triglyceride-rich lipoproteins and their remnants in the rat', *J. Biol. Chem.*, **255**, 5475–5480.

Witte, L. D., Kaplan, D. L., Nossel, H. L., Lages, B. A., Weiss, H. J., and Goodman, D. S. (1978). 'Studies of the release from human platelets of the growth factor for cultured human arterial smooth muscle cells', *Circ. Res.*, **42**, 402–409.

Wychulis, A. R., Spittell, J. A. Jr., and Wallace, R. B. (1970). 'Popliteal aneurysms', *Surgery*, **68**, 942–951.

Yao, J. S. T., and Berger, J. J. (1974). 'Application of ultrasound to arterial and venous diagnosis', *Surg. Clin. North Am.*, **54**, 23–38.

14

The Cardiovascular System

14.1

The Cardiovascular System

B. O. Williams

EPIDEMIOLOGY OF HEART DISEASE IN OLD AGE

Mortality

Heart disease is increasingly common with advancing age and remains the most important single cause of death in old age, in both sexes, worldwide (Table 1) (Burch, 1978; World Health Organization, 1974). In patients over the age of 65 years, heart disease accounts for more than 70 per cent. of all cardiovascular deaths in many countries including the United States and the United Kingdom (Rodstein, 1979; Scottish Health Service, 1981). Between the years 1975 and 1979, in Scotland, death rates in the elderly from all forms of heart disease remained steady in females but increased in males due to an increased mortality rate in men over the age of 85 years in 1979 (Fig. 1) (Scottish Health Service, 1981). The mortality rate from cardiac disease in males was double the rate in females in the 65 to 74 year age group but the male mortality rate was

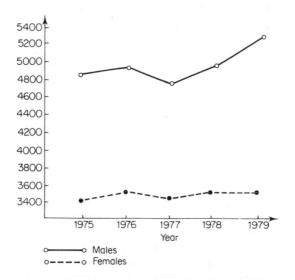

Figure 1   Mortality rate per 100,000 population in 65 years and over in Scotland (ICD 390–429)

61 per cent. more in the 75 to 84 year age group and only 42 per cent. more over the age of 85 years.

The most important form of heart disease is ischaemic heart disease (Burch, 1978; Scottish Health Service, 1981) (Table 2). A recent fall in mortality rates for ischaemic heart disease in the United States, Canada, Australia, and Finland (World Health Organization, 1965–1977) has been followed by a similar fall in Scotland, but not in men or women under the age of 65 years (Scottish Health Service, 1981). There has been a recent fall in the mortality from ischaemic heart disease in men and

Table 1   Ranked causes of death worldwide in subjects 65 years and over. (From World Health Organization, 1974)

Rank	Cause of death
1	Heart disease
2	Stroke
3	Neoplasia
4	Pneumonia
5	Chest infections

women over 75 years of age although the incidence of ischaemic heart disease does rise dramatically with age and women develop myocardial infarction about 10 years on average after men (Konu, 1977). In 1979 mortality due to ischaemic heart disease in the population in Scotland over 65 years accounted for 73 per cent. of all deaths due to ischaemic heart disease (Scottish Health Service, 1981).

Prevalence

A high prevalence of heart disease has been observed in numerous surveys of elderly population groups (Acheson and Acheson, 1958; Droller and Pemberton, 1953; Kennedy, Andrews and Caird, 1977; Kitchin, Lowther, and Milne, 1973; Martin and Millard, 1973). Community surveys have shown a high prevalence of heart disease in relatively fit elderly subjects living at home; 40 per cent. in the age group of 65 to 74 years and 50 per cent. in the age group of 75 years and over had undoubted evidence of heart disease (Table 3) (Kennedy, Andrews, and Caird, 1977).

If ischaemic heart disease is defined by angina pectoris or a past history of myocardial infarction and/or an abnormal Q/QS ECG pattern, then its prevalence is about 20 per cent. in men and 12 per cent. in women over the age of 65 years (Acheson and Acheson, 1958; Kennedy, Andrews, and Caird, 1977; Kitchin, Lowther, and Milne, 1973). Hypertensive heart disease defined as a blood pressure of 180/110 mmHg or more, in addition to electrocardiographic evidence of left ventricular hypertrophy, is present in 8 to 13 per cent. of men and 12 to 16 per cent. of women over the age of 65 years (Kennedy, Andrews, and Caird, 1977).

The prevalence of rheumatic heart disease is less than 5 per cent. in the population over the age of 65 years (Droller and Pemberton, 1953; Kennedy, Andrews, and Caird, 1977) and pulmonary heart disease is relatively uncommon and virtually confined to men (Kennedy, Andrews, and Caird, 1977).

Pathological electrocardiograms are commonly found in symptomatic and asymptomatic elderly subjects (Campbell, Caird, and Jackson, 1974; Cullen, Murphy and Cumpston, 1974; Kitchin, Lowther, and Milne, 1973; Mihalick and Fisch, 1974; Ostrander *et al.*, 1965). Electrocardiographic evidence of cardiac abnormality is present in from 40 to 60 per cent. of apparently fit old people (Campbell, Caird, and Jackson, 1974). About 3 to 10 per cent. of the elderly have Q/QS abnormalities and despite the variation in the reported frequency of T-wave changes, T-wave flattening with or without inversion is a significant abnormality in old age (Caird, Campbell, and Jackson, 1974). Left ventricular hypertrophy is more common in women and right ventricular hypertrophy more common in men. First-degree atrioventricular block is present in 3 per cent. but higher degrees of block are relatively uncommon. Ventricular conduction defects are common. Right bundle branch block is more common than left bundle branch block in the elderly living at home, but the most frequently encountered conduction defect is left anterior hemiblock with or without right bundle branch block (Kitchin, Lowther, and Milne, 1973). In one 5-year longitudinal study of 70 year old subjects, a significant increase in the prevalence of pathological Q waves, left bundle branch block, atrial fibrillation, and first-degree atrioventricular block was observed. Q waves, pronounced ST segment depression, and negative T waves were associated with an increase in mortality in both sexes (Hedenrud *et al.*, 1980).

Table 2   Deaths from heart disease in patients 65 years and over in Scotland in 1979. (From Scottish Health Service, 1981, p. 49)

Age (years)	Total deaths due to heart disease[a]		Ischaemic (%)		Hypertensive (%)		Rheumatic (%)	
	M	F	M	F	M	F	M	F
65–74	4,195	2,945	90.6	82.6	1.7	3.4	0.9	2.7
75–84	3,037	4,009	80.8	75.6	2.2	3.1	0.6	1.2
85+	931	2,215	67.3	56.5	2.5	3.4	0.1	0.6

[a]ICD 390–429.

Table 3   Prevalence of heart disease in relatively fit edlerly population living at home. (From Kennedy, Andrews, and Caird, 1977)

| Age (years) | 65–74 | | 75+ | | |
Sex	M	F	M	F	Total
No. of subjects	102	167	79	153	501
Ischaemic	21	29	20	31	101 (20%)
Hypertensive	1	9	3	15	28 (6%)
Valvular	0	8	3	11	22 (4%)
Pulmonary	2	0	1	0	3 (0.6%)
Mixed ischaemic and hypertensive	1	3	3	4	11 (2%)
Unclassifiable	14	8	14	17	53 (11%)
Total definite heart disease	39 (38%)	57 (34%)	44 (56%)	78 (51%)	218 (43%)
Doubtful heart disease	10	4	1	13	28 (6%)
No heart disease	53 (52%)	106 (64%)	34 (43%)	62 (61%)	255 (51%)

Morbidity

Relatively little information is available about the morbidity associated with heart disease in old age (Caird and Kennedy, 1976). The prevalence (Klainer, Gibson, and White, 1965) and the incidence of cardiac failure (McKee *et al.*, 1971) increase with age. Heart disease has been shown to be a major contributory factor to a loss of independence in disabled elderly subjects living at home (Akhtar *et al.*, 1973) and the most frequent reason for the hospitalization of the elderly population (Gerstenblith, 1980).

Elderly cardiac hospital inpatients utilize 70 per cent. more hospital beds than the 45 to 65 year age group with heart disease and by the time of discharge elderly patients have spent more than twice as long in hospital (Table 4) (Scottish Health Service, 1981). Morbidity statistics from general practice (Royal College of General Practitioners, 1979) show an increase in episode rates for cardiac disorders with age in both sexes but elderly females have more episodes of cardiac disorders than their male counterparts over the age of 65 years and this becomes more apparent over the age of 75 years (Fig. 2).

Table 4   Beds used daily per 100,000 of the population in Scotland and mean duration of stay in 1979. Heart disease ICD (390–429). (From Scottish Health Service, 1981·).

Age (years)	Daily beds used	Mean stay in days (discharges)
15–45	208	8
45–65	2,086	10
65+	3,536	21

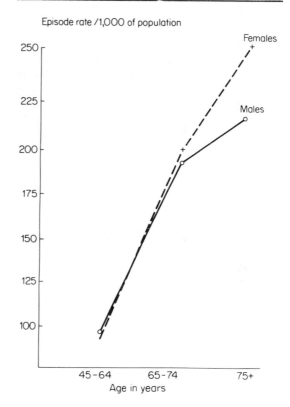

Episode rate /1,000 of population

Figure 2   Morbidity statistics for general practice cardiac diseases (ICD 390–429). (From Royal College of General Practitioners, 1979)

ISCHAEMIC HEART DISEASE: MYOCARDIAL INFARCTION

The prognostic significance of risk factors or predictors of ischaemic heart disease in the elderly differ in many respects from the young and middle aged. Most known risk factors have a lesser effect on mortality, i.e. the life expectancy compared to that of others of the same age and sex is diminished less than that of younger population groups (Rodstein, 1980).

Obesity

Increased relative body weight has not been confirmed as a risk factor (Kennedy, Andrews, and Caird, 1977; Konu, 1977) although there is a relationship in elderly men between obesity and ischaemic heart disease in association with elevated systolic blood pressure levels, diabetes, and a reduced serum high density lipoprotein cholesterol level (Gordon *et al.*, 1977).

Diabetes Mellitus

Diabetes mellitus is a significant risk factor for atherosclerotic disorders in both sexes (Vavrik, 1974) and especially for myocardial infarction (Konu, 1977). Although the blood sugar level was not related to the prevalence of ischaemic heart disease in one study (Kennedy, Andrews, and Caird, 1977) it did appear to be a strong risk factor for elderly females in a major prospective study (Gordon *et al.*, 1977).

Serum Lipids

The evidence for the association between serum total cholesterol and ischaemic heart disease is inconclusive. Serum total cholesterol was not associated with ischaemic heart disease in two studies (Gofman, Young, and Tandy, 1966; Kennedy, Andrews, and Caird, 1977) but was an apparent risk factor for ischaemic heart disease in elderly men (Horsey, Livesley, and Dickerson, 1980), myocardial infarction in both sexes (Konu, 1977), and atherosclerotic cardiovascular diseases in both sexes, particularly in association with diabetes or hypertension (Vavrik, 1974). Serum triglycerides were observed to be an important risk factor for ischaemic heart disease in association with diabetes mellitus in elderly women but not in men (Gordon *et al.*, 1977), and a further study showed no association with myocardial infarction (Konu, 1977). Although there is doubt about a relationship between serum total cholesterol and ischaemic heart disease in old age, there appears to be a positive association of

risk with the serum low-density lipoprotein cholesterol level and a negative association of risk with the serum high-density lipoprotein cholesterol level in both sexes (Gordon *et al.*, 1977).

Sex

Although male sex is a major risk factor for ischaemic heart disease in the young and middle aged this is not so in the elderly (Konu, 1977) and the prevalence rate in men is only 10 to 20 per cent. higher in old age (Kitchin, Lowther, and Milne, 1973).

Hypertension

Atherosclerotic disease in old age is associated with systolic and/or diastolic hypertension (Vavrik, 1974) and a raised blood pressure is a risk factor for ischaemic heart disease in both sexes, at least up to the age of 75 years and for older females (Gordon *et al.*, 1977). Kannel and Gordon (1978) have stressed the importance of hypertension as a risk factor but this has not been confirmed by other workers (Kennedy, Andrews, and Caird, 1977; Kitchin, Lowther, and Milne, 1973; Konu, 1977).

Cigarette Smoking

Cigarette smoking has been considered to be a weaker risk factor for ischaemic heart disease with increasing age and not a risk factor over the age of 65 years (Gofman, Young, and Tandy, 1966). Cigarette consumption was not related to the incidence of myocardial infarction in one study (Konu, 1977) but the prevalence of ischaemic heart disease was related to the level of cigarette smoking and the estimated total lifelong cigarette consumption in an elderly population at home (Kennedy *et al*, 1977).

Although it is possible to predict the development of ischaemic heart disease in the elderly using established risk factors there is no evidence as yet that intervention will necessarily modify the risks. The apparent weaker association between risk factors and ischaemic heart disease in older populations may be due to the fact that young or middle aged individuals who are most affected by these risk factors do not survive beyond middle age, viz. 'exhaustion of the susceptibles', and although single-risk factors may play a less important role in old age, a combination of these factors and the duration of them may combine to modify the natural history of ischaemic heart disease in later life.

CHANGES IN CARDIAC FUNCTION IN OLD AGE

Heart Rate

The resting heart rate alters very little with age (Strandell, 1964) but there is a reduction in the 'intrinsic heart rate', i.e. the heart rate after cardiac pharmacological denervation by simultaneous cholinergic and adrenergic blockade (Jose, 1966). The elderly have a known resistance to beta-adrenergic mediated responses to exercise and isoprenaline (Bertel *et al.*, 1980) and there is an age-related fall in maximum heart rates on exercise (Astrand, Astrand, and Rodahl, 1959; Robinson, 1938). The initial demonstration of reduced beta-adrenoceptors on human lymphocyte membranes (Schocken and Roth, 1977) has been disputed (Abrass and Scarpace, 1981), but it did raise the possibility that these receptors might be reduced in other sites such as the heart and peripheral blood vessels and a decrease in beta-receptors or sensitivity of these receptors might produce an apparent age-associated loss of adrenergic responsiveness.

Cardiac Output

Resting cardiac output and stroke volume index fall with age (Brandfonbrener, Landowne, and Shock, 1955) but the cardiac output can rise considerably with stress due to increases in the stroke volume and the heart rate (Strandell, 1964) and during exercise, the increase in cardiac output with increasing workload is the same in the old as in the young (Strandell, 1976), although the mean cardiac output at any workload is less in the elderly than in the young.

The mechanisms for the reduction in cardiac output in normal old age are not clear, but as there is little change in the resting heart rate the stroke volume must be reduced. The magnitude of the stroke volume is influenced by factors related to diastolic filling, distensibility

of the ventricles, arterial blood pressure, and myocardial contractility.

Systolic pressure load increases with age (Landowne, Brandfonbrener, and Shock, 1955; Master, Dublin, and Marks, 1950) and there is also evidence of increased filling pressure in the left heart. The left ventricular ejection fraction does not appear to alter with age at rest but is reduced in elderly subjects on exercise (Port *et al.*, 1980). Age-related changes in left ventricular function may be due to increased rigidity of the myocardium and reduced compliance (Strandell, 1976) or a decline in the myocardial contractile response (Gerstenblith, Lakatta, and Weisfeldt, 1976). It is important to remember that otherwise silent cardiac disease and, in particular, ischaemic heart disease may underlie apparent age-associated decline in left ventricular efficiency.

PATHOLOGY OF THE CARDIO-VASCULAR SYSTEM IN OLD AGE

In studies of the elderly circulation it must be realized that many pathological changes are present in the majority of elderly subjects, e.g. coronary atherosclerosis, but these should be regarded as diseases and not normal age changes (Pomerance, 1981).

Age Changes

The heart size does not change with age alone (Pomerance, 1981) but remains proportional to the body weight (Smith, 1928). Any apparent increase in heart weight is usually due to ischaemic heart disease (Hodkinson, Pomerance, and Hodkinson, 1979). Myocardial age changes include an increase in fat, especially in the interatrial septum, slight increases in the amount of collagen in the interventricular septum (Lenkiewicz, Davies, and Rosen, 1972) and an increase in the collagen and elastic tissue in the atria (Davies and Pomerance, 1972). Basophilic degeneration of the myocardium is usually present (Pomerance, 1981) and the quantity of lipofuscin in the myocardial fibres increases and leads to a degree of brown atrophy (Fig. 3) (McMillan and Lev, 1962).

There is a loss of muscle cells from the sinoatrial node with an associated relative increase in connective tissue (Davies and Pom-

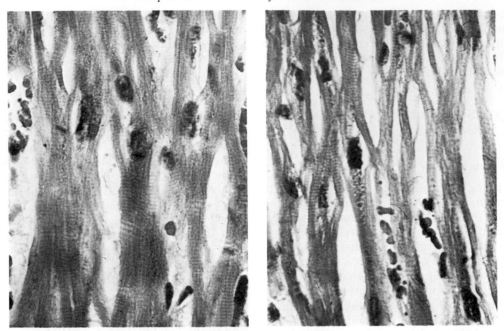

Figure 3   Brown atrophy of heart (H/E ×400). Myocardial fibres on the right are atrophic in comparison to normal fibres on the left. Numerous granules of lipofuscin are present. (By permission of Dr R. A. Burnett, Stobhill Hospital, Glasgow)

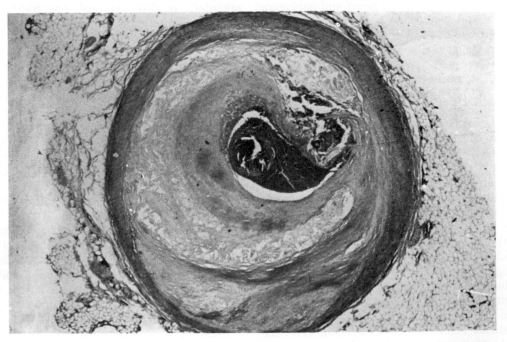

Figure 4   Coronary artery (×20). Lumen severely narrowed by atheroma. Recent haemorrhage into a plaque with surface thrombosis. (By permission of Dr R. A. Burnett, Stobhill Hosptial, Glasgow)

erance, 1972; Lev, 1954). The aetiology of this fibrosis is unclear and not apparently related to vascular disease (Hutchins, 1980). There is little change in the atrioventricular node and the bundle of His (Erickson and Lev, 1952).

Changes in the endocardium are probably related to mechanical factors which produce thickening over the atria and the atrial surfaces of the atrioventricular valves with the development of small nodules along the lines of apposition of the valves (Pomerance, 1967). Yellow lipid deposits appear on the ventricular surface of the anterior mitral valve cusp in the third or fourth decade and accumulate with age (Pomerance, 1967). Fine calcification develops in the aortic cusp bases in the fifth decade and in the mitral ring in the sixth decade (Sell and Scully, 1965).

Pathological Changes

The incidence of most cardiac disorders and especially ischaemic heart disease increase with age and a variety of heart diseases occur predominantly or exclusively in the old (Table 5) (Noble and Rothbaum, 1981).

Table 5 Heart diseases predominantly or exclusively in the elderly. (Adapted from Noble and Rothbaum, 1981)

A. Senile primary cardiac amyloidosis
B. Calcific degenerative disease
    Mitral valve ring calcification
    Aortic valve sclerosis – cusp calcification
    Calcific aortic stenosis
C. Primary mucoid degenerative valve disease
    Mitral regurgitation – the floppy mitral valve
    Aortic regurgitation
D. Conductive system disease
    Sclerodegeneration of the conducting system
      (Lenegre's disease)
    Fibrosis or calcification of the conducting system
      from adjacent structures (Lev's disease)
E. External cardiac rupture complicating myocardial
    infarction
F. Non-bacterial thrombotic endocarditis

Myocardial Disorders

Ischaemic heart disease. In post-mortem studies, a high clinically unsuspected prevalence of ischaemic lesions has been observed and approximately 30 per cent. of all elderly patients have evidence of ischaemic heart disease (see Fig. 4) (Pomerance, 1981).

Age-related microscopic foci of fibrosis are commonly demonstrated (see Fig. 5) in the myocardium but these are not necessarily ischaemic in origin and are probably the result of small foci of earlier myocardial inflammation (Schwartz and Mitchell, 1962).

Extensive fibrosed myocardial infarcts with no previous relevant clinical history are uncommon findings at post-mortem examinations except in old age and external cardiac rupture is a complication of myocardial infarction which is virtually only encountered in elderly patients (Pomerance, 1981).

Senile primary cardiac amyloidosis. This disorder is rarely found in patients under the age of 70 years and its prevalence increases with age over 70 (Wright and Calkins, 1975). Senile cardiac amyloid disease (see Fig. 6) has been demonstrated at post-mortem studies in 50 per cent. of subjects over the age of 65 years and in 84 per cent. over the age of 90 years. Women are more likely to be affected but less severely so than men (Hodkinson and Pomerance, 1977). There is often no macroscopic evidence to suggest the presence of amyloidosis.

Microscopically, the earliest deposits are seen in the atrial capillaries and with increasing accumulation there is resultant pressure atrophy of the myocardium and macroscopic nodular deposits in the atrial endocardium (Pomerance, 1981). Conducting tissues are rarely affected in the disease but in advanced cases deposits may occur in the valves. Extra-cardiac deposits may be found in the lungs and in the small vessel walls of other organs (Pomerance, 1981; Wright and Calkins, 1975).

Hypertrophic cardiomyopathy. Congestive and secondary forms of cardiomyopathy are uncommon but hypertrophic cardiomyopathy is not uncommon in old age (Berger, Rethy, and Goldberg, 1979; Davies, Pomerance and Teare, 1974) and is associated with hypertension (Petrin and Tavel, 1979). Females are more commonly affected but may have a less severe form of the disease (Krasnow and Stein, 1978). Hypertrophy of the septum and left ventricular wall is associated with a characteristic subaortic fibrous band which is diagnostic of hypertrophic cardiomyopathy.

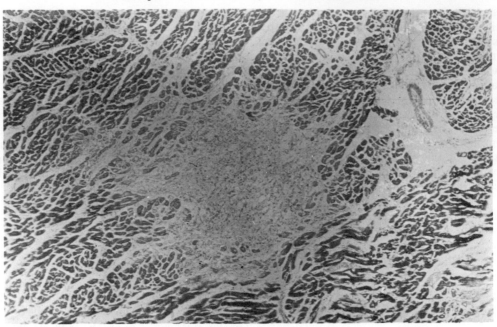

Figure 5   Focal myocardial scarring (H/E ×60). (By permission of Dr R. A. Burnett, Stobhill Hospital, Glasgow)

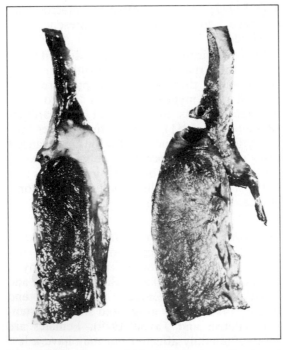

Figure 6 Cardiac amyloid. Sections from hearts cut through the A-V ring. Specimen on the left is normal. Specimen on the right shows enlargement with pallor of the myocadium due to extensive amyloid deposition. (By permission of Dr R. A. Burnett, Stobhill Hospital, Glasgow)

Valve Disorders

Mitral valve ring calcification Degenerative calcification affects the mitral valve ring. Nodules develop from focal calcification and the valve ring becomes rigid with resultant mitral valve regurgitation. Advanced disease may be associated with calcified masses and the exposed calcium forms a site of thrombus formation with a danger of embolization (Korn, De Sanctis, and Sell, 1962). The condition is more common in women (Simon and Liu, 1954) and the clinical importance of mitral ring calcification is related to its severity. Minor degrees are of no clinical significance but massive mitral ring calcification may be a cause of congestive cardiac failure (Korn, De Sanctis, and Sell, 1962) and may be associated with conduction disturbances (Lev, 1964).

Mucoid degeneration – The floppy mitral valve. In this common valve disorder, mucoid degeneration results in softening of the fibrosa with expansion of the valve cusps, stretching of the chordae tendinae, and systolic prolapse of the valve into the left atrium with associated mitral regurgitation (Pomerance, 1981). The incidence of this disorder increases with age (Davies, Moore, and Braimbridge, 1978).

Primarily, the valve cusps are expanded and the mitral valve ring may be dilated (Davies, Moore, and Braimbridge, 1978) with elongation of the chordae tendinae. Complications include rupture of the chordae tendinae, infective endocarditis, heart failure, and unexplained death.

Chronic rheumatic mitral valve disease. The post-mortem prevalence of chronic rheumatic heart disease is falling in the elderly (Pomerance, 1981). Mitral valve pathological changes range from minor degrees of cusp scarring with slight stenosis to grossly thickened distorted cusps associated with severe mitral stenosis and regurgitation.

Aortic valve disease. Degenerative calcific disease is an age-related condition which affects the aortic valve cusps. Most cases have minimal distortion of the valve, viz. aortic sclerosis, but the more severe form is responsible for the majority of cases of aortic stenosis in old age (Pomerance, 1972). Rheumatic disease is associated with thickening and contraction of the cusps with fused commissures and calcification may occur (Fig. 7).

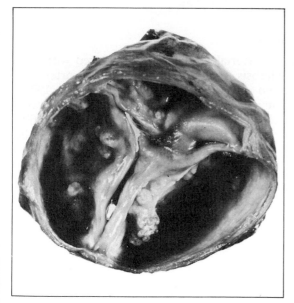

Figure 7   Calcific aortic stenosis. (By permission of Dr R. A. Burnett, Stobhill Hospital, Glasgow)

Infective endocarditis. Infective endocarditis is increasingly becoming a disease of the elderly, who often have no known valve disease (Schnurr *et al.*, 1977), probably due to a reduction in the incidence of rheumatic fever, the use of antibiotics, and increasing survival into old age when degenerative diseases become more prevalent (Pomerance, 1981). The pathological features of the disease are friable, nodular vegetations which occur on the atrial surfaces of atrioventricular valves, the ventricular surfaces of the aortic valves (Fig. 8), or on the jet lesions in valvular regurgitation. The other valves are rarely affected. The vegetations consist of fibrin, red cells, white cells, and microorganisms and the cusps are inflamed and necrotic with associated small abscesses in the myocardium.

Infective endocarditis may occur in rheumatic, degenerative, or congenital abnormalities, in particular in the bicuspid aortic valve. Foreign material, e.g. pacemaker wires or prosthetic valves, may become infected but in the elderly the largest single group of cases have no apparent underlying abnormality (Applefield and Hornick, 1974; Schnurr *et al.*, 1977; Thell, Martin, and Edwards, 1975).

Non-bacterial thrombotic endocarditis (Fig. 9) is common in the elderly because of its relationship to wasting diseases and is usually associated with terminal states (Pomerance, 1981). The pathology is similar to that of infective forms of the disease but the inflammatory reaction and microorganisms are absent and the underlying aortic or mitral valve cusps remain intact (see Chapter 9).

SYMPTOMS AND SIGNS IN CARDIAC DISEASE

Symptoms

The analysis of symptoms in ill elderly patients is often made especially difficult by the presence of multiple pathology and mental confusion which may be associated with acute illness or may be due to underlying chronic brain failure.

Breathlessness as a cardiac symptom may be modified in the elderly by restricted exercise tolerance due to arthritis or neuromuscular disorders. Episodic breathlessness at night is

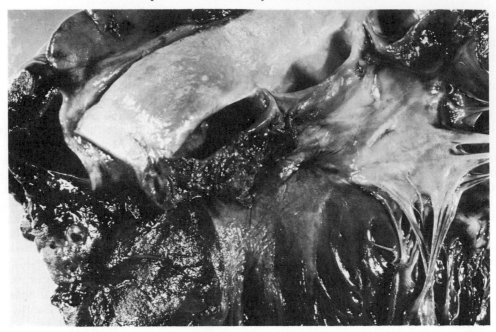

Figure 8   Acute bacterial endocarditis on aortic valve. (By permission of Dr R. A. Burnett, Stobhill Hospital, Glasgow)

suggestive of paroxysmal nocturnal dyspnoea and underlying left heart failure.

Cardiac pain is usually less commanding or even absent in elderly subjects with ischaemic heart disease. Angina may be less likely due to other causes of reduced activity or exercise tolerance. The reasons for the reduced incidence of cardiac pain in the elderly are not clear. Tolerance to cutaneous pain increases and tolerance to deep pain appears to decrease with age (Woodrow *et al.*, 1972), but is it possible that afferent denervation of the heart may be responsible with an age-related reduction in sensory nerve endings (Caird and Dall, 1978), or that symptoms of confusion or breathlessness may cloud the elderly subject's perception of pain. Cardiac ischaemia in old age may be due to disease of the smaller coronary artery vessels and the resulting ischaemic damaged areas of myocardium may be less extensive with less painful effects.

Ankle swelling may be due to congestive heart failure but by itself is more likely to be due to chronic venous insufficiency or hypoproteinaemia. Excessive fatigue may be a prominent symptom in elderly subjects with heart disease and may mask other more classical cardiovascular symptoms. Confusion may

be due to reduced cerebral perfusion as a result of hypotension or a fall in the cardiac output. Syncope may be associated with postural hypotension, Stokes–Adams attacks, transient dysrhythmias, myocardial infarction, or pulmonary embolism.

Signs

The arterial pulse rate is unaltered with age. Sclerosis of the radial and brachial arteries is of no special clinical significance (Caird, 1976). The slow rising pulse of severe aortic stenosis and the collapsing pulse of aortic regurgitation may be identified, although the former may be masked by an age related increase in the rate of the arterial upstroke due to increased stiffness of the vessel wall (Freis *et al.*, 1966). The finding of pulsus alternans in the presence of venous hypertension is evidence of severe cardiac failure and pulsus paradoxus indicates cardiac tamponade.

The significance of the arterial blood pressure is discussed elsewhere (page 00) but an important aspect of measurement is to take the blood pressure in the supine and erect positions to exclude significant blood pressure drop on standing. Normal asymptomatic el-

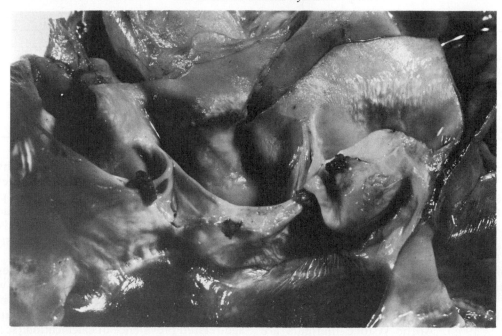

Figure 9   Non-bacterial thrombotic (marantic) endocarditis. Note 'wear and tear' thickening of cusps.
(By permission of Dr R. A. Burnett, Stobhill Hospital, Glasgow)

derly subjects often have a fall of 20 mmHg in systolic blood pressure on standing up (Caird, Andrews, and Kennedy, 1973) and symptoms are unusual unless the systolic pressure falls below 110 mmHg (Caird, 1979).

The venous pulse is often easier to detect in the elderly due to atrophy of the skin and subcutaneous tissues. Obstruction of the venous return in the left innominate vessel is often present and this 'pseudo-obstruction' is due to elongation and unfolding of the aorta. This phenomenon disappears on deep inspiration but occasionally is bilateral and may mimic the venous hypertension of congestive heart failure unless respiratory manoeuvres are performed. The A and V peaks and X and Y nadirs are the same in the jugular venous pulse as in younger subjects. Increased intensity of the A wave usually indicates resistance to right ventricular filling and pulmonary hypertension. Cannon A waves suggest the presence of atrioventricular dissociation. Prominent CV waves suggest tricuspid valve regurgitation and are usually accompanied by systolic hepatic pulsation.

Praecordial palpation will usually help determine enlargement of the ventricles and identify abnormal pulsation, e.g. left ventric-

ular dyskinesia. The apex beat may be displaced by chest deformities due to kyphoscoliosis or by left ventricular enlargement. The character of the apex beat is more important than the site and is forceful in left ventricular hypertrophy but diffuse in left ventricular dilatation. Severe right ventricular hypertrophy is uncommon in old age but a palpable, exaggerated, right ventricular impulse at the left sternal border can be detected in pulmonary hypertension due to rheumatic mitral valve disease or atrial septal defect.

Diastolic murmurs are always abnormal and are usually due to mitral stenosis or aortic regurgitation but systolic murmurs may be detected in as many as 60 per cent. of otherwise cardiovascular normal elderly subjects (Bethel and Crow, 1963; Griffiths and Sheldon, 1975). Systolic murmurs show an increased prevalence with age and are more common in women (Table 6). Most are due to multiple aortic or mitral minor valve abnormalities largely due to calcific degenerative change.

Innocent systolic murmurs are usually due to dilatation of the aorta, minimal fibrotic fusion of one or more commissures of the aortic valve or thickening or calcification of the aortic cusps, viz. aortic sclerosis (Perez *et al.*, 1976).

Table 6   Causes of systolic murmurs in the elderly

Common	Less Common	Rare
Aortic sclerosis	Calcific tricuspid aortic stenosis	Ruptured chordae tendinae
Aortic dilatation	Mitral anterior cusp nodularity	Tricuspid regurgitation
Mitral annulus calcification	Rheumatic mitral regurgitation	Congenital bicuspid aortic valve
Functional	Mitral valve prolapse – mucoid	Atrial septal defect
Fever	degeneration	Idiopathic hypertrophic subaortic
Anaemia	Papillary muscle dysfunction	stenosis
Hyperthyroidism	Supraventricular dysrhythmias	

The murmur is in early or mid systole with an early peak unlike the late peaking of aortic stenosis; it is usually grade 1 or 2 on a scale of 6, loudest in the second or third right or left intercostal spaces with minimal transmission to the right carotid artery and there is no palpable thrill (Vittal, Luisada, and Rao, 1976).

It is often difficult to differentiate on auscultation between aortic and mitral valve murmurs due to kyphoscoliosis and the elderly patient's difficulty in breath-holding (Leading Article, 1968). Aortic systolic murmurs are usually ejection or non-pansystolic and heard at the second right intercostal space with radiation to the right carotid artery and left sternal border, but they may be louder at the apex. Mitral systolic murmurs are usually pansystolic, best heard at the apex, and radiate to the left axilla, but they may be atypical and best detected at the base of the heart.

Systolic murmurs may be temporary and associated with supraventricular tachycardias, atrial fibrillation, fever, anaemia, and hyperthyroidism. Severe aortic stenosis is an unusual cause in the elderly (Leading Article, 1975).

INVESTIGATION OF CARDIAC DISORDERS IN THE ELDERLY

The Chest Radiograph

There are frequent difficulties in interpreting chest radiographs in elderly patients with suspected heart disease. The cardiothoracic ratio is said to increase with age, in the absence of heart disease, over the age of 40 years in females and 55 years in males and ratios of 54 per cent. may be considered as normal in women over the age of 80 years (Cowan, 1959, 1964), although this has been disputed by Rabushka, Melamed, and Melamed, (1968) who observed that elderly subjects who had ratios of more than 50 per cent. usually had hypertension or organic heart disease. Age-related kyphoscoliosis or sternal depression may partly account for an apparent increase in cardiac size (Cowan, 1965). Enlargement of the atria can usually be identified and has the same significance as in the young or middle aged.

The aorta and brachiocephalic arteries are more elongated and tortuous with age which makes them appear more prominent. Unfolding of the aorta is often associated with an age-related prevalence of calcification (see Fig. 10), particularly in elderly women, especially in the left lower quadrant of the aortic knuckle where it represents calcified atheroma, the plaque being related to the insertion of the ductus arteriosus (Caird and Dall, 1978). Linear calcification may be present in atheromatous plaques in the descending aorta. Cardiac calcification may occur in the myocardium,

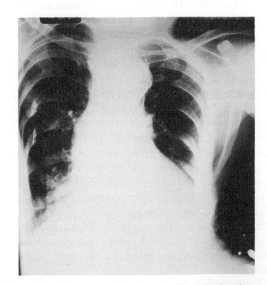

Figure 10   Posteroanterior chest radiograph showing calcification in the arch of the aorta in a 90 year old paient with fractures of the fifth and sixth ribs on the right side

usually as a result of transmural myocardial infarction, in the coronary arteries in areas of adhesive pericarditis, and in thrombus in the left atrium.

Calcification in the cardiac valves is evidence of significant valvular disease and image intensification may elucidate calcification in the aortic valve (Caird, 1976). Lateral radiographs may help identify areas of calcification, particularly in the presence of costal cartilage or tracheobronchial calcification.

There are no known age-related radiological changes in the pulmonary vasculature. Calcification of the pulmonary artery is usually secondary to longstanding pulmonary arterial hypertension or calcification of pulmonary thromboemboli (Schwarten, 1981).

The Electrocardiogram (ECG)

The ECG is a valuable aid to the investigation of cardiac disease in the old although many ECG abnormalities are common in the elderly (Campbell, Caird, and Jackson, 1974) and there is an increased incidence of abnormality with advancing age (Fisch, 1981). There is little evidence that ECG abnormalities are normal age-related variants in old age or that a different coding for normality should be defined.

The PR interval is said to increase with age (Harlan *et al.*, 1967; Simonson, 1972) but this has not been confirmed in studies in old age (Clark and Craven, 1981; Mihalick and Fisch, 1974).

Probable insignificant ECG findings in the elderly include left axis deviation without evidence of left anterior hemiblock, counter-clockwise rotation, minor degrees of clockwise rotation, and incomplete right bundle branch block. The significance of voltage changes of left ventricular hypertrophy without ST-T abnormality is not clear (Caird, Campbell, and Jackson, 1974). Significant changes include Q/QS patterns, ST-T patterns including T-wave flattening, left ventricular hypertrophy in association with ST/T changes, left bundle branch block, and right bundle branch block; these ECG abnormalities are associated with increased cardiovascular morbidity and mortality (Caird, Campbell, and Jackson, 1974).

The ECG is of great value in elucidating dysrhythmias and may be of assistance in the diagnosis of metabolic disorders including hypothyroidism and potassium and calcium imbalance.

Continuous telemetric ECG monitoring is helpful in diagnosing transient dysrhythmias in elderly patients with intermittent symptoms which may be associated with underlying cardiac disease or digoxin toxicity (Taylor, Kennedy, and Caird, 1974). Ambulatory telemetric ECG monitoring has been shown to be helpful in assessing drug therapy in elderly patients with chronic atrial fibrillation (Wang *et al.*, 1980).

The Echocardiogram (Echo)

Echocardiography is a useful non-invasive technique for analysing aspects of left ventricular function, for visualizing the anatomy of the aortic valve and aortic root and abnormalities of the mitral valve (Hess, Hallam, and Wann, 1981).

M-mode echocardiography is useful for measuring the ejection fraction and left ventricular systolic and diastolic volumes and cross-sectional or two-dimensional techniques produce real-time tomographic images of the heart and are useful in assessing left ventricular dyskinesia (Hess, Hallam, and Wann, 1981).

Echocardiographic studies in cardiovascular normal elderly subjects have shown that ageing in itself does not affect left ventricular cavity dimensions, fractional shortening, or the velocity of circumferential fibre shortening (Gerstenblith *et al.*, 1977) but there is an age-related thickening of the posterior wall of the left ventricle (Gerstenblith *et al.*, 1977; Sjögren, 1971) and increase in the aortic root diameter (Gardin *et al.*, 1977; Gerstenblith *et al.*, 1977) associated with reduced compliance of the left ventricle.

Although the echocardiogram may be useful in determining the site of the valvular abnormality in aortic valve disease, the M-mode technique cannot differentiate haemodynamically between severe aortic stenosis and aortic sclerosis (Hess, Hallam, and Wann, 1981), but this technique may be more sensitive in detecting mitral calcification than radiological methods and may be useful in detecting the presence of valvular vegetations (Hess, Hallam, and Wann, 1981).

The Phonocardiogram (PCG)

Studies of phonocardiography in the elderly have largely shown that the characteristics of the heart sounds are unaltered and commonly occurring systolic murmurs tend to be of the ejection type (Aravanis and Harris, 1958; Bethel and Crow, 1963; Bruns and Van der Hauwert, 1958; Davison and Friedman, 1968).

The main use of phonocardiography is in clarifying the nature of physical signs of uncertain clinical significance. The PCG can distinguish between a split first heart sound and loud fourth heart sound (Caird, 1976) and can assist in differentiating between aortic sclerosis and aortic stenosis with haemodynamic obstruction (Aravanis and Luisada, 1957). The opening snap of mitral stenosis and the different types of gallop rhythm can be identified.

The Apexcardiogram (ACG)

The ACG records the movement of the chest wall over the cardiac impulse and for a satisfactory recording a clearly palpable apex beat is necessary and the patient should be calm (Caird, Kennedy, and Kelly, 1973). Qualitative changes of left ventricular hypertrophy and dilatation can be displayed (Caird, 1976) and quantitative information about atrial and ventricular electromechanical intervals can be obtained (Caird, Kennedy, and Kelly, 1973). Simultaneous recordings of the ACG and the PCG are useful in the investigation of heart disease in the elderly (Caird, Kennedy, and Kelly, 1973).

Other Investigations

Systolic time intervals can be used to measure the stroke volume in the elderly (Caird, 1976). Impedance cardiography has been used to study the cardiac output in elderly subjects at rest (Luisada, Bhat, and Knighten, 1980; Williams and Caird, 1980) and during postural stress testing (Lennox and Williams, 1980; Thangarajah *et al.*, 1980).

Radionuclide methods involving peripheral venous injection and blood sampling and external praecordial counting have been employed to validate systolic time interval and impedance measurements of cardiac output

and ejection fraction (Latour, De la Fuente, and Caird, 1980; Williams and Caird, 1980).

More invasive investigations such as cardiac catheterization and angiocardiography are used only when cardiac surgical intervention is proposed, as, for example, in myocardial revascularization or valve replacement when an accurate assessment of the coronary circulation and left ventricular function is necessary.

DYSRHYTHMIAS

Cardiac Dysrhythmias

Cardiac dysrhythmias result from electrophysiological mechanisms of abnormal electrical impulse formation and or abnormal impulse conduction. Ambulatory ECG monitoring studies have shown a high incidence of transient cardiac dysrhythmias in elderly subjects (Clee *et al.*, 1979; Glasser, Clark, and Applebaum, 1979) with or without symptoms and particularly in patients with cardiac disease (Rodrigues Dos Santos and Lye, 1980).

Ageing myocardium is more vulnerable to biochemical insults which produce irritability, e.g. hypoxia or hypokalaemia. Age-related changes of reduced cardiac output and reduced coronary arterial blood flow may impair cardiac function, and cardiac dysrhythmias which might be relatively benign in young adults may precipitate cardiac failure and death in the elderly (Harris, 1970).

Therapy of dysrhythmias is aimed at termination of the abnormal rhythm which may herald electrical or haemodynamic hazards, longer term prophylaxis against recurrence, and the management of any associated diseases or underlying cardiac disorders.

Occasional atrial or ventricular ectopic beats are present in 40 per cent. of apparently healthy elderly people (Kennedy and Caird, 1972) and are of little clinical significance. Frequent ectopic activity is less common and may be due to cardiac disease, metabolic disorders, hypoxia or digoxin toxicity.

Supraventricular Dysrythmias

Sinus arrhythmia is common in old age (Harris, 1976) and may be phasic with an increased rate associated with inspiration.

Atrial dysrhythmias are common and increase in frequency with age (Harris, 1976). Sinus bradycardia with a heart rate of less than 60 per minute may be physiological or may be due to pathology of the sinoatrial node. Causes include raised intracranial pressure, hypothyroidism, obstructive jaundice, myocardial infarction, sinoatrial dysfunction (sick sinus syndrome), carotid sinus hypersensitivity, or the effects of drugs, e.g. digoxin or beta-blockers. Treatment of sinus bradycardia is required during acute myocardial infarction or when symptoms of reduced cardiac output are present. Precipitating causes must be removed or treated and atropine or isoprenaline may be required as a temporary measure. Long-term drug therapy is rarely effective and permanent cardiac pacemaking may be required.

Sinus tachycardia with heart rates over 100 beats per minute may be due to extracardiac causes, e.g. fever, infection, anxiety, pulmonary embolism, anaemia, hyperthyroidism, metabolic upsets, hypoxia, hypovolaemic states, and cardiac causes, e.g. acute myocardial infarction or heart failure. Occasionally sinus tachycardia is present in otherwise healthy subjects (Baurnfeind *et al.*, 1979). Treatment is usually confined to management of underlying causes.

Atrial fibrillation is the most frequent dysrhythmia, after multiple ectopic beats, observed in old age. Its presence may constitute an unfavourable prognostic feature in congestive cardiac failure, especially if hypertension is present (Bedford and Caird, 1960). Atrial fibrillation does not, however, carry the same serious significance as in the young in the absence of clinically demonstrable heart disease and is often coterminous with its precipitating cause. The prevalence of atrial fibrillation varies from 2 to 3 per cent. in healthy elderly subjects (Campbell, Caird, and Jackson, 1974) to 15 per cent. in hospitalized elderly patients (Bedford and Caird, 1960). The dysrhythmia may be temporary, paroxysmal, or chronic (Table 7) and the temporary form is often associated with acute illnesses like myocardial infarction, pulmonary embolism, or infections. Established atrial fibrillation is associated with varying combinations of pacemaker cell losses in the sinus node and fibrosis of the internodal atrial myocardium and chronic atrial dilatation may be accelerated by ischaemic, rheumatic, or

amyloid heart disease (Davies, 1976). Compared to younger populations rheumatic heart disease is an unlikely cause of atrial fibrillation in the elderly but this dysrhythmia in response to hyperthyroidism occurs almost exclusively in elderly subjects (Staffurth, Gibberd, and Hitton, 1965) and it may be the predominant clinical presentation of 'apathetic hyperthyroidism'.

Table 7   Causes of atrial fibrillation in the elderly

Temporary	Chronic
Infections	Ischaemic heart disease
Fever	Hypertension
Stress	Thyrotoxicosis
Acidosis	Amyloid
Hypoxia	Rheumatic heart disease
Hypokalaemia	Atrial septal defect
Myocardial infarction	Constrictive pericarditis
Pulmonary embolism	Pericardial malignant
Pericarditis	disease

Lone atrial fibrillation without evidence of heart disease is found mainly in elderly men, has no adverse effects on survival, and symptoms are uncommon (Evans and Swann, 1954).

Elderly patients with atrial fibrillation may be asymptomatic or may suffer from palpitation or breathlessness, confusion, syncope, or manifestations of peripheral arterial emboli. The irregular radial pulse may be associated with a pulse deficit, a single, jugular venous wave, or variable intensity of the first heart sound and the ECG is diagnostic. Congestive cardiac failure may occur.

In atrial fibrillation with a normal ventricular rate and no adverse haemodynamic consequences, no treatment is necessary. Fast ventricular rates require treatment and spontaneous reversion to sinus rhythm may occur if underlying causes are controlled (Table 7). Fast atrial fibrillation with or without cardiac failure requires urgent treatment (Anderson, 1976) and it is in patients with atrial fibrillation and congestive cardiac failure that the action of cardiac glycosides are seen to the best advantage (Opie, 1980). Digoxin reduces the ventricular rate and improves coronary circulation, myocardial oxygenation, and ventricular filling. There is an associated increase in the force and velocity of myocardial contraction with improved cardiac output. The aim is to maintain the heart rate between 60 and 80

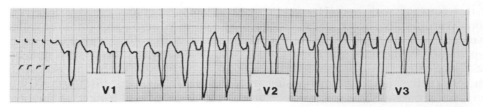

Figre 11   Chest leads V₁, V₂, and V₃ in the electrocardiogram of an 83 year old male with supraventricular tachycardia

beats per minute (for aspects of practical digitalization see the treatment of cardiac failure on page 000). Poor control of the ventricular rate may suggest underlying thyrotoxicosis or cardiac amyloid disease and the addition of a beta-adrenergic blocking agent, e.g. 40 to 160 mg of propranolol daily or 15 mg of pindolol. daily in divided doses may improve ventricular rate control (Wang *et al.*, 1980). Digitalization is preferable to electrical cardioversion in the elderly because the benefits of cardioversion on cardiac efficiency are not clear and the recurrence rate of atrial fibrillation is high (Rodstein, 1979). Most older patients tolerate controlled atrial fibrillation but cardioversion is indicated if cardiac failure or the ventricular rate cannot be controlled by medical measures or if recurrent peripheral emboli are a problem (Harris, 1976).

Atrial flutter has a similar aetiology to atrial fibrillation and is usually associated with underlying organic heart disease. Treatment is usually digitalization and the flutter rhythm may be converted to sinus rhythm or atrial fibrillation. Other useful drugs include beta-blocking agents, verapamil, disopyramide, quinidine, or procainamide.

Paroxysmal supraventricular tachycardia is due to paroxysmal atrial tachycardia or paroxysmal junctional tachycardia and these are difficult to differentiate by ECG (see Fig. 11). This dysrhythmia is usually associated in elderly subjects with ischaemic heart disease, digoxin toxicity, the Wolff–Parkinson–White syndrome, or malignant disease of the mediastinum or pericardium. Chronic supraventricular tachycardia is usually related to digoxin intoxication or malignant pericardial infiltration. Paroxysmal supraventricular tachycardia is less well tolerated in the elderly and more often precipitates heart failure or myocardial ischaemia (Heger, 1981). Treatment may include vagal stimulation using carotid sinus massage or the Valsalva manoeuvre. Digitalization may be required and other useful drugs include beta-blocking agents and disopyramide. Direct current cardioversion may be indicated if the dysrhythmia is life threatening. Maintenance therapy can be successfully achieved with digoxin, beta-blockade, or quinidine.

Paroxysmal atrial tachycardia with 2 : 1 or 3 : 1 atrioventricular block is usually due to digoxin toxicity but may occur in organic heart disease. If digoxin therapy is implicated, it should be withdrawn and potassium depletion should be slowly corrected. If further treatment is required, beta-blocking agents or phenytoin may be effective. When digoxin therapy is not the cause, digitalization is indicated in this dysrhythmia.

Multifocal atrial tachycardia usually occurs in elderly patients with clinical heart disease or severe chronic lung disease (Clark, 1977). Treatment of the underlying disorder is indicated and this may include correction of respiratory disorders, electrolyte imbalance, or metabolic disorders.

Sick sinus syndrome or sinoatrial disorder is common in the elderly (Harris, 1976) and occurs in two main forms either with predominant bradyarrhythmias or alternating tachycardia and bradycardia with long periods of asystole following termination of tachycardia. Sinoatrial disorder is associated with degenerative changes in the sinoatrial node which may prevent adequate impulse formation and often also with an abnormally unresponsive atrioventricular node and the pacing impulse may arise in the sinus node, atria, or atrioventricular node. There may be periods of arrest at a variety of supraventricular levels and clinical manifestations range from no symptoms to unexplained falls, bradycardia, atrial fibrillation with a slow ventricular response, or

Stokes–Adams attacks. The course of this disorder is largely unknown but it appears to be a relatively benign condition and permanent pacing is only necessary if symptoms are troublesome (Shaw, Holman, and Gowers, 1980).

Ventricular Dysrhythmias

Multiple ventricular ectopic beats may be precipitated by stress, smoking, or coffee drinking and are usually associated with organic heart disease in the elderly. Multiple or multifocal ectopic activity often herald the more serious dysrhythmias of ventricular tachycardia or ventricular fibrillation in acute myocardial infarction or digoxin toxicity and treatment is indicated in these circumstances. Immediate treatment with intravenous lignocaine, a bolus of 50 or 100 mg, followed by an infusion rate of 2 mg per minute, is often effective and largely free from side-effects, although excessive doses may produce confusion and aggravate hypotension and careful ECG monitoring is required. Mexiletine or procainamide may be used for lignocaine-resistant ventricular ectopic activity. Ventricular tachycardia, when it is producing disturbance of consciousness or cardiac failure, should be treated by synchronized shock and correction of metabolic acidosis. When ventricular tachycardia is recurrent, a number of agents can be used including phenytoin or disopyramide but the latter should be avoided if congestive cardiac failure or gross cardiomegaly is present as its profound negative inotropic effect may depress atrioventricular conduction, produce hypotension, and aggravate heart failure.

Primary ventricular fibrillation is a complication of acute myocardial infarction in 4 per cent. of the elderly treated in coronary care units (Chaturvedi *et al.*, 1972; Williams *et al.*, 1976). Treatment requires urgent unsynchronized electrical shock in full doses.

CONDUCTION DEFECTS

Cardiac conduction defects are common in the elderly population (Ostrander *et al.*, 1965; Kitchin, Lowther, and Milne, 1973; Cullen, Murphy, and Cumpston, 1974 and Campbell, Caird, and Jackson, 1974). Treatment is generally directed at the management of associated causes or if symptoms occur.

Sinoatrial block is an ECG diagnosis of complete absence of one cardiac cycle (Fig. 12). The significance of this abnormality in the elderly is not clear and no treatment is required.

Bundle Branch Block

Right bundle branch block is more common than left bundle branch block in old age (Campbell, Caird, and Jackson, 1974). The pathology of the bundle branch blocks appears to be related to a variety of factors including age-related mechanical wear and tear, hypertension, ischaemic heart disease, and ventricular hypertrophy (Davies, 1976).

Although right bundle branch block may be associated with ischaemic heart disease, pulmonary heart disease, atrial septal defect, and congenital anomalies of the conduction system, the conduction defect may be present with no obvious cause in old people. Coexisting left bundle branch abnormalities are present in about half of affected individuals (Campbell, Caird, and Jackson, 1974). The major clinical finding is of wide and often fixed splitting of the second heart sound and symptoms are unusual.

Left bundle branch block is usually associated with significant organic heart disease, e.g. ischaemic disease, aortic stenosis, or hyperten-

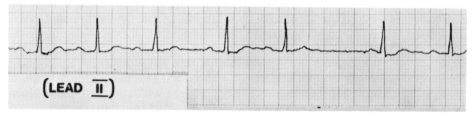

Figure 12   Asymptomatic first-degree heart block and sinoatrial block in an 80 year old male with Parkinsonism

sion. Clinical features include symptoms of the associated cardiac disorder and the auscultatory finding of reversed splitting of the second heart sound, more pronounced on expiration.

Left anterior hemiblock (Rosenbaum, Elizari, and Lazzari, 1970) describes block in the anterior division of the left bundle branch and is characterized by the ECG presence of left axis deviation of more than $-30°$ in the frontal plane. The significance of this conduction abnormality in old age is not clear but it is not associated with any apparent reduction in life expectancy (Caird, Campbell, and Jackson, 1974).

The bundle branch blocks are not, in themselves, associated with symptoms but they may progress to complete heart block and Stokes–Adams attacks necessitating transvenous artificial pacing.

Atrioventricular Block

This conduction defect is defined in three degrees or grades. First-degree or latent heart block is an ECG abnormality where the P – R interval is prolonged beyond the upper limit of normal, 0.22 second. This abnormality has been noted in 2 per cent. of ECGs of otherwise healthy old people (Campbell, Caird, and Jackson, 1974; Fisch *et al.*, 1957; Kennedy and Caird, 1972). Although this conduction defect may be associated with digoxin toxicity or acute myocardial infarction, in most cases the cause is unknown and its prognostic significance is doubtful (Rodstein, Brown, and Wolloch, 1968).

Second-degree heart block occurs as either Mobitz type I (Wenckebach) where the P – R interval progressively lengthens until a ventricular beat fails to occur or as Mobitz type II where the P – R interval remains constant but dropped beats occur periodically; if this is occasional then the pulse will be irregular but if the conduction occurs as 2 : 1 or 3 : 1 then a regular bradycardia will be clinically apparent. Coronary artery disease is the most likely cause in the elderly.

Third-degree or complete heart block occurs when there is no conduction between the atria and ventricles and each is controlled by its own pacemaker. Associated causes include ischaemic heart disease, chronic fibrosis of both bundle branches, cardiomyopathy, or calcific aortic or mitral valve disease (Davies, 1976).

In acute inferior myocardial infarction the atrioventricular node may be temporarily inhibited due to ischaemia or inflammatory oedema (Davies, 1971). The initial mortality may be 30 per cent. or more but most of the survivors revert to normal sinus rhythm within a few days. Atrioventricular block in anterior myocardial infarction is often associated with major damage to both bundle branches and widespread anteroseptal extension (Davies, 1976).

Symptoms in acute or chronic heart block are due to bradycardia (usually less than 40 beats per minute) and critical reduction in the cardiac output with poor cerebral perfusion or to ventricular asystole and less often ventricular tachycardia or fibrillation. Stokes–Adams attacks are characterized by transient syncopal episodes associated with ventricular asystole, bradycardias, or supraventricular or ventricular tachycardias. The clinical signs of complete heart block include regular bradycardia which is associated with cannon waves in the venous pulse, variable intensity of the first heart sound, and an ejection systolic murmur may be present.

The objectives of treatment of complete heart block or lesser degrees of block are to increase the ventricular rate to reduce the likelihood of Stokes–Adams attacks and prevent cardiac failure, and as prophylaxis against life-threatening ventricular dysrhythmias. In acute complete heart block an isoprenaline intravenous infusion may increase the ventricular rate in a dosage regimen of 0.02 to 0.10 μg/kg of body weight per minute. Continuous, supervised ECG monitoring is required as there are always dangers of precipitating ventricular fibrillation or hypotension which may be heralded by an increase in ventricular ectopic activity. The effect of oral isoprenaline (30 mg of saventrine, every 8 hours) in chronic states is unpredictable and often ineffective and in these circumstances a trial of transvenous endocardial pacemaking is indicated with implantation of a permanent pacemaker as necessary (Figs 13 and 14). Pacing the asymptomatic elderly patient with complete heart block is a difficult clinical problem. Expert cardiological advice should be sought and it is probably not necessary to advise permanent pacing if the

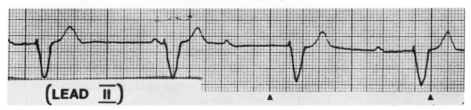

Figure 13   Lead II in the electrocardiogram of an 86 year old female with complete heart block and a permanent bipolar endocardial pacemaker

conduction defect is localized to the atrioventricular node and if the ventricular rate accelerates with atropine or exercise (Leading Article, 1979b). A common problem encountered is the elderly patient with chronic confusion and complete heart block. There is some evidence that chronic complete heart block can cause an ischaemic encephalopathy resulting in dementia and this may sometimes remit with the institution of permanent pacing (Sulg *et al.*, 1969). A trial of pacing is indicated but the trial must continue for at least 1 week to determine if permanent pacemaking is indicated (Stout, 1980).

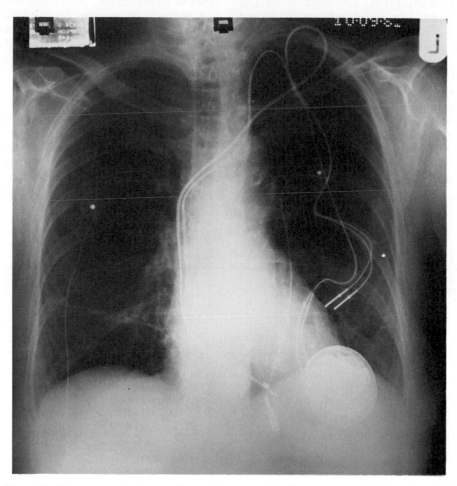

Figure 14   Posteroanterior chest radiograph demonstrating the permanent bipolar endocardial pacemaker

Once permanent pacing is established in elderly patients with complete heart block, the prognosis relates to the associated underlying heart disease (Ginks, Leatham, and Siddons, 1979).

HYPERTENSION

Hypertension, defined as a systolic blood pressure of 160 mmHg or more, a diastolic pessure of 95 mmHg or more, or both, is present in up to 60 per cent. of people over the age of 60 years (Anderson and Cowan, 1959; Stamler *et al.*, 1976). Systemic arterial blood pressure does not necessarily rise with age. In developed societies there is a tendency for most people's systolic pressures to rise with age and for diastolic pressure to remain stable (Anderson and Cowan, 1972), but there is no rise apparent in more primitive cultures (Page and Sidd, 1972).

Hypertension is an important risk factor for cardiovascular morbidity and mortality in males and females at any age (Kannel and Gordon, 1978; Koch-Weser, 1979). Isolated systolic hypertension carries a significant risk (Colandrea *et al.*, 1970; Gubner, 1962; Kannel *et al.*, 1981), especially over 180 mmHg (Shekelle, Ostfield, and Klawans, 1974), and is a better predictor of cardiovascular risk over the age of 60 years (Kannel, Gordon, and Schwartz, 1971).

Aetiology

Most elderly patients with high blood pressure are essential hypertensives. The cause of essential or primary hypertension remains elusive but all of these patients have an increased peripheral resistance (Kirkendall and Hammond, 1980) which may be related in some cases to altered baroreceptor functions. A small minority of patients will have secondary hypertension and most of these patients have chronic renal disease (Table 8). Renal artery stenosis may be unilateral or bilateral and is usually due to atheromatous disease. Hypothyroidism is associated with hypertension and systolic hypertension may occur in thyrotoxicosis. Endocrine rarities associated with hypertension are rare in old age and occasional cases of hypertension associated with coarctation of the aorta may be detected over the age of 60 years. Drug-induced hypertension may occur during therapy with sympathomimetic amines or anti-inflammatory preparations.

Clinical Features

The majority of elderly hypertensives are asymptomatic but a history suggestive of previous renal disease including urinary tract infection or haematuria may be elicited and iatrogenic causes for a raised blood pressure must be excluded. Endocrine causes may be

Table 8   Causes of hypertension

I Primary or essential		
II Secondary	Renal	Chronic pyelonephritis
		Chronic glomerulonephritis
		Collagen diseases
		Renal artery stenosis
		Polycystic disease
		Analgesic nephropathy
	Drug related	Sympathomimetic amines
		Steroids
		Phenylbutazone
		Indomethacin
		Tricyclic antidepressants
		Carbenoxolone
	Endocrine	Hypothyroidism
		Thyrotoxicosis
		Conn's syndrome
		Cushing's syndrome
		Phaeochromocytoma
	Coarctation of the aorta	

suggested if symptoms of polyuria and polydipsia or paroxysmal attacks of sweating and pallor associated with palpitation are present.

Marked blood pressure lability may occur in the elderly (Colandrea *et al.*, 1970) and casual measurements of blood pressure can be particularly unreliable. Three readings at separate visits should be taken after 5 minutes of quiet rest in the erect and supine positions to confirm the presence of hypertension. The blood pressure must be taken in both arms and peripheral pulses examined to exclude coarctation of the aorta. General physical examination must exclude endocrine disorders and abdominal examination may reveal an enlarged polycystic kidney. Auscultation of abdominal bruits are of little diagnostic help in the elderly. Signs of hypertensive end organ damage include left ventricular enlargement, cardiac failure, left ventricular failure, and retinal changes.

Malignant hypertension is rare (Kincaid-Smith, McMichael, and Murphy, 1958) but not unknown in the elderly and this disorder may or may not be associated with very high levels of blood pressure. Fundoscopy will show evidence of haemorrhages and soft exudates with or without papilloedema. Proteinuria is often present.

Special Investigations

Useful investigations of the elderly hypertensive patient include those of serum urea, electrolytes, and creatinine, thyroid function tests, blood sugar and serum uric acid tests. Chest radiograph and the electrocardiogram may show evidence of hypertensive heart damage like left ventricular hypertrophy with ST-T changes. Urinalysis will exclude proteinuria or evidence of infection. The likelihood of detecting a treatable cause of hypertension in the elderly patient is small and more specialized investigation is only justified if there is any clear evidence of a primary underlying cause. Intravenous urography and split renal function tests with renal arteriography and renin studies are indicated if renal artery stenosis is suspected, but only in patients who would otherwise be fit for surgical intervention. Intravenous urography might also be indicated if malignant hypertension was present or if the hypertension was resistant to a three-drug regimen.

Benefits of Antihypertensive Therapy

There is little available evidence that lowering the blood pressure in elderly hypertensives will necessarily confer any benefits. Controlled studies have shown a reduction in mortality in the very old (Priddle *et al.*, 1968) and in the 60 to 69 year old age group (Hypertension Detection and Follow-Up Program Cooperative Group, 1979) and a further study (Veterans Administration Co-operative Study Group, 1972) has suggested that antihypertensive therapy may have a beneficial effect in the elderly, particularly if a major vascular complication was apparent before the start of treatment. The benefits of antihypertensive therapy in elderly stroke patients are not clear (Carter, 1970; Hypertension–Stroke Cooperative Study Group, 1974).

The problem of isolated systolic hypertension in the elderly is a difficult one. The risks of systolic hypertension are established (Colandrea *et al.*, 1970; Gubner, 1962; Shekelle, Ostfield, and Klawans, 1974) and the condition is common (Anderson and Cowan, 1959), but as yet there is no evidence to support the use of antihypertensive treatment in elderly patients with a normal diastolic blood pressure level.

Adverse reactions to antihypertensive drugs have been reported as more common in the elderly (Williamson, 1979). Arterial baroreceptor sensitivity decreases with age (Gross, 1970) and the renal capacity to conserve sodium and water is impaired (Swales, 1979); these factors may result in a reduced capacity to modify circulatory control when antihypertensive stresses are introduced. Injudicious or excessive reduction of the blood pressure may have unfortunate results in the elderly (Jackson *et al.*, 1976) but a significant reduction of blood pressure may be achieved gently and gradually without major side-effects (Amery *et al*, 1978a; Priddle *et al*, 1968). Older hypertensives appear to successfully autoregulate the circulation to the vital organs if the blood pressure reduction is gradually reduced to normal levels (Koch-Weser, 1979).

Management

Clinical assessment of the elderly hypertensive should include consideration of other cardiovascular risk factors, e.g. cigarette smoking, alcohol intake, and the presence of diabetes mellitus, although these risk factors are probably of less importance than in younger patients (Kannel and Gordon, 1978). The elderly subject should be advised to reduce cigarette consumption, moderate alcohol intake, and avoid extra salt at meals. Dietary weight reduction might be indicated in obese patients.

Drug Treatment

Various levels of systolic and diastolic blood pressures have been proposed as acceptable maximum levels in the elderly (Table 9). Evidence of existing hypertensive end organ damage, especially left ventricular hypertrophy or cardiac failure, may influence the physician towards drug treatment, and relative contraindications include hypertensive vascular dementia (Caird, 1977), the presence of severe postural hypotension, and expected poor drug compliance.

Table 9   Recommended levels of blood pressure for antihypertensive treatment in the elderly

Reference	Systolic BP (mm)	Diastolic BP (mm)
Kennedy (1976)		>105
Chrysant, Frolich, and Papper (1976)		> 95
Caird (1977)	>180	>100
Simpson (1978)		>105
Moore-Smith (1980)	>180	>105
O'Malley and O'Brien (1980)	>160	>100
Bannan, Beevers, and Wright (1980)		>105
Radin and Black (1981)	>160	> 95

The adrenergic-neurone blocking agents guanethidine, bethanidine and debrisoquin should be avoided due to their tendency to produce troublesome postural hypotension and reserpine is contraindicated in elderly patients due to its tendency to produce depression.

When the decision to treat has been made, and taking due consideration of any other drug treatment already required for other medical problems, the first line of antihypertensive therapy should be a thiazide diuretic, a beta-adrenergic blocking agent, or a combination preparation of both agents.

Thiazide diuretics, e.g. 5 to 10 mg of bendrofluazide daily or 50 to 100 mg of hydrochlorothiazide daily, act by reducing the blood volume and have a peripheral vasodilating effect. A blood pressure reduction of 10 to 15 mmHg is usually obtained. Potassium supplements are often necessary as the elderly are more sensitive to the potassium-losing effect of thiazides as their dietary potassium intake is reduced and their capacity for renal conservation is impaired (Caird, 1977). The potassium imbalance problem may be ameliorated by using a thiazide combined with a potassium sparing agent, e.g. hydrochlorothiazide and amiloride (moduretic) (Kennedy and MacFarlane, 1972), hydrochlorothiazide and triamterene (dyazide) (Amery et al., 1978a), or hydroflumethiazide and spironolactone (aldactide). Side-effects include a tendency to reduced glucose tolerance (Amery et al., 1978b) and a rise in the serum uric acid, but secondary gout is rare. Susceptible patients with problems of mobility may develop nocturia and urinary incontinence. Provided that small doses are introduced gradually, postural hypotension should not be a problem and rare side-effects include photosensitivity, blood dyscrazias, and acute pancreatitis.

Beta-adrenergic blockers inhibit competitively the action of circulating catecholamines on beta-receptors but their actual hypotensive mechanism is not yet established (Watkins et al., 1980). The response of elderly patients to beta-blockers is reduced (Opie, 1980). Contraindications to therapy include frank heart failure or a history of bronchospasm or heart block. Several preparations are available and once-daily dosage is usually satisfactory to control the blood pressure and maintain patient compliance (Frick and Kala, 1980). A suitable treatment schedule would be 40 to 160 mg of propranolol daily or 100 to 300 mg of metoprolol daily. Side-effects are usually minor but the drug dosage may require reduction or withdrawal if problems of bronchospasm, vivid dreams, cardiac failure, cold extremities, or worsening intermittent claudication become apparent.

Adverse reactions to propranolol have been reported as occurring more frequently in the elderly, but not significantly so (Greenblatt and Koch-Weser, 1973), and their sensitivity to propranolol is decreased (Feely and Stevenson, 1979), but this may be offset in clinical management by an age-related increase in circulating plasma propranolol levels for fixed doses of the beta-blocker (Castleden and George, 1979).

A combination of a beta-blocker and a diuretic may have an additive or synergistic effect in lowering the blood pressure (Petrie *et al.*, 1975) and the rationale for combined beta-blockade and diuretic therapy is based on reducing the recumbent pressure without exaggeration of the postural blood pressure drop, retaining an adequate hypotensive effect while reducing adverse effects, utilizing the properties of one agent to overcome the unwanted action of the other, and improving patient compliance (Dollery, 1977). A fixed combination of 10 mg of pindolol and 5 mg of clopamide reduces the blood pressure in elderly hypertensives by an average of 34/20 mmHg without problems of bradycardia or postural hypotension (Cameron and Crowder, 1981).

Methyldopa acts by reducing the sympathetic output from the brain stem vasomotor centre and has a lesser effect on the peripheral sympathetic nerves resulting in reduction of the peripheral resistance. Side-effects are usually dose-related and drowsiness, postural hypotension, dry mouth, nasal congestion, and fluid retention are not problems when total daily doses of 250 mg to 2 g are added to diuretic therapy in the elderly (Amery *et al.*, 1978a). Methyldopa may be indicated in elderly hypertensives when beta-blockers or diuretics are contraindicated, e.g. obstructive airways disease, diabetes, or gout.

Most elderly hypertensives will achieve satisfactory blood pressure control with thiazides and/or beta-blockers but a minority may require a third-line additional drug. Hydrallazine acts by producing arteriolar dilatation and it may increase arterial compliance, distensibility, and in small doses may be of value in the treatment of isolated or predominant systolic hypertension (O'Malley and O'Brien, 1980). Side-effects of a lupus erythematosus like syndrome or acute rheumatoid state, reflex tachycardia, palpitation, fluid retention, facial flushing, headache, and nasal congestion are less likely if the total daily dose is kept between 10 and 200 mg in divided doses (Kirkendall and Hammond, 1980). There are as yet no clear recommendations for the use of other current antihypertensive drugs like prazosin, clonidine, labetalol, or minoxidil in elderly patients.

Postural Hypotension (See Chapter 16.14)

Postural blood pressure drop is known to be common in the elderly and its prevalence increases with age (Caird, Andrews, and Kennedy, 1973). Studies have shown postural blood pressure drop to be present in 11 to 24 per cent. of otherwise healthy elderly people and 10 to 17 per cent. of geriatric medical admissions who were able to stand on admission to hospital (Table 10).

Table 10   Prevalence of postural blood pressure drop in the elderly

Patients	Postural blood pressure drop (%)	Study
Otherwise healthy	11	Rodstein and Zeman (1957)
Elderly at home	24	Caird, Andrews, and Kennedy (1973)
Untreated elderly hypertensives	11	EWPHE
Geriatric unit admissions	17	Johnson *et al.* (1965)
Geriatric unit admissions	10	Lennox and Williams (1980)

Most elderly people tolerate postural blood pressure drop unless some other stress is introduced. Prolonged bed-rest will tend to produce some degree of cardiovascular deconditioning and difficulty in maintaining the blood pressure on standing. Other aggravating factors (Table 11) include hypovolaemia, acute myocardial infarction, anaemia, or biochemical upsets, and neurological disorders are common associations. Many drugs interfere with circulatory reflexes (Barraclough and Sharpey-Schafer, 1963) (Table 12) and together they constitute the commonest cause of symptomatic postural hypotension in the elderly (Lennox and Williams, 1980).

ISCHAEMIC HEART DISEASE

Angina Pectoris

Anginal pain is often less commanding in the elderly and this may be due to limited physical activity or an altered pain perception. Pain

Table 11　Factors predisposing to postural blood pressure drop in the elderly

Age	Hypovolaemia	Parkinsonism
Prolonged bed rest	Hyponatraemia	Cerebrovascular disease
Varicose veins	Hypokalaemia	Spinal cord lesions
Alcohol abuse	Anaemia	Polyneuropathy
Drugs	Infections	Tabes dorsalis
	Myocardial infarction	Idiopathic orthostatic hypotension
	Diabetes mellitus	

Table 12　Drugs associated with postural hypotension

Phenothiazines	Diuretics
Barbiturates	Antihypertensives
Benzodiazepines	Levodopa
Butyrophenones	Antihistamines
Monoamine oxidase inhibitors	
Tricyclic antidepressants	

may be associated with breathlessness and cessation of exercise and may result in undue fatigue. The pain is usually effort-induced but can occur at rest or in bed. Radiation may occur to the arms, neck, back, or jaw and angina may present as headache or as epigastric pain relieved by antacids. Physical signs may be absent but clinical features of left ventricular dysfunction, hypothyroidism, anaemia, or aortic valve disease may be present. Investigation should include full blood count, thyroid function tests, electrocardiogram, and chest radiograph.

Management should include advice about weight reduction, tobacco avoidance, and appropriate regular exercise, always avoiding sudden exertion or isometric strain. The drug of choice is 0.5 mg of glyceryl trinitrate. This is a vasodilator but probably acts by reducing cardiac work. Tablets can be chewed and allowed to lie in the buccal mucosa until the pain is relieved and then swallowed, but they are most effective if taken prophylactically. Tolerance to headache and facial flushing usually occurs and long-acting or slow-release preparations are available (5 mg of isosorbide dinitrate). However, excessive use of glyceryl trinitrate is a potential cause of postural hypotension.

Failure of pain control with nitrates is an indication for beta-adrenergic blockade which acts by reduction of the sympathetic drive and myocardial oxygen consumption. Propranolol may be administered orally in divided dosage in a total of 40 to 480 mg each day but relative contraindications include bradycardia or atrioventricular conduction disorders and evidence of significant left ventricular dysfunction.

Nifedipine, a vasodilator and calcium antagonist, shows promise in the treatment of intractable angina in the elderly (Rothbaum, 1981), especially if beta-blocking agents are contraindicated. This compound is administered orally in doses of 10 mg thrice daily and side-effects include headache, dizziness, tremor, gastrointestinal upset, and skin flushing. Oral verapamil is another therapeutic option but it must be used with caution in the presence of conducting system disease. Perhexiline maleate may be used in patients with intractable angina but this drug's use is limited by its tendency to produce liver function upset and peripheral neuropathy.

Aortocoronary bypass surgery may offer dramatic relief of symptoms in elderly patients with intractable angina pectoris. Advanced age should not exclude a patient from consideration for myocardial revascularization procedures (Ashor et al., 1973; Gann et al., 1977; Hamby et al., 1973). Symptomatic benefit occurs in 70 to 96 per cent. of older patients with angina which is resistant to medical measures (Gann et al., 1977; Tucker et al., 1977). Operative mortality is higher in the elderly (Jolly, Isch and Shumacker, 1981; Tucker et al., 1977) (Table 13) and post-operative complications are more common. Mortality rates in the elderly are, however, reducing due to earlier surgical intervention before left ventricular damage becomes severe and to improved surgical techniques (Ashor et al., 1973; Berman et al., 1980; Meyer et al., 1975). Survival rates for those elderly patients who leave hospital approximate to survival rates for the general population of the same age (Stephenson, MacVaugh, and Edmunds, 1978). The main prognostic factors for surgical success are related to the adequacy of left ventricular function and the

Table 13   Coronary artery bypass grafting for intractable angina pectoris. Mortality in the elderly

Reference	Age of patients (years)	Numbers of patients	Operative mortality (%)	Late mortality (%)
Ashor et al. (1973)	≥65	78	3	4
Barnhorst et al. (1974)	>65	27	0	3.7
Meyer et al. (1975)	≥70	24	12.6	
Tucker et al. (1977)	>70	67	4.5	6
Gann et al. (1977)	>70	30	6.7	
Stephenson, MacVaugh, and Edmunds (1978)	≥70	25	0	
Berman et al. (1980)	>70	17	17.6%	0
Jolly, Isch, and Shumacker (1981)	>70	71	12.6%	

suitability of the distal coronary arterial tree for venous bypass grafting (Jolly, Isch, and Shumacker, 1981).

ACUTE MYOCARDIAL INFARCTION

The presenting clinical features of acute myocardial infarction may be very variable in elderly patients. Painless infarction is common (Pathy, 1967; Rodstein, 1956) although chest pain is the commanding feature in elderly patients admitted to coronary care units (Williams et al., 1976). Breathlessness and acute confusion are common symptoms (Pathy, 1967) and other major presentations may include sudden death, syncope, stroke (Chin, Kaminski, and Rout, 1977), or giddiness. Less common symptoms include palpitation, vomiting, or sweating. Acute myocardial infarction should be suspected in any elderly person who has a sudden unexplained behavioural change, poor cerebral perfusion or unexplained abdominal pain or hypotension.

The diagnosis may be based on the history and physical examination in the extremely ill patient. The patient may be cold and sweating with a mild pyrexia. The pulse may be normal or there may be a tachycardia or bradycardia and the blood pressure may be raised initially and fall over the first few days. The minority of elderly patients are shocked. The apex beat may be displaced outwards reflecting left ventricular enlargement and an abnormal systolic pulsation at the left sternal border may be due to paradoxical protrusion of the infarcted anterior wall of the left ventricle. The heart sounds may be normal or quiet and a fourth, atrial heart sound may be detected. A transient pericardial friction rub may be heard on the second or third day and a soft pansystolic mitral murmur is often present due to papillary muscle dysfunction or left ventricular dilatation.

The diagnosis is most usefully confirmed by standard 12-lead electrocardiograms taken serially over 3 days, and cardiac enzyme studies may clarify doubtful ECG changes.

Complications

The majority of elderly patients with acute myocardial infarction have dysrhythmias or conduction abnormalities but only a minority of these are of clinical significance.

Severity of myocardial infarction increases with age (Semple and Williams, 1976) and the complications of conduction defects and atrial fibrillation or flutter are more common in older patients as are the shock picture, pulmonary oedema, and congestive cardiac failure, all recognized strong determinants of severity and mortality (Table 14).

Management

Most deaths probably occur before admission to hospital. The majority of elderly survivors with uncomplicated acute myocardial infarction are probably best managed at home (Colling et al., 1976; Hill, Hampton, and Mitchell, 1978; Mather et al., 1976) but hospital admission is indicated if the patient continues to have symptomatic bradycardia, an unstable cardiac state after three hours, heart failure, hypotension, or has been resuscitated from a cardiac arrest. Social factors are important; the patient may prefer to stay at home or the home circumstances may be unsuitable for domiciliary medical and nursing care.

Adequate, rapid pain relief is important to

Table 14   Complications of acute myocardial infarction in a coronary care unit. (Adapted from Semple and Williams, 1976)

Complication	Age (years)		
	<60 (%)	60–70 (%)	≥70 (%)
Heart block and conduction defects	20.0	22.2	34.6
Atrial fibrillation or flutter	5.3	11.6	14.4
Ventricular fibrillation	5.3	5.8	3.8
Shock picture	13.8	15.3	25.0
Pulmonary oedema	47.1	59.2	74.0
Congestive cardiac failure	6.2	11.1	22.1
Pericarditis	10.5	10.6	8.7

achieve and 5 to 10 mg of morphine or 2.5 to 5 mg diamorphine should be given intravenously. A proportion of elderly individuals may, however, have an emetic or a vagal response and opiate toxicity may occur with larger or repeated doses (Caradoc–Davies, 1981). In the anxious patient, general sedation may be achieved with 10 mg of oral chlordiazepoxide or 2 to 5 mg of diazepam which have a satisfactory anxiolytic action without an excessive hypnotic effect in the short term.

Bed-rest is required for a few days only and in mild, uncomplicated cases the patient should normally be up and walking by the end of the first week. There is little merit in complete bed-rest for the very old and they can be managed, from the onset of the attack, in a suitable chair. Prolonged bed-rest will promote constipation, venous thrombosis, hypostatic pneumonia, and impairment of the normal physiological regulating mechanisms with cardiovascular deconditioning and postural hypotension.

Routine anticoagulant therapy does not influence early mortality in myocardial infarction but it may protect against thromboembolism. Short-term parenteral heparin therapy should be given to high-risk elderly patients after severe infarction, in prolonged bed-rest, with obesity, or where a previous history of venous disease is elicited (Mitchell, 1981). Heparin can be administered in full doses of 40,000 units in continuous infusion in 24 hours or in a low-dose subcutaneous regimen of 5,000 units every 8 hours (Belch et al., 1981). Anticoagulant regimens can be stopped when the patient is fully ambulant and contraindications to therapy include active ulceration of the gastrointestinal tract, severe renal or hepatic disease, anaemia, pericarditis, acute stroke, or significant systemic hypertension.

Bladder care may be a particular problem in the male. The use of potent diuretics, atropine, and enforced bed-rest may promote urinary retention. The risks of constipation and faecal impaction can be reduced by the use of a daily oral laxative of the stool-softening and lubricant type. Diet should be in a soft digestible form and assistance in feeding should be discouraged in all but the most disabled.

Treatment of Complications
(See the Treatment of Dysrhythmias and Conduction Defects, pages 472 to 478).

The special aims of the coronary care unit are to reduce mortality by the rapid treatment of complications and to minimize resultant cardiovascular disability in the survivors.

Sinus tachycardia and bradycardia are common and are often reversed by analgesia. Significant ventricular ectopic activity may be prevented with lignocaine or disopyramide and supraventricular dysrhythmias respond to digoxin. Heart failure can be controlled by loop diuretics, vasodilators, and digoxin in appropriate circumstances. Cardiac arrest in primary ventricular fibrillation responds as well in the elderly as in younger patients to immediate unsynchronized electrical shock in full doses (400 J) (Chaturvedi et al., 1972; Linn and Yurt, 1970; Williams et al., 1976).

The main indication for transvenous cardiac pacing is ventricular bradycardia that does not respond to atropine or isoprenaline. Cardiogenic shock and cardiac failure are more common in the elderly (Table 14) and pump failure still eludes a successful method of management in most infarct patients and remains the major cause of death in the coronary unit.

Rehabilitation

The aim of rehabilitation in the elderly coronary patient is to return him to the activities normal for his age and avoid unnecessary invalidism. Efficient medical care in the early stages of the illness is unfortunately rarely matched by adequate attention to the social and emotional aspects of the illness. The elderly patient and his relatives are often unduly pessimistic about recovery chances. Older infarct patients have an increased tendency to continuing disability, especially anxiety, depression, dyspnoea, and fatigue leading to reduced exercise tolerance (Peach and Pathy, 1979). Sudden physical or mental stress situations should be avoided but graded walking exercises will improve physical fitness and counteract angina and depressive symptoms.

Secondary Prevention

The prophylactic benefits of long-term oral anticoagulant therapy after acute myocardial infarction are not entirely clear (International Anticoagulant Review Group, 1970) but in one study a reduced reinfarction rate and mortality rate was noted over a 2-year period in selected elderly patients with good anticoagulant control (Sixty Plus Reinfarction Study Research Group, 1980).

The role of beta-adrenergic blockers as long-term prophylactics in elderly infarct patients is not yet clear. In one study of alprenolol there was no apparent reduction in mortality after myocardial infarction in patients over 65 years of age (Anderson *et al.*, 1979) but in a more recent study using 10 mg of timolol twice daily there was a noted reduction in mortality and the reinfarction rate in men up to the age of 75 years (Norwegian Multicenter Study Group, 1981).

There is no clear evidence that aspirin in conventional or lower dosage can reduce mortality after myocardial infarction (Mitchell, 1980) and as yet there are no firm recommendations for the use of aspirin or similar platelet antiaggregant agents as secondary prevention measures in the survivors of acute myocardial infarction (International Society and Federation of Cardiology, 1981).

Prognosis

Age is a major adverse prognostic factor in acute myocardial infarction (Marchionni *et al.*, 1981; Norris *et al*, 1969; Williams *et al.*, 1976). Mortality increases with age but is not sex related (Norris *et al.*, 1969; Peel *et al.*, 1962) (Table 15).

Table 15 Hospital mortality in acute myocardial infarction. (From Semple and Williams, 1976)

	Age in years		
	<60	*60–70*	*⩾70*
CCU mortality (%)	9.5	15.3	26
Total hospital mortality (%)	15.2	19	37.5

The elderly benefit as much as their younger counterparts from admission to coronary care units (Chaturvedi *et al.*, 1972; Williams *et al.*, 1976) and haemodynamic monitoring in the coronary care unit has led to a significant reduction in mortality (Marchionni *et al.*, 1981). Adverse prognostic factors relate to poor left ventricular performance and the fact that the elderly are more liable to cardiovascular complications related to respiratory problems, renal failure, or other metabolic upsets (Marchionni *et al.*, 1981).

The long-term survival of elderly infarct patients is better relative to their natural expected mortality than younger patients (Biörck, Sievers, and Blomqvist, 1958; Librach *et al.*, 1976). In elderly patients who survive the first 3 months after an acute myocardial infarct, the expected survival at 3 years is 71 per cent. (Pathy and Peach, 1981).

VALVULAR DISEASE

Rheumatic Fever and Rheumatic Heart Disease

The incidence of rheumatic fever is declining (Sievers and Hall, 1971) and it is characteristically a disorder of children and young adults. Uncommon in the elderly, acute rheumatic fever may be recurrent and is often characterized by a protracted course, slight fever, and a low incidence of cardiac damage (Kjörstad, 1957). It is usually a recurrence of the disease in patients with known rheumatic heart disease. Acute rheumatic fever should be considered as the diagnosis in older patients with tachycardia, unexplained pyrexia, arthralgia, and a poor response to digoxin if atrial fibrillation is present (Harris, 1970).

Classical clinical signs may be absent and the course of the disease resembles that of younger patients with a good response to salicylates. Joint lesions may be more persistent and disabling in the elderly (Harris, 1970).

The prevalence of rheumatic heart disease in the general elderly population is 2 to 3 per cent. and 4 per cent. in elderly hospital patients (Bedford and Caird, 1960; Droller and Pemberton, 1953; Kennedy, Andrews, and Caird, 1977; Pomerance, 1976). Rheumatic heart disease is usually acquired before the third decade but related clinical problems predominate, later, in middle age. Mild or moderate chronic rheumatic heart disease in old age is usually associated with minimal valvular lesions, breathlessness, and cyanosis. Coexisting ischaemic heart disease, hypertensive disease, and the development of atrial fibrillation tend to aggravate the rheumatic condition and cardiac failure may result. The mitral valve is most often involved, the aortic valve next, and other valves are rarely affected.

Mitral Valve Disease

Mitral Stenosis

More than half of those elderly patients with rheumatic heart disease have no history of rheumatic markers in early life (Bedford and Caird, 1960). The dominant lesion is mitral stenosis and half have evidence of aortic valve involvement (Bedford and Caird, 1960). Clinical features become apparent when the left atrial pressure rises sufficiently to produce pulmonary venous congestion. Breathlessness on exertion may be associated with attacks of haemoptysis, winter bronchitis, and paroxysmal nocturnal dyspnoea.

Clinical signs may include peripheral cyanosis or a malar flush and atrial fibrillation is present in a third of elderly patients seen in

hospital (Bedford and Caird, 1960). The pulse is usually of small volume and the apex beat is of a tapping character due to a palpable first heart sound. Diastolic and/or presystolic thrills may be present. On auscultation the first heart sound may be loud but the second heart sound is usually normal unless pulmonary hypertension is present. The opening snap may be difficult to detect due to a tendency to stiffness and calcification of the valve cusps in old age. The classical auscultatory finding is a rumbling diastolic murmur which is maximal in intensity just internal to the apex and which is often very localized. Presystolic accentuation of the murmur may be heard in patients in sinus rhythm.

The electrocardiogram shows evidence of left atrial hypertrophy and P mitrale, in sinus rhythm, and right ventricular hypertrophy if pulmonary hypertension coexists. Chest radiograph signs include left atrial enlargement (see Fig. 15), which may be best demonstrated by displacement of the barium-filled oesophagus, and in pulmonary hypertension the right ventricle is enlarged and the main pulmonary artery is dilated. Calcification may be detected in the mitral valve and the left ventricle and aorta appear to be small.

The M mode echocardiogram (Figs 16 and 17) permits assessment of the thickness of the mitral leaflets and the degree of left atrial enlargement. Two-dimensional echocardiography can give a quantification of the degree of mitral valve stenosis (Martin *et al.*, 1979).

Complications of mitral stenosis include atrial fibrillation, in most cases at some time, pulmonary hypertension, pulmonary infarction, attacks of winter bronchitis, and systemic embolization which tends to occur at the onset of atrial fibrillation or at the time of rhythm changes. Left heart failure and congestive cardiac failure may occur. Infective endocarditis is a rare complication of pure mitral stenosis. The prognosis depends on the severity of the lesion, the development of pulmonary hypertension and atrial dysrhythmias, the presence of other valve defects and other forms of heart disease, and the development of cardiac failure.

Mitral Regurgitation

Rheumatic mitral regurgitation is not usually

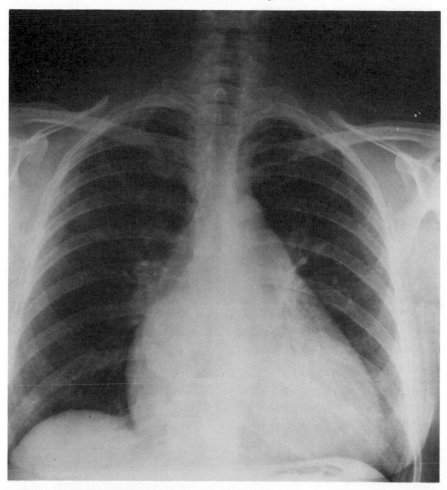

Figure 15 Posteroanterior chest radiograph showing evidence of mitral stenosis (note the double shadow at the right heart border due to left atrial enlargement) in a 73 year old female with rheumatic mitral valve disease

associated with symptoms unless heart failure or other complications supervene. Atrial fibrillation, systemic embolization, winter bronchitis, and haemoptysis may occur, although less often than in pure mitral stenosis. Infective endocarditis is especially common even if the valve lesion is trivial. The arterial pulse is usually small and may have a slightly collapsing character. Atrial fibrillation may be present and left ventricular enlargement may be detected. A systolic thrill may be palpated in severe cases. On auscultation, the first heart sound is usually normal or diminished in intensity. The classical finding is of a loud or soft pansystolic blowing murmur, best heard at the apex; this may radiate to the axilla or the left sternal border. A loud third heart sound and even a short mid-diastolic murmur may be heard due to rapid ventricular filling in severe cases.

The electrocardiogram shows evidence of left ventricular hypertrophy and the P mitrale pattern may be present in sinus rhythm. Chest radiograph shows evidence of left atrial and left ventricular enlargement.

Anticoagulants in Rheumatic Mitral Valve Disease

There is an age-related increased risk of systemic embolization in rheumatic mitral valve disease (Coulshed *et al.*, 1970) and the single most important risk factor for embolism is

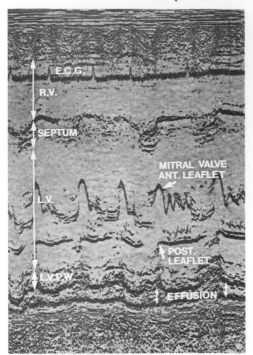

Figure 16   M mode echocardiogram in a 78 year old male with atrial flutter, pericardial effusion, and relatively normal mitral valve. (R.V., right ventricular cavity; septum, inter-ventricular septum; L.V., left ventricular cavity; L.V. P.W., posterior wall of left ventricle). (By permission of Dr M.Been, Stobhill Hospital, Glasgow)

atrial fibrillation (Coulshed *et al.*, 1970; Fleming and Bailey, 1971), although embolism can occur in sinus rhythm with no evidence of atrial dysrhythmias. There is a strong case for long term oral anticoagulation in all patients with more than minimal mitral stenosis, regardless of the cardiac rhythm (Fleming and Bailey, 1971), but the increased risk of bleeding complications in patients over 65 years tends to produce a greater reluctance of physicians to maintain elderly patients on long-term oral anticoagulants (Malcolm, 1980) and there are no clear recommendations for their use.

Other Forms of Mitral Regurgitation

Mitral annulus calcification. This is usually asymptomatic and a radiological diagnosis, the intracardiac calcification best seen in the lateral chest radiograph. More common in elderly women (Osterberger *et al.*, 1981; Simon and Liu, 1954), this non-inflammatory calcification can produce severe haemodynamic abnormalities of the mitral valve (Korn, De Sanctis, and Sell, 1962). Varying degrees of mitral regurgitation may result. Calcified masses may rarely produce obstruction of the valve and functional mitral stenosis may occur due to

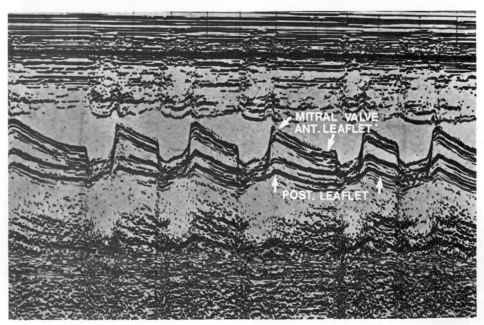

Figure 17   M mode echocardiogram in an 85 year old female with calcified mitral stenosis. (By permission of Dr M. Been, Stobhill Hospital, Glasgow)

severe ring calcification interfering with normal diastolic relaxation (Osterberger *et al.*, 1981).

Mitral cusp mucoid degeneration. This is often asymptomatic but clinical features may include chest pain, palpitation, or syncope, and congestive cardiac failure or infective endocarditis may occur (Tresch *et al.*, 1979). Systolic prolapse of the valve may be associated with a midsystolic click and/or a late systolic murmur heard at the apex and the left sternal border. Regurgitation is usually mild and there are no diagnostic changes in the electrocardiogram or chest radiograph (Tresch *et al.*, 1979). Mitral valve prolapse can be confirmed by echocardiography but as yet the natural history and prognosis of this condition are not clear.

Papillary muscle dysfunction. This occurs in ischaemic heart disease, usually after acute myocardial infarction, but it can occur secondary to reversible ischaemia (Goodwin, 1968). Mild mitral regurgitation usually results but severe acute regurgitation may occur if one of the heads of a papillary muscle ruptures. Papillary muscle dysfunction should be suspected in the elderly coronary patient who develops a late or pansystolic murmur during or after recovery from acute infarction.

Ruptured chordae tendinae. This may occur as a primary disorder of unknown aetiology in the elderly (Selzer *et al.*, 1967). Usually the presentation is of severe mitral regurgitation and acute pulmonary oedema in association with a normal electrocardiogram. Echocardiography is helpful and may demonstrate abnormal valve movement. Secondary forms occur in preexisting abnormalities of the mitral valve mechanisms like mitral valve prolapse, infective endocarditis, or rheumatic heart disease.

Left atrial myxoma. This is an unusual diagnosis in old age (Goodwin, 1963), but it should be suspected if rapidly developing features of mitral valve obstruction are associated with syncope, variable mitral systolic and diastolic murmurs, systemic emboli, and a raised ESR. Diagnosis can be confirmed with two-dimensional echocardiography (Perry *et al.*, 1981). Management includes angiocardiography and

cardiac surgical intervention in elderly subjects who are otherwise good operative risks.

Mitral regurgitation may also occur due to dilatation of the valve ring, without disease of the cusps, in left ventricular failure, most often in severe hypertensive heart disease (Leonard, 1979). This form of functional mitral incompetence is usually reversible with treatment of the underlying cause.

Surgery of the Mitral Valve

Mitral valve surgery is indicated in selected elderly cardiac patients when medical management does not produce satisfactory control of symptoms of the valve lesion or of associated cardiac failure. Open mitral valvotomy is rarely attempted in elderly patients due to calcific disease of the valve mechanisms, but mitral valve replacement has become safer in recent years (Jolly *et al*, 1981). Operative mortality is now 9–17 per cent. (Canepa-Anson and Emanuel, 1979; Jolly, Isch, and Shumacker, 1981; Quinlan, Cohn and Collins, 1975), although emergency surgery increases the risk of mortality (Table 16). Most deaths are due to cardiac failure. The elderly tolerate mitral valve replacement less well in cases of mitral regurgitation than in mitral stenosis (Stephenson, MacVaugh, and Edmunds, 1978).

Table 16 Operative mortality in mitral valve replacement 1977–1979. (From Jolly, Isch, and Shumacker, 1981)

Age (years)	Number of patients	Mortality (%)
All ages	124	4.7
65–70	13	15.0
70+	12	17.0

Aortic Valve Disease

Left ventricular outflow obstruction may be supravalvar, valvar, or subvalvar. Aortic valve stenosis may be congenital when the valve is usually bicuspid or unicuspid, and fibrosis and calcification produce outflow obstruction, or acquired due to postinflammatory commissural adhesion and fibrous thickening or heavy calcific deposition and rigidity (Pomerance, 1976). A minority of cases in old age are due to rheumatic heart disease and in these patients mitral valve disease usually coexists; aortic stenosis occurs in about 4 per cent. of old people (Bedford and Caird, 1960; Kennedy, Andrews, and Caird, 1977; Pomerance, 1976) and is more frequent in men under the age of 80 years and women over the age of 80. All forms of aortic stenosis are similar clinically.

The patient may be asymptomatic or present with dyspnoea, angina, or exertional syncope which is later in the natural history of the disorder and indicates more severe outflow obstruction. Left ventricular failure and congestive cardiac failure are late complications and sudden death may occur even in a symptom free patient with a normal electrocardiogram. Clinical signs include a small volume, slow rising pulse, low pulse pressure, and left ventricular hypertrophy. A systolic thrill may be palpable at the base. A loud, harsh, ejection systolic murmur is usually best heard at the second right interspace and can radiate to the apex, left sternal border, and neck vessels. The second heart sound may be quiet and reversed splitting may occur. In more than half of patients with aortic stenosis a soft diastolic murmur may be heard and an ejection click may precede the systolic murmur. In subvalvar obstruction the ejection click is absent and there is usually no calcification of the aortic valve. The main diagnostic difficulty is in differentiating aortic sclerosis from aortic stenosis, but in the latter the murmur is louder and is associated with left ventricular hypertrophy and reversed splitting of the second heart sound.

The electrocardiogram shows evidence of left ventricular hypertrophy with ST and T changes. Chest radiographs show signs of left ventricular enlargement, especially if aortic regurgitation or left ventricular failure are present. In systolic murmurs which are difficult to elucidate in the elderly, phonocardiography and carotid systolic time interval tracings are helpful in excluding severe aortic stenosis (Flohr, Weir, and Chesler, 1981).

Idiopathic Hypertrophic Subaortic Stenosis (IHSS)

This form of subvalvar obstructive hypertrophic cardiomyopathy occurs when there is generalized left ventricular hypertrophy and disproportionate septal hypertrophy (Goodwin, 1970). Malaligned papillary muscles produce traction on the anterior mitral leaflet which is pulled against the hypertrophied septum in midsystole, resulting in dynamic obstruction to the left ventricular outflow tract. This condition is more common in the elderly than was previously thought (Berger, Rethy, and Goldberg, 1979; Davies, Pomerance, and Teare, 1974; Petrin and Tavel, 1979). Patients usually have no relevant family history, females predominate, and there is an association with hypertension (Petrin and Tavel, 1979). Symptoms may be absent but the clinical presentation may include angina and dyspnoea on exertion; syncope is uncommon. Most patients with IHSS at diagnosis have had murmurs for less than five years. The classical sign is of a loud systolic murmur loudest along the lower left sternal border or at the apex. Left ventricular enlargement is usually present and a loud fourth heart sound may be heard. The diagnosis is confirmed by phonocardiography (Tavel, 1968) and/or echocardiography (Berger, Rethy, and Goldberg, 1979).

Diagnosis of IHSS should be considered in elderly hypertensive females who develop a late-onset systolic murmur. The importance of an accurate diagnosis lies in the fact that marked symptomatic improvement can be gained with propranolol (Berger, Rethy, and Goldberg, 1979) and digoxin, nitroglycerin, and the excessive use of diuretics may be harmful. Surgery may be indicated if medical treatment fails to produce a satisfactory response in the elderly (Kafetz, 1981; Koch *et al.*, 1980).

Aortic Regurgitation

Aortic valve incompetence and regurgitation may rarely occur acutely in the elderly as a result of aortic dissection or due to valve perforation as a complication of infective endocarditis. Chronic regurgitation is commonly due to calcific disease of the valve mechanism and less common causes include deformity of the cusps due to congenital or rheumatic heart disease or postendocarditis or dilatation of the valve ring due to syphilis or ankylosing spondylitis.

Isolated aortic incompetence in the elderly is of unknown aetiology (Bedford and Caird, 1960) and is related to dilatation of the aorta with increased aortic ring circumference and no major abnormality of the aortic valve. This valve disorder is present in about 1 per cent.

of the elderly population (Kennedy, Andrews, and Caird, 1977; Pomerance, 1976) but is usually asymptomatic, the pulse and pulse pressure are normal, and clinical evidence of left ventricular enlargement is rarely present. The prognosis is good and cardiac failure is not a common complication.

Aortic regurgitation acquired in early life is compatible with survival into old age. Symptoms include reduced exercise tolerance and breathlessness, angina, and palpitations. Cardiac failure may occur. In syphilitic aortitis the patient is usually an elderly male without a past history of syphilis but clinical or laboratory evidence of neurosyphilis is often present (Bedford and Caird, 1960). Physical signs of aortic regurgitation include a high pitched early diastolic murmur, best heard along the middle or lower left sternal border. An ejection systolic murmur may be present without underlying aortic stenosis. Severe cases may have a collapsing pulse, increased pulse pressure, and prominent pulsation of the carotid arteries. The electrocardiogram shows evidence of left ventricular hypertrophy and the chest radiograph and echocardiogram shows early enlargement of the left ventricular and atrial cavities. In syphilitic aortitis, irregular dilatation of the aorta may be associated with aneurysm formation and calcification of the ascending aorta.

Surgery of the Aortic Valve

Surgical treatment of aortic stenosis is very effective and it may improve the quality of life and improve the survival of selected elderly patients whose symptoms are troublesome. Operative mortality for aortic valve replacement in patients over 65 years of age is of the order of 2.5 to 18 per cent. (Table 17); how-ever, emergency surgery greatly increases operative deaths (Canepa-Anson and Emanuel, 1979; Quinlan, Cohn, and Collins, 1975) and elderly patients tend to come late to surgery, at a time when the severity of their lesion adversely affects surgical risk. Postoperative complications of atrial dysrhythmias and respiratory problems are more common in the elderly and death is most often due to heart failure. Late survival can be very good, how-ever, and in one study 86 per cent. of operative survivors after valve replacement for aortic stenosis were alive at a mean follow-up period of 43.5 months (Canepa-Anson and Emanuel, 1979). The indications for aortic valve surgery in the elderly are the same as in any other age group (De Bono, English, and Milstein, 1978).

Tricuspid Valve Disease

Tricuspid stenosis is uncommon in old age and is usually part of multiple valve defects in rheumatic heart disease (Bedford and Caird, 1960) or rarely carcinoid disease. The diagnosis rests on evidence of marked elevation of the venous pressure with hepatomegaly and no evidence of cardiac failure. Electrocardiographic evidence includes tall peaked P waves of right atrial hypertrophy in patients in sinus rhythm and right atrial enlargement may be noted on the chest radiograph.

Tricuspid regurgitation is commonly a complication of right-sided heart failure when the right ventricular and right atrial pressures are grossly elevated. Physical signs include a large positive systolic wave in the venous pulse associated with a pansystolic murmur best heard at the lower left sternal border and accentuated on inspiration. Other causes of tricuspid regurgitation are rare in old age.

Table 17   Operative mortality in aortic valve replacement in elderly patients

Reference	Number of patients	Age	Operative mortality (%)
Barnhorst *et al*. (1974)	160	65+	11
Quinlan, Cohn, and Collins (1975)	39	65+	18
Smith *et al*, (1976a)	58	65+	17
De Bono, English, and Milstein (1978)	40	65+	2.5
Stephenson, MacVaugh, and Edmunds (1978)	27	70+	11
Canepa-Anson and Emanuel (1979)	21	70+	5
Jolly, Isch, and Shumacker (1981)	16	70+	7

Pulmonary Valve Disease

Pulmonary valve murmurs are uncommon in old age and may be due to atrial septal defect or rarely in severe pulmonary hypertension, complicating mitral valve disease, or chronic respiratory disorders.

Multiple Valve Disease

Pathological involvement of two or more valves is not uncommon in old age (Bedford and Caird, 1960). Combined mitral and aortic regurgitation was found in 29 per cent. of cases of rheumatic heart disease (Bedford and Caird, 1960). Surgical treatment is associated with a high operative mortality (Oh *et al.*, 1973) but the 5 year survival approaches 50 per cent. (Starr and Lawson, 1976).

CONGENITAL HEART DISEASE

Very few patients with major congenital heart lesions will survive into old age without earlier corrective surgery. The only congenital lesion which permits long-term survival is an ostium secundum defect in the atrial septum (Colmers, 1958; Coulshed and Littler, 1957; Cooley, Hallman, and Hammam, 1966) Perloff and Lindgren, 1974). Occasional cases of patent ductus arteriosus, coarctation of the aorta, and pulmonic stenosis survive to old age (Cooley, Hallman, and Hammam, 1966; Perloff and Lindgren, 1974), but the majority have symptoms before the age of 60 years.

The clinical features of atrial septal defect are the same as in younger patients. Atrial fibrillation is usually present (Fig. 18) (Ellis, Brandenburg, and Swan, 1960; Wood, 1968) and other physical signs include the parasternal heave of right ventricular hypertrophy and a loud ejection systolic murmur, best heard at the second left interspace and associated with wide splitting of the second heart sound. Tricuspid regurgitation may be present. The electrocardiogram shows evidence of right bundle branch block, which is usually complete, and the chest radiograph shows signs of cardiomegaly with gross enlargement of the main pulmonary arteries, indicating pulmonary hypertension (Fig. 19).

The incidence of serious cardiac disability or death increases with advancing age (Markman, Howitt, and Wade, 1965) and deterioration is due to atrial dysrhythmias, recurrent bronchitis, pulmonary hypertension, pulmonary infarction, and heart failure. Medical treatment should be aimed at controlling cardiac failure and atrial dysrhythmias and protecting against recurrent bronchitis with long-term antibiotic therapy.

Surgical corrections of congenital heart defects in patients over 60 years are rarely performed but successful repairs of atrial septal defects have been achieved in small numbers of elderly patients with marked symptomatic benefit (Cooley, Hallman, and Hammam, 1966; Ellis, Brandenburg, and Swan, 1960; Jolly, Isch, and Shumacker, 1981).

PULMONARY EMBOLISM

Pulmonary thromboembolic disease is very common in old age (Towbin, 1954) and is a frequent cause of death in elderly hospital in-patients. Predisposing factors include anaemia, cardiac failure (Bedford and Caird, 1960), obesity, immobility, fractured femur (Sevitt and Gallagher, 1959), chronic venous disease in the legs, and hemiplegia (Byrne and O'Neil, 1952; Denham, Farran, and James, 1973; Warlow, Ogston, and Douglas, 1972). The sources

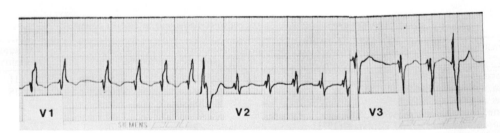

Figure 18 Electrocardiograhic chest leads V₁, V₂, and V₃ showing atrial fibrillation, and complete right bundle branch block in a male patient of 67 years with atrial septal defect

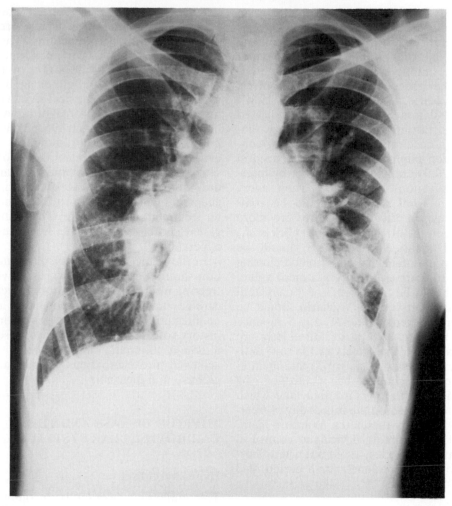

Figure 19   Posteroanterior chest radiograph demonstrating cardiomegaly and pulmonary hypertension in the 67 year old male patient with atrial septal defect

of emboli are thrombi in the leg or pelvic veins or the right atrium, in atrial fibrillation.

Massive and almost invariably fatal pulmonary embolism occurs when more than 50 per cent. of the pulmonary circulation is obstructed by emboli, a condition which is usually heralded by smaller emboli which are often undiagnosed. The patient may be shocked and extremely breathless and cyanosed. Less severe forms may be asymptomatic or may be associated with varying degrees of breathlessness, pleuritic chest pain, haemoptysis, or fever. Clinical signs may include an increase in the respiratory rate, unexplained sinus tachycardia or atrial fibrillation or flutter of sudden onset, a pleural rub or segmental lung collapse, consolidation, or pleural effusion.

The chest radiograph may be normal but linear or wedge-shaped shadows may be present in association with evidence of pleural effusion. The electrocardiogram may be normal or the classical S_1 Q_3 T_3 pattern may be present. Increasing clockwise rotation of the heart may occur in association with an RSR pattern in leads V_1 and V_2. Arterial blood gas analysis may show evidence of hypoxaemia and hypocapnia with reduced gas transfer.

The clinical features are often non-specific and may become apparent at some time after the onset of the condition. Pulmonary arteriography (Le Quesne, 1974) and non-invasive isotope lung scanning are useful in diagnosis and characteristic disturbances of regional lung perfusion and ventilation may be demonstrated, i.e. multiple segmental perfusion defects in the absence of ventilation defects (Fazio and Jones, 1975; Williams *et al.*, 1974).

Anticoagulation is the treatment indicated for venous thrombosis and pulmonary embolus. High-dose intravenous heparin by constant infusion pump should be commenced in a dose of 20,000 units in 24 hours or by intermittent intravenous doses of 10,000 units every 4 hours and oral warfarin should be commenced concurrently. The elderly are more susceptible to the effects of heparin (Jick *et al.*, 1968) and maintenance dosage should be adjusted to maintain the whole blood clotting time at 2 to 3 times the pretreatment value. Heparin should be given for 3 or 4 days until warfarin takes its effect. Warfarin should be administered in reduced doses, e.g. 5 mg once daily for the first 3 days, as the elderly are more sensitive to the effects of the oral anticoagulant (O'Malley *et al.*, 1977) and maintenance dosage should be controlled by measurement of the prothrombin time which should be estimated on the fourth day of treatment and regularly thereafter. Warfarin maintenance dosage is more difficult to control in elderly patients (Eccles, 1975) but where feasible it should be continued for a period of 3 months.

PULMONARY HEART DISEASE

Pulmonary heart disease is unusual in old age and usually occurs in elderly males (Kennedy, Andrews, and Caird, 1977). Frequently associated with other forms of cardiac disease, pulmonary heart disease, is usually due to chronic obstructive airways disease and less often to pulmonary fibrosis, pulmonary vascular obliterative disease or kyphoscoliosis (Hanley, 1976). It is rarely encountered over the age of 75 years.

Chronic cor pulmonale may be diagnosed in the absence of cardiac failure by evidence of right ventricular hypertrophy in patients with a long history of chronic respiratory disease. The patient is usually a male and clinical features include breathlessness, central cyanosis, and tachycardia with evidence of airways ob-

struction and markedly reduced exercise tolerance. Cardiac failure is usually precipitated by intercurrent chest infections. The electrocardiographic signs of cor pulmonale are a P pulmonale, right axis deviation of the mean QRS frontal vector and either an RS pattern in the chest leads or classical right ventricular hypertrophy in lead V_1 or right bundle branch block (Caird and Wilcken, 1962; Millard, 1967; Wood, 1968). The chest radiograph may show evidence of chronic bronchitis and/or emphysema and with the development of cardiac failure there is enlargement of the right heart chambers which may return to normal size after treatment of the failure. The arterial blood gases show evidence of hypoxaemia and hypercapnia.

In the management of cor pulmonale attention should be directed towards preventing or treating intercurrent respiratory infections and cardiac failure. Cor pulmonale is usually a manifestation of the later stages of the natural history of obstructive airways disease and although dramatic improvements may be achieved in exacerbations, the disease is progressive and incurable.

THYROID DISEASE AND THE CARDIOVASCULAR SYSTEM

Hyperthyroidism

This endocrine disorder is uncommon in the elderly (Locke, 1967) but the incidence of cardiac involvement increases with age (Wedgewood, 1976). Hyperthyroidism is associated with a high incidence of atrial fibrillation and this incidence increases with age (Lazarus and Harden, 1969; Locke, 1967; Staffurth, Gibberd, and Hitton, 1965). The dysrhythmia may be paroxysmal or established and 50 per cent. of elderly patients revert to sinus rhythm when they are rendered euthyroid (Lazarus and Harden, 1969). Sinus tachycardia may be associated with an elevated systolic blood pressure and the pulse pressure is usually raised. Left ventricular hypertrophy may occur (Pomerance, 1976) and cardiac failure is likely to develop, especially in patients with other forms of heart disease (Harris, 1970). Hyperthyroid patients with atrial fibrillation have a risk of systemic embolization and long term oral anticoagulation should be considered if the dysrhythmia persists in the euthyroid state or if an embolism has occurred (Staffurth, Gibberd, and Tang Fui, 1977).

The treatment of choice for elderly hyperthyroid patients with atrial fibrillation is radioiodine therapy (Sandler and Wilson, 1959; Staffurth, Gibberd, and Hitton, 1965) but half of these elderly patients require more than one dose (Lazarus and Harden, 1969) and there may be an undue delay in the control of symptoms with radioiodine (Staffurth and Young, 1967). Additional swift, therapeutic response may be achieved with antithyroid preparations, e.g. 15 mg of carbimazole q.i.d., or symptomatic improvement may occur in elderly hyperthyroid patients who receive 160 mg of propranolol daily in divided doses despite the known reduced sensitivity to the effects of beta-blockers in the elderly (Feely and Stevenson, 1979).

Hypothyroidism

Bradycardia is traditionally associated with hypothyroidism but only occurs in the minority of affected patients (Wayne, 1960). Cardiac enlargement may be due to myxoedematous infiltration of the myocardium, associated hypertension, ischaemic heart disease, or pericardial effusion, the latter demonstrated readily by echocardiography. The hypothyroid state is associated with a significant increased risk of ischaemic heart disease (Steinberg, 1968; Vanhaelst *et al.*, 1967) and cardiac failure may occur. The electrocardiogram shows evidence of low-voltage complexes and flat or inverted T waves which usually revert to normal after treatment with thyroxine (Wood, 1968). Great care must be exercised in the administration of thyroxine replacement therapy in elderly hypothyroid patients as their cardiovascular systems appear to be particularly sensitive to the effects of thyroxine.

ANAEMIA AND THE HEART

Anaemia in the elderly may be associated with tachycardia and anginal pain may be precipitated in asymptomatic ischaemic heart disease. Cardiac failure may complicate anaemia but this state is unusual unless the haemoglobin has fallen to levels below 7 grams per 100 ml.

Approximately 7 per cent. of cases of cardiac failure in the elderly are caused by or complicated by anaemia (Bedford and Caird, 1956). Clinical features of severe anaemia and congestive cardiac failure of the high-output type include warm peripheries, tachycardia, normal cardiac size, unless other forms of cardiac disease are present, and ejection systolic or diastolic flow murmurs. Anaemia is usually due to iron deficiency states or megaloblastosis.

Anaemic elderly subjects with iron deficiency anaemia and high-output cardiac failure usually require blood transfusion and packed cells from one litre of blood administered over 6 to 8 hours is usually well tolerated. Further small transfusions, combined with a loop diuretic, may be required every two or three days until the haemoglobin reaches 10 grams per 100 ml (Bedford and Caird, 1960).

Elderly patients with megaloblastic anaemia will normally respond to the appropriate haematinic supplements but severe iron deficiency and potassium depletion may occur as a result of markedly increased red cell formation and iron and potassium supplements should be given (Lawson, Murray, and Parker, 1972).

In anaemic states the prognosis of cardiac failure is generally that of associated anaemia (Bedford and Caird, 1960).

PAGET'S DISEASE OF BONE AND THE CARDIOVASCULAR SYSTEM

Paget's disease of bone appears to be a primary disorder of osteoclastic activity associated with markedly increased bone turnover (Singer *et al.*, 1978). Extensive disease of the bones is associated with a physiological arteriovenous shunt (Edholm, Howarth, and McMichael, 1945) which is probably the result of rapid blood flow through an enormously dilated capillary bed (Rhodes *et al.*, 1972). The cardiac output is increased and cardiac failure may occur, usually in elderly patients with widespread clinical evidence of the disease and other forms of heart disease (Suchett-Kaye, 1970). Metastatic calcification of the valve rings may occur with extension of the calcification to the interventricular septum and associated conduction defects (Harrison and Lennox, 1948).

High-output cardiac failure associated with Paget's disease of bone is an indication for prolonged calcitonin therapy (Hosking, 1981;

Woodhouse, Crosbie, and Mohamedally, 1975) as the cardiac output is reduced to normal levels and symptomatic improvement can be expected (Woodhouse, Crosbie,and Mohamedally, 1975).

SENILE CARDIAC AMYLOIDOSIS

This condition is usually diagnosed at postmortem as the clinical diagnosis in life is rarely made or suspected in elderly patients (Hodkinson and Pomerance, 1977; Wright and Calkins, 1975). A form of primary amyloidosis, this disorder ranges in severity from microscopic deposits confined to the atrial subendocardium to the rare state of diffuse, extensive amyloidosis and associated extracardiac deposits (Wright and Calkins, 1975). The pathogenesis of senile cardiac amyloidosis is not known and milder forms have no associated clinical abnormalities. Clinical features are related to the degree of cardiac involvement and include atrial fibrillation, cardiac enlargement, and cardiac failure (Hodkinson and Pomerance, 1977). The serum alkaline phosphatase may be elevated (Hodkinson and Pomerance, 1974) but there are no specific electrocardiographic abnormalities and there is no association with ischaemic or valvular heart disease, diabetes mellitus, hypertension, or tendency to digoxin toxicity (Hodkinson and Pomerance, 1977; Wright and Calkins, 1975).

ALCOHOLIC HEART DISEASE

Alcoholic heart disease is manifest in three ways (Brigden and Robinson, 1964) as beri-beri heart disease, which is very rare, as dysrhythmias, particularly atrial fibrillation, and thirdly as congestive cardiac failure.

Beri-beri is due to severe deficiency of vitamin B_1. Cardiovascular manifestations include a hyperkinetic circulation, vasodilatation, cardiac enlargement, and pulmonary arterial dilatation. Heart failure may develop suddenly and be rapidly fatal. The clinical response to the standard treatment of cardiac failure is often poor but dramatic, rapid improvement will occur with parenteral thiamine supplements.

Alcoholic patients may have a high red cell mean corpuscular volume (Wu, Chanarin, and Levi, 1974) and it probably requires 10 years of high alcohol intake to produce serious cardiac damage (Levi *et al.*, 1977). When frank heart failure develops the prognosis is poor.

PERICARDIAL DISEASE

Transient Acute Pericarditis

This condition occurs in 10 per cent. of elderly patients with classical acute myocardial infarction (Fig. 20) (Semple and Williams, 1976). Other forms of pericarditis are rare in old age but the disorder may occur in association with viral illnesses, left lower lobe pneumonia, or uraemia. The most common cause of pericarditis in old age is extension of malignant disease of the bronchus or breast. Clinical features include pulsus paradoxus and marked elevation of the venous pressure, and the presence of a pericardial effusion is best confirmed by echocardiography.

Chronic Constrictive Pericarditis

This is a rare condition which usually presents with gross venous pressure elevation, a low pulse pressure, hepatomegaly, ascites, and oedema but no radiological evidence of cardiac enlargement and pericardial calcification can be observed in approximately half of affected patients.

Classical electrocardiographic changes include T-wave flattening or inversion in some or all of the leads associated with low voltage throughout. Pericardiectomy may be indicated and can have successful results in elderly patients (Portal *et al.*, 1966).

CARDIAC FAILURE

The prevalence of heart failure increases with age (Klainer, Gibson, and White, 1965) and in most elderly patients cardiac decompensation is associated with a multiplicity of cardiac pathology (Hodkinson and Pomerance, 1979; Pomerance, 1965).

Left Heart Failure

Left heart failure and pulmonary oedema are usually due to ischaemic heart disease, hypertension, aortic or mitral valve disease, and 74

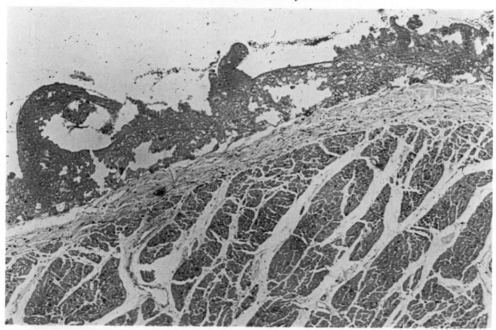

Figure 20 Acute fibrinous pericarditis (H/E ×40). (By permission of Dr R. A. Burnett, Stobhill Hospital, Glasgow)

per cent. of elderly coronary patients develop acute pulmonary oedema as a complication of acute myocardial infarction (Semple and Williams, 1976). Clinical manifestations are due to pulmonary hypertension and increased lung stiffness. Symptoms include effort dyspnoea, paroxysmal nocturnal dyspnoea, and orthopnoea and physical signs include tachycardia, pulsus alternans, gallop rhythm, and bronchospasm associated with bilateral lung crepitations. Signs of hypertensive or valvular disease may be present. Chest radiography shows evidence of cardiac enlargement and pulmonary congestion, and Kerley's lines may be present.

Right Heart Failure

Congestive cardiac failure (Fig. 21) is most commonly the result of right heart failure but it may complicate chronic pulmonary disease or multiple pulmonary emboli. Symptoms include breathlessness and fatigue, the latter often dominating the presentation in old age. Ankle swelling is an early feature and nausea, vomiting, and abdominal pain may result from gastrointestinal and hepatic venous congestion. Confusion may occur as a result of poor cerebral perfusion and hypoxaemia. Clinical signs include ankle and sacral oedema, smooth hepatomegaly, symmetrical bilateral raised venous pressure in all phases of respiration, and a positive hepatojugular reflex. Lung signs may include bilateral crepitations and pleural effusions.

Congestive cardiac failure is a syndrome and where possible the underlying cause or causes should be elucidated and precipitants, e.g. respiratory infection, dysrhythmia, myocardial infarction, or pulmonary embolism, should be managed appropriately (Table 18). Failure may be precipitated or aggravated by fluid retention due to salt excess or to a variety of drugs including steroids and non-steroidal anti-inflammatory preparations.

Management of Acute Left Heart Failure

Acute left heart failure with pulmonary oedema is a medical emergency and should be treated urgently. Pulmonary oedema will be relieved by intravenous injections of loop diuretics e.g. 40 to 80 mg of frusemide, 2 mg of bumetanide, or 50 mg of ethacrynic acid. Bronchospasm can be relieved by parenteral bronchodilators, e.g. 250 mg of aminophylline.

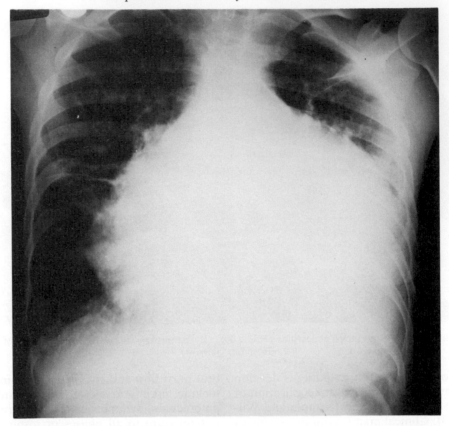

Figure 21   Posteroanterior chest radiograph of an 87 year old female with gross congestive cardiac failure

High-flow humidified oxygen should be administered by a face mask if the elderly patient has no evidence of chronic obstructive airways disease and if he will tolerate the procedure. Morphine (10 mg subcutaneously) has a useful sedative effect, controls dyspnoea, and hyperventilation. Dysrhythmias should be controlled and temporary digitalization may be required.

Management of Cardiac Failure

Bed-rest or chair-rest with elevated legs is important in the treatment regimen of cardiac failure as diuresis will be promoted if exercise is restricted. The elderly patient should not walk until free from oedema.

Oxygen therapy is useful if it can be tolerated by face mask or nasal cannulae. Stringent restriction of fluid or salt intakes are unnecessary but there should be no added salt at mealtimes.

Diuretic Therapy

High efficacy loop diuretics, e.g. frusemide, bumetanide, or ethacrynic acid, should be used in the early stages of treatment of moderate or severe cardiac failure, but maintenance therapy or treatment of milder cases can be achieved with medium efficacy thiazide preparations. Low efficacy agents, e.g. potassium-sparing triamterene or amiloride or the aldosterone antagonist spironolactone, should be administered in combination with high or medium efficacy diuretics.

Diuretics in heart failure will decrease the circulating blood volume and the resultant reduction in the cardiac venous return will reduce the preload factor. Loop diuretics may also dilate peripheral vessels and reduce cardiac workload accordingly.

Side-effects include urinary incontinence or retention, hypokalaemia, dilutional hyponat-

Table 18 Precipitants for cardiac failure

Myocardial infarction	Infection	*Drug effect*
Pulmonary embolism	Anaemia	Digitalis toxicity
Dysrhythmia	Hyperthyroidism	Injudicious thyroxine
Sudden hypertension	Overexertion	replacement
Myocarditis		Beta blockers
		Fluid retention
		(a) Steroids
		(b) Carbenoxolone
		(c) Non-steroidal anti-inflammatory preparations

raemia, reduced glucose tolerance, postural hypotension, hyperuricaemia, and hypocalcaemia. Rare adverse effects include necrotizing vasculitis, cholestatic jaundice, skin rashes, blood dyscrazias, pancreatitis, and diarrhoea.

Potassium Supplements

All diuretics, apart from potassium-sparing agents and aldosterone antagonists, can cause hypokalaemia which can impair cardiac function, increase the cardiac sensitivity to digitalis, cause postural hypotension, and may be associated with muscle weakness (MacLennan, 1981). Elderly cardiac patients are more susceptible to the hypokalaemic effects of diuretics as their total body potassium levels are reduced (Ibrahim *et al.*, 1978; MacLennan, Lye, and May, 1977) and many elderly subjects have inadequate dietary potassium intakes (Dall, Paulose, and Ferguson, 1971; Judge *et al.*, 1974). Potassium depletion should be avoided by providing oral potassium supplements or combining high or medium potency diuretics with spironolactone or potassium-sparing agents. Careful monitoring of the serum potassium is necessary to avoid the dangers of hyperkalaemia.

Digitalis Therapy

Digoxin is now the most widely used of the digitalis glycoside group of compounds which have an inotropic effect in the failing heart (Opie, 1980). The major indication for digoxin is in congestive cardiac failure with atrial fibrillation but the value of the cardiac glycosides in the treatment of patients with cardiac failure in sinus rhythm is controversial; in this situation digoxin has a short-lived inotropic action (Smith and Haber, 1973) and may improve cardiac function on exercise (Murray *et al.*,

1981), but maintenance digoxin probably confers no lasting benefit (Johnston and McDevitt, 1979; Leading Article 1979a; McHaffie *et al.*, 1978). The majority of elderly patients in sinus rhythm on maintenance digoxin therapy can have the digoxin withdrawn, particularly if the plasma digoxin level is less than 0.8 ng/ml. (Dall, 1970; Johnston and McDevitt, 1979).

Digoxin is absorbed rapidly after oral ingestion and therapeutic serum levels are reached within 1 hour and are maintained for 6 hours or more. Most of the drug is eliminated by glomerular filtration which falls with age and as digoxin clearance in the elderly is equivalent to the creatinine clearance (Roberts and Caird, 1976) the half-life of the drug is prolonged (Ewy *et al.*, 1969). Parenteral digoxin is rarely justified unless the patient has swallowing difficulties or compliance is a problem. Intramuscular digoxin is painful due to muscle necrosis and intravenous administration may be indicated in life threatening circumstances.

An oral loading dose of 0.75 mg or 0.5 mg with 0.25 mg maintenance daily should produce serum digoxin concentrations within the therapeutic range (1 to 2 ng/ml) without risk of toxicity within 48 hours when renal function is normal or near normal (Caird and Kennedy, 1977). If renal function is impaired, i.e. serum urea of more than 12 mmol/l or serum creatinine of more than 175 mmol/l, a loading dose of 0.5 mg followed by maintenance with 0.125 mg daily should be appropriate (Roberts and Caird, 1976). A maintenance dose of 0.0625 mg is rarely adequate in the elderly (Whiting *et al.*, 1978).

Most of the toxic effects of digitalis therapy occur in elderly patients with advanced heart disease and atrial fibrillation who are receiving injudicious maintenance doses. Sensitivity to digitalis may be altered by a variety of factors (Table 19) and toxicity is more likely in the presence of poor renal function, severe hypokalaemia, hypercalcaemia, hypothyroidism, or after acute myocardial infarction.

Table 19 Factors affecting sensitivity to digitalis therapy

Increased sensitivity	Reduced sensitivity
Increased age	Hyperkalaemia
Renal failure	Hypocalcaemia
Hypokalaemia	Hyperthyroidism
Hypercalcaemia	Chronic ischaemic heart
Hypothyroidism	disease
Acute myocardial	
infarction	
Hypoxaemia	
Hypomagnesaemia	
Quinidine	

Recently, due to improved awareness of the problems of toxicity and more judicious prescribing of digitalis, there has been a reduction in the incidence of toxic effects in patients with heart disease (Henry *et al.*, 1981). The value of plasma digoxin concentrations, particularly for the diagnosis of toxicity, has been questioned (Ingelfinger and Goldman, 1976), but toxic manifestations are uncommon unless the serum digoxin exceeds 2.5 ng/ml. Severe anorexia and other gastrointestinal symptoms may predominate in the elderly, particularly in females (Henry *et al.*, 1981). Confusion may be the major presenting feature (Church and Marriott, 1959; Dall, 1965). Gynaecomastia and xanthopsia are rare.

Cardiac dysrhythmias are common manifestations of digitalis toxicity in the elderly (Chung, 1970; Dall, 1965). Almost any dysrhythmia or degree of atrioventricular block can occur. The commonest cardiac toxic manifestations are ventricular bigeminy and trigeminy but multifocal ventricular ectopic activity may occur and paroxysmal atrial tachycardia is typically associated with atrioventricular block.

If digitalis intoxication is suspected, the cardiac glycoside should be withdrawn, potassium supplements administered to correct hypokalaemia, and dysrhythmias managed appropriately (Bremner, Third, and Lawrie, 1977). Lignocaine or phenytoin should correct ventricular tachyarrhythmias, supraventricular tachycardia will respond to beta-blockade, and cardioversion should only be used as a last resort. Digoxin antibody therapy may be a

valuable aid to the management of severe digoxin toxicity (Smith *et al.*, 1976b).

Vasodilator Therapy

In heart failure, pulmonary venous hypertension is usually associated with a reduction in the cardiac output and a raised left ventricular filling pressure which results in widespread sympathetic discharge, an increase in heart rate, and myocardial contractility. Arteriolar resistance vessels constrict and concomitant venous constriction reduces the venous capacity and leads to an increase in the cardiac venous return. Vasodilators can improve cardiac performance in patients with acute and chronic heart failure (Chatterjee and Parmley, 1977). Most of these drugs have no direct myocardial inotropic effect and their primary actions are on the precapillary resistance bed and postcapillary capacitance bed. Vasodilators increase venous capacitance and reduce the intracardiac blood volume and decrease the systemic and pulmonary venous pressures (preload). Arteriolar resistance is reduced with pressure unloading effect on the heart (afterload).

Intravenous infusions of phentolamine (Majid, Sharma, and Taylor, 1971) and sodium nitroprusside (Guiha *et al.*, 1974) produce marked improvement in acute and chronic heart failure but this method of treatment is only practicable in the short term and in intensive care areas. Most nitrites produce a significant reduction in the pulmonary and systemic venous pressures and they are useful in relieving venous congestion, but they have little effect on the cardiac output and are therefore not so effective in low cardiac output states (Chaterjee and Parmley, 1977). Sublingual nitroglycerin is short acting but useful in acute left heart failure (Gold, Leinbach, and Sanders, 1972). Nitroglycerin ointment lasts for 3 to 5 hours (Taylor *et al.*, 1975) and sublingual isosorbide dinitrate needs frequent administration to maintain a reduction in the preload (Williams *et al.*, 1977).

Oral hydralazine reduces the afterload and produces a sustained increase in the cardiac output (Chaterjee *et al.*, 1976; Franciosa, Pierpoint, and Cohn, 1977). Longer term therapy may be used in combination with nitrites (Massie *et al.*, 1981).

Theoretically, combined reduction of pre-load and afterload is desirable in heart failure and oral prazosin, the alpha-adrenergic blocking agent, has proved useful in the management of refractory heart failure (Stein *et al.*, 1981) although tachyphylaxis may be an early development (Elkayam *et al.*, 1979; Packer *et al.*, 1979; Stein *et al.*, 1981).

Side-effects of the vasodilators are not usually a problem in the short-term therapy of acutely ill patients but venodilators may reduce pulmonary venous congestion and relieve dyspnoea at the expense of aggravating fatigue and they may produce wide, unpredictable swings in the blood pressure during changes in posture.

Oral pirbuterol, a beta-agonist with vasodilator activity and positive inotropic effects (Dawson *et al.*, 1981), and captopril, a converting enzyme inhibitor (Turini *et al.*, 1979), improve cardiac performance in cardiac failure with few side-effects in the short term.

Vasodilators have marked beneficial effects in improving cardiac function and relieving symptoms in severe heart failure which is resistant to standard therapy, but there is as yet little evidence that there is a long-term benefit for most cardiac patients (Leading Article, 1981; Walsh and Greenberg, 1981).

Elderly patients in cardiac failure should first be managed with diuretic therapy and digitalis when appropriate, and early institution of vasodilator therapy may have a gentler effect on preload and afterload than full doses of diuretics and digoxin (Frankl, 1981).

In acute heart failure and if no haemodynamic monitoring facilities are available then a mixed preload/afterload reducing agent, e.g. prazosin, should be administered (Taylor, 1981).

REFERENCES

Abrass, I. B., and Scarpace, P. J. (1981). 'Human lymphocyte beta-adrenergic receptors are unaltered with age', *J. Gerontol.*, **36**, 298–301.

Acheson, R. M., and Acheson, E. D. (1958). 'Coronary and other heart disease in a group of Irish males aged 65–85', *Br. J. Prev. Soc. Med.*, **12**, 147–153.

Akhtar, A. J., Broe, G. A., Crombie, A., McLean, W. M. R., Andrews, G. R., and Caird, F. I. (1973). 'Disability and dependence in the elderly at home', *Age Ageing*, **2**, 102–110.

Amery, A., Berthaux, P., Birkenhager, W., *et al.* (1978a). 'Anti-hypertensive therapy in patients above 60 years. Fourth interim report of the European Working Party on high blood pressure in the elderly: E.W.P.H.E.', *Clin. Sci. Mol. Med.*, **55**, 263–270.

Amery, A., Berthaux, P., Bulpitt, C., *et al.* (1978b). 'Glucose intolerance during diuretic therapy: Results of trial by the European Working Party on hypertension in the elderly', *Lancet*, **1**, 681–683.

Anderson, M. P., Bechsgaard, P., Frederiksen, J., Hansen, D. A., Jürgensen, H. J., Nielsen, B., Pedersen, F., Pederson-Bjergaard, O., and Rasmussen, S. L. (1979). 'Effect of alprenolol on mortality among patients with definite or suspected acute myocardial infarction', *Lancet*, **2**, 865–868.

Anderson, W. F. (1976). *Practical Management of the Elderly*, 3rd. ed., Blackwell, Oxford, London, Edinburgh, Melbourne.

Anderson, W. F., and Cowan, N. R. (1959). 'Arterial pressure in healthy older people', *Clin. Sci.*, **18**, 103–117.

Anderson, W. F., and Cowan, N. R. (1972). 'Arterial blood pressure in healthy older people', *Gerontol. Clin.*, **14**, 129–136.

Applefield, M. M., and Hornick, R. B. (1974). 'Infective endocarditis in patients over age 60', *Am. Heart J.*, **88**, 90–94.

Aravanis, C., and Harris, R. (1958). 'The normal phonocardiogram of the aged', *Dis. Chest*, **33**, 214–219.

Aravanis, C., and Luisada, A. (1957). 'Obstructive and relative aortic stenosis', *Am. Heart J.*, **54**, 32–41.

Ashor, G. W., Meyer, B. W., Lindesmith, G. G., Stiles, Q. R., Walker, G. H., and Tucker, B. L. (1973). 'Coronary artery disease. Surgery in 100 patients 65 years of age and older', *Arch. Surg.*, **107**, 30–33.

Astrand, I., Astrand, P. O., and Rodahl, K. (1959). 'Maximal heart rate during work in older men', *J. Appl. Physiol.*, **14**, 562–566.

Bannan, L. T., Beevers, D. G., and Wright, N. (1980). 'A B C of blood pressure reduction; the size of the problem', *Br. Med. J.*, **280**, 921–923.

Barnhorst, D. A., Giuliani, E. R., Pluth, J. R., Danielson, G. K., Wallace, R. B., and McGoon, D. C. (1974). 'Open-heart surgery in patients more than 65 years old', *Ann. Thorac. Surg.*, **18**, 81–90.

Barraclough, M. A., and Sharpey-Schafer, E. P. (1963). 'Hypotension from absent circulatory reflexes', *Lancet*, **1**, 1121–1126.

Baurnfeind, R. A., Amat-Y-Leon, F., Dhingra, R. C., Kehoe, R., Wyndham, C., and Rosen, K. M.

(1979). 'Chronic nonparoxysmal sinus tachycardia in otherwise healthy persons', *Ann. Intern. Med.*, **91**, 702–710.

Bedford, P. D., and Caird, F. I. (1956). 'Congestive heart failure in the elderly', *Quart. J. Med.*, **25**, 407–426.

Bedford, P. D., and Caird, F. I. (1960). *Valvular Disease of the Heart in Old Age*, J. and A. Churchill Ltd, London.

Belch, J. J., Lowe, G. D. O., Ward, A. G., Forbes, C. D., and Prentice, C. R. M. (1981). 'Prevention of deep vein thrombosis in medical patients by low-dose heparin', *Scott. Med. J.*, **26**, 115–117.

Berger, M., Rethy, C., and Goldberg, E. (1979). 'Unsuspected hypertrophic subaortic stenosis in the elderly diagnosed by echocardiography', *J. Am. Geriatr. Soc.*, **27**, 178–182.

Berman, N. D., Tirone, D. E., Lipton, I. H., and Lenkei, S. C. (1980). 'Surgical procedures involving cardiopulmonary bypass in patients aged 70 or older', *J. Am. Geriatr. Soc.*, **28**, 29–32.

Bertel, O., Bühler, F. R., Kiowski, W., and Lütold, B. E. (1980). 'Decreased beta-adrenoreceptor responsiveness as related to age, blood pressure and plasma catecholamines in patients with essential hypertension', *Hypertension*, **2**, 130–138.

Bethel, C. S., and Crow, E. W. (1963). 'Heart sounds in the aged', *Am. J. Cardiol.*, **11**, 763–767.

Biörck, G., Sievers, J., and Blomqvist, G. (1958). 'Studies on myocardial infarction in Malmo (III)', *Acta. Med. Scand.*, **162**, 81–97.

Brandfonbrener, M., Landowne, M., and Shock, N. W. (1955). 'Changes in cardiac output with age', *Circulation*, **12**, 557–566.

Bremner, W. F., Third, J. L. H. C., and Lawrie, T. D. V. (1977). 'Massive digoxin ingestion. Report of a case and review of currently available therapies', *Br. Heart J.*, **39**, 688–692.

Brigden, W., and Robinson, J. (1964). 'Alcoholic heart disease', *Br. Med. J.*, **2**, 1283–1289.

Bruns, D. L., and Van der Hauwert, L. G. (1958). 'The aortic systolic murmur developing with increasing age', *Br. Heart J.*, **20**, 370–378.

Burch, P. R. J. (1978). 'Coronary heart disease: Risk factors and ageing', *Gerontology*, **24**, 123–155.

Byrne, J. J., and O'Neil, E. E. (1952). 'Fatal pulmonary emboli', *Am. J. Surg.*, **83**, 47–49.

Caird, F. I. (1976). 'Clinical examination and investigation of the heart', in *Cardiology in Old Age* (Eds F. I. Caird, J. L. C. Dall, and R. D. Kennedy), pp. 127–142, Plenum Press, New York and London.

Caird, F. I. (1977). 'Treatment of hypertension in the elderly', *Prescribers Jr.*, **17**, 52–58.

Caird, F. I. (1979). 'Postural hypotension in the elderly', in *Drugs and the Elderly* (Eds J. Crooks

and I. H. Stevenson), pp. 263–265, Macmillan Press, London and Basingstoke.

Caird, F. I., Andrews, G. R., and Kennedy, R. D. (1973). 'Effect of posture on blood pressure in the elderly', *Br. Heart J.*, **35**, 527–530.

Caird, F. I., Campbell, A. E., and Jackson, T. F. M. (1974). 'Significance of abnormalities of electrocardiogram in old people', *Br. Heart J.*, **36**, 1012–1018.

Caird, F. I., and Dall, J. L. C. (1978). 'The cardiovascular system', in *Textbook of Geriatric Medicine and Gerontology* (Ed. J. C. Brocklehurst), pp. 125–157, Churchill Livingstone, Edinburgh, London, New York.

Caird, F. I., and Kennedy, R. D. (1976). 'Epidemiology of heart disease in old age', in *Cardiology in Old Age* (Eds F. I. Caird, J. L. C. Dall, and R. D. Kennedy), pp. 1–10, Plenum Press, New York and London.

Caird, F. I., and Kennedy, R. D. (1977). 'Digitalisation and digitalis detoxication in the elderly', *Age Ageing*, **6**, 21–28.

Caird, F. I., Kennedy, R. D., and Kelly, J. C. C. (1973). 'Combined apex-cardiography and phonocardiography in investigation of heart disease in the elderly', *Gerontol. Clin.*, **15**, 366–377.

Caird, F. I., and Wilcken, D. E. L. (1962). 'The electrocardiogram in chronic bronchitis with generalized obstructive lung disease', *Am. J. Cardiol.*, **10**, 5–13.

Cameron, E. G. M., and Crowder, D. (1981). 'Viskaldix in the treatment of essential hypertension. A study on hospital out-patients', *Practitioner*, **225**, 581–585.

Campbell, A., Caird, F. I., and Jackson, T. F. M. (1974). 'Prevalence of abnormalities of electrocardiogram in old people', *Br. Heart J.*, **36**, 1005–1011.

Canepa-Anson, R., and Emanuel, R. W. (1979). 'Elective aortic and mitral valve surgery in patients over 70 years of age', *Br. Heart J.*, **41**, 493–497.

Caradoc-Davies, T. H. (1981). 'Opiate toxicity in elderly patients', *Br. Med. J.*, **283**, 905–906.

Carter, A. B. (1970). 'Hypotensive therapy in stroke survivors', *Lancet*, **1**, 485–489.

Castleden, C. M., and George, C. F. (1979). 'The effect of ageing on the hepatic clearance of propranolol', *Br. J. Clin. Pharmacol.*, **7**, 49–54.

Chatterjee, K., and Parmley, W. W. (1977). 'Vasodilator treatment for acute and chronic heart failure', *Br. Heart J.*, **39**, 706–720.

Chatterjee, K., Parmley, W. W., Massie, B., Greenberg, G., Werner, J., Klausner, S., and Norman, A. (1976). 'Oral hydralazine therapy for chronic refractory cardiac failure', *Circulation*, **54**, 879–883.

Chaturvedi, N. C., Shivalingappa, G., Shanks, B.,

McKay, A., Cumming, K., Walsh, M. J., Scaria, K., Lynas, P., Courtney, D., Barber, J. M., and Boyle, D. Mc. (1972). 'Myocardial infarction in the elderly', *Lancet*, **1**, 280–282.

Chin, P. L., Kaminski, J., and Rout, M. (1977). 'Myocardial infarction coincident with cerebrovascular accidents in the elderly', *Age Ageing*, **6**, 29–37.

Chrysant, S. G., Frohlich, E. D., and Papper, S. (1976). 'Why hypertension is so prevalent in the elderly – and how to treat it', *Geriatrics*, **31**, 101–108.

Chung, E. K. (1970). 'Digitalis-induced cardiac arrhythmias', *Am. Heart J.*, **79**, 845–848.

Church, G., and Marriott, J. L. (1959). 'Digitalis delirium', *Circulation*, **20**, 549–553.

Clark, A. N. G., (1977). 'Multifocal atrial tachycardia (MAT)', *Gerontology*, **23**, 445–451.

Clark, A. N. G. and Craven, A. H. (1981). 'PR interval in the aged', *Age Ageing*, **10**, 157–164.

Clee, M. D., Smith, N., McNeill, F. P., and Wright, D. S. (1979). 'Dysrhythmias in apparently healthy elderly subjects', *Age Ageing*, **8**, 173–176.

Colandrea, M. A., Friedman, G. D., Nichaman, M. Z., and Lynd, C. S. (1970). 'Systolic hypertension in the elderly: An epidemiologic assessment', *Circulation*, **41**, 239–245.

Colling, A., Dellipiani, A. W., Donaldson, R. J., and MacCormack, P. (1976). 'Teeside Coronary Survey: An epidemiological study of acute attacks of myocardial infarction', *Br. Med. J.*, **2**, 1169–1172.

Colmers, R. A. (1958). 'Atrial septal defects in elderly patients', *Am. J. Cardiol.*, **1**, 768–773.

Cooley, D. A., Hallman, G. L., and Hammam, A. S. (1966). 'Congenital cardiovascular anomalies in adults', *Am. J. Cardiol.*, **17**, 303–309.

Coulshed, N., Epstein, E. J., McKendrick, C. S., Galloway, R. W., and Walker, E. (1970). 'Systemic embolism in mitral valve disease', *Br. Heart J.*, **32**, 26–34.

Coulshed, N., and Littler, T. R. (1957). 'Atrial septal defect in the aged', *Br. Med. J.*, **1**, 76–80.

Cowan, N. R. (1959). 'The heart lung coefficient in older people', *Br. Heart J.*, **11**, 238–242.

Cowan, N. R. (1964). 'The heart lung coefficient and the transverse diameter of the heart', *Br. Heart J.*, **26**, 116–120.

Cowan, N. R. (1965). 'The frontal cardiac silhouette in older people', *Br. Heart J.*, **27**, 231–235.

Cullen, K. J., Murphy, B. P., and Cumpston, G. N. (1974). 'Electrocardiograms in the Busselton population', *Aust. Ń.Z. J. Med.*, **4**, 325–330.

Dall, J. L. C. (1965). 'Digitalis intoxication in elderly patients', *Lancet*, **1**, 194–195.

Dall, J. L. C. (1970). 'Maintenance digoxin in elderly patients', *Br. Med. J.*, **2**, 705–706.

Dall, J. L. C., Paulose, S., and Ferguson, J. A. (1971). 'Potassium intake of elderly patients in hospital', *Gerontol. Clin.*, **13**, 114–118.

Davies, M. J. (1971). *Pathology of Conducting Tissue of the Heart*, Butterworth, London.

Davies, M. J. (1976). 'Pathology of the conduction system', in *Cardiology in Old Age* (Eds F. I. Caird, J. L. C. Dall, and R. D. Kennedy), pp. 57–80, Plenum Press, New York and London.

Davies, M. J., Moore, B. P., and Braimbridge, M. V. (1978). 'The floppy mitral valve. Study of incidence, pathology and complications in surgical, necropsy and forensic material', *Br. Heart J.*, **40**, 468–481.

Davies, M. J., and Pomerance, A. (1972). 'Quantitative study of ageing changes in the human sinoatrial node and internodal tracts', *Br. Heart J.*, **34**, 150–152.

Davies, M. J., Pomerance, A., and Teare, R. D. (1974). 'Pathological features of hypertrophic obstructive cardiomyopathy (HOCM)', *J. Clin. Pathol.*, **27**, 529–535.

Davison, E. T., and Friedman, S. A. (1968). 'Significance of systolic murmurs in the aged', *New Engl. J. Med.*, **279**, 225–230.

Dawson, J. R., Canepa-Anson, R., Kuan, P., Whitaker, N. H. G., Carnie, J., Warnes, C., Reuben, S. R., Poole-Wilson, P. A., and Sutton, G. C. (1981). 'Treatment of chronic heart failure with pirbuterol: Acute haemo-dynamic responses', *Br. Med. J.*, **282**, 1423–1426.

De Bono, A. H. B., English, T. A. H., and Milstein, B. B. (1978). 'Heart valve replacement in the elderly', *Br. Med. J.*, **2**, 917–919.

Denham, M. J., Farran, H., and James, G. (1973). 'The value of 125 I fibrinogen in the diagnosis of deep venous thrombosis in hemiplegia', *Age Ageing*, **2**, 207–210.

Dollery, C. T. (1977). 'Pharmacological basis for combination therapy of hypertension', *Ann. Rev. Pharmacol. Toxicol.*, **17**, 311–323.

Droller, H., and Pemberton, J. (1953). 'Cardiovascular disease in a random sample of elderly people', *Br. Heart J.*, **15**, 199–204.

Eccles, J. T. (1975). 'Control of warfarin treatment in the elderly', *Age Ageing*, **4**, 161–165.

Edholm, O. G., Howarth, S., and McMichael, J. (1945). 'Heart failure and bone blood flow in osteitis deformans', *Clin. Sci.*, **5**, 249–260.

Elkayam, U., Lejemtel, T. H., Mathur, M., Ribner, H. S., Frishman, W. H., Strom, J., and Sonnenblick, E. H. (1979). 'Marked early attenuation of haemodynamic effects of oral prazosin therapy in chronic congestive heart failure', *Am. J. Cardiol.*, **44**, 540–545.

Ellis, F. H. J. R., Brandenburg, R. O., and Swan, H. J. C. (1960). 'Defect of the atrial septum in the elderly', *New Engl. J. Med.*, **262**, 219–224.

Erickson, E. E., and Lev, M. (1952). 'Aging

changes in the human atrio-ventricular node, bundle, and bundle branches', *J. Gerontol.*, **7**, 1–12.

Evans, W., and Swann, P. (1954). 'Lone auricular fibrillation', *Br. Heart J.*, **16**, 189–194.

Ewy, G. A., Kapadia, G. G., Yao, L., Lullin, M., and Marcus, F. I. (1969). 'Digoxin metabolism in the elderly', *Circulation*, **39**, 449–453.

Fazio, F., and Jones, T. (1975). 'Assessment of regional ventilation by continuous inhalation of radioactive Krypton – 81 m', *Br. Med. J.*, **3**, 673–676.

Feely, J., and Stevenson, I. H. (1979). 'The influence of ageing on propranolol concentration, binding and efficacy in hyperthyroid patients', *J. Clin. Exper. Gerontol.*, **1**, 173–184.

Fisch, C. (1981). 'The electrocardiogram in the aged', in *Geriatric Cardiology* (Eds R. J. Noble and D. A. Rothbaum), pp. 65–74, F. A. Davis Co., Philadelphia.

Fisch, C., Genovese, P. D., Dyke, R. W., Laramore, W., and Marvel, R. J. (1957). 'The electrocardiogram in persons over 70', *Geriatrics*, **12**, 616–620.

Fleming, H. A., and Bailey, S. M. (1971). 'Mitral valve disease, systemic embolism and anticoagulants', *Postgrad. Med. J.*, **47**, 599–604.

Flohr, K. H., Weir, E. K., and Chesler, E. (1981). 'Diagnosis of aortic stenosis in older age groups using external carotid pulse recording and phonocardiography', *Br. Heart J.*, **45**, 577–582.

Franciosa, J. A., Pierpoint, G., and Cohn, J. N. (1977). 'Haemodynamic improvement after oral hydralazine in left ventricular failure', *Ann. Intern. Med.*, **86**, 388–393.

Frankl, W. S. (1981). 'Recognition and management of congestive heart failure', *Geriatrics*, **6**, 92–102.

Freis, E. D., Heath, W. C., Luchsinger, P. C., and Snell, R. E. (1966). 'Changes in the carotid pulse which occur with age and hypertension', *Am. Heart J.*, **71**, 757–765.

Frick, M. H., and Kala, R. (1980). 'Once daily versus twice daily beta-blockers, effects on arrhythmias and hypertension', *Lancet*, **2**, 588.

Gann, D., Colin, C., Hildner, F. J., Samet, P., Yahr, W. Z., and Greenberg, J. J. (1977). 'Coronary artery bypass surgery in patients seventy years of age and older', *J. Thorac. and Cardiovasc. Surg.*, **73**, 237–241.

Gardin, J. M., Henry, W. L., Savage, D. D., and Epstein, S. E. (1977). 'Echocardiographic evaluation of an older population without clinically apparent heart disease', *Am. J. Cardiol.*, **39**, 277.

Gerstenblith, G. (1980). 'Noninvasive assessment of cardiac function in the elderly' in *The Aging Heart* (Aging Vol. 12) (Ed. M. L. Weisfeldt), pp. 247–267, Raven Press, New York.

Gerstenblith, G., Frederikson, J., Yin, F. C. P.,

Fortuin, N. J., Lakatta, E. G., and Weisfeldt, M. L. (1977). 'Echocardiographic assessment of a normal adult aging population', *Circulation*, **56**, 273–278.

Gerstenblith, G., Lakatta, E. G., and Weisfeldt, M. (1976). 'Age changes in myocardial function and exercise response', *Prog. Cardiovasc. Dis.*, **19**, 1–21.

Ginks, W., Leatham, A., and Siddons, H. (1979). 'Prognosis of patients paced for chronic atrioventricular block', *Br. Heart J.*, **41**, 633–636.

Glasser, S. P., Clark, P. I., and Applebaum, H. J. (1979). 'Occurrence of frequent complex arrhythmias detected by ambulatory monitoring findings in an apparently healthy asymptomatic elderly population', *Chest*, **75**, 565–568.

Gofman, J. W., Young, W., and Tandy, R. (1966). 'Ischaemic heart disease, atherosclerosis and longevity', *Circulation*, **34**, 679–697.

Gold, H. K., Leinbach, R. C., and Sanders, C. A. (1972). 'Use of sublingual nitroglycerin in congestive failure following acute myocardial infarction', *Circulation*, **46**, 839–845.

Goodwin, J. F. (1963). 'Diagnosis of left atrial myxoma', *Lancet*, **1**, 464–468.

Goodwin, J. F. (1968). 'Mitral regurgitation in congestive cardiomyopathy', *Postgrad. Med. J.*, **44**, 62–65.

Goodwin, J. F. (1970). 'Congestive and hypertrophic cardiomyopathies', *Lancet*, **1**, 731–739.

Gordon, T., Castelli, W. P., Hjortland, M. C., Kannel, W. B., and Dawber, T. R. (1977). 'Predicting coronary heart disease in middle aged and older persons', *JAMA*, **238**, 497–499.

Greenblatt, D. J., and Koch-Weser, J. (1973). 'Adverse reactions to propranolol in hospitalized medical patients: A report from the Boston Collaborative Drug Surveillance Programme', *Am. Heart J.*, **86**, 478–484.

Griffiths, R. A., and Sheldon, M. G. (1975). 'The clinical significance of systolic murmurs in the elderly', *Age Ageing*, **4**, 99–104.

Gross, M. (1970). 'The effect of posture on subjects with cerebrovascular disease', *Quart. J. Med.*, **39**, 485–493.

Gubner, R. S. (1962). 'Systolic hypertension: A pathogenic entity. Significance and therapeutic considerations', *Am. J. Cardiol.*, **9**, 773–776.

Guiha, N. H., Cohn, J. N., Mikulig, E., Franciosa, J. A., and Limas, C. J. (1974). 'Treatment of refractory heart failure with infusion of nitroprusside', *New Engl. J. Med.*, **291**, 587–592.

Hamby, R. E., Wisoff, B. G., Kolker, P., and Hartstein, M. (1973). 'Intractable angina pectoris in the 65 to 79 year age group: A surgical approach', *Chest*, **64**, 46–50.

Hanley, T. (1976). 'Pulmonary heart disease', in *Cardiology in Old Age* (Eds F. I. Caird, J. L. C.

Dall, and R. D. Kennedy), pp. 209–230, Plenum Press, New York and London.

Harlan, W. R., Graybeil, A., Mitchell, R. E., Oberman, A., and Osborne, R. K. (1967). 'Serial electrocardiograms: Their reliability and prognostic validity during a 24 year period', *J. Chron. Dis.*, **20**, 853–867.

Harris, R. (1970). *The Management of Geriatric Cardiovascular Disease* (Ed. R. Harris), J. B. Lippincott Co., Philadelphia and Toronto.

Harris, R. (1976). 'Cardiac arrhythmias in the aged', in *Cardiology in Old Age* (Eds F. I. Caird, J. L. C. Dall, and R. D. Kennedy), pp. 315–346, Plenum Press, New York and London.

Harrison, C. V., and Lennox, B. (1948). 'Heart block in osteitis deformans', *Br. Heart J.*, **10**, 167–176.

Hedenrud, B., Landahl, S., Mellström, D., Rundgren, A., Roupe, S., and Steen, B. (1980). 'Electrocardiogram at age 70 and 75. A longitudinal population study. I. General presentation of findings', *J. Clin. Exp. Geront.*, **2**, 231–243.

Heger, J. J. (1981). 'Cardiac arrhythmias in the elderly', in *Geriatric Cardiology* (Eds R. J. Noble and D. A. Rothbaum), pp. 145–159, F. A. Davis Co., Philadelphia.

Henry, D. A., Lawson, D. H., Lowe, J. M., and Whiting, B. (1981). 'The changing pattern of toxicity to digoxin', *Postgrad. Med. J.*, **57**, 358–362.

Hess, T. R., Hallam, C. C., and Wann, L. S. (1981). 'Echocardiography in the elderly', in *Geriatric Cardiology* (Eds R. J. Noble and D. A. Rothbaum), pp. 95–104, F. A. Davis Co., Philadelphia.

Hill, J. D., Hampton, J. R., and Mitchell, J. R. A. (1978). 'A randomised trial of home versus hospital management for patients with suspected myocardial infarction', *Lancet*, **1**, 837–841.

Hodkinson, H. M., and Pomerance, A. (1974). 'Cardiac amyloidosis in the elderly: Associated elevation of serum alkaline phosphatase', *Age Ageing*, **3**, 76–78.

Hodkinson, H. M., and Pomerance, A. (1977). 'The clinical significance of senile cardiac amyloidosis: A prospective clinicopathological study', *Quart. J. Med.*, **46**, 381–387.

Hodkinson, H. M., and Pomerance, A. (1979). 'The clinical pathology of heart failure and atrial fibrillation in old age'. *Postgrad. Med. J.*, **55**, 251–254.

Hodkinson, I., Pomerance, A., and Hodkinson, H. M. (1979). 'Heart size in the elderly: A clinicopathological study', *J. Royal Soc. Med.*, **72**, 13–16.

Horsey, J., Livesley, B., and Dickerson, J. W. T. (1980). 'Aged men and ischaemic heart disease: Serum cholesterol and triglyceride levels', *Age Ageing*, **9**, 154–156.

Hosking, D. J. (1981). 'Paget's disease of bone', *Br. Med. J.*, **283**, 686–688.

Hutchins, G. M. (1980). 'Structure of the aging heart', in *The Aging Heart* (Aging Vol. 12) (Ed. M. L. Weisfeldt), pp. 7–23, Raven Press, New York.

Hypertension Detection and Follow-up Program Cooperative Group (1979). 'Five year findings of the hypertension detection and follow-up program. II, Mortality by race, sex and age', *JAMA*, **242**, 2572–2577.

Hypertension–Stroke Cooperative Study Group (1974). 'Effect of antihypertensive treatment on stroke recurrence', *JAMA*, **229**, 409–418.

Ibrahim, I. K., Ritch, A. E. S., MacLennan, W. J., and May, T. (1978). 'Are potassium supplements for the elderly necessary?', *Age Ageing*, **7**, 165–170.

Ingelfinger, J. A., and Goldman, P. (1976). 'The serum digitalis concentration – does it diagnose digitalis toxicity?', *New Engl. J. Med.*, **294**, 867–870.

International Anticoagulant Review Group (1970). 'Collaborative analysis of long-term anticoagulant administration after acute myocardial infarction', *Lancet*, **1**, 203–209.

International Society and Federation of Cardiology, Scientific Councils on Arteriosclerosis, Epidemiology and Prevention, and Rehabilitation (1981). 'Secondary prevention in survivors of myocardial infarction', *Br. Med. J.*, **282**, 894–896.

Jackson, G., Pierscianowski, T. A., Mahon, W., and Condon, J. (1976). 'Inappropriate antihypertensive therapy in the elderly', *Lancet*, **2**, 1317–1318.

Jick, H., Slone, D., Borda, I. T., and Shapiro, S. (1968). 'Efficacy and toxicity of heparin in relation to age and sex', *New Engl. J. Med.*, **279**, 284–286.

Johnson, R. H., Smith, A. C., Spalding, J. M. K., and Wollner, L. (1965). 'Effect of posture on blood pressure in elderly patients', *Lancet*, **i**, 731–733.

Johnston, G. D., and McDevitt, D. G. (1979). 'Is maintenance digoxin necessary in patients with sinus rhythm?', *Lancet*, **1**, 567–570.

Jolly, W. W., Isch, J. H., and Shumacker, H. B. (1981). 'Cardiac surgery in the elderly, in *Geriatric Cardiology* (Eds R. J. Noble and D. A. Rothbaum), pp. 195–210, F. A. Davis Co., Philadelphia.

Jose, A. D. (1966). 'Effects of combined sympathetic and parasympathetic blockade on heart rate', *Am. J. Cardiol.*, **18**, 476–478.

Judge, T. G., Caird, F. I., Leask, R. G. S., and MacLeod, C. (1974). 'Dietary intake and urinary excretion of potassium in the elderly', *Age Ageing*, **3**, 167–173.

Kafetz, K. (1981). 'Surgical treatment of hypertrophic obstructive cardiomyopathy in the elderly', *Postgrad. Med. J.*, **57**, 604–606.

Kannel, W. B., and Gordon, T. (1978). 'Evaluation of the cardiovascular risk in the elderly; the Framingham Study', *Bull. N.Y. Acad. Med.*, **54**, 573–591.

Kannel, W. B., Gordon, T., and Schwartz, M. J. (1971). 'Systolic versus diastolic blood pressure and risk of coronary heart disease – the Framingham Study', *Am. J. Cardiol.*, **27**, 335–346.

Kannel, W. B., Wolf, P. A., McGee, D. L., Dawber, T. R., McNamara, P., and Castelli, W. P. (1981). 'Systolic blood pressure, arterial rigidity and risk of stroke', *JAMA*, **245**, 1225–1229.

Kennedy, R. D. (1976). 'High blood pressure and its management', in *Cardiology in Old Age* (Eds F. I. Caird, J. L. C. Dall, and R. D. Kennedy), pp. 177–191, Plenum, New York and London.

Kennedy, R. D., Andrews, G. R., and Caird, F. I. (1977). 'Ischaemic heart disease in the elderly', *Br. Heart J.*, **39**, 1121–1127.

Kennedy, R. D., and Caird, F. I. (1972). 'Application of the Minnesota code to population studies of the electrocardiogram in the elderly', *Gerontol. Clin.*, **14**, 5–16.

Kennedy, R. D., and MacFarlane, J. P. R. (1972). 'The effects of amiloride during diuretic therapy in elderly subjects', *Age Ageing*, **1**, 103–110.

Kincaid-Smith, P., McMichael, J., and Murphy, E. A. (1958). 'The clinical course and pathology of hypertension with papilloedema (malignant hypertension)', *Quart. J. Med.*, **27**, 117–153.

Kitchin, A. H., Lowther, C. P., and Milne, J. S. (1973). 'Prevalence of clinical and electrocardiographic evidence of ischaemic heart disease in the older population', *Br. Heart J.*, **35**, 946–953.

Kirkendall, W. M., and Hammond, J. J. (1980). 'Hypertension in the elderly', *Arch. Intern. Med.*, **140**, 1155–1161.

Kjörstad, H. (1957). 'Rheumatic fever in the aged', *Acta. Med. Scand.*, **158**, 337–349.

Klainer, L. M., Gibson, T. C., and White, K. L. (1965). 'The epidemiology of cardiac failure', *J. Chronic Dis.*, **18**, 797–814.

Koch, J. P., Maron, B. J., Epstein, S. E., and Morrow, A. G. (1980). 'Results of operation for obstructive hypertrophic cardiomyopathy in the elderly', *Am. J. Cardiol.*, **46**, 963–966.

Koch-Weser, J. (1979). 'Treatment of hypertension in the elderly', in *Drugs and the Elderly* (Eds J. Crooks and I. H. Stevenson), pp. 247–262, MacMillan, London.

Konu, V. (1977). 'Myocardial infarction in the elderly', *Acta. Med. Scand. (Suppl.)*, **604**, 9–68.

Korn, D., De Sanctis, R. W., and Sell, S. (1962). 'Massive calcification of the mitral annulus: A clinico-pathological study of 14 cases', *New Engl. J. Med.*, **267**, 900–909.

Krasnow, N., and Stein, R. A. (1978). 'Hypertrophic cardiomyopathy in the aged', *Am. Heart J.*, **96**, 326–336.

Landowne, M., Brandfonbrener, M., and Shock, N. W. (1955). 'Relation of age to certain measures of performance of heart and circulation', *Circulation*, **12**, 567–576.

Latour, J., De la Fuente, R., and Caird, F. I. (1980). 'Measurement of ejection fraction in the elderly', *Age Ageing*, **9**, 157–164.

Lawson, D. H., Murray, A. M., and Parker, J. L. W. (1972). 'Early mortality in the megaloblastic anaemias', *Quart. J. Med.*, **41**, 1–14.

Lazarus, J. H., and Harden, R. McG. (1969). 'Thyrotoxicosis in the elderly', *Gerontol. Clin.*, **11**, 371–378.

Leading Article (1968). 'Systolic murmurs in the elderly', *Br. Med. J.*, **4**, 530–531.

Leading Article (1975). 'Systolic murmurs in the elderly', *Br. Med. J.*, **4**, 69–70.

Leading Article (1979a). 'Digoxin in sinus rhythm', *Br. Med. J.*, **1**, 1103–1104.

Leading Article (1979b). 'Asymptomatic complete heart block', *Br. Med. J.*, **2**, 1245–1246.

Leading Article (1981). 'Long term vasodilator therapy for heart failure', *Lancet*, **1**, 1350–1351.

Lenkiewicz, J. E., Davies, M. J., and Rosen, D. (1972). 'Collagen in human myocardium as a function of age', *Cardiovasc. Res.*, **6**, 549–555.

Lennox, I. M., and Williams, B. O. (1980). 'Postural hypotension in the elderly', *J. Clin. Exp. Gerontol.*, **2**, 313–329.

Leonard, J. C. (1979). 'Valvar heart disease. Mitral valve disease', *Br. J. Hosp. Med.*, **22**, 204–212.

Le Quesne, L. P. (1974). 'Relation between deep vein thrombosis and pulmonary embolism in surgical patients', *New Engl. J. Med.*, **291**, 1292–1294.

Lev, M. (1954). 'Aging changes in the human sinoatrial node', *J. Gerontol.*, **9**, 1–9.

Lev, M. (1964). 'Anatomic basis for atrio-ventricular block', *Am. J. Med.*, **37**, 742–748.

Levi, G. F., Quadri, A., Ratti, S., and Basagni, M. (1977). 'Preclinical abnormality of left ventricular function in chronic alcoholics', *Br. Heart J.*, **39**, 35–37.

Librach, G., Schadel, M., Seltzer, M., Hart, A., and Yellin, N. (1976). 'Immediate and long term prognosis of acute myocardial infarction in the aged', *J. Chron. Dis.*, **29**, 483–495.

Linn, B. S., and Yurt, R. W. (1970). 'Cardiac arrest among geriatric patients', *Br. Med. J.*, **2**, 25–27.

Locke, W. (1967). 'Hyperthyroidism in the aged', *Geriatrics*, **22**, 11, 173–174.

Luisada, A. A., Bhat, P. K., and Knighten, V. (1980). 'Changes of cardiac output caused by aging: An impedance cardiographic study', *Angiology*, **31**, 75–81.

McHaffie, D., Purcell, H., Mitchell-Heggs, P., and Guz, A. (1978). 'The clinical value of digoxin in patients with heart failure and sinus rhythm', *Quart. J. Med.*, **47**, 401–419.

McKee, P. A., Castelli, W. P., McNamara, P. M., and Kannel, W. B. (1971). 'The natural history of congestive heart failure: The Framingham Study', *New Engl. J. Med.*, **285**, 1441–1446.

MacLennan, W. J. (1981). 'The problem of potassium', in *Advanced Geriatric Medicine*, (Eds F. I. Caird and J. Grimley Evans), Vol. 1, pp. 67–72, Pitman, London.

MacLennan, W. J., Lye, M. D. W., and May, T. (1977). 'The effect of potassium supplements on total body potassium levels in the elderly', *Age Ageing*, **6**, 46–50.

McMillan, J. B., and Lev, M. (1962). 'The ageing heart. Myocardium and epicardium', in *Biological Aspects of Ageing* (Ed. N. Shock), Columbia University Press, New York.

Majid, D. A., Sharma, B., and Taylor, S. H. (1971). 'Phentolamine for vasodilator treatment of severe heart failure', *Lancet*, **2**, 719–724.

Malcolm, A. D. (1980). 'Anticoagulants for heart disease', *Br. J. Hosp. Med.*, **23**, 606–615.

Marchionni, N., Pini, R., Vannucci, A., Calamandrei, M., Conti, A., Di Bari, M., Greppi, B., and Antonini, F. M. (1981). 'Intensive care for the elderly with acute myocardial infarction', *J. Clin. Exp. Gerontol.*, **3**, 47–62.

Markman, P., Howitt, G., and Wade, E. G. (1965). 'Atrial septal defect in the middle aged and elderly', *Quart. J. Med.*, **34**, 409–425.

Martin, A., and Millard, P. H. (1973). 'Cardiovascular assessment in the elderly', *Age Ageing*, **2**, 211–217.

Martin, R. P., Rakowski, H., Kleinman, J. H., Beaver, W., London, E., and Popp, R. L. (1979). 'Reliability and reproducibility of two dimensional echocardiographic measurement of the stenotic mitral valve orifice area', *Am. J. Cardiol.*, **43**, 560–568.

Massie, B., Ports, T., Chatterjee, K., Parmley, W., Ostland, J., O'Young, J., and Haughom, F. (1981). 'Long term vasodilator therapy for heart failure: Clinical response and its relationship to hemodynamic measurements', *Circulation*, **63**, 269–278.

Master, A. M., Dublin, L. I., and Marks, H. H. (1950). 'Normal blood pressure range and its clinical implications', *JAMA*, **143**, 1464–1470.

Mather, H. G., Morgan, D. C., Pearson, N. G., Read, K. L. Q., Shaw, D. B., Steed, G. R., Thorne, M. G., Lawrence, C. J., and Riley, I. S. (1976). 'Myocardial infarction: A comparison be-

tween home and hospital care for patients', *Br. Med. J.*, **1**, 925–929.

Meyer, J., Wukasch, D. C., Seybold-Epting, W., Chiariello, L., Reul, G. J., Jr., Sandiford, F. M., Hallman, G. L., and Cooley, D. A. (1975). 'Coronary artery bypass in patients over 70 years of age', *Am. J. Cardiol.*, **36**, 342–345.

Mihalick, M. J., and Fisch, C. (1974). 'Electrocardiographic findings in the aged', *Am. Heart J.*, **87**, 117–128.

Millard, F. J. C. (1967). 'The electrocardiogram in chronic lung disease', *Br. Heart J.*, **29**, 43–50.

Mitchell, J. R. A. (1980). 'Secondary prevention of myocardial infarction – the present state of the A.R.T.', *Br. Med. J.*, **280**, 1128–1130.

Mitchell, J. R. A. (1981). 'Anticoagulants in coronary heart disease – retrospect and prospect', *Lancet*, **1**, 257–262.

Moore-Smith, B. (1980). 'The management of hypertension in the elderly', in *The Treatment of Medical Problems in the Elderly* (Ed. M. J. Denham), pp. 117–158, MTP Press, Lancaster, England.

Murray, R. G., Tweddel, A. C., Bastian, B. C., Pearson, D., Martin, W., Lorimer, A. R., Hutton, I., and Lawrie, T. D. V. (1981). 'Clinical value of digitalis treatment in cardiac failure', *Br. Heart J.*, **45**, 343.

Noble, R. J., and Rothbaum, D. A. (1981). 'History and physical examination', in *Geriatric Cardiology* (Eds R. J. Noble and D. A. Rothbaum), pp. 55–64, F. A. Davis Co., Philadelphia.

Norris, R. M., Brandt, P. W. T., Caughey, D. E., Lee, A. J., and Scott, P. J. (1969). 'A new coronary prognostic index', *Lancet*, **1**, 274–278.

Norwegian Multicenter Study Group (1981). 'Timolol induced reduction in mortality and reinfarction in patients surviving acute myocardial infarction', *New Engl. J. Med.*, **304**, 801–807.

Oh, W., Hickman, R., Emanuel, R., McDonald, L., Somerville, J., Ross, D., Ross, K., and Gonzalez-Lavin, L. (1973). 'Heart valve surgery in 114 patients over the age of 60', *Br. Heart J.*, **35**, 174–180.

O'Malley, K., and O'Brien, E. (1980). 'Management of hypertension in the elderly', *New Engl. J. Med.*, **302**, 1397–1401.

O'Malley, K., Stevenson, I. H., Ward, C. A., Wood, A. J. J., and Crooks, J. (1977). 'Determinants of anticoagulant control in patients receiving warfarin', *Br. J. Clin. Pharmacol.*, **4**, 309–314.

Opie, L. H. (1980). 'Beta-blocking agents', in *Drugs and the Heart* (Ed. L. H. Opie), Lancet, London.

Osterberger, L. E., Goldstein, S., Khaja, F., and Lakier, J. B. (1981). 'Functional mitral stenosis in patients with massive mitral annular calcification', *Circulation*, **64**, 472–476.

Ostrander, L. D., Brandt, R. L., Kjelsberg, M. O., and Epstein, F. H. (1965). 'Electrocardiographic findings among the adult population of a total natural community, Tecumseh, Michigan', *Circulation*, **31**, 888–897.

Packer, M., Meller, J., Gorlin, R., and Herman, M. V. (1979). 'Haemodynamic and clinical tachyphylaxis to prazosin-mediated afterload reduction in severe chronic and congestive cardiac failure', *Circulation*, **59**, 531–540.

Page, L. P., and Sidd, J. J. (1972). 'Medical management of arterial hypertension', *New Engl. J. Med.*, **287**, 960–967.

Pathy, M. S. (1967). 'Clinical presentation of myocardial infarction in the elderly', *Br. Heart J.*, **29**, 190–199.

Pathy, M. S., and Peach, H. (1981). 'Change in disability status as a predictor of long term survival after myocardial infarction in the elderly', *Age Ageing*, **10**, 174–178.

Peach, H., and Pathy, M. S. J. (1979). 'Disability in the elderly after myocardial infarction', *J. R. Coll. Physicians, Lond.*, **13**, 154–157.

Peel, A. A. F., Semple, T., Wang, I., Lancaster, W. M., and Dall, J. L. G. (1962). 'A coronary prognostic index for grading the severity of infarction', *Br. Heart J.*, **24**, 745–760.

Perez, G. L., Jacob, M., Bhat, P. K., Rao, D. B., and Luisada, A. A. (1976). 'Incidence of murmurs in the aging heart', *J. Am. Geriatr. Soc.*, **14**, 29–31.

Perloff, J. K., and Lindgren, K. M. (1974). 'Adult survival in congenital heart disease', *Geriatrics*, **29** (4), 94–104.

Perry, L. S., King, J. F., Zeft, H. J., Manley, J. C., Gross, C. M., and Wann, L. S. (1981). 'Two-dimensional echocardiography in the diagnosis of left atrial myxoma', *Br. Heart J.*, **45**, 667–671.

Petrie, J. C., Galloway, D. B., Webster, J., Simpson, W. T., and Lewis, J. A. (1975). 'Atenolol and bendrofluazide in hypertension', *Br. Med. J.*, **4**, 133–135.

Petrin, T. J., and Tavel, M. E. (1979). 'Idiopathic hypertrophic subaortic stenosis as observed in a large community hospital: Relation to age and history of hypertension', *J. Am. Geriatr. Soc.*, **27**, 43–46.

Pomerance, A. (1965). 'Pathology of the heart with and without cardiac failure in the aged', *Br. Heart J.*, **27**, 697–710.

Pomerance, A. (1967). 'Ageing changes in human heart valves', *Br. Heart J.*, **29**, 222–231.

Pomerance, A. (1972). 'Pathogenesis of aortic stenosis and its relation to age', *Br. Heart J.*, **34**, 569–574.

Pomerance, A. (1976). 'Pathology of the myocardium and valves', in *Cardiology in Old Age* (Eds F. I. Caird, J. L. C. Dall, and R. D. Kennedy), pp. 11–55, Plenum Press, New York and London.

Pomerance, A. (1981). 'Cardiac pathology in the elderly', in *Geriatric Cardiology* (Eds R. J. Noble and D. A. Rothbaum), pp. 9–54, F. A. Davis Co., Philadelphia.

Port, S., Cobb, F. R., Coleman, E., and Jones, R. H. (1980). 'Effect of age on the response of the left ventricular ejection fraction to exercise', *New Engl. J. Med.*, **303**, 1134–1137.

Portal, R. W., Besterman, E. M. M., Chambers, R. J., Sellors, T. H., and Sommerville, W. (1966). 'Prognosis after operation for constrictive pericarditis', *Br. Med. J.*, **1**, 563–569.

Priddle, W. W., Liu, S. F., Breithaupt, D. J., and Grant, P. G. (1968). 'Amelioration of high blood pressure in the elderly', *J. Am. Geriatr. Soc.*, **16**, 887–892.

Quinlan, R., Cohn, L. H., and Collins, J. J., Jr (1975). 'Determinants of survival following cardiac operations in elderly patients', *Chest*, **68**, 498–500.

Rabushka, S. E., Melamed, J. L., and Melamed, M. E. (1968). 'A radiologic survey', *Geriatrics*, **23**, 136–141.

Radin, A. M., and Black, H. R. (1981). 'Hypertension in the elderly: The time has come to treat', *J. Am. Geriatr. Soc.*, **29**, 193–200.

Rhodes, B. A., Grayson, N. D., Hamilton, C. R., White, R. I., Giargiana, F. A., and Wagner, H. N., Jr (1972). 'Absence of anatomic arteriovenous shunts in Paget's disease of bone', *New Engl. J. Med.*, **287**, 686–689.

Roberts, M. A., and Caird, F. I. (1976). 'Steady-state kinetics of digoxin in the elderly', *Age Ageing*, **5**, 214–223.

Robinson, S. (1938). 'Experimental studies of physical fitness in relation to age', *Arbeits. Physiologie.*, **10**, 251–323.

Rodrigues Dos Santos, A. G., and Lye, M. (1980). 'Transient cardiac arrhythmias in healthy elderly individuals: How relevant are they?' *J. Clin. Exp. Gerontol.*, **2**, 245–258.

Rodstein, M. (1956). 'The characteristics of non-fatal myocardial infarction in the aged', *Arch. Intern. Med.*, **98**, 84–90.

Rodstein, M. (1979). 'Heart disease in the aged', in *Clinical Geriatrics*, (Ed. I. Rossmann), 2nd. ed., pp. 181–203, J. B. Lippincott Company, Philadelphia and Toronto.

Rodstein, M. (1980). 'Ischemic and hypertensive heart disease in the aged: Prognostic and therapeutic factors', *J. Am. Geriatr. Soc.*, **28**, 388–397.

Rodstein, M., Brown, M., and Wolloch, L. (1968). 'First degree atrioventricular heart block in the aged', *Geriatrics*, **23**, 159–165.

Rodstein, M., and Zeman, F. D. (1957). 'Postural blood pressure changes in the elderly', *J. Chron. Dis.*, **6**, 581–588.

Rosenbaum, M. B., Elizari, M. V., and Lazzari, J. O. (1970). *The Hemiblocks*, Tampa Tracings, Oldsmar, Florida.

Rothbaum, D. A. (1981). 'Coronary artery disease', in *Geriatric Cardiology* (Eds R. J. Noble and D. A. Rothbaum), pp. 105–118, F. A. Davis Co., Philadelphia.

Royal College of General Practitioners. Office of Population Censuses and Surveys, Department of Health and Social Security (1979). *Morbidity Statistics from General Practice, 1971–72. Second National Study*, pp. 51–52, HMSO, London.

Sandler, G., and Wilson, G. M. (1959). 'The nature and prognosis of heart disease in thyrotoxicosis', *Quart. J. Med.*, **28**, 347–369.

Schnurr, L. P., Ball, A. P., Geddes, A. M., Gray, J., and McGhie, D. (1977). 'Bacterial endocarditis in England in the 1970s: A review of 70 patients', *Quart. J. Med.*, **46**, 499–512.

Schocken, D. D., and Roth, G. S. (1977). 'Reduced beta-adrenergic receptor concentrations in ageing man', *Nature*, **267**, 856–858.

Schwarten, D. E. (1981). 'Radiologic examination of the heart', in *Geriatric Cardiology* (Eds R. J. Noble and D. A. Rothbaum), pp. 75–93, F. A. Davis Co., Philadelphia.

Schwartz, C. J., and Mitchell, J. R. A. (1962). 'The relation between myocardial lesions and coronary artery disease', *Br. Heart J.*, **24**, 761–786.

Scottish Health Service, Common Services Agency, Information Services Division (1981). *Scottish Health Statistics, 1979*, Vol. 2, HMSO, Edinburgh.

Sell, S., and Scully, R. E. (1965). 'Ageing changes in the aortic and mitral valves; histologic and histochemical studies, with observations on the pathogenesis of calcific aortic stenosis and calcification of the mitral annulus', *Am. J. Pathol.*, **46**, 345–365.

Selzer, A., Kelly, J. J., Jr, Vannitamby, M., Walker, P., Gerbode, F., and Kerth, W. J. (1967). 'The syndrome of mitral insufficiency due to isolated rupture of the chordae tendinae', *Am. J. Med.*, **43**, 822–836.

Semple, T., and Williams, B. O. (1976). 'Coronary care for the elderly', in *Cardiology in Old Age* (Eds F. I. Caird, J. L. C. Dall, and R. D. Kennedy), pp. 297–313, Plenum Press, New York and London.

Sevitt, S., and Gallagher, N. G. (1959). 'Prevention of venous thrombosis and pulmonary embolism in injured patients', *Lancet*, **2**, 981–989.

Shaw, D. B., Holman, R. R., and Gowers, J. I. (1980). 'Survival in sinoatrial disorder (sick-sinus syndrome)', *Br. Med. J.*, **280**, 139–141.

Shekelle, R., Ostfield, A., and Klawans, H. (1974). 'Hypertension and risk of stroke in an elderly population', *Stroke*, **5**, 71–75.

Sievers, J., and Hall, P. (1971). 'Incidence of rheumatic fever', *Br. Heart J.*, **33**, 833–836.

Simon, M. A., and Liu, F. (1954). 'Calcification of mitral valve annulus and its relationship to functional valvular disturbance', *Am. Heart J.*, **48**, 497–505.

Simonson, E. (1972). 'The effect of age on the electrocardiogram', *Am. J. Cardiol.*, **29**, 64–72.

Simpson, F. O. (1978). 'Hypertension', *Br. Med. J.*, **2**, 882–883.

Singer, F. R., Schiller, A. L., Pyle, E. B., and Krane, S. M. (1978). 'Paget's disease of bone', in *Metabolic Bone Disease* (Eds L. V. Avioli and S. M. Krane), Vol. 2, pp. 489–575, Academic Press, New York.

Sixty Plus Reinfarction Study Research Group (1980). 'A double blind trial to assess long term oral anticoagulant therapy in elderly patients after myocardial infarction', *Lancet*, **2**, 989–994.

Sjögren, A. L. (1971). 'Left ventricular wall thickness determined by ultrasound in 100 subjects without heart disease', *Chest*, **60**, 341–346.

Smith, H. L. (1928). 'The relation of the weight of the heart to the weight of the body and the weight of the heart to age', *Am. Heart J.*, **4**, 79–93.

Smith, J. M., Lindsay, W. G., Lillehei, R. C., and Nicoloff, D. M. (1976a). 'Cardiac surgery in geriatric patients', *Surgery*, **80**, 443–448.

Smith, T. W., and Haber, E. (1973). 'Digitalis', *New Engl. J. Med.*, **289**, 945–950, 1010–1014, 1063–1072, 1125–1129.

Smith, T. W., Haber, E., Yeatman, L., and Butler, V. P. (1976b). 'Reversal of advanced digoxin intoxication with F_{AB} fragments of digoxin specific antibodies', *New Engl. J. Med.*, **294**, 797–800.

Staffurth, J. S., Gibberd, M. C., and Hitton, P. J. (1965). 'Atrial fibrillation in thyrotoxicosis treated with radioiodine', *Postgrad. Med. J.*, **41**, 663–671.

Staffurth, J. S., Gibberd, M. C., and Tang Fui, S. Ng (1977). 'Arterial embolism in thyrotoxicosis with atrial fibrillation', *Br. Med. J.*, **2**, 688–690.

Staffurth, J. S., and Young, J. (1967). 'Delay in control of thyrotoxicosis after treatment with radioactive iodine', *J. Clin. Endoc.*, **27**, 1062–1064.

Stamler, J., Stamler, R., Riedlinger, W. F., Algera, G., and Roberts, R. H. (1976). 'Hypertension screening of 1 million Americans. Community hypertension evaluation clinic (CHEC) program of 1973 through 1974', *JAMA*, **235**, 2299–2306.

Starr, A., and Lawson, R. (1976). 'Cardiac surgery in the elderly', in *Cardiology in Old Age* (Eds F. I. Caird, J. L. C. Dall, and R. D. Kennedy), pp. 369–396, Plenum Press, New York and London.

Steinberg, A. D. (1968). 'Myxedema and coronary

artery disease – a comparative autopsy study', *Ann. Intern. Med.*, **68**, 338–344.

Stephenson, L. W., MacVaugh, H., and Edmunds, L. H., Jr (1978). 'Surgery using cardiopulmonary bypass in the elderly', *Circulation*, **58**, 250–254.

Stein, L., Foster, P. R., Friedman, A. W., Statza, J., and McHenry, P. L. (1981). 'Acute and chronic haemodynamic effects of prazosin in left ventricular failure', *Br. Heart J.*, **45**, 186–192.

Stout, R. W. (1980). 'Treatment of cardiovascular disease in the elderly', in *The Treatment of Medical Problems in the Elderly* (Ed. M. J. Denham), pp. 77–115, MTP Press Ltd, Lancaster, England.

Strandell, T. (1964). 'Heart rate, arterial lactate concentration and oxygen uptake during exercise in old men compared with young men', *Acta. Physiol. Scand.*, **60**, 197–216.

Strandell, T. (1976). 'Cardiac output in old age', in *Cardiology in Old Age* (Eds F. I. Caird, J. L. C. Dall, and R. D. Kennedy), pp. 81–100, Plenum Press, New York and London.

Suchett-Kaye, A. I. (1970). 'Paget's disease of bone', *Geront. Clin.*, **12**, 241–255.

Sulg, I. A., Cronqvist, S., Schüller, H., and Ingvar, D. H. (1969). 'The effect of intracardial pacemaker therapy on cerebral blood flow and electroencephalogram in patients with complete atrioventricular block', *Circulation*, **39**, 487–494.

Swales, J. D. (1979). 'Pathophysiology of blood pressure in the elderly', *Age Ageing*, **8**, 104–109.

Tavel, M. E. (1968). 'Clinical phonocardiography. Its use in diagnosis of idiopathic hypertrophic subaortic stenosis', *JAMA*, **203**, 285–286.

Taylor, B. B., Kennedy, R. D., and Caird, F. I. (1974). 'Digoxin studies in the elderly', *Age Ageing*, **3**, 79–84.

Taylor, S. H. (1981). 'Vasodilator treatment of heart failure', *Practitioner*, **225**, 1419–1429.

Taylor, W. R., Forrester, J. S., Magnusson, P., Takano, T., Chatterjee, K., and Swan, H. J. G. (1975), *Circulation*, **52**, Suppl. II, 36.

Thangarajah, N., Hames, T., Mubako, H., Patel, J., and MacLennan, W. J. (1980). 'The use of impedance cardiography in the young and elderly during postural stress', *Age Ageing*, **9**, 235–240.

Thell, R., Martin, F. H., and Edwards, J. E. (1975). 'Bacterial endocarditis in subjects 60 years of age and older', *Circulation*, **51**, 174–182.

Towbin, A. (1954). 'Pulmonary embolism. Incidence and significance', *JAMA*, **156**, 209–215.

Tresch, D. D., Siegel, R., Keelan, M. H., Jr, Gross, C. M., and Brooks, H. L. (1979). 'Mitral valve prolapse in the elderly', *J. Am. Geriatr. Soc.*, **27**, 421–424.

Tucker, B. L., Lindesmith, G. G., Stiles, Q. R., Hughes, R. K., and Meyer, B. W. (1977). 'Myocardial revascularization in patients 70 years of age and older', *West J. Med.*, **126**, 179–183.

Turini, G. A., Brunner, H. R., Gribic, M., Waeber, B., and Gauras, H. (1979). 'Improvement of chronic congestive heart failure by oral captopril', *Lancet*, **1**, 1213–1215.

Vanhaelst, L., Neve, P., Chailly, P., and Bastenie, P. A. (1967). 'Coronary–artery disease in hypothyroidism', *Lancet*, **2**, 800–802.

Vavrik, M. (1974). 'High risk factors and atherosclerotic cardiovascular diseases in the aged', *J. Am. Geriatr. Soc.*, **12**, 203–207.

Veterans Administration Co-operative Study Group on Antihypertensive Agents (1972). 'Effects of treatment on morbidity in hypertension. III. Influence of age, diastolic pressure and prior cardiovascular disease; further analysis of side effects', *Circulation*, **45**, 991–1004.

Vittal, B. S., Luisada, A. A., and Rao, D. B. (1976). 'Importance of aortic dilatation in the genesis of the innocent systolic ejection murmur of the aged', *J. Am. Geriatr. Soc.*, **14**, 366–370.

Walsh, W. F., and Greenberg, B. H. (1981). 'Results of long term vasodilator therapy in patients with refractory congestive heart failure', *Circulation*, **64**, 499–505.

Wang, R., Camm, J., Ward, D., Washington, H., and Martin, A. (1980). 'Treatment of chronic atrial fibrillation in the elderly, assessed by ambulatory electrocardiographic monitoring', *J. Am. Geriatr. Soc.*, **28**, 529–534.

Warlow, C., Ogston, D., and Douglas, A. S. (1972). 'Venous thrombosis following strokes', *Lancet*, **1**, 1305–1306.

Watkins, J., Carl Abbott, E., Hensby, C. N., Webster, J., and Dollery, C. T. (1980). 'Attenuation of hypotensive effect of propranolol and thiazide diuretics by indomethacin', *Br. Med. J.*, **281**, 702–705.

Wayne, E. J. (1960). 'Clinical and metabolic studies in thyroid disease', *Br. Med. J.*, **1**, 78–90.

Wedgewood, J. (1976). 'Remediable heart disease', in *Cardiology in Old Age* (Eds F. I. Caird, J. L. C. Dall, and R. D. Kennedy), pp. 249–265, Plenum Press, New York and London.

Whiting, B., Wandless, I., Sumner, D. J., and Goldberg, A. (1978). 'Computer assisted review of digoxin therapy in the elderly', *Br. Heart J.*, **40**, 8–13.

Williams, B. O., Begg, T. B., Semple, T., and McGuinness, J. B. (1976). 'The elderly in a coronary unit', *Br. Med. J.*, **2**, 451–453.

Williams, B. O., and Caird, F. I. (1980). 'Impedance cardiography and cardiac output in the elderly', *Age Ageing*, **9**, 47–52.

Williams, D. O., Bommer, W. J., Miller, R. R., Amsterdam, E. A., and Mason, D. T. (1977). 'Hemodynamic assessment of oral peripheral vasodilator therapy in chronic congestive heart failure: Prolonged effectiveness of isosorbide dinitrate', *Am. J. Cardiol.*, **39**, 84–90.

Williams, O., Lyall, J., Vernon, M., and Croft, D. N. (1974). 'Ventilation – Perfusion lung scanning for pulmonary emboli', *Br. Med. J.*, **1**, 600–602.

Williamson, J. (1979). 'Adverse reactions to prescribed drugs in the elderly', in *Drugs and the Elderly* (Eds J. Crooks and I. H. Stevenson), pp. 239–246, Macmillan Press Ltd, London.

Wood, P. (1968). *Disease of the Heart and Circulation*, Eyre and Spottiswoode, London.

Woodhouse, N. J. Y., Crosbie, W. A., and Mohamedally, S. M. (1975). 'Cardiac output in Paget's disease: Response to long term salmon calcitonin therapy', *Br. Med. J.*, **4**, 686.

Woodrow, K. M., Friedman, G. D., Siegelaub, A. B., and Collen, M. F. (1972). 'Pain tolerance: Differences according to age, sex and race', *Psychosomatic Med.*, **34**, 548–556.

World Health Organization (1965–1977). *World Health Statistics Annuals*, WHO, Geneva.

World Health Organization (1974). *World Health Statistics Report*, **27** (9), 563.

Wright, J. R., and Calkins, E. (1975). 'Amyloid in the aged heart : Frequency and clinical significance', *J. Am. Geriatr. Soc.*, **23**, 97–103.

Wu, A., Chanarin, I., and Levi, A. J. (1974). 'Macrocytosis of chronic alcoholism', *Lancet*, **i**, 829–831.

15

The Respiratory System

Principles and Practice of Geriatric Medicine
Edited by M. S. J. Pathy
© 1985 John Wiley & Sons Ltd

15.1

The Respiratory System

B. H. Davies

INTRODUCTION

The burden of respiratory disease increases with advancing age. The normal ageing of the respiratory system contributes only slightly, compared to the powerful effects of environmental and personal respiratory insults, recurrent infection and disordered immune responses. These factors combine to produce serious and often long-term disability, which becomes a major challenge to the physician involved in the therapy and rehabilitation of the respiratory patient.

Only rarely will elderly patients with a respiratory illness present with a single well-defined disease, more commonly there will be a complex interaction of different respiratory illnesses within the same patient. As a result of this complexity, the presentation and management of the elderly respiratory patient will tax the diagnostic and therapeutic resources of the physician.

NORMAL AGE-ASSOCIATED CHANGES OF THE RESPIRATORY SYSTEM

Anatomical Changes

Superficial examination of the aged lung resembles the emphysematous lung, they are more voluminous and microscopic examination reveals alteration of the normal geometry. There is enlargement of the alveolar ducts and respiratory bronchioles with a resulting increase in alveolar duct air and a reduction in alveolar air. The alveoli become shallower and flatter and there is a loss of tissue within each alveolus, probably due to a loss of the capillary bed. There is an increase in elastin with age, accumulating preferentially in the pleura and around pulmonary vessels and bronchi. The net effect is a reduction in alveolar surface area, decreasing by 4 per cent. per decade from a mean of 75 m^2 at 30 years (Mauderly, 1978; Niewoehner and Kleinerman, 1964; Thurlbeck and Angus, 1975). In addition to these structural changes in pulmonary architecture, there are subtle changes in responsiveness centrally by the respiratory centre and changes in configuration and mechanical properties of the chest wall, such that there is an increasing degree of kyphoscoliosis with increased calcification of the costal cartilages (Semine and Damon, 1975).

Physiological Change

Lung volume/pressure characteristics change dramatically from birth to death. The changes reflect both alterations in the lungs and chest wall, which occur at different rates and often in different directions. With increasing age, the chest wall becomes stiffer and the lungs more distensible since after maturity the elastic recoil gradually decreases and the lungs become slightly more compliant. The decrease in elastic recoil is approximately 0.25 mm H$_2$O per year (at 50 per cent. total lung capacity or TLC) (Fig. 1). This observation accounts not only for some of the age-related changes in

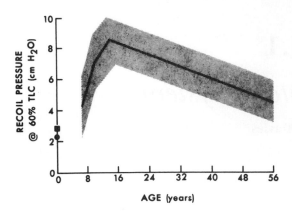

Figure 1   The effect of age on recoil pressure of the lungs. (From Murray, 1981)

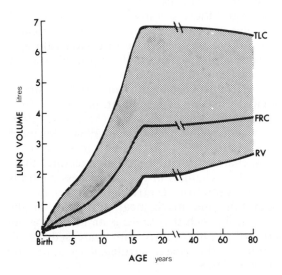

Figure 2   The effect of age on static lung volumes of the lungs. (From Murray, 1976)

lung volumes but for changes in expiratory flow rates and arterial PO_2 as well (Knudson *et al.*, 1977; Murray, 1981; Turner, Mead, and Wohl, 1968). What exact change occurs to elastic fibres during ageing is unclear, but it is likely that although elastin increases with age, the location or structure of the fibres may be abnormal. The effect on lung volumes is such that the vital capacity decreases to approximately 75 per cent. of its value in the seventh decade compared to the age of 17 years and residual volume (RV) increases nearly 50 per

cent. during this time. The TLC remains virtually constant when related to height (Fig. 2).

Ventilatory mechanics also alter with age, there is a decline in forced expiratory volume in one second (FEV_1) and specific airways conductance (Sgaw), the decline in FEV_1 being some 32 ml per year in males and 25 ml per year in females from the age of 25 years (Morris, Mosk, and Johnson, 1971). There is evidence of differences in the chronological age at which the various functions decline, with vital capacity remaining stable when expiratory flow rates are decreasing (Hurwitz, Liben, and Becklake, 1980). This may reflect not only changes in elastic recoil in the elderly but also cause airways in the dependent regions of the lung to prematurely close during expiration (LeBlanc, Ruff, and Milic-Emili, 1970). Gas is therefore trapped distal to sites of closure and poor mixing of inspired air results. This abnormality is mainly responsible for the age-related changes in arterial PO_2 and alveolar-arterial PO_2 differences (Davis *et al.*, 1980; Gibson *et al.*, 1976; Muiesan, Sobrini, and Grassi, 1971). Gas transfer is also influenced by age; with the loss of lung tissue with advancing age, the reduction in alveolar-capillary surface area produces a fall in the transfer factor for carbon monoxide ranging from 0.20 to 0.32 ml per minute per mmHg per year for men and 0.06 to 0.18 ml per minute per mmHg for women per year of adult life (Georges, Saumon, and Leiseau, 1978).

Among the most important physiological changes is a progressive reduction in arterial PO_2. The combination of premature airway closure and loss of elastic recoil results in ventilation-perfusion mismatching. This effect is added to by changes in cardiac output (Sorbini *et al.*, 1968).

A nomogram for the calculation of expected arterial oxygen tension in relation to age has been produced (Table 1), the arterial oxygen tension falling to a mean of 75 mmHg in the seventh decade (Morris, Mosk, and Johnson, 1971).

Table 1   Nomogram for calculation of expected arterial oxygen tension in relation to age

$PaO_2 = 109$ mmHg $- 0.43 \times$ (age in years)
or
$PaO_2 = 14.5$ KPa $- 0.057 \times$ (age in years)

The arterial PCO_2 remains remarkably constant at 40 mmHg mean, during adult life, in spite of a reduction in CO_2 sensitivity. The control of ventilation undergoes profound changes in the elderly. It is unclear whether this is due to an alteration in sensory perception, altered central neuronal processing, chest wall stiffness, or less neuromuscular inspiratory output. Recent evidence suggests there is no difference in respiratory timing control; nor is it attributable to changes in mechanics (Peterson *et al.*, 1981). There are substantial differences in ventilatory responses to both hypoxia and hypercapnia, being reduced by 50 per cent. from those values in the young adult (Dill, Hillyard, and Miller, 1980; Kronenberg and Drage, 1973).

Immunological Changes

The normal respiratory system is sterile beyond the first segmental bronchial division. To achieve this state requires a complex and integrated defence system. Mechanical reflexes such as cough, an intact mucous barrier with normal tracheobronchial ciliary activity, combine with immunological responses in an ill-understood but effective barrier to the penetration of foreign antigens.

That age affects at least some of these components is now recognized. Bronchial mucociliary transport is significantly lower in subjects over 54 years (Puchelle, Zohm, and Bertrand, 1979), and this occurs also in non-smokers (Wanner, 1977). There are significant alterations in tracheal mucous velocity, being slower in non-smoking elderly subjects (Wanner, 1977). Systemic immunologic responses also change with age both in terms of peripheral lymphocyte reactivity and cutaneous recall skin test responses (Goodwin, Searles, and Tung, 1982). That this change in immune response may be significant has been detailed by Makinodan (1978). Systemic antibody responses in vitro are impaired (Del Fraissy, 1980). Both the proportion of T lymphocytes and macrophages in the systemic circulation decline with age (Clot, Chamasson, and Bouchier, 1972). These changes in immunological response and control are important and probably explain not only the increased frequency of severe bacterial infection but also the poor response and higher mortality seen in the eld-

erly, particularly in pneumococcal pneumonia (Emmerling, 1979; Macfarlane *et al.*, 1982). More subtle immunological changes may be responsible for the increased prevalence of chronic fibrosing lung diseases in the elderly. Detailed studies of immunological responses in the bronchoalveolar immune system are still needed.

Metabolic Changes

Little is known concerning the metabolic activities of the lung in the elderly. That the endothelial cells of the pulmonary circulation are metabolically active and can either further metabolize to active, e.g. Angiotensin I, or inactive, e.g. Dopamine, substances has been established in younger adults. Whether subtle changes in metabolic control may be responsible for some cases of asthma or emphysema has not been established (Bakhle and Vane, 1977). Similarly, it has not been established whether in the ageing lung failure to deactivate may produce abnormal systemic states, e.g. blood pressure control (Block and Stalcup, 1981).

Response to Drugs

Ageing is associated with changes both in the metabolic pathway of drugs when used systemically and also an increased incidence of drug related respiratory toxicity. Important respiratory drugs such as isoniazid and theophylline are metabolized differently in the elderly (Krivoy and Alroy, 1980); as a result toxicity is often enhanced. Further study is required of the effect of age and pulmonary disease on drug disposition and metabolism (Greenblatt, Sellers, and Shader, 1982). More specifically, drugs may have an adverse effect on the respiratory system in many ways. Asthma may be induced in atopic subjects, particularly as a general response to antibiotics, iron-dextran, or iodine containing contrast media. Idiosyncratic reactions to aspirin and many other non-steroidal anti-inflammatory agents may present as asthma. Beta adrenoreceptor blocking agents are potentially dangerous in all wheezing patients and are particularly troublesome in that respiratory deterioration may be delayed some months after therapy is initiated. The use of Timolol eye drops in the elderly has been associated with severe asthma (Jones and Ekberg, 1979). Pulmonary parenchymal disease due to drugs is increasing. The changes range from pulmonary oedema (nitrofurantoin, methotrexate) or pulmonary fibrosis (busulphan, cyclophosphamide) (Sostman, Motthoy, and Putman, 1977). Rarely a granulomatous infiltration with eosinophilia may be seen (Demeter, Ahman, and Tomashefski, 1979). Parenchymal infection (superinfection) resulting from the use of immunosuppressants or broad-spectrum antibiotics is an increasing problem. Although bacteria, fungi, or pneumocystis are the most common organisms involved, tubercle in its cryptic miliary form may be reactivated (Bode, Pare, and Fraser, 1974; Feld, Bodey, and Gröschel, 1976).

THE EPIDEMIOLOGY OF RESPIRATORY DISEASE IN THE ELDERLY

The burden of chronic respiratory disease in the elderly is shared between chronic bronchitis and emphysema, neoplasia, and lung infections, particularly pneumonia. Black and Pole (1975) have described an index of 'burden' in which the number of inpatient days in hospital, the outpatient referrals, consultations with the family doctor, days of sickness benefit among workers, and the mortality expressed as loss of

life expectancy are weighted and the burden calculated. In the United Kingdom, respiratory disease with a burden of 13.5 per cent. is second only to mental disease and handicap (13.6 per cent.). This chronic burden is also carried through to mortality statistics where neoplasia, pneumonia, and chronic bronchitis account for the majority of cases. The proportion of deaths due to respiratory diseases is highest in the first year of life (approximately 30 per cent.) falling to 5% in late adolescence and early adult life. From the fifth decade there is a steady rise and in those over 85 it accounts for 25 per cent. of all deaths. In the last 15 years, the death-rates for all causes (after standardizing for age) has fallen and that due to most of the respiratory diseases has fallen even more rapidly with the exception of bronchogenic carcinoma and pneumonia (Fig. 3).

Chronic Bronchitis and Emphysema

Although difficulties exist in terminology, chronic bronchitis and emphysema represent an often intolerable burden on the elderly patient (Royal College of Physicians, 1981). In the United Kingdom it has been estimated that 40,000 patients over 60 years require help with some item of daily living as a result of this disease. In the United Staes 3.3 per cent. of all

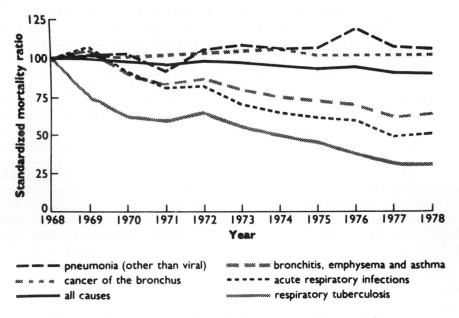

Figure 3   Standardized mortality ratios for respiratory diseases of all ages

disablement is due to chronic bronchitis (Tager and Speizer, 1975). In the elderly the prevalence of chronic bronchitis is difficult to estimate for age alone is associated with a significant increase in the prevalence of morning cough in non-smokers in an urban area, being twice as common in 60 to 70 year patients as in 30 to 40 year patients (Gulsvik, 1979).

Hospital admissions for chronic bronchitis and emphysema have fallen steadily, as has the associated mortality. Yet still 10 per cent. of all medical beds in the United Kingdom are occupied by chest cases, half of whom have chronic bronchitis and emphysema. This apparent fall is not fully explained by the decrease in pollution, either personal or environmental, and other smoking associated diseases have continued to increase (Fig. 3). In a now-dated survey it has been found that 8 per cent. of men and 3 per cent. of women suffer from chronic bronchitis with effort dyspnoea (College of General Practitioners, 1961).

The response to this burden is inadequate (Fletcher and Pato, 1977). Emphasis on prophylaxis with cessation of cigarettes continues to yield only slow responses. Preventive measures against acute episodes are seldom effective; therapy is symptomatic. Respiratory health visitors attached to local chest units could be tried—to counsel and educate. The use of respiratory aids, provision of more economic oxygen delivery systems, and more aggressive bronchodilator regimens should all be considered (Medical Research Council Working Party, 1981).

Carcinoma of the Respiratory Tract

This tragic epidemic of the twentieth century has had a profound effect on mortality rates in the elderly, particularly of men but with increasing rates now also in women. Rare until the beginning of this century, by 1930 it was obvious that rates were increasing so that it is now the commonest malignancy in men and will soon overtake breast as the commonest in women (Fig. 4) (Silverberg, 1980). Approximately 200,000 deaths occur annually in the United States and more than 30,000 in the United Kingdom. The incidence in men is highest in the 65 to 70 years age group and in women around 70 years (Fig. 4). Cancer of the lung accounts for almost 9 and 3 per cent. of all deaths in men and women, respectively. The increase in cigarette consumption parallels the increase in lung cancer rates, the role of air pollution and occupational factors being small (with the exception of asbestos exposure). The increased risk with increasing cigarette consumption is indicated in Table 2. Cessation of smoking is associated with a rapid decline in incidence, reaching the level of non-smokers after 13 years of abstinence in smokers of less than 20 cigarettes a day. It is therefore important, with increasing life expectancy, that the elderly are counselled vigorously against continuing smoking (Benjamin, 1977; Doll, 1970).

Table 2   Death due to lung cancer in relation to cigarette smoking

Number of cigarettes/ day	0	10–20	20–40	>40
Number of deaths/ 1000,000	3.4	54.3	143.9	217.3

Pulmonary Infection

Pneumonic illness remains a serious problem in the elderly. In most series of community-acquired pneumonia, the elderly do less well in terms of mortality, complications, and severity of disease. Of deaths, 80 per cent. are in the over 60's, the incidence of bacteraemia is greater, and empyema, lung abscess are all more common (Macfarlane *et al.*, 1982). The rapid rise in pneumonia as the cause of death in the seventh decade appears to be due to a change in certification (Fig. 5). In many patients this is a terminal event after succumbing to other diseases. However, recent evidence suggests that there may be a true increase in nosocomial pneumonia in elderly hospital patients (Mylotte and Bearn, 1981). The underlying alterations in the defence of the respiratory tract have been indicated previously but a common associated feature in the elderly is the aspiration of oropharyngeal flora during sleep. That this may occur in otherwise healthy patients has only recently been recognized (Huxley *et al.*, 1978).

Tuberculosis

The reduction of tuberculosis from its previous pivotal role as a major killer to that of an

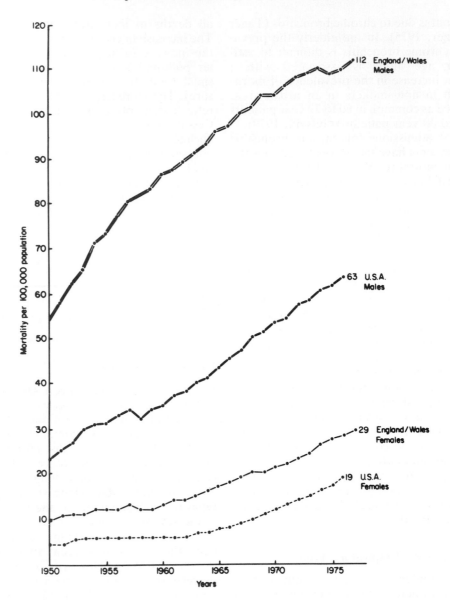

Figure 4   Death rates from bronchogenic carcinoma in the United States and England
and Wales

infrequent, often misdiagnosed, infection has been one of the successes of this century. In the less economically developed countries it remains a scourge; in India the prevalence is 1,500 to 2,000 per 100,000 while in England and Wales notifications for 1978–79 were 16.4 per 100,000.

As the prevalence has declined in the United Kingdom so the disease pattern has altered so that most infective cases, i.e. cavitatory smear positive pulmonary disease, occur in elderly white males (MRC Tuberculosis and Chest Disease Unit, 1980; Stead, 1981). As pulmonary disease declines, so the relative importance of acute miliary tuberculosis increases, for in the elderly, cryptic miliary tuberculosis often causes diagnostic confusion and may be first diagnosed at postmortem.

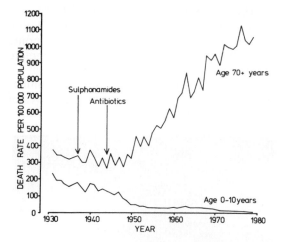

Figure 5   Death rates for pneumonia in the elderly and paediatric age range. (From Flenley, 1981. Reproduced by permission of Professor David Flenley)

Asthma

Asthma is a serious, often undiagnosed, cause of morbidity in the elderly. Difficulties in diagnosis arise because there is a lack of allergic characteristics and chronic bronchitis simulates many clinical features. Recent evidence suggests that asthma in the elderly is common; in one study 6.5 per cent. of those over 70 years have features of asthma (Burr *et al.*, 1979). It appears more prevalent in men than women (5.1 per cent. compared to 1.8 per cent.) and in terms of spirometry more severe. Few of these subjects had asthma that had started in childhood and in some patients the disease may remit spontaneously.

ACUTE RESPIRATORY DISEASE IN THE ELDERLY

Respiratory emergencies constitute a large proportion of geriatric emergencies in both family practice and hospital medicine (Dawson, 1980). The physician is rarely faced with a simple situation, especially in hospital practice, where historically there may be a number of different respiratory diseases, each with a different mode of onset and progression within the same patient. The careful history from both patient and closest relative is invaluable, the meticulous physical examination essential; however, in the face of non-specific symptoms, and difficult physical signs, investigative aids, particularly the chest radiograph, become necessary to diagnosis. Indeed, an effective approach to acute respiratory disease is to base a differential diagnosis on the chest radiograph and relate the clinical history, signs, and other tests to this illness and so produce a diagnosis. A classification of radiographic change is shown in Table 3.

Table 3   Radiographic classification of acute respiratory disease in the elderly

A. Homogenous opaque hemithorax	1. Pulmonary collapse 2. Pleural effusion 3. Collapse/consolidation
B. Partial opacification of the hemithorax	1. Lobar consolidation 2. Lobar atelectasis 3. Lobar masses 4. Pleural effusion
C. Diffuse pulmonary infiltrates	1. Miliary 2. Mid zone 3. Lower zone 4. Perihilar 5. Random
D. Cavitatory disease	1. Infective 2. Neoplastic 3. Infarction 4. Pneumoconiosis 5. Bullae
E. Unilateral hyperlucency	1. Pneumothorax 2. Lung cysts and bullae 3. Pulmonary embolism 4. Check valve bronchial obstruction
F. Bilateral hyperlucency	1. Chronic bronchitis and emphysema 2. Asthma 3. Pulmonary emboli
G. Mediastinal masses	1. Lymph nodes 2. Thymus 3. Thyroid 4. Aneurysms 5. Hiatus hernia
H. Ribs and diaphragm	1. Traumatic fractures 2. Secondary deposits 3. Rupture of diaphragm 4. Herniae

The Diagnosis and Management of the Homogenous Opaque Hemithorax

The radiographic presence of an opaque, homogenous hemithorax is usually caused by one of the diseases in Table 4. Clinically, tracheal deviation is an important sign. It is rare for significant loss of lung volume to occur in pleural effusions, except when there is an associated empyema or it is secondary to longstanding tuberculosis. A valuable aid in diffi-

Table 4   The differential diagnosis of an opaque, homogenous hemithorax

Pulmonary collapse	Carcinoma of the bronchus
	Secondary lymph node compression
	Bronchial adenomas
	Foreign bodies
	Primary tuberculosis
Pleural effusion	Postpneumonic
	Tuberculosis
	Malignancy
	Pulmonary infarction
	Trauma
	Subdiaphragmatic infection
	Oesophageal rupture
Collapse/consolidation	Necrotizing pneumonia
	Alveolar cell carcinoma
	Aspiration pneumonia
	Proximal bronchial carcinoma

cult cases is an overpenetrated posteroanterior view which may reveal a bronchostenosis, a hilar mass, or carinal widening, as well as indicating the tracheal position. Unfortunately, by far the commonest cause of hemithorax opacification is a proximal main bronchus carcinoma (Fig. 6). Evidence of spread to the mediastinum and pleura is common and the patients are rarely operable, with submucosal spread close to the carina being all too common. Foreign bodies occur infrequently and there is usually a history of inhalation. Strictures due to past infection such as tubercle rarely produce recent complete pulmonary collapse. Pleural effusions involving the hemithorax are usually caused by malignancy, extension from primary tumours in the bronchus, breast, colon, and stomach are common. Less so is a primary tumour of the pleura, a mesothelioma; this is usually associated with asbestos exposure and commonly produces a scoliosis to the side of the lesion (Antman, 1982).

A growing problem is the severe empyema, a not uncommon result of severe or poorly treated pneumonia, simulating pleural malignancy with weight loss, obtundation and confusion being clinically evident (Schwartz *et al.*, 1973). It is rare for effusions due to rheumatoid arthritis, heart failure, or hypoproteinaemia to occupy the whole hemithorax although effusions associated with pancreatitis may be mas-

sive (Leff, Hopwell, and Costello, 1978).

The mixed picture of collapse/consolidation is commonly seen in bronchogenic carcinoma where distal infection occurs before complete collapse (Fennesay, 1975). Pneumococcal lobar pneumonia may rarely present as a unilateral opacity with the distinguishing features of an air bronchogram.

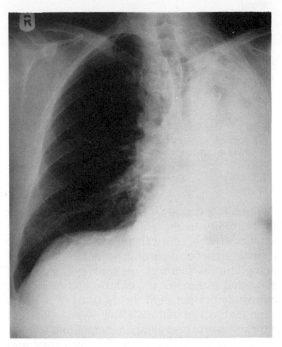

Figure 6   Opacification of hemithorax by collapse due to bronchogenic carcinoma

Management

The compromised pulmonary reserve of the elderly is usually badly affected by further loss of lung volume and general supportive measures such as oxygen and physiotherapy may be necessary until diagnosis is established. Sputum cytology should precede invasive techniques as 80 per cent of proximal carcinomas yield malignant cells when three sputum specimens are examined (Oswald *et al.*, 1971). Fibreoptic bronchoscopy now offers a simple, generally safe, method of direct examination of the tracheobronchial tree. Operative intervention for proximal carcinoma in the elderly is rarely possible due to the poor respiratory function of many of the patients (Ali and Ewer, 1980). In those patients suitable for operation, careful search for metastases is necessary and simple screening techniques, such as barium swallow, useful. Prednisolone (30 mg daily) may be commenced while radiation therapy is initiated, limiting the oedematous response. The more uncommon causes of pulmonary collapse will be revealed either at bronchoscopy (adenoma) or clinically by peripheral lymphadenopathy or splenomegaly. Very rarely mediastinoscopy may need to be considered for mediastinal masses if CAT scanning is unrewarding (Heitzman, 1981).

Where a pleural effusion is suspected, aspiration and pleural biopsy will often reveal the diagnosis, occasionally with the help of ultrasound. The fluid should be cultured particularly for tubercle and anaerobic bacilli, protein, amylase, and glucose levels may be valuable, and microscopy for pus and malignant cells rewarding. An empyema of this size is usually postpneumonic or from a subdiaphragmatic source. Aggressive management is mandatory with intercostal intubation, systemic penicillin with gentamycin, and where indicated metronidazole, the first line of therapy. If response does not occur quickly, decortication may be necessary (Benfield, 1981). Palliative therapy for malignant effusions is now effective. There is little place for repeated aspiration, and ablation of the pleural space should be performed with nitrogen mustard, tetracycline, or *Corynebacterium parvum* (Miller, Hunter, and Howe, 1980). Rarely ablation of the pleural space by instillation of kaolin may be necessary; this is painful and requires general anaesthesia.

The Diagnosis and Management of Partial Opacification of the Hemithorax

The differential diagnosis of partial hemithorax opacification is large and the main causes are outlined in Table 5. Three anatomical areas are potentially involved; pulmonary, pleural, and mediastinal (Fig. 7). The radiographic characteristics are often diagnostic, the pleural effusion with its well defined margins in the lower zone; lobar consolidation without associated pulmonary collapse is seen in pneumonia, pulmonary infarction, neoplasia (especially alveolar cell carcinoma), and radiation pneumonitis. Lobar collapse is usually due to bronchogenic carcinoma but other causes

Table 5 Partial opacification of the hemithorax – differentail diagnosis

Lobar consolidation	Viral, aspiration or bacterial pneumonia
	Pulmonary infarction
	Tumour infiltration
	Radiation pneumonitis
Lobar atelectasis	Primary bronchogenic carcinoma
	Previous tubercle
	Recurrent pneumonia
	Adenoma
	Foreign body
Lobar masses	Neoplasia
	Lung abscess
	Hydatid disease
	Aspergilloma
	Pulmonary infarction
Pleural effusions	Infection
	Neoplasms
	Pulmonary embolism
	Trauma

may be rarely found. The large intralobar mass can occasionally simulate a consolidation but tomography will usually differentiate the slowly growing squamous cell or adenocarcinoma.

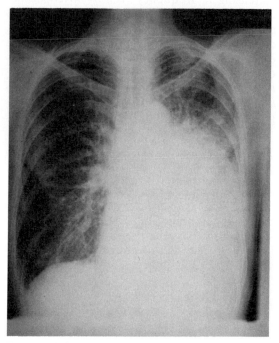

Figure 7 Partial opacification of hemithorax due to lobar pneumonia

Management

Clinically the presence of fever, bronchial breathing, and purulent sputum will suggest pneumonia. A diagnostic aspiration should be carried out in all basal shadows of uncertain location. The sedimentation rate if very high will suggest arteritis or tumour; precipitin lines to *Aspergillus fumigatus* suggests mycetoma. Invasive procedures such as bronchoscopy and lung biopsy may be necessary.

Diffuse Radiographic Pulmonary Disease

The differential diagnosis of diffuse lung disease is vast. No certain method exists, short of lung biopsy, to eliminate the more obscure causes but a simple radiographic classification can be helpful (Table 6).

1. Differential Diagnosis of Miliary Infiltrates

Miliary infiltration usually implies blood borne dissemination. The pattern is of an even, 1.5 to 2.5 mm nodular change, often discrete, infiltrate throughout the lung fields. Miliary tubercle is the foremost cause but acute allergic alveolitis and cytomegalovirus infections are increasing in frequency. Rarely mycoplasma, drug hypersensitivity, or leukaemic infiltrates may simulate miliary shadowing. Clinically, choridal tubercles are very rare, the diagnosis of miliary tubercle usually requiring a biopsy of liver, bone marrow, or lung. Other appropriate tests will include precipitins to alveolitis antigens, cytomegalovirus titres, and cold agglutinins (Fulmer, 1982).

2. Differential Diagnosis of Mid and Upper Zone Infiltrates

This distribution in the elderly is uncommon, occupational causes are most frequent, but bronchopneumonic tubercle and ankylosing spondylitis may be seen rarely. Sarcoid (chronic), allergic alveolitis (chronic). and drug reactions are infrequent (Fig. 8).

3. Differential Diagnosis of Lower Zone Infiltrates

Lower zone infiltrates are common in the elderly, often as a result of aspiration pneumonia.

Table 6   Diffuse radiographic pulmonary disease in the elderly – differential diagnosis

1. *Miliary infiltrates*
   Miliary tuberculosis
   Acute allergic alveolitis
   Cytomegalovirus infection
   Mycoplasma
   Leukaemic infiltrates
   Drug hypersensitivity
2. *Mid and upper zone infiltrates*
   Bronchopneumonic tuberculosis
   Pneumoconiosis
   Ankylosing spondylitis
   Chronic sarcoidosis
   Chronic allergic alveolitis
   Drug hypersensitivity
   – Nitrofurantoin
   – Bleomycin
   – Sulphasalazine
3. *Lower zone infiltrates*
   Aspiration pneumonia
   Cryptogenic fibrosing alveolitis
   Pulmonary fibrosis with collagen diseases
   Asbestosis
   Bronchiectasis
   Pulmonary oedema
   Drug hypersensitivity
4. *Infiltrates radiating from the hila*
   Acute pulmonary oedema
   Lymphangitis carcinomatosis
   Severe viral pneumonia
   Drug hypersensitivity
   – Bleomycin
   – Methotrexate
   Pulmonary haemorrhage
   Pneumocystis carrini pneumonia
5. *Random bilateral infiltrates*
   Bronchopneumonic tubercle
   Aspiration pneumonia
   Pulmonary infarction
   Pulmonary oedema
   Secondary malignancy
   Alveolar cell carcinoma
   Pulmonary eosinophilia

In association with finger clubbing and basal crackles, they suggest cryptogenic fibrosing alveolitis and, with rheumatoid or scleroderma, an associated pulmonary fibrosis (Crystal *et al*, 1981). Other causes are rare and are suggested by occupational history or physical signs (Fig. 9).

4. Differential Diagnosis or Perihilar Infiltrates

This dramatic radiographic picture is due usually to pulmonary oedema or lymphangitis carcinomatosis. Rarely pneumocystis carinii

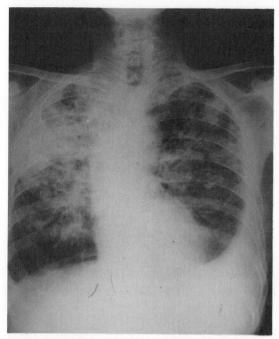

Figure 8 Mid and upper zone infiltrates due to tuberculosis

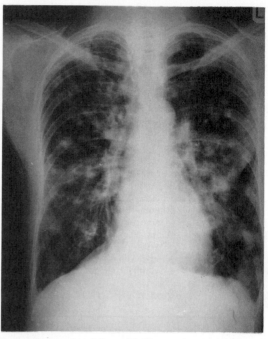

Figure 10 Random bilateral infiltrates due to alveolar cell carcinoma

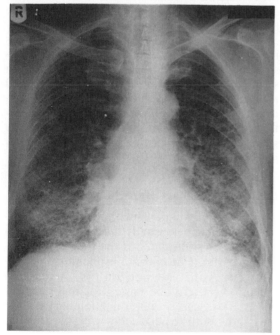

Figure 9 Lower zone infiltrates due to cryptogenic fibrosing alveolitis

pneumonia may present as a complication of cytotoxic chemotherapy or immunological deficiency.

5. Differential Diagnosis of Random Bilateral Infiltrates

This radiographic pattern is of bilateral infiltrates which are not symmetrical and are often coalescent. Tubercle, severe pneumonia (especially aspiration, influenzal, or *Legionella*), secondary malignancy, and atypical pulmonary oedema are the most common (Fig. 10).

Management of Diffuse Lung Disease

The general approach to the patient with diffuse lung disease is that discussed by Crofton and Douglas (1981) and Turner-Warwick and Strickland (1981). Using the above radiographic classification, the presence of four features is assessed. Fever suggests an infective aetiology, especially acute or cryptic miliary tuberculosis in miliary infiltrates (Proudfoot *et al.*, 1969), pneumonia in lower zone infiltrates, lymphangitis in perihilar infiltrates. Dyspnoea tends to be associated with fibrosing lung diseases, pulmonary oedema, infection, or drug reactions. Weight loss will suggest superinfection with bacteria, fungi, or viruses (Williams, Knick, and Remington, 1976) or pulmonary toxicity from drugs (Sostman, Motthey, and Putman, 1977). Physical examination may reveal clubbing, suggesting pulmonary fibrosis or neoplasia; marked sputum production suggests bronchiectasis or alveolar cell carcinoma.

Investigations which are helpful in the differential diagnosis of diffuse lung disease are shown in Table 7. Transbronchial biopsy remains the invasive procedure of choice (Zavala, 1978).

Table 7   Relevant investigations in patients with diffues radiographic infiltrates

Full blood count	Rheumatoid factor	Full lung function
Sedimentation rate	Antinuclear factor	Sputum cytology
Liver function	Viral serology	Sputum culture
Protein electrophoresis	Cold agglutinins	Mantoux test
Urea	Precipitins	Electrocardiogram
Electrolytes		

Cavitatory Radiographic Disease

The delayed presentation of respiratory disease in the elderly predisposes to progression of pneumonias to cavitation, but there is a wide differential diagnosis (Table 8). Bilateral cavitatory disease should suggest tuberculosis, especially in the elderly white male (Fig. 11). Sputum smear is positive in the majority of cases confirming the diagnosis. Fulminating necrotizing pneumonia may become bilateral and other causes such as bronchiectasis, cavitated progressive massive fibrosis, or pulmonary infarction will need to be eliminated.

Table 8   Cavitatory radiographic disease

Infective	Necrotizing pneumonia
	Primary lung abscess
	Tuberculosis
	Aspergilloma
	Nocardiosis
Tumours	Primary bronchogenic carcinoma
	Metastatic carcinoma
Collagen-vascular	Wegener's granulomatosis
	Rheumatoid nodule
	Progressive massive fibrosis
Vascular	Pulmonary infarction
Structural disease	Bullae
	Traumatic lung cysts
	Bronchiectasis

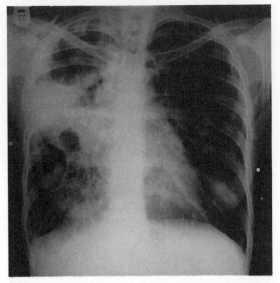

Figure 11   Cavitatory shadowing due to *Klebsiella pneumoniae*

Unilateral cavitatory disease suggests a pneumonia distal to a stenotic bronchial lesion or a necrotizing pneumonia, particularly *Klebsiella* or anaerobic organisms which may produce a lung abscess (Bartlett, 1979).

The problem of superinfection pneumonia is increasing in the hospital environment with associated rapid clinical deterioration, sputum stain positive for gram negative organisms and progressive radiographic shadowing. Mortality, even with antibiotic therapy in combination, is high. Delayed clearing of cavitatory shadows usually indicates a need for bronchoscopy (Weinstein, 1980).

Bilateral Pulmonary Hyperlucency

The majority of patients with bilateral pulmonary hyperlucency usually have asthma, with preservation, until late, of the pulmonary perfusion pattern, or chronic bronchitis and emphysema with attenuation of peripheral perfusion pattern and large proximal pulmonary arteries. Rarely bilateral pulmonary emboli may show both hyperlucency with basal linear or wedge-shaped shadows.

The Management of Acute Severe Asthma

The diagnostic difficulties of asthma in the elderly are formidable; there is usually little spontaneous variation in dyspnoea, it is often severe, and the nocturnal attacks may simulate pulmonary oedema. Peak flow rates or spirometry may show little variation with minimal responses to bronchodilators, and only a response to corticosteroids may suggest the diagnosis. It is significantly underdiagnosed and many patients are labelled bronchitic or in heart failure (Burr *et al.*, 1979).

The history will usually extend over some months, the acute attack reflecting exhaustion as much as increase in airways obstruction. Various oral bronchodilators have usually been prescribed with little effect; a short course of corticosteroids of inadequate dose may have been tried and often multiple antibiotic courses. Clinically it is important to assess the extent of exhaustion; this is often reflected in a high arterial $PaCO_2$ and careful monitoring of blood gas change is crucial to successful management.

The physical signs in the deteriorating patient change from an alert cooperative patient to a tired, often agitated state where the patient lies back in bed, the chin sags, and respiratory movements are confined to the upper chest. The sustained tachycardia of 120 beats per minute or greater usually reflects the hypoxaemia and the peak flow rate is often unrecordable except on low-flow models. The chest radiograph usually shows hyperlucency, occasionally collapse due to plugging, or a pneumothorax. Biochemical analysis shows a low potassium level and the urea may rise with clinical dehydration. The therapy of acute severe asthma is that of maintaining a safe arterial PaO_2 until the bronchoconstriction and inflammatory reactions are controlled. Oxygen by 24% Ventimask should be begun and careful monitoring of blood gases continued, adjusting inspiratory oxygen concentrations as required. The clinical dehydration should be treated with at least 3 litres of intravenous fluid in the initial 24 hours, supplementary potassium, 50 mmol/24 h, is added because of the effect of corticosteroids, salbutamol, and dehydration on potassium concentration (Nogrady, Hartley, and Seaton, 1977). The use of intravenous hydrocortisone with oral prednisolone supplements is necessary (500 mg. hydrocortisone 6 hourly until clinical improvement, 40 mg. prednisolone until control is obtained). The use of intravenous bronchodilators is necessary initially but there seems little place for intravenous aminophylline in this age group: many patients have taken sustained release oral theophyllines prior to admission and overdosage occurs easily and side-effects are often severe. Salbutamol (6 to 8 µg/kg over 15 min) is effective and safe; it may be repeated hourly or more frequently if clinical deterioration occurs. Little evidence exists to suggest that combining salbutamol and theophyllines is beneficial (Handslip, Dart, and Davies, 1982). With frequent PFR measurements, responsiveness to inhaled salbutamol (5 mg by nebulizer) can be assessed and when more than 15 per cent improvement is noted, i-v bronchodilators discontinued (Walters *et al.*, 1981). Infection as a precipitant is common, but the role of bacteria is controversial; ampicillin is generally satisfactory. The use of antacids, prophylactic cimetidine or ranitidine, and oral potassium should all be considered in view of the high steroid dosage.

Generally patients do well and after a day are improving with expectoration of plugs and increasing flow rates. Nocturnal or early morning dipping of PFR may be treated with sustained release theophyllines and as the oral prednisolone is reduced so inhaled corticosteroids are commenced. Combining such prophylactic therapy with inhaled salbutamol and ipratropium often produces gratifying control. The discharge of the patient depends less on cessation of symptoms and signs but more on PFR, as lung function changes may persist for some days (McFadden, Kisei, and De Groot, 1973). A PFR of 60 per cent of predicted is probably safe for consideration of discharge (Seaton, 1978).

The Worsening Asthmatic

The failure to respond to the above therapy or the progressive deterioration in asthmatics is indicated by increasing pulse rates and pulsus paradoxicus, hypoxaemia becomes marked, and hypercapnia ensues. Ventilation becomes mandatory. Rapid rehydration with 'Haemocell' or dextran maintains plasma volume during intubation after preoxygenation. Complete paralysis is maintained and a constant volume ventilator used. The high inspiratory pressures may contribute to pneumothoraces or mediastinal emphysema and salbutamol i-v should be continued. Rarely lavage by bronchoscopy may be indicated.

Such clinical states are often due to failure to seek early medical help, poor awareness of the severity of the attack, and underusage of corticosteroids (Macdonald, Seaton, and Williams, 1976).

Hypercapnic, Hypoxic Respiratory Failure Due to Chronic Bronchitis and Emphysema

This common geriatric emergency is an often-repeated problem in these patients (Geboes, 1979). The classical complaints of cough, sputum, and increasing dyspnoea and wheeze often antedate the first episode of respiratory failure by many years. The importance of sleep apnoea is now recognized as contributing to the hypoxaemia but most admissions are related to recent infection, often with *Haemophilus influenzae or Streptolocaccus pneumoniae* (Phillipson, 1978). Rarely a pneumothorax, general anaesthesia, abdominal surgery, or a cough fracture may be the precipitating cause. The rise in $PaCO_2$ above 50 mmHg and falling PaO_2 below 60 on air confirms the clinical diagnosis. Confusion and drowsiness rarely develop with $PaCO_2$ levels below 65 mmHg. The pulse is bounding and tremor marked. Cor pulmonale may be evident on clinical examination and 'p' pulmonale with right ventricular hypertrophy present on ECG (Hugh-Jones and Whimster, 1978). General supportive measures with controlled inspired oxygen (24 per cent initial concentration) and physiotherapy are essential. Infection should be treated but the role of bacteria is controversial (Tager and Speizer, 1975). Bronchodilators, both intravenous and nebulized, should be given and then corticosteroids if no improvement is obtained. The right heart failure is controlled with diuretics and digoxin may be indicated (Burrows, Kettel, and Niden, 1972).

Respiratory stimulants (e.g. Doxapram) are useful in the deteriorating patient and may both postpone artificial ventilation and allow better cooperation during physiotherapy (Moser, Shibel, and Beamen, 1973). The ventilation of the patient in hypercapnic hypoxic respiratory failure should not be undertaken lightly. It is rare to successfully ventilate the house-bound respiratory cripple and if commenced should follow the general principles of the severe asthmatic (Asmundsson and Kilburn, 1974).

Unilateral Pulmonary Hyperlucency

Unilateral pulmonary hyperlucency is usually due to a pneumothorax (Table 9); the clinical picture of dyspnoea, chest pain, and diminished air entry may not be clinically evident and the patient may be confused and in shock. Further, the radiographic detection of the hairline shadow of the collapsed lung may be difficult to separate when there are associated emphysematous bullae. Inspiration and expiration films may be necessary (Watt, 1978). Rarely the unilateral hyperlucency is due to a large pulmonary embolism reducing the vascularity, but usually there is elevation of the diaphragm, a small pleural effusion, and linear atelectasis. Uncommonly a 'check valve' effect may be seen due to bronchogenic tumour where the distal lung expands to compress the underlying normal lung. The management of pneumothoraces in the elderly is dependent on the degree of lung collapse and its physiological effects. Small pneumothoraces with few symptoms and a well-maintained PaO_2 (above 70 mmHg) can be treated conservatively with rest, supplementary high-flow oxygen, and observation. When dyspnoea supervenes and the PaO_2 falls below 70 mmHg active therapy is necessary. Intercostal intubation alone tends to be prolonged and active initiation of pleuritis with tetracycline (400 to 750 mg in 50 ml of sterile saline) is useful and effective (Goldszer *et al.*, 1979). Rarely surgical intervention by poudrage with kaolin or pleurectomy is indicated.

Table 9 Pneumothoraces in the elderly

LOCAL PULMONARY DISEASE
   Cavitatory or severe pneumonia
   Lung abscess
   Tuberculosis
   Bronchogenic carcinoma
DIFFUSE PULMONARY DISEASE
   Emphysema
   Asthma
   Pulmonary fibrosis
PENETRATING OR SEVERE THORACIC CAGE
   TRAUMA
IATROGENIC
   Artificial ventilation
   Thoracocentesis

PNEUMONIA IN THE ELDERLY

The investigation and management of the elderly pneumonia patient is complicated by the problem of accompanying underlying illness. Epidemiologically there is an increasing mortality from pneumonia with age (Fig. 5). The underlying reasons have been discussed (epidemiology), both depressed immunity and associated illness being relevant. The increased incidence of gram-negative bacterial pneumonia is associated with aspiration, this in turn is influenced by cerebrovascular disease and oesophageal motility. The diagnosis of bacterial pneumonia is more difficult than in the younger patient, there is a lack of cough, toxic confusion predominates, and dehydration occurs early. The early onset of bacteraemia, the increased risk of empyema, and meningitis contribute to the increased mortality (Macfarlane, Finch, and Ward, 1982; Mylotte and Bearn, 1981). *Klebsiella pneumoniae* occurs with increased frequency in the elderly, particularly the institutionalized or hospitalized patient, the incidence of colonization with gram-negative bacilli increasing with age and with debility and chronic disease (Phair, Kauffman, and Bjornson, 1978; Valenti, Jenzen, and Bentley, 1978). Pneumococcal pneumonia is more lethal in the elderly (Macfarlane, Finch, and Ward, 1982), accounting for up to 30 per cent of all community-acquired pneumonias and also as a nosocomial pneumonia. Therapy for bacterial pneumonia in the elderly also poses specific problems: some antibiotics are particularly toxic in the aged, the dose must often be modified because of renal impairment, and there is a wider range of pathogens with a more fulminant course.

Clinical Features

The classical features of pleuritic chest pain, cough, and purulent or blood-stained sputum are uncommon; the toxic confusional state with changes in social behaviour, intellect, and awareness occur progressively in the evolving patient. Extrapulmonary manifestations of pneumococcal meningitis may be masked by an apparent toxic state and the development of pericarditis attributed to ischaemic heart disease.

Progression of the pneumonia may produce further lung damage and abscess formation or rapidly extend to the pleura and produce an empyema (Benfield, 1981). The underlying chronic bronchitis and emphysema deteriorates further and acute respiratory failure supervenes.

Clinical signs are often limited, the patchy bronchial breathing in associating with toxic confusion being most common, but severe dehydration, meningism, or pericardial friction rubs may be present.

The radiographic picture is often severe with lobar consolidation, basal infiltrates, or necrotizing cavitation being most common (Jay, Johanson, and Pierce, 1975). The radiographic pattern may be helpful in establishing an aetiological organism (Table 10) (Fig. 12). Blood cultures are commonly positive in pneumococcal infections, a low white blood cell count in *Klebsiella* or *Legionella* infection, a leukaemoid reaction in tubercle. Gram staining of sputum is valuable, transtracheal aspiration should generally be avoided.

Table 10   Patterns of chest radiograph abnormalities in pneumonia

Lobar	1. Preservation of lobe	– pneumococcal
	2. Bulging of fissure	– staphylococci, klebsiella
	3. Associated collapse	– neoplasm
Segmental	1. With cavitation	– gram negative organisms anaerobes
	2. Basal	– aspiration; subdiaphragmatic focus
Widespread segmental	1. Septicaemia	
	2. Cavitation	– tuberculosis
	3. Viral or Mycoplasma	

Treatment

Early appropriate antibiotic therapy can dramatically improve the patient with community-acquired pneumococcal pneumonia. Benzyl penicillin remains the antibiotic of choice. The use of broad-spectrum antibiotics is not indicated for they encourage resistant organisms and predispose to nosocomial infection. The pulmonary and systemic com-

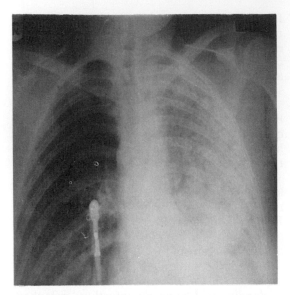

Figure 12   Pneumonia due to *Pneumococcus*

plications of pneumonia must be energetically sought with thoracocentesis, ultrasound, and other appropriate investigations.

Dehydration must be corrected adequately and central venous pressure monitoring may be performed if cardiac disease is suspected; underlying airways obstruction should be treated vigorously with nebulized bronchodilators and postured physiotherapy encouraged. Aspiration pneumonia is best avoided by the use of H-2 antagonists and antacids; antibiotics should be given preferably on the result of sputum culture; metronidazole is often effective with benzyl penicillin.

Nosocomial infection still carries a high mortality in spite of newer antibiotics; restriction of broad-spectrum antibiotics in clinical use reduces the incidence. Staphylococcal infections respond to flucloxacillin, although a second agent may be necessary such as clindamycin or fucidin. *Klebsiella* will usually respond to gentamycin with cefuroxine. Chloramphenicol remains a useful drug in bronchopneumonia with no specified causative organism.

Prophylaxis

The use of influenza vaccine in high-risk groups may be indicated as an annual vaccination. The place of pneumococcal vaccination in the elderly is currently undergoing investigation. The majority of isolates are included in the vaccine (Valenti, Jenzen, and Bentley, 1978) and the vaccine is immunogenic in the elderly. There may well be a role for this vaccine in institutionalized and high-risk groups.

PULMONARY REHABILITATION

There is a growing awareness that the respiratory cripple may significantly improve both the disordered physiology and psychology associated with severe respiratory disease by the use of an individually tailored programme. This programme requires emphasis on correct diagnosis, emotional and physical support, and appropriate therapy. Patients with severe airways obstruction respond best and there is evidence that programmed exercise improves effort tolerance (Cockcroft, Saunders, and Berry, 1981) and careful oxygen therapy alters both hospital admission rates and mortality (Medical Research Council Working Party, 1981). There will be an increasing need for an integrated response involving the family, physiotherapist, and physician to meet this challenge.

REFERENCES

Ali, M. K., and Ewer, M. S. (1980). 'Preoperative cardiopulmonary evaluation of patients undergoing surgery for lung cancer', *Cancer Bull.*, **32**, 100–104.

Antman, K. H. (1982). 'Malignant mesothelioma', *New Engl. J. Med.*, **303**, 200–202.

Asmundsson, T., and Kilburn, K. H. (1974). 'Survival after acute respiratory failure', *Ann. Intern. Med.*, **80**, 54–57.

Bakhle, Y. S., and Vane, J. R. (1977). *Metabolic Functions of the Lung*, Marcel Dekker, New York.

Bartlett, J. G. (1979). 'Anaerobic bacterial pneumonitis', *Am. Rev. Resp. Dis.*, **119**, 19–23.

Benfield, G. F. A. (1981). 'Recent trends in empyema thoracis', *Br. J. Dis. Chest*, **75**, 358–366.

Benjamin, B. (1977). 'Trends and differentials in lung cancer mortality', *W. H. Stat. Rep.*, **30**, 118–136.

Black, D. A. K., and Pole, J. D. (1975). 'Priorities in biochemical research: Indices of burden', *Br. J. Prev. Soc. Med.*, **29**, 222–227.

Block, E. R., and Stalcup, S. A. (1981). 'Metabolic functions of the lung', *Chest*, **81**, 215–223.

Bode, F. R., Pare, J. A. P., and Fraser, R. G.

(1974). 'Pulmonary diseases in the compromised host', *Medicine*, **53**, 255–293.

Burr, M. L., Charles, T. J., Roy, K., and Seaton, A. (1979). 'Asthma in the elderly: An epidemiological survey', *Br. Med. J.*, **1**, 1041–1044.

Burrows, B., Kettel, L. J., and Niden, A. H. (1972). 'Patterns of cardiovascular dysfunction in chronic obstructive lung disease', *New Engl. J. Med.*, **286**, 912–918.

Clot, J., Chamasson, E., and Bouchier, J. (1972). 'Age dependent changes of human blood lymphocyte subpopulations', *Clin. Exp. Immunol.*, **32**, 346–352.

Cockcroft, A. E., Saunders, M. J., and Berry, G. (1981). 'Randomised controlled trial of rehabilitation in chronic respiratory disability', *Thorax*, **36**, 200–203.

College of General Practitioners (1961). 'Chronic bronchitis in Great Britain', *Br. Med. J.*, **2**, 973–979.

Crofton, J., and Douglas, A. (1981). *Respiratory Diseases*, Blackwell Scientific Publications, Oxford.

Crystal, R. G., Godek, E., Ferrans, R. J., Fulmer, J. D., Line, E. R., and Hunninghake, G. W. (1981). 'Interstitial lung disease: Current concepts of pathogenesis, staging and therapy', *Am. J. Med.*, **70**, 542–568.

Davis, C., Campbell, E. J. M., Openshaw, P., Pride, N. B., and Woodruff, G. (1980). 'Importance of airway closure in limiting maximal expiration in normal man', *J. Appl. Physiol.*, **48**, 695–701.

Dawson, J. P. (1980). 'Consultations and treatment in the elderly', *Practitioner*, **224**, 466–467.

Del Fraissy, J. F. (1980). 'Age related impairment of the in vitro antibody response in the human', *Clin. Exp. Immunol.*, **39**, 208–214.

Demeter, S. L., Ahman, M., and Tomashefski, J. F. (1979). 'Drug induced pulmonary disease', *Clev. Clin.*, **46**, 89–124.

Dill, D. B., Hillyard, S. D., and Miller, J. (1980). 'Vital capacity, exercise performance and blood gases at altitude as related to age', *J. Appl. Physiol.*, **48**, 6–9.

Doll, R. (1970). 'Partial steps towards the prevention of bronchial carcinoma', *Scot. Med. J.*, **15**, 433–438.

Emmerling, P. (1979). 'Age related defence against infection with intra-cellular pathogens', *Gerontology*, **25**, 327–336.

Feld, R., Bodey, G. P., and Gröschel, D. (1974). 'Mycobacterioses in patients with malignant diseases', *Arch. Intern. Med.*, **136**, 67–70.

Fennesay, J. J. (1975). 'The radiology of lung cancer', *Med. Clin. N. Am.*, **59**, 95–120.

Flenley, D. C. (1981). *Respiratory Medicine*, Fig. 41, Baillier-Tindall.

Fletcher, C., and Pato, R. (1977). 'The natural history of chronic airflow obstruction', *Br. Med. J.*, **1**, 1645–1648.

Fulmer, J. D. (1982). 'An introduction to the interstitial lung diseases', *Clin. Chest Med.*, **3**, 457–474.

Geboes, K. (1979). 'Emergency admissions of aged people in a general hospital', *Acta. Clin. Belg.*, **34**, 288–295.

Georges, G. A., Saumon, G., and Loiseau, A. (1978). 'The relationship of age to pulmonary membrane conductance and capillary blood volume', *Am. Rev. Resp. Dis.*, **117**, 1069–1078.

Gibson, G. J., Pride, N. B., O'Cain, C., and Quagliato, R. (1976). 'Sex and age differences in pulmonary mechanics in normal non-smoking subjects', *J. Appl. Physiol.*, **41**, 20–25.

Goldszer, R. C., Bennett, J., Van Campen, J., and Rudnitzky, J. (1979). 'Intrapleural tetracycline for spontaneous pneumothorax', *JAMA*, **241**, 724–727.

Goodwin, J. S., Searles, R. P., and Tung, S. K. (1982). 'Immunological responses of a healthy population', *Clin. Exp. Immunol.*, **48**, 403–410.

Greenblatt, D. J., Sellers, E. M., and Shader, R. I. (1982). 'Drug disposition in old age', *New Engl. J. Med.*, **306**, 1081–1088.

Gulsvik, A. (1979). 'Prevalence of respiratory symptoms in the City of Oslo', *Scand. J. Resp. Dis.*, **60**, 275–285.

Handslip, P. D. J., Dart, A., and Davies, B. H. (1982). 'Intravenous salbutamol and aminophylline in asthma: A search for synergy', *Thorax*, **36**, 741–744.

Heitzman, E. R. (1981). 'Computed tomography of the thorax – current perspectives', *Am. J. Rad.*, **136**, 2–12.

Hugh-Jones, P., and Whimster, W. (1978). 'The aetiology and management of disabling emphysema', *Am. Rev. Resp. Dis.*, **117**, 343–378.

Hurwitz, J. A., Liben, A., and Becklake, M. R. (1980). 'Lung function in young adults – evidence for differences in the chronological age at which various functions start to decline', *Thorax*, **35**, 615–619.

Huxley, E. J., Vinslov, J., Gray, W. R., and Pierce, A. K. (1978). 'Pharyngeal aspiration in normal adults and patients with depressed consciousness', *Am. J. Med.*, **64**, 564–568.

Jay, S. J., Johanson, W. G., and Pierce, A. K. (1975). 'The radiographic resolution of strep. pneumoniae pneumonia', *New Engl. J. Med.*, **293**, 798–801.

Jones, F. L. Jr., and Ekberg, N. L. (1979). 'Exacerbation of asthma by Timolol', *New Engl. J. Med.*, **301**, 270.

Knudson, R. J., Clark, D. F., Kennedy, T. C., and Knudson, D. E. (1977). 'Effect of ageing alone on mechanical properties of the normal adult human lung', *J. Appl. Physiol.*, **43**, 1054–1062.

Krivoy, N., and Alroy, G. (1980). 'Oral theophylline in the elderly', *Respiration*, **40**, 233–236.

Kronenberg, R. S., and Drage, C. W. (1973). 'Attenuation of the ventilatory and heart rate responses to hypoxia and hypercapnia with ageing in normal men', *J. Clin. Invest.*, **52**, 1812–1819.

LeBlanc, P., Ruff, F., and Milic-Emili, J. (1970). 'Effects of age and body position on "airway closure" in man'. *J. Appl. Physiol.*, **28**, 448–451.

Leff, A., Hopwell, P. C., and Costello, J. (1978). 'Pleural effusion from malignancy', *Ann. Intern. Med.*, **88**, 532–537.

Macdonald, J. B., Seaton, A., and Williams, D. A. (1976). 'Asthma deaths in Cardiff-1963–74: 90 deaths outside hospital', *Br. Med. J.*, **1**, 1493–1495.

McFadden, E. R. Jr., Kiser, R., and De Groot, W. J. (1973). 'Acute bronchial asthma', *New Engl. J. Med.*, **288**, 221–225.

Macfarlane, J. T., Finch, R. G., Ward, M. J., and Mourae, A. D. (1982). 'Hospital study of adult community acquired pneumonia', *Lancet*, **2**, 255–257.

Makinodan, T. (1978). 'Mechanism of senescence of immune response', *Fed. Proc.*, **37**, 1239–1240.

Mauderly, J. L. (1978). 'Effect of age on pulmonary structure and function of immature and adult animals and man', *Fed. Proc.*, **38**, 173–177.

Medical Research Council Tuberculosis and Chest Disease Unit (1980). 'National survey of tuberculosis notifications in England and Wales 1978–9, *Br. Med. J.*, **281**, 895–898.

Medical Research Council Working Party (1981). 'Long term domiciliary oxygen therapy in chronic hypoxic cor pulmonale complicating chronic bronchitis and emphysema', *Lancet*, **1**, 681–686.

Miller, J. W., Hunter, A. M., and Horne, N. W. (1980). 'Intrapleural immunotherapy with *Corynebacterium parvum* in recurrent malignant pleural effusions', *Thorax*, **35**, 856–858.

Morris, J. F., Mosk, A., and Johnson, L. C., (1971). 'Spirometric standards for healthy nonsmoking adults', *Am. Rev. Resp. Dis.*, **103**, 57–67.

Moser, K. M., Shibel, E. M., and Beamon, A. J. (1973). 'Acute respiratory failure in obstructive lung disease', *JAMA*, **225**, 705–708.

Muiesan, G., Sorbini, C. A., and Grassi, V. (1971). 'Respiratory function in the aged', *Bull. Physiopath. Resp. (Nancy)*, **7**, 973–1009.

Murray, J. F. (1976). *The Normal Lung*, Saunders, Philadelphia.

Murray, J. F. (1981). 'The biological principles of disease', in *Pathophysiology*, (Eds L. D. Smith and S. O. Thier), Saunders, London.

Mylotte, J. M., and Bearn, T. R. (1981). 'Comparison of community acquired and nosocomial

pneumococcal bacteraemia', *Am. Rev. Resp. Dis.*, **123**, 265–268.

Niewoehner, D. E., and Kleinerman, J. (1964). 'Morphologic basis of pulmonary resistance in the human lung and effects of ageing', *J. Appl. Physiol.*, **36**, 412–418.

Nogrady, S. G., Hartley, J. R. P., and Seaton, A. (1977). 'Metabolic effects of intravenous salbutamol in the course of acute severe asthma', *Thorax*, **32**, 559–562.

Oswald, N. C., Hinson, K. F. W., Conti, G., and Miller, A. D. (1971). 'The diagnosis of primary lung cancer with special reference to sputum cytology', *Thorax*, **26**, 623–631.

Peterson, D. D., Pack, A. I., Silage, D. A., and Fishman, A. P. (1981). 'Effects of ageing on the ventilatory and occlusion pressure responses to hypoxia and hypercapnia', *Am. Rev. Resp. Dis.*, **124**, 387–391.

Phair, J. P., Kauffman, C. A., and Bjornson, A. (1978). 'Investigation of host defence mechanisms in the aged as determinants of nosocomial colonisation and pneumonia', *J. Reticuloendothel. Soc.*, **23**, 397–405.

Phillipson, E. A. (1978). 'Control of breathing during sleep', *Am. Rev. Resp. Dis.*, **118**, 909–939.

Proudfoot, A. T., Akhtor, A. J., Douglas, A. C., and Horne, N. W. (1969). 'Miliary tuberculosis in adults'. *Br. Med. J.*, **2**, 273–276.

Puchelle, E., Zohm, J. M., and Bertrand, A. (1979). 'Influence of age on bronchial mucociliary transport', *Scand. J. Resp. Dis.*, **60**, 307–313.

Royal College of Physicians (1981). 'Disabling chest disease – Prevention and care', *J. R. Coll. Phys. of Lond.*, **15**, 69–87.

Schwartz, K. M., O'Toole, R. D., Risher, R. H., and Sullivan, K. N. (1973). 'Anaerobic empyema thoracis', *Arch. Intern. Med.*, **131**, 521–527.

Seaton, A. (1978). 'The management of recurrent severe asthma', in *Advanced Medicine* D. J. (Ed. Wetherall), 14th ed., Pitman Medical, London.

Semine, A. A., and Damon, A. (1975). 'Costochondral ossification and ageing in five populations', *Hum. Biol.*, **47**, 101–116.

Silverberg, E. (1980). 'Cancer statistics 1980', *Ca.*, **30**, 23–38.

Sorbini, C. A., Grassi, V., Solinos, E., and Muiesan, G. (1968). 'Arterial oxygen tension in relation to age in healthy subjects', *Respiration*, **25**, 3–13.

Sostman, H. D., Motthoy, R. A., and Putman, C. E. (1977). 'Cytotoxic drug induced lung disease', *Am. J. Med.*, **62**, 608–615.

Stead, W. W. (1981). 'Tuberculosis among elderly persons: An outbreak in a nursing home', *Am. Intern. Med.*, **94**, 606–610.

Tager, I. B., and Speizer, F. (1975). 'The role of

infection in chronic bronchitis', *New Engl. J. Med.*, **292**, 563–571.

Thurlbeck, W. M., and Angus, G. E. (1975). 'Growth and ageing of normal human lung', *Chest*, **67** (Suppl), 3s–7s.

Turner, J. M., Mead, J., and Wohl, M. E. (1968). 'Elasticity of human lungs in relation to age', *J. Appl. Physiol.*, **25**, 664–671.

Turner-Warwick, M., and Strickland, B. (1981). 'Diagnosis of diffuse disorders of the lung', in *Thoracic Medicine* (Ed. P. Emerson), Butterworths, London.

Valenti, W. M., Jenzer, M., and Bentley, D. (1978). 'Type-specific penumococcal respiratory disease in the elderly and clinically ill', *Am. Rev. Resp. Dis.*, **117**, 233–238.

Walters, E. H., Cockcroft, A., Griffiths, T., Rocchiccioli, K., and Davies, B. H. (1981). 'Optimal dose of salbutamol respiratory solution: Comparison of three doses with plasma levels', *Thorax*, **36**, 625–628.

Wanner, A. (1977). 'Clinical aspects of muco-ciliary transport', *Am. Rev. Resp. Dis.*, **116**, 73–125.

Watt, A. G. (1978). 'Spontaneous pneumothorax: A review of 210 consecutive admissions to Royal Perth Hospital', *Med. J. Aust.*, **1**, 186–191.

Weinstein, L. (1980). 'The "new" pneumonia: The doctor's dilemma', *Ann. Intern. Med.*, **92**, 559–561.

Williams, D. M., Krick, J. A., and Remington, J. S. (1976). 'Pulmonary infection in the compromised host', *Am. Rev. Resp. Dis.*, **114**, 359–394; 593–627.

Zavala, D. C. (1978). 'Transbronchial biopsy in diffuse lung disease', *Chest*, **75**, 727–733.

16

Disorders of the
Nervous System

16.1

Neuropathology of Ageing

Gillian Cole

INTRODUCTION

With increasing age changes occur within the brain, as they do to a greater or lesser extent in other organs. The first section in this chapter deals with the morphological changes which occur in the brains of elderly subjects whose intellectual functions have been unimpaired during life. Many long and painstaking investigations have been carried out in relation to ageing and the brain, and any discussion of 'normal' ageing cannot help but overlap with that most common and devastating of disorders: Alzheimer's disease and senile dementia of the Alzheimer type. The morphological changes which separate so-called 'normal' ageing and dementia are identical, and the only point of distinction is quantitative. Furthermore, these changes cannot wholly be called specific for ageing, since they have been described in other less common disease processes, and in younger patients. Much progress has been made in this field of research, and one of the most important concepts to emerge is that dementia is no longer attributed merely to 'senile decay'; it is a disease process and therefore potentially treatable and hopefully preventable within the foreseeable future.

The second section in this chapter is concerned with the neuropathology of the dementias and non-dementing diseases of the aged. Conditions which are not exclusive to the elderly but are more common in this group have been included.

THE AGEING BRAIN

Macroscopic Appearance of the Ageing Brain

With increasing age the coverings of the brain become thickened and fibrous. The dura is often found to be firmly adherent to the skull vault, and the leptomeninges appear somewhat opaque and thickened. This change is often more apparent over the convexities of the hemispheres.

Some degree of atrophy of the brain is common, and this is reflected in reduced brain weight and volume, shrinkage of grey and white matter components, and often an increase in the size of the ventricles.

A variable shrinkage of the cortical gyri, with widening of the sulci between them, is best appreciated by stripping of the leptomeninges, and is usually most prominent in the fronto-temporal region. A coronal section through an atrophic brain will demonstrate gyral atrophy, widened sulci, and fissures, especially the lateral fissure. Because of loss of white matter the ventricles undergo compensatory enlargement of variable degree, which is usually most obvious in the lateral ventricles.

Brain Weight

Adult brain weight decreases with age and the ventricles become larger, although there is considerable variation within the ageing brain. The figures given by workers in this field vary according to their method and selection of material. The brain weight of a young male adult is about 1,400 g and by the fifth decade is reduced to around 1,375 g, and subsequently to 1,200 to 1,300 g. The female brain weighs on an average 100 g less in adult life (Corsellis, 1976).

The majority of studies show reasonable correlation, with a larger weight loss recorded in those over 60 years of age. No really large series of figures exist for the brain weights of the intellectually normal aged population, and in some studies weight loss is not as great as other workers have shown. Tomlinson (1979) makes the important point that it is easy to include early undetected senile dementias in such studies.

The use of computerized axial tomography (CAT) is proving a valuable method for assessing the degree of cortical atrophy and ventricular enlargement in living subjects. Huckman, Fox, and Topel (1975) reported the results of a study involving a series of abnormal (senile dementia) brains and normal elderly brains. Within the normal group, atrophy was present in 25 per cent., slightly enlarged ventricles were found in 10 per cent., and moderate to severe enlargement in 10 per cent. In Tomlinson's study of 28 intellectually normal aged brains, the incidence of ventricular enlargement tended to be higher. Tomlinson attributed this to the deliberate inclusion of cases of stroke in his series (Tomlinson, Blessed, and Roth, 1968).

Davis and Wright (1977) devised an accurate method of measuring the volume of the cranial cavity and of the brain at autopsy; these normally bear a constant relationship to each other. Brain atrophy is reflected by observing any deviation from this relationship. The authors found a remarkably consistent atrophy among the neurologically normal group of 33 patients over 70 years of age, with only 4 cases within the normal range of brain volume/cavity volume percentage ratio for those under 50 years. They do state, however, that no systematic measures of mental function were available for their cases.

While a considerable variation exists within the ageing brain, there is most often weight loss, reflected by brain atrophy and ventricular size. As more sophisticated and accurate methods of study continue, those areas of uncer-

tainty such as the relationship between brain atrophy and ventricular size are likely to be clarified.

Microscopic Changes in the Ageing Brain

The cortical atrophy described above is reflected histologically by changes in the architecture of the neurones and a decrease in their numbers. Commonly seen neuronal changes include a non-specific cell shrinkage with some loss of Nissl substance.

Lipofuscin

There is an increase in the amount of lipofuscin (an acid-fast lipopigment) within the neuronal cytoplasm. This accumulation of lipofuscin is not ubiquitous, since neurones in different sites and with different functions vary considerably in the amount of lipofuscin they normally possess. Shrinkage of the neurone may give a false impression of pigment increase. The Purkinje cells of the cerebellum, for instance, possess very little lipofuscin, while large amounts may be found in some of the cranial and motor spinal nuclei, and in parts of the thalamus. The function of lipofuscin is discussed in Chapter 16.2.

Hirano Bodies

These are eosinophilic, rod-like inclusions found within neurones, mainly in the region of Sommer's sector in the hippocampus. They may be found in the normal aged brain and in many degenerative conditions. Their electron microscopic features are described by Hirano and coworkers (1968).

Neuronal Cell Loss

Unlike most other cells in the human body, the neurone cannot undergo cell division, and thus once destroyed cannot be replaced. It has been estimated that the brain contains in excess of 20 thousand million neurones. There is now no doubt that at least in some areas of the brain the numbers of neurones decline with increasing age. The technical difficulties in accurately counting neurones or other cells in the brain are intimidating. This problem is gradually being overcome by new techniques, which include the use of computerized equipment.

Earlier studies are few, and one of the most important is the work of Brody (1955), whose time consuming and careful study, which involved counting cells in specific cortical areas, demonstrated a decrease in neurones with increasing age, and this was particularly marked in the superior temporal gyrus. In a later study (Brody, 1970), a marked loss of nuerones was noted in the superior frontal gyrus and the precentral gyrus, while there was a far less significant decrease in the postcentral gyrus and inferior temporal gyrus. A carefully controlled study by Henderson, Tomlinson, and Weightman (1975) compared the results of cell counting in the cerebral cortex by a traditional method using photomicrographs, and by the use of an image analyser. It is gratifying that although the manual counts yielded higher numbers for total cells, and smaller numbers for large cells, there was high correlation between the two methods. The time saved by the use of the image analyser is of course a tremendous advantage.

In a later study Tomlinson and Henderson (1976) confirmed a notable loss of neurones in various sites of the cerebral cortex in old age. In most sites examined this was as high as between 40 and 50 per cent. The patients over the age of 65 were nearly all examined during life and were found to be intellectually normal.

Quantitative biochemical methods (De Kosky and Bass, 1980) demonstrated that cell loss in the frontal cortex of aged demented patients did not differ significantly from that found in age matched controls. This is in keeping with the findings of Terry and coworkers (1977) that there are no significant cell count differences between the normal aged and senile brain.

There are marked variations in neurone loss in the different sites of the brain in which cell counts have been estimated. Hall, Miller, and Corsellis (1975) confirmed by systematic measurements and Purkinje cell counts in 90 cerebellums that the Purkinje cell population dropped by an average of 2.5 per cent. per decade, over the age span from 0 to 100 years, but there were not unexpected wide individual variations.

In some brainstem nuclei there appears to be a remarkable consistency of neurone population, with little or no fall-out in old age. No loss of neurones has been found to occur in old age in the ventral cochlear nucleus (Konigsmark and Murphy, 1972), nor the sixth nerve nucleus (Vijayashankar and Brody, 1977).

The neurones of the inferior olivary nucleus appear to remain consistent even into extreme old age (Monagle and Brody, 1974). In a study of the nucleus of the locus ceruleus, Brody (1978) reports that after the age of 65 years there is a marked decrease in cell number, which in the majority of cases was about 40 per cent. The nuclear cells of the locus ceruleus are rich in monoamine oxidase inhibitors, which are concerned with the suppression of REM sleep. The pertinent suggestion that this cell decrease may explain alterations of sleep patterns in the elderly is of considerable interest.

From these and ongoing studies it is clear that neuronal loss varies from insignificant to marked according to the site examined. That there is no significant difference in cell counts in the brains of 'normal' ageing or senile dements implies that neuronal cell depletion *per se* is not the aetiologic factor of importance in senile dementia.

Astrocytes

In the ageing brain it is extremely common to find an increase in astrocytic glial fibre formation. This increased gliosis may be well demonstrated with a phosphotungstic acid haemotoxylin (PTAH) stain. Gliosis may be particularly prominent in the subpial cortex, periventricular regions, and surrounding small vessels. It may also be marked in the inferior olivary nucleus and dentate nucleus. The astrocytes may appear more prominent in these affected sites.

No significant changes associated with ageing are known to occur in the oligodendroglial or microglial cells.

Corpora Amylacea

Occasional corpora amylacea may be found in the brains of relatively young adults, but they are present in increasing numbers from middle age and are invariably present in the brains of aged individuals. These familiar structures may be found anywhere in the brain, but are particularly common in the subpial area of the cerebral cortex, in the white matter near the ependymal lining of the ventricles, and in a perivascular situation, especially in the white matter. They may be found in large numbers in degenerating white matter, and in many other pathological conditions for example, in the vicinity of an old area of softening. Quantitative studies in relation to their increase in number with age and in various pathological conditions are not yet available (Tomlinson, 1979).

cea appear as rounded structures varying in diameter from about 7 to 20 μm. On haematoxylin and eosin (H/E) stains they consist of amorphous basophilic material, which often stains more intensely in the centre (Fig. 1). They stain positively with many different agents including methyl violet and are metachromatic with toluidine blue. Electron microscopic studies (Ramsay, 1965) demonstrate that they are contained within the processes of fibrous astrocytes. Their chemical structure, which appears to be composed mainly of a glycogen-like substance, has been analysed by Stam and Roukema (1973).

Neuraxonal Dystrophy

Swellings on the axon terminals, both in the central and peripheral nervous system, lead to the formation of axonal spheroids. These may be found in various pathological conditions, particularly as a result of cerebral trauma, but they are also regularly found in certain sites in normal ageing. Viewed under the light microscope on H/E, they appear as eosinophilic or paler hyaline, spheroid, or ovoid structures, measuring from 15 to120 μm across. With increasing age they become more intensely eosinophilic. They eventually undergo further degenerative changes, which may lead to an apparently empty space, but until this time are strongly argyrophilic. Their histochemical structure is of a major protein component with amino acid content and small amounts of phospholipids and carbohydrates (Jellinger, 1973).

The electron microscopic appearance shows that many of the spheroids are partially or totally surrounded by myelin sheaths, though these may be thinned. They are filled with varying amounts of tubulomembranous structures, neurofilaments, abnormal mitochondria, and electron-dense round to ovoid structures.

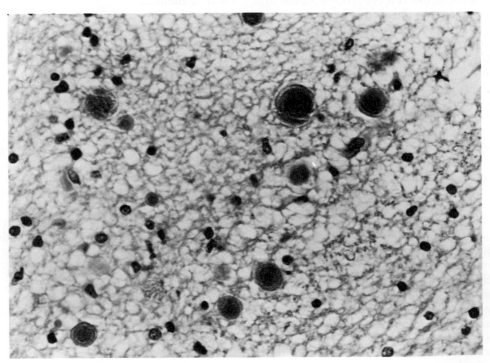

Figure 1   Corpora amylacea in the periventricular area of the brain (H/E ×400)

In normal ageing the formation of spheroids occurs in certain sites, and they are most commonly present in the gracile nucleus. To a lesser degree the substantia nigra, globus pallidus, and anterior horn cells may be affected. The main areas of involvement have been quantitatively studied by a number of workers and are found to increase in number with advancing age.

It seems likely that the formation of these axonal spheroids may lead to impaired synaptic and axon transport mechanisms. Involvement of synapses of somatosensory neurones and in afferent pathways of motor regulation sites, namely the gracile nucleus and substantia nigra suggests an effect on movement coordination, and senile dorsal column ataxia might be attributed to such a process (Seitelberger, 1980).

Cortical Dendrites

Age-related changes within the dendritic processes of the neurones have been demonstrated by a number of workers, using the Golgi technique. The branches of the dendritic system normally contain small protuberances or spines, and studies on rat visual cortex have revealed a gradual, continuous loss of spines which occurs with age (Feldman, 1976). Studies on human cortex include that of Scheibel and coworkers (1976a and 1976b), who have shown that in the aged there is an increasing loss of dendritic spines, followed by loss of dendritic processes, which first affects the horizontal branches. This change is accompanied by swellings on the dendrites, particularly at branching points, and between the apical shaft and parent cell body. Eventually there is loss of affected neurones and replacement gliosis. These investigators studied the prefrontal and temporal cortex and found the third pyramidal layer to be most affected. The importance of diminished synaptic connections as a result of distortion and loss of dendrites is emphasized by Scheibel (1978), and in particular its relation to decreased intellectual function in senile dementia, where the changes are reported to be more severe than in normal ageing. Buell and Coleman (1981) carried out quantitative studies of the parahippocampal gyrus, and demonstrated that clinically normal aged individuals had longer and more branched dendrites than either adults with a mean age of 51 or

those with senile dementia. Their observation was that neurological deterioration associated with normal advancing age was not reflected in the reduced extent of single neurones and that neurones continue to elaborate dendritic material into the tenth decade. In senile dementia the authors found no evidence of continued growth, but nor did they find profound loss of dendrites. Buell and Coleman suggest that the dendritic system may not be directly affected in senile dementia, but that the cause may be biochemical (e.g. neurotransmitter dysfunction) or that there is a threshold effect in which dendritic growth in normal ageing may compensate for neuronal loss and other changes. Compensation for the more severe changes in senile dementia might be ineffective. The fact that dendritic changes were found in all their groups is at variance with the findings of Scheibel and coworkers, and with some other quantitative studies on aged rat cortex. Differences in the findings by various investigators may be explained by a number of factors which include the technique used in quantitative and qualitative methodology, the experimental material used, and the difficulties inherent in the application of the sensitive, and sometimes capricious, Golgi technique to autopsy material. This does not detract from the value of the investigations, and further studies will surely elucidate these interesting and important issues.

Cerebrovascular Changes and Ageing

Certain changes occur within the cerebrovascular system as age advances, but do not result in any obvious neurological disease. Atherosclerosis is the most common cerebrovascular disease to affect the elderly, although not exclusive to the ageing population. This and other conditions which may cause neurological disease will be discussed later.

Histology

The capillaries of the central nervous system (CNS) have the same basic histological appearance as elsewhere in the body. They differ in the absence of a reticulin envelope and the presence of a covering by the foot plates of the astrocytes. The cerebral arteries have a thinner media than arteries elsewhere in the body and possess a well developed internal elastic lamina, but no external elastic layer.

With increasing age the cerebral vessels of the meninges and brain and spinal cord show mild changes. They are slightly thickened and the media of the arteries tend to become hyalinized and more fibrous. Within the media of some vessels deposition of calcium, iron, and other minerals may be evident. This is most commonly seen in the vessels of the basal ganglia, particularly the putamen and globus pallidus, the hippocampus, and cerebellum. The perforating cortical arteries, arterioles, capillaries, and venules tend to coil or show a 'corkscrew' effect, which is apparent with each advancing decade (Fang, 1976).

Amyloid

On light microscopy, with an H/E stain, amyloid stains as a pale pink amorphous substance. Its origin remains obscure, but it may be positively identified by the characteristic staining properties, the best known of which is the Congo red stain which gives a green fluorescence with polarized light. Its appearance on electron microscopy is that of long unbranched fibrils. These fibrils are composed of polypeptide chains.

The CNS is rarely affected by familial, primary, or secondary amyloidosis, but it is well recognized that amyloid may accumulate in certain organs of aged human beings. In patients over 70 years of age Wright and coworkers, (1969) demonstrated amyloid in 63 per cent. of brains, while 37 per cent. had cardiac amyloid, 50 per cent. had aortic amyloid, and 30 per cent pancreatic amyloid. These were the organs most commonly affected, and the frequency with which it was found was significantly higher in older patients when compared to a 30 to 70 year age group.

Amyloid Angiopathy

Scholtz (1938) described the amyloid like deposits in the media and adventitia of cerebral arterioles of older subjects. This phenomenon has since been quite extensively studied, and the amyloid nature of the deposits have been confirmed by electron microscopic studies (Terry and Wisniewski, 1972). Amyloid most frequently involves the arterioles and precapillaries, and in severe cases the veins may also be affected. The incidence of amyloid angiopathy is found to rise with age, and appears to be higher in demented patients (Morimatsu *et al.*, 1975).

The Choroid Plexus in Ageing

With increasing age amyloid has been found in the small vessels of the choroid plexus. Interstitial fibrosis is quite common and calcification of concentric, laminated bodies, sometimes referred to as psammoma bodies, are often present. Few quantitative studies have been done, but most pathologists have the impression that stromal and vascular calcification are seen with more frequency in the elderly. Simple choroid plexus cysts, rarely larger than about 1 cm, are not uncommonly found at autopsy among older age groups.

Pineal Gland

Small cysts are a fairly common autopsy finding in the pineal gland. Larger examples in later life are attributed to a degenerative process in the central core of fibrillary glial cells (Russell and Rubinstein, 1971). They are rarely large enough to cause symptoms. Calcified psammoma bodies are commonly seen after the first decade.

In a study of the relationship of the weight of the pineal gland to age and malignancy, Rodin and Overall (1967) found a size and weight increase with maturity and ageing. The parenchymal cells (pineocytes) were reported to remain similar in size from 2 to 91 years. Findings were not dissimilar in the patients who had died of cancer.

The Pituitary Gland

The average weight of the human pituitary gland is maximal in the fourth decade. Weight loss is said to be mainly from the anterior lobe and slowly declines with age, until 70 years, after which the loss is more rapid. References for the source of these figures, including a report on a slight increase in the percentage of basophils in old age, is given by Lockett (1976).

Neurofibrillary Degeneration

This change was first described by Alzheimer at the beginning of the century. On light microscopy the neurofibrillary tangle (NFT) is not readily detected on routine H/E stains, but is well demonstrated with the use of silver impregnations, such as the von Braunmühl stain. The alteration mainly occurs within certain areas of the cerebral cortex, particularly the medial temporal area and deeper grey matter. They are found in less common sites in some specific pathological conditions. The affected neurones have a dramatic appearance. Thickened and distorted fibrils course through the neuronal cytoplasm and assume a variety of bizarre shapes, such as loops, skeins, and thickened triangular bands (Fig. 2). Eventually the nucleus and cytoplasm are obscured.

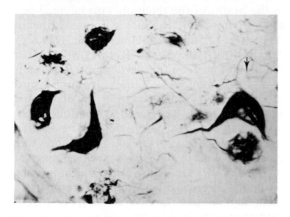

Figure 2   Neurofibrillary tangles in cerebral cortex showing thickened, distorted fibrils within the neuronal cytoplasm (arrow). Senile plaques are also present (von Braunmühl ×630)

The electron microscopic appearance has been studied in detail by many workers which include Kidd (1964), Terry (1963), Terry and Wisniewski (1970, 1972), and Wisniewski, Narang, and Terry (1976). Ultrastructurally the NFT is made up of paired helical filaments, which on longitudinal section are about 22 nm wide and have a constriction at intervals varying from 60 to 80 nm. These abnormal filaments are morphologically unlike any of the normal neurofibres; namely neurotubules, neurofilaments, and microfilaments (Iqbal *et al.*, 1980). It has been shown that there is a depletion of normal microtubules in the affected neurones. These tangled filaments fill most of the peri-karyon and displace the organelles normally present in that site. There is some uncertainty as to whether the tangled structures are actually of tubular or filamentous origin, since immunocytochemical studies have produced conflicting results. Recent studies demonstrate that the protein within the NFT is antigenically related to either the protein of normal neurofilament or neurotubulin (Eng *et al.*, 1980, Gambetti *et al.*, 1980, Grundke-Iqbal *et al,*, 1979.). Its unique and exact identity is not yet certain. The subject of neuronal fibrous proteins is reviewed by Shelanski and Selkoe (1981). Neither the pathogenesis of the NFT nor the precise effect of its formation is fully established, but there seems little doubt that normal metabolic and transport mechanisms must be impaired.

The Senile Plaque

These structures were first described by Blocq and Marinesco (1892). They are commonly associated with the presence of NFT in Alzheimer's disease, but either may predominate. The senile plaque (SP) is frequently found in small numbers in the ageing brain. It occurs most often in the cerebral cortex, particularly in the depths of the sulci, but may also be seen in similar sites to the NFT. On light microscopy they are not detectable with routine H/E stains, but are easily demonstrated with a variety of silver impregnation techniques, such as the von Braunmühl method. They are then seen as rounded, argyrophilic foci of granular and fibrillary structures (Fig. 3). They vary in diameter from 5 to 100 μm (Corsellis, 1976) and may coalesce.

In many of the plaques the central core stains positively for amyloid. The electron microscopic features have been described by many investigators, and there is general agreement concerning their ultrastructure (Terry, 1980; Terry and Wisniewski, 1972; Wisniewski and Terry, 1976). The plaque consists of three major elements: degenerating neuronal processes, reactive glial cells, and amyloid. The predominating element in a particular plaque determines its appearance on light microscopy. There are three major classes of plaque; viz. primitive, classical (or mature), and the burnt-out plaque. The primitive plaque consists of abnormal small neurites (axons and

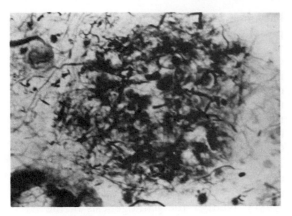

Figure 3 Senile plaque in the cerebral cortex showing a rounded argyrophilic mass of altered fibrillar and granular material (von Braunmühl ×630)

dendrites), many of which are presynaptic terminals. The neurites are packed with abnormal degenerating mitochondria. As the number of neurites increase, small amounts of amyloid are detectable. The classical or mature plaque contains a central core of amyloid which is surrounded by altered neurites containing degenerate mitochondria, acid phosphatase containing dense bodies, and abnormal fibrillar material. This fibrillar material is identical to the paired helical filaments described in the NFT. Macrophages containing lipofuscin, smaller amounts of cellular debris, and occasional astrocytic processes are present. The burnt out plaque consists almost entirely of amyloid, with maybe occasional macrophages and astrocytic processes surrounding it. The degenerating neurites are no longer visible at this stage.

The causal significance of senile plaque formation and amyloid deposition is uncertain. It has been suggested that the escape of antigen–antibody complexes from cerebral blood vessels might lead to the deposition of amyloid and perhaps damage neurites and initiate plaque formation. There is a possibility that the amyloid within senile plaques is derived from IgG (Ishii and Maga, 1976), which suggests that immunological factors are involved.

Animal Studies

Studies have been carried out on a variety of animals for the presence of ageing changes. Dayan (1971) examined the brains of 147 dif-

ferent species of aged animals and birds. He was unable to detect any senile plaques or neurofibrillary tanges in any of the species. He records the presence of a single corpora amylacea in an aged dog. Wisniewski and coworkers, (1970) found some senile plaques in the brains of dogs, which except for the absence of paired helical filaments were indentical to those found in the human brain. Similar plaques to those found in the dog have been found in the brains of aged rhesus monkeys (Wisniewski, Ghetti, and Terry 1973).

Senile plaques and nuerofibrillary tangles are found in the normal human ageing brain and many studies have been made in relation to their frequency and site of distribution. It has been demonstrated that there is a marked quantitative difference between the numbers and distribution of plaques and tangles found in the brains of the mentally normal aged person and those of Alzheimer's disease and senile dementia of the Alzheimer type (SDAT). Tomlinson, Blessed, and Roth (1968) showed that NFTs were either absent or present in very small numbers in the cortex or deeper grey matter of elderly people who had been specifically tested and found to be intellectually normal until shortly before death. The anterior temporal lobe was the only site where they could be found in significant numbers, and the main sites of predilection were the hippocampus and amygdaloid nucleus. In comparison demented subjects had NFT and senile plaque formation which was far more frequent and widespread (Tomlinson, Blessed, and Roth, 1970). Further studies by Tomlinson (1972) revealed that sparse numbers of NFT were found in about 5 per cent. of apparently normal individuals in the hippocampus by the fifth decade. By the seventh decade almost 60 per cent. had some involvement, and by the tenth decade nearly all cases showed some NFT. Senile plaques were present in small numbers in 15 per cent. of subjects in the fifth decade, in over 50 per cent in the seventh decade, and in 75 per cent. by the ninth decade. Dayan (1970) demonstrated a statistically significant relationship between increasing age and frequency of plaques and NFT in the frontal cortex and hippocampus of normal individuals between 30 and 89 years.

Terry (1978) comments on the possibility that there is a continuous spectrum between normality and dementia that because of factors which may be endo- or exogenous, a concentration of lesions is attained, resulting in functional loss with the clinical picture varying from mild forgetfulness to dementia.

Granulovacuolar Degeneration

With very few exceptions this change occurs only in the cytoplasm of the hippocampal neurones. On routine H/E stains under light microscopy, granulovacuolar degeneration is clearly seen. It is characterized by one or several clear vacuoles in the cytoplasm of the neurone, within which a central granule is visible. The granules are argyrophilic (Fig. 4). Electron microscopic studies reveal them to be bounded by a unit membrane containing clear material and a core of dense, finely granular matter. Granulovacuolar degeneration may be found in the normal ageing brain, but is present in much larger numbers of hippocampal neurones in SDAT and Alzheimer's disease. Quantitative studies on normal and demented brains have demonstrated a positive correlation with age during the sixth to ninth decades,

and in Alzheimer's disease the density of affected cells is very much higher than that of age-matched controls. In the latter group it is rare for more than 9 per cent of cells to be involved (Ball and Lo, 1977; Tomlinson and Kitchener, 1972; Woodard, 1962, 1966).

Neurofibrillary Tangles, Senile Plaques, and Granulovacuolar Change

The NFT, senile plaque, and granulovacuolar degeneration are all degenerative changes which are relatively non-specific. Apart from normal ageing they may be seen in large numbers in Alzheimer's disease and SDAT, and indeed the histological diagnosis is untenable in their absence. Neurofibrillary tangles, senile plaques, and granulovacuolar degeneration are invariably present in the brains of patients with Down's syndrome who are over the age of 40 (Olsen and Shaw, 1969). In dementia pugilistica, NFTs are found which are identical to those in Alzheimer's disease (Corsellis, Bruton, and Freeman-Browne, 1973), but for unknown reasons there is a peculiar sparsity of plaques in the cases examined. Neurofibrillary

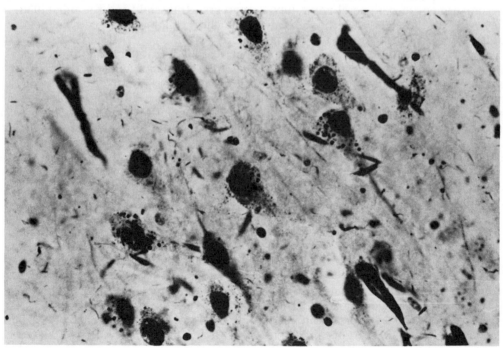

Figure 4   Granulovacuolar degeneration within the hippocampal pyramidal neurones. There are densely staining granules within cytoplasmic vacuoles. Some neurofibrillary tanges are present (von Braunmühl ×375)

tangles are seen in postencephalitic Parkinsonism, the Guam–Parkinsonism dementia complex, and occasionally in cases of subacute sclerosing panencephalitis. In supranuclear palsy, NFTs are present in affected areas of the brain, but are quite different ultrastructurally.

AGEING OF THE SPINAL CORD AND PERIPHERAL NERVES

Within the spinal cord age-related changes are similar to, but less frequent than, those of the brain. However, neurofibrillary tangles, senile plaques, and granulovacuolar change do not occur in the spinal cord. Mild atherosclerotic changes may be evident in the spinal arteries, but amyloid angiopathy has not been reported. Corpora amylacea are found in increasing numbers in the white matter of the cord, especially near the pial surface and surrounding blood vessels. Neuroaxonal spheroids are quite frequently present, particularly within the gracile nucleus, and this may be reflected by mild gliosis and myelin pallor of the gracile columns (Dayan, 1978). Gliosis is increased within the subependymal regions of the cord.

Some impairment of peripheral nerve function may occur in the elderly which is not attributable to a specific disorder. Several investigators have demonstrated evidence of segmental demyelination, indicating Schwann cell damage, and Wallerian-type degeneration, indicating axonal damage. Such changes are usually mild, but are apparent in teased fibre preparations and common in subjects over 60 years of age (Arnold and Harriman, 1970). Slowing of peripheral and central nerve conduction in elderly people has been demonstrated by Dorfman and Bosley (1979).

AGEING AND NEUROLOGICAL DISEASE

The Dementias

Numerous conditions may lead to, or are commonly associated with, dementia. Many of these, such as metabolic disorders, brain infections, intracranial tumours, are not confined to the elderly, and discussion of them is not included in this chapter. The most important forms of dementia associated with ageing are Alzheimer's disease, SDAT, and multi-infarct dementia. The rarer dementias associated with ageing are discussed.

Included in this section are non-dementing neurological disorders of the elderly, and those diseases which are not age associated but more commonly present in that age group. Some of the rare system degenerations may occur in elderly patients, but a full discussion of them is beyond the scope of this chapter. Reference to such disorders may be found in *Greenfield's Neuropathology* (Blackwood and Corsellis, 1976).

Alzheimer's Disease

In 1907 Alzheimer reported the case of a 51 year old woman with dementia. The histopathological findings in the brain that he described, namely the presence of abundant neurofibrillary tangles and senile plaque formation, were identical to those later described in senile dementia. There has been a good deal of controversy as to whether Alzheimer's (presenile) dementia, as originally described by him, can justifiably be considered a different disease from senile dementia. Among earlier workers, Rothschild and Kasanin (1936) stated that the pathological process tended to be more severe in Alzheimer's disease. It has been argued that clinical differences distinguish the two conditions, but these are far from clear-cut and are not apparent in severe cases. The only obvious difference relates to age of onset, and many investigators felt there was no valid basis for separating a pathologically and clinically identical disease occurring in the presenium (usually considered to be under 65 years) from those in an older age group (Neumann and Cohn, 1953; Newton, 1947; Raskin and Ehrenberg, 1956). At present it is regarded as a single disease entity by the majority of investigators. Among others, Terry (1978) has pointed out that those patients with the presenile form are younger and therefore less prone to diseases affecting the elderly. Consequently they live longer and may have a greater concentration of brain lesions. Following the Workshop Conference on Alzheimer's disease, 'Senile Dementia and Related Disorders', Katzman, Terry, and Bick (1978) reported on the recommended terminology by the working committees. It was agreed that the conditions present with almost identical clinical and pathological manifestations, but that 'unknown aetiological factors might be operative in, for example a 50 year old as compared to an 80 year old'. The commission recommended that the disorder in the presenile age group be termed Alzheimer's disease and in the senile age group be termed senile dementia of the Alzheimer type (SDAT).

Clinical Features

In brief, the clinical picture is that of a slowly progressive mental deterioration, with memory defect, disorientation, and confusion, eventually leading to profound dementia. Focal symptoms are quite often present.

Pathological Changes

The brain is atrophic and may weigh as little as 950 g. The leptomeninges are often opaque and thickened. Cortical atrophy with widening of the sulci may be particularly apparent in the frontal region, and the temporal lobes may be severely involved, particularly in the hippocampal region. Variation in the degree of atrophy mainly depends on how long the disease was present before death. Coronal sections of the brain reveal a usually marked enlargement of the ventricles (Fig. 5) and the narrowed atrophic cortex can be appreciated. The deeper grey matter structures may be smaller than usual.

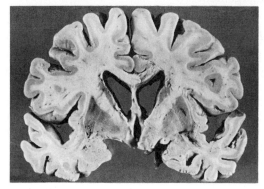

Figure 5 Alzheimer's disease. Coronal section of brain showing marked frontotemporal atrophy. Note the shrunken gyri, widened sulci, and enlarged ventricles

Light Microscopic Findings

The outstanding histological feature is the presence of abundant senile plaques and neurofibrillary tangles. The detailed structures of these have already been described. They are intensely argyrophilic and best demonstrated by the use of a silver stain. The senile plaques and neurofibrillary tangles are present throughout the cortex, in varying intensities. Some plaques may be confluent, and hence appear larger than usual, and plaques may be particularly numerous in the depths of the sulci. Both tangles and plaques are often seen in greatest intensity in the hippocampus and amygdaloid nucleus. Neurofibrillary tangles and senile plaques may be present in more or less equal numbers, or one may predominate over the other. There are numerous reports on the increased frequency of these changes when compared with the brain of the intellectually normal aged person (see above). Neurofibrillary tangles in smaller numbers have occasionally been reported in the hypothalamus, basal ganglia, and occasionally in the brainstem. Granulovacuolar degeneration is present in large numbers of the hippocampal pyramidal neurones. A number of workers have demonstrated a far greater number of affected cells than in the intellectually normal aged brain (see above).

Neuronal loss in the cortex may be difficult to assess, and reference has already been made to some of the recent studies, where the evidence suggests that there is no significant difference between nerve cell loss in Alzheimer's disease, SDAT, and 'normal' ageing. Certain nuclei and specific areas may, however, show more cell loss than age matched controls. Tomlinson, Irving, and Blessed (1981) believe there is some evidence for a greater loss of neurones in the locus coeruleus in severe cases of SDAT. The amygdaloid nucleus has been studied by Herzog and Kemper (1980), who demonstrated a significant decrease in volumetric and cell packing density when comparing SDAT with age matched controls.

Other changes in the neurone include those associated with normal ageing. Increased amounts of lipofuscin within the neuronal cytoplasm, has been shown to be no greater than in a control group (Mann and Sinclair, 1978). There is an increased amount of gliosis in the subpial and subependymal areas and in the inferior olivary nuclei. Amyloid angiopathy may be prominent in some cases of Alzheimer's disease, and this change has been found to be more frequent in the hippocampus in demented than in non-demented cases. Hirano bodies are found with increased frequency in the hippocampal pyramidal layer in cases of Alzheimer's disease and SDAT than in normal subjects of the same age group.

There is evidence that dendritic arborization is less extensive in Alzheimer's disease and SDAT. That other degenerative processes affect nerve endings in Alzheimer's disease and SDAT is demonstrated by the presence of presynaptic material in senile plaques. A considerable number of investigators have demonstrated how these changes are reflected in various neurotransmitters. Choline acetyl transferase (CAT), which is a marker for cholinergic neurones, is reduced in Alzheimer's disease and SDAT, and has been shown to correlate with the reduction in the amount of acetylcholine synthesis. Cholinergic neurones are implicated in memory processes and memory disorder is an important clinical feature of the disease.

Genetic Factors

Familial cases are reported in the literature. Wheelan (1959) reported a family with a sibship of 10, in which there were 2 proven and 3 probable cases of Alzheimer's disease. There is a relatively high incidence of senile dementia for the parents of Alzheimer's disease and of Alzheimer's disease in the offspring of senile dementia (Constantinides, 1978). A number of families have been reported in which Alzheimer's disease appeared to be dominantly inherited, and such families are distinguished by the regular manifestation of the gene (Pratt, 1967). The occurrence of Alzheimer's disease in twins is rare. Davidson and Robertson (1955) reported monozygotic twin sisters discordant for the disease, and Hunter, Dayan, and Wilson (1972) cited their case as the second reported incidence of monozygotic twins discordant for Alzheimer's disease. Cook, Schneck, and Clark (1981) recently reported identical female twins with Alzheimer's disease. Recent investigations into the role of HLA and B antigens have shown no significant

association with senile dementia (Snowden, Woodrow, and Copeland, 1981).

Pick's Disease

This rare type of dementia usually occurs between the ages of 40 and 60 years. The clinical manifestations are those of progressive dementia, but memory is unimpaired. Certain focal neurological signs such as dysphasia, apraxia, and disturbances of gait in the later stages are frequent accompaniments of the disorder. There is a considerable amount of evidence for a Mendelian dominant mode of inheritance (Sjogren, Sjogren, and Lindgren, 1952).

Pathological Appearances

The brain weight may be decreased to 1,000 g or less, and the main feature is marked, circumscribed cortical atrophy, which mainly involves the frontotemporal regions, often bilaterally or to a varying degree in both hemispheres. When the temporal lobe is involved the hippocampus is characteristically spared, which may correlate with the preservation of memory. The cortical atrophy is evident, with markedly widened sulci, and the crowns of the gyri are severely affected giving the 'knife blade' type of atrophy. Coronal sections of the brain indicate that the white matter is also affected by the atrophic process, as the junction of cortex and white matter are no longer clearly defined. The deep grey matter may also be affected, and in particular the caudate nucleus. The lateral ventricles show marked enlargement.

Microscopic Appearances

There is marked neuronal loss, which is often greatest in the upper cortical layers, but the pattern is variable. The affected areas show a marked increase in gliosis. The presence of 'Pick cells' is a distinctive feature in many, but not all cases. This consists of a spherical swelling of the neuronal cell body; the cytoplasm is pale on H/E stains and the nucleus may be displaced towards the cell membrane. Some of these cells contain a rounded homogeneous argyrophilic mass within the cytoplasm, which can be seen distinctly with silver preparations such as the von Braunmühl stain (Fig. 6).

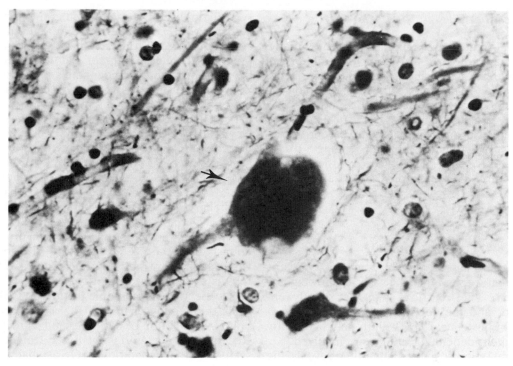

Figure 6   Pick's disease. There is a large argyrophilic mass within a swollen cortical neurone (von Braunmühl ×630)

Affected cells may be present among the small neurones of the cortex and in some of the large pyramidal neurones, and they have been described in the neurones of the basal ganglia and brainstem. Electron microscopic studies of these inclusions reveal that they contain ribosomes, vesicles, lipochromes, microtubules, and neurofilaments (Malamud and Hirano, 1974).

The main distinction from Alzheimer's disease is the presence of 'Pick's cells', and the absence of NFT and SP. Occasional cases have been described with these changes but they are uncommon.

Creutzfeldt Jakob Disease (Spongiform Encephalopathy)

This is a rare form of dementia which usually occurs in middle age and affects both sexes equally. It has been shown beyond doubt that the illness is caused by a transmissible agent, and this has promoted an important advance in scientific attitudes concerning the dementias in later life. Cerebral biopsy tissue from a pa-

tient with Creutzfeldt Jakob disease (CJD) was inoculated into the brain of a chimpanzee (Gibbs *et al.*, 1968), with the subsequent development of an identical disorder in the chimpanzee – both clinically and pathologically. Further work has demonstrated that CJD can be passaged from one chimpanzee to another (Gibbs and Gajdusek, 1969), and similarly in the New World monkey (Gajdusek and Gibbs, 1971). In 1974 Duffy and coworkers reported the transmission of the illness from the transplanted cornea of a patient with CJD to the recipient. Transmissible agents have been shown to cause kuru in man, scrapie in sheep, and mink encephalopathy, with the production of lesions pathologically similar to CJD in the central nervous system. The transmissible agent is commonly referred to as a slow virus, yet it does not behave like any known virus. It produces no inflammatory response in the CNS, nor does it evoke an antibody response. The exact nature of these agents remains uncertain. The subject is discussed in more detail by Gibbs, Gajdusek and Masters (1978).

Clinical Features

In brief the disease is characterized by initially vague symptoms, which include abnormal behaviour, apathy and loss of memory. Delusions may occur, and a variety of neurological signs may become evident, such as motor signs, ataxia, spasticity, and characteristically the development of myoclonic jerks. There is a progressive dementia finally leading to a vegetative state. The course of the disease from early symptomatology to fatal termination may vary from as little as 4 months to about 2 years.

Pathology

The brain may be atrophic, but this is a variable feature, and in some cases brain weight is normal. The ventricles may be slightly enlarged, and the deep grey matter, basal ganglia, brainstem, or cerebellum may be slightly shrunken, depending on the site involved.

Light microscopic examination reveals the basic lesion to be one of neuronal loss, and marked hypertrophy of astrocytes with gliosis in the affected parts of the cortex and other areas. A spongiose change is frequently seen in the grey matter and is variable in degree. (Fig. 7).

Variation in the sites affected in the nervous system, with consequently different clinical symptoms has led to nosological confusion. A presenile dementia with cortical blindness has been described (Heidenhain's syndrome) where the brunt of the disease falls on the occipital cortex. Other variants with myoclonus epilepsy were described by Jones and Nevin (1954). Foley and Denny-Brown (1955) described a condition which they named 'subacute progressive encephalopathy with bulbar myoclonus', and Brownell and Oppenheimer (1965) described an ataxic form of subacute cerebellar degeneration which they considered to be a variant of CJD. It is generally considered that the variation in clinical presentation is explained by the varying sites in the CNS which show pathological change and that CJD is a single disease entity.

The electron microscopic picture in CJD reveals the spongy change to be a membrane-bound vacuolation of neurones and astrocytes. Reactive astrocytes do not differ from those seen in other conditions. Occasionally distended neuronal processes contain an accumulation of mitochondria, dense bodies, and synaptic vesicles which have dense cores (Malamud and Hirano, 1974B).

CJD is a decidely uncommon disorder, but is probably not as rare as is thought. Corsellis

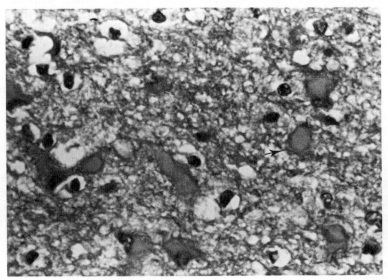

Figure 7   Creutzfeldt Jakob disease. Temporal cortex showing loss of neurones, hypertrophied astrocytes (arrow), and widespread spongiose dengeneration (H/E ×409)

(1976) has pointed out that the diagnosis may be difficult and that many cases go unreported. The disease occurs world wide, and epidemiological studies have not demonstrated the pattern of an infectious disease.

It has been reported occasionally among spouses and within families. Precautions in the handling of material from suspected CJD is necessary, and recommendations for those involved in such procedures are given by Gajdusek and coworkers, (1977).

Diseases of the Basal Ganglia

A number of disorders of the basal ganglia and brainstem are more commonly seen in the elderly. Extrapyramidal disease may present clinically as Parkinsonism with akinetic movement, muscular rigidity, and tremor, or with abnormal voluntary movements (dyskinesia). In a discussion of the classification of extrapyramidal disease Marsden (1981) observes that these two categories appear to be 'opposite poles of the spectrum of extrapyramidal disorders' and he refers to the observation that patients with Parkinson's disease may, when treated with L dopa, develop dyskinesia in place of their akinetic rigid syndrome, and patients with dyskinesia, such as in Huntington's chorea, have their signs decreased by dopamine antagonists, but develop drug-induced Parkinsonism.

Parkinson's Disease

Idiopathic Parkinson's disease is a progressive disorder which most commonly occurs in late middle age. The clinical features are well known. It affects both sexes and in some families there is an increased tendency to develop the disease, and genetic factors have been implicated (Heston, 1980). Dementia may develop in Parkinson's disease, but is not present in all cases. Lieberman and coworkers, (1979) give the incidence of dementia in Parkinson's disease as 32 per cent. in their series of 520 patients, and 10 times higher than among controls. They suggest that Parkinson's disease with dementia may represent a different disorder from those without dementia. Heston concluded that since the dementia is associated with severe Parkinson's disease, it was not necessary to postulate any further explanation.

Pathology

Externally the brain is usually of normal appearance. Cortical atrophy if present is not usually marked. Sections of the midbrain commonly show a varying decrease of the normal pigmentation of the substantia nigra. This may be readily appreciated with the naked eye (Fig. 8).

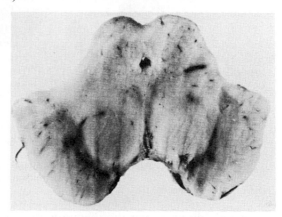

Figure 8   Parkinson's disease. Section of midbrain showing pallor of the substantia nigra, especially in the lateral aspects (H/E ×1.5). (Reproduced by permission of C. S. Treip fromTreip, 1978).

On microscopic examination the characteristic changes are classically found in the central part of the substantia nigra, with pigmented (melanin) cell loss, pallor, or decrease of many remaining pigmented cells and a varying amount of gliosis. Incontinence of pigment may also be seen with pigment lying free in the parenchyma. The typical Lewy inclusion bodies are found in varying numbers within the cytoplasm of the neurones. They consist of rounded, hyaline masses, surrounded by a lighter halo (Fig. 9). They may be single or multiple and vary in size from 5 to 25 μm. Lewy bodies may be found in many other pigmented nuclei in the brain stem, besides the substantia nigra and locus ceruleus. Den Hartog Jager and Bethlem (1960) found Lewy bodies in 14 nuclei of the diencephalon and brainstem, in which they had not previously been described. They confirmed that Lewy bodies had a predilection for pigmented cells in the brainstem and also reported their presence in sympathetic ganglia.

Lewy bodies are found in nearly all cases of

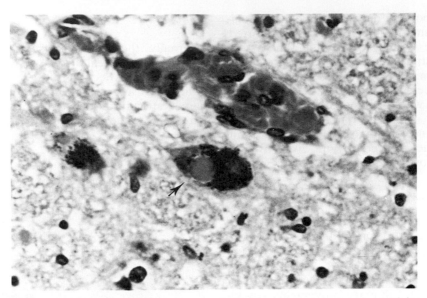

Figure 9   Parkinson's disease. Substantia nigra with a pigmented neurone containing a spherical intracytoplasmic Lewy inclusion body (arrow)

Parkinson's disease, and the diagnosis of idiopathic Parkinsonism must be seriously questioned if they are not. They are occasionally seen in control material and may be a preclinical manifestation of the disease. Atherosclerotic lesions within the basal ganglia may be demonstrated in elderly people and have been implicated by some authors as a cause of Parkinson's disease. There is scant neuropathological confirmation that such lesions can produce the classical clinical picture of Parkinsonism, and the more favoured view is that atherosclerotic lesions may coexist with Parkinson's disease, rather than cause it.

Biochemical Changes

The basic abnormality is a depletion of dopamine in those areas of the brain normally innervated by dopaminergic neurones, especially the striato nigral pathway. There is a lesser depletion of noradrenaline and changes in other systems such as those in 5-hydroxytryptamine, gamma amino butyric acid, and acetylcholine pathways (see Chapter 16.2).

Postencephalitic Parkinsonism

This form of encephalitis, which is generally assumed to be a virus disease, has rarely been reported since the epidemics in the 1920s. It is not particularly associated with ageing, but surviving cases may be found in the older age groups. Clinically such patients may show the typical features of Parkinsonism, but there are clear histological differences from the idiopathic form. Neurofibrillary tangles are found within the pigmented nuclei and deep grey matter, and Lewy bodies are rarely present. The destruction within, and subsequent gliosis in, the substantia nigra is more intense. Cases have been described with no history of encephalitis, but the typical pathological picture suggests that other neurotropic viruses may occasionally involve the substantia nigra. It is of interest that Gamboa and coworkers (1974) found influenza A antigen in the brains of 6 cases of postencephalitic Parkinsonism, but were unable to demonstrate it in control cases with the idiopathic form of Parkinson's disease.

Parkinsonism – Dementia Complex of Guam

This rare disease was described by Hirano, Malamud, and Kurland in 1961. It is confined to the Chamorro population of Guam and usually manifests in the fourth and fifth decades, with a male predominance of about 3:1. The disease is characterized by a progressive dementia and Parkinsonism, and ends fatally within 4 years. In many families it is associated with a locally common form of amyotrophic lateral sclerosis, which differs clinically and pathologically from the classic form. In some patients the two conditions are combined. They are now generally regarded as variants of the same disease.

Pathology

Hirano, Malamud, and Kurland (1961) described the pathological features in 17 cases. Cortical atrophy is present and most prominent in the frontal and temporal lobes. There is pallor of the substantia nigra and locus ceruleus. On light microscopy the prominent feature is the presence of numerous neurofibrillary tangles which are identical to those seen in Alzheimer's disease. In the affected areas there is accompanying neuronal loss and gliosis. The sites involved include the cerebral cortex, hippocampi, hypothalamus, thalamus, globus pallidus, and substantia nigra and tectum of the midbrian.

Striatonigral Degeneration

This rare condition presents clinically as idiopathic Parkinson's disease, between the fifth and seventh decades, but the pathological lesions found in the brain are different. Lewy bodies are not present and the characteristic lesions consist of cell loss and gliosis in the striatum, especially the putamen and substantia nigra. Adams, Bogart, and Van der Eecken (1964) first described this disease and since then a number of cases have been reported. The disease is regarded by some authors as a single entity, but some cases with pontocerebellar atrophy have shown clinical Parkinsonism, combined with the lesions of striatonigral degeneration.

Shy–Drager Syndrome

This uncommon disorder presents with progressive autonomic failure. Shy and Drager (1960) reviewed a number of cases with this syndrome and gave the first neuroanatomical description of a case. The syndrome is characterized by postural hypotension, impotence, anhidrosis, urinary incontinence, muscular rigidity, and tremor. Shy and Drager described widespread neuronal degeneration in many areas, which included most commonly the substantia nigra, caudate nucleus, inferior olives, dorsal vagal nuclei, the locus ceruleus and the intermediolateral columns of the thoracic spinal cord. Autonomic disturbances of sympathetic function have been attributed to the loss of intermediolateral (preganglionic) cells within the cord (Johnson *et al.*, 1966). In a controlled count in this area of 7 cases, Bannister and Oppenheimer (1972) found a marked loss of these cells. The Shy–Drager syndrome has been reported in association with two diseases, namely idiopathic Parkinson's disease and multiple system atrophy of the pontocerebellar or striatonigral type.

Progressive Supranuclear Palsy

This progressive brain disease was first recognized as a clinically and pathologically separate disease entity by Steele, Richardson, and Olszewski in 1964. The disease usually starts in the fifth to seventh decades; the characteristic clinical syndrome is of supranuclear ophthalmoplegia with vertical gaze being mainly affected, dysarthria, dystonia of the neck and upper trunk, and less commonly cerebellar and pyramidal symptoms. The disease is accompanied by a mild 'subcortical' dementia, which can be distinguished clinically from cortical dementia (Albert, Feldman, and Willis, 1974). In their original account all 9 cases described by Steele, Richardson, and Olszewski were males. Since then it has become evident that the disease occurs in both sexes, but is about twice as common in males. The pathological changes are highly characteristic. The chief sites affected are the subthalamic nucleus, globus pallidus, red nucleus, substantia nigra, periaqueductal grey matter, tectum of the mid-brain, and the dentate nucleus in the cerebellum. The affected areas show variable neuronal cell loss, gliosis, and numerous neurofibrillary tangles, which on electron microscopic examination are found to show consistent difference in structure from those associated with Alzheimer's disease. In addition, some neurones show granulovacuolar degeneration, and it is the only condition in which they are found in sites other than hippocampal pyramidal neurones (cf. Alzheimer's disease). The aetiology of the disease is unknown.

Huntington's Disease

Huntington's disease usually has an onset in the 30 to 45 year old groups, with an average duration of 10 to 15 years, and is thus commonly seen in older patients. It has rarely been reported with an onset in much younger and much older patients. The disease is dominantly inherited, and it is therefore important that the diagnosis is confirmed histologically, from the aspect of genetic counselling. The disease is characterized by progressive choreiform movements and dementia.

Pathology

The brain is usually small with a varying degree of cortical atrophy, which is usually most prominent in the frontal and parietal lobes and may be severe. On coronal sections the characteristic atrophy of the caudate nucleus results in a concave outline of the normally convex head of the caudate nucleus, in the anterior part of the lateral ventricles (Fig. 10). The putamen is small and atrophic, and so to a lesser extent is the globus pallidus. There is a variable degree of white matter shrinkage. The brainstem may be of normal size or rather small.

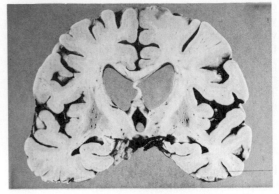

Figure 10 Huntington's disease. Coronal section through frontotemporal region. The ventricles are markedly enlarged and there is severe atrophy of the caudate nucleus and putamen. The cortex is atrophic

Under the light microscope the chief abnormalities are detectable in the caudate nucleus and putamen, and are characterized by a severe loss of mainly small neurones, with astrocytic proliferation and gliosis in the affected areas (Fig. 11). In general these changes tend to be most severe in the superior and posterior parts of the caudate nucleus and putamen, but cases in which changes predominate in one or the other are not uncommon. The pallidum is less severely affected, and the changes tend to be more prominent in its outer segment. Cell loss in other basal ganglia and in the brainstem have occasionally been described, and

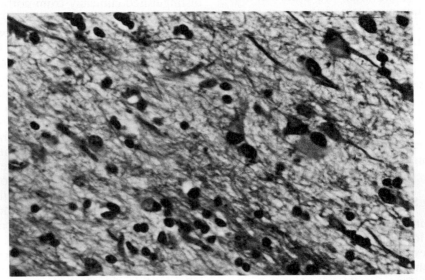

Figure 11 Huntington's disease. Caudate nucleus showing neuronal loss and hypertrophied astrocytes with glial fibre formation (PTAH ×400)

rarely in the dentate nucleus of the cerebellum. Cortical atrophy is reflected by neuronal loss and gliosis, and is reported to be more prominent in the third cortical layer. Non-specific changes such as shrinkage of neurones and increased amounts of lipofuscin are of variable degree.

The biochemical abnormalities in Huntington's disease are discussed in Chapter 16.2. Briefly there is an increase in dopamine concentration in the putamen, caudate nucleus, and substantia nigra. Gamma aminobutyric acid (GABA) is decreased in the same sites, and glutamic acid decarboxylase production for the synthesis of GABA is decreased in the caudate nucleus, putamen, and pallidum.

Motor Neurone Disease

The variable clinical features of this disease are well known. Motor neurone disease is a disorder of middle aged and elderly people, with a rising incidence from the fifth decade. The pathological features are reviewed by Oppenheimer (1976), but will be briefly considered here.

The basic pathological lesion is a loss of large motor cells and resultant gliosis. The clinical symptoms vary according to the severity and involvement of the sites affected, and this is reflected in the nomenclature of the older literature. Progressive muscular atrophy, progressive bulbar palsy, and amyotrophic lateral sclerosis are now generally accepted to be one disease; in Britain, motor neurone disease (MND) is the term most often used for all variants.

The Spinal Cord

Classically there is a loss of large motor cells from the anterior horns, and remaining cells may be shrunken and pyknotic. Neuronoplagia, i.e. phagocytosis of dead nerve cells by microglial phagocytes, may be evident. Similar changes are found in the motor nuclei of the hypoglossal, facial and trigeminal nerves, and the nuclei ambigui. The anterior spinal nerve roots tend to be thin and atrophic. Examination of affected muscles will show the typical features of neurogenic atrophy. The pyramidal tracts (both crossed and uncrossed) show variable degrees of degeneration, with myelin loss

and gliosis. The degeneration may be traced upwards via the cerebral peduncles and posterior part of the internal capsule to the pre- and post-central gyrus, which may show considerable pyramidal cell loss. In other cases degeneration may extend only to the cervical cord or medulla.

There may be a diffuse loss of myelin in the anterior and lateral columns, in addition to the ventral and lateral corticospinal tracts. The posterior columns remain intact. Familial cases of MND have been reported quite frequently, with indentical clinical pathological features, as already described.

Virus Disease in the Elderly

Herpes Zoster

Although by no means restricted to the elderly, herpes zoster is far more common in this age group. This is ascribed to decreased immunological competence in the elderly. It is generally believed that all patients with herpes zoster have had varicella in the past, and it has been shown that detectable serum antibody gradually disappears, after the age of 50 years (Juel-Jensen, 1973), and thus the latent virus is no longer held in check. Local trauma or systemic illness appears to be a precipitating factor in some cases.

Pathology

The site of infection is the posterior root ganglion (commonly the upper cervical, thoracic, or first lumbar ganglion) and the trigeminal ganglion is the most commonly affected of the cranial nerves. The pathological changes affect the sensory neurones within the ganglia, the nerve root, and the nerve serving it, and finally the corresponding dermatome displays the typical vesicular skin eruption. The ganglion is swollen and congested, and in severe cases may be haemorrhagic. Lymphocytic infiltration is present within and around the affected ganglion and necrosis may be seen. The neurones in the vicinity show degenerative changes with loss of Nissl substance, eosinophilic cytoplasm and neuronophagia (Hume-Adams, 1976). Inflammation may extend into the root and spinal nerve for a short distance, and may even spread into the surrounding tissues. In mild cases resolution is usually complete, but severe infections may result in fibrosis, and the persistent and painful postherpetic neuralgia which sometimes develops is attributed to this. In patients dying during the acute stage, changes are reported in the affected level of the spinal cord or brainstem in cases of trigeminal zoster. These consist mainly of neuronophagia, perivascular lymphocytic cuffing, and chromatolysis of neurones. Generalized encephalomyelitis is a rare complication and involvement of the motor nerves is uncommon.

Neurological Non-Metastatic Effects of Malignant Disease

The incidence of malignant disease rises with age, and therefore the non-metastatic neurological manifestations are briefly discussed. Rarely neurological disorders may occur in the presence of carcinoma, which cannot be attributed to metastatic spread, or other secondary metabolic or nutritional factors. Carcinoma of the bronchus, which may be of surprisingly small size, is the most commonly associated malignancy, but carcinoma of other sites and lymphomas have been implicated. The pathogenesis is thought to be one of altered immune response with increased susceptibility to infections, particularly viral infections, or an autoimmune mechanism. The lesions affect different parts of the nervous system and may involve a single site or a combination of sites. Mental confusion may be prominent in some cases. The pathological features may include an encephalitis with predominant involvement of the limbic system, a bulbar encephalitis affecting the lower brainstem, myelitis affecting the anterior horn cells, ganglioradiculitis involving the posterior root ganglia, and cortical cerebellar degeneration. The subject is covered in detail by Thomas Smith (1976).

Normal Pressure Hydrocephalus

This uncommon disorder was first reported by Adams and coworkers (1965). The clinical features are characterized by dementia, unsteadiness of gait, and urinary incontinence. Most patients are in the 60 to 70 year age group. The three patients that Adams and coworkers, described ranged between 62 and 66 years. The

ventricles are enlarged, but the intraventricular pressure is not raised above normal (under 100 mm). The importance of this condition is that it is treatable, and such patients can benefit considerably from CSF shunting procedures. In some cases the aetiological factor cannot be identified, and in others hydrocephalus has been found to follow subarachnoid haemorrhage, or meningitis, with consequent scarring and obstruction within the CSF pathways. The actual mechanism of normal pressure hydrocephalus is poorly understood. Possible pathophysiological mechanisms are discussed by Adams (1980).

Cerebrovascular Disease

The incidence of cerebrovascular disease (CVD) rises rapidly with increasing age (Hutchinson and Acheson, 1975) and is a major cause of neurological disease in the elderly. By far the most common complications of CVD are cerebral infarction and cerebral haemorrhage. CVD may also be an important cause of dementia in the aged. The disease accounts for a substantial number of deaths. In a relatively stable population CVD is responsible for about 15 per cent of all deaths, of which around 9 per cent are caused by cerebral infarction, 4.5 per cent. by cerebral haemorrhage, and 1.5 per cent. by subarachnoid haemorrhage (Yates, 1976).

Pathology

The major cause of cerebral infarction is vascular occlusion from atherosclerosis, superimposed thrombosis, and embolus. Cerebral haemorrhage is frequently associated with hypertension, but changes of atherosclerosis may commonly accompany hypertension. The pathogenesis of stroke disease is fully covered in Chapter 16.8.

Atherosclerosis

The aetiology of atheroma cannot be discussed here, but there still remains some divergence of thought regarding its pathogenesis. Within the brain atheroma affects the large arteries, the basilar verebral system, the anterior, middle, and posterior cerebral arteries, being the most commonly affected. The internal carotid and vertebral arteries in the neck may be involved, and infarction of the middle cerebral artery territory may be secondary to atheroma of the internal carotid arteries. The affected vessel contains patchy yellowish opacities of the wall, which are quite obvious macroscopically. In severe cases the whole artery may be elongated and tortuous, with a markedly reduced lumen. After the initial plaque is formed on the intimal wall, subsequent progression is mainly by deposition of thrombus upon its surface. The thrombus becomes organized and endothelium proliferates over its surface. Within the depth of the plaque cholesterol and fatty degenerative changes are present. The media degenerates and undergoes fibrous replacement, and there is splitting of the internal elastic lamina (Fig. 12). The process of thrombosis upon the internal surface of the plaque may reduce the lumen considerably but rarely totally occludes it. Circulation through the vessel may be further compromised by superimposed thrombus.

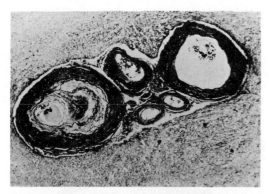

Figure 12 Atherosclerosis. Arteries and arterioles in basal ganglia. Note narrowing of lumen by atheromatous plaque, reduplication and splitting of lamina, and hypertrophied media (Weigert's elastic Van Gieson stain ×240)

Cerebral Infarction

Occlusion of a vessel by whatever mechanism or any event, such as a profound drop in blood pressure in a patient with an already compromised vascular system, usually results in infarction or death of the tissue within the area of supply of the affected vessel. The extent and type of infarction is dependent on a variety of factors (see Chapter 16.8).

A recent ischaemic infarction will result in a swollen softened area within the brain, which if death occurs within 24 hours may not be readily detectable before fixation of the brain. Microscopically early brain infarcts reveal ischaemic change of peripherally situated neurones, disintegration and necrosis of parenchyma and brain cells, and small areas of haemorrhage, and in the first three days acute inflammatory cell infiltration may be brisk. The astrocytes within the area swell, and proliferation occurs about the third day. Microglial phagocytes appear between the second and fifth day and assume the familiar swollen and foamy appearance of Gitter cells. Phagocytosis and astrocytic glial proliferation may continue for months. The eventual result is an area of scarring (Fig. 13) consisting of cystic necrosis, surrounded and traversed by glial fibres. A brownish discoloration is produced by haemosiderin pigment.

Other Lesions Associated with Atherosclerosis and Hypertension

If atherosclerosis is widespread, small irregular softenings are frequently found situated in the pons especially, but also in the central white matter and basal ganglia. Such lesions are found in the vicinity of a diseased artery, and microscopically consist of cystic spaces, sometimes with numerous swollen phagocytes, and variable gliosis which is accentuated in the perivascular area. Such areas are associated with occlusion of small arteries. Haemosiderin-laden phagocytes may be prominent, and indicate recent small haemorrhages, the latter more commonly being associated with hypertension.

Cystic cavities (lacunes) visible to the naked eye may be seen, particularly in the basal ganglia and also in the central white matter. Microscopically these cavities surround normal looking vessels. They are attributed to hypertension which results in spiral elongation and distortion of vessels. This leads to separation from surrounding brain tissue and its subsequent disintegration.

Cerebral Haemorrhage and Hypertension

Cerebral haemorrhage is frequently associated with hypertension and occurs most commonly in the region of supply of the lenticulostriate artery to the basal ganglia. When massive the

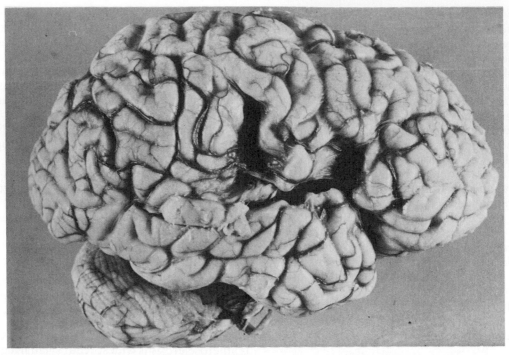

Figure 13   Brain showing depressed cystic scar of old infarct in the distribution of the middle cerebral artery

haemorrhage ruptures into the ventricular system and sometimes extends into the subarachnoid space. It is accompanied by swelling of the affected hemisphere and often the secondary pressure effects of an intracranial space-occupying mass. Less commonly the deep cerebellar white matter and the pons and midbrain are the site of massive haemorrhage.

Small haemorrhages usually about 1 to 2.5 cm in diameter may occur anywhere within the brain. They may be seen as rounded haematomas in the cortical or subcortical regions. When involving white matter they are finally converted to a pigmented slit-like scar, and small haemorrhagic lesions such as this are important in the pathogenesis of minor strokes.

Microscopically the cerebral arteries exhibit changes secondary to hypertension. The vessels are thickened by medial hypertrophy and fibrosis. The internal elastica may show eccentric splitting and duplication, and there is fibrosis of the intima and adventitia. Atherosclerotic changes are variable.

For many years it has been suggested that the formation of miliary microaneurysms (Fig. 14) and their rupture play an important role in the small haemorrhages of hypertensive brains (see Chapter 16.8). Several workers have confirmed and demonstrated their presence by post-mortem angiography (Cole and Yates, 1967; Ross-Russell, 1963).

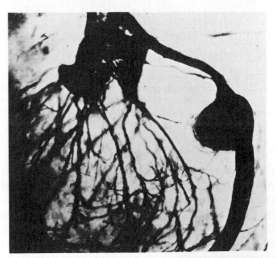

Figure 14   Microaneurysm measuring 800 μm in diameter on long penetrating artery from parietal cortex of 71 year old hypertensive man. (From Ross-Russell, 1963. Reproduced by permission of Oxford University Press)

Vascular Disease and Dementia

Cerebral atherosclerosis has tended to be over diagnosed as a cause of dementia in the elderly. Many elderly brains show quite marked atherosclerotic changes at autopsy, yet their possessors have been known to be intellectually normal during life. Massive cerebral infarction as a complication of atherosclerosis may result in dementia, but more often dementia is caused by small vessel disease, with multiple emboli resulting in numerous small infarcts and cystic spaces. Commonly caused by hypertension, this pathological change results in considerable destruction of cerebral tissue. The preferred terminology for this condition is multi-infarct dementia.

Vascular Disease of the Spinal Cord

Atheroma of the spinal cord arteries of sufficient degree to cause symptoms is extremely rare. Occlusion by thrombus of the spinal part of the anterior spinal artery may result in infarction, and the clinical syndrome is well documented. The cause in most cases has been attributed to minor trauma, such as spondylosis, leading to compression of the anterior spinal artery and its branches (Hughes, 1976). The various complications resulting from spondylosis are somewhat more common in older age groups. Other rare vascular conditions affecting the spinal cord, such as spinal thrombophlebitis, complications of dissecting aneurysm of the aorta, and vascular malformations, are not specifically associated with ageing.

Giant Cell Arteritis

This disease affects elderly people and is uncommon under the age of 55 years. The artery most frequently affected is the superficial temporal artery, but any artery may be affected. Within the central nervous system involved vessels include the intracerebral arteries, the central retinal artery, and the internal carotids. The disease may be generalized and the cause is unknown.

The pathological features are characterized by an inflammation of the whole thickness of an affected segment of artery. In the early stages the wall is infiltrated by leucocytes, but this is later replaced by a granulomatous lesion, consisting of giant cells of the foreign body type and chronic inflammatory cells. The internal elastic lamina is fragmented, and there is fibrous replacement of the media and intimal fibrosis. The result is a scarred, narrowed lumen, and occlusion by thrombus may lead to infarction of the area supplied.

REFERENCES

Adams, R. D. (1980). 'Altered cerebrospinal fluid dynamics in relation to dementia and aging', in *Aging of the Brain and Dementia Aging* Vol. 13 (Eds L. Amaducci, A. N. Davison, and P. Antuono), pp. 217–225, Raven Press, New York.

Adams, R. D., Bogaert, L. van and Van der Eecken, H. (1964). 'Strato-nigral degeneration', *J. Neuropathol. Exp. Neurol.*, **23**, 584–608.

Adams, R. D., Fisher, C. M., Hakin, S., Ojemann, R. G. and Sweet, W. H. (1965). 'Symptomatic occult hydrocephalus with "normal" cerebrospinal fluid pressure. A treatable syndrome', *New Engl. J. Med.*, **273**, 117–126.

Albert, M. L., Feldman, R. G., and Willis, A. L. (1974). 'The "subcortical dementia" of progressive supranuclear palsy', *J. Neurol. Neurosurg. Psychiatry*, **37**, 121–130.

Arnold, N. and Harriman, D. G. F. (1970). 'The incidence of abnormality in contral human peripheral nerves studied by single axon dissection', *J. Neurol. Neurosurg. Psychiatry*, **33**, 55–61.

Ball, M. J., and Lo, P. (1977). 'Granulovacuolar degeneration in the ageing brain and in dementia', *J. Neuropathol. Exp. Neurol.*, **36**, 474–487.

Bannister, R., and Oppenheimer, D. R. (1972). 'Degenerative diseases of the nervous system associated with autonomic failure', *Brain*, **95**, 457–474.

Blackwood, W., and Corsellis, J. A. N. (Eds) (1976). *Greenfield's neuropathology*, 3rd ed., Edward Arnold, London.

Blocq, P., and Marinosco, G. (1892). 'Sur les le'sions et la pathogénié de l'epilepsie dite essentielle', *Semaine médicale (Paris)*, **12**, 445–446.

Brody, H. (1955). 'Organisation of the cerebral cortex. A study of ageing in the human cerebral cortex', *J. Comp. Neurol.*, **102**, 511–556.

Brody, H. (1970). 'Structural changes in the ageing nervous system'. *Interdiscipl. Topics Gerontol.*, **7**, 9–21.

Brody, H. (1978). 'Cell counts in cerebral cortex and brainstem', in *Aging*, Vol. 7, *Alzheimers Disease: Senile Dementia and Related Disorders* (Eds R. Katzman, R. D. Terry, and K. L. Bick), pp. 345–351, Raven Press, New York.

Brownell, B., and Oppenheimer, D. (1965). 'An ataxic form of subacute presenile polioencephalopathy (Creutzfeldt Jakob disease)', *J. Neurol. Neurosurg. Psychiatry*, **28**, 350–361.

Buell, S. J., and Coleman, P. D. (1981). 'Quantitative evidence for selective dendritic growth in normal human ageing, but not in senile dementia', *Brain Res.*, **214**, 23–41.

Cole, F. M., and Yates, P. O. (1967). 'The occurrence and significance of intracerebral microaneurysms', *J. Pathol. Bacteriol.*, **93**, 393–411.

Constantinides, J. (1978). 'Is Alzheimer's disease a major form of senile dementia? Clinical, anatomical and genetic data', in *Aging*, Vol. 7, *Alzheimer's Disease, Senile Dementia and Related Disorders*. (Eds R. Katzman, R. D. Terry, and K. L. Bick), pp. 15–25, Raven Press, New York.

Cook, R. H., Schneck, S. A., and Clark, D. B. (1981). 'Twins with Alzheimer's disease', *Arch. Neurol.*, **38**, 300–301.

Corsellis, J. A. N. (1976). 'Ageing and the dementias', in *Greenfield's Neuropathology* (Eds W. Blackwood and J. A. N. Corsellis), 3rd ed. pp. 796–848, Edward Arnold, London.

Corsellis, J. A. N., Bruton, C. J., and Freeman-Browne, D. (1973). 'The aftermath of boxing', *Psychol. Med.*, **3**, 270–303.

Davidson, E. A., and Robertson, E. E. (1955). 'Alzheimer's disease with acne rosacea in one of identical twins', *J. Neurol. Neurosurg. Psychiatry*, **18**, 72–77.

Davis, P. J. M., and Wright, E. A. (1977). 'A new method for measuring cranial cavity volume and its application to the assessment of cerebral atrophy at autopsy', *Neuropathol. Appl. Neurobiol.*, **3**, 341–358.

Dayan, A. D. (1970). 'Quantitative studies on the aged human brain. 1. Senile plaques and neurofibrillary tangles in "normal" patient'. *Acta Neuropathol. (Berl.)*, **16**, 85–94.

Dayan, A. D. (1971). 'Comparative neuropathology of ageing: Studies on the brain of 47 species of vertebrates', *Brain*, **94**, 31–42.

Dayan, A. D. (1978). 'Neuropathology of aging', in *Textbook of Geriatric Medicine and Gerontology* (Ed. J. C. Brocklehurst), 2nd ed. pp., 158–185, Churchill Livingstone, Edinburgh, London, and New York.

DeKosky, S. T., and Bass, N. H. (1980). 'Effects of aging and senile dementia on the microchemical pathology of human cerebral cortex', in *Aging of the Brain and Dementia*, Vol. 13, *Aging* (Eds L. Amaducci, A. N. Davison, and P. Antuono), pp. 33–37, Raven Press, New York.

Den Hartog Jager, W. A., and Bethlem, J. (1960). 'The distribution of Lewy bodies in the central and autonomic nervous systems in idiopathic paralysis agitans', *J. Neurol. Neurosurg. Psychiatry*, **23**, 283–290.

Dorfman, L. J., and Bosley, T. M. (1979). 'Age-related changes in peripheral and central nerve conduction in man', *Neurology*, **29**, 38–44.

Duffy, P., Wolf, J., Collins, G., DeVoe, A. G., Streeten, B., and Cowen, D. (1974). 'Possible person to person transmission of Creutzfeldt Jakob disease' *New Engl. J. Med.*, **290**, 692–693.

Eng, L. F., Forno, L. S., Bigbee, J. W., and Forno, K. L. (1980). 'Immunocytochemical localization of glial fibrillary acidic protein and tubulin in Alzheimer's disease brain biopsy tissue', in *Aging*, Vol. 13, *Aging of the Brain* (Eds L. Amaducci, A. N. Davison, and P. Antuono), pp. 49–54, Raven Press, New York.

Fang, H. C. (1976). 'Observations on aging characteristics of cerebral blood vessels, macroscopic and microscopic features', in *Neurobiology of Aging* (Eds R. D. Terry and S. Gershon), pp. 155–166, Raven Press, New York.

Feldman, M. (1976). 'Aging changes in the morphology of cortical dendrites', in *Neurobiology of Aging* (Eds R. D. Terry and S. Gershon), pp. 211–227, Churchill Livingstone, London, New York.

Foley, J. M., and Denny-Brown, D. (1955). 'Subacute progressive encephalopathy with bulbar myoclonus', Excerpta Medica, Section VIII, *Neurol. Psychiatr.*, **8**, 782–784.

Gajdusek, D. C., and Gibbs, C. J. (1971). 'Transmission of two subacute, spongiform encephalopathies of man (Kuru and Creutzfeldt Jakob disease', *Nature*, **230**, 588–589.

Gajdusek, D. C., Gibbs, C. J. Jr, Asher, D. M. Brown, P., Diwan, A. Hoffman, P., Nemo, G., Rohwer, R., and White, L. (1977). 'Precautions in medical care and in handing material from patients with transmissible virus dementias', *New Engl. J. Med.*, **297**, 1253–1258.

Gambetti, P., Velosco, M. E., Dahl, D., Bignami, Amico, Roessman, U., and Sindely, S. (1980). 'Alzheimer's neurofibrillary tangles: An immunohistochemical study', in *Aging*, Vol. 13, *Aging of the Brain* (Eds L. Amaducci, A. N. Davison and P. Antuono), pp. 55–63, Raven Press, New York.

Gamboa, E. T., Wolf, A., Yahr, M. D., Harter, D. H., Duffy, P. E., Barden, H., and Hsu, K. C. (1974). 'Influenza virus antigen in postencephalitic Parkinsonism brain', *Arch. Neurol.*, **31**, 228–332.

Gibbs, C. J., and Gajdusek, D. C. (1969). 'Infection as the etiology of spongiform encephalopathy (Creutzfeldt Jacob) disease', *Science*, **165**, 1023–1025.

Gibbs, C. J., Gajdusek, D. C., Asher, D. M., Alpers, M. P., Beck, E., Daniel, P. M., and Matthews, W. B. (1968). 'Creutzfeldt Jakob Disease: Transmission to the chimpanzee', *Science*, **161**, 388–389.

Gibbs, C. J., Gajdusek, D. C., and Masters, C. L. (1978). 'Considerations of transmissible and chronic infections with a summary of the clinical, pathological and virological characteristics of kuru, Creutzfeldt Jakob disease and scrapie', in *Senile Dementia: A Biochemical Approach* (Ed. K. Nardy), pp. 115–130, Elsevier/North-Holland, New York and Amsterdam.

Grundke-Iqbal, I., Johnson, A., Wisnewski, H. M., Terry, R. D. and Iqbal, K. (1979). 'Evidence that Alzheimer neurofibrillary tangles originate from neurotubules', *Lancet*, **1**, 578–580.

Hall, T. C., Miller, A. K. H., and Corsellis, J. A. N. (1975). 'Variations in the human Purkinje cell population according to age and sex', *Neuropathol. Appl. Neurobiol.*, **1**, 267–292.

Henderson, G., Tomlinson, B. E., and Weightman, D. (1975). 'Cell counts in the human cerebral cortex using a traditional and an automatic method', *J. Neurol. Sci.*, **25**, 129–144.

Herzog, A. G., and Kemper, T. L. (1980). 'Amygdaloid changes in aging and dementia', *Arch. Neurol.*, **37**, 625–629.

Heston, L. H. (1980). 'Dementia associated with Parkinson's disease: A genetic study', *J. Neurol. Neurosurg. Psychiatry*, **43**, 846–848.

Hirano, A., Dembitzer, H. M., Kurland, L. T., and Zimmerman, H. M. (1968). 'The fine structure of some intraganglionic alterations', *J. Neuropathol. Exp. Neurol.*, **26**, 167–182.

Hirano, A., Malamud, N., and Kurland, L. T. (1961). 'Parkinsonism–dementia complex, an endemic disease on the Island of Guam', *Brain*, **84**, 662–679.

Huckman, M. S., Fox, J., and Topel, J. (1975). 'The validity of criteria for the evaluation of cerebral atrophy by computerized tomography', *Radiology*, **116**, 85–95.

Hughes, J. T. (1976). 'Diseases of the spine and spinal cord', in *Greenfield's Neuropathology* (Eds W. Blackwood and J. A. N. Corsellis), 3rd ed., pp. 652–687, Edward Arnold, London.

Hume-Adams, J. (1976). 'Virus diseases of the nervous system', in *Greenfield's Neuropathology* (Eds W. Blackwood and J. A. N. Corsellis), 3rd ed., pp. 292–326, Edward Arnold, London.

Hunter, R., Dayan, A. D., and Wilson, J. (1972). 'Alzheimer's disease in one monozygotic twin', *J. Neurol. Neurosurg. Psychiatry*, **35**, 707–710.

Hutchinson, E. C., and Acheson, E. J. (1975). In *Strokes: Natural History, Pathology and Surgical Treatment – Major Problems in Neurology.* (Ed. John N. Walton), Vol. 4, p. 110, W. B. Saunders, London, Philadelphia, Toronto.

Iqbal, K., Grundke-Iqbal, I., Johnson, A., and Wisniewski, H. M. (1980). 'Neurofibrous proteins in ageing and dementia', in *Aging,* vol. 13, Aging of the Brain and Dementia (Eds L. Amaducci,

A. N. Davison, and P. Antuono), pp. 39–46, Raven Press, New York.

Ishii, T., and Maga, S. (1976). 'Immuno-electron microscopic localization of immunoglobulin is in amyloid fibrils of senile plaques', *Acta Neuropathol. (Berl.)*, **36**, 243–249.

Jellinger, K. (1973). 'Neuraxonal dystrophy: Its natural history and related disorders', in *Progress in Neuropathology* (Ed. H. M. Zimmerman), Vol. 2, p. 129, Grune and Stratton, New York.

Johnson, R. H., Lee, D. de J., Oppenheimer, D. R. and Spalding, J. M. K. (1966). 'Autonomic failure with orthostatic hypotension due to intermedio lateral column degeneration', *Quart. J. Med.*, **35**, 276–292.

Jones, D. and Nevin, S. (1954). 'Rapidly progressive cerebral degeneration (subacute vascular encephalopathy) with mental disorder, focal disturbances and myoclonic epilepsy', *J. Neurol. Psychiatry*, **17**, 148–159.

Juel-Jensen, B. E. (1973). 'Herpes simplex and zoster', *Br. Med. J.*, **1**, 406–410.

Katzman, R., Terry, R. D., and Bick, K. L. (1978). 'Recommendations of the nosology, epidemiology, and etiology and pathophysiology commissions of the workshop – Conference on Alzheimer's Disease, Senile Dementia and Related Disorders'. in *Alzheimers Disease: Senile Dementia and Related Disorders* (Eds R. Katzman, R. D. Terry, and K. L. Bick), pp. 579–585, Raven Press, New York.

Kidd, M. (1964). 'Alzheimer's disease: an electron microscopic study', *Brain*, **87**, 307–321.

Konigsmark, B. W., and Murphy, E. A. (1972). 'Volume of ventral cochlear nucleus in man: Its relationship to neuronal population and age', *J. Neuropathol. Exp. Neurol.*, **31**, 304–316.

Lieberman, A., Dziatolowski, M., Kupersmith, M., Serby, M., Goodfold, A., Korein, J., and Goldstein, M. (1979). 'Dementia in Parkinson Disease', *Ann. Neurol.*, **6**, 355–359.

Lockett, M. F. (1976). 'Aging of the adenohypophysis in relation to renal aging', in *Hypothalamus, Pituitary and Aging.* (Eds Arthur V. Everitt and John A. Burgess), pp. 282–296, Charles C. Thomas, New York.

Malamud, N., and Hirano, A. (1974). In *Atlas of Neuropathology*, 2nd revised ed. pp. 330–338, University of California Press, Berkeley, Los Angeles, London.

Mann, D. M., and Sinclair, K. G. N. (1978). 'The quantitative assessment of lipofuscin pigment, cytoplasmic RNA and nucleolar volume in senile dementia'. *Neuropathol. Appl. Neurobiol.*, **4**, 129–135.

Marsden, C. D. (1981). 'Extrapyramidal diseases', in *The Molecular Basis of Neuropathology* (Eds

A. N. Davison and R. H. S. Thompson), pp. 345–383, Edward Arnold, London.

Monagle, R. B., and Brody, H. (1974). 'The effects of age upon the main nucleus of the inferior olive in the human', *J. Comp. Neurol.*, **155**, 61–66.

Morimatsu, M., Hirai, S., Muramatsu, A. and Yoshikawa, M. (1975). 'Senile degenerative brain lesions and dementia' *J. Am. Geriatr. Soc.*, **23**, 390–406.

Neumann, M. A. and Cohn, R. (1953). 'Incidence of Alzheimer's disease in a large mental hospital', *Arch. Neurol. Psychiatry*, **69**, 615–536.

Newton, R. D. (1947). 'Identity of Alzheimer's disease and senile dementia and their relationship to senility', *J. Ment. Sci.*, **94**, 225–249.

Olsen, M. I., and Shaw, C. (1969). 'Presenile dementia and Alzheimer's disease in mongolism', *Brain*, **92**, 147–145.

Oppenheimer, D.R. (1976). 'Diseases of the basal ganglia, cerebellum and motor neurons', in *Greenfield's Neuropathology* (Eds. W. Blackwood and J. A. N. Corsellis), 3rd ed., pp. 608–651, Edward Arnold, London.

Pratt, R. T. C. (1967). In *The Genetics of Neurological Disorders* (Eds. J. A. Fraser-Roberts), p. 75, Oxford University Press, London.

Ramsay, H. J. (1965). 'Ultrastructure of corpora amylacea', *J. Neuropathol. Exp. Neurol.*, **24**, 25–39.

Raskin, N., and Ehrenberg, R. (1956). 'Senescence, senility and Alzheimer's disease', *Am. J. Psychiatry*, **113**, 133–137.

Rodin, A. E., and Overall, J. (1967). 'Statistical relationships of the weight of the human pineal to age and malignancy', *Cancer*, **20**, 1203.

Ross-Russell, R. W. (1963). 'Observations on intracerebral aneurysms', *Brain*, **86**, 425–442.

Rothschild, D., and Kasanin, J. (1936). 'Clinico pathological study of Alzheimer's disease: Relationship to senile condition', *Arch. Neurol. Psychiatry*, **36**, 293–321.

Russell, D., and Rubinstein, L. J. (1971). In *Pathology of Tumours of the Nervous System*, 3rd ed., p. 217, Edward Arnold, London.

Scheibel, A. B. (1978). 'Structural aspects of the ageing brain: Spine systems and the dendritic arbor', In *Alzehimer's Disease: Senile Dementia and Related Disorders* (Eds R. Katzman, R. D. Terry, and K. L. Bick), pp. 353–373, Raven Press, New York.

Scheibel, M. E., Lindsay, R. D., Tomiyasu, U., and Scheibel, A. B. (1976A) 'Progressive dendritic changes in the aging human limbic system', *Exp. Neurol.*, **47**, 392–403.

Scheibel, M. E., Linday, R. D., Tomiyasu, U. and Scheibel, A. B. (1976B). *Exp. Neurol.*, **53**, 420–430.

Scholtz, W. (1938). 'Studien zut Pathologie der Hirngefässe. II. Die drusige Entartung der Hirnarterien und Capillaren', *Zeitschrift für die gesamte Neurologie und Psychiatrie*, **162**, 694–715.

Seitelberger, F. (1980). 'Dementia associated with aging processes: A functional neuropathologic study', in *Aging*, Vol. 13, *Aging of the Brain and Dementia* (Eds L. Amaducci, A. N. Davison, and P. Antuono), pp. 239–244, Raven Press, New York.

Shelanski, M. L., and Selkoe, D. J. (1981). 'Protein changes in the ageing brain' in *The Molecular Basis of Neuropathology*. (Eds A. N. Davison and R. H. S. Thompson), Arnold, London.

Shy, G. M., and Drager, G. A. (1960). 'A neurological syndrome associated with orthostatic hypertension', *Arch. Neurol.*, **2**, 511–527.

Sjogren, T., Sjogren, H., and Lindgren, A. (1952). 'Morbus Alzheimer and Morbus Pick: Genetic, chemical and anatomical study', *Acta Psychiatra. Neurologica Scand.*, *Suppl.*, **82**.

Snowden, P. R., Woodrow, J. C., and Copeland, J. R. M. (1981). 'HLA antigens in senile dementia and multiple infarct dementia', *Age Ageing*, **10**, 259–263.

Stam, F. C., and Roukema, P. A. (1973). 'Histochemical and biochemical aspects of corpora amylacea', *Acta Neuropathol (Berl.)*, **25**, 95–102.

Steele, J. C., Richardson, J. C., and Olszewski, J. (1964). 'Progressive supranuclear palsy', *Arch. Neurol.*, **10**, 333–359.

Terry, R. D. (1963). 'The fine structure of the neurofibrillary tangle in Alzheimer's disease', *J. Neuropathol. Exp. Neurol.*, **22**, 629–642.

Terry, R. D. (1978). 'Ageing, senile dementia and Alzheimer's disease', in *Alzheimer's Disease: Senile Dementia and Related Disorders* (Eds R. Katzman, R. D. Terry, and K. L. Bick), pp. 11–14, Raven Press, New York.

Terry, R. D. (1980). 'Structural changes in senile dementia of the Alzheimer type', in *Aging*, Vol. 13, *Aging of the Brain and Dementia* (Eds L. Amaducci, A. N. Davison, and P. Antuono), pp. 23–32, Raven Press, New York.

Terry, R. D., Fitzgerald, C., Peck, A., Millner, J. and Farmer, P. (1977). 'Cortical cell counts in senile dementia', *J. Neurol. Exp. Neuropathol.*, **36**, 633.

Terry, R. D., and Wisniewski, H. M. (1970). 'The ultrastructure of the neurofibrillary tangle and the senile plaque', in *Ciba Foundation Symposium on Alzheimer's Disease and Related Conditions* (Eds G. E. Wolstenholme and M. O'Connor), Churchill,London.

Terry, R. D., and Wisniewski, H. M. (1972). 'Ultrastructure of senile dementia and of experimental analogs', in *Aging and the Brain – Advances in Behavioural Biology* (Ed. C. Gaitz), Plenum Press, New York, London.

Thomas Smith, W. (1976). 'Nutritional deficiencies and disorders'. In *Greenfield's Neuropathology* (Eds W. Blackwood and J. A. N. Corsellis), 3rd ed., pp. 194–237, Edward Arnold, London.

Tomlinson, B. E. (1972). 'Morphological brain changes in non demented old people', in *Ageing of the Central Nervous System* (Eds H. M. Von Praag and A. F. Kalverboer), pp. 38–57, De Ervon F. Bohn, New York.

Tomlinson, B. E. (1979). 'The ageing brain', in *Recent Advances in Neuropathology* (Eds W. Thomas-Smith and J. B. Cavanagh), pp. 129–159, Churchill Livingstone, Edinburgh, London and New York.

Tomlinson, B. E., Blessed, G., and Roth, M. (1968). 'Observations on the brains of non-demented old people', *J. Neurol. Sci.*, **7**, 331–356.

Tomlinson, B. E., Blessed, G. and Roth, M. (1970). 'Observations on the brains of demented old people'. *J. Neurol. Sci.*, **2**, 205–242.

Tomlinson, B. E., and Henderson, G. (1976). 'Some quantitative cerebral findings in normal and demented old people', in *Neurobiology of Aging* (Eds Robert Terry and Samuel Gershon), pp. 183–209, Raven Press, New York.

Tomlinson, B. E., Irving, D., and Blessed, G. (1981). 'Cell loss in the locus coeruleus in senile dementia of Alzheimer type', *J. Neurol. Sci.*, **49**, 419–428.

Tomlinson, B. E., and Kitchener, D. (1972). 'Granulovacuolar degeneration of hippocampal pyramidal cells', *J. Pathol.*, **106**, 165–185.

Treip, C. S. (1978). *A Colour Atlas of Neuropathology*. Wolfe Medical Publications, London.

Vijayashankar, N., and Brody, H. (1977). 'A study of ageing in the human abducens nucleus', *J. Comp. Neurol.*, **173**, 433–437.

Wheelan, L. (1959). 'Familial Alzheimer's disease', *Ann. Hum. Genet.*, **23**, 300–310.

Wisniewski, H. M., Ghetti, B., and Terry, R. D. (1973). 'Neuritic (senile) plaques and filamentous changes in aged rhesus monkeys', *J. Neuropathol. Exp. Neurol.*, **32**, 566–584.

Wisniewski, H. M., Narang, H. K., and Terry, R. D. (1976). 'Neurofibrillary tangles of paired helical filaments', *J. Neurol. Sci.*, **27**, 173–181.

Wisniewski, H. M., Raine, A. B., Kay, W. J., and Terry, R. D. (1970). 'Senile plaques and cerebral amyloidosis in aged dogs: A histochemical study', *Lab. Invest.*, **23**, 287–296.

Wisniewski, H. M., and Terry, R. D. (1976). 'Neuropathology of the ageing brain', in *Neurobiology of Aging* (Eds R. D. Terry and S. Gershon), pp. 265–280, Raven Press, New York.

Woodard, J. C. (1962). 'Clinico-pathological significance of granulovacuolar degeneration in Alzehimer's disease', *J. Neuropathol. Exp. Neurol.*, **21**, 85–91.

Woodard, J. C. (1966). 'Alzheimer's disease in late adult life', *Am. J. Path.*, **49**, 1157–1165.

Wright, J. R., Calkins, E., Breen, W. J., Stolte, G. and Schultz, R. T. (1969). 'Relationship of amyloid to ageing', *Medicine*, **48**, 39–56.

Yates, P. O. (1976). 'Vascular disease of the central nervous system', in *Greenfield's Neuropathology* (Eds W. Blackwood and J. A. N. Corsellis), 3rd ed., pp. 86–147, Edward Arnold, London.

Principles and Practice of Geriatric Medicine
Edited by M. S. J. Pathy
© 1985 John Wiley & Sons Ltd

16.2

Neurochemistry of Ageing

T. Samorajski, Katherine Persson

INTRODUCTION

The knowledge that neurotransmitter and neuromodulator substances influence behaviour in general and diseases in particular has attracted interest to the neurochemical aspects of human ageing including such age-related diseases as Parkinsonism, Huntington's chorea, and senile dementia of the Alzheimer type. This chapter is a brief review of current information about neurochemical changes in the brain consequent to the normal ageing process and the mechanisms by which age-related diseases influence behaviour.

Most gerontologists consider ageing to be an orderly progression of a developmental lifespan programme. With increasing age, however, many physiological functions decline and susceptibility to disease increases. Thus, older individuals face the prospect of death, usually from complications of a disease that might have been of only minor consequence to younger persons.

Although the incidence of severe brain disease in the elderly is fairly low compared to disease incidence in other organs (Slater and Roth, 1969), many extracerebral conditions affect the brain indirectly, by toxins or by disturbances of cell oxygenation or nourishment. Consequently, 'normal' tissue from elderly individuals is rarely available for chemical study. Post-mortem conditions and regional differences in the brain may complicate the interpretation of data. Much is known about the pathological symptoms encountered by elderly individuals, but the relationship between disease susceptibility and ageing remains largely unknown.

Because of the many technical problems associated with using human tissue, much of the neurochemical investigation of ageing is done with animals, mainly rodents, or other animals selected on the basis of a relatively short lifespan. For some neurochemical comparisons, age-related differences in animal brain may not be relevant to humans (Samorajski and Rolsten, 1973). Consequently, the applicability of animal data to the human condition is limited. It is tempting to speculate that something about our central nervous system and our longer lifespan distinguishes us from lower animals.

Another problem of ageing studies concerns the fact that how well and how long we live is the result of an interaction at the cellular level between genetic programme and environment. We still do not know the extent to which these two factors influence individual differences in ageing populations.

In spite of some obvious limitations, many of the more stable constituents of human brain can be measured. Useful information about changes in protein, amino acids, lipid constituents, and even neurotransmitter substances and their enzymes can be obtained if the samples are carefully selected, properly prepared and stored. The information thus gained suggests that there is surprisingly little obvious chemical change in the brain during adolescence. Changes usually are seen very late in life, probably associated with a diffuse or generalized loss of neurones and alterations in the interstitial and connecting process of the neuropil. Age-related brain diseases, may, however, have more specific focus and show major morphological and neurochemical changes in the regions involved. Parkinsonism, for example, affects primarily the cells of the basal ganglia and is characterized by a major decline in dopamine.

Taken together, the studies indicate that neurochemical changes vary in both rate and time in different mammalian species and according to the severity of pathology, if present.

NORMAL AGEING

Changes in most organs of the body involve diminishing cell division and a gradual replacement of parenchymal cells with connective tissue, including a preponderance of fat cells. Yet, except for blood vessels, the brain has no connective tissue; death of postmitotic neurones is associated with proliferation of metabolically active glial elements (Samorajski and Rolsten, 1973). Consequently, the quantitative aspects of the ageing changes in brain and the rest of the body differ significantly.

Comparisons of the chemical composition of isolated brain and major body components of young and old human beings are shown in Fig. 1. In old age, the body gains lipid content while intracellular water, carbohydrate, protein, and minerals are lost. The increase of lipid at the expense of metabolically more active substances may account for the greater susceptibility and duration of action of many therapeutic drugs administered to aged persons.

The brain contains relatively more water than do the major organs and a smaller quantity of lipid, carbohydrate, protein, and inorganic substances than the whole body at similar age levels (Samorajski, 1980). With ageing the brain content of lipid, carbohydrate, protein, and mineral remains the same or declines only slightly. The brain's water content rises with age, primarily because of a 5 per cent. increase of extracellular water. Decline of weight and change in some chemical constituents of the human brain with age are summarized in Table 1 in ranked order. The values are rough esti-

Major Body Components

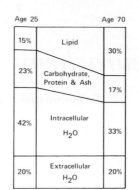
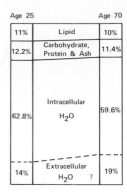

Figure 1 Age and distribution of major components of human body and brain. (Reprinted by permission from Figure 9–1, page 147 in *Psychopharmacology of Aging* by Carl Eisdorfer and William E. Fann (Eds). Copyright 1980, Spectrum Publications, Inc., New York)

mates in some cases, and they may differ markedly in both rate and timing from one brain region to another.

Water Content

Free water comprises the highest proportion of each brain region's weight, ranging from 70 to 90 per cent. depending on the ratio of white to grey matter. Tilney and Rosette (1931) reported that the water content of cerebral hemispheres and cerebellum increases from maturity to senescence, whereas the brainstem, which has less water, shows little or no change during the same period, probably because of its relatively higher proportion of myelin and fewer cellular constituents. The increase in water content in the cerebrum and cerebellum with age is presumably caused by an enlarged extracellular compartment (Bondareff, 1976) that results from death of neurones (Brody, 1955). For these reasons, biochemical parameters for brain regions are often expressed as dry weight or by using DNA or the protein content as reference.

Total Lipids

Lipids, which account for one-half of the dry weight of the human brain, are important constituents of cell membranes which form the matrix of all cells. The predominant lipid-containing element is the myelin sheath. Continuous changes in the amount of lipid present and the fatty acid composition (acyl group) of lipids have been observed as a consequence of ageing (Horrocks, Van Rollins, and Yates, 1981). Lipid content in human brain increases during development, remains relatively constant during maturity, and declines in later life. Decreases in lipid metabolism also occur with age, possibly because of lowered enzyme activity. The enzyme 2', 3'-cyclic nucleotide 3'-phosphodiesterase, which is generally accepted as an index of myelination, decreases in subcortical white matter at a rate of 0.2 per cent. per year per gram of tissue (Toews, Horrocks, and King, 1976). In agreement with these chemical observations, morphologists have shown a loss of myelin with sparing of axons in many regions of the central nervous system (Wisniewski and Terry, 1973). Further loss of lipid and basic myelin protein probably results from death of cortical neurones and consequent degeneration of axons and their associated myelin sheaths.

Concentrations of most lipids in human brain decrease at nearly constant rates after the age of 50 but at different rates for different classes of lipids. Losses ranging from 10 to 20 per cent. between 40 and 70 years of age, occur in cerebroside sulphates, ethanolamine plasmalogens, cerebrosides, sphingomyelins, cholesterol, and serine glycerophospholipids. Other phospholipids, including choline glycerophospholipids and phosphatidyl ethanolamine, decrease little or not at all with age (Table 2).

In addition to the decrease of total lipid content of the human brain, significant ageing changes occur in the fatty acid (acyl group) composition of brain lipids. A time-dependent change in the acyl group composition of the phospholipids (long-chain fatty acid moieties linked to phosphate groups) in the myelin sheath may be one of the mechanisms of ageing in the mammalian brain (Sun and Samorajski, 1973). Some drugs believed to stimulate cerebral metabolism also have marked effects on lipid metabolism in older animals.

Although specific acyl group profiles are associated with each phospholipid, the most significant age-related differences are found in ethanolamine phosphoglyceride (EPG), a ma-

Table 1 Rank order, decline of weight[a], and change in main chemical constituents of average male and female human brain between 25 and 75 years of age. (Reprinted by permission from Table 9–1, page 150 in *Psychopharmacology of Aging* by Carl Eisdorfer and William E. Fann (Eds). Copyright 1980, Spectrum Publications, Inc., New York)

	Rank	25 Years		75 Years	
		1,320 g	Weight (%)	1,200 g	Weight (%)
H_2O[a]	1	1,019.0	77.2	936.0	78.0
Total lipids and lipid complexes[b]	2	115.8	11.8	114.0	9.5
Protein and peptides[c]	3	18.8	9.0	86.4	7.2
Inorganic salts[d]: cations – Na, K, Ca, Mg anions – Cl HCO₃ metals – Cu, Mn, Zn, Fe, Al	4	16.5	1.1	?	?
Free amino acids[e]	5	9.2	0.7	8.4	0.7(?)
Nucleic acids[f]	6	6.3	0.48	6.4	0.54
RNA		5.2	0.40	5.3	0.45
DNA		1.1	0.8	1.1	0.09
Carbohydrates (glycogen)[g]	7	1.6	0.13	?	?

[a]Bürger (1957).
[b]Calculated from equations of Rouser and Yamamoto (1969).
[c]From Bürger (1957) and Himwich (1971).
[d]Tower (1969).
[e]Robinson and Williams (1965) for adult human brain; Davis and Himwich (1975) for 75 year old human based on extrapolation from monkey brain.
[f]Samorajski and Rolsten (1973), based on analysis of frontal cortex.
[g]Kirsch and Leitner (1967).

Table 2 Relative decreases in lipid concentrations in male human brains during ageing. These values were calculated using the equations of Rouser and Yamamoto (1969). Concentration values are given in millimoles per kilogram fresh weight. Phosphatidyl ethanolamines include diacyl and alkylacyl types. Reproduced with permission from Horrocks, Van Rollins, and Yates, 1981, by Edward Arnold Publishers)

Lipid	Concentration Age 40	Loss (%) Age 70	Loss (%) Age 100
Cholesterol	66.2	11	17
Cerebrosides	22.9	14	24
Cerebroside sulphates	7.9	19	48
Lipid phosphorus	69.9	7	11
Choline glycerophospholipids	20.8	5	8
Ethanolamine plasmalogens	15.4	18	29
Phosphatidyl ethanolamines	9.2	2	3
Serine glycerophospholipids	11.9	10	16
Spingomyelins	10.0	12	20

jor brain phospholipid. Ethanolamine phosphoglyceride, which constitutes about 40 percent. of the myelin phospholipids, contains most of the unsaturated acyl group found in myelin (Sun and Samorajski, 1973). The acyl group composition of EPG in myelin from three age groups of mice, rhesus monkeys, and humans were studied by Samorajski and Rolsten (1973) and Sun and Samorajski (1973), who found that the older age groups of all three species had a higher proportions of monoenes (mainly 18:1 and 20:1) and lower proportions of polyenes (mainly 20:4 and 22:4). A decrease with age also occurs in polyunsaturated acyl groups of EPG isolated from frontal grey matter (Bowen, Smith, and Davison 1973). In addition to an increased ratio of saturated to unsaturated acyl groups, the chain length of some fatty acids may increase with age, particularly in the glycolipids (Dhopeshwarkar and Mead, 1975). Considered together, the changes in the acyl group composition of myelin phospholipid are small, but they may be important in determining the functional properties of myelin and other types of membranes during ageing.

Lipid Complexes (Lipofuscin Pigment and Ceroid)

Lipofuscin

The progressive accumulation of intraneuronal lipid pigment (lipofuscin) with age in both normal and diseased brain tissue (Fig. 2) has aroused the interest of many investigators.

Some researchers (Samorajski, Ordy, and Keefe 1965; Zeman, 1971) suggested that the pigmented material might damage cells by disturbing cell geometry and that, if the distortion were severe, cellular activity might be disturbed. Other investigators maintained that the pigment is inert and not harmful to cells (Hyden and Lindstrom, 1950; Tcheng, 1964). Yet another concept of the possible significance of pigment accumulation was expressed by Siakotos and Armstrong (1975), who suggested that lipid pigments may facilitate cell activity by chelating toxic products of metabolism or providing a matrix for immobilizing active enzymes. From these conflicting opinions, it is clear that there is no uniform opinion regarding the functional significance of lipofuscin pigment.

Ceroid

A substance closely related to lipofuscin has been found in the liver of rats maintained on low protein diets (Lillie *et al.*, 1942) and in neurons of patients with Batten–Spielmeyer–Vogt syndrome (Zeman *et al.*, 1970) and Kuf's disease (Boehme *et al.*, 1971). Histochemical studies showed the material to be waxy, and hence it is called 'ceroid'. Although both lipofuscin and ceroid are fluorescent and share many histochemical properties, they differ in density, cationic content, and their excitation and emission maxima are slightly different (Siakotos *et al.*, 1970). Ceroid accumulation is associated with severe cell loss and atrophy in the brain. The accumulation of lipofuscin is

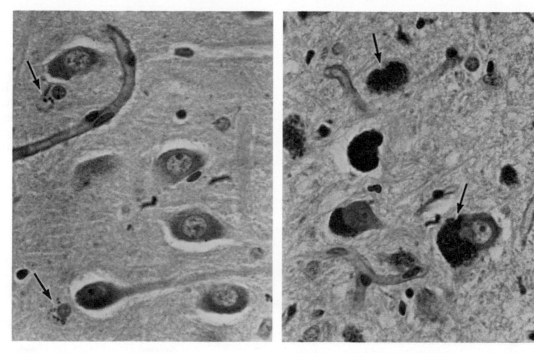

Figure 2   Lipofuscin pigment granules (arrows) in cytoplasm of glial cells in CA1 zone of hippocampus (left) and in neurons of layer 6 from lateral geniculate body of a 74 year old women with left-eye enucleation at the age of 71. Neurons of hippocampus are devoid of pigment (×400)

not related to atrophy or cell loss to the same degree as ceroid, even in syndromes in which marked increases of lipofuscin pigment are seen (Siakotos *et al.*, 1972).

Siakotos, and coworkers (1970) were the first to isolate lipofuscin and ceroid in sufficient quantities for chemical identification. Lysosomal enzymes are present in lipofuscin and ceroid of human brain, suggesting a lysosomal origin or association. Lipofuscin contains a low proportion of normal phospholipids and a relatively larger quantity of non-polar lipid polymer. Ceroid contains a higher proportion of normal phospholipids and acidic polymer. Lipofuscin also contains more zinc than does ceroid, but the latter contains more calcium, iron, and copper (Siakotos *et al.*, 1972).

Further studies by Taubold, Siakotos, and Perkins (1975) showed that lipofuscin contains cholesterol (3%), cholesterol esters (9%), mixed lipids including some polymers (68%), a colourless polymer (8%), and a coloured polymer (12%). Gas–liquid chromatographic analysis suggested the presence of a complex lipid whose unsaturated fatty acids had undergone oxidation and polymerization. Thus, lipofuscin appears to be a heterogeneous substance consisting mainly of polymeric lipid, with phospholipids, amino acids, zinc, and lysosomal enzymes as the predominant constituents.

Wolf and coworkers (1977) isolated the fluorescent and nonfluorescent fractions of ceroid from the brain of a patient with Batten's disease. The lipid soluble material, which was not fluorescent, was made up of cholesterol, free fatty acids, and phospholipids, qualitatively similar to lipofuscin. The fluorescent portion, however, was a retinoyl complex and appeared not to be derived from peroxidized polyunsaturated fatty acids as in lipofuscin. This may account for some of the differences in the physical properties of intraneuronal lipofuscin and ceroid. Further knowledge of the origin, genesis, and distribution of ceroid and lipofuscin with ageing may provide deeper insights into the significance of these materials on the process of ageing in the brain.

Proteins and Peptides

Proteins

Proteins consist of a vast number of complex molecular structures which have diverse functions and an elaborate mechanism for regulating their synthesis. MacArthur and Doisey (1919), among the first to study protein content in human brain, reported that protein content was about 15 per cent. lower in a 67-year-old brain than in one 35 years old. Subsequent studies by Bürger (1957) and Hoch-Ligeti (1963) confirmed that protein content in human brain decreases with age. Recent studies of the brains of mature and old rhesus monkeys by Davis and Himwich (1975) also revealed an age-related decrease in protein content in most areas of the brain examined, the most significant decline (about 10 per cent.) occurring in the pons, thalamus, caudate, and occipital cortex. White matter (corpus callosum) of monkey brain showed no significant change in protein content between 3 and 16 years of age.

Studies of the brain-specific proteins S-100 and 14–3–2 and of the enzyme carbonic anhydrase in animal and human brains revealed that S-100 and carbonic anhydrase increased with age in most of the regions examined (Cicero *et al.*, 1972; Perez and Moore, 1970; Wintzerith *et al.*, 1978). When 14–3–2 neuronal protein was measured in various areas of human brain, no correlation with age was found. Since S-100 protein and carbonic anhydrase are associated with glia, an increase in these constituents may indicate an increase in the glial population with age. An increase with age of S-100 and carbonic anhydrase may also represent a net gain of these constituents in glial cells. Both fibrous and protoplasmic astrocytes accumulate filaments and possibly glycogen with age (Raine, 1976). Thus, an increase in brain-specific protein S-100 and carbonic anhydrase may represent a change in the metabolic state of the glial and/or glial proliferation in response to ageing.

Many enzymes associated with subcellular organelles have been measured in human brain. Meier-Ruge and coworkers (1978) found that most enzymes of the glycolytic pathway were not significantly altered with age. They noted, however, that the two key enzymes of the Embden–Meyerhof pathway, hexokinase and phosphofructokinase (fructose-6-phosphate kinase), were significantly changed; soluble hexokinase increased and phosphofructokinase decreased significantly with age (Fig. 3). Meier-Ruge, and coworkers (1978) proposed that the decrease in phosphofructokinase activity might impair glucose degration and citric acid cycle function, resulting in reduced synthesis of the energy carrier adensoine triphosphatase (ATP). This hypothesis is presented schematically in Fig. 4.

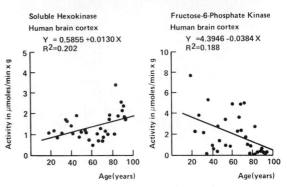

Figure 3 Age-related changes in hexokinase and fructose-6-phosphate kinase (phosphofructokinase) of human brain cortex. (From Meier-Ruge *et al.*, 1978. Reproduced by permission of Elsevier North-Holland Biomedical Press)

Enzymes involved in the catabolism of catecholamines, principally of norepinephrine, are currently a focus of research because of the possible link between altered amine metabolism and depression. Robinson and coworkers (1972) found a marked increase in monoamine oxidase (MAO) levels with age in human hindbrain; Megna and DeGiacomo (1973) and Samorajski and Rolsten (1973) also reported the age-related increase in this enzyme's activity in several different regions of the brain. Other enzymes associated with the metabolism of the monoamines and the neurotransmitters acetylcholine and gamma aminobutyric acid (GABA) have been investigated in many brain areas. With age, the enzymes glutamic acid decarboxylase (GAD), dopa decarboxylase (DDC), tyrosine hydroxylase (TH), and choline acetyl transferase (CAT) declined in some regions, and not in others. The enzymes catechol-*o*-methyltransferase (COMT) and acetylcholinesterase (ACE) showed little or no change with age in all of the brain areas examined. These results are summarized in Table 3.

Glycolytic Pathway

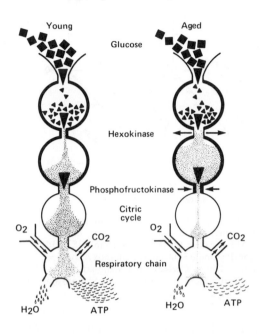

Figure 4 Schematic representation of glycolytic pathway illustrating rate-limiting effects of age-induced alteration of hexokinase and fructose-6-phosphate kinase (phosphofructokinase) on energy production in brain. (From Meier-Ruge *et al.*, 1978. Reproduced by permission of Elsevier North-Holland Biomedical Press)

Table 3 Changes in neurotransmitter enzymes of human brain associated with ageing. (Adapted from Samorajski, 1980)

Enzyme	Type of change	Reference
MAO	Increase in hindbrain, frontal cortex, and caudate	Robinson *et al.*, 1971; Samorajski and Rolsten, 1973
COMT	No change; decrease in caudate	Robinson *et al.*, 1977; Samorajski and Rolsten, 1973
GAD	Decrease in thalamus and temporal lobe	McGeer and McGeer, 1976; Bowen *et al.*, 1977
DDC and TH	Decrease in basal ganglia and amygdala	McGeer and McGeer, 1976
CAT	Decrease in caudate, cortex, and hippocampus	McGeer and McGeer, 1975; Perry *et al.*, 1977
ACE	No change	Samorajski and Rolsten, 1973

Abbreviations: MAO, monoamine oxidase; COMT, catechol-o-methyltransferase; GAD, glumatic acid decarboxylase; DDC, dopa decarboxylase; TH, tyrosine hydroxylase; CAT, choline acetyltransferase; ACE, acetylcholinesterase.

Changes in neurotransmitter-linked enzymes might lead to an alteration in the level of neurotransmitter present and/or a quantitative change in the concentration of its metabolites. Only a small number of human brain samples have been studied for life-span changes in neurotransmitter substances and their metabolites. Bertler (1961), comparing dopamine (DA) content of the caudate nucleus and putamen at senescence (over 70 years of age) with that at maturity (43 to 60 years), reported a decline. Carlsson and Winblad (1976) also found an age-related decrease of DA in the basal ganglia of human brain. A significant decline in norepinephrine (NE) has also been reported in human hindbrain (Robinson, 1975), yet the content of hindbrain serotonin (5-HT) and of the 5-HT metabolite 5-hydroxyindole acetic acid did not vary significantly with age (Fig. 5).

Peptides

Powerful new techniques have become available for characterizing peptides and detecting their presence in the central nervous system. Of the peptides which have only two or three amino acids, glutathione, sarcosine, carnosine, *N*-acetyl-*L*-aspartic acid, homocarnosine, and related peptides are widely distributed in mammalian brain; their levels are generally higher in adulthood than at birth (Davis and Himwich, 1975), but little is known about their distribution in the aged animal and human brain. Except for tripeptide glutathione (which has many functions), the role of these peptides has not been clearly defined. Most promising is the work of Pisano, (1969) with imidazolyl dipeptides (homocarnosine and related peptides) which are in some way related to two types of progressive disorders of the central nervous system. Whether or not biochemical disturbances of any of these peptides cause neurological disorders associated with ageing remains to be learned.

Other peptides containing five or more amino acids function as neurotransmitters in some neuronal systems or perform modulatory or regulatory roles in the function of other neurons. Many of these neuronal peptides (neuropeptides) are confined to the hypothalamic-pituitary axis and may act only as neurohormones on pituitary cells and peripheral organs.

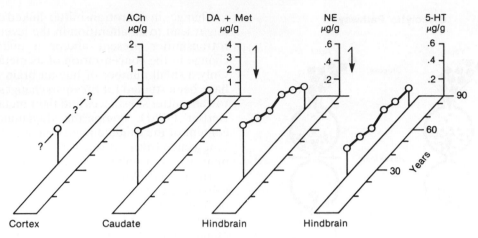

Figure 5   Lifespan changes in brain neurotransmitters. Neurotransmitter values for human brains are from regions with the highest content or are the only values available. Arrows indicate direction and degree of change with age if significant. Mean values for norepinephrine (NE) and serontonin (5-HT) are from Nies *et al.* (1973). Values for dopamine (DA) plus 3-methoxytyramine (MeT), a decomposition product of dopamine, are derived from Carlsson and Winblad (1976). Data for acetylcholine (ACL) are from Tower (1969). (Reproduced by permission of Samorajski *et al.*, 1980, and Librairie de l'Université, Georg and Cie S.A., Geneve)

Physiologically active neuronal peptides widely distributed throughout the brain include methionine-enkephalin (met-enkephalin), leucine-enkephalin (leu-enkephalin), substance P, β-endorphin, neurotensin, somatostatin, thyrotropin-releasing hormone (TRH), bradykinin, cholecystokinin, bombesin, vasopressin, oxytocin, vasoactive intestinal peptide (VIP), angiotensin II, and an α-MSH-like compound (McGeer and McGeer, 1980). Other neuropeptides are being identified and they will undoubtedly be added to the list. The distribution of these peptides in the brain suggests their influence on mood and emotion and many have potent behavioural effects.

Of great current interest are the enkephalins, endogenous pentapeptides that bind to the same sites in brain as do morphine and other opiates. The generic name for materials with opiate-like activity is 'endorphin'. The enkephalins are two of several endorphins in the brain. Three longer-chain peptides, known as α-, β- and λ-endorphins, are regarded as fragments of the 91 amino acid molecule β-lipoprotein. The globus pallidus has the highest concentration of enkephalin of any brain regions thus far examined (Gros *et al.*, 1978) and presumably plays a role in extrapyramidal function. Administration of opioids to rats induces hypokinesia, catalepsy, and muscular rigidity. This action can be inhibited with such agents as apomorphine that block opiate receptors on dopaminergic afferents to the striatum and other brain areas. The opiod peptides may also have a major role in the mechanism of pain sensitivity and memory functions (McGeer and McGeer, 1980). The possible involvement of endorphins in memory, mood, and emotion make them attractive agents for studies of senile dementia and other disturbances often associated with old age.

Although there is no direct evidence that the neuropeptides figure importantly in ageing, the hypothesis is an attractive one to explore. A small number of studies have concentrated on possible age-related changes in brain neuropeptide levels, revealing decreases in ACTH and β-endorphin in hypothalamus and basal ganglia of rat brain (Barden *et al.*, 1981, Gambert *et al.*, 1980) increases in met[5]-enkephalin, and no change in substance P, somatostatin, and neurotensin (Buck, Burks, and Yamamura, 1982). A significant reduction with age in substance P in the putamen but not in the caudate, frontal cortex, hypothalamus, or thalamus has been found, as have significant decreases of neurotensin in nigral pars compacta and pars reticulata. Somatostatin levels were not altered with age in any of the regions studied. These results associate substance P and neurotensin with the functional state of the substantia nigra, and they suggest major differences in ageing in the brains of rodents and human beings.

The effects of neuropeptide and hormone modulators on cognition and affect of the elderly have been studied with animal models, which revealed that vasopressin and ACTH moities are effective, to a variable degree, in improving attention span, motivation, retrieval, acquisition of memory and consolidation (Bartus, 1983; Pigache, 1983; Tinklenberg, 1983; Weingartner, 1983). Attempts to show significant behavioural improvement with neuropeptide administration to demented elderly individuals have, however, been generally disappointing. Recent efforts to modify the ACTH moiety to enhance its potency and possibly blood–brain barrier penetrability also have failed to produce significant improvements in mood and memory (Pigache, 1983). Undoubtedly, many of the obstacles to adequate treatment of dementia will disappear when a more precise definition of the chemistry of mood, memory, and emotion becomes available.

Inorganic Salts

The relatively small proportions of inorganic constituents in brain should not be taken as an indication of their functional unimportance. Reception, conduction, and synaptic transmission involve changes in ionic permeability that depend on membrane-bound calcium and sodium–potassium transport, together with energy-dependent systems. The most widely distributed minerals (macrominerals) sodium, potassium, calcium, magnesium, phosphorus, and chlorine are structural components of tissue; they are present in body fluids and are essential to the function of all cells. Their concentration is somewhat variable in living cells, but it still can be expressed in grams per kilogram or concentration (micromoles) per gram of fresh tissue. The remaining inorganic constitutents are present in much lower concentrations (milligrams or micrograms per kilogram of tissue), hence the name 'trace' elements. Trace elements proven to be essential to two or more species include iron, iodine, chromium, copper, zinc, and selenium (Mertz, 1981). Two non-essential trace elements are of

particular interest to neurochemists: aluminium because of its cytotoxic effects and association with Alzheimer's neurofibrillary tangles, and lithium because of its use in the treatment of depression. Additional trace elements may be added to the list by future research.

Macrominerals are distributed throughout the brain. The grey matter of most mammalian species contains about 100 μmoles of potassium, 60 μmoles of sodium, 2 μmoles of calcium, and 5 μmoles of magnesium per gram of fresh tissue. The total anionic equivalent in grey matter provided by chloride, bicarbonate, sulphates and phosphates is about 60 μmoles per gram of fresh tissue (Tower, 1969). Few data are available for mineral content of brain regions in relation to ageing because of the lack, until recently, of adequate analytic methods. There is, however, an abundance of older information on whole-brain homogenates (Korenchevsky, 1961). These studies have found decreases in potassium, calcium, magnesium, sulphur and phosphorus, and no change in sodium between maturity and old age.

Essential trace elements range in function from having relatively weak ionic effects to highly specific associations with proteins known as metalloenzymes. All or most of the enzymes regulating DNA replication, repair, and transcription are zinc metalloenzymes (Mildvan and Loeb, 1979). Burnet (1981) has suggested that dementia may represent the cascading effects of error-prone or ineffective DNA-handling of enzymes in neurones, presumably from an age-associated loss of ability to make zinc available for insertion into newly synthesized enzyme. Iron, copper, and selenium associated with the enzymes catalase, superoxide desmutase, and glutathione peroxidase, respectively, control the level of intracellular free-radical formation. Enzyme assays and protein metabolism studies of liver and other body organs of rodents have been a frequent focus of ageing studies. Unfortunately, except for studies of superoxide desmutase (SODase, superoxide; superperoxide oxidoreductase, EC 1.15 1.1), there has been little effort to study age-related changes of metalloenzymes in primate or human brain.

Recent research with superoxide desmutase suggests that by catalyzing the removal of superoxide radicals, this metalloenzyme (zinc) may be a major intracellular protective agent against oxygen toxicity. It has been suggested that free radical damage involving oxygen contributes to ageing (Harman, 1971). Superoxide desmutase has been found in all anatomical brain regions and subcellular fractions.

Despite the importance of SODase in the destruction of superoxide free radicals in tissue, its role in ageing is still controversial. There are reports that the specific activity of SODase in the brain of rats and mice remains unchanged with age (Reiss and Gershon, 1976), decreases with age (Massie, Aiello, and Iodice 1979), and is normal in lymphocytes and erythrocytes isolated from patients with Werner's syndrome (Marklund, Lordhensson, and Bäck 1981), a disease often regarded as a progeroid condition. Consequently, the relevance of changes in SODase activity as a cause or consequence of ageing is not certain.

A more compelling role for SODase in ageing has been suggested by Tolmasoff, Ono, and Cutler (1980), who examined the possible role of this enzyme in determining the lifespan of primate species. They found a significant positive correlation between the ratio of SODase-specific activity to metabolic rate in the liver, brain, and heart and the maximum lifespan potential for these species. This correlation suggests that longer-lived species, such as humans, have better protection against the byproducts of oxygen metabolism than do those with shorter lives. Further, tissue levels of SODase may be subject to experimental manipulation. Exposure of adult rats to 85 per cent. oxygen for 8 days caused an increase in SODase activity in lungs and to a lesser degree in brain (Crapo and Tierney, 1974). Therapeutic manipulation of SODase activity in brain and other tissues may be a worthwhile problem for research on ageing.

In view of the selective learning–memory deficits that occur in the early stages of aluminium-induced encephalopathy in animals and the morphological similarity of experimental and Alzheimer–Pick neurofibrillary inclusions, several investigators have examined aluminium content in human brain. Atomic absorption studies by Crapper (1976) revealed elevated concentrations of aluminium in some brain regions of persons who had Alzheimer's disease. Increased tissue concentrations were associated with neurofibrillary degeneration

and not senile plaques. Increased aluminium deposition and dementia may also occur with renal failure (Arieff *et al.*, 1979).

There is considerable species variability to aluminium neurotoxicity (King, De Boni, and Crapper 1975), and not all pathologic manifestations of Alzheimer's disease can be explained entirely on the basis of aluminium accumulation in the brain (Crapper, Karlick, and DeBoni 1978).

Another trace element of interest is lithium because it is often effective in the treatment of manic-depressive illness. Depression affects all age groups, but especially the elderly (Gaitz, 1973). Although treatment is similar for all age groups, several considerations may be important for the older patient. The half-life of lithium in middle-aged persons is about 24 hours, in contrast to 26 to 48 hours in older patients. An older person may therefore reach an adequate dosage level with a smaller amount of drug sooner than a younger person. The elderly are more vulnerable to lithium than younger persons (Prockop, 1976).

Research has demonstrated the role of zinc in protein and nucleic acid metabolism, the role of copper, iron, and selenium in protection against hydrogen peroxide, and the role of chromium in glucose metabolism. Aluminium and lithium seem to be involved in Alzheimer's disease and depression, respectively. No doubt other inorganic constituents and their functions in the brain will be elaborated in the future. Such information may enhance understanding of the role of inorganic constituents in the ageing process of the brain and of the methods by which biochemical reactions may be modulated to improve brain function.

Free Amino Acids

Brain amino acids participate in the metabolism of proteins, in intermediary metabolism associated with the tricarboxylic acid cycle, and in neurotransmission. Amino acids of relatively low concentration, whose main function is the metabolism of protein, include leucine, isoleucine, threonine, serine, cysteine, methionine, arganine, and histidine. The glutamic acid group, which includes aspartic acid, gamma aminobutyric acid (GABA), glutamine, and alanine, forms about 70 per cent.

of the total amino acid pool in the brain and functions as an energy source for the tricarboxylic acid cycle. The glutamic acid group plus taurine may also function as neurotransmitters. Experimental studies have revealed that glutamic and aspartic acids act as neuroexcitants and GABA, glycine, alanine, and taurine as neuroinhibitors in the mammalian brain.

The developmental pattern of the amino acids in early life has been thoroughly studied, and increases in the levels of brain amino acids have been associated with structural and functional maturation. The few researchers who have measured amino acid levels in human brain in relation to ageing have found relatively little consistent change. For example, Prensky and Moser's (1967) investigations of amino acid composition of proteolipids in frontal grey matter revealed a decline with age in aspartic acid and increases in isoleucine and arganine. Glutamic acid was decreased and histidine increased in frontal white matter. Studies in humans are complicated by the fact that glutamic acid decarboxylase and other enzymes associated with neurotransmitter systems are sensitive to post-mortem changes (McGeer and McGeer, 1976). These enzymes may also be affected by drugs used for the treatment of terminal conditions in the elderly (Iversen *et al.*, 1978).

To avoid some of these difficulties, Davis

and Himwich, (1975) investigated the amino acid composition of discrete brain regions of young and old rhesus monkeys. The investigators noted significant differences between anatomical regions and, depending on the region examined, found amino acid levels increased, decreased, or unchanged with age. A few typical examples of amino acid levels in selected brain regions are shown in Fig. 6. Although the changes in monkey brain, as in human brain, are not consistent, it may be inferred from the results of amino acid studies that some change occurs in the homeostasis of the ageing brain. If severe enough, such a change might alter intermediary metabolism, the chemical composition of neurons and glial cells, and the process of neurotransmission and compartmentation in the primate brain.

Nucleic Acids

Regional variations in deoxyribonucleic acid (DNA) and ribonucleic acid (RNA) concentrations in relation to age have been examined in animal and human brain. Although there are disagreements among researchers, RNA cytoplasmic content in mammalian neurones is usually reported as declining with age (Mann, Yates and Stamp, 1978) while the content of DNA in most brain regions remains fairly constant or increases slightly (Samorajski and Rolsten, 1973). The decrease in RNA and increase in DNA and the subsequent lowering of the RNA/DNA ratio with age has been interpreted as a loss of neurons (Samorajski and Rolsten, 1973). We have already cited the fact that glial-specific S-100 protein and carbonic anhydrase increases with age. Taken together, these observations suggest an increase in glial density in relation to the number of surviving neurones in the ageing brain.

Uemura and Hartmann (1978) reported that RNA content in individual cortical cell bodies in human brain decreased from 27.15 to 17.97 pg per cell between 66 and 80 years of age. Further, RNA content and volume of cell body in demented patients were like those of normal patients at similar ages. Thus, in terms of RNA content in individual cortical cell bodies, there seems to be no neurochemical criterion that characterizes senile dementia in comparison to changes that occur during normal ageing.

Many studies have been done on the tran-

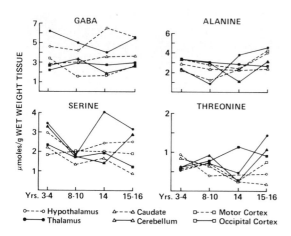

Figure 6 Gamma aminobutyric acid (GABA), alanine, serine, and threonine in monkey brain regions at different ages. SEM was within 11 per cent. (From Davis and Himwich, 1975. Reproduced by permission of Plenum Press, New York)

scriptional properties of neuronal and glial chromatin during ageing. The basis for such research is the belief that numerous cellular and biochemical parameters, which vary as a function of age, reflect modifications of the genetic readout information encoded in chromosomal DNA. The results of the studies are generally consistent with the view that the nucleoprotein complex stabilizes progressively with age. Herrmann (1975) has presented evidence suggesting that increased chromatin stabilization may result from an irreversible crosslinking of amino acid sequences in the mammalian genome.

Recently DNA-bound histones have become a focus of interest because they are the major regulators of the outflow of genetic information from the nucleus to the cytoplasm. Sarkander (1983) showed that neuronal chromatin of old rats (30 months) contain a lower proportion of transcriptional DNA sequences than chromatin isolated from younger rats (12 months old). Further, the rates of histone acetylization, RNA chain elongation, and utilization of RNA sites was increased in old rats. More importantly perhaps, they noted that the rate of change in the structure and transcription of DNA in neurones of the brain parallels species lifespan. From such findings comes the inference that changes at the genetic level occupy a central role in ageing.

Carbohydrates

Glucose is the main carbon source of many brain molecules and normally the sole substrate for the brain's energy metabolism (Maker, Clarke, and Lajtha, 1976; Sokoloff, 1976). Although it is likely that glycogen is stored in neurones in quantities too small to support neuronal metabolism for more than a few seconds, significant quantitative changes may occur with age in the amount of glycogen stored in the protoplasmic astrocytes (Fig. 7). Significant lifespan changes may occur also in the concentration and composition of extracellular glycoprotein and glycosaminoglycan (mucopolysaccharide) (Bondareff, Breen, and Weinstein 1975; Margolis *et al.*, 1975, 1976). The increase of these substances in the brain with ageing may reduce the movement of nutrients through the intercellular space and across plasma membranes, the outer aspect of which carries many oligosaccharides attached to protein chains of the membrane (Marchesi, 1975). The exact relationship between extracellular glycoprotein and the process of neuronal ageing remains unknown. One possibility is that ageing processes in the neurones interior may trigger an increase in oligosaccharide side-chains, signalling that these cells are approaching retirement.

Radiolabelled methods have been applied to

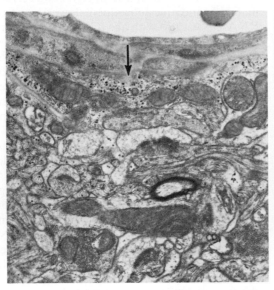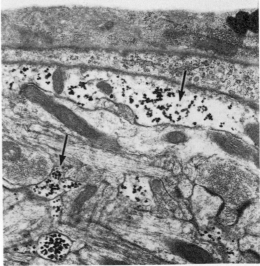

Figure 7   Comparison of glycogen distribution in electron micrographs of protoplasmic astrocytes of mice at 5 months (left) and 34 months (right) of age ($\times 10,000$)

study the effects of ageing on local rates of cerebral glucose utilization. Because the rate of glucose utilization has been found closely coupled with functional activity (Sokoloff, 1977), changes in local cerebral energy metabolism may be used to identify regions of the brain which might have altered functional activity in relation to ageing. Position emission tomography (PET) is proving to be useful for in vivo quantitative measurement of regional radiolabelled glucose utilization. Preliminary investigations of human ageing and of senile dementia of the Alzheimer type (SDAT) indicate that SDAT patients had significantly lower rates (35 to 45 per cent.) than age-matched controls (Leon *et al.*, 1981). There was a strong correlation between the degree of reduction of glucose utilization and cognitive impairment. PET techniques provided a unique means of studying in vivo brain changes related to ageing and senile dementia. Positron emission tomography, combined with computed tomography (CT) densities, may also prove useful for identifying brain regions related to cognitive processes and for evaluating the effects of drugs on specific brain pathways.

NEUROCHEMICAL PATHOLOGY OF AGEING

Depression

Although at no age are persons immune to mental disease, emotional problems increase with age. Depression is probably the most common mental disorder (Goldfarb, 1975). There are many hypotheses regarding etiology. The common neurochemical features of depression are altered catecholamine function, neuronal sodium accumulation, and possibly altered hormone levels (Lipton, and Nemeroff, 1978; Ordy and Kaack, 1975). A great deal of evidence suggests that depressive illness is associated with a depletion of norepinephrine (NE) and probably of serotonin (5-HT) in the brain. It will be recalled that there is an age-related increase of MAO in the brain (Table 3), which breaks down 5-HT and NE to 5-hydroxyidole acetic acid (5-HIAA) and 4-hydroxy 3-methoxy D-mandelic acid (VMA) and related metabolites, respectively. Drugs with marked antidepressant properties inhibit MAO or prevent the re-uptake of discharged NE and 5-HT by nerve endings. Such findings are evidence of a possible change in neurotransmitter and neuroreceptor mechanisms in depression and possibly of other age-related disorders of the brain.

Other common neurological disorders of late life include Alzheimer's disease, Parkinson's disease, Huntington's chorea, and various degrees of mental deterioration, often associated with memory impairment. In Alzheimer's and the closely related Pick's disease, a gradual and progressive dementia occurs in middle to late life. Both have a pathological substrate of cerebral atrophy accompanied by plaques, intracytoplasmic neurofibrillary tangles and, occasionally, granulovacuolar degeneration, especially in the hippocampus and cortex. The neurochemical defect may be diffuse and possibly associated with cholinergic deficiencies in presynaptic components. Spillane and coworkers (1977) examined cortical biopsies removed at craniotomy and found that choline acetyltransferase (CAT) activity was reduced by over 50 per cent. in Alzheimer cases compared to age-matched controls. Perry and coworkers (1977) found that CAT activity decreased with age in normal persons and was most pronounced in the hippocampus. Even greater reduction of enzyme activity was found in the hippocampus of demented patients compared to age-matched controls.

Cholinergic receptors in the hippocampus in normal ageing and senile dementia of the Alzheimer type have been investigated by Nordberg and coworkers (1982). They reported that the number of muscarinic and nicotinic receptor binding sites in the human hippocampus decreases with age, primarily in the anterior part of the hippocampus. In addition, Nordberg *et al.*, (1981) measured cholinergic receptors in the hippocampus of patients with Alzheimer's disease and infarct dementia. In agreement with other studies, they found no change in the number of muscarinic binding sites of the hippocampus in the Alzheimer patients compared to age-matched controls. A selective decrease in hippocampal choline acetyltransferase activity in chronic alcoholic patients (Nordberg *et al.*, 1980) and Alzheimer's disease (Perry and Perry, 1980) has also been reported. Interestingly, Nordberg and coworkers (182) found a decreased number of muscarinic binding sites in the hippocampus of patients with multi-infarct dementia, indicating a cholinergic involvement in this disease as well.

In other disorders the defect may occur in a discrete cortical or subcortical region of the brain. Parkinsonism, for example, has been associated with degeneration of the nigrostriatal dopaminergic system (see Chapter 16.13). Decreased catecholamines (dopamine, norepinephrine, and serotonin) and increased cholinergic functions (choline acetyltransferase) have been reported in most constituents of the basal ganglia (for a review, see Samorajski and Hartford, 1980). In Huntington's chorea, recent post-mortem biochemical and pharmacological studies of human brain suggest that choreic movements associated with this disease are also mediated by the dopaminergic nigrostriatal pathway. Early indications of a selective loss of GABA-containing interneurons in the basal ganglia have not been supported and it now seems that many different types of striatal cell populations are involved. Evidence is growing that chorea arises from an imbalance of the effects of dopamine, acetylcholine, and GABA released from nerve terminals in the basal ganglia (Spokes, 1981). Nerve terminals releasing noradrenalin, serotonin, glutamate, and neuropeptides may be involved also in extrapyramidal control of muscles (Fig. 8). Yet Parkinsonism and Huntington's chorea, although they involve different combinations of neurotransmitter systems, have the common

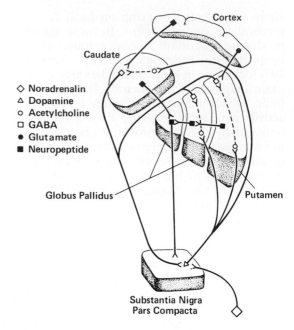

○ Noradrenalin
△ Dopamine
○ Acetylcholine
□ GABA
● Glutamate
■ Neuropeptide

Figure 8 Proposed neurochemical pathways in the basal ganglia. Imbalances among neurotransmitters may be associated with Huntington's disease. (Adapted from Spokes, 1981)

functional feature of mental deterioration and progressive movement disorders. This illustrates the complexity that confronts researchers. Table 4 summarizes the major known chemical defects in cortical and subcortical regions of some primary genetic and postmaturity disorders associated with ageing.

Table 4 Neurochemistry of major neurological disorders in late life

Disorder	Effects on brain	Area(s) and neurochemical defect
Alzheimer's disease	Disorientation and defective memory	*Cortex:* increased cerebroside hexosamine, acid polysaccarides, aluminium[a]; decreased ethanolamine phospholipid[b,c], ganglioside, ATPase[d], and CAT[e]
		Hippocampus: reduced CAT[f]
Parkinson's disease	Akinesia, tremor, rigidity	*Basal ganglia:* decreased dopamine, serotonin, and possibly norepinephrine[g], increased CAT and ACE[h]
Huntington's chorea	Involuntary movements, failing intellect	*Basal ganglia:* decreased total protein, phospholipid, lecithin; increased sphingomyelin, cholesterol, RNA, and strontium[i,j,k]. Imbalance among dopamine, norepinephrine, acetylcholine, GABA, glutamate, and neuropeptide[l]

Abbreviations: ATPase, adenosinetriphosphatase; CAT, choline acetyltransferase; ACE, acetylcholinesterase; RNA, ribonucleic acid; GABA, gamma amino butyric acid.
References: [a]Crapper, Krishnan, and Dalton, 1973; [b]Suzuki, Katyman, and Korey, 1965; [c]Suzuki and Chen, 1966; [d]Shelanski, 1976; [e]Perry *et al.*, 1981; [f]Bowen *et al.*, 1976; [g]Hornykiewicz, 1973; [h]Woert, 1976; [i]Borri *et al.*, 1967; [l]Embree, Bass, and Pope, 1972; [k]Bird and Iversen, 1974; [l]Spokes, 1981.

NUTRITION AND NEUROCHEMISTRY OF AGEING

Even though the nutritional needs of the elderly have not been precisely defined, many studies have examined the effects of various dietary supplements on general health, mental function, and longevity. Some encouraging results have come from the use of the cholinergic precursors lecithin and choline. The rationale for increasing acetylcholine synthesis with precursor therapy is the decline in the cholinergic system that has been reported in normal ageing (Drachman, 1981), with an even more pronounced decline in the age-related pathologies of Huntington's chorea, Alzheimer's disease, tardive dyskinesia, Gilles de la Tourette syndrome, and Friedreich's ataxia (Barbeau, 1978). Thirty to 60 per cent. of patients with these disorders have experienced some clinical improvements from choline and lecithin supplementation, depending on the disorder, dose, and the regime followed (Barbeau, 1978). Cholinergic function may also be related to short-term memory. Bartus and Dean (1981) reported short-term memory improvement in rodents and rhesus monkeys administered a combination of choline and physostigmine (a cholinergic agonist). There is, therefore, some evidence to justify further investigation into the use of cholinergic precursor strategy in treating patients for senile dementia.

Trace element supplementation may also play a significant role in nutrition in the elderly. Indirect evidence summarized by Hsu (1979) suggests that the diets of some elderly persons may be deficient in chromium, zinc, and other trace elements. A marked decline of chromium concentration with age was reported in human tissue samples of kidneys, liver, aorta, and spleen (Schroeder, 1968). Subjects who received chromium supplements often displayed an improved glucose tolerance (Levine, Streetan, and Doisy, 1968), indicating that the dietary chromium intake may be inadequate in an ageing population and, further, that normal carbohydrate metabolism requires chromium. Adequate levels of chromium may be crucial for brain function as neuronal carbohydrate metabolism depends almost totally on the availability of glucose.

Few topics in nutrition are more controversial than vitamins and, among those believed to influence the ageing process, perhaps none has drawn more attention than vitamin E. Large dosages of vitamin E are often prescribed as cures for a wide variety of circulatory, reproductive, and nervous system conditions as well as to protect against ageing (Horwitt, 1977). In clinical practice, one can find few cases of vitamin E deficiency because it is prevalent in the normal diet. New knowledge of oxidants and biological 'protector systems has again catalysed interest in the use of vitamin E and other antioxidants as a means of providing protection against free-radical peroxidative damage to the fatty acid constituents of biologic membranes. Studies with rodents generally support the hypothesis that vitamin E alone or in combination with any number of antioxidants, including selenium, 2-mercaptoethylamine, butylated hydroxytoluene, ethoxyquin, santoquin, and dihydroquaiaretic acid, increases the mean lifespan of experimental animals (Harman and Eddy, 1979).

The mechanism by which antioxidants stabilize membranes is not yet known, but discoveries of positive benefits seem to be dispelling some of the 'enigma' associated with vitamin E. Meanwhile, more work needs to be done on the role of antioxidants on the ageing process in terms of protecting membranes from peroxidative damage. Emerging hints of the utility of the vitamin for a wide variety of disorders affecting humans will undoubtedly stimulate new research.

COMMENT

The neurochemical findings of decreases in total lipids and proteins in normal ageing of the human brain correlate with some degree of neuronal loss, gliosis, and damage at the synaptic level. Such changes may make the brain increasingly susceptible to exogenous substances and to disease. Characteristic of many diseases of the brain are further neuronal loss, gliosis, and the appearance of plaques, tangles, and the accumulation of various inclusions, each with its characteristic chemistry. Vascular disease may affect brain-barrier systems and transport of oxygen and nutrients to the nerve cells, resulting in additional functional decline that may or may not be associated with neuronal loss.

Evidence from morphological and biochemical investigations suggests that the breakdown of neuronal integrating mechanisms during normal ageing is the sum of alterations that have occurred throughout the brain. By contrast, disease processes associated with ageing and resulting in a specific functional decline may be the expression of change in a discrete area of the brain. Advances in our knowledge of the role of specific neurotransmitters on mood and behaviour may further clarify the physiological and psychological events that accompany ageing.

Of all substances measured in the ageing human brain, the glycolytic enzymes hexokinase and phosphofructokinase and the neurotransmitter systems seem to be particularly vulnerable to ageing and pathology. The occurrence of diseases late in life may be interpreted as adding yet another echelon of functional change to the already accelerating defects of some molecular mechanisms in the brain.

New techniques for studying brain chemistry with positive emission tomography (PET) promise greater flexibility and precision for probing neurochemical events in the living brain. Thus, the time may soon arrive when conditions of health and disease may be studied in the ageing brain under conditions of varying emotional states.

ACKNOWLEDGEMENTS

We acknowledge Drs J. M. Ordy, Lloyd Horrocks and Kenneth Brizzee for helpful comments. We are indebted to Lore Feldman, Les Goekler and Lisa Hatfield for technical expertise in preparing this manuscript.

REFERENCES

Arieff, A. I., Cooper, J. D., Armstrong, D., and Lazarowitz, V. C. (1979). 'Dementia, renal failure and brain aluminum', *Ann. Intern. Med.,* **90**, 741–747.

Barbeau, A. (1978). 'Emerging treatments: Replacement therapy with choline or lecithin in neurological diseases', *Can. J. Neurol. Sci.* **5**, 157–160.

Barden, N., Dupont, A., Labrie, F., Merand, Y., Rouleau, D., Vaudry, H., and Boissier, J. R. (1981). 'Age-dependent changes in the β-endorphin content of discrete rat brain nuclei', *Brain Res.* **208**, 209–212.

Bartus, R. (1983). 'Neuropeptide effects on behavior and neurotransmitter function in aged rodents and primates', in *Neuropeptide and Hormone Modulation of Brain Function, Homeostasis, and Behavior* (Eds J. R. Sladek, J. M. Ordy, and B. Reisberg), Raven Press, New York (in press).

Bartus, R. T., and Dean, R. L. (1981). 'Age related memory loss and drug therapy: Possible directions based on animal models', in *Aging*, Vol. 17, *Brain Neurotransmitters and Receptors in Aging and Age-Related Disorders* (Eds S. J. Enna, T. Samorajski, and B. Beer), pp. 209–223, Raven Press, New York.

Bertler, A. (1961). 'Occurrence and localization of catecholamines in the human brain', *Acta Physiol. Scand.* **51**, 97–107.

Bird, E. D., and Iverson, L. L. (1974). 'Huntington's chorea: Post-mortem measurement of glutamic acid decarboxylase, choline acetyltransferase and dopamine in basal ganglia', *Brain,* **97**, 457–472.

Boehme, D., Cottrell, J. C., Leonberg, S. C., and Zeman, W. (1971). 'A dominant form of neuronal ceroidlipofuscinosis', *Brain,* **94**, 745–760.

Bondareff, W. (1976). 'Extracellular space in the aging cerebrum', in *Aging*, Vol. 3, *Neurobiology of Aging* (Eds R. D. Terry and S. Gershon), pp. 167–175, Raven Press, New York.

Bondareff, W., Breen, M., and Weinstein, H. G. (1975). 'Changes in the neuronal micorenvironment associated with aging', in *Advances in Behavioural Biology*, Vol. 16, *Neurobiology of Aging* (Eds J. M. Ordy and K. R. Brizzee), pp. 485–503, Plenum Press, New York.

Borri, P. F., Opden Velde, W. M., Hooghivinkel, G. J. M., and Bruyn, G. W. (1967). 'Biochemical studies in Huntington's chorea. VI. Composition of striatal neutral lipids, phospholipids, glycolipids, fatty acids and amino acids', *Neurol (NY),* **17**, 172–178.

Bowen, D. M., Smith, C. B., and Davison, A. N. (1973). 'Molecular changes in senile dementia', *Brain,* **96**, 849–856.

Bowen, D. M., Smith, C. B., White, P., and Davison, A. N. (1976). 'Neurotransmitter-related enzymes and indices of hypoxia in senile dementia and other abiotrophies', *Brain,* **99**, 459–496.

Bowen, D. M., Smith, C. B., White, P., Goodhardt, M. J., Spillane, A., Flack, R. H. A., and Davison, A. N. (1977). 'Chemical pathology of the organic dementias, Part 1. Validity of biochemical measurements on human post-mortem brain specimens', *Brain,* **100**, 397–426.

Brody, H. (1955). 'Organization of the cerebral cortex. III. A study of aging in the human cerebral cortex', *J. Comp. Neurol.*, **102**, 511–556.

Buck, S. H., Burks, T. F., and Yamamura, H. I.(1982). 'Neuropeptide alterations in the central nervous system in aging',*Geroutology*, **28** (Suppl. 1), 25–34

Bürger, M. (1957). 'Die chemische biomorphose des menschlichen gehirns. Abhandlungen der sächsischen akademie der wissenschaften, Leipzig', *Mathematischnaturwissen schaflliche Klasse*, **45**, 1–62.

Burnet, F. M. (1981). 'A possible role of zinc in the pathology of dementia', *Lancet*, **1**, 186–188.

Carlsson, A., and Winblad, B. (1976). 'Influence of age and time interval between death and autopsy of dopamine and 3-methoxytyramine levels in human basal ganglia', *J. Neural. Transm.* **38**, 271–276.

Cicero, T. J., Ferrendelli, J. A., Suntzeff, V., and Moore, B. W. (1972). 'Regional changes in CNS levels of the S-100 and 14–3–2 proteins during development and aging of the mouse', *J. Neurochem.*, **19**, 2119–2125.

Crapo, J. D., and Tierney, D. F. (1974). 'Superoxide desmutase and pulmonary oxygen toxicity', *Am. J. Physiol.*, **226**, 1401–1407.

Crapper, D. R. (1976). 'Functional consequences of neurofibrillary degeneration', in *Aging,* Vol.3, *Neurobiology of Aging* (Eds R. D. Terry and S. Gershon), pp. 405–432, Raven Press, New York.

Crapper, D. R., Karlik, S., and De Boni, U. (1978). 'Aluminum and other metals in senile (Alzheimer) dementia', in *Aging,* Vol. 7, *Alzheimer's Disease: Senile Dementia and Related Disorders* (Eds R. Katzman, R. D. Terry and K. L. Bick), pp. 471–485, Raven Press, New York.

Crapper, D. R., Krishnan, S. S., and Dalton, A. J. (1973). 'Brain aluminum distribution in Alzheimer's disease and experimental neurofibrillary degeneration', *Science*, **180**, 511–513.

Davis, J., and Himwich, W. A. (1975). 'Neurochemistry of the developing and aging mammalian brain', in *Advances in Behavioral Biology*, Vol. 16, *Neurobiology of Aging* (Eds J. M. Ordy and K. R. Brizzee), pp. 329–357, Plenum Press, New York.

Dhopeshwarkar, G. A., and Mead, J. F. (1975). 'Age and lipids of the central nervous system: Lipid metabolism in the developing brain', in *Aging*, Vol. 1, *Clinical Morphologic, and Neurochemical Aspects in the Aging Central Nervous System* (Eds H. Brody, D. Harman and J. M. Ordy), pp. 119–132, Raven Press, New York.

Drachman, D. A. (1981). 'The cholinergic system, memory, and aging', in *Aging*, Vol. 17, *Brain Neurotransmitters and Receptors in Aging and Age-Related Disorders* (Eds S. J. Enna, T. Samorajski and B. Beer), pp. 255–268, Raven Press, New York.

Eisdorfer, C., and Fann, W. E. (Eds) (1980). *Psychopharmacology of Aging*, Spectrum Publications, New York.

Embree, L. J., Bass, N. H., and Pope, A. (1972). 'Biochemisty of middle and late life dementias', in *Handbook of Neurochemistry* (Ed. A. Lajtha), Vol. 7, pp. 329–369, Plenum Press, New York.

Gaitz, C. M. (1973). 'Mental disorders: Diagnosis and treatment', in *Theory and Therapeutics of Aging* (Ed. E. W. Busse), pp. 72–82, Mecom Press, New York.

Gambert, S. R., Garthwaite, T. L., Pontzer, C. H. and Hagen, T. C. (1980), 'Age-related changes in central nervous system beta-endorphin and ACTH', *Neuroendocrinology*, **31**, 252–255.

Goldfarb, A. (1975). 'Depression in the old and aged', in *The Nature and Treatment of Depression* (Eds F. Flach and S. Graghi), pp. 119–144, John Wiley and Sons, New York.

Gros, C., Pradelles, P., Humbert, J., Dray, F., Le Gal La Salle, G., and Ben-Ari, Y. (1978). 'Regional distribution of metenkephalin within the amygdaloid complex and red nucleus of the stria terminalis', *Neurosci. Lett.*, **10**, 193–196.

Harman, D. (1971). 'Free radical theory of aging: Effect of the amount and degree of unsaturation of dietary fat on mortality rate', *J. Gerontol.*, **26**, 451–457.

Harman, D., and Eddy, D. E. (1979). 'Free radical theory of aging: Beneficial effect of adding antioxidants to the maternal mouse diet on life span of offspring; possible explanation of the sex difference in longevity', *Age*, **2**, 109–122.

Herrmann, R. L. (1975). 'Age-related changes in nucleic acids and protein synthesis', in *Advances in Behavioral Biology*, Vol. 16, *Neurobiology of Aging* (Eds J. M. Ordy and K. R. Brizzee), pp. 307–327, Plenum Press, New York.

Himwich, W. A. (1971). 'Biochemical processes of nervous system development', in *The Biopsychology of Development* (Eds E. Tobach, L. R. Aronson and E. Shaw), pp. 173–194, Academic Press, New York.

Hoch-Ligeti, C. (1963). 'Effects of aging on the central nervous system', *J. Am. Geriat. Soc.*, **11**, 403–408.

Hornykiewicz, O. (1973). 'Metabolism of dopamine and L-dopa in human brain', in *Frontiers in Catecholamine Research* (Eds E. Usdin and S. H. Snyder), pp. 1101–1107, Pergamon Press, New York.

Horrocks, L. A., Van Rollins, M., and Yates, A. J. (1981). 'Lipid changes in the ageing brain', in *The Molecular Basis of Neuropathology* (Eds R. H. S. Thompson and A. N. Davison), pp. 601–630, Edward Arnold Publishers Ltd, London.

Horwitt, M. K. (1977). 'Vitamin E', *Nutr. Rev.*, **35**, 57–62.

Hsu, J. M. (1979). 'Current knowledge on zinc, copper and chromium in aging', Wld. Rv. Nutr. Diet, **33**, 42–69.

Hyden, H., and Lindstrom, B. (1950). 'Microspectrographic studies on the yellow pigment in nerve cells', *Discuss. Faraday Soc.*, **9**, 436–441.

Iversen, L. L., Bird, E., Spokes, E., Nicholson, P., and Suckling, C. J. (1978). 'Agonist specificity of GABA binding sites in human brain and GABA in Huntington's disease and schizophrenia', in *GABA Neurotransmitters* (Eds P. Krogsgaard-Larsen and J. Scheel-Kruger), pp. 179–190, Alfred Benzon Symp., XII, Munksgaard.

King, G. A., De Boni, U., and Crapper, D. R. (1975). 'Effect of aluminum upon condition avoidance response acquisition in the absence of neurofibrillary degeneration', *Pharmacol. Biochem. Behav.*, **3**, 1003–1009.

Kirsch, W. M., and Leitner, J. W. (1967). 'Glycolytic metabolites and cofactors in human cerebral cortex and white matter during complete ischaemia', *Brain Res.*, **4**, 358–368.

Korenchevsky, V. (1961). 'Chemical changes with ageing', in *Physiological and Pathological Aging* (Ed. G. H. Bourne), pp. 87–159, Hafner Publishing, New York.

Leon, M. J. de, Ferris, S. H., George, A. E. Rosenbloom, S., Reisberg, B., Christman, D. R., Fowler, J., Gentes, C., Emmerich, M., and Wolf, A. (1981). 'Position emission tomography and computed tomography evaluations of regional brain metabolism in senile dementia', *Age*, **4** (Abs.), 146.

Levine, R. A., Streetan, D. P. H., and Doisy, R. (1968). 'Effects of oral chromium supplementation on the glucose tolerance of elderly human subjects', *Metabolism*, **17**, 114–125.

Lillie, R. D., Ashburn, L. L., Sebrell, W. H., Daft, F. S., and Lawry, J. V. (1942). 'Histogenesis and repair of the hepatic cirrhosis in rats produced on low choline diets and preventable with choline', *U.S. Public Health Report*, **57**, 502–507.

Lipton, M. A., and Nemeroff, C. B. (1978). 'The biology of aging and its role in depression', in *Aging: The Processs and the People* (Eds. G. Usdin and C. J. Hofling), pp. 47–95, Brunner/Mazel, New York.

MacArthur, C. G., and Doisey, E. A. (1919). 'Quantitative chemical changes in the human brain during growth', *J. Comp. Neurol.*, **30**, 445–486.

McGeer, E. G., and McGeer, P. L. (1975). 'Age changes in the human for some enzymes associated with metabolism of catecholamines, GABA and acetylcholine', in *Advances in Behavioral Biology*, Vol. 16, *Neurobiology of Aging* (Eds J. M.

Ordy and K. R. Brizzee), pp. 287–305, Plenum Press, New York.

McGeer, P. L., and McGeer, E. G. (1976). 'Enzymes associated with the metabolism of catecholamines, acetylcholine, and GABA in human controls and patients with Parkinson's disease and Huntington's chorea', *J. Neurochem.*, **26**, 65–76.

McGeer, P. L. and McGeer, E. G. (1980). 'Chemistry of mood and emotion', *Ann. Rev. Psychol.*, **31**, 273–307.

Maker, H. S., Clarke, D. D., and Lajtha, A. L. (1976). 'Intermediary metabolism of carbohydrates and amino acids', in *Basic Neurochemistry* (Eds G. J. Siegel, R. W. Albers, R. Katzman, and B. W. Agranoff), 2nd ed., pp. 279–307, Little, Brown and Co., Boston.

Mann, D. M. A., Yates, P. O., and Stamp, J. E. (1978). 'The relationship between lipofuscin pigment and ageing in the human nervous system', *J. Neurol. Sci.*, **37**, 83–93.

Marchesi, V. (1975). 'The structure and orientation of a membrane protein', in *Cell Membranes; Biochemistry, Cell Biology and Pathology* (Eds G. Weissmann and R. Claiborne), pp. 45–53, HP Publishing Co., New York.

Margolis, R. V., Margolis, R. K., Chang, L. B., and Preti, C. (1975). 'Glycosaminoglycans of brain during development', *Biochemistry*, **14**, 85–88.

Margolis, R. K., Preti, C., Lai, D., and Margolis, R. V. (1976). 'Developmental changes in brain glycoproteins', *Brain Res.*, **112**, 363–369.

Marklund, S., Nordensson, I., and Bäck, O. (1981). 'Normal CuZn superoxide desmutase, Mn superoxide desmutase, catalase and glutathione peroxidase in Werner's syndrome', *J. Gerontol.*, **36**, 405–409.

Massie, H. R., Aiello, V. R., and Iodice, A. A. (1979). 'Changes with age in copper and superoxide desmutase levels in brains of C57BL/6J mice', *Mech. Ageing. Dev.*, **10**, 93–99.

Megna, G., and DeGiacomo, P. (1973). 'Le attivita delle monoaminossidasi cerebrali nell'uomo: Rilievi in relazione ad eta, sesso e pathologie mentali', *Acta. Neurol.*, **28**, 459–465.

Meier-Ruge, W., Hunziker, O., Iwangoff, P., Reichlmeier, K., and Sandoz, P. (1978). 'Alterations of morphological and neurochemical parameters of the brain due to normal aging', in *Senile Dementia: A Biomedical Approach* (Ed. K. Nandy), pp. 33–44, Elsevier North-Holland Biomedical Press, Amsterdam.

Mertz, W. (1981). 'The essential trace elements', *Science*, **213**, 1332–1338.

Mildvan, A. S., and Loeb, L. A. (1979). 'The role of metal ions in the mechanisms of DNA and RNA polymeroses', *CRC Crit. Rev. Biochem.*, **6**, 819–844.

Nies, A., Robinson, D. S., Davis, J. M., and Ravaris, C. L. (1973). 'Changes in monoamine oxidase with aging', in *Psychopharmacology of
Aging* (Eds C.Eisdorfer and W.E. Fann), pp. 41–
54, Plenum Press, New York.

Nordberg, A., Adolfsson, R., Aquilonius, S-M.,
Marklund, S., Oreland, L., and Winblad, B.
(1980). 'Brain enzymes and acetylcholine recep-
tors in dementia of Alzheimer type and chronic
alcohol abuse', in *Aging*, Vol. 13, *Aging of the
Brain and Dementia* (Eds L. Amaducci, A. N.
Davison, and P. Antnono), pp. 169–171, Raven
Press, New York.

Nordberg, A., Adolfsson, R., Marcusson, J., and
Winblad, B. (1982). 'Cholinergic receptors in the
hippocampus in normal ageing and dementia of
Alzheimer type', in *Cellular and Molecular Mech-
anisms of Aging in the Nervous System*, (Eds E.
Filogamo, E. Giacobini, and A. Vernadakis),
Vol. 18, pp. 23–245, Raven Press, New York.

Ordy, J. M., and Kaack, B. (1975). 'Neurochemical
changes in composition, metabolism and neurotransmitters in the human brain with age', in *Advances in Behavioral Biology*, Vol. 16,
Neurobiology of Aging (Eds J. M. Ordy and K.
R. Brizzee), pp. 253–285, Plenum Press, New
York.

Perez, V. L., and Moore, B. W. (1970). 'Biochemistry of the nervous system in aging', *Interdispl.
Topics Gerontol.*, **7**, 22–45.

Perry, E. K., Gibson, P. H., Blessed, G., Perry, R.
H., and Tomlinson, B. E. (1977). 'Neurotrans-
mitter enzyme abnormalities in senile dementia',
J. Neurol. Sci., **34**, 247–265.

Perry, E. K., and Perry, R. H. (1980). 'The cholinergic system in Alzheimer's disease', in *Biochemistry of Dementia* (Ed. P. J. Roberts), pp. 135–
183, John Wiley and Sons, New York.

Perry, E. K., Tomlinson, B. E., Blessed, G., Perry,
R. H., Cross, A. J., and Crow, T. J. (1981).
'Neuropathological and biochemical observations
on the noradrenergic system in Alzheimer's disease', *J. Neurol. Sci.*, **51**, 279–287.

Pigache, R. (1984). 'Effects of ACTH moieties on
cognition and affect in elderly', in *Neuropeptide
and Hormone Modulation of Brain Function,
Homeostasis and Behavior* (Eds J. R. Sladek,
J. M. Ordy, and B. Reisberg), Raven Press, New
York (in press).

Pisano, J. J. (1969). 'Peptides', in *Handbook of
Neurochemistry*, Vol. 1, *Chemical Architecture of
the Nervous System* (Ed. A. Lajtha), pp. 53–74,
Plenum Press, New York.

Prensky, A. L., and Moser, H. W. (1967). 'Changes
in the amino acid composition of proteolipids of
white matter during maturation of the human nervous system', *J. Neurochem.*, **14**, 117–121.

Prockop, L. D. (1976). 'Lithium: Research and

therapeutic profile in affective disorders', in *The
Biomedical Role of Trace Elements in Aging* (Eds
J. M. Hsu, R. L. Davis, and R. W. Neithamer),
pp. 209–219, Eckerd College Gerontology Center, St Petersburg.

Raine, C. S. (1976). 'Neurocellular anatomy', in
Basic Neurochemistry (Eds G. J. Siegel, R. W.
Albers, R. Katzman, and B. W. Agranoff), 2nd
ed., pp. 5–33, Little, Brown and Co., Boston.

Reiss, V. and Gershon, D. (1976). 'Comparison of
cytoplasmic superoxide desmutase in liver, heart,
and brain of aging rats and mice', *Biochem. Biophys. Res. Co-mun.*, **73**, 255–262.

Robinson, D. S. (1975). 'Changes in monoamine
oxidase and monoamines with human development and aging', *Fed. Proc.*, **34**, 103–107.

Robinson, D. S., Davis, J. M., Nies, A., Ravaris,
C. L., and Sylvester, D. (1971). 'Relation of sex
and aging to monoamine oxidase activity of human brain, plasma, and platelets', *Arch. Gen.
Psychiatry*, **24**, 536–539.

Robinson, D. S., Davis, J. M., Nies, A., Colburn,
R. W., Davis, J. N., Bourne, H. R., Bunney, W.
E., Shaw, D. M., and Coppen, A. J. (1972).
'Ageing, monoamines and monoamine-oxidase
levels', *Lancet, 1*, 290–291.

Robinson, D. S., Sourkes, T. L., Nies, A., Harris,
L. S., Spector, S., Bartlett, D. L., and Kaye, I.
S. (1977). 'Monoamine metabolism in human
brain', *Arch. Gen. Psychiatry*, **34**, 89–92.

Robinson, N. and Williams, C. B. (1965). 'Amino
acids in human brain', *Clin. Chim. Acta.*, **12**, 311–
317.

Rouser, G., and Yamamoto, A. (1969). 'Lipids', in
Handbook of Neurochemistry, Vol. 1, *Chemical
Architecture of the Nervous System* (Ed. A.
Lajtha), pp. 121–169, Plenum Press, New York.

Samorajski, T. (1980). 'Neurochemical changes in
the aging human and non-human primate brain',
in *Psychopharmacology of Aging* (Eds C. Eisdorfer and W. E. Fann), pp. 145–168, Spectrum Publications, New York.

Samorajski, T., and Hartford, J. (1980). 'Brain
physiology of aging', in *Handbook of Geriatric
Psychiatry* (Eds E. W. Busse and D. G. Blazer),
pp. 46–82, Van Nostrand Reinhold Co., New
York.

Samorajski, T., Hicks, P. B., and Ordy, J. M.
(1980). 'Metabolism of other neurotransmitters in
degenerative syndromes associated with aging', in
États Déficitaires Cérébraux Liés À L'Âge
(Ed. R. Tissot), pp. 125–152, Georg et CIE S.
A., Genève.

Samorajski, T., Ordy, J. M., and Keefe, J. R.
(1965). 'The fine structure of lipofuscin age pigment in the nervous system of aged mice', *J. Cell.
Biol.*, **26**, 779–795.

Samorajski, T., and Rolsten, C. (1973). 'Age and

regional differences in the chemical composition of brains of mice, monkeys and humans', in *Progress in Brain Research*, Vol. 40, *Neurobiological Aspects of Maturation and Aging* (Ed. D. H. Ford), pp. 253–265, Elsevier, New York.

Sarkander, H.-I., (1983). 'Age-dependent changes in the organization and regulation of transcriptionally active neuronal, and monostrocytes glial chromation, in *Brain Aging and Neuropharmacology* (Eds J. Cervós-Navarro and H.-I. Sarkander), pp. 301–327, Raven Press, New York.

Schroeder, H. A. (1968). 'The role of chromium in mammalian nutrition', *Am. J. Clin. Nutr.,* **21**, 230–244.

Shelanski, M. L. (1976). 'Neurochemistry of aging: Review and prospectus', in *Aging*, Vol. 3, *Neurobiology of Aging* (Eds R. D. Terry and S. Gershon), pp. 339–349, Raven Press, New York.

Siakotos, A. N., and Armstrong, D. (1975). 'Age pigment, a biochemical indicator of intracellular aging', in *Advances in Behavioral Biology*, Vol. 16, *Neurobiology of Aging* (Eds J. M. Ordy and K. R. Brizzee), pp. 369–399, Plenum Press, New York.

Siakotos, A. N., Goebel, H. H., Patel, V., Watanabe, I., and Zeman, W. (1972). 'The morphogenesis and biochemical characteristics of ceroid isolated from cases of neuronal ceroid-lipofuscinosis', in *Advances in Experimental Medicine and Biology* (Eds B. W. Volk and S. M. Aronson), pp. 53–61, Plenum Press, New York.

Siakotos, A. N., Watanabe, I., Saito, A. L., and Fleischer, S. (1970). 'Procedures for the isolation of two distinct lipopigments from human brain lipofuscin and ceroid', *Biochemical Medicine*, **4**, 361–375.

Slater, E., and Roth, M. (1969). 'Ageing and the mental diseases of the aged', in *Clinical Psychiatry, 3rd ed.*, (Eds E. Slater and M. Roth), pp. 539–544, The Williams and Wilkins Company, Baltimore.

Sokoloff, L. (1976). 'Circulation and energy metabolism of the brain', in *Basic Neurochemistry*, (Eds G. J. Siegel, R. W. Albers, R. Katzman, and B. W. Agranoff), 2nd ed., pp. 388–413, Little, Brown and Co., Boston.

Sokoloff, L. (1977). 'Relation between physiological function and energy metabolism in the central nervous system', *J. Neurochem.,* **29**, 13–26.

Spillane, J. A., White, P., Goodhardt, M. J., Flack, R. H. A., Bowen, D. M., and Davison, A. N. (1977). 'Selective vulnerability of neurons in organic dementia', *Nature*, **266**, 558–559.

Spokes, E. G. S. (1981). 'The neurochemistry of Huntington's chorea', *Trends in Neurosciences,* **4**, 115–118.

Sun, G. Y., and Samorajski, T. (1973). 'Age differences in the acyl group composition of phosphoglycerides in myelin isolated from the brain of the rhesus monkey', *Biochim. Biophys. Acta.,* **316**, 19–27.

Suzuki K., and Chen, G. (1966). 'Chemical studies on Jakob–Creutzfeldt disease', *J. Neuropathol. Exp. Neurol.,* **25**, 396–408.

Suzuki K., Katzman, R., and Korey, S. F. (1965). 'Chemical studies on Alzheimer's disease', *J. Neuropathol. Exp. Neurol.,* **24**, 211–224.

Taubold, R. D., Siakotos, A. N., and Perkins, E. G. (1975). 'Studies on chemical nature of lipofuscin (age pigment) isolated from normal human brain', *Lipids,* **10**, 383–390.

Tcheng, K. T. (1964). 'Some observations on the lipofuscin pigments in the pyramidal and Purkinje cells of the monkey', *J. Hirnforsch.,* **6**, 323–326.

Tilney, F. and Rosett, J. (1931). 'The value of brain lipoids as an index of brain development', *Bull. Neurol. Inst. N.Y.,* **1**, 28–71.

Tinklenberg, J. (1984). 'Vasopressin effects on cognition and affects in the elderly', in *Neuropeptide and Hormone Modulation of Brain Function, Homeostasis and Behavior* (Eds J. R. Sladek, J. M. Ordy, and B. Reisberg), Raven Press, New York (in press).

Toews, A. D., Horrocks, L. A. and King, J. S. (1976). 'Simultaneous isolation of purified microsomal and myelin fractions from rat spinal cord', *J. Neurochem.,* **27**, 25–31.

Tolmasoff, J. M., Ono, T., and Cutler, R. G. (1980). 'Superoxide desmutase: Correlations with life-span and specific metabolic rate in primate species', *Proc. Natl. Acad. Sci., U.S.A.,* **77**, 2777–2781.

Tower, D. B. (1969). 'Inorganic constituents', in *Handbook of Neurochemistry*, Vol. 1, *Chemical Architecture of the Nervous System* (Ed. A. Lajtha), pp. 1–24, Plenum Press, New York.

Uemura, E., and Hartmann, H. A. (1978). 'RNA content and volume of nerve cell bodies in human brain. 1. Prefrontal cortex in aging normal and demented patients', *J. Neuropathol. Exp. Neurol.,* **37**, 487–496.

Weingartner, H. (1984). 'Effects of neuropeptides on cognition in normal young and aged subjects', in *Neuropeptide and Hormone Modulation of Brain Function, Homeostasis, and Behavior* (Eds J. R. Sladek, J. M. Ordy, and B. Reisberg), Raven Press, New York (in press).

Wintzerith, M., Labourdette, G., Delaunoy, J. P., and Mandel, P. (1978). 'Nucleic acids, total and glial protein changes in rat brain with aging', *Age,* **1**, 125–129.

Wisniewski, H. M., and Terry, R. D. (1973). 'Morphology of the aging brain, human and animal', *Prog. Brain Res.,* **40**, 167–186.

Woert, M. H. van (1976). 'Parkinson's disease, Tardive dyskinesia, and Huntington's chorea', in *Bi-*

ology of Cholinergic Function (Eds A. M. Goldberg and I. Hanin), pp. 583–601, Raven Press, New York.

Wolfe, L. S., Ng Ying Kin, N. M. K., Baker, R. R., Carpenter, S., and Andermann, F. (1977). 'Identification of retinoyl complexes as the auto-fluorescent component of the neuronal storage material in Batten disease', *Science*, **195**, 1360–1362.

Zeman, W. (1971). 'The neuronal ceroid-lipofuscinosis Batten–Vogt syndrome. A model for human aging?', *Adv. Geront. Res.*, **3**, 147–169.

Zeman, W., Donahue, S., Dyken, P., and Green, J. (1970). 'The neuronal ceroid lipofuscinoses (Batten–Vogt syndrome)' in *Handbook of Clinical Neurology* (Eds P. J. Vinken and G. W. Bruyn), pp. 588–679, North-Holland Publishing, Amsterdam.

Principles and Practice of Geriatric Medicine
Edited by M. S. J. Pathy
© 1985 John Wiley & Sons Ltd

16.3

Psychology of Ageing

J. E. Birren, Anita M. Woods

The purpose of this chapter is to characterize normal age-related changes that occur in psychological functioning across the life span. This look at the psychology of ageing can be seen as the study of the transformation or changes that occur in the behaviour of the relatively healthy adult living under representative environmental conditions. Individuals who have unusual health problems, genetic disorders, or who live under uncommon environmental circumstances do not represent the typical pattern of ageing to be expected of most persons. Knowledge of age-related normal psychological changes provides a basis for judgements of deviation from the norm in relation to disease or malfunctioning and is essential for both assessment and diagnosis and for the evaluation of therapeutic efficacy.

THREE AGES

An integrated picture of normal psychological change with age is made difficult by the fact that the individual's subsystems do not all change in the same manner and at the same rate. A behavioural definition of ageing has been offered by Birren and Renner (1980) in their statement that 'aging refers to the regular changes that occur in mature, genetically representative organisms living under representative environmental conditions as they advance in chronological age' (p. 4). It is important to keep in mind, however, that three general dimensions of the individual should be distinguished – biological age, psychological age, and social age.

The first of these dimensions represents the biological age of the individual, i.e., the extent to which the individual is biologically younger or older than his or her chronological age and, therefore, the likely number of years of life remaining. Clearly one can be biologically older or younger than one's chronological age. Biological ageing implies a decremental viewpoint; i.e., it refers to our biological vulnerability as a function of inherent processes which increase susceptibility to disease with age and increase the likelihood of death. It is presumed that the fundamental biological changes reduce one's probability of survival and range of adaptability to environmental change (Handler, 1960).

Somewhat related to biological age is psychological age, which refers to one's adaptive behavioural capacities. Adaptive behavioural capacities, such as perception, memory, learning, and creativity must to some extent be a function of biological involution associated with decreased power of survival and adjustment. However, a decrease in an organism's biological vigour and potential for survival may not be accompanied by a decrease in capacity for reasoning and abstraction. It is most likely that at the extremes of poor health one finds a close dependence of psychological capacities on biological processes.

In reasonably healthy adults, there is only a loose coupling between health and behaviour and many observe an increasing psychological competence, even with concomitant decreases in biological adaptability. In this sense one's psychological age can be 'younger' than one's biological age. In yet another domain, that of social functioning, one may find the individual growing older in such a way that many of his or her social roles are met with increasing effectiveness.

It appears useful to differentiate the biological age, psychological age, and social age of an individual. Each domain has its patterns and unique relationships, and while the three ages of mankind are to some extent interdependent, there is also a degree of autonomy of function among them. If we propose three age-related dimensions of man—biological, psychological, and social—then it is appropriate to distinguish three underlying constellations of change (Birren and Schroots, 1981). Underlying biological age are the processes of senescence which determine the probability of survival with the passage of time. Underlying social age are the processes of eldering which determine our passage into the succession of roles expected for our age in a particular society. Underlying psychological age are the processes of geronting which determine our effectiveness in adapting to both environmental and internal changes. Geronting implies the existence of an executive nervous system which has multiple capacities such as learning and memory, and can plan and execute choices in behaviour.

NORMAL AND PATHOLOGICAL PROCESSES DISTINGUISHED

Many of the changes found in very old people are appropriately attributed to disease and not to their age. Senile dementia of the Alzheimer's type found in older adults is not biologically typical of older members of the species. Ageing refers to those changes that occur in every person albeit at a different rate or at a different chronological age. The psychology of ageing, however, must focus upon concepts of mental health as well as physical health. If there are difficulties in defining physical health in terms of an optimum state of biochemical, psychological, and morphological well-being, one can see how much more difficult it is to define mental health. Even here it is desirable to make the effort, however, because further understanding of what is normal and the control of undesirable deviations from the norm are essential.

Criteria for mental health have been discussed by many sources, but have not been much elaborated with regard to the older adult. Generally, good mental health is marked by: (a) a positive attitude towards the self, or self-acceptance, (b) integration of the personality into a harmonious unit, (c) relative personal autonomy, (d) an accurate perception of reality that is congruent with others judged to be functioning in a healthy manner, (e) adaptation to environmental demands, and (f) movement towards transcendence or the obviation of limitations of function (Birren and Renner, 1981).

There are many changes to which the individual must react with the passage of time. It is expected that a mentally healthy individual can adapt to the physical changes of age affecting appearance, vision, and hearing, as well as to the process of bereavement which results from losses of loved ones. Reactions of pain, sadness, and unhappiness to such changes are to be expected, which emphasizes the pertinence of the following comments: 'There is a danger in confusing the mental disorders with suffering and mental health with happiness. A person who is clinically depressed is unhappy and suffers, but one can be unhappy and suffer without being clinically depressed, and indeed, without any impairment in the capacity to act within the confines of one's natural abilities' (Williams, 1972, p. 4).

Lurking in this comment is the idea of adaptation in relation to one's natural abilities. Thus good mental health is that which leads individuals to maximize their potentials. This further suggests that the mentally healthy older adult can adapt in such a way that his or her self-esteem and self-confidence remain high and that they continue to demonstrate pursuit of goals and a purpose in life despite the physical changes and psychological losses which may occur. In contrast to this are the mentally ill elderly, who are unable to achieve a sustaining balance of exchange with their environment despite an abundance of available resources.

Schaie points out that students who are interested in adult development should understand 'that while further growth will occur beyond mid-life, such growth does not necessarily imply continued behavioral differentiation' (Schaie, 1981, p. 201). However, he points out that individual differences in behaviour will automatically increase with advancing age. Presumably this will occur even if due only to the variations in environmental resources and learning experiences available to the older person. The fact that individual differences are greater in an old compared with a young population is an important point to be kept in mind by the professional person for use as an intellectual defence against the stereotypes of old age.

INTEGRATION AND LIFE REVIEW

Among the better known authors, Jung (1962) described a shift from the middle aged person to the older as one which initiates a change from outer direction and achievement-striving to a greater preoccupation with the inner life.

Similar to Jung, Hall (1922) pointed out that every older person should deliberately pass his life review in the sense that the later years were appropriately directed towards integration of one's life experiences. It is too soon to suggest that it is a universal experience to integrate one's life in the later years, but clearly there is evidence that there is a trend towards such reintegrated behaviour with age.

Butler (1963) pointed to the tendency of older adults to review their lives. The significant point then is the fact that a tendency for life review should not be regarded as an abnormal preoccupation, but as a constructive act on the part of older persons. The distinction between repetitive reminiscing and constructive integration is one that can be sensitive in the life of an older person because younger persons often become impatient and close their ears to the integrative efforts of older persons. This may be particularly true of a person faced with a terminal illness who needs his or her life to be accepted as it has been lived. Buhler (1968) also thought that the process of adding up one's life was the goal of a normally ageing adult with fulfilment being derived from the process of integration.

It seems reasonable that there may be a somewhat higher proportion of integrators with age—those persons who attempt to derive meaning from the way life has been lived. On the other hand, there will probably be those persons who spend their lives as they have lived them—through styles of denial. These changing rhythms of the life must, however, be importantly influenced by the culture. In times of economic hardship and social stress the drive to survive probably preoccupies attention that might have been directed towards some form of integration.

Earlier work by Cumming and Henry (1961) suggested that it was normal for older adults to disengage from society and for society to disengage from the individual. The so-called disengagement theory pointed to a mutual withdrawal of activities and roles and a reduction of emotional involvement by the older adult. One implication was that those who successfully disengaged had a higher morale than those who did not disengage. Contradictory evidence was presented by Havighurst, Neugarten and Tobin (1968) who indicated that life satisfaction tended to be greater in older persons who were active and engaged, in contrast to those who were disengaged. Havighurst (1968) thought that the issue was not one of a process of engagement or disengagement but a continuing process of adaptation. Here the individual plays a self-constructing role in adapting to the biological and social changes that occur. It is not unreasonable, then, that one of the ways of adapting to later life is by reintegrating experience.

A point to emphasize here, however, is that the older person may find some disconcerting tendencies to dream of old events and relationships (Butler, 1963). Old events take on a new saliency towards the end of life. Some guidance may be necessary for older individuals going through this stage, whether from informal supports, such as family members or spiritual advisors, or from professional supports in the form of psychologists, psychiatrists or social workers.

PERSONALITY

Personality traits may be even more influenced by cohort differences than those of intellectual abilities. A 25-year longitudinal study reported by Woodruff and Birren (1975) indicated remarkably stable results on a measure of intelligence. It was noted, however, that if subjects were asked to check as mature adults what they were like as undergraduates, there was an understatement of the level of maturity that the subjects showed when they had taken the test 25 years earlier. In other words, there is a change with age in the view of the self that is different from the measurement of personality itself. There may also be changes in cultural bias in self-revelation on a test of personality, with current youngsters being more willing to indicate responses that at an earlier period would have been felt socially negative or reflected badly on the self. Measured personality traits on personality questionnaires, which include many aspects of values and attitudes, show considerable stability over the adult life.

Botwinick (1978), however, has raised systematically the question of whether older adults are not less willing to take risks. Thus, with age there may be a general trend to be conservative in judgement situations. This may not be entirely irrational, however, in that a lower willingness to risk may be a result of perception of greater consequences of wrong decisions. For example, the loss of a small amount of money by an older adult on a horse race might have greater consequences since the money is less likely to be as replaceable as it would be for a young adult.

The tendency for older adults to be self-doubting was shown in studies by Klein (1972). In group situations older adults were more influenced by others; i.e., older adults tended to bring their perceptions or reports of their perceptions more in line with a group opinion. Klein tested perceptual judgements in older adults both in group situations and singly. A surprising result was that the older individuals tended to show accuracy in perceptual tests when tested alone, but were more influenced by other opinions in groups. This would suggest that they do not regard themselves as being as competent as young adults see themselves. An attempt by Klein to test this factor directly did result in improved performance; i.e., when Klein gave older persons reassurance about the level of their performance, they significantly raised their level of resistance to group opinions.

MORALE

Although depression may increase with age, data suggest that the average person in late life is by no means depressed. A study by Flannagan (1978) of representative cohorts of 1,000 each of 30 year olds, 50 year olds, and 70 year olds indicated that there were only slight differences between the 50 year olds and 70 year olds with regard to their view of the quality of their lives. About 85 per cent. indicated that the quality of their lives was good, very good, or excellent.

The Flannagan study yielded three clusters of factors that were important to all persons with regard to quality of life. The first of these clusters included material comforts, work, and health. These factors could be seen as relatively impersonal contributions to one's quality of life. The second cluster included close friends and socializing, and appears to involve some degree of personal intimacy. The third cluster included learning, creative expression, and the opportunity to use one's capacities.

Another study of age-related subjective feelings of well-being was made by Harris and coworkers (1975). In this study, 4,254 persons were interviewed in their households and were considered representative of the American public over the age of 18. Approximately 23 per cent. of persons over the age of 65 indicated that their greatest problem was fear of crime, while 12 per cent. pointed to loneliness.

Twenty-three per cent. of individuals over the age of 65 agreed with the statement, 'This is the dreariest time of my life.' This can be compared with 13 per cent. of persons under 65 who agreed with this same statement. It would seem, therefore, that there is a rise in the percentage of persons who have unfavourable morale in the later years, but this by no means constitutes anywhere near the majority of these persons. This survey report ended with the statement 'Not only do four out of five older people look back on their past with satisfaction, three out of four feel that their present is as interesting as it ever was, and over half are making plans for their future. Granted, life could be happier for 45 per cent. of older people, but an even higher 49 per cent. of those under 65 feel the same' (Harris *et al.*, 1975, p. 151).

In conclusion, the attribution of poor morale and a high level of loneliness to older persons is not justified. Poor morale as a reaction to loneliness is not typical of older persons. Indeed, the surveys reported here would seem to point to the fact that a satisfied acceptance of the past, an anticipation of the future, and a desire to grow through learning would better characterize the older normal adult population.

COMPETENCE

Individuals competent in living an independent life are not only influenced by external factors such as the nature of the physical and social environment but also by attitudes towards the self. Bengtson (1973) notes a positive cycle of events, leading to increased competence, which involves self-labelling as able and the internalization of the self as being an effective agent. According to the survey of Harris and coworkers (1975), the majority of persons over 65 regard themselves as being very good at getting things done, while only 35 per cent. of the general public views persons over 65 as being capable. It would seem that the general public of persons under the age of 65 have a somewhat more negative view about the efficiency and competency of persons over 65 than do the over 65 persons themselves. It would thus appear that most older persons are more self-confident than the general public image. The important point is that there is a widespread negative anticipation of growing older and the negative views must be unlearned as one enters this phase of life. This also has implications for the mental health of persons in the middle years in which middle aged adults object to or resent the idea of growing old because of the negative image of the circumstances of life for persons over 65. The general picture among persons over 65 is that they are deriving considerable satisfaction from their present lives and are looking forward to the future. Considerable research evidence shows that there is no particular life style that has an outstandingly high proportion of persons who age 'successfully' (Williams and Wirths, 1965).

One of the important, yet relatively undeveloped, topics in the psychology of ageing is that of the attainment of a high level of competence in the later years which may be referred to as wisdom. Generally, students of intellectual function have studied, as did Piaget, the development of cognitive capacities and reasoning in children. The attribution of wisdom can be looked upon as a sign of social approval, a signal to older persons one admires or likes. Such social attribution is not neces-

sarily related to any inherent qualities of the older adult. However, given the allusions of many centuries of comments about wise older adults, it would appear that some adults pass through life and not only accumulate valuable experience but can manipulate such experience in relation to current demands as to be both effective and admired for their effectiveness. Clayton and Birren (1980) have reviewed the historic background of wisdom and have reported empirical research. One of the characteristics of wisdom, according to the description given by Clayton and Birren, may be a tendency towards a reflective mode of thought in older persons. This may in turn be aided by mellowing of the temperament in which one is slightly more detached and thus prone to act reflectively. Lowenthal, Thurnher and Chiriboga (1975) describe a re-integrative stage at the onset of old age which may reflect this stage of wisdom.

INTELLIGENCE

How one reports and how one interprets age changes in intellectual functions depends to a great extent on one's model of intellectual processes. The simplest model of intelligence holds that it is composed of two factors, one being verbal (e.g., the Mill Hill Vocabulary Test) and the other being non-verbal (e.g., the Raven Progressive Matrices). Another two-factor approach is that of Horn and Cattel (1967) who have proposed two kinds of intellectual function – 'crystallized' abilities which are thought to reflect learning and experience, and 'fluid' abilities which reflect the neuroanatomic integrity of the central nervous system.

A more differentiated view of intelligence such as that of Guilford (1967) or Thurstone and Thurstone (1949) emphasizes the interaction of many factors, each of which might differentially change with age. Regardless of what model of intellect one uses, performance on verbal tests tends not to decline with age, but in fact may rise. This is true whether one looks at cross-sectional data adjusted for educational level, sequential studies, or other designs. Apparently, the healthy nervous system continues to store information with age. On the average, the older adult demonstrates a higher level of performance on a vocabulary test than does a young adult. Schaie (1980) reported that by the age of 67 performance on a verbal meaning test was 17 per cent. higher than at the age of 25. Thus the norm is for one's vocabulary to continue to grow with age, so that a healthy older adult whose vocabulary falls below the mean for a young adult should be viewed with suspicion. This statement has to be qualified, of course, in terms of the educational level of the subject (Birren and Morrison, 1961).

Botwinick (1977) called the rise in verbal performance with age and the decline in perceptual–integrative performance a classic ageing pattern. While a decline in performance related to perceptual functions and manipulative skills with age is often noted, the seriousness of these phenomena is not as great as if a low vocabulary score were found. Because this function is well maintained in later life, loss of stored information with age is suggestive of some threat to the integrity of the central nervous system.

The most significant factor influencing intelligence test performance over the life span appears to be the health status of the individual. In particular, rapid changes in cognitive performance for an individual should always be regarded as potentially significant indicators of deteriorating physical health.

Alpaugh and Birren (1977) found age differences in measures of both divergent thinking and preference for complexity. They suggested that both divergent thinking and motivation decline with age. Kogan (1974) has found relatively complex relationships between cognitive style and ageing and has also provided an interesting review on creativity and cognitive style, emphasizing the complexities of research in this area.

With regard to specific abilities, there seems to be a consensus that intellectual tasks involving a speed component usually tend to show age decrements in most individuals fairly early, usually in the thirties. Abilities that are commonly utilized in everyday life tend to be rather insensitive to this age-related speed factor. This includes not only vocabulary tests as usually scored (see Botwinick and Storandt, 1974; Botwinick, West, and Storandt, 1975) but also tasks such as arithmetic facility, which is both non-verbal and highly speeded and also extensively practised. The tasks which remain at the centre of controversy are those that char-

acterize fluid intelligence such as figural induction or letter series tasks. These show rather different patterns cross-sectionally and longitudinally. Horn and Donaldson (1976), while conceding that some individuals may avoid declines to a substantial extent, argue that others may be showing losses in the period of 20 to 50 years. However, various longitudinal studies show that most individuals who continue in such studies show little or no decline until the early sixties. Clearly, the possibility of differential patterns of development should be carefully scrutinized, and if such patterns are found to be common, identification of possible mechanisms (health, life style, longevity, and cohort) should be pursued.

MEMORY

Even in normal ageing there is usually a subjective perception of decline in the ability to acquire and remember information. The high frequency of memory complaints in normal aged persons coupled with the diagnostic value of memory testing in the assessment of pathology make this one of the most important areas of research in ageing today. Perhaps in no other area of the psychology of ageing is the distinction between normal performance and impaired performance so critical for the determination of present and future levels of functioning and well-being.

The bulk of human memory and ageing research has grown from an information-processing approach to the acquisition and remembering of information. This model assumes that the 'rememberer' actively participates in the process, and therefore one's cognitive strategies and their effectiveness for remembering are a major focus of investigation.

A number of studies have investigated the capacity of primary memory, a short-term store from which information is lost if not rehearsed. These studies have usually focused on how many letters, words, or digits a person can recall in correct serial order. Results of such studies have generally not found age differences; or if they have, those differences have been small in magnitude (Botwinick and Storandt, 1974; Craik, 1968). In a recent review of the memory and ageing literature, Craik

(1977) concluded that age differences in primary memory capacity are minimal if the tasks do not require cognitive manipulation to reorganize the information at the input level. In more demanding situations, however, where adults are required to restructure input, primary memory capacity may be reduced and may result in significant age differences in the amount of information available for storage in subsequent stages of process (Hartley, Harber, and Walsh, 1980).

Age differences are apparent in secondary memory, the repository for newly learned information (Fozard, 1980). One of the most replicated findings in memory and ageing research is that when the amount of information to be remembered exceeds the limits of primary memory, older people are not able to recall as much of that information as are younger people.

Therefore, much of the recent research on memory and ageing has concentrated on understanding the nature and causes of age-related deficits in secondary memory. Several major lines of research have found it useful to differentiate between acquisition, storage, and retrieval operations when hypothesizing about the age differences in secondary memory. As there is apparently little evidence that long-term retention is impaired in older people, not much attention is now directed towards the storage stage of memory as the possible locus of age-related deficits (Craik, 1977). Most interest is now focused on the acquisition and retrieval stages.

Attempts to determine whether the memory decrements in older people reflect mainly an acquisition deficiency (in which the information is not available in memory) or a retrieval deficiency (in which the information is available but is not accessible at the time of recall) have met with mixed results. The extensive literature on this problem was reviewed by Craik (1977) and Smith (1980) who concluded that retrieval difficulty may contribute to the age differences in the recall of information, but is not the sole cause. Furthermore, issue has been taken with this research approach in that it may be impossible to study these two stages independently of each other.

Another line of research has focused on the organizational processes used by older and younger learners. This approach has not produced consistent results, but there seems to be a trend towards finding that older people do not organize input spontaneously. Other findings indicate that when they are instructed to organize or are taught organizational strategies, older people sometimes enhance their memory performance, but the magnitude of the age difference is still significant.

Another research approach on memory and ageing suggests that younger and older people do not encode information the same way, which manifests itself in performance variables. The levels-of-processing approach hypothesized by Craik and Lockhart (1972) permits a closer look at encoding processes. Events that are processed more deeply and elaborately through the use of orienting tasks (e.g., semantic processing versus phonemic processing) are assumed to be able to be recalled more readily than events not processed as deeply or elaborately. A summary of this literature by Smith (1980) suggests that not only might the processing deficit in older people be a function of their lack of spontaneously engaging in semantic processing but it may also reflect the inability to maximize the benefits of semantic processing.

PERCEPTION

The recent focus of perceptual research on ageing has been on the study of adult age differences in the capacity to take in new information and to attend selectively to this new information. Recent evidence suggests that older persons are at a disadvantage in tasks requiring the processing of briefly presented information (Hoyer and Plude, 1980; Kline and Orme-Rogers, 1978; Walsh, 1976). Such findings necessitate consideration of the concept of attention and its role in perceptual processes.

Investigations of age-related differences in the capacity of attention are concerned with the quantity of information to which attention can be allocated at any given moment. Adult age differences are found in tasks requiring attention to be divided (a) between two input sources, (b) between stimulus input and rehearsal, and (c) between rehearsing and retrieving or responding (Craik, 1977; Craik and Simon, 1980; Hoyer and Plude, 1980). There is now renewed interest in the question of adult age differences in selective attention—the ability to separate relevant from irrelevant information. A number of studies using different paradigms have demonstrated such age-related differences in selective attention, with deficits found in the older person's ability to extract the relevant bits from a body of information (Hoyer, Rebok, and Sved, 1979; Rabbitt, 1965).

In general, information-processing limitations are imposed by time and space. All perceptual processes take time, as the flow of information proceeds through a sequence of stages, each marked by greater abstraction. The issue of space deals with how much information can be handled at any one moment. Most conceptualizations of human information processing see the first, most peripheral level of analysis to take place at the sensory receptor site. It is at this point that environmental information is 'translated' into some kind of code and then transmitted to 'higher' levels of processing. Perceptual processes operate on this information, and some theorists suggest that attentional mechanisms guide the processing of that information (Hoyer and Plude, 1980).

Most scientists in the field of perception will agree that the distinctions among sensation, attention, and perception are a little arbitrary. However, age-related limits on processing have been found at each of these levels of analysis (Fozard *et al.*, 1977; Kline and Orme-Rogers, 1978; Kline & Szafran, 1975; Kline & Orme-Rogers, 1978; Walsh, 1976; Welford, 1980). Successful attempts to link age-related processing limits to underlying mechanisms and specific loci are revitalizing research on ageing and perception. Unlike our knowledge of processing limits in the peripheral sensory systems, however, the precise locus of the slowing in higher order levels of processing has yet to be determined. That this slowing in central processing time occurs as a function of age can be attested to by countless studies in the literature. Kline and Szafran (1975), in the conclusion to their study on the time it takes the visual system to recover from stimulation, stated the case well as follows: '. . . there is, with increasing adult age, a significant increase in the time needed to process completely a single perceptual event.' They also suggested that this slowing limits the number of perceptual events that the senescent visual system handles per unit of time.

Perceptual ageing research is in need of further inquiry related to how the content of perceptual experience changes as we grow older. Such factors as attitudes or expectations, related perhaps to 'perceptual style,' may influence age-related differences in perception between individuals. It is possible that higher order processes that are unique to the individual in terms of selectivity may be able to play a compensatory role in the perceptual experience of the ageing individual.

VISION

Important structural changes that affect visual processing are the decrease in pupil diameter and the thickening and yellowing of the crystalline lens with advancing age. These changes impose limits on the amount of light reaching the retina. Thus, beginning at the most peripheral level of analysis of incoming information, the older adult functions with age-imposed limits on his processing capacity.

Perhaps the most common change in vision with age is that of accommodation. Changes in the elasticity of the lens result in a lessened ability to shorten or lengthen the focal length of the lens to accommodate to an object being viewed at varying distances. The consistency of the change with age in accommodation has prompted some investigators to believe that age changes in visual accommodation are part of some more fundamental general biological process with ageing. That seems somewhat unlikely, however, since the age changes in accommodation tend to level out at some time in the seventies, but individuals may live 30 or more years beyond the age of reaching the maximum rigidity of the lens.

While the aged iris still responds to changes in illumination, its resting diameter is smaller, admitting less light. Thus older people gain relatively more in visual acuity than do younger people as the illumination is raised. The smaller pupil also affects the amount of light reaching the eye under conditions of extreme low illumination requiring dark adaptation.

There are other changes in the eye of significance for individuals, but they are best viewed as consequences of diseases affecting the optic structures and functions and not as normal changes that all persons will experience.

HEARING

There is a widely experienced change in audition involving a differential loss of acuity with advancing age. This loss affects high-tone sensitivity in particular, and there is some question as to whether this loss, termed presbycusis, is a normal biological change with age. Crosscultural studies of age-related hearing changes indicate that environmental conditions have some impact on this decrease in acuity. It is sufficiently widespread, however, to be a likely accompaniment of advancing age for many older persons.

There can be a secondary involvement of hearing loss with other aspects of behaviour. Schaie, Baltes, and Strother (1964) reported a correlation between hearing impairment and intellectual functioning in men. It has also been suggested that a tendency to paranoia in selected older adults is exacerbated by hearing loss.

It is important, however, to make a distinction as to when the behavioural consequences are secondary and when they are a primary consequence of a change in the central nervous system itself. In some instances speech perception is not improved by a hearing aid because the central mechanisms for processing information are themselves defective. A true secondary effect occurs, for example, when the peripheral auditory structures of the ear are contributing to the changes in auditory acuity while the integrity of the brain itself is left unimpaired in processing information. This is a key issue of whether to attribute behaviour change in a particular older person to a change in the peripheral structure or jointly to a central factor.

In one case, the information does not get into the nervous system for processing. In the other case, the information may get in but it is not interpreted. Nowhere is this issue of peripheral versus central involvement more significant than in the role of slowness of behaviour with age.

SLOWNESS IN BEHAVIOUR

A large volume of literature, with observations now almost spanning 100 years, has shown that there is a general tendency towards slowing of behaviour with age. Earlier considerations of the facts of slowing were often interpreted as reflecting motor deficits. One might be slow because joints are stiff and the neural muscular contractions sluggish. The data suggest, however, that there is a large core of common variance in slowing such that one may speak of a generalized slowness with advancing age as well as specific factors of slowness associated with particular structures.

A 20 per cent. increase in simple reaction time has been noted between 20 year olds and 60 year olds (Welford, 1977). A study of age differences in speed of simple reaction time responses of the finger, jaw, and foot indicated that the amount of slowing was about the same for the three different response modes (Birren and Botwinick, 1955). This clearly suggests that the slowness under the experimental conditions was due to the nervous system itself and not to the special properties of the neuromuscular response.

In related studies, it was found that measurements of different types of speed in old subjects would yield a significantly large general speed factor. Further, Botwinick and Storandt (1974) looked at psychological test results and identified four major speed-related factors. They came to the conclusion that memory tasks which require repeated sequential processing of information are most sensitive to changes in cognitive speed. Clearly, then, memory as manifested is not insulated from an effect of cognitive processing speed. In fact, both the storage and the retrieval processes are influenced by an age change in behavioural speed.

Botwinick and Storandt (1974) noted that this general speed component affected simple movements as well as tasks which contained a large element of cognition. The authors further observed from their results that age differences in speed of responses were not limited to simple motor aspects of tasks, but involved to an even greater extent verbal processes. The results in general support the view of others that older subjects tend to show a characteristically slower response speed, whereas young adult subjects are more task specific in their response speed (Birren, Riegel, and Morrison, 1962).

A review of the literature seems to support this conclusion that with age there is an emergent, limiting factor in the speed of task completion—a general decline in the speed of behaviour. This is an important inference and bears upon the issue as to the basis of the correlations between speed of response, hearing sensitivity, and intellectual function. In the case of intelligence the question is whether the primary change is in the intellectual ability which then results secondarily in the slowing of information processing, or whether the slowing of information processing is the antecedent giving rise to the lower intellectual performance. While the age difference in the speed of response was first noted and measured in simple stimuli and responses, it was later found in complex behaviours including measurements of intellectual abilities.

One of the more interesting features of intellectual tests given to older adults is that the intercorrelations among different measures tend to rise. This raises the question as to whether there is high stability in the structure of intellectual abilities with age. In a confirmatory design reported by Cunningham (1974), he noted that 'the general conclusion resulting from the data analysis so far is that the interrelationship among cognitive variables, as represented in the factor structure, appeared to be changing with age, and that these differences were most pronounced for highly speeded variables.'

The implication here is that with age the limitation on speed of information processing emerges and increasingly begins to limit the performance of a wide range of intellectual tasks.

Schaie and his associates have pointed out that it is necessary to the analysis of data of these sorts to separate the contributions of ontogenetic changes in individuals, cohort differences, and the effects of time of measurement. Most studies do not permit the separation of such effects; thus the general results associated with age are inextricable confounds of different sources of variance. With regard to a possible ontogenetic change in speed of cognitive processes, the data of Schaie and Parham (1977) in a cohort-sequential design reported the declines as early as the age of 39 for word fluency.

Another look at behavioural speed was conducted by Walsh and Thompson (1978) who examined peripheral processing changes with age using a visual masking task. Their results clearly indicated that there is slowing in peripheral processing speed, but also that there is slowing in central perceptual processing speed (Williams, 1978). The implication of such findings for human performance is that one should be aware that slowness in behaviour is not limited to a slowness in peripheral input or output mechanisms, but is importantly involved in cognitive processes across a wide range of information processing, such as retrieval of information from long-term store.

If there is a slowing of processing with age, then the scanning of information both in short- and long-term storage would be influenced. In the case of long-term storage, what would appear as a defect in memory may be a problem of access, particularly when searching for many items in a complex array. This is more usually illustrated in the case of scanning items in short-term memory. Anders and Fozard (1973) looked at the increased differences in retrieving items in short term store in relation to the size of the set of items in short-term memory. There appears to be a slowness in retrieving items from short term memory in older persons compared with young, but as the number of items in the short-term memory to be scanned increases, the slowness is further manifested. What then may appear to be a change in the rate of decay of short-term storage may in fact be a slowness in scanning time which is manifested as a pseudo-memory decay time.

Although the older view of the age-related changes in behaviour held that speed was psychomotor in character and that memory was cognitive, research indicates that slowness can exercise a limiting effect upon memory and other cognitive processes.

PSYCHOPHYSIOLOGY

One of the rapidly expanding areas of research in the psychology of ageing is that of event-related electrical potentials. Earlier research in the psychophysiology of ageing gave emphasis to such variables as blood pressure, pulse, and skin resistance. There is a new thrust in attempting to link sensory-evoked potentials as well as contingent negative variation to age-related behaviours. Implicit in the new look in research is the belief that such electrical phenomena are related to or are indicators of cognitive processing, attention, and arousal. The potentials are divided up between those occurring in the first 100 milliseconds after the stimulus, those occurring between 100 and 300 milliseconds, and those occurring after 300 milliseconds. The positive potentials recorded after 300 milliseconds appear to be associated with attention (Bowman, 1980). Results show that with age the early components are increased in amplitude whereas the components after 100 milliseconds are decreased in amplitude (Marsh and Thompson, 1977). The effects of age on event related potentials has been most significant in instances where the subjects are required to engage in active cognitive processing in contrast to passive processing. In addition to amplitude, latency of the wave components has also been found to change with age (Dreschler 1978; Schenkenberg, 1970). The latency of late components in event related potentials show larger age differences. A reduction in central inhibition has been credited for the increase in amplitude of response in the early components of the event-related potential (Dreschler, 1978; Dustman and Beck, 1969; Shagass, 1972).

The contingent negative variation (CNV) is a slow negative shift in electrical potential that occurs in the time interval between two stimuli that are contingently related, as in a reaction time experiment which consists of a warning signal followed by a fixed period before the signal to which the subject should respond. The CNV is thought to reflect the development of expectation or the preparation of a response to an expected stimulus or event. Distraction reduces the amplitude of the CNV. Under some experimental conditions investigators have reported no age differences in the amplitude of the CNV while others have reported age differences. The inconsistencies in the findings have been discussed by Smith, Thompson, and Michalewski (1980). The interpretation is that age differences are shown under conditions of passive processing or stimulation, whereas under active stimulation the elderly and the young show the same levels of cortical excitability. This leads to the important inference that the cortical variable is an arousal state and that there may be a decreased capacity in the elderly to sustain arousal levels.

Earlier in the experimental literature on the psychology of ageing, older subjects were thought to have a diminished ability to develop and maintain intentional sets. Tecce and co-workers (1980a, 1980b) linked the evidence of a reduced CNV phenomena and a lessened capacity to switch attention. It would appear that the CNV, as measured in reaction time and cognitive processing, offers a tool to analyse age differences in performance. This experimental paradigm may not only limit extraneous sources of variance but may help us to begin to attribute ageing phenomena to mechanisms in focused anatomical sites and transmitter systems within the brain.

The literature leaves us with the impression that under conditions of appropriate stimulation older subjects can sustain a high arousal level and show minimum age differences in electrical potentials. The differences in performance may result not from a change in the primary information transmitting system of the brain but in a modulating system, e.g., the norepinephrine system.

HEALTH BEHAVIOUR RELATIONSHIPS

Much research evidence has been collected showing important relationships between behavioural capacities or competence and health variables. Behaviour is influenced by health and, in turn, health is influenced by behaviour. Long term dietary behaviours, for example, involved in the ingestion of foodstuffs including caffeine, alcohol, and other components of the diet can have long-term negative outcomes. As in many other areas, the study of nutrition and behaviour has concentrated its efforts on young organisms. Little evidence is thus available at the present time about relationships throughout development (Miller, 1981).

While attention is often paid by the general public to the questions of nutrition and ageing, not much is known to separate behaviours which are inherently related to the age of the organism from those which are consequences of life-long dietary habits. For the most part, relationships between nutrition and brain function are grossly altered by the diets of experimental animals and/or humans. Fernstrom (1981), who contributed to the 1980 working Conference on Nutrition and Behavior, has commented: 'Little information is available concerning the impact of normal vagaries of nutrition on brain function and behavior in

well-nourished individuals.' Of great significance to those working with an elderly population is his further comment that 'relatively
little information is available concerning nutrition–drug interaction, where the drugs are
themselves nutrients that affect brain functions
or are compounds whose efficacy within the
body is influenced by diet composition' (Fernstrom, 1981, p. 59).

In contrast to the absence of significant literature on the relationship of age, behaviour
and nutrition, there is a growing body of literature on exercise physiology and ageing.
While it is widely accepted that cognition, personality, and motor functions may be influenced by cardiovascular and cerebrovascular
status, another pathway of influence to consider is via the physical activity patterns of
individuals pursuing physical fitness. It is worth
while in observing these relationships to consider the association between the speed of
behaviour and physical fitness or activity level.

One of the correlates of a high level of physical activity is an increased sense of well-being.
Research by Tredway (1978) pointed out that
there is a correlation between the mood of the
individual and whether they engage in active
exercise (e.g., calisthenics or running) in contrast to a control group. A recent study by
Woods (1981) on age differences in the effect
of physical activity on information-processing
speed demonstrated that reaction-time slowing
with age varies with the physical fitness level
and can be modified by induced neuromuscular
activation (e.g., pedalling an exercycle while
responding to stimuli).

The speed of behaviour as epitomized in reaction time measurements seems to be correlated with age and the presence of
cardiovascular or cerebrovascular disease, and
is influenced by physical fitness and activity
level. Thus, measurements in speed of response are useful in assessing the individual
both for diagnostic purposes and also for
assessing effects of therapeutic regimes. The
study of ocular-motor reaction time in dementia in relation to controls indicates a significant
relationship between speed of behaviour and
the integrity of the nervous system (Pirozzolo
and Hansch, 1981). An earlier review of the
literature also indicated that the speed of performance on such simple tasks as writing or
addition also discriminates between the 'nor-

mal' elderly and those older individuals with
organic brain disease (Birren, Woods, and
Williams, 1979).

Relationships between the speed of behaviour, age, physical fitness, and cardiovascular
and cerebrovascular disease raises the question
as to the pathways underlying these relationships. A study by Bondareff, Mountjoy, and
Roth (1982) compared tissues from brains of
old patients who died from dementing disease
with control material. It is worthy to note that
a large difference was obtained in the cell
counts in the nucleus of the ascending recti-
cular system through the locus ceruleus.
Apparently, patients with dementing disease
show a significant loss of cells in this important
nucleus. The consequences are a change in the
level of arousal of cortical neurons via this
pathway. Slowness of behaviour also appears
to be associated with damage to the frontal
lobes. In such instances slowing may appear as
apathy and unresponsiveness (Lezak, 1976).
Focal brain damage with a resulting reduction
in slowness of behaviour would seem to be of
a different character than that produced by a
diffused radiating system such as the ascending
reticular system. It is possible that there is a
tendency with age to a loss of cells in the locus
ceruleus (Brody, 1976). This neuclus radiates
norepinephrine-secreting axons throughout the
cerebrum and the cerebellum. It is thus in a
critical position to modulate the response to all
stimuli and be a general contributor to the
slowness of old age.

PSYCHOBIOLOGY

The future of the psychology of ageing may
indeed be involved with differential changes in
neurotransmitter systems such as dopamine,
norepinephrine, seritonin, and gaba (Davis
and Himwich, 1975; Samorajski, Rosten, and
Ordy, 1971). Both the absolute levels of neurotransmitters and also their levels relate to
one another and may be related to age changes
in behaviour. This aspect of the neurosciences
is just in its infancy, but has great promise.
The extent to which physical activity, such as
running, influences the level of neurotransmitters directly or indirectly is, of course, the subject for future research. Given the
observations that physical conditioning facilitates the secretion of endorphines (Carr *et al.*,

1981), it has been suggested that there may be a feedback loop in the human between the level of physical activity, endorphine, perceived well-being, and cognitive functioning.

Other chapters in this volume will examine some of the structural alterations which occur with ageing, such as subcellular alterations and metabolic changes. These alterations manifest themselves at the behavioural level as a decrease in sensory, learning, and motor functions, with a decrease in the speed of response being one of the most characteristic changes. The changes in actual numbers of neurons and glial cells during ageing remains a controversial subject, with conflicting findings probably resulting from the many variables that must be taken into consideration before any valid conclusions can be drawn.

A series of recent investigations by the Berkeley Neuroanatomy Group (Diamond and Connor, 1981) have yielded some exciting observations related to the potential of ageing cerebral cells in rats. Initial investigations of the changes in neuron number and size and glial number in the medial occipital cortex demonstrated that the greatest decrease in density of neurons and two types of glia occurred before 108 days of age, with a non-significant decrease after this time to 650 days of age.

Following these findings of an insignificant cell loss until very old age, the ageing dendrite became the next focus of study. Dendritic density, total dendritic branching, and total spine density per unit length were similar in the 90 and 630 day old animals. Increases occurring in the later phases of development seem to follow a predetermined, non-abberrent pattern. The functional significance of these findings could be explored by behavioural testing, as in the tasks run by Cummins and coworkers (1963) in their findings that enriched animals make fewer errors on behavioural test measures.

This lack of a significant loss of neurons in ageing rat brains, along with the growth of dendrites in old animals, offer encouraging trends towards the potential of the ageing brain. 'Aging apparently has the biological potential to be a positive event under optimum conditions' (Diamond and Connor, 1981).

REFERENCES

Alpaugh, P. K., and Birren, J. E. (1977). 'Variables affecting creative contributions across the adult life span', *Hum. Dev., 20,* 240–248.

Anders, T. R., and Fozard, J. L. (1973). 'Effects of age upon retrieval from primary and secondary memory', *Dev. Psychol.,* 1973, **9,** 411–415.

Bengtson, V. L. (1973). *The Social Psychology of Aging,* Bobbs-Merrill, New York.

Birren, J. E., and Botwinick, J. (1955). 'Speed of response as a function of perceptual difficulty and age'. *J. Gerontology,* **10,** 433–436.

Birren, J. E., and Morrison, D. F. (1961). 'Analysis of the WAIS subtests in relation to age and education', *J. Gerontology.,* **16,** 363–369.

Birren, J. E., and Renner, V. J. (1980). 'Concepts and issues of mental health and aging', in *Handbook of Mental Health and Aging* p. 3–33 (Eds. J. E. Birren, and R. B. Sloane), Prentice-Hall, Englewood Cliffs, New Jersey.

Birren, J. E., and Renner, V. J. (1981). 'Concepts and criteria of mental health and aging'. *Am. J. Orthopsychiatry,* **51,** 242–254.

Birren, J. E., Riegel, K. F., and Morrison, D. F. (1962). 'Age differences in response speed as a function of controlled variations of stimulus conditions: Evidence of a general speed factor', *Gerontologia,* **6,** 1–18.

Birren, J. E., and Schroots, J. J. F. (1980). 'A psychological point of view toward human aging and adaptability', in *Adaptability and Aging. Proceedings of the Ninth International Conference of Social Gerontology*, Quebec, Canada, August 1980, pp. 43–54.

Birren, J. E., Woods, A. M., and Williams, M. V. (1979). 'Speed of behavior as an indicator of age changes and the integrity of the nervous system', in *Bayer Symposium* p. 10–44 (Eds. F. Hoffmeister and C. Mueller), No. VII, Springer-Verlag, Berlin.

Bondareff W., Mountjoy, C. Q., and Roth, M. (1982). 'Loss of neurons of origin of the adrenergic projection to cerebral cortex (nucleus locus ceruleus) in senile dementia', *Neurology,* **32,** 164–168.

Botwinick, J. (1977). 'Intellectual abilities', in *Handbook of the Psychology of Aging.* (Eds. J. E. Birren and K. W. Schaie), p. 580–605 Van Nostrand Reinhold, New York.

Botwinick, J. (1978). *Aging and Behavior.* New York: Springer, New York.

Botwinick, J., and Storandt, M. (1974). *Memory, Related Functions and Age*, Charles C. Thomas, Springfield, Illinois.

Botwinick, J., West, R., and Storandt, M. (1975). 'Qualitative vocabulary test responses and age', *J. Gerontol*, **30,** 574–576.

Bowman, T. E. (1980). 'Electrocortical and behavioral aspects of visuospatial processing and cognitive orientation in young, middle aged and elderly females', Unpublished doctoral dissertation, University of Southern California.

Brody, H. (1976). 'An examination of cerebral cortex and brainstem aging', in *Neurobiology of Aging* (Eds. R. D. Terry and S. Gershon) p. 177–182 Raven Press, New York.

Buhler, C. (1968). 'Fulfilment and failure of life', in *The Course of Human Life* (Eds. C. Buhler and F. Massarik). p. 400–403 Springer, New York.

Butler, R. N. (1963). 'The life review: An interpretation of reminiscence in the aged', *Psychiatry,* **26**, 65–76.

Carr, D. B., Bullen, B. A., Skrinar, G. S., Arnold, M. A., Rosenblatt, M., Beitins, I. Z., Martin, J. B., and McArthur, J. W. (1981). 'Physical conditioning facilitates the exercised-induced secretion of beta-endorphin and beta-lipotropin in women' *New Engl. J. Med.,* **305**: (10), 560–563.

Clayton, V. P., and Birren, J. E. (1980). 'The development of wisdom across the life-span. A reexamination of an ancient topic', in *Life-Span Development and Behavior* (Eds. P. B. Baltes and O. G. Brim, Jr.), p. 103–135 Vol. 3, Academic Press, New York.

Craik, F. I. M. (1968). 'Short-term memory and the aging process', in *Human Aging and Behavior,* (Ed. G. A. Talland), p. 131–168 Academic Press, New York.

Craik, F. I. M. (1977). 'Age differences in human memory', in *Handbook of the Psychology of Aging* (Eds. J. E. Birren and K. W. Schaie), p. 384–420 Van Nostrand Reinhold, New York.

Craik, F. I. M., and Lockhart, R. S. (1972). 'Levels of processing: A framework for memory research', *J. Verb. Learn. Verb. Behav.,* **11**, 671–684.

Craik, F. I. M., and Simon, E. (1980). Age differences in memory: 'The roles of attention and depth of processing in *New Directions in Memory and Aging: Proceedings of the George A. Talland Memorial Conference* (Eds. L. W. Poon, J. L. Fozard, L. S. Cermak, D. Arenberg, and L. W. Thompson), p. 95–112 Lawrence Erlbaum, New Jersey.

Cumming, E., and Henry, W. E. (1961). *Growing Old: The Process of Disengagement*, Basic Books, New York.

Cummins, R. A., Walsh, R. N., Budtz-Olsen, O. E., Konstantinos, T., and Horsfall, F. R. (1973). 'Environmentally induced changes in the brains of elderly rats', *Nature,* **243**, 516–518.

Cunningham, W. R. (1974). 'Age changes in the factor structure of human abilities', Unpublished doctoral dissertation, University of Southern California.

Davis, J. M., and Himwick, W. A. (1975). 'Neu-

rochemistry of the developing and aging mammalian brain', in *Neurobiol. Aging* (Eds. J. M. Ordy, and K. R. Brizzee) Plenum, New York.

Diamond, M. C., and Connor, J. R., (1981). 'A search for the potential of the aging brain'. in *Brain Neurotransmitters and Receptors in Aging and Age Related Disorders*. (Eds. J. M. Enna, T. Samorajski, and B. Beer) p. 43–58 Raven Press, New York.

Dreschler, F. (1978). 'Quantitative analysis of neurophysiological processes of the aging CNS', *J. Neurol.,* **218**, 197–213.

Dustman, R. E., and Beck, E. C. (1969). 'The effects of maturation and aging on the waveform of visually evoked potentials', *Electroencephalogr. Clin. Neurophysiol.,* **26**, 2–11.

Fernstrom, J. D. (1981). 'Nutrition, brain function, and behavior', in *Nutrutional Behavior* (Ed. S. E. Miller), pp. 59–68, Franklin Institute, Philadelphia.

Flannagan, J. C. (1978). 'A research approach to improving our quality of life', *Am. Psychol.,* **33**, 138–147.

Fozard, J. L. (1980). 'The time for remembering.' in *Aging in the 1980s.* (Ed. L. W. Poon), p. 273–287 The American Psychological Association, Washington D.C.

Fozard, J. L., Wolf, E., Bell, B., McFarland, R. A., Podalsky, S. (1977). 'Visual perception and communication', in *Handbook of the Psychology of Aging* (Eds. J. E. Birren and K. W. Schaie), p. 497–534 Van Nostrand Reinhold, New York.

Guilford, J. P. (1967). *The Nature of Human Intelligence*, McGraw-Hill, New York.

Hall, G. S. (1922). *Senescence*, Appleton-Century Crofts, New York.

Handler, P. (1960). 'Radiation and aging', in *Aging*, (Ed. N. W. Shock) p. 190–223 American Association for the Advancement of Science, Washington D.C.

Harris, L., *et al. (1975). The Myth and Reality of Aging in America*, The National Council on Aging, Washington, D.C.

Hartley, J. T., Harber, J. O., and Walsh, D. A. (1980). 'Contemporary issues and new directions in adult development of learning and memory', in *Aging in the 1980s* (Ed. L. W. Poon), p. 239–252 The American Psychological Association, Washington D.C.

Havighurst, R. J. (1968). 'A social-psychological perspective on aging', *Gerontologist,* **8**, 67–71.

Havighurst, R. J., Neugarten, B. L., and Tobin, S. S. (1968). 'Disengagement and patterns of aging', in *Middle Age and Aging* (Ed. B. L. Neugarten) p. 161–177 University of Chicago Press, Chicago, Illinois.

Horn, J. L., and Cattel, R. B. (1967). 'Age differences in fluid and crystallized intelligence', *Acta.*

Psychol., **26**, 107–129.

Horn, J. L., and Donaldson, G. (1976). 'On the myth of intellectual decline', *Am. Psychol.,* **31**, 701–719.

Hoyer, W., and Plude, D. (1980). 'Attentional and perceptual processes in the study of cognitive aging', in *Aging in the 1980s: Psychological Issues* (Ed. L. W. Poon), p. 227–238 The American Psychological Association, Washington, D.C.

Hoyer, W. J., Rebok, G. W., and Sved, S. M. (1979). 'Effects of varying irrelevant information on adult age differences in problem solving', *Gerontol.* **34**, 553–560.

Jung, C. G. (1962). *Modern Man in Search of a Soul*, Translated by W. S. Dell and C. F. Baynes, Routledge & Kegan Paul, London.

Klein, R. C. (1972). 'Age, sex, and task difficulty as predictors of social conformity', *J. Geron.,* **27**, 229–236.

Kline, D. W., and Orme-Rogers, C. (1978). 'Examination of stimulus persistance as the basis for superior visual identification performance among older adults', *J. Geront.,* **33**, 76–81.

Kline, D. W., and Szafran, J. (1975). 'Age differences in backward monoptic visual masking', *J. Geront.,* **30**, 307–311.

Kogan, N. (1974). 'Categorizing and conceptualizing styles in younger and older adults', *Hum. Dev.,* **17**, 218–230.

Lezak, M. D. (1976). *Neuropsychological Assessment.* Oxford University Press, London.

Lowenthal, M. F., Thurnher, M., and Chiriboga, D. *Four Stages of Life: A Psychosocial Study of Women and Men Facing Transition*, Jossey-Bass, San Francisco.

Marsh, G. R., and Thompson, L. W. (1977). 'Psychophysiology of aging', in *Handbook of the Psychology of Aging* (Eds. J. E. Birren and K. W. Schaie) p. 219–248 Van Nostrand Reinhold, New York.

Miller, S. A. (Ed.) (1981). *Nutrition and Behavior,* (1981). The Franklin Institute, Philadelphia.

Pirozzolo, F. J., and Hansch, E. C. (1981). 'Oculomotor reaction time in dementia reflects degree of cerebral dysfunction', *Science,* **214**, 349–350.

Rabbitt, P. M. A. (1965). 'An age-decrement in the ability to ignore irrelevant information', *J. Gerontol.,* **20**, 233–238.

Samorajski, T., Rolsten, C., and Ordy, J. M. (1971). 'Changes in behavior, brain, and neuroendocrine chemistry with age and stress in C57B1/10 male mice', *J. Gerontol.,* 1971, **26**, 168–175.

Schaie, K. W. (1980). 'Intelligence and problem solving', in *Handbook of Aging and Mental Health* (Eds. J. E. Birren and R. B. Sloane), p. 262–284 Prentice-Hall, Englewood Cliffs, New Jersey.

Schaie, K. W. (1981). 'Psychological changes from midlife to early old age; implications for the maintenance of mental health', *J. Orthopsychiat.,* **51**, 199–218.

Schaie, K. W., Baltes, P. B., and Strother, C. R. (1964). 'A study of auditory sensitivity in advanced age' *J. Gerontol.,* **19**, 453–457.

Schaie, K. S., and Parham, I. A. (1976). 'Stability of adult personality traits: Fact or fable?; *J. Personal. Soc. Psychol.,* **13**, 649–653.

Schenkenberg, T. (1970). 'Visual, auditory and somatosensory evoked responses of normal subjects from childhood to senescence', Unpublished doctoral dissertation, University of Utah.

Shagass, C. (1972). *Evoked Brain Potentials in Psychiatry*, Plenum Press, New York.

Smith, A. D. (1980). 'Introduction to cognitive issues: Advances in the cognitive psychology of aging', in *Aging in the 1980s* (Ed. L. W. Poon) p. 223–225 The American Psychological Association, Washington D.C.

Smith, D. B. D., Thompson, L. W., and Michalewski, H. J. (1980). 'Averaged evoked potential research in adult-aging-status and prospects', *Aging in the 1980s: Psychological Issues* (Ed. L. W. Poon) p. 135–151 The American Psychological Association, Washington, D.C.

Tecce, J. J., Yrchik, D. A., Meinbresse, D., and Cole, J. O. (1980a). 'CNV rebound and aging: I. Attention functions', in *Motivation, Motor and Sensory Processes of the Brain: Electrical Potentials, Behavior and Clinical Use* (Eds. H. H. Kornhuber and L. Deeche), Elsevier Biomedical Press, p. 552–561 New York.

Tecce, J. J., Yrchik, D. A., Meinbresse, D., Dessonville, C. L., Clifford T. S., and Cole, J. O. (1980b). 'CNV rebound and aging: II. Type A and B CNV shapes', in *Motivation, Motor and Sensory Processes of the Brain: Electrical Potentials, Behavior and Clinical Use* (Eds. H. H. Kornhuben and l. Deeche), p. 562–573 Elsevier Biomedical Press, New York.

Thurstone, L. L., and Thurstone, T. G. (1949). *SRA Primary Mental Abilities*, Science Research Associates, Chicago.

Tredway, V. A., 'Mood and exercise in older adults' (1978). Unpublished doctoral dissertation, University of Southern California.

Walsh, D. (1976) 'Age differences in central perceptual processing: Adichoptic backward masking investigation', *J. Gerontol.,* **31**, 178–185.

Walsh, D. A., and Thompson, L. W. (1978). 'Age differences in visual sensory memory', *J. Gerontol.,* **33**, 383–387.

Welford, A. T. (1977). 'Motor performance', in *Handbook of the Psychology of Aging* (Eds. J. E. Birren and K. W. Schaie), p. 450–496 Van Nostrand Reinhold, New York.

Welford, A. T. (1980). 'Sensory, perceptual, and motor processes in older adults', *Handbook of Aging and Mental Health* (Eds. J. E. Birren & R. B. Sloane), Prentice-Hall, Englewood Cliffs, New Jersey. p. 192–213.

Williams, M. V. (1978). 'Age differences in speed of perceptual processes: Comparison of three centrally acting masks', Unpublished doctoral dissertation, University of Southern California.

Williams, R. H. (1972). *Perspectives in the Field of Mental Health,* National Institute of Mental Health, Rockville Maryland.

Williams, R. H., & Wirths, C. C. (1965) *Lives Through the Years.* Atherton Press, New York.

Woodruff, D. S., and Birren, J. E. (Eds.) (1975). *Aging: Scientific Perspectives and Social Issues,* Van Nostrand, New York.

Woods, A. M. (1981). 'Age differences in the effect of physical activity and postural changes on information processing speed', Unpublished doctoral dissertation, University of Southern California.

Principles and Practice of Geriatric Medicine
Edited by M. S. J. Pathy
© 1985 John Wiley & Sons Ltd

16.4

The Clinical Psychology of the Elderly

Ann D. M. Davies, A. G. Crisp

INTRODUCTION

It is only fairly recently that psychologists have begun to work collaboratively with geriatricians, yet it is clear that psychological factors play a crucial part in the care of the elderly. Psychological resources or deficits influence a person's response to a disease process and to rehabilitation. Additionally, ill health frequently precipitates behavioural or interpersonal problems (Lipowski, 1975). This chapter attempts to show the scope and variety of psychological work with the elderly. Four major areas will be discussed: (a) assessment issues; (b) rehabilitation; (c) the design of environments to support independence; (d) adjustment and coping issues.

ASSESSMENT ISSUES

The Case for Formal Assessment

Assessment is the process of collecting and combining information about the characteristics of individuals and situations to allow decisions to be made. Decision-making is itself a cognitive process prone to certain types of errors. Humans generalize from inadequate evidence, place too much weight on vivid details and under-use information based on populations (Nisbett and Ross, 1980). An informal report at a case conference that Mrs A. is 'aggressive' may derive from a single incident under exceptional circumstances. It does not say whether other observers would class Mrs A's

behaviour in this way or how often and in what situations 'aggressive' acts must be performed to justify the description. The case for formal assessment is that it helps to reduce bias and error. The assessment procedure should specify: (a) the purpose (who assesses whom and for what reason); (b) the information to be included and excluded; (c) the criteria by which it is decided a characteristic is displayed; (d) how information is to be quantified and compared with existing norms; (e) how generalizable the procedure is, over time (retest reliability), over testers (inter-rater agreement) and over situations; (f) the validity of the procedure, i.e. the extent to which the data and decision rules can be demonstrated to be relevant to the decision at hand.

Methods of Assessment

An ideal assessment procedure is acceptable to the elderly person's cohort and culture, is easily administered, and produces evidence relevant to the decision to be made. It should discriminate between people of differing levels of functioning and be sensitive to change (Raskin and Jarvik, 1979). There are many methods of assessment: interviewing, observation, testing, and self-ratings. Each has a range of utility, but also limitations. Information, however collected, is partial, so inference is always necessary. Interviews are based mainly on verbal behaviour at a point in time, within a clearly controlled setting; nurses' ratings are based on longer intervals and cover more of the subject's life behaviours, but nurses tend to notice behaviours that directly affect physical care and may fail to report psychological symptoms such as passivity, social withdrawal, or anxiety (Hefferin and Hunter, 1975). Self-report assessments are quick and cheap and provide information not readily obtainable otherwise (e.g. subjective response), but they cannot be used validly with the intellectually impaired or those lacking in insight. It is also known that the personal evaluations of old people tend to minimize or deny problems (Carp and Carp, 1981). Self-report and interview data should therefore be supplemented by other evidence. Discrepancies occur in the information yielded by different assessment methods. Kuriansky and coworkers (1976), for example, collected data on activities of daily living. Actual performance scores did not correlate with elderly subjects' self-ratings of 'dependency'. Kahn and coworkers (1975) found memory complaints in the old unrelated to memory dysfunction as measured by psychometric tests and the two symptoms had different diagnostic implications. Finally, Maddox and Douglas (1973) showed that subjective health reports differed from assessments based on physical examination.

Generalizability

Assessment procedures should meet certain standards of generalizability (reliability and validity). The questions are: 'Can the observations be generalized across subjects, observers, settings, occasions and behaviours?' If the purpose of assessment is to monitor the effectiveness of a drug (e.g. Lloyd-Evans, Brocklehurst, and Palmer, 1978) or to measure change (e.g. Davies, 1972), the crucial generalizability issue is the repeatability of the test: test measurements should be stable in the absence of true change. A test of low reliability shows fluctuations unrelated to true change – so one may wrongly attribute a score change to the effects of treatment or time. Longer tests are more reliable than short, so there are dangers in abbreviating existing measures. Arising from the fact that tests are never perfectly reliable (the correlation between test and retest is less than one), individuals with extremely low initial scores tend to show most gain on retest and those with the highest initial

socre, greatest loss. These statistical effects have to be taken into account before gains in score are attributed to treatment. The assessment procedure must be sensitive enough to distribute the scores of people at different levels of functioning. If an entire group fails or obtains near-perfect marks, the test is of inappropriate level and improvements or decrements cannot be measured unambiguously.

Cognitive Assessment

The term 'cognition' covers a range of mental processes from information processing carried out over periods of milliseconds to the construction of complex systems of knowledge about the world and awareness of our place in it. 'Attending to a conversation' or 'remembering an appointment' are both examples of cognition. Much more needs to be known about cognitive processes before tests develop beyond the level of crude indicators (Rabbitt, 1982).

Most cognitive assessments of the elderly in a clinical context are carried out to make a diagnostic or placement decision. Very rarely there is a call for assessment of IQ (although a short form of the Weschler adult intelligence scale exists for use with old people; Britton and Savage, 1966). Assessment instruments vary in their comprehensiveness. Full neuropsychological assessment provides information on comprehension, memory, language, visual recognition, use of gesture, and purposeful movement (Christensen, 1979; Goodglass and Kaplan, 1972). Such assessments may be diagnostically useful and will also reveal the presence of difficulties which have implications for placement, e.g. severe dressing apraxias. At the other end of the range there are brief mental status questionnaires used in the context of diagnosing brain failure (Hodkinson, 1972; Kahn *et al.*, 1960). These identify gross deficits in memory and orientation but sample a very limited range of abilities and do not detect mild impairment. The set test (Isaacs and Ahktar, 1972; Isaacs and Kenny, 1973) asks the elderly person to list colours, etc., within categories or sets. Potentially this provides a measure of memory and attention over a wider range of ability but normative data on mentally impaired people is, as yet, poor. The Kendrick battery consists of a digit-copying and an object-learning test (Gibson and Kendrick, 1979) and distinguishes between dementing and non-dementing psychiatric patients. The pattern misclassifies a substantial proportion of long-term care patients, however (Gibson, Moyes, and Kendrick, 1980).

One of the major difficulties in assessing for intellectual deterioration is that premorbid functioning must usually be inferred. Nelson and McKenna (1975) suggest that current reading age provides an estimate of previous intelligence. Nelson has developed a reading list based on non-phonetic spellings (e.g. ache). Success depends on the person having previously known the word and the score allows an estimate of premorbid intelligence. Prospective measurement of deterioration requires tests to be repeated over a period of weeks or months: ideally, parallel forms should be used.

Poor performance in an elderly person may be due to sensorimotor or motivational deficits. Materials must be large, easy to manipulate, and presented in the context of familiar and meaningful activities. Prior familiarization with test procedures raises an elderly person's score (Binks and Davies, 1981). Instructions must be slow and clear. Old people respond cautiously so a test format that allows omissions will unduly penalize. Fear of evaluation sometimes lowers performance. Langer and coworkers (1979) found that nursing home residents do better on a memory test when it was presented as 'a new activity' rather than as a test. Factors such as motivation, anxiety, or fatigue are of course part of the elderly person's total test picture but if inferences about cognitive capacity are to be made, it is important to make allowance for those 'modifiers' (Botwinick, 1977).

Competence Assessment

Competence or skill assessment is concerned with what a person is able to do within the context of the resources provided by a particular environment. This type of assessment is central to decisions concerning placement and is often also the first stage in treatment. The question 'Will Mrs A. be able to cook meals for herself in her basement kitchen' encompasses two issues: firstly Mrs A.'s characteristics – her cognitive and motor skills and her interests in relation to cooking—and sec-

ondly the special circumstances of her kitchen. In a different setting (e.g. using an electric rather than a gas cooker) Mrs A.'s competence to cook may be different. Competence assessment should be based on detailed observation of behaviour in its 'ecological setting'. More usually an attempt is made to match an individual's profile of behaviours to the criteria of admission to a desired placement. One difficulty is that the context in which information is collected (e.g. an admission ward) may differ in important ways from the target environment (a housing scheme) and if this is so assessment will be of limited validity. Generalizability over raters is also important; behaviours and characteristics must be rated similarly by different observers. Providing precise verbal descriptions of behaviours (e.g. 'incontinent of urine more than once a day') helps to raise agreement, whereas use of vague labels such as 'good' or 'fair' results in different staff interpreting the scale in different ways. A variety of behaviour rating scales exists (Hall, 1980). Most, unfortunately, focus on deficiencies rather than skills. The CAPE Behaviour Rating Scale (Pattie and Gilleard, 1979) has items for bathing, walking, incontinence, confusion, etc., grouped into four scales – physical disability, apathy, communication difficulties, and social disturbance. The geriatrician, however, has also to focus on an old person's usable resources – skills, support systems, interests, and perceived opportunities. It is perhaps a measure of the 'custodialism' of many wards that such factors are not considered relevant in screening. It is worth pointing out that people within the same diagnostic category may vary widely in their competence in a given environment.

Functional Analysis

Functional analysis is an assessment strategy which has as its goal identification and control of the factors that cause and maintain behaviour (Kiernan, 1974). It entails an individual analysis of specific behaviours (rather than the global behaviours covered by the rating scales described above) and assumes continuity of assessment and treatment. The assessment procedure is an attempt to describe a behaviour in terms of the classes of variable associated with its occurrence, especially the stimuli in the environment that set off the behaviour (the antecedants or discriminative stimuli, S_D) and those that follow it (the consequences or reinforcing stimuli, S_R). Behavioural 'deficits' or 'excesses' are regarded as attributable to stimuli within the person's current environment or past history. The functional significance of discriminating and reinforcing stimuli is assessed through close observation of the form, severity, and consequences of the behaviours and from this analysis treatment goals are set. If, for example, an old person is said to require 'some assistance' in dressing (CAPE scale item 1) a functional analysis would start from the actual act of dressing. Close observation during a baseline phase would suggest whether the behaviour can be inferred to be due to: (a) impairment of fine movement leading to difficulty with buttons, hooks, etc.; (b) dressing in the wrong order or inappropriately; (c) mild motor impairment plus manifestations of severe anxiety; (d) attention and conversation from care staff during dressing. Each of these points to a treatment programme but the action taken – providing velcro fasteners, supervision, anxiety management training, or staff attention at times other than dressing—depends on the 'behaviour diagnosis' (Kanfer and Saslow, 1969). Hypotheses about functionally important factors are tested through intervention (treatment). The consequences are monitored and if 'treatment' has no effect, the hypotheses are reformulated. Various designs allow the clinician to test formally whether an intervention with an individual has been successful (Hersen and Barlow, 1976).

The behavioural literature suggests four ways in which age-related behaviour deficits or excesses may arise.

Inadequate or Inappropriate Reinforcement Contingencies

An effective reinforcing stimulus strengthens a behaviour and occasions it to occur more frequently. In later life, behavioural inadequacies arise in circumstances deficient in reinforcing events. Death of a spouse, for instance, removes a powerful source of social and material reinforcement (e.g. social approval within a confiding relationship, domestic ser-

vices, etc.). Behaviours previously maintained by this reinforcement (e.g. activity patterns) are likely to change in consequence. In some institutional environments the total amount of available reinforcement is low and this is associated with apathy, low morale, and depression. As described below in the section on environmental issues, staff behaviour may actually strengthen passive and dependent behaviour and allow independent and purposeful behaviour to extinguish.

Inadequate Stimulus Conditions

To be maintained, a behaviour requires appropriate antecedent conditions (those stimuli habitually associated with initiation of the behaviour). The availability of 'setting' stimuli alters with age, however. In part this is a function of sensory impairments (Corso, 1977; Fozard et al., 1977). These limit access to primary sources of information and consequently reduce the scope of intellectual activity (Gray and Isaacs, 1979). Hearing losses are particularly significant in this respect. They are associated with depression and may cause the appearance of confusion. Chronic physical conditions such as bronchitis and rheumatism have similar functional consequences in that they result in reduced physical mobility and social participation. Behaviours which are only initiated in a social setting (e.g. appropriate conversational activity) will occur less often so that social skills deteriorate. Ecological studies suggest that even healthy elderly people have access to a very limited number of social settings (Barker and Barker, 1961). If reduced social activity is due to environmental circumstances such as retirement, poor health, or loss of friends (Dickens and Perlman, 1981; Lowenthal and Boler, 1965; Miller and Beer, 1977) rather than being intrinsic to the ageing process, it should be amenable to modification by environmental intervention. Studies of withdrawn, unresponsive behaviour in the institutionalized elderly have shown that this is directly responsive to a change in stimulus conditions. McClannahan (1973), for instance, increased engagement in activities by prompting initial participation and by announcing the activities using cues which compensated for sight and hearing loss.

Reinforcement of Inappropriate or Maladaptive Behaviour

Problem behaviour in the elderly may arise consequent upon inadvertent reinforcement by others. Self-injurious behaviour in institutional settings is of this type (Mishara and Kastenbaum, 1973). Care staff cannot ignore potentially dangerous behaviours such as self-injury, wandering (Snyder *et al.*, 1978), and falling (Overstall, 1978). The literature has largely neglected, however, the important part social contingencies play in developing and maintaining these problems. Studies of other client groups suggest that positive reinforcement of other more adaptive behaviours is the treatment of choice (Baumeister and Rollings, 1976; Crisp and Coll, 1980).

Excessive Contingent Negative Experiences

Behaviour that is followed by persistent negative or aversive experiences diminishes in frequency and may disappear from the repertoire. Accordingly, behaviour deficits arise in older people as a consequence of negative attitudes expressed by society towards them. Studies suggest, for instance, that despite physiological changes in older women and men, there is no evidence of limitation in their ability to function sexually (Ludeman, 1981). The idea of sexual relationships between elderly persons is, however, found to be particularly shocking and is actively discouraged (Eastman, 1979), resulting in a decline in sexual interest and activity in old age.

A thorough functional analysis of the behaviour of an elderly person may be guided by the four paradigms discussed above. It is important, however, not to consider behaviour solely in terms of deficit paradigms but to review, also, individual strengths and resources.

REHABILITATION: INDIVIDUAL TREATMENT ISSUES

Goal-Planning

Goal-planning is fundamental to systematic care and makes possible the evaluation of interventions (Davies and Crisp, 1980). Performance goals specify who will do what, under what conditions, and with what degrees of success. They specify the attainments the elderly person will have achieved when that stage of therapeutic rehabilitation is reached, and do so precisely, so that everyone concerned knows that the goal has been attained. For example, 'On five mornings each week Mrs A. will complete, without help, the exercises prescribed by the physiotherapist and will walk the length of the ward with a Zimmer aid.' The performance goal in this example specifies the precondition for achievement (e.g. access to the physiotherapist and a Zimmer aid). The goal should also specify the consequence of non-attainment (e.g. not returning home, transfer to a continuing care setting). Specifying the consequence draws attention to other services that may be needed and influences the likelihood of the goal being reached.

Eliminative goals state which behaviours are to be decreased in frequency, e.g. disruptive behaviours. They state what the person will not be doing when the stage of rehabilitation is complete. While elimination of undesirable behaviour contributes indirectly to rehabilitation, goals stated in positive terms are superior. It is preferable to increase behaviours incompatible with the problem behaviour than to suppress the problem itself. Goldiamond (1974) argues that a 'constructional' approach is less coercive and better respects an individual's rights. While one can observe directly what does occur it is not possible to observe the absence of behaviour. Monitoring the effectiveness of a procedure is therefore easier when positive performance goals are set.

Targets for Intervention

Skills necessary for independent daily living have received much attention since these are prone to deteriorate in old age, either as a consequence of severe physical incapacity or changes in the environments which have prompted and maintained them in the past. The degree to which elderly people are able to undertake basic activities of daily living determines their independence in the community and the nature of the day and residential support services needed should independent living cease to be possible. Studies suggest that self-toileting, mobility, washing, dressing, and feeding skills are important indices of functional capacity. In a study of one hundred consecutive admissions to sheltered housing, residential homes, and long-stay hospital beds, it was reported that 81 per cent. of subjects could be correctly classified on the basis of three dependency variables: daytime incontinence of urine, the ability to prepare a hot drink, and the ability to get into and out of bed (Alexander and Eldon, 1979). Self-toileting training, mealtime behaviour, and mobility have been the subject of experimental scrutiny and will be discussed here, illustrating the general trend of behavioural work in this area.

Self-Toileting

Many elderly persons, both at home and in residential care settings, urinate in their clothing during the day. Milne (1976) reviewed prevalence studies suggesting that between 13 and 48 per cent. of institutionalized elderly and between 1.6 and 42 per cent. of the elderly living in the community manifest this problem. The considerable variability reflects in part different definitions of incontinence and assessment techniques.

There is virtually no research on the self-toileting behaviour of normal elderly individuals. A functional analysis, however, suggests that self-toileting in adult years is not solely a matter of control or responding to bladder and bowel pressures. Rather is it a complex, socially learned process, which can be hindered by cognitive impairment and exposure to institutional environments as well as by physical changes.

One of the most influential attempts at a theoretical analysis of the social environmental aspects of self-toileting behaviour is that of Ellis (1963), who adopted a social learning paradigm. The analysis presented in Fig. 1 is based upon Ellis's initial formulation. Here S_D refers to the discriminative stimulus, the detection of tension in the bladder; R_E refers to the response, elimination; and S_{R+}, the positive reinforcing stimulus, refers to the reduction in bladder tension as a consequence of R_E.

However, before training, i.e. before appropriate social controls have been established,

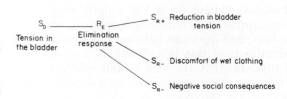

Figure 1 Before toilet training: positive and negative consequences

there are also negative reinforcing stimuli present, these are the presence of wet clothing following R_E and also negative social consequences (referred to as S_{R-} in Fig. 1).

Once self-toileting skills have been learned (or relearned) the elimination response should occur in response to an appropriate (i.e. socially sanctioned) context of cues rather than to bladder tension, S_D. A period of postponement of the response to S_D is also introduced into the model to accommodate the additional behaviours that training establishes. These are shown in Fig. 2. Here S_D again refers to tension in the bladder; R_A refers to approach responses; S_{RA} refers to cues generated by these approach responses. These cues combine with those from the environment; S_T refers to cues generated by the toilet area, R_U refers to undressing responses, R_P to postural changes, and R_E refers to the elimination response.

Each of the events and relationships in this model can be subjected to a finer grain analysis

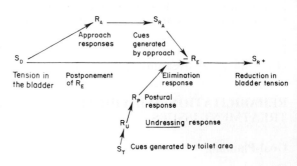

Figure 2 Self toileting established

but the model outlined is sufficient to show that there is a complex chain of events between the onset of bladder tension cues and the responses, locomotor behaviours, and elimination—a complexity not represented in models based on laboratory urodynamic investigations alone. A definition of urinary incontinence which emphasizes loss of control either during the bladder-filling or postponement phases effectively excludes from consideration a number of factors which are significant in the loss of self-toileting skills, particularly in the institutionalized elderly. A much wider definition of incontinence is demanded by the social learning model. This model clarifies the relationship between the various behavioural components of self-toileting and interruptions in any of the stimulus–response links can result in the elderly urinating in their clothing. Important factors include delays in recognizing bladder tension, difficulties in reaching the toilet, failure to recognize the toilet area, and difficulties in undressing. An environment that places barriers to mobility, either through distance or through organizational policies (e.g. having to call an attendant), reduces the likelihood of competent self-toileting. These factors are especially important at night-time. Once failures of self-toileting occur at night (perhaps associated with drug use or with difficulty in reaching the toilet) daytime failures are more likely to occur.

The model has important implications for assessment and therapeutic intervention. In addition to urodynamic assessment it is necessary to incorporate data on (a) how and when the need to urinate arises in the patient's normal living environment; (b) the patient's mobility skills; (c) the ability to recognize appropriate locations; (d) undressing and dressing skills; (e) the time taken to carry out these activities in relation to the ability to postpone the elimination response; (f) assessment of the environment in which the elderly person resides with a view to locating barriers to independent self-toileting. Only on the basis of such a comprehensive assessment can a therapeutic programme be developed which is directed at all the patient's needs.

Finally, the social learning model suggests points of intervention whereby retraining may be initiated. One approach involves determin-

ing the temporal locus of S_D, i.e. attempting to detect or predict the time at which an incontinent episode is likely to occur in relation to fluid intake and prompting self-toileting or toilet training at this time. Such an approach has been recommended by Spiro (1978) and has been used successfully by Collins and Plaska (1975) in a study of nocturnal enuresis among residents of a nursing home. An alternative approach has involved manipulating reinforcement contingencies, i.e. intervening at point S_{R+} in the model. Such approaches involve periodically checking the patient's clothing, rewarding the patient if dry, and applying mild aversive contingencies if the patient's clothing is found to be soiled. This approach also involves reinforcing the patient when appropriate self-toileting is observed. This strategy does not appear to be as powerful as other techniques. It has been used in studies by Pollock and Liberman (1974), Atthowe (1972), and Grosicki (1968). Both positive and negative outcomes have been reported.

The feasibility of intervening at point S_T in the model has been explored with demented elderly patients based upon work of Azrin and Foxx (1971). The patient is toileted at arbitrarily set invervals irrespective of the fullness of the bladder and remains for extended periods in or near the toilet in order to strengthen cues elicited by the toilet area over the elimination response. Positive reinforcement and mild aversive techniques are also employed. Results are limited but they do suggest that the procedure is effective in re-establishing independent self-toileting (Sanavio, 1981).

Research has also given some consideration to the treatment of incontinence which has arisen from primarily physical causes and in which social and environmental aspects are of secondary importance. Classical conditioning techniques have been applied to the treatment of urinary incontinence, specifically spastic neurogenic bladder (Ince, 1980). Biofeedback techniques have been used in the context of detrusor instability (Cadozo et al., 1980b), urinary retention and urinary incontinence (Wear, Wear, and Cleeland, 1979), and fecal incontinence (Engel, Nikoomanesh, and Schuster, 1974).

A number of psychological approaches are

therefore potentially available to the clinician for reestablishing continent behaviour. However, research to date is limited and inconclusive.

Mealtime Behaviours

In an observational study of feeding skills and mealtime arrangements in a continuing care setting for elderly patients, 12 out of a group of 22 residents were found to possess inadequate feeding skills (Davies and Snaith, 1980a). In addition, the study reported that certain features of the care regime, notably ward organization, hospital management practices, and catering policy were contributing to the unsatisfactory mealtime skills and arrangements observed.

Self-feeding skills and associated mealtime behaviours such as social interaction are, however, responsive to training and environmental interventions. Indeed, self-feeding is usually regarded as one of the easiest skills to establish since food is an effective reinforcer for most patients. When self-feeding skills are very limited or non-existent, manual guidance with positive reinforcement is the most effective procedure. It consists of manually prompting the patient's hand through the eating sequence while reinforcing progress by social and other forms of reinforcement. Baltes and Zerbe (1976) report studies in which two subjects (a 67 year old woman and a 79 year old man) were encouraged to increase self-feeding responses from a near-zero level to an average of 14.3 and 20 responses per session, respectively, by means of prompting, shaping, and reinforcement contingent upon correct self-feeding. Geiger and Johnson (1974) report the use of similar procedures to increase the frequency of correct eating behaviour (defined as the complete consumption of a main meal, together with two other courses). Six subjects (aged 69 to 91 years) participated in this study, the number of meals eaten correctly rising from an average of 12 to 70 per cent. during treatment.

Social as well as perceptual motor skills are involved in mealtime behaviour. Correct feeding is prompted and maintained by social and environmental factors and, conversely, interaction at mealtimes responds to changes in the physical environment. Seating patients around tables set appropriately with cutlery, glasses, and jugs not only encourages conversation but also prompts patients to help each other. Self-feeding skills are less likely to deteriorate under these conditions than if meals are eaten in solitude beside a bed or on trays placed in front of wheelchairs (Davies and Snaith, 1980b; Melin and Gotestam, 1981).

Mobility Training

A number of studies have disclosed the close relationship between age and disability. The survey of *Handicapped and Impaired in Great Britain* (Harris, Cox, and Smith, 1971) estimated that 1 in 5 men and women aged 65 to 74 and about 1 in 3 men and 1 in 5 women aged 75 and above had some form of impairment. Strokes, arthritic conditions, and other causes of impairment which result in the restriction of motor activity figure prominently among the elderly in community and institutional settings.

Although the literature is limited a number of studies have reported ways in which physical mobility in the elderly may be improved. Motivational problems have received most attention: stroke patients in particular are often described as poorly motivated. One of the earliest studies of this kind was that of Garmezy and Harris (1953) who explored the use of rewards on the performance of a motor task by cerebral palsied children. An increase in speed was reported when reinforcement was used but this did not generalize to occasions when reinforcement was withheld. Goodkin (1966) has listed a number of steps for using behavioural procedures in this area:

(a) Observe and record the patient's behaviour.
(b) Define specifically the behaviours to be increased in frequency and those to be decreased.
(c) Establish both positive and negative reinforcers which are powerful enough to change the client's behaviour.

Using these procedures, Goodkin reports a study in which an elderly female client was motivated to use her wheelchair. Following an assessment of baseline performance and the use of positive attention and feedback, wheelchair use increased considerably. MacDonald and Butler (1974) report similar procedures to increase walking in two elderly residents of a nursing home who were normally transported in a wheelchair. During treatment, standing and walking were prompted with social praise and conversation used as reinforcers. Similarly, Libb and Clements (1969) used reinforcement to increase the participation of a group of elderly residents of a nursing home in an exercise programme. Trombley (1966) and Trotter and Inman (1968) emphasize the value of reinforcement in increasing participation in physiotherapy. Fordyce (1976) gives detailed examples of programmes suitable for use with patients with various disorders of gait. One point to note in mobility studies is that 'motivation' is not a unitary concept but itself requires analysis for each individual. The interests and preferences of each 'poorly motivated' elderly person must be investigated to ascertain what stimuli and events are valued enough 'to make them worth working for'. Such motivation may be highly idiosyncratic so an analysis of valued objects and activities is an essential part of training.

ENVIRONMENTAL ISSUES

The Goals of Care

The term 'environment' refers to the arrangement of objects in space and to characteristics of the social world, including encouragement and social reinforcement. Environments must be evaluated in the context of treatment goals. If the objective is: 'Mrs A. is to be enabled to feed, dress, and toilet herself at home' a 'therapeutic' environment will be that setting and regime that maximizes the chance of the goal being reached (Canter and Canter, 1979). A regime in which nurses serve Mrs A.'s meals, help her to her feet, and dispense medication may be 'antitherapeutic' in that the probability of goal attainment is reduced. This discussion assumes that the aims of institutional care are:

(a) 'normalization', i.e. the provision of the least restrictive environment, one that uses resources so that the elderly person can engage in activities previously valued (Miller, 1977);

(b) the provision of a 'prosthetic' environment, namely one designed to compensate for sensori-motor and cognitive deficits;

(c) the support of a person's individual treatment.

If normalization is to be promoted, the environment must permit a range of options to suit individual needs. Although social and physical activity declines among the 'normal' elderly, home-centred activity and passive pursuits increase (Gordon and Gaitz, 1977). Old people who report involvement also express more life satisfaction. It is therefore reasonable to suppose that environments designed to promote social interaction and participation will benefit most old people.

An environment designed to promote individualized treatment demands a style of care very different from one primarily designed to deliver smooth and standardized routine care. Greater interchangeability of roles is required so that the person on duty performs those tasks that 'need to be done' rather than only those assigned by job description, e.g. a cleaner may be expected to reinforce the conversation of withdrawn patients. This type of management is particularly important in long-term care settings, where the risk of losing manipulative and social skills is greatest. Organizational flexibility is commoner in smaller establishments than large (Slagsvold, 1981).

Designing Environments to Promote Independent Living Skills

The arrangement of space (walls, windows, and partitions), the use of furniture and equipment, the size of an establishment and its ambient conditions, critically affect the extent to which independent living skills are promoted. The layout of a building may enable the maintenance of a sense of direction; a dayroom may be furnished so that social interaction is highly likely, a chair may be provided that is easy to rise from, or the effort of doing so may be such as to reduce the sitter's motivation to try.

As people age they undergo sensori-motor changes. They have difficulty in seeing in low levels of illumination and are slow to adapt to sudden changes, especially in tasks requiring control of movement. Thus falls frequently occur on leaving a toilet area or on the initial step of a descending flight of stairs facing a window (Fozard, 1981). Raising ambient illumination may reduce accidents and disorientation and encourage greater mobility.

Changes in auditory discrimination with age also have design implications; speech intelligibility is affected by distracting noise, so background music and television is likely to reduce conversation; differential loss for high tones suggests that buzzers are to be preferred for call systems; conversations need to be louder, so rooms in which private matters are discussed need high sound containment.

Barriers in the environment severely constrain the elderly person's activities. Cot sides on beds, restraining chairs, use of wheelchairs for ambulant people, and lack of access to toilet and kitchen facilities thwart independent living skills. Since the elderly are significantly smaller in stature (Stoudt, 1981), bed height should be such that the person's feet touch the ground from a seated position so that sliding off is unnecessary. Heights convenient for nursing staff raise the risk of falls for old people and deter them from leaving bed, especially at night, thereby contributing to problems of motivation and incontinence.

A door locked at a high level to curb a wanderer may prevent the free passage of other patients, requiring them to ask staff for permission to pass, increasing dependency, and reducing motivation. Design features influence all users of an environment, not only those for whom modifications are planned (Raschko, 1974; DHSS, 1980).

Increasing Privacy and Regulation of Social Contact

People outside institutions have needs for casual and intimate conversation and solitude. Stress results when control over interaction is not possible and anxiety, depression, and withdrawal may result (Zimring, 1981). Altman (1975) suggest that 'privacy' is not excluding others but is rather regulating social contacts to and from others. The old person has fewer resources to govern this process; sensori-motor slowing means that escape from unwanted contacts is difficult. Territorial behaviour is a basic regulatory process and is exercised into extreme old age. Fairhurst (1976) showed that

geriatric patients utilized handbags, Zimmer walking aids, and corner positions to maximize the domain that was 'theirs' and defence of the territory took precedence over interaction. It is therefore important to provide elderly people with space they can regard as their own to be used as the base from which social excursions are made. Old people with access to personal space are more sociable in public areas (De Long, 1970). A wish to regulate social interaction probably underlies the finding that lounges at the end of corridors tend to be under-used: their social commitment is great and retreat is difficult (Lawton, 1974). Control over social interaction is increased by making encounters more predictable, i.e. by reducing the number of potential users of a space so that it is easier to recognize acquaintances and detect intruders. Designs which subdivide living spaces into semiprivate areas (courtyards, corridors, etc.) reduce the information an elderly person has to process and promote friendships, since we get to know best those near us whom we see often.

The size of group affects the feelings of attachment between members and the likelihood of conversation (O'Donnell, 1980). Most studies show that there will be more interaction in small lounges for 6 to 8 persons than in lounges designed for 25 to 40. Most studies show that with more than 12 members mutal interaction is reduced: large lounges designed for 25 to 40 people discourage social mixing. Distances are too great for casual discourse. When chairs are placed side by side round walls it is hard to see facial expression and so cues for suitable conversation are reduced, especially for those with hearing problems. There will be more interaction in small lounges for 6 to 8 persons (Lipman and Slater, 1979) or, in larger rooms, if chairs are grouped around tables (Melin and Gotestam, 1981; Peterson *et al.*, 1977), an effect which influences both the sociable and socially isolated (Davies and Snaith, 1980a). Wilkin, Hughes and Evans (1981) report that residential homes may tolerate around a third of confused residents without affecting social interaction adversely. Chairs placed close to centres of visual activity attract onlookers and can become the setting for conversations (Lawton, 1974). Social activity is increased by placing seats near an existing focus of attention, in entrance halls and corridors, as well as settings explicitly designated as lounges. Provision of tables, desks, and magazines in various locations permits control over the extent to which people make themselves available to others. Television and other sources of sound, however, preempt choice and are better placed in special partitioned and carpeted areas.

By personalization of shared bedroom areas using photos and mementos, staff see an old person less as a medical condition and more as a person (Millard and Smith, 1981). This also enhances a sense of self-identity and continuity with the past (Slater and Gill, 1981).

Increasing Engagement in Activity

Upon entering an institution the scope for independent activity is reduced and skills may deteriorate for lack of practice. A need arises to 'activate' or 'engage' the person, either by devolving self-care to residents (Marston and Gupta, 1977) or by increasing recreational activity (Jenkins, Lunt and Powell 1977; McClannahan and Risley, 1975; McCormack and Whitehead, 1981; Powell *et al.*, 1979; Quilitch, 1974). Engagement can be increased dramatically, even in the severely disabled, by providing a range of suitable materials, demonstrating and prompting and reinforcing their use. It is important to match patients and materials, starting at a level of difficulty allowing early success. Inactivity in the old is partly environmentally determined and is not solely due to inherent deficits in motivation and functioning. This is important, because care staff frequently assume the inactive elderly cannot or do not wish to be active.

Reducing Dependency

Problems arise from joint expectations of authorities, staff, and residents that care staff are there to provide physical services—to 'do things for' the elderly person. Nurse training in particular emphasizes bodily care: nurses tend not to notice or record aspects of patients' psychological state. Talking to patients or joining their activities is assigned low priority. These trends persist even with increased staff to patient ratios (Hefferin and Hunter, 1975; Savage and Widdowson, 1974). In a series of observational studies, Baltes and her colleagues showed that staff differentially support dependent behaviour. When elderly nursing home residents behaved in a dependent manner (e.g. asking or waiting to be helped) staff responded by supporting dependence; when residents behaved independently staff were also more likely to be supportive of dependent rather than independent behaviour (Baltes, Burgess, and Stewart, 1980; Barton, Baltes, and Orzech, 1980). Under these circumstances the frequency of independent behaviour is reduced. Supporting independent behaviour is difficult because there are stereotypes of appropriate care-giving behaviour and many routines are quicker if completed by staff (e.g. transporting in a wheelchair rather than encouraging walking). Staff are reinforced for supporting dependency, a serious challenge for the organization of a geriatric service. What is required is: (a) an agreed objective: that its purpose is to provide independence; (b) an awareness of the actual behaviour of care staff and the consequences for patient behaviours; (c) the provision of discriminative and reinforcing stimuli for staff to support the elderly person's independent behaviour. There have been a number of attempts to change the type and extent of staff–patient interaction. Merely instructing staff in appropriate behaviour has little effect (Katz, Johnson, and Gelfand, 1972). Staff discussion groups and films, the approval of supervisors, direct payments, written or graphic feedback, and telephone reminders have been used with varying results (Melin, 1981; Montegar *et al.*, 1977; Sand and Berni, 1974; Stoffelmayr, Lindsay and Taylor, 1979; Melin, 1981). It seems that manipulating the reinforcement of staff is insufficient to tackle this complex problem. Change is also needed in antecedent management policies, e.g. in the organization of workloads and clarifying the risks that staff may legitimately allow patients to take (Norman, 1979).

Increasing Orientation

Orientation is the ability to relate to the environment, to know who one is, and where one is in place and time. 'Wayfinding' refers to orientation within a spatial location and involves selecting and storing information about landmarks and the relationships between them. Important self-assessments are based on wayfinding. We feel incompetent or anxious when lost (Zimring, 1981). Being able to see through or out of a setting helps spatial orientation so windows and transoms should be low. There should be distinctive landmarks at choice points, and visual cues such as signposts, colour codes, and pictograms to indicate the functions of important locations such as toilets, reception areas, and dining areas. Appropriate lighting and furniture also helps. Redundant cuing using several modalities benefits the visually disabled, e.g. changes in the texture of floor and wall coverings, the penetration of distinctive sounds and smells, etc. It should not be assumed that the cues provided can be used without training. Colour coding requires new learning and interference from previous associations may have to be overcome: symbol and picture cues are easier, especially for the mentally impaired (Klisz and Dye, 1981). Hanley (1981) trained ward orientation by taking patients to a location, describing, it and coaching them as to its name. Although wayfinding improved above a baseline level, there was no generalization to other locations or starting points.

Reality orientation (RO) is a broader technique which aims to increase orientation for place, time, and person. In 'classroom RO' patients are rehearsed in salient facts about their lives, using aids such as notices, calendars, and materials to stimulate group discussions (Drummond, Kirchoff, and Scarbrough, 1978; Hanley, McGuire, and Boyd, 1981). Evaluation of RO has proved difficult. Small improvements have been reported, especially with the mildy impaired, on some of the cognitive measures monitored (Schwenk, 1979), but typically there is no marked generalization towards behaviours (Citrin and Dixon, 1977; Harris and Ivory, 1976; Woods, 1979; Zepelin, Wolfe, and Kleinplatz, 1981). The main demonstrated benefit of classroom RO is that it improves staff morale and attitudes towards the elderly (Smith and Barker, 1972). The aim of '24 hour RO' is to teach staff to communicate effectively with the elderly confused person, providing accurate information while keeping instructions brief and clear. There have been no systematic studies of the ways staff and patients' interactions change when such a programme is introduced. Clearly RO can increase the attention and stimulation patients receive, and is best regarded as a way of legitimizing staff–patient contact by providing a distinctive kind of patient management.

Increasing Control and Autonomy: The Structure of the Patient's Day

The term 'control' refers to the belief that one has at one's disposal a response that can influence the outcome of an event (Thompson, 1981). The belief is strengthened by providing choices, making the environment predictable, and supplying information relevant to decision-making. Kahana (1980) found that morale in the elderly is higher when individual perferences for control are matched by the environment. Desire for control is not absolute: in conditions of risk, control is relinquished if another person is believed capable of limiting maximum danger. For this reason some people wish to know nothing of what is going on during medical procedures. Under these circumstances those who habitually believe that outcomes are determined by external factors are less anxious than those who believe that outcomes depend on their own efforts (Miller, 1979). In situations of minimum risk, internal locus of control is related to positive self-concept, especially in elderly men (Reid, Haas, and Hawkins, 1977). Institutional policies encouraging control increase self-esteem for most elderly people. This is important in long-term care. Those entering have typically failed in maintaining an autonomous existence and personal competence, and self-esteem may be low (Lawton, 1980).

Residents can be given control in a variety of ways: options over furniture, clothing, activities, and meals. In structuring the day a balance must be sought between predictability and choice. Predictability without choice induces a feeling of helplessness; unpredictability also undermines control. The aim should be to structure the day providing choices comparable to those available to elderly people in their own homes rather than focusing on administrative events such as duty shifts. This policy implies early morning wakening only for those who need it individually, an after-lunch nap on the bed for most people, a last main meal of the day in the evening, and a bedtime which is not too early and flexible enough to allow those who wish to stay up late to do so (DHSS,

1976). Bulk organization of care in washing, toileting and meal service should be reexamined since these entail fruitless waiting while others are receiving attention.

Little is known of the optimal duration for activity sessions. Short sessions are desirable for those of limited attention span or for those with behaviour problems – who may pass as 'acceptable' if they are not too long in the company of any one group. A change of location for different activities provides stimulation in a restricted world, reducing interference between different types of learning. Some activities conflict even if pursued within even a large central space. Adequate boundaries are needed between areas designed for physical activity and for activities needing freedom from distraction.

Evaluating Institutional Environments

Evaluation is important to compare institutions, see whether they change over time, and investigate which features are associated with desired outcomes. Evaluation requires examination both of physical features and organizational policies. Moos and Lemke (1980) have developed the Multi Phasic Environmental Assessment Procedure for use in care settings for the elderly (see Raphael and Mandeville, 1979, for a survey of opinions about hospital environments). Donabedian (1966) suggests three dimensions along which the quality of an environment can be assessed: (a) the structure of care (variables associated with facilities, equipment, and staffing); (b) the process of care (what happens and in what order, how problems are defined and treatment carried out); (c) the outcomes (mortality, morbidity, social functioning, patient satisfaction, etc.). Structural assessments alone (e.g. surveys of building and staffing) can be misleading. Slagsvold (1981), for instance, found that large high-cost nursing homes in Norway provided better facilities than small homes, but when processes of care were examined there was a clear advantage to smaller establishments. Kushlik and Blunden (1974) argue that the behaviour of clients themselves is the appropriate index of quality of care. 'Outputs' such as the proportion of people engaged in activity provide evidence of the quality of life of residents and indirect evidence of quality of care,

since appropriate facilities and staff policies are assumed to promote adaptive behaviour in residents (Kushlik and Blunden, 1974; Davies and Knapp, 1981). This viewpoint presupposes that 'outputs' like engagement are for the most part environmentally determined. They may, however, also be determined by individual characteristics and preferences, in which case additional concurrent information is required.

Environmental assessment is best seen as a process of identifying problems of care. Jacobs, Christoffel, and Dixon (1976) discuss four generalized types: (a) problems of care arising from environmental factors (poor facilities, lack of supplies, lack of reinforcement for junior staff), solutions requiring changes of designs and policy; (b) problems arising from lack of knowledge or skill about what should be done (training and education are needed); (c) problems because probationers lack feedback about the consequences of their decisions, e.g. success of placements (improved communication between care staff is required); (d) problems of care arising from apathy (these require action to increase motivation, e.g. by rewarding good practice and fostering 'good reputations' among peers). Once a problem has been identified and action to solve it initiated a solution will not necessarily be reached. Interventions may have deleterious side-effects (Kahn, 1977). Hence an evaluation of quality of care needs to be ongoing. An evaluation of environments is an integral part of monitoring the effectiveness of treatment.

ADJUSTMENT AND COPING

Stressful Life Events in Old Age

There is an extensive literature which seeks to demonstrate a causal relationship between stressful life events and physical or psychological illness (Dohrendwend and Dohrendwend, 1974; Renner and Birren, 1980). A stressor is a stimulus external or internal to the person which is construed as threatening, e.g. a bereavement, accident, or a bodily change signifying illness. The way a stressor is appraised depends on the person's behavioural competence and coping resources, their perceived control over the event, and factors associated with personality and physiological reactivity. The eventual health outcome depends on whether normal coping processes reduce the threat, whether social supports are available, and whether events are isolated or compounded by long-term difficulties.

Coping responses have two functions: firstly, to reduce the threat of the event either by changing the environment or changing oneself, and, secondly, to combat symptoms of anxiety and depression that have been aroused. If normal coping processes fail there may be more drastic attempts at adjustment, including the development of pathological symptoms, demand for legitimized illness status, or attempts at suicide (Miller and Ingham, 1980). Cochrane and Sobol (1980) suggest that most people have a hierarchy of coping mechanisms. At the first level there are defence mechanisms such as denial or reappraisal which allow events to be misperceived or reinterpreted to reduce their impact. An objective loss may be seen as 'for the best', devalued, or simply put out of mind. At the second level there are stress opposing experiences such as previous or current positive events. These do not directly prevent stressors but make them more bearable. Elderly people have fewer positive current life events so their adjustment to current stressors may depend heavily on previous successes and on continuing sources of life satisfaction. A third adjustment resource is the presence of an intimate personal relationship. Wider social support systems (friends and neighbours) may also help.

Research suggests that the elderly utilize all three coping mechanisms. Although elderly people are more likely to experience events such as bereavements and serious illness, it is not known whether their impact is greater. Neugarten and Hagestad (1976) suggest that expected events (those perceived as being 'on time' at that stage of the life-cycle) are less threatening. Sands and Parker (1980) found that for elderly people death-related events are less stressful and Palmore and coworkers, (1979) found that in this age group illness has surprisingly little effect on social and psychological adaptation, though it does affect physical functioning. Events occurring singly had few negative effects but there was a cumulative effect, especially for those with poor social resources. In a survey of elderly people in the community Linn, Hunter, and Harris (1980) found that those with depressive symptomatology had experienced more deaths and accidents among relatives and friends and had been involved in more arguments. Murphy (1982) also found more severe life events in a depressed elderly group than in controls. Absence of a confiding relationship was associated with vulnerability to depression if a severe event occurred, but two-thirds of those without a confidant had never had one, suggesting that lifelong adjustment patterns are involved. If a life event changes social roles most elderly people have fewer opportunities for rebuilding resources. Relocation and bereavement are thus of potentially greater significance.

Coping with Relocation

The term relocation is used to refer to changes in living situation, including moving house (Carp, 1968), entering an institution (Lieberman, 1961), and moves within or between institutions (Killian, 1970). Not surprisingly it has been hard to come to firm conclusions from studies covering such a wide range. Early fears were that relocation was associated with increased mortality in the year after the move and that the move itself might be harmful (Aldrich and Mendkoff, 1963). Coffman (1981) in an extensive methodological review has concluded, however, that there is no general mortality effect. Concentration on this variable may have retarded understanding of other aspects of adjustment to institutional life. There are three stages in relocation: (a) decision and preparation; (b) the impact of the move itself; (c) the settling-in process (Yawney and Slover, 1973). The success of relocation depends on factors related to each of these: whether the move is voluntary or involuntary, the state of physical and mental health at the time of the move, and the degree of predictability and control within the new environment (Bourestom and Pastalan, 1981; Schulz and Brenner, 1977). Borup (1981) has described a number of precepts of good practice to help elderly people reduce and cope with stress accompanying relocation. Willingness to move is an important determinant of successful adjustment and preparation is particularly important for the reluctant. Visits to the new environment should be arranged prior to the move and the patient's family involved.

During the move itself and the settling in period the environment should be made as predictable as possible. Information about those aspects which require adjustment should be given and care staff should provide activities which test coping skills yet allow experiences of success. Empirical studies are scarce but Krantz and Schulz (1980) found that providing elderly people with relevant information and control over their environment significantly improved subjective health and active behaviour. Rodin and her colleagues designed studies to see whether declines in alterness and activity level associated with relocation could be reversed (Rodin, 1980). By increasing the choice and control patients had over their new environment, teaching explicit coping skills and substituting environmental explanations for the negative attributions patients made about their problems, significant positive changes in health and behavioural coping were obtained relative to controls.

Bereavement

Widowhood has been described as the single most disruptive crisis of all transitions in the life cycle (Hendricks and Hendricks, 1981). Rowlands (1977) found death of a significant other a factor predicting mortality, especially in men, but it is not clear whether it is bereavement itself or concomitant environment events that are detrimental. Parkes (1972) suggests that mourning is itself a powerful source of stress which frequently results in physical and mental illness. Various stages of mourning have been proposed (Bowlby, 1980; Matz, 1979; Parkes, 1972). Lindemann (1944), for instance, identified five basic phases: (a) a cluster of somatic symptoms; (b) preoccupation with the image of the deceased; (c) feelings of guilt; (d) hostile reactions, irritability, and anger; (e) loss of pattern of conduct. However, there is virtually no empirical evidence to support stage theories and no norms exist for the amount of mourning that may be regarded as 'healthy'. The effects of 'anticipatory grieving' are also unclear. With a sample of mean age 61 years, Clayton and coworkers, (1973) found no difference in prevalence of postbereavement symptoms depending on whether the terminal illness was long or short, but Gerber and coworkers, (1975a) report that those who had

nursed through a lengthy illness had poorer medical adjustment. Glick, Weiss, and Parkes, (1974) emphasize that the way in which news of impending death is broken affects ultimate adjustment. Information should be given over a period of time, where possible, so there is no single 'occasion'. There should be frequent opportunities for discussion, as distress may lead to distortion in what is assimilated and meetings should be timed so that the family member does not have to return directly to the bedside.

Psychological adjustment of the elderly bereaved appears variable (Atchley, 1975). Heyman and Gianturco (1973) found surprisingly little disruption in social networks, activities, emotional stability, and health change in a longitudinal study of 41 elderly people married at the time of first testing but subsequently seen at an average 21 months after the death. Palmore and coworkers, (1979) confirms this. Although widowhood can precipitate isolation, people widowed in late life have had more opportunity to anticipate changed social roles. As Bowlby (1980) points out, however, there is no age after which a person may not respond to loss by disordered mourning.

Most therapeutic approaches focus on emotional support, permitting expression of grief, formation of new social roles, and immediate practical problems. There is some evidence that brief counselling along these lines reduces medical problems in the elderly bereaved during the first 6 months relative to controls (Gerber *et al.*, 1975b).

Gauthier and Marshall (1977) presented a cognitive behavioural analysis of grief. They emphasize the role of reinforcement in extending or prolonging the grief experience. On the basis of this analysis they report the successful treatment of four patients with chronic grief. The treatment involved working with members of the patient's social network with a view to restructuring their responses to the patient's grieving by reinforcing non-grieving behaviour and presenting mild aversive consequences for grief-related depressive behaviour. Flooding techniques were also used to enable the patient to vividly experience images of the deceased.

A study by Flannery (1974) reports the successful treatment of a 77 year old patient manifesting grief-related somatic and mood disorders. The therapist differentially reinforced the patient's positive statements about himself, ignored negative statements, and prompted and shaped the discussion of grief-related topics. Treatment was conducted within the framework of a behavioural contract in which the continuity of therapeutic sessions was contingent upon the patient observing all steps of the contract. A study by Hussian and Lawrence (1981) reports the successful application of problem-solving training (Goldfried and Davison, 1976) with a group of depressed institutionalized elderly patients. It is not clear whether patients with grief-related mood disorders were included in the study; however, this approach and the previous strategies clearly have potential value for intervention in this area.

Helping the Family Cope with an Infirm Elderly Person

Most empirical studies of family life emphasize that family ties remain strong throughout life (Shanas, 1977; Sussman, 1976). Among the healthy, elderly transactions with adult children tend to be asymmetrical, being in the direction of old to young. Old people prefer giving to taking and tend to minimize such disagreement as may occur (Knipscheer and Bevers, 1981). The onset of chronic illness and disability calls for a major reappraisal of established roles which Blenkner (1965) refers to as the assumption of 'filial responsibility'. Children have to cope practically and emotionally with the dependence of one on whom they have previously depended. The goal must be to make life as satisfactory as possible for both generations (Robinson and Thurnher, 1979). Studies of the rare cases of abuse and commoner cases of neglect suggest that some families, however, are unsuited to being caretakers of highly dependent older members and have a real unwillingness to assume it (Hickey and Douglass, 1981; Stevenson, 1981). It is not clear to what extent this is rooted in past hostility or current difficulties, but sudden unwanted dependency is a trigger, especially if demands for services are regarded as illegitimate or unacceptable. It is important to recognize these relatively rare cases and also to spread the load of care for willing but overburdened caretakers faced with conflicts of responsibility.

Relative Support Groups

Although controlled outcome studies are lacking, several case studies report that relatives find support groups helpful (Fuller *et al.*, 1979; Leeming and Luke, 1977; Safford, 1980). Three main aims of such groups can be identified: (a) education; (b) support from professionals; (c) exchange of information and support between group members.

As part of an educational programme the group should have information on the patient's condition covering its course, likely outcome, and management. Without knowledge, relatives may harbour unrealistic expectations and feel anger or guilt if hopes are not realized. It is important that relatives of mentally impaired patients appreciate that 'their' patient has little insight and that annoying behaviours such as memory lapses, self-neglect, or persistent questioning are part of a progressive disease process. Stroke relatives need information on the acute and chronic aspects of the condition, on the role of rehabilitation, and the possibility of further strokes. Simple explanations of puzzling symptoms such as visual agnosia or unilateral neglect may be required. There is a role, too, for general health education on changes of life style and the maintenance of self-care skills.

Support from professionals covers both practical aid (e.g. laundry services, holiday respite) and counselling. The type of support appropriate will depend on current difficulties. Relatives of both mentally impaired and stroke patients face daunting problems of emotional adjustment. With each there must be adjustment of patterns of activity and dependence within the family. Relatives may be very disturbed by failures to communicate effectively with an impaired family member. Difficulties of this sort appear to be more distressing to relatives than physical burdens of incontinence and nursing care. Gilleard, Watt, and Boyd (1981) report that 'perceived burden' is associated with the patient's attention-demanding behaviour. Relatives therefore need guidance in detecting factors in the environment triggering or reinforcing such incidents. Many find the social isolation imposed by care of an infirm elderly person hard to accept (Gilhooly, 1980). A support group may provide the impetus to leave the patient for short periods if sitter services can be arranged and this increases the social world of the caregiver, lessening their perceived load. Relatives will benefit from professional concern for their own welfare, especially from communication of the fact that their difficulties are appreciated.

The regular meeting of a group presents opportunities for mutual support. Exchanges of experiences and information are helpful provided that care is taken to see that relatives do not become discouraged. It may be necessary to emphasize that although members share similar responsibilities, their specific problems differ. A problem-solving focus to the group is helpful. Specific goals set within a behavioural framework focus on whichever problem is most salient to the caregiver (e.g. 'make arrangements so that a friend can be visited for 2 hours before the next meeting'). Reports back to the group and approval for targets attained provide reinforcement for problem-solving behaviour. In suitable cases, relatives may be helped to intervene directly in modifying their patient's problem behaviours. Thus Davies (1981) taught a wife to reduce a stroke patient's complaining behaviour by differentially prompting and reinforcing positive reminiscences and Dapcich-Miura and Hovell (1979) describe a programme supervised by a daughter to increase the compliance of an elderly man to a complex rehabilitation regime.

CONCLUSIONS

Clinical psychology has traditionally been associated with psychometric assessment having its origins in the mental testing movement, and evaluation still plays an important part in the psychologist's work. However, the role has changed. Emphasis is now placed upon therapeutic research, the management and treatment of patients, and the design of therapeutic environments. In this chapter we have described some of these new developments, emphasizing their therapeutic implications. There are many gaps in our presentation, however. The behavioural approach has been applied to many further problem areas (Patterson and Jackson, 1980). We have not described the various psychotherapeutic approaches available (Sparacino, 1978); nor have we discussed research on the modification of intellectual deficits (Baltes and Baltes, 1980). There is a wide range of intervention strategies potentially available to the clinician in addition to those discussed. Many of these approaches still rest upon flimsy empirical foundations. There needs to be an intensification of research effort with a view to identifying those procedures that will have lasting therapeutic value. Every discipline has false alarms. Given a sound empirical base, research and development should concentrate on intervention in those settings in which the elderly naturally reside with the naturally occurring resources, reinforcers, and agents of change. The implication of clinical psychology for policy decision regarding the care of the elderly should not be overlooked.

REFERENCES

Aldrich, C. K., and Mendkoff, E. (1963). 'Relocation of the aged and disabled: A mortality study', *J. Am. Geriat. Soc.,* **11**, 185–194.

Alexander, J. R., and Eldon, A. (1979). 'Characteristics of elderly people admitted to hospital, Part III. Homes, and sheltered housing', *Epidemiol. Community Health,* **33**, 91–95.

Altman, I. (1975). *The Environment and Social Behavior: Privacy, Personal Space, Territory, Crowding,* Brooks/Cole, Monterey, California.

Atchley, R. C. (1975). 'Dimensions of widowhood in later life', *Gerontologist,* **15**, 176–178.

Atthowe, J. M. (1972). 'Controlling nocturnal enuresis in severely disabled and chronic patients'. *Behav. Ther.,* **3**, 232–239.

Azrin, N. H., and Foxx, R. M. (1971). 'A rapid method of toilet training the institutionally retarded', *J. Appl. Behav. Anal.,* **4**, 89–99.

Baltes, M. M., Burgess, R. L., and Stewart, R. B. (1980). 'Independence and dependence in self-care behaviors in nursing home residents: An operant-observational study', *Int. J. Behav. Dev.,* **3**, 489–500.

Baltes, M. M., and Zerbe, M. B. (1976). 'Independence training in nursing home residents', *Gerontologist,* **16**, 428–432.

Baltes, P. B., and Baltes, M. M. (1980). 'Plasticity and variability in psychological aging: Methodological and theoretical issues', in *Determining the Effects of Aging on the Central Nervous System.* (Ed. G. E. Gurski), A. G. Schering, Berlin.

Barker, R. R., and Barker, L. S. (1961). 'The psychological ecology of old people in Midwest, Kansas and Yoredale, Yorkshire', *J. Gerontol.,* **16**, 144–149.

Barton, E. M., Baltes, M. M., and Orzech, M. J. (1980). 'Etiology of dependence in older nursing home residents during morning care: The role of staff behavior', *J. Pers. Soc. Psychol.*, **38**, 423–431.

Baumeister, A. A., and Rollings, J. P. (1976). 'Self-injurious behaviour', in *International Review of Research in Mental Retardation* (Ed. N. R. Ellis), Vol. 8, Academic, New York.

Binks, M. G., and Davies, A. D. M. (1981). 'The set test as a clinical sign of senile dementia: A review', *Proc. Twelfth Int. Cong.Gerontol., Hamburg*, **1**, 284.

Blenkner, M. (1965). 'Social work and family relationships in later life with some thoughts on filial maturity', in *Social Structure and the Family*. (Eds. E. Shanas and G. F. Streib), Prentice-Hall, Englewood Cliffs, New Jersey.

Borup, J. H. (1981). 'Relocation: Attitudes, information network and problems encountered', *Gerontologist*, **21**, 501–511.

Botwinick, J. (1977). 'Intellectual abilities', in *Handbook of the Psychology of Aging* (Eds J. E. Birren and K. W. Schaie), Van Nostrand Reinhold, New York.

Bourestom, N., and Pastalan, L. (1981). 'The effects of relocation on the elderly', *Gerontologist*, **21**, 4–7.

Bowlby, J. (1980). *Attachment and Loss*, Vol. 3, *'Loss, Sadness and Depression*, Hogarth Press, London.

Britton, P. G., and Savage, R. D. (1966). 'A short form of the W.A.I.S. for use with aged', *Br. J. Psychiatry*, **112**, 417–418.

Cadozo, L., Stanton, S. L., Hefner, J. and Allan, V. 'Biofeedback in the treatment of detrusor instability', *Br. J. Urology*, **50**, 250–254.

Canter, D., and Canter, S. (1979). *Designing for Therapeutic Environments: A Review of Research*, John Wiley, Chichester.

Carp, F. M. (1968). 'Effects of improved housing on the lives of older people', in *Middle-age and Aging* (Ed. B. Neugarten), University of Chicago Press.

Carp, F. M., and Carp, A. (1981). 'It may not be the answer, it may be the question', *Res. Aging*, **3**, 85–100.

Christensen, A.-L. (1979). *Luria's Neuropsychological Investigation*, 2nd ed., Munksgaard, Copenhagen.

Citrin, R. S., and Dixon, D. N. (1977). 'Reality orientation: A mileu therapy used in an institution for the aged', *Gerontologist*, **17**, 39–43.

Clayton, P. J., Halikas, J. A., Maurice, N. L., and Robins, E. (1973). 'Anticipatory grief and widowhood', *Br. J. Psychiatry*, **122**, 47–51.

Cochrane, R., and Sobol, M. (1980). 'Life stresses and psychological consequences', in *Psychological Problems: The Social Context* (Eds. P. Feldman and J. Orford), John Wiley, Chichester.

Coffman, T. L. (1981). 'Relocation and survival of institutionalized aged: A re-examination of the evidence', *Gerontologist*, **21**, 483–500.

Collins, R. W., and Plaska, T. (1975). 'Mowrer's conditioning treatment for eneuresis applied to geriatric residents of a nursing home', *Behav. Ther.*, **6**, 632–638.

Corso, J. F. (1977). 'Auditory perception and communication', in *Handbook of the Psychology of Aging* (Eds J. E. Birren and K. W. Schaie), Van Nostrand Reinhold, New York.

Crisp, A. G., and Coll, P. (1980). 'Modification of self-injurious behaviour in a profoundly retarded child by differentially reinforcing incompatible behaviour', *Br. J. Ment. Subnorm.*, **26**, 2, 81–88.

Dapcich-Miura, E., and Hovell, M. F. (1979). 'Contingency management of adherence to a complex medical regimen in an elderly heart patient', *Behav. Ther.*, **10**, 193–201.

Davies, A. D. M. (1972). 'The effects of age, sex and occupation on selected psychological and physical variables: Some preliminary results of a longitudinal study', in *Ageing of the Central Nervous System: Biological and Psychological Aspects* (Eds. H. M. van Praag and A. F. Kalverboer), De Erven F. Bohn, Haarlem.

Davies, A. D. M. (1981). 'Neither wife nor widow: An intervention with the wife of a chronically handicapped man during hospital visits', *Behav. Res. Ther.*, **19**, 449–451.

Davies, A. D. M., and Crisp, A. G. (1980). 'Setting performance goals in geriatric nursing', *J. Adv. Nurs.*, **5**, 381–388.

Davies, A. D. M., and Snaith, P. A. (1980a). 'The social behaviour of geriatric patients at mealtimes: An observational and an intervention study', *Age Ageing*, **9**, 93–99.

Davies, A. D. M., and Snaith, P. A. (1980b). 'Mealtime problems in a continuing care hospital for the elderly', *Age Ageing*, **9**, 100–105.

Davies, B., and Knapp, M. (1981). *'Old People's Homes and the Production of Welfare'*, Routledge and Kegan Paul, London.

De Long, A. J. (1970). 'The micro-spatial structure of the older person: Some implications of planning the social and spatial environment', in *Spatial Behavior of Older People* (Eds L. A. Pastalan, and D. H. Carson, The University of Michigan – Wayne State University, Institute of Gerontology, Ann Arbor, Michigan.

Department of Health and Social Security (1976). *The Organization of the In-Patient's Day*, H.M.S.O., London.

Department of Health and Social Security and the Welsh Office (1980). 'Hospital accommodation for elderly people', 'Health Building Note no. 37 (mimeo), July 1980.

Dickens, W. J., and Perlman, D. (1981). 'Friendship over the life-cycle', in *Personal Relationships 2: Developing Personal Relationships (Eds. S. Duck and R. Gilmour)*, Academic Press, London.

Dohrendwend, B. S., and Dohrendwend, B. P. (Eds) (1974). *Stressful Life Events: Their Nature and Effects*, John Wiley, New York.

Donabedian, A. (1966). 'Evaluating the quality of medical care', *Mil. Mem. Fund Quart*, **44**, 166–203.

Drummond, L., Kirchoff, L., and Scarbrough, D. R. (1978). 'A practical guide to reality orientation: A treatment approach for confusion and disorientation', *Gerontologist*, **18**, 568–573.

Eastman, M. (1979). 'O yes they do!', *New Life*, **6**, 10–15.

Ellis, N. R. (1963). 'Toilet training and the severely defective patient: An S-R reinforcement analysis', *Am. J. Ment. Defic.*, **68**, 98–103.

Engel, B. T., Nikoomanesh, P., and Schuster, M. M. (1974). 'Operant conditioning of rectosphincteric responses in the treatment of fecal incontinence', *New Engl. J. Med.*, **1974**, March 21, 646–649.

Fairhurst, E. (1976). 'Personal space, non-verbal communication and rehabilitation', Paper presented to The British Sociological Conference on Sociology, Health and Illness, Manchester, 6–9 April.

Flannery, R. B. (1974). 'Behavior modification of geriatric grief: A transactional analysis', *Int. J. Aging Hum. Dev.*, **5**, 197–202.

Fordyce, W. E. (1976). *Behavioral Methods for Chronic Pain and Illness'*, C. V. Mosby Co., Saint Louis.

Fozard, J. L. (1981). 'Person–environment relationships in adulthood: Implications for human factors engineering', *Hum. Factors*, **23**, 7–27.

Fozard, J. L., Wolf, E., Bell, B., McFarland, R., and Podolsky, S. (1977). 'Visual perception and communication', in *Handbook of the Psychology of Aging* (Eds J. E. Birren and K. W. Schaie), Van Nostrand Reinhold, New York.

Fuller, J., Ward, E., Evans, A., Massam, K., and Gardner, A. (1979). 'Dementia: Support groups for relatives', *Br. Med. J.*, **1**, 1684–1685.

Garmezy, N., and Harris, J. G. (1953). 'Motor performance of cerebral palsied children as a function of their success in achieving material rewards', *Child Dev.*, **24**, 287–299.

Gauthier, J., and Marshall, W. L. (1977). 'Grief: A cognitive-behavioural analysis', *Cog. Ther. Res.*, **1**, 39–44.

Geiger, O. G., and Johnson, L. A. (1974). 'Positive education for elderly persons: Correct eating through reinforcement', *Gerontologist*, **14**, 432–436.

Gerber, I., Rusalem, R., Hannon, N., Battin, D., and Arkin, A. (1975a). 'Anticipatory grief and aged widows and widowers', *J. Gerontol.*, **30**, 225–229.

Gerber, I., Wiener, A., Battin, D., and Arkin, A. M. (1975b). 'Brief therapy to the aged bereaved', in *Bereavement: Its Psychosocial Aspects*. Columbia University Press, New York. Eds B. Schoenberg, I. Gerber, A. Wiener, A. H. Kutscher, D. Peretz, and A. C. Carr.

Gibson, A. J., and Kendrick, D. C. (1979). *The Kendrick Battery for the Detection of Dementia in the Elderly*, NFER Publishing Co., Windsor.

Gibson, A. J., Moyes, I. C. A., and Kendrick, D. (1980). 'Cognitive assessment of the elderly long-stay patient', *Br. J. Psychiatry*, **137**, 551–557.

Gilhooly, M. L. M. (1980). 'The social dimensions of dementia', Paper presented at The British Psychological Society Annual Conference, Aberdeen, Scotland, 30 March 1980.

Gilleard, C. J., Watt, G., and Boyd, W. D. (1981). 'Problems of caring for the elderly mentally infirm at home', Paper presented at the twelfth International Congress of Gerontology, Hamburg.

Glick, I. O., Weiss, R. S., and Parkes, C. M. (1974). *The First Year of Bereavement*, John Wiley, New York.

Goldfried, M. R., and Davison, G. C. (1976). *Clinical Behaviour Therapy*, Holt, Rinehart and Winston, New York.

Goldiamond, I. (1974). 'Towards a constructional approach to social problems', *Behaviorism*, **2**, 1–84.

Goodglass, H., and Kaplan, E. (1972). *The Assessment of Aphasia and Related Disorders*, Lea and Febiger, Philadelphia.

Goodkin, R. (1966). 'Case studies in behavioral research in rehabilitation', *Percept. Mot. Skills*, **23**, 171–182.

Gordon, C., and Gaitz, C. M. (1977). 'Leisure and lives: Personal expressivity across the life span', in *Handbook of Aging and the Social Sciences*, (Eds R. H. Binstock and E. Shanas), Van Nostrand Rheinhold. New York.

Gray, B., and Isaacs, B. (1979). *Care of the Elderly Mentally Infirm*, Tavistock Publications, London.

Grosicki, J. P. (1968). 'Effect of operant conditioning on modification of incontinence in neuropsychiatric geriatric patients', *Nurs. Res.j* **17**, 304–311.

Hall, J. N. (1980). 'Ward rating scales for long-stay patients: A review', *Psychol. Med.*, **10**, 277–288.

Hanley, I. G. (1981). 'The use of signposts and active training to modify ward disorientation in elderly patients', *J. Behav. Ther. Exp. Psychiatry*, **23**, 241–248.

Hanley, I. G., McGuire, R. J., and Boyd, W. D. (1981). 'Reality orientation and dementia: A controlled trial of two approaches', *Br. J. Psychiatry*, **138**, 10–14.

Harris, A. I., Cox, E., and Smith, C. R. W. (1971). *Handicapped and Impaired in Great Britain*, HMSO, London.

Harris, C. S., and Ivory, P. B. (1976). 'An outcome evaluation of reality orientation therapy with geriatric patients in a state mental hospital', *Gerontologist*, **16**, 496–503.

Hefferin, E. A., and Hunter, R. E. (1975). 'Nursing observation and care planning for the hospitalized aged', *Gerontologist*, **15**, 57–60.

Hendricks, J., and Hendricks, C. D. (1981). *Aging in Mass Society: Myths and Realities*, 2nd ed., Winthrop Publications, Cambridge, Massachusetts.

Hersen, M., and Barlow, D. (1976). *Single-Case Experimental Designs: Strategies for Studying Behavior Change*. Pergamon, New York.

Heyman, D. K., and Gianturco, D. T. (1973). 'Long-term adaptation by the elderly to bereavement', *J. Gerontol.*, **28**, 359–362.

Hickey, T., and Douglass, R. L. (1981). 'Neglect and abuse of older family members: Professionals' perspectives and case experiences', *Gerontologist*, **21**, 171–176.

Hodkinson, H. M. (1972). 'Evaluation of a mental test score for assessment of mental impairment in the elderly', *Age Ageing*, **1**, 233–238.

Hussian, R. A., and Lawrence, P. S. (1981). 'Social reinforcement of activity and problem-solving training in the treatment of depressed institutionalized elderly patients', *Cog. Ther. Res.*, **5**, 57–69.

Ince, L. P. (1980). 'Spinal cord learning', in *Behavioral Psychology in Rehabilitation Medicine: Clinical Applications*, William and Wilkins, Baltimore and London.

Isaacs, B., and Ahktar, A. J. (1972). 'The set test: A rapid test of mental function in old people', *Age Ageing*, **1**, 222–226.

Isaacs, B., and Kenny, A. T. (1973). 'The set test as an aid to the detection of dementia in old people', *Br. J. Psychiatry*, **123**, 467–470.

Jacobs, C. M., Christoffel, T. H., and Dixon, N. (1976). *Measuring the Quality of Patient Care: The Rationale for Outcome Audit*, Ballinger Publishing Co., Cambridge, Massachusetts.

Jenkins, J., Lunt, B., and Powell, L. (1977). 'Increasing engagement in activity of residents in old peoples' homes by providing recreational materials', *Behav. Res. Ther.*, **15**, 429–434.

Kahana, E. (1980). 'A congruence model of person-environment interaction', In *Aging and the Environment: Directions and Perspectives* (Eds M. P. Lawton, P. G. Windley, and T. O. Byerts), Garland STPM Press.

Kahn, R. L. (1977). 'Perspectives in the evaluation of psychological mental health problems for the aged', in *Geropsychology: A Model of Training and Clinical Service* (Ed. W. D. Gentry), Ballinger Publishing Co., Cambridge, Massachusetts.

Kahn, R. L., Goldfarb, A. I., Pollack, M., and Peck, A. (1960). 'Brief objective measures for the determination of mental status in the elderly', *Am. J. Psychiatry*, **117**, 326–328.

Kahn, R. L., Zarit, S., Hilbert, N. M., and Neiderehe, G. (1975). 'Memory complaint and impairment in the aged: The effect of depression and altered brain functioning', *Arch. Gen. Psychiatry*, **32**, 1569–1573.

Kanfer, F. H., and Saslow, G. (1969). 'Behavioral diagnosis', in *Behavior Therapy: Appraisal and Status* (Ed. C. M. Franks), pp. 417–444, McGraw-Hill, New York.

Katz, R. C., Johnson, C. A., and Gelfand, S. (1972). 'Modifying the dispensing of reinforcers: Some implications for behaviour modification with hospitalized patients', *Behav. Ther.*, **3**, 579–588.

Kiernan, C. (1974). 'Behaviour modification'. in *Mental Deficiency* (Eds A. M. Clake and A. D. B. Clarke), 3rd ed., Methuen, London.

Killian, E. C. (1970). 'Effect of geriatric transfers on mortality rates', *Social Work*, **15**, 19–26.

Klisz, D. K., and Dye, C. J. (1981). 'Learning ability for two spatial orientation systems in elderly nursing home residents', *Educational Gerontology*, **6**, 307–316.

Knipscheer, K., and Bevers, A. (1981). 'Older parents and their middle-aged children: Symmetry or asymmetry in their relationship', Paper presented at the Twelfth International Congress of Gerontology, Hamburg.

Krantz, D. S., and Schulz, R. (1980). 'A model of life crisis, control and health outcomes: Cardiac rehabilitation and relocation of the elderly', in *Advances in Environmental Psychology*, Vol. 2, *Applications of Personal Control*, (Eds A. E. Baum and J. E. Singer, Erlbaum Associates, Hillsdale, New Jersey.

Kuriansky, J. B., Gurland, B. J., Fleiss, J. L., and Cowan, D. W. (1976). 'The assessment of self-care capacity in geriatric psychiatric patients by objective and subjective methods', *J. Clin. Psychol.*, **32**, 95–102.

Kushlik, A., and Blunden, R. (1974). 'Proposals for the setting up and evaluation of an experimental service for the elderly: A document for discussion', Research Report No. 107, Health Care Evaluation Research Team, Winchester.

Langer, E., Rodin, J., Beck, P., Weinman, C., and Spitzer, L. (1979). 'Environmental determinants of memory impairment in late adulthood', *J. Pers. Soc. Psychol.*, **37**, 2003–2013.

Lawton, M. P. (1974). 'The human being and the institutional building', in *Designing for Human Behavior* (Eds J. Lang, C. Burnette, W. Moleski and D. Vachon, Stroudsberg, Dowden Hutchinson and Ross, Pennsylvania.

Lawton, M. P. (1980). *Environment and Aging*, Brooks/Cole, Monterey, California.

Lazarus, L. W., Stafford, B., Cooper, K., Cohler, B., and Dysken, M. (1981). 'A pilot study of an Alzheimer patient's relatives discussion group', *Gerontologist*, **21**, 353–358.

Leeming, J. T., and Luke, A. (1977). 'Multi-disciplinary meetings with relatives of elderly hospital patients in continuing-care wards', *Age Ageing*, **6**, 1–5.

Libb, J. W., and Clements, C. B. (1969). 'Token reinforcement in an exercise programme for hospital geriatrics', *Percept. Mot. Skills*, **28**, 957–958.

Lieberman, M. A. (1961). 'The relationship of mortality rates to entrance to a home for the aged', *Geriatrics*, **16**, 515–519.

Lindemann, E. (1944). 'Symptomatology and management of acute grief', *Am. J. Psychiatry*, **101**, 141–148.

Linn, M. W., Hunter, K., and Harris, R. (1980). 'Symptoms of depression and recent life events in the community elderly', *J. Clin. Psychol.*, **36**, 675–682.

Lipman, A., and Slater, R. (1979). 'Homes for old people: Towards a positive environment', in *Designing for Therapeutic Environments* (Eds D. Canter and S. Canter), John Wiley, Chichester.

Lipowski, Z. J. (1975). 'Physical illness, the patient and his environment: Psychosocial foundations of medicine', *American Handbook of Psychiatry*, **4**, 1–42.

Lloyd-Evans, S., Brocklehurst, J. C., and Palmer, M. K. (1978). 'Assessment of drug therapy in chronic brain failure' *Gerontol.*, **24**, 304–311.

Lowenthal, M. F., and Boler, D. (1965). 'Voluntary vs involuntary social withdrawal', *J. Gerontol.*, **20**, 363–371.

Ludeman, K. (1981). 'Sexuality of the older person: Review of the literature', *Gerontologist*, **21**, 203–208.

McClannahan, L. E. (1973). 'Therapeutic and prosthetic living environments for nursing home residents', *Gerontologist*, **13**, 424–429.

McClannahan, L. E., and Risley, T. R. (1975). 'Design of living environments for nursing home residents: Increasing participation in recreational activities'. *J. Appl. Behav. Anal.*, **8**, 261–268.

McCormack, D., and Whitehead, A. (1981). 'The effect of providing recreational activities on the engagement level of long-stay geriatric patients', *Age Ageing*, **10**, 287–291.

MacDonald, M. L., and Butler, A. K. (1974). 'Reversal of helplessness: Producing walking behavior in nursing home wheelchair residents using behavior modification procedures', *J. Gerontol.*, **29**, 97–101.

Maddox, G. L., and Douglas, E. B. (1973). 'Self-assessment of health: A longitudinal study of elderly subjects', *J. Health Soc. Behav.*, **14**, 87–93.

Marston, N., and Gupta, H. (1977). 'Interesting the old', *Community Care*, **1977**, 16 Nov.

Matz, M. (1979). 'Helping families cope with grief', in *Helping Clients with Special Concerns* (Eds S. Eisenberg and L. E. Paterson. Rand McNally, Chicago.

Melin, E. (1981). 'How to stimulate the persons who take care of the old patients', Paper presented at Twelfth International Congress of Gerontology, Hamburg.

Melin, L., and Gotestam, K. G. (1981). 'The effects of rearranging ward routines on communication and eating behaviours of psychogeriatric patients', *J. Appl. Behav. Anal.*, **14**, 47–51.

Millard, P. H., and Smith, C. B. (1981). 'Personal belongings – a positive effect?', *Gerontologist*, **21**, 85–90.

Miller, D. B., and Beer, S. (1977). 'Patterns of friendship among patients in a nursing home setting', *Gerontologist*, **17**, 269–275.

Miller E. (1977). *Abnormal Ageing: The Psychology of Senile and Presenile Dementia*, John Wiley, London.

Miller, P. M., and Ingham, J. G. (1980). 'Reflections on the life-events-to-illness link with some preliminary findings', in *Stress and Anxiety* (Eds I. G. Sarason and C. D. Spielberger), Vol. 6, John Wiley, New York.

Miller S. M. (1979). 'Controllability and human stress: Method, evidence and theory', *Behav. Res. Ther.*, **17**, 287–304.

Milne, J. S. (1976). 'Prevalence of incontinence in the elderly age groups', in *Incontinence in the Elderly* (Ed. F. L. Willington), Academic Press, London.

Mishara, B. L., and Kastenbaum, R. (1973). 'Self-injurious behavior and environmental change in the institutionalized elderly', *Int. J. Aging Hum. Dev.*, **4**, 133–145.

Montegar, C. A., Reid, D. H., Madsen, C. H., and Ewell, M. D. (1977). 'Increasing institutional staff to resident interactions through in-service training and supervisor approval', *Behav. Ther.*, **8**, 533–540.

Moos, R. H., and Lemke, S. (1980). 'The multiphasic environmental procedure: A method for comprehensively evaluating sheltered care settings', in *Community Mental Health: A Behavioral/Ecological Perspective* (Eds A. Jeger and B. Slotnick), Plenum, New York.

Murphy, E. (1982). 'Social origins of depression in old age', *Br. J. Psychiatry*, **141**, 135–142.

Nelson, H. E., and McKenna, P. (1975). 'The use of current reading ability in the assessment of dementia', *Br. J. Soc. Clin. Psychol.*, **14**, 259–267.

Neugarten, B. L., and Hagestad, G. O. (1976). 'Age and the life course', in *Handbook of Aging and the Social Sciences* (Eds R. H. Binstock and E. Shanas), Van Nostrand Reinhold, New York.

Nisbett, R., and Ross, L. (1980). *Human Inference: Strategies and Shortcomings of Social Judgement,* Prentice Hall, Englewood Cliffs.

Norman, A. J. (1979). *Rights and Risks: A Discussion Document on Civil Liberty in Old Age*, National Corporation for the Care of Old People, London.

O'Donnell, C. R. (1980). 'Environmental design and the prevention of psychological problems', in *Psychological Problems: The Social Context*, (Eds P. Feldman and J. Orford), John Wiley, Chichester.

Overstall, P. W. (1978). 'Falls in the elderly – epidemiology, aetiology and management', in *Recent Advances in Geriatric Medicine*, (Ed. Bernard Isaacs), Churchill Livingstone, London.

Palmore, E., Cleveland, W. P., Nowlin, J. B., Ramm, D., and Siegler, I. C. (1979). 'Stress and adaptation in later life', *J. Gerontol.*, **34**, 841–851.

Parkes, C. M. (1972). *Bereavement: Studies of Grief in Adult Life*, Tavistock Publications, London.

Patterson, R. L., and Jackson, G. M. (1980). 'Behavior modification with the elderly', in *Progress in Behavior Modification*, (Eds M. Hersen, R. M. Eisler, and P. M. Miller), Vol. 9, Academic Press, New York.

Pattie, A. H., and Gilleard, C. J. (1979). *Manual of the Clifton Assessment Procedures for the Elderly,* Hodder and Stoughton, Sevenoaks, Kent.

Peterson, R. F., Knapp, T. J., Rosen, J. C., and Pither, B. F. (1977). 'The effects of furniture arrangements on the behaviour of geriatric patients', *Behav. Ther.*, **8**, 464–467.

Pollock, D. D., and Liberman, R. P. (1974). 'Behavior therapy of incontinence in demented in-patients', *Gerontologist*, **14**, 488–491.

Powell, L., Felce, D., Jenkins, J., and Lunt, B. (1979). 'Increasing engagment in a home for the elderly by providing an indoor gardening activity', *Behav. Res. Ther.*, **17**, 127–135.

Quilitch, H. F. (1974). 'Purposeful activity increased on a geriatric ward through programmed recreation', *J. Am. Geriatr. Soc.*, **22**, 226–229.

Rabbitt, P. M. A. (1982). 'How to assess the elderly? An experimental psychologist's view', *Br. J. Clin. Psychol.*, **21**, 55–60.

Raphael, W., and Mandeville, J. (1979). *Old People in Hospital,* King Edward's Hospital Fund, London.

Raschko, Betty Ann (1974). 'Physiological and behavioral characteristics of the elderly: A basis for design criteria for interior space and furnishings', *Rehabil. Lit.*, **35**, 10–31.

Raskin, A., and Jarvik, L. F. (1979). *Psychiatric Symptoms and Cognitive Loss in the Elderly: Evaluation and Assessment Techniques,* John Wiley, New York.

Reid, D. W., Haas, G., and Hawkins, D. (1977). 'Locus of desired control and positive self-concept in the elderly', *J. Gerontol.*, **35**, 395–402.

Renner, V. J., and Birren, J. E. (1980). 'Stress: Physiological and psychological mechanisms', in *Handbook of Mental Health and Aging* (Eds J. E. Birren and R. B. Sloane), Prentice-Hall, Englewood Cliffs, New Jersey.

Robinson, B., and Thurnher, M. (1979). 'Taking care of aged parents: A family cycle transition', *Gerontologist,* **19**, 586–593.

Rodin, J. (1980). 'Managing the stress of aging: The role of control and coping', in *Coping and Health,* (Eds S. Levine and U. Holger', Plenum Press, London.

Rowlands, K. F. (1977). 'Environmental events predicting death for the elderly', *Psychol. Bull.*, **84**, 349–372.

Safford, F. (1980). 'A program for families of the mentally impaired elderly', *Gerontologist,* **20**, 656–660.

Sanavio, E. (1981). 'Toilet retraining psychogeriatric residents', *Behav. Modif.*, **5**, 417–427.

Sand, P., and Berni, R. (1974). 'An incentive contract for nursing home sides', *Am. J. Nurs.*, **74**, 1646–1648.

Sands, J. D., and Parker, J. (1980). 'A cross-sectional study of the perceived stressfulness of several life events', *Int. J. Aging Hum. Dev.*, **10**, 325–341.

Savage, B. J., and Widdowson, T. (1974). 'Revising the use of nursing resources', *Nursing Times,* 1372–1374.

Schulz, R., and Brenner, G. (1977). 'Relocation of the aged: A review and theoretical analysis', *J. Gerontol.*, **32**, 323–333.

Schwenk, M. A. (1979). 'Reality orientation for the institutionalized aged: Does it help?', *Gerontologist*, **19**, 373–377.

Shanas, E. (1977). 'The elderly: Family bureaucracy and family help patterns', Paper presented at the Institute de la Vie Conference, Vichy, France.

Slagsvold, B. (1981). 'The relationship between size, cost and quality in nursing homes', Paper presented at the Twelfth International Congress of Gerontology, Hamburg.

Slater, R., and Gill, A. (1981). 'Environmental personalization in institutional settings', Paper presented at the Twelfth International Congress of Gerontology, Hamburg.

Smith, B. J., and Barker, H. R. (1972). 'Influence of a reality orientation training program on the attitude of trainees', *Gerontologist,* **12**, 262–264.

Snyder, L. H., Rupprecht, P., Pyrek, J., Brekus, S., and Moss, T. (1978). 'Wandering', *Gerontologist,* **18**, 272–280.

Sparacino, J. (1978). 'Individual psychotherapy with the aged: A selective review', *Int. J. Aging Hum. Dev.,* **9**, 197–220.

Spiro, L. R. (1978). 'Bladder training for the incontinent', *J. Gerontol. Nurs.,* **4**, 28–35.

Stevenson, O. (1981). 'Caring and dependency', in *The Impact of Ageing* (Ed. D. Hobman), Croom Helm, London.

Stoffelmayr, B. E., Lindsay, W., and Taylor, V. (1979). 'Maintenance of staff behavior', *Behav. Res. Ther.,* **17**, 271–273.

Stoudt, H. W. (1981). 'The anthropometry of the elderly', *Hum. Factors,* **23**, 29–37.

Sussman, M. (1976). 'The family life of old people', in *Handbook of Aging and the Social Sciences* (Eds R. H. Binstock and E. Shanas), Van Nostrand Reinhold, New York.

Thompson, S. C. (1981). 'Will it hurt less if I can control it? A complex answer to a simple question', *Psychol. Bull.* **90**, 89–101.

Trombley, C. (1966). 'Principles of operant conditioning related to training of arthritic quadriplegic patients', *Am. J. Occup. Ther.,* **20**, 217–220.

Trotter, A., and Inman, D. (1968). 'The use of positive reinforcement in physical therapy', *Phys. Ther.,* **48**, 347–352.

Wear, J. B., Wear, R. B., and Cleeland, C. (1979). 'Biofeedback in urology using urodynamics: Preliminary observations', *J. Urol.,* **121**, 464–468.

Wilkin, D., Hughes, B., and Evans, G. (1981). 'Integration of confused and lucid elderly people in institutional care: Effects on levels of activity and communication', Paper presented at the Twelfth International Congress of Gerontology, Hamburg.

Woods, R. T. (1979). 'Reality orientation and staff attention: A controlled study', *Br. J. Psychiatry,* **134**, 502–507.

Yawney, B. A., and Slover, D. L. (1973). 'Relocation of the elderly', *Social Work,* **18**, 86–95.

Zepelin, H., Wolfe, C. S., and Kleinplatz, F. (1981). 'Evaluation of a year-long reality orientation program', *J. Gerontol.,* **36**, 70–77.

Zimring, C. M. (1981). 'Stress and the designed environment', *J. Soc. Iss.,* **37**, 145–171.

Principles and Practice of Geriatric Medicine
Edited by M. S. J. Pathy
© 1985 John Wiley & Sons Ltd

16.5

Neurological Disorders of the Elderly

R. A. Griffiths

INFLUENCE OF AGE ON NEUROLOGICAL SIGNS

Neurological function declines with increasing age. As with many other body systems, the original emphasis on chronological ageing has gradually given way to a recognition of the importance of multiple pathology, often age-related but not necessarily unique to the elderly (Allison, 1962; Critchley, 1931; Critchley, 1956; Howell, 1949; Hurwitz and Swallow, 1971; Klawans *et al.*, 1971; Kokmen *et al.*, 1977; Locke and Galaburda; 1978 Newman, Dovenmuehle, and Busse, 1960; Prakash and Stern, 1973; Skre, 1972;).

Impaired vision, hearing, taste and smell; ptosis and miosis; poor optical convergence and inappropriate pupil reactions; diminished upward conjugate deviation of the eyes; absent abdominal reflexes; absent tendo Achillis and other reflexes; impaired vibration, tactile and pain sensation have all been attributed to ageing (Critchley 1931; Critchley, 1956, Howell, 1949; Skre, 1972).

It must never be accepted that abnormal physical signs in the elderly are due to ageing alone. With increasing awareness that they may have a pathological basis, a diligent search must be made for other signs of various syndromes which occur and for the responsible disease process. Epidemiological and demographical surveys of individual signs have pointed the way to a more comprehensive approach which must include statistical correlation to determine constellations of signs and to observe progress to definitive diseases.

Loss of ankle jerks is common in old age and this loss is age-related (Bhatia and Irvine, 1973; Milne and Williamson 1972). If tendo Achillis reflexes are absent then other tendon reflexes may be absent also, particularly the knee jerks. Bilateral absence of tendo Achillis reflexes and knee jerks is significantly related to weakness of both legs. Loss of vibration sense in the lower limbs is often accompanied by loss of position sense and there is an association between loss of position sense and vibration sensation, and loss of tendo Achillis reflexes and knee jerks. The loss of these signs is related to diabetes and hypertension and probably represents the manifestations of peripheral neuropathy.

The plantar reflexes are rarely affected by age alone (Klawans *et al.*, 1971). As usually elicited, by a light scratch, the latency of the abdominal reflexes is increased with increasing age. If a painful stimulus is used, the latency period is constant and unaffected by age (Magladery *et al.*, 1960).

Many signs and reflexes have been described as concomitants of dementia and are said to represent a return to a more primitive state. A positive palmomental reflex is age-related and more common in dementia (Otomo, 1965). It can occur without evidence of any neurological disease and in normal persons the EMG is nearly always positive, so it has very little practical importance. Snout and sucking reflexes are common in severe Alzheimer's disease. These responses have no particular value in localizing cerebral lesions (Paulson, 1977) and are not essential to the diagnosis of a particular pathological dementing disease.

ALZHEIMER'S DISEASE

Bradykinesia, rigidity, and dementia have multiple causes and are common in old people. The early signs of these conditions may be interpreted, in isolation, as age related. Sixty per cent. of patients with Alzheimer's disease have Parkinsonian signs and up to 50 per cent. of patients with Parkinson's disease develop dementia, which is commoner in old patients who deteriorate more rapidly and have cerebral atrophy (Danielczyk, Riederer, and Seeman, 1980; Gottfries *et al.*, 1980; Pearce, 1974). However, such patients may have the physical manifestations of Alzheimer's disease, which is a continuous spectrum with Parkinsonism or dementia as the presenting features – both being present in the final stages of the disease.

The symptoms and course of Alzheimer's disease are considered to be pathognomonic (Rothschild and Kasanin, 1936; Sjögren, 1952; Sourander and Sjögren, 1970) although it may be necessary to exclude other causes (Haase, 1977). Facetiousness (moria) is sometimes seen in the early stages of the disease. Aspontaneity and short periods of purposeless restlessness may occur. The akinesia–rigidity syndrome is often observed in this early stage. Spacial disorientation is usually more obvious than temporal disorientation – probably associated with direct facial staring and visual agnosia – and is possibly due to disease of the frontal lobes or tracts between parietal and temporal lobes.

In the intermediate stage so-called focal signs occur but as they always occur in conjunction with manifestations of intellectual deterioration they should not be given undue emphasis and significance. Asemia may manifest itself as dysphasia, dyslexia, and dysgraphia. Apraxia and agnosia indicate cerebral involvement which should be taken in the context of global disintegration. Repetitive utterances (logoclonia) and perseveration may occur in this period.

In the final stage, cerebral seizures, forced laughing and crying, laughing attacks, the Klüver–Bucy syndrome (Pilleri, 1966), incontinence, return of primitive reflexes, and pelvi–crural contracture characterize the state of amentia and loss of quality of consciousness. Sjögren (1952) considered that the early akinesia–rigidity problems were frontal lobe in origin but, in the later stages, extrapyramidal rigidity was due to basal ganglia disease. He pointed out that the Parkinsonian features of Alzheimer's disease have led many to a mistaken diagnosis of Parkinson's disease. These patients do not have tremor or pill-rolling movements.

In the early stages of the disease gait is often affected – patients are unable to coordinate and maintain the rhythm of walking. Initiation of walking may be slow due to the momentary locking of the motor phase – walking is thus deliberate, slow, unsteady, and without pulsion phenomena. Unsteadiness is not made worse by closing the eyes. The whole body is stiff, the arms being stiff but flexed. The disturbance has been attributed to a direct or indirect lesion of the prefrontal cortex. Pearce (1974) found, in the early stages, that there was slight flexion of the neck, elbows, and hips, and resistance to passive movement was common. This resistance, though falling short of rigidity or spasticity, was akin to gegenhalten. Early facial masking and, later, forward staring with brief eye movements and inability to sustain lateral or vertical gaze or eye closure may be of central origin. In later stages the gait becomes marche à petit pas as basal ganglia degeneration occurs. Mild bilateral facial paresis of upper motor neurone type is common.

ARTERIOSCLEROTIC PARKINSONISM AND SENILE PARKINSONISM

Kleist (1927) pointed out the relationship of psychiatric and neurological motor negativism in the catatonic manifestations of psychiatric and neurological disease. He distinguished motor resistance from the opposition and contradictory action of psychiatric disorders, naming the former 'gegenhalten'. This motor negativism is manifest in the antigravity muscles and has a similar distribution pattern to decerebrate rigidity – in extension of the neck, flexion of the jaw, hand grip, adduction of the arms and legs, and extension of the knees.

When pressure is exerted against these movements, resistance is encountered which varies directly with the applied force – and increases with repetitive movement. Kleist's cases had cerebral arteriosclerosis and widespread état lacunaire, particularly of basal ganglia and thalamus, but he considered lesions of the thalamus essential to the physical condition. Several of these patients had a degree of frontal lobe atrophy or damage.

Various syndromes of cerebrovascular disease, often incomplete initially, merge into a state of Parkinsonism manifest by bradykinesia and rigidity but without tremor, athetosis, or chorea (Critchley, 1929). These syndromes have a basis of marche à petit pas with immobile facies and rigidity, sometimes associated with pseudo-bulbar symptoms, pseudo-bulbar palsy, pyramidal signs, and cerebellar signs. As originally described by Critchley they are, obviously, not only due to arteriosclerosis but include degenerative diseases of the brain. Alzheimer's disease, Gowers' simple senile paraplegia, and Jakob's senile rigidity are obviously included in the overall description (Critchley, 1929; Gowers, 1892a). The pathology of arteriosclerotic Parkinsonism described by Critchley is varied and includes état criblé due to spiralled elongation of small arteries due to raised blood pressure (Yates, 1976), microscopic area of haemorrhage or softening, cerebral atrophy, gliosis, neuronal loss, neurofibrillary tangles, senile plaques, and demyelination of frontopontine tracts. In all cases the corpus striatum, particularly the globus pallidus, is affected.

The facies, though fixed, is bewildered, and emotional responses are prompt and often excessive. Posture is less flexed than in Parkinson's disease and the gait is characteristically marche à petit pas. There may be a tendency to fall backwards with concurrent plantar flexion (clawing) of toes. Climbing stairs is more normal but descending stairs is hesitant.

Muscle tone is increased but is not characteristic of pyramidal spasticity or ordinary extrapyramidal rigidity. The rigidity is lead-pipe in character, greater in the limbs than in the trunk, and more evident with proximal movement than distal movement. The rigidity is not equal between extension and flexion but is greater in antigravity muscles, i.e. arm flexion and leg extension. It can be briefly summarized as rigidity grafted on the spastic attitude. The rigidity varies directly with the force applied. The patient may overcompensate by voluntary movement or seems to oppose the examiner.

If the patient's attention is distracted the rigidity is more easily assessed. The characteristic opposition or counterpull has been described by Kleist (1927) and is demonstrated by fixation contraction of passively or actively shortened muscles (Foerster, 1921). In the advanced stage of the condition, a movement at one joint is associated with involuntary movement of the others, e.g. dorsiflexion of the foot produces flexion of the knee and hip and flexion of the head produces flexion of the legs.

The muscles may feel harder than normal and when the condition is present, it is invariably found in the legs, which consequently appear more well developed.

There is no diminution of motor power and no paresis of gross movements, but fine movements are impaired. Alternating movements are slow and irregular – pronation and supination of hands is slow but the arms are relatively fixed, unlike cerebellar disease where the elbows and arms move simultaneously.

Bradykinesia and poverty of movement resemble classical Parkinson's disease but are less marked in arteriosclerotic Parkinsonism.

Associated movements may be present (Wilson, 1925). Synergistic movements, though slow, are still retained in arteriosclerotic Parkinsonism. Movements of cooperation such as arm swinging are not abolished although they differ from the normal in the lack of movement of the elbow. Imitative synkinesia in most conditions is bilateral and equal, but one limb may be more affected than the other in arteriosclerosis. Catatonia is a characteristic feature of arteriosclerotic Parkinsonism and may be adopted spontaneously.

Speech is characteristically monotonous; pseudo-bulbar types also have a nasal quality and the cerebellar types a scanning quality. Poverty of speech occurs at a later stage and may amount to mutism, particularly if dementia is present.

The tendon reflexes will depend on the degree of pyramidal involvement. They may be slow in response and decline. If plantar responses are extensor in character, without obvious cause, it is worth searching for evidence of arteriosclerotic Parkinsonism. The plantars may be extensor when the legs are extended and flexor when the legs are flexed (Buzzard and Barnes, 1906).

Physical changes usually precede mental

changes, particularly in mild cases, but may predominate at an early stage. Global deterioration is difficult to differentiate from other causes of dementia. Arteriosclerotic (multi-infarct) dementia is identifiable and simple criteria may help in diagnosis (Hachinski, Lasen, and Marshall 1974; Harrison *et al.*, 1979).

Although the onset of arteriosclerotic Parkinsonism is usually insidious, it may date from a mild stroke. Deterioration is usually more rapid and step-like than Parkinson's disease or Alzheimer's disease. All these conditions terminate in amentia and paraplegia in flexion (Yakovlev, 1954).

CORTEX AND BASAL GANGLIA

The cerebral cortex has a profound influence on posture. The decorticate state produces flexion rigidity of arms and extensor rigidity of legs (Davis, 1925). Decerebrate rigidity from lesions at the pretectal level produces extension of arms and legs with pronation and flexion of hands and inversion and extension of feet.

Denny-Brown (1962) determined the status of the basal ganglia in the maintenance of posture. This consideration did not conflict with the concept of the basal ganglia and the control of movement in that movement itself can be considered as a change in posture. From post-mortem and experimental studies he determined two basic patterns of control:

(a) Lesions of the striatum (caudate nucleus and putamen) produce flexion rigidity of arms and legs when the patient is lying down, which changes to rigid flexion of upper limbs and rigid extension of lower limbs when the patient is lifted from contact with the bed into a more vertical position. This is the striatal syndrome or hemiplegic dystonia (dystonia = fixed attitude).

(b) Lesions of the globus pallidus produce tremor and progressive flexion rigidity of arms and legs which is worse when the patient is lying down. This is the pallidal syndrome or progressive dystonia in flexion.

Although these syndromes are associated with specific areas of basal ganglia pathology they are more likely to be due to loss of corticostriate and corticopallidal fibre systems. Cortical lesions in area 6 produce some rigidity of the pallidal type. If spasticity is added to dystonia this rigidity in both the syndromes described becomes more severe.

Denny-Brown (1962) differentiated between paralysis agitans and arteriosclerotic Parkinsonism in that the former has the characteristic tremor and the latter rigidity and bradykinesia, but there is every degree of transition between the two states.

Arteriosclerosis affects the putamen particularly, there are small areas of softening and état criblé. Tremor is less evident with damage to the putamen but lesions of the globus pallidus are more often associated with tremor. Arteriosclerotic rigidity has a hemiplegic pattern, it is greater in flexion of the arms and extension of the legs, and in severe cases there is pseudo-bulbar palsy.

In paralysis agitans, passive plasticity (rigidity) appears first in the flexors of the upper limb. Rigidity is always associated with a change of posture and adoption of an attitude of flexion; attempted movement away from this position produces increasing resistance. Terminally this loss of plasticity is associated with paraplegia in flexion; at this stage tremor is much less evident.

Rigidity is a reaction to passive applied motion; it has a plastic quality and presents a constant resistance throughout the whole range of applied movement. It is usually more prominent in flexor muscles. It can be overcome by willed relaxation and EMG recordings are then silent over 5 to 10 degrees of movement. Over a larger range of movement contraction of the stretched muscle occurs.

Plastic rigidity is due to the recruiting of motor units which then drop out at the same time as others are recruited. Thus the number of motor units discharging during stretch is small and fairly constant. This is in contrast to spasticity when an increasing number of motor units respond increasingly to a maximum when they cease firing and the so-called lengthening reaction occurs. In rigidity the lengthening reaction is not coordinated and occur progressively in individual motor units. Cogwheeling occurs with synchronization of individual motor units, which then contract together and relax together.

A fixed attitude (dystonia) is accompanied by increasing resistance against movement away from the adopted position. In the early stages of dystonia, EMG recordings are indistinguishable from Parkinsonian rigidity but when fully developed the motor units do not show a lengthening reaction when the muscle is stretched – they continue to discharge and more motor units are recruited. This resistance increases with increasing stretch. The terminal stage of Parkinsonism, paraplegia in flexion, is accompanied by a steady activity of motor units proportional to the degree to which the posture is maintained – the pallidal syndrome.

In studies of cortical lesions, Denny-Brown (1962) describes two physiological responses – exploratory and avoiding – which are behavioural antagonists. Medial frontal lobe lesions facilitate exploration and lessen tactile evading reactions. Consequently, grasping, sucking, and stiffening of a limb in response to touch (gegenhalten) occur. Parietal lobe lesions facilitate avoiding reactions which result in a catatonic persistence of attitude – flexion and stiffening of the limbs and extension of fingers. When the cortical lesion produces diminution of exploratory or evading reactions a subcortical, simpler representation may become evident. The instinctive grasp response to touch may be lost and the grasp reflex, needing a coarser stimulus which is proprioceptive, replaces it. This proprioceptive grasp reflex is mediated by the gamma motor system. Lesions of the posterior cortex release a response to visual stimulus manifest as perseveration of gaze. The basal ganglia are involved in these subcortical reactions.

TREMOR

Tremor is an involuntary oscillation dependent on muscle activity. If the central and peripheral nervous systems are intact it may hardly be visible but can be suitably amplified and recorded (Sinclair Honour, and Griffiths 1977). It is multifactorial in origin and represents a motor homeostasis from which rapid reflex and voluntary movement can occur (Marsden, 1978). Subclinical physiological tremor is increased by cold (shivering), exhaustion, or fear, but pathological tremors are generally of central origin and help to identify the anatomical site of nervous system disease.

Physiological Tremor

Frequency and amplitude of physiological tremor increases from proximal to distal parts of the limb. In the finger, basic mechanical tremor frequency is 25 Hz, in the hand 9 Hz, and in the forearm 2 Hz (Joyce and Rack, 1974; Stiles and Randall, 1967). On this is superimposed a neurogenic input of 10 Hz which tends to be filtered off at the elbow and fingers but is augmented by the natural mechanical frequency of the wrists. It is, therefore, convenient to consider tremor as an oscillator (neural element) exciting a tuned circuit (mechanical element) (Marshall and Walsh, 1956). The neural element is determined by the rate of firing of motor units (Gillies, 1972; Milner-Brown, Stein, and Yemm, 1973a, 1973b), inhibition by Renshaw cells and Golgi tendon organs (Elble and Randall, 1976; Veale, Rees, and Mark, 1973), and oscillations in the stretch reflex servoloop (Hagbarth and Young, 1979; Lippold, 1970; Young and Hagbarth, 1980). The frequency of physiological tremor is 8 to 12 Hz, particularly with the arms extended, and frequency decreases in the elderly (Griffiths *et al.*, 1981; Marsden *et al.*, 1969; Marshall, 1961). The amplitude of physiological tremor is directly proportional to the force of muscle contraction (Hammond, Merton, and Sutton, 1956) and EMG recordings show that in physiological tremor agonists and antagonists act together (Shahani and Young, 1976).

Beta-adrenergic receptors in muscle are concerned with the production of physiological tremor. Intra-arterial adrenaline and isoprenaline increase the amplitude of physiological tremor but noradrenaline and tyramine have no effect. The effect is blocked by propranolol (Marsden *et al.*, 1967; Marsden, Meadows, and Lowe 1969).

Benign Essential Tremor

Exaggerated physiological tremor of 8 to 12 Hz which is minimal at rest but visible with posture and action occurs in a variety of conditions (Struppler, Velho-Groneberg, and Claussen, 1976). Among these conditions are anxiety, fatigue, shivering, phaeochromocytoma, hypoglycaemia, thyrotoxicosis, infusions of adrenaline and isoprenaline, levodopa, thyroxine, heavy metals (mercury, lead, manganese), lithium, adrenergic bronchodilators (salbutamol, terbutaline), dexamphetamine, caffeine, phenothiazines, reserpine, tricyclic antidepressants, anticonvulsants (phenytoin, sodium valproate) (Hyman, Dennis, and Sinclair, 1979), and alcohol withdrawal (Lefebvre-D'Amour, Shahani, and Young, 1978). Many of these tremors respond to treatment of the precipitating cause but persistence of tremor occasionally indicates permanent damage.

The decreases of frequency of physiological tremor and essential tremor with age (Marshall, 1962) suggest that a basic physiological abnormality exists and that essential tremor is merely an exaggerated form of physiological tremor. However, two types of essential tremor are recognizable, one with the same frequency as physiological tremor and the other usually below 6.5 Hz (Critchley, 1949; Findley and Gresty, 1981). In this context, apart from the classical resting tremor of 3 to 7 Hz in Parkinson's disease, both physiological and essential tremors are also found (Shahani and Young, 1976), and alcoholic patients have physiological tremor greater than 8 Hz or action tremor less than 8 Hz (Lefebvre-D'Amour, Shahani, and Young 1978), but the latter may well be cerebellar in origin.

The characteristics of benign essential tremor are that it has a regular sinusoidal movement on tremorgrams and is associated with synchronous EMG activity of both agonists and antagonists. The pathology is unknown (Critchley, 1949). It is often familial (Dana, 1887) and is inherited as an autosomal dominant. It shows anticipation in occurring at a younger age in succeeding generations and has a tendency to die out (Larsson and Sjögren, 1960). It may not occur until later life when it is known as senile tremor, but the characteristics are the same as in younger familial patients.

Essential tremor usually begins in the upper limbs, often in the right hand first, arms, head, legs, chin, tongue, face; palate, larynx, eyelids and eyes may also be affected. It is relieved during sleep and made worse by stress or excitement and the execution of fine movements. The patient's hand writing shows this exacerbation of tremor well and differs from that of Parkinson's disease in that there is no micrographia.

Although essential tremor is a monosymptomatic disorder it can occur in conjunction with other physical signs and diseases (Critchley, 1949).

Five per cent. of subjects with benign essential tremor eventually develop Parkinson's disease (Lance and McLeod, 1981). Some patients with essential tremor also have alternating activity of agonists and antagonists on EMG records which may indicate that the pattern is not specific for Parkinson's disease (Findley and Gresty, 1981), but these patients may in fact be the ones who progress to Parkinson's disease (Lance, Schwab, and Peterson, 1963).

No specific pathological lesion has been found to account for benign essential tremor. Beta-2 adrenergic drugs exacerbate physiological tremor by a peripheral action which is blocked by appropriate beta-2 blockade. Beta-1, lipid soluble, blocking drugs would seem to have a central action in reducing benign essential tremor. Propranolol is effective peripherally and centrally and small doses are effective in the elderly (Griffiths and Good, 1982; Murray, 1981).

Tremor of 8 to 12 Hz may be dependent on the inferior olive. The neurons of the inferior olive fire in rhythmical bursts and harmaline, an alkaloid which increases the synchronicity of inferior olivary neuronal firing, also exaggerates tremor at this frequency by impulses carried by the olivocerebellar fibres and thence to anterior horn motoneurons (Llinas and Volkind, 1973).

Parkinsonian Tremor

The classical tremor of Parkinson's disease (Fig. 1) has a frequency of 3 to 7 Hz at rest, characterized by alternating activity of agonists and antagonists (Jung, 1941; Lance, Schwab, and Peterson, 1963). It disappears with optimum relaxation and sleep and can often be controlled voluntarily. It disappears on posture and action in mild cases. Lance and coworkers (Lance *et al.*, 1963; Lance and McLeod, 1981) stressed the importance of accentuated physiological tremor at 8 to 12 Hz which replaces the classical tremor on movement. It is associated with synchronous contraction of agonists and antagonists, and is often responsible for the frequency of the cogwheel phenomenon. It has been shown (Findley and Gresty, 1981; Gresty

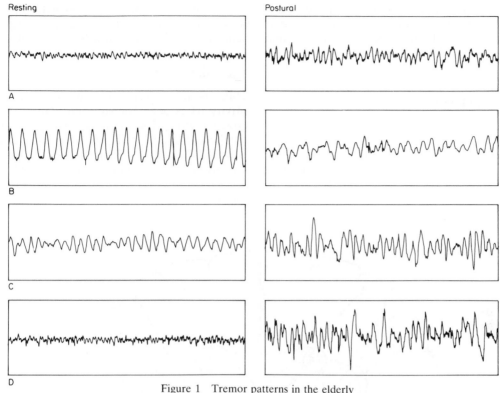

Figure 1   Tremor patterns in the elderly
A–Normal   C–Senile Parkinsonism
B–Parkinson's disease   D–Benign Essential Tremor

Reproduced by permission of *Geriatric Medicine*

and Findley, 1981) by spectral analysis and Fourier transformation that the fundamental frequencies of Parkinson's disease are 4 to 5 Hz for symptomatic resting tremor with an additional higher frequency of 6 Hz of low amplitude and not usually clinically detectable; there is symptomatic postural and action tremor also of 6 Hz and a cogwheel frequency of 6 Hz. They observed that the 6 Hz tremor in hemiParkinsonism was different from the postural physiological tremor on the unaffected side in that the latter had a higher frequency of 8 to 10 Hz.

It is possible that classical Parkinsonian resting tremor is generated in the cortico-strio-pallido-thalamo-cortical loop, driven by the dentato-thalamic connection. This is normally inhibited by the substantia nigra (Fig. 2). Lesions in the cerebral cortex (Bucy and Case, 1939; Klemme, 1940), globus pallidus (Guiot and Brion 1953), ventro lateral nucleus of thalamus (Hassler, 1955), and pyramidal tract (Oliver, 1949; Putnam, 1938) abolish Parkinsonian tremor. James Parkinson himself (Parkinson, 1817) observed that tremor disappeared on the hemiplegic side of a patient with paralysis agitans who sustained a stroke.

Cerebellar Tremor

There are two components to this tremor; one is an action tremor observed during movement of the upper limb and the other is a postural tremor, when movement has achieved its goal, which really involves the base of the limb. The frequency of action tremor is 5 per second and the frequency of postural tremor is 3 per second. There is no tremor at rest. The neocerebellum is linked with the opposite cerebral cortex and tremor is produced by lesions of this part of the cerebellum, i.e. the cerebellar hemispheres. The cerebellum may also have some controlling influence on the amplitude of other tremors. Intention tremor can be abolished by stereotactic lesions in the ventro-lateral nucleus of the thalamus. In mercury poisoning the action tremor of 5 per second is associated with a selective loss of the granular layer of the cerebellum (Kurland, Faros, and Siedler, 1960; Rondot, Jedynak, and Ferrey, 1978).

SPECIAL SENSES

Vision and Hearing

Vision deteriorates with age from many causes (Fozard *et al.*, 1977), as does hearing (Gacec and Schuknecht, 1969; Spoor, 1967). These are considered elsewhere.

Caloric nystagmus decreases with age after 60 years and correlates with high-frequency hearing loss (Brunner and Norris, 1971).

Taste and Smell

There is an age-related decrease in taste sensitivity (Cooper, Blaish, and Zubek, 1959; Grzegorczyk, Jones, and Mistretta, 1979; Hughes, 1969) due to a progressive loss of taste buds (El-Baradi and Bourne, 1951). Olfactory sensitivity declines with age (Moncrieff, 1966) due to atrophy of olfactory bulb fibres (Smith, 1942).

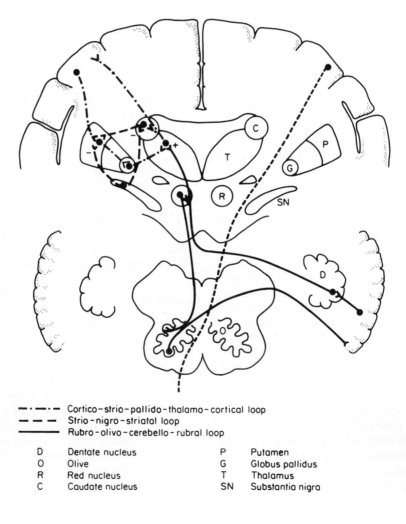

— · — · — Cortico–strio–pallido–thalamo–cortical loop
— — — Strio–nigro–striatal loop
———— Rubro–olivo–cerebello–rubral loop

D	Dentate nucleus	P	Putamen
O	Olive	G	Globus pallidus
R	Red nucleus	T	Thalamus
C	Caudate nucleus	SN	Substantia nigra

Figure 2   Tremorgenic pathways. (Reproduced by permission of *Geriatric Medicine*)

PERIPHERAL SENSATION

The classical concept that each type of peripheral sense organ is concerned in the appreciation of a specific sensory modality has been
gradually supplanted by a classification of receptors according to function, viz. mechanoreceptors, thermoreceptors and polymodal
nociceptors, and proprioceptors. Mechano-
reception is concerned with pressure, touch,
vibration, and tickle; receptors which detect
velocity (Meissner corpuscle, hair follicle receptors), acceleration (Pacinian corpuscles)
which respond maximally to vibration at 200
Hz, and threshold (free nerve endings); and
their densities in the skin (Schmidt, 1978).

In the elderly it is difficult to test sensory
modalities easily by the clinical methods used
in younger patients but these should not be
neglected. Touch, pain, and vibration deserve
special consideration. Temperature sensation
does not seem to have been particularly studied in the elderly.

Sensory complaints are common in the elderly. Formication and paraesthesia occur,
postherpetic neuralgia is more intractable
(Critchley, 1931), and leg cramps are common.

Pain

There is diminished sensitivity to pin-prick in
old age (Procacci *et al.*, 1970) but there are no
changes in cutaneous nerve networks to explain this (Cauna, 1964).

Vibrotactile Sensation

Studies of touch alone would be unrewarding
in the elderly and there are no studies in depth
of this aspect of peripheral sensation. Mechanoreceptors, however, can be tested by vibration.

Vibration is not a sensory entity and depends
on primary sensation of touch and rapid
changes in pressure. Normally the threshold
for perception is higher in the toes than in the
fingers. Reduced vibration sensation accompanies peripheral neuritis, diabetes mellitus,
and pernicious anaemia (Cosh, 1953) and hypersensitivity to vibration has been found in
hemi-Parkinsonism on the affected side in the
early stages of classical paralysis agitans, and

in postencephalitic and post-traumatic Parkinsonism (Gordon, 1945).

Vibrotactile sensation is dependent on two
types of receptor. Below 50 Hz these are
Meissner's corpuscles and others, and for frequencies above 50 Hz, Pacinian corpuscles –
but there may be a variety of receptors (Verrillo, 1980). At all ages the lowest thresholds
occur at approximately 200 to 250 Hz. The
palaesthesiometer (Corso, 1971; Lindblom,
1981) has a set frequency of 100 Hz and this,
although not the appropriate frequency for
measuring the lowest thresholds, fits the descending parts of the vibration perception logarithmic threshold curve which are parallel at
all ages (Fig. 3). The threshold for appreciation
of vibration increases with age in the frequency
range served by Pacinian corpuscles and is particularly marked as frequency of vibration increases after the nadir of the curve. There are
changes in number and structure of Pacinian
corpuscles with age (Cauna, 1964).

The threshold is increased in diabetics, being
equivalent to an age change of 20 years and
this is independent of the duration or severity
(Mirsky, Futterman, and Broh-Kahn, 1953;
Steinberg and Graber 1963). The threshold is
increased in the presence of peripheral arteriosclerosis, being equivalent to an age change
of 10 years. The threshold is also increased on
the hemiplegic side after a stroke, the upper
limb being more affected than the lower limb
(Zankel, 1969).

Vibration sensation is not lost with lesions
of the posterior columns but rather the ability
to carry out tasks involving simultaneous
analysis of spatial and temporal characteristics
of stimuli (Wall and Noordenbos, 1977).

THE EYES

Drooping of the upper lids is common in the
elderly; there is laxity of the levator palpebrae
and degeneration of supportive tissue. There
is also degeneration of the iris and a relative
parasympathetic preponderance. Thus senile
ptosis and miosis should not stimulate a search
for hidden disease unless other physical signs
are present.

Diminution of upward conjugage deviation
of the eyes, but not of downward deviation, is
age related in the absence of neurological disease (Chamberlain, 1970); by 70 years this

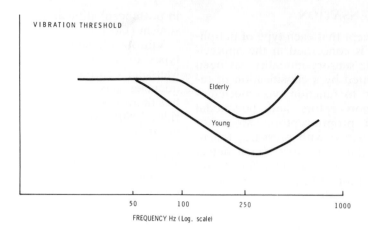

Figure 3   The vibration perception logarithmic threshold curve. (Adapted from Verrillo, 1980. Reproduced by permission of R. T. Verrillo)

movement is reduced in 50 per cent. of individuals. It may be due to muscle disuse since patients with kyphosis tend to have reasonably good upward conjugate deviation. Alone, it should not be considered to be significant.

Horner's Syndrome

This group of physical signs (Horner, 1869), complete or incomplete, is often present in other syndromes (Jaffe, 1951a, 1951b). Commonly considered to consist of ptosis, miosis, enophthalmos, and loss of sweating on the ipsilateral side of the face, it is often accompanied by increased facial temperature and tear secretion and occasionally cataract. The sympathetic tract for the dilator pupillae originates in the hypothalamus, passes caudally in the lateral tegmentum of the midbrain, pons, and medulla to the intermediolateral cell columns of C8, T1, and T2. The preganglionic fibres leave the cord at this level and pass via the anterior roots and white rami to the superior cervical ganglion. The postganglionic fibres pass along the common carotid artery to its bifurcation. Thence, the vasomotor and sudomotor fibres pass along the external carotid artery; the pupillodilator and fibres to nonstriated muscle in the upper lid pass along the internal carotid artery to join the first division of the trigeminal nerve (Fig. 4).

Thus lesions of the brainstem, cervical cord, nerve roots C8–T2, superior cervical ganglion, or common carotid artery may give rise to Horner's syndrome. Lesions distal to the carotid bifurcation will not produce loss of sweating. The degree of miosis is said to vary with site of the lesion, being maximal when C8 and T1 roots are involved – an accurate indication of completeness is failure of the pupil to dilate when cocaine is applied locally. If the postganglionic course is affected, i.e. peripheral to the superior cervical ganglion, adrenaline dilates the pupil markedly, but if the lesion is central to the superior cervical ganglion adrenaline has little or no effect. The dilator effect is due to increased receptor sensitivity following degeneration of the postganglionic fibres.

Unilateral Horner's syndrome can accompany:

(a) Wallenberg's lateral medullary syndrome – occlusion of the posterior-inferior cerebellar artery.
(b) Raedar's syndrome – pain in trigeminal territory and Horner's syndrome without sweating and usually due to lesions affecting the internal carotid artery fibres.
(c) Pancoast's syndrome – pain in shoulder and arm, wasting of small muscles of hand and Horner's syndrome – usually an apical carcinoma of lung.
(d) Payne's syndrome (Payne, 1981) – hoarse voice, ipsilateral diaphragmatic paralysis,

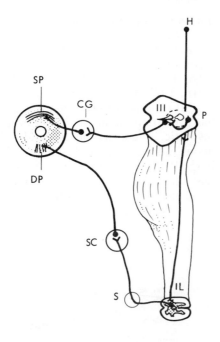

Figure 4   Autonomic control of the pupil

PARASYMPATHETIC
P- Pretectal nucleus
III- III Nerve nucleus
CG-Ciliary ganglion
SP- Sphincter pupillae

SYMPATHETIC
H- Hypothalamus
IL- Intermedio-lateral cell column
SC- Superior cervical ganglion
DP- Dilator pupillae
S - Sympathetic ganglion

shoulder pain, and Horner's syndrome, due to malignant disease related to the fifth cervical nerve root.
(e) Cervical spondylosis – often with root signs.

Unilateral Horner's syndrome alone is rarely of great significance and a search for a cause will probably only reveal cervical spondylosis.

Impaired Upward Conjugate Deviation

Parinaud's syndrome (Parinaud, 1883) is characterized by paralysis of conjugate upward deviation of the eyes but is often accompanied by diplopia, ptosis, nystagmus, and papilloedema. It may be due to a tumour of the pineal, cerebrovascular disease, and inflammation. The additional features and progression distinguish it from the age-related diminution in upward conjugate deviation. This physical sign is also found in the early stages of progressive supranuclear palsy but other signs point to the diagnosis.

Seventy-five per cent. of patients with Parkinson's disease have significant defect of eye movement, the commonest being deficient up-ward conjugate gaze. Apart from paralysis of upward conjugate deviation and a positive glabellar tap sign, patients with Parkinsonism may have infrequent blinking, blepharoclonus, blepharospasm, lid retraction, ptosis, poor convergence and accommodation, convergence spasm and nystagmus (Corin, Elizan, and Bender, 1972; Smith, 1966). In hydrocephalus there may be diminished upward conjugate deviation of the eyes with large sluggish pupils but this is uncommon in communicating hydrocephalus (Swash, 1976). Diminished upward conjugate deviation indicates a lesion in the posterior commissure or the pretectal region. It is not uncommon in the elderly with Alzheimer's disease and accompanying Parkinsonian signs, and occurs often with chronic subdural haematoma.

Glabella Reflex

Consideration should be given to the simple glabella reflex, the glabellar tap sign, and the more sophisticated analysis of both by electromyography (EMG).

Reflex blinking from tapping the forehead was first described by Walker Overend in 1896

(Overend, 1896). Wartenberg (1945) noted that the reflex could be evoked by light, sound, visual threat, and touching the palate.

Myerson (1944) found that repeated tapping on the glabella produced repeated reflex blinking in postencephalitic Parkinsonism, though not constant in arteriosclerotic and senile forms, the normal response being cessation of blinking after the first few taps – habituation. Garland (1952, 1955) considered that this positive response to repeated tapping, which he found in 79 per cent. of patients, was diagnostic of the Parkinsonian state. It has since been shown that this positive glabellar tap sign is

not as specific and occurs in Alzheimer's disease, cerebrovascular disease, other cerebral diseases, the neurologically normal, and with increasing age (Pearce, Aziz, and Gallagher, 1968; Pearce and Miller, 1973; Prakash and Stern, 1973; Wright and Boyd, 1964).

EMG studies showed that the glabella reflex has two components, an initial proprioceptive, myotatic, oligosynaptic R1 and a later cutaneous nociceptive, polysynaptic R2 (Kugelberg, 1952). R3 with a latency of 75 to 90 ms has been found in young subjects but is of small amplitude and duration. There is increasing evidence that R1 is also cutaneous; the

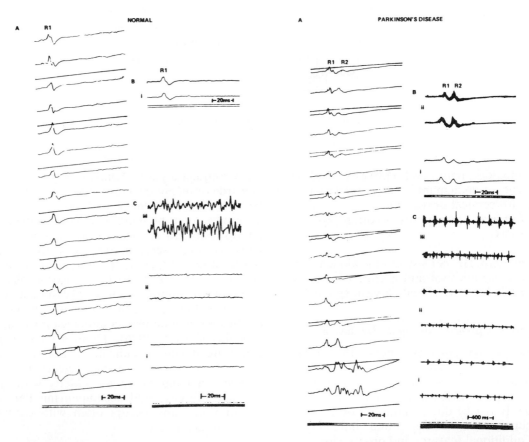

Figure 5   EMG recordings from orbicularis oculi (right above left throughout)
A   Series of responses (1, 3, 5, 7, etc., from bottom) to tapping of glabella
Bi   Average of 16 responses, from A
  ii   Superimposition of 16 responses
Ci   Eyes open
  ii   Eyes lightly closed
  iii Eyes firmly closed
The EMG recording of a normal patient shows rapid habituation of R2. In Parkinson's disease R2 does not habituate. The EMG recording C shows blepharoclonus of 4.5 to 6.5 per second in the patient with Parkinson's disease

Jendrassik manoeuvre has no effect on the amplitude of R1 and vibration does not invoke a tonic response or reduce R1 amplitude as it does in the H reflex. There is no Renshaw recurrent inhibition of R1. This indicates that the motoneuron pool is devoid of a gamma system (Penders and Delwaide, 1973; Shahani and Young, 1973). Blinking, itself, corresponds to the R2. If elicited by tapping the glabella, both components are present; if elicited by electrical stimulation of the supraorbital nerve, R1 is not present in the recording on the opposite (contralateral) side. Habituation of the glabellar tap sign is manifested by progressive diminution of R2 and increased latency (Fig. 5) and is dependent on the strength and rate of presentation of the stimulus (Thompson and Spencer, 1966). Normally the R2 habituates after 2 or 3 taps on the glabella and is a quasi-purposeful reaction to a stimulus which on repetition has proved to be innocuous. The cerebral cortex is concerned in habituation. Fear, stress, and distraction reduce habituation but concentration on the manoeuvre itself increases habituation (Boelhouwer and Brunia, 1977; Gregoric, 1973; Penders and Delwaide, 1973). R1 and R2 are reduced during sleep (Ferrari and Messina, 1972). In coma R2 decreases and may disappear completely (Kimura, 1973; Lyon, Kimura, and McCormick, 1972). Thus cortical activation increases R1 and R2 and cortical depression diminishes them; but it is probable that this is mediated via an inhibitory mechanism in the midbrain reticular formation.

Trigeminal rhizotomy abolishes both responses. Trigeminal tractotomy modifies the R2 response (Kugelberg, 1952) (Fig. 6). The R2 is delayed in Wallenberg's lateral medullary syndrome (Kimura and Lyon, 1972), multiple sclerosis with pontine signs (Kimura, 1970), and internuclear ophthalmoplegia (Namerow and Etemadi, 1970). In hemiparesis on the affected side the R2 is small, of long duration, and rapidly habituates (Dehen *et al.*, 1976; Rushworth, 1962). R1 is variable, sometimes of larger amplitude, though often reduced in amplitude.

As elicited clinically the gabella tap reflex in peripheral facial palsy shows diminution of response on the affected side but may be exaggerated if the lesion is central (Wartenberg, 1945). Patients with Bell's palsy show in-

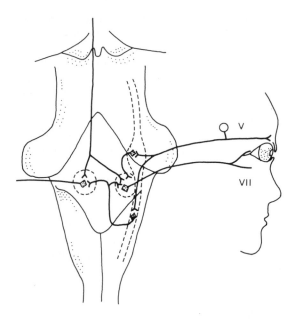

Figure 6   Pathways for glabella reflex

creased latency of R1, particularly, and R2. R1 is absent in the early stages of Bell's palsy; if R2 is detectable in the early stages prognosis is good (Schenck and Manz, 1973).

The corneal reflex is not altered with age; it is abolished or has increased latency if there is brain stem damage (Magladery and Teasdall, 1961). The corneal reflex EMG shows a bilateral R2 response but no R1 (Rushworth, 1962).

In Parkinson's disease, the latency of R2 is shorter, the amplitude is increased, and habituation does not occur (Kimura, 1973; Rushworth, 1962). The pattern is similar in senile chorea and tardive dyskinesia (Ferguson, Lenman, and Johnston, 1978). In the treatment of Parkinsonism, habituation of R2 is increased, i.e. a return to normal, by levodopa and amantadine but not by anticholinergic drugs (Klawans and Goodwin, 1969; Messina, Di Rosa, and Tomasello, 1972; Penders and Delwaide, 1971).Chlorpromazine produces the same changes as are found in Parkinson's disease (Rushworth, 1962). Diazepam reduces the R2 response (Kimura, 1973). The R2 response differs from normal and Parkinson's disease in patients with Huntington's chorea. The amplitude and duration are decreased, latency is increased, and habituation is rapid (Estaban and Giménez-Roldán, 1975). This is the opposite of Parkinson's disease and possibly reflects the increased concentration of dopamine in the basal ganglia in Huntington's chorea (Bird and Iversen, 1974). Treatment of Parkinson's disease with levodopa produces the same effects and, of course, choreic movements are an indication of toxic effects.

The EMG responses of the glabellar tap sign in Parkinsonism and hemiplegia would suggest that if cortical and basal ganglia disease were present, a variety, ranging between the two, might be found. This would obviously influence the clinical response to repeated tapping on the glabella and should be taken into account when interpreting negative results in patients with Parkinsonism as they may well have cerebral disease as well.

LOCALIZATION

Corneomandibular Reflex

Although somewhat neglected, this sign is indicative of supranuclear trigeminal disorder (Wartenberg, 1948). The elicitation of the corneal reflex is accompanied by movement of the jaw to the opposite side. It is found bilaterally in dementia and old age (Paulson and Gottlieb 1968), amyotrophic lateral sclerosis, état lacunaire, and on the hemiplegic side of patients after strokes.

Perseveration

The inappropriate repetition of movement or speech is often associated with aphasia, even after recovery, but it can occur when a patient is fatigued. It is considered to be due to lesions of the dominant parietal and inferior temporal lobes. It may interfere with communication to an extent that the patient may be considered to be demented. It also occurs with diffuse brain disease but even in this context may be considered to have localizing characteristics. Continued observation of the patient during examination will often reveal it. Specific testing can be simply made by asking the patient to close his eyes and then open them; if then asked to put out his tongue he will close his eyes again (Allison, 1966; Allison and Hurwitz, 1967).

Impersistence

The inability to maintain a motor act is often seen in diffuse brain disease but occurs characteristically with lesions of the non-dominant parietal lobe. It can be elicited by asking the patient to protrude his tongue or to look to one side; although able to complete the act the patient is unable to maintain the position even if repeatedly urged to do so. (Ben-Yishay *et al.*, 1968; Fisher, 1956).

Grasp Reflex

The grasp reflex is elicited by firm pressure with the testing fingers across the palm from the ulnar to the radial side. The fingers clasp but the thumb is often extended; once elicited, increased stimulus increases the response. It has two components; the first is tactile and the second is proprioceptive.

Medial frontal lobe lesions facilitate the tactile response which triggers the proprioceptive response, representing release of a more primitive subcortical mechanism. If the lateral aspect of the parietal lobe is damaged then a light stimulus will lead to extension of the fingers and withdrawal of the hand. Apart from cortical lesions, these reactions can be produced by lesions of the basal ganglia and represent, respectively, exploratory and evading reactions (Denny-Brown, 1962).

Clinically a unilateral grasp reflex indicates a lesion in the contralateral frontal cortex.

PARKINSONISM AND DEMENTIA IN DEGENERATIVE NEUROLOGICAL DISEASE

Akinesia rigidity syndromes other than Parkinson's disease do not usually have marked visible tremor of the Parkinsonian type of 5 to 7 per second. Some of these conditions terminate with problems of communication due to anarthria and aphonia and possibly secondary dementia. This must be distinguished from Alzheimer's disease with Parkinsonian features.

Other degenerative conditions have an affinity, both clinical and pathological, to the akinesia rigidity diseases and are included in this description for convenience:

(a) Multiple system atrophy

Olivo-ponto-cerebellar atrophy
Striato-nigral degeneration
(b) Progressive supranuclear palsy
(c) Cerebellar cortical degeneration
(d) Familial spastic paraplegia
(e) Motor neuron disease
(See Table 1)

Multiple System Atrophy

Historically, olivo-ponto-cerebellar atrophy (OPCA) and striato-nigral degeneration (SND) are separate diseases, but common clinical signs and pathological changes often associated with the Shy–Drager syndrome (Shy, and Drager, 1960) have promoted a concept of multiple system atrophy (MSA) (Graham, and Oppenheimer, 1969; Spokés, Bannister, and Oppenheimer, 1979) which has merit in including not only classical presentation of these conditions but also mixed forms often presenting atypically.

Pathologically these conditions are 'degenerative' because they are of unknown aetiology and because such a description is convenient until a common primary disease process is identified. In this context they have similarities with other conditions which present as Parkinsonian syndromes or terminate with dementia and paraplegia in flexion. The pathological lesions are cell loss and gliosis but the Lewy bodies characteristic of Parkinson's disease (PD) are not found.

Olivo-Ponto-Cerebellar Atrophy

Familial cases of the Menzel type (Menzel, 1891, which can be classified into familial, dominant, and recessive groups (Konigsmark and Weiner, 1970), are unlikely to occur in the elderly; the Dejerine–Thomas type (Dejerine, and Thomas, 1900) is rare but may be easily misdiagnosed until identified at post-mortem examination.

Macroscopically there is atrophy of the cerebellar cortex, middle cerebellar peduncles, partial atrophy of the inferior cerebellar peduncles, atrophy of the ventral aspect of the pons and of the olives. Microscopically there is loss of neurons in the pons and olives and there is loss of Purkinje cells and basket cells in the cerebellar cortex. There is fibrillary astrocytosis in the regions of cell loss; the cerebellar white matter is demyelinated and this

extends back to the middle and inferior cerebellar peduncles.

The basal ganglia and thalamus are also involved in neuronal loss and gliosis. The substantia nigra often shows cell loss, neuronophagia, and pigment incontinence as in PD, but no Lewy bodies which are the hallmark of PD. In the cerebral cortex some cases show hyaline vacuolar degeneration and gliosis of the prefrontal and temporal neocortex but usually the cerebral cortex is spared. There is sometimes degeneration in the posterior columns and spinocerebellar tracts in the spinal chord.

Clinically OPCA starts with disturbance of gait and balance. The gait is characteristic of cerebellar disease, being broad-based with a tendency to fall when turning; later it may become a Parkinsonian marche à petit pas. In the early stages falls occur but vertigo is rare. Upper limb ataxia begins later when intention tremor and dysdiadokokinesia can be demonstrated. There is progressive deterioration of handwriting. Slow scanning speech may present early in the disease but as Parkinsonian features develop the speech may be slow. The eyes may become prominent and fixed and nystagmus may be present in about half of the cases. As the disease progresses, cerebellar hypotonia is replaced by extra pyramidal rigidity and mask-like facies is evident. A tremor of head and limbs similar to benign essential tremor may be present in the early stages but later the characteristic resting tremor of PD may appear. Extra pyramidal manifestations usually manifest themselves within 5 years of the onset of the disease. Pyramidal tract signs sometimes occur in the late stages and the plantar responses may become extensor. Intellectual deterioration is a late change but incontinence of urine may present early in the disease (Critchley, and Greenfield, 1948; Dejerine, and Thomas, 1900; Eadie, 1975c).

Striato-Nigral Degeneration

In 1961 a disease entity similar to PD was described (Adams, van Bogaert, and van der Eecken, 1961, 1964). Pathologically there is a degeneration of the caudate nucleus, putamen, globus pallidus, and substantia nigra with macroscopic shrinking and change of colour.

There is neuronal loss which is severe in the putamen but also present in the caudate nucleus and substantia nigra with a replacement fibrillary astrocytosis; shrinkage of the globus pallidus is due to loss of striato-pallidal fibres. No Lewy bodies are found in the substantia nigra and the changes are essentially those of OPCA. There are no senile plaques in the cerebral cortex.

Clinically the predominant signs are gradually developing rigidity and bradykinesia with Parkinsonian tremor in some cases. It affects one side of the body first but when both sides are affected, as the disease progresses, bulbar signs appear; there is difficulty in chewing and swallowing and speech becomes flat, weak, and hesitant. The face, posture, and gait are Parkinsonian. Micrographia and loss of associated movements occurs. Intellectual deterioration and depression occur but are not really different from PD (Adams, 1968).

Shy–Drager Syndrome

This syndrome of progressive autonomic failure comprises orthostatic hypotension, atonic bladder, urinary and rectal incontinence, decreased sweating and impotence, and Parkinsonism. Many patients suffer from transient ischaemic attacks due to postural hypotension which is made worse with levodopa, and progressive ataxia. Pathological studies have shown that these patients have PD with Lewy bodies, or SND and/or OPCA. Clinically the patients who have Lewy body disease may show very little indication of clinical PD (Bannister, and Oppenheimer, 1982; Oppenheimer, 1980; Spokes, Bannister, and Oppenheimer, 1979). The cause of the autonomic failure has been identified as a loss of cells in the intermediolateral cell column of the spinal cord (Bannister, and Oppenheimer, 1972; Graham, and Oppenheimer, 1969; Johnson *et al.*, 1966). Sphincter disturbances are due to lesions of Onuf's nucleus (Onufrowicz, 1900; Sung, Mastri, and Segal, 1979), a group of cells in the sacral intermediolateral cell column.

Progressive Supranuclear Palsy

The neuropathology and clinical features of progressive supranuclear palsy (PSP) were first identified as a diagnostic entity by Steele, Ri-

chardson, and Olzewski in 1964. Similar cases had been reported before this (Alajouanine, Delafontaine, and Lacan, 1926; Chavany, van Bogaert, and Godlewski, 1951; Cornil, and Kissel, 1929; Posey, 1904; Verhaart, 1958). Before 1964 there were probably other patients with PSP who were classified as atypical Parkinsonism, presenile dementia, or arteriopathic degeneration (Steele, 1972), and since 1964 many cases have been reported (Dalziel, and Griffiths, 1977).

Macroscopically the brain may show little evidence of the disease apart from some pallor and slight shrinkage of the structures affected. Microscopically there is loss of neurones, myelinated fibres, and astrocytic gliosis. Affected neurons contain neurofibrillary tangles but these are different morphologically from those of Alzheimer's disease (Powell, London, and Lampert, 1974). The brainstem and cerebellum are involved, particularly the substantia nigra, the globus pallidus, the subthalamic nuclei, the dentate nuclei, the reticular formation of the midbrain, and the pretectal region. This has been termed 'heterogeneous system degeneration of the central nervous system' (Verhaart, 1958) and has some of the characteristics of MSA.

The disease occurs sporadically and sex distribution is equal (Dix, Harrison, and Lewis, 1971); the onset is insidious and usually starts in the sixth decade. It is progressive with death occurring on an average within 6 years. PSP usually presents with a disturbance of gait, unsteadiness, and frequent falls. In 40 per cent. visual disturbance is the first complaint and because disturbance of upward conjugate deviation does not present too much disability the presenting symptom is an inability to look downwards. Pseudo-bulbar symptoms may present early including dysphagia, dysarthria, and emotional lability.

The classical condition as originally described (Steele, Richardon, and Olszewski, 1964) is quite distinct from Parkinson's disease but some subsequent reports have included cases with more prominent Parkinsonian features and it has been suggested that there is a spectrum between the two diseases (Corin, Elizan, and Bender, 1972). However, pathologically Parkinson's disease is characterized by Lewy bodies in the substantia nigra, which is not the case in PSP.

The characteristic feature of PSP is supranuclear ophthalmoplegia. There is defective vertical conjugate gaze initially with, later, involvement of lateral gaze and/or convergence. Doll's head eye movements are usually preserved (Bielschowsky, 1935). Often patients are unaware of their inability to look downwards but complain of vague visual disturbance (Messert, and van Nuis, 1966). Occular motor dysfunction is not specific to PSP and has been reported in as many as 75 per cent. of patients with PD, although it is less marked than in the former (Corin, Elizan, and Bender, 1972). Doll's head eye movements depend on pursuit, fixation, vestibular and neck reflexes, and may be lost in severe cases of PSP. This is not strictly a supranuclear manifestation but is indicative of more widespread involvement. Disturbances of conjugate deviation are not usually accompanied by any complaint of diplopia and are considered to be due to lesions in the pretectal region. More extensive involvement, including nuclear ophthalmoplegia (Blumenthal, and Miller, 1969; Ishino *et al.*, 1974) and internuclear ophthalmoplegia (Mastaglia, and Grainger, 1975), can occur, when diplopia may well be a symptom. Ptosis and retraction of the upper lids may be present (Behrman *et al.*, 1969).

Characteristically there is a dystonic rigidity of the neck and upper trunk, but this may not occur until the later stages of the disease. This axial rigidity is prominent in the early stages and later spreads to involve the limbs.

Pseudo-bulbar signs always develop. Dysarthria and dysphagia accompanied by generalized rigidity lead to an increased risk of aspiration pneumonia which is the most frequent cause of death. The jaw and facial reflexes are usually increased and the facies is deeply furrowed and spastic.

Dementia is said to be the presenting complaint in 33 per cent. of cases (Dix, Harrison, and Lewis, 1971) but is usually not severe. This dementia has been considered to be of 'subcortical' type (Albert, Feldman, and Willis, 1974) and is characterized by forgetfulness, slowing of thought processes, emotional or personality changes, and impaired ability to manipulate acquired knowledge. Dementia, however, should not be diagnosed purely because the patient is unable to communicate and some patients retain reasonable mentation un-

til late in the disease (Dalziel, and Griffiths, 1977).

There are several negative features which assist in the differential diagnosis from PD; tremor is not usually present, associated arm movements during walking are preserved, and the posture usually remains erect until the rigidity becomes severe.

Levodopa has been used in the management of these patients with varying, but usually limited, success (De Renzi, and Vignolo, 1969; Gilbert, and Feldman, 1969; Gross, 1969; Jenkins, 1969; Klawans, 1969; Mastaglia *et al.*, 1973; Sacks, 1969; Wagshul, and Daroff, 1969). There is usually some improvement in rigidity and general mobility but very little improvement in eye movements.

Cerebellar Cortical Degeneration

In the elderly these conditions can be familial (Holmes, 1907) or sporadic (Marie, Foix, and Alajouanine, 1922) or acquired. Clinically they present as pure cerebellar diseases with ataxia and, later, intention tremor but the final stages, when patients are confined to bed, may present a difficulty in diagnosis and inability to communicate may produce an erroneous diagnosis of dementia.

Familial cases were originally described by Holmes (1907) as cerebello-olivary atrophy. The disease always involves the cerebellar cortex with secondary changes in the olives; many families have been described and the pathology and clinical picture reviewed (Eadie, 1975b; Greenfield, 1954). Although considered to be an autosomal dominant inheritance there have been sibships without affected parents and in one family heterozygous females were affected more severely than males (Richter, 1950). Overall the sexes are affected equally.

The disease usually starts in the fifth decade and lasts from 10 to 25 years. Gait is usually affected first, being broad-based and staggering, with a tendency to fall, indicating bilateral cerebellar disease. Ataxia later extends to the arms with intention tremor, dysdiadokokinesia and hypotonia. Dysarthria is cerebellar in type — scanning, slurred, and sometimes explosive. Occasionally nodding tremor of the head and nystagmus develop. Dementia and incontinence are said to occur in the later stages of the disease. Occasionally pyramidal and Parkinsonian features are present, particularly in the later stages when the patient is confined to bed.

Macroscopically the paleocerebellum is affected with atrophy, particularly, of the vermis and superior folia. Microscopically there is always degeneration and loss of Purkinje cells and often loss of cells in the inferior olives which have olivo-cerebellar projections to the primarily affected Purkinje cells. Purkinje cell axons and olivary cell axons are lost, with demyelination, in the cerebellar white matter and inferior cerebellar peduncles, respectively. A fibrillary astrocytosis is often present. In some cases, neurofibrillary changes or senile plaques have been described in the cerebral cortex but it must be remembered that these may also be due to the age of patients and/or concomitant Alzheimer's disease.

Sporadic cases are essentially the same as familial cases, differing only in that a family history cannot be obtained.

Acquired cerebellar cortical degeneration may be due to alcoholism, remote malignancy, hypothyroidism, or toxins such as heavy metals or anticonvulsants.

Cerebellar degeneration due to alcoholism was described clinically and pathologically by André-Thomas (1905). The problem has been reviewed by Mancall (1975) and is probably increasing in frequency. Certainly it is the commonest cause of acquired cerebellar degeneration. Males are affected more than females in a ratio of 10:1. Peak incidence is in the fifth decade. Associated Wernicke–Korsakoff syndrome, polyneuropathy, amblyopia, and loss of body weight are common and hepatic cirrhosis is inevitable. Macroscopically the superior vermis and the antero-superior folia of the cerebellar hemisphere are somewhat shrunken. Microscopically, Purkinje cells, molecular layer cells, and granule cells are lost. There is a fibrillary astrocytosis in the areas affected. Similar changes in the deep cerebellar nuclei are probably secondary. Secondary involvement of the inferior olives occurs. A cerebellar gait is the usual presenting problem, followed by cerebellar ataxia of upper limbs and slurring of speech. The progress of the disease is rapid and usually plateaus out within a year.

Cerebellar degeneration due to remote malignancy is considered elsewhere (page 641). It usually affects all four limbs and trunk equally and may remit with treatment of the primary carcinoma.

Cerebellar disease and its relationship to hypothyroidism was conclusively defined in 1960 (Jellinek, and Kelly, 1960). The pathology was described by Price, and Netsky (1966) but post-mortem examination results are scanty. There is moderate loss of Purkinje cells, particularly in the vermis. Microglial proliferation is present and glycogen-containing bodies termed myxoedema bodies are present.

Cerebellar signs have been described in lead, manganese, and mercurial poisoning. Organic industrial solvents can also be implicated. Reversible cerebellar ataxia is produced by a variety of drugs — nitrazepam, glutethimide, 5-fluorourcil and diphenylhydantoin (phenytoin).

It is important for any patient presenting with cerebellar signs to eliminate any remediable causes. It is said that half of the cases of clinical cerebellar cortical atrophy are associated with malignancy, but the malignant process may not be identified until post-mortem.

Familial Spastic Paraplegia

Strümpell (1880, 1886, 1904), described familial spastic paraplegia (FSP) with spasticity confined to the legs in patients in middle age, one of whom lived to be 69 years old. Since then, various family types have been described. Essentially there is degeneration of the corticospinal tracts and, to a lesser extent, the posterior columns and sometimes the spinocerebellar tracts. There is sometimes loss of Betz cells in the cerebral cortex and motor neurons in the anterior horns of the spinal cord. Microscopically there is loss of fibres, demyelination, and fibrilliary astrocyiosis. The degeneration of the corticospinal tract is caudal to the medullary decussation, and degeneration of the posterior columns is greater in the fasciculus gracilis.

There are pure forms of the familial disease but other families have been described (Sutherland, 1975) with impaired mentation, epilepsy, optic atrophy, extrapyramidal manifestations, ataxia, amyotrophy, muscle dystrophy, and cardiac abnormalities.

Clinically, in adults, there is gradually increasing spasticity, loss of vibration sensation, and later position sense in the legs. Deterioration is usually gradual for 10 years and then the condition tends to plateau. With the spasticity there is relatively little loss of power, knee and ankle reflexes are increased, and the plantar responses are extensor.

Sanger Brown (1892) described a family affected with spasticity of the legs and cerebellar ataxia of the arms. This condition of hereditary spastic ataxia (HSA) provides a link between FSP, OPCA, and Friedreich's ataxia (Eadie, 1975a), but very few patients survived to old age.

Motor Neurone Disease

The three types of motor neurone disease (MND) generally accepted are:

(a) Amyotrophic lateral sclerosis (ALS) (Charcot and Joffroy, 1868), characterized by degeneration of the anterior horn cells and pyramidal tracts, weakness, exaggerated reflexes and extensor plantar responses, and pseudo-bulbar palsy.

(b) Spinal motor neurone disease (SMND) (Aran, 1850; Cruveilhier, 1853, Duchenne, 1853) characterized by degeneration of anterior horn cells in the spinal cord, weakness, wasting and fasciculation of muscles, loss of reflexes.

(c) Progressive bulbar palsy (PBP) (Duchenne, 1860), characterized by degeneration of 'anterior horn' cells in the medulla, weakness and wasting of the tongue, facial muscles, palatal and laryngeal muscles, fasciculation of tongue.

Since the original descriptions of the disease and that of Gowers (1892b) only moderate advances have been made in understanding the aetiology of the disease and no treatment has been shown to improve the prognosis. The literature, including historical backgrounds to the eponymous classifications, was reviewed in 1975 (Bonduelle, 1975; Colmant, 1975; Norris, 1975), and the complicated nosology was reviewed and summarized (Hudson, 1981; Kurtzke, 1982) particularly with reference to conditions such as Guam disease and autosomal dominant inheritance in some families.

MND is not transmissible to rhesus monkeys (Gibbs, and Gajdusek, 1968). Neurotoxins; substituted fluoropyrimidines and actinomycin D (Koenig, 1968), organophosphorus and organomercuric compounds, and isoniazid (Cavanagh, 1968) produce a comparative pathological condition in experimental animals. Histochemical studies have not shown any specific biochemical abnormality except 'progressive inhibition of DNA directed mRNA synthesis in affected neurons' (Mann, and Yates, 1974) which indicated the primary site of action of any pathogen.

In the Guam type of ALS it is possible that lathyrism due to cycadin from the nut *Cycas circinalis* is the cause of what has been thought to be a familial form of ALS associated with a Parkinsonian dementia syndrome. This arouses speculation that sporadic forms may be due to azoxy or nitrosamine-like agents (Kurland, 1977).

Macroscopically there is shrinkage of the corticospinal tracts, anterior nerve roots, and muscles. Occasionally shrinkage of the precentral gyri can be observed. Microscopically there is degeneration and loss of Betz cells and anterior horn cells, loss of fibres and demyelination in the pyramidal tracts, and sometimes, to a lesser extent, degeneration of spinocerebellar tracts. These changes are accompanied by fibrillary astrocytosis. The XII nerve nuclei are nearly always involved and, to a lesser and variable extent, motor nuclei of XI, X, IX, VII, and V nerves. Although VI, IV, and III motor nuclei are usually spared, degenerative changes were noted by Mann and Yates (Mann, and Yates, 1974), particularly loss of RNA from the III nerve motor neurones. The pyramidal tracts are particularly affected in the posterior part of the internal capsule, the middle third of the cerebral peduncles, pyramids, and corticospinal tracts. The pyramidal tract degeneration is more severe at lower levels (Brownell, Oppenheimer, and Hughes, 1970; Davison, 1941) and may be a transneuronal degeneration (Bertrand, and von Bogaert, 1925). MND has been considered as 'part of the spectrum of a particular type of multiple system atrophy analagous to olivo-ponto-cerebellar atrophy' (Brownell, Oppenheimer, and Hughes, 1970). There is loss of motor fibres and demyelination in the anterior nerve roots and peripheral nerves with neurogenic atrophy of muscles, i.e. groups of atrophic fibres with large numbers of marginal nuclei alongside groups of normal or slightly enlarged fibres. From muscle biopsy studies there is evidence of collateral innervation in cases with ALS but not SMND (Butler *et al.*, 1977), and this, combined with muscle fibre hypertrophy, appears to correlate with a better prognosis.

The disease is distributed uniformly throughout the world, males being affected more than females in a ratio of 3:2. Incidence and mortality rate are somewhat greater than 1 per 100,000 and the prevalence is somewhat less than 5 per 100,000. Mean age of survival is 3 to 4 years. Injury and operation in the 5 years before the onset of symptoms has been found to have some significance (Kurtzke, 1982). The mean age of onset, from the onset of motor symptoms, is in the fifth decade.

Clinically amyotrophy affects the thenar eminence first and spreads centripetally in the arms and shoulders. The legs are affected later. Fasciculation of muscle may precede weakness and atrophy. Cramps, which may be the presenting symptom, disappear as muscular atrophy increases. Pyramidal signs are not consistent although pyramidal tracts are affected post-mortem. The presence of increased tendon reflexes accompanying muscle wasting is of diagnostic value. Extensor plantar reflexes and increased tendon reflexes are found particularly in the lower limbs but the plantar reflexes are often flexor. Progressive bulbar symptoms and signs are prognostic and are the presage of death due to inhalation pneumonia. Apart from PBP, pseudo-bulbar palsy may be present, indicated by increased jaw-jerk and a corneomandibular reflex (Gordon and Bender, 1971), and if pseudo-bulbar palsy presents then it is often overtaken by bulbar palsy as the disease progresses. Bulbar signs, both lower motor neurone and upper motor neurone in type, can often be found before bulbar symptoms develop and should always be sought.

There is a pseudo-polyneuritic form of MND which is characterized by paresis, initially of the dorsi-flexors of the foot, and a steppage gait. As the disease advances there is paralysis and wasting of leg muscles, particularly the antero-lateral group, and progressive loss of ankle and knee jerks. Pyramidal signs are concealed by the amyotrophy. This may be confused with the cauda equina syndrome but there is no sensory loss.

In elderly patients there may be a slight pallor of the posterior columns and a faint spinal halo which may be responsible for some of the abnormal pathological findings which have been described in some cases. This, and peripheral neuropathy, would account for some symptoms and signs which have been considered to be variants of the disease. Dementia and Parkinsonism are characteristics of Alzheimer's disease which may also affect some patients and must be differentiated from syndromes including these conditions. Myasthenic syndromes have been described with some response to prostigmine (Mulder, Lambert, and Eaton, 1959). Atrophy of small muscles of the hands occurs in the elderly (Lhermitte, and Nicolas, 1925; Marie, and Foix, 1912) but does not usually cause any difficulty in diagnosis.

ALS, dementia, and Parkinsonism constitute a complex of disease presentations which show neuronal loss, degeneration of the substantia nigra without Lewy bodies, and astrocytic gliosis. They are different from Alzheimer's disease, Creutzfeldt–Jakob disease, and Pick's disease, and Bonduelle (1975) considers these to be extensions of ALS and favours a genetic origin of these diseases. Familial types of ALS occur about a decade earlier than sporadic cases and have a dominant inheritance (Kurland and Mulder, 1955). Encephalomyelitis due to remote carcinoma can produce an MND syndrome (p. 651).

Cervical myelopathy due to spinal arterial lesions can imitate ALS but sensory changes will be found and the XII nerve nucleus is not affected. Aetiologically arteriosclerosis has been thought to have an association with amyotrophic lateral sclerosis but this is probably coincidental. The territory supplied by the anterior spinal artery supplies the anterior horns and the ventral and lateral tracts (Gillilan, 1958) and is particularly susceptible to arteriosclerosis (Jellinger, 1967), but progressive generalized amyotrophy is uncommon (Wells, 1966) and, since spinothalamic tracts are also involved, sensory deficits can be detected (Zeitlin, and Lichtenstein, 1936). Aortic disease can present as progressive MND (Hughes, and Brownell, 1966).

Electromyography produces changes which are a consequence of denervation and generation of collaterals from surviving motor neurons. Fasciculation (motor unit) and fibrillation (motor fibre) potentials are found. Fasciculation indicates motor unit discharges, which are no more variable in shape in MND muscle than in normal muscle although the interval between them is larger in MND. Fibrillation potentials are observed more frequently in weaker muscles. Collateral regeneration produces a larger motor unit potential and as the disease progresses these become wider.

Clinical signs and neuropathological lesions in degenerative neurological diseases are summarized in Table 1.

NORMAL PRESSURE HYDROCEPHALUS

This was first defined as a clinical condition amenable to treatment in 1965 (Adams *et al.*, 1965; Hakim, and Adams, 1965). Normal pressure hydrocephalus (NPH) comprises a syndrome of dementia with gait disturbance and urinary incontinence associated with ventricular dilatation of the brain and a cerebrospinal fluid (CSF) pressure of less than 200 mm of CSF; up-to-date reviews of this condition are available (Briggs, 1978; Katzman, 1977; Ojemann, 1972).

Five per cent. of patients admitted to hospital with dementia have NPH with a maximum incidence at 55 to 65 years. There are, therefore, few cases among the elderly demented but it has been surmised that this may be due to inadequate diagnosis. In about

Table 1   Clinical signs and neuropathological lesions

	MSA		PSP	CCD	FSP	MND
	OPCA	SND				
Clinical						
Limb ataxia	+	0	0	+	0	0
Hyperreflexia	±F	0	±	±	+	+
Extensor plantars	±F	0	±	0	+	+
Extrapyramidal signs	+	+	+	±	∓	∓F
Optic Atrophy	∓F	0	0	0	∓	0
Nystagmus	+F	0	0	±	0	0
Paralysis of vertical gaze	∓	∓	+	0	∓	0
Pathology						
Cerebral cortex	∓	∓	∓	∓	∓	±F
Basal ganglia	±	+	+	0	0	∓F
Substantia nigra	+	+	+	0	∓	∓F
Cerebellar cortex	+	∓	∓	+	∓	0
Cerebellar nuclei	+	∓	+	±	0	0
Olives	+	∓	0	+	0	0
Nuclei pontis	+	∓	±	0	0	0
Posterior columns	±F	?	?	0	+	∓F
Spinocerebellar tracts	±F	?	?	0	∓	±
Corticospinal tracts	±F	?	?	0	+	+
Anterior horn cells	±	?	∓	0	∓	+
Intermediolateral cell column	±	+	?	?	?	?

MSA	Multiple system atrophy	+	Common
OPCA	Olivo-ponto-cerebellar atrophy	± or ∓	Occasional
SND	Striato-nigral degeneration	0	Absent
PSP	Progressive supranuclear palsy	?	Not known
CCD	Cerebellar cortical degeneration	F	Familial (usually)
FSP	Familial spastic paraplegia		
MND	Motor neuron disease		

one-third of patients there is no precipitating cause, but the cause is identifiable in others:

Subarachnoid haemorrhage (Folz, and Ward, 1956)

Meningitis (Hill, Lougheed, and Barnett, 1967)

Trauma (Bannister, Gilford, and Kocen, 1967)

Tumour (Adams *et al.*, 1965)

Aqueduct stenosis (LeMay, and New, 1970)

Ectasia of the basilar artery (Ekbom, Greitz, and Kugelberg, 1969)

Paget's disease (Dohrmann, and Elrick, 1982; Friedman, Slaver, and Klawans, 1971)

In most cases there is scarring in the subarachnoid space, basal cisterns, and supratentorial space, in cases following subarachnoid haemorrhage, meningitis, and trauma, and in idiopathic cases. Degeneration of the arachnoid granulations and fibrosis occurs in the elderly and has been thought to account for some ventricular dilatation in old age (Wolf, 1959).

Symptoms and Signs

Mental Changes

Mental changes usually appear first and consist of apathy and mild short-term memory impairment, paranoia, delirium, and inappropriate laughing and crying. In the early stages these mental changes may fluctuate from day to day (Adams, 1966). Impairment of the ability to calculate may be an early problem but dysphasia develops later, progressing gradually to asemia as a state of akinetic mutisum develops. Dysarthria is rare but the speech may become slow and quiet.

Disturbance of Gait

Disturbance of gait usually develops after the onset of mental symptoms. It is a spastic ataxia, often with difficulty in initiating movement (i.e. an apraxia of gait; see Messert, and Baker, 1966) which is associated with a tonic foot (grasp) reflex (Botez *et al.*, 1975). Sometimes the gait is marche à petit pas. Reflexes in the legs are increased and the plantar reflexes eventually become extensor. Parkinson-

ian features, rigidity, bradykinesia, and tremor sometimes occur (Jakobs *et al.*, 1976) and present some difficulty in diagnosis. It has been suggested that the spastic paraplegia is due to the fact that the corticospinal fibres subserving leg movements pass over the lateral ventricle and are thus susceptible to damage due to dilatation, while face and arm corticospinal fibres are separated from the lateral ventricle and protected by the caudate nucleus (Yakovlev, 1947). Parkinsonian features are often found in the early stages of Alzheimer's disease and have been considered to be due to frontal lobe lesions (Sjögren, 1952), although Parkinsonism developing later in Alzheimer's disease is due to damage to the basal ganglia. In the later stages of NPH grasp reflexes and other primitive reflexes can be demonstrated.

The spastic paraparesis may resemble the myelopathy due to cervical spondylosis and present some difficulty in differential diagnosis (Fischer, 1977).

Urinary Incontinence

Urinary incontinence is usually the last of the triad of clinical features to develop. Characteristically it does not worry the patient or cause any concern. It is considered to be an 'anosognosia of micturition' (Adams, 1975) and in this context patients with lesions of the frontal lobe lose control of micturition (Andrew and Nathan, 1964).

CSF Pressure

The basic concept of CSF circulation was developed by Dandy (Dandy, 1919; Dandy, and Blackfan, 1913), but questions of detail still remain (Davson, 1967; Davson, Hollingsworth, and Segal, 1970), particularly in the case of hydrocephalus (Milhorat, 1972).

CSF is secreted into the ventricles from the choroid plexuses. Production of CSF is reduced by acetazolamide and is aided by arterial pulsation in the choroid plexuses. Some element of filtration occurs since large molecules do not enter the CSF. The vascular endothelium forms this blood–CSF barrier. The fluid passes out of the ventricles via the foramina of Lushka and Magendie into the subarachnoid space and is then absorbed into the venous system via the arachnoid villi because the hydrostatic pressure of the CSF is higher than that of the venous drainage. There may be some absorption via the Virchow–Robin spaces and pial capillaries. The normal volume of CSF is 140 ml, the specific gravity is 1005, and it is produced at a rate of 0.35 ml/min, which does not change in hydrocephalus. The rate of absorption is linearly related to the intraventricular pressure and is not affected by acetazolamide (Cutler *et al.*, 1968; Lorenzo, Page, and Watters, 1970). In NPH this relationship is partially lost (Lorenzo, Bresnan and Barlow, 1974).

Obstruction within the ventricles produces internal hydrocephalus, while obstruction outside the ventricles, in the cisterns and subarachnoid space, produces communicating hydrocephalus — NPH is one aspect of this latter problem. In NPH it was originally thought that there was an initial rise in intraventricular pressure but as the ventricle increased in size and its internal surface area also increased, the pressure decreased in proportion to the increase in surface area (according to Pascal's law $P \propto 1/r$ of pressure relationships and radius in a sphere; see Hakim and Adams, 1965). This theory has been disproved and alternative routes of absorption of CSF develop (Geschwind, 1968). The ependyma becomes flattened and extracellular cerebral odema occurs, resulting in periventricular atrophy and degeneration (Milhorat *et al.*, 1970).

Briggs (1978) has reviewed the problem of CSF pressure, particularly in NPH. Intracranial pressure (ICP) is not stable and lumbar puncture pressure does not always mirror ICP. ICP monitoring has shown variations in pressure in both normals and patients with raised ICP:

(a) A waves (plateau waves) showing large maintained increases in pressure occur in patients with pathologically raised ICP are associated with hydrocephalic attacks and can be terminated by voluntary hyperventilation.

(b) B waves (Fig. 7) occur normally during sleep at a rate of 1 or 2 per minute and might influence the progress of NPH.

(c) C waves correspond to Traube–Herring–Mayer fluctuations of blood pressure.

In NPH, although lumbar puncture pressure is normal, ICP is raised. Some patients have moderately raised flat ICP recordings on a 24 hour monitoring; others, with a slightly higher ICP, show irregular recordings with B waves (see Fig. 7) and occasionally develop A waves — and the term NPH should be altered to 'episodically raised pressure hydrocephalus'.

Diagnosis

Diagnosis depends on recognition of the classical triad of dementia, gait disturbance, and incontinence. Radioisotope-labelled serum albumin cisternography (RISA scan) has been used widely in confirmation of the diagnosis. This is injected by lumbar puncture and passes the basal cisterns over the cerebral hemispheres to reach the sagittal sinus in 24 hours and does not normally enter the ventricles. In NPH, RISA rapidly enters the ventricles and radioactivity persists for up to 72 hours and cannot be detected over the cerebral hemispheres. It is presumed that the subarachnoid or arachnoid granulation fibrosis prevents passage over the cerebral hemispheres and the RISA enters the fourth ventricle. However, some patients meeting these criteria do not

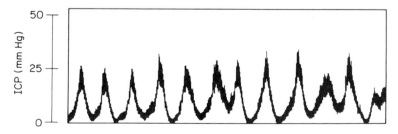

Figure 7   Normal pressure hydrocephalus, lateral ventricular pressure recordings. Classical B waves of 25 mmHg are superimposed on zero pressure for a period of 6 min. (Reproduced by permission of Mr Michael Briggs)

improve with ventricle shunts, and some patients with Alzheimer's disease show the typical changes of NPH on RISA scan. A computerized tomography (CT) scan shows dilated ventricles and normal cortical surface in NPH but even in conjunction with an RISA scan is not an infallible method of diagnosis and certainly not an infallible predictor of response to ventricular shunting.

Other methods of investigation are by air encephalography, lumbar spinal infusion with measurement of CSF pressure, and brain biopsy; but no single test has proved to be completely reliable. It was noted in the description of early cases that there was improvement of the patients' clinical condition with repeated lumbar puncture and withdrawal of CSF (Hakim, and Adams, 1965). Briggs (1978) recommends that suspected patients should have lumbar puncture on three consecutive days and that 10 to 20 ml of CSF should be removed on each occasion. Only patients showing clinical improvement should be investigated further. ICP monitoring will then determine which patients should be selected for shunting.

INTRACRANIAL TUMOURS

The approximate average annual incidence of primary brain tumours is 10 per 100,000 (Kurland, 1980). There is a rapid and continual increase in incidence after the age of 40 years (Annegers *et al.*, 1980).

Brain tumours are classified according to tissue of origin (Zülch, 1979). The term glioma embraces all tumours of neuroglial origin (astrocytes, oligodendrocytes, ependymal cells) and constitutes 40 per cent. of cerebral tumours in the adult. Meningiomas account for 15 per cent. of intracranial tumours and cerebral metastases probably account for about 30 per cent. Pituitary adenomas and craniopharyngiomas together account for about 10 per cent in adults.

Clinical Characteristics

The mode of presentation is often specific but combinations can occur (Thomas, 1983):
(a) General, e.g. mental deterioration or epilepsy.
(b) Focal, e.g. hemiparesis.

(c) Raised intracranial pressure, headaches, vomiting, papilloedema.

Meningiomas sometimes produce intermittent symptoms (Daly, Svien, and Yoss, 1961). Development of symptoms may be rapid with glioblastomas and metastases. Meningiomas, accoustic neuromas, and pituitary adenomas develop slowly. The presenting condition may be progressive dementia, particularly with tumours of the frontal lobes or corpus callosum.

Approximately 10 to 15 per cent. of elderly patients with epileptic seizures have cerebral tumours (Roberts, Godfrey, and Caird, 1982). Hemiparesis due to a tumour is not usually difficult to distinguish from that due to a stroke despite the fact that sudden hemorrhage can occur in a tumour with resultant rapid development of a hemiplegia and coma. In a patient with hemiplegia in whom a tumour is suspected, the gradual deterioration rather than improvement will confirm a tumour, while, conversely, hemiplegia due to stroke tends to improve. Treatment with dexamethasone will generally improve the clinical status of a patient with a tumour but has practically no effect on the hemiplegia due to a stroke (Matthews, 1978).

Focal presentation may be visual due to involvement of any part of the optic tracts. Dysphasia and ataxia may sometimes be of focal importance. Sixth nerve and third nerve palsies, and extensor plantar responses, may be due to a tumour but care should be taken in attributing them to a tumour at a particular site; they are often due to stretching or pressure from an expanding tumour on the opposite side of the brain.

Headache, vomiting, and papilloedema are not as common modes of presentation with increasing age, probably due to reduction in cerebral volume. Apathy, lethargy, confusion, impaired mobility, and incontinence have been attributed to raised intracranial pressure in the elderly (Turner, and Caird, 1982).

Diagnosis and Treatment

A computerized axial tomography (CAT) scan is essential to confirm the diagnosis and to exclude other disease. Brain biopsy may be necessary in some cases. Dexamethasone, 4 mg three times daily for 3 or 4 days, with gradual reduction afterwards to control symptoms, has value in diagnosis, preparation for operation, and palliation.

NEUROLOGICAL EFFECTS OF MALIGNANT DISEASE

The concept of neurological manifestations of malignant disease developed gradually but was not fully recognized until after World War II when it reached the status of respectability by the association of peripheral sensory neuropathy with carcinoma of the bronchus (Denny-Brown, 1948).

Carcinomatous neuropathy, neuromyopathy, and myopathy; Brain, and Henson, 1958; Henson, Russel, and Wilkinson, 1954, were accepted designations of disease but require more specific taxonomy dependent on clinical and pathological correlations (Brain, 1965; Henson, 1970). These non-metastatic neurological syndromes are, however, rare in malignant disease and association is not supported statistically; but, in reverse, there are associations which cannot be ignored, perhaps the most obvious being that approximately half the patients with acquired progressive cortical cerebellar degeneration have malignant disease (Henson, 1970). They can occur long before a malignant process is manifest and, indeed, can occur in the absence of malignant disease. The various syndromes described are found in elderly patients and when identified should stimulate investigation for occult neoplasm (Fig. 8):

Progressive multifocal leukoencephalopathy
Encephalopathy due to abnormal polypeptides and metabolic changes
Encephalomyelitis
   (a) Limbic encephalitis
   (b) Bulbar encephalitis
   (c) Cerebellar encephalitis
   (d) Ganglioneuronitis (ganglioradiculitis)
   (e) Motor neuronitis
Cortical cerebellar degeneration
Peripheral neuropathy
Dermatomyositis
Eaton–Lambert syndrome

Encephalopathy

Progressive multifocal leukoencephalopathy (Richardson's disease) occurs in patients with reticuloendothelial malignant disease (Åström, Mancall, and Richardson, 1958; Richardson, 1965, 1970) and is characterized by multiple spreading areas of demyelination in the cerebral hemispheres, brainstem, cerebellum, and sometimes the spinal cord, surrounded by deformed oligodendrocytes containing virus particles, and giant astrocytes (Cavanagh *et al.*, 1959; Richardson, 1965). It is probable that it is due to infection with a papova virus (Padgett *et al.*, 1971; Weiner *et al.*, 1972; ZuRhein, and Chou, 1965). However, it cannot be overemphasized that this disease is rare. It never occurs in healthy individuals and rarely is it prolonged, usually lasting a few weeks or months before death occurs. Neurological manifestations vary from presentation with hemiplegia, visual field defects, aphasia, and cerebellar signs to progressive dementia without focal neurological signs, but inevitably the condition progresses to a comatose state with generalized neurological signs. Grand mal and myoclonus occur occasionally during the course of the disease. The disease is difficult to diagnose in life except by the circumstances presaging its development; the CSF is normal and the EEG shows non-specific slow-wave activity. It occurs in other diseases with altered immune responses other than malignancy.

Encephalopathy can be due to endocrine and metabolic abnormalities consequent on production of abnormal proteins with endocrine like actions by neoplastic tissue. Hypercalcaemia, hyperadrenalism, hypoglycaemia, and hyponatraemia with water intoxication are well-established effects which may present with confusion. Pellagra and the Wernicke–Korsakoff syndrome and vitamin B12 deficiency may result from malnutrition due to various consequences of malignant disease (Henson, and Urich, 1979; Rees, 1978).

Encephalomyelitis

This condition comprises limbic encephalitis, cerebellar encephalitis, bulbar encephalomyelitis, myelitis affecting anterior horn cells, and ganglioneuronitis affecting the posterior root ganglia with Wallerian degeneration in the posterior columns and peripheral nerves. There is loss of nerve cells, microglial proliferation, and perivascular round-cell infiltration (Henson and Urich, 1979). A predominantly limbic form with dementia, toxic psychosis, and epilepsy occurs (Henson, Hoffman, and Urich, 1965; Corsellis, Goldberg, and Norton, 1968); the EEG shows slow waves and spikes over the temporal lobes and a CAT scan is necessary to exclude secondary deposits. The bulbar form is characterized by vertigo, ataxia, nystagmus, and bulbar palsy. The spinal form shows the effects of progressive anterior horn cell disease

and ganglioneuronitis is manifest by sensory neuropathy; this sensory neuronopathy and motor neuronopathy may be combined (Henson, and Urich, 1970). The CSF may show an increase in lymphocytes in the acute stage, protein is often raised, and the Lange curve is paretic. Brain-specific complement-fixing antibodies are found in serum and CSF (Croft *et al.*, 1965; Wilkinson, 1964). In peripheral neu-

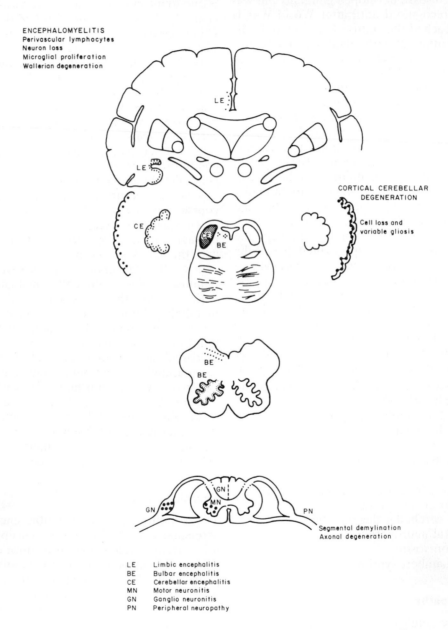

Figure 8   Pathological changes in the central nervous system due to malignant disease

ropathy the CSF protein may be raised and arouse a suspicion of the Guillain–Barré syndrome. Cerebellar encephalitis seems a more appropriate term for the cerebellar lesion than the original designation of this condition as 'subacute cerebellar degeneration' (Brain, Daniel, and Greenfield 1951; Henson, and Urich, 1979).

These conditions may occur separately or in various combinations. They usually occur as a result of oat cell carcinoma of the bronchus which is of neurectodermal origin — which suggests an immune reaction common to the carcinoma and the central nervous system.

Cerebellar Degeneration

This may occur as an 'inflammatory' condition in association with encephalomyelitis and was first described by Greenfield (1934), but there is a cortical cerebellar degeneration which is associated with carcinoma and where degeneration of the cerebellum is the primary neurological manifestation with only minimal secondary changes in its connections. This may be subacute but the cerebellum may appear atrophic with loss of Purkinje cells and gliosis (Brain, Daniel, and Greenfield, 1951; Henson and Urich, 1979). Progressive clinical signs of cerebellar disease occur. The CSF may contain excess lymphocytes and protein with a paretic type of Lange curve of the type associated with encephalomyelitis, but this is unusual in cortical cerebellar degeneration. Subclinical cerebellar cortical degeneration is common in all carcinomas, involving loss of Purkinje cells in

carcinoma of the ovary and granule cells in others (Schmid, and Riede, 1974).

Peripheral Neuropathy

Several types of peripheral neuropathy (Fig. 9) have been described (Bruyn, 1979; Croft, Urich, and Wilkinson, 1967; Croft, and Wilkinson, 1965; Denny-Brown, 1948; Henson, and Urich, 1970) associated with carcinoma of the bronchus, ovary, breast, and stomach and with reticuloendothelial disorders. Neuropathy may be the presenting condition and cancer may be an important cause of chronic progressive polyneuropathy in the elderly (Newman, and Gugino, 1964) — although not age related (Croft, and Wilkinson, 1965). Although clinical signs may be present in approximately 5 per cent. of patients, electrophysiological changes are present in 30 to 40 per cent. (Hildebrand, and Coërs, 1967; Trojaborg, Frantzen, and Andersen, 1969).

The commonest type is sensorimotor distal symmetrical neuropathy (Croft, and Wilkinson, 1965) similar to Guillain–Barré disease (Henson, and Urich, 1970), and the CSF protein may be increased, a factor which makes the diagnosis difficult unless the premonitory symptoms of the Guillain–Barré disease have been identified. It may be mild in terminally ill patients and some of the signs are not uncommon in old age; it may precede by many months the identification of a neoplasm, which may itself only be discovered at post-mortem examination. Pure sensory neuropathy may be difficult to distinguish from sensory neurono-

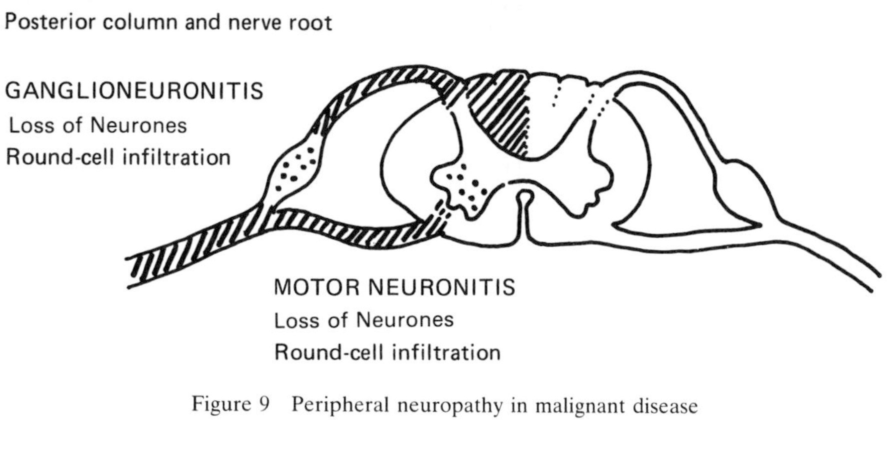

WALLERIAN DEGENERATION
Posterior column and nerve root

GANGLIONEURONITIS
Loss of Neurones
Round-cell infiltration

MOTOR NEURONITIS
Loss of Neurones
Round-cell infiltration

Figure 9   Peripheral neuropathy in malignant disease

pathy, the latter being one aspect of encephalomyelitis, which is due to degeneration of neurones of the posterior root ganglia with perivascular round-cell infiltration and is often accompanied by proximal muscle changes due to anterior horn cell disease. Sensory neuropathy due to ganglioneuronitis is characterized by distal paraesthesia, shooting pains, impairment of all sensory modalities, posterior column ataxia, impaired tendon reflexes, and pseudo-athetosis.

Neuromuscular Effects

There is doubt as to whether a true carcinomatous myopathy occurs (Rowland, and Schotland, 1965). Dermatomyositis is characterized by diffuse oedematous erythema of the face, thorax, and anterior aspects of joints, being accompanied by proximal limb weakness, often with pain and tenderness of the muscles. Dysphagia and dysarthria sometimes occur but ocular muscles are spared. Neoplasms are more common in older patients with dermatomyositis (Arundell, Wilkinson, and Haserick, 1960) and the breast, stomach, bronchus, uterus, and ovary are the most frequent sites. As with other manifestations of occult cancer, dermatomyositis may precede the discovery of a neoplasm which may only be found at post-mortem examination.

The Eaton–Lambert myasthenic syndrome is associated with carcinoma of the bronchus (Eaton, and Lamber, 1957; Lambert, and Rooke, 1965). This is characterized by weakness and slowness of movement and limb pain. The condition differs from myasthenia gravis in the absence of cranial muscle involvement, diminution of tendon reflexes, and characterisitc response to tetanic nerve stimulation by an increase in amplitude of action potentials instead of a decrease as in myasthenia gravis (Fig. 10). The miniature end-plate potentials are reduced in amplitude but are normal in frequency in myasthenia gravis (Elmqvist *et al.*, 1964), which is due to a reduction in the number of receptor sites (Fambrough, Drachman, and Satyamurti, 1973); in the Eaton–Lambert syndrome, miniature end-plate potentials are normal, the abnormality being that the number of quanta of acetylcholine released by each nerve impulse is reduced (Elmqvist, and Lambert, 1968) (Fig. 11). The condition probably has an autoimmune basis due to the production of an autoantibody to tumour proteins which may bind to the nerve terminal (Lang *et al.*, 1981).

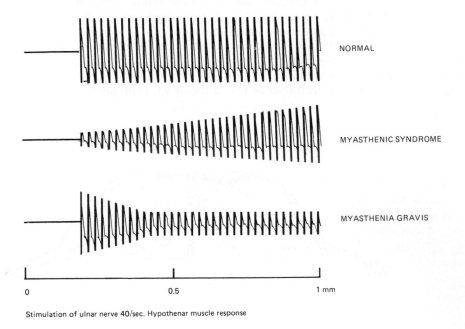

NORMAL

MYASTHENIC SYNDROME

MYASTHENIA GRAVIS

0   0.5   1 mm

Stimulation of ulnar nerve 40/sec. Hypothenar muscle response

Figure 10   Electromyograms in myasthenic syndromes

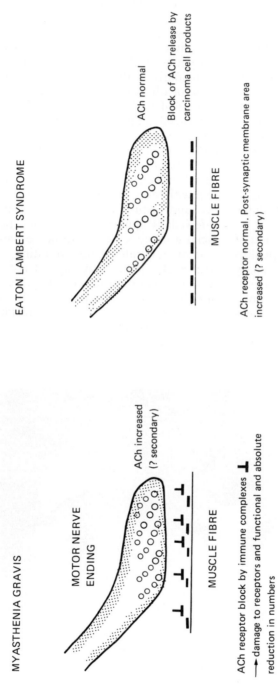

EATON LAMBERT SYNDROME

ACh normal

Block of ACh release by carcinoma cell products

MUSCLE FIBRE

ACh receptor normal. Post-synaptic membrane area increased (? secondary)

Tetanic stimulation gradually overcomes defective ACh release → increasing responses

MYASTHENIA GRAVIS

MOTOR NERVE ENDING

ACh increased (? secondary)

MUSCLE FIBRE

ACh receptor block by immune complexes → damage to receptors and functional and absolute reduction in numbers

Tetanic stimulation produces small regular responses

Figure 11 Neurotramsitter abnormalities in myasthenic syndromes

HERPES INFECTIONS OF THE CENTRAL NERVOUS SYSTEM

Herpes Simplex Encephalitis

Herpes simplex virus (HSV) exists in two forms, type 1 and type 2, which can be distinguished by growth characteristics, physical properties, and serology (Juel-Jensen, and MacCallum, 1972). Primary infection with type 1 virus produces oral and pharyngeal lesions and is the commonest form of primary HSV infection. HSV encephalitis in adults is often a primary infection with type 1 virus. Localized encephalitis suggests a neural route of infection via the olfactory or trigeminal nerve but generalized infection of the brain is probably due to viraemia (Tomlinson, and MacCallum, 1969).

Although HSV encephalitis is uncommon, it is the commonest type of virus encephalitis found in adults in the Western world. Primary infection or secondary infection from a persistent mucocutaneous source are both possible. Recurrent mucocutaneous lesions are not accompanied by a rise in antibody titre but in the early stages of encephalitis there is a rise in antibody in the blood and antibody also appears in the CSF (Illis, and Gostling, 1972).

Pathologically there is asymmetrical swelling of the cerebrum with areas of necrosis, particularly in the temporal lobes and limbic cortex (Fig. 12), but other regions of the brain are also involved to a lesser degree. The necrosis is asymmetrical but bilateral lesions are found, particularly in the limbic cortex. Early lesions show death of neurones and a proliferation of microglial and round cells, with perivascular round-cell infiltration, in the brain and meninges. Inclusion bodies may be found, particularly in the early stages (Adams, 1976).

In about one-fifth of cases there is a prodromal influenza-like illness. The majority present with fever, headache, personality changes, fits, and disturbances of consciousness. After a few days aphasia, hemianopia, hemiplegia, facial weakness, and third nerve palsy, unilateral or generalized fits, vomiting, and coma with neck rigidity may suggest a cerebral abscess or a cerebral tumour. Papilloedema may also be present at this stage. If the patient survives there is usually severe residual neurological disability — the most common being marked memory loss (Adams, and Miller,

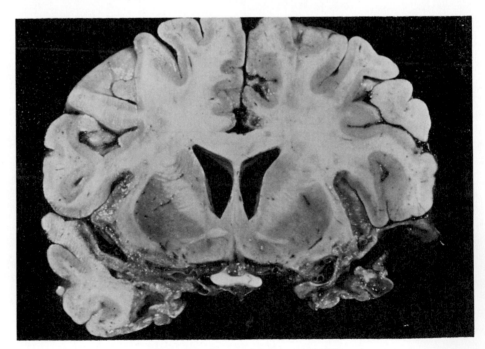

Figure 12 Herpes simplex encephalitis

1973; Illis, 1977; Juel-Jensen, and MacCallum, 1972; Matthews, 1975; Oxbury, and MacCallum, 1973).

A computerized axial tomography (CAT) scan may be helpful in diagnosis and will exclude brain abscess and tumour. However, if the CAT scan is undertaken at an early stage in the disease it may well be negative and should be repeated (Clavaria, du Boulay, and Moseley, 1976; Enzmann *et al.*, 1978). Carotid angiography is helpful, showing early venous filling and a plethora of vessels in affected areas (Sheldon, 1973).

The electroencephalogram (EEG), though usually of limited value, may be helpful occasionally. There is slowing of background activity with periodic delta wave activity and focal sharp waves and spikes. The changes may particularly involve one temporal region. Similar EEG changes also occur in Creutzfeltd–Jakob disease and other viral encephalitides, but are different from the very slow delta activity of cerebral abscess (Cobb, 1975; Upton, and Gumpert, 1970).

It should be evident that the CAT scan and EEG should be performed before lumbar puncture. The CSF pressure is often raised, there is usually an increase in cells (greater than 50 per cmm with lymphocyte predominance), and the protein may be more than 100 mg/dl in about one-third of patients. However, low values and negative findings are not uncommon (Whitley *et al.*, 1982). Brain biopsy tissue and CSF cells should be examined by immunofluorescence and tissue culture (Dayan, and Stokes, 1973; Flewett, 1973) but negative findings should not delay treatment. Brain biopsy is a *sine qua non* in diagnosis and should be taken from the most severely affected temporal lobe or the right temporal lobe if there is no obvious localization.

The ESR is usually raised and there may be a periheral polymorph leucocytosis and lymphocytosis with thrombocytopenia. Blood and CSF should be taken as soon as possible and repeated for viral antibody estimation to show a rising titre.

Idoxuridine has been used systemically in anecdotal cases but, in controlled trials, has been shown to be of little value and dangerous. It produces marrow depression, abnormal liver function tests, and gastrointestinal tract haemorrhages. For these reasons cytosine arabinoside has been used in preference to idoxuridine. Adenine arabinoside has also been used with some effect (Landry, Booss, and Hsiung, 1982) but it is considered by many that it does not affect the outcome of the illness. Acyclovir is currently being evaluated in the treatment of HSV encephalitis (Elion, 1982), but it is questionable whether antiviral drugs, so far, have been effective in the treatment of this disease. Active treatment of cerebral oedema may well be the deciding factor in the determination of recovery. In this respect, vidarabine may be problematic as it needs large amounts of intravenous fluid for its administration and additional diuretics may be needed to remove excess fluid. The aggressive use of mannitol in the treatment of cerebral oedema, which has been used in conjunction with antiviral agents, may well have been the most effective treatment in cases which have recovered. On the supposition that HSV encephalitis might be the result more of a hypersensitivity response than a local cytopathic effect of the virus, steroids and ACTH have been used, but there is increasing evidence that steroids are actually harmful.

Trigeminal Neuralgia

Symptoms usually start in the sixth decade but can begin much later. Spastic paraplegia with unilateral or bilateral trigeminal neuralgia forms one of the syndromes of multiple sclerosis. This has led to a suspicion that herpes zoster might be implicated in the development of multiple sclerosis, but this has been confidently refuted (Beebe, and Kutzke, 1969). The characteristic pain can result from compression of the V cranial nerve by a tumour, neurofibromatosis, or Paget's disease and in association with facial hemiatrophy, facial myoclonus, or peroneal muscular atrophy (Brain, and Walton, 1969). In many cases, however, no underlying pathology is detected.

There is some evidence that HSV is implicated in the aetiology. Section of the sensory root of the Gasserian ganglion for trigeminal neuralgia has been followed by herpetic lesions of the second and third division of the V nerve from which HSV was isolated (Carton, and Kilbourne, 1952); previous section of the postganglionic fibres prevented this occurring. Patients with recurrent trigeminal neuralgia followed by the cutaneous lesions of herpes have been recorded frequently (Behrman, and Knight, 1954). Juel-Jensen, and MacCallum (1972) found antibody to HSV in all female patients with trigeminal neuralgia which was significantly different from matched controls; they did not, however, find any significant difference in men.

Carbamazepine, phenytoin, and clonazepam usually relieve the condition. If full control with carbamazepine is achieved, this often allows the dosage to be reduced and the drug may then be needed only on rare occasions. If the condition is intractable to drugs then thermocoagulation of the sensory root will achieve relief, even in the aged (Sweet and Wepsic, 1974).

Herpes Zoster

Zoster or shingles (Fig. 13) refers to the cutaneous eruption and associated pain which characterizes the condition (Greek: *herpein* — to creep, *zoster* — girdle) but the varicella-zoster virus (VZV) causes other nervous system manifestations.

It was first demonstrated by von Baerensprung (1863) that the cutaneous eruption was accompanied by lesions in the corresponding posterior root ganglion. Head and Campbell (1900) confirmed this and noted that the ganglia most effected were C2-4 and T2-LI. Usually one ganglion is involved but adjacent ganglia may be less severely affected. In the cranial nerves, the Gasserian ganglion is most often involved, producing particularly zoster of the ophthalmic division, and although it has been described in the geniculate ganglion this is extremely rare.

Kundratitz (1925) produced varicella-like lesions by intradermal injection of vesicle fluid from patients with zoster. A virus was isolated from a patient with zoster by Weller and Stoddard (1952), and Weller and Coons (1954) found that the viruses of zoster and varicella were indistinguishable. The virus has a similar size and structure to HSV (Almeida, Howatson, and Williams, 1962) and has been identified in the trigeminal nerve and ganglion (Esiri and Tomlinson, 1972), the spinal cord in myelitis following zoster of T10 (Hogan, and Krigman, 1973), and in the brain in VZV encephalomyelitis (McCormick *et al.*, 1969).

McCarthy (1972) found that the disease has its highest incidence between the sixth and eighth decades and postulated that after an

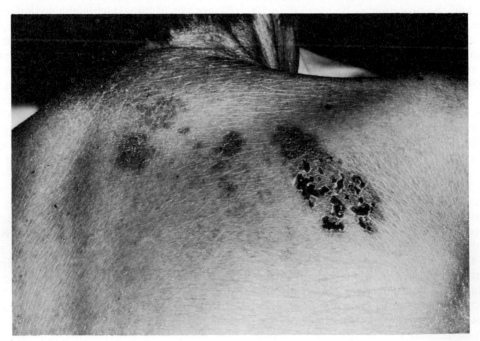

Figure 13 Herpes zoster. Lesions affecting right T1 and T2 with weakness of the right shoulder.

attack of varicella the virus persists in a form which preserves the virus genome intact and that zoster occurs when restriction on replication is removed. The pathway taken by the virus to and from sensory ganglia is through the Schwann cells. Reactivation produces an acute necrotizing inflammatory response in the posterior root ganglion, the virus passes peripherally in the sensory nerve, producing a neuritis, and when it reaches the skin a vesicular rash like chicken-pox occurs (Hope-Simpson, 1965). Reactivation is often preceded by some precipitating factor in the two weeks prior to the onset of the condition (Juel-Jensen, 1970; Juel-Jensen, and MacCallum, 1972):

Precipitating factor	Associated factors
Physical trauma: injuries, burns, operations	Myeloma
Cold	Lymphosarcoma
Frontal sinusitis (ophthalmic zoster)	Hodgkin's disease
Chemicals, steroid creams, shampoos	Lymphocytic leukaemia
Ultraviolet light	Carcinomatosis
X-rays	Cytotoxic drugs
Emotion	
Artificial fever	

The factors which provoke zoster probably produce hyperaemia of peripheral nerves or ganglia and in this context the sensory ganglion has the most abundant vascular supply of the central nervous system.

In the acute stage of the disease the ganglion is swollen, congested, and may be haemorrhagic. Microscopically there is inflammation and lymphocytic infiltration with a few plasma cells and polymorphs. Necrosis may occur. Type A intranuclear inclusion bodies may be found. This inflammation extends into the posterior nerve root and into the spinal nerve. At the level of the affected ganglion there is often perivascular cuffing by lymphocytes in the dorsal horn and sometimes in the ventral horn of the spinal cord, with microglial proliferation. In encephalomyelitis there is similar widespread involvement of the brain. The posterior columns can become demyelinated. After the acute phase, fibrosis of peripheral nerves occurs and is associated with postherpetic neuralgia.

Pain

Pain usually precedes the development of the rash and can be the only manifestation. Postherpetic pain can be very disabling, particularly after ophthalmic zoster and in the elderly. Acute inflammation probably accounts for the early pain and postherpetic pain is probably due to fibrosis of peripheral nerves (Adams, 1976; Juel–Jensen, and MacCallum, 1972). Occasionally there may be sensory loss in the territory of the sensory root affected. Idoxuridine in dimethylsulphoxide applied locally to the vesicles has proved an effective method of reducing postherpetic pain, and vidarabine and acyclovir given systemically have also proved effective.

Encephalomyelitis

This usually follows the rash and is not particularly related to cranial nerve zoster. Headache, fever, vomiting, and confusion are the usual symptoms with occasionally fits, and there are signs of meningeal irritation. Focal signs are uncommon but occasionally hemiparesis, facial palsy, and ataxia occur. Following recovery there may be some memory impairment but this is not as severe as that following HSV encephalomyelitis. The mortality rate is as high as 50 per cent., but probably benign cases of meningoencephalitis are not reported and may not have had appropriate investigations.

The EEG may show decreased alpha activity and the CSF shows an increase in cells, particularly lymphocytes, with increased protein. In some cases a rise of complement-fixing antibody to the virus has been shown in the CSF.

These patients should be treated with vidarabine or acyclovir and mannitol (Juel-Jensen and MacCallum, 1972; McKendall, and Klawans, 1978).

Myelitis

Involvement of the posterior columns and the anterior horns of the spinal cord is common (Denny-Brown, Adams, and Fitzgerald, 1944; Head, and Campbell, 1900; Lhermitte, and Nicolas, 1924) and severe myelitis may develop (Hogan, and Krigman, 1973). Segmental motor weakness (Fig. 13) occurs about 3 to 11 days after the rash but only one or two muscles of the myotome are usually affected and there may be considerable separation of the dermatomes and myotomes (Broadbent, 1866; Taterka and O'Sullivan, 1943; Thomas, and Howard, 1972); however, recovery is good (Gupta, Helal, and Kiely, 1969).

Diaphragmatic paralysis occurs with zoster affecting C5 and C6 (Brostoff, 1966). Constipation and urinary retention with an atonic ulcerated bladder due to thoracolumbar and sacral posterior root involvement, respectively, can also occur (Juel-Jensen, and MacCallum, 1972; Rankin, and Sutton, 1969; Richmond, 1974) but, in the elderly, constipation is usually due to analgesics.

Polyneuropathy

This, too, follows the rash but may be delayed for up to 2 months. It is of Guillain–Barré type with the CSF protein considerably raised and a minimal increase in cells. The neuropathy is symmetrical and in half the cases there is associated cranial nerve involvement (Dayan, Ogul, and Graveson, 1972).

Cranial Nerves

Involvement of sensory and motor cranial nerves has been frequently described and discussed (Juel–Jensen, and MacCallum, 1972; McKendall, and Klawans, 1978). The disease undoubtedly affects cranial nerve sensory ganglia but motor signs are due to localized 'anterior horn' cell involvement and motor neuritis; zoster of occiput and neck may be accompanied by cranial motor nerve manifestations (Thomas, and Howard, 1972).

Retrobulbar neuritis, optic neuritis, and optic atrophy, and insidious optic neuritis may occur. Oculomotor, trochlear, and abducens nerve paralyses occur in association with trigeminal zoster affecting, particularly, the ophthalmic division. Ptosis, either unilateral or bilateral, can occur.

Trigeminal zoster is the most common, accounting for 95 per cent. of lesions affecting the cranial nerves, and the ophthalmic division is affected in two-thirds of cases. If the nasociliary branch of the ophthalmic division is also involved, then conjunctivitis occurs with the possibility of the development or keratitis and iridocyclitis — when the pain may be intense. If the eye is threatened then vidarabine is mandatory. The motor division of the V nerve can also be affected.

Facial paralysis may be indistinguishable from Bell's palsy but may be associated with zoster lesions of the ear. The Ramsay Hunt syndrome (Durham, 1960; Hunt, 1907a, 1907b, 1909) consists of pain in the external auditory meatus and pinna with herpes of the tympanic membrane, internal auditory meatus and pinna, combined with facial palsy. Loss of taste may occur in the anterior two-thirds of the tongue. Hunt considered that the geniculate ganglion was involved and that swelling of the ganglion produced pressure on the motor fibres of the VII nerve. However, Hunt himself failed to confirm the syndrome he described pathologically, and zoster of the ear is due to involvement of branches of either C2 or trigeminal nerve. In practically all the cases which have come to pathological examination there is neuritis of the facial nerve and, if it occurs, the Ramsay Hunt syndrome is rare (Alkesic, Budzilovich, and Lieberman, 1973; Denny–Brown, Adams, and Fitzgerald, 1944). The facial palsy represents a motor concomitant of zoster similar to that found in the limbs. The eighth nerve is rarely involved but neuritis has been described with inflammation of the cochlea.

Antibiotic treatment is now so well established that vidarabine or acylovir is nearly always required for zoster of the V cranial nerve, motor zoster, sacral zoster, encephalomyelitis, and immunosuppressed patients (Juel-Jensen, 1982; Timbury, 1982).

PERIPHERAL NEUROPATHY

In the peripheral nervous system, neurones and their axons are invested by Schwann cells which elaborate myelin around the axons and maintain their viability (Hall, 1978). The production of myelin is directly influenced by the axon (Weinberg and Spencer, 1976). The blood supply of peripheral nerves comes from a longitudinal anastomosis of arterioles and drains into an anastomosis of venules in the perineurium; these communicate with a longitudinal capillary anastomotic network in the endoneurium. The perineurium is a lamellated cellular sheath which forms a diffusion barrier for the peripheral nerve. The endoneurial capillaries have endothelial cells which are zipped together to form tight junctions — similar to the 'blood–brain barrier' of the central nervous system — but it is deficient in the dorsal roots and autonomic ganglia. The perineurial diffusion barrier and the blood–nerve barrier regulate the composition of the endoneurial fluid and are obviously significant in regulating the access of toxic substances to the peripheral nerve (Olsson, 1975; Thomas, 1981; Thomas, and Olsson, 1975).

There is a significant decrease in the number of myelinated fibres in peripheral nerves with increasing age (O'Sullivan, and Swallow, 1968; Swallow, 1966; Tohgi, Tsukagoshi, and Toyokura, 1977) and there is evidence that this also involves unmyelinated fibres (Ochoa, and Mair, 1969). There is also an age-related loss of myelinated fibres in the dorsal and ventral nerve roots (Corbin, and Gardner, 1937). Studies of individual myelinated axons from peripheral nerves of subjects without peripheral neuropathy, chronic disease or cardiac failure with oedema, show that, in the normal elderly, there is a preponderance of fibres with short internodal length, increased segmental demyelination and Wallerian-type degeneration (Arnold, and Harriman, 1970; Lascelles, and Thomas, 1966).

In peripheral myelinated nerve fibres, internodal length is directly proportional to axon diameter, the velocity of conduction being proportional to the external diameter of the myelinated fibre (Hursh, 1939). Conduction velocity of both motor and sensory fibres in peripheral nerves decreases with increasing age and general deterioration, including dementia (Kaeser, 1970). It is associated with increased duration and reduced amplitude of the motor action potential and sensory action potential, and is due to loss of large fibres and demyelination/remyelination (Buchthal, and Rosenfalck, 1966; Cruz Martinez *et al.*, 1978; Dorfman, and Bosley, 1979; Wagman, and Lesse, 1952).

Minor degrees of peripheral neuropathy are common in the elderly and are manifest by loss of vibrotactile sensation, decreased motor power, and loss of reflexes, particularly in the legs. Some of these changes may be age related and due to a loss of peripheral nerve fibres and anterior horn cells. Others may be a consequence of entrapment, particularly by osteoarthrosis of cervical and lumbar spine.

The commonest causes of peripheral neuropathy in the elderly are diabetes mellitus, peripheral vascular disease, drugs, alcoholism, and malignancy (Argov, and Mastaglia, 1979; Croft, Urich, and Wilkinson, 1966; Huang, 1981; Mirsky, Futterman, and Broh-Kahn, 1953; Steinberg, and Graber, 1963). Classification into mononeuritis multiplex, axonal degeneration, segmental demyelination, and entrapment neuropathies (McLeod, 1982) provides a pathological basis in considering individual patients, but can only be complimentary to a good medical history, examination, and simple investigation. Electrophysiological studies and nerve biopsy are often essential to elucidate the primary cause. In the elderly, it must be remembered that malnutrition, malabsorption, impaired renal function, and multiple aetiology should all be taken into consideration.

Neuropathologically, the peripheral neuropathies are classified according to the identifiable lesion and the accompanying neurophysiological changes (Table 2):

(a) The neurone and its processes may be affected — neuronopathies and axonopathies — and the latter may be proximal or distal or both (Thomas, 1981).

(b) Segmental demyelination due to disease of Schwann cell or myelin.

(c) Wallerian degeneration (Waller, 1850) was originally applied to the degeneration of the distal part of a transected peripheral nerve fibre, and the proximal changes to the nearest node of Ranvier. The term has been extended to include any degeneration in an axon which has been separated from its cell body in either the peripheral or central nervous systems. If the cell body and axon remain continuous as in the 'dying-back' phenomenon, the similar degenerative changes are called 'Walleian-type' degeneration (Urich, 1976). Isolated vascular occlusions can produce this condition, i.e. mononeuritis multiplex.

Damage to the neurone may manifest itself in the distal part of the axon (Cavanagh, 1964) as a 'dying-back' process and the proximal part of the axon in the posterior columns (Prineas, 1969a, 1969b), and may progress until cell

Table 2   Classification of peripheral
neuropathy

Axonal degeneration	Segmental demyelination
Medical conditions	
Diabetes mellitus	Diabetes mellitus
Some drugs	Some drugs
Alcohol	Guillain–Barré syndrome
Gold, arsenic	Relapsing polyneuritis
Acromegaly	Peroneal muscular atrophy
Amyloid disease	
Vitamin B1 and B12	
deficiency	
Neoplasms	
Neurophysiology	
Slightly reduced conduction velocity	Greatly reduced conduction velocity
Variable motor unit potentials	Normal motor unit potentials
Positive sharp waves	No sharp waves
Fasciculation	No fasciculation

Mononeuritis multiplex

(*Medical conditions*)

Diabetes mellitus
Polyarteritis nodosa
Rheumatoid arthritis
Systemic lupus erythematosis
Sarcoidosis
Amyloidosis
Immunization

death occurs, or the process may be arrested and followed by regeneration. Secondary breakdown of myelin may occur with changes in Schwann cells similar to Wallerian degeneration (Urich, 1976). Degenerating fibres conduct at normal velocity until conduction fails; there is a reduction in maximal conduction velocity in these conditions which is presumably due to failure in conduction in large diameter fibres (Hopkins and Gilliatt, 1971). When nerve fibres regenerate after axonal degeneration, the internodal distances are shortened and conduction velocity may be reduced to 75 per cent. of that in normal nerves (Cragg, and Thomas, 1964).

In segmental demyelination the axon remains more or less intact. It may be due to disease of the Schwann cell or myelin. In the early stages there is widening of the node of Ranvier but whole internodes may be affected. When recovery takes place, remyelination shows as irregular internodes and thinner myelin. Conduction velocity is severely impaired in segmental demyelination. This slowing is due to decreased resistance and increased capacitance at the internodes (Rasminsky, and Sears, 1972).

Demyelination may be due to endoneurial vascular changes, damage to Schwann cells, or direct effects on myelin. One type of peroneal muscular atrophy is associated with segmental demyelination of large fibres and sensory impairment for light–touch, vibration, and position sense, with preservation of pain and temperature sensation; the other is due to neuronal degeneration in anterior horns and dorsal root ganglia (Thomas, 1975). In the Guillain–Barré syndrome, macrophages make a direct attack on the peripheral nerve myelin (Asbury, Arnason, and Adams, 1969) and the condition presents as acute segmental demyelination.

The paraproteinaemias, macroglobulinaemia (8 per cent.) and multiple myeloma (3 per cent.), are sometimes associated with peripheral neuropathy of various types, some of which are associated with deposition of amyloid in peripheral nerve tissue. Secondary amyloid does not usually produce peripheral neuropathy but sporadic cases of primary amyloid neuropathy can occur in the elderly. They are characterized by loss of small myelinated and unmyelinated fibres with loss of pain and temperature sensation but preservation of light–touch, position, and vibration sensation (Dyck, and Lambert, 1969; Thomas, and King, 1974).

Neuronopathies and axonopathies are due to changes in cell metabolism and axonal conduction, many of which can be drug induced (Argov, and Mastaglia, 1979; Thomas, 1981) (see Table 3).

Chronic relapsing polyneuritis is similar to the Guillain–Barré syndrome and it is possible that the disease processes are essentially the same though different temporally (Matthews, Howell, and Hughes, 1970). Some patients with chronic relapsing polyneuritis respond to steroids but dependence on steroids often results (Austin, 1958). Chronicity is associated with the HLA-B8 antigen and chronicity may

Table 3   Drug-induced neuropathy

Antimicrobial drugs	Cardiovascular drugs
Streptomycin	Hydralazine
Ethambutol	Amiodarone
Isoniazid	Disopyramide
Nitrofurantoin	Clofibrate
Metronidazole	
Sulphonamides	
Amphotericin	
Antineoplastic drugs	*Antirheumatic drugs*
Vincristine	Gold
Chlorambucil	Indomethacin
Mustine	Phenylbutazone
	Others
	Phenytoin
	Chlorpropamide
	Propylthiouracil

be related to the host-immune response and may be genetically determined (McLeod, 1982).

VITAMIN B12 NEUROPATHY AND SUBACUTE COMBINED DEGENERATION OF THE CORD

The neurological changes due to vitamin B12 deficiency can be considered as a central–peripheral distal axonopathy with secondary Wallerian degeneration. The serum level of vitamin B12 falls with age (Boger *et al.*, 1955). Both vitamin B12 deficiency and folate deficiency produce an identical megaloblastic anaemia. Folate becomes metabolically trapped as methyl tetrahydrofolate (methyl-THFA) which cannot be utilized in the absence of vitamin B12 (adenosylcobalamin) (see Fig. 14). (See Table 4 for the different forms of vitamin B12). Subacute combined degeneration (SACD) of the cord does not occur in simple folate deficiency. The anaemia of vitamin B12 deficiency responds to folate but SACD does not respond — and may be exacerbated. It has been shown that methionine prevents the expected development of SACD in monkeys (Scott *et al.*, 1981; Scott and Weir, 1981).

The first comprehensive clinical and pathological description of the neurological condition was published in 1900 (Russell, Batten,

and Collier, 1900) and the term subacute combined degeneration of the cord was used. The term vitamin B12 neuropathy was introduced by Richmond and Davidson (1958) and showed that the wider neurological condition was not necessarily associated with pernicious anaemia.

In SACD there is degeneration of long tracts in the spinal cord. The posterior columns, particularly the fasciculus gracilis, and the spinocerebellar tracts are affected in the upper cervical cord and medulla, and in the lumbar regions the corticospinal tracts are particularly affected, the lesions showing maximal severity in the midthoracic cord where the only intact fibres may be those in direct relationship to the central grey matter (Smith, 1976). The demyelination is of Wallerian type. Peripheral nerves are often affected and there is loss of myelin sheaths.

Clinically the disease presents with paraesthia in the feet, ataxia, and spastic paraparesis. There may be involvement of the arms but spastic paraplegia of the legs with anaesthesia spreading to the trunk is usually predominant.

Cigarette smoking increases the relative amount of cyanocobalamin in the plasma and since this is less closely bound to plasma proteins than other forms of vitamin B12 it is excreted more readily in the urine. In pernicious anaemia and tobacco amblyopia, the total cobalamin concentration of plasma is lowered, but in both the concentration of cyanocobalamin is raised. Chronic retrobulbar neuritis may be a consequence, with loss of visual acuity and sometimes temporal pallor of the

Table 4   Forms of vitamin B12

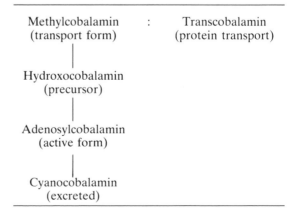

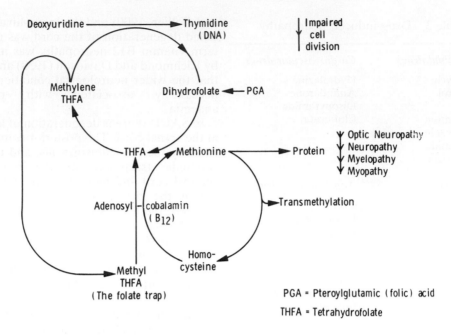

Figure 14   Vitamin B12 and folic acid interaction

fundi (Chisholm, 1979). Colour vision may also be affected (blue/yellow discrimination), which is related to smoking and age (Chisholm, 1972).

Memory impairment may occur in vitamin B12 deficiency; hallucinations, mania, and paranoia — megaloblastic madness — may be precipitated by giving folic acid to patients with pernicious anaemia (Smith and Oliver, 1967). In this context folic acid deficiency can produce psychiatric disorders, particularly in the elderly (Girdwood, 1968).

ENTRAPMENT NEUROPATHIES

Early symptoms of compression neuropathies are positive, pain and paraesthesia, rather than negative, weakness and sensory loss. Anatomical diagnosis can be confirmed by electrophysiology but pathogenesis may be in some doubt (Downie, 1982). Compression may be simple due to swelling or inflammation of fibrous, osseous, or muscular bands and tunnels but multiple factors may be involved in the production of a particular entrapment syndrome, e.g. spondylosis, diabetes mellitus, ischaemia, and generalized polyneuropathy (Upton, and McComas, 1973). The entrapment lesion can vary from transient physiological block, through axonal transection to complete nerve transection (Ochoa, Fowler, and Gilliatt, 1972; Seddon, 1943).

Systemic diseases such as myxoedema, acromegaly, rheumatoid arthritis, Raynaud's disease, and fluid retention facilitate the development of symmetrical bilateral entrapment syndromes.

Upper Limb

Ulnar Nerve

A wide carrying angle of the elbow, particularly in females, may predispose to chronic traction on the nerve. The ulnar nerve is particularly susceptible to the effects of external pressure behind the medial humeral epicondyle when the partially flexed elbow rests on a hard surface with the wrist pronated. Active flexion of the elbow tightens the two heads of the arcuate ligament of the flexor carpi ulnaris, thus increasing ischaemia of the nerve in the cubital tunnel (Wadsworth, 1977).

There is usually paraesthesia of the little finger and ulnar half of the ring finger, which is made worse by full elbow flexion maintained for 5 minutes (Wadsworth, 1980). The interossei and hypothenar muscles are weak and wasted. Downie (1982) considers that sensory loss on the ulnar half of the ring finger, clearly distinguishable from the radial half, favours an ulnar nerve lesion rather than a root, plexus, or cord lesion and that definite weakness of the terminal phalanx of the little finger (flexor digitorum profundus) indicates an ulnar nerve lesion at the elbow. Anterior transposition of the ulnar nerve would seem to be the treatment of choice.

Compression of the ulnar nerve at the wrist is usually due to repeated hand injury. The deep palmar branch is usually involved which results in weakness and wasting of interossei, but the hypothenar muscles are spared.

Median Nerve

At the elbow, entrapment of the median nerve may occur at three sites:
(a) above the elbow where occasionally the nerve passes through an atavistic supracondylar foramen;
(b) when the nerve passes between the two heads of pronator teres;
(c) at the origin of the interosseous branch (Nigst and Dick, 1979).

Aching in the forearm and local tenderness at the entrapment site may occur. Paraesthesia and sensory loss may occur but weakness of long flexors of the wrist and fingers distinguishes the level from that of the carpal tunnel syndrome. Lesions of the anterior interosseous nerve are characterized by weak flexion of the tip of the thumb and index finger when attempting to form an 'O' with these digits (Spinner, 1970).

The carpal tunnel syndrome epitomizes all the facets of these conditions. It was first described in 1913 (Marie and Foix, 1913) and increasingly recognized after World War II (Brain, Wright, and Wilkinson, 1947). Local, systemic, and dynamic factors are involved (Downie, 1965; Inglis, Straub, and Williams, 1972).

Burning paraesthesia in the hand, not necessarily localized to the median nerve territory, may radiate centripetally to forearm, elbow, and even shoulder. There is weakness of abductor pollicis brevis. This condition

should be confirmed by nerve conduction studies, particularly before surgical decompression.

Radial Nerve

Entrapment may occur in the radial tunnel. External compression at this site produces wrist drop, weakness of the brachioradialis, wrist and finger extensors, with sensory loss of the interdigital cleft between thumb and index finger. If only the posterior interosseous branch is involved then there is weakness of finger extension alone.

In the upper limb, extrapment neuropathies have been described for the suprascapular, dorsal scapular, and lung thoracic nerves.

Lower Limb

Lateral Popliteal Nerve

Usually compression is external at the point where the nerve is related to the neck of the fibula and the origin of peroneus longus. Repetitive inversion movements of the foot produce traction on the nerve in this 'fibular tunnel' with resultant paraesthesia of the lateral aspect of the calf. Loss of weight conduces to foot drop from external compression (Woltman, 1930).

Lateral Cutaneous Nervous Thigh

Entrapment of this nerve where it passes under the lateral end of the inguinal ligament occurs in obese patients. The result is 'meralgia paraesthetica', pain, and paraesthesia of the lateral aspect of the thigh. Sensory loss has a clear-cut medial border which overlies the middle of the quadriceps, and the knee jerk is unimpaired — which distinguishes it from L3 root lesions (Downie, 1982).

Tarsal Tunnel Syndrome

Although described in 1960 (Kopell, and Thompson, 1960) this syndrome is relatively uncommon. Burning paraesthesia of the plantar surface of the foot, accompanied by weakness of intrinsic foot muscles and tenderness of the posterior tibial nerve as it passes below the medial malleolus, deep to the flexor retinaculum, constitutes the full syndrome. It is exaggerated by walking and prolonged standing.

MYOPATHIES IN THE ELDERLY

Muscle Fibres

Muscle fibres contain myofibrils (Fig. 15) consisting of myofilaments of myosin and actin. The myofilaments are surrounded by sarcoplasm containing nuclei, mitochondria, glycogen, and enzymes, and the whole is invested by the sarcolemma. Invaginations of the sarcolemma form a complex system of tubules, the T tubules and the logitudinal sarcoplasmic reticulum, which are concerned with synchronous depolarization and are associated with calcium release. This calcium activates myosin ATPase with release of energy for muscle contraction, which is due to sliding of myosin and actin filaments over each other (Bradley, 1975; Huxley, 1971). High-energy phosphate is provided by ATP which itself is the product of either anaerobic glycolysis in the extramitochondrial phase of the sarcoplasm or aerobic metabolism of pyruvate and long-chain free fatty acids in the mitochondria. Myopathies due to deficiencies of enzymes involved in these metabolic processes characteristically produce muscle stiffness, weaknes and cramp, myoglobinuria, and raised serum creatine phosphokinase on exercise. Although most of these specific enzyme deficiency myopathies occur in children or young adults, there are some late-onset types (Kost, and Verity, 1980; Morgan-Hughes, 1982).

Table 5   Myopathies in the elderly

MUSCULAR DYSTROPHIES

Limb-girdle syndrome
Facioscapulohumeral syndrome
Scapuloperoneal syndrome
Dystrophia myotonica
Progressive external ophthalmoplegia

INFLAMMATORY MYOPATHIES

Polymyositis
Dermatomyositis
Polymyalgia rheumatica
Granulomatous myositis
Viral myositis

PERIODIC PARALYSES

Primary and secondary

ENDOCRINE AND METABOLIC MYOPATHIES

Thyroid disease
Osteomalacia and hyperparathyroidism
Pituitary disease
Steroid myopathy

TOXIC MYOPATHIES

In man the differentiation into red narrow and white broad fibres (Table 6) is not possible but fibre type and physiology show the same

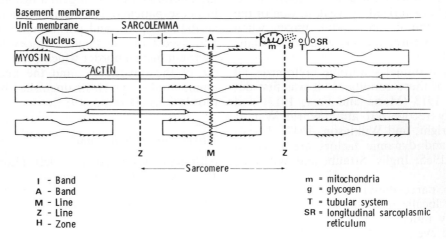

I - Band
A - Band
M - Line
Z - Line
H - Zone

m = mitochondria
g = glycogen
T = tubular system
SR = longitudinal sarcoplasmic reticulum

Figure 15   Myofibril

Table 6   Muscle fibres

	Type 1	Type 2
	Red, narrow	White, broad (Ranvier 1873)
	Myoglobin +++	Myoglobin +
	Slow twitch	Fast twitch (Ranvier 1874)
	Tonic movement (posture)	Phasic movement (Reflex)
	Resistent to fatigue	Susceptible to fatigue
	Mitochondria +++	Mitochondria +
	Sarcoplasmic reticulum +	Sarcoplasmic reticulum ++
	Oxidative respiration	Glycolytic respiration
Staining		
ATPase pH 9.4	+	+++
NADH – TR	+++	+

correlation in men as in animals (Warmolts and Engel, 1972). Each motor nerve fibre serves an individual motor unit, the fibres of which are distributed randomly in a checkerboard pattern in peripheral muscle and are all of the same type. The motoneurone itself determines the type of fibre. If a motoneurone dies then its muscle fibres atrophy but are reinnervated by sprouting from neighbouring motoneurones. This results in type grouping of contiguous muscle fibres (Kugelberg, Edström, and Abbruzze, 1970). In peripheral neuropathy there is atrophy of type 1 and type 2 fibres; in addition, type grouping occurs in chronic neuropathy (Carroll and Brooke, 1978).

Disuse atrophy of muscle, which may be due to various disorders including upper motor neurone lesions, produces type 2 atrophy (see Fig. 16). Stretch and contractiltiy are the primary stimuli for incorporation of protein and maintenance of muscle (Goldberg, and Goodman, 1969) and, if stimuli are absent, atrophy results. Type 2 muscle fibres are particularly concerned with voluntary movement and selective type 2 atrophy may occur. However, type 2 atrophy is the commonest seen and is not very specific.

In amyotrophic lateral sclerosis there is denervation atrophy with smallness and angulation of type 1 and type 2 fibres plus hypertrophy of some type 2 fibres.

In pathological muscle there is a tendency to type 1 predominance which is probably due to change in function of motor units from voluntary, phasic, fast twitch (type 2) to tonic, slow twitch (type 1) (Bradley, 1975). Fibre size is variable with scattered small fibres, some hypertrophic fibres, and muscle fibre splitting.

Table 7   Muscle biopsy

Denervation	*Myopathy* (and chronic denervation)
Single fibre atrophy	Scattered small fibres
Group atrophy	Fibre splitting
Angular fibres (<90°)	Multiple central nuclei
Type grouping	Hypertrophic fibres
Type 1 atrophy	*Type 2 atrophy*
Dystrophia myotonica	Common; often non-specific
Limb-girdle syndromes	Females; sedentary males
Rheumatoid arthritis	Upper motoneurone lesion
	Myasthenia gravis
	Steroids

Electromyography (motor unit potentials)	
Denervation	*Myopathy* (and chronic denervation)
Large amplitude	Small amplitude
Long duration	Short duration
Polyphasic	Polyphasic
Fibrillation potentials at rest	No fibrillation potentials at rest
Reduced interference (maximal contraction)	

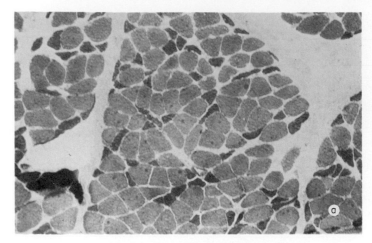

(a) Type 2 atrophy ATPase pH 9.4

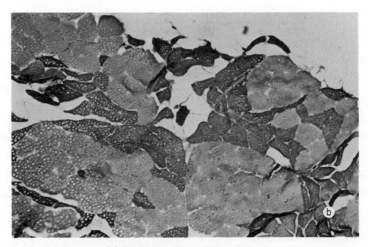

(b) Type grouping ATPase pH 9.4

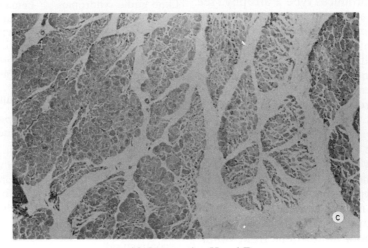

(c) Denervation H and E

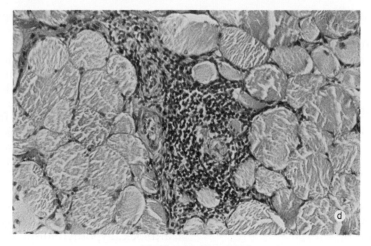

(d) Myositis H and E

Figure 16   Muscle biopsy. (Reproduced by permission of Dr Margaret Esiri)

Facioscapulohumeral dystrophy (FSHD) shows considerable variation in severity and may be so slowly progressive that it may not shorten life. The muscle shows variation of fibre size from very small fibres to hypertrophic forms, the latter often of type 2.

In dystrophia myotonica there is a primary abnormality in the sarcolemma which produces partial depolarization and the muscle fibre membrane is leaky to sodium. There is an increase in the number of internal nuclei and atrophy of type 1 fibres.

Ageing Muscle

In old age, there is a decrease in muscle strength and atrophy of muscle which resembles progressive muscular dystrophy (Verzár, 1959) but is due to changes in motor units (Gutmann, and Hanzlíková, 1976); and a decrease in muscular work capability due to diminished efficiency in muscle energy metabolism (Ermini, 1976).

Changes in muscle in the elderly may be secondary to changes in the motoneurones or diminished mobility. Senile muscle atrophy is a specific entity due to changes in the neuromuscular junction and morphological changes in muscle fibres. Changes in the motor endplate are different from those due to denervation (Gutmann, and Hanzlíková, 1972).

The earliest change is in the motor endplate.

The synaptic cleft is widened and infoldings of the receptor site are reduced. These changes occur before there is any loss of spinal motoneurones. It proceeds to random loss of muscle fibres. There is, however, grouped atrophy as well and neurogenic factors may be of greatest importance (Gutmann, and Hanzlíková, 1976; Jennekens, Tomlinson, and Walton, 1971; Serratrice, Roux, and Aquaron, 1968). Neurogenic muscle degeneration may depend on the length of axon. In limb muscles, age-related degeneration starts earliest in the longest axons. It is accompanied by sprouting from adjacent healthy subterminal fibres, from the nodes of Ranvier (Harriman, Taverner, and Woolf, 1970).

Ovoid swellings, axonic spheres, occur in subterminal axons; they are seen in distal muscle at a comparatively early age and proximal muscle from middle age onwards (Harriman, 1976). Atrophy of muscle fibres is accompanied by clusters of sarcolemma nuclei. Some fibres show compensatory hypertrophy. There is an increase in the number of muscle nuclei which may be due to ageing or denervation. Concentric muscle fibrils, 'ring binden', occur in ageing muscle and also in many muscular dystrophies (Schotland, Spiro, and Carmel, 1966).

The EMG shows temporal dispersion within the motor unit, increased duration of the motor potential, and an increased number of polyphasic potentials (Carlson, Alston, and Feldman, 1964; Peterson, and Kugelberg, 1949), which is probably due to sprouting but there is loss of functioning motor units (Campbell, McComas, and Petito, 1973).

Muscular Dystrophies

A muscular dystrophy is a progressive, genetically determined, primary degenerative myopathy (Walton, 1961) (see Table 6).

The Duchenne type of muscular dystrophy (Duchenne, 1868) does not occur in the elderly and survival of patients with the Becker, milder, form (Becker, and Kiener, 1955) to old age is unusual.

Limb-girdle syndromes may be of several types. Both myopathic and neuropathic forms probably occur (Bradley, 1975, 1979). Late-onset cases (Nevin, 1936) may include patients with polymyositis (Bradley, 1979).

There are several forms of the autosomal recessive limb-girdle muscular dystrophy (LGMD) which either begin in the pelvic girdle (Leyden–Möbius type) or shoulder girdle (Erb type) and do not affect the facial muscles until the disease is very advanced (Walton, and Nattrass, 1954). The tongue and masseters are not affected in either LGMD or FSHD, and in older patients the serum CPK, although raised, is not as high as in younger patients, in both conditions.

Facioscapulohumeral dystrophy (FSHD) is less common and more benign than LGMD. Landouzy and Dejerine (1884) acknowledged the description by Duchenne (1868) of FSHD, in his paper on the eponymous pseudo-hypertrophic muscular dystrophy. One of the patients described by Landouzy and Dejerine was still alive at 85 years of age (Justin-Besançon *et al.*, 1964). The condition is an autosomal dominant disorder. Facial weakness and winging of scapulae are the characteristic features. Muscle biopsy may show only minimal type 1 fibre atrophy.

The scapuloperoneal syndrome may be neurogenic and of autosomal dominant inheritence or myopathic with X-linked inheritance. Clinically the condition presents as the Erb type of shoulder-girdle syndrome plus peroneal muscular atrophy (Carroll, 1979; Davidenkow, 1939). Clinically there is mild shoulder-girdle weakness, severe weakness of anterior tibial and peroneal muscles, and hypertrophy of the extensor digitorum brevis.

Dystrophia myotonica is an autosomal dominant disorder presenting clinically with myotonia localized to forearms and tongue, weakness of facial muscles with ptosis, atrophy of sternomastoids, progressive peripheral muscular dystrophy, cataracts, frontal balding, gonadal atrophy, and progressive mental deterioration (Roses, Harper, and Bossen, 1979; Walton, 1964). Afflicted individuals may present with varying degrees of severity dependent on age. In the elderly, cataracts may be the presenting feature. Dystrophia myotonica is a multisystem disease and can present with heartblock, hypothyroidism, dysphagia, hypersomnolence, and muscle stiffness. The diagnosis may be delayed for years. The IgG may be low.

Progressive external ophthalmoplegia may occur in isolation or in association with limb muscle weakness. Ptosis often precedes ophthalmoparesis which is followed by shoulder-girdle and pelvic-girdle muscle weakness. There is an autosomal dominant condition — oculopharyngeal dystrophy — which is characterized by progressive ptosis and loss of extra ocular movement, and which is accompanied by dysphagia, which occurs in later life (Rowland, 1975; Victor, Hayes, and Adams, 1962). The pathological changes in affected muscle are similar to those seen in elderly patients (Rebeiz, Caulfield, and Adams, 1969; Rebeiz *et al.*, 1972). These conditions are important in the differential diagnosis of other neurological diseases, e.g. myasthenia gravis and progressive supranuclear palsy.

Inflammatory myopathies

Polymyositis and dermatomyositis are characterized by weakness of neck flexors and limb girdle muscles progressing over several weeks or months. Muscle pain and tenderness may be present but are often absent. In dermatomyositis there is a lilac-tinged erythema of butterfly distribution on the face which also involves the periorbital region, shoulders, and extensor surfaces of hands and other joints. Serum creatine phosphokinase (CPK) and adolase are raised but the ESR is usually normal. The EMG shows short small polyphasic motor units, fibrillation potentials, and positive sharp waves. Muscle biopsy shows necrosis and phagocytosis in the perifascicular region, perifascicular atrophy, regeneration, and infiltration of connective tissue with round cells which may be perivascular. Polymyositis and dermatomyositis may be associated with other autoimmune diseases, systemic sclerosis, lupus erythematosis, and rheumatoid arthritis; and, particularly in the elderly, with malignant disease. In pure forms of the disease and in those associated with immune disorders there is evidence that the disease is due to an autoimmune process induced by mononuclear cells of thymic origin (Edwards *et al.*, 1981; Hudgson, and Walton, 1979; Morgan-Hughes, 1979).

Polymyalgia rheumatica (see Chapter 25.1) occurs in patients over 60 years of age and is characterized by muscle pain and stiffness in the shoulder-girdle muscles which is worse on waking and is associated with a raised ESR and normal CPK. The muscle biopsy may show type 2 fibre atrophy. The EMG is normal. The danger of this condition is in its association with temporal arteritis.

Granulomatous myositis may be due to sarcoidosis or polyarteritis nodosa. Sarcoidosis usually produces a slowly progressive limb-girdle weakness and polyarteritis nodosa is a particularly painful myopathy with patchy muscle infarction (Gardner-Thorpe, 1972).

Viral myositis is usually due to Echo or Coxsackie infections. The condition is characterized by severe muscle pain in limb-girdle and trunk muscles without weakness.

Periodic Paralyses

Familial periodic paralyses due to autosomal dominant inheritance and associated with hypo-, hyper-, and normokalaemia occur in children and young adults. It has been postulated that they are due to changes in sodium pump mechanisms in the sarcolemma, resulting in increased sodium and water in muscles during an attack (Bradley, 1975). The paralysis is a flaccid symmetrical weakness with areflexia. Secondary hypokalaemia can occur as a result of renal, endocrine, or gastrointestinal tract disease. Periodic weakness may occur in either familial or secondary cases after exercise, a heavy meal, anxiety, and cold. In familial cases the attacks gradually become less severe as the patient gets older (Boruma, and

Schipperheyn, 1979).

Potassium depletion in the elderly is a result of reduced physical activity, low potassium intake, stress, diuretics, laxatives, chronic renal failure, hypomagnesaemia, and iron, folate, or vitamin B12 deficiency (MacLennan, 1981). Although the serum potassium concentration does not adequately reflect the total body potassium, hypokalaemia is usually manifested by cardiac effects, dysrhythmias, and ECG changes, postural hypotension, depression, constipation; and muscle weakness, paralysis, and rhabdomyolysis (MacLennan, 1981).

Muscular weakness is a common presenting symptom in primary aldosteronism and periodic attacks of weakness can occur in this condition (Conn, 1955; Conn, Knopf, and Nesbit, 1964).

Endocrine and Metabolic Myopathies

Thyroid Disease (see Chapter 21)

Weakness was recognized as a symptom of hyperthyroidism in the classical description of the disease (Graves, 1835) and is found in 80 per cent. of patients (Havard *et al.*, 1963). The shoulder-girdle is particularly affected but progressive distal muscle weakness may be followed by 'acute thyrotoxic myopathy' characterized by bulbar symptoms of ptosis, dysphagia, and dysarthria accompanied by diarrhoea, vomiting, and atrial fibrillation.

Weakness is found in 40 per cent. of patients with hypothyroidism (Ramsay, 1974). A characteristic myopathy has been described (Norris and Panner, 1966). Myalgia is an early symptom, which is made worse when treatment is initiated. Proximal muscle weakness, stiffness, cramps, myotonia, and hypertrophy characterize the fully developed condition. The Achilles tendon reflex time is increased in 77 per cent. of patients with myxoedema (Lambert *et al.*, 1951). Myoedema, mounding after muscle percussion, occurs in some patients with hypothyroidism; it is painless and lasts for about one minute but is electrically silent (Salick, Colachis, and Pearson, 1968).

Pituitary Disease

In acromegaly, limb-girdle weakness is not uncommon and may be accompanied by raised serum CPK and hypertrophy of muscle fibres with high glycogen content (Mastaglia, Barwick, and Hall, 1970). The carpal tunnel syndrome is common (Pickett *et al.*, 1975).

Cushing's syndrome is often accompanied by limb-girdle weakness (Cushing, 1932; Müller, and Kugelberg, 1959). Undoubtedly this is due to steroid myopathy but severe myopathy follows adrenalectomy for Cushing's syndrome and is associated with high plasma ACTH; excessive lipid is found in type 1 fibres (Prineas *et al.*, 1968).

Osteomalacia and Hyperparathyroidism (see Chapter 25.2)

Proximal muscle weakness can occur with osteomalacia due to practically any cause. Muscle wasting is only ever slight and tendon reflexes may be increased; bone pain and tenderness are common and increase the disability (Schott, and Wills, 1976). Muscle weakness is more common in osteomalacia than it is in primary hyperparathyroidism (Smith, and Stern, 1967, 1969). The myopathy of hyperparathyroidism is similar to that of osteomalacia (Patten *et al.*, 1974) but the relationship is not clear; nor is the mechanism by which disordered calcium metabolism in these conditions produces the myopathy (Stern and Fagan, 1979).

Steroid Myopathy

This condition is a proximal myopathy indistinguishable from the myopathy of Cushing's syndrome (Perkoff *et al.*, 1959). There is type 2 fibre atrophy and the EMG shows classical myopathic features — short duration, low amplitude, polyphasic potentials — 9-alpha fluorine-substituted synthetic steroids seem to be more likely to produce myopathy. Stopping the drug usually produces recovery in up to one year and phenytoin has a value in preventing and treating steroid myopathy (Stern and Fagan, 1979).

Toxic Myopathies

Toxic myopathies are often associated with myoglobinuria and form a continuum from acute rhabdomyolysis, with severe muscle pain and tenderness, flaccid quadriparesis with areflexia, raised serum CPK, gross myoglobinuria, and renal failure; through acute/subacute painful proximal myopathy with proximal pain and tenderness, weakness and diminished reflexes; to subacute/chronic painless proximal myopathy with weakness, wasting and diminished reflexes, with normal CPK, and no myoglobinuria. Alcohol produces all these forms. Many drugs have been implicated in these disorders. Myasthenic and myotonic syndromes have also been described (Lane, and Mastaglia, 1978; Penn, 1979).

TRANSIENT GLOBAL AMNESIA

Originally described by Bender (1956), this syndrome of transient global amnesia (TGA) became more generally recognized following the description by Fisher, and Adams (1958, 1964).

Most attacks are single and usually occur in patients over the age of 50 years. The onset is sudden with repetitive stereotyped queries but retention of insight and identity. There is retrograde amnesia, initially for hours or days, and continuing loss of memory for all new information for possibly a few hours. The patient is confused and restless initially and despite recapitulation of the events occurring during the period of amnesia there remains a memory vacuum. The retrograde amnesia decreases over a period of time and may remit completely, but amnesia remains for the period of the attack itself. Immediate memory, recall, as tested by digit span, is unimpaired; thus, essentially, the attack affects recent memory but not immediate and remote memory (Shuttleworth and Morris, 1966). Motor performance is unimpaired during the attack and does not have the characteristics of the automatism of psychomotor epilepsy. The memory impairment is not associated with confabulation or other manifestations of Korsakow's syndrome, and differs from hysteria in that personal identity is retained. The attacks are similar to head injury but none can be detected and they are usually isolated phenomena.

The differential diagnosis is from toxi-confusional states, epilepsy, head injury, alcoholism, hypoglycaemia, encephalitis, migraine, and hysteria (Godwin-Austin, 1982).

TGA is usually benign and confined to a single attack but repeated episodes occur in some patients (Lou, 1968), and familial cases have been reported (Corston, and Godwin-Austin, 1982).

The EEG is usually normal but abnormalities over the temporal lobes have been described (Tharp, 1969) and there may be paroxysmal sharp and slow waves, particularly on the left (Wandless, 1981).

The memory loss has the characteristic pattern of the axial amnesic syndrome resulting from bilateral medial temporal lobe lesions affecting the hippocampus but not the mamillo-thalamic system (Ponsford, and Donnan, 1980; Scoville and Milner, 1957).

The posterior cerebral artery supplies the occipital lobe and the medial and basal parts of the temporal lobe, including the hippocampus. Bilateral posterior cerebral artery occlusions produce a permanent amnesic syndrome characterized by an inability to acquire new knowledge, a degree of retrograde amnesia but no long-term memory loss, with adequate intellectual function and no clouding of consciousness. In addition patients have considerable bilateral field defects with sparing of central vision (middle cerebral artery) and sparing of the pupillary light reflexes. Amnesia with alexia and without agraphia (often with colour agnosia) can follow a left posterior cerebral artery occlusion and may be temporary or permanent. Left temporal lobectomy can produce temporary or permanent amnesia (Benson, Marsden, and Meadows, 1974). However, there is some continuing doubt that isolated lesions of the left temporal lobe can produce amnesia.

Essentially the aetiology has been considered to be either ischaemic or epileptic (Whitty, 1977). However, the aetiology may be varied, to some extent, depending on the age of the patient.

Aetiology

(a) Cerebrovascular arteriosclerosis and temporary ischaemic attacks (Bolwig, 1968; Evans, 1966; Jensen, and Olivarus, 1980; Longridge, Hachinski, and Barber, 1979; Matthew, and Meyer, 1974)
(b) Epilepsy (Cantor, 1971; Deisenhammer, 1981; Fisher, 1982; Fisher, and Adams, 1964)
(c) Migraine (Caplan *et al.*, 1981; Evans, 1966; Gilbert, and Benson, 1972)

(d) Associated with brain tumour (Findler *et al.*, 1983)
(e) Cerebral angiography (Cochran *et al.*, 1982)
(f) Cardiac dysrhythmia (Dugan, Lordgren, and O'Leary, 1981; Greenlee, Crampton, and Miller, 1975)
(g) Diazepam intoxication (Gilbert and Benson, 1972)

Although TGA was originally considered to be a benign condition, and possibly cases associated with migraine carry a better prognosis, it has been shown that TGAs may be associated with transient ischaemic attacks of the vertebrobasilar system, completed stroke (Jensen, and Olivarus, 1980; Matthew, and Meyer, 1974), and, particularly in the more elderly, recurrent TGAs may lead to dementia.

SPECIAL INVESTIGATIONS

Brain Scanning

Scintiscan with 99^mTc pertechnetate remains a useful screening investigation despite the development of more sophisticated methods. Cerebral infarction is detectable between 2 and 8 weeks after onset (Glasgow *et al.*, 1965). Acute subdural haematoma, like acute infarction, is not easily detected but chronic subdural haematoma is detected in 90 per cent. of cases. Of space-occupying lesions 80 to 90 per cent. are recognized by scintiscan (MacDonald, 1981 Roberts, and Caird 1982).

Computerized Axial Tomography (CAT) Scan

This was developed in 1973 (Hounsfield, 1973) and has fully justified its early evaluation (Ambrose, 1973). Infarction, haemorrhage, and tumours are detectable and distinguishable by this technique (Cronquist *et al.*, 1975; Gawler *et al.*, 1974; Hayward, and O'Reilly, 1976; Yock, and Marshall, 1975). Intravenous sodium iothalamate contrast has improved its value in the identification of some lesions (Ambrose, Gooding, and Richardson, 1975) by increasing the density of vascular tissue. Infarction can be identified within 48 hours. Acute subdural haematomas are usually visible on the CAT scan but chronic subdural haematomas may have the same density as brain

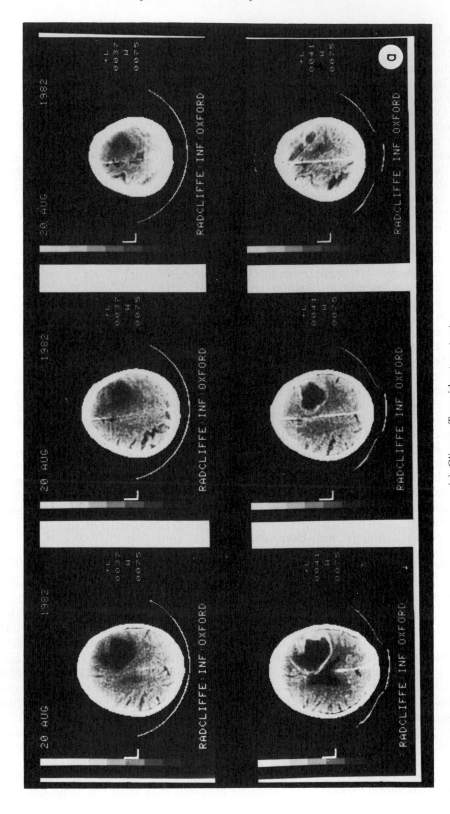

(a) Glioma. Top without contrast
Bottom with contrast

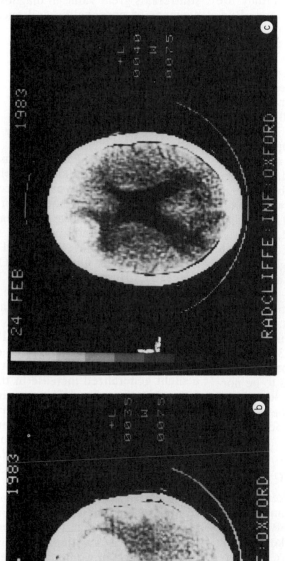

(c) Left frontal haematoma. Without contrast

(b) Meningioma (from anterior part of falx)

Figure 17 Computerized axial tomography. (Reproduced by permission of Dr Philip Sheldon)

and may be missed, particularly if they are bilateral (Galbraith *et al.*, 1976; Garcia-Bunuel, 1979). The pattern of haemorrhage is invaluable in identifying the source, particularly from aneurysms on the circle of Willis. Intracerebral haematomas can be identified and drained. It is increasingly recognized that clinical diagnoses are subject to error and many such, of infarction, are actually due to haemorrhage.

Ventricular size and cortical atrophy tend to increase with increasing age in the normal elderly (Barron, Jacobs, and Kinkel, 1976; Jacoby, Levy, and Dawson, 1980), but there is a more definite relationship between brain atrophy and cognitive impairment (Jacoby and Levy, 1980a; Roberts, and Caird, 1976). A type of endogenous depression of late life is associated with ventricular enlargement but not cortical atrophy (Jacoby, and Levy, 1980b).

In dementia the CAT scan identifies 10 per cent. of patients who have a 'treatable' structural lesion, 38 per cent. with cerebral atrophy (presumably Alzheimer's disease), 35 per cent. with cerebral infarction, and 16 per cent. of patients in whom the brain appears to be normal, suggesting another cause for 'dementia' (Bradshaw, Thomson, and Campbell, 1983). A degree of cerebral atrophy may occur without clinical dementia.

Nuclear Magnetic Resonance (NMR)

NMR imaging was being undertaken experimentally in the 1950s but clinical imaging, as such, did not really emerge until 1980 (Bydder, 1983; Holland, Moore, and Hawkes, 1980). Apart from the possibility to more accurate diagnosis of lesions identified by the CAT scan, this technique permits more accurate definition of structures in the brainstem and posterior fossa and is able to differentiate between grey and white matter, thus facilitating the diagnosis of degenerative brain disease (Doyle *et al.*, 1981).

Electroencephalography and Evoked Potentials

Although the electroencephalogram (EEG) has, in many respects, been superceded by the computerized axial tomography (CAT) scan it still retains great value in diagnoses and management of encephalitic and encephalopathic disorders:

Epilepsy
Virus encephalitis
Jacob–Creutzfeldt disease
Huntington's chorea
Alzheimer's disease
Progressive supranuclear palsy

The four classical EEG rhythms are present, but modified, in the elderly. Alpha rhythm (8 to 13 Hz), from the parieto-occipital areas, shows a decrease in frequency of 0.5 to 1 Hz each decade after the age of 60 years, but never falls below 8 Hz and is of lower frequency in males than in females (Busse, and Wang, 1979; McGeorge, 1981; Obrist, 1954; Otomo, 1966; Silverman, Busse, and Barnes, 1955; Wang, Obrist, and Busse, 1970). Voltage, persistence, and reactivity of alpha rhythm also decrease with age (Spehlman, 1981), as does alpha blocking (Otomo, and Tsubaki, 1966).

Theta activity (4 to 7 Hz) and delta activity (0 to 3 Hz) can occur normally at any site and a slight generalized increase in theta waves is normal in those aged 75 years and over; but many elderly show episodic, irregular, slow activity in the theta and delta range, particularly in the temporal areas, predominantly the left anterior temporal (Busse *et al.*, 1954; Obrist, 1954; Obrist, Eisdorfer, and Kleemeier, 1962; Obrist *et al.*, 1963).

Beta activity (>13 Hz) is common in the frontal region but can occur normally in all areas. Incidence and persistence of beta rhythm increases with increasing age and is more common in women than men (Hubbard, Sunde, and Goldensohn, 1976; Silverman, Busse, and Barnes, 1955).

General illness can produce slowing, particularly of alpha activity. In dementia, the basic frequency is usually less than 8 Hz and is related to the severity of intellectual impairment (Roberts, McGeorge, and Caird, 1978), and focal slow waves superimposed on this slow background activity suggest arteriosclerosis as a cause of the dementia.

Slowing of alpha activity is related to decreased cerebral oxygen consumption and cerebral blood flow, which indicate decreased cerebral metabolism (Obrist *et al.*, 1963).

In the elderly, diffuse, slow, and mixed abnormal EEGs are associated with low blood pressure and decompensated heart disease; normal EEGs are associated with mild hypertension (Obrist *et al.*, 1963; Wang and Busse, 1974). In this context, however, sustained severe hypertension is associated with intellectual impairment (Wilkie, and Eisdorfer, 1971).

In dementia, the episodic irregular theta and delta activity of the temporal areas, and predominantly the left side, found in the normal ageing patient, is much more accentuated and spreads from the anterior temporal areas to the mid and posterior temporal areas (Barnes, Busse, and Friedman, 1956). Continuous generalized theta activity and generalized delta waves also occur in dementia, and life expectancy is related to the degree of slowing (Müller, Grad, and Engelsmann, 1975).

Persistence and amplitude of beta activity may be excessive in patients who are taking sedatives, e.g. barbiturates and benzodiazepines, and with anxiety. Fast activity disappears in very old age but this is probably due to cerebral atrophy.

Large space-occupying lesions produce localized non-specific slowing of the alpha rhythm. Meningiomas are often associated with spike activity. Cerebral infarction is manifest by localized loss of activity. Cerebral abscesses show slow delta waves.

Spike and wave activity associated with a fit is diagnostic of epilepsy. Spike and wave paroxysms may occur in the interictal state and confirm the diagnosis, but they can be found in patients without clinical epilepsy.

In metabolic and toxic encephalopathic disorders, hepatic, renal, and hypoglycaemic, there is a tendency to marked slowing which correlates with the severity and level of consciousness. Asynchronous slow waves are common in Parkinson's disease and Alzheimer's disease. Bisynchronous slow waves occur in developed progressive supranuclear palsy (Su, and Goldensohn, 1973). In encephalitic disorders there is similar slowing, but activity tends to be of a high amplitude (Mitchell, 1983).

Huntington's chorea is characterized by a flat, featureless record and loss of any alpha rhythm. Jacob–Creutzfeldt disease is accompanied by generalized slow waves of a high amplitude at a rate of 1 Hz.

Evoked potentials, visual, auditory, and somato-sensory, have been shown to be of great help in the early diagnosis of multiple sclerosis, but their value would be limited in the elderly with multiple sensory and neurological problems (Mastaglia, and Carroll, 1982) although they may have value in patients with dementia (Goodin, Squires, and Starr, 1978).

REFERENCES

Adams, J. H. (1976). 'Virus diseases of the nervous system', in *Greenfield's Neuropathology* (Eds W. Blackwood and J. A. N. Corsellis), pp. 292–326, Edward Arnold, London.

Adams, H., and Miller, D. (1973). 'Herpes simplex encephalitis: A clinical and pathological analysis of twenty-two cases', *Postgrad. Med. J.*, **49**, 393–397.

Adams, R. D. (1966). 'Further observations on normal pressure hydrocephalus', *Proc. Roy. Soc. Med.*, **59**, 1135–1140.

Adams, R. D. (1968). 'The striatonigral degenerations', in *Handbook of Neurology* (Eds P. J. Vinken and G. W. Bruyn), Vol. 6, pp. 694–702, North-Holland, Amsterdam.

Adams, R. D. (1975). 'Recent observations on normal pressure hydrocephalus', *Schweiz. Arch. Neurol. Neurochir. Psychiatr.*, **116**, 7–15.

Adams, R. D., van Bogaert, L., and Van der Eecken, H. (1961). 'Dégénérescences nigro-striées et cèrèbello-nigro-striées', *Psychiatria et Neurologia (Basel)*, **142**, 219–259.

Adams, R. D., van Bogaert, L., and Van der Eecken, H. (1964). 'Striato-nigral degeneration', *J. Neuropath. Exp. Neurol.*, **23**, 584–608.

Adams, R. D., Fisher, C. M., Hakim, S., Ojemann, R. G., and Sweet, W. H. (1965). 'Symptomatic occult hydrocephalus with "normal" cerebrospinal-fluid pressure. A treatable syndrome', *New Engl. J. Med.*, **273**, 117–126.

Alajouanine, T., Delafontaine, P., and Lacan, J. (1926). 'Fixité du regard par hypertonie, prédominant dans le sens vertical avec conservation des mouvements automatico-réflexes', *Rev. Neurol.*, **33**(ii), 410–419.

Albert, M. L., Feldman, R. G., and Willis, A. L. (1974). 'The "subcortical dementia" of progressive supranuclear palsy', *J. Neurol. Neurosurg. Psychiatr.*, **37**, 121–130.

Alkesic, S. M., Budzilovich, G. N., and Lieberman, A. N. (1973). 'Herpes zoster oticus and facial paralysis (Ramsay Hunt syndrome): Clinicopathologic study and review of literature', *J. Neurol. Sci.*, **20**, 149–159.

Allison, R. S. (1962). *The Senile Brain. A Clinical Study*, Edward Arnold, London.

Allison, R. S. (1966). 'Perseveration as a sign of diffuse and focal brain damage', *Br. Med. J.*, 2, 1027–1032, 1095–1101.

Allison, R. S., and Hurwitz, L. J. (1967). 'On perseveration in aphasics', *Brain*, 90, 429–448.

Almeida, J. D., Howatson, A. F., and Williams, M. G. (1962). 'Morphology of varicella (chickenpox) virus', *Virology*, 16, 353–355.

Ambrose, J. (1973). 'Computerised transverse axial scanning (tomography). 2. Clinical application', *Br. J. Radiol.*, 46, 1023–1047.

Ambrose, J., Gooding, M. R., and Richardson, A. E. (1975). 'Sodium iothalamate as an aid to diagnosis of intracranial lesions by computerised transverse axial scanning', *Lancet*, 2, 669–674.

André-Thomas, (1905). 'Atrophie lamellaire des cellules de Purkinje', *Rev. Neurol.*, 13, 917–924.

Andrew, J., and Nathan, P. W. (1964). 'Lesions of the anterior frontal lobes and disturbances of micturition and defaecation', *Brain*, 87, 233–262.

Annegers, J. F., Schoenberg, B. S., Okazaki, H., and Kurland, L. T. (1980). 'Primary intracranial neoplasms in Rochester, Minnesota', in *Clinical Neuroepidemiology* (Ed. F. Clifford Rose), pp. 366–371, Pitman, Tunbridge Wells.

Aran, F. A. (1850). 'Recherches sur un maladie non encore décrite du système musculaire: Atrophie musculaire progressive', *Arch. Gén. Méd.*, 4 Ser. 24, 172–214.

Argov, Z., and Mastaglia, F. L. (1979). 'Drug-induced peripheral neuropathies', *Br. Med. J.*, 1, 663–666.

Arnold, N., and Harriman, D. G. F. (1970). 'The incidence of abnormality in control human peripheral nerves studied by single axon dissection', *J. Neurol. Neurosurg. Psychiat.*, 33, 55–61.

Arundell, F. D., Wilkinson, R. D., and Haserick, J. R. (1960). 'Dermatomyositis and malignant neoplasms in adults', *Arch. Derm.*, 82, 722–725.

Asbury, A. K., Arnason, B. G., and Adams, R. D. (1969). 'The inflammatory lesion in idiopathic polyneuritis: Its role in pathogenesis', *Medicine (Baltimore)*, 48, 173–215.

Aström, K-E., Mancall, E. L., and Richardson, E. P. (1958). 'Progressive multifocal leukoencephalopathy, a hitherto unrecognised complication of chronic lymphatic leukaemia and Hodgkin's disease', *Brain*, 81, 93–111.

Austin, J. H. (1958). 'Recurrent polyneuropathies and their corticosteroid treatment', *Brain*, 81, 157–192.

Baerensprung, von (1863). 'Beiträge zur Kenntnifs der Zoster (Dritte Folge)', *Charité-Annales*, 11, 96–116.

Bannister, R., Gilford, E., and Kocen, R. (1967). 'Isotope encephalography in the diagnosis of de-mentia due to communicating hydrocephalus', *Lancet*, 2, 1014–1017.

Bannister, R., and Oppenheimer, D. R. (1972). 'Degenerative dieases of the nervous system associated with autonomic failure', *Brain*, 95, 457–474.

Bannister, R., and Oppenheimer, D. R. (1982). 'Parkinsonism, system degeneration and autonomic failure', in *Movement Disorders. Neurology*, 2, (Eds C. D. Marsden and S. Fahn), pp. 174–190, Butterworths, London.

Barnes, R. H., Busse, E. W., and Friedman, E. L. (1956). 'The psychological functioning of aged individuals with normal and abnormal electroencephalograms: A study of hospitalized individuals', *J. Nerv. Ment. Dis.*, 124, 583–593.

Barron, S. A., Jacobs, L., and Kinkel, W. R. (1976). 'Changes in size of normal lateral ventricles during aging determined by computerized tomography', *Neurology*, 26, 1011–1013.

Becker, P. E., and Kiener, F. (1955). 'Eine neue X-chromasomale Muskeldystrophie', *Archiv. für Psychiatrie und Nervenkrank*, 193, 427–448.

Beebe, J. W., and Kutzke, J. F. (1969). 'Herpes zoster and multiple sclerosis', *Br. Med. J.*, IV, 303.

Behrman, S., Caroll, J. D. Janota, I., and Matthews, W. B. (1969). 'Progressive supranuclear palsy. Clinico-pathological study of four cases', *Brain*, 92, 663–678.

Behrman, S., and Knight, G. (1954). 'Herpes simplex associated with trigeminal neuralgia', *Neurology*, 4, 525–530.

Bender, M. B. (1956). 'Syndrome of isolated episode of confusion with amnesia', *Journal of the Hillside Hospital*, 5, 212–215.

Benson, D. F., Marsden, C. D., and Meadows, J. C. (1974). 'The amnesic syndrome of posterior cerebral artery occlusion', *Acta. Neurol. Scand.*, 50, 133–145.

Ben-Yishay, Y., Diller, L., Gerstman, L., and Haas, A. (1968). 'The relationship between impersistence, intellectual function and outcome of rehabilitation in patients with left hemiplegia', *Neurology (Minneap.)*, 18, 852–861.

Bertrand, I., and van Bogaert, L. (1925). 'Rapport sur la sclérose latéralle amyotrophique. Anatomie pathalogique', *Rev. Neurol.*, 1779–806.

Bhatia, S. P., and Irvine, R. E. (1973). 'Electrical recording of the ankle jerk in old age', *Geront. Clin. (Basel)*, 15, 357–360.

Bielschowsky, A. (1935). 'Lectures on motor anomalies of the eyes. III. Paralyses of the conjugate movements of the eyes', *Arch. Ophthalmol.*, 13, 569–583.

Bird, E. D., and Iversen, L. L. (1974). 'Huntington's chorea, post-mortem measurement of glutamic acid decarboxylase, choline acetyltransferase and dopamine in basal ganglia', *Brain,* **97**, 457–472.

Blumenthal, H., and Miller, C. (1969). 'Motor nuclear involvement in progressive supranuclear palsy', *Arch. Neurol.*, **20**, 362–367.

Boelhouwer, A. J. W., and Brunia, C. H. M. (1977). 'Blink reflexes and the state of arousal', *J. Neurol. Neurosurg. Psychiatry*, **40**, 58–63.

Boger, W. P., Wright, L. D., Strickland, S. C., Gylfe, J. S., and Ciminera, J. L. (1955). 'Vitamin B12: Correlation of serum concentration and age', *Proc. Soc. Expl. Biol. (NY)*, **89**, 375–378.

Bolwig, T. G. (1968). 'Transient flobal amnesia', *Acta. Neurol. Scand.*, **44**, 101–106.

Bonduelle, M. (1975). 'Amyotrophic lateral sclerosis', in *Handbook of Clinical Neurology* (Eds P. J. Vinken and G. W. Bruyn), Vol. 22, pp. 281–338, North-Holland, Amsterdam.

Boruma, O. J. S., and Schipperheyn, J. J. (1979). 'Periodic paralysis', in *Handbook of Clinical Neurology* (Eds P. J. Vinken and G. W. Bruyn), Vol. 41, pp. 147–174, North-Holland, Amsterdam.

Botez, M. I., Léveillé, J., Berube, L., and Botez-Marquard, T. (1975). 'Occult disorders of cerebrospinal fluid dynamics. Early diagnosis criteria', *Eur. Neurol.*, **13**, 203–223.

Bradley, W. G. (1975). 'Inherited disease of skeletal muscle', in *Recent Advances in Clinical Neurology* (Ed. W. B. Matthews), Vol. 1, pp. 284–331, Churchill Livingstone, Edinburgh.

Bradley, W. G. (1979), 'The limb-girdle syndromes', in *Handbook of Clinical Neurology* (Eds P. J. Vinken and G. W. Bruyn), Vol. 40, pp. 433–469, North-Holland, Amsterdam.

Bradshaw, J. R., Thomson, J. L. G., and Campbell, M. J. (1983). 'Computed tomography in the investigation of dementia', *Br. Med. J.*, **286**, 277–280.

Brain, W. R. (1965). 'Introduction', in *The Remote Effects of Cancer on the Nervous System* (Eds W. R. Brain and F. H. Norres), pp. 1–4, Grune and Stratton, New York.

Brain, W. R., Daniel, P. M., and Greenfield, J. G. (1951). 'Subacute cortical cerebellar degeneration and its relation to carcinoma', *J. Neurol. Neurosurg. Psychiat.*, **14**, 59–75.

Brain, W. R., and Henson, R. A. (1958). 'Neurological syndromes associated with carcinoma', *Lancet*, **2**, 971–974.

Brain, W. R., and Walton, J. N. (1969). *Brain's Diseases of the Nervous System*, VIIth ed., pp. 160–164, Oxford University Press, London.

Brain, W. R., Wright, A. D., and Wilkinson, M. (1947). 'Spontaneous compression of both median nerves in the carpal tunnel', *Lancet*, **1**, 277–282.

Briggs, M. (1978). 'Raised intracranial pressure with particular reference to normal pressure hydrocephalus', in *Recent Advances in Clinical Neurol-*ogy, **2**, (Eds W. B. Matthews and G. H. Glaser), pp. 129–143, Churchill Livingstone, Edinburgh.

Broadbent, W. H. (1866). 'Case of herpetic eruption in the course of the branches of the brachial plexus, followed by partial paralysis in corresponding motor nerves', *Br. Med. J.*, **2**, 460.

Brostoff, J. (1966). 'Diaphragmatic paralysis after herpes zoster', *Br. Med. J.*, **2**, 1571–1572.

Brown, S. (1892). 'On hereditary ataxy, with a series of twenty-one cases', *Brain*, **15**, 250–268.

Brownell, B., Oppenheimer, D. R., and Hughes, J. T. (1970). 'The central nervous system in motor neurone disease', *J. Neurol. Neurosurg. Psuchiat.*, **33**, 338–357.

Brunner, A., and Norris, T. W. (1971). 'Age-related changes in caloric nystagmus', *Acta. Otolaryngol. (Stockh.)*, **282**(Suppl.), 5–24.

Bruyn, G. W. (1979). 'Carcinomatous polyneuropathy', in *Handbook of Clinical Neurology* (Eds F. J. Vinken, G. W. Bruyn), Vol. 38, pp. 679–693, North-Holland, Amsterdam.

Buchthal, F., and Rosenfalck, A. (1966). 'Evoked action potentials and conduction volocity in human sensory nerves', *Brain Res.*, **3**, 1–122.

Bucy, P. C., and Case, T. J. (1939). 'Tremor. Physiologic mechanism and abolition by surgical means', *Arch. Neurol.*, **41**, 721–746.

Busse, E. W., Barnes, R. H., Silverman, A. J., Shy, M. G., Thaler, M., and Frost, L. L. (1954). 'Studies of the processes of ageing: Factors that influence the psyche of elderly persons', *Am. J. Psychiat.*, **110**, 897–903.

Busse, E. W., and Wang, H. S. (1979). 'The electroencephalographic changes in late life: A longitudinal study', *J. Clin. Exp. Geront.*, **1**, 145–158.

Butler, R. C., Gawel, M., Rose, F. C., and Sloper, J. C. (1977). 'Muscle biopsy in motor neurone disease', in *Motor Neurone Disease* (Ed. F. Clifford Rose), pp. 79–93, Pitman, London.

Buzzard, E. F., and Barnes S. (1906). 'A case of chronic progressive double hemiplegia', *Rev. Neurol. Psychiat.*, **4**, 182–191.

Bydder, G. M. (1983). 'Clinical nuclear magnetic resonance in aging', *Br. J. Hosp. Med.*, **29**(4), 348–356.

Campbell, M. J., McComas, A. J., and Petito, F. (1973). 'Physiological changes in ageing muscles', *J. Neurol. Neurosurg. Psychiat.*, **36**, 174–182.

Cantor, F. K. (1971). 'Transient global amnesia and temporal lobe seizures', *Neurology (Minneap.)*, **21**, 430–431.

Caplan, L., Chedru, F., Lhermitte, F., and Mayman, C. (1981). 'Transient global manesia in migraine', *Neurology (NY)*, **31**, 1167–1170.

Carlson, K. E., Alston, W., and Feldman, D. J. (1964). 'Electromyographic study of ageing in skeletal muscle', *Am. J. Phys. Med.*, **43**, 141–145.

Carroll, J. E. (1979). 'Facioscapulohumeral and scapuloperoneal syndromes', in *Handbook of Clinical Neurology* (Eds P. J. Vinken and G. W. Bruyn), Vol. 40, pp. 415–431, North-Holland, Amsterdam.

Carroll, J. E., and Brooke, M. H. (1978). 'Pathophysiology of diseases affecting muscle', in *Neurological Pathophysiology* (Eds S. G. Eliasson, A. L. Prensky, and W. B. Hardin), 2nd ed., pp. 83–108, Oxford University Press, New York.

Carton, C. A., and Kilbourne, E. D. (1952). 'Activation of latent herpes simplex by trigeminal and sensory root section', *New Engl. J. Med.*, **246**, 172–176.

Cauna, N. (1964). 'The effects of ageing on the receptor organs of the human dermis', in *Aging*, Vol 6, *Advances in Biology of Skin* (Ed. W. Montagna), pp. 63–96, Pergamon, New York.

Cavanagh, J. B. (1964). 'The significance of the 'dying-back' process in experimental and human neurological disease', *Int. Rev. Exptl. Pathol.*, **7**, 219–267.

Cavanagh, J. B. (1968). 'Organo-phosphorus neurotoxicity and the 'dying back process', in *Motor Neuron Diseases* (Eds F. H. Norris and L. T. Kurland), pp. 292–300, Grune and Stratton, New York.

Cavanagh, J. B., Greenbaum, D., Marshall, A. H. E., and Rubinstein, L. J. (1959). 'Cerebral demyelination associated with disorders of the reticuloendothelial system', *Lancet*, **2**, 524–529.

Chamberlain, W. (1970). 'Restriction in upward gaze with advancing age', *Trans. Am. Ophthalmol. Soc.*, **68**, 233–244.

Charcot, J. M., and Joffroy, A. (1869). 'Deux cas d'atrophie musculaire progressive avec lésions de la substance grise et des faisceaux antérolatéraux de la moelle épinière', *Arch. Physiol. (Paris)*, **2**, 354–367, 629–649, 744–760.

Chavany, J. A., van Bogaert, L., and Godlewski, S. (1951). 'Sur un syndrome de rigidité à prédominance axiale, avec perturbation des automatismes oculo-palpebraux d'origine encéphalitique', *Presse Med.*, **59**, 958–962.

Chisholm, I. A. (1972). 'The dyschromatopsia of pernicious anaemia', *Mod. Probl. Ophthal.*, **11**, 130–135.

Chisholm, I. A. (1979). 'Anaemia: General and neuro-ophthalmic features', in *Handbook of Clinical Neurology* (Eds P. J. Vinken and G. W. Bruyn), Vol. 38, pp. 15–32, North-Holland, Amsterdam.

Clavaria, L. E., du Boulay, G. H., and Moseley, I. F. (1976). 'Intracranial infections: Investigation by computerized axial tomography', *Neuroradiology*, **12**, 59–71.

Cobb, W. A. (1975). 'Electroencephalographic changes in viral encephalitis', in *Viral Diseases of the Nervous System* (Ed. L. S. Illis), pp. 76–89, Bailliere Tindall, London.

Cochran, J. W., Morrell, F., Huckman, M. S., and Cochran, E. J. (1982). 'Transient global manesia after cerebral angiography. Report of seven cases', *Arch. Neurol.*, **39**, 593–594.

Colmant, H. J. (1975). 'Progressive bulbar palsy in adults', in *Handbook of Clinical Neurology* (Eds P. J. Vinken and G. W. Bruyn), Vol. 22, pp. 111–156, North-Holland, Amsterdam.

Conn, J. W. (1955). 'Primary aldosteronism, a new clinical syndrome', *J. Lab. Clin. Med*, **45**, 6–17.

Conn, J. W., Knopf, R. F., and Nesbit, R. M. (1964). 'Clinical characteristics of primary aldosteronism for an analysis of 145 cases', *Am. J. Surg.*, **107**, 159–172.

Cooper, R. M., Blaish, I., and Zubek, J. P. (1959). 'The effect of age on taste sensitivity', *J. Gerontol.*, **14**, 56–58.

Corbin, K. B., and Gardner, E. D. (1937). 'Decrease in number of myelinated fibres in human spinal roots with age', *Anat. Rec.*, **68**, 63–74.

Corin, M. S., Elizan, T. S., and Bender, M. B. (1972). 'Oculomotor function in patients with Parkinson's disease', *J. Neurol. Sci.*, **15**, 251–265.

Cornil, L., and Kissel, P. (1929). 'Syndrome extrapyramidal avec paralysie verticale du regard et conservation des mouvements automatico-réflexes', *Rev. Neurol.*, **36**(i), 1189–1191.

Corsellis, J. A. N., Goldberg, G. J., and Norton, A. R. (1968). 'Limbic encephalitis and its association with carcinoma', *Brain*, **91**, 481–496.

Corso, J. F. (1971). 'Sensory processes and age effects in adults', *J. Gerontol.*, **26**, 90–105.

Corston, R. N., and Godwin-Austin, R. B. (1982). 'Transient global amnesia in four brothers', *J. Neurol. Neurosurg. Psychiat.*, **45**, 375–377.

Cosh, J. A. (1953). 'Studies on the nature of vibration sense', *Clin. Sci.*, **12**, 131–151.

Cragg, B., and Thomas, P. K. (1964). 'The conduction velocity of regenerated peripheral nereve', *J. Physiol.*, **171**, 164–175.

Critchley, M. (1929). 'Arteriosclerotic Parkinsonism', *Brain*, **52**, 23–83.

Critchley, M. (1931). 'The neurology of old age', *Lancet*, **1**, 1119–1127, 1221–1230, 1331–1337.

Critchley, M. (1949). 'Observations on essential (heredofamilial) tremor', *Brain*, **72**(2), 113–139.

Critchley, M. (1956). 'Neurological changes in the aged', *J. Chronic Dis.*, **3**, 459–477.

Critchley, M., and Greenfield, J. G. (1948). 'Olivo-ponto-cerebellar atrophy', *Brain*, **71**, 343–364.

Croft, P. B., Henson, R. A., Urich, H., and Wilkinson, P. C. (1965). 'Sensory neuropathy with bronchial carcinoma. A study of four cases showing serological abnormalities', *Brain*, **88**, 501–514.

Croft, P. B., Urich, H., and Wilkinson, M. (1967). 'Peripheral neuropathy of sensorimotor type associated with malignant disease', *Brain*, **90**, 31–66.

Croft, P. B., and Wilkinson, M. (1965). 'The incidence of carcinomatous neuropathy with special reference to carcinoma of the lung and the breast', in *The Remote Effects of Cancer on the Nervous System* (Eds W. R. Brain and F. H. Norres), pp. 44–54, Grune and Stratton, New York.

Cronquist, S., Brismar, J., Kjellin, K., and Söderström, C. F. (1975). 'Computer-assisted axial tomography in cerebrovascular lesions', *Acta. Radiol.*, **16**, 135–145.

Cruveilhier, J. (1853). 'Sur la paralysie musculaire progressive atrophique', *Arch. Gén. Méd.*, 5 Ser. **1**, 561–603.

Cruz Martinez, A., Barrio, M., Perez Conde, M. C., and Gutierrez, A. M. (1978). 'Electrophysiological aspects of sensory conduction velocity in healthy adults', *J. Neurol. Neurosurg. Psychiat.*, **41**(12), 1092–1096.

Cushing, H. (1932). 'The basophil adenomas of the pituitary body and their clinical manifestations (pituitary basophilism)', *Bull. Johns Hopkins Hosp.*, **50**, 137–195.

Cutler, R. W. P., Page, L., Galicich, J., and Watters, G. V. (1968). 'Formation and absorption of cerebrospinal fluid in man', *Brain*, **91**, 707–720.

Dana, C. L. (1887). 'Hereditary tremor, a hitherto undescribed form of motor neurosis', *Am. J. Med. Sci.*, **94**, 386–393.

Dandy, W. E. (1919). 'Experimental hydrocephalus', *Ann. Surg.*, **70**, 129–142.

Dandy, W. E., and Blackfan, K. D. (1913). An experimental and clinical study of internal hydrocephalus', JAMA, **61**, 2216–2217.

Danielczyk, W., Riederer, P., and Seemann, D. (1980). 'Benign and malignant types of Parkinson's disease: Clinical and patho-physiological characterization', *J. Neural. Transm. (Suppl.)*, **16**, 199–210.

Daly, D. D., Svien, H. J., and Yoss, R. E. (1961). 'Intermittent cerebral symptoms with meningiomas', *Arch. Neurol.*, **5**, 287–293.

Dalziel, J. A., and Griffiths, R. A. (1977). 'Progressive supranuclear palsy', *Age and Ageing*, **6**, 185–191.

Davidenkow, S. (1939). 'Scapulo-peroneal amyotrophy', *Arch. Neurol. Psychiat. (Chicago)*, **41**, 694–701.

Davis, L. E. (1925). 'Decerebrate rigidity in man', *Arch. Neurol. Psychiat. (Chicago)*, **13**, 569–579.

Davison, C. (1941). 'Amyotrophic lateral sclerosis. Origin and extent of the upper motor neurone lesion', *Arch. Neurol. (Chicago)*, **46**, 1039–1056.

Davson, H. (1967). *Physiology of the Cerebrospinal Fluid*, Churchill, London.

Davson, H., Hollingsworth, G., and Segal, M. B. (1970). 'The mechanism of drainage of the cerebrospinal fluid', *Brain*, **93**, 665–678.

Dayan, A. D., Ogul, E., and Graveson, G. S. (1972). 'Polyneuritis and herpes zoster', *J. Neurol. Neurosurg. Psychiat.*, **35**, 170–175.

Dayan, A. D., and Stokes, M. I. (1973). 'Rapid diagnosis of encephalitis by immunofluorescent examination of cerebrospinal fluid cells', *Lancet*, **1**, 177–179.

Dehen, H., Willer, J. C., Bathien, N., and Cambier, J. (1976). 'Blink reflex in hemiplegia', *Electroenceph. Clin. Neurophys.*, **40**, 393–400.

Deisenhammer, E. (1981). 'Transient global manesia as an epileptic manifestation', *J. Neurol.*, **225**, 289–292.

Dejerine, J., and Thomas, A. (1900). 'L'atrophie olivo-ponto-cérébelleuse', *Nouv. Iconogr. Salpêt.*, **13**, 330–370.

Denny-Brown, D. (1948). 'Primary sensory neuropathy with muscular changes associated with carcinoma', *J. Neurol. Neurosurg. Psychiat.*, **11**, 73–87.

Denny-Brown, D. (1962). *The Basal Ganglia*, Oxford University Press.

Denny-Brown, D., Adams, R. D., and Fitzgerald, P. J. (1944). 'Pathological features of herpes zoster: A note on "geniculate herpes"', *Arch. Neurol. Psychiat. (Chicago)*, **51**, 216–231.

De Renzi, E., and Vignolo, L. A. (1969). 'L-dopa for progressive supranuclear palsy', *Lancet*, **2**, 1360.

Dix, M. R., Harrison, M. J. G., and Lewis, P. D. (1971). 'Progressive supranuclear palsy. A report of 9 cases with particular reference to the mechanism of the oculomotor disorder', *J. Neurol. Sci.*, **13**, 237–256.

Dohrmann, P. J., and Elrick, W. L. (1982). 'Dementia and hydrocephalus in Paget's disease: A case report', *J. Neurol. Neurosurg. Psychiat.*, **45**, 835–837.

Dorfman, L. J., and Bosley, T. M. (1979). 'Age-related changes in peripheral and central nerve conduction in man', *Neurology*, **29**(1), 38–44.

Downie, A. W. (1965). ' "Misery in the hand" — the carpal tunnel syndrome', *North Carolina Med. J.*, **26**, 487–493.

Downie, A. (1982). 'Peripheral nerve compression syndromes', in *Recent Advances in Clinical Neurology* (Eds W. B. Matthews and G. H. Glaser), Vol. 3, pp. 47–66, Churchill Livingstone, Edinburgh.

Doyle, F. H., Pennock, J. M., Orr, J. S., Gore, J. C., Bydder, G. M., Steiner, R. E., Young, I. R., Clow, H., Bailes, D. R., Burl, M., Gilderdale, D. J., and Walters, P. E. (1981). 'Imaging of the brain by nuclear magnetic resonance', *Lancet*, **2**, 53–57.

Duchenne, G. (1853). 'Étude comparée des lésions anatomiques dans l'atrophie musculaire progressive et dans la paralysie générale', *Union. Méd.*, **7**, 202.

Duchenne, G. (1860). 'Paralysis musculaire progressive de la langue, due voile du palais et des lèvres', *Arch. Gén. Méd.*, **16**, 283–296.

Duchenne, G. B. (1868). 'Recherches sur la paralysie musculaire pseudohypertrophique, ou paralysie myosclérosique', *Arch. Gén. Méd.* (6 Ser.), **11**, 5–25, 179–209, 305–321, 421–443, 552–588, 868.

Dugan, T. M., Nordgren, R. E., and O'Leary, P. (1981). 'Transient global amnesia associated with bradycardia and temporal lobe spikes', *Cortex*, **17**, 633–638.

Durham, R. H. (1960). *Encyclopedia of Medical Syndromes*, p. 261, Harper and Row, New York.

Dyck, P. J., and Lambert, E. H. (1969). 'Dissociated sensation in amyloidosis', *Arch. Neurol.*, **20**, 490–507.

Eadie, M. J. (1975a). 'Hereditary spastic ataxia', in *Handbook of Clinical Neurology* (Eds P. J. Vinken and G. W. Bruyn), Vol. 21, pp. 365–381, North-Holland, Amsterdam.

Eadie, M. J. (1975b). 'Cerebello-olivary atrophy (Holmes type)', in *Handbook of Clinical Neurology* (Eds P. J. Vinken and G. W. Bruyn), Vol. 21, pp. 403–414, North-Holland, Amsterdam.

Eadie, M. J. (1975c). 'Olivo-ponto-cerebellar atrophy (Dejerine–Thomas type)' in *Handbook of Neurology* (Eds P. J. Vinken and G. W. Bruyn), Vol. 21, pp. 415–431, North-Holland, Amsterdam.

Eaton, L. M., and Lambert, E. H. (1957). 'Electromyography and electric stimulation of nerves in diseases of motor unit: Observations on myasthenic syndrome associated with malignant tumours', JAMA, **163**, 1117–1124.

Edwards, R. H. T., Isenberg, D. A., Wiles, C. M., Young, A., and Snaith, M. L. (1981). 'The investigation of inflammatory myopathy', *J. Ray. Coll. Phys. Lond.*, **15**, 19–24.

Ekbom, K., Greitz, T., and Kugelberg, E. (1969). 'Hydrocephalus due to ectasia of the basilar artery', *J. Neurol. Sci.*, **8**, 465–477.

El-Baradi, A. F., and Bourne, G. H. (1951). 'Theory of tastes and odours', *Science*, **113**, 660–661.

Elble, R. J., and Randall, J. E. (1976). 'Motor-unit activity responsible for 8- to 12-Hz component of human physiological finger tremor', *J. Neurophysiol.*, **39**, 370–383.

Elion, G. B. (1982). 'Mechanism of action, pharmacology and clinical efficacy of acyclovir', in *Herpesvirus, Clinical, Pharmacological and Basic Aspects* (Eds H. Shiota, Y-C. Cheng, and W. H. Prussof), pp. 229–235, Excerpta Medica, Amsterdam.

Elmqvist, D., Hofmann, W. W., Kugelberg, J., and Quastel, D. M. J. (1964). 'An electrophysiological investigation of neuromuscular transmission in myasthenia gravis', *J. Physiol.*, **174**, 417–434.

Elmqvist, D., and Lambert, E. H. (1968). 'Detailed analysis of neuromuscular transmission in a patient with the myasthenic syndrome, sometimes associated with bronchogenic carcinoma', *Mayo Clin. Proc.*, **43**, 689–713.

Enzmann, D. R., Ranson, B., Norman, D., and Talberth, E. (1978). 'Computed tomography of herpes simplex encephalitis', *Neuroradiology*, **129**, 419–425.

Ermini, M. (1976). 'Aging changes in mammalian skeletal muscle', *Gerontology*, **22**, 301–316.

Esiri, M., and Tomlinson, A. H. (1972). 'Herpes zoster. Demonstration of virus in trigeminal nerve and ganglion by immunofluorescence and electron microscopy', *J. Neurol. Sci.*, **15**, 35–48.

Estaban, A., and Giménez-Roldán, S. (1975). 'Blink reflexes in Huntington's chorea and Parkinson's Disease', *Acta. Neurol. Scand.*, **52**, 145–157.

Evans, J. H. (1966). 'Transient loss of memory, an organic mental syndrome', *Brain*, **89**, 539–548.

Fambrough, D. M., Drachman, D. B., and Satyamurti, S. (1973). 'Neuromuscular junction in myasthenia gravis: Decreased acetylcholine receptors', *Science*, **182**, 293–295.

Ferguson, I. T., Lenman, J. A. R., and Johnston, B. B. (1978). 'Habituation of the orbicularis oculi reflex in dementia and dyskinetic states', *J. Neurol. Neurosurg. Psychiatry*, **41**, 824–828.

Ferrari, E., and Messina, C. (1972). 'Blink reflexes during sleep and wakefulness in man', *Electroenceph. Clin. Neurophysiol.*, **32**, 55–62.

Findler, G., Feinsod, M., Lijovetzky, G., and Hadani, M. (1983). 'Transient global amnesia associated with a single metastasis in the non-dominant hemisphere, Case Report', *J. Neurosurg.*, **58**, 303–305.

Findley, L. T., and Gresty, M. A. (1981). 'Tremor', *Br. J. Hosp. Med.*, **26**, 16–32.

Fischer, C. M. (1977). 'The clinical picture in occult hydrocephalus', *Clin. Neurosurg.*, **24**, 270–284.

Fisher, C. M. (1982). 'Transient global amnesia. Precipitating activities and other observations', *Arch. Neurol.*, **39**, 605–608.

Fisher, C. M., and Adams, R. D. (1958). 'Transient global amnesia', *Trans. Am. Neurol. Assoc.*, **83**, 143–146.

Fisher, C. M., and Adams, R. D. (1964). 'Transient global amnesia', *Acta. Neurol. Scand.*, **40** (Suppl.), 9. 1–83.

Fisher, M. (1956). 'Left hemiplegia and motor impersistence', *J. Nerv. Ment. Dis.*, **123**, 201–218.

Flewett, T. H. (1973). 'The rapid diagnosis of

herpes simplex encephalitis', *Postgrad. Med. J.*, **49**, 398–400.

Foerster, O. (1921). 'Zur Analyse u. Pathophysiologie der striären Bewegungsstörungen', *Zeitschrift für die gesamte Neurologie und Psychiatrie, 73*, 1–169.

Foltz, E. L., and Ward, A. A. (1956). 'Communicating hydrocephalus from subarachnoid bleeding', *J. Neurosurg.*, **13**, 546–566.

Fozard, J. L., Wolf, E., Bell, B., McFarland, R. A., and Podoloky, S. (1977). 'Visual perception and communication' In *Handbook of the Psychology of Ageing* (Eds J. E. Birren and K. W. Schaie), pp. 497–534 Van Nostrand Reinhold, New York.

Friedman, P., Slaver, K., and Klawans, H. L. (1971). 'Neurologic manifestations of Paget's disease of the skull', *Dis. Nerv. Syst.*, **32**, 809–817.

Gacec, R. R., and Schuknecht, H. F. (1969). 'Pathology of presbycusis', *Int. Audiology, 8*, 199–209.

Galbraith, S., Blaiklock, C. T., Jennett, B., and Steven, J. L. (1976). 'The reliability of computerized transaxial tomography in diagnosing acute traumatic intracranial haematoma', *Br. J. Surg.*, **63**, 157.

Garcia-Bunel, L. (1979). 'Computerized tomography and subdural haematomas', *Lancet*, **1**, 110.

Gardner-Thorpe, C. (1972). 'Muscle weakness due to sarcoid myopathy: 6 case reports and an evaluation of steroid therapy', *Neurology (Minneap.)*, **22**, 917–928.

Garland, H. G. (1952). 'Parkinsonism', *Br. Med. J.*, **2**, 153–155.

Garland, H. G. (1955). 'Some clinical aspects of Parkinsonism', *Proc. Roy. Soc. Med.*, **48**, 867–868.

Gawler, J., Bull, J. W. D., Du Boulay, G. H., and Marshall, J. (1974). 'Computer-Assisted Tomography (EMI Scanner). Its place in investigation of suspected intracranial tumours', *Lancet*, **2**, 419–423.

Geschwind, N. (1968). 'The mechanisms of normal pressure hydrocephalus', *J. Neurol. Sci.*, **7**, 481–493.

Gibbs, C. J., and Gajdusek, D. C. (1968). 'Kuru — a prototype of subacute infectious disease of the nervous system as a model for the study of amyotrophic lateral sclerosis', in *Motor Neuron Diseases* (Eds F. H. Norris and L. T. Kurland), pp. 269–279, Grune and Stratton, New York.

Gilbert, J. J., and Benson, D. F. (1972). 'Transient global amnesia: Report of two cases with definite etiologies', *J. Nerv. Ment. Dis.*, **154**, 461–464.

Gilbert, J. J., and Feldman, R. G. (1969). 'L-dopa for progressive supranuclear palsy', *Lancet*, **2**, 494.

Gillies, J. D. (1972). 'Motor unit discharge patterns during isometric contraction in man', *J. Physiol. (Lond.)*, **223**, 36–37.

Gillilan, L. A. (1958). 'The arterial blood supply of the human spinal cord', *J. Comp. Neurol.*, **110**, 75–100.

Girdwood, R. H. (1968). 'Abnormalities of vitamin B12 and folic acid metabolism — their influence on the nervous system', *Proc. Nutr. Soc.*, **27**, 101–107.

Glasgow, J. L., Currier, R. D., Goodrich, J. K., and Tutor, F. T. (1965). 'Brain scans at varied intervals following CVA', *J. Nucl. Med.*, **6**, 902–916.

Godwin-Austin, R. B. (1982). 'Where am I?', *Br. Med. J.*, **285**, 85–86.

Goldberg, A. L., and Goodman, H. M. (1969). 'Effects of disuse and denervation on amino-acid transport by skeletal muscle', *Am. J. Physiol.*, **216**, 1116–1119.

Goodin, D. S., Squires, K. C., and Starr, A. (1978). 'Long latency event-related components of the auditory evoked potential in dementia', *Brain*, **101**, 635–648.

Gordon, A. (1945). 'Vibration sense as a differential diagnostic sign in doubtful cases of Parkinsonian syndrome', *J. Nerv. Ment. Dis.*, **101**, 589–590.

Gordon, R. M., and Bender, M. B. (1971). 'The corneomandibular reflex', *J. Neurol. Neurosurg. Psychiat.*, **34**, 236–242.

Gottfries, C. G., Adolfsson, R., Aquilonius, S-M., Carlsson, A., Oreland, L., Svennerholm, L., and Winblad, B. (1980). 'Parkinsonism and dementia disorders of Alzheimer type: Similarities and differences', in *Parkinson's Disease. Current Progress, Problems and Management* (Eds U. K. Rinne, M. Klingler, and G. Stamm), pp. 197–208, Elsevier North Holland, Amsterdam.

Gowers, W. R. (1892a). *A Manual of Diseases of the Nervous System* Vol. 1, 2nd ed. pp 470–471, Churchill, London.

Gowers, W. R. (1892b). 'Chronic spinal muscular atrophy', in *Diseases of the Nervous System*, Vol. 1, 2nd ed., pp. 471–498, Churchill, London.

Graham, J. G., and Oppenheimer, D. R. (1969). 'Orthostatic hypotension and nicotine sensitivity in a case of multiple system atrophy', *J. Neurol. Neurosurg. Psychiat.*, **32**, 28–34.

Graves, R. J. (1835). 'Clinical lectures', *Lond. Med. Surg. J.*, **7**, 516–520.

Greenfield, J. G. (1954). *The Spino-Cerebellar Degenerations*, Blackwell, Oxford.

Greenfield, J. G. (1934). 'Subacute spinocerebellar degeneration occurring in elderly patients', *Brain*, **57**, 161–176.

Greenlee, J. E., Crampton, R. S., and Miller, J. Q. (1975). 'Transient global amnesia associated with cardiac arrhythmia and digitalis intoxication', *Stroke*, **6**, 513–516.

Gregoric, M. (1973). 'Habituation of the blink reflex', in *New Developments in Electromyography and Clinical Neurophysiology*, (Ed. J. Desmedt), vol. 3, pp. 673–677, Karger, Basel.

Gresty, M. A., and Findley, L. J. (1981). 'Tremors in Parkinson's disease', in *Research Progress in Parkinson's Disease* (Eds F. C. Rose and R. Capildeo) pp. 75–87, Pitman, Bath.

Griffiths, R. A., Dalziel, J. A., Sinclair, K. G. A., Dennis, P. D., and Good, W. R. (1981). 'Tremor and senile Parkinsonism', *J. Gerontol.*, **36**(2), 170–175.

Griffiths, R. A., and Good, W. R. (1982). 'The pharmacology of tremor', *Geriatr. Med.*, **XII**, 41–49.

Gross, M. (1969). 'L-dopa for progressive supranuclear palsy', *Lancet*, **2**, 1359.

Grzegorczyk, P. B., Jones, S. W., and Mistretta, C. M. (1979). 'Age-related differences in salt taste acuity', *J. Gerontol.*, **34**, 834–840.

Guiot, G., and Brion, S. (1953). 'Traitment des mouvements anormaux par la coagulation pallidale', *Rev. Neurol.*, **89**, 578–580.

Gupta, S. K., Helal, R. H., and Kiely, P. (1969). 'The prognosis in zoster paralysis', *J. Bone Joint Surg.*, **51B**, 593–603.

Gutmann, E., and Hanzlíková, V. (1972). *Age Changes in the Neuromuscular System*, Scientechnica, Bristol.

Gutmann, E., and Hanzlíková, V. (1976). 'Fast and slow motor units in ageing', *Gerontology*, **22**, 280–300.

Haase, G. R. (1977). 'Diseases presenting as dementia', in *Dementia* (Ed. C. E. Wells), 2nd ed., pp. 27–67, F. A. Davis, Philadelphia.

Hachinski, V. C., Lassen, N. A., and Marshall, J. (1974). 'Multi-infarct dementia: A cause of mental deterioration in the elderly', *Lancet*, **2**, 207–210.

Hagbarth, K-E., and Young, R. R. (1979). 'Participation of the stretch reflex in human physiological tremor', *Brain*, **102**, 509–526.

Hakim, S., and Adams, R. D. (1965). 'The special clinical problem of symptomatic hydrocephalus with normal cerebrospinal fluid pressure', *J. Neurol. Sci.*, **2**, 307–327.

Hall, S. M. (1978). 'The Schwann cell: A reappraisal of its role in the peripheral nervous system', *Neuropathol. Appl. Neurobiol.*, **4**, 165–176.

Hammond, P. H., Merton, P. A., and Sutton, C. G. (1956). 'Nervous gradation of muscular contraction', *Br. Med. Bull.*, **12**, 214–218.

Harriman, D. G. F. (1976). 'Muscle', in *Greenfield's Neuropathology* (Eds W. Blackwood and J. A. N. Corsellis), pp. 849–902, Edward Arnold, London.

Harriman, D. G. F., Taverner, D., and Woolf, A. L. (1970). 'Ekbom's syndrome and burning paraesthesiae. A biopsy study by vital staining and electron microscopy of the intramuscular innervation with a note on age changes in motor nerve endings in distal muscles', *Brain*, **93**, 393–406.

Harrison, M. J. G., Thomas, D. J., Du Boulay, G. H., and Marshall, J. (1979). 'Multi-infarct dementia', *J. Neurol. Sci.*, **40**, 97–103.

Hassler, R. (1955). 'The influence of stimulations and coagulations in the human thalamus on the tremor at rest and its physiopathologic mechanism', in *Proceedings of the Second International Congress of Neuropathology*, pp. 637–643, Excerpta Medica, London, Amsterdam.

Havard, C. W. H., Campbell, E. D. R., Ross, H. B., and Spence, A. W. (1963). 'Electromyographic and histological findings in the muscles of patients with thyrotoxicosis', *Q. J. Med.*, **32**, 145–163.

Hayward, R. D., and O'Reilly, G. V. A. (1976). 'Intracerebral haemorrhage: Accuracy of computerized axial scanning in predicting the underlying aetiology', *Lancet*, **1**, 1–4.

Head, H., and Campbell, A. W. (1900). 'The pathology of herpes zoster and its bearing on sensory localisation', *Brain*, **23**, 353–523.

Henson, R. A. (1970). 'Non-metastatic neurological manifestations of malignant disease', in *Modern Trends in Neurology* (Ed. D. Williams), Vol. 5, pp. 209–225, Butterworths, London.

Henson, R. A., Hoffman, H. L., and Urich, H. (1965). 'Encephalomyelitis with carcinoma', *Brain*, **88**, 449–464.

Henson, R. A., Russel, D. S., and Wilkinson, M. (1954). 'Carcinomatous neuropathy and myopathy. A clinical and pathological study', *Brain*, **77**, 82–121.

Henson, R. A., and Urich, H. (1970). 'Peripheral neuropathy associated with malignant disease', in *Handbook of Clinical Neurology* (Eds P. J. Vinken and G. W. Bruyn), Vol. 8, pp. 131–148, North-Holland, Amsterdam.

Henson, R. A., and Urich, H. (1979). 'Remote effects of malignant disease: Certain intracranial disorders', in *Handbook of Clinical Neurology* (Eds F. J. Vinken and G. W. Bruyn), Vol. 38, pp. 625–668, North-Holland, Amsterdam.

Hildebrand, J., and Cöers, C. (1967). 'The neuromuscular function in patients with malignant tumours', *Brain*, **90**, 67–82,

Hill, M. E., Lougheed, W. M., and Barnett, H. J. M. (1967). 'A treatable form of dementia due to normal-pressure communicating hydrocephalus', *Can. Med. Assoc. J.*, **97**, 1309–1320.

Hogan, E. L., and Krigman, M. R. (1973). 'Herpes zoster myelitis. Evidence for viral infection of spinal cord', *Arch. Neurol. (Chicago)*, **29**, 309–313.

Holland, G. N., Moore, W. S., and Hawkes, R. C. (1980). 'Nuclear magnetic resonance tomography of the brain', *J. Comput. Assist. Tomogr.*, **4**, 1–3.

Holmes, G. (1907). 'A form of familial degeneration of the cerebellum', *Brain*, **30**, 466–489.

Hope-Simpson, R. E. (1965). 'The nature of herpes zoster: A long term study and a new hypothesis', *Proc. Roy. Soc. Med.*, **58**, 9–20.

Hopkins, A. P., and Gilliatt, R. W. (1971). 'Motor and sensory nerve conduction velocity in the baboon; normal values and changes during acrylamide neuropathy', *J. Neurol. Neurosurg. Psychiat.*, **34**, 415–426.

Horner, F. (1869). 'Uber eine Form von Ptosis', *Klin. Mbl. Augenheilk.*, **7**, 193–198.

Hounsfield, G. N. (1973). 'Computerised transverse axial scanning (tomography). 1. Description of system', *Br. J. Radiol.*, **46**, 1016–1022.

Howell, T. H. (1949). 'Senile deterioration of the central nervous system', *Br. Med. J.*, **1**, 56–58.

Huang, C-Y. (1981). 'Peripheral neuropathy in the elderly: A clinical and electrophysiologic study', *J. Am. Geriatr. Soc.*, **29**(2), 49–54.

Hubbard, O., Sunde, D., and Goldensohn, E. S. (1976). 'The EEG in centenarians', *Electroenceph. Clin. Neurophys.*, **40**, 407–417.

Hudgson, P., and Walton, J. N. (1979). 'Polymyositis and other inflammatory myopathies', in *Handbook of Clinical Neurology* (Eds P. J. Vinken and G. N. Bruyn), Vol. 41, pp. 51–93, North-Holland, Amsterdam.

Hudson, A. N. (1981). 'Amyotrophic lateral sclerosis and its association with dementia, parkinsonism and other neurological disorders: A review', *Brain*, **104**, 217–247.

Hughes, G. (1969). 'Changes in taste sensitivity with advancing age', *Geront. Clin. (Basel)*, **11**, 224–230.

Hughes, J. T., and Brownell, B. (1966). 'Spinal cord ischaemia due to arteriosclerosis', *Arch. Neurol. (Chicago)*, **15**, 189–202.

Hunt, J. R. (1907a). 'On herpetic inflammation of the geniculate ganglion. A new syndrome and its complications', *J. Nerv. Ment. Dis.*, **34**, 73–96.

Hunt, J. R. (1907b). 'Herpetic inflammation of the geniculate ganglion. A new syndrome and its aural complications', *Arch. Otol.*, **36**, 371–380.

Hunt, J. R. (1909). 'The paralytic consequences of herpes zoster of the cephalic extremity', JAMA, **53**, 1456–1457.

Hursh, J. B. (1939). 'Conduction velocity and diameter of nerve fibres', *Am. J. Physiol.*, **127**, 131–139.

Hurwitz, L. J., and Swallow, M. (1971). 'An introduction to the neurology of ageing', *Geront. Clin. (Basel)*, **13**, 97–113.

Huxley, A. F. (1971). 'The activation of striated muscle and its mechanical response', *Proc. Roy. Soc. B*, **178**, 1–27.

Hyman, N. M., Dennis, P. D., and Sinclair, K. G.

A. (1979). 'Tremor due to sodium valproate', *Neurology,* **29**, 1177–1180.

Illis, L. S. (1977). 'Encephalitis', *Br. J. Hosp. Med.*, **18**, 412–422.

Illis, L. S., and Gostling, J. V. T. (1972). *Herpes Simplex Encephalitis*, Scientechnica, Bristol.

Inglis, A. E., Straub, L. R., and Williams, C. S. (1972). Median nerve neuropathy at the wrist', *Clin. Orthop.*, **83**, 48–54.

Ishino, H., Higashi, H., Kuroda, S., Yabuki, S., Hayahara, T., and Otsuki, S. (1974). 'Motor nuclear involvement in progressive supranuclear palsy', *J. Neurol. Sci.*, **22**, 235–244.

Jacobs, L., Conti, D., Kinkel, W. R., and Manning, E. J. (1976). ' "Normal pressure" hydrocephalus', *JAMA*, **235**, 510–512.

Jacoby, R. J., and Levy, R. (1980a). 'Computed tomography in the elderly. 2. Senile dementia: Diagnosis and functional impairment', *Br. J. Psychiat.*, **136**, 256–259.

Jacoby, R. J., and Levy, R. (1980b). 'Computed tomography in the elderly. 3. Affective disorder'. *Br. J. Psychiat.*, **136**, 270–275.

Jacoby, R., Levy, R., and Dawson, J. M. (1980). 'Computed tomography in the elderly. 1. The normal population'. *Br. J. Psychiat.*, **136**, 249–255.

Jaffe N. (1951a), 'Horner's syndrome', *Am. J. Ophthalmol.*, **34**(2), 1182–1183.

Jaffe N. (1951b), 'Localization of lesions causing Horner's syndrome', *Arch. Ophthalmol.*, **44**, 714–728.

Jellinek, E. H., and Kelly, R. E. (1960). 'Cerebellar syndrome in myxoedema', *Lancet*, **2**, 225–227.

Jellinger, K. (1967). 'Spinal cord arteriosclerosis and progressive vascular myelopathy', *J. Neurol. Neurosurg. Psychiat.*, **30**, 195–206.

Jenkins, R. (1969). 'L-dopa for progressive supranuclear palsy', *Lancet*, **2**, 742.

Jennekens, F. G. I., Tomlinson, B. E., and Walton, J. N. (1971). 'Histochemical aspects of five limb muscles in old age', *J. Neurol. Sci.*, **14**, 259–276.

Jensen, T. S., and Olivarus, B. de F. (1980). 'Transient global amnesia as a manifestation of transient cerebral ischaemia', *Acta Neurol. Scandinav.*, **61**, 115–124.

Johnson, R. H., Lee, G. de J., Oppenheimer, D. R., and Spalding, J. M. K. (1966). 'Autonomic failure with orthostatic hypotension due to intermediolateral column degeneration', *Quart. J. Med.*, **35**, 276–292.

Joyce, G. C., and Rack, P. M. H. (1974). 'The effects of load and force on tremor at the normal human elbow joint', *J. Physiol.*, **240**, 375–396.

Juel-Jensen, B. E. (1970). 'The natural history of shingles: Events associated with reactivation of varicella-zoster virus', *J. Roy. Coll. Gen. Prac.*, **20**, 323–327.

Juel-Jensen, B. E. (1982). Personal communication.

Juel-Jensen, B. E., and MacCallum, F. O. (1972). *Herpes Simplex, Varicella and Zoster*, Heinemann, London.

Jung, R. (1941). 'Physiologische Untersuchungen über den Parkinsonon tremor und andere Zitterformen bein Menschen', *Z. gest. Neurol. Psychiat.*, **173**, 263–332.

Justin-Besançon, L., Pequignot, H., Contamin, F., Delauvierre, P., and Rolland, P. (1964). 'Myopathie de type Landouzy-Dejerine. Présentation d'une observation historique', *Revue Neurologique*, **110**, 56–57.

Kaeser, H. E. (1970). 'Nerve conduction velocity measurements', in *Handbook of Clinical Neurology* (Eds P. J. Vinken and G. W. Bruyn), Vol. 7, pp. 116–196, North-Holland, Amsterdam.

Katzman, R. (1977). 'Normal pressure hydrocephalus', in *Dementia* (Ed. C. E. Wells), 2nd ed. pp. 69–92, F. A. Davis, Philadelphia.

Kimura, J. (1970). 'Alterations of the orbicularis oculi reflex by pontine lesions. Study in multiple sclerosis', *Arch. Neurol.*, **22**, 156–161.

Kimura, J. (1973). 'The blink reflex as a test for brain-stem and higher central nervous system function', in *New Developments in Electromyography and Clinical Neurophysiology*, (Ed. J. Desmedt), Vol. 3, pp. 682–691, Karger, Basel.

Kimura, J., and Lyon, L. W. (1972). 'Orbicularis oculi reflex in the Wallenberg syndrome: alteration of the late reflex by lesions of the spinal tract and nucleus of the trigeminal nerve', *J. Neurol. Neurosurg. Psychiatry*, **35**, 228–233.

Klawans, H. (1969). 'L-dopa for progressive supranuclear palsy', *Lancet*, **2**, 1359.

Klawans, H. L., and Goodwin, J. A. (1969). 'Reversal of glabellar reflex in Parkinsonism by L-dopa', *J. Neurol. Neurosurg. Psychiatry*, **32**, 423–427.

Klawans, H. L., Tufo, H. M., Ostfeld, A. M., Shekelle, R. B., and Kilbridge, J. A. (1971). 'Neurological Examination in an elderly population', *Dis. Nerv. Syst.*, **32**, 274–279.

Kleist, K. (1927). 'Gegenhalten (motorischer Negativismus) Zwangsgreifen u. Thalamus Opticus'. *Monatsschrift für Psychiatrie und Neurologie*, **65**, 317–396.

Klemme, R. M. (1940). 'Surgical treatment of dystonia, paralysis agitans and athetosis', *Arch. Neurol. Psychiat. (Chicago)*, **44**, 926.

Koenig, H. (1968). 'Neurobiological effects of agents which alter nucleic acid metabolism', in *Motor Neuron Diseases* (Eds F. H. Norris and L. T. Kurland), pp. 347–368, Grune and Stratton.

Kokmen, E., Bossemeyer, R. W., Barney, J., and Williams, W. J. (1977). 'Neurological manifestations of ageing', *J. Gerontol.*, **32**, 411–419.

Konigsmark, B. W., and Weiner, L. P. (1970). 'The olivopontocerebellar atrophies: A review', *Medicine (Baltimore)*, **49**, 227–241.

Kopell, H. P., and Thompson, W. A. L. (1960). 'Peripheral entrapment neuropathies of the lower extremity', *New Engl. J. Med.*, **262**, 56–60.

Kost, G. J., and Verity, M. A. (1980). 'A new variant of late-onset myophosphorylase deficiency', *Muscle Nerve*, **3**, 195–201.

Kugelberg, E. (1952). 'Facial reflexes', *Brain*, **75**, 385–396.

Kugelberg, E., Edström, L., and Abbruzze, M. (1970). 'Mapping of motor units in experimentally reinervated rat muscle', *J. Neurol. Neurosurg. Psychiat.*, **33**, 319–329.

Kundratitz, K. (1925). 'Experimentelle Übertragung von Herpes zoster auf den Menschen und die Beziehungen von Herpes zoster zu Varicellen'. *Monatschr. Kinderh.*, **29**, 516–523.

Kurland, L. T. (1977). 'Epidemiology of amyotrophic lateral sclerosis with emphasis on antecedent events from case-control comparisons', in *Motor Neurone Disease* (Ed. F. Clifford Rose), pp. 14–29, Pitman, London.

Kurland, L. T. (1980). 'The contribution of the Mayo Clinic centralized diagnostic index to neuroepidemiology in the United States', in *Clinical Neuroepidemiology* (Ed. F. Clifford Rose), pp. 37–46, Pitman, Tunbridge Wells.

Kurland, L. T., and Mulder, D. W. (1955). 'Epidemiological investigation of amyotrophic lateral sclerosis. 2. Familial aggregations indicative of dominant inheritance', *Neurology (Minneap.)*, **5**, 182–196, 249–268.

Kurland, L. T., Faros, S. N., and Siedler, H. (1960). 'Minamata disease. The outbreak of a neurologic disorder in Minamata, Japan, and its relationship to the injestion of seafood contaminated by mercuric compounds', *World Neurol.*, **1**, 370–395.

Kurtzke, J. F. (1982). 'Motor neurone(e) disease', *Br. Med. J.*, **284**, 141–142.

Lambert, E. H., and Rooke, E. D. (1965). 'Myasthenia state and lung cancer', in *The Remote Effects of Carcinoma on the Nervous System* (Eds W. R. Brain and F. H. Norres), pp. 67–80, Grune and Stratton, New York.

Lambert, E. H., Underdahl, L. O., Beckett, S., and Mederos, L. O. (1951). 'A study of the ankle jerk in myxoedema', *J. Clin. Endocr.*, **11**, 1186–1205.

Lance, J. W., and McLeod, J. (1981). *A Physiological Approach to Clinical Neurology*, 3rd ed., Butterworths, London.

Lance, J. W., Schwab, R. S., and Peterson, E. A. (1963). 'Action tremor and the cogwheel phenomenon in Parkinson's disease', *Brain*, **86**, 95–110.

Landouzy, L., and Dejerine, J. (1884). 'De la myopathie atrophique progressive (myopathie héréditaire) débutant, dans l'enfance, par la face, sans altération due système nerveuse', *Comptes rendus hebdomadaires des séances de l'Academie des sciences (CR Acad. Sci. (Paris))*, **98**, 53–55.

Landry, M. L., Booss, J., and Hsiung, G. D. (1982). 'Duration of vidarabine therapy in biopsy-negative herpes simplex encephalitis', *JAMA*, **247**, 332–334.

Lane, R. J. M., and Mastaglia, F. L. (1978). 'Drug-induced myopathies in man', *Lancet*, **2**, 562–565.

Lang, B., Newsom-Davis, J., Wray, D., and Vincent, A. (1981). 'Autoimmune aetiology for myasthenia (Eaton–Lambert) syndrome', *Lancet*, **2**, 224–226.

Larsson, T., and Sjögren, T. (1960). 'Essential tremor. A clinical and genetic population study', *Acta. Psychiat. Neurol. (Scand.)*, **144**(Suppl.), 36, 11–175.

Lascelles, R. G., and Thomas, P. K. (1966). 'Changes due to age in internodal length in the sural nerve in man', *J. Neurol. Neurosurg. Psychiat.*, **29**, 40–44.

Lefebvre-D'Amour, M., Shahani, B. T., and Young, R. R. (1978). 'Tremor in alcoholic patients', in *Physiological Tremor, Pathological Tremors and Clonus* (Ed. J. E. Desmedt), pp. 160–164, Karger, Basel.

LeMay, M., and New, P. D. J. (1970). 'Radiological diagnosis of occult normal pressure hydrocephalus', *Radiology*, **96**, 347–358.

Lhermitte, J., and Nicolas, M. (1924). 'Les lésions spinales du zona: La myelite zosterienne', *Rev. Neurol.*, **1**, 361–364.

Lhermitte, J., and Nicolas, M. (1925). 'Les amyotrophies de la main chez le vieillard. Étude anatamo-clinique', *Encéphale*, **20**, 701–712.

Lindblom, U. (1981). 'Quantative testing of sensibility including pain,' *Clinical Newophysol.* (Eds. E. Stalberg and R. R. Young). pp. 168–190, Butterworth London.

Lippold, O. C. J. (1970) 'Oscillation in the stretch reflex arc and the origin of the rhythmical 8–12 c/ s component of physiological tremor', *J. Physiol.*, **206**, 359–382.

Llinas, R., and Volkind, R. A. (1973). 'The olivocerebellar system: Functional properties as revealed by harmaline-induced tremor', *Exp. Brain. Res.*, **18**, 69–87.

Locke, S., and Galaburda, A. M. (1978). 'Neurological disorders of the elderly', in *Clinical Aspects of Ageing* (Ed. W. Reichel), pp. 133–138, Williams and Wilkins, Baltimore.

Longridge, N. S., Hachinski, V., and Barber, H. O. (1979). 'Brain stem dysfunction in transient global amnesia', *Stroke*, **10**, 473–474.

Lorenzo, A. V., Bresnan, M. J., and Barlow, C. F. (1974). 'Cerebrospinal fluid absorption deficit in normal pressure hydrocephalus', *Arch. Neurol.*, **30**, 387–393.

Lorenzo, A. V., Page, L. K., and Watters, G. V. (1970). 'Relationship between cerebrospinal fluid formation, absorption and pressure in human hydrocephalus', *Brain*, **93**, 679–692.

Lou, H. O. C. (1968). 'Repeated episodes of transient global amnesia', *Acta. Neurol. Scand.*, **44**, 612–618.

Lyon, L. W., Kimura, J., and McCormick, W. F. (1972). 'Orbicularis oculi reflex in coma: Clinical, electrophysiological and pathological considerations'. *J. Neurol. Neurosurg. Psychiatry*, **35**, 582–588.

McCarthy, K. (1972). 'Varicella-zoster and related viruses', *J. Clin. Path.*, **25**, (Suppl. 6), 46–50.

McCormick, W. F., Rodnitsky, R. L., Schocher, S. S., and McKee, A. P. (1969). 'Varicella-zoster encephalomyelitis. A morphological and virologic study', *Arch. Neurol.*, **21**, 559–570.

MacDonald, J. B. (1981). 'The scintiscan', in *Advanced Geriatric Medicine* (Eds F. I. Caird and J. Grimley Evans), Vol. 1, pp. 84–87, Pitman, London.

McGeorge, A. P. (1981). 'The electroencephalogram', in *Advanced Geriatric Medicine* (Eds F. I. Caird and J. Grimley Evans), Vol. 1, pp. 80–83, Pitman, London.

McKendall, R. R., and Klawans, H. J. (1978). 'Nervous system complications of varicella-zoster virus', in *Textbook of Clinical Neurology* (Eds P. J. Vinken and G. W. Bruyn), Vol. 34, pp. 161–183, North-Holland, Amsterdam.

MacLennan, W. J. (1981). 'The problem of potassium', in *Advanced Geriatric Medicine* (Eds F. I. Caird and J. G. Evans), Vol. 1, pp. 67–72, Pitman, London.

McLeod, J. G. (1982). 'Neuropathies and myopathies', in *Neurological Disorders in the Elderly* (Ed. F. I. Caird), pp. 163–181, John Wright, Bristol.

Mancall, E. L. (1975). 'Late (acquired) cortical cerebellar atrophy', in *Handbook of Clinical Neurology* (Eds P. J. Vinken and G. W. Bruyn), Vol. 21, pp. 477–508, North-Holland, Amsterdam.

Magladery, J. W., and Teasdall, R. D. (1961). 'Corneal reflexes', *Arch. Neurol.*, **5**, 269–274.

Magladery, J. W., Teasdall, R. D., French, J. H., and Busch, E. S. (1960). 'Cutaneous reflex changes in development and ageing', *Arch. Neurol.*, **3**, 1–9.

Mann, D. M. A., and Yates, P. O. (1974). 'Motor neurone disease: The nature of the pathogenic mechanism', *J. Neurol. Neurosurg. Psychiat.*, **37**, 1036–1046.

Marsden, C. D. (1978). 'The mechanisms of physiological tremor and their significance for pathological tremors', in *Physiological Tremor, Pathological Tremors and Clonus* (Ed. J. E. Desmedt), pp. 1–16, Karger, Basel.

Marsden, C. D., Foley, T. H., Owen, D. A. L., and McAllister, R. G. (1967). 'Peripheral beta-adrenergic receptors concerned with tremor', *Clin. Sci.*, **33**, 53–65.

Marsden, C. D., Meadows, J. C., Lange, G. W., and Watson, R. S. (1969). 'Variation in human physiological finger tremor, with particular reference to changes with age', *Electroencephalogr. Clin. Neurophysiol.*, **27**, 169–178.

Marsden, C. D., Meadows, J. C., and Lowe, R. D. (1969). 'The influence of noradrenaline, tyramine and the activation of sympathetic nerves on physiological tremor', *Clin Sci.*, **37**, 243–252.

Marshall, J. (1961). 'The effect of ageing upon physiological tremor', *J. Neurol. Neurosurg. Psychiatry*, **24**, 14–17.

Marshall, J. (1962). 'Observations on essential tremor', *J. Neurol. Neurosurg. Psychiatry*, **25**, 122–125.

Marshall, J., and Walsh, E. G. (1956). 'Physiological tremor', *J. Neurol. Neurosurg. Psychiatry*, **19**, 260–267.

Marie, P., and Foix, C. (1912). 'L' atrophie isolée non progressive des petits muscles de la main. Téphromalacie antériure', *Nouv. Icongr. Salpêtrière*, **25**, 353–363, 427–453.

Marie, P., and Foix, C. (1913). 'Atrophie isolée de l'éminence thénar d'origine nevritique. Role du ligament annulaire anterieur de carpe dans la pathogénie de la lésion', *Rev. Neurol. Paris*, **26**, 647–649.

Marie, P., Foix, C., and Alajouanine, T. (1922). 'De l'atrophie cérébelleuse tardive à prédominance corticale', *Rev. Neurol.*, **38**, 849–885, 1082–1111.

Mastaglia, F. L., and Carroll, W. M. (1982). 'Evoked potentials in neurological diagnosis', *Br. Med. J.*, **285**, 1678–1679.

Mastaglia, F. L., Barwick, D. D., and Hall, R. (1970). 'Myopathy in acromegaly', *Lancet*, **2**, 907–909.

Mastaglia, F. L., and Grainger, K. M. R. (1975). 'Internuclear ophthalmoplegia in progressive supranuclear palsy', *J. Neurol. Sci.*, **25**, 303–308.

Mastaglia, F. L., Grainger, K., Kee, F., Sadka, M., and Lefroy, R. (1973). 'Progressive supranuclear palsy. Clinical and electro-physiological observations in 11 cases', *Proc. Aust. Assoc. Neurol.*, **10**, 35–44.

Matthew, N. T., and Meyer, J. S. (1974). 'Pathogenesis and natural history of transient global amnesia', *Stoke*, **5**, 303–311.

Matthews, W. B. (1975). 'Virus infections', in *Recent Advances in Clinical Neurology*, 1 (Ed. W. B. Matthews), pp. 163–186, Churchill Livingstone, Edinburgh.

Matthews, W. B. (1978). 'The treatment of acute ischaemic stroke', in *Recent Advances in Clinical Neurology* **2**, (Eds W. B. Matthews and G. H. Glaser), pp. 9–14, Churchill Livingstone, Edinburgh.

Matthews, W. B., Howell, D. A., and Hughes, R. C. (1970). 'Relapsing corticosteroid-dependent polyneuritis', *J. Neurol. Neurosurg. Psychiat.*, **33**, 330–337.

Menzel, P. (1891). 'Beitrag zur Kenntniss der hereditären Ataxie und Kleinhirnatrophie', *Arch. Psychiat. Nervenkr.*, **22**, 160–190.

Messert, B., and Baker, N. H. (1966). 'Syndrome of progressive spastic ataxia and apraxia associated with occult hydrocephalus', *Neurology (Minneap.)*, **16**, 440–452.

Messina, C., Di Rosa, A. E., and Tomasello, F. (1972). 'Habituation of blink reflexes in Parkinsonian patients under levodopa and amantadine treatment', *J. Neurol. Sci.*, **17**, 141–148.

Messert, B., and van Nuis, C. (1966). 'A syndrome of paralysis of downward gaze, dysarthria, pseudobulbar palsy, axial rigidity of neck and trunk and dementia', *J. Nerv. Ment. Dis.*, **143**, 47–54.

Milhorat, T. H. (1972). *Hydrocephalus and the Cerebrospinal Fluid*, Williams and Wilkins, Baltimore.

Milhorat, T. H., Clark, R. G., Hammock, M. K., and McGrath, P. P. (1970). 'Structural, ultrastructural, and permeability changes in the ependyma and surrounding brain favouring equilibration in progressive hydrocephalus', *Arch. Neurol.*, **22**, 397–407.

Milne, J. S., and Williamson, J. (1972). 'The ankle jerk in older people', *Geront. Clin. (Basel)*, **14**, 86–88.

Milner-Brown, H. S., Stein, R. B., and Yemm, R. (1973a). 'Changes in firing rate of human motor units during linearly changing voluntary contraction', *J. Physiol.* **230**, 371–390.

Milner-Brown, H. S., Stein, R. B., and Yemm, R. (1973b). 'The orderly recruitment of human motor units during voluntary isometric contractions', *J. Physiol.*, **230**, 359–370.

Mirsky, I. A., Futterman, P., and Broh-Kahn, R. H. (1953). 'The quantitive measurement of vibratory perception in subjects with and without diabetes mellitus', *J. Lab. Clin. Med.*, **41**, 221–235.

Mitchell, J. D. (1983). 'EEG and evoked potential techniques', *Hospital Update*, **9**, 443–454.

Moncrieff, R. W. (1966). 'Changes in olfactory preference with age', *Rev. Laryngol. Otol. Rhinol. (Bord.)*, **86**, 895–904.

Morgan-Hughes, J. A. (1979). 'Painful disorders of the muscle', *Br. J. Hosp. Med.*, **22**, 360–365.

Morgan-Hughes, J. A. (1982). 'Defects in energy pathways of skeletal muscle', in *Recent Advances in Clinical Neurology* (Eds W. B. Matthews and G. H. Glaser), Vol. 3, pp. 1–46, Churchill Livingstone, Edinburgh.

Mulder, D. W., Lambert, E. H., and Eaton, L. M. (1959). 'Myasthenic syndrome in patients with amyotrophic lateral sclerosis', *Neurology*, **9**, 627–631.

Müller, H. F., Grad, B., and Engelsmann, F. (1975). 'Biological and psychological predictors of survival in a psychogeriatric population', *J. Geront.*, **30**, 47–52.

Müller, R., and Kugelberg, E. (1959). 'Myopathy in Cushing's syndrome', *J. Neurol. Neurosurg. Psychiat.*, **22**, 314–319.

Murray, T. J. (1981). 'Essential tremor', in *Disorders of Movement* (Ed. A. Barbeau), pp. 151–170, MTP Press, Lancaster.

Myerson, A. (1944). 'Tap and thrust responses in Parkinson's disease', *Arch. Neurol. Psychiat.*, **51**, 480.

Namerow, N. S., and Etemadi, A. (1970). 'The orbicularis oculi reflex in multiple sclerosis', *Neurology,* **20**, 1200–1203.

Nevin, S. (1936). 'Two cases of muscular degeneration occurring in late adult life, with a review of the recorded cases of late progressive muscular dystrophy (late progressive myopathy)' *Quart. J. Med.*, **17**, 51–68.

Newman, G., Dovenmuehle, R. H., and Busse, E. W. (1960). 'Alterations in neurologic status with Age', *J. Am. Geriatr. Soc.,* **8**, 915–917.

Newman, M. K., and Gugino, R. J. (1964). 'Neuropathies and myopathies associated with occult malignancies', *JAMA*, **190**, 575–577.

Nigst, H., and Dick, W. (1979). 'Syndromes of compression of the median nerve in the proximal forearm (pronator teres syndrome; anterior interosseous syndrome), *Arch. Orthopaed, Traum. Surg.*, **93**, 307–312.

Norris, F. H. (1975). 'Adult spinal motor neuron disease. Progressive muscular atrophy (Aran's disease) in relation to amyotrophic lateral sclerosis', in *Handbook of Clinical Neurology* (Eds P. J. Vinken and G. W. Bruyn), Vol. 22, pp. 1–56, North-Holland, Amsterdam.

Norris, F. H., and Panner, B. J. (1966). 'Hypothyroid myopathy. Clinical, electromyographical and ultrastructural observations', *Arch. Neurol. (Chicago)*, **14**, 574–589.

Obrist, W. D. (1954). 'The electroencephalogram of normal aged adults', *Electroenceph. Clin. Neurophys.*, **6**, 235–244.

Obrist, W. D., Busse, W. D., Eisdorfer, C., and Kleemeier, R. W. (1962). 'Relation of the electroencephalograph to intellectual function in senescence', *J. Geront.*, **17**, 197–206.

Obrist, W. D., Sokoloff, L., Lassen, N. A., Lane, M. H., Butler, R. N., and Feinberg, I. (1963). 'Relationship of EEG to cerebral blood flow and metabolism in old age', *Electroenceph. Clin. Neurophys.*, **15**, 610–619.

Ochoa, J., Fowler, T. J., and Gilliatt, R. W. (1972). 'Anatomical changes in peripheral nerves compressed by a pneumatic tourniquet', *J. Anatom.*, **113**, 443–455.

Ochoa, J., and Mair, W. G. P. (1969). 'The normal sural nerve in man. II. Changes in the axons and Schwann cells due to aging', *Acta. Neuropath. (Berlin).*, **13**, 217–239.

Ojemann, R. G. (1972). 'Normal pressure hydrocephalus', in *Scientific Foundations of Neurology* (Eds M. Critchley, J. L. O'Leary, and B. Jennett), pp. 302–308, Heinemann, London.

Oliver, L. C. (1949). 'Surgery in Parkinson's disease. Division of the lateral pyramidal tract for tremor. Report on 48 operations', *Lancet,* **1**, 910–913.

Olsson, Y. (1975). 'Vascular permeability in the peripheral nervous system', in *Peripheral Neuropathy* (Eds P. J. Dyck, P. K. Thomas, and E. H. Lambert), pp. 120–190, W. B. Saunders, Philadelphia.

Onufrowicz, B. (1900). 'On the arrangement and function of the cell groups of the sacral region of the spinal cord in man', *Arch. Neurol. Psychopath.*, **3**, 387–412.

Oppenheimer, D. R. (1980). 'Lateral horn cells in progressive autonomic failure', *J. Neurol. Sci.,* **46**, 393–404.

O'Sullivan, D. J., and Swallow, M. (1968). 'The fibre size and content of the radial and sural nerves', *J. Neurol. Neurosurg. Psychiat.*, **31**, 464–470.

Otomo, E. (1965). 'The palmomental reflex in the aged', *Geriatrics,* **20**, 901–905.

Otomo, E. (1966). 'Electroencephalography in old age: Dominant alpha pattern', *Electroenceph. Clin. Neurophys.*, **21**, 489–491.

Otomo, E., and Tsubaki, T. (1966). 'Electroencephalography in subjects sixty years and over', *Electroenceph. Clin. Neurophys.*, **20**, 77–82.

Overend, W. (1896). 'Preliminary note on a new cranial reflex', *Lancet,* **1**, 619.

Oxbury, J. M., and MacCallum, F. O. (1973). 'Herpes simplex virus encephalitis', *Postgrad. Med. J.*, **49**, 387–389.

Padgett, B. L., Walker, D. L., ZuRhein, G. M., and Eckroade, R. J. (1971). 'Cultivation of Papova-like virus from human brain with progressive multifocal leukoencephalopathy', *Lancet,* **1**, 1257–1260.

Parinaud, H. (1883). 'Paralysie des mouvements associes des yeux', *Arch. de Neurol.,* **5**, 145–172.

Parkinson, J. (1817). *An Essay on the Shaking Palsy*, Sherwood, Neely and Jones, London.

Patten, B. M., Bilezikian, J. P., Mallett, L. E., Prince, A., Engel, W. K., and Aurbach, G. D. (1974). 'Neuromuscular disease in primary hyperparathyroidism', *Ann. Intern. Med.*, **80**, 182–193.

Paulson, G. W. (1977). 'The neurological examination in dementia', in *Dementia* (Ed. C. E. Wells), 2nd ed., pp. 169–188, F. A. Davis, Philadelphia.

Paulson, G., and Gottlieb, G. (1968). 'Developmental reflexes'. The reappearance of foetal and neonatal reflexes in aged patients', *Brain*, 91, 37–52.

Payne, C. M. E. (1981). 'Newly recognized syndrome in the neck: Horner's syndrome with ipsilateral vocal cord and phrenic nerve palsies', *J. Roy. Soc. Med.*, 74, 814–818.

Pearce, J. (1974). 'The extrapyramidal disorder of Alzheimer's disease', *Eur. Neurol.*, 12, 94–103.

Pearce, J., Aziz, H., and Gallagher, J. C. (1968). 'Primitive reflex activity in primary and symptomatic parkinsonism', *J. Neurol. Neurosurg. Psychiatry*, 31, 501–508.

Pearce, J., and Miller, E. (1973). *'Clinical Aspects of Dementia'*, Baillière Tindall, London.

Penders, C. A., and Delwaide, P. J. (1971). 'Blink reflex studies in patients with Parkinsonism before and during therapy', *J. Neurol. Neurosurg. Psychiatry*, 34, 674–678.

Penders, C. A., and Delwaide, P. J. (1973). 'Physiologic approach to the human blink reflex', in *New Developments in Electromyography and Clinical Neurophysiology*, (Ed. J. Desmedt), Vol. 3, pp. 649–657, Karger, Basel.

Penn, A. S. (1979). 'Myoglobin and myoglobinuria', in *Handbook of Clinical Neurology* (Eds P. J. Vinken and G. W. Bruyn), Vol. 41, pp. 259–285, North-Holland, Amsterdam.

Perkoff, G. T., Silber, R., Tyler, F. H., Cartwright, G. E., and Wintrobe, M. M. (1959). 'Studies in disorder of muscle. Part XII. Myopathy due to the administration of therapeutic amounts of 17-hydroxycorticoids', *Am. J. Med.*, 26, 891–898.

Peterson, I., and Kugelberg, E. (1949). 'Duration and form of action potentials in the normal human muscle', *J. Neurol. Neurosurg. Psychiat.*, 12, 124–128.

Pickett, J. B. E., Layzer, R. B., Levin, S. R., Schneider, V., Campbell, M. J., and Sumner, A. J. (1975). 'Neuromuscular complications of acromegaly', *Neurology (Minneap.)*, 25, 638–645.

Pilleri, G. (1966). 'The Kluver–Bucy syndrome in man', *Psychiat. Neurol. (Basel)*, 152, 65–103.

Ponsford, J. L., and Donnan, G. A. (1980). 'Transient global amnesia — a hippocampal phenomenon', *J. Neurol. Neurosurg. Psychiat.*, 43, 285–287.

Posey, W. C. (1904). 'Paralysis of the upward movements of the eyes', *Ann. Ophthalmol.*, 13, 523–531.

Powell, H. C., London, G. W., and Lampert, P. W. (1974). 'Neurofibrillary tangles in progressive supranuclear palsy', *J. Neuropath. Exp. Neurol.*, 33, 98–106.

Prakash, C., and Stern, G. (1973). 'Neurological signs in the elderly', *Age Ageing*, 2, 24–27.

Price, T. R., and Netsky, M. G. (1966). 'Myxoedema and ataxia. Cerebellar alterations and neural myxoedema bodies', *Neurology (Minneap.)*, 16, 957–962.

Prineas, J. W. (1969a). 'The pathogenesis of dying-back polyneuropathies. Part 1. An ultrastructural study of experimental tri-ortho-cresyl phosphate intoxication in the cat', *J. Neuropath Exp. Neurol.*, 28, 571–597.

Prineas, J. W. (1969b). 'The pathogenesis of dying-back polyneuropathies. Part II. An ultrastructural study of experimental acrylamide intoxication in the cat', *J. Neuropath. Exp. Neurol.*, 28, 598–621.

Prineas, J., Hall, R., Barwick, D. D., and Watson, A. J. (1968). 'Myopathy associated with pigmentation following adrenalectomy for Cushing's syndrome', *Quart. J. Med.*, 37, 63–77.

Procacci, P., Bozza, G., Buzzelli, G., and Della Corte, M. (1970). 'A cutaneous pricking pain threshold in old age', *Geront. Clin. (Basel)*, 12, 213–218.

Putnam, T. J. (1938). 'Relief from unilateral paralysis agitans by section of the pyramidal tract', *Arch. Neurol.*, 40, 1049–1050.

Ramsay, L. D. (1974). *Thyroid Disease and Muscle Dysfunction*, Heinemann, London.

Rankin, J. T., and Sutton, R. A. L. (1969). 'Herpes zoster causing retention of urine', *Br. J. Urol.*, 41, 238–243.

Ranvier, L. (1873). 'Propriétés et structures différentes des muscles rouges et des muscles blancs chez les lapins et chez les rates', *CR Soc. Biol. (Paris)*, 77, 1030–1043.

Ranvier, L. (1874). 'De quelques faits relatifs à l'histologie et à la physiologie des muscles striés', *Arch. Physiol. Norm. Path.*, *Deusciène Ser* 1, 5–15.

Rasminsky, M., and Sears, T. A. (1972). 'Internodal conduction in undissected demyelinated nerve fibres', *J. Physiol.*, 227, 322–350.

Rebeiz, J. J., Caulfield, J. B., and Adams, R. D. (1969). 'Oculopharyngeal dystrophy. A presenescent myopathy. A clinico-pathological study', in *Progress in Neuroophthalmology, Proc. Second. Int. Cong. Neuro-Genetics and Neuroophthalmology* (Eds J. R. Brunette and A. Barbeau), Vol. 2, pp. 12–31, Excerpta Medica, Amsterdam.

Rebeiz, J. J., Moore, M. J., Holden, E. M., and Adams, R. D. (1972). 'Variations in muscle status with age and systemic disease', *Acta. Neuropath. (Berlin)*, 22, 127–144.

Rees, L. H. (1978). 'Endocrine manifestations of cancer', *Medicine*, 10, 485–490.

Richardson, E. P. (1965). 'Progressive multifocal leukoencephalopathy', in *The Remote Effects of*

Cancer on the Nervous System (Eds W. R. Brain and F. H. Norres), pp. 6–16, Grune and Stratton, New York.

Richardson, E. P. (1970). 'Progressive multifocal leukoencephalopathy', in *Handbook of Clinical Neurology* (Eds P. J. Vinken and G. W. Bruyn), Vol. 9, pp. 485–499, North-Holland, Amsterdam.

Richmond, J., and Davidson, S. (1958). 'Subacute combined degeneration of the spinal cord in non-Addisonian megaloblastic anaemia', *Quart. J. Med.*, **27**, 517–531.

Richmond, W. (1974). 'The genito-urinary manifestations of herpes zoster: Three case reports and a review of the literature', *Br. J. Urol.*, **46**, 193–200.

Richter, R. B. (1950). 'Late cortical cerebellar atrophy. A form of hereditary cerebellar ataxia', *Am. J. Hum. Genet.*, **2**, 1–29.

Roberts, M. A., and Caird, F. I. (1976). 'Computerized tomography and intellectual impairment in the elderly', *J. Neurol. Neurosurg. Psychiat.*, **39**, 986–989.

Roberts, M. A., and Caird, F. I. (1982). 'Investigation of neurological disorders', in *Neurological Disorders in the Elderly* (Ed. F. I. Caird), pp. 52–66, John Wright, Bristol.

Roberts, M. A., Godfrey, J. W., and Caird, F. I. (1982) 'Epileptic seizures in the elderly: 1. Aetiology and type of seizure', *Age Ageing*, **11**, 24–28.

Roberts, M. A., McGeorge, A. P., and Caird, F. I. (1978). 'Electroencephalography and computerised tomography in vascular and non-vascular dementia in old age', *J. Neurol. Neurosurg. Psychiat.*, **41**, 903–906.

Rondot, P., Jedynak, C. P., and Ferrey, G. (1978). 'Pathological tremors: Nosological correlations', in *Physiological Tremor, Pathological Tremors and Clonus* (Ed. J. E. Desmedt), pp. 95–113, Karger, Basel.

Roses, A. D., Harper, P. S., and Bossen, E. H. (1979). In *Handbook of Clinical Neurology* (Eds P. J. Vinken and G. W. Bruyn), Vol. 40, pp. 485–532, North-Holland, Amsterdam.

Rothschild, D., and Kasanin, J. (1936). 'Clinicopathologic study of Alzheimer's disease', *Arch. Neurol. Psychiat. (Chicago)*, **36**, 293–321.

Rowland, L. P. (1975). 'Progressive external ophthalmoplegia', in *Handbook of Clinical Neurology* (Eds P. J. Vinken and G. W. Bruyn), Vol. 22, pp. 177–302, North-Holland, Amsterdam.

Rowland, L. P., and Schotland, D. L. (1965). 'Neoplasms and muscle disease', in *The Remote Effects of Cancer on the Nervous System* (Eds W. R. Brain and F. H. Norres), pp. 83–97, Grune and Stratton, New York.

Rushworth, G. (1962). 'Observations on blink reflexes', *J. Neurol. Neurosurg. Psychiatry,* **25**, 93–108.

Russell, J. S. R., Batten, F. E., and Collier, J. (1900). 'Subacute combined degeneration of the spinal cord', *Brain*, **23**, 39–110.

Sacks, O. W. (1969). 'L-dopa for progressive supranuclear palsy', *Lancet*, **2**, 591–592.

Salick, A. I., Colachis, S. C., and Pearson, C. M. (1968). 'Myxoedema myopathy: Clinical, electrodiagnostic and pathologic findings in advanced case', *Arch. Phys. Med. Rehab.*, **49**, 230–237.

Schenck, E., and Manz, F. (1973). 'The blink reflex in Bell's palsy', in *New Developments in Electromyography and Clinical Neurophysiology* (Ed. J. Desmedt), Vol. 3, pp. 678–681, Karger, Basel.

Schmid, A. H., and Riede, U. N. (1974). 'A morphometric study of the cerebellar cortex from patients with carcinoma. A contribution on quantitative aspects in carcinotoxic cerebellar atrophy', *Acta. Neuropath. (Berlin)*, **28**, 343–352.

Schmidt, R. F. (1978). *Fundamentals of Sensory Physiology,* Springer-Verlag, Berlin, Heidelberg.

Schotland, D. L., Spiro, D., and Carmel, P. (1966). 'Ultrastructural studies of ring fibres in human muscle disease', *J. Neuropath. Exp. Neurol.*, **25**, 431–442.

Schott, G. D., and Wills, M. R. (1976). 'Muscle weakness in osteomalacia', *Lancet*, **1**, 626–629.

Scott, J. M., Dinn, J. J., Wilson, P., and Weir, D. G. (1981). 'Pathogenesis of subacute combined degeneration: A result of methyl group deficiency', *Lancet*, **2**, 334–337.

Scott, J. M., and Weir, D. G. (1981). 'The methyl folate trap', *Lancet*, **2**, 337–340.

Scoville, W. B., and Milner, B. (1957). 'Loss of recent memory after bilateral hippocampal lesions', *J. Neurol. Neurosurg. Psychiat.*, **20**, 11–21.

Seddon, H. J. (1943). 'Three types of nerve injury', *Brain*, **66**, 237–288.

Serratrice, G., Roux, H., and Aquaron, R. (1968). 'Proximal muscular weakness in elderly subjects', *J. Neurol. Sci.*, **7**, 275–299.

Shahani, B. T., and Young, R. R. (1973). 'Blink reflexes in orbicularis oculi', in *New Developments in Electromyography and Clinical Neurophysiology* (Ed. J. Desmedt), Vol. 3, pp. 641–648, Karger, Basel.

Shahani, B. T., and Young, R. R. (1976). 'Physiological and pharmacological aids in the differential diagnosis of tremor', *J. Neurol. Neurosurg. Psychiatry*, **39**, 772–783.

Sheldon, P. W. G. (1973). 'Specific angiographic changes in acute herpes simplex encephalitis', *J. Neurol. Neurosurg. Psychiat.*, **36**, 888.

Shuttleworth, E. C., and Morris, C. E. (1966). 'The transient global amnesia syndrome. A deficit in the second stage of memory in man', *Arch. Neurol.*, **15**, 515–520.

Shy, G. M., and Drager, G. A. (1960). 'A neurological syndrome associated with orthostatic hypotension', *Arch. Neurol. (Chicago)*, **2**, 511–527.

Silverman, A. J., Busse, E. W., and Barnes, R. H. (1955). 'Studies in the process of ageing: Electroencephalographic findings in 400 elderly subjects', *Electroenceph. Clin. Neurophys.*, **7**, 67–74.

Sinclair, K. G. A., Honour, A. J., and Griffiths, R. A. (1977). 'A simple method of measuring tremor using a variable – capacitance transducer', *Age Ageing*, **6**, 168–174.

Sjögren, H. (1952). 'Clinical analysis of morbus Alzheimer and morbus pick', *Acta. Psychiat. Neurol. Scand.*, **82** (Suppl.), 67–115.

Skre, H. (1972). 'Neurological signs in a normal population', *Acta. Neurol. Scand.*, **48**, 575–606.

Smith, C. G. (1942). 'Age incidence of atrophy of olfactory nerves in man', *J. Comp. Neurol.*, **77**, 589–595.

Smith, J. L. (1966). 'Ocular signs of Parkinsonism', *J. Neurosurg.*, **24**, 284–285.

Smith, R., and Oliver, R. A. M. (1967). 'Sudden onset of psychosis in association with vitamin B12 deficiency', *Br. Med. J.*, **3**, 34.

Smith, R., and Stern, G. (1967). 'Myopathy, osteomalacia and hyperparathyroidism', *Brain*, **90**, 593–602.

Smith, R., and Stern, G. (1969). 'Muscular weakness in osteomalacia and hyperparathyroidism', *J. Neurol. Sci.*, **8**, 511–520.

Smith W. T. (1976). 'Nutritional deficiencies and disorders', in *Greenfield's Neuropathology* (Eds W. Blackwood and J. A. N. Corsellis), pp. 194–237, Edward Arnold, London.

Sourander, P., and Sjögren, H. (1970). 'The concept of Alzheimer's Disease and its clinical implications'. in *Alzheimer's Disease and Related Conditions*, (Eds G. E. W. Wolstenholme and M. O'Connor), pp. 11–36, Churchill, London.

Spehlman, R. (1981). *EEG Primer*, Elsevier/North-Holland, Amsterdam.

Spinner, M. (1970). 'The anterior interosseous nerve syndrome: With special attention to its variations', *J. Bone Joint Surg.*, **52A**, 84–94.

Spokes, E. G. S., Bannister, R., and Oppenheimer, D. R. (1979). 'Multiple system atrophy with autonomic failure — clinical, histological and neurochemical observations on four cases', *J. Neurol. Sci.*, **43**, 59–82.

Spoor, A. (1967). 'Presbycusis values in relation to noise induced hearing loss', *Int. Audiology*, **6**, 48–57.

Steel, J. C. (1972). 'Progressive supranuclear palsy', *Brain*, **95**, 693–704.

Steele, J. C., Richardson, J. C., and Olszewski, J. (1964). 'Progressive supranuclear palsy', *Arch Neural. (Chicago)*, **10**, 333–359.

Steinberg, F. U., and Graber, A. L. (1963). 'The

effect of age and peripheral circulation on the perception of vibration', *Arch. Phys. Med.*, **44**, 645–650.

Stern, L. Z., and Fagan, J. M. (1979). 'The endocrine myopathies', in *Handbook of Clinical Neurology* (Eds P. J. Vinken and G. W. Bruyn), Vol. 41, pp. 235–258, North-Holland, Amsterdam.

Stiles, R. N., and Randall, J. E. (1967). 'Mechanical factors in human tremor frequency' *J. Appl. Physiol.*, **23**, 324–330.

Strümpell, A. (1880). 'Beiträge zur Pathologie des Rückenmarks', *Archiv. für Psychiatrie*, **10**, 676–717.

Strümpell, A. (1886). 'Ueber eine bestimmte Form der primären combinirten Systemerkrankung des Rückenmarks', *Archiv. für Psychiatrie*, **17**, 217–238.

Strümpell, A. (1904). 'Die primäre Seitenstrangsklerose (Spastiche Spinoparalyse)', *Deutsche Zeitschrift für Nervenheilkunde*, **27**, 291–239.

Struppler, A., Velho-Groneberg, P., and Claussen, M. (1976). 'Clinic and pathophysiology of tremor'. in *Advances in Parkinsonism* (Eds W. Birkmayer, and O. Hornykiewicz), pp. 287–302, Roche, Basle.

Su, P. C., and Goldensohn, E. S. (1973). 'Progressive supranuclear palsy', *Arch. Neurol.*, **29**, 183–186.

Sung, J. H., Mastri, A. R., and Segal, E. (1979). 'Pathology of Shy–Drager syndrome', *J. Neuropath. Exp. Neurol.*, **38**, 353–368.

Sutherland, J. M. (1975). 'Familial spastic paraplegia', in *Handbook of Clinical Neurology* (Eds P. J. Vinken and G. W. Bruyn), Vol. 22, pp. 421–431, North-Holland, Amsterdam.

Swallow, M. (1966). 'Fibre size and content of the anterior tibial nerve of the foot', *J. Neurol. Neurosurg. Psychiat.*, **29**, 205–213.

Swash, M. (1976). 'Disorders of ocular movement in hydrocephalus', *Proc. Roy. Soc. Med.*, **69**, 480–484.

Sweet, W. H., and Wepsic, J. C. (1974). 'Controlled thermocoagulation of trigeminal ganglion and rootlets for differential destruction of pain fibres', *J. Neurosurg.*, **40**, 143–156.

Taterka, J. H., and O'Sullivan, M. E. (1943). 'The motor complications of herpes zoster', *JAMA*, **122**, 737–739.

Tharp, B. R. (1969). 'The electroencephalogram in transient global amnesia', *Electroenceph. Clin. Neurophysiol.*, **26**, 96–99.

Thomas, D. G. T. (1983). 'Brain tumours', *Br. J. Hosp. Med.*, 29/2, 148–158.

Thomas, J. E., and Howard, F. M. (1972). 'Segmental zoster paresis — a disease profile', *Neurology (Minneap.)*, **22**, 459–466.

Thomas, P. K. (1975). 'Peripheral neuropathy', in *Recent Advances in Clinical Neurology* (Ed. W.

B. Matthews), pp. 253–283, Churchill Livingstone, Edinburgh.

Thomas, P. K. (1981). 'Peripheral neuropathy', in *The Molecular Basis of Neuropathology* (Eds A. N. Davison and R. H. S. Thompson), pp. 412–441, Edward Arnold, London.

Thomas, P. K., and King, R. H. M. (1974). 'Peripheral nerve changes in amyloid neuropathy', *Brain*, **97**, 395–406.

Thomas, P. K., and Olsson, Y. (1975). 'Microscopic anatomy and function of the connective tissue components of peripheral nerve', in *Peripheral Neuropathy* (Eds P. J. Dyck, P. K. Thomas, and E. H. Lambert), pp. 168–189, W. B. Saunders, Philadelphia.

Thompson, R. F., and Spencer, W. A. (1966). 'Habituations: a model phenomenon for the study of neuronal substrates of behaviour', *Physiol. Rev.* **73**, 16–43.

Timbury, M. C. (1982). 'Acyclovir', *Br. Med. J.*, **285**, 1223–1224.

Toghi, H., Tsukagoshi, H., and Toyokura, Y. (1977). 'Quantitative changes with age in normal sural nerves', *Acta. Neuropath. (Berlin)*, **38**(3), 213–220.

Tomlinson, A. H., and MacCallum, F. O. (1969). 'Herpes simplex encephalitis — virological diagnosis', in *Virus Diseases and the Nervous System* (Eds C. W. M. Whitty, J. T. Hughes, and F. O. MacCallum), pp. 21–27, Blackwell, Oxford.

Trojaborg, W., Frantzen, E., and Andersen, I. (1969). 'Peripheral neuropathy and myopathy associated with carcinoma of the lung', *Brain*, **92**, 71–82.

Turner, J. W., and Caird, F. I. (1982). 'Intracranial tumour', in *Neurological Disorders in the Elderly* (Eds F. I. Caird and J. A. Simpson), pp. 231–234, Wright, Bristol.

Upton, A. R. M., and Gumpert, J. (1970). 'Electroencephalography in diagnosis of herpes simplex encephalitis', *Lancet*, **1**, 650–652.

Upton, A. R. M., and McComas, A. J. (1973). 'The double crush in nerve-entrapment syndromes', *Lancet*, **2**, 359–362.

Urich, H. (1976). 'Diseases of peripheral nerves', in *Greenfield's Neuropathology* (Eds W. Blackwood and J. A. N. Corsellis), 3rd ed., pp. 688–770, Edward Arnold, London.

Veale, J. L., Rees, R., and Mark, R. F. (1973). 'Renshaw cell activity in normal and spastic man', in *New Developments in Electromyography and Clinical Neurophysiology* (Ed. J. E. Desmedt), pp. 523–547, Karger, Basel.

Verhaart, W. J. C. (1958). 'Degeneration of the brain stem reticular formation, other parts of the brain stem and the cerebellum. An example of hererogenous systemic degeneration of the central nervous system', *J. Neuropath. Exp. Neurol.*, **17**, 382–391.

Verrillo, R. T. (1980). 'Age related changes in the sensitivity to vibration', *J. Gerontol.* **35**, 185–193.

Verzár, F. (1959). 'Muscular dystrophy and old age', *Geront. Clin.*, **1**, 41–51.

Victor, M., Hayes, R., and Adams, R. D. (1962). 'Oculopharyngeal muscular dystrophy: A familial disease of late life characterised by dysphagia and progressive ptosis of the eyelids', *New Engl. J. Med.*, **267**, 1267–1272.

Wadsworth, T. G. (1977). 'The external compression syndrome of the ulnar nerve at the cubital tunnel', *Clin. Orthop.*, **124**, 189–204.

Wadsworth, T. G. (1980). *The elbow*, Chap. 8, Churchill Livingstone, Edinburgh.

Wagman, I. H., and Lesse, H. (1952). 'Maximum conduction velocities of motor fibers of ulnar nerve in human subjects of various ages and sizes', *J. Neurophysiol.*, **15**, 235–244.

Wagshul, A., and Daroff, R. B. (1969). 'L-dopa for progressive supranuclear palsy', *Lancet*, **2**, 105–106.

Wall, P. D., and Noordenbos, W. (1977). 'Sensory functions which remain in man after complete transaction of dorsal columns', *Brain*, **100**, 641–653.

Waller, A. (1850). 'Experiments on the section of the glossopharyngeal and hypoglossal nerves of the frog, and observations on the alterations produced thereby in the structure of their primitive fibres', *Phil. Trans. Roy. Soc. Lond. Series B*, **140**, 423–429.

Walton, J. N., and Nattrass, F. J. (1954). 'On the classification, natural history and treatment of the myopathies', *Brain*, **77**, 170–231.

Walton, J. N. (1961). 'Muscular dystrophy and its relation to other myopathies', *Res. Publ. Assoc. Nerv. Ment. Dis.*, **38**, 378–395.

Walton, J. N. (1964). 'Progressive muscular dystrophy', in *Disorders of Voluntary Muscle* (Ed. J. N. Walton), pp. 276–304, Churchill, London.

Wandless, I. (1981). 'Transient global amnesia', *Gerontology*, **27**, 334–339.

Wang, H. S., Obrist, W. D., and Busse, E. W. (1970). 'Neurophysiological correlates of the intellectual function of elderly patients living in the community', *Amer. J. Psychiat.*, **126**, 1205–1212.

Wang, H. S., and Busse, E. W. (1974). 'Heart disease and brain impairment among aged persons', in *Normal Aging* (Ed. E. Palmore), Vol. II, pp. 160–167, Duke University Press, Durham, N. C.

Warmolts, J. R., and Engel, W. K. (1972). 'Open-biopsy electromyography. 1. Correlation of motor unit behaviour with histochemical muscle fiber type in human limb muscle', *Arch. Neurol.*, **27**, 512–517.

Wartenberg, R. (1945). 'Orbicularis oculi reflex', in *The Examination of Reflexes*, pp. 25–34, Yearbook Publishers, Chicago.

Wartenberg, R. (1948). 'Winking-jaw phenomenon', *Arch. Neurol. Psychiat.*, **59**, 734–753.

Weinberg, H., and Spencer, P. S. (1976). 'Studies on the control of myelinogenesis. II. Evidence for neuronal regulation of myelin production', *Brain Res.*, **117**, 363–378.

Weiner, L. P., Herndon, R. M., Narayan, O., Johnson, R. T., Shah, K., Rubinstein, L. J. Preziosi, T. J., and Conley, F. K. (1972). 'Isolation of virus related to SV40 from patients with progressive multifocal leukoencephalopathy', *New Engl. J. Med.*, **286**, 385–390.

Weller, T. H., and Coons, A. H. (1954). 'Fluorescent antibody studies with agents of varicella and herpes zoster *propogated* in vitro', *Proc. Soc. Exp. Biol. Med.*, **86**, 789–794.

Weller, T. H., and Stoddard, M. B. (1952). 'Intranuclear inclusion bodies in cultures of human tissue inoculated with varicella vesicle fluid', *J. Immunol.*, **68**, 311–319.

Wells, C. E. C. (1966). 'Clinical aspects of spinovascular disease', *Proc. Roy. Soc. Med.*, **59**, 790–796.

Whitley, R. J., Soong, S-J., Linneman, C., Lui, C., Pazin, G., and Alford, C. A. (1982). 'Herpes simplex encephalitis. Clinical assessment', *JAMA*, **247**, 317–320.

Whitty, C. W. M. (1977). 'Transient global amnesia', in *Amnesia* (Eds C. W. M. Whitty and O. L. Zangwill), 2nd ed., pp. 93–103, Butterworths, London.

Wilkie, F. L., and Eisdorfer, C. (1971). 'Intelligence and blood pressure in the aged', *Science*, **172**, 959–962.

Wilkinson, P. C. (1964). 'Serological findings in carcinomatous neuropathy', *Lancet*, **1**, 1301–1303.

Wilson, S. A. K. (1925). 'Disorders of motility and of muscle tone', *Lancet*, **2**, 1–10, 53–62, 169–178, 215–219, 268–276.

Wolf, A. (1959). 'Clinical neuropathology in relation to the process of ageing', in *The Process of Ageing in the Nervous System* (Eds J. E. Birren, H. A. Innis, and W. F. Windle), pp. 175–182, C. C. Thomas, Springfield, Illinois.

Woltman, H. W. (1930). 'Pressure as a factor in the development of neuritis of the ulnar and common peroneal nerves in bedridden patients', *Am. J. Med. Sci.*, **179**, 528–532.

Wright, W. B., and Boyd, R. V. (1964). 'The glabellar tap sign in elderly patients', *Geront. Clin. (Basel)*, **64**, 124–128.

Yakovlev, P. I. (1947). 'Paraplegias of hydrocephalics. A clinical note and interpretation', *Am. J. Ment. Defic.*, **51**, 561–576.

Yakovlev, P. I. (1954). 'Paraplegia in flexion of cerebral origin', *J. Neuropathol. Exp. Neurol.*, **13**, 267–296.

Yates, P. O. (1976). 'Vascular disease of the central nervous system', in *Greenfield's Neuropathology* (Eds W. Blackwood and J. A. N. Corsellis), 3rd ed., pp. 86–147, Edward Arnold, Edinburgh.

Yock, D. H., and Marshall, W. H. (1975). 'Recent ischaemic brain infarcts at computerized tomography: Appearances pre- and post-contrast infusion', *Radiology*, **117**, 599–608.

Young, R. R., and Hagbarth, K-E. (1980). 'Physiological tremor enhanced by manoeuvres affecting the segmental stretch reflex', *J. Neurol. Neurosurg. Psychiatry*, **43**, 248–256.

Zankel, H. T. (1969). 'Pallesthesia studies in stroke patients', *South. Med. J.*, **62**, 8–11.

Zeitlin, H., and Lichtenstein, B. W. (1936). 'Occlusion of the anterior spinal artery', *Arch. Neurol. Psychiat. (Chicago)*, **36**, 96–111.

Zülch, K. J. (1979). *Histological Typing of Tumours of the Central Nervous System*. WHO, International Classification of Tumours No. 21, WHO, Geneva.

ZuRhein, G. M., and Chou, S-M. (1965). 'Particles resembling Papova virus in human cerebral demyelinating disease', *Science*, **148**, 1477–1479.

Principles and Practice of Geriatric Medicine
Edited by M. S. J. Pathy
© 1985 John Wiley & Sons Ltd

16.6

Gait and Balance

B. Isaacs

INTRODUCTION

The standard clinical examination of the hospital patient takes place with the subject in bed. Observation of the gait and recording of the findings in the case report are unusual. This is anomalous, especially in older patients in whom difficulty in walking is a frequent presenting symptom. Balance is tested by Romberg's Test when neurological disease is suspected, but is not routinely observed or recorded in elderly patients, even when admission has been necessitated by a balance disorder. This is rather like clerking a patient admitted with breathlessness and swelling of the ankles without recording the heart sounds.

Much can be learned about diagnosis, functional assessment and prognosis by the simple observation of gait and balance. The measurement of gait characteristics, such as speed and length of step, presents no technical difficulties, but is little used in clinical practice. Clinical scales of balance are rarely used. More complex methods of gait and balance measurement are confined to research laboratories, but are beginning to demonstrate their potential value to the clinician.

In this section the methods of measurement of gait and balance, and their clinical applications, will be described.

GAIT ANALYSIS

Gait analysis has its own terminology and the following definitions will be used:

A stride is the distance in the line of progression between two successive contacts of the heel of the same foot with the ground.

A step is the distance in the line of progression between the point of contact of the heel of one foot with the ground and the point of contact of the other heel.

Stride length and step length are measured in relation to the line of progression.

Stride width is the sum of the perpendicular distance between the midpoint of each foot in turn while it is resting on the ground, and the line of progression.

Frequency of stepping (also known as Cadence) is the number of steps in unit time.

Step time and stride time are the times taken for the completion of one step and one stride respectively.

In the course of each step there is a stance phase in which part of the foot is in contact with the ground and a swing phase in which no part of the foot is in contact with the ground. The stance phase normally begins with 'heel on', and ends with 'toe off', i.e. the last contact of the toe with the ground. In the course of each stride there is a period of double support when at least part of each foot is in contact with the ground. From the measurement of the time and distance factors the following additional parameters can be determined:

Time and distance symmetry is the ratio of right step time to left step time and of right step distance to left step distance. These are affected by neurological and orthopaedic conditions, e.g. hemiplegia, osteoarthritis of the hip.

Step-to-step and stride-to-stride variability is obtained by dividing the standard deviation of the length of the step or stride by the mean. This gives a measure of 'error' in the generation of successive steps, which may be related to diffuse brain damage.

The double-support time can be measured as a period of time or as a proportion of total stride time, in which case it is known as the 'double-support ratio'. An increase in the double support ratio is a sensitive indicator of impaired stability.

The step length to body height ratio gives a better basis of comparison of step length in young and old than does the step length itself, since old people are generally shorter than young ones.

MEASUREMENT OF GAIT

Complex apparatus is necessary for the determination of some of these parameters. However, speed, step length, and frequency, which are valuable measures, can be determined with a stop watch in any ward or physiotherapy department merely by timing the patient walking over a short measured distance and counting the steps taken. Large increases in step-to-step variability and the double-support ratio and large deviations from symmetry can be observed without instrumentation and should be recorded.

Laboratory methods of measuring the time and distance factors are not generally available. The earlier work was done with cinematography (Marey, 1874) and cyclography (Murray, Drought, and Kory, 1964). This work involved attaching markers to thinly clad or naked subjects, collecting large amounts of information, painstakingly measuring and analysing it, and then not always being quite

sure what to do with it. Modern refinements include the use of television cameras and other opto electronic methods with computerized analysis of the co ordinates of the positions of the markers (Woltring, 1974).

In the Department of Geriatric Medicine of the University of Birmingham a simpler system has been developed which gives direct measurement of the time and distance factors without imposing restrictions on the subject (Nayak *et al.*, 1982).

Other methods of gait analysis involve measurements of the forces acting through the legs – much used in the development of prostheses and artificial limbs (Smidt and Wadsworth, 1973); studies of the angles at the hip, knee, and ankle joints during walking (Grieve, 1968); electromyographic studies of the sequence of firing of the muscles involved in leg movement (Rozin, 1971); and studies of energy consumption during walking (Ralston, 1976). These have a limited clinical application and will not be further discussed.

Some physiotherapists have used with success the Benesh system of notation of movement (McGuiness-Scott, 1980), originally designed with the needs of choreography in mind. This may have useful applications in the analysis and correction of the hemiplegic gait.

NORMAL WALKING

Normal walking is initiated without undue pelvic tilt. The arms swing reciprocally and do not shoot out to the sides or grab at furniture. The head is held erect without spinal curvature. Stepping is regular without stagger or stumble movements. The feet are clear of the ground during each step. Initial contact is made with the heel and the foot then moves over until 'toe-off'.

CLINICAL OBSERVATION OF GAIT IN THE ELDERLY

The clinical observation of gait should be conducted in a well-dressed, properly-shod patient initially sitting in a suitably supportive chair of correct height and with the right type of arms. The walking area should be uncluttered by furniture, should be brightly illuminated, and should have a neutral floor pattern without stripes or shine. Anxious attendants should not hover around the patient.

This contrasts with the circumstances in some wards where patients may be asked to rise from unsuitable chairs while wearing pyjamas which are in danger of falling down or carrying catheter bags, and with ill-fitting slippers and no socks.

The doctor can quickly train himself to estimate speed, step length, and stepping frequency and to note the patterns characteristic of hemiplegia, Parkinson's disease, osteoarthritis of the hips, cerebellar ataxia, balance disorders, and muscle weakness. Of the innumerable points to be noted the following are clinically significant:

(a) The symmetry of step length gives a clue to hemiplegia or arthritis.

(b) The pelvic tilt is increased in hip joint disease and diminished in Parkinsonism. It is best observed by looking at the movement of the shoulders.

(c) The stride width is increased in cerebellar disease and in arthritis but not in the unstable.

(d) Arm movement becomes uncoupled at a stepping frequency of less than 0.75 Hz (Craik, Herman, and Finley, 1976) and is absent in Parkinsonism even at higher stepping frequencies.

(e) Trunk posture. Forward flexion of the upper dorsal spine and of the head is characteristic of patients with unstable balance. These patients also show irregularity of foot placement and visible prolongation of double support.

CLINICAL APPLICATIONS OF GAIT ANALYSIS

Geriatricians are accustomed to looking at a patient's gait and deciding what is wrong with him and whether he is recovering. There is probably a great deal of scope for improving the accuracy of these observations by measurement.

Normal values for the gait of ordinary people are listed in Table 1. The main parameters are as follows:

Table 1. Provisional table of midrange normal values for time and distance components of gait. (From Gabell 1983).

		[Age range]	
		25–59	70–70
Velocity	m/s	1.3	1.2
Step frequency	Hz	1.8	1.8
Step length	m	0.8	0.65
Stride width	m	0.08	0.10
Step length variability	%	4	10
Step length symmetry	R/L or L/R	1.03	1.20
Double support ratio	%	10	12

(a) Speed—in excess of 0.5 m.

(b) Step length—in excess of 0.5 m (i.e. the step length is greater than two foot-lengths, meaning that daylight is visible between the heel of the leading foot and the toe of the trailing foot).

(c) Stepping frequency—between 1.25 and 2.25 Hz.

(d) Step width—not greater than 0.1 m.

(e) Step-to-step varability—not greater than 10 per cent.

(f) Double-support ratio—not greater than 12 per cent.

In addition to the grosser changes which can be detected in disease states, gait analysis has revealed the following:

(a) Impaired vision and impaired illumination cause slowing of the gait, shortening of the step, and an increase of the double-support ratio.
(b) A period of rest before walking is associated with irregularity, expressed as increased step-to-step variability.
(c) Females perform less well than males on all gait parameters, and this effect is particularly noticeable during the wearing of high heels. Women who have worn high heels for much of their life perform less well than men, even when they are wearing 'sensible' shoes.

(d) Fully ambulant demented patients show significant differences in all gait parameters from age-matched mentally normal controls (Visser, 1983).

BALANCE

The centre of mass of the human body varies in position as the parts of the body are moved in relation to one another. For maintenance of the upright posture during standing it is required that the vertical line through the centre of mass should fall within the support base. Movement of this line towards the edge of the support base is detected by a large number of sensors – visual, vestibular and proprioceptive. The information which they provide is transmitted to brain centres whose integrated activity results in the transmission of finely graded instructions to the muscles of the neck, trunk, and limbs with the aim of restoring the line of pressure to the centre of the support base. If this does not suffice to prevent a fall, alternative strategies are called upon, namely 'sweeping' movements of the trunk and upper limbs to shift the position of the centre of mass and staggering movements of the lower limbs to alter the position of the support base.

Balance can be studied clinically by observing sway, sweep, and stagger during rising from a chair, standing, walking, and turning.

Sway

In the normal subject with feet slightly apart and eyes open, the anteroposterior sway is usually just visible and there are no sweeping or staggering movements. Sway is somewhat increased when the feet are placed close together. A slight displacement, as by the sudden application of gentle pressure to the sternum, produces increased sway in normal people and sweeping or staggering responses in those with abnormal balance (Njiokiktjien and De Rijke, 1972). Closing the eyes causes little or no change in sway in normals, but produces a substantial increase in patients with proprioceptive loss (classically in tabes dorsalis) who are largely dependent on vision to detect and correct sway.

In elderly subjects with impaired vision closure of the eyes may diminish sway (reversed Romberg ratio), presumably because closing

the eyes eliminates a source of confusion in the information.

Anteroposterior sway is usually greater than lateral sway but the latter is increased asymmetrically in patients with unilateral vestibular disease.

Quantification of Sway

The Wright ataxiameter (Wright, 1971) is a cheap and portable instrument which gives a rough measure of sway in one plane at a time; it provided much of our knowledge of sway in old age (Overstall *et al.*, 1977). More fundamental work in sway has been done using force platforms (Snijders and Verduin, 1973). These are complex and expensive transducer systems, from which can be derived a measurement of the total movement of the centre of mass in unit time – known as the mean sway path – which gives a good approximation of the degree of balance disorder (Nayak *et al.*, 1982) and an analysis of the frequency of the oscillations of which the observed sway is compounded, which may help in localizing the central nervous structure whose malfunction is responsible for the disturbance of balance (Seliktar *et al.*, 1978).

In patients with a complaint of vertigo or with hearing loss or tinnitus, vestibular function tests can be helpful in localizing peripheral vestibular lesions and distinguishing them from central lesions. Electronystagmography on a change of head position gives a quick, comfortable, and sensitive test for detecting these lesions.

GAIT AND BALANCE

Getting out of bed, rising from a chair, walking, turning, and sitting down – all essential activities of a normal day – are highly sensitive to disturbances of balance. Fear of falling is a greater obstacle to activity than is pain or limitation of joint movement.

Disturbances of balance, however generated, are reflected in the gait pattern. The main adaptation to a balance disorder is shortening of the step length, accompanied by slowing of the gait and increase in the double-support ratio. Where in addition there is interference with the proprioceptive loop control of stepping, the stepping pattern becomes irregular with a great increase in step-to-step variability (Guimaraes and Isaacs, 1980). Any sensation of instability during walking is reflected in the development of sweeping, clutching, and grabbing movements of the arms. This pattern is particularly noticeable in people who have fallen repeatedly or who have lain for long periods on the ground after falling, and who suffer severe loss of confidence in their walking ability. The term 'post-fall syndrome' has provisionally been given to this appearance (Murphy and Isaacs, 1982) and this diagnosis carries a grave prognosis. Less severe forms of the syndrome can be treated and the patient may revert to normal.

Even more significant may be the clinical finding of normal balance in a patient with a history of recurrent falls. If carelessness and distractability can be excluded as the cause of such falls, the suspicion must be high that the falls are due not to a balance disturbance but to an alteration in the blood flow through some pathway in the balance mechanism, possibly as a result of episodic cardiac dysrhythmia.

CONCLUSION

The laboratory analysis of gait and balance in old people is still at an early stage and present techniques are too complex for clinical use. The information derived from the laborabory, however, shows that some estimate of speed, stepping frequency, step length, and sway should form part of the routine clinical examination of the elderly, together with a description of the gait and the pattern of rising from a chair and standing. This information can guide the clinician towards a correct diagnosis and to the evaluation of functional deficiency.

REFERENCES

Craik, R., Herman, R., and Finley, F. R. (1976). 'Human solutions for locomotion: II – Interlimb co-ordinates', *Adv. Behav. Biol.,* **18**, 51–64.

Gabell, A. (1983). 'Relationships between gait and balance', MSc Thesis, University of Birmingham.

Grieve, D. W. (1968). 'Gait patterns and the speed of walking', *Biomed. Eng.,* **3**, 119–122.

Guimaraes, R. M., and Isaacs, B. (1980). 'Characteristics of the gait in old people who fall', *Int. Rehabil. Med.,* **2**, 4.

McGuinness-Scott, J. (1980). 'Benesh notation: An introduction to recording clinical data'., *Physiotherapy,* **66** (8), 268–270.

Marey, E. J. (1874). *Animal mechanisms*, Henry S. King, London.

Murphy, J., and Isaacs, B. (1982). 'The post-fall syndrome: a study of 36 elderly patients'. *Gerontology,* **28**, 265–270.

Murray, M. P., Drought, A. B., and Kory, R. L. (1964). 'Walking patterns of normal men', *J. Bone Joint Surg. (Am.),* **46**, 335–360.

Nayak, U. S. L., Gabell, A., Simons, M. A., and Isaacs, B. (1982). 'Measurement of gait and balance in the elderly', *J. Am. Geriatr. Soc.,* **30**, 516–520.

Njiokiktjien, C. J., and De Rijke, N. (1972). 'The recording of Romberg's test and its application in neurology', *Agressologie (Paris),* **13c**, 1–7.

Overstall, P. W., Exton-Smith, A. N., Imms, F. J., and Johnson, A. L. (1977). 'Falls in the elderly related to postural imbalance', *Br. Med. J.,* **1**, 261–264.

Ralston, H. J. (1976). 'Energetics of human walking', *Ad. Behav. Biol.,* **18**, 77–98.

Rozin, R. (1971). 'Investigation of gait', *Electromyogr. Clin. Neurophysiol.,* **11**, 183–190.

Seliktar, A., Susau, Z., Najenson, T., and Solzi, P. (1978). 'Dynamic features of standing and their correlation with neurological disorders', *Scand. J. Rehabil. Med.,* **10**, 59–64.

Smidt, G. L., and Wadsworth, J. B. (1973). 'Flow reaction forces during gait: Comparison of patients with hip disease and normal subjects', *Phys. Ther.,* **53**, 1056–1062.

Snijders, C. J., and Verduin, M. (1973). 'Stabilograph: An accurate instrument for sciences interested in postural equilibrium', *Agressologie (Paris),* **14c**, 15–20.

Visser, H. (1983). 'Gait and balance in senile dementia of Alzheimer's type', *Age and Aging,* **12**, 296–301.

Woltring, H. D. (1974). 'New possibilities of human motion studies by real time light spot position measurements'. *Biotelem. Patient Monit.,* **1**, 132–146.

Wright, B. M. (1971). 'A simple mechanical ataxiameter', *J. Physiol.,* **218**, 27–28.

16.7

Falls

P. W. Overstall

EPIDEMIOLOGY

Falls are one of the commonest problems of old age. Random surveys of old people living at home show that about 20 per cent. of men and 40 per cent. of women give a history of a fall during the previous months (Exton-Smith, 1977; Prudham and Evans, 1981; Sheldon, 1960). The proportion who fall increases with age (see Fig. 1). A decline in the prevalence of falls was noted among very old men by Exton-Smith (1977) and among women of the same age by Prudham and Evans (1981). This may represent the survival of an exceptionally fit elite or be an artefact due to the relatively small numbers available for study at that age.

The majority of falls go unreported, and less than 3 per cent. a year of the elderly who fall at home sustain an injury requiring medical attention (Gray, 1966; Waller, 1978). Nonetheless, the numbers involved are sufficiently large to ensure that a hospital serving a catchment area of 210,000 inhabitants with 33,000 aged 60 years or over might expect to have 16 beds continuously occupied by elderly persons admitted because of a fall (Lucht, 1971).

Within the protected environment of a residential home the rate of severe falls may be as high as 11 per cent. per year (Gryfe, Amies, and Ashley, 1977), which reflects the often poor state of health of the residents and raises

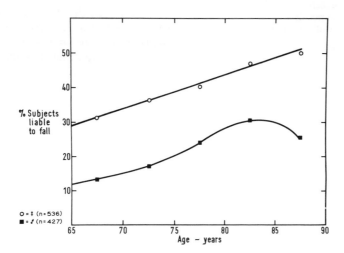

Figure 1   Age incidence of falls. (From Exton-Smith, 1977. Reproduced by permission of The Royal Society of Medicine)

doubts about the usefulness of improving home safety as a means of preventing falls.

Site and Time of Fall

The majority of serious falls occur by day indoors, or within the immediate environs of the house (Brocklehurst *et al.*, 1976; Lucht, 1971; Wild, Nayak, and Isaacs, 1981). Most falls on stairs occur when the person is descending, and many more accidents occur on straight, single flights than on U-shaped two-flight stairs (Svanström, 1974). In institutions falls are most common in the first week after admission and during times of maximum activity, despite adequate supervision (Sehested and Severin-Nielsen, 1977). A low fall rate may reflect low activity and overprotectiveness by the staff (Morris and Isaacs, 1980).

CLINICAL PRESENTATION

A precise classification of falls based on aetiology is not yet possible. This is partly due to ignorance of the underlying alterations in balance control, but also because it is usual to find pathological impairment in a number of areas, any or all of which may be relevant to the fall. A simple, but clinically useful approach is shown in Table 1.

Table 1   Classification of falls

Trips and accidents
Falls not due to external hazard:
Fall following change in position
Spontaneous fall when walking or standing
Any fall may be initiated by:
Postural hypotension
Cardiac syncope
Drugs
Acute illness
Organic brain disease
Head rotation or vertigo
Poor vision
Osteomalacia
Psychological factors

Trips and Accidents

Trips and accidents account for about 45 per cent. of falls (Overstall *et al.*, 1977; Sheldon, 1960). The prevalence of this type of fall declines with increasing age (Exton-Smith, 1977). In a study in which 82 per cent. of those who fell were over the age of 75, Wild, Nayak, and Isaacs, (1981) found that tripping was uncommon. This study was of patients who had reported a fall to their general practitioner and since most trips do not cause injury such events were likely to be under-represented. The relation between falls due to trips and age probably reflects the greater mobility of the young who get out of doors more, and in whom the occasional trip or accidental fall does not shake their confidence unduly and does not restrict their activities.

It is probably true that those who trip are more posturally stable and, by implication, less debilitated than those who fall for other reasons, such as loss of balance, drop attacks, and after rising from a chair. This is supported by the finding that postural sway when standing is the same in those who fall because of a trip as non-fallers, compared with significantly increased sway among other fallers (Overstall *et al.*, 1977). We do not know whether this active group of trippers and accidental fallers maintain their mobility and confidence, and have a lower mortality than other fallers, although there is indirect evidence that they do (Wild, Nayak, and Isaacs, 1981). If mortality is lower in this group it will be important to ask whether it is their higher level of physical activity which protects them or whether the amount of activity reflects their better general health.

Falls Not Due to External Hazards

Characteristically the patient is at a loss to explain why she fell. Remarks such as, 'It just happened', 'Down I went', or 'I lost my balance', are often heard. Some try to rationalize it by saying, 'I must have tripped', which rarely means that they actually did trip. Similarly, patients who say that they felt giddy at the time are frequently describing a sense of unsteadiness and a fear of falling rather than true vertigo.

It has already been mentioned that the balance of these patients measured as postural sway is impaired when compared with non-fallers or those who have tripped. Precisely where the impairment lies is not always apparent, but it is helpful to recall that maintenance of the upright position depends on vision, proprioception, the labyrinths, and a stable base. The extrapyramidal system, cerebellum, and cortical centres coordinate the whole process, and the clinician must try to decide which areas are critically affected. There is considerable reserve in the overall system and any one of the sources of postural information may be lost with little of consequence. For example, patients with bilateral ablation of the labyrinths will walk steadily and will continue even when blindfolded, but if they then step on to uneven ground and lose the stability of their base, they immediately fall (Martin, 1967a).

Many elderly patients are in a similar position. A person may have a long-standing unilateral labyrinthine lesion due to, say, Ménière's disease, which, on its own, is not particularly troublesome. In addition, he may have cervical spondylosis with loss of the important proprioceptive information normally provided by the cervical mechanoreceptors. He then gets out of bed in the middle of the night without turning on the light and falls because, deprived of visual cues, he has passed the critical point where his balance can be maintained. This 'final straw' syndrome is frequently observed among elderly fallers, and it is not difficult to understand why a fall is so often the consequence of a chest infection, heart failure, or the use of a powerful hypnotic. Patients who fall for no apparent reason may be divided into subgroups according to the displacing force required; thus a fall following a change in position requires more force than a spontaneous fall when walking or standing, and patients in this latter group may be those who are most frail.

Fall Following Change of Posture

Not all patients who feel unsteady and then fall after rising from the sitting or lying position have postural hypotension. Rising, walking, and even standing are inherently unstable positions, and require coordinated and effective action from the antigravity muscles if balance is to be maintained. For many old persons, the rise from the relative safety of their chair is one of the most hazardous moments of their day.

Spontaneous Fall When Walking or Standing

These are often falls which puzzle and frighten the sufferer most. Unexpectedly and for no apparent reason the patient will say, 'My legs gave way'. On close questioning it may be possible to detect a loss of concentration at the critical moment. For instance, a patient busy making tea fell when she was interrupted by a ring at the door. Similarly another, while walking along the street, her mind on her shopping list, fell when hailed by a friend across the street. One could postulate that these falls are the result of an age-related slowing of central decision-making processes, and the consequent difficulty that some old persons have of coping with a rapidly changing situation or a sudden increase in mental data that require attention (Welford, 1977).

Falling at a time when the patient is hurrying to the lavatory is commonly reported (Sehested and Severin-Nielsen, 1977), and presumably results from loss of attention due to the pressing needs of an unstable bladder.

Falls during awkward movements, such as carrying a loaded tray through a narrow doorway or turning rapidly, emphasize that such patients have little postural reserve and that, unlike younger persons, the speed of their reflexes is insufficient to save them once balance is lost. Obesity and arthritis of the spine, hips, and knees reduce nimbleness and increase the likelihood of a fall once a person is unstable.

Drop Attacks

These are usually described as a separate phenomenon, although it is doubtful if they differ fundamentally from the falls described in the preceding section. They are, by definition, unexpected falls without loss of consciousness or neurological sequelae, and the patient is frequently unable to stand afterwards unless helped. They are estimated to be responsible for between 12 and 25 per cent. of falls in the elderly (Overstall *et al.*, 1977; Sheldon, 1960) and are largely confined to women (Stevens and Matthews, 1973), although with advancing age the number of men affected does increase (Exton-Smith, 1977).

The aetiology remains uncertain. Vertebrobasilar insufficiency is the usual explanation, but this was excluded by Stevens and Matthews (1973) and brainstem ischaemia is an uncommon finding in elderly patients investigated in a vestibular clinic (Overstall, Hazell, and Johnson, 1981). Although drop attacks may follow transient ischaemia in the vertebrovasilar territory due to occlusion of the vertebral arteries by cervical osteophytes or emboli, this is relatively rare, and the diagnosis is best avoided unless there is supporting evidence of brainstem dysfunction such as dysarthria, diplopia, or homonymous hemianopia.

It seems unlikely that drop attacks can be attributed to a single cause, and close examination of these patients shows that many of them have a variety of postural defects. When investigated, they are invariably found to have vestibular disorders (Hazell, 1979) and their postural sway is increased (Overstall *et al.*, 1977). Why drop attacks should occur on some occasions and not on others is unclear. Possibilities include transient and minor physical ill-health, cardiac arrhythmias, drug side-effects related to the plasma elimination half-life and the time of the last dose, and psychological upsets. The female prepondrance has not yet been satisfactorily explained.

INITIATING OR AGGRAVATING FACTORS

Postural Hypotension

This should be sought even in patients who do not complain of dizziness or loss of balance when rising from the sitting or lying position. It is present in up to 24 per cent. of persons aged 65 or over (Caird, Andrews, and Kennedy, 1973) but many are asymptomatic. Patients with postural hypotension who fall have greater body sway than aged matched controls. However, there is probably no causal relationship between the drop in blood pressure and increased sway, and it is likely that the majority of elderly patients with postural hypotension have multiple central nervous system defects (Overstall, Johnson, and Exton-Smith, 1978). In practice, the majority of these patients will improve when hypotensive drugs and tranquillizers are stopped and physiotherapy improves mobility.

Cardiac Syncope

A fall associated with loss of consciousness raises the possibility of cardiac syncope. The patient may use the word 'blackout', but this is unreliable, and it is better to ask whether she can remember hitting the floor. Preceding palpitations, dizziness, chest pain, and dyspnoea can be useful clues, and a reliable witness is invaluable. Sometimes the episode mimics an epileptic fit.

Livesley and Atkinson (1974) reported that 50 per cent. of falls observed in 76 elderly patients were a result of unstable cardiac rhythm. Most clinicians would think that was an over-estimate, but if there is serious doubt over the diagnosis, the patient should undergo continuous ambulatory cardiac monitoring.

Drugs

Drugs may cause falls through a variety of mechanisms, but the common problem is dullness and slowing due to hypnotics and tranquillizers. Fallers are more likely than controls to have taken a sedative during the previous 24 hours, but this may reflect the fact that their health is generally poorer (Wild, Nayak, and Isaacs, 1981). Prudham and Evans (1981) found that a significantly increased proportion of fallers had taken tranquillizers, but not hypnotics, compared with non-fallers.

Long-acting hypnotics can cause considerable hangover, daytime confusion, and falls. Barbiturates are notorious (Gibson, 1966; Macdonald and Macdonald, 1977), but nitrazepam (Evans and Jarvis, 1972; Greenblatt and Allen, 1978) and flurazepam (Greenblatt, Allen, and Shader, 1977; Oswald, 1979) can be equally troublesome, and the ill-effects may only be apparent after several weeks of continuous use.

Alcohol should not be forgotten as a cause of falls (Waller, 1978), although fallers do not appear to differ from non-fallers in their consumption of alcohol (Prudham and Evans, 1981).

Hypoglycaemia may cause falls in patients taking chlorpropamide (Schen and Benaroya, 1976).

Acute Illness

A fall may be the presenting feature of a serious illness such as a chest infection, cerebral infarct, diarrhoea, gastrointestinal haemorrhage, or cardiac failure (Howell, 1971). Falls are common in patients who have a toxic confusion.

Organic Brain Disease

Pathology involving the sensori-motor cortex, cerebellum, or basal ganglia is likely to impair postural control, and the commonest conditions that do so are senile dementia of the Alzheimer type (SDAT) cerebrovascular disease, particularly the multi-infarct variety, and Parkinsonism. Falls are a common feature of these conditions, sometimes at an early stage before the clinical diagnosis is obvious. There is, however, very little information on the relation between anatomical changes and impaired balance, although poor postural control is a well described feature of basal ganglia disease (Martin, 1967b) and elderly fallers have lower mental test scores than controls (Isaacs, 1978; Wild, Nayak, and Issacs, 1981).

We need to know how important cerebrovascular disease and hypertension are as causes of falls, since preventative measures could be helpful. For a long time it was assumed that declining IQ scores were a normal accompaniment of ageing, until it was shown that untreated hypertensives did less well on intelligence testing than those who were free of disease or whose hypertension was medically controlled. Other experiments have shown a direct correlation between reduced cerebral oxygenation and impaired mental performance (Eisdorfer, 1977). It would not be surprising if a similar relationship was shown between mild cerebral ischaemia and falls.

Head Rotation and Vertigo

Turning the head is blamed by 5 per cent. and giddiness by another 9 per cent. of old persons for their falls. Both groups have increased postural sway compared with controls (Overstall *et al.*, 1977). Either group may have true vertigo, but this is relatively unusual, and non-fallers are as likely to complain of it as fallers. What these patients are commonly describing is a feeling of disequilibrium, and fallers report this more frequently than non-fallers (Prudham and Evans, 1981). The increased sway indicates poor postural reserve, and the likelihood is that even minor changes in equilibrium will cause a fall.

Vertigo after rotating or extending the neck is usually said to be the result of vertebrobasilar ischaemia, but the evidence for this, except in a small minority of cases, is negligible. What is more likely is that the patient has cervical mechanoreceptor dysfunction or a peripheral vestibular lesion or both.

The contribution of the mechanoreceptors in the apophyseal joints of the cervical spine to postural control has been described by Wyke (1979). He emphasizes that even in the presence of a normally functioning vestibular system, the loss of afferent input from these mechanoreceptors for any reason (degenerative, infective, or traumatic) causes clinically significant disturbances such as vertigo, nystagmus, and ataxia.

Central vestibular lesions are found in 50 per cent. and peripheral lesions in 34 per cent. of elderly referrals to a specialist clinic (Overstall, Hazell, and Johnson, 1981). Although this was a selected group of patients, the impression is that vestibular lesions are common, but are frequently undetected without special investigations.

Vision

A minor reduction in visual acuity in persons over the age of 75 is associated with femoral neck fractures (Brocklehurst *et al.*, 1976) and fallers, particularly those over the age of 70 years, have significantly poorer vision than non-fallers (Wilder-Smith and Thorp, 1981). There is, however, no difference between fallers and non-fallers in their use of spectacles (Prudham and Evans, 1981).

Postural sway when standing increases when the eyes are closed. Both peripheral and central vision are important for maintaining steady balance, and it has been shown that patients with a vestibular defect rely on vision more than normal persons to maintain their balance (Begbie, 1967). Martin (1976b) has also shown how vision can, to a great extent, compensate for the lack of vestibular function. Patients completely devoid of vestibular function may lead fairly normal lives, but become unsteady in darkness, in fog, if the surface is at all uneven, or when they are descending stairs. Even minor reductions in visual acuity may therefore have an important effect on balance in old people who already have reduced afferent information from other parts of the balance system.

Osteomalacia

Osteomalacia should be suspected in patients who complain of falls and difficulty in walking, particularly if they have poor sunlight exposure, are taking anticonvulsant drugs, or have a history of gastrectomy or renal disease.

Psychological Factors

Tiredness, restlessness, undue haste, and unexplained errors of judgement are frequently present at the time of a fall (Gray, 1966; Svanström, 1974). Depression with psychomotor retardation may result in misperception of environmental danger or an inappropriate response (Jacobson, 1974).

DIAGNOSIS

The old instruction to take a proper history is particularly valuable in patients who fall. One needs an exact description of the events leading up to the fall: whether there was a change in posture, head rotation, true vertigo, a sense of disequilibrium, palpitations, or loss of consciousness. A drug history and assessment of the patients' mental state are mandatory. Mild dementia is easily missed unless looked for, and the diagnosis has major relevance for future management.

The patient should be asked about ear disease, the presence of deafness, and tinnitus. Although tinnitus indicates a vestibular lesion, it is of no further localizing value. The patient's gait and balance with eyes open and closed should be observed, and the lying and standing blood pressure measured.

Backward leaning suggests Parkinson's disease, cerebrovascular disease, or SDAT and is presumably due to involvement of the basal ganglia, although it may indicate an apraxia or an altered perception of spatial relationships. It is sometimes seen in neurologically normal patients who have been confined to bed for a long time. Leaning to one side during walking suggests a vestibular or cerebellar lesion.

There may be an easily recognized gait, such as the 'marche à petits pas' due to multiple cerebral infarcts, or what is sometimes known as the 3F syndrome (fear of further falling) where the patient makes exaggerated and fearful efforts to clutch on to furniture, lunges for a chair long before she has reached it, and constantly calls out that she is going to fall (although rarely does so).

Limited neck movements are found in most old people and may be relevant if limitation is severe or there are other postural defects. Nystagmus should be looked for when the neck is flexed, extended, and rotated. Visual acuity and fields should be assessed.

MANAGEMENT

Improving general health, treating obvious problems, and stopping harmful drugs are the first steps. Thereafter the aim is to improve confidence and mobility. How one goes about it depends largely on the skills and enthusiasm available locally, since there is no overwhelming evidence that any particular therapeutic approach is better than another.

An active department of geriatric medicine should encourage early referral, particularly from accident and emergency departments. Prompt assessment and treatment is likely to prevent the catastrophic decline that so often affects old persons once their balance and confidence is lost. Treatment may be started in hospital, day hospital, or through a domiciliary physiotherapist, and regular follow-up should be arranged for those at risk.

Advice to Patients

The patient should be given an explanation of the nature of her postural impairment, and warned that falls are often the result of the 'final straw'. Thus she should make full use of vision and never move about at night without the lights on. Descending poorly lit stairs and walking on uneven ground are particularly dangerous. Getting in and out of bed and chairs, and turning should be done cautiously. Sedative drugs and alcohol should be avoided, and every effort made to remain active and maintain mobility. If living alone, she should be advised on the installation of an alarm.

General Measures

Elderly persons who have had falls respond enthusiastically to a daily programme of balance exercises, but objective evidence of improvement is difficult to demonstrate (Overstall and Kinsman, unpublished results).

The exercises (Table 2) take about 10 minutes, and after the patient has been shown how to do them she continues them on her own each day at home. Initially the therapist corrects faulty posture and teaches safe ways of getting

Table 2 Balance exercises
(Repeat each exercise 10 times.) (From Overstall, 1970. Reproduced with permission of the editor of the *Journal of the American Geriatrics Society*)

1. (a) Stand, with finger support, first on one leg and then the other.
   (b) Repeat, counting to 10, on each leg.
   (c) Repeat, counting to 20, on each leg.
2. (a) Sit on a dining chair, turn, and look to left and then to right.
   (b) Repeat with arms abducted.
   (c) Touch the left foot with the right hand, and then the right foot with the left hand.
3. (a) While sitting, pick up an object from the floor, straighten up, and then replace it on the floor.
4. (a) Stand and slowly pick up an object from a table; place it on a chair and then back on the table.
   (b) Repeat, but this time slowly place the object on the floor.

in and out of a bed and chair, and as mobility increases, so confidence gradually improves.

A stick or walking aid is often a great help in improving the patient's sense of security, but she must be taught how to use it properly, and once it has served its purpose and she is walking with confidence, it should be withdrawn.

The patient should be taught how to get up off the floor in case she has another fall (Fig. 2), and a home visit by an occupational therapist to advise on safety is desirable. However, external hazards are not usually an important cause of falls. An alarm system can give great psychological support (particularly to relatives). However, it needs to be carefully assessed and the patient asked about her attitude, since installed alarms are rarely used by those who fall (Wild, Nayak, and Isaacs, 1981). The main reasons given as to why these alarms are not used are that the systems are technically faulty, inconvenient, and difficult to use, or psychologically unacceptable (Feeney,

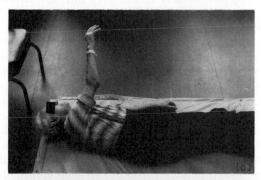
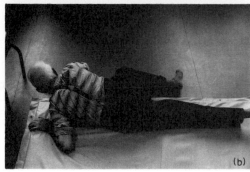
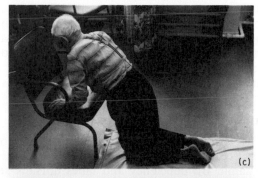
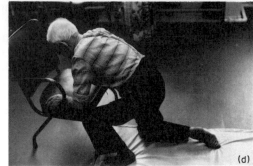

Figure 2 Instructions to patient for getting up after a fall

(a) Remain calm and concentrate on rolling over. Turn head in the direction of roll, and bring the arm and knee over together.
(b) Push up with the arms to get into the all-fours position and crawl to the nearest chair.

(c) Approach the chair from the front and put your hands on the seat.
(d) Bend your best knee (i.e. the strongest and least arthritic), push up, and twist round to sit in the chair.

Galen, and Gallagher, 1975). Some old people say that they do not use their alarms because they do not want to be a nuisance and disturb anyone.

Vestibular Lesions

Peripheral lesions usually respond well to drugs such as 15 to 30 mg of cinnarizine three times daily or 8 mg of betahistine three times daily. If no improvement is seen within 3 weeks, there is little point in continuing the drug and referral for specialist advice should be considered. Surgery (e.g. decompression of the endolymphatic sac) for Ménière's disease is often helpful.

Central vestibular lesions are not improved by drugs, and powerful vestibular sedatives such as the phenothiazines are best avoided, since they may make the patient feel worse.

The Cooksey–Cawthorne exercises (Cooksey, 1946) can be valuable where there is disabling vertigo. The aim is to increase the patient's tolerance of unequal balance between the two ears, and should be performed for at least 5 minutes three times daily. The patient is advised to seek out head positions and movements that cause vertigo as far as can be tolerated, since the more frequently vertigo is induced the more rapidly tolerance develops.

Ataxia

This is likely to be due to a cerebellar lesion or to cord compression by cervical spondylosis. Vitamin B$_{12}$ deficiency and tabes dorsalis are rare, but it is important that they are not missed.

The aim with these patients is to teach normal movements and stimulate awareness of balance and posture through constant repetition. Frenkel's exercises (which were originally designed for tabetic patients) encourage the patient to use his eyes and ears as subtitutes for other afferent information, and to move in precise rhythmic patterns to counting (Frenkel, 1917).

Cervical Spondylosis

The usual problem is disordered mechanoreceptor function, and the patient should be encouraged to rely on vision to compensate for lost afferent input. Extreme neck movements which are known to produce giddiness should be avoided, but it is best not to put the patient into a cervical collar, since this may make things worse, particularly in the dark. Gentle exercises to improve the range of neck movements should be done daily, as well as general balance exercises to improve mobility and confidence.

Poor Vision

Patients with multiple postural defects may be considerably helped if their vision acuity is improved by appropriate spectacles or cataract extraction. Biofocal lenses are occasionally confusing and troublesome to old people and may need to be changed. For patients with poor vision, a stick or walking frame may provide guidance and a visual point of reference.

PROGNOSIS

Falls, particularly in the very old, are usually a sign of serious ill-health. In one series, a quarter of those with falls had died within a year, five times as many as in the control group. Of those who lay on the floor for more than one hour after their fall, half were dead within 6 months. Mortality was greatest in those who were house-bound or immobile, had abnormal gait and balance, had an impaired mental test score, and were incontinent (Wild, Nayak, and Isaacs, 1981). Despite this poor outlook for a minority of patients, worthwhile improvements can usually be achieved in the remainder.

REFERENCES

Begbie, G. H. (1967). 'Some problems of postural sway', in *Myotatic, Kinesthetic and Vestibular Mechanisms, CIBA Foundation Symposium*, (Eds A. V. S. de Reuck and J. Knight), pp. 80–92, Churchill, London.

Brocklehurst, J. C., Exton-Smith, A. N., Lempert Barber, S. M., Hunt, L., and Palmer, M. (1976). 'Fracture of the femur in old age; a two centre study of associated clinical factors and the cause of the fall', *Age Aging, 7*, 7–15.

Caird, F. I., Andrews, G. R., and Kennedy, R. D. (1973). 'Effect of posture on blood pressure in the elderly', *Br. Heart J., 35*, 527–530.

Cooksey, F. S. (1946). 'Rehabilitation in vestibular injuries', *Proc. Roy. Soc. Med.,* **39**, 273–275.

Eisdorfer, C. (1977). 'Intelligence and cognition in the aged'. in *Behaviour and Adaptation in Late Life* (Eds E. W. Busse and E. Pfeiffer), pp. 219–220. Little, Brown & Co., Boston.

Evans, J. G., and Jarvis, E. H. (1972). 'Nitrazepam and the elderly', *Br. Med. J.,* **4**, 487.

Exton-Smith, A. N. (1977). 'Functional consequences of ageing; clinical manifestations', in *Care of the Elderly: Meeting the Challenge of Dependency* (Eds A. N. Exton-Smith and J. G. Evans), pp. 41–57, Academic Press, London.

Feeney, R. J., Galer, M. D. and Gallagher, M. M. (1975). *Alarm Systems for Elderly and Disabled People*, Institute for Consumer Ergonomics Ltd. University of Technology, Loughborough.

Frenkel, H. S. (1917). 'The treatment of tabetic ataxia by means of systematic exercise', 2nd ed, Heinemann, London.

Gibson, I. I. J. M. (1966). 'Barbiturate delirium', *Practitioner,* **197**, 345–347.

Gray, B. (1966). *Home Accidents among Older People*, Royal Society for the Prevention of Accidents, London.

Greenblatt, D. J., and Allen, M. D. (1978). 'Toxicity of nitrazepam in the elderly', *Brit. J. Clin. Pharmacol,* **5**, 407–413.

Greenblatt, D. J., Allen, M. D., and Shader, R. I. (1977). 'Toxicity of high dose flurazepam in the elderly', *Clin. Pharmacol. Ther.,* **21**, 355–361.

Gryfe, C. I., Amies, A., and Ashley, M. J. (1977). 'A longitudinal study of falls in an elderly population. I. Incidence and morbidity', *Age Ageing,* **6**, 201–211.

Hazell, J. W. P. (1979). 'Vestibular problems of balance', *Age Ageing,* **8**, 258–260.

Howell, T. H. (1971). 'Premonitory falls', *Practitioner,* **206**, 666–667.

Isaacs, B. (1978). 'Are falls a manifestation of brain failure', *Age Ageing,* **7**(Suppl.), 97–105.

Jacobson, S. B. (1974). 'Accidents in aged', *NY State J. Med.,* **74**, 2417–2420.

Livesley, B., and Atkinson, L. (1974). 'Repeated falls in the elderly', *Mod. Geriatr.,* **4** (11), 458–467.

Lucht, U. (1971). 'A prospective study of accidental falls and resulting injuries in the home among elderly people', *Acta. Soc. Med. Scand.,* **2**, 105–120.

Macdonald, J. B., and Macdonald, E. T. (1977). 'Nocturnal femoral fracture and continuing widespread use of barbiturate hypnotics', *Br. Med. J.,* **2**, 483–485.

Martin, J. P. (1967a). 'Role of the vestibular system in the control of posture and movement in man', in *Myotatic, Kinesthetic and Vestibular Mechanisms. CIBA Foundation Symposium* (Eds A. V. S. de Reuck and J. Knight), pp. 92–96, Churchill, London.

Martin, J. P. (1967b). *The Basal Ganglia and Posture*, Pitman, London.

Morris, E. V., and Isaacs, B. (1980). 'The prevention of falls in a geriatric hospital', *Age Ageing,* **9**, 181–185.

Oswald, I. (1979). 'The why and how of hypnotic drugs', *Br. Med. J.,* **1**, 1167–1168.

Overstall, P. W. (1980). 'Prevention of falls in the elderly', *J. Am. Ger. Soc.,* **XXVIII**, 481–484.

Overstall, P. W., Hazell, J. W. P., and Johnson, A. L. (1981). 'Vertigo in the elderly', *Age Ageing,* **10**, 105–109.

Overstall, P. W., Imms, F., Exton-Smith, A. N., and Johnson, A. L. (1977). 'Falls in the elderly related to postural imbalance', *Br. Med. J.,* **1**, 261–264.

Overstall, P. W., Johnson, A. L., and Exton-Snith, A. N. (1978). 'Instability and falls in the elderly'., *Age Ageing,* **7**(Suppl.), 92–96.

Overstall, P. W., and Kinsman, R. (unpublished result). 'Balance exercises for elderly fallers'.

Prudham, D., and Evans, J. G. (1981). 'Factors associated with falls in the elderly; a community study', *Age Ageing,* **10**, 141–146.

Schen, R. J., and Benaroya, Y. (1976). 'Hypoglycaemic coma due to chlorpropamide; observations on twenty-two patients', *Age Ageing,* **5**, 31–36.

Sehested, P., and Severin-Nielsen, T. (1977). 'Falls by hospitalized elderly patients; causes, prevention', *Geriatrics*, April **1977**, 101–108.

Sheldon, J. H. (1960). 'On the natural history of falls in old age', *Br. Med. J.,* **2**, 1685–1690.

Stevens, D. L., and Matthews, W. B. (1973). 'Cryptogenic drop attacks: An affliction of women', *Br. Med. J.,* **1**, 439–442.

Svanström, L. (1974). 'Falls on stairs: An epidemiological accident study', *Scand. J. Soc. Med.,* **2**, 113–120.

Waller, J. A. (1978). 'Falls among the elderly – human and environmental factors', *Accid. Anal. Prev.,* **10**, 21–33.

Welford, A. T. (1977). 'Causes of slowing of performance with age', in *Interdisciplinary Topics in Gerontology* (Ed. I. R. Mackay), Vol. 11, p. 43, Karger, Basle.

Wild, D., Nayak, U. S. L., and Isaacs, B. (1981). 'How dangerous are falls in old people at home?', *Br. Med. J.,* **282**, 266–268.

Wilder-Smith, O. H. G., and Thorp, T. A. S. (1981). 'How dangerous are falls in old people at home?', *Br. Med. J.,* **282**, 2132–2133.

Wyke, B. (1979). 'Cervical articular contributions to posture and gait: Their relations to senile disequilibrium', *Age Ageing,* **8**, 251–258.

Principles and Practice of Geriatric Medicine
Edited by M. S. J. Pathy
© 1985 John Wiley & Sons Ltd

16.8

The Epidemiology and Pathogenesis of Stroke and Transient Ischaemic Attacks

P. O. Yates

BLOOD SUPPLY TO THE BRAIN

The brain is supplied with blood by the internal carotid and vertebral arteries which through the basilar artery and the circle of Willis form an anastomotic net of great flexibility. Obviously, the system has evolved to allow for temporary occlusion of one or more of the extracranial cerebral arteries in the neck during movement. It is equally useful in the aged when such occlusion may occur temporarily or permanently through disease; in some people who have a perfect anastomotic system even one internal carotid or one vertebral artery may supply sufficient blood to the brain for survival where the other three major arteries are obstructed by disease.

In such cases blood supply to the brain is often augmented by retrograde flow from the external carotid along branches of the internal carotid such as the ophthalmic. However, the circle of Willis itself shows considerable variation in the size and completeness of its component vessels, only 20 per cent. being of optimal pattern (Riggs and Rupp, 1963).

The arterial distribution from the circle follows three general paths. The central branches perforate the base and hypothalamic areas; the short circumferential branches supply the thalamus and other basal ganglia; the long circumferential vessels run on the surface to supply the cortex and underlying white matter. There is little or no anastomosis of the first two groups of arteries except at the arteriole and capillary level, but quite large communications exist between the anterior, middle, and posterior arteries on the surface of the brain. This allows survival of the peripheral parts of the territory supplied by any one of these major channels should its main trunk be occluded.

Similarly, the branches from vertebral and basilar arteries form paramedian and short circumferential systems which show little connection with each other and supply deeper brain stem and cerebellar nuclei, and long circumferential branches, the superior, anterior and posterior inferior cerebellar arteries that run over the surface of the cerebellum supplying the cortex and nearby white matter. These latter vessels have a number of large anastomotic channels between each other.

SUBDIVISION OF CEREBROVASCULAR DISEASE

Clinically it is often convenient to consider cerebrovascular disease in three subdivisions: firstly, as major strokes often resulting in death or major disability; secondly, as minor strokes with relatively minor neurological disability and nearly full recovery; thirdly, as transient ischaemic attacks (TIA) involving short lived disability of any cerebral function with apparent complete recovery and sometimes frequent repetition of an identical attack.

Such a classification lacks a basis of pathological correlation and therefore any logical indication of therapy, prevention, and prognosis other than general nursing care. All three types of stroke may be caused by obstructive vascular disease leading to ischaemia or to disruptive disease producing haemorrhage and tissue displacement. However, things are not quite so clear-cut because rupture of an artery or aneurysm may provoke vascular spasm at some distance with resultant ischaemia; and a ruptured artery can rarely supply effectively the territory beyond the point of haemorrhage.

DISEASE OF EXTRACRANIAL ARTERIES

Obstructive cerebral arterial disease in the elderly is almost always due to atherosclerosis with thrombotic complications or to embolism. Other much rarer conditions occasionally cause problems: temporal giant cell arteritis may affect medium-sized cerebral arteries (Cromptom, 1959); polyarteritis nodosa and various granulomatous arteritides such as Takayasu's disease (Nasu, 1963) have been reported at all ages.

Atherosclerosis is as Crawford (1960) defined it a 'widely prevalent arterial lesion characterized by patchy thickening of the intima, the thickenings comprising accumulations of fat and layers of collagen and like fibres'. There are many hypotheses as to its nature and aetiology. It seems probable that focal damage to the endothelial cell lining occurs because of (a) imperfect streamlining, (b) attachment of antigen–antibody complexes, (c) pulses of increased nor-epinephrine levels, (d) raised carbon monoxide levels in cigarette smokers. Platelets adhere at the site of damage (Woolf *et al.*, 1968) and by their presence stimulate a monoclonal proliferation of smooth muscle cells from the media which are capable of type III collagen production. At the same time the defect in the endothelial lining, imperfectly repaired, allows the seepage of plasma lipids into the plaques. There are a number of complications that ensue and that have special significance for the cerebral circulation.

Firstly, atheromatous plaques once formed are the site of frequent small mural thrombus formation which when dislodged by the blood stream or neck movement may temporarily obstruct distal vessels and through the effects of ischaemia give rise to one variety of transient ischaemic attack. Such platelet and fibrin emboli have been observed slowly traversing the only easily visible part of the cerebral circulation (the retinal vessels), and the occurrence of transient amblyopia is well documented (Russell, 1961).

Pathogenesis

It is useful to consider the pathogenesis of obstructive cerebrovascular disease in terms of the large mainly extracranial carotid and vertebral arteries, the major intracranial arteries, and the intracerebral vessels. Atherothrombotic narrowing and occlusion of one or more of the vessels in the neck is twice as common in men aged 50 to 70 as in women. (Hultquist, 1942). He reported occlusion to be present at routine hospital autopsy in about 5 per cent. of cases. Stenosis with potential thrombus formation in an internal carotid artery is clinically more important than complete occlusion which, if confined to the cervical part of a single vessel, does not usually produce clinical symptoms. The significance of stenosis and occlusion of these major vessels lies in the fact that the disease process is likely to affect more than one vessel (Hutchinson and Yates, 1957), extending to the limit the anastomotic potential of the intracranial cerebral arteries. Thus such patients may survive with perhaps only a single vertebral or carotid artery supplying the whole cerebrovascular tree and are extremely vulnerable to further insults, whether these be a fall of blood pressure, an episode of hypoglycaemia, or an acute blood loss as from a peptic ulcer or trauma.

The internal carotid sinus is, perhaps because of its imperfect hydrodynamics, one of the earliest sites in the body for the development of atheroma. Plaques here are especially liable to the complication of sudden haemorrhagic dissection and expansion of the lesion which may occur a number of times before final occlusion of the arterial lumen. Each haemorrhage will provoke a spasm of the arterial wall of varying duration and may activate a sinus reflex fall of blood pressure. Debris from these haemorrhages readily calcifies, forming a rigid non-compressible structure so that the carotid sinus receptor nerves that lie outside the atheromatous plaque may be unusually sensitive to the examining finger of the physician.

A fall of blood pressure is only significant if it results in a reduction of cerebral blood flow. In the normal physiological state and in young hypertensives cerebral blood flow is controlled by autoregulatory methods based on the reactivity of arterioles in such a way that it remains constant over a mean arterial pressure of 60 to 140 mmHg (Strandgaard *et al.*, 1973). Below this range cerebral blood flow is reduced. However, in hypertensives the autoregulatory mechanism is shifted to a higher level; the lowest tolerable mean pressure may be over 100 mmHg in such patients.

There is increasing evidence that patients whose cerebrovascular tree is compromised by disease are liable to attacks of cerebral ischaemia and even infarction if the blood pressure is reduced suddenly from their personal norm (Ledingham and Rajagopalan, 1979). Attempts to reduce the blood pressure for therapeutic or preventative reasons must proceed slowly and with caution in the elderly.

The basilar artery is formed by the confluence of the two vertebral arteries and joins the circle of Willis via the posterior cerebral arteries. Its branches supply the vital brainstem and posterior hypothalamic nuclei, including, for example, the locus caeruleus and dorsal nucleus of the vagus, which through noradrenalin transmitters appear to have some control of the microcirculation of the whole of the central nervous system (Swanson and Hartman, 1980). Therefore, disease of the vertebral vessels should always be looked for not only in focal hindbrain syndromes but also where a generalized cerebral dysfunction is found.

The cervical course of the vertebral arteries through the lateral masses of the cervical vertebrae is well protected from trauma and extreme neck movement in the young, but is very vulnerable in the middle aged and elderly. The distorting effect of osteoarthritic changes in the neurocentral joints, the collapse of the intervertebral discs, together with artherosclerotic changes in the arteries may be sufficient to cause temporary obstruction following certain movements of the neck. Attacks of syncope, tinnitus, dizziness, and ataxia in the elderly may often have such a cause.

Iatrogenic problems are well known to follow attempts to treat the arthritic and osteophytic changes of cervical spondylosis by manipulative techniques. Thrombosis of the vertebral arteries causing death has been reported as an unhappy complication (Pratt-Thomas and Berger, 1947).

'STEAL' SYNDROMES

Severe atheroma of the aortic arch with extension to obstruct the origins of subclavian or innominate arteries obviously contributes to the whole picture of cerebrovascular insufficiency. Its special importance may be to cause the 'subclavian steal syndrome' (Reivich *et al.*, 1961). If the obstruction is proximal to the mouth of the vertebral artery then the blood supply to the arm which cannot flow directly from the aorta might depend on retrograde flow down this vessel, thus 'stealing' blood from the basilar artery and circle of Willis. Energetic exercise of the arm with rapid opening of the vessels in the muscles increases the blood demand up to fourfold and reduces the blood pressure in the circle of Willis precipitating clinical signs of cerebral ischaemia.

Wherever anastomotic channels of any size are available similar reversals of flow from the cerebral circulation may be found. For example, if the common carotid artery is occluded below the bifurcation then the flow in the internal carotid may be reversed to supply the external carotid. Within the skull similar 'internal steal' situations may occur between one major cerebral artery and another.

A slightly different situation is found in the surviving brain tissue around an infarct or haemorrhage where blood flow studies have shown an inappropriately rich arterial flow (Hachinski, Lassen, and Marshall, 1974). It seems that blood vessels in these areas may show loss of tone and responsiveness, which by reducing peripheral resistance causes a local excessive flow. There will be a fall in the perfusion pressure elsewhere in the territory of the parent artery. Excessive flow because of electrolyte and acid/base imbalance may be as deleterious to neuronal function as ischaemia. It is usually a temporary phenomenon but may persist for months.

Occlusion of individual intracranial arteries occasionally results from atheroma and local thrombosis but more commonly by embolism from larger proximal arteries or from the heart. Of course, in a case of generalized arterial disease occlusion of a particular intracranial artery is only the most obvious lesion; atheroma may restrict collateral supply and emboli may be multiple.

Anastomotic arteries, when required for collateral supply, hypertrophy in young humans when a major artery such as an internal carotid has been obstructed, usually by trauma or ligation. Similarly, the 'theft' of blood through the shunt of an arteriovenous malformation will, in the young, cause great hypertrophy of feeder vessels. However, in the old human this facility seems no longer to be available at a time when disease would make it desirable, even life-saving.

The most common cerebral infarct occurs in the territory of the middle cerebral artery. Atherosclerotic narrowing of the middle cerebral artery is often seen at autopsy but local thrombosis and occlusion is not common. In a series of cases where 47 large infarcts were found in the middle cerebral territory, Lhermitte, Gautier, and Derousene (1970) reported that in 6 cases no local arterial occlusion was found but in these and 20 other cases the internal carotid artery was blocked. Half of the 47 infarcts resulted from embolic occlusion from a diseased heart or major extracranial artery. When a large artery such as one of the main arteries of a hemisphere is obstructed the zone of damage usually lies well within the artery's apparent territory. The earliest change is swelling of both grey and white matter as capillary integrity is lost. Very early infarction can often only be appreciated as an area of 'softening' to the feel. Where there is a good collateral blood supply the lesion will be haemorrhagic. This is more usually the case where the cause of the obstruction is an embolus and where atheromatous disease is not widespread.

The question of the relative vulnerability to ischaemia of the various cells and tissues of the nervous system is still not certain. There is no doubt that the metabolism and function of neurones stops within 5 to 10 minutes and recovery of their function (which might be essential to the unsupported survival of the patient) may take days or even 2 to 3 weeks. Experimental studies of precisely timed periods of ischaemia usually fail to take account of the production of capillary sludging and microthrombi which, though transient, may prolong the period of ischaemia. There is increasing experimental evidence that where small vessel blood remains fluid as by preheparinization and the microcirculation is thus able to restart immediately at the end of an ischaemic period, then neurones may function after quite long periods of is-

chaemia (Hossmann and Hossmann, 1973). An additional factor is the metabolic demand by nerve cells which is greatly increased in epileptic attacks and significantly decreased during barbiturate therapy.

DISEASE OF INTRACRANIAL AND INTRACEREBRAL ARTERIES

Arteries penetrating brain tissue are all small and thin walled, having very little medial coat and no external elastic lamina. They do not show atherosclerotic changes and in the absence of hypertension are rarely occluded except by small emboli. These are usually thrombotic in origin but occasionally cholesterol crystals and other debris from ulcerated atheromas in larger proximal vessels. In cases of moderate to severe trauma, whether or not bones are broken, fat emboli arise and this is especially a problem when surgical procedures to correct a fractured femur in elderly people is delayed for 2 to 3 days. The infarcts that result, although small and even microscopic, are frequently numerous.

Atherosclerotic dementia, now commonly called multi-infarct dementia, is a result of small intracerebral vessel disease. This is not usually due to an atherosclerotic process with thrombosis but to multiple embolism and even more commonly to the effects of hypertension on small central arteries.

In young people the arteries of the brain respond to a moderate but persistent rise in blood pressure by an appropriate hypertrophy of the muscular medial coat, as do vessels elsewhere in the body (Cook and Yates, 1972). In the elderly, focal loss of the muscle coat occurs with or without hypertension and small intracerebral vessels are converted to tubes of unreactive collagen with occasional defects in the internal elastic lamina. Tone is lost because of the loss of the medial muscle and such small arteries become elongated and dilated, taking up a tortuous path divorced to a large extent from the neighbouring brain tissue.

From time to time the endothelial lining of such small but stretched vessels is disrupted and plasma or even whole blood permeates the collagen of the wall to produce a hyaline appearance; a number of them become occluded by platelet/fibrin thrombus.

These changes in small arteries are most obvious in the paramedian penetrating vessels that run directly from the basilar artery into the pons and midbrain or from the circle of Willis and its large branches into the basal ganglia and hypothalamus. It is in these areas that numerous small infarcts and cystic spaces are to be seen in the brains of elderly hypertensive people.

The loss of tissue in cases of multi-infarct dementia, scattered widely as it may be, is usually over 50 ml in total and this implies an equivalent reduction in cerebral blood flow. However, the paralysis of vasoregulatory mechanisms in the adjacent surviving tissue allows an increase in flow so it is doubtful whether measurements of total or even regional flow will help to differentiate this type of dementia from Alzheimer's disease.

The changes that follow rapid or excessive rises of blood pressure where the mean pressure may be for some time above 140 mmHg cause failure of the tonic vasoregulatory mechanism of the cerebral arterioles and frequent small ruptures occur; thus a generalized state of cerebral oedema, fibrinous exudation, and petechial haemorrhage is found with the usual clinical picture of severe headache, impairment of consciousness, convulsions, and various focal neurological deficits. Such a hypertensive encephalopathy, when it occurs in the aged, may be followed in those who survive by a persistent but variable dementia.

Examination of the brain of elderly hypertensive patients will frequently reveal the presence of a number of 'stroke' lesions, many more than in a normotensive case. Cole and Yates (1968) carefully examined the brains from 100 hypertensive and 100 age- and sex-matched normotensive people dying in hospital from a wide variety of causes. They found that a quarter of the normotensives had suffered old or recent cerebral infarcts, large and small, or cystic scars. About a quarter of the hypertensives also showed evidence of cerebral infarction; a further quarter showed old or recent haemorrhagic lesions or pigmented cysts. Only a few hypertensive patients had a mixture of infarcts and haemorrhages.

An interesting finding was the number of small, non-fatal lesions of a size producing mordibity and multi-infarct dementia. In the 100 normotensives, 17 brains showed an average of 5 small (>1 cm) infarcts. The 100 brains

from hypertensive patients showed a similar number of lesions per case but many more cases were affected; 18 cases had an average of 5 small infarcts but an additional 23 cases showed an average of 5 small haemorrhages. These figures draw attention to the fact that haemorrhages are a very common cause of small as well as large strokes, a phenomenon appreciated only by pathologists until the CAT scanner made the differentiation of small infarcts and haemorrhages possible during life. These haemorrhages result from the rupture of small (500 μm to 2 mm) aneurysms found on intracerebral arteries of hypertensive people. Such aneurysms were first described by Charcot and Bouchard (1868) but their true incidence was not fully appreciated until Russell (1963) and Cole and Yates (1967) studied many brains by post-mortem angiography.

Cole and Yates found that 46 per cent. of hypertensive brains each showed an average of 20 microaneurysms. Only 2 of 21 patients under 50 had any; of those aged over 65, more than half had aneurysms. Of an age- and sex-matched 'normotensive' group Cole and Yates found only 7 per cent. with aneurysms, all had diastolic pressures over 100 mmHg, and all were over 65 years. All patients with large or small, recent or old haemorrhages in the brain showed microaneurysms. They were found in the basal ganglia, pons, and cerebellum and noticeably in cortical gyral white matter – a frequent site for 1 to 2 cm slit haemorrhages.

These intracerebral aneurysms have a very similar histological picture to that of the saccular (so-called congenital) aneurysms of the circle of Willis, but, of course, on a much smaller scale. There is a breach of the elastic membrane and focal loss of medial muscle; remaining collagen stretches to form the sac. As indicated above, increasing age as well as hypertension is clearly important in producing this phenomenon. Whether this age factor is the focal loss of smooth muscle or increasing 'brittleness' of elastic is not known. There is some evidence that the larger saccular aneurysms of the circle of Willis are predisposed to rupture by inadequately structured type III collagen in some people (Pope *et al.*, 1981).

Apart from the obvious complications of rupture these small sacs may thrombose and by occluding the vessel itself produce small infarcts. Most surveys from Europe and North

America found subarachnoid haemorrhage to be about 12 per 100 of all cerebrovascular disease, which would suggest it accounts for about 2 per 100 of all deaths in those countries.

The cooperative study between a large number of centres in the United States and one in England found that only about half of their 5,000 or so cases were due to rupture of an aneurysm of the circle of Willis, many of the rest being secondary to an intracerebral haemorrhage. About two-thirds of all cases show significant hypertension and, as we all know, the modal age for presentation with subarachnoid haemorrhage is around 55 years. Few pathologists today are prepared to accept the old idea of Forbus (1930) that congenital medial defects are the basis of the circle of Willis aneurysms. These vascular defects are also frequent at sites both intra- and extracranially where berry aneurysms do not occur, so some additional factor must be present. Certainly I believe that almost a half of all cases of subarachnoid haemorrhage should be considered with hypertensive cerebral haemorrhage as having a similar basis in intracerebral microaneurysms. Many of these involved cortical arteries, rupture of which would surely produce subarachnoid haemorrhage.

TRANSIENT ISCHAEMIC ATTACKS

The name transient ischaemic attack (TIA) refers strictly to a clinical condition whose aetiology is assumed to be a temporary failure of blood supply. What is by definition transient is the episode of cerebral dysfunction from which complete recovery is expected within minutes or at longest 23 hours. I suspect that not all cases labelled as TIAs fulfil this requirement absolutely and that quite a proportion have some residual disability, perhaps revealed only by very careful examination before and after an attack. There is increasing evidence that after some TIAs there is long-term histopathological and pathophysiological change of a focal nature.

The symptoms of these attacks have a rapid onset and are usually maximal by 5 or 10 min, disappearing within 30 min. Return to normal is often as swift as the loss of function. In a report of a cooperative study of over 1,000 patients from 10 centres in the United States, Dyken, Conneally, and Haerer (1977) found

that for attacks in the vertebrobasilar territory the mean duration was 8 minutes; for those in either carotid area it was 14 minutes. I think that the pathogenesis of such episodes is probably very different from that of the more prolonged attack where recovery may take 24 hours. Similarly, there is probably a very wide spectrum of TIAs ranging from those cases where a large number of small events occur over many months or years, most of which are hardly recognizable clinically because of the small area or clinically silent nature of the nervous tissue involved, to those that have only one or two attacks leading to a major stroke (Marshall, 1964).

The transient attacks which a neurologist or even a primary care physician records are almost certainly a small fraction of the real number of such events. The prevalence appears to vary for people over 65 years of age who have had no permanent stroke from 18 per 1,000 in Georgia (Karp *et al.*, 1973) to 63 per 1,000 in Illinois (Ostfeldt *et al.*, 1973). The annual incidence for people of middle age is around 1 per 1,000 (Heyman *et al.*, 1974).

Whatever the mechanism of production of TIAs, there seems to be some prognostic significance in their occurrence, for definite stroke is seen in approximately 10 per cent. of patients within a year of the first attack (Rees *et al.*, 1970) and approximately 30 per cent. in a 3 to 8 year follow-up (Heyman *et al.*, 1974). Most of these completed strokes were probably due to cerebral infarction, although it is not clear that all patients had autopsy examination; the unreliability of the clinical diagnosis of the pathology of a small stroke is notorious to pathologists and, with increasing use of the CAT scanner, to radiologists also.

We know from the regional cerebral blood flow studies report by Rees and coworkers in 1970 that persistent focal changes in flow may be present 90 days after a clinically transient attack – obviously it was the signs and symptoms that were transient and not the attack on the tissues, which appears to have had more permanent effects. It is probable that what has happened in these cases is a permanent loss of autonomic control of small arteries in such an area. There is some evidence to show that the internal cerebral arteries are innervated by a central adrenergic system arising in the locus caeruleus in the brainstem. This system may not only control local blood flow but may also allow variations in the blood–brain barrier function of the vascular endothelial cells. It is, of course, quite separate from the more widely understood vasomotor control of cerebral arteries outside brain tissue which are to some extent under the influence of the superior cervical ganglion. Persistent disturbance of vasomotor control close to an old small infarct or haemorrhage would provide a locus minores resistentes, which during hemodynamic upset (e.g. a sudden rise or fall of systemic blood pressure) would be a site for transient attacks repeatedly of a similar clinical presentation. However, it is true that deliberately lowering the blood pressure in these patients by tilt tables and other devices only rarely precipitates an attack.

There are many reports in which the significance of hypertension has been dismissed largely because of the lack of a suitable hypothesis by which it could be implicated. It remains a fact that approximately half of a large series of patients with TIAs were hypertensive. The hypertensive has obvious disease of small intracerebral arteries exemplified in the production of microaneurysms. This is especially so after age 50. The aneurysm sac sometimes occludes by thrombosis, and, if the small parent artery is involved, an infarct of 1 to 2 cm may be found in basal cerebral regions or in the brainstem or cerebellum. Sometimes the beginning of such an affair appears to have been rupture and a small haemorrhage, raising the possibility that substances may be released around the vessel that could produce spasm of the artery itself, e.g. serotonin from platelets (Zervas *et al.*, 1973) or prostaglandin F_2 (La Torre *et al.*, 1974). Thus a much greater field of temporary ischaemia would be produced than might eventually be destroyed by necrosis.

Sources for emboli in the heart and great vessels are well known, as is the frequent association of myocardial infarction with its dangerous mural thrombus and small strokes or TIAs (approximately a third of TIA patients have ischaemic heart disease) (Marshall and Wilkinson, 1971).

The relevance of atheromatous stenotic lesions of the carotid and vertebral arteries is obvious. Surgical endarterectomy of the internal carotid sinus atheromatous plaque is said to give complete relief from TIAs in more than 50 per cent. of the cases with carotid stenosis. Perhaps the conversion from turbulent to laminar flow through the sinus allows the new endothelium to withstand further thrombosis.

More striking emboli, when seen in the retina and those that usually leave permanent sequelae, are derived from the contents of atheromatous plaques that have been dissected by rupture of the overlying intima. It seems doubtful if this crystalline debris often produces really significant infarcts except where function is especially vulnerable to small lesions, as in the retina. In 1961 Hollenhurst reported retinal arterial obstruction by crystals of cholesterol in 11 per cent. of 235 patients with symptoms of carotid system disease and 5 per cent. of those with vertebrovasilar disease. Twenty per cent. of 35 patients who underwent carotid endarterectomy had such retinal emboli.

When emboli lodge in peripheral cerebral arteries there is a possibility that they may fragment and pass through the capillary bed. Whether this happens depends on the amount of fibrin incorporated into the thrombus and the speed of fibrinolysis, for platelets by themselves do not form very tough permanent aggregations.

Many have reported the passage of pale clumps through the retinal vessels, and Miller Fisher in 1959 referred to such observations that were made as early as 1870. His own patient had attacks of monocular blindness with recovery, and the emboli took 65 minutes to clear the retinal vascular tree. McBrien, Bradley, and Ashton showed in 1963 that these emboli were almost pure platelet aggregations. Time is obviously very important in producing symptoms, and Skovborg and Lauritzen (1965) watched several emboli pass through the retina much more rapidly, each taking only approximately 2 minutes, without producing symptoms.

Undoubtedly these platelet collections form very commonly after a high-fat meal, a time which Mustard (1957) showed to have increased coagulation activity. I want to draw attention to the fact that a high-fat diet is often associated with intake of cow milk protein. Immune complexes produced in response to such foreign protein are now thought to be important in damaging vascular endothelium and allowing platelet attachment. Indeed, some believe that this phenomenon, which may be observed early in childhood, is the real basis for atheromatous disease, which then develops along the lines indicated by Rokitansky (1853) and Duguid (1948).

Rundles and Kimbell (1969) reminded us that 16 per cent. of the population have redundant loops of internal carotid artery and these kinky vessels might be obstructed by neck turning. If the circulation is already compromised by occlusion of a major vessel, general events may produce fleeting focal disability. The site of abnormal function depends very much on the anastomotic potential of the circle of Willis and of the junctions between cortical surface arteries. In a patient with one carotid artery occluded, sudden anaemia and hypotension caused by intermittent gastrointestinal haemorrhage might produce focal rather than general cerebral dysfunction, as might the episodic failure of cardiac output associated with cardiac dysrhythmias (Walter, Reid, and Wenger 1970). As many as one-fourth of patients with TIAs may belong to this hemodynamic group. McAllen and Marshall (1973) reported cessation of TIAs after cardiac control by a pacemaker.

Cerebral blood flow is greatly influenced by the blood viscosity, in which the red blood cell is a major factor. In the Framingham survey men with haemoglobin levels above 15 g/dl had approximately twice the incidence of cerebral infarction. It seems that in some patients with TIAs a high haematocrit is an important factor. A group of workers in London (Thomas *et al.*, 1977) treated such a group of patients by venesection sufficient to lower the mean haematocrit from 49 to 43. Of course, the haemoglobin level also fell by just over 2 g/dl, and the oxygen-carrying capacity of the blood fell by 13 per cent. Cerebral blood flow, however, was increased by 50 per cent. Five patients with carotid TIAs remained free of attacks for at least 5 months, as did 3 out of 4 patients with vertebrobasilar TIAs. Perhaps many of our patients, at least in the Western world, would benefit from regular venesection – the 'bleeding and cupping' so popular over a hundred years ago when every good physician carried a jar of leeches on his rounds.

Nor can one ignore hypoglycaemia, as in the case reported by Portnoy (1965), where tran-

sient left hemiparesis occurred during hypoglycaemia in a man with right-sided internal carotid stenosis. After endarterectomy he had no further attacks, even when he was hypoglycaemic. It has already been mentioned that the internal carotid sinus reflex may be a cause of sudden hypotension, especially when made hypersensitive to external pressure by the presence of calcified atheroma or by a recent haematoma expanding the plaque. The neurologist's palpating finger has probably produced many an ischaemic attack that, fortunately, is usually transient.

Finally, one must remember that episodes of cerebral dysfunction of vascular origin are part of a spectrum that cannot always be divided into sharp clinical entities with names such as TIA, small stroke, stroke with full recovery, mild or moderate stroke, completed stroke, and finally death.

REFERENCES

Charcot, J. M., and Bouchard, C. (1886). 'Nouvelles recherches sur la pathogénie del' hémorrhagie cérébrale', *Archives de Physiologie Normale et de Pathologie*, **1**, 110–127, 643–665.

Cole, F. M., and Yates, P. O. (1967). 'The occurrence and significance of intracerebral microaneurysms', *J. Path. Bact.*, **93**, 393–411.

Cole, F. M., and Yates, P. O. (1968). 'Comparative incidence of cerebrovascular lesions in normotensive and hypertensive patients', *Neurology (Minneap.)*, **18**, 255–259.

Cook, T. A., and Yates, P. O. (1972). 'A histometric study of cerebral and renal arteries in normotensives and chronic hypertensives', *J. Pathol.*, **108**, 129–135.

Crawford, T. (1960). 'Some aspects of the pathology of atherosclerosis', *Proc. R. Soc. Med.*, **53**, 9–12.

Crompton, M. R. (1959). 'The visual changes in temporal (giant cell) arteritis', *Brain*, **82**, 377–390.

Duguid, J. B. (1984). 'Thrombosis as a factor in the pathogenesis of aortic atherosclerosis', *J. Path. Bact.*, **60**, 57–61.

Dyken, M. L., Conneally, M., and Haerer A. F. (1977). 'Co-operative study of hospital frequency and character of transient ischemic attacks', *J A M A*, **237**, 882–886.

Forbus, W. D. (1930). 'On the origin of miliary aneurysms of the superficial cerebral arteries', *Bull. Johns Hopk. Hosp.*, **47**, 239–284.

Hachinski, V. C., Lassen, N. A., and Marshall, J. (1974). 'Multi-infarct dementia', *Lancet*, **2**, 207–210.

Heyman, A., Leviton, A., Millikan, C. H., Nefzger, M. D., Ostfeldt A. M., Sahs, A. L., Stallones, R. A., and Whisnant, J. P. (1974). 'Report of the Joint Committee for Stroke Facilities. XI. Transient focal cerebral ischemia epidemiological and clinical aspects', *Stroke*, **5**, 277–287.

Hollenhurst, R. W. (1961). 'Significance of bright plaques in the retinal arterioles', *J A M A*, **178**, 23–29.

Hossmann, V., and Hossmann, K. A. (1973). 'Return of neuronal functions after prolonged cardiac arrest', *Brain Res.*, **60**, 423–438.

Hultquist, G. T. (1942). *Uber Thrombose und Embolie der Arteria Carotidis und Hierbei Vorkommende Gehirnveranderungen*, Fischer, Jena, Stockholm.

Hutchinson, E. C., and Yates, P. O. (1957). 'Carotico-vertebral stenosis', *Lancet*, **i**, 2–5.

Karp, H. R., Heyman, A., Heydon, S., Bartel, A. G., Tyroler, H. A., and Hames, C. G. (1973). 'Transient cerebral ischemia', *J A M A*, **225**, 125–128.

La Torre, E., Patrono, C., Fortuna, A., and Grossi-Belloni, D. (1974). 'Role of prostaglandin F_2 in human cerebral vasospasm', *J. Neurosurg.*, **41**, 293–299.

Ledingham, J. G. G., and Rajagopalan, B. (1979). 'Cerebral complications in the treatment of accelerated hypertension', *Q. J. Med.*, **48**, 25.

Lhermitte, F., Gautier, J. C., and Derousené, C. (1970). 'Nature of occlusions of the middle cerebral artery', *Neurology (Minneap.)*, **20**, 82–88.

McAllen, P. M., and Marshall, J. (1973). 'Cardiac dysrhythmia and transient cerebral ischaemic attacks', *Lancet*, **i**, 1212–1214.

McBrien, D. J., Bradley, R. D., and Ashton, N. (1963). 'The nature of retinal emboli in stenosis of the internal carotid artery', *Lancet*, **i**, 697–699.

Marshall, J. (1964). 'Transient ischaemic cerebrovascular attacks', *Q. J. Med.*, **33**, 309–324.

Marshall, J., and Wilkinson, I. M. S. (1971). 'The prognosis of carotid transient ischaemic attacks in patients with normal angiograms', *Brain*, **94**, 395–402.

Miller Fisher, C. (1959). 'Observations of the fundus oculi in transient monocular blindness', *Neurology (Minneap.)*, **9**, 333–347.

Mustard, J. F. (1957). 'Increased activity of the coagulation mechanism during alimentary lipaemia: Its significance with regard to thrombosis and atherosclerosis', *J. Can. Med. Assoc.*, **77**, 308–314.

Nasu, T. (1963). 'Pathology of pulseless disease', *Angiology*, **14**, 225–242.

Ostfeldt, A. M., Shekelle, R. B., and Klawans, H. L. (1973). 'Transient ischemic attacks and risk of stroke in an elderly poor population', *Stroke*, **4**, 980–986.

Pope, F. M., Nicholls, A. C., Narsisi, P., Bartlett, J., Neil-Dwyer, G., and Doshi, B. (1981). 'Some patients with cerebral aneurysms are deficient in type III collagen', *Lancet*, **1**, 973–975.

Portnoy, H. D. (1965). 'Transient ischaemic attacks produced by carotid stenosis and hypoglycaemia', *Neurology (Minneap.)*, **15**, 830–832.

Pratt-Thomas, H. R., and Berger, K. E. (1947). 'Cerebellar and spinal injuries after chiropractic manipulation', *J A M A*, **133**, 600–603.

Rees, J. E., Du Boulay, G. H. Bull, J. W. D., Marshall, J., Ross Russel, R. W., ans Symon, L. (1970) 'Regional cerebral blood flow in transient ischaemic attacks', *Lancet*, **ii**, 1210–1213.

Reivich, M., Holling, H. E., Roberts, B., and Toole, J. F. (1961). 'Reversal of blood flow through the vertebral artery and its effect on cerebral circulation', *N. Engl. J. Med.*, **265**, 878–885.

Rokintansky, A. (1853). *A Manual of Pathological Anatomy* (translated by G. E. Day), The Sydenham Society, London.

Riggs, H. E., and Rupp, C. (1963). 'Variation in the form of circle of Willis', *Arch. Neurol. (Chicago)*, **8**, 8–14.

Rundles, W. R., and Kimbell, F. D. (1969). 'The kinked carotid syndrome', *Angiology*, **20**, 177–194.

Russell, W. R. (1961). 'Observations on the retinal blood vessels in monocular blindness', *Lancet*, **2**, 1422–1428.

Russell, W. R. (1963). 'Observations on intracerebral aneurysms', *Brain*, **86**, 425–442.

Skovborg, F., and Lauritzen, E. (1965). 'Symptomless retinal embolism', *Lancet*, **2**, 361–362.

Strandgaard, S., Oleson, J., Skinhøj, E., and Lassen, N. A. (1973). 'Autoregulation of brain circulation in severe arterial hypertension', *Br. Med. J.*, **i**, 507–510.

Swanson, L. W., and Hartman, B. K. (1980). 'Biochemical specificity in central pathways related to peripheral and intracerebral homeostatic function', *Neurosci Lett.*, **16**, 55–60.

Thomas, D. J., Du Boulay, G. H., Marshall, J., Pearson, T. C., Russell, R. W., Symon, L., Wethersley-Mein, G., and Zilkha, E. (1977). 'Effect of haematocrit on cerebral blood flow in man', *Lancet*, **2**, 941–943.

Walter, P. F., Reid, S. D., and Wenger, N. K. (1970). 'Transient cerebral ischemia due to arrhythmia', *Ann. Intern. Med.*, **72**, 471–474.

Woolf, N., Bradley, J. P. W., Crawford, T., and Carstairs, K. C. (1968). 'Experimental mural thrombi in the pig aorta. The early natural history', *Br. J. Exp. Path.*, **49**, 257–264.

Zervas, N. T., Kuwayama, A., Rosoff, C. B. and Salzman, E. W. (1973). 'Cerebral arterial spasm. Modification by inhibition of platelet function', *Arch. Neurol.*, **28**, 400–404.

Principles and Practice of Geriatric Medicine
Edited by M. S. J. Pathy
© 1985 John Wiley & Sons Ltd

16.9

Clinical Aspects and Medical Management of Stroke Disease in the Elderly

Davis Coakley

Interest in cerebrovascular disease has increased considerably during the past decade. Significant advances have been made in investigative techniques, more emphasis has been placed on treatment during the acute stage and units specializing in stroke rehabilitation have been developed around the world. Despite all this research and interest, however, many important questions about the investigation and treatment of stroke and threatened stroke remain unanswered.

THREATENED STROKE – TRANSIENT ISCHAEMIC ATTACKS

A transient ischaemic attack (TIA) may be the harbinger of a stroke. The majority of studies show that 15 to 25 per cent. of patients with untreated TIA develop cerebral infarction. There is also a very high risk of serious heart disease; in fact the latter is a more common cause of death than stroke (Simonsen *et al.*, 1981). About 30 per cent. of hospital stroke admissions and 10 per cent. of stroke cases in the community describe previous TIAs (Harrison, 1980). Unfortunately, it is not possible to predict which patients with TIA will subsequently develop a stroke but patients with multiple episodes within a short period are particularly at risk. Carotid TIAs are more sinister than those in the vertebrobasilar territory.

Aetiology of Transient Ischaemic Attacks

Most transient ischaemic attacks are thought to be due to embolization of platelet, fibrin, or atheromatous debris from an atherosclerotic plaque in the carotid or vertebrobasilar tree. Rapid fragmentation of these emboli allow subsequent restoration of blood flow (see Chapter 16.8).

The heart is another potential source of emboli. Mural thrombi may form within 2 months of a myocardial infarction but akinetic segments of the myocardium may be a source for embolus formation indefinitely. Rheumatic heart disease, bacterial and non-bacterial endocarditis, atrial myxomata, and myxomatous degeneration of the mitral valve may all give rise to transient ischaemic episodes. Myxomatous degeneration of the mitral valve once thought benign is now known to cause progressive mitral regurgitation and cardiac arrhythmias. The condition may be found in both young and old but Barnett, Boughner, and Cooper (1978) found a particularly high incidence (40 per cent.) in a group of young adults who had a stroke and/or a transient ischaemic attack. Cerebral blood flow falls even with modestly elevated haematocrits and vertebrobasilar and carotid TIA have been reported in polycythaemia rubra vera. Hyperviscosity due to paraproteinaemias may also be associated with episodes of cerebral ischaemia.

Haemodynamic factors are probably much more important in the genesis of transient ischaemic attacks in elderly patients with generalized atherosclerosis than in patients of a younger age group (Helps, 1979). Variations in cerebral autoregulation may explain why some elderly people with minor falls of systemic arterial pressure develop clinical signs of cerebral ischaemia whereas others with greater falls in blood pressure remain asymptomatic (Wollner *et al.*, 1979). Naritomi, Sakai, and Meyer, (1979) in a study of the pathogenesis of transient ischaemic attacks within the vertebrobasilar arterial system implicated haemodynamic factors and dysautoregulation. Long-term ECG monitoring in patients with cerebrovascular insufficiency has led to more awareness of dysrhythmia as a cause of focal or generalized neurological symptoms (McHenry, Toole, and Miller, 1976). Ueda, Toole, and McHenry (1979) found that cardiac dysrhythmia is likely to cause TIA more frequently in patients over the age of 60 than in a younger age group. Haemodynamically significant arrhythmias were observed in 32 per cent. of patients with TIA in a study by Luxon *et al.*, (1980) but in only 3% of an age-and sex-matched control group. Antiarrhythmic therapy resulted in marked symptomatic improvement in some of their patients.

Giant cell arteritis should always be considered, especially in patients presenting with transient episodes of blindness. Stroke is responsible for about 50 per cent. of deaths due to giant cell arteritis. The vertebral arteries are usually more severely involved than the carotid arteries (Pathy, 1982).

Lacunar infarction may be heralded by transient events in 60 per cent. of cases (Barnett, 1980). As discussed later these lacunes may give rise to TIAs with pure motor or pure sensory symptoms.

Very occasionally a patient with an intracranial space occupying lesion such as a subdural haematoma or a neoplasm may present as a TIA (Fig. 1). Welsh *et al.*, (1979) reported four cases with chronic subdural haematoma presenting as transient neurological deficits and it is of relevance that three of their patients were in the geriatric age group. Moreover, two of their elderly patients also had carotid bruits.

The combination of degenerative cervical disc changes and osteoarthrosis of the cervical diathrodial joints increase the vulnerability of the vertebral arteries to compression as they traverse the vertebral canal, with possible resultant vertebrobasilar ischaemia. Constricting periarterial fibrosis associated with cervical osteoarthritic spurs may also be a factor in compression. Vertebral artery compression can be converted to complete obstruction by rotating the head. Patients with evidence of severe cervical atherosclerosis may develop transient neurological symptoms, mainly dysarthria and nystagmus on rotation and extension of the neck. The consequences of stenosis or occlusion of the vertebral artery may range

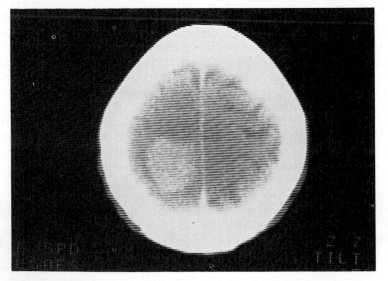

Figure 1 CT. scan of a patient who presented initially with a transient ischaemic attack. The scan shows a uniform mass of high attenuation in the left parietal area. The patient had a meningioma. (Photograph by courtesy of Dr T. O'Dwyer)

from symptomless or insignificant to catastrophic, depending on the integrity and calibre of the opposite vertebral artery, the adequacy of the cardiac output, the systemic blood pressure, and the presence of absence of a functional collateral circulation (Pathy, 1982). Very occasionally symptoms of vertebrobasilar ischaemia may be due to stenosis of the subclavian artery proximal to the origin of the vertebral artery with reversal of blood flow down the ipsilateral vertebral artery to supply blood to the upper limb (the subclavian steal syndrome).

Clinical Presentation

It is not always possible to distinguish clinically between carotid or vertebrobasilar insufficiency. Some patients have symptoms relating to both vascular territories.

Symptoms and signs which implicate the carotid tree reflect involvement of the cerbral hemisphere and eye. The sensorimotor disturbance is contralateral whereas the eye disturbance is ipsilateral, The eye and brain are rarely involved simultaneously. Transient monocular blindness is the most common ocular manifestation (amaurosis fugax) and it is often the first warning sign of problems in the carotid tree. Classically the patient describes the event as a shade falling over his field of vision until complete loss of sight occurs. Abrupt generalized blurring or a wedge-shaped visual loss are rarer presentations. Whereas eye involvement usually presents in a fairly stereotyped way, cerebral hemisphere involvement can present in several different ways. The middle cerebral artery territory is most often involved, and ischaemia of its distal branches usually presents as weakness of the contralateral arm and hand. There are many other presentations which implicate the carotid tree and these include various combinations of sensorimotor manifestations involving the face and upper and lower limbs. The episode may only involve the lips or fingers and it may be dismissed by the patient as not being of any significance. Occasionally the patient may become aphasic or present with other manifestations of temporoparietal ischaemia during a transient ischaemic episode.

Episodes of vertigo, ataxia, diplopia, scintillating scotomata, dysarthria, dysphagia, circumoral paraesthesia, nausea and vomiting, and neurological signs involving alternately one or both sides of the body are manifestations of transient ischaemic attacks in the vertebrobasilar territory. The variable involvement of brain stem occipital lobes and part of a temporal lobe determines the wide spectrum of clinical presentation. Visual features are common and these in combination with giddiness, ataxia, and nausea form a frequent combination of symptoms. There may also be occipital headache and this may often be intense. Drop attacks (Chapter 16.7) may also occur but as many other conditions can lead to falls it is difficult to make this diagnosis with confidence in the absence of other features of vertebrobasilar ischaemia. Brust *et al.*, (1979) found autopsy evidence which suggests that at least some drop attacks are caused by transient ischaemia of the corticospinal tracts.

Transient Global Amnesia

Complete loss of memory usually for a few hours is the typical presentation of a patient with transient global amnesia. The patient has retrograde amnesia for a period of days, weeks, or even years during an attack. Apart from a period of amnesia for the episode itself memory returns to normal after the event. During the attack there is no impainment in the state of consciousness, or evidence of seijure activity or impairment of motor, sensory, or reflex systems. The condition tends to occur in older people with generalized vascular disease.

Transient global amnesia has been associated with vertebrobasilar insufficiency and more specifically with hippocampal ischaemia (Longridge, Hachinski, and Barber, 1979). In the past it is has been considered as an essentially benign condition. However, it now appears that some patients, particularly those in whom the transient global amnesia is accompanied by other manifestations of vertebrobasilar insufficiency, have a greatly increased risk of developing a stroke or permanent memory impairment (Jensen and Olivarius, 1980).

Investigations

General assessment and routine investigations may bring to light remediable conditions such as orthostatic hypotension, polycythaemia, arteritis, and other aetiological factors mentioned previously.

Detailed radiography of the cervical spine with anteroposterior, lateral, and oblique views will be necessary in patients with vertebrobasilar problems. More specialized investigations such as echocardiography will be indicated in some cases of TIA. Ambulatory electrocardiographic monitoring should be carried out on all patients if possible. In an ideal world all patients would also have a CT scan to rule out the possibility of a subdural haematoma but they should certainly have one if there is a history of a head injury or clinical features which raise the suspicion of a haematoma (Welsh *et al.*, 1979).

A large number of non-invasive techniques have been developed for use in assessing carotid flow (Gawler, 1979). They include opthalmodynamometry, facial thermometry, oculopneumoplethysmography, velocity wave form analysis of the carotid pulse, and various Doppler techniques (Fig. 2). These tests are particularly useful when dealing with elderly patients as they are safe and relatively easy to perform. One has to be aware, however, that their sensitivity is limited and atheromatous plaques may be missed.

Arteriography is indicated if surgery is contemplated. Arteriography is performed by injecting contrast material into a catheter with its tip in the ascending aorta and selective catheterization of the neck vessels (Figs. 3, 4 and 5). Complications depend very much on the centre performing the technique and rates as low as zero to as high as 28 per cent. have been reported (Faught, Trader, and Hanna, 1979). Increased risk of complications occurs in the following conditions, multiple myeloma, diabetes, inpaired renal function, congestive cardiac failure, recent or impending myocardial infarction, dehydration and advance age.

Intravenous Digital Subtraction Arteriography is a new technique whereby the arterial system can be visualized by injecting contrast intravenously (Fig. 6). This method is ob-

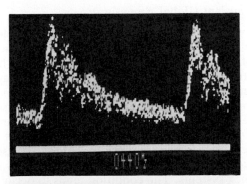

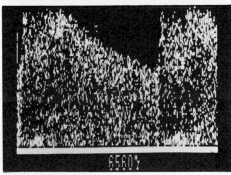

Figure 2 Direct continuous wave Doppler evaluation. (a) Spectral analysis of normal internal carotid artery showing concentration of intensity of the spectrum along the upper border of the frequency envelope. (b) Spectural analysis from a patient with severe internal carotid stenosis showing spectural broadening with the majority of the signal amplitudes at the lower frequencies. (Photograph by courtesy of Miss W. Kingston)

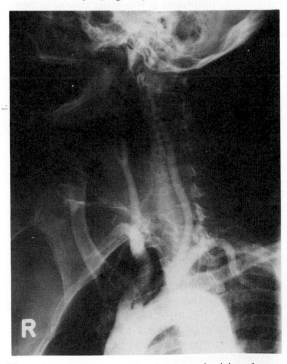

Figure 3 Arch aortogram showing normal origins of great vessels and carotid bifurcations. (Photograph by courtesy of Dr M. Molloy)

viously less hazardous than arterial catheterization and is eminently suitable for demonstrating the carotid bifurcation. The safety and simplicity of intravenous digital arteriography make it possible to screen patients with transient ischaemic attacks and non-symptomatic carotid bruits. As contrast is injected intravenously the examination can be performed on an outpatient basis. The economical benefit in film cost alone is also significant (about one-tenth of the cost of a conventional arteriogram). Intravenous digital subraction arteriography is still at the developmental stage. However, it will undoubtedly play an increasing role in demonstrating flow rates, stenoses, and atheroma in the arterial system in the future.

Management

Although transient ischaemic attacks are important harbingers of completed strokes it is now realized that cardiac disease and hyper-

tension are significant factors in bringing about subsequent completed strokes and death (Loeb, Priano, and Albano, 1978). Careful attention should therefore be paid to the cardiovascular system and hypertension should be controlled. Any haemodynamic factors or other relevant abnormalities discovered during investigation should be treated appropriately (see elsewhere under relevant sections). The management of those patients whose symptoms are due to carotid or vertebrobasilar microemboli is still very controversial.

Vascular surgeons advocate the merits of carotid endarterectomy whereas physicians tend in general to adopt a more conservative approach and advocate medication. In the latter situation the choice is between anticoagulation and antiplatelet drugs.

Carotid Endarterectomy

In this operation stenosing or ulcerating atheromatous lesions at the bifurcation of the common carotid artery are removed. It is a

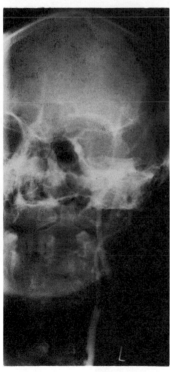

Figure 4 Selective left common arteriogram in a patient with right-sided TIAs. There is an atheromatous ulcerating plaque in the common carotid and a 90 per cent. stenosis just distal to the origin of the internal carotid. (Photograph by courtesy of Dr M. Molloy)

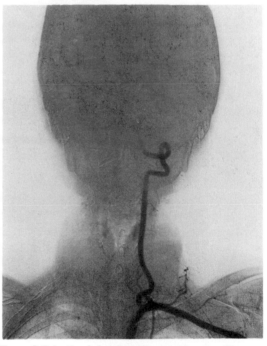

Figure 5 Selective left subclavian arteriogram. There are marked atheromatous changes and stenoses in the left subclavian proximal to the origin of the vertebral artery. There is an 80 per cent. stenosis at the origin of the vertebral artery. (Photograph by courtesy of Dr M. Molloy)

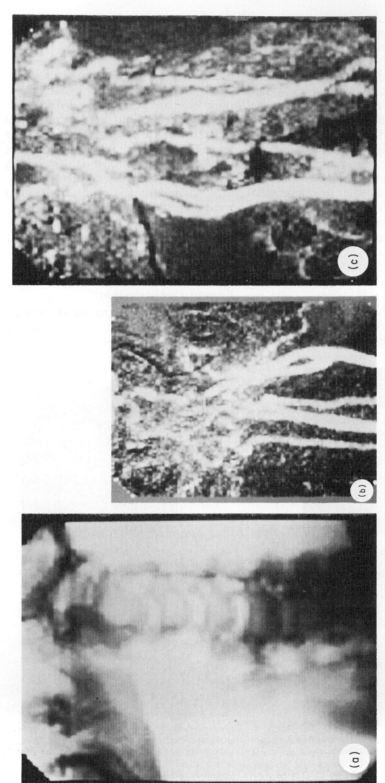

Figure 6 Intravenous digital subtraction arteriography. image (a) is a digitalized mask image from a fluoroscopic screen. Images B and C are subtracted digitalized fluoroscopic images showing normal carotid bifurcations on both sides (b) left side and (c) right side in a patient complaining of Ts. These images were obtained following 40 cc of intravenous contrast medium, i.e. the same amount used for an intravenous pyelogram examination. The examination can be performed on ar, outpatient basis. (Photograph by courtesy of Dr M. Molloy)

well-established procedure which is performed in many centres throughout the world. Yet to date there is no totally convincing statistical evidence which would compel physicians to recommend this operation for patients suitable for surgery (Barnett, 1979). Toole *et al.*, (1978) found that patients with TIA had the same result if untreated, medically treated, or surgically treated when followed up for 5.5 years. Now, however, the results of surgery are improving with better techniques and the emphasis of medical treatment has switched from anticoagulation to antiplatelet therapy. Further trials are necessary and some are in progress.

Results depend very much on the expertise of the surgeon (Hertzer, 1978). The combined perioperative serious morbidity (e.g. stroke and myocardial infarction) and mortality rate should be less than 5 per cent. Every doctor who refers patients for surgery should know the local morbidity and mortality figures for both investigation and surgery. The risks of carotid endarterectomy increases if the patients have other signs of atherosclerosis. Age itself is not necessarily a contraindication to operation when the patient's general condition does not pose an undue hazard. Surgery should not be considered in the presence of multiple risk factors such as a history of hypertension, myocardial infarction, and congestive failure in patients over 65 (Robertson and Watridge, 1979, Thompson and Talkington 1979).

Extracranial–Intracranial Anastomoses

Since the first successful anastomosis between the superficial temporal artery and a branch of the middle cerebral artery (Yasargil 1969) there has been a growing interest in the use of extracranial–intracranial anastomoses in the treatment of cerebrovascular disease. The ideal case for this procedure is a patient who presents with transient ischaemic attacks and who is found to have stenosis of the middle cerebral artery (Editorial, 1979). Other indications for this surgery remain uncertain and controlled studies are currently being undertaken to evaluate its place in the treatment and presentation of stroke. In good hands the operation is remarkably free of complications (Lumley, 1980). As vertebral artery stenosis rarely leads to infarction, preventive reconstructive surgery is usually not practical. Whether microsurgical procedures involving the occipital artery and posterior inferior cerebellar arteries have a place in treatment remains to be determined.

Anticoagulation

There have been a number of conflicting reports about the effectiveness of anticoagulation in preventing transient ischaemic attacks or strokes and a definitive study has yet to be carried out (Perkin, 1979). Anticoagulation may decrease the incidence of stroke, especially in the first few months after the initial transient episode (Whisnant, Metsumoto, and Elveback, 1973). Cerebral haemorrhage is a very serious complication of therapy (Olsson *et al* 1980) and elderly hypertensive patients are particularly at risk. There are often serious problems in ensuring adequate control in the elderly and this limits the use of anticoagulants in this group. In a situation where a patient continued to have further transient episodes despite antiplatelet drugs a trial of anticoagulation should be considered if there is no specific contraindication. If possible therapy should not be continued beyond 12 months as most haemorrhagic complications appear to occur after this time, perhaps because the patient becomes careless with the medication (Sandok *et al.*, 1978).

Antiplatelet Drugs

The core of an arterial thrombus is made up of masses of platelets and these are surrounded by leucocytes and fibrin. Platelet aggregation may thus be the initial step in arterial thrombus formation (Mitchell, 1979). In recent years a considerable amount of research has been carried out using drugs such as aspirin and dipyridamole, which modify platelet function. These drugs are given in the hope of inhibiting platelet aggregation and preventing the adherence of platelets to an area of damaged endothelium. Aspirin has been found to be of benefit in threatened stroke, but only in men. Moreover the benefit has been modest (Canadian Cooperative Study Group, 1978). Aspirin and dipyridamole both inhibit platelet function in different ways and experimental evidence suggests that the two agents may have a synergistic effect. There is uncertainty about the optimum dose of aspirin when used alone (Masotti *et al.*, 1979) or in combination with dipyridamole (Moncada and Korbut, 1978). An American/Canadian trial is currently evaluating the benefits of combined therapy using aspirin 1,200 mg daily and dipyridamole 300 mg daily (Barnett, 1980). In most trials to date the dose of aspirin was 1,300 mg daily in divided doses. In the elderly a b.d. dosage would be reasonable and enteric-coated aspirin is an effective platelet antiaggregant which gives reasonable blood levels. There are several clinical trials of platelet-active drugs currently in progress so that in due course more light may be thrown on what is at present a very confusing aspect of therapy. However, antiplatelet drugs appear to be far from ideal therapy. They are particularly disappointing in patients with evidence of widespread atheroma (Barnett, 1979). The majority of patients, whether treated or untreated, cease to have transient ischaemic attacks within 2 years but the increased risk of myocardial infarction and stroke remains.

The Asymptomatic Carotid Bruit

Most bruits heard in the neck of elderly subjects arise in the external carotid or the praecordium. The prevalence of carotid bruits increases with age and they are more common in hypertensive subjects (Wilkinson *et al.*, 1979). Studies on asymptomatic bruit, presumed but not documented to reflect internal carotid artery stenosis indicate an incidence of about 4 per cent. of the population over 50 (Mohr, 1982*a*). In a community survey Wilkinson and coworkers (1979) evaluated the significance of asymptomatic bruits while taking account of age, sex, systolic blood pressure, and prior heart disease. Of these variables only age and systolic blood pressure were significant in the prediction of stroke, but each of them including bruits was a significant predictor of vascular disease mortality. The Framingham study found that carotid bruit made a significant independent contribution to stroke risk but they observed that more often than not the stroke occurred in another vascular territory (Wolf *et al-*, 1979). Humphries and coworkers (1976) found that patients with asymptomatic bruits were not at greater risk than an aged matched control population without bruits.

The risk of stroke in this group is probably not great enough to warrant surgery (Harrison, 1980) and Barnett (1980) has advocated the conservative approach of anti-platelet therapy. However, surgeons claim that those with severe stenosis have a higher risk of carotid stroke and that all patients with asymptomatic bruits should be investigated initially by non-invasive means. The high-risk patients could then be selected for further investigation and possible endarterectomy (Thompson and Talkington, 1979). Durward and coworkers (1982) followed patients who had undergone unilateral carotid operations but who also had significant stenosis on the opposite side. The incidence of stroke in the territory of a significant asymptomatic carotid plaque was low (3 per cent.) during the follow up period. In fact, it was higher in the territory of the previously operated carotid artery (5 per cent.). There was a 4 per cent. incidence of stroke involving the vertebrobasilar territory. In view of their findings Durward and coworkers advocated that patients with asymptomatic bruits should be reviewed regularly and that surgery should be contemplated only when symptoms appear.

STROKE

When assessing a patient with clinical features suggesting stroke the clinician must ask himself three basic questions: is it a stroke, where is the lesion, and what is the aetiology? Too often stroke is thought of as an obvious diagnosis needing little in the way of clinical expertise and minimal investigation. If this approach is adopted remediable conditions will be missed with dire consequences for the patient.

Is it a Stroke?

Some patients are unconscious or semiconscious when first seen. Under these circumstances focal neurological signs may not be as apparent as they would be in a conscious patient. Careful examination of the face and limbs will usually determine whether a hemiplegia is present. Unilateral puffing of the cheek on expiration indicates facial paralysis on that side. If the limbs are lifted and allowed to fall the flaccid hemiplegic limbs will fall to the bed more heavily than uninvolved limbs. There may be other signs such as absence of limb withdrawal on painful stimulation, depressed reflexes, and a Babinski response.

However, neurological signs suggesting an intracranial lesion in an elderly person should not automatically lead to a diagnosis of a vascular lesion. Several other conditions should be considered and they can usually be excluded by a careful clinical assessment and simple biochemical tests. They include head injury, epilepsy, hyperglycaemia and hypoglycaemia, hypothyroidism, hypothermia, drug overdosage, hepatic and renal failure, arteritis, meningitis, cerebral abscess, subdural haematoma, and a neoplasm.

Neurological abnormalities of sudden onset usually imply a cerebrovascular accident but neurological signs can also develop rapidly with hypoglycaemia. Insulin-dependent diabetics and elderly patients on long-acting oral medication are particularly at risk. Hyperosmolar non-ketotic diabetic coma can present with neurological signs and delay in diagnosis probably contributes to the high mortality of this condition. The elderly patient found unconscious on the floor with a scalp wound is another cause of diagnostic uncertainty. All but very serious head injuries are unlikely to produce focal signs at the onset so if there is evidence of an obvious hemiplegia the probability of an antecedent cerebrovascular accident is high (Marshall, 1976).

Meningitis has been described as the most silent neurological abnormality of old age (Carter, 1979) and the fact that the diagnosis is often made late in the course of the illness contributes to the poor prognosis of the condition in this age group. They may present with malaise and clouding of consciousness but headache and neck stiffness may be minimal or absent. If there is the slightest suspicion of meningitis a lumbar puncture is indicated provided there is no papilloedema (Coakley, 1981).

It is also important to consider subdural haematoma as therapy must be instituted promptly. Dronfield, Mead, and Langman (1977) reviewed the presenting features of all patients with a subdural haematoma who were admitted to hospital wards over a 5-year period in Nottingham. Hemiparesis was the most common neurological abnormality and in the majority of cases it was contralateral to the haematoma. The hemiparesis is usually mild

when compared with the depth of coma. Other focal neurological signs included dysphasia, unilateral pupillary dilatation, extensor plantar responses, papilloedema, and homonymous hemianopia.

If a 'stroke' is not complete within 12 hours the possibility of a space-occupying lesion should be suspected (Editorial, 1978). Two of the most significant features of a space occupying lesion in the elderly are progressive mental and/or focal neurological symptoms. If patients presenting with atypical features are investigated the likelihood of misdiagnosing a tumour as a vascular stroke in the elderly is probably low. Twomey (1978) examined the records of 1,009 patients diagnosed as a vascular stroke in the geriatric unit at Northwick Park Hospital, London, over a 7-year period. Only four of these patients were subsequently found to have a brain tumour, i.e. 0.4 per cent. of all strokes.

A source of infection elsewhere in the body should alert one to the possibility of an intracranial abscess. There may be a persistent low-grade fever, together with signs of a space-occupying lesion.

Where is the Lesion?

As part of the routine assessment of any patient with a stroke an effort should be made to determine the vascular territory involved and particularly to distinguish between carotid and vertebrobasilar involvement.

The Carotid Tree

Internal carotid artery. If the anterior and middle cerebral territories are involved with internal carotid occlusion massive infarction results. The patient has a dense hemiplegia and if the lesion is on the dominant side he is aphasic. Cerebral oedema may lead to coma. More usually the anterior cerebral artery receives blood from the anterior communicating artery and under these circumstances it is difficult to distinguish between internal carotid and middle cerebral artery occlusion.

Middle cerebral artery. A vascular accident involving the main trunk of the middle cerebral artery in the dominant hemisphere produces a contralateral hemiplegia affecting mainly the upper limb and face, hemianopia, expressive dysphasia, and cortical sensory loss. An extensive infarct will also produce a receptive dysphasia, dyslexia, right–left disorientation, dyscalculia, and dyspraxia. Involvement of the non-dominant hemisphere will produce a contralateral hemiplegia but it may also lead to neglect of the opposite side of the body and dyspraxia. The clinical picture varies when only branches of the middle cerebral are involved and coma is less likely to occur as the infarct is smaller. Hemiparesis may be the dominant feature but occasionally hemianaesthesia is the major finding.

The Anterior Cerebral Artery

Infarction in the territory of this artery produces a contralateral hemiplegia, cortical sensory loss, and frequently aphasia. The weakness affects the leg more than the arm. Mental impairment may be a prominent feature. Urinary incontinence also occurs and it may be particularly persistent with non-dominant hemisphere lesions. The patient may also show a lack of concern about the social consequences of the incontinence (Adams, 1974).

The Vertebrobasilar Tree

The basilar artery. The basilar artery supplies the vital centres in the brainstem and occlusion of the main trunk produces coma, small pupils, and usually early death. There is bulbar palsy and a flaccid quadraplegia. A very distressing condition known as akinetic mutism results when the patient retains consciousness but is incapable of responding to stimulation other than by following a moving object with his eyes.

Occlusion of the smaller branches of the basilar artery will produce a range of clinical presentations. These include ipsilateral cranial nerve palsies with contralateral weakness and sensory impairment. Vertigo, deafness, ataxia, dysphagia, dysarthria, and diplopia are other clinical features which may be found. Occlusion of the cerebellar arteries gives rise to nuclear lesions, sensory deficits, Horner's syndrome, and cerebellar ataxia. Involvement of the posterior inferior cerebellar artery is associated with sudden onset of vomiting, vertigo, and dysphagia.

Physical signs include ipsilateral cerebellar signs and contralateral hemianalgesia most frequently involving the modalities of pain and temperature. There may also be an ipsilateral Horner's syndrome. These clinical features (lateral medullary syndrome) may also be found in patients who have occluded the vertebral artery. Most patients who develop the lateral medullary syndrome survive and usually do not develop subsequent posterior circulation strokes (Caplan, 1981).

Posterior cerebral artery. The posterior cerebral artery apart from supplying mid brain structures also supplies the temporal lobe and the cortex of the occipital lobe. Occlusion of this artery gives rise to a variety of clinical presentations including an isolated homonymous hemianopia, visual agnosia, amnesia, and mild paraparesis accompanied by a dense hemianaesthesia which may be associated with spontaneous unilateral pain (thalamic pain). Skew deviation of the eyes, paresis of vertical eye movement, and poorly reactive pupils are evidence of mid-brain involvement which if it is extensive will result in deep coma and decerebrate posturing.

What is the Aetiology?

Several studies have shown how difficult it can be to distinguish clinically between cerebral thrombosis, haemorrhage, and embolism. In a recent Swedish study the bedside diagnosis turned out to be correct in 69 per cent. but in 24 per cent. the diagnosis had to be altered after hospital investigation and in the remaining 7 per cent. no definite preliminary and/or final diagnosis could be made (Von Arbin *et al.*, 1981).

Cerebral Infarction

Cerebral infarction accounts for over 80 per cent. of strokes and it can be due to large artery thrombosis, small vessel pathology leading to lacunar infarction, or cerebral embolism.

Large vessel thrombosis. The clinical signs associated with large vessel thrombosis are typically gradual in onset. The thrombosis usually forms on atherosclerotic plaques and these are found most commonly at the branching of blood vessels. The sites most frequently involved are the internal carotid artery at the carotid sinus, the bifurcation of the middle cerebral artery, the junction of the vertebral and basilar arteries, the posterior cerebral artery as it winds around the cerebral peduncle, and the anterior cerebral artery as it curves over the corpus callosum.

Lacunar infarction. Lacune is a neuropathological term for a small area of softening in the brain. These lesions are associated with lipohyalanosis or atheroma of the small penetrating arteries in the brain. The onset of a stroke due to a lacunar lesion may be very abrupt. The clinical diagnosis of lacunar syndrome is suggested by the following presentations: a pure motor hemiplegia, a pure sensory stroke, the dysarthria-clumsy hand syndrome, and homolateral ataxia with crural paresis. Hypertension is usually present and patients generally make a good recovery. However, it is now realized that although the clinical features suggest a lacunar lesion they are not specific and they have been reported in some patients who were found to have large cortical lesions on CT scanning. These latter patients tended to be older than those with lacunes and not hypertensive (Nelson *et al.*, 1980).

Cerebral Embolism

Embolism is now recognized as a common cause of infarction in older patients yet it is usually not possible to diagnose it with certainty on clinical grounds. Atheromatous plaques on the walls of the great vessels and the internal carotid, and cardiac lesions are the sources of these emboli. Atrial fibrillation with rheumatic heart disease is the classical cardiac condition associated with embolization. However, available evidence now suggests that atrial fibrillation without rheumatic heart disease is an important source of emboli in the elderly. The Framingham study has shown that patients with rheumatic heart disease had a seventeenfold increased risk of stroke compared to the general population and those with chronic idiopathic atrial fibrillation had a 5.6-fold increase (Wolf *et al.*, 1978). Darling, Austen, and Linton (1967) found that atrial fibrillation with atherosclerosis was a significant cause of systemic embolization in the older age

group. More recently other arrhythmias including chronic sinoatrial disorder have also been associated with embolus formation (Fairfax, Lambert, and Leatham, 1976).

In most cases of cerebral embolism the onset is sudden with maximum deficit at the beginning, however, the onset may be gradual in some cases. Approximately 12 per cent. have a seizure at onset and headache occurs in 25 per cent. of patients with emboli but it is usually mild (Easton and Sherman, 1980).

Intracerebral Haemorrhage

A primary intracerebral bleed is more likely to occur in patients with a long history of hypertension. The haemorrhages usually result from rupture of microaneurysms (Charcot–Bouchard aneurysms) on the striate arteries. The onset is usually abrupt with headache and vomiting followed by loss of consciousness, neck rigidity, and a dense hemiplegia. The onset, however, may be less dramatic and more gradual if the blood is contained within the brain parenchyma. In this situation the CSF may be clear and a mistaken diagnosis of cerebral infarction could be made. In the Harvard stroke study a clinical diagnosis of embolism had to be changed in 5 per cent. to intracerebral haemorrhage after more detailed investigation (Mohr *et al.*, 1978).

The diagnosis of cerebellar haematoma should always be considered in a patient who presents with headache, vertigo, and vomiting. Cerebellar ataxia may not be convincing and the patient's condition may deteriorate without the severe hemiplegia and deviation of the eyes associated with oedema of the hemisphere.

Subarachnoid haemorrhage. It is a common misconception that the occurrence of a subarachnoid is rare in old age. The incidence does not decline with age and death from a ruptured Berry aneurysm is commonest in the sixth and seventh decades. Subarachnoid haemorrhage accounts for about 40 per cent. of all new cases of intracranial haemorrhages (Kurtzke, 1976). A hemiplegia is present in about 20 per cent of the patients; however, it is usually not as dense and the level of consciousness is not as deep as that seen in the majority of cases with a primary intracerebral bleed.

Investigating Stroke

Careful clinical assessment and routine haematological tests will exclude many of the conditions such as polycythaemia and giant cell arteritis which may precipitate or mimic a stroke. Syphilitic arteritis if suspected should be eliminated by serological tests but it is now very rare. Specific cardiac investigations may be indicated on the basis of the clinical examination and an ECG should always be performed to rule out a myocardial infarction. When embolism is suspected continuous ECG monitoring may reveal an arrhythmia and an echocardiogram may demonstrate valvular abnormalities, thrombus formation, tumour, or akinetic segments of the myocardium.

Most of the specialized investigations carried out after stroke are not without risk and the physician must decide in each individual case if the information sought is worth the risk involved.

Cerebrospinal Fluid

Lumbar puncture should be undertaken when specific information obtainable only from the CSF is required and when the need for this information is great enough to justify the risk. The procedure should be carried out with a fine bore needle as this diminishes the risk of subsequent CSF leakage. If the CSF is examined using a spectrophotometer it is possible to distinguish between bilirubin compounds derived from haemorrhage and those present in the CSF following the barrier damage consequent on infarction. Using this technique Kjellin and Soderstrom (1974) claimed they could distinguish haemorrhage from infarction within 5 to 6 hours of the stroke.

Skull X-Ray

A skull X-ray is indicated, particularly in those patients with symptoms suggesting a space-occupying lesion and those who have had a head injury. There may be evidence of raised intra-cranial pressure, pineal shift, areas of abnormal calcification or rarefaction or a fracture. Calcification may be seen in the carotid syphons.

Electroencephalography (EEG)

Although this procedure is tolerated better by the elderly than scanning (Critchley, 1978) its use in stroke patients is limited as the changes found are usually non specific. After infarction focal change may be observed mainly over the temporal lobe as the majority of infarcts occur in the territory of the middle cerebral artery. Normal records are common with small brain-stem vascular lesions (Harrison, 1976).

Echoencephalography

This non-invasive procedure is particularly useful in identifying the position of midline structures. A diagnosis of intracerebral haemorrhage or a space-occupying lesion is favoured if there is a significant shift in the first 24 hours. The majority of patients with cerebral haemorrhage have records showing a shift of more than 3 mm. In patients with cerebral infarction a shift may occur as cerebral oedema develops.

Brain Scan

This is another non-invasive technique. The brain is scanned after the intravenous injection of a radioactive isotope (Fig. 7). It is a useful investigation if a neoplasm is suspected as the scan may be positive from the onset and the lesion will be seen to increase in size and density with serial recordings. A subdural haematoma is suggested if there is a crescentic peripheral area of uptake.

Dynamic scans which image the arrival of isotope with the gamma camera during the first 60 seconds after intravenous injection will detect carotid occlusion if present as well as demonstrating any abnormalities in the cerebral circulation.

Computerized Axial Tomography

Gawler (1979) has argued that computerized tomography is the investigation of first choice in all patients with stroke and that it should be to the brain what a chest X-ray is to the lung. He claims that unless it is freely available, patients suitable for surgical management will be overlooked and that the argument that the investigation is too expensive is a financial and

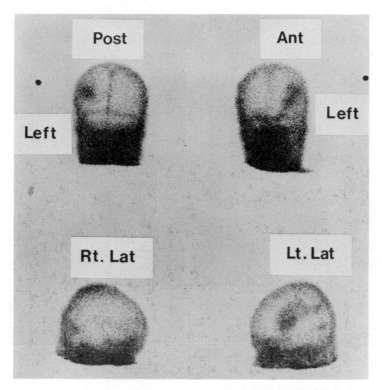

Figure 7　Isotope brain scan of a stroke patient showing extensive infarction in the distribution of the right middle cerebral artery. (Photograph by courtesy of Dr P. Freyne)

not a medical one. A cerebral haemorrhage is shown as a high-density area and it can be detected immediately after a stroke (Fig. 8). Cerebral infarction is shown as a low density area (Fig. 9) and it becomes detectable within 4 to 8 hours (Boysen and Poulson, 1980).

Cerebral haematomas are being diagnosed more frequently since the advent of CT scanning and as a result the mortality of this condition has declined from 51 to 26 per cent. (Weisberg, 1979). CT scanning is useful before anticoagulation for a progressing stroke or a transient ischaemic attack as it is not uncommon that a clinical diagnosis has to be rejected when the CT scan demonstrates a small haematoma (Boysen and Poulson, 1980). CT scan is also of great value when a subdural haematoma is suspected (Caird, 1979). However, it is important to realize that CT scanning is not infallible (West and Coakley, 1982). Chronic subdural haematomas may become isodense

with brain and can be missed, particularly if they are bilateral so that there is no significant shift of midline structures (Cameron, 1978; Greenhouse and Barr, 1979). Small haemorrhages may also be missed, particularly if they occur in the brainstem.

Regional Cerebral Blood Flow

Regional cerebral blood flow can now be measured by atraumatic isotope techniques using intravenous and inhalation techniques (Tolonen *et al.*, 1980). These techniques are usually used for research purposes and although they may provide valuable information they are not commonly used in routine evaluation of patients with cerebral vascular disease.

Three-dimensional measurements of cerebral blood flow can now be made using the

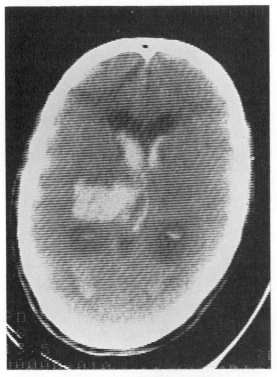

Figure 8 CT scan showing characteristic appearances of a spontaneous hypertensive haemorrhage. There is an irregular high attenuating mass in the left basal ganglia. The haemorrhage has extended into the ventricles and there is also evidence of acute hydrocephalus. (Photographs by courtesy of Dr T. O'Dwyer)

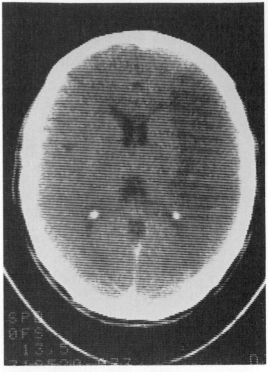

Figure 9 CT scan showing characteristic features of a non-haemorrhagic infarct in the right middle cerebral artery. There is a large low density area involving grey and white matter on the right side and there is also some ventricular compression indicating some slight mass effect. (Photograph by courtesy of Dr T. O'Dwyer)

recently developed photon emission computer assisted tomography (ECAT). It is too early yet to evaluate the role of this technique in routine investigations but it would certainly appear to be a major advance in the investigation of cerebral haemodynamics.

Angiology

This investigation should only be contemplated when surgery is under serious consideration. It is sometimes necessary when the possibility of a space-occupying lesion such as a subdural haematoma is suspected but cannot be confirmed by non-invasive techniques. It is also indicated after subarachnoid haemorrhage if the neurosurgeon considers the patient suitable for subsequent surgery.

MANAGEMENT OF STROKE

Home or Hospital

Whether the stroke patient should be treated at home or in hospital has been a matter of debate (Mulley and Arie 1978). As recently as 1978 Brocklehurst and coworkers found in a survey of 135 stroke patients in Manchester that only 40 per cent were admitted to hospital on the day of the stroke. The decision whether or not to admit appeared to be influenced primarily by social factors such as whether the patient was living alone or with relatives who could not cope. A patient with a minor stroke or TIA can be investigated as an outpatient provided it can be done promptly. The family of an aged patient with an extremely poor prognosis may wish to nurse the patient at home (Wright and Robson, 1980). In general, however, unless home care facilities are very good with access to domicillary consultation, adequate nursing, domicillary physiotherapy, and occupational therapy, other patients should be referred to hospital. In some areas home care is very inadequate and many stroke patients are neglected and they have little contact with doctor, nurse, or therapist (Isaacs, Neville, and Rushford, 1976).

Hospital admission makes it easier to diagnose and treat remediable conditions and to ensure that the acute stage of the illness is managed appropriately. The rehabilitation team can be involved on the first day of admission. The admission of stroke patients to general hospitals is more likely to stimulate research and interest in stroke disease.

Blower and Ali (1979) have pointed out that although the greater deficit in stroke care occurs in the rehabilitation phase, the acute care and investigation phase can usually be improved in most hospitals. These authors describe a comprehensive stroke unit in Greenwich which provides integrated care with investigation and rehabilitation from the first day of admission.

Immediate Prognosis

Between one-third and one-half of the patients admitted die within the first 3 weeks and of the survivors about one-quarter will be confidently independent, one-half will be able to walk independently using an aid and have limited personal independence, and one-quarter will remain heavily dependent. The mortality rate increases with age. Drowsiness and coma on admission are associated with a high mortality rate and the majority who remain deeply comatose following admission die within 48 hours (Marquardsen, 1969). Failure of conjugate gaze towards the side of the limb weakness is also an indication of a poor prognosis for survival when combined with a dense hemiplegia (Oxbury, Greenhall, and Grainger, 1975). The onset of pupillary changes and impairment of the oculovestibular reflexes are other ominous signs. Marked suppression of minute eye movement activity carries a particularly grave prognosis (Coakley, 1984; Coakley and Thomas 1977).

Patient Care

It has been shown that the mortality rate in acute stroke is as low on general wards with good nursing standards as on special intensive care units (Kennedy *et al.*, 1970).

Regular observations of vital signs and neurological status should be made. Airways obstruction must be prevented, particularly in obtunded patients and those with bulbar palsy. A nasogastric tube should be inserted. Intravenous fluids may be necessary in the first 48 hours and Sambrook, Hutchinson, and Aber (1973) have emphasized the importance of good water and electrolyte balance in patients with a reduced level of consciousness. The syndrome of inappropriate ADH (antidiuretic hormone) secretion (SIADH) may occur in some patients during the acute phase.

Urine output should be monitored carefully. An indwelling catheter is usually necessary for incontinent females but unless there is retention condom drainage is most suitable for men. The catheter or condom should be removed at the earliest opportunity and bowel and bladder training should commence. Careful attention should be given to bowel function and impaction should be prevented (Canning, 1974).

The prevention of pressure sores is one of the most important aspects of care during the acute stage. Regular turning is one of the oldest and most efficient ways of preventing prolonged excess pressure on tissue. At least two nurses are always required for turning a patient if shearing stresses are to be avoided. However, the initial deep tissue damage may occur before the patient reaches the ward. Patients who lie for long periods on casualty trolleys and X-ray tables have been shown to be particularly at risk (Dyson, 1978). Coakley and Rhodes (1982) have developed a pad (Jobst protection Pad) which is strapped to the patient at the time of first admission and which is worn continuously during the acute phase of the stroke. Special beds which may impair mobility (e.g. water beds) or impede chest expansion (net beds) or which isolate the patient should not be used. The heels and ankles should be protected and a bed cradle will prevent limb immobilization by tightly tucked bed clothes.

A patient regaining consciousness after a stroke may find himself aphasic, hemiplegic, and in a strange environment. He should be given a very careful explanation of what has happened to him and his treatment programme should be outlined. Isolation should be avoided and it is best not to nurse a stroke patient in a single room, especially during the early phase of his disability (Kenly and Watson 1979).

The physiotherapist should be involved on the first day of admission. Treatment should concentrate while the patient is unconscious on chest care, correct positioning, and passive movements of the limbs. The patient should start sitting out of bed when consciousness returns. A good team relationship between nursing and therapy staff is essential from the very beginning if patients are to make optimum progress during rehabilitation (see Chapter 29).

Hypertension

The autoregulatory mechanisms controlling cerebral blood pressure may be impaired after a cerebrovascular accident. A transient increase in diastolic pressure of 110 to 120 mmHg during the first 48 hours is not unusual in subjects who have been normotensive previously. Treatment is unnecessary in this situation. Oxbury (1975) recommends treatment with IM hydrallazine if the diastolic pressure is above 130 mmHg on several consecutive readings. The older the patient is, the more cautious one should be about any attempts to lower blood pressure in the acute phase of stroke. A marked fall in blood pressure will be accompanied by a fall in cerebral perfusion which may lead to a worsening of the stroke (Britton, de Faire, and Helmers, 1980). Malignant hypertension, although a definite indication for prompt treatment, is very rare in old age (Caird and Dall, 1978).

Myocardial Infarction and Acute Stroke

A stroke may be the presenting feature of a myocardial infarction in old age (Pathy, 1967). Chin, Kaminsky, and Rout (1977) found an incidence of 12.7 per cent. of acute myocardial infarction in a 3-year prospective study of acute cerebrovascular accidents admitted to a geriatric unit within 72 hours of onset. Grant and Dowey (1980) found a similar percentage in a 10-year retrospective study of acute stroke patients admitted to a medical unit in Dublin. The prognosis for patients with myocardial infarction and stroke is extremely poor. The mortality was 53 per cent. in the first study and 76.6 per cent. in the second.

Specific Therapy

Cerebral Oedema

In recent years therapeutic endeavour has concentrated mainly on efforts to prevent the clinical deterioration associated with the development of cerebral oedema. This deterioration generally occurs between the second and seventh day after infarction. If deterioration occurs on the first day it is likely to be due to progression of the stroke. After 10 days deterioration it is again unlikely to be due to cerebral oedema unless there has been further infarction.

Gradual impairment of consciousness is the most common clinical sign of oedema. The neurological deficit may worsen. It is important to appreciate that pupillary dilation is seen in less than 25 per cent. of patients during herniation and papilloedema is rare. Rising blood pressure and declining pulse rate, which are usually associated with increased intracranial pressure from various other causes are not usually seen with ischaemic oedema (Sherman and Easton, 1980).

Steroid therapy. Dexamethasone has been found to be very beneficial when treating the oedema associated with cerebral neoplasia. However, although Patten and coworkers (1972) found dexamethasone to be of value in acute stroke more recent studies have not reached the same conclusion (Mulley, Wilcox, and Mitchell, 1978; Santambrogio *et al.*, 1978). The discrepancy between the poor response in stroke and the dramatic effects observed with neoplasia may be explained by the different nature of the oedema in both situations. The oedema associated with tumours is principally extracellular and due to loss of blood flow autoregulation in the surrounding brain subjected to the pressure of the expanding lesion. This *vasogenic* oedema responds well to steroids. The intracellular or *cytotoxic* oedema associated with cerebral infarction does not appear to respond to steriod therapy. It may be that improvements observed in some patients with stroke have been due to an effect on the vasogenic oedema produced by the mass effect of massive infarction (O'Brien, 1979). Parsons-Smith (1979) claims that the disappointing results with steroids in stroke are due mainly to the fact that in many of the trials patients were either observed for 24 hours or subjected to delayful investigations before treatment was initiated. There may also be subgroups with stroke who would benefit more than others from steroid therapy. Parsons-Smith (1979) recommends 10 mg i.v. of dexamethasone as soon as the diagnosis of stroke is made and 4 mg i.m. every 6 hours should be continued for at least 3 days. If the patient deteriorates on withdrawal of the therapy higher doses may be used.

Meyer and coworkers (1971) and Mathew and coworkers (1972) found glycerol to be of value in the acute phase of cerebral infarction. Beneficial secondary effects which have been claimed for glycerol include enhancement of cerebral metabolism, increase in blood flow, platelet antiaggregation and ADH inhibition (Buonanno and Toole 1981). Glycerol must be given slowly to avoid rebound pressure. A 10% solution may be given by slow intravenous drip over 4 to 6 hours twice daily and it is usually administered for about 4 days. It may also be given orally every 2 hours to a total dose of 2 gm/kg body weight. Despite the early favourable reports, studies later in the decade, as in the case of steroid therapy, were less enthusiastic (Gelmers, 1975; Larsson, Marinovich, and Barber, 1976). Fawer and coworkers (1978) found that glycerol improved motor and sensory functions in patients with moderate disability but patients with severe disability were not improved at all.

Less hazardous techniques for measuring local cerebral blood flow and monitoring intracranial pressure are being developed and these will allow more exact assessment of oedema and its consequences following stroke. These advances should also eventually result in an agreed and rational approach to therapy (Anderson and Cranford, 1979).

Cerebral Blood Flow Modification

Vasodilation. Some vasodilators such as CO_2 and papaverine which increase cerebral blood flow have not been shown to be of value in treating acute cerebral ischaemia (Editorial, 1971). Yamamato and coworkers (1980) found that cerebral vasodilator response to hypercarbia is mildly impaired by the atherosclerosis of normal ageing but greatly impaired in patients with symptomatic ischaemia and vertebrobasilar insufficiency.

Vasoconstriction. Aminophylline constricts normal cortical vessels and this blood, in theory, may be diverted to the ischaemic areas where there is vasoparalysis (Boysen and Poulsen 1980). Although Geismar, Marquardsen, and Sylvest (1976) found an initial significant improvement in stroke patients treated with aminophylline, at subsequent assessment the survival rate, length of stay in hospital, and social readaption were not significantly different from the control group. Britton and coworkers (1980) concluded that aminophylline had no significant effect on cerebral infarction with the serum theophylline levels in the therapeutic range recommended for patients with asthma.

Reducing Blood Viscosity

Patients with a high haematocrit have an increased whole blood viscosity. The Framingham study has shown that the group with the least risk of developing a stroke had normal blood pressure and a low haematocrit. Those with high normal haematocrits had an increased risk of stroke (Kannell *et al.*, 1972).

Low molecular weight dextran has been shown to reverse the intravascular sludging of red cells thereby reducing blood viscosity and increasing capillary flow. Two studies (Gilroy, Barnhart, and Meyer, 1969; Matthews and *et al.*, (1976) found that low molecular weight dextran decreased the mortality in the acute stage of stroke. However, Matthews and coworkers (1976) noted that the survivors were severely disabled and after 6 months no significant benefit from treatment could be demonstrated.

Anticoagulation

Anticoagulants are used in treating patients who have had a cerebral embolus in the hope of preventing a recurrence. In patients with rheumatic heart disease or mural thrombus this is most likely to occur in the months immediately after the initial episode. It may be difficult to ensure compliance in some elderly patients but a serious attempt should be made to keep the patient anticoagulated for at least 6 months. After this the risk of a further episode decreases substantially (Adams *et al.*, 1974, Easton and Sherman, 1980).

There have been reservations expressed about a policy of immediate anticoagulation following cerebral embolism lest the infarct should become haemorrhagic. However, as the recurrence rate is the highest immediately after the cerebral embolism anticoagulation should be initiated with Heparin (provided there are no specific contraindications) in all patients with cerebral embolism in whom the CSF is not haemorrhagic and the neurological deficit is not massive and persistent beyond 24 hours (Easton and Sherman 1980; Marshall, 1976).

Anticoagulants have been used in the treatment of progressive strokes in the hope of arresting their development. However, unless one has investigated the patient to exclude a cerebral haemorrhage in this situation anticoagulation could have disastrous consequences.

Surgery

Operations on occluded or severely stenosed carotid arteries during the acute stage of stroke have yielded very poor results. A cerebellar haematoma or a subcortical haematoma with evidence of increasing intracranial pressure are indications for surgery in selected patients.

Stupor continuing for more than a week after a stroke may be due to an intracerebral haematoma and some of these patients, of whatever age, are suitable for operation (Caird, 1979). One requires the facilities of a neurosurgery unit to distinguish superficial haematomas from the more deeply seated haematomas (Oxbury, 1975).

Following a subarachnoid haemorrhage patients who are considered well enough for surgery should be assessed by a neurosurgeon. Angiography and surgery are contraindicated if the patient is in coma as the risks are greatly increased. Patients who are suitable should be operated on as early as possible as the risk of rebleed is greatest in the first 2 weeks. Nukui and coworkers (1977) have reported favourable results using modern microsurgical techniques in patients over the age of 60 who were in good health before their subarachnoid haemorrhage. The value of antifibrinolytic agents to reduce the risk of rebleeding after subarachnoid haemorrhage has not been proven in double blind studies (Kaste and Ramsay, 1979; Van Rossum *et al.*, 1977).

Deep Venous Thrombosis and Stroke

There is a high incidence of DVT in immobilized patients despite physiotherapy including leg and breathing exercises and a policy of early mobilization. Radioactive isotope techniques have revealed that about 50 per cent. of stroke patients develop a deep vein thrombosis (Denham *et al.*, 1973; Gibberd, Gould, and Marks, 1976). Thrombosis can occur on the normal side but it usually occurs in the paralysed limb. Although there may be local changes in venous blood flow due to the impairment of muscle pumping action total limb flow is either normal or even increased in hemiplegic limbs (Warlow, 1978). Changes in haemostasis including a rise in the platelet count and circulating platelet aggregates and an increase in the plasma fibrinogen occur in the acute stage of stroke (Warlow, 1978). Deep venous thrombosis, however, can occur in stroke patients without these changes. Prolonged pressure on the calf leading to vein wall damage may be an important factor in initiating thrombosis.

Small quantities of heparin in amounts that will not diminish the whole blood clotting time or otherwise induce detectable coagulation disorders can provide anticoagulation protection. McCarthy and coworkers (1977) and Gelmers (1980) found a reduction in the incidence of deep venous thrombosis when using low-dose heparin in patients with cerebral infarction.

Deterioration due to a pulmonary embolus following a stroke is often attributed to a further stroke or to a chest infection (Adams, 1974; Denham *et al.*, 1973). Because of the danger of intracranial haemorrhage there is a reluctance to use full anticoagulation for established deep venous thrombosis in the absence of definite evidence of pulmonary emboli. This again emphasizes the importance of adequate investigation facilities to distinguish between cerebral infarction and haemorrhage. However, the preponderance of pulmonary emboli arise in stroke patients without evidence of clinical venous thrombosis. Miyamoto and Miller (1980) reduced the incidence of pulmonary emboli dramatically in patients with cerebral infarction undergoing rehabilitation in their unit. All patients were screened about 10 days to 2 weeks after the stroke and if the iodine–125 fibrinogen leg scan was positive they were fully anticoagulated.

REFERENCES

Adams, G. F. (1974). *Cerebrovascular Disability and the Ageing Brain*, Churchill Livingstone, Edinburgh.

Adams, G. F., Hutchinson, M., Merrett, J. D., and Pollock A. M. (1974). 'Mitral stenosis and cerebral embolism: Survival in patients treated with and without anticoagulants', *J. Neurol. Neurosurg. and Psychiatr.*, **37**, 378–383.

Anderson, D. C., and Cranford, R. E. (1979). 'Cortico steroids in ischaemic stroke', *Stroke, 10*, 68–71.

Barnett, H. J. M. (1979). 'The pathophysiology of transient cerebral ischaemic attacks', *Med. Clin. North Am.*, **63**, 649–679.

Barnett, H. J. M. (1980). 'Prevention of stroke', *Am. J. Med.*, **69**, 803–805.

Barnett, H. J. M., Boughner, D. R., and Cooper, P. E. (1978). 'Further evidence relating cerebral ischaemic events to prolapsing mitral valve', *Abstract. Ann. Neurol.*, **4**, 163–164.

Benhamou, A. C., Kieffer, E., Tricot, J. F., Maraval, M., Lethoai, H., Benhamou, M., Boespflug, O. and Natoli, J. (1981). 'Carotid artery surgery in patients over 70 years of age' *Int. Surg.*, **66**, 199–202.

Blower, P., and Ali, S. (1979). 'A stroke unit in a district general hospital: The Greenwich experience', *Br. Med. J.*, **2**, 644–646.

Boysen, G., and Poulson, O. B. (1980). 'Recent advances in the diagnosis of cerebrovascular disease', *Acta. Neurol. Scand. Suppl.*, **78**, 62, 49–59.

Britton, M., de Faire, U., and Helmers, C. (1980). 'Hazards of therapy for excessive hypertension in acute stroke', *Acta. Med. Scand.*, **207** (4), 253–257.

Britton, M., de Faire, U., Helmers, C., Miah, K., and Rane, A. (1980). 'Lack of effect of theophylline on the outcome of acute cerebral infarction', *Acta. Neurol. Scand.*, **62**, 116–123.

Brocklehurst, J. C., Andrew, K., Morris, P., Richards, B. R., and Laycock, P. L. (1978). 'Why admit stroke patients to hospital', *Age and Ageing*, **7** (2), 100–108.

Brust, J. C. M., Plank, C. R., Heatton, E. B., and Sanchez, G. F. (1979). 'The pathology of drop attacks: A case report', *Neurology (Minneap.)*, **29**, 786–790.

Buonanno, F., and Toole, J. F. (1981). 'Management of patients with established (completed) cerebral infarction', *Stroke, 12* (1), 7–16.

Caird, F. G. (1979). 'Investigation of the elderly patient with stroke', *Age Ageing, Suppl.*, **8**, 44–49.

Caird, F. G., and Dall, J. L. C. (1978). 'The cardiovascular system', in *Textbook of Geriatric Medicine and Gerontology* (Ed. J. C. Brocklehurst), Churchill Livingstone, Edinburgh.

Cameron, M. M. (1978). 'Chronic subdural haematoma: A review of 114 cases', *J. Neurol., Neurosurg. Psychiatr.*, **41** (9), 834–839.

Canadian Cooperative Study Group (1978). 'A randomized trial of aspirin and sulphinpyrazone in threatened stroke'., *New Engl. J. Med.*, **299**, 53–59.

Canning, M. (1974). 'Care of the unconscious patient', *Nursing Mirror*, Aug. 9th, 61.

Caplan, L. R. (1981). 'Vertebrobasilar disease – Time for a new strategy', *Stroke, 12* (1), 111–114.

Carter, A. B. (1979). 'The neurologic aspects of ageing', in *Clinical Geriatrics* (Ed. I. Rossman), Lippincott, Philadelphia.

Chin, P. L., Kaminski, J., and Rout, M. (1977). 'Myocardial infarction coincident with cerebrovascular accidents in the elderly', *Age Ageing*, **6** (1), 29–37.

Coakley, D. (1981). 'Acute stroke and other neurological emergencies in old age', in *Acute Geriatric Medicine* (Ed. D. Coakley), Croom Helm, London, and PSG, Littleton, Massachusetts.

Coakley, D. (1985). '*Minute eye movement and brain stem function*, CRC Press, Florida.

Coakley, D., and Rhodes, J. (1982). 'Pressure sores: A new approach to prevention', *Geriatric Medicine*, **12** (3), 54–55.

Coakley, D., and Thomas, J. G. (1977). 'The ocular microtremor record and the prognosis of the unconscious patient', *Lancet*, **1**, 512–515.

Critchley, E. M. R. (1978). 'Electro-encephalography today', *J. R. Soc. Med.*, **71**, 473–476.

Darling, R. C., Austen, W. G., and Linton, R. R. (1967). 'The value of 125g fibrinogen in the diagnosis of deep venous thombosis in hemiplegia', *Age Ageing*, **2**, 207–210.

Denham, M. J., Farran, H. and James, G. (1973. 'The value of 125 Fibrinogen in the diagnosis of deep venous thrombosis in hemiplegia', *Age and Ageing*, **2**, 207–210.

Dronfield, M. W., Mead, G. M., and Langman, M. J. S. (1977). 'Survival and death from subdural haematoma on medical wards', *Postgrad. Med. J.*, **53**, 57–60.

Durward, O. J., Ferguson, G. G. and Barr, H.W.K. (1982). 'The natural history of asymptomatic carotid bifurcation plaques', *Stroke*, **13**, 4, 459–464.

Dyson, R. (1978). 'Bedsores – the injuries hospital staff inflict on patients', *Nursing Mirror,* **140**, 24, 30.

Easton, J. D., and Sherman, D. G. (1980). 'Management of cerebral embolism of cardiac origin', *Stroke*, **11**, 433–442.

'Editorial (1971). 'Cerebral vasodilators', *Br. Med. J.*, **2**, 702–703.

'Editorial (1978). 'Investigating stroke', *Br. Med. J.*, 11503.

Editorial, (1979). 'Extracranial – intracranial anastomoses', *Lancet*, **1**, 1384–1385.

Fairfax, A. J., Lambert, C. D., and Leatham, A. (1976). 'Systemic emoblism in chronic sino-atrial disorder', *New Engl. J. Med.*, **295**, 190–192.

Faught, E., Trader, S. D., and Hanna, G. R. (1979). 'Cerebral complications of angiography for transient ischaemia and stroke: Prediction of risk', *Neurology*, **29**, 4–15.

Fawer, R., Justafre, J. C., Berger, J. P., and Schelling, J. C. (1978). 'Intravenous glycerol in cerebral infarction: A controlled 4 month trial', *Stroke*, **9**, 484–486.

Gawler, J. (1979). 'New diagnostic methods', *Practitioner*, **223**, 806–811.

Geismar, P., Marquardsen, J., and Sylvest, J. (1976). 'Controlled trial of intravenous aminophylline in acute cerebral infarction', *Acta. Neurol. Scand.*, **54**(2), 173–180.

Gelmers, H. J. (1975). 'Effect of glycerol treatment on the natural history of acute cerebral infarction', *Clin. Neurol. Neurosurg.*, **78** (14), 277–282.

Gelmers, H. J. (1980). 'Effects of low-dose subcutaneous heparin on the occurrence of deep vein thrombosis in patients with ischaemic stroke', *Acta. Neurol. Scand.*, **61**, 313–318.

Gibberd, F. B., Gould, S. R., and Marks, P. (1976). 'Incidence of deep vein thrombosis and leg oedema in patients with strokes', *J. Neurol. Neurosurg. Psychiatr.*, **39**, 1222–1251.

Gilroy, J., Barnhart, M. I., and Meyer, J. S. (1969). 'Treatment of acute stroke with Dextran 40', *J. Am. Med. Assoc.*, **210** (2), 293–298.

Grant, A. P., and Dowey, K. E. (1980). 'The association of acute stroke and myocardial infarction in elderly', *Ir. Med. J.*, **149** (1), 15–18.

Greenhouse, A. H., and Barr, J. W. (1979). 'The

bilateral isodense subdural hematoma on computerized tomographic scan', *Arch. Neurol.*, **36**, 305–307.

Harrison, M. J. G. (1976). 'The investigation of strokes', in Cerebral Arterial Disease (Ed. R. W. Ross Russell), Churchill Livingstone, Edinburgh.

Harrison, M. J. G. (1980). 'Surgery for ischaemic stroke', *Br. J. Hosp. Med.*, **23**, 108–112.

Helps, E. P. W. (1979). 'Transient ischaemic attacks: Guide to management', *Geriatr. Med.*, **9** (5), 41–45.

Hertzer, N. R. (1978). 'Carotid endartectomy and common sense', *Surg. Gynaecol. Obstet.*, **147** (2), 235–236.

Humphries, A. W., Young, J. R., Santilli, R. N., *et al.*, (1976). 'Unoperated, asymptomatic significant internal carotid artery stenosis: A review of 182 instances', *Surgery*, **80**, 695–698.

Isaacs, B., Neville, Y., and Rushford, J. (1976). 'The striken, the social consequences of stroke', *Age Ageing.*, **5**, 188–192.

Jensen, T. S., and Olivarius, B. (1980). 'Transient global amnesia as a manifestation of transient cerebral ischaemia', *Acta. Neurol. Scand.*, **61**, 115–124.

Kannell, W. B., Gordon, T., Wolf, P. A. and McNamara, P. (1972). 'Haemoglobin and the risk of cerebral infarction: the Framingham study', *Stroke*, **3**, 409–20.

Kaste, M., and Ramsay, M. (1979). 'Transexamic acid in subarchnoid haemorrhage. A double-blind study', *Stroke,* **10**, 519–522.

Kenly, M., and Watson, J. E. (1979). 'Nursing', in *Disorders of the Nervous System in Medical-Surgical Nursing and Related Physiology* (Ed. J. Watson), W. B. Saunders, Philadelphia.

Kennedy, F. B., Pozen, T. J., Gabelman, E. H., *et al.* (1970). 'Stroke intensive care – an appraisal', *Am. Heart J.*, **80**, 188–196.

Kjellin, K. G., and Soderstrom, C. E. (1974). 'Diagnostic significance of C.S.F. spectrophotometry in cerebrovascular disease', *J. Neurol. Sci.*, **23**, 359–369.

Kurtzke, J. F. (1976). *The Distribution of Cerebrovascular Disease in Stroke* (Eds F. J. Gillingham, C. Maudsley and A. E. Williams), Churchill Livingstone. Edinburgh.

Larsson, O., Marinovich, N., and Barber, K. (1976). 'Double blind trial of glycerol therapy in early stroke', *Lancet*, **1**, 832–834.

Loeb, C., Priano, A., and Albano, C. (1978). 'Clinical features and long-term follow up of patients with reversible ischaemic attacks', *Acta. Neurol. Scand.*, **57**, 471–480.

Longridge, N. S., Hachinski, V., and Barber, H. O. (1979). 'Brain stem dysfunction in transient global amnesia', *Stroke*, **10**, 473–474.

Lumley, J. S. P. (1980). 'Cerebral revascularization

in stroke prophylaxis', *Ann. R. Coll. Surg. Engl.*, **62**, 335–343.

Luxon, L. M., *et al.* (1980). 'Controlled study of 24 hour ambulatory electrocardiographic monitoring in patients with transient neurological symptoms', *J. Neurol. Neurosurg. Psychiatr.* **43** (1), 37–41.

McCarthy, S. T., Turner, J. J., Robertson, D., Hawkey, C. J., and Macey, D. J. (1977). 'Low-dose heparin as a prophylaxis against deep vein thrombosis after acute stroke', *Lancet*, **2**, 800–801.

McHenry, L. C., Toole, J. F., and Miller, H. S. (1976). 'Longterm E.C.G. monitoring in patients with cerebrovascular insufficiency', *Stroke, 7*, 264–269.

Marquardsen, J. (1960). 'The natural history of acute cerebrovascular disease', *Acta. Neurol. Scand.* **45**, Suppl. 38, 192.

Marshall, J. (1976). 'Clinical diagnosis of completed stroke', in *Cerebral Arterial Disease* (Ed. R. W. Ross Russell), Churchill Livingstone, Edinburgh.

Masotti, G., Galanti, G., Poggesi, L., Abbrate, R., and Neri Serneri, G. C. (1979). 'Differential inhibition of prostacyclin production and platelet aggregation by aspirin', *Lancet, 2*, 1213–1216.

Mathew, N. T., Meyer, J. S., Rivera, V. M., *et al.* (1972). 'Double blind evaluation of glycerol therapy in acute cerebral infarction', *Lancet, 2*, 1327–1329.

Matthews, W. B., Oxbury, J. M., Grainger, K. M. R., and Greenhall, R. C. D. (1976). 'A blind controlled trial of Dextran 40 in the treatment of ischaemic stroke', *Brain*, **99**, 193–206.

Meyer, J. S., Charney, J. Z., Rivera, V. M., and Mathew, N. T. (1971). 'Treatment with glycerol of cerebral oedema due to acute cerebral infarction', *Lancet, ii*, 993–1001.

Millikan, C. H. and McDowell, F. H. (1980). 'Treatment of progressing stroke', in *Current Concepts in Cerebrovascular Disease* (Eds. F. McDowell, E. H. Sonnenblick, M. Lesh.), Grune and Stratton, New York, London.

Mitchell, J. R. A. (1979). 'Does aspirin prevent stroke?', *Practitioner*, **223**, 668–672.

Miyamoto, A. T., and Miller, L. S. (1980). 'Pulmonary embolism in stroke: Prevention by early heparinization of venous thrombosis detected by iodine–125 fibrinogen leg scans', *Arch. Phys. Med. Rehab*, **61**, 584–587.

Mohr, J. P. (1982a). 'Asymptomatic carotid artery disease', *Stroke*, **13**, 4, 431–432.

Mohr, J. P. (1982b). 'Lacunes', *Stroke*, **13**, 1, 3–11.

Mohr, J. P., Caplan, L. R., Melski, J. W., Goldstein, R. J., Duncan, G. W., Kistler, J. P., Pessin, S., and Bleich, H. L. (1978). 'The Harvard Cooperative Stroke Registry: A prospective registry', *Neurology*, **28**, 754–762.

Moncada, S., and Korbut, R. (1978). 'Dipyridamole and other phosphodiesterase inhibitors act as antithrombotic agents by potentiating endogenous prostacyclin', *Lancet*, **1**, 1286–1289.

Mulley, G., and Arie, T. (1978). 'Treating stroke: Home or hospital', *Br. Med. J.*, **2**, 1321–1322.

Mulley, G., and Wilcox, R. G., and Mitchell, J. R. A. (1978). 'Dexamethasone in acute stroke', *Br. Med. J.* ,2, 994–996.

Naritomi, H., Sakai, F., and Meyer, J. S. (1979). 'Pathogenesis of transient ischaemic attacks within the vertebrobasilar system'. *Arch. Neurol.*, **36**, 121–128.

Nelson, R. F., Pullicino, P. Kendall, B. E., and Marshall, J. (1980). 'Computed tomography in patients presenting with lacunar syndromes', *Stroke, 11* (3), 256–261.

Nukui, H., Nagaya, T., Tanaka, S., *et al.* (1977). 'The indication for surgical treatment in patients over 60 years of age with ruptured intracranial aneurysm'. *Jpn. Neurol. Med-Chir*, **17** (11), 6, 525–532.

O'Brien, M. D. (1979). 'Ischaemic cerebral oedema – A review', *Stroke, 10* (6), 623–628.

Olsson, J. E., Brechter, C., Backlund, H., Krook, H., Muller, R., Nitelius, E., Olssonn, O., and Tornberg, A. (1980). 'Anticoagulant vs anti-platelet therapy as prophylactic against cerebral infarction in transient ischaemic attacks', *Stroke*, **1980**, II (1), 4–9.

Oxbury, J. M. (1975). 'Treatment of stroke', *Br. Med. J.*, **4**, 450–452.

Oxbury, J. M., Greenhall, R. C. D., and Grainger, K. M. R. (1975). 'Predicting the outcome of stroke: Acute stage after cerebral infarction', *Br. Med. J.*, **3**, 125–127.

Parsons-Smith, B. G. (1979). 'First aid for acute cerebral stroke'. *Practitioner*, **223**, 553–557.

Pathy, M. S. (1967). 'Clinical presentation of myocardial infarction in the elderly', *Br. Heart J.*, **19**, 290–299.

Pathy, M. S. (1982). 'Vertebrobasilar syndrome', in *Geriatrics* (Ed. 1). Platt, Vol. 1, pp. 431–451, Springer-Verlag, Berlin, Heidelberg, and New York.

Patten, B. M., Mendell, J., Bruun, B. Curtin, W., and Carter, S. (1972). 'Double blind study of the effects of dexamethasone on acute stroke', *Neurology (Minneap.)*, **22**, 377–383.

Perkin, G. D. (1979). 'Anticoagulants in transient ischaemic attacks', in *Progress in Stroke Research* (Eds R. M. Greenhalgh and F. Clifford Rose), Pitman Medical, London.

Sambrook, M. A., Hutchinson, E. C., and Aber, G. M. (1973). 'Metabolic studies in subarachnoid haemorrhage and strokes – II. Serial changes in cerebrospinal fluid and plasma urea electrolytes and osmolality', *Brain*, **96**, 191–202.

Sandok, B. A., Furhan, A. J., Whisnant, J. P., and

Suncht, T. M. (1978). 'Guidelines for the management of transient ischaemic attacks', *Mayo Clin. Proc.,* **53** (10), 665.

Santambrogio, S., Martinotti, R., Sardella, F., *et al.* (1978). 'Is there a real treatment for stroke? Clinical and statistical comparison of different treatments in 300 patients', *Stroke,* **9** (2), 130–132.

Sherman, D. G., and Easton, J. D. (1980). 'Cerebral oedema in stroke', *Postgrad. Med.,* **68** (1), 107–120.

Simonsen, N., Christiansen, H. D., Hettberg, A., Marquardsen, J., Pedersen, H. E., and Sorensen, P. S. (1981). 'Longterm prognosis after transient ischaemic attacks', *Acta. Neurol. Scand.* **63**, 156–168.

Thompson, J. E., and Talkington, C. M. (1979). 'Carotid surgery for cerebral ischaemia', *Surg. Clin. North Am.,* **59** (4), 539–553.

Tolonen, U., Ahonen, T., Kallanranta, E., Hokkanen, E., Koskinen, M., and Kuikka, J. (1980). 'Evaluation of cerebral infarctions of the carotid area by an intra venous xenon and technetium method', *Acta. Neurol. Scand.,* **61**, 137–145.

Toole, J. F., Yuson, C. P., Janeway, R., Johnston, F., Davis, C., Cordell, A. R., and Howard, G. (1978). 'Transient ischaemic attacks: A prospective study of 225 patients'. *Neurology.,* **28** (8), 746–753.

Twomey, C. (1978). 'Brain tumours in the elderly', *Age Ageing,* **7**, 138–145.

Ueda, K., Toole, J. F., and McHenry, L. C. (1979). 'Carotid and vertebrobasilar transient ischaemic attacks: Clinical and angiographic correlation', *Neurology,* **29**, 1094–1101.

Van Rossum, J., Winzen, A. R., Endtz, L. J., Schoen, J. H. R., and de Jonge, H. (1977). 'Effect of transexamic acid on rebleeding after subarachnoid haemorrhage: A double-blind controlled clinical trial', *Ann. Neurol.,* **2**, 242–245.

Von Arbin, M., Britton, M., de Faire, U., Helmers, C., Miah, K., and Murray, V. (1981). 'Accuracy of bedside diagnosis in stroke', *Stroke,* **12** (3), 288–293.

Warlow, C. (1978). 'Venous thrombo embolism after stroke', *Am. Heart J.,* **96** (3), 283–285.

Weisberg, L. A. (1979). 'Computerized tomography in intracranial haemorrhage', *Arch. Neurol.,* **36**, 422–426.

Welsh, J. E., Tyson, G. W., Winn, H. R., and Jane, J. A. (1979). 'Chronic subdural hematoma presenting as transient neurological deficits', *Stroke,* **10**, 564–567.

West, B., and Coakley, D. (1982). 'Art and artifact in Diagnosis', *Geriatric Medicine,* **xiii** (1), 28.

Whisnant, J. P., Metsumoto, N., and Elveback, L. R. (1973). 'The effect of anticoagulation therapy on the prognosis of patients with transient cerebral ischaemic attacks in a community'., *Mayo Clin. Proc.,* **48**, 844.

Wilkinson, W. E., Heyman, A., Heyden, S., Bartel, A., Tyroler, H. A., Karp, H., and Hames, C. G. (1979). 'Risk of stroke and death due to vascular disease in persons with asymptomatic cervical arterial bruits', *Stroke,* **10**, 490.

Wolf, P. A., Dawber, T. R., Thomas, H. E., and Kannel, W. B. (1978). 'Epidemiologic assessment of chronic atrial fibrillation and risk of stroke: The Framingham Study', *Neurology (Minneap.),* **28**, 973–977.

Wolf, P. A., Kannel, W. B., Gordon, T., McNamara, P. M., and Dawber, T. R. (1979). 'Asymptomatic carotid bruit and risk of stroke: The Framingham Study (abstract)'. *Stroke,* **10** (1), 96.

Wollner, L., McCarthy, S. T., Soper, N. D. W., and Macy, D. J. (1979). 'Failure of cerebral autoregulation as a cause of brain dysfunction in the elderly', *Br. Med. J.,* **1**, 1117–1118.

Wright, W. B., and Robson, P. (1980). 'Crisis procedure for stroke at home', *Lancet,* **2**, 249–250.

Yamamoto, M., Meyer, J. S., Sakai, F., and Yamaguchi, F. (1980). 'Ageing and cerebral vasodilator responses to hypercarbia', *Arch. Neurol.,* **37**, 489–496.

Yasargil, M. G. (1969). 'Anastomosis between the superficial temporal artery and a branch of the middle cerebral artery', in *Microsurgery applied to Neurosurgery,* pp. 105–115, Georg Thieme Verlag', Stuttgart.

Principles and Practice of Geriatric Medicine
Edited by M. S. J. Pathy
© 1985 John Wiley & Sons Ltd

16.10

Subdural Haematoma

M. S. J. Pathy

SUBDURAL SPACE

The normally potential subdural space is maintained in its usual state by the varying pressure of the cerebral hemispheres against the dura. In the supine position a pressure of approximately 10 mmHg falls in the erect position and rises when coughing or straining due to fluctuations in the intracranial venous pressure. Intracranial hypotension from any cause will reduce the pressure on the opposing dural surfaces.

Direct or indirect head injury may result in bleeding into the subdural space. Tearing of cortical veins or arteries with formation of an acute subdural haematoma is commonly due to severe trauma. The concomitant concussion to the underlying brain tissue may be of greater significance than the haemorrhage. Clinical evidence of subdural bleeding is usually evident within 48 hours and commonly presents with progressive clouding of consciousness. Hemiplegia with contralateral pupillary dilation may ensue.

A subacute subdural haematoma develops after significant head injury with or without loss of consciousness. The features of rising intracranial pressure develop over the next few days to two weeks. The clinically acute and subacute subdural haematomata are seen at all ages and are associated with abundant evidence of brain damage which have no distinctive features in old age and will not be discussed further.

CHRONIC SUBDURAL HAEMATOMA

A chronic subdural haematoma is clinically defined as occurring three weeks after a head injury. The chronological dividing line from a subacute haematoma is arbitary and pathological findings indicate that the fibroblastic changes so characteristic of the chronic state begin to take place within a few hours of blood accumulating in the subdural space.

Rougerie and Caldera (1955) suggested that bleeding might occur between the layers of the dura rather than in the subdural space. Re-examination of this earlier work by electron microscopy lends support to this contention (Friede and Schachenmayr, 1978).

Chronic subdural haematoma occurs particularly in infancy and old age. It often follows minor trauma and is commonly due to tearing of a vein traversing the subdural space (Pudenz and Shelden, 1946; Rabe, Flynn, and Dodge, 1962). Waga and coworkers (1972) recorded a history of head injury in 96 per cent. of elderly Japanese subjects, but experience in the United Kingdom is in keeping with the findings of So (1976), who noted evidence of head injury in only 20 per cent. of elderly patients. About 50 per cent of subdural haematoma are bilateral.

The low intracranial pressure associated with cerebral atrophy in later life or following a lumbar puncture (Arseni, Ionescu, and Dinu, 1970), dehydration from disease (Fontan *et al.*, 1963; Klein, 1963), or iatrogenic causes (Marshall and Hinman, 1962; Mardešić and Cigit, 1965) increases the likelihood of a subdural bleed. Other predisposing factors are many, and include bleeding disorders (Edson *et al.*, 1973; Talmant *et al.*, 1967) and anticoagulant therapy (Chawla, 1968). In many reports anticoagulants have been incriminated in 12 to 14 per cent. of subdural haematoma (Bret *et al.*, 1976; Lizuka 1972; Sreerama *et al.*, 1973; Wiener and Nathanson, 1962) but selectivity of patients to specialised referral centres often distorts apparent incidence.

Pathophysiology of Chronic Subdural Haematoma

A chronic subdural haematoma is characterized by its defined encapsulation between the dura mater and arachnoid (De Reuk, Roels, and Vander Eecken, 1976). The presence of blood, or more specifically of fibrin or fibrin degradation products in the subdural space, stimulates an early fibroblastic reaction in both layers of the dura with complete encapsulation of the haemorrhage within about 14 days (Apfelbaum, Guthkelch, and Shulman 1974). Thin-wall vascular channels grow from the fibroblastic dural capsule (neomembrane).

The late increase in size of a chronic subdural haematoma was postulated by Gardner (1932) to be due to an osmotic gradient drawing CSF into the subdural haematoma. Zollinger and Gross (1934) considered that osmotic pressure differences resulted in fluid transfer from the capillaries of the neomembrane into the subdural sac but Weir (1980) found no colloid osmotic pressure difference in subdural fluid and venous blood of 20 patients.

In the early part of this century, Trotter (1914) believed that the enlargement of a chronic subdural haematoma was due to repeated bleeding. This view has now been substantiated by the recovery of [57]Cr- labelled red cells from chronic subdural haematoma 24 hours after i.v. administration (Ito *et al.*, 1976). It now seems clear that the late increase in size of chronic subdural haematoma is a consequence of repeated microhaemorrhages from the highly permeable new sinusoidal-type vessels which proliferate from a thickened haematoma capsule. This bleeding is facilitated by local hyperfibrinolysis (Ito, Komai, and Yamamoto, 1975; Ito *et al.*, 1976; and Komai *et al.*, 1977; Yamamoto *et al.*, 1974).

Clinical Features

A history of head injury is frequently overlooked in old people because it is minimal or unavailable due to forgetfulness, confusion, drug therapy, or alcohol (Table 1).

The frequent presence of a degree of cere-

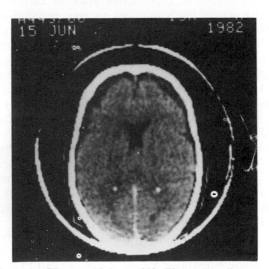

Figure 1   CT scan, 15 June 1982. The septum lies centrally. A halo of low density over both frontal lobes is due to the presence of bilateral frontal subdural haematomas

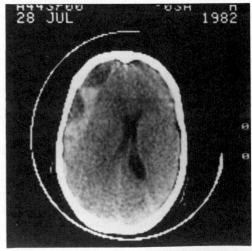

Figure 2   28 July 1982. The septum is well displaced to the right of the midline by an extensive subdural lying over both frontal poles but containing fresh blood on the left side only

Table 1   Some features of 114 patients with subdural haematoma. (From Cameron, 1978. Reproduced by permission of the *Journal of Neurology Neurosurgery and Psychiatry*)

Total patient group (114)	Subacute (44)	Chronic (70)	Percentage of total
Male	26	56	72
Female	18	14	28
Average age	56	56	—
History of head injury	32	40	63
Fluctuation in symptoms or signs	7	21	24
In coma by the time of surgery	12	3	13
Bilateral haematomas evacuated	1	12	11

bral atrophy in old age may allow the subdural haematoma to be tolerated for long periods and it may remain asymptomatic. The initial haematoma itself may produce little brain damage. It is the frequency of recurrent bleeding from the new vessels which proliferate from the encapsulating membrane that often generates symptoms (Fig. 1 and 2) and possibly leads to a fatal outcome in the absence of surgical intervention. Thus the onset of symptoms may be late or insidious or non-specific (McKissock, Richardson, and Bloom, 1960; Perlmutter, 1961; Glover, and Weiss, Raskind *et al.*, 1972), but sometimes rapidly progressive with or without a long period of prior clinical quiescence.

Intracranial pressure may be normal or only moderately raised and infrequently fluctuating levels of consciousness may oscillate between normal alertness or slight drowsiness to coma. As the condition progresses, periods of drowsiness become more frequent and prominent, but coma is commonly a terminal event.

Episodic or established confusion may be misinterpreted in the elderly (Table 1) with consequent devastating delay in diagnosis and treatment (So, 1976). Memory disorders may be prominent. Headache and paresis or mild hemiplegia (Table 2) which may fluctuate over time commonly occur. Gait disorders have been prominent in some studies (Waga *et al.*, 1972). Choreiform movements are a rare manifestation of chronic subdural haematoma (Bae, Vates, and Kenton, 1980; Gilmore and Brenner 1979).

Localized neurological deficits such as cranial nerve palsies, cortical sensory loss, and dysphasia are uncommon. The occasional

Table 2   Most common clinical findings in 114 patients with subdural haematoma. (From Cameron, 1978. Reproduced by permission of the *Journal of Neurology, Neurosurgery and Psychiatry*)

Clinical findings	Subacute	Chronic	Percentage of total
Hemiparesis (45 patients)			40
Ipsilateral to haematoma	11	7	16
Contralateral to haematoma	10	17	24
Personality or intellectual change	11	23	30
Papilloedema (23 patients)			20
With headache and vomiting	1	6	6
With hemiparesis	2	7	8
With coma	4	3	6
Coma (15 patients)	12	3	13
Unilateral pupillary dilation	5	1	5
Headache (48 patients)			
With other neurological findings			38
Alone			5

occurrence of a chronic subdural haematoma in the posterior fossa (Achslough, 1952; Fisher, Kim, and Sachs, 1958 Gross, 1955; Murthy, Deshpande, and Reddy, 1980 Pourpre, Tournoux, and Rebuffat, 1957) may lead to cerebellar and brainstem symptoms and signs or sometimes persistent vomiting. Catatonia (Woods, 1980) and presentations simulating transient ischaemic attacks (Robin, Maxwell, and Pitkethly, 1978) are rare manifestations of subdural haematoma.

Diagnosis

A high index of clinical awareness is the cardinal diagnostic requirement in elderly patients with unexplained neuropsychiatric symptoms or signs or altered states of consciousness or hemiplegia with additional unexplained features.

Computerized Tomography (CT)

The CT scan is the single most effective method of identifying a subdural haematoma. In the acute phase the haematoma is generally hyperdense in relation to the surrounding brain, isodense in the subacute stage, and hypodense in 70 per cent. of chronic phase patients (Scotti *et al.*, 1977). Isodense haematomas, particularly when bilateral, may give rise to diagnostic difficulties. However, a midline shift and the characteristic deformity of the ventricles usually permits a CT diagnosis in the isodense scan (Moeller and Erickson, 1979). Visible displacement of cortical sulci in patients with isodense chronic subdural haematoma is an important feature (Kim, Hemmati, and Weinberg, 1978). Bilateral isodense haematomas without midline displacement are suggested by bilaterally small ventricles with a characteristic configuration (Marcu and Becker, 1977). Using high-resolution CT scanning, Barmeir and Dubowitz (1981) found that medial displacement of the grey–white matter interface was visible in 96.3 per cent. of patients with isodense haematomas.

Other Diagnostic Methods

Where CT facilities are not available, scinti-scanning will demonstrate the majority of chronic subdural haematomas. Echo encephalography gives diagnostic information in about a half of affected patients (Hurwitz, Halpern, and Leopold, 1974; So, 1976). Guarino (1982) has suggested that ausculation of the skull while percussing over its surface provides reliable diagnostic information, but these findings require confirmation.

Treatment

Associated bleeding disorders should be treated where possible and predisposing drugs, e.g. anticoagulants, discontinued.

Rarely, resolution of the encapsulated fluid may be spontaneous (Bender, 1960; Chokroverty and Mayo, 1968). Symptoms may subside following the administration of mannitol and/or steroids, but resolution and recovery may take several weeks. Markwalder (1981) marshals cogent evidence for the benefits of evacuation of the haematoma through burr holes, a procedure which is well tolerated even in advanced age. Markwalder and coworkers (1981) demonstrated that simple burr hole removal of the subdural fluid was curative despite leaving the entire neocapillary network *in situ*. They suggest that by removal of haemorrhagic fluid which contains anticlotting factors, the self-perpetuating cycle of microhaemorrhages from the capillaries of the neomembrane is interrupted. Preoperative reduced cerebral blood flow has been shown to improve after evacuation of haematoma in a group of elderly patients (Brodersen and Gjerris, 1975). Joshy (1982) has clearly shown by repeated CT scanning that there is a residual collection of subdural fluid a week after burrhole evacuation, but that by the eighth to twelfth week resolution of the subdural collection takes place with invariable full expansion of the brain. It is probable that reduction of the subdural pressure by even partial evacuation of the haematoma (Tabaddor and Shulman, 1977) enhances the probability of spontaneous resolution (Gannum, Cook, and Browder, 1962). Small haematomas can be successfully treated with steroids provided progress is monitored by repeated CT scanning (Victoratus and Bligh, 1981). However, it is clear that for the great majority of symptomatic old people, early burr hole craniostomy with drainage is the appropriate treatment.

REFERENCES

Achslough, J. (1952). 'Hématome sous-dural chronique de la fosse cérébrale postérieure, *Acta. Neurol et psychiat. Belg.*, **52**, 790–794.

Apfelbaum, R. I., Guthkelch, A. N., and Shulman, K. (1974). 'Experimental production of subdural haematomas', *J. Neurosurg.*, **20**, 336–346.

Arseni, C., Ionescu, S., and Dinu, M. (1970). 'Intracranial hypotension: An etiological factor of subdural hematoma (chronic subdural hematoma following spinal subarachnoid block anesthesia)', *Rev. Roum. Neurol.*, **7**, 283–286.

Bae, S. H., Vates, T. S., Jr, and Kenton, E. J. III (1980). 'Generalized chorea associated with chronic subdural hematomas', *Ann Neural.*, **8**, 449–450.

Barmeir, E., and Dubowitz, B. (1981). 'Grey–white matter interface. (G-WM1) displacement: A new sign in the computed tomographic diagnosis of subtle subdural hematomas', *Clin. Radiol.*, **32**, 393–396.

Bender, M. D. (1960). 'Recovery from subdural hematoma without surgery', *J. Mt, Sinai. Hosp.* **27**, 52–58.

Bret, P., Lecuire, J., Lapras, C., Deruty, R., Desgeorges, M., and Proudhon, J. L. (1976). 'Subdural hematomas and anticoagulant therapy', *Neurochirurgie*, **22**, 603–620.

Brodersen, P., and Gjerris, F. (1975). 'Regional cerebral blood flow in patients with chronic subdural hematomas', *Acta Neurol. Scand.*, **51**, 233–239.

Cameron, M. M. (1978). 'Chronic subdural haematoma: A review of 114 cases', *J. Neurol. Neurosurg. Psychiat.*, **41**, 834–839.

Chawla, J. C. (1968). 'Subdural haemorrhage: A complication of anti-coagulant therapy', *Guys Hosp. Rep.*, **117**, 75–78.

Chokroverty, S., and Mayo, C. M. (1968). 'Spontaneous resolution of subdural haematoma', *Dis. Nerv. Syst.*, **29**, 704–706.

De Reuk, J., Röels, H., and Vander Eecken, H. (1976). 'Complications of the chronic subdural hematoma', *Clin. Neurol. Neurosurg.*, **79**, 203–210.

Edson, J. R., McArthur, J. R., Branda, R. F., *et al.* (1973). 'Successful management of subdural hematoma in a hemophiliac with an antifactor VIII antibody', *Blood*, **41**, 113–122.

Fisher, R. G., Kim, J. K., and Sachs, E. (1958). 'Complications in posterior fossa due to occipital trauma – their operability'. *JAMA*, **167**, 176–182.

Fontan, A., Verger, P., and Battin, J. J., *et al.* (1963). 'Hématome sousdural du nourrisson et déshydration avec hyponatriémie', *J. Med. Bordeaux*, **140**, 589–595.

Friede, R. L., and Schachenmayr, W. (1978). 'The origin of subdural neomembranes. 1. Fine structure of the dura-arachnoid interface in man', *Am. J. Pathol.*, **92**, 53–68.

Gannum, W. E., Cook, A. W., and Browder, E. J. (1962). 'Resolving subdural collections', *J. Neurosurg.*, **19**, 865–869.

Gardner, W. J. (1932). 'Traumatic subdural hematoma with particular reference to the latent period', *Arch. Neurol. Psychiat.*, **27**, 847–858.

Gilmore, P. C., and Brenner, R. P. (1979). 'Chorea: A late complication of a subdural hematoma', *Neurol.*, **20**, 1044–1045.

Gross, S. W. (1955). 'Posterior fossa hematomas', *J. Mt Sinai. Hosp.*, **22**, 286–289.

Guarino, J. R. (1982). 'Auscultatory percussion of the head', *Br. Med. J.*, **284**, 1075–1077.

Hurwitz, S. R., Halpern, S. E., and Leopold, G. (1974). 'Brain scans and encephalography in the diagnosis of chronic subdural hematoma', *J. Neurol.*, **40**, 347–350.

Ito, H., Komai, T., and Yamamoto, S. (1975). 'Fibrin and fibrinogen degradation products in chronic subdural hematoma', *Neurol. Med. Chir. (Tokyo)*, **15**, 51–55.

Ito, H., Yamamoto, S., Komai, T., *et al.* (1976). 'Role of local hyperfibrinolysis in the etiology of chronic subdural hematoma', *J. Neurosurg.*, **45**, 26–31.

Kim, K. S., Hemmati, M., and Weinberg, P. E. (1978). 'Computed tomography in isodense subdural hematoma', *Radiol*, **128**, 71–74.

Klein, M. R. (1963). 'L'hématome sous-dural du nourrisson', *Neurochirurgie*, **6**, 152–163.

Komai, T., Ho, H, and Yamashina, T., *et al.* (1977). 'Etiology of chronic subdural hematoma – role of local hyperfibrinolysis', *Neurol. Med. Chir.*, **17** (Pt 2), 499–505.

Lizuka, J. (1972). 'Intracranial and intraspinal haematomas associated with anti-coagulant therapy'. *Neurochirurgie. (Stuttg.)* **15**, 15–25.

McKissock, W., Richardson, A., and Bloom, W. H. (1960). 'Subdural haematoma: A review of 389 cases', *Lancet*, **1**, 1365–1369.

Marcu, H., and Becker, H. (1977). 'Computed-tomography of bilateral isodense chronic subdural hematomas', *Neuroradiol*, **14**, 81–83.

Mardešić, D., and Cigit, S. (1965). 'Subduralni hematom poslije hipontremičke dehidracije dojenc-'ta', *Lijecn Vjesn.*, **87**, 753–760.

Markwalder, T. M. (1981). 'Chronic subdural haematomas: A review', *J. Neurosurg.*, **54**, 637–645.

Markwalder, T. M., Steinsiepe, K., Rohner, M., Reichenback, W., and Markwalder, H. (1981). 'The course of chronic subdural haematomas after burr-hole craniostomy and closed system drainage', *J. Neurosurg.*, **55**, 390–396.

Marshall, S., and Hinman, F. Jr., (1962). 'Subdural

hematoma following administration of urea for diagnosis of hypertension', *JAMA, 182*, 813–814.

Moeller, A., and Erickson, K. (1979). 'Computed tomography of iso-attentuating subdural hematomas', *Radiol., 130*, 149–152.

Murthy, V. s., Deshpade, D. H., and Reddy, G. N. N. (1980). 'Chronic subdural hematoma in the cerebello pontine angle', *Surg. Neurol, 14*, 227–229.

Joshy, M., Moussa A. L. (1982). 'The impact of computed tomography on the treatment of chronic subdural haematoma', *J. Neurol. Neurosurg. Psychiat., 45*, 1156–1158.

Perlmutter, I. (1961). 'Subdural haematoma in older patients', *JAMA, 176*, 212–214.

Pourpre, Tournoux, and Rebuffat, (1957). 'Hématome de la fosse postérieure', *Neurochirurgie, 3*, 200–202.

Pundenz, R. D., and Shelden, C. H. (1946). 'The Lucite Calvarium – a method for the direct observation of the brain', *J. Neurosurg., 3*, 487–505.

Rabe, E. F., Flynn, R. E., and Dodge, P. R. (1962). 'A study of subdural effusions in an infant with particular reference to the mechanism of their persistence', *Neurol. (Minneap.), 12*, 79–92.

Raskind, R., Glover, M. B., and Weiss, S. R. (1972). 'Chronic subdural hematoma in the elderly: A challenge in diagnosis and treatment', *J. Am. Geriat. Soc., 20*, 330–334.

Robin, J. J., Maxwell, J. A., and Pilkethly, D. T. (1978). 'Chronic subdural hematoma simulating transient ischemic attacks', (Letter), *Ann. Neurol., 4*(2), 154.

Rougerie, J., and Caldera, R. (1955). 'L'hématome chronique du nourrisson. Étude clinique et bases thérapeutiques', *Neurochirurgie, 2*, 38–57.

Scotti, G., Terbrugge, K., and Melancon, D., *et al.* (1977). 'Evaluation of the age of subdural hematomas by computerized tomography'., *J. Neurosurg., 47*, 311–315.

So, S. C. (1976). 'Chronic subdural haematoma in the elderly', *Aust. N.Z. J. Surg., 46*, 167–169.

Sreerama, V., Ivan, L. P., Dennery, J. M., and Richard, M. T. (1973). 'Neurological complications of anticoagulant therapy'., *Can. Med. Assoc. J., 108*, 305–307.

Tabaddor, K., and Shulman, K. (1977). 'Definitive treatment of chronic subdural haematoma by twist-drill craniostomy and closed system drainage', *J. Neurosurg. 46*. 220–226.

Talmant, J. C., Collet, M., and Sartre, R., *et al.* (1967). 'Les hémorragies du système nerveux central au cours des lencoses aiguës. (A propos d'une localization rare révélatrice de l'affection', *Sem. Hosp. Paris, 43*, 3022–3026.

Trotter, W. (1914). 'Chronic subdural haemorrhage of traumatic origin and its relation to pachymeningitis haemorrhagica interna', *Br. J. Surg., 2*, 271–291.

Victoratus, G. C., and Bligh, A. S. (1981). 'A more systematic management of subdural haematoma with aid of CT scan', *Surg. Neurol., 15*, 158–160.

Waga, S., Ohtsubo, K., Ishikawa, D., and Handa, H. (1972). 'Chronic subdural haematoma in the aged', *Neurologia Medico. Chirurgica (Tokyo), 12*, 84–90.

Weir, B. (1980). 'Oncotic pressure of subdural fluids', *J. Neurosurg., 53*, 512–515.

Wiener, L. M., and Nathanson, M. (1962). 'The relationship of subdural hematoma to anticoagulant therapy', *Arch. Neurol. (Chicago), 6*, 282–286.

Woods, S. W. (1980). 'Catatonia in a patient with subdural haematomas', *Am. J. Psychiat., 8*, 983–984.

Yamamoto, S., Ito, H., and Mizukoshi, H., *et al.* (1974). 'Hemorrhage from the outer membrane of chronic subdural hematoma', *Neurol. Surg. (Tokyo), 2*, 239–242.

Zollinger, R., and Gross, R. E. (1934). 'Traumatic subdural hematoma: An explanation of the late onset of pressure symptoms', *JAMA, 103*, 245–249.

16.11

Spinal Cord Ischaemia

M.S.J. Pathy

Spinal cord vascular disease is uncommon in relation to cerebrovascular disease, though its frequency has been underrated.

Our basic understanding of the arterial blood supply to the spinal cord is largely based on the anatomical studies of Adamkiewicz (1881, 1882) and his fellow anatomist, Kadyi (1889) in Cracow and Tanon (1908) in Paris. Their findings were extended and codified by Suh and Alexander (1939) and Herren and Alexander (1939). The finer details of the spinal cord circulation have been emerging over the last 40 years (Di Chiro and Fried, 1971; Djindjian, 1970; Dommisse, 1975 Lazorthes, 1962; Lazorthes, 1972; Turnbull, 1971, 1972, 1973;), but appreciation of the precise circulatory haemodynamics does not compare with current knowledge on the cerebral circulation.

The early embryonic segmental vascular pattern undergoes drastic modification with foetal development. The anterior two-thirds of the cord are essentially supplied by the anterior spinal artery which is a series of anastomotic links receiving reinforcement from 2 to 17 radicular arteries (Tureen, 1938); most commonly there are between 6 and 10 radicular feeders (Gillilan, 1958; Suh and Alexander, 1939). The anterior spinal artery is formed from branches of the two vertebral arteries and runs caudally in the anterior median fissure to be supplemented in the neck by branches from the deep cervical and ascending cervical arteries, in the dorsal region by 1 to 3 branches from the fourth and/or fifth intercostal arteries and in the thoracolumbar region mainly by the artery of Adamkiewicz (arteria Magna). The level of these anastomoses shows considerable individual variation.

Blood flows in both caudal and rostal directions in the anterior spinal artery, and generally in opposite converging directions from adjacent pairs of anterior radicular arteries. The blood supply to the anterior two-thirds of the cord is potentially tenuous where the upper and lower bloodstream meet to form watershed zones (Henson and Parsons, 1967) (Fig. 1). Zülch (1976) suggests that 10 per cent. of subjects who have a minimum blood supply of only 2 to 3 major anterior radicular arteries have watershed areas which are potentially vulnerable to spinovascular insufficiency, particularly at the T4 level.

The posterior third of the cord is supplied by two posterior spinal arteries which are reinforced by posterior radicular vessels along their length.

The direction of blood flow in anterior and posterior spinal arteries may be reversed by altered physiological demands or by pathological changes. The blood supply to the cord is kept constant by autoregulatory mechanisms as in the brain. Blood flow changes appropriately in response to alterations in blood pressure and CO_2 tension (Kindt, 1972), but the ability to autoregulate may be lost in post-traumatic ischaemia (Senter and Venes, 1979) or in hypercarbia (Flohr, Pöll, and Brock, 1971).

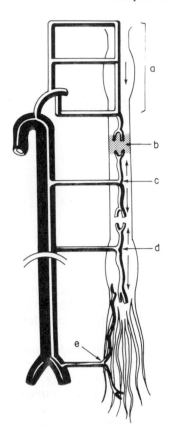

(Reproduced by permission of the *Quarterly Journal of Medicine*)

Figure 1   The arterial supply of the spinal cord.
a   Cervical and upper thoracic cord supplied by branches of vertebral, ascending cervical and superior intercostal arteries
b   'Wateshed' at level of fourth thoracic segment
c   Midthoracic cord supplied from a single intercostal artery
d   Thoracolumbar region supplied by a large vessel near the diaphragm (arteria magna)
e   Cauda equina supplied from lower lumbar, ilio-lumbar, and lateral sacral arteries, which occasionally supply the distal part of the cord also

Henson, R. A. and Parsons, M. (1967).

SPINAL VENOUS SYSTEM

The veins lie parallel to the arteries on and within the cord. The anterior spinal vein runs posterior to the anterior spinal artery and one or two main posterior veins run longitudinally on the posterior surface of the cord. There are abundant venous connections both within the cord and on the surface and with the pial plexi and veins of the epidural space. The final drainage is mainly into the azygos and jugular systems via segmental intervertebral veins.

VASCULAR DISORDERS OF THE CORD

The experimental findings of Niels Stensen (1669) preceded clinical observations on the interruption of the arterial supply to the spinal cord by almost two centuries. During his study on the muscle function in the dogfish Stensen was able to produce reversible paralysis of the tail of the fish by occluding the descending aorta. Subsequent experimental and clinical work has shown that the aorta must usually be compressed above the renal arteries to produce paraplegia (Adams and van Geertruyden, 1956).

SPINOVASCULAR INSUFFICIENCY

This may be discussed from a clinical or anatomical viewpoint. Though an anatomical rubric is used here for descriptive convenience, it will be appreciated that blood flow inadequacy to the spinal cord can be a phenomenon common to or transgressing both intra- and extraspinal arteries including the aorta.

The site and magnitude of ischaemic change in the spinal cord is greatly influenced by the level, number, and size of the radiculomedullary arteries which anastomose with the anterior spinal artery. The watershed areas receiving blood from adjacent radiculomedullary feeders are particularly vulnerable to ischaemia. The recent experimental neuropathological study of Zivin, de Girolami, and Hurwitz (1982) throws considerable light on the pathophysiology of spinal cord ischaemia. They were able to produce a spectrum of neurological deficits ranging from permanent paraplegia to transient paraparesis with complete recovery by temporarily ligating the spinal artery of rabbits.

Spinovascular insufficiency may be a sequela of many unrelated disorders which include cervical spondylosis (Chapter 16.12), trauma, tumours, granulomatous conditions, embolic and haemodynamic phenomena, atheroma, and diseases associated with arteritis. Intervertebral disc embolism is rare (Srigley *et al.*,

1981). In the first half of this century syphilis was the commonest single cause but it is now rare in the United Kingdom. Atherosclerosis is currently among the leading causes of spinal ischaemia (Henson and Parsons, 1967), but Silver and Buxton (1974) emphasize the high incidence of myocardial infarction in spinal stroke and suggest that this is due to the critical lowering of spinal artery perfusion pressure in the vulnerable watershed areas. Foshburg and Brewer (1976) believe that dissecting aneurysms of the aorta are probably the commonest cause of acute vascular injury of the spinal cord. Long-tract neural conduction has been found to be relatively resistant to the ischaemic effects of the experimental reduction of spinal blood flow to 20 to 25 per cent. of normal blood flow (Kobrine, Evans, and Rizzoli, 1979).

Anterior Spinal Artery

The anterior spinal artery supplies the anterior two thirds of the cord; thrombosis of this vessel was first reported by Spiller (1909). The ischaemic event is more commonly heralded by segmental or root pain rather than by girdle pain so often quoted. Pain is often intense and is followed after a variable interval of one to several hours by flaccid paraplegia or quadriplegia depending on the level of obstruction. Rarely the paralysis is abrupt and prodromal symptoms are absent (Beck, 1952; Baasch, Maier, and Plancherel, 1958; Beck, 1952). Initial retention of urine is commonly followed by urinary and faecal incontinence. The paretic muscles exhibit wasting and fasciculation at an early stage due to anterior horn cell destruction. Pyramidal features develop later, but spasticity is often slight.

Loss of pain and temperature sensation with a defined upper level is an early finding, but posterior column modalities remain intact. The sensory deficits frequently improve with time (Silver and Buxton, 1974). Cervicomedullary infarction may give rise to a Horner's syndrome (Pariser and Lasagna, 1949), vertical nystagmus (O'Brien and Bender, 1945), and occasionally hypoglossal paralysis with ipsilateral paralysis of the tongue (Davison, 1937; Gillian, 1964).

Occlusion of an anterior radicular artery may produce features indistinguishable from those of anterior spinal artery occlusion (Hogan and Romanul, 1966).

Transient ischaemic attacks involving the spinal cord may be isolated episodes heralding cord infarction and closely parallel the situation in the cerebrovascular system (Henson and Parsons, 1967; Zivin, de Girolami, and Hurwitz, 1982).

Posterior Spinal Artery

Isolated occlusion of the posterior spinal artery is rare (Périer *et al.* 1960; Williamson, 1894) due to an adequate collateral system. The predominant clinical findings are segmental anaesthesia, loss of proprioception, vibration and tactile discrimination, ataxia, and areflexia. Most commonly there is involvement of the circumflex collateral arteries with consequent lateral or anterior zone neurological features (Dhaene, 1961; Garcin, Gadleurski, and Randot, 1962; Hetzel, 1960; Périer *et al.* 1960).

Aorta

Le Gallois (1830) noted reversibility of motor paresis due to cord ischaemia induced by temporary aortic ligation. Experimental occlusion of the aorta of cats for less than 15 minutes gives rise to temporary paraplegia, but aortic occlusion exceeding 20 minutes leads to permanent paraplegia (Tureen, 1936).

A galaxy of clinical descriptions and syndromes have been ascribed to spinal cord ischaemia resulting from atherosclerotic narrowing of the ostia of the intercostal and lumbar branches of the aorta.

The origins of the thoracic and lumbar segmental arteries may be acutely obstructed by a dissecting aneurysm of the aorta giving rise to a spinal stroke (Kalischer, 1914; Sethi, Hughes, and Takaro, 1974; Thompson, 1956). Spinal trauma (Hughes, 1964), or thrombotic (Lueth, 1940; Ratinov and Jimenez-Pabon, 1961) or embolic (Rudar, Urbanke, and Radonic, 1962; Silver and Buxton, 1974) occlusion of the abdominal aorta, traumatic aortic aneurysm (Conti *et al.*, 1982), and, in recent years, surgery involving the aorta (Hughes, 1964; Pasternak, Boyd, and Ellis, 1972) may give rise to a spinal stroke. Though suprarenal aortic surgery is more likely to be associated with spinal cord infarction, Ferguson and coworkers (1975) have reviewed the serious spinal cord ischaemic effects of infrarenal abdominal aortic surgery.

The clinical features may encompass the extremes of abrupt permanent paraplegia to mild sensory deficits. Intermittant claudication associated with muscle wasting (Leriche syndrome; Leriche, 1940) may be a manifestation of occlusion of the abdominal aorta (Kekwick, McDonald, and Semple, 1952).

Little has been added to Dejerine's (1911) graphic description of intermittant cord ischaemia in which he describes the progressive spastic weakness and numbness of the lower limbs on walking which subside with resting, only to recur repeatedly on recommencing activity. Sphincter disturbances, increased reflexes, and extensor plantar responses may be transient accompaniments of the exercise-induced motor and sensory phenomena.

Chronic Myelopathy

The possibility that chronic myelopathy may be due to aortic atheroma was muted by Marie and Foix (1912). Further cases were reported by Winkelman and Eckel (1932), Keschner and Davison (1933), Alajouanine and Hornet (1937), and Jellinger (1964). The clinical picture may resemble motor neurone disease with muscle wasting and slowly progressive paraplegia (Neumayer, 1965; Skinhøj, 1954). The atheromatous change is mainly in the aorta, but may involve the arteries of the spinal cord (Gruner and Lapresle, 1962).

Prognosis

Where paralysis is complete and persists for several days, recovery is absent or minimal. If the brunt of the motor deficit is in one limb, recovery is moderate or, less often, complete. In transient episodes of paraparesis, immediate recovery is normally complete, but the likelihood of a subsequent established spinal stroke exists. The chronic progressive myelopathic presentation has a better prognosis than motor neurone disease (Zülch, 1976).

Treatment

The incidence of cord ischaemia following vascular surgery within the body cavity has fallen considerably with greater awareness of the an-atomical and haemodynamic vulnerability of the cord, (El-Toraei and Juler, 1979).

The maintenance of adequate cardiac output after myocardial infarction and avoidance of drug overdosage will lessen the risk of acute cord ischaemia.

Primary predisposing factors will clearly require active treatment.

When complete infarction of the anterior two-thirds of the cord occurs, the treatment of the patient will be the management of paraplegia. Care of the bowels, the management of urinary incontinence (Chapter 26.3), and the prevention of pressure sores (Chapter 20.2) requires considerable understanding and skill. Physical treatment is directed towards improving upper limb and trunk power aimed at achieving wheelchair independence.

Antiplatelet agents such as aspirin, dipyridamole, or sulphinpyrazone may be considered where transient cord ischaemia is recurrent, but the efficacy of these agents in this condition awaits confirmation.

SPINAL VEINS

Spinal vein thrombosis is commonly secondary to inflammatory, neoplastic, or traumatic conditions of the vertebral column. Septicaemia and pelvic thrombophlebitis are significant antecedants and polycythaemia may be a predisposing factor (Grunberg, Blair, and Rawcliffe, 1950).

Extensive haemorrhagic cord infarction with spinal thrombophlebitis (Wyss, 1898) are the characteristic pathological findings.

The white matter of the cord is initially involved in various occlusions with subsequent involvement of the grey matter occurring later and probably as a secondary phenomenon (Gillilan, 1970; Greenfield and Turner, 1939). In her authoritative study on the veins of the spinal cord, Gillilan (1970) points out that the posterolateral white matter and lateral corticospinal tract are involved at the outset and only as the process extends do the lateral spinothalamic and spinocerebellar tracts become involved. These findings are in keeping with the clinical description of dissociated or complete sensory loss at and below the level of the lesion associated with progressive paraparesis.

Experimental occlusion of the posterior

spinal veins in rhesus monkeys produces gliosis associated with demyelination confined to the posterior columns (Doppman, Girton, and Popovsky, 1979).

The clinical picture may be dominated in the initial phase by associated disease. Back pain may be intense and signs of rapidly progressive transverse myelopathy are common (Hughes, 1971), though it seems likely that evidence of minor localized spinal venous occlusion may pass unrecognized when it is secondary to more florid precipitating disease.

SPINAL EPIDURAL AND SUBDURAL HAEMATOMA

Epidural Haematoma

Unlike the intracranial dura which is firmly attached to the adjacent bony surfaces, the spinal dura is traditionally considered to be separated from the vertebral periostium by a loose meshwork of fat and venous channels.

The external lamina of the dura mater lines the vertebral canal but its intimate attachment to the vertebral periostium, posterior longitudinal ligament, and ligamenta flava prevents its separate distinction except in early infancy (Bruyn and Bosma, 1976). In practice, the internal lamina is accepted as the definitive dura mater. The epidural fat content is greater in the dorsolumbar region than in the cervical portion of the vertebral canal, but in both regions it diminishes with age.

The epidural vertebral venous plexus is of considerable prominence. The venous pressure in this plexus intimately parallels the CSF pressure (Verjaal, 1947). Bruyn and Bosma consider the size and extent of the internal vertebral venous plexus to be a reflection of its role as a circulatory volume–pressure regulating system accommodating alterations in intracranial, intraspinal, intrathoracic, and intra-abdominal volume pressure status.

Epidural haematomas are considerably more common than haematomas in the spinal subdural space. They may occur at any level, though only 25 per cent. occur in the cervical region (Correa and Beasley, 1978).

Aetiology

Trauma, bleeding disorders (Edelson, Chernik, and Posner, 1974), and coagulopathies may be causal factors. About a third of epidural bleeds are associated with anticoagulant therapy (Harik, Raichle, and Reis, 1971). Lumbar puncture may tear an epidural vein or arteriole and produce significant bleeding (Laglia *et al.*, 1978). In about a half of the cases bleeding is spontaneous and no cause is found (Bruyn and Bosma, 1976).

Clinical Features

Acute back pain, symmetrical paraparesis, or tetraparesis developing within hours and rapidly becoming total, and sensory loss are cardinal symptoms. Rarely pain is absent (Senelick, Norwood, and Cohen, 1976). The level of sensory loss depends on the site of the haematoma. If it is compressing the conus medullaris the sensory loss is typically to the level of the groins (Vapalahti and Kuurne, 1975). Tendon reflexes are usually diminished or absent and the plantars are most commonly flexor. Early loss of bowel and bladder function occurs. Spontaneous recovery occurs rarely and only one case of recurrent paraplegia with eventual full recovery is currently recorded (Hernandez, Vinuela, and Feasby, 1982).

Diagnosis

Urgent myelography is critical.

Treatment

Any anticoagulant drug should be discontinued and bleeding and coagulation disorders treated where possible.

Early surgical evacuation of the blood clot is essential and commonly results in rapid resolution of symptoms (Markham, Lynge, and Stahlman, 1967). If surgical decompression is delayed for over 36 hours, the probability of recovery falls below 50 per cent. (McQuarrie, 1978).

Subdural Haematoma

The aetiological associations, clinical manifestations, and management closely parallel epidural haematomas. Marsden, Breuer, and Schoene (1979) suggest that a proportion of subdural haematomas originate from a spinal subarachnoid bleed. Subdural bleeding following lumbar puncture most commonly occurs in thrombocytopenic patients (Edelson, Chernick, and Posner, 1974). Occipital headache, neck stiffness, and vomiting may rarely occur in spinal subdural haematoma as a consequence of intracranial extension of an associated spinal subarachnoid haemorrhage (Vinters, Barnett, and Kaufmann, 1980). As with epidural haematomas, the prognosis is good only if the condition is diagnosed promptly and the clot evacuated before severe spinal cord compression and subsequent ischaemic necrosis occurs (Russell, Maroun, and Jacob, 1981). A platelet infusion should be given to thrombocytopenic patients.

Spinal Subarachnoid Haemorrhage

Bleeding in this plane may result from lumbar puncture for diagnostic or anaesthetic reasons. More commonly subarachnoid haemorrhage is spontaneous and arises from a spinal angioma (Henson and Croft, 1956). These vascular malformations can remain clinically silent until old age despite being surprisingly large (Pennybacker, 1958). Other recorded associations with subarachnoid bleeding include intraspinal tumours, mainly ependymomas (Djindjian *et al.*, 1978; Henson and Croft, 1956) and neoplasms of the conus medullaris and ·cauda equina (Rice *et al.*, 1978), polyarteritis nodosa (Henson and Croft, 1956), systemic lupus erythematosis (Fody, Netsky, and Mark, 1980), and Sjögren' syndrome (Alexander *et al.*, 1981).

Intense backache may herald the presence of blood in the subarachnoid space, but occipital headache, neck stiffness, and photophobia can dominate the scene. Due to the diluting effect of the CSF, a space-occupying haematoma is rare, but it may occur and compress the spinal cord or the cauda equina (Marsden, Breuer and Schoene, 1979; Plotkin, Ronthal, and Froman, 1966; Rengachary and Murphy, 1974).

Treatment

Mangement is directed towards the underlying precipitating cause. Usually no specific treatment is required other than bed-rest until the bleeding subsides. Surgical evacuation of the clot is required if compressive symptomatic features develop.

CAUDA EQUINA CLAUDICATION

In a series of studies between 1949 and 1955 Verbiest (1949, 1950, 1954, 1955) described the occurrence and effects of structural narrowing of the lumbar vertebral canal. An anteroposterior diameter of 10 mm or less is common in symptomatic cases. Schatzker and Pennal (1968) stressed the importance of associated shallowness of the nerve root-containing lateral recesses in the production of symptoms. Verbiest subdivided patients with small spinal canals into those where the stenosis was the sole cause of neural compression (absolute stenosis) and those where additional encroachment of the canal was necessary to produce symptoms. An age distribution of 50 to 85 years was recorded in half the patients. The causes of spinal stenosis may be classified into (a) developmental, (b) degenerative, (c) spondylolisthesis, (d) spondylotic spondylolisthesis, (e) traumatic, (f) iatrogenic (Schatzker and Pennal, 1968). Wilson (1969) points to the close correlation between cauda equina claudication and anteroposterior narrowing of the lumbar spinal canal secondary to enlarged apophyseal joints, thickened ligamenta flava, and encroachment by intravertebral disks or marginal osteophytes.

Blau and Logue (1961) discussed six elderly patients with symptoms of intermittent claudication on exercise due to compression of the cauda equina by chronic central protrusion of a lumbar intervertebral disk.

Increased dilatation and prominence of the vessels of the spinal cord of the mouse follow electrically induced repetitive hind limb exercise (Blau and Rushworth, 1958). Blau and Logue (1961) postulated that when patients with cauda equina claudication walk, similar dilatation of the vessels of the cauda equina occurs. In the presence of nerve root compression by a disk protrusion, adequate vasodilatation of the cauda equina vessels cannot take place and symptoms of ischaemic neuritis occurs.

The rate of oxygen uptake by peripheral nerves is proportional to the frequency of nerve stimulation and impulse transmission (Cranfield, Brink, and Bronk, 1957). Evans (1964) suggests that this is a more probable explanation for the relative ischaemia of active cauda equina roots during exercise.

All patients with cauda equina claudication develop symptoms while walking, but Wilson (1969) identified two subgroups:

(a) those where posture or body movement predominantly precipitates symptoms and
(b) a smaller group in whom symptoms are intimately related to exercise.

Clinical Presentation

The general picture is characterized by significant sensory symptoms causally related to posture or to exercise. Paraesthesiae and pain which is cold or burning or in severe cases graphically described as searing, is located in the lumbar region, buttocks, or thighs. Sensory manifestations may commence in the feet and progress upwards to the buttocks (Blau and Logue, 1961). Less commonly pain is indistinguishable from sciatica due to nerve root compression from a herniated lumbar intervertebral disk (Macnab, 1971). Exercise-induced symptoms tend to occur after a constant quantum of walking and rapidly subside with rest. Weakness of the legs may accompany sensory features. Where postural factors predominate, activities associated with sustained extension of the spine precipitate symptoms and forward flexion and squatting produces relief (Brish, Lèrner, and Braham, 1964). In both groups pain can radiate diffusely around the pelvis and thighs and may be severe.

Neurological signs are often inconspicuous. Deep tendon reflexes are usually diminished or absent in the lower limbs. Muscle wasting is absent or slight and occurs in the glutei, hamstrings, and calves, but is often difficult to determine in old people. Loss of superficial sensation or hyperaesthesia may be evident over the fifth lumbar and first sacral dermatomes.

Investigation

Myelography may show posterior or posterolateral indentations (Schatzker and Pennal, 1968).

Treatment

Non-steroidal anti-inflammatory drugs and epidural cortisone should be tried. A lumbosacral brace may reduce symptoms where postural factors are significant.

Laminectomy with partial facetectomy produces gratifying results in younger patients, but where lumber spondylosis predominates in old age conservative management is appropriate.

REFERENCES

Adamkiewicz, A. (1881). 'Die Blutegafässe des menschlichen Rückenmarkes. I. Teil. Die Gefässe der Rückenmarkes substanz', *Sber. Akad. Wiss. Wien. math-nat. K1,* **84** (3), 469–502.

Adamkiewicz, A. (1882). 'Die Blutgefässe des menschlichen Rückenmarkes. II. Die Gefässe des Rückenmarkes Oberflässche', *Sber. Akad. Wiss. Wien. math-nat. K1,* **85** (3), 101–130.

Adams, H. D., and van Geertruyden, H. H. (1956). 'Neurologic complications of aortic surgery', *Ann. Surg.,* **44,** 574–610.

Alajouanine, T., and Hornet, T. (1937). 'Le ramollissement aigu de la möelle (un cas anatomoclinique ayant évolué sous l'aspect d'une lésion médullaire transverse aigue chez une femme âgée, artérioscléreuse), *Rev. Neurol.,* **67,** 400–407.

Alexander, E. L., Craft, C., Dorsch, C., Moser, R. L., Provost, T. T., and Alexander, G. E. (1981). 'Necrotizing arteritis and spinal subarachnoid hemorrhage in Sjögren Syndrome', *Ann. Neurol.,* **11,** 632–635.

Baasch, E., Maier, C., and Plancherel, P. (1958). 'Diagnosis and therapy of occlusion of the anterior ventral spinal artery', *Schweiz. Arch. Neur. Psychiat.,* **82,** 182–188.

Beck, K. (1952). 'Das Syndrom des Verschlusses der Vorderen Spinalarterien'. *Deutsche Ztschr. Nervenk.* **167.** 164–186.

Blau, J. N., and Logue, V. (1961). 'Intermittant claudication of the cauda equina. An unusual syndrome resulting from central protrusion of a lumbar intervertebral disc', *Lancet,* **1,** 1081–1086.

Blau, J. N., and Rushworth, G. (1958). 'Observations on the blood vessels of the spinal cord and their response to motor activity', *Brain,* **81,** 354–363.

Brish. A., Lèrner, M. A., and Braham, J. (1964). 'Intermittent claudication from compression of the cauda equina by a narrowed spinal canal', *J. Neurosurg.,* **21,** 207–211.

Bruyn, G. W., and Bosma, N. J. (1976). 'Spinal extradural hematoma', in *Handbook of Clinical Neurology* (Eds P. J. Vinken and G. W. Bruyn),. Vol. 26, pp. 1–30, North Holland, Amsterdam.

Conti, V. R., Calverley, J., Safley, W. L., Estes, M., and Williams, E. H. (1982). 'Anterior spinal artery syndrome with chronic traumatic aortic aneurysm', *Ann. Thorac. Surg.*, **133**, 81–85.

Correa, A. V., and Beasley, B. A. (1978). 'Spontaneous cervical epidural hematoma with complete recovery', *Surg. Neurol.*, **10**, 227–228.

Cranfield, P. F., Brink, F., and Bronk, D. W. (1957). 'The oxygen uptake of the peripheral nerve of the rat', *J. Neurochem.*, **1**, 245–249.

Davison, C. (1937). 'Syndrome of anterior spinal artery of medulla oblongata', *Arch. Neurol. Psychiat.*, **37**, 91–107.

Dejerine, J. (1911). 'La claudication intermittente de la moelle épiniére', *Paris Presse Méd.*, **19**, 981–984.

Dhaene, R. (1961). 'Softening of the spinal cord in the region of the anterior spinal artery', *Acta. Neurol. Belg.*, **61**, 223–239.

Di Chiro, G., and Fried, L. C. (1971). 'Blood flow currents in spinal cord arteries', *Neurology (Minneap.)*, **21**, 1088–1096.

Djindjian, M., Djindjian, R., Hondart, R., and Hurth, M. (1978). 'Subarachnoid hemorrhage due to intraspinal tumours', *Surg. Neurol.*, **9**, 223–229.

Djindjian, R. (1970). *Angiography of the Spinal Cord*, University Park Press, Baltimore.

Dommisse, G. F. (1975). *The Arteries and Veins of the Human Spinal Cord from Birth*, Churchill Livingstone, Edinburgh.

Doppman, J. L., Girton, M., Popovsky, M. A. (1979). 'Acute occlusion of the posterior spinal vein. Experimental study in monkeys', *J. Neurosurg.*, **51**, 201–205.

Edelson, R. N., Chernik, N., and Posner, J. B. (1974). 'Spinal subdural hematomas complicating lumbar puncture', *Arch. Neurol.*, **31**, 134–137.

El-Toraei, I., and Juler, G. (1979). 'Ischemic myelopathy', *Angiology*, **30**, 81–94.

Evans, J. G. (1964). 'Neurogenic intermittent claudication', *Br. Med. J.*, **2**, 985–987.

Ferguson, L. R. J., Bergan, J. M., Conn, J., Jr, and Yao, J. S. (1975). 'Spinal ischemia following abdominal aortic surgery', *Ann. Surg.*, **181**, 267–272.

Flohr, H., Pöll, W., and Brock. M. (1971). 'Regulation of Spinal cord blood flow', in *Brain and Blood Flow* (Ed. R. W. R. Russell), pp. 406–409, Pitman Medical and Scientific Publishing Co., London.

Fody, E. P., Netsky, M. G., and Mark. R. E. (1980). 'Subarachnoid spinal hemorrhage in a case of systemic lupus erythematosus', *Arch. Neurol.*, **37**, 173–174.

Foshburg, R. G., and Brewer, L. A. (1976). 'Arterial vascular injury to the spinal cord', in *Handbook of Clinical Neurology* (Eds P. J. Vinken and G. W. Bruyn), Vol. 26 (Part II), pp. 63–79, North-Holland, Amsterdam.

Garcin, R., Godlewski, S., and Rondot, P. (1962). 'Etude clinique des medullopathies d'origine vasculaire', *Rev. Neurol.*, **106**, 558–591.

Gillilan, L. A. (1958). 'The arterial blood supply of the human spinal cord', *J. Comp. Neurol.*, **110**, 75–103.

Gillilan, L. A. (1964). 'The correlation of the blood supply to the human brain stem with clinical brain stem lesions', *J. Neuropath. Exp. Neurol.*, **23**, 78–108.

Gillilan, L. A. (1970). 'Veins of the spinal cord. Anatomic details; suggested clinical applications', *Neurology*, **20**, 860–868.

Greenfield, J. G., and Turner, J. W. A. (1939). 'Acute and subacute myelitis', *Brain*, **62**, 227–252.

Grundberg, A., Blair, J. L., and Rawcliffe, R. M. (1950). 'Unusual neurological symptoms in polycythaemia rubra vera', *Edinburgh Med. J.*, **57**, 305–308.

Gruner, J., and Lapresle, J. (1962). 'Etude anatomo-pathologique des medullopathies d'origine vasculaire', *Rev. Neurol.*, **106**, 592–631.

Harik, S. I., Raichle, M. E., and Reis, D. J. (1971). 'Spontaneously remitting spinal epidural hematoma in a patient on anticoagulants', *New Engl. J. Med.*, **284**, 1355–1357.

Henson, R. A., and Croft, P. B. (1956). 'Spontaneous spinal subarachnoid haemorrhage', *Q. J. Med.*, **25**, 53–66.

Henson, R. A., and Parsons, M. (1967). 'Ischaemic lesions of the spinal cord: An illustrated review', *Q. J. Med.*, **142**, 205–222.

Hernandez, D., Vinuela, F., and Feasby, T. E. (1982). 'Recurrent paraplegia with total recovery from spontaneous spinal epidural hematoma', *Ann. Neurol.*, **11**, 623–624.

Herren, R. Y., and Alexander, L. (1939). 'Sulcal and intrinsic blood vessels of the human spinal cord', *Arch. Neurol. Psychiat.*, **41**, 678–687.

Hetzel, H. (1960). 'Thrombotic occlusion of the ventral radicular artery, the anterior spinal artery and the posterior spinal artery', *Dtsch. Z. Nervenheilk.*, **180**, 301–316.

Hogan, E. L., and Romanul, F. C. (1966). 'Spinal cord infarction occurring during insertion of aortic graft', *Neurol. (Minneap.)*, **16**, 67–74.

Hughes, J. T. (1964). 'Spinal cord infarction due to aortic trauma', *Br. Med. J.*, **2**, 356.

Hughes, J. T. (1971). 'Venous infarction of the spinal cord', *Neurol. (Minneap.)*, **21**, 794–800.

Jellinger, K. (1964). 'Zur Morphologie und Pathogenese arterieller Durchblutungsstörungen des Rückenmarkes', *Wien. Klin, Wschr.*, **76**, 109–114.

Kalischer, O. (1914). 'Demonstration eines präparates (aneurysma dissecans der aorta mit paraplegie)' *Berl. Klin. Wschr.* **51**. 1286–1287.

Kadyi, H. (1889). *Uber die Blutgefasse des men-*

schlichen Ruckenmarkes, pp. 1–144. Gubrnwicz and Schmidt, Lemberg.

Kekwick, A., McDonald, L., and Semple, R. (1952). 'Obliterative disease of abdominal aorta and iliac arteries with intermittent claudication', *Quart. J. Med.*, **21**, 185–200.

Keschner, M., and Davison, C. (1933). 'Myelitic and myelopathic lesions; arteriosclerotic and arteritic myelopathy', *Arch. Neurol. Psychiat.*, **29**, 702–705.

Kindt, G. W. (1972). 'Autoregulation of spinal cord blood flow', *Eur. Neurol.*, **6**, 19–23.

Kobrine, A. I., Evans, D. E., and Rizzoli, H. V. (1979). 'The effects of ischaemia on the long tract neural conduction in the spinal cord', *J. Neurosurg.*, **50**, 639–644.

Laglia, A. G., Eisenberg, R. L., Weinstein, P. R., and Mani, R. L. (1978). 'Spinal epidural hematoma after lumbar puncture in liver disease', *Ann. Intern. Med.*, **88**, 515–516.

Lazorthes, G. (1962). 'La vascularization de la möelle épiniére', *Rev. Neurol.*, **106**, 535–556.

Lazorthes, G. (1972). 'Pathology, classification and clinical aspects of vascular diseases of the spinal cord', in *Handbook of Clinical Neurology*, Vol. 12. Chap. 19, pp. 492–506, (Eds P. J. Vinken and G. W. Bruyn) North Holland, Amsterdam.

Le Gallois, J. J. C. (1830). *Experiences sur le Principe de la Vie*, Hautel, Paris.

Leriche, R. (1940). 'De la résection du carefour aortico-iliaque avec double sympathectomie lombaire pour thrombose arteritique de l'aorte. Le syndrome de l'oblitération terminoaortique par arteinte', *Press Méd.*, **48**, 33–604.

Lueth, H. C. (1940). 'Thrombosis of the abdominal aorta; a report of four cases showing the variability of symptoms', *Ann. Intern. Med.*, **13**, 1167–1173.

Macnab, I. (1971). 'Negative disc exploration. An analysis of the causes of nerve-root involvement in sixty-eight patients', *J. Bone Joint Surg.*, **53A**, 891–903.

McQuarrie, I. G. (1978). 'Recovery from paraplegia caused by spontaneous spinal epidural hematoma', *Neurol. (Minneap.)*, **28**, 224–228.

Marie, P., and Foix, C. (1912). 'L'atrophie isolée non progressive Des petits muscles de la main Fréquence relative et pathogénie. Téphromalacie antérieure Poliomyélite, nevrite radiculaire ou non radiculaire', *Nouv. Iconcgr. Salpet.*, **25**, 353–363.

Markham, J. W., Lynge, H. H., and Stahlman, G. E. B. (1967). 'The syndrome of spontaneous epidural hematoma', *J. Neurosurg.*, **26**, 334–342.

Marsden, J. C., Breuer, A. C., and Schoene, W. C. (1979). 'Spinal subarachnoid hematomas: Clue to a source of bleeding in traumatic lumbar puncture', **29**, 872–876.

Neumayer, E. (1965). 'Die vasculare Myelopathie', in *Anstaltsneurologie* (Ed. W. Birkmayer), p. 147, Springer-Verlag, Wien.

O'Brien, F. H., and Bender, M. B. (1945). 'Localizing value of vertical nystagmus', *Arch. Neurol. Psychiat.*, **54**, 378–380.

Pariser, S., and Lasagna, L. (1949). 'Occlusion of anterior spinal artery', Case Report. *J. Mt. Sinai. Hosp.*, **16**, 128–131.

Pasternak, B. M., Boyd, D. P., and Ellis, H. F. (1972). 'Spinal cord injury after procedures on the aorta', *Surg. Gynecol. Obstet.*, **135**, 29–34.

Pennylacker, J. (1958). 'Discussion on vascular disease of the spinal cord', *Proc. Roy. Soc. Med.*, **51**, 547–550.

Périer, D., Demanet, J. C., Henneaux, J., and Vincente, A. N. (1960). 'Does a syndrome of the posterior spinal arteries exist? Apropos of 2 anatomo-clinical observations', *Rev. Neurol. (Paris)*, **103**, 396–409.

Plotkin, R., Ronthal, M., and Froman, C. (1966). 'Spontaneous spinal subarachnoid hemorrhage. Report of 3 cases', *J. Neurosurg.*, **25**, 443–446.

Ratinov, G., and Jimenez-Pabon, E. (1961). 'Intermittent spinal ischemia', *Neurol. (Minneap.)*, **11**, 546–549.

Rengachary, S. S., and Murphy, D. (1974). 'Subarachnoid hematoma following lumbar puncture causing compression of the cauda equina', Case Report, *J. Neurosurg.*, **41**, 252–254.

Rice, J. F., Shields, C. B., Morris, C. F., and Neely, B. D. (1978). 'Spinal subarachnoid hemorrhage during myelography', Case Report, *J. Neurosurg.*, **48**, 645–648.

Rudar, M., Urbanke, A., and Radonic, M. (1962). 'Occlusion of the abdominal aorta with dysfunction of the spinal cord', *Ann. Int. Med.*, **56**, 490–494.

Russell, N., Maroun, F. B., and Jacob, J. C. (1981). 'Spinal subdural hematoma in association with anticoagulant therapy', *Can. J. Neurol. Sci.*, **8**, 87–89.

Schatzker, J., and Pennal, G. F. (1968). 'Spinal stenosis, a cause of cauda equina compression', *J. Bone Joint Surg.*, **50B**, 606–618.

Senelick, R. C., Norwood, C. W., and Cohen, G. H. (1976). 'Painless' spinal epidural hematoma during anticoagulant therapy', *Neurol. (Minneap.)*, **26**, 213–225.

Senter, H. J., and Venes, J. L. (1979). 'Loss of autoregulation of post traumatic ischemia following experimental spinal cord trauma', *J. Neurosurg.*, **50**, 198–206.

Sethi, G. K., Hughes, R. K., and Takaro, T. (1974). 'Dissecting aortic aneurysms' (Collective review), *Ann. Thorac. Surg.*, **18**, 201–215.

Silver, J. R., and Buxton, P. H. (1974). 'Spinal stroke', *Brain*, **97**, 539–550.

Skinhøj, E. (1954). 'Arteriosclerosis of spinal cord; 3 cases of pure syndrome of spinal artery', *Acta. Psychiat. Scand.*, **29**, 139–144.

Spiller, W. G. (1909). 'Thrombosis of the cervical anterior median spinal artery: Syphilitic acute anterior poliomyelitis', *J. Nerv. Ment. Dis.*, **36**, 601–613.

Srigley, J. R., Lambert, C. D., Bilbao, J. M., and Pritzker, K. P. H. (1981). 'Spinal cord infarction secondary to intervertebral disc embolism', *Ann. Neurol.*, **9**, 296–301.

Stensen, N. (Stenonius, N.) (1669). *Elementorum Myologiae Specimen sen Musculi Descriptro Geometuca*, Apnd. Johan. Janssonium a Waesberge and Viduamm Amsterdam.

Suh, T. H., and Alexander, L. (1939). 'Vascular system of the human spinal cord', *Arch. Neurol. Psychiat.*, **41**, 659–677.

Tanon, L. (1908). 'Les arteres de la möelle dorsolumbaire. Considerations anatomiques et cliniques', *Thesis*, **98**, (Ed. Vigot), Paris.

Thompson, G. B. (1956). 'Dissecting aortic aneurysm with infarction of spinal cord', *Brain*, **79**, 111–118.

Tureen, L. L. (1936). 'Effect of experimental temporary vascular occlusion on spinal cord; correlation between structural and functional changes', *Arch. Neurol. Psychiat.*, **35**, 789–807.

Tureen, L. L. (1938). 'Circulation of the spinal cord and the effect of vascular occlusion', *Res. Publ. Ass. Res. Nerv. Ment. Dis.*, **18**, 394–437.

Turnbull, I. M. (1971). 'Microvasculature of the human spinal cord', *J. Neurosurg.*, **35**, 141–147.

Turnbull, I. M. (1972). 'Blood supply of the spinal cord', in *Handbook of Clinical Neurology* (Eds P. J. Vinken and G. W. Bruyn), Vol. 12, Chap. 18, pp. 478–491, North Holland, Amsterdam.

Turnbull, I. M. (1973). 'Blood supply of the spinal cord: Normal and pathological considerations', *Clin. Neurosurg.*, **20**, 56–84.

Vapalahti, M., and Kuurne, T. (1975). 'Acute paraplegia caused by a spontaneous extradural hematoma of the conus medullaris area', *Acta. Chir. Scand.*, **141**, 484–487.

Verbiest, H. (1949). 'Sur certaines fonnes rares de compression de la queue de cheval', in *Hommage a Clovis Vincent*, pp. 161–174, Maloine, Paris.

Verbiest, H. (1950). 'Primaire stenose van het Lumbale Wervelkanaal bij Volwassenen Een Niekw Ziektebeeld', *Ned. Tijdschr. Geneesk.*, **94**, 2415–2433.

Verbiest, H. (1954). 'A radicular syndrome from developmental narrowing of the lumbar vertebral canal', *J. Bone Joint Surg.*, **36B**, 230–237.

Verbiest, H. (1955). 'Further experiences on the pathological influence of a developmental narrowness of the bony lumbar vertebral canal', *J. Bone Joint Surg.*, **37B**, 576–583.

Verjaal, A. (1947). 'Physiologie en Pathologie van de Liquordruk', *Geneesk. Bl*, **41**, 529–571.

Vinters, H. V., Barnett, H. J. M., and Kaufmann, J. C. E. (1980). 'Subdural hematoma of the spinal cord and widespread subarachnoid hemorrhage complicating anticoagulant therapy', *Stroke*, **11**, 459–464.

Williamson, R. T. (1894). 'On the relation of the spinal diseases to the distribution of lesions of the blood vessels to the spinal cord', *Med. Chron.*, **2**, 161–178; 262–273; 328–336.

Wilson, C. B. (1969). 'Significance of the small lumbar spinal canal: Cauda equina compression syndromes due to spondylosis', *J. Neurosurg.*, **31**, 499–506.

Winkelman, N. W., and Eckel, J. L. (1932). 'Focal lesions of spinal cord due to vascular disease', *JAMA*, **99**, 1919–1926.

16.12

Cervical Spondylosis

M. S. J. Pathy

Cervical spondylosis, predominantly a disorder of middle and old age, is a chronic condition of the cervical disks, often loosely denoted as degenerative, and associated with reactionary osteophytic new bone formation, though Verbiest (1973) doubts an absolute correlation between osteophyte formation and disc degeneration. The condition is to be distinguished from intervertebral disk herniation, (Brain, Knight, and Bull; Key, 1838), although secondary spondylosis may be a late sequela of a disk protrusion (O'Connell, 1956).

The water content of the disk, especially the nucleus pulposus, gradually diminishes with age (Coventry, Ghormley, and Kernohan, 1945; Püschel, 1930). The reduction in mucoid gel and subsequent fibrous replacement of the nucleus pulposus contributes to the loss of intervertebral space with alteration of the characteristic ball rolling movement of one cervical vertebra upon another (Keyes and Compere, 1932). Thinning of the cervical intervertebral disk produces increasing proximity and eventual contact of the neurocentral joints; further disk narrowing can then only take place anteriorly with loss of normal cervical lordosis (Macnab, 1975) (Fig. 1). Osteoarthrosis of the diarthrodial apophyseal (Fig. 2) and neurocentral joints is so often associated with intervertebral disk changes that it is traditional and reasonable clinical practice to include these joint changes within the description of cervical spondylosis.

Osteophytes form at the margins of the thinning disks and posterior osteophytes can produce transverse bars which may seriously encroach on the sagittal diameter of the spinal canal. Osteophytic spurs from the apophyseal and the neurocentral joints may compromise the intravertebral foraminal dimensions and compress the corresponding nerve roots; further root constriction may result from dural sheath fibrosis (Frykholm, 1951). Osteophytes stabilize adjacent vertebrae and increase the weight-bearing surface area of the vertebral end plates (Hoff and Wilson, 1976).

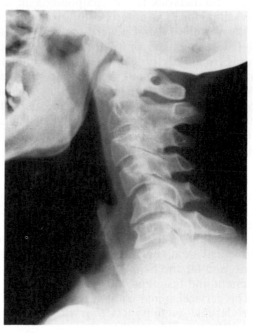

Figure 1   Loss of normal cervical lordosis

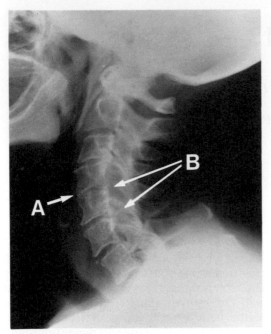

Figure 2   Cervical spondulosis.
A Marked narrowing of disk spaces
B Marked involvement of apophyseal joints

The spatial relationship of the cervical spinal cord and its nerve roots to the surrounding bony vertebral cage largely determines the potential for nervous tissue compression in the cervical region. The anteroposterior dimension of the vertebral canal is very variable and at C4–C7 has a range of 12 to 22 mm with an average diameter of 17 mm (Wolf, Khilnani, and Malis, 1956), but Payne and Spillane (1957) found the average sagittal diameter at C6 to be a little over 14 mm. Murone and City (1974) noted that Japanese men have smaller cervical spinal canals than European adults. The sagittal dimension of the spinal canal may be 2 to 3 mm narrower when the neck is extended than when flexed (Bechar *et al.*, 1971). There is less variability in spinal cord size and an average sagittal dimension of 10 mm at C1 was found by Lowman and Finkelstein (1942). The remaining canal space is occupied by cerebrospinal fluid, dura, peridural venous network, and fat and by the posterior longitudinal ligament and ligamenta flava.

The cervical spinal column is endowed with considerable mobility (Bechar *et al.*, 1971), and although the spinal cord is anchored laterally by the dentate ligament, it moves rostro-caudally during flexion and extension of the neck. This may be of major significance if the sagittal diameter of the canal is seriously compromised.

Seventy-five per cent. of patients over the age of 65 have radiological evidence of cervical disk degeneration. Although symptoms are most commonly absent or minimal, even in the presence of advanced spondylotic changes, significant correlation does exist between the radiological severity of spondylosis and the symptoms and signs of neurological or vertebral artery involvement (Pallis, Jones, and Spillane, 1954). Pain in the neck or the cervical muscles may result from changes in the apophyseal or neurocentral joints. Brachial radiculitis, characteristic headache, vertigo, myelopathy, vertebrobasilar ischaemia (see Chapter 16.11), drop attacks, and syncope, are among the common presenting features of cervical spondylosis (Brain, 1963). This chapter is concerned with disorders of the cervical nerve roots (radiculopathy) and spinal cord (myelopathy) associated with cervical spondylosis.

SPONDYLOTIC RADICULOPATHY

The cervical intervertebral foramina are bounded posterolaterally by the apophyseal joints and anteromedially by the neurocentral joints and (in some circumstances) by the intervertebral disks. Compression of the spinal nerve roots entering the foramina by osteophytes has been considered the principal cause of radiculopathy (Pallis, Jones, and Spillane, 1954), but no radiological difference has been demonstrated between patients with spondylotic radiculopathy and those with spondylosis only (Brooker and Barter, 1965; Friedenberg and Miller, 1963). However, during neck extension foraminal size is reduced due in part to dynamic vertebral subluxation and to exaggerated lordosis (Hadley, 1956; Waltz, 1967). The combination of foraminal encroachment by osteophytes and generous vertebral mobility may produce symptomatic nerve root compression during cervical flexion and extension. However, root sleeve fibrosis (Frykholm, 1947) may account for some cases where radiological evidence of foraminal encroachment is absent. Affected nerve roots are hypersensitive to mechanical deformation or altered tension (Smyth and Wright, 1958) and ventral root stimulation may produce pain akin to the traditionally appreciated dorsal root pain (Frykholm, 1951).

Clinical Features

Commonly the disorder presents with recurrent pain and stiffness in the neck aggravated by cervical movement. Associated crepitus may be obvious to both patient and observer. The neck is often held in a fixed and sometimes laterally flexed position. Localized pain in the neck is possibly related to osteoarthrosis of the affected diarthrodial joints although abnormal intervertebral movement due to ligamentous laxity may cause neck pain (Verbiest, 1973). Tender zones are detectable over the paraspinal muscles. Headache is often persistent and nagging in character and occipital in site, but often radiates to the forehead. The range of movement in the cervical spine is diminished, particularly lateral flexion and rotation. More clearly related to the radiculopathy is the boring segmental pain and paraesthesia in the upper limb, including the shoulder and scapula or, if C6-C7 roots are involved, in the anterior chest to simulate ischaemic cardiac pain. Acute episodes of radicular pain may at times intervene on a background of chronic aching discomfort and may be associated with related muscle weakness and wasting. The small muscles of the hands and flexors of the wrists and fingers are most commonly affected due to the predominant involvement of the lower cervical vertebrae. Muscle fasciculation is rare. Depending on the nerve root compressed, the biceps, triceps, or supinator tendon reflexes may be lost. An inverted radial reflex indicates involvement of the fifth spinal segment and may be associated with other evidence of cervical myelopathy. All modalities of sensation may be impaired over the affected dermatome.

Cervical Spondylotic Myelopathy

This condition is one of the commonest diseases affecting the spinal cord in old age (Brain, 1954).

Aetiology

The precise mechanism of cord damage is uncertain, but several factors contribute in greater or lesser degree to the development of spondylotic myelopathy. A narrow spinal canal with a sagittal diameter of less than 14 mm is a characteristic finding (Payne and Spillane, 1957). The anteroposterior canal diameter is least when the neck is extended. This dynamic reduction in canal size is further augmented by bulging and thickening of the ligamenta flava (Breig, 1960; Penning, 1968; Taylor, 1953) and infolding of the dura (Breig, 1960) on neck flexion. The cervical cord may be proximated to spondylotic bars anteriorly by the dentate ligaments (Kahn, 1947), which could provide a potential risk of-recurrent trauma during cervical movements (Bedford, Bosanquet, and Russell, 1952). Posterior spondylotic bars are particularly likely to lead to cord compression in those subjects with constitutionally narrow vertebral canals. Burrows (1963) found the sagittal diameter at the level of the middle of the vertebral body to be significantly less in patients with spondylotic myelopathy than in unaffected controls. Spondylotic changes are most prominent at C5/6 and less often at C4/5 (Crandall and Batzdorf, 1966). Degenerative changes in the intervertebral disks and posterior articulations may lead to vertebral subluxation (Hadley, 1956), which frequently occurs above spondylotic fused vertebrae (Stoops and King, 1962). These changes increase the likelihood of intermittent cord compression during flexion and extension movements of the neck. A combination of vertebral subluxation and hyperlordosis makes significant inroads into available spinal canal space (Epstein *et al.*, 1970). Calcification (Kamura *et al.*, 1979) or infolding (Adornato and Glasberg, 1980) of the ligamenta subflava, calcification of the posterior longitudinal ligament (Hanai, Adachi, and Ogasawara, 1977; Murakami, Muroga, and Sobue, 1978; Nagashima, 1972; Tsukimoto, 1960) – predominantly a disease of middle age and elderly Japanese (Table 1) – arthrotic hypertrophy of the apophyseal joints and laminae (Epstein *et al.*, 1978) and Paget's disease may sufficiently compromise the cervical spinal canal to give rise to cord compression. Primary cervical spondylolisthesis is extremely rare, but secondary spondylolisthesis may occur in association with cervical disk degeneration and lead to cord compression (Figs. 3 and 4). Rheumatoid arthritis involving the cervical spine may be complicated by subaxial subluxation leading to myelopathy (Ball and Sharp, 1971; Bland, 1974; Boyle, 1971; Park, O'Neill, and McCall, 1979) and Halla and Fallahi (1981) draw attention to the need for early diagnosis and surgical intervention to prevent progressive and permanent cord damage.

Table 1   Clinical presentation of 26 patients with ossification in the posterior longitudinal ligament. (From Hanai, Adachi, and Ogasawara, 1977. Reproduced by permission of the *Journal of Bone and Joint surgery*

Pain in the neck or arm	26/26	100 per cent.
Numbness and coldness of the arms and legs	25/26	96 per cent.
Weakness or heaviness of the arms or legs	23/26	81 per cent.
Urinary or intestinal symptoms	14/26	54 per cent.

Evidence of spinal cord compression is lacking in some cases and a substantial body of opinion favours a vascular factor in the pathogenesis of cervical myelopathy (Allen, 1952; Barré, 1924; Brain, 1948; Chakravorty, 1969; Clarke, 1955; Mair and Druckman, 1953; Mayfield, 1979; Morton, 1950; Taylor, 1964). Osteophytic compression may involve the anterior spinal artery, but Chakravorty points out that there is often only one anterior radicular artery and less often two or three radicular vessels. Radicular artery involvement may profoundly impair the integrity of the anterior two-thirds of the cord. The radicular artery and intervertebral portion of the vertebral artery may be compressed by spondylotic induced fibrosis of the peridural tissues (Chakravorty, 1969) or the dural sheaths (Frykholm, 1951) which these vessels traverse. However, the natural history of cervical radiculopathy is

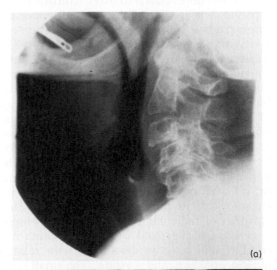

(a)

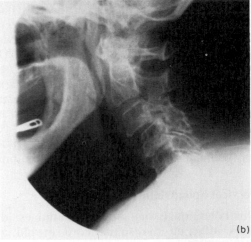

(b)

Figure 4   Cineradiography of patient in Fig. 3. Virtually no movement occurs below C3. Major movement on flexion and extension occurs at the cranio-verebral junction, as can be seen by comparing the distance between the occiput and the arch of C1 at the limits of these movements

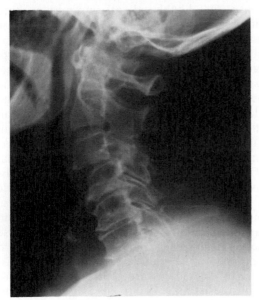

Figure 3   Patient with cervical myelopathy due to cord compression. C3 is subluxed forward on C4 and at this level the canal is markedly narrowed

rarely complicated by myelopathy (Lees and Turner, 1963; Nurick, 1970) and Wilson and coworkers (1969) were unable to produce experimental cervical myelopathy in dogs by interrupting the anterior spinal and radicular arteries. Repeated movement and stretching of the cord over bony spondylotic ridges may have a critical effect on the anterior circulation of the cord (Turnbull, Breig, and Hassler, 1966). Cord ischaemia may result from osteophytic compression of the spinal venous plexus at foraminal level (Brain, Northfield, and Wilkinson, 1952).

Gooding (1974) hypothesized that root sleeve fibrosis associated with degenerative changes in the apophyseal and intervertebral joints might lead to recurrent spasm in the lateral spinal arteries and possible loss of local segmental autoregulation with consequential cervical cord ischaemia.

Symptoms

The divers aetiological possibilities and variable pathological localizations in grey or white matter and anterior, lateral, or posterior columns engender a wide variety of clinical manifestations. A history extending over a year is common and has been reported in over half of a large series of patients referred for neurosurgical opinion (Gonzalez-Feria and Peraita-Peraita, 1975), but it may vary from 2 months to 10 years (Phillips, 1975). Typically the presenting feature of cervical myelopathy is an insidiously developing spastic paraparesis which is rarely complete even in the late stages of the disorder. Complaints are predominantly of heaviness, tiredness, stiffness, or weakness in the legs, particularly on walking, and often considered by the patient to be features of advancing age. Symptoms may be acutely precipitated by trauma or following undue cervical extension during anaesthesia. Radiculopathy uncommonly accompanies myelopathy (Phillips, 1975), but paraesthesiae due to cord involvement occur in over a third of patients. Vibration sense is impaired in 37 per cent. and positional sense in 14 per cent. of cases but it may be difficult to distinguish these findings from age-related changes in the individual elderly patient. Impairment of pain and temperature sensation is less common, although it may occur more often when kyphosis is

marked (Adams and Logue, 1971). There is often a mixture of upper and lower motor neurone features. Nurick (1970) believes that complete sparing of the upper limbs is exceedingly rare in cervical myelopathy. Motor weakness with wasting of the shoulder girdle, deltoid, and triceps and of the small muscles of the hand with clumsiness for fine movement is not infrequent. Muscle tone is increased and, if the anterior horn cells for the corresponding segment are intact, the tendon jerks are usually brisk. The triceps jerk is most commonly diminished or lost due to the frequent involvement of the sixth cervical segment. The radial reflex may be inverted due to the fifth cervical segment involvement (Wilkinson, 1976). The confirmation of the normal jaw jerk in the presence of increased tendon reflexes in the upper limb is of considerable diagnostic value in excluding midbrain lesions. In the lower limbs, the spastic paraparesis is associated with hyperreflexia and extensor plantar responses. The abdominal reflexes are often diminished or absent, but this finding has little diagnostic value in old age. The H-reflex in the upper extremity correlates closely with the degree of spastic paralyses (Okamoto *et al.*, 1980). The paraplegia or less commonly quadriplegia is rarely severe enough to produce the bed-fast or chair-fast state. Rarely ataxia is a presenting feature due to predominant posterior column involvement. Disturbance of micturition is unusual and only found late in the disorder.

Muscle fasciculation is uncommon, particularly in the upper limbs. Generally muscle wasting is minimal in the lower limbs, but rarely it may be marked and associated with overt fasciculation.

Diagnosis

Diagnostic difficulties may result from disorders which share neurological symptoms with cervical spondylosis, or more often in old age, because of the concurrence of symptomatic cervical spondylosis and these other disorders.

Entrapment neuropathy of the median nerve and costoclavicular syndrome may give rise to a combination of sensory disturbance and muscle wasting in the upper limbs; the radial localization of wasting in the hand of the former and the mixture of small muscle wasting in the hand with ulnar forearm sensory impairment in the latter are often the distinguishing features. Motor neurone disease produces more profound muscle wasting and the prominent fasciculation is rare in spondylotic myelopathy. The presence of an exaggerated jaw jerk confirms involvement above the cervical spinal cord.

Radiology

Despite the frequency of radiological evidence of cervical osteoarthrosis in the general population over the age of 55 (Lawrence, de Graaf, and Laine, 1963) careful radiological examination of the cervical spine (McRae, 1960; Pallis, Jones, and Spillane, 1954) demonstrates the positive value of this investigation in the overall assessment of cervical spondylosis.

The neurocentral joints are demonstrated on the antero-posterior radiograph but the lateral radiograph is perhaps the most generally useful routine view. It demonstrates the alignment of the spine and the height of the disks. The apophyseal joint can also be seen on lateral views although the off-lateral view (Paris and Young, 1967) provides more information on the outline of this joint. Anterior and posterior osteophytes can also be detected in this view. The anteroposterior diameter can be measured from the posterior aspect of the vertebral body to the cortical line of the spinous process (Wolf, khilnani, and Malis, 1956). The cord is highly vulnerable if this diameter is 10 mm or less and it is probably under increased risk of compression if the sagittal diameter is from 10 to 13 mm.

Lateral views in flexion and extension may show up a critical reduction in canal dimension and demonstrate subluxation. The intervertebral foramen are visualized by an oblique view.

Positive contrast myelography visualizes infringement of bony and soft tissue on the spinal cord and also normally outlines the nerve root sheaths. Pneumomyelography may provide additional localizing information in cervical spondylotic myelopathy (Crandall and Hanafree, 1964) but in practice few centres use this technique. Cineradiography demonstrates dynamic compressive features. Hinshaw, and co-workers (1979) have shown cervical spinal aniography to be of value in accurately localizing vertical discogenic compressive lesions

preparatory to surgical intervention in younger patients.

Calcification of the posterior longitudinal ligament is well recognized on a plain lateral radiograph and its dimension by axial transverse tomography (Hanai, Adachi and Ogasawara (1977)) but computed tomographic finding correlate more closely with the clinical features of myelopathy (Yamamoto *et al.*, 1979)).

CSF

Queckenstedt's test may be positive when the neck is flexed or extended but normal with the head in a neutral position (Northfield and Osmond-Clark, 1967). The protein level is rarely raised to the levels seen in spinal tumours and the characteristically normal white cell count may be of value in the differential diagnosis (Nurick, 1975).

Treatment (see also Chapter 25.3)

Radiculopathy

Immobilization of the neck is the cardinal ingredient of management where pain predominates. When pain is acute and severe, 2 or 3 days of bed-rest with 10 to 15 lb (4.5 to 7 kg) traction with the neck initially in the position of greatest comfort and, as muscle spasm diminishes, slight flexion of the neck is preferred. For the great majority of patients a light, well-fitting, adjustable collar or a well-moulded plastozote collar worn for about 4 to 6 weeks is the single most useful procedure. Prolonged use of a collar is not to be recommended. Where pain is moderate, simple analgesics suffice, but with more severe discomfort the non-steroidal anti-inflammatory drugs administered for about 2 weeks are effective and side-effects are relatively slight when given for this brief period. Heat via a gel pack or short- or microwave diathermy is helpful. Manipulation with manual traction (Cryiax, 1948) has given dramatic relief in some patients, but several instances of paraplegia are reported following injudicious manipulation. Patients should be advised to avoid undue physical activity involving the upper limbs and the carrying of heavy objects during the acute phase.

When pain has subsided, the muscles of the shoulder girdle and neck should be strengthened by active resisted exercises followed by relaxation exercises.

Surgery. Intractable pain is exceptional and, therefore, only rarely is surgery required where severe presistent pain fails to respond to medical or physical endeavours. Progressive neurological disorder may more often require surgical intervention.

Verbiest (1973) believes that foraminal decompression by the lateral approach with an interbody fusion procedure to maintain stability gives the most appropriate results, but Adams' view (1976) that the surgical method used should be tailored to suit the extent, mechanism, and localization of the radiculopathy expresses current opinion as a broad generalization.

Myelopathy

Effective immobilization of the cervical spine in a well-fitting cervical collar appears to arrest the progress of the disorder in over 40 per cent. of cases (Bradshaw, 1957; Wilkinson, 1976). The benefits of various surgical manoeuvres are to some extent clouded by the uncertain pathogenesis of the myelopathy in any series of cases.

Early reports indicated that laminectomy and anterior interbody fusion gave comparable results but subsequent studies suggested that anterior fusion gave significantly better results than laminectomy (Crandall and Batzdorf, 1966). In a long-term follow-up Gregorius, Estin, and Crandall (1976) found that while the very elderly do not always improve following surgery, those treated by anterior interbody fusion generally progressively improved, whereas after any form of laminectomy disability worsened after an initial period of improvement. However, more recently, Lunsford, Biosionette, and Zorub (1980) were unable to demonstrate that anterior surgery produced long-term results surpassing those attained by conservative treatment (Gorter, 1976; Lees and Turner, 1963; Nurick, 1972).

For the vast majority of elderly patients with cervical myelopathy treatment is symptomatic: 53 per cent. of patients may improve without treatment (Lees and Turner, 1963). The man-

agement of urinary incontinence and prevention of pressure sores may become relevant in a small proportion of cases, but most patients can be reassured that though the condition will fluctuate for a period it will eventually stabilize. The avoidance of unnecessary bed-rest for intercurrent disorders is critical if mobility is to be safeguarded. Where spasticity is marked, slowly increasing doses of dantrolene sodium may be of value.

REFERENCES

Adams, C. (1976). 'Cervical spondylotic radiculopathy and myelopathy', in *Handbook of Clinical Neurology* (Eds. P. J. Vinken and G. W. Bruyn), Vol. 25, Chap. 9, pp. 97–112, North Holland, Amsterdam.

Adams, C. B. T., and Logue, V. (1971). 'Studies in cervical spondylotic myelopathy. II. Observations on the movement and contour of the cervical spine in relation to the neural complications of cervical spondylosis', *Brain,* **94**, 569–586.

Adornato, B. T., and Glasberg, M. R. (1980). 'Diseases of the spinal cord', in *Neurology. Science and Practice of Clinical Medicine (Ed. R. N. Rosenberg), Vol. 5, pp. 392–433, Grune and Stratton, New York.*

Allen K. I. (1952). 'Neuropathies caused by bony spurs in the cervical spine with special reference to surgical treatment', J. Neurol. Neurosurg. Psychiat., **15**, 30–36.

Ball, J., and Sharp, J. (1971). 'Rheumatoid arthritis of the cervical spine', in *Modern Trends in Rheumatology*, Vol. 2, pp. 117–138, Butterworths, London.

Barré, J. (1924). 'Pyramidal lesions and vertebral arthritis', *Médicine, Paris,* **5**, 358–360.

Bechar, M., Front, D., Bornstein, B., and Matz, S. (1971). 'Cervical myelopathy caused by narrowing of the cervical spinal canal. The value of X-ray examination of the cervical spinal column in extension', *Clin. Radiol.,* **22**, 63–68.

Bedford, P. D., Bosanquet, F. D., and Russell, R. W. (1952). 'Degeneration of the spinal cord associated with cervical spondylosis', *Lancet,* **2**, 55–59.

Bland, J. H. (1974). 'Rheumatoid arthritis of the cervical spine', *J. Rheumatol.,* **1**, 319–341.

Boyle, A. C. (1971). 'The rheumatoid neck', *Proc. Roy. Soc. Med.,* **64**, 1161–1165.

Brain, W. R. (1954). 'Cervical spondylosis', *Ann. Int. Med.,* **41**, 439–446.

Brain, W. R. (1963). 'Some unsolved problems of cervical spondylosis', *Br. Med. J.,* **1**, 771–777.

Brain, W. R., Knight, G. C., and Bull, J. W. D. (1948). 'Discussion on rupture of the intervertebral disc in the cervical region', *Proc. Roy. Soc. Med.*, **41**, 509–516.

Brain, W. R., Northfield, R. W. C., and Wilkinson, M. (1952). 'Neurological manifestations of cervical spondylosis', *Brain*, **75**, 187–225.

Breig, A. (1960). *Biomechanics of the Central Nervous System*, Almquist and Wiksell, Stockholm.

Brooker, A. E., and Barter, A. W. (1965). 'Cervical spondylosis. Clinical study with comparative radiology', *Brain*, **88**, 925–936.

Burrows, E. H. (1963). 'The sagittal diameter of the spinal canal in cervical spondylosis', *Clin. Radiol*, **14**, 77–86.

Chakravorty, M. S. (1969). 'Arterial supply of the cervical spinal cord and its relation to the cervical myelopathy in spondylosis', *Ann. Roy. Coll. Surg. Engl.*, **45**, 232–251.

Clarke, E. (1955). 'Cervical myelopathy; common neurological disorder', *Lancet*, **1**, 171–176.

Coventry, M. B., Ghormley, R. K., and Kernohan, J. W. (1945). 'The intervertebral disc: Its microscopic anatomy and pathology. Part 1. Anatomy, development and physiology', *J. Bone Joint Surg.*, **27A**, 105–112.

Crandall, P. H., and Batzdorf, U. (1966). 'Cervical spondylotic myelopathy', *J. Neurosurg.*, **25**, 57–66.

Crandall, P. H., and Hanafee (1964). 'Cervical spondylotic myelopathy studied by air myelography', *Am. J. Roentgenol.*, **94**, 1260–1269.

Cyriax, J. (1948). *Deep Massage and Manipulation Illustrated*, 3rd ed., Baillière Tindall, London.

Epstein, J. A., Carras, R., Epstein, B. S., and Levine, L. S. (1970). 'Myelopathy in cervical spondylosis with vertebral subluxation and hyperlordosis', *J. Neurosurg.*, **32**, 421–426.

Epstein, J. A., Epstein, B. S., Lavine, L. S., Carras, R., and Rosenthal, A. D. (1978). 'Cervical myeloradiculopathy caused by arthrotic hypertrophy of the posterior facets and laminae', *J. Neurosurg.*, **49**, 387–392.

Friedenberg, Z. B., and Miller, W. T. (1963). 'Degenerative disc disease of the cervical spine', *J. Bone Joint Surg.*, **45A**, 1171–1178.

Frykholm, R. J. (1947). 'Deformities of dural pouches and strictures of dural sheaths in cervical region producing nerve-root compression; contribution to etiology and operative treatment of brachial neuralgia', *J. Neurosurg.*, **4**, 403–413.

Frykholm, R. (1951). 'Cervical nerve root compression resulting from disc degeneration and root-sleeve fibrosis. A clinical investigation', *Acta. Chir. Scand.*, (Suppl.), **160**, 1–149.

Gonzalez-Feria, L., and Peraita-Peraita, P. (1975). 'Cervical spondylotic myelopathy', *Clin. Neurol. Neurosurg.*, **78**, 19–33.

Gooding, M. R. (1974). 'Pathogenesis of myelopathy in cervical spondylosis', *Lancet* **II**, 1180–1181.

Gorter, K. (1976). 'Influence of laminectomy on the course of cervical myelopathy', *Acta. Neurochir.*, **33**, 265–281.

Gregorius, F. K., Estrin, T., and Crandall, P. H. (1976). 'Cervical spondylotic radiculopathy and myelopathy. A long term follow up study', *Arch. Neurol.*, **33**, 618–625.

Hadley, L. A. (1956). *The Spine: Anatomico-Radiographic Studies, Development and the Cervical Region*, Charles C. Thomas, Illinois.

Halla, J. T., and Fallahi, S. (1981). 'Cervical discovertebral destruction, subaxial subluxation and myelopathy in a patient with rheumatoid arthritis', *Arth. Rheum.*, **24**, 944–947.

Hanai, K., Adachi, H., and Ogasawara, H. (1977). 'Axial transverse tomography of the cervical spine narrowed by ossification of the posterior longitudinal ligament', *J. Bone Joint Surg.*, **59-B**, 481–484.

Hinshaw, D. B., Yamada, S., Hasso, A. N., and Thompson, J. R. (1979). 'Cervical spinal angiography in midline spondylosis', *Surg. Neurol.*, **12**, 15–19.

Hoff, J. T., and Wilson, C. B. (1976). 'The pathophysiology of cervical spondylotic radiculopathy', in *Clinical Neurasurgery. Proceedings of Congress of Neurological Surgeons, Denver, Colorado*. The Williams and Wilkins Co., Baltimore.

Kahn, E. A. (1947). 'The role of the dentate ligaments in spinal cord compression and the syndrome of lateral sclerosis', *J. Neurosurg.*, **4**, 191–199.

Kamura, K., Nanko, S., Furukawa, T., Mannen, T., and Toyokura, Y. (1979). 'Cervical radicomyelopathy due to calcified ligamenta flava', *Ann. Neurol.*, **5**, 193–195.

Key, C. A. (1838). 'On paraplegia depending on disease of the ligaments of the spine',. *Guy's Hosp. Rep.*, **3**, 17–34.

Keyes, D. C., and Compere, E. L. (1932). 'The normal and pathological physiology of the nucleus pulposus of the intervertebral disc. An anatomical, clinical and experimental study', *J. Bone Joint. Surg.*, **14**, 897–939.

Lawrence, J. S., de Graaff, R., and Laine, V. A. I. (1963). In *The Epidemiology of Chronic Rheumatism* (Eds. J. H. Kellgren, M. R. Jeffrey, and J. Ball), Vol. 1, p. 98, Blackwell Scientific Publications, Oxford.

Lees, F., and Turner, J. W. A. (1963). 'Natural history and prognosis of cervical spondylosis', *Br. Med. J.*, **2**, 1607–1610.

Lowman, R., and Finkelstein, H. (1942). 'Air myelography for demonstration of the cervical spinal cord', *Radiology*, **39**, 700.

Lunsford, L. C., Bissionette, P. A. C., and Zorub,

D. S. (1980). 'Anterior surgery for disc disease. Part 2: Treatment of cervical spondylotic myelopathy in 32 cases', *J. Neurosurg.*, **53**, 12–19.

Macnab, I. (1975). 'Cervical spondylosis', *Clin. Orthop.*, **109**, 69–77.

McRae, D. L. (1960). 'The significance of abnormalities of the cervical spine', *Am. J. Roentgenol.*, **84**, 3–25.

Mair, W. G. P., and Druckman, R. (1953). 'The pathology of spinal cord lesions and their relations to the clinical features in protrusion of the cervical intervertebral discs. (A report of 4 cases)', *Brain*, **76**, 70–91.

Mayfield, F. H. (1979). 'Cervical spondylotic radiculopathy and myelopathy', *Adv. Neurol.*, **22**, 307–321.

Morton, D. E. (1950). 'Anatomical study of human spinal column, with emphasis on degenerative changes in cervical region', *Yale J. Biol. Med.*, **23**, 126–146.

Murakami, N., Muroga, T., and Sobue, I. (1978). 'Cervical myelopathy due to ossification of the posterior longitudinal ligament', *Arch. Neurol.*, **35**, 33–46.

Murone, I., and City, N. (1974). 'The importance of the sagittal diameters of the cervical spinal canal in relation to spondylosis and myelopathy', *J. Bone Joint Surg.*, **56**, 30–36.

Nagashima, C. (1972). 'Cervical myelopathy due to ossification of the posterior longitudinal ligament', *J. Neurosurg.*, **37**, 653–660.

Northfield, D.W.C., and Osmond-Clarke, H. (1967). In *Cervical Sondylosis and other Diseases of the Cervical Spine* (Eds Lord Brain and M. Wilkinson), p. 207, Heinemann, London.

Nurick, S. (1970). 'The natural history of the neurological complications of cervical spondylosis', D. M. Thesis, University of Oxford.

Nurick, S. (1972). 'The pathogenesis of spinal cord disorder associated with cervical spondylosis', *Brain*, **95**, 87–100.

Nurick, S. (1975). 'The cervical spine and paraplegia', in *Modern Trends in Neurology* (Ed. D. Williams), Chap. 9, pp. 167–182, Butterworths, London and Boston.

O'Connell, J. E. A. (1956). 'Cervical spondylosis', *Proc. Roy. Soc. Med.*, **49**, 202–208.

Okamoto, N., Murakami, Y., Baba, I., and Kubo, T. (1980). 'H-reflex of the upper extremities in cervical myelopathy', *Int. Orthop.*, **4**, 193–203.

Pallis, C., Jones, A. M., and Spillane, J. D. (1954). 'Cervical spondylosis; incidence and implications', *Brain*, **77**, 274–289.

Paris, F. A., and Young, A. C. (1967). Quoted from A.C. Young, 'Radiology of the cervical spine', in *Cervical Spondylosis* (Eds. W. R. Brain and M. Wilkinson) pp. 133–196, William Heineman, London.

Park, W. M., O'Neill, M. O., and McCall, I. V. (1979). 'The radiology of rheumatoid involvement of the cervical spine', *Skeletal. Radiol.*, **4**, 1–7.

Payne, E. E., and Spillane, J. D. (1957). 'The cervical spine. An anatomicopathological study in 70 specimens (using a special technique) with particular reference to the problem of cervical spondylosis', *Brain*, **80**, 571–596.

Penning, L. (1968). 'Discussion on vascular disease of the spinal cord', *Proc. Roy. Soc. Med.*, **51**, 547–550.

Phillips, D. G. (1975). 'Upper limb involvement in cervical spondylosis', *J. Neurol. Neurosurg. Psychiat.*, **38**, 386–390.

Püschel, J. (1930). 'Der Wassergehalt normaler und degenerieter Zwischenwirbelscheiben', *Beitr. Path. Anat.*, **84**, 123–130.

Smyth, M. J., and Wright. V. (1958). 'Sciatica and the intervertebral disc. An experimental study', *J. Bone Joint Surg.*, **40A**, 1401–1418.

Stoops, W. L., and King, R. B. (1962). 'Neural complications of cervical spondylosis, their response to laminectomy and foramenotomy', *J. Neurosurg.*, **19**, 986–999.

Taylor, A. R. (1953). 'Mechanism and treatment of spinal cord disorders associated with cervical spondylosis', *Lancet*, **1953**, 717–720.

Taylor, A. R. (1964). 'Vascular factors in the myelopathy associated with cervical spondylosis', *Neurol. (Minneap.)*, **14**, 62–68.

Tsukimoto, H. (1960). 'A case report: Autopsy of syndrome of compression of spinal cord owing to ossification within spinal canal of cervical spine', *Arch. Jap. Chir.*, **29**, 1003–1007.

Turnbull, I. M., Breig, A., and Hassler, O. (1966). 'Blood supply of the cervical spinal cord in man', *J. Neurosurg.*, **24**, 951–965.

Verbiest, H. (1973). 'The management of cervical spondylosis', *Clin. Neurosurg.*, **20**, 262–294.

Waltz, T. A. (1967). 'Physical factors in the production of myelopathy of cervical spondylosis', *Brain*, **90**, 395–404.

Wilkinson, M. (1976). 'The clinical aspects of myelopathy due to cervical spondylosis', *Acta. Neurol. Belg.*, **76**, 276–278.

Wilson, C. B., Bertan, V., Norrell, H. A., Jr, and Hakuda, S. (1969). 'Experimental cervical myelopathy', *Arch. Neurol. Chicago.*, **21**, 571–589.

Wolf, B. S., Khilnani, M., and Malis, L. (1956). 'The sagittal diameter of the bony cervical spinal canal and its significance in cervical spondylosis', *J. Mt Sinai Hosp.*, **23**, 283–292.

Yamamoto, I., Kageyama, N., Nakamura, K., and Takahashi, T. (1979). 'Computed tomography in ossification of the posterior longitudinal ligament in the cervical spine', *Surg. Neurol.*, **12**, 414–418.

16.13

Parkinson's Disease

Marion Hildick-Smith

EPIDEMIOLOGY

Parkinson's disease is one of the commonest neurological conditions both in Britain and America. Its prevalence, i.e. the number of cases per unit population on a given date, has been assessed in several studies (Brewis *et al.*, 1962; Garland, 1952; Kurland, 1958) at rates varying from 59 to 187 per 100,000 population. The higher figure results from Kurland's relatively complete study and is more likely to be the correct one. The prevalence of Parkinson's disease has been shown by several workers (Brewis *et al.*, 1962; Gudmundsson, 1967; Kurland, 1958) to increase with age, being 500 per 100,000 of the population over 50 years old and about 1,000 per 100,000 in those aged 60 or more.

The suggestion that a significant percentage of cases of idiopathic Parkinsonism may show a positive family history of the disease has not subsequently been confirmed (Yahr, 1982).

The cause of idiopathic Parkinsonism is unknown. One theory is that it may be due to a primary deficiency in those cells in the hypothalamus which are responsible for MSH (melanocyte-stimulating hormone) release. An alternative is that the disease may be due to a virus such as the herpes simplex virus or to a heavy metal accumulation.

Symptomatic Parkinsonism can either be 'arteriosclerotic' (Critchley, 1929), postencephalitic (now becoming rarer), or drug-induced. Typical symptoms sometimes occur as part of a generalized neurological condition such as senile dementia of the Alzheimer type.

ALTERATIONS IN NATURAL HISTORY WITH TREATMENT

In the 15 years between 1949 and 1964 there was a noticeable increase in the proportion of elderly people with Parkinsonism attending neurological clinics (Hoehn and Yahr, 1967). Later, as the benefits of levodopa treatment came into effect, Parkinsonian patients survived longer (Rinne, 1978; Sweet and McDowell, 1975). It was shown by Birkmayer *et al.*, (1974) that this increased longevity was of particular importance in the very old. For example, patients aged 80 to 90 might have their death from the condition postponed from 2 to 6 years after its onset.

Parkinson's disease is now largely a disease of the elderly. A recent small epidemiological study (Godwin-Austen *et al.*, 1982) has shown that 58 per cent. of sufferers are aged 70 or over. In this age group women patients outnumber the men, and a significant number are widowed and living alone.

One of the benefits of levodopa therapy has been that patients remain mobile for a longer period, with their disability improved by almost 50 per cent. However, the underlying progress of the disease is masked, not halted. The patient now lives long enough to develop more advanced features of the condition, e.g. dementia or postural instability, which are very difficult to treat.

PATHOLOGY

The exact nature, site, and extent of the lesions

responsible for this condition are still not clear, though the loss of melanin pigment from the substantia nigra has long been known (Greenfield and Bosanquet, 1953). Changes have also been found in the globus pallidus, putamen, and caudate nucleus, and less severe alterations in the locus caeruleus and in the pigmented cells of the dorsal nucleus of the vagus, while the presence of Lewy bodies (neurones with hyaline inclusions) is increasingly recognized as a positive indication of the disease.

There is overlap in pathology between Parkinsonism and Alzheimer's disease (SDAT) (see Chapter 16.5). In one autopsy study by Boller *et al*. (1979) the prevalence of Alzheimer changes (senile plaques and fibrillary tangles) and of dementia among patients with Parkinsonism (33 per cent.) was over 6 times that of an age-matched population (6.1 per cent.). A similar study by Hakim and Mathieson (1979) confirms the higher incidence of dementia in Parkinsonism on clinical and histological data and suggests the simultaneous presence of Alzheimer's disease in an elderly group of patients. Survival in demented Parkinsonian patients is shorter than in those who are mentally clear.

NEUROCHEMISTRY

Our understanding of the neurochemical changes in this condition is far from complete, despite much detailed study. Original work by Ehringer and Hornykiewicz (1960) showed a deficiency of dopamine in the substantia nigra which was later correlated (Bernheimer *et al*., 1965) with the degree of cell loss. Clinical work (Birkmayer and Hornykiewicz, 1961) showed that intravenous injections of levodopa given to 20 Parkinsonian patients led to dramatic short-term improvement in their symptoms. At this stage it appeared that Parkinsonian symptoms were due to a simple deficiency of dopaminergic (inhibitory) mechanisms in the basal ganglia, allowing the cholinergic (excitatory) mechanisms to predominate. Neurochemical balance could be restored by increasing the dopamine or decreasing the acetyl choline effect.

Our present understanding of what happens at the synaptic level is that synthesized dopamine is stored in the presynaptic neurone (see Fig. 1). One messenger which acts across the synapse is adenyl cyclase and this stimulates the D_1 receptors in the postsynaptic neurone. A second set of receptors (D_2) is not linked by adenyl cyclase and these may be more important in Parkinsonism. Later work has suggested that there may be up to 4 dopamine receptors.

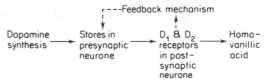

D_1 does depend on adenyl cyclase

D_2 does not depend on adenyl cyclase

Figure 1   Dopaminergic synapse

It has gradually become clear that all manifestations of Parkinsonism cannot be explained by simple dopamine deficiency. The progress of the disease proved not to be halted by dopamine replacement, and the response to levodopa treatment failed after an average period of 5 years. The reasons for this failure are not clear. One theory is the development of hypersensitivity at the receptor site, showing itself as levodopa-induced dyskinesia (Parkes, 1981). Another suggestion is that the brain loses the ability to synthesize and store the dopamine from its precursor amino acids (Marsden, 1980).

Dopamine agonists are substances which act either directly on the postsynaptic dopamine receptors or indirectly via the release of adenyl cyclase. They can theoretically work even when the levodopa response has failed. Bromocriptine has been the most successful of this group and may act as a partial direct agonist, though evidence conflicts about whether it also stimulates adenyl cyclase. Newer drugs such as lisuride may stimulate D_2 receptors, while deprenyl acts by decreasing the degradation of dopamine and hence 'sparing' its effect.

In normal ageing, choline acetyl transferase (CAT) activity in the brain declines (Bowen and Davison, 1978), as may receptor binding of acetyl choline. Theoretically, therefore, one might expect levodopa to be even more effective in the elderly in restoring the dopamine–acetyl choline balance.

Although dopamine deficiency is the most

important and constant biochemical lesion in Parkinson's disease, the roles of other neurotransmitters may have some importance. The concentrations of GABA (gamma amino butyric acid), GAD (glutamic acid decarboxylase), serotonin, noradrenaline, and the peptide angiotensin are also reduced in parts of the Parkinsonian brain, though none of these substances has yet found a useful role in therapy and the changes may be of secondary consequence.

Neurochemically there is much in common between Parkinsonism and dementia (SDAT). Memory seems to be a cholinergic function and in SDAT both acetyl choline and dopamine are decreased. In Parkinsonian patients dementia may perhaps have been precipitated prematurely by dopaminergic or anticholinergic drugs. In Parkinsonism the neurochemical changes are predominantly in the basal ganglia; in SDAT they are generalized. Both conditions may result from damage to the isodendtritic core and its ascending projections (Rossor, 1981). Comparing the neurotransmitter changes in ageing and in dementia Carlsson *et al.* (1980) suggest that dementia shows the characteristics of accelerated ageing.

DIFFICULTIES IN DIAGNOSIS IN THE ELDERLY

Many of the characteristic signs and symptoms of Parkinsonism represent a caricature of the ageing process, for e.g. stooping posture, slow movements, shuffling gait, tremulous hands, and some dulling of the intellect. It is not surprising, therefore, that many patients do not report their problems and the onus is on the doctor to keep this treatable condition in mind, since the diagnosis is often made at the first glance.

Contrariwise, some doctors are too ready to diagnose Parkinsonism as the cause of stuttering gait and indistinct speech following a series of small strokes, and to keep such patients on inappropriate medication (White and Barnes, 1981).

When Parkinsonism begins unilaterally, misdiagnosis as a hemiplegia may prevent appropriate treatment. This is particularly likely to occur if the characteristic tremor is absent. Slowness in writing could be due to Parkinsonism, or to arthritic hands. Parkinsonism affect-

ing primarily the autonomic functions, with flushing, heat intolerance, seborrhoea, may make the patient appear hyperthyroid – while a slow, withdrawn patient may look hypothyroid or depressed.

Problems with swallowing may often occur late in the disease, accompanied by weight loss, suggesting a diagnosis of carcinoma of the cesophagus. The patient may recover well when the abnormal contractions of the oesophagus (secondary to Parkinsonian changes in the vagal nucleus) respond to dopamine treatment.

CLINICAL FEATURES

Many elderly patients, on the other hand, will present with the classical signs and symptoms described by James Parkinson – rhythmic tremor, flexed posture, monotonous voice, and tendency to falls. Similarly many will have the muscular rigidity (cogwheel or leadpipe in type) and the immobile mask-like face which is now regarded as typical but which did not feature in the original description. Characteristic problems which arise from Parkinsonian bradykinesia include difficulty in doing up buttons, cutting up meat, or signing a pension book. Rigidity in trunk muscles may lead to inability to roll over in bed. Difficulty in initiating movements leads to problems getting out of a chair or bed, while characteristic 'freezing' episodes may occur on encountering an obstacle (such as a doorway or the edge of a carpet). It is worth while asking leading questions, if necessary, to elicit many of these characteristic disabilities.

CONDITIONS AFFECTING TREATMENT

There are special problems in treating Parkinson's disease in an elderly patient. In addition to the usual caution with dosage (because of altered pharmacokinetics in the old), attention to other conditions needing concurrent treatment, to increased likelihood of adverse drug reactions, and problems of drug compliance are critically important.

Prostatism or glaucoma will affect the choice of treatment, as anticholinergic drugs may be contraindicated. Postural hypotension may worsen on treatment, especially if the patient is suffering from the Shy–Drager syndrome.

Recent myocardial infarction or arrhythmia is less often a reason for discontinuing anti-Parkinsonian drugs now that combined preparations like Sinemet and Madopar are available. Peptic ulcer sufferers need to take care with these drugs as occasional bleeding has occurred. Malignant malanoma may be activated by these drugs.

It is important to note prolonged or recent medication with phenothiazines like chlorpromazine or prochlorperazine, and butyrophenones such as haloperidol.

These drugs can cause Parkinsonism by blocking the postsynaptic neurones. Dopamine is then ineffective and treatment should be by stopping the offending drug and giving an anticholinergic agent. It is now suggested that psychiatrists who have attempted to solve this problem by giving long-term anticholinergic treatment along with the major tranquillizers may have been doing their patients a disservice (Franz, 1975). The anticholinergics are effective only in controlling, not in preventing, the Parkinsonian symptoms, and meanwhile they may be masking the onset of an irreversible drug-induced tardive dyskinesia.

Probably the most important condition affecting treatment is long-term mental confusion, and the neurochemical and pathological overlap between Parkinsonism and SDAT is confirmed in clinical studies (Gottfries *et al.*, 1980., Martin *et al.*, 1973; Parkes *et al.*, 1974 Pearce, 1974). Controversy has existed for 100 years (Ball, 1882) about whether the intellect is affected in Parkinson's disease. The incidence of dementia in recent surveys of Parkinsonian patients has varied from 11 to 53 per cent. (Celesia and Wannamaker, 1972; Mindham, Marsden, and Parkes, 1976; Pollock and Hornabrook, 1966), and in a carefully age-matched study Loranger *et al.* (1972) found 36 per cent. of elderly Parkinsonian patients were intellectually impaired.

There is equal controversy over whether preexisting dementia should preclude levodopa treatment for Parkinsonism (Broe and Caird, 1973; Drachman and Stahl, 1975; Sacks *et al.*, 1970). Most physicians treating the elderly would now attempt treatment with slowly increasing doses of levodopa (Hildick-Smith, 1976b; Sutcliffe, 1973; Vignalou and Beck, 1973) now using a combined preparation. Confusional side-effects are twice as likely in the elderly so care with dosage is important. As confusion is a central side-effect, not a peripheral one, addition of a dopa decarboxylase inhibitor does not reduce its incidence.

The recent successful trial of levodopa in a small number of demented patients without Parkinsonism (Lewis, Ballinger, and Presly, 1978) offers further evidence of the overlap between the two conditions.

EXAMINATION BEFORE TREATMENT

The most important single examination before treatment is to assess the patient's mental state by a questionnaire such as the one used by Hodkinson (1972). It is important to introduce the questions tactfully and to ensure that the patient is not deaf, dysphasic, unduly depressed, nor oversedated, nor confused by drug therapy. These factors can influence the mental score, as may an intercurrent illness, infection, or other cause of a toxic confusional state. It is vital, therefore, to find out from relatives whether the present confusion is of short-term or has insidiously progressed over several years, and to exclude other causes of dementia.

In some patients it is difficult to separate the signs and symptoms of Parkinsonism from those of cerebrovascular disease/dementia. Signs of pyramidal tract damage, e.g. supranuclear palsy, or of frontal lobe involvement, e.g. primitive reflex responses, provide diagnostic clues. In other patients the Parkinsonian picture may be the prelude to a more relentless neurological condition. Examples of this are (a) nigrostriatal degeneration (which cannot be confidently diagnosed in life); (b) Steele-Richardson syndrome, where there is progressive palsy of conjugate ocular movements; (c) olivoponto cerebellar degeneration where cerebellar signs may later appear; and (d) Shy–Drager syndrome where autonomic failure leading to profound orthostatic hypotension may be a prominent feature.

In any chronically disabling condition it is important to have some objective measurements of disability before treatment.

Bradykinesia may be measured by timing the patient signing his name and address. The patient can also be timed walking a defined distance (e.g. 15 to 20 feet), noting length of step, armswing, posture, and any hesitation or imbalance on turning or negotiating an obstacle.

Functional assessments of ability to get in and out of bed, roll over in bed, do up buttons, and cut up meat give an overall impression of the patient's independence before and during treatment.

TREATMENT OF NON-DISABLING PARKINSONISM

A small proportion of patients have benign Parkinsonism (Hoehn and Yahr, 1967) and are not severely disabled for 20 years or more. Others who have the more usual prognosis of slowly increasing disability and death within 5 to 10 years first present at a stage where they have recognizably Parkinsonian facies or tremor but are not yet disabled by this or by any bradykinesia. For these patients modern teaching would be to keep levodopa treatment until it is really needed and manage this stage of the disease by other means. It is seldom reasonable, however, to delay starting treatment in an elderly patient.

The importance of regular walking and exercise has long been recognized in Parkinsonism, as has the fact that bed-rest for any intercurrent illness makes it more difficult for the patient to regain his mobility. Therapists have devised regimes of leg, trunk, and shoulder exercises (Davis, 1977), but controlled trials of physiotherapy are recent (Franklyn *et al.*, 1981; Gibberd *et al.*, 1981), partly because of the many difficulties inherent in standardizing and evaluating treatment. Equipment such as the polarized light goniometer and the video cassette recorder has enabled more precise assessment of the underlying gait disturbance (Flewitt, Capildeo and Rose, 1981) and directed attention to the possibility of improving 'heel-strike' by practice and by alteration to the shoes. Many patients will need walking aids as their disease progresses, and a suitable one is the Delta aid shown in the photograph (Fig. 2).

Measures like raising the height of a chair and bed, and of fastening clothing with zips or velcro (instead of buttons) may help to maintain the patient's independence. Beattie and Caird (1980) found that elderly Parkinsonian patients living at home were underprovided with equipment for daily living, aids for bath-

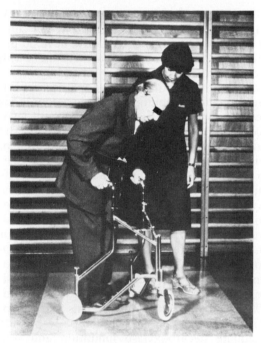

Figure 2   Elderly patient using a Delta aid

ing and feeding being particularly necessary in the later disabled stages.

First studies by speech therapists suggested that their efforts may be of limited avail in established Parkinson's disease (Perry and Das, 1981), but a later study was more promising (Scott and Caird, 1981).

The antihistaminic agent orphenadrine (disipal) may be useful in a dose of 100 to 300 mg a day, as it reduces rigidity and has a mildly alerting and euphoriant action. Occasionally a beta-blocker such as propranolol (inderal) may help in Parkinsonian tremor.

The Parkinson's Disease Society produces booklets (Godwin-Austen, 1971; *Parkinsons Disease Day to Day*, Godwin-Austen and Hildick-Smith 1983 *Parkinson's Disease – a General Practitioners' Guide*) which are informative and up-to-date, and meetings of local branches of the Society can be supportive and combat the social isolation felt by many patients and their families (Singer, 1973).

TREATMENT OF DISABLING PARKINSON'S DISEASE

Levodopa is the treatment of choice once there is significant disability (Caird and Williamson,

1978; Hildick-Smith, 1976a; Sutcliffe, 1973; Vignalou and Beck, 1973). Up to 85 per cent. of patients, including the elderly, have 50 per cent. objective improvement on treatment with a combined preparation (Fig 3a and b).

Sinemet (a mixture of the dopa decarboxylase inhibitor carbidopa with levodopa) has been shown to be superior to the pure levodopa (Marsden, Parkes, and Rees, 1973). The carbidopa blocks the wasteful metabolism of levodopa outside the brain, enabling dosages to be reduced four-to fivefold while side-effects on heart and gut are reduced. Sinemet is now available as sinemet 275 (carbidopa 25, levodopa 250 mg), sinemet 110 (10:100), and sinemet plus (25:100). An average daily total for an elderly patient might be 500 mg of levodopa. Those taking less than 750 mg a day of sinemet 110 might benefit by changing to sinemet plus, starting at 1 tablet t.d.s. (Hoehn, 1980; Nibbelink *et al.*, 1981), This latter preparation contains enough carbidopa to provide adequate decarboxylase inhibition and stop persistent nausea.

Madopar (a mixture of the dopa decarboxylase inhibitor benserazide with four parts of levodopa) is roughly equivalent to sinemet in effectiveness (Barbeau *et al.*, 1972; Diamond, Markham, and Treciokas, 1978; Korten *et al.*, 1975). It is available as madopar 250 (benserazide 50, levodopa 200 mgm), 125 (25:100), or 62.5 (12.5 : 50) and has produced less nausea during initial treatment (Rinne and Molsa, 1979).

When levodopa and the combined preparations were first introduced the tendency was to increase doses to the near-dyskinetic levels which produced maximum short-term benefit. Recent studies suggest that the levodopa benefit period (normally 4–5 years or so) depends partly on the advance of the disease process and partly on the total accumulated levodopa dosage, and that drug dosage should be as low as possible in the patient's long-term interest. Timing of the dosage can be altered – e.g. patients may take one of their tablets before physical or social effort. Fatigue was troublesome in 47 per cent. of patients who replied to the Parkinson's Disease Society questionnaire (Oxtoby, 1981). Some sufferers wake refreshed after sleep and can wait an hour or so before medication. More commonly the tablets

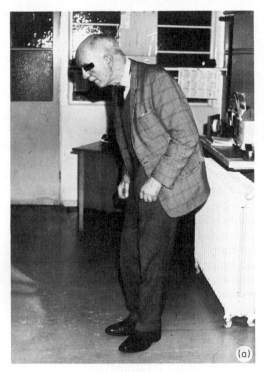 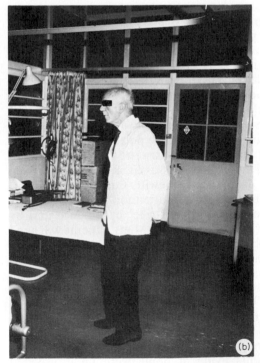

Figure 3   Elderly patient (a) before and (b) after treatment with sinemt

are needed on waking when the serum level of levodopa is low.

Depression is a frequent accompaniment to Parkinsonism (Mindham, Marsden, and Parkes, 1976) and needs careful treatment. A tetracyclic preparation such as mianserin should be chosen if cardiac and anticholinergic side-effects are to be avoided. Sometimes a tricyclic such as amitryptiline may be chosen for its anticholinergic action if nocturnal incontinence is a problem. The antidepressant nomifensine should theoretically be beneficial because it acts to inhibit dopamine uptake; however, the drug seems to have no signficant effect in Parkinsonism, though it might be useful for concurrent depression.

DECOMPENSATED PARKINSONISM

After some years the response to levodopa begins to fade (Hunter *et al.*, 1973; Shaw, Lees, and Stern, 1980). Addition of an anticholinergic may be helpful in younger patients (Hughes *et al.*, 1971) but is liable to cause confusion in elderly ones (Caird and Williamson, 1978). If response fades after 2½ to 3 hours (end-of-dose deterioration), the patient can try to alter timings within the same daily total or can risk the dyskinesias which may occur when the total daily intake is increased.

'On–off' episodes, sudden unpredictable variations in response to levodopa (Marsden and Parkes, 1976) are distressing and occur in up to 50 per cent. of patients after 6 years. This side-effect seems to be less common in the elderly, possibly because they receive lower levodopa dosages. Alternatively the old may have a relatively benign form of the condition or may die before reaching this stage of the disease.

The present place of the dopamine agonist bromocriptine is in this stage of levodopa failure (Calne *et al.*, 1978), as its longer half-life smooths out the uneven levodopa response and enables the patient to regain benefit on a lower, less toxic, levodopa dose for up to 2 years. Starting with a dose of 1.25 mg per day, the average dose needed by elderly patients is 10 to 20 mg. The first daily dose of bromocriptine is usually given with the morning Sinemet or Madopar since bromocriptine takes about 2 hours to act.

The possible role of bromocriptine as first treatment for disabling Parkinsonism continues under investigation at maximally tolerated (Lees and Stern, 1981) and low doses (Teychenne *et al.*, 1981). The drug appears only rarely to cause dyskinesias, but is less potent than levodopa. It may take 15 to 22 weeks (Teychenne *et al.*, 1981) to achieve 39 per cent. overall improvement in the patient's condition, but when it fails after 2 years levodopa is ineffective (Lees and Stern, 1981). Low dose régimes (starting from 1.25 mg once or twice a day, increasing by weekly increments to 10 to 20 mg a day) suit elderly patients and give rise to less confusion, nausea, and hallucinations.

Bromocriptine is only partially successful, but is the best of the long-acting dopamine agonists presently available, as many of those tried have shown unacceptable toxicity. Pergolide in doses of 2 to 5 mg a day can enable the levodopa dosage to be reduced (Liebermann *et al.*, 1979). Lisuride in doses of 0.6 to 4.8 mg daily (given with an antiemetic such as domperidone) may be able to prolong benefit for some months after bromocriptine has been abandoned (Schachter *et al.*, 1979). Deprenyl enabled levodopa dosages to be reduced (Birkmayer, 1978) but benefit was not maintained after a few months. Supplies are now more readily available and this drug should prove valuable in levodopa failure.

An alternative approach to diminishing control is a drug 'holiday' (Sweet *et al.*, 1972). By withdrawing all or part of the levodopa treatment for a week or so in hospital it was hoped that the patient's nigrostriatal neurones would regain sensitivity to the drug. While some workers report regained benefit on levodopa for 6 to 12 months (Weiner *et al.*, 1981), others confirmed the dangers of immobility during the withdrawal period (Direnfeld *et al.*, 1980) and the concept seems unlikely to be of benefit to the old.

TERMINAL PARKINSONISM

The introduction of levodopa treatment has reduced the excess mortality of Parkinson's disease from 2.9 to 1.85 times normal (Hoehn and Yahr, 1967; Rinne, 1978). The patients' last months of life, when all significant drug benefit has failed, continue to demand every care and skill from doctors, nurses, and relatives, so that death can be as peaceful and dignified as possible. Confusional symptoms or agitation due to complex and multiple drug therapy may be helped by removing all but the most essential medication. While overinvestigation must be avoided, it is essential to treat any condition causing the patient distress. Many patients and families will welcome the help of their own clergymen or of the hospital chaplain.

CONCLUSION

Elderly patients have shared with others the benefits of treatment with combined levodopa preparations for Parkinsonism, and may particularly benefit from the present tendency towards low-dosage regimes. Further understanding of the mechanism of levodopa failure and experimentation with newer drugs and régimes should give additional benefits in the next decade or two.

REFERENCES

Ball, B. (1882). 'De l'insanité dans la paralysie agitante', *Encéphale*, **2**, 22–32.

Barbeau, A., Mars, H., Botez, M. I., and Joubert, M. (1972). 'Levodopa combined with peripheral decarboxylase inhibition in Parkinson's disease', *Canad. Med. Assoc. J.*, **106**, 1169–1174.

Beattie, A., and Caird, F. I. (1980). 'The occupational therapist and the patient with Parkinson's disease', *Br. Med. J.*, **280**, 1354–1355.

Bernheimer, H., Birkmayer, W., Hornykiewicz, O., Jellinger, K., and Seitelberger, F. (1965). 'Zur Differenzierung des Parkinsön-Syndroms'. in *Proceedings of 8th International Congress of Neurology*, pp. 145–148, Medical Academy, Vienna.

Birkmayer, W. (1978). 'Longterm treatment with L-deprenyl', *J. Neural. Trans.*, **43**, 239–244.

Birkmayer, W., and Hornykiewicz, O. (1961). 'Der L 3, 4 dioxyphenylalanin (=DOPA) Effekt bei der Parkinsonakinese', *Wien. Klin. Wochenschr.*, **73**, 787–788.

Birkmayer, W., Ambrozi, L., Neumayer, E., and Riederer, P. (1974). 'Longevity in Parkinson's disease treated with L-dopa', *Clin. Neurol. Neurosurg.*, **1**, 15–19.

Boller, F., Mizutani, T., Roessman, U., and Gambetti, P. (1979). 'Parkinson's disease, dementia and Alzheimer disease: clinicopathological correlations', *Ann. Neurol.*, **7**, 329–335.

Bowen, D. M., and Davison, A. N. (1978). 'Biochemical changes in the normal ageing brain', in *Recent Advances in Geriatric Medicine* (Ed. B.

Isaacs), pp. 54–59, Churchill Livingstone, Edinburgh, London, and New York.

Brewis, M., Poskanzer, D. C., Rolland, C., and Miller, H. (1962). 'Neurological disease in an English city', *Acta. Neurol. Scand.*, **42**, (Suppl. 24), 31–36.

Broe, G. A., and Caird, F.I. (1973). 'Levodopa for Parkinsonism in elderly and demented patients', *Med. J. Aust.*, **1**, 630–635.

Caird, F. I., and Williamson, J. (1978). 'Drugs for Parkinson's disease', *Lancet*, **1**, 986.

Calne, D. B., Plotkin, C., Williams, A. C., Nutt. J. G., Neophytides, A., and Teychenne, P. F. (1978). 'Longterm treatment of Parkinsonism with bromocriptine', *Lancet*, **1**, 735–738.

Carlsson, A., Gottfries, C-G., Svennerholm, L., Adolfsson, R., Oreland, L., Winblad, B., and Aquilonius, S-M. (1980). 'Neurotransmitters in human brain analysed postmortem', in *Parkinson's Disease Current Progress, Problems and Management* (Eds U.K. Rinne, M. Klinger, and G. Stamm), pp. 121–133, Elsevier North Holland Biomedical Press, Amsterdam and New York.

Celesia, G. C., and Wannamaker, W. M. (1972). 'Psychiatric disturbances in Parkinson's disease', *Dis. Nerv. Syst.*, **33**, 577–583.

Critchley, M. (1929). 'Arteriosclerotic Parkinsonism', *Brain*, **52**, 23–83.

Davis, J. C. (1977). 'Team management of Parkinson's disease', *Am. J. Occup. Ther.*, **31**, 300–308.

Diamond, S. G., Markham, C. H., and Treciokas, L. J. (1978). 'A double blind comparison of levodopa, madopar and sinement in Parkinson's disease', *Ann. Neurol.*, **3**, 267–272.

Direnfeld, L. K., Feldman, R. G., Alexander, M. P., and Kelly-Hayes, M. (1980). 'Is L-dopa holiday useful?, *Neurol.*, **30**, 785–788.

Drachman, D. A., and Stahl, S. (1975). 'Extrapyramidal dementia and levodopa', *Lancet*, **1**, 809.

Ehringer, H., and Hornykiewicz, O. (1960). 'Verteilung von Noradrenalin und Dopamin im Gehirn des Menschen und ihr Verhalten bei Erkrankungen des extrapyramidalen Systems', *Klin. Wochenschr.*, **38**, 1236–1239.

Flewitt, B., Capildeo, R., and Rose, F. C. (1981). 'Physiotherapy and assessment in Parkinson's disease using the polarized light goniometer', in *Research Progress in Parkinson's Disease* (Eds F. C. Rose and R. Capildeo), pp. 404–413, Pitman, London.

Franklyn, S., Kohout, L. J., Stern, G. M., and Dunning, M. (1981). 'Physiotherapy in Parkinson's disease', in *Research Progress in Parkinson's Disease* (Eds F. C. Rose and R. Capildeo), pp 397–400 Pitman London.

Franz, D. N. (1975). 'Drugs for Parkinson's disease: centrally acting muscle relaxants', in *The Pharmacological Basis of Therapeutics* (Eds L. J.

Goodman and A. Gilman), pp. 227–244, Macmillan, New York.

Garland, H. G. (1952). 'Parkinsonism', *Br. Med. J.*, **1**, 153–155.

Gibberd, F. B., Page, N. G. R., Spencer, K. M., Kinnear, E., and Hawksworth, J. B. (1981). 'Controlled trial of physiotherapy and occupational therapy for Parkinson's disease', *Br. Med. J.*, **282**, 1196.

Godwin-Austen, R. B. (1971). *Parkinson's Disease* and *Parkinson's Disease Day to Day*. Booklets for patients and their families, published by the Parkinson's Disease Society, 81 Queen's Road, London.

Godwin-Austin, R. B., and Hildick-Smith, M. (1983) Parkinson's Disease – a general practitioners' guide. Franklin Scientific Products. London.

Godwin-Austen, R. B., Lee, P. N., Marmot, M. G., and Stern, G. M. (1982). 'Smoking and Parkinson's disease', *J. Neurol., Neurosurg., and Psychiat.*, **45**, 577–581.

Gottfries, C. G., Adolfsson, R., Aquilonius, S. M., Carlsson, A., Oreland, L., Svennerholm, L., and Winblad, B. (1980). 'Parkinsonism and dementia disorders of Alzheimer type: similarities and differences', in *Parkinson's Disease. Current Progress; Problems and Management*. (Eds U. K. Rinne, M. Klinger, and G. P. Stamm), pp. 197–208, Elsevier North Holland Biomedical Press, Amsterdam and New York.

Greenfield, J. G., and Bosanquet, F. D. (1953). 'The brainstem lesions in Parkinsonism', *J. Neurol. Neurosurg. Psychiat.*, **16**, 213–226.

Gudmundsson, K. R. (1967). 'A clinical survey of Parkinsonism in Iceland', *Acta. Neurol. Scand.*, **43** (Suppl. 33), 1–61.

Hakim, A. M., and Mathieson, G. (1979). 'Dementia in Parkinson's disease: a neuropathologic study', *Neurology*, **29**, 1209–1214.

Hildick-Smith, M. (1976a). 'Alternatives to levodopa', *Br. Med. J.*, **1**, 1406.

Hildick-Smith, M. (1976b). 'Assessing dementia in the older Parkinsonian patient', *Mod. Geriatr.*, **6**, 33–39.

Hodkinson, H. M. (1972). 'Evaluation of a mental test score for assessment of mental impairment in the elderly', *Age Ageing*, **1**, 233–238.

Hoehn, M. M. (1980). 'Increased dosage of carbidopa in patients with Parkinson's disease receiving low doses of levodopa', *Arch. Neurol.*, **37**, 146–149.

Hoehn, M. M., and Yahr, M. D. (1967). 'Parkinsonism: onset, progression and mortality', *Neurology.*, **17**, 427–442.

Hughes, R. C., Polgar, J. G., Weightman, D., and Walton, J. N. (1971). 'L-dopa in Parkinsonism – the effects of withdrawal of anticholinergic drugs',

Br. Med. J., **2**, 487–491.

Hunter, K. R., Laurence, D. R., Shaw, K. M., and Stern, G. M. (1973). 'Sustained levodopa therapy in Parkinsonism', *Lancet*, **2**, 929–931.

Korten, J. J., Keyser, A., Joosten, M. G., and Gabreels, F. J. M. (1975). 'Madopar vs. Sinemet', *Eur. Neurol.*, **13**, 65–71.

Kurland, L. T. (1958). 'Pathogenesis and treatment of Parkinsonism' (Ed. W. S. Fields), pp. 5–49, Charles C. Thomas, Springfield, Ill.

Lees, A. J., and Stern, G. M. (1981). 'Sustained bromocriptine therapy in previously untreated patients with Parkinson's disease', *Research and Clinical Forums*, **3**, 29–32.

Lewis, C., Ballinger, B. R., and Presly, A. S. (1978). 'Trial of levodopa in senile dementia', *Br. Med. J.*, **1**, 550.

Liebermann, A. N., Liebowitz, M., Neophytides, A., Kupersmith, M., Mehl, S., Kleinberg, D., Serby, M., and Goldstein, M. (1979). 'Pergolide and lisuride for Parkinson's disease', *Lancet*, **2**, 1129–1130.

Loranger, A. W., Goodell, H., McDowell, F. H., Lee, J. E., and Sweet, R. D. (1972). 'Intellectual impairment in Parkinson's syndrome', *Brain*, **95**, 405–412.

Marsden, C. D. (1980). 'On–off' phenomena in Parkinson's Disease', in *Parkinson's Disease, Current Progress, Problems and Management* (Eds U. K. Rinne, M. Klinger, and G. Stamm), pp. 241–254, Elsevier North Holland Biomedical Press, Amsterdam and New York.

Marsden, C. D., and Parkes, J. D. (1976). 'On–off' effects in patients with Parkinson's disease on chronic levodopa therapy', *Lancet*, **1**, 292–296.

Marsden, C. D., Parkes, J. D., and Rees, J. E. (1973). 'A year's comparison of treatment of patients with Parkinson's disease with levodopa combined with carbidopa versus treatment with levodopa alone', *Lancet*, **2**, 1459–1462.

Martin, W. E., Loewenson, R. B., Resch, J. A., and Baker, A. B. (1973). 'Parkinson's disease. Clinical analysis of 100 patients', *Neurology*, **23**, 783–790.

Mindham, R. H. S., Marsden, C. D., and Parkes, J. D. (1976). 'Psychiatric symptoms during L-dopa therapy for Parkinson's disease and their relationship to physical disability'. *Psychol. Med.*, **6**, 23–33.

Nibbelink, D. W., Bauer, R., Hoehn, M., Muenter, M., Stellar, S., and Berman, R. (1981). 'Sinemet 25: 100' in *Research Progress in Parkinson's Disease* (Eds F. C. Rose and R. Capildeo), pp. 226–232, Pitman, London.

Oxtoby, M. (1981). *Survey of Patients in contact with the Parkinson's Disease Society*, Parkinson's Disease Society, London.

Parkes, J. D. (1981). 'Dyskinesias', in *Research*

Progress in Parkinson's Disease (Eds F. C. Rose and R. Capildeo), pp. 254–264, Pitman, London.

Parkes, J. D., Marsden, C. D., Rees, J. E., Curzon, G., Katamaneni, B. D., Knill-Jones, R., Akbar, A., Das, S., and Kataria, M. (1974). 'Parkinson's disease, cerebral arteriosclerosis and senile dementia', *Q. J. Med.*, **43**, 49–61.

Parkinson's Disease Day by Day. A further booklet published by the Parkinson's Disease Society, London.

Pearce, J. (1974). 'Mental changes in Parkinsonism', *Br. Med. J.*, **2**, 445.

Perry, A. R., and Das, P. K. (1981). 'Speech assessment of patients with Parkinson's disease', in *Research Progress in Parkinson's disease* (Eds F. C. Rose and R. Capildeo), pp. 373–383, Pitman Medical, London.

Pollock, M., and Hornabrook, R. W. (1966). 'The prevalence, natural history and dementia of Parkinsonism', *Brain*, **89**, 429–448.

Rinne, U. K. (1978). 'Recent advances in research on Parkinsonism', *Acta. Neurol. Scand.*, **67** (Suppl. 57), 77–113.

Rinne, U. K., and Molsa, P. (1979). 'Levodopa with benserazide or carbidopa in Parkinson's disease', *Neurology*, **29**, 1584–1589.

Rossor, M- N. (1981). 'Parkinson's disease and Alzeheimer's disease as disorders of the isodendritic core', *Bri. Med. J.*, **283**, 1588–1590.

Sacks, O. W., Messeloff, C., Schartz, W., Goldfarb, A., and Kohl, M. (1970). 'Effects of L-dopa in patients with dementia', *Lancet*, **1**, 1231.

Schachter, M., Blackstock, J., Dick, J. P. R., George, R. J. D., Marsden, C. D., and Parkes, J. D. (1979). 'Lisuride in Parkinson's disease', *Lancet*, **2**, 1129.

Scott, S., and Caird, F. I. (1981). 'Speed therapy for patients with Parkinson's disease', *Bri. Med. J.*, **280**, 1354–1355

Shaw, K. M., Lees, A. J., and Stern, G. M. (1980). 'The impact of treatment with levodopa on Parkinson's disease', *Q. J. Med.*, **49**, (195), 283–293.

Singer, E. (1973). 'Social costs of Parkinson's disease', *J. Chron. Dis.*, **26**, 243–254.

Sutcliffe, R. L. G. (1973). 'L-dopa therapy in elderly patients with Parkinsonism', *Age Ageing.*, **2**, 34–38.

Sweet, R. D., Lee, J. E., Spiegel, H. E., McDowell, F. (1972). 'Enhanced response to low doses of levodopa after withdrawal from chronic treatment', *Neurology.*, **22**, 520–525.

Sweet, R. D., and McDowell, F. H. (1975). 'Five years' treatment of Parkinson's disease with levodopa: therapeutic results and survival of 100 patients', *Ann. Intern. Med.*, **83**, 456–463.

Teychenne, P. F. Bergsrud, D., Racy, A., and Vern, B. (1981). 'Lowdose bromocriptine therapy in Parkinson's disease', *Research and Clinical Forums*, **3**, 37–47.

Vignalou, J., and Beck, H. (1973). 'La L-dopa chez 122 Parkinsoniens de plus de 70 ans', *Gerontol. Clin.*, **15**, 50–64.

Weiner, W. J., Koller, W. C., Perlik, S., Nausieda, P. A., and Klawans, H. L. (1981). 'The role of transient levodopa withdrawal (drug holiday) in the management of Parkinson's disease', in *Research Progress in Parkinson's Disease* (Eds F. C. Rose and R. Capildeo), pp. 275–281, Pitman Medical, London.

White, N. J., and Barnes, T. R. E. (1981). 'Senile Parkinsonism, a survey of current treatment', *Age Ageing*, **10**, 81–86.

Yahr, M. (1982). *In Parkinsonism Recent Advances*, p. 4, International Medicine Supplement 3, Franklyn Scientific Publications, London.

16.14

The Autonomic Nervous System

A. N. Exton-Smith

A salient characteristic of ageing is impairment of homeostasis leading to a diminished ability of the organism to react to environmental and other forms of stress. Even in extreme old age homeostasis may still be maintained under resting conditions, but when the organism is subjected to stress disturbances of physiological balance may readily occur and the time for recovery after cessation of the displacing stimulus is usually prolonged in the older person. Types of stress which require complex physiological adjustments are extremes of environmental temperature, physical exercise, hypoxia, trauma, and disease and with advancing age there is a progressive deterioration in the ability to adapt to these. Both the neural and endocrine systems play a major role in regulating the reactions of the organism to changes in the environment and it seems likely that impairment in function of the autonomic nervous system makes a major contribution to the decline in efficiency of homeostatic regulation. It has long been known that many functions within the central nervous system show a deterioration with advancing age, but only recently has it been recognized that an age-related decline in physiological performance also occurs in the autonomic nervous system.

In the elderly many of the manifestations of autonomic dysfunction arise from diffuse multisystem defects and they include postural hypotension, impaired thermoregulatory capacity, sweating abnormalities, decreased lachrymation, pupillary abnormalities, gastrointestinal disorders, and disturbances of bladder function. The most important clinical syndromes are postural hypotension and hypothermia. The increasing prevalence of these conditions with advancing age can be attributed to the effects of physiological impairment of function in the autonomic nervous system and to its involvement in a number of pathological processes which are common in old age.

PHYSIOLOGY OF AUTONOMIC CONTROL

The chemical transmitters in the nervous system include acetylcholine, 5-hydroxytryptamine (5HT), dopamine, adrenaline, and noradrenaline. The principal transmitter at the autonomic ganglia is acetylcholine and its action at this site is not paralysed by atropine. Ganglion blocking agents such as hexamethonium and mecamylamine are believed to act by competing for acetylcholine and preventing it from reaching the receptor. Since the parasympathetic ganglia are also cholinergic the bulbosacral outflow is affected by ganglion blocking drugs. Acetylcholine is the neurotransmitter at the postganglionic nerve endings of the parasympathetic system, and some sympathetic nerve endings, namely the sudomotor fibres supplying the eccrine glands which form the majority of the sweat glands, and at some vasodilator fibres to the muscles. Atropine paralyses these actions of acetylcholine. Noradrenaline is the principal transmitter substance for the postganglionic sympathetic nervous system. The adrenoreceptors are of two types which are differentiated on the basis of the relative potencies of adrenergic agents. Noradrenaline predominantly stimulates alpha receptors; its effects include vasoconstriction, intestinal relaxation, and pupillary dilation. These actions are blocked by phentolamine and phenoxybenzamine. The beta receptors are stimulated by isoprenaline and both alpha and beta receptors are stimulated by adrenaline. The main effects of beta receptor stimulation are vasodilation, especially in the muscles, and an increase in the rate and force of cardiac contraction with a tendency to develop arrhythmias and bronchial dilatation. Propranolol and other beta-blocking agents inhibit these actions.

It is now believed that dopamine is an important neurotransmitter in the autonomic nervous system as well as in the central nervous system since it has been found in significant amounts in the autonomic ganglia and nerves (Thorner, 1975). Dopamine receptors are stimulated by dopaminergic agonists including apomorphine and bromocriptine and they are blocked by dopaminergic antagonists such as phenothiazines and metoclopramide and to a lesser extent by the adrenoceptor antagonists. The specific dopamine effects can be demonstrated by first blocking the alpha and beta receptors and then administering dopamine agonists. The latter can then be blocked by dopamine antagonists. In Parkinsonism, deficiency of dopamine may lead to the unopposed action of acetylcholine with peripheral manifestations such as greasy skin, excessive sweating, and vasomotor instability. These effects are reversed by the administration of L-dopa or dopamine receptor stimulating drugs such as bromocriptine.

Neurochemical Changes with Ageing

There have been few studies of the effect of ageing on neurotransmission in the autonomic nervous system. Frolkis and coworkers (1973) investigated acetylcholine metabolism in adult and old rats, rabbits, and cats at sites of acetylcholine action, namely, the vascular receptors, the nervous centres especially in the hypothalamic area, the autonomic ganglia, and the cholinergic peripheral effector system. The biosynthesis and hydrolysis of acetylcholine were found to decrease with increasing age;

thus there was a decrease in acetyltransferase and cholinesterase activity but an increase in the sensitivity of cholinoreceptor protein to acetylcholine. Repeated stimulation led to weakening of the reactions and rapid exhaustion of the reflexes from the vascular chemoreceptor sites. Since the number of receptors is diminished in old age the overall effect was reduction in the functional efficiency of the autonomic reflex arcs. Frolkis (1968) found that a stimulus with a potential of 0.35 V caused bradycardia on stimulating the vagus in young rats, but a potential of 0.53 V was required to produce a similar effect in old rats. The excitability of autonomic ganglia also appears to decline in old animals and the number of impulses the ganglia can transmit per second decreases. These age-related changes in the autonomic ganglia may contribute to the sluggish initiation of autonomic reflexes which have been observed in elderly people during tests of thermoregulatory function (Collins, Easton, and Exton-Smith, 1981) with a reduction in the ability of the peripheral effector system to respond to central stimulation.

Pharmacodynamic Changes with Ageing

There are two main pharmacodynamic changes which have been described, namely, a decrease in the number of some specific receptors leading to a reduction in intrinsic sensitivity to drugs and an increased target organ sensitivity possibly associated with diminished innervation (Collins, 1982). There have been few studies of change in receptor sensitivity in older people. Vestal, Wood, and Shaw (1979) have demonstrated that there was an age-related increase in the dose of isoprenaline required to increase heart rate by 25 beats a minute and that the blocking of this action by propranolol was decreased in older subjects. The authors attributed these findings to a reduction in the number of receptors with increasing age.

Associated with the decline in parasympathetic and sympathetic nervous effects with age there appears to be a concurrent increase in the sensitivity of target organs to transmitter substances. Although not proven these changes with ageing can be regarded as comparable to the effects of denervation at postganglionic sites and this peripheral denervation sensitivity is at least partially due to the proliferation of receptors which occurs after denervation.

Bannister and coworkers (1979) have demonstrated exaggerated responses to noradrenaline infusion in patients with widespread autonomic failure; this peripheral postganglionic hypersensitivity appears to be highly selective for sympathomimetic amines.

With increasing age there is probably a differential change in vascular chemoreceptor and baroreceptor reflexes; chemoreceptors become increasingly sensitive whereas baro reflexes become weaker. This difference may be due to increased chemical sensitivity on the one hand and to a reduction in the mechanical efficiency of vascular stretch receptors on the other (Timiras, 1972). Thus in old age regulatory control is maintained since the increased sensitivity to chemical mediators compensates for the impaired efficiency of baroreceptor reflexes.

PHYSIOLOGICAL IMPAIRMENT OF FUNCTION

Several studies indicate that impairment of autonomic function is common in older people even in the absence of disease.

Cardiovascular Reflexes

Caird, Andrews, and Kennedy (1973) in a survey of old people living at home found that the incidence of postural hypotension increases with age. A fall of 20 mmHg or more in systolic blood pressure was observed in 16 per cent. of subjects aged 65 to 74 years and in 30 per cent. of those aged 75 and over. They believe that autonomic dysfunction is the underlying cause and this commonly interacts with other factors (see page 784). Gross (1970) also found that impairment of circulatory reflexes increases in frequency with advancing age, as manifested by abnormality of the blood pressure response to the Valsalva manoeuvre. Strandell (1964) observed the mean increase in heart rate on standing in middle aged and elderly subjects was 10 to 15 beats per minute compared with approximately 20 beats per minute in young adults. Bristow and coworkers (1969) recorded the reflex bradycardia produced by the rise in pressure following intravenous injection of phenylephrine (25 to 100 μg) and they found

a diminished baro reflex sensitivity with increasing age. It was believed that this was due to decreased distensibility of the arterial wall at the baro reflex site in old age.

Thermoregulatory Responses

Fox and coworkers (1973b) measured body temperatures in a random sample of 1,020 people aged 65 and over living at home in Great Britain during the first 3 months of 1972. Lowering of deep body temperature as measured by the urine temperature was significantly correlated with advancing age. In 10 per cent. of subjects the deep body temperature was less than 35.5 °C and these individuals were thought to have some degree of thermoregulatory failure as shown by an inability to maintain an adequate core-peripheral temperature gradient. The mean difference between the urine temperature and the hand temperature in this group was 2.9 °C compared with 4.6 °C for those in the normal temperature group whose deep body temperatures were 36.0 °C and above. This possibility was confirmed when a 15 per cent. subsample of the 1,000 participants in the Camden survey which was also conducted in the first three months of 1972 were submitted to thermoregulatory function tests involving the measurement of physiological responses to a cycle of neutral, cool, and warm environments created by a specially designed air-conditioned test-bed. It was found that shivering occurred during the cooling period in 12 per cent. of the subjects as compared with 30 per cent. in a group of young adults. Sweating occurred in all the young subjects but only in about half the elderly during the period of warming.

Abnormal peripheral blood flow patterns on cooling and warming (see Fig. 1) were found in 56 per cent. of the men and 45 per cent. of the women. These abnormal patterns were found to be rare in the young control subjects.

When tests of thermoregulatory function were repeated 4 years later in 45 of the subjects a significantly higher proportion had low resting peripheral blood flow (less than 5 ml per 100 ml hand tissue per minute) and a higher proportion had a non-constrictor response on cooling (Collins *et al.*, 1977).

Forty-three per cent. of those with abnormal vasomotor responses to cooling and only 10 per cent. of those with normal responses were found to have postural hypotension with a fall in systolic pressure greater than 20 mmHg. In the group with a normal peripheral blood flow pattern it was found that there was a significant increase in the deep body temperature required to initiate sweating on warming compared with the level in the first study.

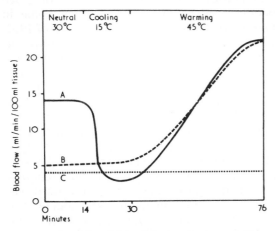

Figure 1 Peripheral blood flow responses of (A) normal, (B) non-constrictor, and (C) non-constrictor/non-dilator people

The main factors responsible for a decline in efficiency of thermoregulation in old age are a decreased basal oxygen consumption associated with a reduced functional cell mass, impairment of physiological mechanisms for heat conservation, e.g. cutaneous vasoconstriction, and a diminished ability to increase heat production by shivering in response to cold stress. Thus older subjects are generally less able to maintain body heat stores during convective cooling (Collins, Easton, and Exton-Smith, 1981). In young adults transient vasoconstrictor responses at rest may be demonstrated in a neutral environment with microelectrode recording of sympathetic activity from cutaneous nerves.

This activity occurs in a rhythmic fashion with a frequency which increases up to about 10 per minute in a cold environment. In elderly subjects photoelectric plethysmograph studies of vasomotor responses in the skin show that these rhythmic blood flow changes are virtually absent in those old people who show a lack of response to cooling when undergoing thermoregulatory tests (Collins, 1982).

PATHOLOGICAL CONDITIONS AFFECTING AUTONOMIC FUNCTION

The autonomic nervous system may be affected by a number of pathological processes and by the action of drugs, of which the more important are listed in Table 1. The most widespread involvement occurs in the Shy–Drager syndrome and although this is a rare disease all the manifestations of autonomic failure are to be found in the clinical picture.

Table 1: Pathological conditions affecting autonomic function

Central disturbances	Autonomic neuropathy
Shy–Drager syndrome	Diabetes mellitus
Parkinsonism	Malignancy
Wernicke's encephalopathy	Amyloidosis
Hypothalamic lesions	Acute infective
Cerebrovascular disease	polyneuropathy
Tabes dorsalis	Vitamin B complex
Paraplegia	deficiency
Chronic alcoholism	Chronic alcoholism
Psychotropic drugs	Peripheral acting drugs

Shy–Drager Syndrome

Shy and Drager (1960) described two cases of a neurological syndrome associated with orthostatic hypotension, defective sweating, and sphincter disturbances with subsequent appearance of somatic neurological manifestations. The pathological changes included widespread degeneration in the medulla, the posterior hypothalamic region, the cerebellum, the third nerve nuclei, the basal ganglia, the autonomic ganglia, the dorsal nucleus of the vagus, with reduction in the number of cells in the anterolateral column of the spinal cord. The neurochemical changes include marked depletion of dopamine and noradrenaline in brain regions which are normally rich in chatecholamines (Spokes, Bannister, and Oppenheimer, (1979).

Thomas and Schirger (1963) described 30 cases of the syndrome in which the presenting feature was orthostatic hypotension. The ages ranged from 42 to 74 years and the condition was three times more common in men than in women. The onset of the somatoneurological manifestations was usually insidious and followed the known onset of postural hypotension by 6 months to 20 years. Eleven patients had features resembling Parkinsonism.

Parkinsonism

Orthostatic hypotension can occur in patients with paralysis agitans. Aminoff and Wilcox (1971) described the clinical feature of 11 Parkinsonian patients in whom autonomic dysfunction was present. Three had the Shy–Drager syndrome in whom autonomic symptoms preceded somatic neurological manifestations, while in 8 patients the autonomic symptoms succeeded the somatic manifestations. Investigation of autonomic function showed a resting blood pressure lower than expected for the patient's age and sex, orthostatic hypotension and increased sensitivity to noradrenaline, impairment of thermoregulatory function, with patchy loss of sweating and abnormal bladder function. Gross, Bannister, and Godwin-Austen (1972) found that in 20 patients under the age of 63 with idiopathic Parkinsonism the Valsalva responses were normal but the percentage fall in the mean blood pressure on passive tilting was significantly greater than in a control group of patients matched for age. L-dopa therapy of patients with uncomplicated Parkinsonism sometimes first reveals evidence of autonomic dysfunction and it is possible that autonomic disturbances in paralysis agitans occur much more frequently than is generally recognized.

Wernicke's Encephalopathy

Birchfield (1964) found the following clinical features in 40 cases of Wernicke's disease: orthostatic hypotension (32), ophthalmoparesis (26), nystagmus (32), ataxia (in all of the 25 patients tested), peripheral neuropathy (29), and Korsakoff's psychosis (28). The condition is due to thiamine deficiency often associated with alcoholism and characteristic petechial haemorrhages are to be found in the walls of the third ventricle, the hypothalamus and mamillary bodies. The hypothalamic lesions in Wernicke's encephalopathy can also lead to hypothermia (Philip and Smith, 1973). The disorder of temperature regulation is often overlooked. The response to thiamine administration in Wernicke's encephalopathy is usually dramatic.

Hypothalamic lesions

Lesions localized in or near the hypothalamus may lead to impairment of temperature regulation, postural hypotension, and disorders of micturition. Abnormalities of body temperature control were present in 13 of 16 patients shown at autopsy to have hypothalamic disease (Bauer, 1954). Some lesions lead to recurrent bouts of hypothermia in either winter or summer, so called intermittent neurogenic hypothermia, (Maclean and Emslie-Smith, 1977). In one case reported by Fox and coworkers (1970) the episodic hypothermia which later progressed into chronic hypothermia was attributable to a lesion in the anterior hypothalamus localized in the anterior preoptic region ventral to the anterior commisure. Fox and coworkers (1973a) have also described intermittent neurogenic hypothermia in diencephalic autonomic epilepsy where episodes may last for only a few hours and where there are inappropriate thermoregulatory responses with profound sweating in cool conditions.

Cerebrovascular Disease

Johnson and coworkers (1965) found that a substantial proportion of the patients in a geriatric department in Oxford suffered from orthostatic hypotension (17 per cent. had a fall in systolic pressure of 20 mmHg or more after standing for 2 minutes). They attributed this to cerebrovascular disease. At autopsy ischaemic lesions were found at many sites in the brain but not in the spinal cord, hypothalamus, or brainstem. Gross (1970) suggested that age and debility rather than cerebrovascular disease might be important factors. Orthostatic hypotension and impairment of thermoregulation may also be due to psychotropic drugs (especially phenothiazines) which are commonly prescribed for patients suffering from the effects of cerebrovascular disease.

Autonomic Neuropathy

Diabetes mellitus is the commonest cause of autonomic neuropathy associated with peripheral neuropathy. In diabetic autonomic neuropathy the symptoms include dizziness and faintness due to postural hypotension, intermittent nocturnal diarrhoea, intermittent vomiting, gastric fullness, dysuria, reduced sweating in the legs and impairment of temperature regulation leading to hypothermia. The incidence of peripheral neuropathy as a complication of diabetes is uncertain and the reported frequency varies from 4 to 93 per cent. (Roberts, 1970). It is even more difficult to estimate the frequency of autonomic involvement. In one series (Rundles, 1945) 25 to 30 per cent. of patients with sensory or motor neuropathy were considered to have autonomic involvement and in another series (Odel *et al.*, 1955) the frequency was greater than 75 per cent.

Sharpey-Schafer and Taylor (1960) investigated 337 patients attending a diabetic clinic and found that 69 had diabetic neuropathy. Of 35 who were studied fully, 17 showed a complete absence of circulatory reflexes and 14 a diminution in response to the Valsalva manoeuvre, tipping, coughing, hyperventilation, and mental arithmetic. Ewing, Campbell, and Clarke, (1976) emphasized that it has a bad prognosis; the mortality in 2½ years in a series of diabetic patients was twice as great when autonomic neuropathy was present compared with those in whom tests of autonomic function were normal. The authors suggested that in diabetes with clinical features of neuropathy simple autonomic function tests provide a good guide to prognosis.

Other Disorders of the Nervous System

Less common causes of autonomic neuropathy include the neuropathy associated with malignant disease (especially carcinoma of the bronchus and pancreas), amyloidosis, and acute infective polyneuropathy (the Guillain–Barré syndrome).

Other diseases of the central nervous system which may lead to autonomic dysfunction include tabes dorsalis (Sharpey-Schafer, 1956), Holmes–Adie syndrome (Croll, Duthie, and MacWilliam, 1935), paraplegia (Johnson, Park, and Frankel, 1971), and chronic alcoholism (Barraclough and Sharpey-Schafer, 1963).

CLINICAL SYNDROMES

The most important clinical manifestations of impaired autonomic function in the elderly are disorders of blood pressure regulation presenting as postural hypotension and disorders of thermoregulation leading to hypothermia and hyperthermia. Autonomic impairment also leads to disturbances of gastrointestinal function and to disorders of bladder function; these aspects are considered elsewhere.

Postural Hypotension

Blood pressure regulation depends on cardiac output and peripheral resistance. The heart rate which influences cardiac output is controlled by baroreceptor reflexes originating from the carotid sinus; a fall in blood pressure leads to cardiac acceleration. Peripheral resistance is dependent on vasoconstrictor tone mediated by the sympathetic nervous system. Normally on standing after lying in the supine position parasympathetic activity decreases, causing cardiac acceleration, and sympathetic activity increases, resulting in constriction of arterioles and veins. About 700 ml of blood leaves the chest and is rapidly pooled in the venous reservoirs in the abdomen and legs. The pressure in the right atrium falls to or below the mean intrathoracic pressure and there is diminished return of blood to the right side of the heart. In a fit young adult systemic arterial pressure drops only transiently on standing and within 15 to 30 seconds the pressure returns to the previous level or slightly above this. In old people, however, homeostasis is less well maintained and in an investigation of old people participating in a hypothermia survey 14 per cent. were found to have postural hypotension with a fall in systolic blood pressure of 20 mmHg or more on standing (Exton-Smith, Green, and Fox, 1975). In a follow-up survey 4 years later the proportion who had postural hypotension was found to have increased (Collins *et al.*, 1977).

Pathogenesis

Autonomic dysfunction leading to postural hypotension may be due to impairment of the afferent part of the baroreceptor reflex arc (Sharpey-Schafer and Taylor, 1960), to lesions in the central structures (Appenzeller and Descarries, 1964), or to impairment of function in the effector system (Bannister, Ardill, and Fenton, 1967) which is responsible for systemic arteriolar constriction and possibly constriction of venous reservoirs.

Ziegler (1980) has investigated the autonomic response to standing by measurement of plasma noradrenaline levels. Standing evokes a diffuse increase in sympathetic nervous activity with enhanced release of noradrenaline. In all young subjects plasma noradrenaline concentration may show a 100 per cent. increase within 5 minutes of standing. Abnormal patterns of change are found in patients with postural hypotension. Thus patients with idiopathic orthostatic hypotension have abnormally low resting levels due to depleted tissue stores and a failure to release noradrenaline in response to tyramine; standing causes hypotension which is not accompanied by an increase in heart rate nor in plasma noradrenaline concentration. These patients and those with postural hypotension due to autonomic neuropathy (e.g. in diabetes) have an increased responsiveness to noradrenaline infusion. Patients with Shy–Drager syndrome have normal resting plasma levels for noradrenaline but no increase in levels on standing.

The causes of autonomic dysfunction leading to an increasing incidence of postural hypotension with age include an age-related decline in physiological mechanisms and the presence of pathological conditions, some of which are listed in Table 1. Wilkins, Culbertson, and Ingelfinger, (1951) have emphasized that failure to control the splanchnic vascular bed may play an important part in the development of postural hypotension. In diabetic patients with evidence of peripheral neuropathy and presumed autonomic neuropathy, demyelination of the greater splanchnic nerve which is a major sympathetic pathway has been demonstrated (Low *et al.*, 1975).

The commonly used drugs which can cause postural hypotension are hypotensive agents, diuretics, L-dopa, and the phenothiazines. In the Glasgow study (Caird, Andrews, and Kennedy, 1973) two or more of the following factors – varicose veins, urinary tract infection, anaemia, hyponatraemia, absent ankle jerks and the use of potentially hypotensive drugs – were present in 50 per cent. of subjects with a fall in systolic pressure of 30 mmHg or more and in 17 per cent. without postural hypotension ($p < 0.01$). This suggests that postural hypotension in relatively healthy old people has more than one cause.

Clinical Features

In many instances postural hypotension is asymptomatic since autoregulation of the cerebral circulation is able to compensate for the fall in systemic arterial pressure. In other cases, when autoregulation fails, possibly as the result of cerebrovascular disease or if the orthostatic fall in blood pressure is excessive, the patient complains of weakness, faintness, dizziness, loss of balance, or blacking out, especially when rising from the lying position. A fall associated with postural hypotension may lead to fracture or to accidental hypothermia when the old person is living in cold conditions. Whenever postural hypotension is discovered a search should be made for somatic neurological involvement, including peripheral neuropathy, pyramidal tract lesions, olivopontocerebellar degeneration, and Parkinsonism. Even in the absence of clinical signs of multiple system degeneration elsewhere in the nervous system it is possible that deterioration in autonomic function is associated with a physiological decline in somatic function. Thus Overstall and coworkers (1977, 1978) have shown that body sway is greater in those old people with postural hypotension compared with age-matched controls, and this increase in sway is unrelated to the level of blood pressure.

Management

Drugs with potentially hypotensive action should be withheld and appropriate treatment should be given to those patients who are found to have a correctable cause of postural hypotension. There are several approaches to the management of severe postural hypotension but most have serious limitations. Pooling of blood on assuming the upright position may be prevented by mechanical means such as the wearing of an antigravity suit.

Although successful this is not usually a practical measure in the elderly. To be effective elastic stockings have to be full length and used in combination with an elastic abdominal support and these measures too are not well tolerated by older patients. The expansion of circulatory blood volume by the use of mineralocorticoid hormones is usually ineffective in severe cases; in moderate postural hypotension it may be effective in large doses (0.5 to 2.0

mg/day of fludrocortisone), but these cause supine hypertension and carry the risk of precipitating cardiac failure or pulmonary oedema. Perkins and Lee (1978) have shown that severe postural hypotension may respond to therapy with the prostaglandin synthetase inhibitor flurbiprofen (50 mg twice daily) combined with fludrocortisone. The patient they describe was able to lead a normal life after 3 months combined therapy whereas prior to treatment she was unable to stand owing to syncope associated with a fall in blood pressure to a level which was unrecordable.

Another approach to treatment is the use of dihydroergotamine. Lang, Jansen, and Pfoff (1975) have reported significant improvement in postural hypotension treated with dihydroergotamine (2 mg 3 times a day). The effects of this drug may be due largely to its powerful and relatively selective action on the capacity reservoirs in the peripheral circulation.

Recently Man In't Veld and Schalekamp (1981) have shown that a beta adrenoreceptor agonist, pindolol, is therapeutically effective in severe postural hypotension. They described 3 patients who were bedridden before treatment; while taking pindolol (15 mg/day) they were able to walk and did not collapse when standing for 15 minutes. Although increase in supine blood pressure occurred this did not reach hypertensive levels. The use of this treatment requires further evaluation in the elderly since the patients they describe were all under the age of 65. Orthostatic drop in blood pressure still occurred but the autoregulation in the cerebral circulation was able to maintain cerebral perfusion.

Accidental Hypothermia

Homeothermy, or the capacity to maintain a stable deep-body temperature, is an evolutionary development found only in birds, man, and other mammals. Ideally all body tissues would be maintained at optimum temperature but this would be difficult to achieve and costly in energy production. Thus in man and other homeothermic animals deep body or 'core' temperature is controlled and the superficial or body 'shell' acts as a variable insulator or heat sink. The heart and circulation provide a heat exchanger system. In a warm environment the blood flow to the skin is increased to promote the transfer of heat to the body surface. Under cool conditions the blood flow is reduced to conserve heat. This vasomotor regulation is capable of maintaining homeothermy only over a limited range of environmental temperatures. As a protection against hyperthermia and hypothermia the additional mechanisms of sweating and shivering are brought into play.

In man, vasomotor control in the skin depends upon vasoconstrictor autonomic nerves and on a vasodilator mechanism. The vasoconstrictor mechanism predominates in the hands and the feet and is only weekly represented in the proximal parts of the limbs and the trunk. Under thermally neutral conditions the blood flow in the hand is within the range 4 to 10 mls/100 ml of hand tissue per minute. In a person who feels cold but who is not shivering blood flow is approximately 1 ml per 100 ml of hand tissue per minute and when the body is heated it may rise to over 40 ml. The stimulus to vasoconstriction arises mainly from the cold receptors in the skin.

Within the vasomotor control zone hand blood flow is very sensitive to small changes in skin temperature in the rest of the body, marked vasoconstriction, and vasodilation being elicited by minor degrees of cooling and warming, respectively. The way in which the vasodilator mechanisms operate is unknown. Active vasodilation begins just before sweating is initiated and is the dominant mechanism for promoting heat loss by increasing transport of the heat to the skin for evaporation by sweating.

Hypothermia is defined as a state of subnormal body temperature in which the deep body temperature falls below 35.0 °C. It became recognized in Great Britain during the 1960s as a problem particularly affecting old people. The term accidental hypothermia is used to imply that the lowering of deep-body temperature is unintentional and it has to be distinguished from hypothermia which is induced therapeutically.

Prevalence

Even up to 15 years ago accidental hypothermia was thought to be a rare condition. It was known to occur in association with certain diseases, e.g. myxoedema, hypopituitarism, and alcoholism. The British Medical Association's Committee on Accidental Hypothermia in the Elderly (BMA, 1964) reviewed the descriptions of cases reported in the literature and concluded that there was no accurate information on the prevalence of the condition. Hospital reports indicated that very few cases were recognized clinically before admission and elderly people with hypothermia suffered a high mortality.

Duguid, Simpson, and Stowers (1961) described 23 cases occurring in Scotland. All the patients were elderly and developed hypothermia indoors. Deep-body temperatures on admission as measured by a rectal thermometer ranged from 22.8 to 31.9 °C. Rosin and Exton-Smith (1964) described 32 patients with hypothermia, half of whom were seen during the very cold winter of 1962–63. With the exception of one, aged 39 years, their ages ranged from 60 to 92 years. Although 10 patients were found lying on the floor the others suffered from lesser degrees of exposure; 10 were in bed at home, 2 were sitting in a chair, 1 developed hypothermia in hospital, and in the remainder a history of events prior to admission could not be obtained.

The largest survey of hypothermia in the elderly is that reported by Maclean and Emslie-Smith (1977). Eighty-five of the 100 consecutive cases of hypothermia were over the age of 60 years. About half of these patients were found lying on the floor after a fall due either to an accident or to an illness. One or more underlying disorders were present in one-fifth of the patients.

The Royal College of Physicians' survey (1966) conducted in ten hospital groups during the months of February, March, and April 1965 established the incidence of hypothermia as 0.68 per cent. of all patients admitted, of whom 42 per cent. were over the age of 65. These results indicate that about 3,800 elderly patients could have been admitted with hypothermia to hospitals in Great Britain during these three winter months. Ten years later a second Royal College of Physicians' survey conducted at two London hospitals in January to April 1975 showed that 3.6 per cent. of patients over the age of 65 admitted to hospital were hypothermic, a prevalence considerably higher than that of the previous College study (Goldman *et al.*, 1977).

Aetiology

As in so many disorders of the elderly multiple factors are involved in the aetiology of accidental hypothermia in old people, and the more important are shown in Table 2.

Table 2   Causes of accidental hypothermia in the elderly

1. *Exogenous* – cold exposure
2. *Endogenous* – (a) Physiological

(i).	impaired thermoregulatory responses
(ii).	impaired temperature perception

(b) Pathological

(i).	endocrine: myxoedema, hypopituitarism, diabetes mellitus
(ii).	neurological: hemiplegia, Parkinsonism, Wernicke's encephalopathy and other hypothalamic lesions
(iii).	locomotor: arthritis and other causes of immobility
(iv).	mental: confusional states, dementia, depression
(v).	infections: bronchopneumonia, septicaemia
(vi).	circulatory: cardiac infarction, pulmonary embolism
(vii).	drugs: phenothiazines, hypnotics and tranquillizers, antidepressants, alcohol
(viii).	miscellaneous: exfoliative dermatitis, steatorrhoea, extensive Paget's disease

Exogenous Factors

Exposure to cold is an overriding cause and the Royal College of Physicians' survey (1966) showed a clear relationship between the incidence of hypothermia and a low environmental temperature. The number of cases rose considerably when the ambient temperature fell below 0 °C. Many elderly people living at home who develop hypothermia have some common characteristics; they usually live alone under cold conditions and their houses lack basic amenities, and they often have impaired mobility, nocturia, insomnia, and liability to falls (Collins *et al.*, 1977; Exton-Smith, 1977; Fox *et al*, 1973b). A common story is of an old person who falls after attempting to get out of bed at night; he remains on the floor for several hours, often partly clad, and is discovered the next day by a neighbour or a home help. Thus the exposure is likely to be longer when the old person lives alone and is socially isolated.

In many cases, however, exposure is minimal, and in some cases some elderly people develop hypothermia under mild weather conditions. Such a patient may be found in bed apparently well covered with clothes. In these instances insufficient body heat is being generated, so that even good external insulation is ineffective, and in the majority of cases endogenous factors are of greater importance than cold exposure.

Endogenous Factors

The high incidence of accidental hypothermia in old people can mainly be accounted for by the physiological decline in thermoregulatory function which has been clearly revealed in both cross-sectional and longitudinal studies (Collins *et al.*, 1977; Fox *et al.*, 1973b). The impairment of thermoregulatory reflexes has also been demonstrated in the survivors of accidental hypothermia (Macmillan *et al.*, 1967); on moderate cooling shivering was absent, the metabolic rate did not rise, and there was defective vasoconstriction. As a result the deep-body temperature fell abnormally and progressively. These patients are at risk of developing further attacks of hypothermia which may be precipitated by moderate cold exposure or by the use of small doses of drugs with a hypothermic action such as the phenothiazines.

Shivering thermogenesis is another component of thermoregulation. Collins, Easton, and Exton-Smith (1981) have investigated the metabolic response to cooling in healthy elderly subjects (mean age 80 years) and in control subjects (mean age 26 years). Using a body-cooling unit air at a temperature of 20 °C was blown over the surface of the body at a velocity of 0.5 m/s for 30 minutes. Shivering which was monitored by an electromyograph and an accelerometer was found to be absent or less intense in the older group.

Mean metabolic heat production rose by 14.4 W/m^2 in the elderly and by 25.1 W/m^2 in the young controls. In general the elderly group were less able to maintain core temperature in the face of cold stress.

In addition to impaired thermoregulatory function many old people have a diminished sensitivity to cold. Tests of digital thermosensation (Collins *et al.*, 1977) show that young people perceive mean temperature differences of about 0.8 °C whereas elderly subjects can discriminate only between mean temperature differences of 2.5 °C. Some are unable to perceive differences of 5 °C or more. Moreover, it has been shown that when old people are given the opportunity of controlling their own thermal environment many of them are less precise in making the necessary temperature adjustments and take longer in attaining the optimum temperature for thermal comfort (Collins, Exton-Smith, and Doré, 1981; Collins and Hoinville, 1981). It is likely that a lesser sensitivity to cold is one of the reasons for the relatively large numbers of old people who appear to be able to tolerate cold conditions without discomfort. Nevertheless such individuals may be at risk of overtaxing the heat-conserving capacity of a failing thermoregulatory system.

Although some old people admitted to hospital suffer from primary accidental hypothermia (i.e. the hypothermia is the result of cold exposure and failing thermoregulation), in the majority pathological conditions are present. Hypothermia associated with myxoedema and hypopituitarism is well known, but diabetes mellitus is the commonest endocrine disorder in most reported series of cases of hypothermia. It most often occurs in diabetic ketoacidosis (Gale and Tattersall, 1978) where the arteriovenous oxygen difference is abnormally low; it seems likely that an important factor in these cases is the depression of metabolic heat production resulting from failure in oxygen utilization. Vasomotor dysfunction due to autonomic neuropathy can contribute to impaired thermoregulation in elderly diabetic patients, but the extent of this is unknown. A stroke may be responsible for the initial fall and cold exposure because the patient remains immobile on the floor. In a number of neurological and locomotor disorders immobility is a factor limiting the amount of heat generated and in Parkinsonism there may be an additional factor of autonomic dysfunction. Patients with confusional states and dementia may be unaware of environmental hazards and there is some evidence for impairment of temperature regulation in dementia. The psychotropic drugs commonly prescribed for these conditions also affect thermoregulation. Bronchopneumonia can precipitate hypothermia and it usually develops insidiously in those suffering from hypothermia due to other causes. Other severe infections, cardiac infarction, and pulmonary embolism can cause an acute derangement of the thermoregulatory mechanisms.

Clinical Features

Appearance. The patient usually has a grey colour due to a mixture of pallor and cyanosis. The skin is cold to the touch not only in exposed parts of the body but also in those parts normally covered; e.g. the axillae and abdominal wall. The puffy facial appearance, the slow cerebration, and a husky voice may be mistaken for myxoedema. The diagnosis can be established by measurement of the rectal temperature using a low reading clinical thermometer which should read down to 25 °C.

Mental symptoms. An acute confusional state is often a salient feature. Drowsiness is usually apparent when the deep body temperature falls below 32 °C. The lower the body temperature the more likely is the patient to be comatose and in the series described by Rosin and Exton-Smith (1964) three-quarters of the patients with rectal temperatures below 27 °C were unconscious.

Nervous system. As the body temperature falls the reflexes become progressively depressed, shivering is usually absent and becomes replaced by muscle hypertonus which gives rise to neck stiffness simulating meningism and to rigidity of the abdominal wall. An involuntary flapping tremor in the arms and legs has been observed in some patients (Rosin and Exton-Smith, 1964).

Cardiovascular system. The heart rate slows in response to cold due to sinus bradycardia or slow atrial fibrillation. The electrocardiogram usually shows some degree of heart block with an increase in PR interval (in patients with sinus rhythm) and there is delay in intraventricular conduction. A pathognomonic sign is the appearance of a 'J' wave shown by a characteristic deflection at the junction of the QRS and ST segment (Osborn, 1953; Emslie-Smith, 1958). The size of the 'J' wave varies from patient to patient and it is not related to the severity of hypothermia; the 'J' wave even in severe hypothermia is often absent altogether. In any one individual the height of the wave diminishes as the patient recovers and the deep-body temperature rises. A fall in arterial blood pressure is an ominous sign.

Respiratory system. In severe hypothermia respirations are slow and shallow which can progress to apnoea, the pO_2 in the arterial blood is low, and the oxygen dissociation curve is shifted so that less oxygen is given up to the tissues at a given partial pressure of oxygen. The effect is to produce tissue anoxia and this may be an important factor influencing prognosis (McNicol and Smith, 1964). When hypopnoea is marked the pCO_2 may be so greatly elevated as to give rise to respiratory failure. Bronchopneumonia may be present without the usual clinical signs and the basal crepitations which are often present may be due to cold injury to the alveoli.

Alimentary system. Gastric dilatation is common and gives rise to the risk of aspiration of gastric contents. Acute ulceration of the stomach can cause haematemesis. Acute pancreatitis is often found at post-mortem examination but during life it is usually overlooked since few of the typical signs are present in the hypothermic patient. It should be suspected if the patient winces when firm pressure is applied to the epigastrium. A rise in the serum amylase was found in 11 of the 15 cases tested by Duguid, Simpson, and Stowers (1961).

Renal system. Renal blood flow and glomerular filtration rate are decreased and tubular function is impaired. Oliguria is common and acute tubular necrosis can occur. This may be due to a combination of ischaemia and the direct effect of cold on the kidneys.

The blood. Haemoglobin and haematocrit may be raised owing to a decrease in plasma volume. A moderate elevation of the white cell count often occurs but a normal or low white cell count does not exclude the possibility of an infection such as bronchopneumonia. Thrombocytopenia is not uncommon and this has been attributed to sequestration of platelets in the liver and spleen; it can give rise to bleeding. Multiple infarcts may occur in the myocardium, viscera, limbs, or pancreas (Duguid, Simpson, and Stowers, 1961).

Metabolism. The blood urea is usually moderately raised and the pattern of serum electrolytes varies according to the degree of renal and respiratory failure. Blood sugar concentrations above 6.7 mmol/l are common; in the absence of diabetes mellitus blood sugar returns to normal as the patient's temperature rises. In the series reported by Mills (1973) none of the non-diabetic patients who subsequently survived and who had an initial blood sugar above 6.7 mmol/l was found to have developed diabetes mellitus. Occasionally profound hypoglycaemia occurs.

Raised serum levels of the muscle enzymes aspartate aminotransferase and hydroxybutyrate dehydrogenase and creatine kinase are often found. Very high levels of these enzymes should lead to the suspicion that hypothermia is secondary to myxoedema; the levels fall to normal when the deep-body temperature rises even before thyroid replacement is started (Maclean, Griffiths, and Emslie-Smith, 1968). When myxoedema is suspected to be an underlying cause of hypothermia the diagnosis of hypothyroidism should be confirmed by assay of serum levels of tri-iodothyronine and thyroxine and by measurement of the serum TSH levels. Low levels of T3 and T4 and raised TSH are typical of primary myxoedema but the extent to which the levels of these hormones are influenced by hypothermia in the absence of myxoedema is not known and caution is required in the interpretation of the results of these assays. Moreover, it is known that serum T3 levels can be depressed in severely ill patients in the absence of hypothyroidism and hypothermia. A raised level of plasma cortisol is frequently found in hypothermia and is a good indicator of the patient's prognosis (Maclean and Browning, 1975a). There is also evidence that cortisol utilization during hypothermia is often very poor and is sometimes absent (Maclean and Browning, 1975b).

Prognosis

There are several factors which influence the outcome of patients suffering from accidental hypothermia. Both surveys carried out on behalf of the Royal College of Physicians (Royal College of Physicians, London 1966; Goldman *et al*, 1977) clearly showed an inverse relationship between the deep-body temperature and mortality. In addition to the severity of hypothermia the outcome is also influenced by its duration; the longer the period during which low deep-body temperatures are maintained the greater the likelihood of serious metabolic disturbances and the development of complications which are irreversible. The nature of the underlying disease responsible for hypothermia has a considerable influence on outcome, especially in elderly patients in whom multiple pathological processes are present (Exton-Smith, 1973). Prognosis is better when the causal disease is reversible or can be readily treated, e.g. when hypothermia is secondary to the administration of phenothiazines or if thiamine deficiency in Wernicke's encephalopathy is corrected.

Management

Ideally a rapid restoration of normal temperature would be the best method of treatment since it should avoid some of the complications resulting from a prolonged hypothermia. Although rapid active surface rewarming can be practised as standard management in fit young adults who suffer from primary hypothermia due to cold immersion or exposure, such a procedure is hazardous in the elderly and frequently leads to circulatory collapse and an 'after drop' in the core temperature which may precipitate cardiac dysrhythmias. It is therefore generally advocated that there should be no active rewarming, the lightly covered patient should be nursed in a cubicle at an ambient temperature of 25 to 30 °C and the body temperature should be allowed to come up very slowly. One of the two therapeutic regimens summarized in Table 3 can be instituted according to the degree of hypothermia.

The measures outlined in these two regimens can be regarded as standard for the majority of cases of accidental hypothermia. For the individual patient, however, more detailed consideration has to be given to the use of some of these measures.

Table 3   Management of accidental hypothermia

Mild hypothermia (deep body temperature 32–35 °C)

1. Room temperature of cubicle 25–30 °C; deep-body temperature allowed to rise at about 0.5 °C/hour
2. Barrier nursing; administration of broad-spectrum antibiotic
3. Controlled oxygen administration by means of a Venturi mask
4. Pulse and blood pressure monitoring; if there is a fall in the blood pressure during the treatment the patient is cooled again temporarily by lowering the room temperature
5. Active measures for the prevention of pressure sores e.g. large cell ripple mattress

Moderate to severe hypothermia (deep-body temperature below 32 °C)

Additional measures to above requiring treatment in an Intensive Care Unit.

1. Institution of positive pressure ventilation to correct hypoxia and to re-expand collapsed alveoli
2. Insertion of central venous catheter for measurement of pressure and administration of warm fluids
3. The correction of dehydration and electrolyte disturbances
4. Loading dose of intravenous prophylactic antibiotic, e.g. ampicillin or cloxacillin
5. Monitoring of deep body temperature either continuously, i.e. thermister in external auditory meatus, or half-hourly (rectal thermometer)
6. ECG monitoring for cardiac dysrhythmias

Oxygen and assisted ventilation. The low arterial pO_2 levels which occur in hypothermia produce tissue anoxia. For patients whose rewarming proceeds satisfactorily the administration of pure oxygen is usually successful in restoring arterial oxygen levels to normal. When there is severe depression of the respiratory centre, especially in hypothermia secondary to psychotropic drugs, anoxia may be the only stimulus driving respiration. In these cases oxygen therapy alone causes apnoea and it is essential to institute artificial ventilation. Ledingham and Mone (1972) have reported good results from the use of intermittent positive pressure ventilation in hypoxic hypothermic patients.

Fluid and electrolyte disturbances. Severe alteration can occur in hypothermia, especially in seriously ill or comatose patients. Monitoring of central venous pressure is essential in order to minimize the risk of pulmonary oedema following intravenous fluid replacement. Abnormal water retention, haemodilution, and very low serum electrolyte concentrations are also features of hypothermia associated with long-standing myxoedema or hypopituitarism. Treatment with intravenous hypertonic saline should be avoided since it may precipitate pulmonary oedema and it may be necessary to use high doses of fludrocortisone (0.5 to 2.0 mg/ day) if there is no response to fluid restriction alone over a period of 2 to 3 days.

If present, hyperkalaemia presents a serious hazard and requires prompt treatment. It can be due to several causes such as renal failure, glycogen depletion, and skeletal muscle damage. The usual electrocardiographic signs are often obscured by the ECG changes due to hypothermia itself. Ventricular fibrillation may occur suddenly or with little warning since hypothermia enhances the toxic effects of potassium (Maclean and Emslie-Smith, 1977). It is best treated through stimulating glycogen synthesis by the intravenous administration of soluble insulin and glucose.

Antibiotics. In many hypothermic patients who die shortly after recovering normal body temperature, extensive bronchopneumonic changes unsuspected during life are found at postmortem examination. Although in comatose patients the routine use of antibiotics to prevent infection is of doubtful value, occult infection is so often already present in hypothermia that it is advisable to use a wide-spectrum antibiotic such as the intravenous administration of ampicillin (or ampicillin combined with cloxacillin) until the deep-body temperature returns to normal levels.

Thyroid hormones and steroids. Thyroid hormones should not be administered to hypothermic patients. Only if there is a strong suspicion from the clinical history or laboratory evidence that hypothermia is due to myxoedema should tri-iodothyronine be given in small doses (10 μg, 2 or 3 times a day).

It is now recognized that the routine use of hydrocortisone is not required for treatment of accidental hypothermia. Maclean and Emslie-Smith (1977) have shown that not only are plasma 11-OHCS levels elevated in most hypothermic patients but utilization of cortisol is impaired. They have also shown that hypotension in hypothermia is not usually associated with low cortisol levels.

Hyperthermia

The adverse effects of high environmental temperatures on a population are seen mainly in the elderly, and mortality in the older age groups increases dramatically during heat waves. Thermoregulatory impairment due to diminished or absent sweating in older people is thought to be one of the factors responsible for heat stroke in hot conditions.

Mortality in Heat Waves

The United States Vital Statistics Report for the Nation for the years 1952 to 1967 reveal that during heat waves persons over the age of 50 show an increase in deaths from all causes beyond the numbers expected and progressively so with advancing years (Ellis, 1972). In the heat waves which occurred in New York City in July 1972 and in August and September 1973 the excess deaths of the aged population were ascribed mainly to ischaemic heart disease and to a lesser extent to cerebrovascular disease (Ellis, Nelson, and Pincus, 1975). Only a very few deaths were certified as due to the effects of heat illness alone. Macpherson, Ofner, and Welch (1967) have shown that in a large home for the aged in Sydney mortality was lowest when the afternoon temperature was between 21 and 26 °C but was 13 per cent. above average when the temperature ranged between 27 and 32 °C. This effect of temperature became more marked in persons over the age of 70 years.

Even in the more moderate climate of the United Kingdom mortality also changes with fluctuations in environmental temperature (OPCS, 1975, 1976). It is lowest when the mean temperature is about 17 to 18 °C and rises with mean temperatures above 20 °C. To investigate these effects of temperature on mortality it is necessary to study daily records since variations are obscured when monthly patterns of mortality are studied; this is probably because when a heat wave leads to a sudden increase in mortality of those at greatest risk fewer die in the immediately succeeding weeks (Lyster, 1976).

Aetiology

Ellis and coworkers (1976) have drawn attention to the relationship between increased mortality in the elderly in hot conditions and impairment of eccrine sweating. An investigation of sweating responses to thermal stimulation and to the intradermal injection of acetylocholine or methacholine in subjects with a mean age of 70 years compared with the responses in young subjects was carried out by Foster and coworkers (1976). In old people there was marked reduction in sweating activity and an increase in the threshold of sweating, both of which are more pronounced in women than in men. An additional factor accounting for the increased vulnerability to heat of elderly people could be the prevalence of cardiovascular and cerebrovascular disease. Ellis (1976) has emphasized the dangers during heat waves of prescriptions of psychotropic drugs, particularly the phenothiazines which interfere with thermoregulation and suppress sweating.

Clinical Features of Heat Stroke

The manifestations of heat stroke in the elderly are different from those occurring in young healthy adults. Levine (1969) has described some of these features in 25 patients whose average rectal temperature on admission was 41.3 °C. Underlying conditions include arteriosclerotic heart disease, congestive cardiac failure, diabetes mellitus, Parkinsonism, and recent or old stroke. A history of prodromal illness was rarely available but some patients complained of weakness, nausea, vomiting, dizziness, headache, breathlessness, anorexia, and a feeling of warmth. Salient clinical features were dehydration with anhydrosis in the majority of patients (84 per cent.), coma with complete unresponsiveness to painful stimuli (72 per cent.), and signs of pulmonary consolidation (76 per cent.), often due to gram-negative staphylococcal infection. Of the 15 patients in whom the serum sodium levels were estimated 6 had concentrations above 150 meq/l. Elderly patients have a diminished ability to combat dehydration because of depressed sensorium, weakness, and failure of the cardiovascular and renal mechanisms for water conservation. The transfer of the heat from the body core to the periphery may also be impaired because of a diminished ability in older people with cardiovascular disease to make the necessary circulatory adjustments.

Management

The reduction of deep-body temperature can be achieved by cold water sponges and iced baths, but the success of rapid external cooling requires vigorous massage to the skin to counteract reflex peripheral vasoconstriction produced by the markedly elevated core-to-shell thermal gradient induced by external cooling. Circulatory shock occurs in many heat stroke victims and intravenous fluids are required to counteract water and/or salt depletion; in addition there is considerable danger of precipitating pulmonary oedema. The prognosis is very poor due often, as in the case of accidental hypothermia, to the serious nature of the underlying diseases which are found in many elderly patients suffering from hyperthermia.

Tests of Autonomic Function

Many investigations of autonomic function which are commonly used in younger subjects are less suitable for the elderly; these include the measurements of cardiovascular responses to static work, apnoeic face immersion, the Valsalva manoeuvre, and cold pressor tests. In the elderly non-invasive techniques which require little physical or mental effort by the subject are more appropriate. Collins and coworkers (1980) have reported the results of investigation of autonomic function by means of three tests:
(a) beat-to-beat variation in the heart rate during postural change,
(b) vasomotor thermoregulatory function, and
(c) lower body negative pressure.

Heart Rate Response to Standing

The heart rate responsiveness on standing is diminished with increasing age; in young adults the increase is reported to be nearly 20 beats per minute and in middle and old age 10 to 15 beats per minute (Strandell, 1964). In young subjects Ewing and coworkers (1978) found that the most pronounced decrease in the rate

response interval on the electrocardiogram usually occurred at the fifteenth beat, followed by a maximum increase in the interval at the thirtieth beat after standing. This response was consistent in young and older controls but was absent in diabetic patients with autonomic neuropathy. The '30:15' ratio may not, however, be a reliable estimate, particularly as the presence of sinus arrhythmia can significantly influence the value of a pre-selected interbeat interval (Oliver, 1978). In the investigations by Collins, and coworkers (1980) comparison of heart rate responses in 9 normal control subjects (mean age of 24 years) with 11 healthy elderly without evidence of postural hypotension or sinus arrhythmia (mean age of 75 years) showed a pronounced flattening of the response in the elderly (see Fig. 2).

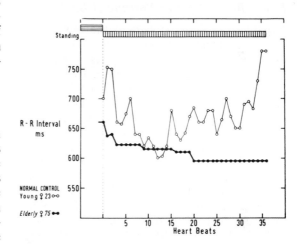

Figure 2   Heart rate response (the rate response interval) on changing from the lying to the standing position in a young subject and an elderly subject

Vasomotor Thermoregulatory Function

A test of thermoregulatory function designed to study temperature control in the zone of vasomotor regulation i.e. between the initiation of sweating or of shivering, has been developed for investigation of elderly patients. The test involves the measurement of physiological responses to a cycle of neutral, cool, and warm environments created by a specially designed air-conditioned test-bed (Fox, 1969) and has proved acceptable to the elderly. One-third of the elderly healthy subjects exhibited abnormal reflex blood flow responses of the hand, mainly as the result of a poor vasoconstrictor response during cooling (Collins *et al.*, 1977). Forty-three per cent. of those with abnormal motor responses to cooling and only 10 per cent. of those with normal responses were found to have postural hypotension indicated by a fall in systolic blood pressure on standing of 20 mmHg or more. In 3 elderly patients who had recovered from episodes of spontaneous hypothermia and in a patient with the Shy–Drager syndrome the constrictor response to cooling was considerably reduced and in addition there was a diminished vasodilator response on warming. It is suggested that a non-constrictor response to cold and postural hypotension are signs indicating an increased liability to hypothermia.

Lower Body Negative Pressure (LBNP)

Negative pressure applied to the lower body causes an increased pooling of blood in the lower extremities and the physiological responses include an increase in heart rate, decreased systolic and mean blood pressure, decreased pulse pressure, a reduction in peripheral and central blood flows, and decreased cardiac output. A progressive LBNP test is well tolerated by elderly people and avoids the practical difficulties inherent in postural tests on relatively immobile patients. Collins and coworkers (1980) have studied the normal pattern of response in young and elderly subjects to a sequence of 2 minute periods of LBNP (-10, -20, -30, -40, and -50 mmHg) separated by 3 minute control intervals. Reduction in systolic blood pressure with little change in diastolic pressure and an increase in heart rate occurred earlier at smaller imposed negative pressures in the elderly than in the young.

The regression of change in blood pressure with change in heart rate during LBNP shows a significant age-related difference in this haemodynamic relationship; a given fall in systolic blood pressure in the elderly is accompanied by a much smaller increment in heart rate (Fig. 3). In the extreme case of a 70 year old woman with the Shy–Drager syndrome there was virtually no change in heart rate, although blood pressure fell precipitously with LBNP. Four elderly patients who were found to have an atonic bladder on urodynamic investigation

also showed a marked intolerance to LBNP. On the other hand those elderly patients whose urinary incontinence was due to detrusor instability were found to have normal blood pressure control for their age during the LBNP test. Three elderly patients with mild hypertension and receiving diuretics and no other hypotensive therapy showed almost no changes in systolic blood pressure, heart rate, and pulse volume during LBNP investigations.

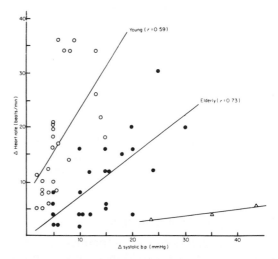

Figure 3 The relationship between increased heart rate and reduction in systolic blood pressure in healthy elderly and young subjects during LBNP tests: ($\circ$) young adults (17 to 35 years), ($\bullet$) elderly (66 to 85 years), and ($\triangle$) a 70 year old patient with Shy–Drager syndrome

REFERENCES

Aminoff, M. J., and Wilcox, C. S. (1971). 'Assessment of autonomic function in patients with Parkinsonian syndrome', *Br. Med. J.*, **iv**, 80–84.

Appenzeller, O., and Descarries, L. (1964). 'Circulatory reflexes in patients with cerebrovascular disease', *New. Engl. J. Med.*, **271**, 820–823.

Bannister, R., Ardill, L., and Fentem, P. (1967). 'Defective autonomic control of blood vessels in idiopathic orthostatic hypotension', *Brain*, **90**, 725–746.

Bannister, R., Davies, B., Holly, E., Rosenthal, T., and Sever, P. (1979). 'Defective cardiovascular reflexes and supersensitivity to sympathomimetic drugs in autonomic failure', *Brain*, **102**, 163–176.

Barraclough, M. A., and Sharpey-Schafer, E. P. (1963). 'Hypotension from absent circulatory reflexes: Effects of alcohol, barbiturates, psychotherapeutic drugs and other mechanisms', *Lancet,* **1**, 1121–1126.

Bauer, H. G. (1954). 'Endocrine and other clinical manifestations of hypothalamic disease: A survey of 60 cases with autopsies', *J. Clin. Endocrinol. Metab.,* **14**, 13–31.

Birchfield, R. I. (1964). 'Postural hypotension in Wernicke's disease', *Am. J. Med.,* **36**, 404–414.

Bristow, J. C., Gribbon, B., Honour, A. J., Pickering, T. G., and Sleight, P. (1969). 'Diminished baroreflex sensitivity in high blood pressure and aging man', *J. Physiol (Lond).,* **202**, 45–46P.

British Medical Association (1964). 'Accidental hypothermia in the elderly', *Br. Med. J.,* **ii**, 1255–1258.

Caird, F. I., Andrews, G. R., and Kennedy, R. D. (1973). 'Effect of posture on blood pressure in the elderly', *Br. Heart J.,* **35**, 527–530.

Collins, K. J. (1982). 'Autonomic failure and the elderly', in *Autonomic Failure* (Ed. R. G. Bannister), Oxford University Press, Oxford.

Collins, K. J., Doré, C., Exton-Smith, A. N., Fox, R. H., MacDonald, I. C., and Woodward, P. M. (1977). 'Accidental hypothermia and impaired temperature homeostasis in the elderly', *Br. Med. J.,* **i**, 353–356.

Collins, K. J., Easton, J. C., and Exton-Smith, A. N. (1981). 'Shivering thermogenesis and vasomotor responses with convective cooling in the elderly', *J. Physiol. (Lond).,* **320**, 76p.

Collins, K. J., Exton-Smith, A. N., James, M. H., and Oliver, D. J. (1980). 'Functional changes in autonomic nervous responses with ageing', *Age Ageing,* **9**, 17–24.

Collins, K. J., Exton-Smith, A. N., and Doré, C. (1981). 'Urban hypothermia: Preferred temperature and thermal perception in old age', *Br. Med. J.,* **282**, 175–177.

Collins, K. J., and Hoinville, E. (1981). 'Temperature requirements in old age', *Building Services Engineering Research and Technology.,* **1**, 165–172.

Croll, W. F., Duthie, R. J., and MacWilliam, J. A. (1935). 'Postural hypotension: Report of a case', *Lancet,* **1**, 194–198.

Duguid, H., Simpson, R. G., and Stowers, J. M. (1961). 'Accidental hypothermia', *Lancet,* **2**, 1213–1219.

Ellis, F. P. (1972). 'Mortality from heat illness and heat-aggravated illness in the United States', *Environ. Res.,* **5**, 1–58.

Ellis, F. P. (1976). 'Heat waves and drugs affecting temperature regulation', *Br. Med. J.,* **iii**, 474.

Ellis, F. P., Exton-Smith, A. N., Foster, K. G. and Weiner, J. S. (1976). 'Mortality during heat waves in very young and very old persons and eccrine sweating', *Isr. J. Med. Sc.,* **12**, 111–116.

Ellis, F. P., Nelson, F., and Pincus, L. (1975). 'Mortality during heat waves in New York City, July 1972 and August–September, 1973', *Environ. Res.,* **10**, 1–13.

Emslie-Smith, D. (1958). 'Accidental hypothermia: A common condition with a pathognomonic ECG', *Lancet,* **2**, 492–495.

Ewing, D. J., Campbell, I. W., and Clarke, B. F. (1976). 'Mortality in diabetic autonomic neuropathy', *Lancet,* **1**, 601–603.

Ewing, D. J., Campbell, I. W., Murray, A., Neilson, J. M. M., and Clarke, B. F. (1978). 'Immediate heart-rate responses to standing: Simple test for autonomic neuropathy in diabetes', *Br. Med. J.,* **i**, 145–147.

Exton-Smith, A. N. (1973). 'Accidental hypothermia', *Br. Med. J.,* **4**, 727.

Exton-Smith, A. N. (1977). 'Functional consequences of ageing: Clinical manifestations', in *Care of the Elderly: Meeting the Challenge of Dependency* (Eds A. N. Exton-Smith and J. Grimley Evans,), Academic Press, London.

Exton-Smith, A. N., Green, M. F., and Fox, R. H. (1975). 'An intensive study of elderly people with particular reference to control of body temperature', in *Proceedings of the Tenth International Congress of Gerontology,* Jerusalem.

Foster, K. G., Ellis, F. P., Doré, C., Exton-Smith, A. N., and Weiner, J. S. (1976). 'Sweat responses in the aged', *Age Ageing,* **5**, 91–101.

Fox, R. H. (1969). 'The controlled-hyperthermia heat tolerance test', in *Human Biology. A Guide to Field Methods* (Eds J. S. Weiner and J. A. Lourie), pp. 359–74, Blackwell, Oxford.

Fox, R. H., Davies, T. W., Marsh, F. P., and Urich, H. (1970). 'Hypothermia in a young man with an anterior hypothalamic lesion', *Lancet,* **2**, 185–188.

Fox, R. H., Wilkins, D. C., Bell, J. A., *et al.* (1973a). 'Spontaneous periodic hypothermia: Diencephalic epilepsy', *Br. Med. J.,* **ii**, 693–695.

Fox, R. H., Woodward, P. M., Exton-Smith, A. N., Green, M. F., Donnison, D. V., and Wicks, M. H. (1973b). 'Body temperatures in the elderly: A national study of physiological, social and environmental conditions', *Br. Med. J.,* **i**, 200–206.

Frolkis, V. V. (1968). 'The autonomic nervous system in the ageing organism', *Triangle,* **8**, 322–328.

Frolkis, V. V., Bezrukov, V. V., Duplenko, Y. P., Shcheglovea, I. V., Shevtchnk, V. G., and Verkhratsky, N. S. (1973). 'Acetylcholine metabolism and cholinergic regulation of functions in aging', *Gerontologia,* **19**, 45–54.

Gale, E. M. and Tattershall, R. B. (1978). 'Hypothermia in a complication of diabetic keto-acidosis'. *Br. Med. J.,* **ii**, 1387–1389.

Goldman, A., Exton-Smith, A. N., Francis, G., and O'Brien, A. (1977). 'Report on a pilot study of low temperature in old people admitted to hospital', *J. Roy. Coll. Physicians, Lond.*, **11**, 291–306.

Gross, M. (1970). 'Circulatory reflexes in cerebral ischaemia involving different vascular territories', *Clin. Sci.*, **38**, 491–502.

Gross, M., Bannister, R., and Godwin-Austen, R. (1972). 'Orthostatic hypotension in Parkinson's disease', *Lancet*, **I**, 174–176.

Johnson, R. H., Smith, A. C., Spalding, J. M. K., and Wollner, L. (1965). 'Effect of posture on blood pressure in elderly patients', *Lancet*, **I**, 731–733.

Johnson, R. H., Park, D. M., and Frankel, H. L. (1971). 'Orthostatic hypotension and the renin-angiotensin system in paraplegia', *Paraplegia*, **9**, 146–152.

Lang, E., Jansen, W., and Pfaff, W. (1975). 'Orthostatische hypotenie bei älteren Menschen', *Med. Klin.*, **70**, 1979.

Ledingham, I. McA., and Mone, J. G. (1972). 'Treatment after exposure to cold', *Lancet*, **1**, 534.

Levine, J. A. (1969). 'Heat stroke in the aged', *Am. J. Med.*, **47**, 251–257.

Low, P. A., Walsh, J. C., Huang, C. Y., and McLeod, J. G. (1975). 'Sympathetic nervous system in diabetic neuropathy – a clinical and pathological study', *Brain*, **98**, 341–356.

Lyster, W. R. (1976). 'Death in summer', *Lancet*, **2**, 469.

Maclean, D., and Browning, M. C. K. (1975a). 'Plasma 11-hydroxycorticosteroid concentrations and prognosis in accidental hypothermia', *Resuscitation*, **3**, 249.

Maclean, D., and Browning, M. C. K. (1975b). 'Cortisol utilization in accidental hypothermia', *Resuscitation*, **3**, 257.

Maclean, D., and Emslie-Smith, D. (1977). *Accidental Hypothermia*, Blackwell, Oxford.

Maclean, D., Griffiths, T. D., and Emslie-Smith, D. (1968). 'Serum enzymes in relation to electrocardiographic changes in accidental hypothermia', *Lancet*, **2**, 1266.

Macmillan, A. L., Corbett, J. L., Johnson, R. H., Smith, A. C., Spalding, J. M. K., and Wollner, L. (1967). 'Temperature regulation in survivors of accidental hypothermia of the elderly', *Lancet*, **2**, 165–169.

McNicol, M. W., and Smith, R. (1964). 'Accidental hypothermia', *Br. Med. J.*, **i**, 19–21.

Macpherson, R. K., Ofner, F., and Welch, J. A. (1967). 'Effect of prevailing air temperature on mortality', *Brit. J. Prev. Soc. Med.*, **21**, 1–17.

Man In't Veld A. J., and Schalekamp, M. A. D. H. (1981). 'Pindolol acts as a beta-adrenoceptor agonist in orthostatic hypotension: Therapeutic implications'. *Br. Med. J.*, **282**, 929.

Mills, G. L. (1973). 'Accidental hypothermia in the elderly', *Brit. J. Hosp. Med.*, **10**, 691–699.

Odel, H.M., Roth, G. M., and Kealing, F. R. (1955). 'Autonomic neuropathy simulating the effects of sympathectomy as a complication of diabetes mellitus', *Diabetes*, **4**, 92–98.

Oliver, D. J. (1978). 'Heart-rate response to standing as a test for autonomic neuropathy', *Br. Med. J.*, **1**, 1349–50.

OPCS (1975, 1976). *Monitor*, Office of Population Censuses and Surveys, London.

Osborn, J. J. (1953). 'Experimental hypothermia: Respiratory and blood pH changes in relation to cardiac function', *Am. J. Physiol.*, **175**, 389–398.

Overstall, P. W., Imms, F. J., Exton-Smith, A. N., and Johnson, A. L. (1977). 'Falls in the elderly related to postural imbalance', *Br. Med. J.*, **1**, 261.

Overstall, P. W., Johnson, A. L., and Exton-Smith, A. N. (1978). 'Instability and falls in the elderly', *Age Ageing*, **7** (Suppl.), 92.

Perkins, C. M., and Lee, M. R. (1978). 'Flurbiprofen and fludrocortisone in severe autonomic neuropathy', *Lancet*, **2**, 1058.

Phillip, G., and Smith, J. F. (1973). 'Hypothermia and Wernicke's encephalopathy', *Lancet*, **2**, 122.

Roberts, A. H. (1970). 'Neurological complications of systemic diseases', *Br. Med. J.*, **i**, 33–35.

Rosin, A., and Exton-Smith, A. N. (1964). 'Clinical features of accidental hypothermia with observations on thyroid function', *Br. Med. J.*, **i**, 16–19.

Royal College of Physicians of London (1966). Report of the Committee on Accidental Hypothermia.

Rundles, R. W. (1945). 'Diabetic neuropathy: General review with report of 125 cases', *Medicine*, **24**, 111–160.

Sharpey-Schafer, E. P. (1956). 'Circulatory reflexes in chronic disease of the afferent nervous system', *J. Physiol. (Lond).*, **134**, 1–10.

Sharpey-Schafer, E. P., and Taylor, P. J. (1960). 'Absent circulatory reflexes in diabetic neuritis', *Lancet*, **1**, 559–562.

Shy, G. M., and Drager, G. A. (1960). 'A neurological syndrome associated with orthostatic hypotension', *Arch. Neurol.*, **2**, 511–527.

Spokes, E. G., Bannister, R., and Oppenheimer, D. R. (1979). 'Multiple system atrophy with autonomic failure: Clinical, histological and neurochemical observations on four cases', *J. Neurol. Sci.*, **43**, 59–82.

Strandell, T. (1964). 'Circulatory studies in healthy old men', *Acta. Med. Scand.*, **175** (Suppl. 414), 1–44.

Thomas, J. E., and Schirger, A. (1963). 'Neurologic manifestations in idiopathic orthostatic hypotension'. *Arch. Neurol.*, **8**, 204–208.

Thorner, M. O. (1975). 'Dopamine is an important neurotransmitter in the autonomic nervous system'. *Lancet,* **1**, 662–664.

Timiras, P. S. (1972). *Developmental Physiology and Ageing,* pp. 502–526, Macmillan, New York.

Vestal, R. E., Wood, A. J., and Shand, D. G. (1979). 'Reduced beta-adrenoreceptor sensitivity in the elderly', *Clin. Pharmacol. Ther.,* **26**, 181–186.

Wilkins, R. W., Culbertson, J. W., and Ingelfinger, F. L. (1951). 'Effect of splanchnic sympathectomy in hypertensive patients', *J. Clin Invest.,* **30**, 312–319.

Ziegler, M. G. (1980). 'Postural hypotension', *Ann. Rev. Med.,* **31**, 239–245.

17

Psychiatry of the Elderly

Principles and Practice of Geriatric Medicine
Edited by M. S. J. Pathy
© 1985 John Wiley & Sons Ltd

17.1

Psychiatry of the Elderly

S. P. Hodgson, D. J. Jolley

THE SIGNIFICANCE OF THE ELDERLY FOR PSYCHIATRY

The metamorphosis of the human condition occasioned by increasing numbers of old people in developed and developing parts of the world is happening as surely and silently as the opening of a flower, perceptible and appreciated only with the help of slow motion photography. More people survive into old age, and the next 30 years will see the very old—75 plus and 85 plus—achieving even greater significance (Fig. 1a and b). While most of the increase in number of old people is attributable to improved life expectation among the young, survival within old age and particularly among disabled old people has also increased (Fig. 2) (Office of Health Economics, 1979).

These changes face us as individuals, families, and society with challenges that are new and unexplored, most especially within aspects of emotional and mental life. Thus they have implications for all those agencies of society that are involved with helping people when personal adjustments break down in response to these changes.

Psychiatric services in Great Britain over the past hundred years have been provided by the mental hospital system: large county asylums offering safety, understanding, and variably enlightened management to the mentally ill set apart for a while (short or long) from the rest of society (Jones and Sidebotham, 1962) Over

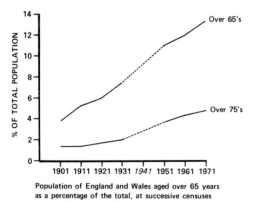

Population of England and Wales aged over 65 years as a percentage of the total, at successive censuses

(a)

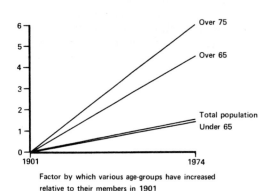

Factor by which various age-groups have increased relative to their members in 1901

(b)

Figure 1   (a) Population of England and Wales aged over 65 years as a percentage of the total, at successive censuses. (b) Factor by which various age groups have increased relative their members in 1901

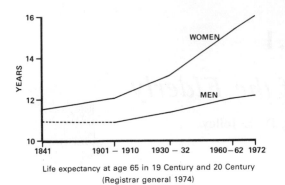

Life expectancy at age 65 in 19 Century and 20 Century
(Registrar general 1974)

Figure 2   Life expectancy at the age of 65 in the nineteenth and twentieth centuries

90 per cent. of all mental illness beds are still provided in these county asylums (DHSS, 1975), despite the move since the 1950s to offer newly avilable forms of assessment and treatment through smaller general hospital psychiatric units and support within the community rather than apart from it (Hawks, 1975). The number of mental illness (mainly mental hospital) beds in England has been reduced from about 105,000 in 1971 to 84,000 in 1976 (a drop of 20 per cent.). The elderly now occupy over 45 per cent. of all mental illness beds and annual admission rates of the elderly have increased by 14 per cent. compared with a 0.6 per cent. increase for under sixty-five's— a twenty-threefold differential in favour of old age (DHSS, 1973a, 1975, 1979). In part this reflects the nature and needs of the mental disorders of old age, which are different in emphasis from those affecting the young. Yet the contribution of old people to psychiatric service clientele varies widely, depending on

the interest and style of work of the service as much as on the needs of the local population (Sainsbury, Costain, and Grad, 1965). General hospital and teaching hospital units admit disproportionately fewer elderly, 14 per cent. as against 20 per cent. of mental hospital admissions (DHSS, 1973a), for they prefer younger clients with more real or supposed potential for cure (Smith, 1961) (Fig. 3). Thus, comparing Wessex with the North West Region, the first admission rates of the over 75 age group to mental institutions in Wessex were twice those in the North West—514 as against 229 per 100,000 population (DHSS, 1979). Within these regions individual mental hospitals (e.g. Herrison and Prestwich Hospitals) reflect these differences: 345 admissions to Herrison (Wessex) compared with 171 to Prestwich (NWRHA) contributing 24 and 14 per cent., respectively, of all admissions for the year 1969 (DHSS 1973b).

As more services become closely involved with their local communities they inevitably come into contact with more old people. These, by virtue of their multidimensional problems, containing physical and social as well as emotional or mental components, bring psychiatry into a progressively closer working relationship with the primary health care services, social service departments and other hospital specialties, especially geriatric medicine (Jolley and Arie, 1978).

CHANGING EXPECTATIONS

Industrial wealth has purchased not only more life, greater life expectation, and greater population size, but also a higher quality of life if

AGES	ALL AGES		OVER 65		UNDER 65	
	1971	1976	1971	1976	1971	1976
ALL UNITS	173,230	178,841 (↑ 3%)	34,383	39,221 (↑ 14%)	138,847	139,620 (↑ 0.6%)
MHs	125,600	121,285 (↓ 3%)	26,625 = 21% of MH admissions		98,975 = 79% of MH admissions	
DGHs	29,083	51802 (↑ 75%)	4,183 = 14% of DGH admissions		24,900 = 86% of DGH admissions	
THs	7,417		741		6,670	
MH = MENTAL HOSPITALS, DGH = DISTRICT GENERAL HOSPITALS, TH = TEACHING HOSPITALS						

Figure 3   Admissions for mental illness in 1971 and 1976 for England by age and type of unit (DHSS, 1973, C, 1979)

this is measured in terms of material comforts and time available for leisure, pleasure, and self-fulfilment (McKeown, 1976). Within the life-time of octogenarians a decent education has become the right of everyone rather than the privilege of a few. Work done is rewarded with equable pay, working hours are strictly controlled, conditions of work are required to meet defined standards, and exploitation which was commonplace is virtually unknown. Even exposure to unemployment is buffered from the naked poverty that it brought in the 1930s. Compulsory retirement may have its drawbacks, but the previous requirement to 'work until you drop, then starve until you die' was not so cosy. Food is more plentiful, is available in richer variety throughout the year, and is more hygienically prepared and packaged. Heating may be safely programmed throughout the house by a timeswitch where it used to be coaxed by fumbling fingers to flicker from damp and sooty coals. Domestic light source has passed from candle power, through oil lamps, the gaselier, to the ubiquitous electric light bulb, summoned by the flick of a switch. Communication over long distances can be achieved in an instant by telephone, radio, or television where long journeys by foot or horsepower would have been the only possibility. Family size has reduced. Mobility of able family members to distant parts of this country and the rest of the world has become commonplace. Women have achieved emancipation and share in the growing expectation of an entertaining, rewarding, and (often) easier life (Jefferys, 1978.)

When problems arise, particularly in association with ill-health, people have come to expect considerate, efficient, and effective response from health services, comparable in quality with that attendant upon their whims or needs from other industries. Yet it is well within the memory of our older citizens that the trials of life were to be accepted and endured by families with little expectation of outside help, which when available was spartan and ignorant by today's standards, even if kind (Blythe, 1969). For the mentally ill 'help' was to be suffered to exist in the community or the workhouse; 'treatment' was removal to the asylum, for those so disordered as to require certification. In hospitals, the efficacy of curtailing illness and its complications has rapidly increased and therewith expectations have changed, among both patients and staff, from the 'care' of L'hopital of the monastries to the 'cure' of modern medicine. Beds, including beds in mental illness hospitals, are not now seen as places of rest but expensive elements of the treatment machinery and must achieve an acceptable 'turnover' or 'throughput'. Patients do not expect to be crushed into overcrowded wards nor to be stripped of dignity nor deprived of their rights and respect as citizens. Where an institution fails to provide the expected standard, such failure is unlikely to be excused as charitable in intent but risks the consequences of exposure and scandal (Committee of Inquiry into Whittingham Hospital, 1972).

Medicine has certainly become much more potent than it was, with an impressive array of medication and hardware that produces effective treatment of many conditions both physical and mental. Yet success with acute exacerbations of illnesses has not rid mankind of the chronic component of many conditions. Indeed, undesirable effects of treatments themselves sometimes give rise to symptoms which pose problems or require endurance. Many of the illnesses, including mental illnesses, suffered by old people have chronic components and the accumulation of these within individuals leads to the characteristic population profile that shows disabilities concentrated in the elderly. Even disabled old people prefer for the most part to live in their own homes and they still, despite the general expectation of an easy life, receive most of the support they need from within their family. An elderly spouse, a daughter living with them or nearby, a sister or brother, daughter-in-law, son, or even 'just a neighbour' may take on a major caring role. Professional support to people at home – by primary health care services; general practitioners working with health visitors, district nurses, and perhaps other auxilliary staff, and by social service departments; social workers, home helps, meals-on-wheels, neighbourhood wardens—has increased tremendously since World War II. These 'domiciliary services' are exposed to the same scrutiny and expectation of high quality, understanding, competence, and efficient delivery as has been associated with the institutional sector. Yet here, in the matrix of interrelated and sometimes opposed wishes and expectations of patient, lay supporters, professional supporters, and advisers, lies great potential for conflict and misunderstanding. A life style that includes considerable personal suffering, risk, inconvenience, and lack of time for leisure or pleasure may be bearable to a 70 year old who has experienced and observed much worse privations within her lifespan and may certainly appear to her to be preferable to the prospect of giving up 'home' for the sterile security and convenience of an institutionalized finale. An attendant daughter-in-law, seeing the progressive unrelenting suffering of her old relative who is determined to live on at home, the risks growing, not diminishing, and her own anxiety unassuaged, may find intolerable the demands this life style makes upon her—precluding such full attention to her growing family, career prospects, and leisure pursuits as she has learned to think is proper within the context of the very different life she herself has known.

PSYCHIATRIC CLINICAL METHOD

Thinking, feeling (emotionally), willing, perceiving, understanding, believing, communicating by words and gestures—these are often complex, subtle, and 'difficult-to-define' phenomena, yet the essence of humanity. When faced with problems which have their origin in these elements of being it is helpful to adopt a consistent strategy for collecting and marshalling information so that logical and useful interpretation of the facts can be made. Varied and interesting these phenomena are, and they deserve the dignity of clear and orderly consideration routinely applied to other clinical symptomatology. Woolly thinking in the face of their complexity renders no good service.

The clinician's burden in determining and evaluating an elderly person's mental state is to gain an understanding of what is normal for that patient and for her peer group, and to clarify what deviation from the individual and/or peer group norm is present. The method used rests securely on obtaining a full and reliable history of the development of the patient and her problem, examination of her current mental state and physical state, supported where necessary by further special investiga-

tions; the key aspects are shown in Fig. 4a and b. It is often preferable to make initial contact with the patient at her own home, by a domiciliary visit. This has a number of advantages including the speed and flexibility with which the clinician can get to the patient. The patient is often more confident and able to demonstrate or discuss her problems without the added fear or confusion produced by the alien territory of hospital or the examination room. In addition a wealth of material evidence of her previous and present life style, including

---

(a) HISTORY

Presenting complaint
History of presenting complaint
Past illnesses – psychiatric
                 medical and surgical
Family history of illnesses – psychiatric
                               medical and surgical
Personal history
Premorbid personality
Drugs: prescribed, non-prescribed, alcohol, tobacco

(b) MENTAL STATE

Appearance – person and personal surroundings
Behaviour
Talk
Mood
Thought
Beliefs – to delusions
Perceptions – to hallucinations
Cognitive functions – concentration and attention
                       orientation
                       memory
                       new learning
                       calculation
                       abstract/conceptual thinking
                       IQ

(c) FORMULATION

Precis of the phenomena
Differential diagnosis
Aetiological factors
Special investigations – physical
                         psychiatric
                         psychological
                         social
Management – immediate
             long term
Predicted outcome – short term
                     long term
Review

Figure 4   Psychiatric history-taking and examination

support from others, be they family or professional, is available at home and difficult to reconstruct in the clinic (Arie and Jolley, 1982). When a domiciliary visit is not practical, e.g. when a patient is already in hospital for another reason, information collected by a social worker colleague is of invaluable help to the clinician.

History

History (Fig. 4a) has to be obtained from a reliable informant other than the patient. This is not to say that the patient's version of developments is to be disregarded, it is all important. Yet her view is coloured and may be distorted by her current mental state. This is obvious when a grossly confused old man presents aspects of battalion life during World War I as current issues. It may be less obvious, but just as pertinent, when a painfully guilt-ridden old lady describes her current woes as the inevitable consequences of misdemenours from her past. An objective analysis may present her as rather less tarnished in reality than the rest of mankind.

Presenting Complaint

Here should be determined, firstly, exactly what has brought the patient to attention. Often it is not she herself who has sought advice but others who care for her have encouraged her, or come to ask for help on her behalf. An understanding of what constitutes the problem identified by the patient and/or her supporters lays the foundation for providing an acceptable remedy. Many fruitless hours and pounds sterling can be spent pursuing false problems that appear interesting or important to the medical man, but are of no consequence to the patient.

History of Presenting Complaint

Here a careful reconstruction of the development of the problem sets out the time sequence of events and changes in experience and/or behaviour of the patient. The occurrence of changes in the social circumstances of the patient and, identification of apparently 'key'

events which have triggered change or seemed to weigh unduly heavily on her mind are important. Indeed, it is probable that extra life events, be they pleasant or unpleasant, are stressful and may be associated with illness (Brown, Harris, and Copeland, 1977). Anniversaries of times good or bad may not be easy to identify but very pertinent. Similarly, the passage into a time of life which is beyond one's parents' lifespan of years, or during which family members have had misfortunes, is stressful, but not always brought out for consideration. Recognized physical illnesses and changes of medication are clearly important events and need to be noted accurately. The order of changes in behaviour and experience and the presence of fluctuations in behaviour between days and within days must all be carefully teased out and catalogued.

Previous Illnesses

Previous physical illnesses should be noted in time sequence with an indication of what management was undertaken at the time (hospital admission, operation, medication). Similarly, previous psychiatric illnesses should be recorded in chronological order together with the treatment received, if any. It may be necessary to further explore and corroborate these accounts by discussion with the general practitioner and access to hospital notes. Previous patterns of illness may be recurring or may colour a newly emerging pathology.

Family Illnesses

It is useful to construct a limited family tree, to include siblings, parents, and children at least. Grandparents and more distant relatives may be mentioned if they have significant illnesses. Familial physical illnesses may contribute to the current problem by their presence or because the patient becomes preoccupied with the possibility that they will occur.

In terms of psychiatric history, familial inheritance of the mental disorders of late life does occur, most notably in some dementing illnesses and also in the functional psychoses of old age, although found here less frequently

than among their equivalents with early onset
(Slater and Cowie, 1971).

Personal History

Old people have lived a long time and thus
they have passed through a series of personal
epochs, and also related to a wider world which
has changed progressively from their infancy
to senium. 'Where were you brought up?'
'What did your father do?' 'How many of you
were there in the family?' These are questions
usually accepted with considerable appetite
and in the response lies the beginning of understanding of what made this individual tick,
and how she has ticked from then on. What
sort of schooling? What sort of job record?
Has she 'made good', or been one of many, or
slipped from grace? Courtship, marriage,
householding, parenthood, retirement, widowhood, perhaps remarriage—a series of situations demanding differing qualities from the
role-holder. No two life stories are the same;
each tale is a source of interest and delight
yielding valuable clues when it comes to un-
ravelling the riddle of the present problem,
experience, or behaviour.

Personality

A good deal of information about the patient's
style of living and style of responding to situations in general and particular terms will have
emerged during the collation of his/her personal history. Ambition or the lack of it will
shout clear from the overall structure. Personality traits may have underlain career choices:
e.g. clerical jobs require neat and tidy minds,
management demands a certain ruthlessness
and ability to make decisions. An inability to
make lasting relationships may lead to failed
marriage and friendships or a rapidly changing
work record. Suspicion of others may lead to
a cold marriage ('emotional divorce') or restless moving from one house to another without
ever establishing 'home'. It is difficult and generally unsatisfactory to produce a 'classification' of personality types, but it is possible to
identify characteristic attitudes and responses,
interests and capacities that provide an accurate reflection of usual personality function for
the individual and within which the changed
aspects can be identified.

Habits

The regular taking of drugs and of smoking
and drinking alcohol are of sufficient significance to deserve a special note, as are any
changes in these habits.

Mental State

While the history of the patient and her problem requires to be corroborated or corrected
by another witness, the 'mental state' (Fig. 4b)
is determined at clinical interview but may take
into account information from other sources,
e.g. nursing staff who are able to make observations over longer periods. It may be necessary to accumulate evidence for the complete
mental state over a number of interviews for
two major reasons. Firstly, nothing is gained
by pressing on, steamroller-like, through a prescribed examination format when the patient's
concentration span has been exceeded. Secondly, a single 'cross-sectional' view of the patient is insufficient data on which to base a
diagnosis and formulation of psychiatric illness
since fluctuations are common and the consistency or variability of the mental state over
time is a vital observation. Time is an important tool in gaining the patient's confidence;
listening and looking are its preferred acces-
sories and questions must be used carefully
only to refine understanding.

General Description

Starting at the outside and working gradually
into the strata of mental function, nothing useful should be disregarded. The state of a house
and garden informs wonderfully about the oc-
cupant's past and present interests and competence. Her appearance, including state of
dress, hair, teeth, use of walking aides,
hearing-aide, evidence of incontinence or continence sets the scene for further examination.
How does she respond to the suggested interview? Can she settle down for a chat or is she
repeatedly wandering off to other matters, or
wringing her hands or shouting at (imaginary)
persecutors?

In addition to a full description of the individual in these terms, many clinicians make
routine use of scales that cover some of the
most common dimensions of behavioural ab-

normality or decline encountered in geriatric psychiatry (Wilkin and Jolley, 1978). This allows crude comparison between the behaviour of groups of patients and can be used to monitor changes in individuals over time.

Talk

Is the flow of talk spontaneous or only when encouraged? Is there pressure of talk, or is speech slow and retarded. Is there evidence of dysphasia, perseveration, flight of ideas, circumstantiality, or other thought disorder? Is articulation impaired, and is the rhythm and timbre of speech controlled? The content of talk may be colourful or gloomy as particular themes dominate conversation; ideas of physical illness, guilt, persecution, riches, family long dead, etc.

Mood (Affect)

It is conveyed in words, ideas, form of speech and tone of voice, facial expression, and bodily posture as well as physical and psychological functioning. Too much melancholy, irritability, hostility, fear, or happiness may be apparent in the major mood disorders and 'blunting' or inappropriateness of affect may be the result of a chronic schizophrenic illness. The organic dementias also impair mood control which may become shallow and unresponsive or give way to 'catastrophic' outbursts under minimal pressure with 'emotional incontinence' demonstrated particularly in arteriosclerotic brain syndromes. Enquiry should be made about interests, appetite, weight, sleep, concentration, and the possibility of variation in mood, which may have a daily pattern.

Thought

The form of thought can be altered in terms of its rate and understandability. Is thinking fast or slow? Are associations running wild or following a logical sequence? Is there intrusion of thoughts from elsewhere? Is there evidence of distractability?

Content

Particular themes may be intruding on thinking to the exclusion of others and preoccupation with or obsessional rumination upon these themes may be dominating mental life and preventing realistic interaction with the world around the patient.

Belief

Unusual beliefs may be held because of the cultural background of the patient. All sorts of old wives' tales persist in the minds of old wives (and husbands), leading them to all manner of strange activities – especially taking potions for their bowels, etc. Sometimes individuals take an element of local tradition and become slave to it – it becomes an overvalued idea. Simple misunderstanding may lead to strange beliefs, but when an abnormal belief is held with unshakeable intensity and is outside the normal cultural and experiential context of the patient it is termed a delusion. Some delusions appear to be secondary to other abnormalities, such as disordered mood (e.g. a severely depressed man may be convinced of his own imagined poverty)and perception (e.g. auditory hallucinations, such as telling a widow she is to be killed and convincing her of this). Other delusions appear to be 'primary', arising 'out-of-the-blue' – in the elderly these may occur in acute organic confusional states but in the absence of coarse brain disease like this they are characteristic of schizophrenia.

Perception

Perceptions that are in themselves accurate may be misinterpreted, as when a patient who is convinced that she is dying of cancer infers from the consultant's action (in failing to discuss her case at the end of the bed) that he has done so to avoid burdening her with the painful truth. When perfectly innocent events or actions are repeatedly felt to be of special significance by a patient—'I can tell from the way people look at me and then turn away'—the patient is experiencing ideas of reference.

False perceptions may be based on real stimuli, sight, sound, etc., and be distorted in the process of perception: e.g. shadows on the curtains being seen as writhing snakes; this is an illusion. Visual illusions are particularly common in acute organic psychosyndromes. Hallucinations occur when false perceptions arise without any recognizable real stimulus, they may occur in any sensory modality but auditory hallucinations are particularly common in the persecutory states of late life.

Obsessional Phenomena

These are thoughts, words, deeds, or feelings that the patient recognizes to be her own but enter consciousness repeatedly. They are recognized as inappropriate or silly in the circumstances and are actively resisted, yet they recur and cause great distress. Thus they are pathological and different in kind from productive checking traits that they are accepted by some 'obsessional' people as part and parcel of their style of living.

Cognitive Function

Changes occur in cognitive function with normal ageing and because pathological dementing and confusional syndromes are quite common in the elderly, examination of cognitive function is very important. It must be carried out carefully and with sensible regard for its limitations. When the patient is temporarily fearful or severely depressed she may also do poorly on formal testing and would be badly served indeed if proffered a diagnostic label suggesting irreversible decline.

Intelligence and educational level. Many elderly people received only an elementary education and some did not have the opportunity to learn to read and write. An estimate of intelligence can be obtained from work records, ability to cope with shopping, government forms, and so on. The patient's vocabulary and arithmetic calculations including the use of new and old currency adds a further dimension.

Orientation. Orientation in time, place, and person should be investigated. Such information is permanently lost only in severe dementing illness but goes early in acute confusional states and generally is lost in the order quoted, i.e. one's identification of self lasts beyond the awareness of place or time.

Memory. Long-term memory generally survives until the later stages of dementing illnesses, or at least may contain sufficient retrievable information to allow the patient to give some correct answers. Thus it is good practice to begin exploring this aspect of memory first. Retrieval of more recently stored (short-term) information may not be so easy and new learning, of material presented at the interview, is a very sensitive test of memory impairment. Indeed, it may be too sensitive for reliable use with many old people, giving false positive identification of 'organicity'.

To circumvent the possibility of worrying the patient with complicated tasks of doubtful value, many centres have produced simple rating scales of memory and orientation (Qureshi and Hodkinson, 1974). These are useful, have good interscale reliability, and one at least has been demonstrated to correlate closely with pathological and biochemical evidence of cerebral impairment (Blessed, Tomlinson, and Roth, 1968). Even so, these scales must be understood and used as measures of performance and not as diagnostic tools. Diagnosis rests on the collation of the breadth of material available from the whole of the history and mental state and not on one simple paper and pencil test!

In addition, a number of other simple and acceptable tests of intellectual function have been produced for research purposes (e.g. the set test of Isaacs and Akhtar, 1972) or for work with more impaired patients. These, too, may be found useful in the clinical setting.

Concentration. This is traditionally measured from the speed taken to perform simple serial intellectual tasks, e.g. rehearsing the months of the year, counter calendar, from December to January, or serial subtractions of 7 starting at 100. These tests can be used with the elderly but should not exhaust the patient.

Abstraction. Tests of abstract thinking, e.g. by the interpretation of proverbs, analysis of differences, and similarities, can be used with the elderly but their interpretation may not be easy, given that educational opportunities were limited 80 years ago.

Further investigation of cognitive function may require the expertise of the clinical psychologist.

Full Physical Examination

This is mandatory, including particular attention to neurological status.

Special Investigations

A full blood picture, urinanalysis, and chest X-ray are justifiable as routine. Wider investigations, in physical, psychological, and social spheres, may be indicated by clinical findings or suspicion.

Formulation

The purpose of the formulation (Fig. 4c) is to present the abnormal phenomena identified in a concise summary together with key aspects of personality and personal context and from these to argue a differential diagnosis and aetiology. Thence a plan of further assessment and investigation can lead on to propose therapeutic interventions, with an estimate of their likely outcome. In addition the formulation provides a scheme which can be reviewed and revised in a methodical way when events (as quite often) take a different turn from those predicted.

CLASSIFICATION OR FRAMEWORK FOR THINKING ABOUT PSYCHIATRIC DISORDERS

British psychiatry has adopted a system of classification based on syndromes that were identified by the meticulous labours of German alienists at and around the turn of the century. Their method was based on systematic study of the mental status of patients presented to them in their mental hospital work and follow-up of these patients, often for a lifetime (Kraepelin, 1909). Psychiatrists first dealt only within hospitals, with lunacy—mental disorder so great that incarceration was required. The development of psychiatry as a medical discipline and the vast development of hospital services led to the possibility of mentally ill folk, not so disturbed that compulsory admission was needed, being permitted to voluntarily seek treatment. The further extension this century of the boundaries of medical services and the concepts of what constitutes doctors'

business has made help available to people whose habitual emotional reactions are disabling.

(i) Eccentric Life Styles and Abnormal Adjustments

Some extraordinary people establish themselves as outside the normal range early in life and remain so. Subnormality of intellect is perhaps the easiest example of this to understand; determined by 'culture' or pathology it renders the person less able than others and vulnerable at times of stress. Similarly people with abnormal personalities consistently behave outside the normal run of mankind, being characteristically more impulsive, more meticulous, more energetic, cyclothymic, depressive, or hypochondriacal depending on their particular bent. Such eccentricities may lead individuals to be prone to neurotic breakdowns. Yet neurotic disorders (usually anxiety, or depression 'understandable' in terms of what has happened to the patient) can and do occur in well-balanced personalities who are found out by major stresses which threaten their adjustment, especially at times of physical illness (Bergmann, 1971).

Functional Psychoses

These represent major departures from the sufferer's usual mode of being, but they occur in clear consciousness and no pathological changes in the brain have been identified sufficiently to account for the changes. These illnesses are the affective psychoses; depressive or bipolar (manic-depressive) psychoses, and the schizophrenic psychoses.

Organic Psychoses

In these psychoses the abnormalities of mental state are attributable to demonstrable organic changes affecting the brain directly or indirectly from bodily disease. They are usefully described as the acute confusional states and subacute confusional states (delirium), and the chronic organic psychosyndromes – the dementias.

The broad categories we have introduced are not mutually exclusive, and indeed they reflect only one kind of classification – a phenomenological division (Fig. 5). The affective disorders, for example, lend themselves to be viewed as a spectrum—the range of symptoms being spread along the neurotic–psychotic axis but not necessarily relating directly to aetiology, or to treatment. Abnormal personalities can certainly suffer severe depressive illness, schizophrenia, or an organic psychosyndrome.

QUANTITATIVE VARIATIONS	QUALITATIVE VARIATIONS
Eccentric adjustments Abnormal personalities	Functional psychoses Organic psychoses Delirium
Neurotic disorders	Dementia
Neurotic Symptoms AFFECTIVE DISORDERS	Psychotic Symptoms

Figure 5 A framework of psychiatric disorders

People with established schizophrenia or manic-depressive illness may dement or become acutely confused. People suffering from progressive dementias may become profoundly depressed, etc. It is important to keep the possibility of such changes and combinations in mind when dealing with elderly patients and to resist the temptation to label all mental abnormality in old people as 'organic' or 'dementia'. A depressed man who has had a stroke certainly has cerebrovascular disease, but his depression can be addressed in its own right, and may well be reversible even though the cerebrovascular disease is not.

RECOGNIZABLE MAIN THEMES

Personality Disorders, Subnormality, and Psychoneuroses

'Personality' is a multidimensional concept encompassing physique, emotional tenor and control, drive, intellect, and more. Eccentricity derives from excess or deficiencies on one or more of these dimensions and thus accommodates disorders of personality ranging from those with positive, outgoing, disruptive features to the obverse—negative, reserved, self-effacing characteristics. In addition, creative genius, high intelligence, or subnormality can be usefully considered along with other life styles that deviate throughout from the stat-

istical norm. Personality which has become established through adolescence into early adult life generally endures into old age unless disrupted by a serious mental illness or brain damage, but ageing carries with it a quietening of drives and emotions, thus 'characters' outstanding through positive, outgoing, aggressive behaviour become less 'troublesome', but the quiet and withdrawn frequently become even more incapacitated and may become a cause for concern. Thus serious personality difficulties constitute a dwindling group of psychiatric referrals in advanced life as emotional maturity and the waning of powerful drives operate in conjunction with social changes that take older people away from the arena of multiple personal contacts that fuel conflict. These same social changes hasten the personally withdrawn character into vulnerability from intensified isolation.

Events such as physical illness or induced social change bring hidden deviance into the light of extended human contact. Illness may mean that interference (treatment) from other people becomes essential. Careful attendants may find themselves abused and bewildered by the demands of a 'patient' who shouts out a child-like insistence on immediate satisfaction (Nurse! Nurse!) but can never be satisfied. Other patterns of abnormality include opinionated, domineering postures that bespeak fierce independence but belie a perverse and clinging dependence; the structure of caring has presented itself as 'meat' to a slumbering but well-practised style which has poisoned relationships in earlier life. Small wonder (to illustrate further) that when her husband died her children kept well away and that a series of potential friends and helpers have retreated in self-defence. Illness is a very powerful 'possession' to such people, for others find retreat taboo in the face of it. In a similar way changed social circumstances such as rehousing into a 'sheltered' housing complex, admission to a residential home, or even modernization of an existing home may provide an arena in which previous personal battles are reenacted.

A number of systems that attempt to classify personality deviations are available (Eysenck, 1952; Schneider, 1923) but frequently prove simplistic and too rigid to accommodate the subtleties and complexities presented by individual deviants. It is best to identify the individual's life themes of attitude, emotion, behaviour, etc., as evidenced by performance in various life situations. This makes it possible to understand current patterns of response and to plan strategies of management that will avoid or reduce predictable consequences for the abnormal personality.

Deviant intellectual ability, especially subnormality, may also 'come to light' consequent upon the demands made of individuals to cope with old age's toll of possible ill-health, relative poverty, living alone, etc. (Nunn *et al.*, 1974). Deviant personalities (including intellects) are associated with vulnerability to neurotic disorders—emotional reactions that are an understandable response to the stress that causes them but pathological in the intensity, duration, and sometimes form of that reaction.

Anxiety State

An anxiety state is characterized by the emotion of fear spread out thin and associated with autonomic nervous system overactivity, sweating, trembling, palpitations, dry mouth, etc., and is rarely seen in pure culture in the elderly. It is usually contaminated by depressive feelings, hypochondriasis, or obsessional symptoms.

Depressive Neurosis

Depressive neurosis is the most common syndrome and includes persistent or variable sadness, weeping, excessive worrying, wakefulness, and bad dreams. There is decline in interests, appetite, and sociability and the ability to concentrate on and gain enjoyment from matters of the moment wanes. Time is spent ruminating on misfortunes or missed fortunes. Such reminiscence and recrimination moves the sufferer nearer to doubt and despair that anything more worth while can be achieved or experienced. Failure to seek help, non-compliance with treatment for intercurrent physical illness, and even self-injury, self-poisoning, or suicide may occur.

Obsessional Symptoms

Obsessional symptoms are not uncommon in old age. Obsessional traits of checking may become more marked and eventually become disabling as no decision can be sustained and the sufferer flounders in a 'folie de doute'. Obsessional-compulsive syndromes sometimes arise in this age group with thoughts, feelings, or behaviour repeatedly taking over consciousness and receiving resistance as they are recognized as foolish and inappropriate, but these are usually evidence of underlying depressive illness or physical disorder.

Hypochondriasis

The morbid preoccupation with ideas and complaints of ill-health may persist as an established personality trait, but arising or intensified in old age it is frequently symptomatic of a depressive or real physical illness.

Hysterical Conversion Symptoms

Hysterical conversion symptoms are seen in the elderly and always indicate the presence of more serious disorders such as depressive states, confusional states, or physical illness.

Roughly 20 per cent. of old people are found to be suffering from neurotic disorders by community surveys (Kay, Beamish, and Roth, 1964) and for about half of these, neurosis has newly arisen with old age (Bergmann, 1971). Thus there is certainly no falling off in prevalence of neurotic disorder in the senium, though it often goes unrecognized (Bergmann, 1981) and is less likely to be referred on for psychiatric advice than similar problems identified among young people. This is probably a reflection of lay as well as medical expectations of normal ageing, yet it deprives many patients of the possibility of help. Bergmann's work, while identifying certain personality types (anxious/hysterical and insecure/rigid) as perhaps predisposing to late onset neurosis, also established beyond doubt that physical illness, especially cardiac disease, much of which had gone unrecognized, underlay the emergence of neurotic symptomatology (Fig. 6). Thus late-onset neurotic syndromes should receive careful medical evaluation. The same study (Bergmann, 1971) also made clear that 'social factors' were of little or no consequence in the aetiology of neurotic disorders and dismissal of such states as 'social disease' is inaccurate and leads to neglect of real potential for effective treatment (Boyd, 1981).

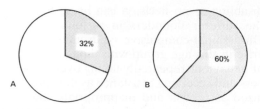

Percentage of people who are moderately / severely physically ill

A = Mentally normal elderly

B = Those with neurotic illness starting after 65 years

Bergmann '71

Figure 6   Distribution of physical and mental illness among the elderly (over 65), showing the percentage of people who are moderately or severely physically ill. (A) Mentally normal elderly and (B) those with neurotic illness starting after 65 years. (From Bergmann, 1971)

Mood Disorders

Depressed Mood

Depressed mood is common among old people at large (Kay, Beamish, and Roth, 1964), among the clients of general practitioners (Shepherd *et al.*, 1981) and social service departments (Goldberg, 1970), among admissions to general medical and geriatric wards (Bergmann and Eastham, 1974), and among patients referred to psychiatrists (Jolley and Arie, 1976). In many instances it is possible to identify stresses that have 'caused' or 'precipitated' the depressed mood. Yet sometimes the cause seems trivial in the face of the severity of the reaction it has provoked and the family history of depression stands out as more important (Fig. 7). Thus it is useful to allow

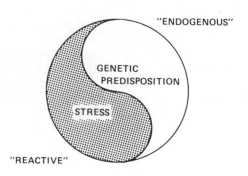

Figure 7   The constitution of mood disorders

depressions a *dimension* 'reactive–endogenous' as well as a dimension of severity (mild–moderate–severe and/or suicidal). In addition some depressed patients, particularly those who are severely depressed, may develop psychotic thinking and delusion-like ideas about themselves or others, and even describe limited hallucinatory experiences. Thus a third dimension, that of psychotism is necessary to describe a depressive state in anything like completeness. It is probable that mild, reactive depressions are most common in the community and in the clienteles of general practitioners and geriatricians, with a skew towards the more severe, more endogenous, more psychotic states in the clientele of psychiatrists. The form of the illness in the more endogenous, or constitutionally based, states may include psychomotor retardation or nonproductive overactivity (agitation). The former can progress to depressive stupor and the latter is usually associated with intense subjective anxiety. Diurnal variation of mood and of psychomotor function, with exacerbation of symptoms in the morning, is common. Appetite is poor, weight is lost, sleep is very poor, and often characterized by early morning wakening. Concentration is impaired and the patient finds it difficult to put her mind successfully to any task.

Psychotic thinking may begin when she dwells unreasonably on minor indiscretions of the past so that these become enlarged out of all proportion and are supposed to be evidence of her guilt and unworthiness. Real achievements and real worth come to be denied and are replaced by convictions that her financial status is insecure, her house and clothing filthy and unusable, and her body in a state of disrepair and decline. Hypochondriacal delusions may be very painful or outrageous; the emaciated depressive is hopelessly convinced he is dying of cancer and nothing can be done to save him; the anorexic woman will not eat and claims her body is already swollen with faeces that cannot and must not pass on out of her as she contains enough sewage to engulf the world. In such extreme cases, nihilistic ideas are not uncommon so that patients will hold views that they are dead, their heart has stopped, kidneys are defunct, no air is entering their lungs, etc. Among these notions, the theme that 'my brain is gone, I've gone senile' is of particular importance as it is not rare and in conjunction with psychomotor retardation and impaired concentration gives rise to a 'pseudodementia' that may be difficult to differentiate from a real dementing process (Post, 1975).

In profound and psychotic depressions sensitive ideas that people are turning away in disgust, or giving each other knowing looks or something similar, are frequently reported and hallucinatory experiences may be described. These are in keeping with the mood and beliefs of the depressed patient. Thus voices whisper short deprecatory comments: 'Disgraceful. Better dead. Filth', etc. A smell of putrefaction may be attributed to rotting flesh. Gnawing sensations in the abdomen may confirm the (supposed) presence of an evil cancer.

In addition a range of other phenomena, obsessional thoughts, social phobias, and hysterical dissociative states including amnestic fugues, may be mobilized by depression.

It is important to bear in mind that patients who have had mood disorders earlier in life may relapse in old age, but generally their illnesses respond to treatment. Similarly depressions arising for the first time in old age may do so in the setting of physical illness, including pathology of the nervous system (e.g. arteriosclerotic brain disease, Parkinsonism), but can be treated successfully independently of the course of the physical illness. The prognosis for depressive states has been transformed by the introduction of effective physical treatments so that most episodes can be brought to partial or complete resolution. This is a wonderful advance compared with the prolonged and progressive gloom to death that was the prospect for senile melancholics a few decades ago (Post, 1978), yet some patients do suffer from recurrent episodes, and others never regain their previous adjustment (Post, 1962). Thus it is important to offer ongoing surveillance and help to such people rather than assume that effective treatment of one episode represents a lifelong cure.

Mania and Hypomania

Mania and hypomania are seen in old people, sometimes as recurrences of illness established earlier in life or, less commonly, arising for the first time. Either way, the presentation may be 'atypical' and less easily recognized than the effusive, dynamic, euphoric equivalent seen in the young. Pressure of talk, flight of ideas, grandiose notions, disinhibition, overactivity, and disregard of the need to eat regularly, take medication, or sleep may all be present to variable degree. Yet the mood may be dominated by irritability or suspicion rather than open generosity and bonhomie. Perplexity, lack of concentration, and mild clouding of consciousness may all rouse the suspicion of an organic psychosyndrome. Paranoid interpretations of other people's lack of enthusiasm for outrageous ventures may suggest a paranoid illness. In addition it is not uncommon for features of severe depression and hypomania to occur in the same patient at the same time giving rise to a mixed affective state (Post, 1965). The prognosis for episodes of hypomania is good with a return to a previous personality probable. Personality may include a degree of cyclothymia and there is, as with the depressive states, the possibility of relapse into further manic or alternative depressive episodes and/or a more permanent deviation of personality towards one extreme of mood or the other.

Paranoid Syndromes

Paranoid ideation is not uncommon in mentally abnormal old people and may be due to a variety of factors. Certain personalities thrive on a degree of suspicion and alienation which seems to fuel them with considerable energy to achieve a great deal, perhaps in terms of career or material gain, but they lack a dimension for making warm, meaningful personal relationships. This may have led them to remain single or pass through one or more unsatisfactory marriages with little sexual warmth. Changes that make it difficult to remain aloof from others or impair the certainty with which observations can be made or stored are very threatening to such people and frequently mobilize ideas of persecution, exploitation, or derision. Thus the loss of a work routine and the isolation that follows through lack of other interests or contacts may be sufficient to move a personality beyond the range of healthy mistrust to pathological suspicion. Impairment of vision, impairment of hearing, and impairment of mobility all make it less easy to be sure what is going on, what is being said, what is or intended. Similarly, a progressively more faulty memory facilitates the emergence of paranoid postures that explain problems in terms of misdeeds done to the patient by others (moving objects, stealing money, etc.) rather than admit mistakes made by herself (put it somewhere safe, but forgot where that was). Major mood swings, hypomanic or depressive, may also mobilize paranoid thinking in predisposed individuals.

Those other persistent persecutory states of old age that are independent of progressive memory decline and not accounted for by a primary mood disorder have been a source of interest, discussion, and disagreement among psychiatrists for the most of this century (Kay, 1963). More recent thinking on the subject has the benefit not only of research but also the follow-through of earlier studies. In general the view now is that splitting these states into a number of categories with differing emphasis in mental state and presumed different prognosis is not justifiable. Post (1966) favours a tripartite descriptive classification into:

1. *Auditory hallucinosis* with auditory hallucinations the main or only abnormal phenomenon described and good preservation of personality.
2. *Paranoid schizophrenia-like states,* with third person auditory hallucinations and paranoid delusions, sensitive ideas of reference, and possibly ideas that the mind or body are being controlled by outside agencies (passivity experiences), but with relative preservation of affect and personality.
3. *Schizophrenia* of late life with more erosion of affect, drive, and personality. Passivity phenomena are well developed in addition to third-person auditory hallucinations and delusions. Even in these states formal thought disorder and catatonic features which are seen in younger schizophrenics are virtually unknown.

There is no skew within this spectrum of symptomatology associated with sensory deficits but a strong family history of schizophrenia is associated with type 3. Types 1 and 2 may be 'situation bound' and removal from the home where such symptoms have developed may lead to their disappearance, at least for a while. In the past all these persistent persecutory states ran a chronic, often progressive course and if they released behaviour that led to hospitalization this would usually mean the patient would stay in hospital for the rest of her days ('she', because these states are much more common among women). With effective medication now available, together with competent community support, most such patients can spend most of their days at home regardles s of the presenting symptomatology.

Schizophrenia does not carry with it a shortened expectation of life, so a considerable number of schizophrenics who have remained ill or relapsed into illness grow old with an established and sometimes progressive abnormal mental state. Even now most such elderly schizophrenics are encountered only in the long-stay wards of mental hospitals. Yet increasingly they and their successors are housed in their own homes, a hostel, or old people's home. They are often much more disabled than patients with late onset syndromes, for their personalities, drive, affect, and thinking have been eroded for much longer and from a time when their impressionable nervous system was more disorganized by the pathology. Florid symptomatology has often faded with age (and treatment) leaving anergic, cold, and thought-disordered shadows. There is now evidence that the more severe forms of schizophrenia do give rise to brain atrophy (Crow *et al.*, 1980), but it is always important to look for the possibility of newly arising and possibly reversible symptom complexes even in these classically 'burned-out' cases.

As with other delineations in the psychiatry of old age the division between affective disorders and the schizophrenia-like illnesses is not absolute and conditions best described as schizoaffective can occur. They show mixed features of schizophrenia and prominent mood abnormality. This is not a large group of patients and it is probable that the course of the illness is more malignant than either that of the mood disorders or the persistent persecutory states (Post, 1971).

Organic Psychosyndromes

While emotional disorders and difficulties in relating to changed circumstances are more common in the old age population at large and even among those old people who come to the attention of doctors, it is the organic psychosyndromes occurring in old age that dominate our thinking both professionally and personally. There are two main syndromes: the acute confusional states (delirium) that may persist to a subacute form, but from which there is the probability of recovery if death does not supervene, and the dementing syndromes which are chronic, often progressive and from which recovery is unlikely. These two are not mutually exclusive; indeed, many patients experience repeated episodes of delirium during the course of a dementia and an episode of delirium may resolve, leaving a patient with a persistent dementia.

Acute Confusional States (*Delirium*) (Jolley, 1981a; Lipowski, 1980)

Acute confusional states usually develop, and declare themselves, very rapidly over a matter of minutes or hours. The picture is characterized by variability over time with exacerbations of the more florid aspects especially likely at night. The most characteristic feature of the mental state is the presence of clouded consciousness evidenced by quickly developed disorientation for time, place, and person. Thinking becomes disorganized, fragmented, and distorted, with content varying as themes from the past and misinterpretations of the present are interlaced with lucid intervals. Thus past memories may well up into the present but new material cannot be learned nor is the experience of delirium generally available to recall in the future. Mood is also variable but fear and anxiety are probably the most common affects and may be very distressing in their intensity. Misinterpretations, illusions, and hallucinations, especially in the visual modality, are characteristic of the syndrome and commonly emerge or are intensified at nighttime. Transient and disorganized abnormal beliefs reflect the patient's alienation from current reality. These are influenced by the patient's previous personality and experience and may give rise to behaviour that produces difficult management situations. In addition, changes in psychomotor activity are part-and-parcel of the delirium syndrome and motor agitation, plucking of the bed clothes or repetitive rehearsal of previous occupational activity may be seen. Speech is also disturbed and may become incoherent.

Delirium is essentially a symptomatic psychosis and an underlying physical illness should always be suspected. Indeed it is usual in the elderly for a number of factors to contribute to the picture and satisfaction at identifying one pathology may be short lived if the other four or five less obvious problems remain operative. Thus while it is important to have in mind a checklist of possible intracranial and systemic troubles, such as outlined in Fig. 8, it is also essential to consider the probable underlying state of the cerebral cortex (is there evidence from the history suggestive of a dementing syndrome predating this acute episode?), the sensory apparatus providing information to it, and the prevailing mood. An established depression may impair concentration and reduce co-operation as well as colour the form and content of delirium. The social milieu can be all important in precipitating, preventing, or resolving an episode of confusion. Transfer from a reassuring home to a clinically austere hospital ward can be sufficient to tip the balance towards confusion. A calm, friendly, clear-cut style of management may provide the basis for a return to reality (Fig. 9).

Thus management falls into two interrelated tasks: on the one hand to identify and treat underlying and causative pathologies and on the other to care for the person during the delirium to minimize its intensity and avoid secondary complications. The first is addressed by careful history-taking, clinical examination, and further investigation where appropriate. The second is based on nursing applied with an understanding of the nature of delirium. Thus care must be taken that the patient is as comfortable as possible, food and drink provided to maintain good nutrition and hydration and avoid hunger and thirst. Parenteral vitamins are often thought to be helpful. Bowels and bladder must be regulated to avoid the discomfort of constipation, retention, or incontinence. Potentially painful lesions must be dressed, and analgesia prescribed where appropriate. If the patient is in hospital, a side room is preferable during the acute phase of delirium for the social milieu can be more easily regulated than that in the general ward. Good lighting obviates confusing shadows. Regular, calm attendants wearing easily identifiable clothing encourage calm and confidence in their patient. It may be necessary to

A. *Intracranial conditions*:

Pressure:	Space-occupying: subdural heamatoma, cerebral abscess, cerebral tumour. Low-pressure hydrocephalus.
Trauma:	Postconcussional states.
Infection:	Encephalitis, meningitis.
Vascular:	Cerebral thrombosis or embolism, hypertensive encephalopathy, subarachnoid haemorrhage.
Convulsion:	Postictal states (including post ECT).

B. *Systemic conditions*:

Infection:	Especially chest infections, urinary tract infections, septicaemia.
Vascular:	Polyarteritis nodosum.
Anoxia:	Anoxic in respiratory failure, stagnant in cardiac insufficiency, anaemic after blood loss, in anaemias, carbon monoxide poisoning.
Metabolic:	Renal failure, hepatic failure, electrolyte and acid–base imbalance. Hypercapnia.
Endocrine:	Under or overactivity of the thyroid, adrenal, pituitary, or parathyroid glands. Diabetes mellitus.
Vitamin deficiencies:	Especially of the B vitamins.
Pharmacy:	It is impossible to overemphasize the importance of drugs in producing unwanted effects on cerebral function. Many drugs have psychotropic activity either directly or by altering the metabolism of other drugs taken concurrently.
Withdrawal syndromes:	Discontinuing powerful cerebral sedatives such as alcohol, barbiturates, or benzodiazepines releases delirium tremens.

Figure 8   Checklist of common physical causes of symptomatic confusional states

use tranquillizers to reduce anxiety and control hallucinations, delusions, and aggressive behaviour. Haloperidol is probably the tranquillizer of choice and should be used in adequate doses, with review of the dose and frequency depending on the patient's response.

As the confusional episode clears, the progress can be greatly facilitated by providing cues to the patient through staff, relatives, newspapers, personal photographs, etc. In addition, as soon as it is reasonable the patient should be allowed to exercise the skills that are recovering. Thus conversations, reading, sitting out of bed, walking, and getting to know the layout of the ward are all therapeutic activities and help in the task of avoiding withdrawal, a bed-fast habit, or other complications of the acute episode.

Delirium is frighteningly clear cut in its outcome—death or recovery in a matter of days (Roth, 1955). It is the syndrome of the assessment ward, where it may be present in 16 per cent. of admissions, but elsewhere it arises sporadically and is rarely encountered in community surveys (Bergmann and Eastham, 1974).

The Dementia Syndrome (Jolley, 1981b, Jolley 1980)

If delirium is the syndrome of the assessment ward, dementia rules quietly, insidiously, but perniciously in all other situations and particularly where old people are grouped together for protective care. Thus it affects 4 per cent. of 65 to 69 year olds, 26 per cent. of 75 to 79 year olds and 60 per cent. of those over 85 years (Nielsen, 1962). On average 5 per cent. of all old people (65 years plus) living at home are severely disabled by a dementia and a further 5 per cent. are less severely impaired. The old-fashioned caring which is available in residential facilities of old people's homes, long-stay geriatric and psychiatric hospital wards attracts greater concentrations, 29, 42, and 49 per cent., respectively, of demented people (Kay, Beamish, and Roth, 1962). The recent device of sheltered housing seems to preferentially exclude dements and this raises doubts about its status as a contribution to caring rather than to economic housing (O'Brien, 1971).

Dementia is a syndrome of 'acquired global

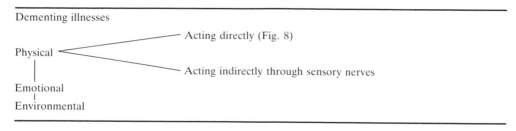

Figure 9　Major factors contributing to confusional states and dementing syndromes in the elderly

impairment of memory and personality but without impairment of consciousness' (Lishman, 1978). As a syndrome it may arise out of one or more of a range of processes and thus has a range of possible outcomes (Stout and Jolley, 1981). Livesley and others (Livesley, 1977; Isaacs and Caird, 1976) have argued against the use of the term 'dementia' as they feel it generates nihilism in the responsible clinician. Yet their alternative terminology 'brain failure' is hardly more optimistic and in seeking comparability with other syndromes of organ failure (renal failure, heart failure, etc.) does the dementing brain the disservice of overlooking the many ways in which it continues to function quite well.

Memory impairment in dementia is much greater than that asssociated with normal ageing and the pattern of memory loss is different (Miller, 1974). In dementia recent memories and the ability to learn new material are the first affected though impersonal information from the past may also be forgotten or misremembered. Personal memories with strong emotional association, even from early childhood, seem to be very strongly held, but even here when an independent account is available it may find fault with the dement's account of things. The range of interests and activities become narrow as ability and mental energy wanes and personality styles become rigidly caricatured. Thus the strict, domineering housewife retains her determination above all else, brooking no argument and demanding immediate compliance. The possessive husband proceeds through intolerance and irritability to a confining and sometimes dangerous jealousy. The well-adjusted, affectionate, and sociable continue to be so, accepting their difficulties and increasing dependence with endearing good humour. Thought content is dominated by the past with scant interest for, nor grasp of, the present. Similarly, the content of conversation is likely to become impoverished, repetitive, and even stereotyped or perseverative. Lack of emotional response may give way to lack of emotional control and catastrophic reactions of rage or despair can be released when the demented person is pushed beyond her (narrowed) limits of competence. Primitive neurological reflexes reemerge and sphincter control may be lost early or late in the process.

Physical appearance often changes markedly so that the patient 'puts on years' in a matter of months, losing stature, weight, and strength and becomes lined and grey. Such patients fall easy prey to intercurrent illnesses, especially chest infections.

Most old people presenting with a dementing syndrome are found to be suffering from one of the major dementing illnesses: senile dementia Alzheimer type (SDAT) or arteriosclerotic dementia (multiple infarct dementia). In many instances other factors are contributory to the dementing syndrome and in some patients these other factors constitute the whole aetiology. Attention to 'contributory factors' is always helpful and occasionally 'curative' (Fig. 9).

Senile dementia (Alzheimer type). This condition is also known by alternative names: presbyophrenia, parenchymatous dementia, primary neuronal dementia, etc. It is the archetypal 'senility' characterized by a slowly progressive deterioration of personality and memory. Women are affected more commonly than men, genetic factors being important in at least some families (Larsson, Sjogren, and Jacobsen, 1963). Interesting associations with chromosomal abnormalities and with Down's syndrome have been reported (Olson and Shaw, 1969) and there is evidence that other parts of the nervous system including the peripheral nerves may also be involved (Levy, 1975). Clinical and histopathological observations have been brought together by Corsellis, Tomlinson, and Blessed (Corsellis, 1977; Blessed, Tomlinson, and Roth, 1968). Their work made it clear that brains of patients suffering from senile dementia contain many more intraneuronal neurofibrillary tangles (of Alzheimer) and silver-staining plaques than do brains of age-matched controls and that the severity of dementia in life correlates broadly with the concentration of senile plaques identified at post-mortem. Electron microscopy suggests that a good deal of cytoarchitecture remains intact but biochemical findings reveal deficiency of choline acetyl transferase (CAT) which is essential to the production of the transmitter substance acetyl choline. Reduction of CAT levels correlates closely with the severity of dementia (Perry, 1980). In addition the neurones from dementing brains are deficient in RNA (Mann, Yates, and Barton, 1977.) Observations from other laboratories have suggested that immunological incompetence may be a factor in senile dementia and there is quite a powerful lobby that would give slow viruses an aetiological role (Sutton and Lord, 1978).

Certainly a great deal of interesting and potentially useful research has been initiated recently, but as yet no treatment at the biological level is available that helpfully influences the progress of the disease. It is now generally felt that histological and biochemical findings suggest that this is one and the same illness as that described in the presenium by Alzheimer, yet within the clinical syndrome there is a range from 'benign forgetfulness' with slow deterioration to an 'Alzheimerized' form in which prietal lobe dysfunctions aphasia, agnosia, together with gait disturbance and epileptic fits, are associated with rapid decline to an early death (McDonald, 1969).

Arteriosclerotic dementia (multiinfarct dementia). This condition is also known by alternative names: cerebrovascular dementia, multiple infarct dementia. It is characterized by a more erratic, stepwise deterioration of function (Fig. 10). Each step is associated with new cerebral infarcts in the brain related to atherosclerotic changes in the blood vessels. Infarcts may occur when small emboli from atheromatous plaques in large neck vessels impact in the small end arteries of the cerebrum (Hachinski, Lassen, and Marshall, 1974), or when cerebral vessels become thrombosed or when systemic blood pressure falls as a result of myocardial infarction or other conditions. Each new infarct is evidenced by acute, sometimes florid clinical changes: monoplegia, dysphasia, epileptic convulsions, etc. Infarcts usually resolve over a period of days or weeks but leave a scar and some deficiency of the cerebral function which that tissue previously served. In addition there is a cumulative loss of personality and memory function amounting to a dementia. Tomlinson, Blessed, and Roth's classic investigations showed that the degree of dementia as measured by tests of memory function correlate strongly with the volume of cerebral cortex infarcted. 'Dementia' is only significant when the volume of cortex lost is in excess of 50 ml (Tomlinson, Blessed, and Roth, 1970.) A number of factors are known to predispose to cerebrovascular dementia, most notably hypertension, and so the control of blood pressure in middle age may prevent its development. In the established case reducing blood stickiness may be helpful. Yet at present it is unusual to be able to influence the course of the condition which differs from senile dementia of the Alzheimer type in its stepwise nature (Fig. 10), in the marked fluctuation in

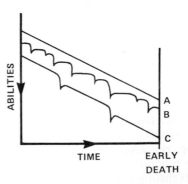

Figure 10 Crude representation of the course of senile dementia and arteriosclerotic dementia where A is senile dementia, B arteriosclerotic dementia, and C combined type

performance that is seen day by day even between episodes of acute infarction, and in the relative preservation of some abilities (represented in non-infarcted areas). Yet the total pattern of deterioration is in the end similar to SDAT and includes decline to an early death, most commonly (as in SDAT) by bronchopneumonia, although myocardial infarction or cerebrovascular accident provide an alternative mode of demise. As both SDAT and arteriosclerotic dementia are common, they may occur in the same patient, producing a mixed picture.

A number of other dementing illnesses may be encountered in geriatric practice and are of theoretical importance. Both Pick's disease and Huntington's chorea are inherited conditions. In Pick's disease frontal lobe function is lost early so that behavioural changes predate memory decline. In Huntington's chorea, too, frontal lobe function deteriorates but the basal ganglia also atrophy to produce a syndrome of abnormal choreiform movements as well as mental change (Office of Health Economics, 1980; Sjogren, Sjogren, and Lingren, 1952). Syphilitic dementia as a delayed consequence of treponemal infection is still encountered ocassionally, but another even rarer condition, Creutzfeld–Jacob disease, has acquired as important standing as a spongiform encephalopathy and the first 'transmissible' dementing illness thought to be produced by a slow-virus-like organism, (Corsellis, 1979; Luxon, Lees, and Greenwood, 1979).

Contributing factors. Other factors (See Figs 8 and 9) commonly contribute to impaired function in elderly 'demented' patients. Sometimes the problem is a physical one: illness may act directly to interfere with cerebral function by the production of toxins, pressure, high temperature, or cerebral dysrhythmia, or they may have indirect influence through the peripheral nerves, producing pain, discomfort, and over-arousal. Contrariwise the impairment of sensory input by failure of the special senses, immobility, or weightlessness induced for nursing purposes (e.g. waterbed) may leave the cerebrum understimulated. Sometimes depression, anxiety, or paranoia may coexist with a dementing illness or be so severe in themselves that they produce an impression of dementia or 'pseudodementia'. Treatment of such 'func-

tional' psychopathology may be very useful to the patient and her supporters even if memory decline persists.

Environmental factors are also very important. Neither poverty nor social disadvantage cause any of the dementing illnesses, but understimulating or suffocating living situations which may prevail on long-stay wards or over-protective households do not allow the best cerebral performance from an impaired brain.—nor do situations of excessive stress which may occur when social failure goes unaided or an elderly person is living with a much more energetic and modern-thinking family.

As with delirium, it is important to seek out the various possible factors contributing to a dementing syndrome in a particular individual: dementing illness, physical illness or disability, sensory impairment, emotional disturbance, and/or social circumstances. The search may reveal pathologies that can be treated quite simply and will help in management. Yet it is important to work very sensitively with the existing supports available to the patient. Medicine has a good deal to offer but in this syndrome family care, social services help, and even offers of time from volunteers have as much if not more importance. Maintenance at home is often a reasonable objective when a spouse or child is available to provide supervision, but they themselves require support. In the absence of such a 24 hour presence in the home few dements can survive for any length of time and all that do so are at considerable risk. Thus placement in residential care or hospital may be necessary and the enlightened management of the milieu there is all important in determining the quality of life for the patient (and her coresidents) (Evans *et al.*, 1981). A number of techniques have been developed to encourage optimal management regimes in institutions (Woods and Britton, 1977). These all take their directives from the lessons taught by relatives, particularly husbands or wives, who manage dements with amazing success by devoting their time, energies, and emotions to the role of 'prosthesis' that fills in for each new defect, encourages each glimmer of ability, and redirects each indiscretion. It is probable that further help in erecting successful prosthetic environments will come from nursing, occupational therapy, physiotherapy, and psychology initiatives, and electronic prostheses may well leaven the load of these humane carers.

PROBLEMATIC BEHAVIOURS

A number of syndromes of abnormal behaviour are seen commonly among old people. They do not in themselves constitute 'psychiatric disorder' though they are frequently attributed to mental illness and in some instances this is a correct assumption.

Alcohol Abuse

While excessive drinking is not uncommon in this country, and is clearly on the increase (Kendell, 1979), this is not a habit usually associated with old age. Yet problems related to alcohol abuse are seen among the elderly and fall into two discernable patterns. Some people have survived into old age despite heavy drinking throughout their lives. They often suffer physical stigmata of their chronic excesses with cirrhosis of the liver, cardiac myopathy, peripheral neuritis, etc. If cut off from their source of supply they are likely to crave alcohol and experience delirium tremens. Other people turn to drink in old age. In this very interesting group women are well represented. They have often had little obvious interest in alcohol in the past; some have expressed strong views against it; while others have reserved it for special occasions. Frequently it is possible to identify precipitating circumstances that have produced, in the first instance, understandable anxiety or depression: loss of a satisfying job, loss of a spouse, deterioration of a favourite neighbourhood, loss of physical prowess. Sometimes there has been evidence of the beginning of a dementing illness before alcohol is taken to excess. It may be that this should be seen as another 'loss' or it may be that the dementia releases a 'forbidden' drive. Late-onset drinkers usually present with problems associated with intoxication—falls, confusion, coma—and come to notice within a few years of the onset of drinking. Serious withdrawal syndromes such as delirium tremens are unusual for the brain has not had time to habituate to higher concentrations of alcohol. The prognosis for late onset drinkers is probably quite good if the underlying problem can be identi-

fied and dealt with by a more appropriate and less hazardous strategy than the bottle.

Drug Abuse

Misuse of drugs, be they stimulants or tranquillizers, is generally associated with the younger generations. Yet some people do abuse medication in old age. In many instances the mechanism is similar to that outlined for late-onset drinkers—a syndrome of response to intolerable losses, especially by illnesses that have led to the prescription of pain relieving or tranquillizing medication. The pattern of gratification or relief from distress by taking pills persists. In addition old people sometimes find themselves the victims of abuse by drugs, which may be prescribed in all good faith but which produce more harm by way of unwanted effects (especially when taken alongside other potent medicines) than the intended good.

Self-Poisoning

Self-poisoning is to be regarded very seriously in the elderly for it is commonly symptomatic of a severe depressive state (Kessel, 1965). The possibility than an overdose was taken by mistake should not be easily accepted. Completed suicide is common in the elderly and usually occurs in a setting of depression (which may have been recognized), physical illness or disability, and/or social isolation. Many patients who kill themselves have been seen by doctors during this preterminal depression, depression which could in some instances have been treated successfully if it had been given the respect it deserved (Shulman, 1978).

Self-Neglect

What is considered 'homely' is very much a matter of personal taste, and what is homely for some is untidy or uninhabitable for others. It is important to be fairly broad-minded when making judgement on the state of an old person's personal habitat. Yet there are certainly homes that reflect very strange versions of living and others that reflect an inability to cope. Many of the old people who emerge from the strangest houses cluttered to the ceilings with collections of oddities and items of idiosyncratic importance appear to be free of major psychiatric disorder (Clark, Mankikar, and Gray, 1975). It takes a sustained effort to create these collections and the most that can be said is that their creators are eccentric, certainly not ill. Paranoid states or chronic schizophrenia may lead a householder to keep closed curtains, invest in numerous locks or alarms, or even armories for self defence. Progressive dementias are evidenced by neglect to clean, to change curtains, to bring in fresh food, and to throw away half-eaten food. This failure brings the sufferer quite quickly to the attention of neighbours, relatives, social services, and doctors. Dementia in combination with unsupervized pets, dogs or cats, can devastate a home in a matter of months. Depressive states produce incapacity more quickly and an anergic depressive may be found sitting in a house which is neat and tidy but without food, drink, or heating. Over a few weeks she fades from her usual busy competence to achieve no disturbance of the household at all, not even the dust.

'Failure to Cooperate'

Failure to accept well-intentioned offers of help, refusal of medication, and failure to make the expected progress after an acute 'set-back' such as physical illness or bereavement is a frequent cause of concern. Sometimes this is based in well-practised bloody-mindedness. Perhaps more often the 'offender' has found advantages and reassurance in a situation of withdrawal or dependency and needs time and guidance to venture out of it. More severe depressive states or paranoid states may also present in this way as may unsuspected mild or moderate degrees of dementia. In addition sensory deficits, particularly deafness, or neurological defects involving the parietal lobes may make comprehension and cooperation very difficult.

Sexual Abberations, Stealing, and Aggression

Sexual aberrations, stealing, and aggression are antisocial acts rarely associated with old age. Where they occur there is often evidence of psychiatric disorder: a transient confusional state, more enduring mood disorder, or paranoid state or a progressive dementia. Common to all is a degree of disinhibition uncommon

within normal ageing. In most instances these underlying pathologies can be helped, if not cured, by appropriate treatment and it is important that this is made available in a non-punitive atmosphere, with help and reassurance to members of the family and other important helpers lest the old man or old lady be judged irretrievably 'beyond the pale'.

Wandering

Though most 'wanderers' are found to be 'lost' because of a confusional state or dementing syndrome, it is not unknown for patients with severe agitation in association with early morning wakening in a depressive illness to be described under this umbrella. Within the organic psychosyndromes the urge to 'move on' is often based on previous practice; the housewife who used to go shopping every day 'just for the walk and to see what's to do' will naturally wish to continue to do so. Otherwise the wish to return to familiar territory or to be away from unusual and unsettling situations is common and understandable. Thus a move to unfamiliar surroundings may precipitate wandering that resolves when the patient returns home. People who have moved house within old age or late middle age may begin to seek their previous home when only mildly demented, but even those who have lived forty years or more in the same marital home may make off in quest of 'home' when severely demented. In this situation home may be the village life of 1900 and quite unattainable. Medication may be useful in reducing anxiety, agitation, and the very drive to wander, but sympathetic, interesting conversation and the offer of alternative activity by acceptable and indefatigable carers are the best for diversion, and diversion is a better objective than arrest.

Incontinence

Incontinence is not essentially a 'psychiatric problem' but incontinence of urine and sometimes of faeces is common in elderly psychiatric patients and psychiatric disorder is common in incontinent patients. The combination of mental disorder and incontinence is not always beyond hope of resolution. Incontinence must be carefully but vigorously investigated in every case and may well be helped by the physical treatments and nursing techniques now available. In addition, mood disorders may be contributing to the lack of drive to keep dry and clean or reducing speed of thought or movement to such an extent that the patient does not get to the toilet although aware of the need. In every situation attention to the patient's self-respect, dignity, and interests are likely to improve sphincter control and help her response to difficulties that remain.

A number of other behavioural syndromes, 'house-bound', 'hysterical', and 'hypochondriacal', have been mentioned earlier in this chapter and the general principle reiterated that such syndromes are not diagnoses in themselves but frequently call attention to underlying personal or emotional or physical difficulties, or a combination of these. Careful investigation of the contributory factors often makes it possible to divine a plan of treatment that helps the patient back towards a more constructive pattern of behaviour.

IMPORTANT CHALLENGES OF OLD AGE

Old age is marked by several major life stresses, some of which are commonly linked with emotional difficulties.

Retirement

Withdrawal or exclusion from the workforce in the early or mid sixties is now almost universal and has become for administrative purposes the portal of old age (Hearnshaw, 1972). For some the losses involved in leaving work are insufferable—loss of routine, loss of constructive activity, loss of companions, loss of status and financial worth. The 'working classes' are, perhaps appropriately, the hardest hit, with restricted resources available to them, and people without interests other than their former occupation find structureless time very threatening. After a short 'holiday' of relaxation and self-congratulation, a period of gloom and emptiness may be marked by symptoms of anxiety, irritability, and depression which usually resolves as adjustment is made to the new life style. Yet it is not uncommon for more morbid reactions to occur and persist, in which case they must be treated as pathological and help offered to facilitate readjustment.

Among the unforeseen problems of retirement are the stresses imposed upon marriages. Life together for 40 of 50 years may have been sustained with happiness and joy or merely mutal tolerance when both partners have time and territory of their own for most of each waking day. When both have nowhere else to go any time of any day the demands on these long-established bonds may become too great to bear without restructuring.

Illness and Disability

The prevalence of disability increases rapidly within old age (Townsend in the Disability Alliance, 1979), and the relationships between physical illness and emotional problems has been emphasized (see Fig. 6) (Bergmann, 1971). Many people take time to accept their altered self-image when faced with serious illness or limitation of their abilities, but most do resolve to find an acceptable lifestyle. When neurotic symptoms become very severe or persist they deserve treatment in their own right and will often become less distressing even though the 'cause' – physical disability, etc.— persists.

Deaths

Dying is now rare outside of old age so that old people frequently face bereavement by death of a husband or wife and the prospect of their own demise in rapid succession. The 'timely' deaths of old age yield less pathological grief than the unexpected, catastrophic loss of a young spouse (Parkes, 1972), yet not everyone has prepared themselves for the event. Very 'close' marriages may have left the remaining partner dangerously isolated and short of social skills and contacts with the rest of the world. Preoccupation with minor or long-tolerated physical infirmity may be symptomatic of a persisting depression and serious, life-threatening depressive states may evolve. Again such pathological reactions require identification and treatment rather than passive 'understanding'. Eventually a new adjustment can usually be achieved and this may even include remarriage, which in itself can present a new hierarchy of challenges and possible pitfalls.

Approaching death is a task taken in their stride by most older people. For some the notching up of birthdays beyond the years achieved by school friends and adversaries becomes a consuming game. Despite the limitations of life, much is found that is worth while, 'Sad to be old, glad to be alive', yet death itself is rarely feared, rather the possibility of pain, discomfort, or exhaustion, especially if this is to be borne alone (Blythe, 1981). The assurance of good medical care and nursing during this unfashionable but inescapable last act is needed and should be provided.

TREATMENT

Treatment programmes must be realistic and take into account the 'whole person' and his her needs rather than pretend that a limited prescription for identified pathology is likely to 'do the trick'. For every individual a hierarchy of approaches should be considered:

(a) to place the patient in the situation (psychological, geographical) likely to encourage her best performance;
(b) to exercise and develop her abilities and potential;
(c) to arrange acceptable prostheses for acquired deficiencies and disabilities;
(d) to prescribe specific treatments;
(e) to monitor progress and review the treatment plan at sensible intervals.

The balance of attention that has to be directed to each of these varies with the strengths/weaknesses of the patient and the nature and severity of the pathological processes identified.

Psychological security is not the same as physical safety. Some old people prefer to be in their own territory, albeit objectively less 'safe', than to be in the 'security' of a strange hospital, subservient to rules and routines not of their own making. Hospital may be to one person a haven from supposed persecutors, to another a helpful, simplified environment in which to reconstruct coping strategies, while for another it removes all the external cues to identity and routine that have thus far enabled them to trace a passage through days and nights of failing memory.

Psychiatric Treatments

Psychological

At the base of every treatment programme is the therapeutic relationship forged between physician and patient. This may seek to venture no further than a simple acknowledgement of mutual respect and trust, assurance of an acceptable goal to therapeutic endeavour, and the exhibition of skill and compassion. Without it little or nothing can be achieved.

Psychotherapy

It may be that emotional relationships with a therapist (individual therapy) or within a group that includes one or more therapist(s) (group therapy) will be used to help a patient come to a new adjustment with herself changed by age, disabilities, and disappointments. Psychotherapeutic aims with the elderly are generally limited and directed to clarification of new roles and possibilities, facilitating disengagement from lost roles and hopes, and may need to include prolonged support because major restructuring of long-established personality traits is unrealistic (Verwoerdt, 1981).

Milieu Therapy

The principle of managing the social environment of patients to provide stimulation and reassurance has been discussed in relation to a cure and chronic organic psychosyndromes. These syndromes make patients particularly vulnerable and responsive to the social milieu, but everyone, especially at times of illness or threat, is influenced by their surroundings and attention must be paid to this, lest neglect leads to unnecessary withdrawal, fear, alienation, etc.

Reality Orientation

Patients who have become disorientated either through rapidly disorganizing illness (delirium) or through understimulation (and institutional care can be very potent in this) may benefit from programmes concerned to emphasize relearning of current orientation. A number of variations on this technique have been developed and all have their advantages and limitations (Powell-Proctor, 1981). Many units have adopted elements of the technique, but it is important not to go overboard for one approach. Aims must be decided by realistic appraisal of patients' potential. Attempting the impossible distresses both therapist and therapized.

Behaviour Therapy

Undesirable behaviour or undesired emotional reactions can sometimes be modified by behaviour therapy using conditioning techniques: operant conditioning, desensitization, implosion. Unwanted behaviours may be extinguished by lack of reward and replaced by healthier, better adapted behaviours encouraged by suitable rewards. Planning and effecting appropriate programmes is the province of the clinical psychologist.

Physical Treatments

Psychotropic Medication

There has been a massive expansion in the number of useful psychotropic drugs available over the past 30 years. They are now the most prescribed medicines in the United Kingdom, bewildering in their claims to potency and sometimes in their effects. Unwanted effects are common in elderly patients so that care in prescribing is important. Low doses may be therapeutic where higher dosage is counterproductive and the possibility of interaction with other prescribed or patent medicines must be borne in mind.

Tranquillizers

Minor tranquillizers, notably the benzodiazepines are very widely prescribed and are useful in states of tension and anxiety. Their place is limited in the elderly as they easily produce confusion, drowsiness, and disinhibition instead of or in addition to the desired effect. If they are used, dosage should be low and held under review.

The major tranquillizers are more useful as long as they are handled with care. This usually means low dosage and anticipating side-effects.

In low dosage anxiety and agitation, which may lead to motor restlessness, can be contained and higher doses can be used to suppress hallucinations (auditory hallucinations are generally easier to control than visual hallucinations, especially in long standing syndromes) and delusional thinking. Some of the phenothiazines have side effects that make them difficult to use in the elderly. Thus chlorpromazine produces drowsiness, unsteadiness, loss of body temperature, as well as having widespread effects on the cardiovascular system and nervous system (Parkinsonism, fits, atropine-like action). Promazine, thioridazine, and perphenazine may be preferable and trifluoperazine has been found to be very effective in persistent persecutory states (Post, 1966). Haloperidol, a butyrophenone, is also useful in controlling anxiety, agitation, and paranoid thinking. Used as an injection in the emergency situation it brings control quickly and with little hazard, although high doses and prolonged use, as with all those major tranquillizers, may produce extrapyramidal symptoms. Drug-induced Parkinsonism can be controlled with anti-Parkinsonism agents such as orphenidrine. These must also be used in low dosage and reviewed. They should not be given prophylactically in anticipation of Parkinsonism as they are very likely to produce a confusional state.

Antidepressants

Tricylic antidepressants have been available for over 20 years and the earliest representatives of their kind, imipramine and amitryptiline, are still drugs of first choice. In the elderly, and particularly the very elderly, they must be used in low dosage (starting with 10 mg b.d. or t.d.s.), building up slowly to a therapeutic level. Even so unwanted effects may be so troublesome that they have to be discontinued. Unwanted effects include cardiovascular effects, hypotension, dysrhythmias, atropine-like effects – constipation, retention of urine, dry mouth, glaucoma, and central nervous system effects with acute confusion and epileptic fits a possibility. Milder tricyclics such as dothiapen may be more successful and the recently introduced tetracyclic antidepressants (e.g. mianserin) are said to be potent and relatively free of side-effects.

'Antidementia' drugs

A surprising number of medicines are marketed with a claim to improve performance in patients suffering from dementing illnesses. Some are said to improve cerebral blood flow, some to facilitate the transfer of nutriments from blood to neurones, and others to stimulate neurones directly. It is probably fair to say that none of these products are of accepted usefulness and some may be harmful by opening up blood flow to regimes other than the brain. All have the potential danger of persuading the physician that he has completed his task by prescribing them.

It is possible that research derived from recent advances in understanding the substrate of the dementias will give rise to a new series of drugs as effective in the dementias as L-dopa has become in Parkinsonism (Rossor, 1981).

Electroplexy (ECT) (Pippard and Ellam, 1981)

Electrically induced convulsions have been used successfully in the treatment of severe mental illnesses since the late 1940s. In the elderly their use is confined to severe mood disorders, usually psychotic depressions where ECT may be life-saving in the face of mute resistance and refusal to eat or drink or active suicidal intent. With careful selection of cases, including evaluation of physical fitness and careful attention to modification of the fit and anaesthesia, this is an important and relatively safe form of treatment. Certainly many cases are encountered where the rapid response achieved with ECT is preferable to the prolonged suffering from depression and risk of multiple side-effects from antidepressant medication.

Compulsory Orders

Most mentally ill old people are able to accept help and treatment voluntarily. Of all admissions in 1976 to mental illness and mental handicap beds only 11.2 per cent. were compulsory (DHSS, 1979), and within our own service for elderly patients only 8 out of 700 managed during a year require compulsory treatment and even then the period of formal detention is usually brief. The 1959 Mental Health Act has been superseded by the Mental Health Act 1983. For most situations a working knowledge of 4 compulsory orders is sufficient. These are Section 5 (previously S 30), Section 4 (previously S 29), Section 2 (previously S 25), and Section 3 (previously S 26).

Section 5 (previously S 30) Patients Already in Hospital. This allows the Responsible Medical Officer (consultant) to detain a patient who is already in hospital (psychiatric or otherwise) for 72 hours from the time he signs the report. The grounds are that the RMO considers the patient to be a danger to himself or to others by reason of mental illness and the report requires only his signiture. The 72 hours allows time for the full application procedure for admission for assessment or treatment to be carried out.

Section 4 (previously S 29) Admission in an Emergency. This allows for one doctor (preferably the GP who has known the patient before) together with the nearest relative *or* an approved social worker to admit a patient to hosptial in an emergency, ie. when even the little delay involved in arranging Section 2 would be too great. The order lasts for 72 hours from the time of admission.

Section 2 (previously S 25) Admission for Assessment. This is the preferred means of compulsory admission. It allows admission for observation and treatment of a 28 day period on the recommendation of 2 doctors, one of whom is 'approved' as having psychiatric expertise. In practise the usual combination is of the patient's GP and the psychiatrist who will be treating the patient. The application is made by the next of kin or by an approved social worker. The patient has a right of appeal to a Mental Health Tribunal within 14 days.

Section 3 (previously S 26) Addmission for Treatment. This is a 6 months order, allowing for treatment of mental illness which has to be described by the 2 doctors recommending admission. The reasons have to be given as to why it is necessary to override the patient's lack of consent.

As for S4, an 'approved' doctor and one

other make the recommendations, and the application is by the nearest relative, or by an approved social worker having first obtained the nearest relatives consent. The patient has a right of appeal to a Mental Health Review Tribunal. (Blueglass, 1983).

Most patients who are dealt with under compulsory powers respond well to treatment that is offered and many are able to return to their homes to continue better adjusted lives. It is very few indeed who require long-term compulsory detention.

AN OUTLINE OF PSYCHOGERIATRIC SERVICES

It has been clear for half a century that the greater number of elderly people in our society would change the practice of psychiatry (Lewis, 1946). That this inevitable change is only now occurring with speed and encouragement bears witness to the recalcitrance of established patterns of practice in the face of declared patterns of need. For a while some psychiatric services turned away from the elderly fearing they might tarnish the new-found image of 'curability' that had become associated with general hospital psychiatry, effective physical treatments and psychotherapy, and community care. In addition the old county asylums, ill-sited and ill-equipped to give appropriate response to the needs of old age, fell foul of scandals arising out of inadequate care. Yet gradually good sense has prevailed and a new breed of psychiatric services for the elderly, or psychogeriatric services, has been appearing with increasing consistency over the past decade (Jolley and Arie, 1976). Each service provides individual features dependent upon local geography and available patterns of care, but a broadly similar structure is discernable in most well-known services (Arie and Jolley, 1982; Dick, 1982). Thus they will respond to the mental health needs arising out of the elderly of a defined catchment population, usually a health district of 200,000 with 28,000 aged 65 years plus. In this way most psychogeriatric services dissociate themselves from caring for chronic psychiatric patients who 'graduate' into old age, but accept the full range of psychiatric disorders that arise within the senium. Patients are seen at home for initial assessment and where further investigation is required either at an outpatient clinic or by inpatient care, this should be in association with a geriatric physician and preferably in a general hospital. A series of guidelines (DHSS, 1970, 1971, 1972) has suggested that 0.3 to 0.4 psychiatric beds for severely demented patients should be provided in addition to the general psychiatry ration of 0.5 beds per 1,000 population, but that functional psychiatric disorders in the elderly should be accommodated within that 0.5 beds. Day care (0.3 to 0.4 places per 1,000 population) for severely demented patients is envisaged as an important addition to the beds. These day hospital places are used mainly as a component of continuing care in contrast to the emphasis on rehabilitation seen in most geriatric day hospitals (Brocklehurst and Tucker, 1980). If day hospital places are sited closely with inpatient facilities they are a particularly useful asset in forging a workable link between institution and community modes of care. In some regions well-designed units with both beds and day places are now being built on sites within the population they serve and promise to confirm the principles of good psychogeriatric practice in their bricks and mortar. Yet even these units depend on adequate and appropriate manning.

Young psychiatrists are finding work in well-organized services attractive and rewarding. Nursing staff need to be able to work with patients who present problems from profound physical dependency to active suicidal intent, to organize a range of investigations, and to work with other disciplines in designing and carrying out treatment programmes among in-patients and day patients. In addition, psychiatric nurses working in the community (CPNs) carry support and treatment out of the unit and feed back information to the rest of the unit on progress, successes, and anxieties outside the safe walls in patients' own homes. Social workers provide a further dimension to the care and treatment that is required by patients and their families and establish the service as part of the 'welfare' available to old people. Many patients can survive at home only with help of home-helps, meals-on-wheels, etc., and some may eventually require residential care either with the local authority or in a private or voluntary home. Occupational therapy, physiotherapy, and the skills of the clinical psychologist are required elements of the psychogeriatric team in its work inside and out of the hospital. Liaison with geriatric medicine is essential, and guidelines on achieving this have been issued jointly by the British Geriatric Society and the Royal College of Psychiatrists (Royal College of Psychiatrists, 1979). Close-working relationships with many other disciplines including general medicine surgery are also important, as are relationships with social service departments and the primary health care teams. Psychiatric problems are so prevalent among old people and the capacity of even the most vigorous psychogeriatric team so limited that its role must be one of enabling and facilitating management rather than taking on and taking away all potential clients. Working with colleagues and other agencies is potentially rewarding but requires elements of mutual understanding and respect before this potential can be realized. Working in teams and coordinating the work of a number of teams to achieve the best management of individual patients and groups of patients is not an easy craft and not one that can be acquired from book work alone (Norman, 1982).

Education and Research

Thus there is a great need for educational facilities to make available to the wide range of agencies involved with caring for old people a basic understanding of the psychiatric disorders of old age. There is a similarly great need for those engaged in psychiatric services to gain up-to-date guidance on the recognition and management of physical disorders as they present in their elderly clients. On every hand there is a need to come to terms with the skills and understanding required when working with colleagues on an equal basis. At present a few brave new ventures, most notably the creation of a Department of Health Care of the Elderly at Nottingham, are attempting to open up these important and interesting issues. It will be sad if these approaches fail to find new advocates for want of finance in the currently grim economic climate surrounding the universities.

The same can be said of research. A number of very promising avenues of investigation into the biological substrate of mental disorders, their association with physical illnesses, and the social factors influencing their course and possible management have been initiated during the past 5 years. Let us hope that further exploration will be possible for it will surely add even more interest and attraction to this already fascinating field and may (especially if conceived in terms applied to current dilemmas) facilitate improvements in the care we are able to offer our patients.

REFERENCES

Arie, T., and Jolley, D. J. (1982). 'Making services work: Organization and style of psychogeriatric services', in *The Psychiatry of Late Life* (Eds R. Levy and F. Post), Blackwell Scientific Publications, Oxford.

Bergmann, K. (1971). 'The neuroses of old age', in *Recent Advances in Psychogeriatrics* (Eds D. W. K. Kay and A. Walk), RMPA.

Bergmann, K. (1981). 'Neurosis in old age', in *Health Care of the Elderly* (Ed. Tom Arie), Croom Helm, London.

Bergmann, K., and Eastham, E. G. (1974). 'Psychogeriatric ascertainment and assessment for treatment in an acute medical ward setting', *Age Ageing*, **3**, 174–188.

Blessed, G., Tomlinson, B. E., and Roth, M. (1968). 'The association between quantitative measures of dementia and senile changes in the cerebral grey matter of elderly subjects', *Br. J. Psychiatry*, **114**, 797–811.

Bluegrass, R. (1983). *A Guide to the Mental Health Act 1983*, Churchill Livingstone, Edinburgh.

Blythe, R. (1969). *Akenfield*, Penguin Books, Middlesex (see *District Nurse*, pp. 229–236).

Blythe, R. (1981). *The View in Winter*, Penguin Books, Middlesex.

Boyd, R. (1981). 'What is a "Social Problem" in Geriatrics?', in *Health Care of the Elderly* (Ed. Tom Arie), Croom Helm, London.

Brocklehurst, J. C., and Tucker, J. S. (1980). 'Progress in geriatric day care', King Edwards Hospital Fund, London.

Brown, G. W., Harris, T., and Copeland, J. R. (1977). 'Depression and loss', *Br. J. Psychiatry*, **130**, 1–18.

Clark, A. N. G., Mankikar, G. D., and Gray, I. (1975). 'Diogenes syndrome', *Lancet,* **1**, 366–369.

Committee of Inquiry into Whittingham Hospital (1972). Cmnd. 4861, HMSO, London.

Corsellis, J. A. N. (1977). 'Observations on the neuropathology of dementia', *Age Ageing,* **6** (Suppl.), 20–29.

Corsellis, J. A. N. (1979). 'On the transmission of dementia: A personal view of the slow virus problem', *Br. J. Psychiatry*, **134**, 553–559.

Crow, T. J., Frith, C. D., Johnstone, E. C., and Owens, D. G. (1980). 'Schizophrenia and cerebral atrophy', *Lancet*, **1**, 1129–1130.

DHSS (1970). *Psychogeriatric Assessment Units*, Circular HM 70, p. 11.

DHSS (1971). *Hospital Services for the Mentally Ill*, Circular HM 71, p. 97.

DHSS (1972). *Services for Mental Illness Related to Old Age*, Circular HM 72, p. 71.

DHSS (1973a). *Psychiatric Hospitals and Units in England and Wales, In-Patient Statistics from the Mental Health Enquiry for the Year 1971*, Statistical Research Report Series No. 6, HMSO, London.

DHSS (1973b). *The Facilities and Services of Psychiatric Hospitals in England and Wales 1971*, Statistical and Research Report Series No. 5, HMSO, London.

DHSS (1973c). 'Psychiatric hospitals and units in England and Wales', in *In-Patient Statistics from the Mental Health Inquiry for 1971*, Statistical and Research Report Series No. 6, HMSO, London.

DHSS (1975). *Censuses of Patients in Mental Hospitals and Units in England and Wales at the End of 1971*, Statistical and Research Report Series No. 10, HMSO, London.

DHSS (1979). *In-Patient Statistics for the Mental Health Enquiry for England 1976*, Statistical and Research Report Series No. 22, HMSO, London.

Dick, D. H. (1982). *The Rising Tide*, Developing services for mental illness in old age, National Health Service Health Advisory Service.

Evans, G., Hughes, B., Wilkin, D., and Jolley, D. (1981). 'The management of mental and physical impairment in non-specialist residential homes for the elderly', Psychogeriatric Unit Research Report No. 4, University Hospital of South manchester.

Eysenck, H. (1952). *The Scientific Study of Personality*, Macmillan, New York.

Goldberg, E. M. (1970). *Helping the Aged*, Allen and Unwin, London.

Gunn, J. (1981). 'Reform of mental health legislation', Editorial, *Br. Med. J.*, **283**, 1487–1488.

Hachinski, V. C., Lassen, N. A., and Marshall, J. (1974). 'Multiple infarct dementia', *Lancet*, **2**, 207–210.

Hawks, D. (1975). 'Community care: An analysis of assumptions', *Br. J. Psychiatry*, **127**, 276–285.

Hearnshaw, L. S. (1972). 'Work and age', *Age Ageing*, **1**, 81–87.

Isaacs, B., and Akhtar, A. J. (1972). 'The set test: A rapid test of mental function in old people', *Age Ageing*, **1**, 222–226.

Isaacs, B., and Caird, F. (1976). 'Brain failure: A contribution to the terminology of mental abnormality in old age', *Age Ageing*, **5**, 241.

Jefferys, M. (1978). 'The elderly in society', in *Text-book of Geriatric Medicine and Gerontology (Ed. J. C. Brocklehurst)*, Churchill Livingstone.

Jolley, D. J. (1981a). 'Acute confusional states in the elderly', in *Acute Geriatric Medicine* (Ed. D. Coakley), Croom Helm, London.

Jolley, D. J. (1981b). 'Dementia: Misfits in need of care', in *Health Care of the Elderly* (Ed. T. Arie) Croom Helm, London.

Jolley, D. J., and Arie, T. (1976). 'Psychiatric services for the elderly: How many beds?', *Br. J. Psychiatry*, **129**, 418–423.

Jolley, D. J., and Arie, T. (1978). 'Organization of Psychogeriatric Services'. *Br. J. Psychiatry*. **132**, 1–11.

Jolley, D. J., and Arie, T. (1980). 'Dementia in old age: An outline of current issues', *Health Trends*, **12**, 1–4.

Jones, K., and Sidebotham, R. (1962). *Mental Hospitals at Work*, Routledge and Kegan-Paul, Henley-on-Thames.

Kay, D. W. K. (1963). 'Late paraphrenia and its bearing on the aetiology of schizophrenia', *Acta Psychiatr. Scand.*, **39**, 159–170.

Kay, D. W. K., Beamish, P., and Roth, M. (1962). 'Some medical and social characteristics of elderly people under state care', Sociol. Rev. Monogr. No. 5, University of Keele.

Kay, D. W. K., Beamish, P., and Roth, M. (1964). 'Old age mental disorders in Newcastle upon Tyne: Part 1: A study of prevalence', *Br. J. Psychiatry*, **110**, 146–158.

Kendell, R. E. (1979). 'Alcoholism: A medical or a political problem?', *Br. Med. J.*, **1**, 367–371.

Kessel, W. I. N. (1965). 'Self poisoning', *Br. Med. J.*, **2**, 1265–1270 and 1336–1340.

Kraepelin, E. (1909). *Psychiatry*, 8th ed, Leipzig.

Larsson, T., Sjogren, T., and Jacobsen, G. (1963). 'Senile dementia', *Acta. Psychiatr. Scand.*, **39** (Suppl.), 167.

Levy, R. (1975). 'The neurophysiology of dementia', in *Contemporary Psychiatry* (Eds T. Silverstone and B. Barraclough), *Br. J. Psychiatry*, Special Publication No. 9.

Lewis, A. (1946). 'Ageing and senility: A major problem for psychiatry', *J. Ment. Sc.*, **92**, 150–170.

Lipowski, Z. J. (1980). 'Delirium updated', *Compr. Psychiatry*, **21** (3), 190–196.

Lishman, W. A. (1978). *Organic Psychiatry*, Blackwell Scientific Publications, Oxford.

Livesley, B. (1977). 'The pathogenesis of brain failure in the elderly', *Age Ageing*, **6** (Suppl.), 9–19.

Luxon, L., Lees, A. J., and Greenwood, R. J. (1979). 'Neurosyphilis today', *Lancet*, **1**, 90–93.

McDonald, C. (1969). 'Clinical heterogeneity in senile dementia', *Br. J. Psychiatry*, **115**, 267–271.

McKeown, T. (1976). *The Modern Rise of Population*, Edward Arnold, London.

Mann, D. M. A., Yates, P. O., and Barton, C. M. (1977). 'Cytophotometric mapping of neuronal changes in senile dementia', *J. Neurol. Neurosurg. Psychiatry*, **40**, 299–302.

Muir Gray, J. A. (1980). 'Section 47', *Age Ageing*, **9**, 205–209.

Nielson, J. (1962). 'Geronto-psychiatric period prevalence investigation in a geographically delimited population', *Acta. Psychiatr. Scand.*, **38**, 307.

Norman, A. (1982). *Mental Illness in old age: Meeting the Challenge*, Policy Studies in Ageing No. 1, Centre for Policy on Ageing.

Nunn, C., Bergmann, K., Britton, P. G., Foster, E. M., Hall, E. M., and Kay, D. W. K. (1974). 'Intelligence and neurosis in old age', *Br. J. Psychiatry*, **124**, 446–452.

O'Brien, T. D. (1971). 'Disease and disability in residential homes for the elderly', M. D. Thesis, Manchester University.

Office of Health Economics (1979). *Dementia in Old Age*.

Office of Health Economics (1980). *Huntington's Chorea*.

Olson, M. I., and Shaw, G. M. (1969). 'Presenile dementia and Alzheimer's disease in mongolism', *Brain*, **92**, 147–156.

Parkes, C. M. (1972). *Bereavement*, Tavistock, London.

Perry, E. K. (1980). 'The cholinergic system in old age and Alzheimer's disease', *Age Ageing*, **9**, 1–8.

Pippard, J., and Ellam, L. (1981). 'Electro convulsive treatment in Great Britain', *Br. J. Psychiatry*. **139**, 563–568.

Post, F. (1962). *The Significance of Affective Symptoms in Old Age*, Oxford University Press, London.

Post, F. (1965). *The Clinical Psychiatry of Late Life*, Pergamon Press, Oxford.

Post, F. (1966). *Persistent Persecutory States of the Elderly*, Pergamon Press, Oxford.

Post, F. (1971). 'Schizo-affective symptomatology in late life', *Br. J. Psychiatry*, **118**, 437–445.

Post, F. (1975). 'Dementia, depression and pseudodementia', in *Psychiatric Aspects of Neurological Disease*, (Eds F. Benson and D. Blumer), Grune and Strattan, New York.

Post, F. (1978). 'Then and now', *Br. J. Psychiatry*, **133**, 83–86.

Powell-Proctor, L. (1981). 'Reality orientation: A treatment of choice?, *Geriatr. Med.*, November **1981**, 88–92.

Qureshi, K. N., and Hodkinson, H. M. (1974). 'Evaluation of a ten-question mental test in the institutionalized elderly', *Age Ageing*, **1**, 152–157.

Rossor, M. N. (1981). 'Parkinson's disease and Alzheimer's disease as disorders of the isodendritic core', *Br. Med. J.*, **283**, 1588–1590.

Roth, M. (1955). 'The natural history of mental disorder in old age', *J. Ment. Sc.*, **101**, 281–296.

Royal College of Psychiatrists (1979). *Guidelines for Collaboration between Geriatric Physicians and Psychiatrists in the Care of the Elderly*, The Bulletin, November, p. 168.

Sainsbury, P., Costain, W. R., and Grad, J. (1965). 'The effects of a community service on the referral and admission rates of elderly psychiatric patients', in *Psychiatric Disorders in the Aged*, W. P. A. Symposium. Geigy, Manchester.

Schneider, K. (1923). *Psychopathic Personalities*, 9th ed. (1950), F. Denticke, Vienna.

Shepherd, M., Cooper, B., Brown, A. C., and Kalton, G. (1981). *Psychiatric Illness in General Practice*, 2nd ed., Oxford University Press, Oxford.

Shulman, K. (1978). 'Suicide and parasuicide in old age', *Age Ageing*, **2**, 201–209.

Slater, E., and Cowie, V. (1971). *The Genetics of Mental Disorders*, Oxford University Press.

Sjogren, T., Sjogren, H., and Lingren, A. G. H. (1952). 'Morbus Alzheimer and Morbus Pick: genetic clinical and patho-anatomical study', *Acta Psychiatr. Scand.*, **82** (Suppl.).

Smith, S. (1961). 'Psychiatry in general hospitals', *Lancet*, **2**, 1158.

Stout, I., and Jolley, D. (1981). 'The dementia syndrome and how to recognize it', *Geriatr. Med.*, February **1981**, 15–18.

Sutton, R. N. P., and Lord, A. (1978). 'Slow viruses and neurological disease', in *Modern Topics in Infection* (Ed. J. Williams), Heinemann, London.

The Disability Alliance (1979). *The Government's Failure to Plan for Disablement in Old Age*, (Principal author Peter Townsend).

Tomlinson, B. E., Blessed, G., and Roth, M. (1970). 'Observations on the brains of demented old people', *J. Neurol. Sci.*, **11**, 205–242.

Verwoerdt, A. (1981). 'Psychotherapy for the elderly', in *Health Care of the Elderly* (Ed. T. Arie), Croom Helm, London.

Wilkin, D., and Jolley, D. J. (1978). 'Mental and physical impairment in the elderly in hospital and residential care', *Nurs. Times.*, **74** (29), 117–120, 124.

Woods, R. T., and Britton, P. G. (1977). 'Psychological approaches to the treatment of the elderly', *Age Ageing*, **8**, 104–108.

18
Special Senses

Principles and Practice of Geriatric Medicine
Edited by M. S. J. Pathy
© 1985 John Wiley & Sons Ltd

18.1

The Eye

P. Graham

EXTERNAL CONDITIONS

A small group of diseases affecting the external eye is seen predominantly in the elderly. These conditions are mostly of a relatively trivial nature, but they are often missed or misunderstood.

Entropion

Senile entropion results from atrophic changes in the lower lid. Fibres of the orbicularis muscle, lacking adequate support, migrate upwards towards the lid margin, causing the lower part of the thin and flexible tarsal plate to lose support. Contraction of the muscle than causes the lid margin to become kinked inwards, so that the lashes rub on the eye, causing considerable discomfort. The condition is not necessarily present continually, and where the history suggests its presence, the deformity can often be provoked by asking the patient to squeeze the lids tightly, when the lid margin may be observed to invert. Correction requires a minor plastic procedure, and a variety of operations is in use – a sure sign that none is entirely free from recurrence. While operation is awaited, relief from the discomfort may be obtained by applying a 2 to 3 mm wide strip of adhesive plaster vertically to keep the lid margin slightly everted.

Ectropion and Epiphora

In its more severe form, ectropion is easily identified as the lower lid is clearly not in apposition to the globe, and indeed the lid may become so far everted that the lower palpebral conjunctiva is exposed and becomes hypertrophic. In the earlier stages, however, at a time when it is easily corrected, it is often overlooked. Ectropion of the medial part of the lower lid leads to the lower lacrimal punctum becoming slightly everted, so that it ceases to dip into the tears collecting at the inner angle. As a result, tears overflow from the most dependent central part of the lid. The eye is then wiped repeatedly, often in a downward direction, accentuating the deformity. At the stage of slight medial eversion only, application of the cautery to the conjunctival surface of the lid below the punctum will often correct the defect and restore normal drainage, whereas the later stages may require more extensive plastic repair.

Watering of the eye in any age group may be due to obstruction of the canaliculus or naso lacrimal duct, but in the elderly an additional cause is watering in the absence of any obstruction on irrigation. It is probable that the cause is a gradual reduction in the efficiency of the 'pumping' action of the orbicularis muscle on the lacrimal sac. This type of epiphora is difficult to relieve.

VISUAL IMPAIRMENT

Table 1 *Common causes of visual failure in the elderly*

Rapid onset	Gradual onset
Retinal detachment	Cataract
Vascular occlusion	Macular degeneration
Ischaemic optic	Chronic glaucoma
neuropathy	Diabetic retinopathy
Acute glaucoma	

Retinal Detachment

The vast majority of retinal detachments are due to the formation of retinal holes, and only this type (rhegmatogenous detachment) is considered. Of the several types of retinal hole, two show an increasing frequency with age.

The arrowhead tear occurs most frequently in the upper temporal quadrant of the retina, and is associated with adhesion of the vitreous to the retina combined with traction due to changes in the vitreous gel as a result of age. These lead to retraction of the vitreous from the retina, which is extremely common from middle age onwards, and in most cases is harmless although it often causes alarm by producing recurring entoptic streaks of light in the peripheral field accompanied by a 'floater' which is due to a small opacity on the posterior vitreous face. The flashes are due to the detached vitreous touching the retina during eye movements, and gradually cease as the gel retracts further. The condition is eponymously named Foster–Moore's syndrome. Although it is only very occasionally a precursor of detachment, it is probably wise to dilate the pupil and examine the retinal periphery carefully.

Round retinal holes form as a result of degenerative processes in the retina, are often multiple, and may be preceded by other ophthalmoscopic signs such as peripheral lattice degeneration. They are in fact not uncommon, being found in 'normal' eyes at autopsy, and although some lead to separation of the retina, this is not invariably the case.

The symptoms of retinal detachment vary. In most cases there is a spreading shadow starting in the periphery of the field, in the quadrant diametrically opposed to the actual detaching retina, sometimes preceded by bright entoptic flashes. When the detachment involves the macular area, the visual failure becomes profound. It is not uncommon, especially in the case of the arrowhead tear, for the formation of the hole to rupture a small blood vessel, leading to haemorrhage into the vitreous which precedes the actual separation of the retina.

The management of these patients depends on whether or not the retina has already detached. If a retinal hole likely to cause detachment is found, then the promotion of inflammatory adhesions between choroid and retina by light coagulation with a laser or xenon arc, or by external application of a cryoprobe, will seal the hole and prevent separation. Such holes are usually symptomatic, causing light flashes or haemorrhage, or are in the sound eye of a patient with detachment, and the simple discovery of an asymptomatic hole on routine examination does not mean that treatment is necessarily advisable.

If detachment has already occurred, adhesion can only be promoted after the retina and choroid have been brought into apposition by one or more of a variety of complex surgical procedures, the selection of which requires considerable experience.

The prognosis for central vision in detachment depends mainly on whether the macula itself has been detached and on the duration of the separation. Even a brief period of macular detachment often leads to some impairment, which increases rapidly with time. Where the macula remains attached, the visual effects may be confined to some loss of visual field.

Vascular Occlusion

Complete occlusion of the central retinal artery is a relatively uncommon event, but transient obstruction of the main vessel or one of its branches is fairly common and gives rise to the temporary obscuration of vision known as amaurosis fugax, which may involve either the whole or only part of the visual field. In complete occlusion, the cause may be either an embolus, arising from atheroma of the great vessels or less commonly from valvular disease of the heart, or thrombosis. It may also be caused by giant-cell arteritis (Chapter 24), although an ischaemic optic neuropathy is more common in this condition. In both cases, spasm may serve to complete an otherwise partial obstruction. Amaurosis fugax is usually due to the passage of friable platelet emboli, and it is remarkable how successive emboli may be observed to pursue a consistent path through the vessels, giving a similar loss of field in each attack. This constant path is presumably determined by haemodynamic factors, such as the streaming of flow in the vessels.

In complete occlusion vision is totally and

very suddenly lost. The central artery may be observed to be attenuated and to contain a fragmented column of blood. Within a few minutes the inner layers of the posterior retina in the area affected lose their transparency and become milky-white except for the fovea, where these layers are thin, so that the typical 'cherry-red spot' is seen. Occasionally in a branch occlusion, the actual embolus may be visible, usually impacted at a bifurcation. The history and appearance leave no doubt as to diagnosis. In contrast, the diagnosis of amaurosis fugax has to be made largely from history, although rarely one may be fortunate enough to be able to observe emboli in transit during an attack.

Treatment of a complete occlusion, especially where the whole retina is involved, is unfortunately rarely effective. Many of these patients are not seen until some hours or even days after the event, by which time, even if circulation is restored, function does not return. In very recent occlusions, it is sometimes possible to move the embolus more peripherally, and thereby limit the permanent damage, by the use of vasodilators, massage of the eye, and even paracentesis of the anterior chamber to lower intraocular pressure and improve blood flow. In most, however, there is substantial permanent loss of vision.

In amaurosis fugax, a search should be made for a possible origin of the emboli. In some cases, this is in the carotid, and endarterectomy may be worth considering, especially if there have been other transient neurological symptoms. In the more common situation where no direct attack on the source of emboli is possible, the long-term use of small doses of aspirin may be of value in reducing platelet stickiness.

Venous occlusion is much more common than arterial obstruction. In most cases, only a portion of the venous drainage is affected, and the obstruction is not always complete. A major factor in the causation of venous obstruction seems to be external pressure upon the vein. This may be from the adjacent artery, since the site of obstruction can frequently be observed to be an arteriovenous crossing, and it is therefore probable that disease of the arterial wall is a factor. Stasis, due to reduction in flow from disease on the arterial side may also play a part, and there is a significant as-

sociation between raised intraocular pressure and the occurrence of venous occlusion.

The clinical picture is variable, depending on whether the obstruction is at the disk or in the branch vein, and also on whether it is partial or complete. There may be no symptoms whatever if the macular area is not involved, and a branch vein occlusion or a partial obstruction at the disk may sometimes be observed during routine ophthalmoscopy. The appearance may vary from no more than an increase in the calibre and tortuosity of the veins through scattered superficial haemorrhages to the gross picture of complete obstruction at the disk, when the veins are enormously dilated and tortuous, the disk swollen and oedematous, and the whole fundus is covered with both superficial and deep haemorrhages. It is worth noting that a picture very similar to that of partial obstruction at the disk may be produced by a general restriction of retinal flow, such as may occur in Takayasu's (or pulseless) disease.

The prognosis in venous occlusion is also very variable. A greater or lesser degree of collateral circulation eventually bypasses the site of obstruction, and these vessels can often be identified ophthalmoscopically. The extent to which function returns is to some extent related to the severity of the initial clinical picture, but is also dependent on the relation of the area affected to the macula. Fluorescein angiography in these patients shows that there may be areas of retina in which the capillary circulation is absent with associated microaneurysms – a picture reminiscent of diabetic retinopathy. These areas of retina become hypoxic and, as in the diabetic, this may provoke the development of highly permeable new vessels with, later, fibrosis and traction. If adjacent to the macula, leakage from these vessels may impair central vision, while they are, like those seen in diabetes, liable to cause preretinal or vitreous haemorrhage. In the worse cases of occlusion at the disk, large areas of retina may become ischaemic, leading to extensive neovascularization, not only of the retina but also in the iris and anterior chamber angle, giving rise to an intractable form of haemorrhagic glaucoma which responds poorly to treatment and may lead to enucleation as the only means of relieving pain.

The likely prognosis can be reasonably

assessed at about 3 months after the onset, by which time collateral circulation will have become established. If little or no recovery of vision has occurred by this time, the prognosis for significant improvement is poor. In cases where there has been complete occlusion of the whole venous drainage and there are large areas of non-perfused retina, consideration should be given to pan-retinal ablation with the xenon-arc coagulator or argon laser in order to prevent the development of neovascular glaucoma. Treatment of areas of non-perfusion close to the macula or of localized neovascular formations must be considered very carefully, and it is advisable to wait for 12 months or more before intervening. Not all localized new vessels bleed, and it is probably wise to wait until the first occurrence of heamorrhage before embarking on treatment. In the past, treatment with anticoagulants has been employed, especially in partial obstruction, but trials have given unconvincing results, although there is some suggestion that they may both reduce the incidence of neovascular glaucoma and provoke vitreous haemorrhage. It is now fairly generally agreed that their use is not indicated in this condition.

Suggested further reading:- Kohner and Schilling, 1976a.

Acute Glaucoma

The main factor in this disease is mechanical, the root of the iris coming into contact with the trabecular tissue in the angle of the anterior chamber. Acute angle closure occurs in the younger subject in association with the shallow anterior chamber and the consequent narrow angle seen in hypermetropes. With increasing age there is a gradual reduction in the depth of the anterior chamber due to growth of the lens (which grows throughout life), so that angle closure glaucoma shows an increasing incidence with age.

External factors also play a part, and attacks may be provoked by dilatation of the pupil in poor light or, paradoxically, by pupillary constriction which, by impeding the flow of aqueous through the pupil, causes forward bowing of the iris ('physiological' iris bombe). It is also well known that the use of mydriatic drugs may provoke attacks, as may emotional stress.

In the typical acute attack there is severe pain, caused by the rapid rise in intraocular pressure, with profound reduction in vision. The pain may involve the whole fifth nerve territory. The eye becomes injected and the cornea becomes oedematous, so that detail of the iris is difficult to see and the pupil is semidilated, inactive, and often non-circular. The eye feels hard on palpation.

Permanent damage to vision will rapidly result from untreated acute glaucoma, and immediate skilled opthalmic assistance is required. The pressure can usually be reduced by the use of osmotic agents orally (glycerol) or intravenously (mannitol), acetazoleamide to reduce aqueous secretion, and miotics. After the pressure has fallen and the eye has settled down, the management is surgical. Most eyes can be rendered safe by the simple procedure of making a small peripheral iridectomy, which widens the angle of the anterior chamber, though in some, permanent damage to the angle may have so impaired natural aqueous outflow that external drainage must be established by filtration surgery.

The typical acute glaucoma may be preceded or replaced by lesser degrees of angle closure, giving attacks, typically in the evenings, of slight discomfort and impairment of vision associated with the characteristic symptom of rainbow haloes around small bright sources of light (not radiating streaks or spokes). These haloes should be distinguished from those which may arise in the early stages of cataract. The latter are usually fainter and are constant over periods of weeks or months, whereas glaucomatous haloes last only a few hours and are unmistakably rainbow in character.

Suggested further reading: Heilmann and Richardson, 1978.

Cataract

Senile cataract is the commonest remediable cause of blindness in the elderly with, as its name implies, a rapidly rising incidence with age. The aetiology remains obscure, though there is no doubt that metabolic factors play a part in its genesis and that there is some hereditary element. It occurs much more commonly in the eyes of diabetic patients (and should not be confused with true diabetic cataract which is rare, of rapid onset, and usually seen in younger patients) and is also a common consequence of miotic therapy for glaucoma; it is much more common and occurs at an earlier age in, for example, the Indian subcontinent than in Europe. The relative importance of heredity, nutritional factors, and other environmental influences in this increased prevalence is not known.

The disease presents in several forms, its initial symptoms depending on the type of cataract. The commonest form, cuneiform cataract, presents ophthalmoscopically as a series of spokes or wedges of opacity, best seen sharply focused against the red reflex of the fundus by using a +10 D lens in the opthalmoscope. Initially these opacities are concealed behind the iris and can be seen only with the pupil dilated, causing no symptoms. This stage is very common in the elderly, and as many of these opacities never progress to the point of serious impairment of vision, needless worry may be caused to patients by mentioning their presence when they are found during routine ophthalmoscopy. Cuneiform cataract usually only increases slowly, and causes a gradual decrease in both distant and near vision, often with increased difficulty in bright light owing to the scattering effect of the opacities.

In contrast to the very slow development of cuneiform cataract, centrally placed opacities cause a more rapid deterioration in vision by virtue of their greater optical effect. In some eyes, the slow increase in refractive index of the lens nucleus becomes pathologically accelerated, causing a rapid increase in the converging power of the lens, leading to myopia, of which the first sign is a deterioration in distant vision together with decreasing dependence on reading glasses. At this stage, the signs on opthalmoscopy are minimal, especially with an undilated pupil, as there is only a slight loss of transparency in the central part of the lens and the vision can still be improved by a change of spectacles. With a dilated pupil the loss of transparency is more obvious by contrast with the clear periphery. Later, usually when the refraction has become 7 to 8 dioptres more myopic than at the onset, the central lens becomes almost opaque, with rapid deterioration in acuity.

The most rapid loss of vision is seen when the cataract occupies the central posterior cortex of the lens, which is close to the nodal point of the optical system of the eye. This is the site of opacities secondary to other intraocular disease, the effects of radiation or steri-

oid therapy, but there is a form of senile cataract producing in its early stages a sheet of opacity in the posterior lens which is known as cupuliform cataract. This causes a rapid fall in acuity, most noticeable in bright light and on reading, both of which lead to pupillary constriction.

All forms of senile cataract eventually end with a completely opaque lens, and in the later stages the degenerate cortex may liquefy, with absorption of water from the aqueous and swelling, leading in some cases to the diffusion of irritant material into the anterior eye, producing a form of uveitis, often with secondary glaucoma. This may require removal of the lens even in circumstances where there is little visual benefit.

The indications for removal of cataract depend very much on the occupation and visual requirements of the patient. Although for many years it has been possible to remove the lens by the intracapsular method at any time in the evolution of cataract, the belief that surgery is impossible until the cataract is 'ripe' (i.e. until most of the lens cortex has become opaque) still persists, and it is necessary to make sure that the patient understands that surgery will be advised as soon as it is likely that aphakic vision will be an improvement rather than a handicap. For a patient who requires good central acuity this may be early, in some cases when vision is still 6/9 or 6/12, but in those who do little reading, the distortion, alteration in magnification, and restriction in visual field inherent in spectacle correction of these eyes, even if modern aspheric lenses are used, can be such a poor exchange for improved central acuity that it may be desirable to defer operation until poor vision is clearly impairing mobility. Unilateral or markedly asymmetrical cataract presents a special problem, as spectacle correction of an aphakic eye is impossible in these circumstances.

The unsatisfactory optical state of the eye when corrected by spectacles after cataract surgery may be somewhat ameliorated by using contact lenses, but this approach is rather limited by the fact that the elderly often have considerable difficulty in tolerating and manipulating contact lenses, even of the soft, extended wear types now available.

Fortunately, at the present time, developments in intraocular surgery have begun to produce a solution to this optical problem, with a return to a modification of the older, extracapsular type of operation in which, instead of removing the whole lens with its capsule intact, the anterior capsule is incised and the contents removed, leaving the equatorial and posterior capsule *in situ*. In its original form this operation was abandoned, as only the hard central nucleus of the lens could be removed, leaving the softer peripheral cortex to disintegrate and slowly absorb, to the accompaniment of considerable irritation and potential complications, often leading to the capsule becoming opaque, the so-called after-cataract. It was with the objective of minimizing the amount of soft cortex that cataracts were allowed to 'ripen'.

Major factors in the revival of extracapsular surgery have been the widespread use of the operating microscope and the development of finely controllable suction/aspiration instrumentation permitting the accurate and controlled removal of all soft lens material under high magnification. Together with this development there has been an increasing use and sophistication of acrylic intraocular lenses, after both intra- and extracapsular surgery. These restore almost normal optics and thereby overcome the problems inherent in spectacle or contact lens correction of aphakia, especially where this is unilateral.

The modern form of extracapsular extraction makes the fixation of intraocular lenses more satisfactory as the lens can be retained in the empty capsule, and there is also hope that it will lead to a decreased incidence of postoperative retinal detachment and the persistent maculopathy which often mars the result of an otherwise successful operation. A careful balance must be struck between the increased difficulty and operative risks of the more complex operations and their potentially much superior functional results, but it is steadily tilting in favour of their advantages, although many surgeons are still reluctant to insert lens implants into both eyes.

Macular Degeneration

Senile macular degeneration is by a large margin the most common cause of intractable blindness in the elderly. There are several different clinical modes of presentation, but all are variants of the same underlying abnormality.

The first ophthalmoscopic sign of the disease may be seen at a fairly early age, though it is rare before the fourth decade. It takes the form of small, localized, and ill-defined white or yellow-white spots, most frequently seen in the macular area although they may occur anywhere in the fundus, known as colloid bodies or drusen. These are small hyaline excrescences on the membrane of Bruch which separates the choroid from the pigment epithelium. Overlying these excrescences, the pigment epthelium becomes thinned, producing the typical small pale spot. The drusen are not necessarily permanent and their distribution may change with time. Where they absorb, the atrophic changes in the pigment epithelium persist and may coalesce to from 'windows' of depigmentation which are visible with the ophthalmoscope. At this stage, which may never be passed, there is no impairment of vision.

The adhesion of the pigment epithelium to Bruch's membrane in these eyes tends to be defective, and eventually areas may actually detach, the space becoming filled with serous fluid. The outer layers of the overlying retina become more remote from their source of blood supply, which is exclusively from the choroid (the outer retina being avascular), and retinal function is impaired. Eventually, permanent atrophic changes occur in both retina and pigment epithelium. This process manifests itself clinically as a reduction in central acuity, often with metamorphopsia – i.e. the distortion of perceived shape due to disturbance of the arrangement of the retinal receptors.

Concurrently with this process of detachment of the pigment epithelium, there is frequently an ingrowth through small defects in Bruch's membrane of small tufts of neovascular tissue from the choroid into the space beneath the pigment epithelium. These vessels are very permeable and may give rise to serous exudation or haemorrhage into this space. Bleeding may rupture through into the potential space between retina and pigment epithelium, and even occasionally through the retina itself, giving preretinal or vitreous haemorrhage. The occurrence of this type of exudative or haemorrhagic process is accompanied by a rapid, profound, and permanent fall in central vision. The area involved gradually resolves into an atrophic, approximately circular scar, giving this variant the name of disciform macular degeneration.

A further variant is the occurrence of a slow atrophic change involving the whole of the macular area in eyes exhibiting drusen. The choroid becomes attenuated and the pigment in the pigment epithelium becomes dispersed and aggregated into ophthalmoscopically visible clumps, while the overlying retina becomes atrophic, with gradual impairment of function. Deterioration of vision in this type of senile macular degeneration is often very slow, but at any time may accelerate owing to the onset of detachment of the pigment epithelium or disciform degeneration. The exact nature of the pathological process which produces this atrophic change (sometimes called 'dry' senile macular degeneration) is uncertain.

All of these forms of degeneration can be diagnosed with the opthalmoscope, but additional information, which may be of value in assessing the possibility of treatment, can be obtained by fluorescein angiography of the fundus, which reveals subretinal neovascular tufts and delineates areas of detached pigment epithelium. Unfortunately, although our understanding of some of the pathological processes concerned in senile macular degeneration has increased considerably, the therapeutic possibilities remain very limited. Though numerous claims have been made for various forms of drug therapy, there is no convincing evidence that any systemic or topical medication affects the course of the disease. The only form of treatment of any value, in a very limited number of patients, is the destruction of subretinal neovascular formations by photocoagulation, preferably using the argon laser, and the treatment of areas of pigment epithelial detachment with the krypton or argon laser to limit their spread. The former is applicable only to those formations which are not so close to the fovea that the treatment itself would destroy central vision, or situated between the fovea and the optic disk, where effective treatment would interrupt the nerve fibre layer, with a similar disastrous effect. This considerably limits the technique, and trials suggest that the most that can be expected is that destruction of suitably placed neovascular formations will at least delay, but probably not prevent, eventual loss of central vision. To be effective at all, treatment must be carried out in the very early stages of visual deterioration, and the number of eyes in which lesions are suitably placed is disappointingly small.

For the majority, where treatment is not possible, management resolves into assisting the patient to make the best use of the remaining vision. These patients understandably believe that the deterioration in vision will progress relentlessly to complete blindness, and it is essential to emphasize that the disease affects central vision only and that peripheral vision will remain intact. The use of magnifying aids is helpful, from the simple magnifying glass to compound spectacle magnifiers which allow high magnification at a reasonable working distance, albeit with a restricted field. Macular degeneration is often combined with some degree of cataract simply because both are common diseases of the elderly eye, and removal of the cataract may well be helpful.

Suggestions for further reading: Ffytche, 1976; Gass, 1977.

Chronic Glaucoma

Chronic glaucoma is a relatively common disease, having a markedly increasing incidence with age. Although loss of vision in one eye is not uncommon, it is not so commonly the primary cause of blindness in both eyes (registrable blindness) as is often believed. In many patients in whom glaucoma is mentioned in the statistics of blindness, the glaucoma is an associated disease, the actual cause of blindness being one of the other prevalent disorders of old age, or the glaucoma is a secondary consequence of other intraocular diseases.

The onset of chronic glaucoma is insidious, with a gradual loss of peripheral visual field. Only at a very late stage is central vision, and therefore the visual acuity, affected. The loss of field is believed on good evidence to be due to ischaemic damage to the intraocular portion of the optic nerve, the circulation in this tissue being influenced by the level of intraocular pressure, although anatomical and general vascular factors probably also play a part. The mean intraocular pressure of glaucomatous eyes is above that for normal eyes, but it is important to realize that there is a very considerable overlap, nerve damage identical to that seen in classical chronic glaucoma with 'raised' pressure occurring in eyes with 'normal' pressure, and eyes being observed with 'abnormal' pressure over many years without damage. It is not possible to set a reliable upper limit for safe pressure.

There is a considerable hereditary tendency in the disease. This is polygenetic, so it does not follow a Mendelian pattern but manifests itself as a substantially increased incidence in immediate relatives.

As a relatively common disease of insidious onset, chronic glaucoma has received attention as a possible target for presymptomatic screening. Initially, it was hoped that measurement of intraocular pressure would serve to detect early cases of the disease. This hope has not been realized, owing to the impossibility of defining 'normal' pressure, as noted above. It is now generally accepted that mass tonometric screening is ineffective and wasteful of resources. Early cases of the disease can often be recognized or suspected by careful observation of the central cup of the optic disk, in particular the ratio of the diameter of the cup to that of the disk itself. A ratio of over 0.6:1.0 is very uncommon in normal eyes, and merits further investigation. Another approach has been to make use of the higher incidence of glaucoma in near relatives by confining screening efforts to the older members of this group. Bearing in mind that loss of vision in both eyes from chronic glaucoma alone is uncommon, the cost-effectiveness of widespread screening is doubtful, and its use could divert scarce ophthalmic resources from more worthwhile work.

The management of glaucoma is based on control of the intraocular pressure to a level at which loss of visual field ceases. This level varies from one patient to another, and the only certain method of assessing the adequacy of control is the monitoring of the state of the visual field at regular intervals. Control of pressure is normally achieved wherever possible by using topical administration of miotic drugs, the first choice usually being pilocarpine, possibly supplemented by adrenaline and in some cases by oral administration of acetazoleamide. More recently the beta-blocking drug timolol has been widely employed in topical form, and has the advantage of avoiding the unpleasant visual effects of the miosis induced by pilocarpine. No single treatment regime suits all patients and the most suitable one must be determined for each individual by trial. In some cases, if adequate control of pressure cannot be achieved by medical means it is necessary to reduce the pressure surgically.

Suggested further reading: Heilmann and Richardson, 1978.

Diabetic Retinopathy

The neovascular form of diabetic retinopathy is seen more commonly in younger patients, usually with insulin-dependent disease. More characteristic of the maturity onset diabetic is a background retinopathy with normal vision, eventually developing into an exudative maculopathy with gradually falling central acuity.

Fluorescein angiography of the macular area in these patients shows areas of capillary nonperfusion, around the edges of which are the typical diabetic exudates, frequently producing partial or complete circinate formations. Where the fovea is included within one of these, treatment is not practicable, as the retina within these areas is no longer capable of function, but where they are eccentrically placed, photocoagulation of the centre of the formation to destroy the hypoxic retina usually leads to resolution of the surrounding exudates and may improve vision or prevent its deterioration. This procedure is best carried out after identification of the areas to be treated by angiography, and to be effective it must be undertaken before vision deteriorates or in the very early stages of visual loss.

Suggested further reading:- Kohner and Schilling, 1976b.

REFERENCES

Ffytche, T. J., (1976). 'Macular Disease' in *Medical Opthalmology* (Ed. F. C. Rose), Chapman of Hall, London.

Gass, D. M. J. (1977). *Stereoscopic Atlas of Macular Diseases*, C. V. Mosby Co., St. Louis.

Heilmann, K., and Richardson, K. T. (1978). *Glaucoma: Conceptions of a Disease*, Georg Thieme, Stuttgart.

Kohner, E. M., and Schilling, J. S., (1976). 'Retina Vein Occlusion', in *Medical Ophthalmology* (Ed. F. C. Rose), Chapman of Hall, London.

Kohner, E. M. and Schilling, J. S. (1976b). 'Treatment of diabetic retinopathy', in *Medical Ophthalmology* (Ed. F. C. Rose), Chapman & Hall, London.

Principles and Practice of Geriatric Medicine
Edited by M. S. J. Pathy
© 1985 John Wiley & Sons Ltd

18.2

The Auditory System

R. Mills

Although examples can always be found in everyday personal experience of individuals who, even in advanced old age, retain 'perfect' hearing, the majority of the elderly suffer from a varying degree of hearing loss. Such change is so normally associated with old age that it is accepted as almost 'a fact of life', and the loss, certainly in our society, is in consequence commonly not afforded the consideration given to other handicaps and infirmities.

The physiologic changes of normal senescence in the auditory system become at some stage advanced enough (and of such a character) to cross a 'borderline' after which the changes become pathological in the clinical and social sense that difficulty in communication arises. Where that 'borderline', admittedly an indistinct and grey area, lies must in part depend upon the nature and extent of structural and functional deficiencies in the auditory apparatus. It will also depend upon other factors – the ability or willingness of the patient to exercise other, particularly visual, sensory systems as aids to the failing faculty of hearing (indeed it depends upon a basic wish to hear at all), and the quality of the auditory information provided by the cocommunicator. In the elderly the particular and usual problem is presbyacusis – the age-related changes which occur in the auditory apparatus and lead variably to hearing difficulty.

PRESBYACUSIS

Presbyacusis is defined as the deafness of ageing. This loss of efficiency and gradual deterio-

ration in the auditory system is compounded, in common with all senescent processes, by both a decrease in viability and an increase in vulnerability of the constituent cells. The hearing loss is a consequence of the functional components of the auditory system failing to keep themselves in good working order, a property determined presumably by genetic and hereditary factors, against the onslaught over the years of potentially noxious agents. Presbyacusis will result from genetic or hereditary factors and their interplay with known or suspected, potentially deleterious, agents active in the cellular environment, although in any case it is presently impossible to distinguish the relative contribution to hearing loss provided by each facet of this equation.

Aetiology

Research into the aetiology of presbyacusis has been largely concerned with examination of the contribution that these potentially deleterious agents may make. Against the background of the, at present, unmeasureable variance of individual susceptibility, no clear-cut answer may be expected.

A number of possible factors have been examined of which the favourite candidate is noise-induced damage—the constant noise, variable in its intensity, present in the environment to which the auditory system is exposed throughout life. Its importance is evoked to explain sex differences in presbyacusis and the differences observed in the hearing of the aged in rural and urban populations (Hinchcliffe,

1959a, 1959b; Rosen *et al.*, 1964 Weston, 1964). However, studies of the hearing loss in ageing subjects with a history of wartime noise exposure suggest the independence of presbyacusis and noise-induced hearing loss (Macrae, 1971). Consideration has also been given to the importance of diet and climatic conditions, but their immediate relevance is complicated by the effect they in turn might have upon cardiovascular disease, another possible aetiological agent (Rosen, 1969; Rosen and Olin, 1965; Weston, 1964).

Incidence

The incidence and extent of hearing loss as a function of ageing is usually measured by changes in the pure tone audiogram.

Since the earliest study by Bunch (1931) the common pattern of a progressive loss in acuity for the higher frequencies occurring with increasing age has been found by numerous investigators. Sampling of suitably selected populations has led to the production of a series of audiometric curves indicating the hearing loss as an average or expected maximum in its degree and distribution throughout the test frequency range that is to be expected at a given age. The Wisconsin Hearing Survey of 1957 is one such source; another useful one, from which an example is given below, is Hinchcliffe's (1959c) paper (Fig. 1).

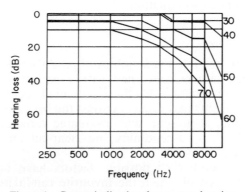

Figure 1 Curves indicating the average hearing loss that might be expected to occur at the given ages (from Hinchcliffe, 1959a)

Fisch (1978) summarizes the results of such studies by stating that 'about one third of the population of 65 years and over suffers from a hearing impairment which can have unfavourable social consequences'.

Pathology and Pathophysiology

Histological study reveals age-related changes (of varying significance in their effect upon hearing) occurring in all parts of the auditory pathway. Lesions are described in the middle ear mechanism, the hair cells, and spiral ganglion cells of the inner ear, and in the neurones of the central pathways. Otopathologists have been concerned not simply with description of such changes in isolation but with establishing them as the pathological correlates of disturbances in auditory function as measured by the available battery of psychoacoustic tests. In studying presbyacusis they have sought the location, extent, and nature of cellular and structural abnormalities lying behind the characteristic audiograms of presbyacusis.

The mainstay to date of such investigation has been the study of suitably prepared and stained specimens of the human temporal bone using the light microscope. Using this technique, Schuknecht (1974a, 1974b), in a series of authoritative studies has defined differing patterns of cellular and structural damage associated with ageing, relating them to specific audiometric changes. These, with the observations of other workers, are considered in detail below.

Middle Ear Changes

It is unlikely that such a degree of conductive hearing loss as might result from age-related changes in the tympanic membrane and ossicular chain is of practical significance (Belal and Stewart, 1974).

Inner Ear Changes

Schuknecht (1974a) describes four types of inner ear deafness associated with ageing, ascribing a particular pathological pattern and characteristic hearing loss to each. They are:
(a) sensory presbyacusis;
(b) neural presbyacusis;
(c) strial presbyacusis;
(d) cochlear conductive presbyacusis.
It is the occurrence in a relatively pure form of each that has allowed the pathological cor-

relate to be established, but analysis of any given case may commonly disclose elements of two or more types coexisting. The functional effects, when this is the case, would appear to be additive (Schucknecht, 1974a).

Sensory presbyacusis. Crowe, Guild, and Polvogt (1934) first described both sensory and neural changes in presbyacusis. The pathological correlate of the sensory form is a loss of hair cells dominantly in the basal turn of the cochlea and, as this region subserves hearing for higher frequencies, the resulting audiogram shows that characteristic – a relatively abrupt high tone loss.

Neural presbyacusis. In this form a loss occurs in the neuronal cells of the spiral ganglion leaving a relatively intact sensory cell population.

Both the site and extent of the neuronal loss are important (Otte, 1968), whether it occurs in that region of the cochlea subserving the speech frequencies and whether it is severe enough to compromise the encoding of speech. Relatively few neurones are needed for the production of a normal pure tone audiogram, so it is characteristic of neuronal presbyacusis that the patient actually suffers a handicap disproportionately worse than the pure tone audiogram may lead one to suspect. The pure tone audiogram may resemble in shape that of sensory presbyacusis but the speech audiogram will be comparatively worse (Fig. 2).

In both sensory and neuronal presbyacusis the basal turn of the cochlea seems to be curiously vulnerable.

Strial presbyacusis. The hearing loss of strial presbyacusis is usually manifest at an earlier age than the other presbyacutic types.

The histological findings are a relatively normal population of hair cells and neurones. The pathology is found in the stria vascularis and consists essentially of atrophic changes in the middle and apical regions of the cochlea (Johnsson and Hawkins, 1972; Takahashi, 1971).

The characteristic audiogram, of which an example is given below (Fig. 3), shows a 'flat' loss throughout the range tested by the pure tone audiogram. Though overall sensitivity is depressed the difficulties with discrimination arising from differing frequency losses is avoided and thus this form responds well to simple overall amplification – a relatively simple provision in hearing aid design.

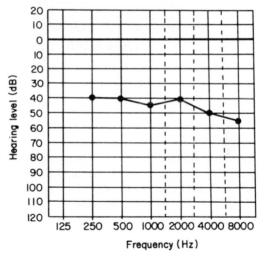

Figure 3 Audiometric curve typical of striae presbyacusis

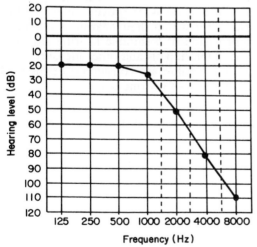

Figure 2 Audiometric curve typical of both neural and sensory presbyacusis. In the former discrimination would be more impaired

Cochlear conductive presbyacusis. A fourth type of audiometric pattern is characterized by a progressive fall-off in sensitivity throughout the test range (Fig. 4), distinguishing it from the audiograms of sensory and neural presbyacusis in which the lower frequencies remain relatively intact (Fig. 2).

In this type the structures implicated in the

pathogenesis of the preceding three types are relatively normal; there is no constant nor significant hair cell or neuronal loss and the stria vascularis appears intact.

Schuknecht (1974a) argues the pathological basis for conductive presbyacusis; at this stage it is reasonable to assume that age-related changes in the mechanical properties of the basilar membrane may be responsible.

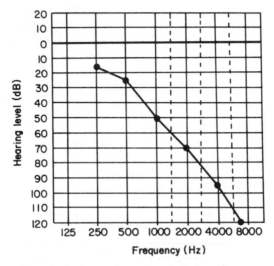

Figure 4   Audiometric curve typical of cochlear conductive presbyacusis

Central Changes

A similarly precise correlation between pathological change and auditory dysfunction as that described for the inner ear has not been achieved in the central pathways.

It is naive to assume that the hearing loss of presbyacusis could be ascribed simply to inner ear changes. Indeed, definite auditory dysfunction (concerned with speech discrimination) associated with ageing and of probable central origin is described by Palva and Joiknen (1970) and Goetzinger and coworkers (1961).

Histological evidence is scarce but Kirikae, Sato, and Skitara (1964) and Hansen and Reske-Nielsen (1965) describe age related degenerative changes within the brainstem nuclei and at cortical level and go some way towards associating them with audiometric findings. The implications of such changes are discussed by Hinchcliffe (1962).

Clinical Characteristics of Presbyacusis

In summary the diagnosis of presbyacusis is based upon the following:
(a) A complaint of gradually increasing bilateral hearing loss, with or without tinnitus, but in the absence of other symptoms referrable to the ear.
(b) The finding of a normal tympanic membrane and, on testing with tuning forks, a Rinne positive response in both ears and a central Weber.
(c) The finding of a pure tone audiogram similar in shape to those illustrated above, or a compound of one or more types. On balance it will usually be of a descending audiometric pattern. It is emphasized that the loss must be *essentially symmetrical* – asymmetry demands further search for other possible pathologies.

Additional testing may reveal:
(a) The finding of a variably impaired speech audiogram depending upon the type and extent of inner ear loss and the possible existence and influence of any central component.
(b) The presence of loudness recruitment commonly, as a result of hair cell disorder, and on occasion tone decay as a function of neuronal loss.

Treatment of Presbyacusis

Though a variety of medical therapies have been tried none is of proven value. In those patients for whom their hearing is a handicap the provision of a suitable hearing aid should be considered. This and other measures which may be of value are considered below in the management of hearing loss.

THE SYMPTOMS OF EAR DISEASE

Presbyacusis is characterized by hearing loss and tinnitus. Other auditory pathologies may place an added burden of hearing loss upon an already compromised system. In clinical practice other symptoms arising from such disease within the auditory system itself or in closely related structures are commonly encountered. It is worth while considering these at this stage – particular emphasis is placed on those aspects relevant to geriatric practice.

Hearing Loss

Traditionally and usefully, hearing loss has been classified as being conductive or sensorineural ('perceptive' in older terminology) in type. In a given pathology or patient they may, of course, coexist.

A sensorineural loss arises from a lesion or dysfunction within the end-organ (cochlea), the VIII nerve trunk, brainstem nuclei, or central auditory pathways to cortical level. The term allows for further subdivision into 'sensory' loss when the lesion lies within the cochlea and 'neural' loss when the fault lies in the remainder of the pathway. A conductive loss arises in consequence of some interference with the normal physiological passage of sound through the external and middle ear.

Detailed questioning of a patient with hearing difficulties will often reveal the specific components contributing to the problem. Not only is the perceived sound too quiet but distortions are also experienced, adding confusing and distracting elements. It is worth considering these elements and their practical consequences in detail.

Diminished Sensitivity and Discrimination

We may test the sensitivity of a patient's hearing by presenting him with a series of signals, usually pure tones, and assessing the least intensity of each at which they can be consistently heard. This series of individual thresholds for given tones forms the basis of the 'hearing test' most commonly used in clinical practice – 'the pure tone audiogram' (PTA).

In clinical practice frequencies between 125 and 8,000 Hz are used and the 'threshold' for each test tone plotted on a standard form; the range of frequencies of particular relevance are those covering the speech range – between 250 and 3,500 Hz in general.

The essential problem arises from the fact that a hearing loss occurs, or proceeds, only very rarely on an even front. It is almost invariable that the loss will affect differing frequencies to differing degrees, leaving certain frequencies more readily heard than others. In practical terms this means that the patient finds difficulty in 'discriminating' one from another the elements of speech composed of differing frequencies. They experience difficulties in speech discrimination.

In the elderly the most commonly encountered abnormality in hearing, as measured on the PTA, is that the higher frequencies are relatively more affected than the lower. The patient is relatively deafer to the elements in speech of higher frequency than he is to the lower; because consonants in speech are generally of higher frequency than the vowels he can hear one speaking but cannot discern what is said. He has lost the elements in speech, namely the consonants, that confer intelligibility, but has retained to a relative degree the vowels which confer audibility. Fortunately the consonants are more readily appreciated by lip reading and so a start may be made in compensation.

A more precise determinant of the degree of difficulty a patient has in hearing speech is the 'speech audiogram', where the patient is presented, in controlled conditions, with words or sentences and his performance is scored. The actual form of this test varies in practice and uses variously sentences or word lists. To a large extent the PTA will reflect or imply what is obtained on a speech test, as one might infer from the preceding comments, but it is not always so and it is the other elements of aberrated function which in large part explain these discrepancies. One should remember also that an elderly or confused patient might well have difficulty in performing these more elaborate tests.

Derangements of Loudness Perception – 'Loudness Recruitment'

This phenomenon, commonly present in presbyacusis, is characteristic of hair cell disorder – i.e. it is a feature of cochlear or sensory hearing loss. It is a major problem, introducing, on occasion, elements of actually physically uncomfortable distortion into the appreciation of sounds and constituting one of the main difficulties to be overcome in the design of hearing aids.

Loudness recruitment may be defined as a disproportionate and increasing growth of loudness with increasing intensity of sound above the patient's threshold. Thus to a patient suffering this phenomenon, an increase in the intensity of a sound from, say, 40 to 50 dB will sound to him disproportionately louder than a similar increment between 30 and 40 dB. (In a normally hearing ear an increase from 30 to 40 dB would seem equally as loud as that between 40 and 50 dB.)

Also, in most normally hearing ears a loud sound becomes uncomfortable, if not actually painful, to the hearer at about 90 to 105 dB. above the threshold for that sound. If loudness recruitment is present then the 'discomfort' level is reached at a level rather lower above threshold. Loudness discomfort with the closely allied phenomenon of loudness recruitment forms the basis for a range of audiological tests designed to localize a hearing loss within the auditory system; if recruitment or loudness discomfort is present it is likely, but not certain, that the loss originates within the cochlea.

In practical terms, recruitment, involving varying frequencies, will distort the sound perceived and compound the problem of discrimination. Loudness discomfort is responsible for a common phenomenon – the raising of one's voice to repeat an obviously misheard remark provokes, if not an actual wince, the comment, 'Don't shout, I'm not deaf'.

Impaired Sound Localization

The ability to localize sound appears to depend upon the analysis of differences between the two ears of three elements in the signal – time, phase, and intensity. The auricles themselves, through their intricate shaping, introduce echoes and thus contribute to localization and in fact can allow the patient with only one hearing ear to yet retain some element of localization. Obviously the greatest difficulty does arise when there is any pronounced assymetry in the sensitivity of the ears.

One must presume that with diminished acuity, with deficiencies in hair cell function introducing elements of recruitment, and with abnormal neural conduction introducing elements of delay in central transmission – all of which are features of presbyacusis – the integration of afferent information is affected.

The elderly patient finds difficulty in localizing and thus discriminating (in another sense) the desired 'signal' in background noise interference and may well thus miss the 'cue in' of a sentence, therefore making nonsense of what he hears and, unless particularly well motivated, giving little incentive to continue listening.

Tinnitus

A patient suffering from tinnitus complains of noise in the head or ears. In its commonly encountered form it is 'subjective' in that no source within the patient himself or the environment is audible to an observer. Very rarely tinnitus may be 'objective' and audible to the observer. The more important causes of this type of tinnitus are vascular in origin and usually pulsatile in nature. They demand careful auscultation of the head and neck with particular attention to the distribution of the main arteries.

Subjective tinnitus is very common. The United States National Health Survey of 1968 disclosed that some 20 per cent. of the adult population admitted this symptom. It is increasingly common with increasing age (Hinchcliffe, 1961; Reed, 1960), certainly to the age of 70, and thus is a usual concommitant of presbyacusis; often, indeed, it is the tinnitus about which the patient primarily complains rather than any element of hearing loss.

It is described usually as a rushing, buzzing, or ringing noise but many variants are encountered. Should it consist of formed words or sentences a psychiatric disturbance is suggested rather than an auditory dysfunction. In fact, excepting the significance of pulsatile tinnitus, the characteristics are of little importance for, from the diagnostic point of view, they do not indicate the nature or site of the causative pathology.

The mechanism of generation of subjective tinnitus remains largely a mystery. It may be present with or without associated hearing loss or demonstrable hearing deficit and pathologies of differing types at all levels within the auditory pathway are considered to be capable of causing it. A unilateral tinnitus requires special attention, as even in the absence of hearing loss it may be an early symptom of serious pathology, e.g. acoustic neuroma.

Useful alleviation of this symptom is only rarely achieved. The physician's role, after exclusion of significant pathology, is primarily one of adequate and patient explanation of its benign nature.

Otalgia

Otalgia may originate within the ear or may be referred from numerous structures in the head and neck.

Pain originating within the ear is usually a consequence of acute inflammation of either the middle ear cleft or skin of the external ear canal. Acute otitis media is unusual in the elderly; at this age infective middle ear disease is usually chronic in nature and characteristically painless. Much more rarely pain may result from the erosion of malignant disease, dural involvement by cholesteatoma, or, in the inner ear, the expansion of an acoustic neuroma. A peculiarly severe pain accompanies myringitis bullosa haemorrhagica, a lesion of presumed viral aetiology which causes haemorrhagic vesiculation of the drum and external meatus.

Referred pain is a common and important phenomenon. A number of cranial nerves send sensory components to the external and middle ear; a lesion elsewhere within their territory may be manifest as otalgia.

In the elderly common causes of such referred pain are cervical osteoarthrosis and temperomandibular joint dysfunction. In both pain may be centred on the ear but they usually show differing radiations – the former with a cervical root distribution, the latter with a preauricular, maxillary, or mandibular pattern. Beware also of the presentation of carcinomata on the base of the tongue, pharynx, or larynx as otalgia – the disease may otherwise often be asymptomatic. Its occurrence is much more likely in a male with a long history of tobacco usage.

Otorrhoea

Particular attention should be paid to the nature of the discharge. Inflammation of the middle ear cleft, as may be expected of inflammation caused by respiratory pathogens, is usually mucopurulent and inoffensive in nature. On the other hand, infections involving the breakdown of keratin are characterized by the offensive odour resulting from protein degradation. Thus the discharge of otitis externa is usually scant and offensive. Cholesteatoma, although a middle ear disease, is essentially a disorder of keratinization and this too produces an offensive discharge.

Bleeding or a blood-stained discharge may occur as an acute event, e.g. in myringitis bullosa haemorrhagica. Chronic discharge, discoloured by blood, is a feature of processes distinguished by the formation of granulation tissue, i.e. chronic inflammation of the middle ear cleft. Rarely, and of particular relevance to the elderly, it may signify malignant change in a chronic suppurative otitis media with the formation of an invasive squamous cell carcinoma. Profuse granulation tissue in a chronic ear should always be considered as a possible malignancy.

Facial Palsy

Facial nerve palsies are usually of idiopathic origin, 'Bell's palsy', which appears to be purely and selectively a whole nerve neuronitis of the VII cranial nerve. However, auditory pathologies of significance causing facial palsies, and encountered in geriatric practice, include herpes zoster oticus, cholesteatoma in chronic suppurative otitis media, and carcinoma of the middle ear.

The most important step in the initial assessment of facial palsy is the exclusion of any middle ear pathologies; such disease, as instanced above, requires immediate and specialized otologic management. It is outside the scope of this chapter to consider the numerous aetiologies of facial palsy and their management. Readers are referred to the relevant chapter in Scott-Browne's *Diseases of the Ear, Nose and Throat* (Groves, 1979).

Disorders of Vestibular Function

Some disorders of the vestibular system are now coming to be recognized as features of the ageing vestibular apparatus, though they do not necessarily have precise correlation with the changes of presbyacusis in the auditory apparatus. A useful analysis and classification of 'the dysequilibrium of ageing' is given by Schuknecht (1974b) who lists the following main types:

(a) cupulolithiasis of ageing;
(b) ampullary dysequilibrium of ageing;
(c) macular dysequilibrium of ageing;
(d) vestibular ataxia of ageing.

THE INVESTIGATION OF HEARING LOSS

The following account in this context can only be brief. It is intended that it should give some idea of the range of audiometric tests used in clinical practice and indicate sources for further reading.

In broad terms tests of auditory function have two aims – to assess the actual extent of any hearing deficit and to determine where, within the auditory system, the fault lies. The second, localizing, function is concerned with placing the lesion in the middle ear, cochlea, or central connections, thus indicating whether the hearing loss is conductive, sensory, or neural in type.

A middle ear loss may be identified in degree and site by the pure tone audiogram where used to measure both air and bone conduction and the actual mechanisms of drum, ossicles, and eustachian tubal function further analysed by tympanometry (see Brooks, 1976).

The investigation of a sensorineural loss usually proceeds through the tests listed below, the pure tone and speech audiograms establishing the overall deficit with the more specialized tests of localization following. To determine whether a given loss is primarily sensory or neural, tests are used which rely upon the demonstration of two phenomena – recruitment, characteristic of cochlear disease, and adaption (tone decay), characteristic of a neuronal lesion.

Pure Tone Audiometry

Excepting presbyacusis and noise-induced hearing loss (where the loss is classically maximal at 4,000 Hz) it is unwise to infer the nature of the causative pathology from the audiometric pattern. The pure tone audiogram indicates the relative severity with which individual frequencies are involved and thus allows, in practical terms, qualified inferences to be drawn as to the likely speech handicap a patient suffers. To some extent also it indicates the likelihood of a hearing aid being of value.

Speech Audiometry

Reference has been separately made to this test because in practical terms it indicates more accurately than the pure tone audiogram the patient's ability to hear and comprehend speech. It is thus the best test to use in assessing the likely benefit to be derived from a hearing aid (and provides a vital measure in the assessment of a patient's suitability for reconstructive ear surgery).

It has a further application as regards localization function. Speech discrimination is compromised, particularly in lesions of the VIII nerve, though, interestingly, it is much less likely to be affected by pathology in the more central parts of the pathway (Noffsinger *et al.*, 1972; Parker, 1968). Stephens (1976) provides a comprehensive review of the application of speech audiometry in the study of central auditory dysfunction.

Tests of Loudness Recruitment

The most commonly used form of this test is Fowler's loudness balance test (Fowler, 1936) for unilateral disease or the loudness discomfort level (Hood and Poole, 1966) for bilateral disease. The stapedius reflex response is also useful in assessing the presence of recruitment (Metz, 1952).

Tests of Adaption

Adaption or tone decay is a phenomenon akin to neuronal fatigue. In the auditory system this is expressed as a response declining in threshold with time for a sustained tone.

The 'tone decay test' commonly used is that described by Carhart (1957) or alternatively the 'Stapedius reflex tone decay test' (Anderson, 1970) may be used in an objective assessment.

Special Tests of Central Auditory Function

A wide range of tests of varied practical and research application are described. Readers are referred to Stephens' excellent review (1976).

Electroneurophysiological Tests of Auditory Function

There is obviously an advantage in tests of auditory function which allow the integrity of the auditory system to be assessed in patients unable or unwilling, for one reason or another, to cooperate in subjective tests. Various techniques allow the electroneurophysiological response initiated by a sound stimulus to be followed from cochlea to auditory cortex. They are valuable in both establishing the auditory threshold, bearing in mind that the stimuli employed are either 'clicks' or pure tones, and in being potentially able to localize lesions within all parts of the auditory pathway.

The theoretical and practical aspects of such tests are considered by Gibson (1978).

THE MANAGEMENT OF HEARING LOSS IN THE ELDERLY

Four main approaches will be considered:
(a) surgical management;
(b) medical management;
(c) hearing aids;
(d) other aids to communication.
In general conductive hearing losses are theoretically amenable to surgical correction whereas, at the present state of knowledge, sensorineural losses are not. A few specific types of sensorineural loss require prompt medical treatment, and in them a reasonable restoration of hearing may be attained, but the vast majority of such are managed with a hearing aid.

A conductive loss arises in consequence of some interference with the normal transmission of sound across the external and middle ear. In these areas the main structural components are epithelium, bone, and connective tissue; all these possess excellent regenerative and healing potential. Functional prostheses, provided they are made of suitably inert material, are well tolerated in the middle ear. These factors combine to allow the useful application of surgery to effect functional repair.

A sensorineural loss is a different matter. The sensory cells and their connecting nerves seem curiously vulnerable to trauma, and as fixed postmitotics possess no regenerative capacity. Surgical intervention cannot be used here to promote or institute useful healing and, at this stage of the art, no prosthetic substitution by surgical means may functionally replace or bypass any defective sensory or neural component. Considerable research however continues in this field (Ballantyne, Evans, and Morrison, 1978).

In the elderly the provision of a hearing aid will in practice constitute the most usual form of management. The sensorineural loss of presbyacusis has so far proved unresponsive to a number of medical treatments and there is, as yet, no place for surgery.

Surgical Management

Though conductive losses are commonly amenable to surgery, they may all equally be expected to benefit from a hearing aid. Hearing aids prove most effective and give less problems when used to overcome conductive rather than sensorineural losses. One of the main factors limiting the successful use of an aid is recruitment resulting from hair cell loss. In a purely conductive loss this, and other distortions, are absent and it is simply a question of amplifying sound to overcome the single handicap of evenly diminished acuity.

In the elderly, where for various reasons one may have reservations about recommending non-essential surgery and where hearing aids provide an excellent alternative in management of a conductive loss, the latter course is usually chosen. However, certain pathologies causing conductive loss may be corrected by 'minimal' surgery possible under local anaesthetic. Stapedectomy for otosclerosis is a good example. Age alone should be no bar to the successful performance of this operation; it has been of value to patients in their eighties. On the other hand, reconstructive surgery to repair extensive damage of drum and ossicles may require lengthy and elaborate repair with uncertain results. A hearing aid provides just as good a functional result and it would seem the logical choice.

Medical Management

Although of rare occurrence, two clinical entities should be mentioned. In the management of both prompt medical treatment is required.

Syphilitic Hearing Loss

Presenting in old age as a manifestation of tertiary or neurosyphilis, immediate treatment with steroids and suitable antibiotic may either restore some degree of hearing or, at least, prevent further deterioration (Morrison, 1975).

'Sudden' Sensorineural Hearing Loss

On occasion patients suffer an inner ear loss, with or without accompanying vestibular symptoms. The loss is usually unilateral, but it may involve both ears, and no specific causative agency is apparent. Two theories are evoked to explain the phenomenon though the evidence is conflicting. Hearing loss is assumed either to be due to infection (caused by as yet unidentified, presumably viral, agents) or it has a vascular basis. Whichever mechanism is considered operative in a given case determines the choice of treatment – steroids in the former case and vasodilator therapy in the latter. In part also the choice is determined by the site of the lesion, as indicated by audiometric findings. The presence of recruitment suggests a cochlear pathology, probably due to vascular factors, but the finding of tone decay is in favour of an inflammatory cause. In the elderly patient the aetiology is more usually vascular. A useful assessment of this problem and its management is provided by Morrison and Booth (1970).

Hearing Aids

A hearing aid is designed to amplify the constituent sounds of human speech to a level perceptible to the wearer. It should ideally do this in a way which avoids the introduction of any element of distortion and it should allow for, and certainly not aggravate, the particular aberrations of hearing peculiar to the wearer – especially any element of recruitment.

This amplification may be attained in two ways:
(a) acoustic amplification;
(b) electronic amplification.
Acoustic aids, such as ear trumpets and 'auricles' are largely now out of fashion. However, the practising physician who has much to do with the elderly deaf may well find the 'speaking tube' of value in communication. It provides useful amplification without significant distortion and is of easy and universal application.

Electronic aids amplify by electronic means and are classified as:
(a) body worn aids, where microphone, power source, and amplifier are worn as a unit on the body;

(b) ear level aids, worn on the head.

In each case they may be either air or bone conduction aids, depending upon the final mode of delivery of the acoustic signal. An air conduction aid employs an ear mould or 'insert', fitting into the external ear canal and delivering the sound thence to the drum, and a bone conduction aid employs a vibrator, in contact with the skull, and thereby transmitting the sound, via bone, essentially to the inner ear. The latter is a less effective mechanism but may have to be employed if, for anatomical reasons, an insert may be impractical or if chronic suppuration of either middle or external ear prevents the use of an insert.

In presbyacusis there will usually be a high frequency loss and it is when this encroaches upon the speech frequency range that social handicap results.

The aid must amplify selectively this part of the range and bring to the patient's hearing those elements of speech composed of higher frequencies – the consonants. Also a spoken sentence contains sounds and words varying in loudness and differing by up to 30 dB with consonants as the quieter elements. There is thus a second reason for amplifying selectively the upper speech frequency range. Comparatively less amplification will be needed for those areas, the low frequency and louder vowel sounds, which are left relatively unscathed by degenerative changes.

The patient with presbyacusis is doubly disadvantaged. He has a selective loss of hearing for consonants which are the quieter elements of speech, and which, most importantly, confer intelligibility.

Recruitment with loudness discomfort is commonly present. In the environment loud noises will naturally and normally occur—the clatter of crockery, doors slamming, dogs barking, etc. Unless some device is incorporated into the aid such sounds along with the desired elements of speech will be amplified to an uncomfortable level. It may actually cause physical discomfort; in any event it will be distracting and act as a positive disincentive to the continued wearing of the aid. An automatic device is needed to cut out such noxious stimuli – an 'automatic volume control'.

If a variant of this same mechanism is employed selectively in the speech range with respect of frequency and volume, it can be used to 'iron out' the abrupt loudness variations caused by recruitment exaggerating the normal fluctuations in intensity encountered in normal speech.

The ideal hearing aid will thus:

(a) Cover the speech range (and on occasion useful information may be provided by extending outside it).

(b) Provide selective amplification for the areas in which the patient's sensitivity is decreased. This is achieved by altering the frequency response of the aid – in general terms the best alteration is provided by a gradual increase in amplification of about 7 dB per octave over the speech range (Knight, 1967).

(c) Selectively amplify the quieter elements of speech, the consonants, certainly to the level of the more audible elements, the lower frequency vowels.

(d) Iron out the extremes of variation in intensity that will be a natural consequence of recruitment.

(e) Protect the wearer from the amplification of loud environmental noise – uncomfortable to the normally hearing, even more so to the deaf with loudness discomfort.

These provisions, (c), (d), and (e) are achieved by automatic volume control of which three basic methods exist:

(a) peak clipping;
(b) compression amplification;
(c) automatic gain control.

Discussion of these elements is outside the scope of this chapter, and the reader is advised, for further information, to consult Ballantyne (1977) and in matters of the design, function, and application of aids Martin (1976) and Markides (1976).

The comments above concern, in theory, the requirements of the 'ideal' aid. The design and efficiency of hearing aids are constantly being improved with advances in electronic engineering. Aids cannot, however, be expected to restore perfect hearing. It is not important in fact that they fail to do this, as their role should be viewed as improving auditory perception, by providing more auditory clues, rather than restoring hearing.

It is vital that, when a patient is to be fitted and provided with an aid, he should understand exactly what it is designed to do, what he can expect of it, and how it is used to best advantage. Realistic advice, uncoloured by undue pessimism, is critical to the successful wearing of an aid. The patient must be encouraged to 'experiment', using it as much as possible initially in all social circumstances, so that he can establish for himself its limitations and find those occasions on which it is of value. Above all he must be encouraged to persist in such efforts.

Ideally an after-care service should be established so that at intervals after provision with an aid the patient has the opportunity to discuss any problems with the physician or speech or hearing therapist. Many problems which discourage the user are simply solved. The electronic functioning of the aid may become defective, the insert may be ill-fitting causing discomfort and auditory feedback (the uncomfortable whistling noise which many associate with the use of an aid), wax may build up in the external ear canal, or the material of which the insert is made may prove irritant. These and other minor points are easily corrected.

Patients often resist the suggested use of an aid believing that it will lead to a more rapid deterioration in their hearing. With the aids commonly employed in the management of presbyacusis firm reassurance may be given on this count, certainly with ear-level models. Very powerful aids, such as those used in the education of the deaf child (and occasionally as body-worn aids in the adult), require caution and specialized advice in this respect.

The usual resistance encountered is that of cosmesis – the wearing of an aid constitutes the public admission of a handicap that an individual would prefer to keep to himself. Much can be done by reassurance; ear-level aids are small and discrete, the hair may be arranged differently, or the aid may be incorporated successfully into spectacles.

Other Aids to Communication

Other aids and services may prove of value in countering the social isolation that follows from hearing loss. They may provide help in the auditory sense by amplifying the output from radio, television, or telephone or they may provide additional visual information, e.g. lights that as warning signals may be fitted to telephone or doorbell. Programmes subtitled for the hard of hearing are increasingly presented nowadays by television services. Lastly, instruction in lip-reading may offer many the advantage necessary to enjoy full benefit from a hearing aid.

Whether an aid, auditory or visual, is used or not, communication with the deaf depends in large part upon the clarity and quality of the speech to which the patient would be attentive and the environment in which he listens. When talking to the deaf, in both professional and social contact, the speaker must enunciate words carefully and talk adequately, but not overly loudly; to talk too loudly is a common fault exacerbating any distortion caused by recruitment and antagonizing through the effects of loudness discomfort. The environment should be free of distracting sights and noise and the patient should be able to see the speaker's face and lips clearly. Gestures, unless controlled and purposive, can be distracting.

Physicians should remember that by the time help is sought for a hearing problem some degree of social isolation is commonly already incurred and it is against this background that any management will be instituted.

BALANCE AND THE VESTIBULAR SYSTEM

A few general observations concerning symptoms of imbalance may be of value to clinicians.

Above all, it takes a particularly articulate patient to describe the symptoms of vestibular disorder – a problem illustrated by the number of terms used in description, e.g. 'dizzy', 'giddy', 'vertigenous'. The likelihood of the patient's meaning and understanding of the term he employs differing from that of the doctor's is high. Particular effort is thus required to establish precisely what the patient means.

It is often valuable to establish whether any particular physical manoeuvre or movement initiates vertigo – characteristic positions bring on the vertigo of cupulolithiasis, or 'benign positional vertigo', and the description of how vertigo is initiated by hyperextension, with possibly other symptoms in addition, points towards vertebro basilar insufficiency.

A prime purpose of the history and physical examination (including special tests) of the vestibular system is to establish whether the lesion lies in the end organ or the more central connections – a situation analagous to the division of hearing loss into sensory or neural elements. This division is useful in both systems in that it directs the physician towards one or other of two differing fields of pathology. Examples of end organ lesions include certain forms of dysequilibrium of ageing (cupulolithiasis and ampullary dysequilibrium), ototoxic vestibular damage, Ménière's disease, and trauma to the temporal bone; central lesions cover the range of vascular insufficiencies, demyelination, tumours, etc.

In traditional teaching the dysfunction caused by a peripheral pathology, i.e. a disorder within the labyrinth itself, is described as 'true vertigo', i.e. the patient feels markedly disorientated, often with the sensation of the environment spinning around him. More central pathologies cause a lesser upset; vague unsteadiness or imbalance is experienced. Though this division is usefully often true, it is erroneous to consider that it is the localization or site of the lesion, whether it is peripheral or central, that is the determinant of the nature of the imbalance suffered – it is rather the fact that the pathologies occurring more commonly in the peripheral field are characterized by sudden onset causing severe functional deficit; the central pathologies, demyelination, or tumours are of more insidious onset, allowing compensation by the central and contralateral vestibular mechanisms to occur pari-passu with only occasional and minor disparity in function between the two sides causing lesser imbalance. It is the nature of the pathology which determines the severity of the upset rather than its localization within the system; e.g. a lateral medullary infarct, through a central lesion, will most certainly cause severe and sudden vertigo.

It would be better to restate traditional teaching by saying that peripheral lesions of the vestibular system are rarely characterized by minimal vestibular symptoms.

The maintenance of equilibrium is dependent upon the integration of sensory afferent information provided by the vestibular, ocular, and proprioceptive systems. The importance of the visual system lies primarily in its role of compensation for vestibular anomalies – one could look upon the usual form of vestibular nystagmus, with its fast and slow component, as composed, in its slow phase, of the anomalous movement induced by vestibular dysfunction, and in its fast phase by the visual correction imposed upon this fault. This ocular compensation is the more vital in coping with peripheral rather than central lesions – removal of ocular fixation characteristically exacerbates any symptom of disorientation and accentuates any nystagmus that might be present when the lesions lie peripherally. In centrally placed lesions removal of optic fixation has either little effect upon the symptoms and signs or may actually alleviate the former and extinguish the latter.

This fact is of value in assessing the history. Specific enquiry should be made of the effect of eye closure and how the patient copes with his imbalance in the dark. This phenomenon, incidentally, also forms the basis of a number of vestibular function tests designed to localize lesions within the system.

A full consideration of the vestibular apparatus as a sensory system in its own right lies outside the scope of this chapter. Readers may find the following authorities and sources of value in further study: Schuknecht. (1974b), Edwards (1973), and Yatsu and Smith (1979).

REFERENCES

Anderson, H., Barr, B., amd Wedenburg, E. (1970). 'Early diagnosis of eighth nerve tumours by acoustic reflexes', *Acta. Otolaryng. (Stokh.)* Supp. 263, 232–237.

Ballantyne, J. (1977). 'Hearing aids', in *Deafness*, Part 3, pp. 61–80, Churchill Livingstone, Edinburgh, London and New York.

Ballantyne, J. C., Evans, E. F., and Morrison, A. W. (1978). 'Electrical auditory stimulation in the management of profound hearing loss', *J. Laryngol. Otology. Suppl.*, **1**, October, 1–[117.

Belal, A., and Stewart, T. (1974). 'Pathological changes in the middle ear joints', *Ann. Otology. Rhinol. Laryngol.*, **83**, 159–166.

Bunch, C. C. (1931). 'Further observations on age variations in auditory acuity'. *Arch. Otolaryngol.*, **13**, 170–180.

Carhart, R. (1957). 'Clinical determination of abnormal auditory adaption', *Arch. Otolaryng.*, **65**, 32–39.

Crowe, S., Guild, S., and Polvogt, L. (1934). 'Observations on pathology of high tone deafness', *Bull. Johns Hopkins Hosp.*, **54**, 315–379.

Edwards, C. H. (1973). 'Disorders of balance', in *Neurology of the Ear, Nose and Throat*, p. 104–182, Butterworths, London.

Fisch, L. (1978). 'The ageing auditory system', in *Textbook of Geriatric Medicine and Gerontology* (Ed. J. C. Brocklehurst), p. 283, Churchill Livingstone, Edinburgh and London.

Fowler, E. P. (1937). 'Measuring sensation of loudness', *Arch. Otolaryng.*, **26**, 514–521.

Gibson, W. P. R. (1978). *The Essentials of Clinical Electric Response Audiometry*, Churchill Livingstone, Edinburgh and London.

Goetzinger, C., Proud, G. O., Dirks, D., and Embrey, J. (1961). 'Study of hearing in advanced age', *Arch. Otolaryngol.*, **73**, 662–674.

Groves, J. (1979). 'Facial paralysis', in *Diseases of the Ear, Nose and Throat* (Ed. W. G. Scott-Browne), Vol. 2, pp. 865–908, Butterworths, London.

Hansen, C., and Reske-Nielsen, E. (1965). 'Cochlear and cerebral pathology in aged patients', *Int. Audiol.*, **7**, 45, and *Arch. Otolaryngol.*, **82**, 115–132.

Hinchcliffe, R. (1959a). 'The threshold of hearing as a function of age', *Acoustica*, **9**, 303–307.

Hinchcliffe, R. (1959b). 'The threshold of hearing of a random sample rural population', *Acta. Otolaryngol.*, **50**, 411–422.

Hinchcliffe, R. (1959c). 'Correction of pure tone audiograms for advancing age', *J. Laryngol. Otololog.*, **73**, 12, 830–832.

Hinchcliffe, R. (1961). 'Prevalence of the commoner ear, nose and throat conditions in the adult rural population of Great Britain', *Brit. J. Prev. Soc. Med.*, **15**, 128–140.

Hinchcliffe, R. (1962). 'The anatomical locus of presbyacusis', *J. Speech and Hearing Disorders*, **27**, 301–311.

Hood, J. D., and Poole, J. (1966). 'Tolerable limit of loudness: its clinical and physiological significance', *J. Acoust. Soc. Amer,.* **40**, 47–53.

Johnsson, L., and Hawkins, J. Jr. (1972) 'Symposium on basic ear research, II. Strial atrophy in clinical and experimental deafness', *Laryngoscope*, **82**, 1105–1125.

Kirikae, I., Sato, I., and Skitara, T. (1964). 'Auditory function in advanced age with reference to the histological changes in the central auditory system', *Laryngoscope*, **74**, 205–220.

Knight, J. J. (1967). 'Redetermination of optimum characteristics for hearing aid with insert telephone', *International Audiology*, **6**, 322–326.

Macrae, T. H. (1971). 'Noise induced hearing loss and presbyacusis', *Audiology*, **10**, 5–15.

Markides, A. (1976). 'Selection of hearing aids', in *Scientific Foundations of Otolaryngology* (Eds R. Hinchcliffe and D. Harrison), pp. 824–830, William Heinemann, London.

Metz, O. (1952). 'Threshold of reflex contractions

of muscles of middle ear and recruitment of loud-ness', *Arch. Otolarung.*, **55**, 536–543.

Morrison, A. W. (1975). 'Late syphilis', in *Management of Sensori-neural Hearing Loss*, pp. 109–144, Butterworths, London and Boston.

Morrison, A. W., and Booth, J. B. (1970). 'Sudden deafness: An otological emergency', *Br. J. Hosp. Med.*, **4**, 287–298.

Martin, M. C. (1976). 'Auditory prostheses', in *Scientific Foundations of Otolaryngology* (Eds R. Hinchcliffe and D. Harrison), pp. 805–823, William Heinemann, London.

Noffsinger, D., Olsen, W. O., Carhart, R., *et al.* (1972). 'Auditory and vestibular aberrations in multiple sclerosis', *Acta. Otolaryng. (Stockh.)* Suppl. 303, 1–63.

Otte, J. (1968). 'Estudio del ganglio espiral y su relacion con la discriminacion', *Rev. Otorinolaring.*, **28**, 89–97.

Palva, A., and Jokinen, K. (1970). 'Presbyacusis, V Filtered speech test', *Acta. Otolaryngol.*, **70**, 232–241.

Parker, W., Decker, R. L., and Richards, N. G. (1968). 'Auditory function and lesions of the pons', *Arch. Otolaryng.*, **87**, 228–240.

Reed, G. (1960). 'An audiometric study of 200 cases of subjective tinnitus', *Arch. Otolaryngol.*, **71**, 84–94.

Rosen, S. (1969). 'Dietary prevention of hearing loss', *IX Int. Congr. Oto. Rhino. Lar. Exerpta Med VIII*, **189**, 134–139.

Rosen, S. and Olin, P. (1965) 'Hearing loss and coronary artery disease'. *Arch. Otolaryng.*, **82**, 236–243.

Rosen, S., Plester, D., El-Mofty, A., and Rosen, H. (1964). 'High frequency audiometry in presbyacusis', *Arch. Otolaryngol.*, **79**, 18–32.

Schuknecht, H. F. (1974a) 'Presbyacusis', in *Pathology of the Ear*, pp. 388–403, Harvard University Press, Cambridge, Massachusetts.

Schuknecht, H. F. (1974b). 'The dysequilibrium of ageing', in *Pathology of the Ear*, pp. 403–409, Harvard University Press, Cambridge, Massachusetts.

Stephens, S. D. G. (1976). In *Application of psychiacoustics to central auditory dysfuction in Scientific Foundations of Otolaryngology* (Eds R. Hinchcliffe and D. Harrison), pp. 352–361, William Heinemann, London.

Takahashi, T. (1971). 'Ultrastructure of the pathologic stria vascularis and spiral prominence in man', *Ann. Otololog. Rhinol. Laryngol.*, **80**, 721–735.

United States National Health Survey (1968). *Hearing States and Ear Examination (1960–1962)*, Ser. 11, No. 32. Nat. Center for Health Statistics.

Weston, T. E. (1964). 'Presbyacusis. A clinical study', *J. Laryngol.*, **78**, 273–286.

Yatsu, F. M. and Smith, J. D. (1979). 'Neurologic aspects of vertigo', in *diseases of the Ear, Nose and Throat*, Vol. 2, pp. 837–864, Butterworths, London.

19
Disorders of Communication

19.1

Disorders of Communication

Joyce Edwards, Ena Davies

INTRODUCTION

Communication difficulties in the elderly population vary tremendously: most people need no special care, can make their own decisions, and state them clearly. It is important to stress this and not to stereotype the elderly as dependent, inarticulate, and deaf (Blythe, 1979; Elder, 1977). However, to be cut off from human communication by the effects of disease, such as a stroke, is so devastating that for the small percentage so handicapped all the services available must be mobilized as a priority.

The term 'communication' (rather than speech) is used throughout in order to emphasize that communication is not confined to speech. It is important to continue speaking to a person when no verbal reply is possible, but it must also be remembered that we constantly communicate non-verbally as we talk. We can also learn to interpret the non-verbal communication of others (body language, gesture language, mechanical forms of communication, etc.) and learn to use alternative methods ourselves. Speech is the goal, of course, but alternative forms may be the means of facilitating verbal communication, or may have to become the only, and viable, means of communication, if speech becomes physically impossible.

The natural process of ageing manifests itself gradually in changes in communication ability. These changes affect the respiratory system (speech and voice are dependent upon breath); the larynx (voice); the ear (hearing and the reception of language); the eyes (visual language); and the central nervous system (language skills and linguistic usage, articulation of speech, cognition, and memory). Elderly people take longer to perceive language, so that there may be a marked time lag in response. Short-term memory may become increasingly affected, although long-term memory may be enhanced. Breakdown in communication is a combination of ageing and pathology, including previous infections and traumas, and further pathologies occurring later in life (such as osteoarthritis) (Beasley and Davis, 1981). Specific problems of communication arise from motor speech disorders, voice disorders, aphasia, and deafness (see Chapter 18.2 on the auditory system). Most people with communication problems are relatively mobile, able to live at home, and attend for therapy as an outpatient. Others may live at home but receive treatment in a day hospital. Some will be hospitalized but eventually become mobile again, perhaps still requiring therapy after returning home. Some will require extended care and thus will be institutionalized.

Given that a person is physically handicapped (e.g. by hemiplegia), speechless, and has difficulty in comprehension, it becomes difficult for professionals and society alike to see that person as a thinking individual with many needs to communicate and with a right to therapy. Why is there a responsibility to provide speech therapy for the elderly? Both professionals and government question the cost of an apparent non-productive end result where there may be little or no observable progress, even degeneration, no return to the workforce, and commonly a short term enjoyment of the successes obtained. The answer relates to the quality of life. It is natural to need some measure of success for our efforts, but optimizing the quality of care by improved communication, even without speech, should be considered reward enough. The comfort and well-being of the person can be dramatically improved, and further regression (and thus increased nursing care) can be arrested. Professionals tend to be overworked in all areas, while the numbers of elderly keep growing; any method which improves communication, and thus eases the difficulties of physical care, should be considered, even where traditional speech therapy is not productive. Speech therapists, like other professionals, have had little specialized training in geriatric medicine, and need to know more about speech and language disorders of the elderly population and general linguistic ageing.

Probably the most challenging problem is the confrontation of death and dying. The ageing process is also, in itself, an extension of the normal processes of grief and loss, with the loss of home, physical competence, independence, speech and hearing, and many loved ones. Professionals working with the elderly cannot deny natural concerns and conflicts in themselves, and must also endeavour to interpret them for the speechless person. The elderly are mostly courageous people who have had productive lives and whose capacity for growth and change enrich us if we respond to them. We are there to help the person to heal him-or herself and to help him or her to face grief and loss, death itself, and to die with dignity—'the last stage of growth' (Kübler-Ross, 1975). This means that each day is precious, as is the two-way communication of appreciation and love, and joy in the youthfulness of helpers. The elderly, like all patients, know their own needs, and can be allowed to help in their own rehabilitation. Communication is fundamental to human beings, and the restoration of even minimal communication restores human dignity and worth of the patient to all carers, including the person and family. The mere presence of the therapist can improve the general care remark-ably; the withdrawal of therapy can result in general abandonment of effort and resultant isolation and misery for the individual. These basic rights must not be violated.

While the percentage of speech problems is small the numbers involved are large. The projected figures indicate that almost all professionals will be required to work with some elderly at some point, and these will include the communicatively impaired. The plans we make for the elderly now will also ultimately be for ourselves. Probably 3 to 4 per cent. of all elderly have verbal communication problems; when deafness is added there will be about 40 to 60 per cent.

PATHOLOGY OF NEUROLOGICAL DISORDERS

Aphasia

The incidence of neurological disorders increases proportionately with advancing years, cerebrovascular disease being the major contributory cause of cerebral infarction, haemorrhage, or embolus. It is generally assumed that 'for almost every right handed and for many left handed adults, the left hemisphere subserves all or most of the functions of language' (Benson, 1979). Damage to the left hemisphere is therefore likely to impair language function, to a greater or lesser degree, giving rise to the syndrome of aphasia. This complex, multifaceted accumulation of symptoms has challenged neurologists and students of aphasia for the past century.

Darley, Aronson, and Brown (1975) define aphasia as 'a multi-modality reduction in the capacity to decode (interpret) and encode (formulate) meaningful linguistic elements, that is words (morphemes), and larger syntactic units. It is manifested in difficulties in listening, reading, speaking and writing'. The classification of aphasia has been based mainly on symptoms, or clusters of symptoms, presented by individual patients. The early localizationists have left a legacy of terminology which still persists today, although many of their hypotheses have been questioned.

The term 'Broca's aphasia' is synonymous with expressive or motor aphasia, and arises from damage to Broca's area – the third frontal convolution of the left hemisphere. It describes the collection of symptoms arising when, in the absence of any impairment of intelligence, the patient exhibits word-finding difficulties, non-fluency in conversational speech, problems in repetition because of an inability to grasp the word, inconsistent articulatory problems, or dissociation between auditory input and speech output. Articulation may be affected by inconsistent errors and, in the more severe forms, the patient may be unable to imitate articulatory patterns. There will also be grammatical errors, more especially with determiners and prepositions. Automatic speech is often intact as the patient is able to reproduce series speech, i.e. days of the week, months of the year, etc. Both reading and writing skills are affected, sometimes to the point of complete failure to read aloud.

Wernicke's contribution to the knowledge of aphasia has been recorded by the classification of Wernicke's aphasia, commonly referred to as sensory or receptive aphasia, arising from damage to Wernicke's area in the posterior part of the superior temporal gyrus. Wernicke's aphasia is more frequently found in the older patient, who exhibits marked difficulty in the comprehension of spoken and written language. The condition is more marked in the inability to understand words in isolation, whereas the patient may be able to comprehend within a contextual framework. More familiar words may be recognized, but there is often selective affect of words in a given semantic class and of specific grammatical constructions. Spoken output will depend on the level of comprehension: if this is limited then meaningful speech will also be limited. Paraphasia is a common characteristic of Wernicke's aphasia, being the fluent production of often meaningless speech and in its most severe form producing a jargon dysphasia.

These problems are paralleled in reading and writing – although the production may be legible, the content may be totally incomprehensible. Despite the severity of the problem, patients with Wernicke's aphasia are often able to imitate body actions (e.g. dancing), but are unable to imitate selective movements (e.g. protrusion of the tongue).

In addition to these major classifications, a variety of distinct categories exist to describe classic features which take precedence over other symptoms:

Anomia

A selective loss of ability to evoke specific words is a characteristic of all aphasics, but when word-finding difficulties are disproportionate to other symptoms the classification of anomia is used.

Apraxia; Dyspraxia

The major differential factor between dysarthria (see the following section) and certain forms of dysphasia is the constancy of the disorder affecting both voluntary and involuntary movements alike. It is this feature of constancy that discriminates dysarthria from dyspraxia, which Nielsen (1962) defines as 'a disturbance in which a patient, without dementia, incoordination, or paralysis, is nevertheless, because of motor incapacity, unable to apply his powers to a voluntary purpose'.

These patients demonstrate difficulties in either evocation of movement or execution of movement. The vegetative functions of chewing, sucking, and swallowing remain intact, but the patient is often unable to protrude the tongue to command, purse the lips, or imitate gesture or movement volitionally, although the movement may occur automatically in context.

Apraxia of speech varies in severity, in its most severe form affecting all oral and articulatory movements, along with other locomotor disorders, making the production of speech movements and patterns impossible.

Apraxia is described by Luria (1966) as a 'loss of kinetic schemes that provide afferent organisation'. The more complex the movement the greater is the difficulty in its performance – hence speech is likely to suffer.

Agnosia

Another major group of acquired neurological disorders is the agnosias. Dejerine (in Brown, 1972) defines agnosia as 'a difficulty of recognition'. Recognition is 'that psychological phenomenon which permits us by the use of one or another of our senses to identify an object under observation with an object previously observed and of which we have registered the memory picture in the form of a mental image'.

In agnosia the loss of recognition is confined to one sense organ, either vision, hearing, or touch being selectively impaired.

Alexia; Agraphia

Among the clusters of symptoms exhibited in aphasia are those of alexia and agraphia. Both may exist as discrete neurological disorders or may coexist with other features of the aphasia syndrome.

Alexia is an acquired disorder in which the ability to read is impaired by brain damage. Unlike dyslexia which is a developmental disorder of children who have problems in learning reading skills, alexia is the loss of reading ability in adults who, prior to the onset of the neurological disorder or trauma, were fluent readers.

Historically the inability to recognize the letters of the alphabet was classified as letter blindness and the inability to read words as word blindness. These terms have been replaced by literal alexia and verbal alexia, respectively. Benson (1979) defines three categories of alexia:

(a) parietal – temporal alexia, frequently referred to as alexia **with** agraphia in which both reading and writing ability is impaired with varying degrees of severity;

(b) occipital alexia where alexia exists in isolation from writing disturbance – an alexia **without** agraphia. Although patients suffering from this condition are able to write they are unable to read or remember what they have written;

(b) frontal alexia often coexists with Broca's aphasia. Patients with frontal alexia show a severe literal alexia and a lesser degree of verbal alexia (Benson, Brown, and Tomlinson, 1971).

Alexia is often accompanied by impairment of writing skills. The majority of patients suffering from aphasia demonstrate some problems with written language mirroring the difficulties they experience with spoken output. The quality of writing may be impaired when hemiplegia forces a change to the use of the non-preferred hand. Visual field defects will also affect the quality of written output. The ability to spell may be affected and the linguistic content bizarre governed by the extent and severity of the disorder.

Global Aphasia

Many patients present with global difficulties in the days immediately post-trauma. There may be considerable spontaneous recovery, but if comprehension of spoken, written, and non-verbal language persists, then the classification of global aphasia is applied.

Finally, Benson (1979) tabulates the syndromes according to the neuroanatomical lesion, but points out that 'totally different pathological states can and do produce identical aphasic syndromes'.

He identifies the following categories:

(1) Perisylvian aphasia syndromes
   (i) Broca aphasia
   (ii) Wernicke aphasia
   (iii) conduction aphasia

(2) Borderzone aphasia syndromes
   (i) Transcortical motor aphasia
   (ii) Aphasia of anterior cerebral artery infarction
   (iii) Transcortical sensory aphasia
   (iv) Mixed transcortical aphasia

(3) Subcortical aphasia syndromes
   (i) Aphasia of Marie's quadrilateral space
   (ii) Thalamic aphasia
   (iii) Striatal aphasia
   (iv) Aphasia from white matter lesions

(4) Non-localizing aphasic syndromes
   (i) Anomic aphasia
   (ii) Gobal aphasia

(5) Alexia
   (i) Parietal-temporal alexia
   (ii) Occipital alexia
   (iii) Frontal alexia

Assessment is obviously of paramount importance to determine the patient's abilities and disabilities. He or she is functioning on residual language skills which will vary enormously from one individual to another, dependent upon the nature, site, and depth of the lesion, the age of onset, the premorbid state, and the psychological adjustment to the handicap.

Standardized tests are available to provide a differential diagnosis. Among those in more frequent use in the United Kingdom are:

(a) An Aphasia Screening Test (Whurr, 1974)

(b) Boston Diagnostic Aphasia Examination (1972 Lea and Febiger, Philadelphia)

(c) Functional Communication Profile (Goodglass and Kaplan, 1972)

(d) Minnesota Test for Differential Diagnosis of Aphasia (Schuell, 1972)

(e) Porch Index of Communicative Ability (Porch, 1967)

(f) Reporter's Test (De Renzi and Ferrari, 1978)

(g) Token Test (De Renzi and Vignolo, 1962)

(h) A new test of Thompson (1983) should also be considered

SPEECH THERAPY WITH THE APHASIC PERSON

Owing to the multiple problems of the elderly aphasic a modified version of conventional speech therapy (Chapey, 1981; Fawcus *et al.*, 1982; Jenkins *et al.*, 1975; Schuell, 1972; Schuell *et al.*, 1974) has been found to be most effective. What would seem rigid and inflexible for the younger stroke person provides structure and security as a framework for therapy with the older person. The initial approach is often greatly assisted by the use of Amer-Ind (American-Indian) gestures (Skelly, 1979), which can be used to facilitate speech rather than replace it and which incorporates work on the apraxia of the unparalysed hand. Relief of the apraxia of the mouth and the facilitation of writing may thus result, thereby simultaneously reinforcing the spoken word. Vocabulary drills utilize rhythm by holding the hand and beating the stressed syllables as a sentence incorporating the word is spoken. The word is first seen as a picture, then seen as a written word, said, spelled, chanted in phrase, sentence, or question, and heard within the context of many other sentences and questions. A basic 50 word Amer-Ind vocabulary may be learned gradually in this way. Reality orientation (Holden and Woods, 1982) and general conversation at the level of comprehension of the individual or group are used routinely.

Individual therapy is usually only suitable in early stages of treatment or with special problems; otherwise groups of two or more persons are considerably more stimulating and motivating. The ideal group includes many helpers, so that each aphasic person has individual help within the group. Amer-Ind groups gradually progress to further vocabulary, such as the first five hundred words of *The Teacher's Word Book* (Thorndike and Lorge, 1959), using 20 words at a time in alphabetical sequences, but continuing the same routine as above (without gestures). Groups can progress in this way to more and more advanced vocabulary, and individuals can progress from group to group according to speed of progress. The ultimate goal should be membership in a stroke club if possible.

By following the same routine each time, the elderly avoid confusion and appear to respond well, even where severe comprehension problems are involved. This structure may be more tedious for the therapist, but the vocabulary framework can gradually be expanded to include considerable language stimulation (various uses of words, humour, the nature of the problem and acceptance, philosophy, etc.) as the group progresses, with appropriate phrases, sentences, questions, and conversation, and the use of the Language Master (LA4) machine (see List of Communication Aids at the end of the chapter) for rhythms, pictures from Learning Development Aids (LA5) and Photographic Teaching Materials (LA10) also add variety. Sheets from conventional material (Speech and Language Rehabilitation, 1980) and writing practice sheets (caligraphy) can be used for home practice and individual work, also involving the use of the unparalysed hand. In the early stages of writing it is often helpful to guide the hand as the person writes.

Many people ask if the speechless person can write down his or her needs, but this is rarely possible unless the problems are confined to the articulation of speech; the elderly person who becomes aphasic following a stroke usually has great difficulty in writing with the unparalysed hand, or in using a mechanical aid, or even indicating pictures on a vocabulary board (LA3). This is because the body apraxia and language difficulties at the cortical level are usually too severe. As function returns verbal ability and hand dexterity usually progress at the same rate.

It is important to give considerable language stimulation as frequently as possible, but only for short periods in order to avoid fatigue. Helpers are a great asset in providing extra stimulation (see the section on helpers).

PATHOLOGY OF NEUROLOGICAL DISORDERS

Dysarthria

In contrast to the language problems exhibited by aphasic patients, the dysarthric patient knows what he or she wishes to say but cannot coordinate the movements of respiration, phonation, articulation, resonance, and prosody in order to produce intelligible speech.

Dysarthria is the collective term for a group of related speech disorders classified by Darley, Aronson, and Brown (1975) according to the site of the lesion and the nature of the deficit.

Spastic Dysarthria

Bilateral upper motor neurone lesion characterized by 'slow, rasping, laboured speech, and each word is prolonged. It is dominant in lower tones and hardly intelligible'. (Parker quoted in Darley *et al*, 1975).

Hypokinetic Dysarthria (Parkinsonism): Extrapyramidal Lesion (see Chapter 16.13)

The characteristics of Parkinson's disease are rigidity, slowness (bradykinesia), and inefficiency of movement (i.e. affecting range and speed), together with tremor and abnormalities of posture and facial immobility. The slowness results in dysarthria (hypokinetic), dysphonia and quiet speech (due to respiration problems and mental state), stammering and palilalia (repetition of words), pitch change and loss of inflection, stress, and rhythm (prosody), causing hesitations, stoppages, and bursts of speed (Dejong, 1967; Scott, 1983; Scott and Williams, 1982). Speech may become inaudible and slow speech may also accelerate (as does the gait) to unintelligibility. Levodopa may improve speech consistent with general physical improvement, but anticholinergic preparations appear ineffective. Too high a dose of levodopa can have an adverse effect on speech by increasing the dysarthria.

Hyperkinetic Dysarthria (Chorea; Dystonia): Extra Pyramidal Lesion

Speech is characterized by hesitation and jerkiness because of the lack of synchrony between respiration, phonation, and articulation. Sudden fluctuations in muscle tone disrupt fluent speech.

Ataxic Dysarthria: Cerebellar Lesion

'Descriptive terms recur in the literature; slow, staccato, slurred, jerky, forced, explosive, irregular, interrupted, drawling, monotonous, . . . and most frequently, scanning' (Darley, Aronson, and Brown, 1975).

Flaccid Dysarthria: Lower Motor Neurone Lesion

Speech quality is dependent upon which nerves are affected. Reduced control of exhalation of voicing and precision of articulation may arise as a result of damage to V trigeminal, VII facial, X vagus, and/or XII hypoglossal, nerves.

Mixed Dysarthrias (Amyotrophic Lateral Sclerosis): Lesions of Multiple Systems

Speech is a mixture of flaccid and spastic dysarthria dependent upon the course of the disease.

As with aphasia, a differential diagnosis based on systematic assessment (Beasley and Davis, 1981; Darley, Aronson, and Brown, 1975; Enderby, 1980; Robertson, 1980) will provide the basis for dysarthria therapy. Assessment may continue during therapy, and reassessment at intervals may be required.

SPEECH THERAPY WITH THE DYSARTHRIC PERSON

The role of the speech therapist in treating the dysarthric patient is very much a part of the team approach, and the method used (e.g. Proprioceptive Neuromuscular Facilitation, PNF) should be integrated with physiotherapy and other treatment and care (see Chapter 29). The approach will be through muscles involved in breathing, chewing and swallowing, and speech, with special attention being paid to posture (Darley, Aronson, and Brown, 1975; Rosenbeck in Beasley and Davis, 1981; Scott and Williams, 1982). Probably an ongoing diagnosis will be done while the therapist is working on the symptoms. Dysarthria therapy with Parkinson's disease problems may also emphasize the rate of speech. If all speech therapy with the elderly has to be defended, no aspect is more controversial than that of the progressive neurological diseases, of which Parkinson's is one of the most numerous. Yet again a case must be made for promoting and maintaining the highest possible level of quality of life and ease of care, and of the patient's right to services. As in the case of strokes, the handicaps resulting from Parkinson's disease are multiple and devastating, with profound psychosocial problems involved, not only for the person concerned but also for the family and carers involved. Drugs, although helpful, cannot be relied upon alone, and a team approach to promote and maintain optimal functioning is required. Short periods of intensive speech therapy will be more effective than convensional versions (Scott, 1983) and early referral is vital.

Where dysarthria is so severe that speech is not intelligible it may be more important to promote and encourage a desire to communicate by means of a mechanical communicator. This makes possible a reasonable channel of communication through the written word by tapping out letters on a small machine resembling a calculator, but with letters in place of numerals (LA2). Such an alternative removes the tension and anxiety of not being understood and frequently facilitates speech by allowing the person to relax. (Nor should we underestimate the powerful effect of the intriguing little machine on onlookers, who thus become curious and immediately begin to communicate with a person they would otherwise ignore.) Where speech remains impossible the person can continue with the machine so long as a hand remains capable of either directly pressing the keys or of holding an aid (such as a closed pen) to do so. Where the voice is too quiet, or entails excessive effort, an amplifier, resembling a hearing aid in reverse, may be useful (LA6 and LA11). Anxiety concerning dependency on aids is usually unfounded: people will always prefer to talk, and do so as soon as they are able to make themselves understood verbally.

The shift of emphasis from speech as the ultimate goal of therapy to that of establishing communication using whatever residual abilities the elderly patient may possess is a far more positive approach to management than pursuing an unattainable goal. Silverman (1980) in the preface to his book states that 'it would be difficult to conceive of a child or adult who is so severely impaired that there would be no non-speech communication system that he or she could use'. Recent advances in non-speech systems offer hope to those who would previously have been classed as non-communicators.

If a technological aid is recommended its availability, acceptability, and portability will be salient to its selection. Maintenance is another important factor to ensure the patient is never without a communication tool.

Careful selection of an appropriate alternative is essential to avoid disappointment on the part of the patient and his family. The selection of the appropriate supplement will depend on the primary assessment of the individual needs, the acceptability of a supplement or augmentative by the patient, time and support for the introduction, and training in the use of the supplement. There will be no one system which will suit all patients. Assessment of abilities to ensure the patient has the necessary skills to use the particular supplement is also required. Acceptability may be dependent upon the time and support that can be offered by family or care-giver. Considerable time may need to be spent in educating the support team to accept a non-speech system – the cooperation of the team is essential to success.

Systems may be classified as aided or unaided. Examples of unaided systems would be gestural (e.g. Amer-Ind) or manual signing (e.g. British or American sign language). The use of pantomimic gestures often emerges as the first step towards the retrieval of communication skills (Schlanger, 1976). Aided systems are those which require some form of visual display which the patient may indicate. These may be simple picture charts, line drawings, symbols, or traditional orthography in the form of alphabet boards or word boards.

The enormous advances in technology have broadened the horizons for the speech and language handicapped. Most aids use traditional orthography to provide a visual display or hard-copy printout (LA2, LA7, LA8, LA13, LA14). Others utilize word boards linked to TV monitor (LA12) and the newest

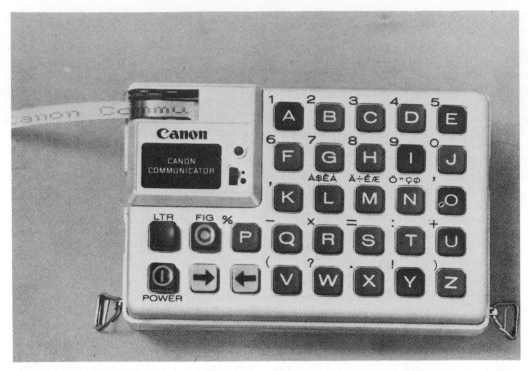

Figure 1   Canon communicator

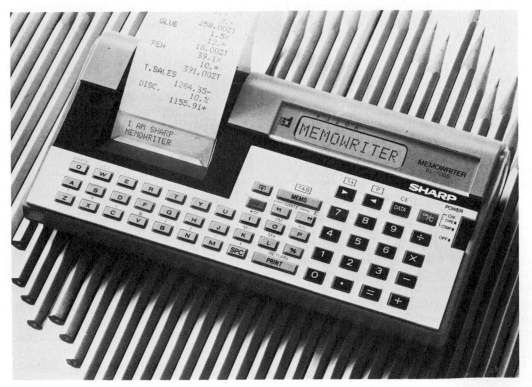

Figure 2   Memowriter

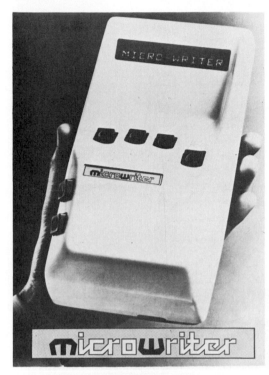

Figure 3   Microwriter

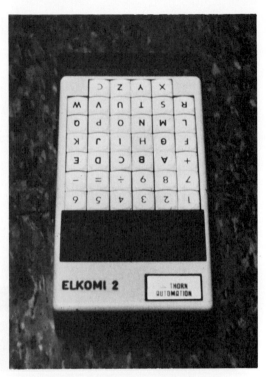

Figure 4   Elkomi 2 communicator

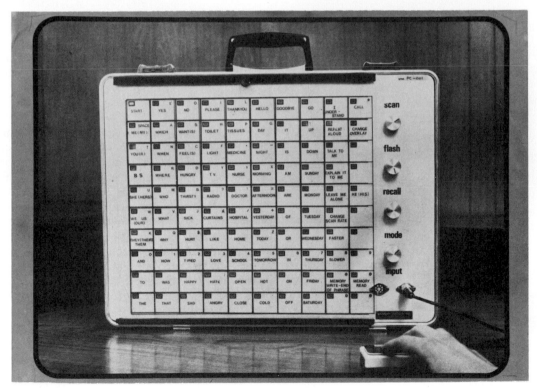

Figure 5   Possum communicator

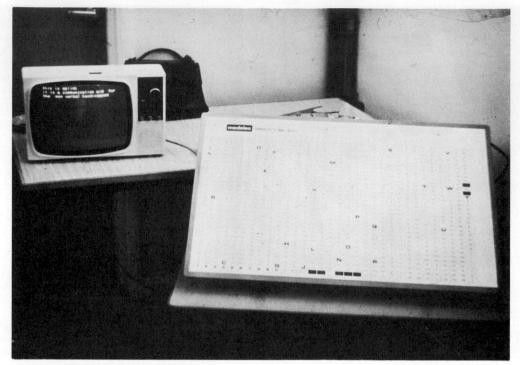

Figure 6 Splink

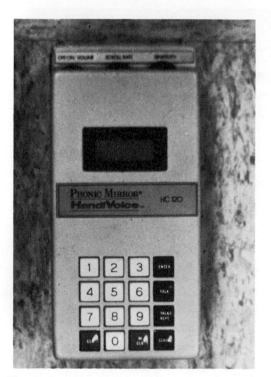

Figure 7 Phonic Mirror Handivoice: synthetic speech

devices incorporate synthetic speech (LA9, LA1).

Chosen appropriately supplements can enhance the communication skills of the elderly.

TEAM APPROACH

How should the health care team (and this should include the family), of which the speech therapist is a part, approach communication problems? Each member needs to understand the following: (a) comprehension problems, which may or may not include various degrees of deafness; (b) expressive problems, including the non-verbal person; (c) chewing and swallowing (and dental hygiene) problems, as the same muscles are used in speech; (d) voice problems; (e) the need for communication: mental stimulation is a great problem for the lonely old person.

Communication can be enhanced by:
(a) Listening, observing, interpreting, emphathizing, and asking oneself '**What** am I communicating?', i.e. by body language, tone of voice, etc. (Börsig and Steinacker, 1982).

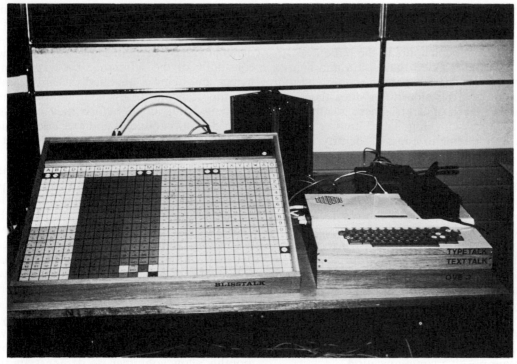

Figure 8   Blisstalk

(b) Using clear, simple, speech with a raised voice (**not** a shout), with the face in a good light, even though the person cannot reply; using **adult** speech and language at all times, although the speech and language is kept simple and with repetition.

(c) Ensuring that dentures, glasses, hearing aid, and other appliances are clean and functioning.

(d) Learning alternative methods to speech (e.g. gesture (Skelly, 1979), pictures (LA3), writing, and mechanical aids) with the help of the speech therapist.

(e) Understanding deafness and the use of hearing aids (with the help of the hearing therapist) (Maurer and Rupp, 1979).

(f) Understanding the effects of background noise which can obliterate efforts to communicate.

(g) Undertaking simple screening procedures (with the help of the speech therapist).

(h) General mental stimulation (orientation to time, place, weather, outside events, family, season, etc.) to **preserve** communication.

Simple screening procedures allow an estimate of the degree of comprehension and expressive speech to be made. For example, questions requiring a simple 'yes' or 'no' answer can be very misleading as a smiling nod can seem appropriate to so many questions. Moreover, automatic routines are often accompanied by gestures which gain the correct response without the person having understood the verbal request. Controlled screening items help to prevent the underestimation or overestimation of the level of language. Underestimating the language of a stroke patient, particularly their comprehension of language, affects management. People react strongly to being talked down to or to having their problems discussed in front of them. The patient becomes upset and displays increasing management difficulties. Their reactions may also be normal ones of fear of a new situation, a special problem to the elderly, resulting in confusion or lack of attention and an appropriate depression. On the other hand, overestimating the level of communication assumes that the person is understanding normally, and expects him or her to follow through with instructions, subsequently labelling them uncooperative when they are unable to do so. Negative reactions from carers then produce more distress behaviours in the patient.

It must be stressed that vision and hearing problems also contribute to the comprehension difficulties of the elderly, as does the rapid, complex speech of carers. There is often boredom, depression, loneliness, and a loss of rights, all leading to a loss of identity, personality, and dignity, with subsequent disorientation. These problems may also be related to the excessive use of drugs. Drugs may be given because there is concern about depression and/or sleeplessness, but they can result in confusion, memory loss, and withdrawal, and, most importantly, they prevent constructive adjustment to problems and response to therapy, especially speech therapy. Lack of response to therapy, and the feeling of progress and wellbeing that should result, leads to a loss of hope of recovery, and so the person is caught in a downward spiral. It is the role of the team to prevent this self-perpetuating situation and to maintain positive communication.

Helpers on the Rehabilitation Team

The role of helpers for speech therapy is a controversial one, but deserves special consideration in relation to communication work with the elderly. To rehabilitate people to sit at home, or in long stay homes and hospitals, only to vegetate and lose speech again seems pointless, and attempts to train other staff in communication methods may be thwarted by staff shortages. Two objections raised by professionals are that, firstly, paid helpers tend to describe themselves to others as therapists, and may work unsupervised, thus implying a training and expertise they do not possess, and, secondly, although paid helpers may be supervised while the therapist is working, who supervises when he or she resigns, is ill, or on leave? Other departments (e.g. occupational therapy) who employ helpers do not have only one therapist at a time to cover clinics, as in speech therapy, and thus always have a qualified person available to supervise. One solution that has proved practicable is to have an official arrangement that the supervisor of a geriatric day hospital, or physiotherapy or occupational therapy department, will take over

the helpers when necessary. This arrangement has the added advantage that helpers often get good experience in other departments, to the benefit of all concerned. They can be reminded constantly of the difference between being a helper and being a qualified therapist, and in the importance of assessment and programme planning being done before they can assist. Clear definition of goals and exact descriptions of working routines should be set out in writing.

Volunteer helpers are equally important in a geriatric communication therapy programme. They may be obtained by various means, e.g. a local branch of the British Red Cross Society, and similar goals should be written up for them. The fundamental difference between volunteers and paid helpers is that a volunteer will have one person only to work with, and for an hour or so a week, whereas paid helpers can work full time on many different aspects of the programme and may be involved with large numbers of persons with strokes. Follow-up sessions of about once monthly allow volunteers to demonstrate their work if progress is to be expected. However, if the goal is to maintain a peak level of achievement only, frequent return is not so important, but helpers do need the regular encouragement of a staff member, if only by telephone contact. The ultimate goal should be for the person to move into a stroke club (Griffith, 1980).

Family members can be used as helpers, of course, when this is suitable, but one advantage of non-related helpers is the lack of emotional involvement. Sometimes it is helpful to involve a relative with other members of a group in order to gain insights without emotional complications, but it must be remembered that relatives do need a break, and this also helps the family. Of greater value perhaps is the formation of family support groups where they can share their concerns and ways of solving problems.

Finally, a comprehensive programme of paid helpers and volunteers for geriatric communication disorders will also require a paid coordinator if the speech therapist is not to be overwhelmed by administration.

In summary, the speech therapy (communication) programme for the elderly includes assessment and diagnosis, and the planning of therapy by team approach to promote and maintain a desire to communicate. Therapy may be conducted in groups or on an individual basis, and is directed towards reaching and maintaining maximum speech and language function, or communication by alternative means. The speech therapist maintains a good speech and language environment by discussion with family members and with all those who treat or care for the individual.

LIST OF COMMUNICATION AIDS

LA 1   Blisstalk: Royal National Institute of Technology, Stockholm, Sweden.

LA 2   Canon Communicator: Canon Business Machines (UK) Ltd, Waddon House, Stafford Road, Croydon.

LA 3   College of Speech Therapists Communication Chart: The College of Speech Therapists, Harold Poster House, 6 Lechmere Road, London, NW2 5BU.

LA 4   Language Master: Bell and Howell A-V Ltd, Alperton House, Bridgewater Road, Wembley, Middlesex, HA0 1EG.

LA 5   Learning Development Aids: Park Works, Norwich Road, Wisbech, Cambridgeshire, PE13 2AX.

LA 6   Medeci Speech Aid Amplifier: Ingrams Hearing Aids Ltd, London Road, Riverhead, Sevenoaks, Kent, TN13 2DN.

LA 7   Memowriter: Sharp Electronics, Retail Distribution.

LA 8   Microwriter Ltd, 7 Old Park Lane, London, W1Y 3LJ.

LA 9   Phonic Mirror Handivoice: P. C. Werth Ltd, Audiology House, 45 Nightingale Lane, Balham, London, SW12 8SU.

LA 10   Photographic Teaching Materials: 23 Horn Street, Buckingham, MK18 3AP.

LA 11   Speech Amplifier: Jedcom Products, 318 Green Lanes, London N4.

LA 12   Splink: Medelec Ltd, Manor Way, Old Woking, Surrey GU22 9JU.

LA 13   Elkomi II Communicator.

LA 14   Possum Communicator: Possum Controls Ltd, Middlegreen Road, Slough, Berks.

REFERENCES

Beasley, D. S., and Davis, G. A. (Eds) (1981). *Aging: Communication Processes and Disorders*, Grune and Stratton, New York.

Benson, D. F. (1979). *Aphasia, Alexia and Agraphia: Clinical Neurology and Neorosurgery Monographs*, Churchill Livingstone, New York.

Benson, D., Brown, J., and Tomlinson, E. (1971). Varieties of Alexia, *Neurology (Minneap.)*, **21**, 951–957.

Blythe, R. (1979). *The View in Winter*, Penguin Books.

Borsig, A., and Steinacker, I. (1982). 'Communication with the patient in the intensive care unit', *Nursing Times (Suppl.)*, March **1982**.

Brown, J. W. (1972). *Aphasia, Apraxia and Agnosia. Clinical and Theoretical Aspects*. Charles C. Thomas, Springfield, Illinois.

Chapey, R. (Ed.) (1981). *Language Intervention Strategies in Adult Aphasia*, Williams and Wilkins.

Darley, F. L., Aronson, A. E., and Brown, J. R. (1975). *Motor Speech Disorders*, W. B. Saunders, Philadelphia.

Dejong, R. N. (1967). *The Neurologic Examination*, 3rd ed., Hoeber, New York.

De Renzi, E., and Vignolo, L. A. (1962). 'The token test: A sensitive test to detect receptive disturbances in aphasics', *Brain*, **85**, 665–678.

De Renzi, E., and Ferrari, C. (1978). 'Reporter's test', *Cortex*, **14**, 2.

Elder, G. (1977). *The Alientated; Growing Old Today*, Writers and Readers Publishing Co-operative.

Enderby, P. (1982). *Frenchay Dysarthria Assessment*, 2nd ed., College Hill Press, California.

Fawcus, M., *et al.* (1982). *Working with Dysphasics*, The Winslow Press Ltd.

Goodglass, H., and Kaplan, E. (1972). *The Assessment of Aphasia and Related Disorders*, Lea and Febiger, Philadelphia.

Griffith, V. E. Chest Heart and Stroke Association Volunteer Stroke Scheme, St Martins, Grimms Hill, Great Missenden, Bucks, HP16 9BG.

Holden, U. P., and Woods, R. T. (1982). *Reality Orientation*, Churchill Livingstone.

Jenkins, J., Jimenez-Pabon, E., Shaw, R. E., and Sefer, J. W. (1975). *Schuell's Aphasia in Adults. Diagnosis, Prognosis and Treatment*, Harper and Row, Maryland.

Kubler-Ross, E. (1975). *Death, The Final Stage of Growth*, Prentice-Hall, Englewood Cliffs, New Jersey.

Luria, A. R. (1966). *Higher Cortical Functions in Man*, Basic Books, New York.

Luria, A. R. (1970) *Traumatic Aphasia*. Mouton, The Hague, Holland.

Maurer, J. F., and Rupp, R. R. (1979). *Hearing and Aging*, Grune and Stratton.

Nielsen, J. M. (1962). *Agnosia, Apraxia, and Aphasia. Their Value in Cerebral Localisation*, Hafner, New York.

Porch, B. (1967). *Porch Index of Communicative Ability*, Palo Alto Consulting Psychologists, California.

Robertson, S. J. (1980). *Test: Dysarthria Profile*, London.

Schlanger, P. H. (1976). 'Training the adult aphasic to pantomime', Paper presented at fifty-first Annual Meeting of American Speech and Hearing Association, Houston.

Schuell, H. (1972). *Minnesota Test for Differential Diagnosis of Aphasia*, University Minnesota Press, Minneapolis.

Schuell, H., Jenkins, J. J., and Jimenez-Pabon, E. (1964). *Aphasia in Adults. Diagnosis, Prognosis and Treatment*, Hoeber, New York.

Scott, S. (1983). 'Communication disorder and its treatment in Parkinson's disease', *Proc. of the nineteenth Congress of the International Assoc. of Logopedics and Phoniatrics*, Folia Phoniatrica, Karger.

Scott, S., and Williams, B. (1982). 'Asking questions about Parkinsonian speech', *Geriatrics*, **12**, 69–72.

Silverman, F. H. (1980). *Communication for the Speechless*, Prentice-Hall, New Jersey.

Skelly, M. (1979). Amer-Ind Gestural Code, Elsevier, New York. (Obtainable from Thomond Books, P.O. Box 85, Limerick, Ireland.)

Speech and Language Rehabilitation (1980). *A Workbook for the Neurologically Impaired*, 2 vols, 2nd ed., The Intersate Publishers. USA.

Thompson, I. (1983). 'Communication deficits in normal and abnormal ageing', In *Proc. of the nineteenth Congress of the International Assoc. of Logopedics and Phoniatrics*, Folia Phoniatrica, Karger.

Thorndike, E. L., and Lorge, I. (1959). *The Teacher's Word Book of 30,000 Words*, Bureau of Publications, New York.

Whurr, R. (1974). *An Aphasia Screening Test*, London.

20

Skin Diseases

Principles and Practice of Geriatric Medicine
Edited by M. S. J. Pathy
© 1985 John Wiley & Sons Ltd

20.1

Skin Disorders

R. Marks

The skin looks and feels different in old age. The well-known wrinkling and bagginess, the duller appearance, and the slightly rougher texture are merely the most obvious changes in the exposed skin. In fact numerous alterations take place during ageing in both structure and function in all of the skin's component parts. In this chapter it is intended to describe these changes in non-diseased skin, indicate the way in which these may cause symptoms, and provide an overview of the impact of skin disease in this age group.

THE EFFECTS OF AGEING ON 'NORMAL' SKIN

Ageing is evident in all skin structures, although it may not be equally evident in all of its components in any one individual. Furthermore, when any measurement of skin structure or function within a population at one point in time is related to age it is usual for there to be a wide scatter of individual observations. These two facts alone make it extremely difficult to determine a person's age accurately by examining the skin. It becomes almost impossible when it is realized that what is frequently called ageing of the skin is mostly the effects of chronic solar damage. It is often very difficult to sort out changes due to true biological ageing from the effects of cumulated environmental injury. As both biological ageing and environmental effects share in causing the appearance of 'ageing' and they are both responsible for disordered skin function they are both deserving of description.

THE EFFECT OF CUMULATIVE ENVIRONMENTAL INJURY ON THE SKIN

By far the most damaging environmental hazard with which the skin has to contend is ultraviolet light (UVL) from the sun. Individuals in places such as Australia, South Africa, and the Southern United States are very much more at risk than those in temperate areas such as North West Europe. But the equation reads 'damage is proportional to dose rate × time of exposure', and even in the comparatively sunless United Kingdom, outdoor workers (e.g. farmers, construction site workers) who spend long periods in the open air can experience severe solar damage in the long term.

The degree of skin pigmentation is of paramount importance in modulating the damaging effects of UVL. Black-skinned people rarely suffer from sunburn or from more serious long-term skin damage due to long-term exposure. In general the darker the complexion the more inherent protection there is. There are also less dramatic and less well-defined unexplained individual and group predispositions to solar damage that do not appear to be based on pigmentation.

By convention, ultraviolet light is subdivided into three broad spectral bands, A, B, and C. Ultraviolet light 'A' (UVA) – so-called long-wave UVL – stretches from a wavelength of about 320 nm to visible blue violet light at about 400 nm. Ultraviolet 'B' (UVB) band encompasses wavelengths from 280 to 320 nm and is known as short-wave UVL. The UVC band is of little practical importance as virtually none reaches the earth because it is filtered out in the atmosphere. UVB appears to be the most significant type of radiation biologically as far as chronic solar damage is concerned, although UVA (the more penetrating rays) may have a lesser role.

Connective Tissue Damage

The most dramatic long-term effect of solar exposure is the degeneration of upper dermal connective tissue. This is only found in sun exposed skin and is present to a much greater degree in light-skinned individuals. It is known as solar elastotic degeneration because the abnormal tissue takes on the staining properties of elastic tissue. The 'elastotic' material may in fact be abnormal collagen rather than a form of elastin and despite much research and considerable disputation the matter has not been resolved. 'Elastotic change' is obvious without elastic stains on ordinary haematoxylin and eosin-stained sections (Fig. 1). The band of degenerate tissue is in the upper and (when severe) mid dermis but for some curious reason leaves the immediate subepidermal zone free. It tends to be more basophilic than normal and the usual fibrillar pattern of the connective tissue gives way to either irregular short chunky wavy strands or amorphous blobs. The connective tissue degeneration causes the majority

of the wrinkling of the skin popularly associated with old age (Fig. 2). Not only is the affected skin wrinkled and even fissured but its elastic properties have changed so that in places it 'sags' (e.g. beneath the chin, under the eyes).

In addition to these textural alterations in

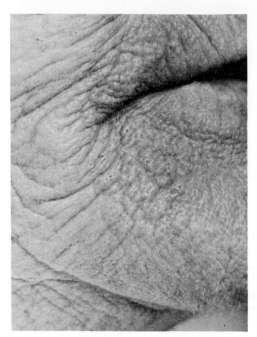

Figure 2 Wrinkling from solar elastosis

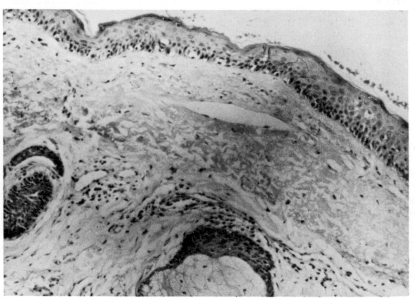

Figure 1 Solar elastosis. Biopsy of elderly subject's skin showing extensive solar elastosis (H and E × 45)

chronically sun-damaged skin its colour tends to change and take on a yellowish-white opaque hue. Elastotic degeneration is responsible for so-called 'sailor's neck' and also most of the wrinkles and other unsightly aberrations that middle aged 'women of fashion' attempt to have removed by 'facelifts'.

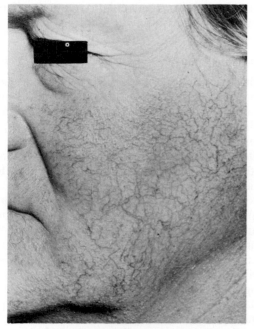

Figure 3   Severe facial telangiectasia

Numerous other changes are found in skin severely affected by this connective tissue change. Widely dilated superficial capillaries (telangiectasia) are sometimes seen and presumably result from loss of mechanical support for the vessel walls (Fig. 3). Curiously persistent and prominent blackheads are quite commonly found periorbitally at the lateral and upper parts of the cheeks. On the arms and dorsa of the hands two findings are commonly found in association with severe solar damage. The first is the well-known irregular purple patches – so-called senile purpura. The other is the appearance of odd angulated and sometimes triradiate scars (Fig. 4). These latter are always 'rationalized' by their owners as being due to some type of trauma but in fact they seem to occur spontaneously.

Attempts at measuring the altered physical properties of sun-damaged skin in vivo in man have been partially successful and confirm the loss of elasticity and tautness that is detectable clinically (Wijn *et al.*, 1979).

Epidermal Neoplasia and Solar Damage

Solar Keratoses (Syn. Senile Keratoses)

The most obvious effect on the epidermis of long-continued sun exposure is the development of preneoplastic and frankly neoplastic

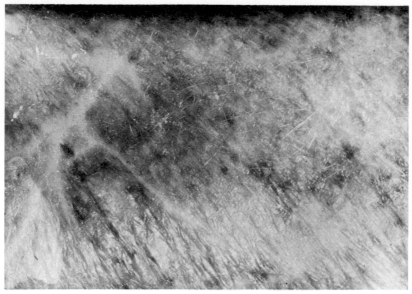

Figure 4   Triradiate scar from solar degeneration

lesions. These lesions can, and sometimes do, arise independently of solar damage but they are very much more frequent when prolonged sun exposure has occurred. It should be noted that chronically sun-exposed skin will have subclinical alterations as well as the more obvious lesions. Early dysplastic changes have been described in the normal-appearing but chronically sun-exposed epidermis between the frank lesions due to solar damage (Pearse and Marks, 1977).

Solar keratoses are the commonest lesions of this sort and these are virtually restricted to the light-exposed sites. Some of these preneoplastic epidermal lesions slowly progress to squamous cell cancers but others appear to regress. Clinically they are apparent as small warty or scaly grey (or sometimes pink) spots or patches (Fig. 5). Treatment for these small lesions will depend on their number and site. Locally destructive treatment with curettage and electrocautery or cryotherapy is often sufficient. Excision is often chosen because this gives a histological diagnosis and is more certain.

Where there are multiple lesions, topical application of 5-fluorouracil may be used. The ointment (5% 5-FU) is applied twice daily for a 10-day period. The affected areas often become quite sore after treatment – and as the drug photosensitizes the skin the patient must be told to avoid sun exposure during the period of treatment.

Recently a therapeutic effect of the retinoids (vitamin A derivatives) for solar keratoses has been described (Moriarty *et al.*, 1982). The long-term result of treatment with the retinoid etretinate (Tigason) of patients who have solar keratoses is not yet known, but clearly this would be a very convenient treatment if the long-term results are satisfactory.

Intraepidermal Epithelioma (Bowen's Disease)

These lesions are squamous cell carcinomas that have not begun to invade but have proliferated within the confines of the epidermis. They are sometimes due to chronic sun exposure but are more often seen on non-exposed sites than solar keratoses and it is assumed that other mechanisms are frequently to blame for these lesions.

Clinically they may have a psoriasiform appearance (Fig. 6) and the diagnosis of Bowen's disease should be suspected when a solitary red plaque with a scaling surface appears on the trunk or limbs of an elderly individual without a previous history of psoriasis. Histologically there may also be a superficial resemblance to psoriasis but the gross cellular atypia and epidermal disorganization make the distinction an easy one. Treatment, after confir-

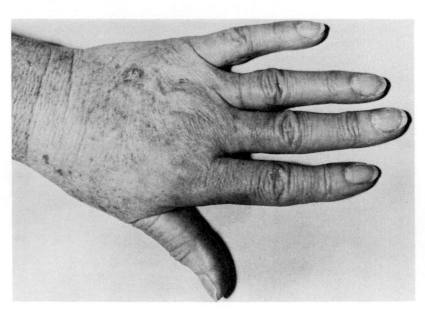

Figure 5   Typical solar keratosis on back of hand

mation by biopsy, is either by surgical removal or by local destruction using electrocautery, cryotherapy, topical chemotherapy (with 5-FU), or by radiotherapy. These lesions may be static or at least only locally malignant for many years and they do not often progress to squamous cell carcinoma with metastasis.

Keratoacanthomata

These odd lesions have been described as 'self-healing squamous cell epitheliomata'. They most often appear on sun-damaged skin but may also occur on the shaded areas. They arise quite rapidly and can reach a diameter of 2 cm or more in just a few weeks. Characteristically they are nodules which have steep walls and a central horny plug (Fig. 7). After reaching their zenith they regress as rapidly as they arise but often leave an area of scarring behind them.

Histologically they may be difficult to distinguish from squamous cell carcinoma and as a rapidly growing lesion of the latter type can resemble a keratoacanthomata clinically, the diagnosis has to be made with care. If the diagnosis can be made confidently the most

appropriate treatment is curettage with diathermy of the base.

Basal Cell Carcinoma (Rodent Ulcer)

These lesions are for the most part locally invasive only, although there are several reported examples where metastasis has occurred (Costanza *et al.*, 1974). They are extremely common and in most skin clinics one or two new patients with basal cell carcinoma (BCC) turn up in each session. The term rodent ulcer presumably refers to their fancied likeness to the bites of rats and probably results from the horrifying large and neglected ulcerated lesions of the face once not uncommon in the poorer sections of the community.

The site most often involved is the face and the commonest type of BCC is the nodule or plaque. They are grey or pearly with a smooth or atrophic surface that may have dilated blood vessels coursing over it (Fig. 8). These lesions gradually enlarge and then ulcerate at the centre. Sometimes this type of lesion contains flecks of brown or black pigmentation and indeed some lesions may be entirely pigmented which can make the diagnosis quite difficult.

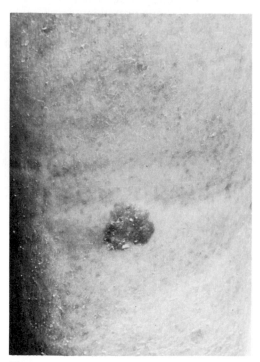

Figure 6   Scaling red patch due to Bowen's disease on back of hand

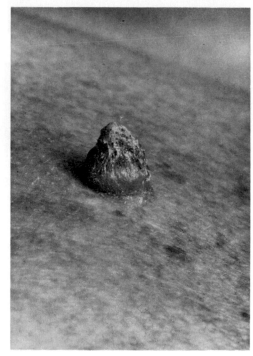

Figure 7   Typical keratoacanthoma

Another type of lesion is known as a 'morphoeic' BCC because of its superficial resemblance to a firm indurated whitish flat patch of morphoea. In these lesions there is a very pronounced fibrotic reaction to the neoplastic epithelium which results in the lesion described.

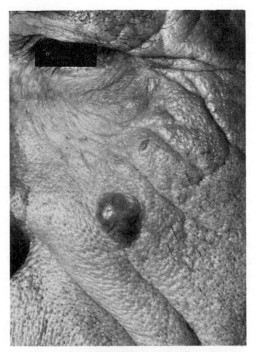

Figure 8   Typical nodular basal cell carcinoma

The diagnosis is usually obvious but should always be confirmed by biopsy. The typical rounded lobules of abnormal basaloid epithelium are usually fairly easy to identify and then the diagnosis is certain (Fig. 9).

Treatment is either by excision, curettage and cautery, or radiotherapy, depending on the site and size of the lesion and the general health of the patient.

Squamous Cell Carcinoma

Squamous cell carcinoma can arise in a solar keratosis or de novo. Although persistent exposure to sunlight is a potent cause of this neoplasm it is by no means the only identifiable cause. These lesions can arise in chronic stasis ulcers and in the scars of lupus vulgaris or lupus erythematosus. Whether this neoplastic transformation is due to the tissue disturbance itself or the previous treatment to the lesion is unknown. Squamous cell cancer can also arise as a result of previous arsenic administration though this is much less frequently seen now. On the penis and at the anal margin transformation of viral warts into frankly neoplastic lesions has been suspected but the evidence for this is still circumstantial. It may also be seen without any obvious provoking cause.

This cancer can present either as an ulcer or a warty nodule or plaque. When the lesion is

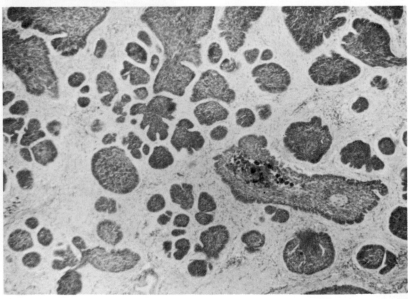

Figure 9   Biopsy of basal cell carcinoma showing lobules of basophilic epidermal cells
(H and E × 45)

ulcerated there is often a rolled everted margin (Fig. 10) and an indurated base. Solitary warty nodules or plaques in the elderly should always be suspected of having a neoplastic origin – especially when the lesion is on the light exposed skin and there is evidence of chronic solar damage. The diagnosis should always be confirmed by biopsy. In general these lesions are slow to metastasize and their prognosis is excellent if treatment is given when the lesions are small. Squamous cell carcinomata of the lips, ears, and genitalia have a more sinister reputation and may metastasize at a much earlier stage in their development.

Treatment is either by surgical excision or by locally destructive measures as described for Bowen's disease.

Seborrhoeic Warts (Syn. Seborrhoeic Keratoses)

Seborrhoeic warts are benign epithelial proliferations that accumulate over the skin surface in old age, like barnacles on a rusting hulk. Their cause is unknown but they tend to occur more frequently in light-exposed areas and it is possible that persistent light exposure plays some part in their formation. They are particularly common over the face but are also commonly seen over the shoulders and mid back as well as the backs of the hands and the forearms. They are warty pigmented structures, and because of this are often mistaken for malignant melanomata. The degree of pigmentation is extremely variable, ranging from jet black to completely unpigmented (Fig. 11).

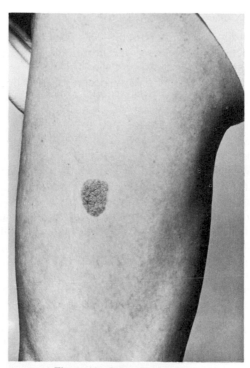

Figure 11   Seborrhoeic wart

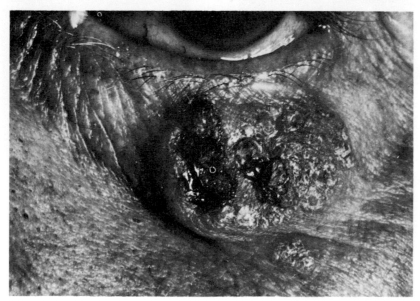

Figure 10   Typical squamous cell carcinoma

If they catch in clothing or become inflamed or are very unsightly, or there is a problem in their identification, it is best to remove them. Curettage and then cautery of the base usually suffices.

Neoplasia of Pigment Cells

Lentigo maligna (Hutchinson's freckle or precancerous melanosis of Dubreuilh) is a premalignant lesion of the pigment cells (melanocytes). It mostly occurs on the light-exposed areas, particularly the face, but sometimes develops on the upper trunk or elsewhere. It is a flat, irregular, brown pigmented area which is often more deeply pigmented in some parts than others (Fig. 12). It spreads slowly over a period of years and causes little harm until, as happens not infrequently, a frank malignant melanoma arises within it. This has a similar prognosis to a malignant melanoma arising de novo and adequate surgical treatment is urgently required. Lentigo maligna itself can either be tackled surgically, if it is in a suitable site, or even removed by some locally destructive form of treatment such as cryotherapy or cautery.

Malignant Melanoma

Malignant melanoma arises more frequently in sun-exposed skin than in non sun-exposed and in the elderly 'sun-battered' individual this possibility should be remembered. It should also be borne in mind that this neoplasm is now more common in all age groups than it once was. A full description is not possible here but any enlarging pigmented lesion should be suspect. Some varieties ulcerate early, others remain non-pigmented at the primary site. The prognosis depends on their depth of invasion and the earlier they are removed the better.

Other Types of Chronic Environmental Injury

Erythema Ab Igne

Persistent exposure to a focal heating source results in marked changes in the skin. Because of the habit of elderly individuals of sitting in front of coal or electric fires it is the front of the lower legs that receives the brunt of the injury. The usual and most benign result is the condition known as erythema ab igne. This is easily recognized from the reticulate brownish pigmentation on the affected site (Fig. 13).

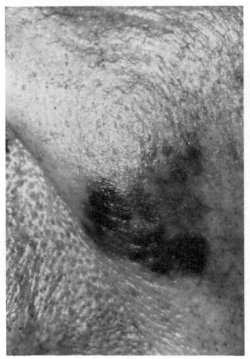

Figure 12   Lentigo maligna on cheek. Note variagate pigmentation

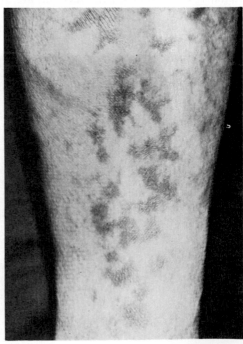

Figure 13   Reticulat pigmentation due to erythema ab igne

Histological examination of the site shows an elastotic degeneration not dissimilar to that seen in chronically sun-exposed sites. In addition the small blood vessels are dilated and distorted and there is evidence of considerable red cell extravasation within the upper dermis. The epidermis itself is obviously abnormal and shows similar but less dramatic alterations than seen in sun-damaged skin (Shahrad and Marks, 1977). Nonetheless, preneoplastic keratoses may occur and even squamous cell carcinoma is occasionally seen. It is interesting to note that chronic heat injury has been incriminated as a carcinogenic stimulus in other situations.

Perniosis (Chilblains)

Repeated exposure to the damp cold with subsequent rapid warming causes an odd persistent vessel dilatation at the periphery and seems to occur most frequently in the United Kingdom. The condition known as perniosis (chilblains) causes itchy bluish-mauve swellings over the toes and less commonly the fingers, ears, buttocks, and elsewhere. They are by no means restricted to the elderly and indeed are not uncommon, for reasons that are not clear, in young, slightly overweight women.

Facial Telangiectasia

A ruddy glow on the cheeks is by no means a reliable marker to good health. It is often present alongside visibly dilated small blood vessels when there has been long continued 'climatic' injury. It seems more common in North West Europe and is probably a reflection of both the susceptibility of the fair-skinned population in this geographic area and the cold winds and chilly winters that the inhabitants experience. It seems to result from disruption of the dermal connective tissue and elastotic degeneration with subsequent loss of mechanical support for the dermal blood vessels. This type of change in the facial skin seems to predispose to the condition known as rosacea (see later).

BIOLOGICAL AGEING IN THE SKIN

The skin surface texture is very obviously altered in the elderly – even in non-light exposed areas. The surface feels somewhat rougher and looks more matt in appearance. We call this sensory combination 'dry skin' and it appears validated when application of water temporarily improves its condition. In fact we really do not know whether the moisture content of the skin is any less in this situation than normal. We link the roughness and transient response to water with dryness because this accords with our sensory experience of inanimate materials. Interestingly, studies of the contour of aged skin shows that it becomes less pronounced in the elderly. The change in surface texture is probably related to physical changes in the stratum corneum. The individual horn cells of the stratum corneum – the corneocytes – enlarge with increasing age (Plewig, 1970). This is curious as the epidermal cells that form them actually appear to shrink in size. The epidermis decreases in thickness with age and its dermoepidermal junction flattens (Marks, 1981). This apparent paradox may be explained as due to a change in geometry of the epidermal cells but at the moment there is no evidence in favour of this suggestion. The changed surface area of corneocytes may reflect the altered cell kinetics of the epidermis in the elderly. Although there has been controversy the results overall suggest that there is a reduced rate of epidermal cell production as a result of the ageing process. Turnover studies of the stratum corneum using dansyl chloride or other fluorescent markers which become substantive to the stratum corneum and then fluoresce, certainly would suggest that there is a diminished 'throughput' of epidermal cells in aged individuals (Baker and Blair, 1968). The pigment-producing cells – the melanocytes – also decrease in size, in number, and in activity with age (Snell and Bischitz, 1963).

The adnexal structures also show marked ageing changes. The sweat glands work less efficiently and the secretory cells develop irregular granules of lipofuchsin whose significance is entirely unknown. There is diminished sweat production in the elderly and this is more marked in men.

The pilosebaceous apparatus shows quite marked alterations with increasing age. Scalp hair shows the most obvious changes. The hair density diminishes so that overall the hair on the scalp seems somewhat more sparse. This should be distinguished from male pattern loss (which is also sometimes seen in women) in which there is a specific pattern of bitemporal recession and loss of hair from the vertex. There is in addition a loss of pigment from the hair shaft. This is curiously variable in its time of appearance in that 'premature' greyness is not at all uncommon. The density of body hair and sexual hair also decreases in old age. The rate of sebum secretion also decreases, though sebaceous glands on the face may hypertrophy paradoxically. The hypertrophied glands then appear as orange or yellow dome-shaped nodules that are often mistaken for basal cell carcinoma.

The dermal connective tissue shares in the general process of attrition seen in the ageing process and seems to undergo alterations quite independent of those changes due to chronic damage from ultraviolet light. Elasticity decreases and in general the skin appears stiffer. Measurements using ultrasound and an X-ray technique show that the dermis becomes increasingly thin with age (Tan *et al.*, 1982). There appears to be a loss of glycosaminoglycan and probably decreasing water content as a consequence. The collagen itself becomes progressively crosslinked and insoluble and this change itself probably also accounts for some of the observed changes in the skin's appearance and properties.

THE PATTERN OF SKIN DISORDER IN THE ELDERLY

Virtually no skin disease is specific to the elderly though the incidence, presentation, and natural history of many disorders change in this age group. In addition the severity and symptomatology may differ in the elderly. The group of disorders that are lumped together as 'eczema' may be regarded as a particularly good example of the changed pattern of skin disease in the elderly. Atopic dermatitis is primarily a disorder of children and young adults, but may occasionally be seen in old age. When it does occur in later life there tends to be less in the way of excoriation and more lichenification with dusky pigmentation at the maximally affected sites. Some patterns of eczema are more frequently seen in the elderly – discoid and asteatotic eczemas for example. It must also be remembered that the skin is a much less efficient protective organ in old age and may respond with an eczematous reaction to comparatively trivial trauma.

Some blistering diseases such as pemphigus, although more common in the elderly, are also not infrequently seen in younger adults. Others, such as dermatitis herpetiformis, are spread throughout all age groups. Although the elderly tend, in general, to be less complaining than younger folk where skin disease is concerned they are often more incapacitated by it. They tolerate erythroderma, due to any cause, badly and may succumb to pneumonia, hypothermia, secondary infection, or cardiac decompensation if this occurs.

The incidence of benign and malignant neoplasms of the skin is markedly different in the elderly, some lesions such as solar keratoses, squamous cell, and basal cell carcinomata being strongly related to the cumulated dose of sunlight over the years. Other lesions such as Campbell de Morgan spots and seborrhoeic warts are of unknown cause but increase in frequency in older age groups.

MANAGEMENT OF SKIN DISORDERS IN THE ELDERLY

Certain points must be borne in mind when it comes to designing treatment schedules for the elderly. Because of diminished mobility it may be almost impossible for an elderly person to apply topical treatment to the feet or to the back. Skin disorders of the hands and feet may be even more disabling in old age than they are in other age groups. Firstly, the diminished elasticity of the stratum corneum will make fissures even more difficult to manage and will delay their healing. Secondly, the depressed potential for healing of the elderly may prolong the disorder, converting a comparatively trivial problem into a major disability. Because of the tendency of the elderly to have 'dry, itchy' skin disorders tend to be irritant in this age group and, whatever else is prescribed, attention should be given to ensuring adequate hydration by the prescription of emollients of one sort or another. Systemic treatments may also present difficulties for the aged. As there is often concomitant renal, hepatic, or gastrointestinal disease, drugs and dosages that would normally be appropriate may well be either dangerous or ineffective. In addition the difficulties that the elderly may experience in attending clinics and outpatients departments may make the usual monitoring of progress of common persistent skin disorders (e.g. psoriasis) quite impossible. Particular care must be exercised with systemic corticosteroids as the water-retaining and protein-losing effects of these compounds may seriously endanger the elderly.

Ichthyotic Disorders and Xeroderma in the Elderly

The group of disorders known collectively as the ichthyoses are characterized by persistent and generalized scaling unassociated with inflammatory change. The large majority of these are the result of an inherited disorder of keratinization and/or desquamation. Autosomal dominant ichthyosis (also known as ichthyosis vulgaris) is by far the commonest of these congenital dermatoses. Although very little is known concerning the metabolic basis of this disease there is more information about two phenotypically similar disorders. The first of these is X-linked recessive ichthyosis which is manifest only in males. There appears to be a deficiency of 'steroid sulphatase' in X-linked ichthyosis which may be directly responsible for the disorderly desquamation observed in this disease (Shapiro *et al.*, 1978; Williams and Elias, 1981). The second of these disorders is Refsum's syndrome, in which there is an abnormality of alpha hydroxylation of branchchain fatty acids. This leads to an accumulation of unusual branch-chained fatty acid containing lipids in all body tissues including the epidermis (Davies *et al.*, 1977). When these two disorders are considered with other evidence of disturbed lipid metabolism in other types of ichthyosis, it becomes plain that lipid metabolism plays an important role in epidermal differentiation. Furthermore, it appears that complex lipids, such as ceramides, are deposited within the intercorneocyte area and may have an important part to play in the barrier function of the stratum corneum. All ichthyotic disorders worsen in old age. The reason for this aggravation of these skin conditions with the passing of the years are complex and not understood in full. As mentioned previously, quite marked changes occur within the epidermis in old age and the whole process of epidermal differentiation alters. The corneocytes increase in surface area and volume and may become somewhat thinner (though there is no direct evidence for this latter point). For a given segment of stratum corneum this results in a decreased volume of intercorneocyte space as compared to a younger stratum corneum with smaller corneocytes. As the intercorneocyte space appears to be important with regard to the penetration of water (transepidermal water loss) and for the control of the orderly release of cells in the process of desquamation it should not be surprising that the skin of the elderly tends to 'dryness and scaliness' and that scaling disorders worsen.

Low temperature and low relative humidity tend to aggravate ichthyotic and other xerodermatous states. This causes considerable discomfort in the elderly in the winter time and is especially troublesome in the north-eastern United States where central heating and frequent bathing also serve to make the condition worse. So-called 'winter itch' and 'bath itch' are very common in such areas and can be difficult to relieve symptomatically.

When a dry scaly skin makes its appearance for the first time in an elderly subject and its onset is relatively sudden the event should be regarded as a danger signal. This so-called 'acquired ichthyosis' may be the marker of malignant disease. The most frequent type of malignant disease to be associated is a reticulosis.

Acquired ichthyosis is also seen in lepromatous leprosy undergoing reaction to treatment and the reason for its appearance in the course of this disease is as much a mystery as it is in Hodgkin's disease. Essential fatty acid deficiency may be seen after intestinal bypass operations and this can also result in a form of acquired ichthyosis. Similarly the condition has been described as a complication of the administration of drugs lowering serum lipids (MER29 and the butyrophenones). In these last two causes of acquired ichthyosis it seems likely that the disturbances of lipid metabolism produced may well be the basis for the disturbance of epidermal differentiation.

In most patients there is little one can do to tackle the underlying cause of the ichthyosis or xerodermatous condition and the aim of the treatment is the relief of symptoms. Emollient creams and lotions can give considerable relief.

Emollient soaps and bath oils may also help. The patient should also be instructed to employ humidifiers in their central heating system and not to scrub the skin or vigorously towel down after bathing or showering.

Acne

Acne is classically, but not exclusively, a disorder of adolescence. For example, it is not particularly uncommon to see quite young infants with acne lesions over the cheeks, chin, and forehead. Acne may also appear for the first time in the latter half of life, although it is unusual for this to happen. When it does occur in the elderly it can be quite extensive and cause much discomfort as the lesions tend to be larger and more numerous. Acne is essentially a disorder of hair follicles and sebum secretion, and as has already been mentioned the sebaceous glands sometimes become hypertrophied in old age. Whether this anomaly or other vagaries of sebaceous gland structure and/or function are involved when acne occurs in old age is unknown.

The formation of large comedones (blackheads) around the eyes in old age has already been described. Similar large and distorted hair follicles with comedone-like plugs occasionally occur over the back in the elderly.

Rosacea

Acne and rosacea are often confused – partially because of the older name for rosacea of 'acne rosacea'. Both disorders occur on the face and both show papules at some point in their history – but that is all they have in common.

Rosacea is a quite common disorder of the facial skin. Typically it occurs more frequently in the middle aged and elderly and seems to be slightly more common in women than in men. It is mostly a disorder of fair-skinned, caucasian types but is also seen in darker types from Southern Europe (Marks, 1976). It is uncommon in peoples from the Indian subcontinent and South East Asia and is distinctly rare in black African peoples.

Rosacea is characterized by facial erythema and telangiectasia affecting the cheeks, chin, nose, and forehead (Fig. 14). It spares the per-

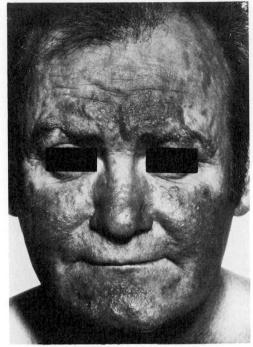

Figure 14   Typical rosacea with erythema and inflamed papules

ioral areas, the hairline, and the nasolabial grooves. Aside from the erythema and telangiectasia, inflammatory papules and pustules occur in crops. The nose may be affected, and in a small proportion (particularly men) shows the alteration known as rhinophyma (Fig. 15). In rhinophyma there is enormous sebaceous gland and dermal fibrovascular hypertrophy. Patients with the disorder complain of discomfort from frequent facial flushing and become quite depressed at the disfigurement caused by the disease.

Microscopically there are marked dermal changes in rosacea, with loss of connective tissue integrity, vascular dilatation, and oedema. If a papule is biopsied large numbers of inflammatory cells may be seen in addition to the connective tissue changes (Marks and Harcourt-Webster, 1969). The disorder is not a folliculitis as was originally believed and the inflammation is often granulomatous in that histiocytes predominate, and in approximately 10 per cent. of cases there are giant cell systems.

Although it is relatively easy to say what does not cause rosacea (Marks, 1968) it is

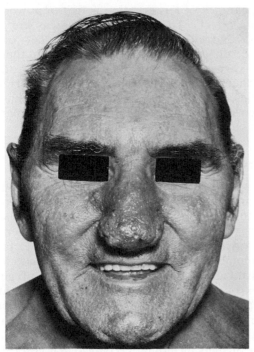

Figure 15　Rhinophyma (gross nasal swelling) and mild rosacea

much more difficult to determine what is the underlying sequence of changes. In addition the problem has become more complex with the realization that there may be an important involvement of immunological mechanisms (Manna, Marks, and Holt, 1982). However, it does appear that dermal connective tissue dystrophy in facial skin caused by environmental influences may be important in the pathogensis of the disease.

As far as treatment is concerned the inflammatory component (i.e. the papules and pustules) responds well to tetracyclines (Marks and Ellis, 1971) and metronidazole (Pye and Burton, 1976). No topical treatment is required.

THE SKIN AND MALIGNANT DISEASE

Squamous cell carcinoma and malignant melanoma have already been briefly discussed and will not be further described. In this section it is intended to cover two topics – skin manifestations of visceral malignancy and cutaneous lymphomas and sarcomas.

Skin Manifestations of Visceral Malignancy

Metastases from carcinoma of the bronchus, kidney, stomach, breast, and prostate not uncommonly present in the skin. The lesions are not easily diagnosed clinically and are often first recognized for what they are after histological examination. The most usual clinical presentation is that of a single or a group of steadily enlarging smooth pink or skin-coloured nodules on the head or trunk.

Acanthosis Nigricans

This is an uncommon skin disorder in which the skin of the flexures becomes thickened, warty, and pigmented. It has to be distinguished from pseudo-acanthosis nigricans which accompanies obesity and in which there may be some darkening and thickening of the axillary, groin, and neck skin. 'True' acanthosis nigricans is marked by other features in addition, including a curious velvety thickening of palmar skin, an increase in numbers and in the degree of pigmentation of seborrhoeic warts, a generalized increase in skin pigmentation, and a thickening of the buccal and lingual mucosae. The condition is particularly associated with adenocarcinoma of the gastrointestinal tract but has also been described as accompanying other types of malignant disease. It has also been described in association with congenital endocrine syndromes – particularly if involving the pituitary gland.

The cause of the link between acanthosis nigricans and malignancy is unknown, but it has been suggested that ectopic hormone production may be responsible. The condition remits if the underlying carcinoma is successfully treated.

Acquired Ichthyosis

When dry, flaky skin appears all over the body for the first time in middle age or in the elderly there is a strong possibility of underlying neoplastic disease. The condition cannot be distinguished from ordinary autosomal dominant ichthyosis although it tends to be more severe. It is also generally more severe than the common 'dry skin' seen in the elderly in winter time or in the course of any moderately severe systemic illness. It has often been described in association with Hodgkin's disease but can also occur with other types of malignant disease.

Necrolytic Migratory Erythema

This fascinating but rare disorder has been recognized only relatively recently as an external sign of a malignant tumour of the pancreatic alpha cells (Kahan, Perez-Figaredo, and Neimanis, 1977). Reddened, slightly raised eroded areas appear over the legs, trunk, and face which gradually extend. Histologically, there is a quite characteristic degenerative change in the upper epidermis. There is no information as to the reason for the association of this curious skin disorder with the rare pancreatic neoplasm. It does not appear to be the result of the increased levels of glucagon found in the syndrome or of the hyperglycaemic state. It may, however, be the result of persistently decreased blood levels of amino acids.

Figurate Erythemas

Under this term is included a number of erythematous rashes in which the raised, reddened areas are either annular or bizarrely polycyclic. One of these is a particularly good 'cutaneous clue' to visceral malignancy. This is the disorder known as erythema gyratum repens. The best description of the strange appearance of this eruption is that of a 'wood grain effect'. The erythematous areas are in loops and whorls which occur in parallel – one inside the other (Fig. 16). It appears that there is a very strong relationship between this odd erythema and carcinoma of the bronchus (Holt and Davies, 1977). Remissions in the rash have been described after removal of the primary tumour.

Dermatomyositis

This is one of the so-called connective tissue disorders, being related to both lupus erythematosus and scleroderma. As its name implies it has both a skin and a muscle component. Polymyositis is virtually the same disorder but without any skin involvement. The muscles involved are predominantly around the limb girdles but other groups can become affected. There is a patchy destructive inflammation in the involved muscles, resulting in weakness and tenderness. The skin demonstrates a variety of signs including the typical mauvish (heliotrope) periocular rash and a dusky erythematious eruption over the backs of the fingers and around the finger nails. Over the joints small necrotic areas appear, due to vascular occlusion. In severely affected patients deposits of calcium occur in the affected muscles and in areas of skin (calcinosis cutis).

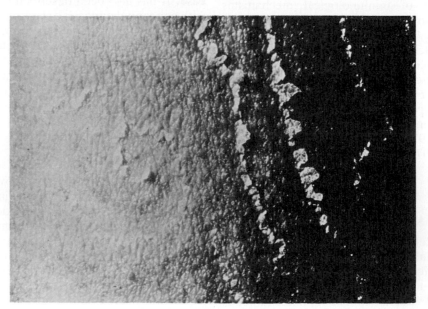

Figure 16   Erythema gyratum repens (note wood grain effect)

The relationship between dermatomyositis and malignancy is less certain than for some of the previously described skin syndromes. It has been suggested that the association is strong when the disorder occurs in postmenopausal women and that then malignancy of the genital tract is especially likely. However, recently some doubt has been cast over the validity of this assumption and the true relationship between dermatomyositis and visceral malignancy must remain *sub judice*.

Bullous Pemphigoid

This blistering disease of the elderly will be described later (page 888). There has also been considerable controversy over the relationship between this disorder and malignant disease (Ahmed, Chu, and Provost, 1977) and it may well be that the source of the disagreement stems from the fact that more than one disease is included under the same title. A good case has been made for the association in a small group of patients but it is difficult to identify these individuals by either clinical examination or laboratory investigation.

Cutaneous Lymphomas

These are common disorders which are not confined to the elderly. They have caused great confusion in the past because of the lack of adequate criteria for their diagnosis.

Mycosis Fungoides

This is an uncommon lymphoma of the T-cell series of lymphocytes which begins in the skin and remains confined to the skin till late in the disorder. Clinically the first signs consist of persistent oval or rounded red patches over the trunk and upper limbs. They may have a slightly scaly surface and are often misdiagnosed as eczema, psoriasis, or ringworm. The patches gradually become thicker and more numerous until they are large lumpy plaques. Later these may erode. The condition is slowly progressive and eventually the patient succumbs from either intercurrent infection or the visceral spread of the disease.

Histologically the characteristic sign is the presence of abnormal mononuclear cells. These are large with a large hyperchromatic nucleus. In the earlier stages of the disease the cells are sparse and may not be recognized in the sample removed. Later on the cells are present in larger numbers and are often seen within the epidermis in small clusters (so called Pautrier microabcesses).

A variety of treatments are available for this lymphoma but unfortunately none of them are curative although they may hold the disease in check for some time. In the early stages PUVA treatment (photochemotherapy with UVA; see Roenigk *et al.*, 1979) has proved extremely helpful for some patients. Later, when the patches are thicker, electron beam therapy has also proved useful. Conventional radiotherapy may also be used. Systemic chemotherapy has not been as successfully employed as in Hodgkin's disease or other lymphomata. However, considerable success has been reported from the use of topical nitrogen mustard.

The Sézary Syndrome

This rare condition is in reality a form of mycosis fungoides as it is believed that the same cell type is involved (Winkelmann, 1974). There is a severely pruritic erythroderma, loss of hair, and thickening of the skin of the face and hands. In the peripheral blood there are abnormal large mononuclear cells with a hyperchromatic convoluted nucleus and a high leukocytosis. The condition is sometimes regarded as a leukaemoid variant of mycosis fungoides.

Treatment with electron beam therapy and chemotherapy has been used but is not often strikingly successful.

Other Cutaneous Lymphomata

There are several other rare lymphomatous conditions affecting the skin, including a localized 'Pagetoid') type of mycosis fungoides and lymphosarcoma. Rarely, deposits of Hodgkin's disease cellular infiltrate may occur in the skin.

Kaposi's Idiopathic Haemorrhagic Sarcoma

This is a rare neoplastic disease of vascular tissue, though the exact cell of origin is uncertain. The disease has been rare in Europe but is more common in parts of Uganda and South Africa, where there are foci of high prevalence. In the past 2 or 3 years it has been described in a highly virulent almost 'epidemic' form among homosexual men, Haitians and recipients of blood transfusions in the United States as part of AIDS. In Europe it remains an unusual disorder which is predominantly seen in aged Jewish men from Russia or Poland and in elderly folk who come from the Po River basin in Italy. However, cases due to AIDS are now appearing on this side of the Atlantic. Clinically the condition usually presents with purplish nodules or plaques on the skin of the lower limbs but lesions may occur at any site. In the European form of the disease it is only slowly progressive but eventually causes death through metastasis.

BLISTERING DISEASES IN THE ELDERLY

The past two decades have seen major advances in the understanding of the blistering disorders. Although among the less common of skin diseases, the devastation that they can cause in the elderly makes their inclusion in this chapter a necessity. The more commonly occurring members of this group of disorders are set out in Table 1.

In addition to those diseases set out in the table there are several disorders which can blis-

Table 1 The major blistering diseases and their age incidence

Disease	Site of Defect	Age incidence
Pemphigus (all varieties)	Intraepidermal	Occurs throughout adult life but more past middle age
Epidermolysis bullosa (all varieties)	Subepidermal	Inherited disease, manifestations begin early
Pemphigoid	Subepidermal	Most common after age of 60
Dermatitis herpetiformis	Subepidermal	All ages may be affected, but not uncommonly first appears in the elderly
Erythema multiforme	Subepidermal	All ages, but can be very severe in the elderly
Herpes zoster	Intraepidermal	More common in the elderly

ter at some stage in their natural history. Acute eczema is one such disorder. Eczema is characterized by the appearance of vesicles due to focal oedema of the epidermis, when this process is exaggerated for one or other reason then blistering may occur. Porphyria cutanea tarda is characterized by skin fragility, hirsutes, skin thickening, and pigmentation on the light-exposed sites. In addition blisters may occur in these areas after a period of sun exposure.

Blistering may also be seen in drug eruptions. Nalidixic acid is a particular drug which may evoke a blistering reaction.

Insect bites and burns can also cause blistering and the latter should be remembered as a cause of localized blistering from 'hot water bottles' or falling asleep in front of the fire, in the elderly individual.

Blisters are also sometimes seen on the legs of grossly oedematous subjects – usually in the course of severe chronic congestive cardiac failure. This is almost entirely confined to the very old.

Pemphigus

This is a chronic blistering disease in which the underlying fault appears to be in the cohesion of the epidermal cells and which has an autoimmune basis. Conventionally the disease is classified according to the site of the epidermal split. The commonest variety is known as pemphigus vulgaris in which the split occurs just above the basal layer of epidermal cells (suprabasal split). Another variety of pemphigus (pemphigus vegetans) is also characterized by splitting above the basal layer but in this very rare type other changes occur within the epidermis as well. If the splitting occurs within the granular cell layer just below the stratum corneum the split is termed 'superficial' or subcorneal. Two varieties of pemphigus possess this type of abnormality. The more common is known as pemphigus foliaceous and a generalized form of this disorder occurs endemically in Brazil (Fogo selvagem). The other variety is termed pemphigus erythematodes and interestingly this has some features in common with lupus erythematosus.

Pathology

As stated above, the disorder is characterized

by the occurrence of splits within the epidermis. At the site of the split, epidermis seems to lose its ability to 'stick together'. Epidermal cells are seen to round up and lose their usual angular appearance – a process called acantholysis (Fig. 17). In superficial pemphigus the split may be so 'high up' in the epidermis that it may be missed and the ragged appearance of the upper epidermis thought to be artefactual.

Immunopathology of Pemphigus

Understanding of the nature of pemphigus has been transformed by the demonstration of circulating antibodies to intercellular areas of the epidermis in more than 90 per cent. of the patients (Chorzelski, Jablonska, and Beutner, 1973). These antibodies are of both IgG and IgM classes and an indirect immunofluorescence test is used to determine their presence diagnostically. They are reactive to the same epidermal site no matter which mammalian species is used to provide the skin as the substrate (indicator) tissue. Indeed monkey oesophagus or guinea pig lip are often used in practice as they are 'technically' convenient. Deposits of IgG and complement components (C3) can be found at the same intercellular site in the skin around the blistering lesions in the large majority of patients. A 'direct' immunofluorescence test is used to detect their presence and this test is also useful in providing confirmation of the diagnosis.

The circulating antibodies are not only of enormous help diagnostically, they also have a prognostic value. Their titre mirrors the severity and activity of the disease quite accurately. In addition a rise in the titre may presage a relapse.

The presence of circulating antibodies and their demonstration at the sites of the disease suggest their involvement in its pathogenesis. Early attempts at reproducing the disease in animals using injections or infusions of human serum containing the antibodies were unsuccessful. More recently the lesion has been induced in vitro in human skin (Schlitz and Michel, 1976) and now there seems little doubt that the antibodies are directly involved in the production of the lesions.

The nature of the antigen is much less certain. It seems to be some component of the glycocalyx of the epidermal cell and ultrastructural findings suggest that this may be part of the desmosomal apparatus.

Epidemiological Aspects

As far as is known, pemphigus occurs in all racial types. There is, however, a curious geographic and ethnic distribution. As mentioned above, one particular variety of superficial

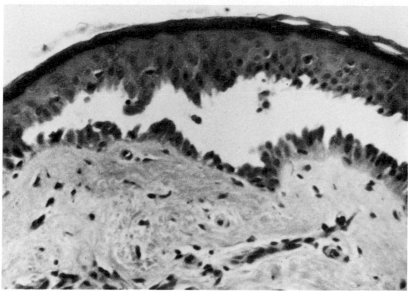

Figure 17 Biopsy from lesion of pemphigus vulgaris. Note suprabasal split (H.E. × 90)

pemphigus – Foga selvagem – is endemic in some parts of Brazil and it has been suggested that it could be due to an arthropod-borne virus. There is a preponderance of certain HLA haplotypes in sufferers from pemphigus – notably DW3 – and pemphigus vulgaris seems to occur more commonly in Jews than would be expected by chance. Also the disease is by no means uncommon in Asiatic peoples and in black Americans. The vagaries of distribution are difficult to explain with a unifying hypothesis and it may be that pemphigus is not one disease but many. In this context it is worth noting that the drug penicillamine can produce a blistering disease that is clinically and histologically virtually identical with spontaneously occurring pemphigus (Marsden *et al.*, 1976).

Clinical Aspects

In about half the patients with pemphigus vulgaris the disease starts in the oral mucosa, and many patients present at the dentists (Chapter 11.1). Other mucosae may be affected including the laryngeal and vaginal. On the skin the disorder usually begins insidiously but there are some patients in whom there is a dramatically sudden onset. Actual blisters are uncommon. Erosions are much more frequently observed (Fig. 18). They may occur anywhere on the skin surface but are more common in the flexural areas initially. Before adequate treatment was available the number and size of the eroded areas gradually increased and the affected individual became increasingly toxic and almost inevitably died (Lever, 1965). The generalized nature of the disturbance is evident from the so-called Nikolwski sign which, although not specific to pemphigus, is quite characteristic of it. If pressure is put on the skin of an affected individual and a shearing stress applied, the skin surface seems to move over the lower parts and a flaccid blister is produced.

The various forms of superficial pemphigus although unpleasant are not quite such vicious diseases. In pemphigus foliaceous moist scaling areas of erythema appear on the upper trunk and in the flexures. Uncommonly very large areas of skin are involved and the patient then becomes as ill as with pemphigus vulgaris. Pemphigus erythematodes is rare, and has clinical and immunopathological features in common with discoid lupus erythematosus. It is a genuine 'overlap' syndrome in that it really does possess features of both diseases.

The successful treatment of pemphigus requires experience. Several options are available. Probably the most frequently employed uses high doses of corticosteroids systemically. Prednisone is given in high enough dose to completely suppress the disease and this may require as much as 150 mg of Prednisone per day. The dose is gradually reduced after the disease has been brought under control. An-

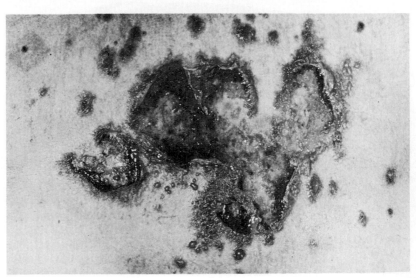

Figure 18   Erosions due to pemphigus vulgaris

other approach to treatment ulilizes immuno-suppressive agents – either methotrexate or azathioprine (Lever, and Schaumberg-Lever, 1977). These drugs take some time to act and it has become usual to start them at the same time as the steroids then reduce the latter after some weeks till only the immunosuppressive is keeping the disease in check.

Gold therapy (as for rheumatoid arthritis) has also been used (Pennys, Eaglestein, and Frost, 1976).

Pemphigus is a most unpleasant disorder and requires sympathy, skill, and experience for a successful outcome. Care must be taken to ensure that the patient does not suffer as much from the treatment as from the disease.

Bullous Pemphigoid

Bullous pemphigoid is predominantly a disease of the elderly and is rarely seen before the age of 55. In the United Kingdom it is more frequently seen than pemphigus, but is nonetheless quite uncommon.

Pathology and Immunopathology

Blisters form beneath the epidermis and it may be difficult to distinguish histologically from other subepidermal blistering diseases including dermatitis herpetiformis, erythema multiforme, and porphyria cutanea tarda. There is usually a prominent upper dermal inflammatory cell infiltrate consisting predominantly of neutrophils and eosinophils.

Immunofluorescent examination of perilesional skin reveals deposits of IgG and the C3 complement component in more than 80 per cent. of patients. In addition there are circulating antibodies in the blood directed against the basement membrane region of the epidermis. Current evidence suggests that these have a pathogenetic role in the disease (Jordon and Provost, 1981).

Clinical Features

Bullous pemphigoid differs from pemphigus in that in most instances it begins quite abruptly. Large tense blisters form anywhere on the skin surface over a day or two. In the mildly affected patients only a few blisters occur, but when the disorder is more severe many large, blood-filled blisters make their appearance.

Although patients with bullous pemphigoid may be unwell and have considerable discomfort from their skin lesions, there is not the same severe systemic disturbance as in pemphigus. The buccal mucosa is much less frequently involved than in pemphigus. Whereas pemphigus goes into remission only after several years, pemphigoid is much more an intermittent problem with two or three episodes spaced over a year or two.

Treatment for pemphigoid is similar in many respects to that for pemphigus, the major difference being that the dose of steroids required to control the appearance of new lesions is usually much less than in pemphigus.

Dermatitis Herpetiformis

Dermatitis herpetiformis (DH) is a chronic remittent vesicular disorder which unlike the previous two blistering diseases is markedly itchy. The age of onset is very variable, but it is certainly not particularly uncommon in old age and there seem to be a group of elderly folk in whom the disease first makes its appearance after the age of 60.

Pathology and Immunopathology

The vesicles form subepidermally as in pemphigoid, but unlike the latter disease there is a characteristic 'prebullous' lesion in which there is accumulation of inflammatory cells, especially neutrophils, at the tips of the dermal papillae (papillary microabcess; Fig. 19). In the upper dermis there is a perivascular lymphocytic infiltrate and fragments of neutrophils.

There are no circulating antibodies to components of skin although there are antibodies to reticulin in approximately 15 per cent. of patients (Fry, 1981). Direct immunofluorescent examination of uninvolved skin reveals deposits of IgA at the papillary tips in about 80 per cent. of patients and a continuous band of IgG in about 20 per cent. (Fry, 1981).

Clinical Aspects

Small vesicles and erythematous urticarial lesions appear over the extensor surfaces of the

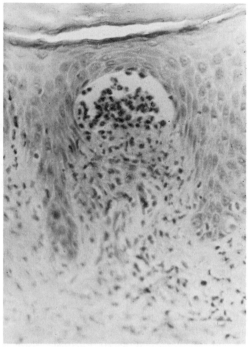

Figure 19 Biopsy from lesion of dermatitis her-petiformis. Note neutrophils in papillary tip abcess (H.E. × 90)

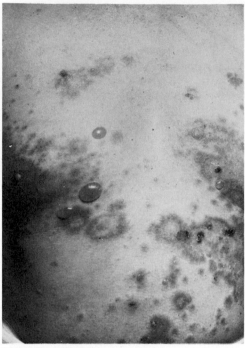

Figure 20 Vesicular and erythematous lesions due to dermatitis herpetiformis

body including the knees, elbows, buttocks, scalp, and shoulders (Fig. 20). As mentioned previously the disorder is intensely itchy.

Interestingly, some two-thirds of patients also appear to suffer from gluten enteropathy of a mild type and abnormal tests of absorption from the gut are not uncommon (Marks *et al.*, 1968). The reason for this association is unclear but it should be noted that patients with DH also have a higher incidence of autoimmune diseases including thyroid disease, pernicious anaemia, and systemic lupus erythematosus.

Dapsone (diamino diphenyl sulphone) and certain other sulphonamide-type drugs have a dramatic suppressive effect on the symptoms and signs of the disease. Most patients respond to 100 mg of dapsone per day or less, but some require as much as 250 or even 300 mg per day. The disease begins to abate after some 12 to 24 hours after treatment and usually relapses some 24 to 48 hours after stopping the drug. A more lasting effect appears to come from a gluten-free diet (Fry *et al.*, 1973), although it may be necessary to continue treatment for more than a year before a therapeutic effect is seen.

INFECTIONS OF THE SKIN AND INFESTATIONS IN THE ELDERLY

Evidence suggests that the immune system functions less well with advancing years. Despite this there does not seem to be an increased prevalence of the common skin infections in the elderly. It seems that the reverse may be the case as far as boils, viral warts, mollusca contagiosa, herpes simplex, and ringworm infections are concerned. It is true, however, that some infections are more devastating when they do occur in older age groups. Cellulitis of the legs and erysipelas are examples of bacterial infection of the skin which can cause severe illness in older people. The latter disorder in particular is noteworthy for its severity. Erysipelas produces severe toxaemia and can also produce severe necrosis of the skin at the site of infection.

Herpes Zoster

Herpes zoster (or shingles) is more common in the elderly. It is a reactivation of varicella (chicken pox), the virus having lain dormant in the dorsal root ganglia until some local or general event triggers it to migrate along the nerve roots and sensory nerves to the skin. The disorder produced is essentially local chicken pox in the area of skin supplied by the affected sensory nerves. There is usually fever and considerable systemic disturbance. The affected skin is at first swollen, red, and tender, with small papulovesicles. The individual spots become in succession frankly vesicular, pustular necrotic, and then crusted (Fig. 21). Often the lesions coalesce to produce quite large areas of necrosis.

Herpes zoster is a painful disease. It is not unusual for the zone affected to feel 'sensitive' and be painful for several days before the illness appears. The pain and discomfort may be intense during the attack. Unfortunately pain and paraesthesia can persist for some considerable time after the rash has subsided, and this can cause great disability.

The disease is especially unpleasant when the ophthalmic branch of the fifth nerve is affected as not only are the forehead and eyelids involved but the conjunctiva is also inflamed. There is photophobia at first but later the eye becomes closed because of swelling of the eyelids.

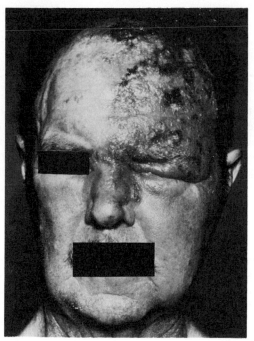

Figure 21   Ophthalmis herpes zoster (shingles)

Patients with zoster should be admitted to hospital unless the attack is a mild one and there is little systemic disturbance. When large areas of skin are involved, skilled and sympathetic nursing is required. It is usual to give analgesics to relieve the pain but it should be remembered that if strong opiate type drugs are administered there is a real danger of addiction. It has also become customary to prescribe an antibiotic to 'prevent secondary infection'. The vesicular, necrotic and inflamed areas certainly look as though they are infected by bacteria but generally they are not, and antibiotics are prescribed more for the doctor's 'comfort' than the patient's wellbeing.

Systemic steroids are favoured by some physicians to prevent post herpatic neuralgia (Eaglestein *et al.*, 1970). Even doses as high as 60 mg of prednisone per day do not seem at aggravate the condition or delay healing as may be expected.

In recent years various antiviral drugs have been submitted to clinical trial and some have appeared to shorten the disease. Topically applied idoxuridine has its supporters but the evidence in its favour is slim. Acyclovir, which has some activity against varicella zoster virus (Collins 1983), has recently become available. An intravenous infusion of acyclovir relieves acute pain and halts the progression of herpes zoster in the elderly and in immunosuppressed patients, but it does not prevent post-herpetic neuralgia (Bean *et al.*, 1982, Peterslund *et al.*, 1981). Evidence of the usefulness of acyclovir in its new oral form is still awaited.

Treatment

See Chapter 16.5.

Infestations

Scabies and louse infestations are by no means uncommon in elderly subjects. Scabies can be difficult to identify if it is not remembered that despite the waning of the epidemic in the late 1960s and early 1970s it is still a common disease. A few tell-tale papules over the elbows, knees, buttocks, or on the genitalia in someone with severe itchiness should heighten one's suspicion and stimulate an intensive look for the scabies burrows on the palms, sides of fingers, soles, and wrists. It can run riot round institutions for the aged as it spreads quite easily by skin-to-skin contact, which although often venereal is by no means always of this type. To be effective, treatment with benzyl benzoate or gammexane applications should be carried out exactly according to the instructions with at least two 'all over' paintings separated by a 24-hour period.

Lice are now much more common than we like to think. The head louse is more prevalent in younger age groups (presumably because of their more prolific hair!). Pubic lice are more frequent in sexually active age groups as they are contracted by venereal contact. Body lice are the least common of this unpleasant parasitic triad and are mainly found in vagrants. It is important to note that lice in the United Kingdom are now resistant to DDT and gammexane and should be treated with malathion or similar compound. The clothes must be 'deloused' when there is infestation by the body louse.

CHRONIC ULCERATION OF THE SKIN

Wound healing processes are depressed in old age and lesions that would heal in younger age groups can persist to form chronically ulcerated areas. Because of their importance gravitational and ischaemic ulcerations and decubitus ulcers will be discussed here, but it should be remembered that there are a wide variety of other causes (Table 2).

Gravitational ulceration

Gravitational ulcers (see Chapter 13.1) occur in the course of the persistent nutritional disturbance of the soft tissues of the lower legs due to venous incompetence and hypertension. The condition is sometimes known as the 'Gravitational syndrome'. The veins of the deep venous system become incompetent (often after venous thrombosis) and communicate the resulting increase in hydrostatic pressure to the superficial veins via the communicating veins. This results in tissue oedema and in perivascular deposits of fibrin (Browse *et al.*, 1977). The hypoxaemia caused by this sequence results in fibrosis and in some situations actual necrosis.

Ulceration of the skin commonly occurs around the medial malleolus and is a relatively

Table 2 Causes of chronic ulceration and their characteristics

Diagnosis	Site involved	Particular features
Gravitational	Around ankle	Odema, pigmentation of surrounding skin, sloughy base
Ischaemic	Anywhere on lower leg or foot	Painful, pallor and atrophy of surrounding skin
Decubitus	Over pressure areas	Deeply penetrating
Neurotropic	Over pressure areas on feet	Deeply penetrating
Diabetic	Over toes particularly	Tend to be sloughy
Haemoglobinopathy	Lower leg	Other signs of the disorder
Syphilitic gumma	Anywhere on skin	Classically 'punched out' appearance
Tuberculous	Anywhere on skin	Surrounding skin has mauve-blue appearance
Squamous cell carcinoma	Anywhere	Ulcer edges are raised and rolled
Pyoderma gangrenosum	Anywhere	May be enormous and rapidly developing
Rheumatoid arthritis	Anywhere, but legs commonly	May be purpuric lesions accompanying

late phenomenon in the sequence of events. Before this happens there is usually oedema of the foot and lower leg and aching discomfort in the affected part. In addition to these early signs, pigmentation of the skin (mostly due to deposits of haemosiderin) and tethering of the skin to the underlying deeper tissues with stiffening are usually present for some time prior to ulceration.

Eczematous change in the skin occurs in some patients. This is sometimes due to the disorder itself and sometimes the result of allergic contact hypersensitivity to topical applications used in treatment. Such substances as neomycin and lanolin often cause this type of contact dermatitis.

Superficial varicosities give little information

concerning the pressure in the deep venous system but they are often present as is a 'venous flare' or network of superficial varicosities at the sides of the foot.

The Gravitational ulcer itself is usually surprisingly painless though may cause discomfort. The base is usually sloughy and the edges tend to be ragged and suffused (Fig. 22). In fact the appearance of the ulcerated lesions is very variable, being dependent on the length of history, the presence of infection, and the success or otherwise of attempts at healing. In some patients there is more than one ulcer and indeed the ulcerated area may encircle the leg.

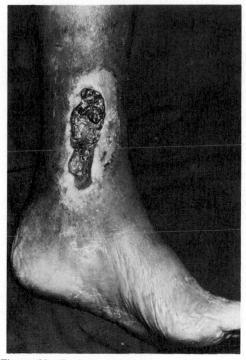

Figure 22 Typical stasis ulcer and other stasis changes

Gravitational ulcers may persist for many years. It is not uncommon for patients to tell you that their ulcer has been present off and on for more than 20 years. Treatment in general is unsatisfactory as even if the ulcer does heal the underlying vascular problem remains, predisposing to further ulceration. Most ulcers can be induced to heal by a combination of bed-rest, leg elevation, adequate support by bandaging, and loss of weight. Some believe that support is of particular importance and use either elasticated stockings or elasticated bandages to supply support to the venous system.

The ulcer itself needs little else other than protection. However, when there is infection present (as there often is) appropriate treatment should be given to prevent further tissue damage. When the infection is mild (as with most patients) little else need be done other than to apply mildly antibacterial washes and/ or lotions. Povidine iodine preparations are quite suitable and may be better than dilute hypochlorite or potassium permanganate solutions. When there is erythema and tenderness of the surrounding skin then systemic antibiotics should be prescribed after taking a bacterial swab to determine the sensitivities of the infecting microorganism. Topical antibiotics should not be used as they are not very efficient in this clinical situation and can sensitize the surrounding skin. If left untreated infected ulcers can cause severe cellulitis with systemic upset and even septicaemia.

It is often helpful to remove pus, crust, and clot by bathing with sterile saline or by use of either streptokinase/streptodornase solution or dextran monomer beads.

A more recent approach to the treatment of the Gravitational syndrome is with fibrinolytic agents such as the anabolic agent Stanozolol. It is expected that these agents will hasten the removal of the perivascular fibrin deposits, allowing more efficient tissue perfusion. Early reports of the use of these drugs suggest that this type of treatment in combination with elasticated support to the affected legs may assist resolution.

Decubitus Ulcers

See Chapter 20.2.

Ischaemic ulcers

Areas of skin necrosis appear at the periphery of regions to which the arterial supply has been compromised. The commonest cause of the underlying arterial disorder is atherosclerosis and the most frequently affected sites are the toes, heels, dorsa of feet, and around the ankles. The surrounding skin is pale, cool, and atrophic with loss of hair and skin markings. The ulcers themselves tend to form and to worsen in cold weather and, unless treatment is instituted, progress till the part involved is irretrievably gangrenous and lost.

Treatment must be directed at improving the arterial perfusion of the affected part and the only certain way of doing this is by surgical removal or bypass of an obstruction. Unfortunately the currently available drugs have little effect on the nutritional blood supply to the skin, but it is hoped that newer prostanoid derivatives and agents influencing tissue levels of prostacycline will have a more substantial effect.

REFERENCES

Ahmed, A. R., Chu, T. M., and Provost, T. T. (1977). 'Bullous pemphigoid: Clinical and serological evaluation for associated malignancy', *Arch. Dermatol.*, **113**, 969.

Baker, H., and Blair, C. P. (1968). 'Cell replacement in the human stratum corneum in old age', *Br. J. Dermatol.*, **80**, 367–372.

Bean, C., Braun, C., Balfour H. H. (1982) 'Acyclovir therapy for acute herpes zoster', *Lancet* **2**, 118–121.

Browse, N. L., Jarrett, P. E. M., Morland, M., and Burnand, K. (1977). 'Treatment of liposclerosis of the leg by fibrinolytic enhancement: A preliminary report', *Br. Med. J.*, **2**, 434–435.

Chorzelski, T. P., Jablonska, S., and Beutner, E. H. (1973). 'Clinical significance of pemphigus antibodies', in *Immunopathology of the Skin* (Eds E. H. Beutner, T. P. Chorzelski, S. F. Bean, and R. E. Jordon), Chap. 2, pp. 25–45, Dowden Hutchinson and Ross, Stroudsburg, Pennsylvania.

Collins P. (1983) 'The spectrum of antiviral activities of acyclovir in vitro and in vivo'. *Antimicrob. Chemother.* **12**, Suppl. B, 19–27.

Costanza, M. E., Dayal, Y., Binder, S., and Nathanson, L. (1974). 'Metastatic basal cell carcinoma'. *Cancer*, **34**, 230–235.

Davies, M. G., Marks, R., Dykes, P. J., and Reynolds, D. (1977). 'Epidermal abnormalities in Refsum's disease', *Br. J. Dermatol.*, **97**, 401–406.

Eaglestein, W. H., Katz, R., and Brown, J. A. (1970). 'The effects of early corticosteroid therapy on the skin eruption and pain of herpes zoster', *JAMA*, **211**, 1681–1683.

Fry, L. (1981). 'Immunopathology of dermatitis herpetiformis', in *The Epidermis in Disease*, (Eds R. Marks and E. Christophers), Chap. 40, pp.561–571, MTP Press, Lancaster.

Fry, L., Seah, P. P., Riches, D. J., *et al.* (1973). 'Clearance of skin lesions in dermatitis herpetiformis after gluten withdrawal', *Lancet*, **1**, 288–291.

Holt, P. J. A., and Davies, M. G. (1977). 'Erythema gyratum repens', *Br. J. Dermatol.*, **96**, 343–347.

Jordon, R. E., and Provost, T. T. (1981). 'Vesiculo bullous skin diseases', in *Comprehensive Immunology*: 7. *Immuno Dermatology* (Eds R. A. Good and S. B. Day), pp. 361–376, Plenum Medical Book Co., New York and London.

Kahan, R. S., Perez-Figaredo, R. A., and Neimanis, A. (1977). 'Necrolytic migratory erythema', *Arch. Dermatol.*, **113**, 792–797.

Lever, W. F. (1965). *Pemphigus and Pemphigoid*, C. C. Thomas, Springfield, Illinois.

Lever, W. F., and Schaumberg-Lever, G. (1977). 'Immunosuppresants and Prednisone in pemphigus vulgaris; Therapeutic results in 63 patients 1961–75', *Arch. Dermatol.*, **113**, 1236–1241.

Manna, V., Marks, R., and Holt, P. J. A. (1982). 'Involvement of immune mechanisms in the pathogenesis of rosacea', *Br. J. Dermatol.*, **107**, 203–208.

Marks, R. (1968). 'Concepts in the pathogenesis of rosacea', *Br. J. Dermatol.*, **80**, 170–177.

Marks, R. (1976). *Common Facial Dermatoses*, John Wright and Sons Ltd, Bristol.

Marks, R. (1981). 'Measurement of biological ageing in human epidermis', *Br. J. Dermatol.*, **104**, 627–633.

Marks, R., and Ellis, J. (1971). 'Comparative effectiveness of tetracycline and ampicillin in rosacea', *Lancet*, **2**, 1049–1052.

Marks, R., and Harcourt-Webster, J. N. (1969). 'Histopathology of rosacea', *Arch. Dermatol.*, **100**, 683–691.

Marks, R., Whittle, M. W., Beard, R. J., Robertson, W. B., and Gold, S. C. (1968). 'Small bowel abnormalities in dermatitis herpetiformis', *Br. Med. J.*, **1**, 552–555.

Marsden, R. A., Ryan, T. J., Vanhegan, R. I., Walshe, M., Hill, H., and Mowat, A. G. (1976). 'Pemphigus foliaceous induced by penicillamine', *Br. Med. J.*, **2**, 1423–1424.

Moriarty, M., Dunn, J., Darragh, A., Lambe, R., and Brick, I. (1982). 'Etretinate in treatment of actinic keratosis', *Lancet*, **1**, 364–365.

Pearse, A. D., and Marks, R. (1977). 'Epidermal proliferation in actinic keratoses and in the epidermis on which they arise', *Br. J. Dermatol.*, **96**, 45–50.

Pennys, N. S., Eaglestein, W. H., and Frost, P. (1976). 'Management of pemphigus with gold compounds', *Arch. Dermatol.*, **112**, 185–187.

Peterslund, N. A., Seiger-Hansen, K., Ipsen, J., Esmann, V., Schonheyder, H., Juhl, H. (1981) 'Acyclovir in herpes zoster', *Lancet* **2**, 827–830.

Plewig, G. (1970). 'Regional differences in cell sizes in the human stratum corneum', *J. Invest. Dermatol.*, **54**, 19–23.

Pye, R. J., and Burton, J. L. (1976). 'Treatment of rosacea by metronidazole', *Lancet*, **1**, 1211–1212.

Roenigk, H. H. Jr., and 16 others (1979). 'Photochemotherapy for psoriasis: A clinical co-operative study of PUVA-48 and PUVA-64', *Arch. Dermatol.*, **115**, 576–579.

Schlitz, J. R., and Michel, B. (1976). 'Production of epidermal acantholysis in normal skin in vitro by the IgG fraction from pemphigus serum', *J. Invest. Dermatol.*, **67**, 254–260.

Shahrad, P., and Marks, R. (1977). 'The wages of warmth: Changes in erythema ab igne', *Br. J. Dermatol.*, **97**, 179–186.

Shapiro, L. J., Weiss, R., Webster, D., and France, J. T. (1978). 'X-linked ichthyosis due to steroid sulphatase deficiency'. *Lancet*, **1**, 70–72.

Snell, R. S., and Bischitz, P. G. (1963). 'The melanocytes and melanin in human abdominal wall skin: A survey made at different ages in both sexes and during pregnancy', *J. Anat. (London)*, **97**, 361–376.

Tan, C. Y., Statham, B., Marks, R., and Payne, P. A. (1982). 'Skin thickness measurement by pulsed ultrasound: Its reproducibility, validation and variability', *Br. J. Dermatol.*, **106**, 657–667.

Wijn, P. F. F., Brakkee, A. J. M., Kuiper, J. P., and Vendrik, A. J. H. (1979). 'The alinear viscoelastic properties of human skin in vivo related to sex and age', in *Bioengineering and the Skin* (Eds R. Marks and P. A. Payne), pp. 135–145, MTP Press, Lancaster.

Williams, M. L., and Elias, P. M. (1981). 'Stratum corneum lipids in disorders of cornification', *J. Clin. Invest.*, **68**, 1404–1410.

Winkelmann, R. K. (1974) 'Symposium on the Sézary cell', *Mayo Clin. Proc.*, **49**, 515–525.

Principles and Practice of Geriatric Medicine
Edited by M. S. J. Pathy
© 1985 John Wiley & Sons Ltd

20.2

Pressure Sores

J. N. Agate

Where ill old patients are nursed there is always a risk of pressure sores. These often painful, often dangerous, complications of many diseases are aptly called 'pressure' sores (ulcers) or bedsores because these indicate the principal cause. The description 'decubitus ulcers' adds nothing to an understanding of these misfortunes, for they are not always contracted while in the lying position. That pressure sores are uncommon in good geriatric wards indicates that staff are aware of the hazards and the causal factors, accept that constant watchfulness and discipline are needed to avoid them, and take pride in their avoidance—and so do most people who nurse older invalids at home. Pressure sores cause pain, unnecessary prolongation of a patient's hospital stay, and even risk to life in the worst cases, yet they are largely preventable. They are not acceptable anywhere, least of all in a hospital. Their management is not just a nursing responsibility though it absorbs much nursing time. Doctors have a duty to understand the causation, to modify their own policies accordingly, to be as watchful as nurses, and to advise the latter positively.

PATHOLOGY

Pressure higher than normal capillary pressure exerted for a sufficient time causes oedema, local thrombosis in small vessels and the microcirculation, and damages vascular endothelium. Just beyond the site of greatest pressure there is also occlusion of vessels by platelets and a further area of risk to tissue (Barton, 1973). Tissue death then results in an open ulcer of epidermal depth, full skin thickness depth, or worse. Pressure persisting over a region where thick muscle, fat, or fascia underlies the skin may lead to a huge 'blind' aseptic mass of necrosis which bursts through the skin, sometimes without apparent warning, leaving a hideous cavity with undermined edges, often several inches across. Experimental work on animals by Husain (1953) showed how ischaemic necrosis occurs in muscles by tissue compression over bony prominences. This was confirmed in human subjects by Pathy (1960), who observed that muscle necrosis may occur at the stage when only skin erythema is visible—hence the subsequent appearance of the aseptic necrotic matter. Once this has burst forth, sepsis penetrating to deeper levels is to be expected. Thermographic studies may indicate in advance where this future tissue destruction is likely to occur, but these are scarcely practicable as routine observations.

CAUSATION

A minority of 'pressure' sores are brought about by repeated rubbing of vulnerable prominences across the sheets by patients who are restless. They might better be called friction burns, but they present similar problems to true pressure sores. The inexpert moving of patients about the bed by failing first to lift them clear, may cause severe shearing stresses and tearing of skin. A heavy patient sitting up

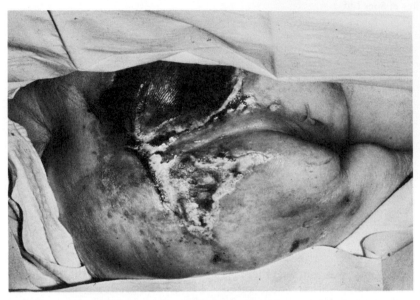

Figure 1

with a back-rest may, in sliding, subject the buttocks to the same shearing stresses. The coefficient of friction is increased when the sheets are wet because of incontinence.

A skin tear or minimal break in any area subject to pressure, maceration of the skin, even repeated incontinence resulting in a patch of erythema or 'urine rash', will predispose to a sore. Incontinence multiplies the risk five-fold. Nevertheless, the prime causal factor is pressure when a major part of the body weight is transmitted between a bony prominence and a relatively hard surface below, compressing the skin and adjacent soft tissues. The most vulnerable points are the sacrum, the heels and dorsal convexity, even the scapular spines in a supine patient, the greater trochanter, knees, iliac crest, and the shoulders in patients in a lateral position. The bed-fast state puts these pressure points at risk, but equally the unrelieved sitting position lays the area under the ischial tuberosities open to hazard. In very frail patients all areas in contact with the sheets may be vulnerable, and so may be the medial aspects of the knees, particularly if there is adductor muscle spasm. Constant vigilance coupled with the drill of turning the patient as often as may be necessary to avoid prolonged pressure is the key to both prevention and cure.

Husain (1953) showed that low pressure for long periods is more damaging than high pressure for short periods. The normal mean capillary pressure is some 20 to 30 mmHg; if all the body area of an average man was available to transmit the weight, the pressure would be about 17 mmHg (Siegal, Vistnes, and Laut, 1973). In some circumstances much higher pressures build up. Thus, lying on a linoleum-covered floor the pressure on sacral skin may exceed 240 mmHg, and the same is true on operating tables (Redfern *et al.*, 1973). At this level of local pressure even quite a short operation could have caused an inescapable pressure sore before the patient regains the ward, while on a standard interior sprung mattress the range of pressures at various prominent points may be from 21 to 71 mmHg, and with a fracture board in addition it reaches 164 mmHg.

Whenever the pressures build up the involuntary reaction of a healthy person while sitting or even while asleep is to fidget and shift position at intervals. Ill people, especially old people, may be immobile, in stupor or coma, under the influence of sedatives, too much in pain to tolerate movement, too muddled or demented to decipher what is amiss, or are otherwise unable to respond appropriately to the warning signals coming from skin under pressure. Others, like paraplegics with sensory loss, may never receive the sensory stimuli centrally and are always gravely at risk from pressure. It is characteristic of many old people to be thus at a multiple disadvantage in the first phases of their illnesses, when the incidence of pressure effects is greatest. The classical experiments of Exton-Smith and Sherwin (1961), with recording apparatus mounted under beds, demonstrated how closely the paucity of old people's movements in bed correlated with their vulnerability to pressure sores. Exton-Smith, Norton, and McLaren, (1962) evolved a simple clinical risk score based on the patient's mental status, degree of activity and mobility, continence and general condition, to predict likely development of pressure sores. This scoring system emphasizes to doctors and nurses the immediate vulnerability of patients, and can be profitably used to improve practices where the pressure sore incidence is unacceptably high.

Nutritional factors, lowered blood pressure (an observation often missed), oedema of tissues, damage to tissues by injections, etc., peripheral vascular insufficiency (often putting the extremeties at extreme risk), and anaemia may contribute significantly to pressure sore development. Nutritional factors include general malnutrition, iron deficiency, perhaps zinc deficiency, for zinc promotes the healing of indolent ulcers (Pories *et al.*, 1967), and ascorbic acid deficiency, which may have reached a clin-

ically recognizable level in some deprived old people. Ascorbic acid stores are known to be sharply lowered following surgical operations in old people (Schwartz, 1970). Hypoproteinaemia delays the healing of pressure sores. Sudden protein deficiency can be caused by active restriction of protein intake in treating renal failure in old people; the massive and suddenly occurring pressure sores (Fig. 1) which result have convinced the author that this is not an acceptable line of treatment for old people, even in established uraemia.

TYPES OF PRESSURE SORES

After the appearance of small skin abrasions, with or without signs of a urine rash, one can expect excoriation and the loss of the epidermis, some bleeding, and exposure of the dermal layers and thus of the sensory nerve endings (Fig. 2). Such a superficial and relatively benign ulcer would be painful and may extend over many square centimetres. Healing should be rapid, nevertheless, if nutrition is adequate, sepsis is prevented, and pressure relieved. A much more severe type of ulcer is that where the full skin thickness is destroyed; a further stage is loss of all the subcutaneous tissues, perhaps down to the bone, in the massive, deep, cavitated ulcer described above. Sometimes the dead tissue persists as a hard

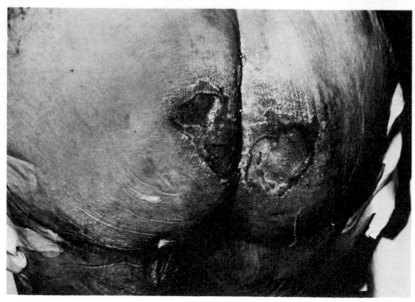

Figure 2

dry black infarcted eschar, which must be removed. Large ulcers of this size, up to 25 cm across and several centimetres deep in the worst cases, are a threat to life, constitute a major open wound which is liable to infection and to cause fluid and serum loss, and is only capable of healing slowly by granulation and with late scarring. Huge infarcted sores can arise with astonishing speed, even overnight, in some circumstances like sudden thrombosis of the inferior vena cava. The rim of a forgotten bedpan caused a massive circular black sore within 12 hours in a stuporose, aged patient.

INCIDENCE

Though brief illnesses barely allow time for pressure sores to develop, one-third of sores develop in the first week of old people's bedfastness, and two-thirds appear within the first two weeks (Exton-Smith, Norton, and McLaren, 1962). A later onset of sores suggests the onset of a fresh disorder, such as hypotension after a 'silent' cardiac infarction. Once it has appeared a deep ulcer may persist for many weeks, threatening life, and the general prognosis of recovery will be related to the speed of appearance, size, and depth of such a pressure sore. Exceptionally in a gravely ill old person skin sores develop at any point of contact with anything.

PREVENTION

General Measures

Common factors in the causation (see above) being acknowledged, the first essential is to identify which patients are at greatest risk and give them special attention. Often it is best to group them together so that a skilled nursing cadre can concentrate on preventative routines at frequent intervals. Treatment of acute illness and management of anaemia, malnutrition, hypotension, and any state leading to immobility must be urgently arranged. Any proposal to use total bed-rest can be questioned, though occasionally it cannot be avoided. Erythema over a pressure area is the danger signal.

The essence of prevention is repeated relief of pressure by regular skilled lifting, turning, and shifting. Where the patient can help in doing this, he must be instructed how to do so, but many seriously ill elderly patients simply cannot unless assisted; the most ill have to be passively lifted and turned. The best intervals for this turning depend on the accumulation of risk factors and must not be haphazard or based on arbitrary routine. It might have to be ordered four-hourly for a 'low risk' patient, but as often as half-hourly in an extremely high risk situation. Turning is from side to side, side to back, back to side, entirely depending on skin areas at risk or those already 'broken'. There is no gainsaying the absolute necessity of regular turning, done by the exercise of skill and muscle power by nurses in pairs, though mechanical devices may help (see below).

The use of a bed cradle is almost obligatory so that the extra pressure of tight bed covers can be avoided. Beds must have good modern sorbo, thick foam or interior sprung mattresses, without fracture boards if possible, but covered by a plastic sheet, and the linen must be clean, smooth, and dry to minimize shearing stresses. The bed should be modern, hydraulically operated, and designed to give every assistance to nursing. Wedge-shaped foam pieces (Lennard pads) under the calves prevent heel contact with the sheets, they may require wrapping round each leg in vulnerable subjects (Fig. 3). Various foam and inflatable rings and simple inflatable air beds have been used, but their value is questionable except occasionally for isolating an existing sore from direct pressure. Sheepskins or their synthetic equivalents probably only reduce shearing stress, but they may marginally improve the local 'microclimate'. Sectionalized deep foam mattresses or gel mattresses and pads redistribute direct pressure by conforming to the body contours and spreading the load widely over the underlying mattress. Specially vulnerable points like heels, ankles, elbows, and knees in arthritic subjects may be protected by foam pads incorporated in elasticated sleeves. Rings on which the heels rest are discredited; they might increase ischaemia by shearing action.

Interesting alternative surfaces for patients to lie upon have been advocated. In the United States plain uncovered sawdust, renewed as appropriate, has been tried, but it is open to understandable aesthetic objections. From Denmark originally came the notion of cush-

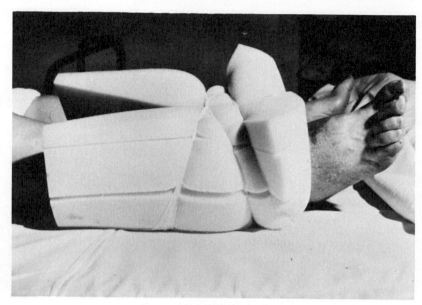

Figure 3

ions and pads of tiny expanded polystyrene sand-like globules, designed to conform to the body contours; but once moulded to a shape they are unyielding, and the system has not found many advocates. The use of a heap of eight feather-filled cushions scattered around on a foam base and replaced every four hours or so gives pressure readings of the order of 35 mmHg.

Mechanical Aids

Since studies were done on the pressure levels set up by various types of floors, beds, operating tables, etc. (Redfern *et al.*, 1973), there has been a steady search for means of relieving pressure mechanically. Any such system, if totally reliable, might relieve nurses of some work and much anxiety. The alternating air pressure mattress ('ripple bed') is designed so that two sets of interdigitating air cells are inflated alternately to move the body weight between them repeatedly, using a pumping cycle of about 10 minutes. In its later large-cell (15 cm) form (Bliss, McLaren, and Exton-Smith, 1966) and with appropriate variable pressure control, it has proved effective. Higher pressure ranges are involved here (e.g. 21 to 77 mmHg), but the automatic mechanical shift of the many points of application of pressure every 10 minutes is highly appropriate. Smaller

ripple pads are used for people sitting in chairs for long periods. The net-bed (the Mecabed, see Fig. 4) suspends the patient on a fine net as if in a hammock, and yet he can be raised, lowered, or rotated from side to side by a single person using two handles. This and other turning frames evolved over the years are liable to restrict spontaneous activity.

The low-air-loss (LAL) patient support system consists of 20 to 24 vertical microporous cushion-like large plastic air cells forming a sectional bed on a hinged frame. Each cell is individually inflated with warm air from a pumping system, and a steady low air loss takes place upwards past the patient, providing a fluid support system at correct humidity and temperature and resulting in low pressure readings under test (Greenfield, 1972; Scales, 1972). For highly vulnerable patients liable to pressure sores, for paraplegics and burns cases, etc., this LAL system is most valuable, but its high cost makes its widespread use impracticable. Fifteen years ago modern water beds were introduced (Russell Grant, 1967). Though bulky, heavy, and immovable, they are highly effective for prevention of pressure sores and for the treatment of severe cases. The patient in effect floats supine on a trough of warmed water, of normal bed dimensions and 30 to 40 cm in depth, but in fact lies upon a tough plastic water-filled envelope. Weight

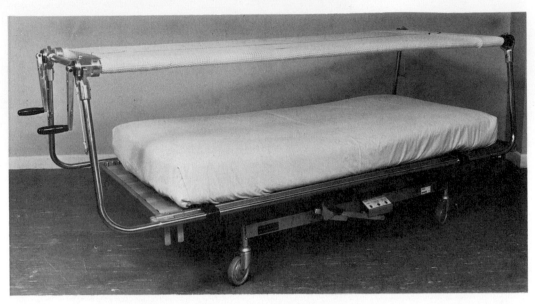

Figure 4   Net-Bed (Mecabed)

distribution is excellent and pressure values are low (19 to 43 mmHg), but not as low as with the LAL bed. In all these mechanical supporting systems the patient is recumbent, but often this may not be desirable. Lifting and other nursing manoeuvres are difficult. Failure of the heating element involves a risk of hypothermia. Other variants on the water bed have been evolved to counter some of these disadvantages; in one (Schatrumpf, 1972) the patient's well-distributed weight is transmitted to a shallow unheated water bath by many plastic balls held down by a plastic membrane. The more recently designed so-called 'fluidized-bead' bed (Thomson *et al.*, 1980) consists of a tank similar to a water bed but filled instead with millions of microspheres of glass of 50 to 150 μm diameter, covered by a filter sheet on which the patient lies or even sits. The microspheres are kept in continuous motion by an upward current of warm pumped air such that the system behaves like fluid but is not wet. This might be the ideal pressure sore nursing milieu, especially since when the air flow is stopped the media immediately becomes 'solid', and the patient is maintained in whatever position he occupied at that moment. This makes turning by one nurse a simple procedure. The high cost of the apparatus severely restricts its availability.

At a practical level the preferred mechanical help for nurses in pressure sore prevention remains the well established ripple bed, with water beds for occasional use in small numbers, and otherwise the various net suspension beds or simple mechanical turning frames.

Mechanical devices are never a substitute for the skill of a conscientious team of nurses.

TREATMENT OF THE SORE

For the superficial ulcer, an occlusive spray (e.g. compound tincture of benzoin) or a water-vapour-transmitting plastic adhesive dressing, and avoidance of further pressure should be enough. Sometimes 0.5% Cetrimide cream on a dressing is advised.

Deep pressure sores have to be regarded as surgical wounds. Once cleaned they can usually be allowed to granulate from below, but this initial cleaning is vital. Full debridement is needed, and since all the sloughing tissue is dead it can be eased out with careful use of forceps and scalpel, without need of anaesthetic. Other ferment aids to cleansing are tripsin powder or the gel of mixed streptokinase and streptodornase ('Varidase') applied to gauze. These are expensive, but effective. A malic, benzoic, and salicyclic acid compound cream ('Aserbine' or 'Malatex') has advocates (Leading Article, 1978). Probably other local lotions, creams, and applications are best avoided.

Deep healing pressure sores with overhanging edges must be kept open for drainage and granulation from below. Normally gauze packing is used. Several synthetic or plastic substances are used to keep the wound supported by a core which encourages drainage away of fluids and pus, and promotes clean granulation. Examples are microscopic beads of dextran dispensed as a sterile powder ('Debrisan'), and more recently a 'Silastic' dressing which is formed as a foam by mixing with a catalyst and is then poured direct into the wound, in the contours of which it sets as a rubbery absorbent dressing (Wood, Williams, and Hughes, 1977). These substances have yet to be fully evaluated. Aniline dyes are still used with effect for local application to some infected pressure sores.

GENERAL MEASURES

Anaemia must be promptly corrected. A high protein intake and even plasma transfusion is indicated in serious intractable cases; therapeutic doses of ascorbic acid appear beneficial. Pories and coworkers (1967) found that zinc encouraged ulcer healing but other authors have disputed its value. It is given as zinc sulphate 220 mg 3 times a day after food and it seems to be non-toxic. The use of anabolic steroids to promote pressure sore healing is not adequately substantiated.

Plastic surgery may be contemplated if epithelialization is delayed, provided the pressure sore has a clean granulating base. The plastic surgical methods in use are rotation flaps and transpositions. These and other treatment methods have lately been reviewed (Orlando, 1981).

It may be said that in spite of the interest shown in the last three decades in pressure sores, and despite the ingenuity of makers of mechanical aids for prevention and treatment, the basic aetiological facts remain inescapable; they are ever present yet easily forgotten. No real substitute has been found for the watchfulness and sheer hard work of nurses, backed up by fully informed and properly motivated doctors. A low incidence of sores in a ward indicates a high quality of fundamental nursing care; a high incidence calls that quality into question. In this respect geriatric teams have an ongoing duty to perform and a mission to conduct among their colleagues.

REFERENCES

Barton, A. A. (1973). 'Pressure sores: an electron microscope and thermographic study', *Mod. Geriat.*, **3**, 8–14.

Bliss, M. R., McLaren, R. and Exton-Smith, A. N. (1966). Department of Health and Social Security Monthly Bulletin No, **25**, pp. 238–268.

Exton-Smith, A. N., Norton, D., and McLaren, R. (1962). *An Investigation of Geriatric Nursing Problems in Hospital*, National Corporation for the Care of Old People, Reprinted 1975, Churchill Livingstone, London.

Exton-Smith, A. N., and Sherwin, R. W. (1961). 'Prevention of pressure sores: significance of bodily movements', *Lancet*, **2**, 1124–1126.

Greenfield, R. A. (1972). 'The L.A.L. bed system', *Nurs. Times*, **68**, 1192–1194.

Husain, T. (1953). 'An experimental study of some pressure effects on tissues, with reference to the bed sore problem', *J. Path. and Bact.*, **66**, 57.

Leading Article (1978). 'Treating pressure sores', *Br. Med. J.*, **1**, 1232.

Orlando, J. (1981). In *Topics in Ageing and Long Term Care*, (Ed. W. Reichel), pp. 127–135, Williams and Wilkins, Baltimore and London.

Pories, W. J., Henzel, J. H., Rob, C. G., and Strain, W. H. (1967). 'Acceleration of wound healing in man with zinc sulphate given by mouth', *Lancet*, **1**, 121–124.

Redfern, S. J., Jenied, P. A., Gillingham, M. E., and Lunn, H. F. (1973). 'Local pressures with ten types of patient support systems', *Lancet*, **2**, 277–280.

Russell Grant, W. (1967). 'Weightlessness in the treatment of bedsores and burns', *Proc. R. Soc. Med.*, **65**, 1065–1066.

Scales, J. T. (1972). 'The L.A.L. patient support system', *Proc. R. Soc. Med.*, **65**, 1065–1066.

Schatrumpf, J. R. (1972). 'New bed for treating pressure sores', *Lancet*, **2**, 1399–1400.

Schwartz, P. L. (1970). 'Ascorbic acid and wound healing', *J. Am. Diet. Assoc.*, **6**, 497–503.

Siegal, R. J., Vistnes, L. M., and Laub, D. R. (1973). 'The use of water beds for the prevention of pressure sores', *Plast. Reconstr. Surg.*, **51**, 31–37.

Thomson, W., Dunkin, L. J., Ryan, D. W., *et al.*, (1980). 'Fluidised-bead bed in the intensive therapy unit', *Lancet*, **1**, 568–570.

Wood, R. A. B., Williams, R. H. P., and Hughes, L. E. (1977). 'Foam elastomar dressing in the management of open granulating wounds', *Br. J. Surg.*, **64**, 554–557.

21

The Endocrine System

21.1

The Endocrine System

M. F. Green

HORMONES AND AGEING

The simple definition of a hormone is a chemical synthesized by an endocrine gland that is then secreted into the bloodstream and circulated to the target organ(s) that it affects. The hormone level and its variation from an acceptable normal functional mean are determined by feedback control of an oscillating dysequilibrium. In reality, hormonal mechanisms are much more complex than the control of secretion, circulation, and effector response. Relationships between hormones and with their target organs are very likely to be affected by ageing and the diseases of old age. Non-bloodstream mediated chemical regulation, especially in the CNS and gut, can also be regarded as hormonal and may be defective in old age.

The production and release of hormones and target organ response to them is usually mediated by enzymes. These are catalyst proteins that control biological reactions throughout the body. Enzymes are also very likely to be affected by age-related 'physiological' deviations as well as the many diseases that tend to affect the elderly.

Some hormones only act by stimulating (or inhibiting) other hormones, e.g. in the CNS/hypothalamic–pituitary axis, or act on clearly defined target organs, e.g. ACTH on the adrenal cortex. Others have widespread metabolic effects, e.g. thyroxine. Hormones act in a variety of ways affecting any or all aspects of RNA/DNA (e.g. replication, transcription, or translation), as well as enzyme levels and effectiveness, and therefore any aspect of cell division, growth, and metabolism. Amino acid hormones from the thyroid and adrenal medulla and peptides from the CNS, parathyroids, and pancreas are usually large molecules and do not penetrate easily into cells. They activate cell membrane receptors, while the gonadal and adrenocortical steroids penetrate through the membrane and directly affect genetic action, because they are lipid soluble.

Hormones that influence the nuclear RNA are not usually fast acting and have been called permissive. They broadly establish the background function of cells, organs, and indeed the general metabolic setting of the whole body. Quicker acting hormones are more immediate and by acting at the cell membrane release preformed intracellular constituents. The sensitivity to immediate hormones is set by the permissive hormones (Holmegaard, 1982).

The intracellular 'second messenger' response to immediate hormones is often, but not always, cyclic-AMP (cyclic adenosine-3', 5'-monophosphate, or cAMP). Calcium and magnesium ions are thought to influence secondary messenger intracellular responses to immediate hormones such as insulin and acetylcholine (ACh). cAMP is the second messenger for TSH, ACTH, parathormone, gonadotrophins, glucagon, and calcitonin. cAMP may be the messenger for arginine vasopressin (AVP) and catecholamine. cAMP and one or two other active intracellular chemicals are able to mediate many unrelated hormonal effects because of differences in the specificity of the cell membrane response to the circulating hormone, and of the nuclear target to the cAMP.

Figures 1 and 2 summarize the many aspects of endocrine biochemistry and hormonal monitoring. All could be affected by 'ageing', homeostatic dysfunction, non-endocrine pathology, and drugs, as well as by standard endocrine diseases. As well as discussing these aspects of geriatric endocrinology in individual sections some general matters must be reviewed first.

Hormones require nutrients, vitamins, trace elements, ions, and cofactors for their synthesis, modulated by enzymes which require similar factors. Peptide hormones in particular are often synthesized in an inactive form and then transformed by hormone/enzyme action into the active hormone. Synthesis and release of hormones and enzymes may often be affected by ageing.

Control of Hormone Production

CNS neurologically modulated negative feedback control of hormone production is influenced by a variety of signals distinct from the simple homeostatic 'servo' response to circulating blood levels of the hormone. These signals include stress, acute and chronic illness, and pain, nutrition, sleep, and physical activity. The signals may be distorted in older people. Deviation may be towards increased sensitivity, e.g. of the hypothalamic osmoreceptor affecting AVP (Helderman *et al.*, 1978), as well as the more likely decreased responsiveness of, for example, pituitary LH response to lowered testosterone levels in older men, and there may be more than just one gonadal target organ failure (Snyder, Reitano, and Utiger, 1975). As well as the recognized negative endocrine feedback system more recent investigation of neuroendocrine oligopeptides that can be releasing or inhibiting has opened up new frontiers. Psychomotor and sensory factors influencing the CNS link in the feedback loop may introduce an element of positive feedforward control (Comfort, 1979).

Little is known about the extent to which vascular or degenerative disease in the CNS (e.g. producing stroke, dementia, and Parkinson's disease) might affect neuroendocrine

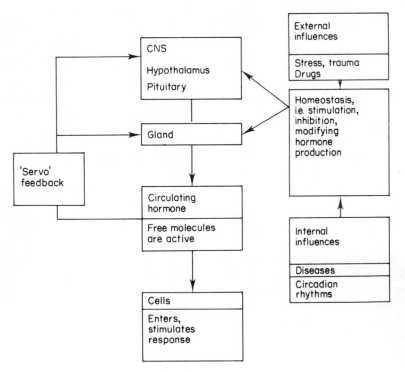

Figure 1   Endocrine control pathways

pathways in the supraoptic and other nuclei, the hypothalamus, and pituitary. Some major homeostatic defects of old age might be at least partly caused by neuroendocrine defects, e.g. affecting blood pressure control, thermo-regulation, and glucose and electrolyte balance.

Disturbed biological (circadian or nyctohemeral) rhythms in the aged might also be due to or cause endocrine abnormality. Reduced clearance might prolong the presence of hormones in the body without necessarily causing serious pathological effects, e.g. the 'raised' or rather sustained levels of plasma cortisol seen during the night in old people without Cushing's Syndrome (Green and Friedman, 1968).

Disturbed amine metabolism and clearance has been thought to be a factor – primarily – rather than merely a marker in depression.

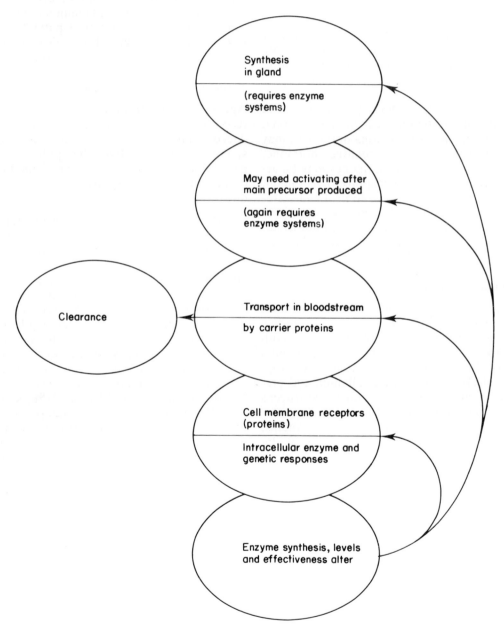

Figure 2   Basic endocrine biochemistry

This is the rationale behind most antidepressant drugs. Other biochemical abnormalities, e.g. of cortisol levels and thyroid function, may just be markers of secondary response, not necessarily pathological. Depression is a common disease in the elderly and further research into neuroendocrinology may be therapeutically helpful in depression as well as in Parkinson's disease and dementia.

Glands

As with other organs there is considerable functional reserve in endocrine glands so that age-related cell loss, fibrosis, lymphatic infiltration, or even frank disease damage may be tolerated.

Particularly in the CNS target organ part of the endocrine system more than one hormone, e.g. inhibiting and/or releasing hormones, may affect production of circulating hormone. Pre-hormones or stored hormones may be activated or released under appropriate stimuli. The chances of deviation of control and secretion are more likely with increasing age as the controlling stimuli and cellular and intracellular enzyme and nucleic acid systems become more likely to be defective.

Hormonal Transport

Biological activity is usually related to the level of free chemical. The level of specific binding proteins may be affected by age, e.g. a tendency to a lowered thyroxine binding globulin (TBG), by disease, subnutrition, and drugs (particularly likely to affect albumin and pre-albumin), and by other hormones. Oestrogens tend to increase, and androgens to decrease, the secretion of specific binding proteins. Obesity, a common finding in the elderly, decreases sex hormone binding globulin.

In passing, obesity may also affect peripheral storage and action of sex hormones in a subtle way, e.g. by influencing the extent to which adrenal androgens are converted to oestrogen in the postmenopausal woman. Obesity may then protect from osteoporosis, although immobility will tend to restore the risk.

Altered protein binding of hormone will also affect the removal of the hormone from the circulation as well as the availability of free/active hormone.

Decreased metabolism and excretion, i.e.

the clearance rate of hormones such as thyroxine and adrenal hormones, is a feature of old age. In normal aged individuals the elegant feedback control merely reduces the amount of hormone produced and maintains homeostasis. In clinical practice the implication is that less hormone may often be needed to restore endocrine normality than in younger people. Many young and middle aged people seem to require up to 0.3 mg a day or even more of L-thyroxine to restore and maintain euthyroidism. Most older hypothyroid patients are at risk of being made unwell if their daily intake exceeds 0.1 to 0.2 mg of L-thyroxine.

Target Cell/Organ Response

Ageing may be strongly related to an altered receptor response to hormones and to a reduced adaptability of receptor–intracellular systems. Kanungo (1980) has published a 4-page table listing changes in animal and human tissue and receptor response, most being in the direction of a decrease with age.

(a) Reduced numbers of cells or general damage to surviving cells may be the simplest explanation for reduced hormone response.

(b) The specific hormone receptors on/in the cell wall may be reduced in number or responsiveness. These protein receptors can be affected by the regulating hormone which determines the receptor concentration in target cells. A low level of oestrogen in female rats correlates with a low level of cerebral oestrogen receptors (Kanungo, Patnaik, and Koul, 1975). Kanungo (1980) gives many other examples of possible age-related changes in hormone receptors. They may be affected by changes in enzyme induction, especially under the influence of steroids (and this includes the effects of neurotransmitters such as ACh), changes in noradrenergic membrane receptors, or in carbohydrate and protein metabolism. Obesity can affect carbohydrate metabolism by an effect on cell membranes producing either mild so-called mature-onset diabetes with substantial amounts of effective insulin still available, or also be a factor in insulin-resistant diabetes. Previous hormone stimulation, e.g. the therapeutic use of corticosteroids, may produce a blunted response due to a reduced receptor number as well as sensitivity (Salomon, Elhanan, and Amir-Zaltsman, 1981). Some stimuli can increase receptor sensitivity, e.g. beta-blockers and opiates.

(c) There may be an age-related alteration in the permeability of the cell wall to the hormone or of the hormone receptor (HR) complex that activates the intracellular second messenger, acetyl transferase (AT), by increasing AT inside the cell membrane. This coupling is defective in pseudo-hypoparathyroidism. The state of the membrane proteins, the level of cofactors such as glyceryl triphosphate (GTP) and magnesium ions, and inhibition from prostaglandins will affect coupling in the cell membrane. There may be more than one HR complex, e.g. that with alpha catecholamines (HR_1) has an opposite effect on AT to that with beta catecholamines (HR_2). Alpha catecholamines include opiate drugs and prostaglandins as well as adrenal catecholamines and ACh; beta catecholamines are TSH, ACTH, PTH, and glucagon.

Drugs such as beta adrenergic blockers and the H_2 blockers, cimetidine and ranitidine, are used to block the normal receptor activity in disease states because they have a high competitive binding affinity for receptors.

(d) The second messenger, usually cAMP, might be reduced or possible be abnormal. Many factors can affect cAMP activity including (1) phosphodiesterase (PDE) activity in turn affected by magnesium and cortisol, by hypothyroidism and drugs including benzodiazepines, thiazides, and sulphonylureas, and by PDE inhibitors such as theophylline and caffeine; the relief of bronchospasm by theophylline and similar drugs is thought to be due to reduced cAMP degradation; (2) alterations in cAMP-dependent protein kinase (PK) with which the cAMP binds; cortisol and possibly insulin affects cAMP–PK binding.

It is difficult to study cAMP intracellularly and homogenates and plasma concentrates have therefore been used. Some cAMP is produced basally and is not hormonally stimulated, but alterations are likely to reflect endocrine function and abnormalities. Many studies, usefully summarized by Holmegaard (1982), show that plasma cAMP is increased in hyperthyroidism, chronic renal failure, cholestatic jaundice, and illness associated with shock and stress (e.g. surgery, myocardial infarction, haemorrhage, infection, and hypoxia), while it is decreased in hypothyroidism and may be increased or decreased in diabetes. Plasma cAMP was not raised in an elderly group studied before herniotomy. This study did suggest a greater variability of cAMP in elderly patients undergoing surgery, perhaps as a result of increased adrenal sensitivity (Blichert-Toft *et al.*, 1979).

This brief discussion of the various mechanisms affecting hormonal stimulus and inhibition on cell function has concentrated on cAMP. In recent years the role of prostaglandins in the disease state and the use of prostaglandin-modifying drugs is also a topic of great interest but beyond the scope of this review. It is clear that the effect of hormones may be partly mediated by prostaglandin-influenced pathways and conversely that prostaglandin abnormalities and prostaglandin-influencing drugs may affect hormone function. This situation is likely to occur in old age. Perhaps the most widely used group of drugs influencing prostaglandins are the non-steroidal anti-inflammatories (NSAIs). These are used in a variety of arthritic and rheumatic conditions and also in malignant disease to alleviate pain and inflammation.

(e) The nuclear response to HR complexes may be altered with age. This will be an obvious consequence of any structural damage that might very well be present in both mitotic and non-mitotic cells in old age. The nuclear membrane might be less permeable to the second messenger, and the final target tissue (the nuclear chromatin material) might be less responsive or produce a faulty metabolic response.

HORMONAL DISORDERS

Hormonal deficiency and excess are relatively common in ill old people. Clear-cut easily recognizable classical endocrine syndromes do occur in the elderly, e.g. ketotic or hyperosmolar diabetes mellitus. However, endocrine dysfunction in the aged does not usually conform to the typical pattern seen in young and middle aged patients. Modified physical and mental symptoms and signs, or atypical or completely non-specific presentations (such as confusion, anorexia and weight loss, and immobility or falls) so often seen in elderly patients, are the usual presentations of endocrinopathies. More problems other than endocrine ones may be present in the same person, especially if conditions such as hormonal/electrolyte/calcium abnormalities associated with cancer or myeloma, or the many disease and drug causes of a low plasma sodium, often loosely grouped together as the 'syndrome of inappropriate ADH secretion – SIADH', are included. Any endocrine abnormality may occur, even in very old people, except those affecting menstruation and fertility (and elderly men can still be fertile).

Even if one does not count all the minor impairments of glucose intolerance so often revealed by biochemical screening that do not always seem to merit hypoglycaemic treatment there is likely to be at least one endocrine/metabolic problem on average in every new elderly inpatient.

The disorders to be considered can be broadly grouped into eleven categories:

1. Diabetes mellitus (see Chapter 23.1).
2. Thyroid dysfunction. This and diabetes are the commonest clinically identifiable hormonal disorders in the elderly. Hyperthyroidism is commoner than thyrotoxicosis. If one broadly groups diseases in old age into (a) those that virtually only occur in the elderly, (b) those that are commoner in old age but do occur in younger people, and (c) those that occasionally occur, but are rare in older age groups, then diabetes and thyroid disease clearly fall into category (b).
3. The inevitable menopause in all menstruating women is, in a sense, by far the commonest geriatric endocrine deficiency state. The effects of rapidly occurring oestrogen lack in women at the menopause and of a slower and later decline in androgens in men, on bones, the cardiovascular system, skin, and other tissues, are complex. Not very much is known about the long-term pros and cons of treating women with replacement oestrogens after the menopause (except to ameliorate the now well-recognized psychological and psychosomatic problems due to the immediate effects of oestrogen decline). Similarly, the use of replacement sex hormones in elderly women and men with bone (or other diseases) is not proven, although topical oestrogens sometimes help 'senile' vulvovaginitis and occasionally urinary incontinence.
4. Hypo- and hypercalcaemia. Bone and renal disease, malnutrition in its broadest sense, i.e. including dietary and absorptive defects, particularly affecting vitamin D, and fluid balance problems, malignancy (cancer and myeloma), and parathyroid abnormalities are probably the commonest causes of disturbed calcium homeostasis.
5. Various abnormalities of electrolytes, e.g. potassium and sodium, and important ions such as magnesium may develop as primary disorders, or more commonly may be secondary to other diseases, e.g. renal failure, or to drugs.
6. Malignant disease is common in old age and may be associated with endocrine abnormalities, usually caused by ectopic (rather than eutopic) hormone production, e.g. SIADH, or be secondary to malnutrition associated with cachexia, or be due to vomiting or dehydration. These various abnormalities can cause serious morbidity and even mortality in their own right.
7. Endocrine abnormalities of the CNS. The rapidly expanding field of neuroendocrinology with its ever-increasing plethora of stimulating, inhibiting, and modifying neurotransmitters (hormones) and prostaglandins has not yet given its full attention to research into this subject and links with the diseases of old age.

   The treatment of Parkinson's disease with L-dopa, bromocriptine, and other centrally acting drugs and research into the pharmacopathology of chronic brain failure (dementia) has raised the hope of a better understanding and even neurotransmitter replacement therapy of cortical and subcortical degeneration, e.g. of cholinergic transmitters, and of depression.
8. Hypothalamic and pituitary–adrenal dis-

ease. These seem to be rare in the elderly. It cannot be emphasized too strongly that diseases of the hypothalamus, pituitary, and target organ can occur; the frequency of primary hypothyroidism should not distract one from considering hypopituitarism as a possible cause of atypical hypothyroidism in an elderly subject. I have seen three new cases of acromegaly in old age during the last 10 years. Mondal and Sinha (1979) reported a 70 year old woman with acromegaly. Mondal and Biswas (1979) have also reported the relatively rare clinical feature of pretobial myxoedema in an elderly patient with thyrotoxicosis.

Any primary or secondary endocrinopathy is theoretically possible, not just hyper- and hypoplasia, but functioning glandular malignancies (i.e. producing eutopic hormones) have been recorded.

9. Drugs. One of the important tenets of geriatric practice is to consider iatrogenic disease as a possible cause of symptoms and signs. The multiple accumulative pathology already alluded to often leads to a reactive polypharmacy, even in a doctor trying to avoid excessive medication, as it is often possible to cure or alleviate many of the diseases revealed by thorough history taking, careful examination and appropriate investigations. Many drugs can cause or aggravate endocrine disease (e.g. diabetogenic diuretics) or produce significant biochemical abnormalities, often with endocrinological consequences, e.g. disturbed potassium or sodium metabolism.

Drugs are also a potent cause of diagnostic confusion because they may affect endocrine function tests (see below).

10. New frontiers. Reference has already been made to the interesting field of neuroendocrinology. A similar field seems to be opening up in the rapid expansion of knowledge about the ubiquitous prostaglandins and about drugs affecting prostaglandin metabolism, as well as in the identification and roles of various gastrointestinal hormones. These two areas raise complex fascinating questions about what is a hormone and what hormonal abnormalities, as yet unidentified, prostaglandin abnormalities may cause in older people.

11. Ageing. Endocrine deficiency is often mentioned when the fascinating question is discussed of whether ageing is inevitably programmed (by organ failure, e.g. of ovaries) or is due to intrinsic cellular processes (e.g. the Hayflick cell division limit), specific disease pathologies, some other cause, or a mixture of reasons. Although ovarian failure is inevitable in all women, it does not lead rapidly to decline and death. There is no evidence that endocrine hyper- or hypofunction or hormonal treatment can prevent, postpone, or reverse ageing. Obviously, endocrine defects may resemble non-specific biological ageing, hypothyroidism being the prime example, but the majority of elderly people do not develop endocrine disease even if they live to be 100; conversely, despite the frequency of endocrine pathology in old age the majority of serious pathology, e.g. degenerative, vascular, or psychiatric, is not due to endocrine disorders.

General Considerations

Before the eleven major categories can be reviewed in detail some further general points must be reiterated.

The multiple pathology characteristic of the elderly means that:

(a) More than one endocrine disorder from any of the categories may occur in the same individual, perhaps due to a common auto-immune defect or underlying malignancy.

(b) There may be a complicated and interdependent relationship between a variety of diseases and drugs, e.g. thyroid disease, heart failure, beta-blockers and diuretics, renal failure, calcium, glucose. More than one disease may contribute to the same symptom or sign.

(c) Common geriatric presentations may be wholly or partly (due to summation or crescendo effects with other diseases) caused by endocrine abnormalities. The usual common feature of these final common pathways is their non-specificity. For instance, hypothyroidism causing vague immobility or instability (possibly leading to falls) due to neuromuscular defect, or myopathy, or weakness due to cerebellar ataxia or depression (the 'gone off her feet' syndrome), or deafness, or confusion/depression (often inaccurately described as senility or 'what can you expect at her age'). Impaired or grossly defective homeostasis, not clearly identifiable as a disease but potentially lethal nonetheless, may be caused, aggravated, or precipitated by endocrine disorders, e.g. hypothermia or postural hypotension.

Endocrine Investigations

Even when a good history can be obtained from a patient, relative, or friend and a thorough multisystem examination is performed, it is customary at any age to confirm a suspected endocrine diagnosis by appropriate tests. Replacement or suppressive hormonal treatment is usually needed for a long time or for the rest of the patient's life, and incorrect treatment can be harmful or just unnecessary and complicate compliance with other necessary medications. When the presentation, as so often in older people, is non-specific and examination unrewarding except to confirm the presence of illness or disability, endocrine tests are accepted as an obligatory part of a biochemical profile. These tests are screening rather than discretionary. Geriatricians have welcomed the general availability of basic auto-analyser/multiple-run tests including urea, electrolytes, proteins, calcium, glucose, and thyroid function. As Hodkinson says, 'The considerable prevalence of treatable diseases which may be present atypically or non-specifically makes it essential that the clinician should master the screening as well as the discretionary methods of evaluating tests results. Furthermore, the frequent disturbances of test results by disease interactions, renal impairment or other metabolic disturbances or drugs mean that interpretation must be especially soundly based' (Hodkinson, 1977). Abnormal results often reveal disease, but there may also be false positives.

There are some important caveats to be considered by the enthusiastic geriatric endocrinologist, especially if he is bent on screening every elderly person who comes his way. Firstly, in the elderly, potential causes of variation in endocrine tests are many and are often affected by nutrition and hydration, by serum proteins (which are often low in the ill elderly), and by renal function. They can also be affected by the way a sample is taken (i.e. by 'cuffing' or postural effects) and sent to the laboratory – a low potassium may become normal or a normal one high if the red cells lyse from delay or even unnecessary warming during delay in transport of an electrolyte sample. Coexistent diseases and/or drugs may also affect results. The non-endocrinologist sometimes forgets the importance of repeated measurements, not just to follow possible ageing or age-related changes from a longitudinal research point of view (rather than cross-sectional point observations) but also because random (possibly due to disease, drug or nutrition) or circadian, diurnal/nyctohemeral, or other rhythmic effects often influence hormone levels very considerably. After all, the nature of simple hormone systems is of a dynamic variation in the circulating hormone level (and of its metabolites or markers), depending on the balance of glandular production, target organ response, and metabolism of the hormone, as well as a controlling servo/feedback response to the controlling hormone. The common finding of a low protein/low serum T4 not necessarily due to hypothyroidism is a well-documented finding and the T4 usually becomes normal as and when the patient recovers. We also see a number of raised rather than low T4s and abnormally high FTIs not due to thyrotoxicosis or any other immediately obvious pathology. These usually return to normal when repeated, especially if the patient improves. If a TRH test has been done it is usually normal.

Hodkinson (see Chapter 7.1 and Hodkinson, 1977) discusses the main technical problems of interpreting screening profile and discretionary tests in the elderly and helps to clarify the problem of normal ranges and false positives and negatives which are particularly difficult to understand when trying to interpret endocrine and biochemical tests in the elderly. It is fairly easy to explain false positives, e.g. a low serum T4 to hypoproteinaemia (usually a low albumin although an age-related low TBG may also be the cause) and not hypothyroidism, but in the presence of multiple pathology accepting a false negative, i.e. a falsely 'normal' result due to disease or drug, could lead to a hypo- or hyperglandular pathology being missed.

At the risk of being too simple it is also important to remember that the endocrine test form usually asks the requesting doctor for details, i.e. clinical information (symptoms and signs), and drugs. One suspects that this section is often inadequately completed. It should also include a reminder to give the times of drug ingestion in relation to the blood test, especially the time of the last dose of thyroid or antidiabetic medication. The staff in endocrine laboratories are usually pleased to suggest possible factors affecting the interpretation of tests, and what further tests might elucidate an unexplained clinical abnormality or how to investigate apparently normal results when endocrine dysfunction is still suspected. They can only help in this way if they are informed or consulted about the reasons for the investigations. The need for clinician/laboratory expert communication is becoming even more important with the increasing number of endocrine tests available. It may also be necessary to liaise specifically with the local laboratory to establish a normal range for the elderly.

There is a particular need for a regularly updated checklist of drug effects on laboratory tests. This problem is well illustrated by two articles which will be discussed in more detail in the section on thyroid dysfunction. In the review of drug effects on *in vitro* thyroid function tests (Wenzel, 1981), some four and a half pages are devoted to drug effects on T4 and T3 and on TSH and TRH tests; the author gives almost 200 references. Many of the drugs mentioned are used in elderly patients. The second article (Kaplan *et al.*, 1982) reviews the relationship between acute illness and thyroid test abnormalities. The authors emphasize the importance of relating medication of a disease to test interpretation.

The final substantial caveat is to remind the reader of the widely accepted principles of screening:

(a) The condition being screened for should be a worthwhile, i.e. an important, problem. Endocrine disorders are important in the elderly.
(b) The condition should be treatable. Most primary and secondary endocrine dis-

orders in the elderly can, and should, be treated.
(c) There should be facilities for diagnosing and treating endocrine disease in the elderly.
(d) The identification of latent or early disease is particularly relevant to the elderly.

Many surveys of the incidence and prevalence of abnormal endocrine test results in the elderly (Hodkinson, 1977; Sewell *et al.*, 1981) are based on hospital populations and may reflect sampling and admission policies.

There are now some normal established ranges for the elderly in the community. These tests will be discussed in more detail in the relevant section but it is interesting to note that:

(a) The range for electrolytes and magnesium seems to be the same for young and old subjects; urea and creatinine, uric acid and alkaline phosphatase appear to show a higher range in the elderly (Leask, Andrews, and Caird, 1973).
(b) There are some statistically significant but relatively minor age-related changes in total protein, albumin, globulin, calcium, and phosphate (Keating *et al.*, 1969), but if elderly men are compared with women they show a relatively lower range of phosphate levels (Hodkinson and McPherson, 1973).
(c) The free thyroxine index has a similar range at all ages, but the TSH is fairly often raised in the elderly, at least up to 20 μU/l in euthyroid subjects (Hodkinson, 1977) although some may have 'prehypothyroidism'.
(d) The general tendency to find slightly raised (suggesting impaired glucose tolerance) or clearly raised (suggesting diabetes) blood glucose levels with increasing age has invoked considerable discussion. This discussion has centered on the possibility that these changes are due to an age-related change of little or no pathological significance, or an increase in true prevalence of diabetes, or a mixture of the two. There is now a general agreement that there is a progressive impairment in glucose tolerance from middle into old age; the literature has been reviewed by Davidson

(1979). The relatively recently introduced laboratory test of glycosylated haemoglobin shows that the percentage of this form of haemoglobin increases progressively and significantly with ageing (Graf, Halter, and Porter, 1978). This rising percentage of glycosylated haemoglobin is thought to correlate with the reaction of red blood cells to increased concentrations of plasma glucose. Despite these very striking biochemical findings, the situation is by no means clear because if commonly accepted criteria for the diagnosis of diabetes are used (particularly the glucose tolerance test) then perhaps more than half the subjects studied over 70 years of age would have diabetes! The subject of diabetes is dealt with in Chapter 20 but these brief remarks are recorded here to illustrate the problem of endocrine screening, and also because other endocrine abnormalities may affect glucose tolerance, e.g. thyroid dysfunction, and also renal impairment and drugs.

Despite the growing literature on endocrine assessment of the elderly, both in ill and fit subjects, not much is known about the anatomy of endocrine glands in the elderly, partly because of the general decline in post-mortem studies. The major definitive work on pathology of the aged was published in 1965 (McKeown, 1965). A clinico-pathological survey from Northwick Park, which will be discussed in detail in the section on thyroid disease (Denham and Wills, 1980), suggests that there is considerable autopsy evidence of anatomical abnormalities in the thyroid gland of elderly subjects. The incidence of thyroid dysfunction is much less, and there is some correlation between nodular goitres and hyperthyroidism, but microscopical abnormalities cannot always be correlated with thyroid function results.

THYROID PHYSIOLOGY AND THYROID FUNCTION TESTS

A brief résumé of the thyroid gland and its control and activity is necessary to understand the complexities of (a) age-related changes in the gland and its function, (b) hyper- and hypothyroidism in older patients, and (c) the influence of a variety of acute and chronic disease and of drugs on both intrinsic thyroid function and thyroid function tests in the elderly.

Levels of circulating thyroid hormone are governed by a simple classical servo/feedback mechanism mediated by the hypothalamic pituitary thyroid axis. Increased or decreased metabolic demand seems to be the main modifier of the feedback working through the CNS or at the tissue level.

Figure 3 illustrates this hormonal axis and Fig. 4a, b, and c summarizes what is known about age-related changes in circulating hormones and thyroid function and their control. Evidence may be insufficient to be dogmatic about what abnormalities may occur and different surveys report low, normal, or high results in aged subjects (patients). Generalizations made from selected groups are of necessity slanted. Results from very ill old people with multiple or atypical pathology, subjected to pharmacy, who are studied when admitted to hospital are unlikely to be relevant to the elderly population generally, especially healthy old people out of hospital. Nevertheless, the problem must be faced because thyroid function tests should be done on ill old people and will need interpretation.

The complexity of these figures illustrates how difficult it can be to be certain about diagnosing endocrine dysfunction in the elderly, especially when the clinical features are not diagnostic and tests only reveal borderline abnormalities. It is certainly not possible to integrate all the observed abnormalities and deviations of the thyroid axis into a coherent pattern in older people. As already indicated the three important areas to review and understand are:

(a) Definite thyroid disease causing morbidity and mortality. Even if the clinical picture is highly suggestive, thyroid function tests are obligatory, even allowing for all the caveats listed subsequently regarding interpretation of these tests. It is important to confirm a diagnosis that may require major treatment for hyperthyroidism by surgery or with radioactive iodine, beta-blockers, or carbimazole or life-long thyroxine replacement therapy for myxoedema.

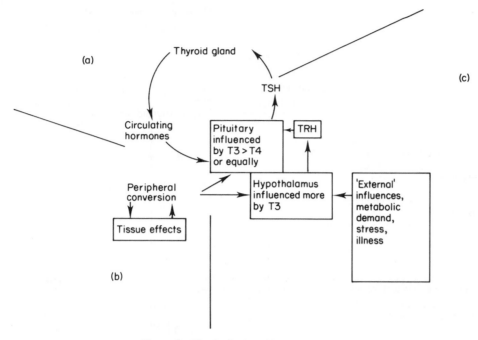

Figure 3   The basic thyroid feedback axis

(b) Age-related changes compensatory for other factors, e.g. disease or drugs. These usually lead to falsely low but sometimes falsely high total or protein-bound T4 levels and a variety of other changes in thyroid function and tests. These are usually of no clinical significance except to confuse the unsuspecting clinician. It is important to call attention to the fact that disease and drug effects could also produce spuriously normal TFTs when hypo- or hyperfunction is present and could obscure the true reason for ill-health in an old person.

(c) Age-related senescence causing or at least associated with abnormal tests and 'pathological' effects not immediately diagnosable as *definite* hyper- or hypothyroidism. The many age-related abnormalities in the hypothalamic pituitary thyroid tissue target organ feedback system are illustrated in Fig. 4. The overall axis can be conveniently divided into three slices starting with the thyroid itself and circulating hormones (Fig. 4a), then the peripheral conversion and clearance mechanisms (Fig. 4b), and finally the CNS hypothalamic–pituitary–thyroid part of the system (Fig. 4c).

Nomenclature

As in all human biochemistry the levo (L-) isomer of thyroid hormones is the normal effective circulating hormone, not the dextro (D-) form. D–T4 has some clinical activity and was used in the past as a slimming aid. However, it is the L-isomers of T4 and T3 that are normally measured and LT4 and LT3 that are used in treating hypothyroidism. In the text T4 and T3 will always refer to the L-isomer.

Other useful standard abbreviations are:

TT4	Total thyroxine
TT3	Total triiodothyronine
FT4	Free thyroxine
FT3	Free triiodothyronine
FT4I	Free thyroxine index
FT3I	Free triiodothyronine index
rT3	Reverse triiodothyronine
TSH	Thyroid-stimulating hormone
TRH	TSH-releasing hormone
TBG	Thyroxine binding globulin
TBPA	Thyroxine binding pre-albumin
I	Iodide
PII	Plasma inorganic iodide
TFTs	Thyroid function tests

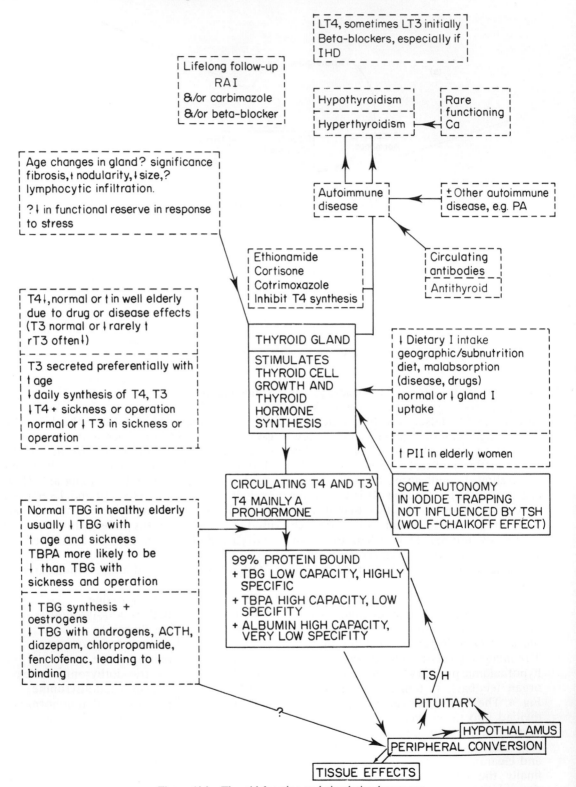

Figure 4(a)   Thyroid function and circulating hormones

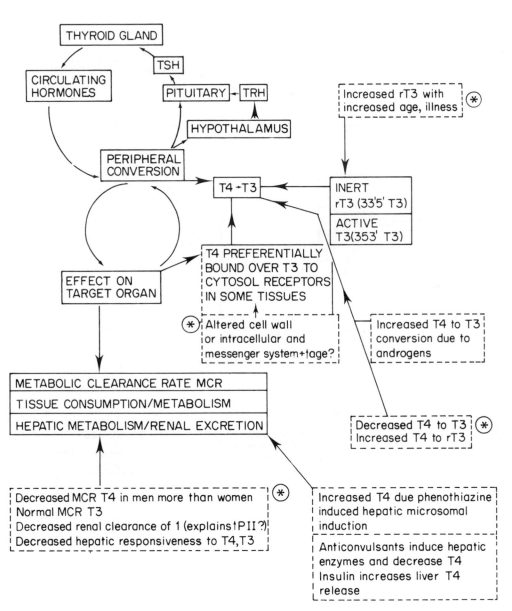

Figure 4(b)   Peripheral conversion and clearance of thyroid hormones

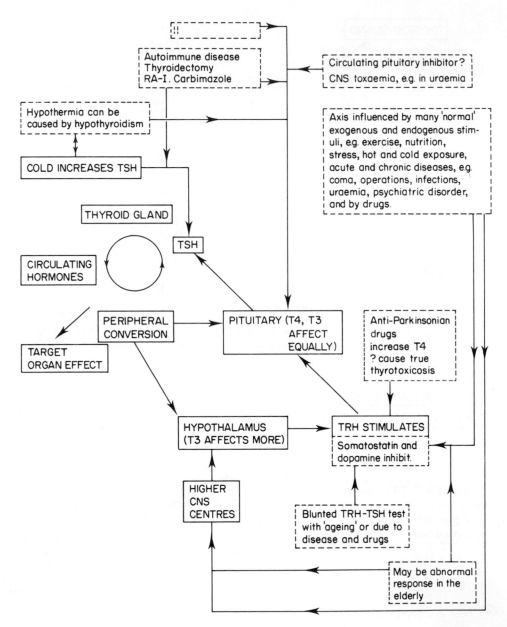

Figure 4(c)   CNS and hypothalamic–pituitary relationships

T4 is the main hormone secreted by the thyroid and is the predominant circulating thyroid hormone, being present at 60 times the T3 level in the peripheral blood. T4 is converted peripherally to T3 by deiodination. T3 is considerably more active and is the main effector hormone. However, orally administered T3 is cleared so rapidly in the body that 8-hourly doses would be needed to maintain euthyroidism. So once-a-day T4 is usually used as maintenance therapy (except in hypothermia due to hypothyroidism) on the assumption that peripheral T4 to T3 conversion is normal (see treatment below).

T4 is 99.96 per cent bound to carrier proteins and T3 is 99.5 per cent protein-bound (Hodkinson, 1977), most T4 and much of the T3 being carried in the blood bound to an α-globulin, thyroxine binding globulin (TBG). Some is bound to pre-albumin and a little to albumin. Age-related and illness and drug-related reductions in these proteins, particularly albumin, are common. Low total T4 and T3 results are often found in ill and medicated old people, and could be due to true hypothyroidism or false positives usually due to hypoprotinaemia (with normal amounts of free active T4 and T3). For the same reasons high normal T4 and T3 could actually reflect hyperthyroidism if carrier proteins are low. More than a fifth of the patients admitted to a busy active geriatric department may have protein abnormalities sufficiently abnormal to affect the standard screening thyroid tests.

The main age-related changes seen in well old people are a fall in T3 production, apparently due to reduced peripheral conversion (deiodination) of T4 to T3. Further reduction in T4 to T3 conversion and an increased production of rT3 may be caused by illness.

FT4 and FT3, and FT4I and FT3I and TSH may also be affected by disease and drugs (see below).

Melmed and Hershman (1982) have summarized the current knowledge about the various parameters and tests of thyroid function in elderly euthyroid, hypo- and hyperthyroid subjects. Figure 5 shows their age-related ranges of TSH, T4 production, T4, and T3, and clearly illustrates changes in old age but also shows the considerable uncertainty of what the normal range is for T4 and T3 in the elderly.

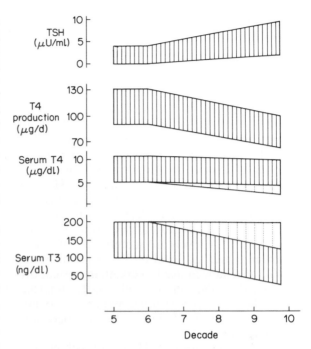

Figure 5 Vertical matching diagrams showing normal ranges of serum TSH, T4, and T3, and the T4 production rate as a function of age. The stippled region shows the range of uncertainty of present data. (From Melmed and Hershman, 1982. Reproduced by permission of Elsevier Publishing Co. Inc.)

Effects of Disease on Thyroid Function and on Thyroid Function Tests

Coexistent disease, so common in the older patient, may affect thyroid function as well as distorting the clinical picture, but more often other disease alters thyroid function tests (TFTs) and confuses the diagnosis (see Chapter 7.1). Table 1 shows some of the many acute and chronic diseases that have been shown to affect TFTs.

Disease often seems to cause (a) a low T3 in the elderly sick, mainly by reduced peripheral T4 to T3 conversion, (b) a low T4 because of low serum proteins (including low albumin and TBG) – a quarter of Hodkinson's (1977) admissions had protein binding abnormalities that could affect simple standard tests – and (c) raised levels of inactive rT3. Other permutations are seen, e.g. low T3 and raised T4 levels (Burrows *et al.*, 1975), and the TSH levels may be low, normal, or high. Impaired secretion of TSH and TSH–TRH response in very ill patients with the low T4 syndrome may be a direct CNS effect producing defective thyroid function rather than just a misleading test due to altered circulating levels of total or bound T4 and T3, and TSH but with adequate tissue stimulation by free hormone. The low T4, impaired TSH picture indicates a poor prognosis (Vierhapper *et al.*, 1982). Kapstein and coworkers (1982) also found reduced TT4 levels correlated with mortality in almost 200 critically ill patients. Conversely, it is important to remember that the raised TSH levels often found in patients with damaged thyroids, e.g. after partial thyroidectomy, are often associated with clinical euthyroidism (Wilkin *et al.*, 1977). T4 levels are sometimes rather low, but an increased level of T3 seems to be the main mechanism used to maintain normal thyroid status. This finding is obviously important in following up thyrotoxic patients who may show raised TSH levels before becoming hypothyroid.

A low T4, normal TSH picture with no definitely diagnostic clinical features of hypothyroidism usually means normal thyroid function, although hypopituitarism can occur in the older age group (Exton-Smith, 1972). A normal total or free T3 level is encouraging but in the sick elderly low T4 syndrome may be associated with low T3, raised rT3 (reverse triiodothyronine). A normal TSH would probably indicate a wait-and-see policy.

(a) The effects of disease on TBG, TSH, T4, and T3 have been reviewed by Friedman and coworkers (1980).

(b) Kaplan and coworkers (1982) found abnormal free T4 levels in 25 per cent and FT4I or TSH abnormal in 16 per cent, but thyroid disease was only present in 3 per cent of a large series of actutely ill patients without known thyroid dysfunction. T4 levels were high, normal, and low, total and free levels were often reduced, TSH levels were normal or slightly raised, and rT3 was usually raised reciprocally to a lowered T3. All the abnormalities tended to return to normal as the clinical state improved. This study does not, of course, resolve the issue of whether these changes represent true thyroid dysfunction, albeit transient, that might impair the response to treatment of other primary conditions. The authors conclude that an accurate thyroid diagnosis in acturely ill patients can usually be made by measuring FT4I and TSH and taking medication into account (see below for drug effects on thyroid function).

(c) Nutritional deficiency is often recorded as

Table 1   Effect of disease on thyroid function (tests)

Disease	Change in T4, T3
Hypothalamic–pituitary deficiency	↓ T4, ↓ T3
Thyroid overactivity (including cancer)	↑ T3, ↑ T3 and ↑ T4
Thyroid underactivity	↓ T3, ↓ T4
Cirrhosis	↑ T4 or ↑ T4 ↑ T3 or ↓ T3
Ulcerative colitis	↑ T3
Acute psychiatric disorder	↑ T4 and FT4I ± ↑ T3
Myocardial infarction, myocarditis, cardiac failure Respiratory infections Septicaemia Peritonitis, pancreatitis, hepatitis Meningitis, encephalitis Nephritis, nephrotic syndrome, chronic renal failure CVA, coma Calcium breast Diabetes acidosis Protein malnutrition, malabsorption Protein-losing enteropathy, carbohydrate deprivation Anaemia, SLE OA	↓ T4 usually may be normal or ↑ T4 ↓ T3 Often ↑ rT3

a cause of altered TFTs. Spencer and co-workers (1983) suggest that fasting leads to an initial rise in FT4, serum TSH is transiently suppressed, TRH levels are unchanged, and TrT3/TT4 fall initially but soon rise again and TSH levels return to normal. The importance of this is that the acuteness of 'starvation' in an ill patient and when TFTs are taken may crucially affect the results obtained.

(d) Myocardial infarction may be associated with a reduced T3 and elevated rT3, the changes being more marked in the 'iller' patients (Wiersinga, Lie, and Touber, 1981). The changes seem to be due to decreased peripheral conversion (deiodination) of T4 to T3, which is the usual explanation for reduced T3 levels in the subjects, and to a lower metabolic clearance of T4. The lowered T3 levels cause a rise in TSH, T4 and T3 then rise, and eventually the swinging endocrine pendulum settles back to normal. Kahana and coworkers (1983) did not feel infarct 'size' was the factor most likely to affect the TFT changes. They found a correlation between cortisol levels and the transient T3, rT3, and TSH changes.

(e) Hypothermia may be due to primary or secondary hypothyroidism. On its own, hypothermia causes a relatively delayed rise in TSH (Fisher and Odell, 1971). Although rapid changes in T4, T3, and rT3 as a consequence of 'illness' (e.g. any precipitating or coexistent disease such as CVA or pneumonia) may occur in hypothermia, T4 has a serum half-life of about 8 days so that hypothermia would not usually affect TFTs in its own right, unless very prolonged.

(f) Investigation of patients with chronic renal failure has shown normal TSH levels, but a blunted TSH–TRH response. Weetman, Weightman, and Scanlon (1981) suggest that a uraemic toxin may interfere with central dopaminergic control. Dopamine physiologically inhibits TSH secretion, and if their conclusion is correct this uraemic poison might be affecting thyroid function rather than just TFTs. It could also be responsible, via CNS pathways, for other uraemic problems such as lethargy and motor abnormalities.

(g) Oppenheimer (1982) has reviewed TFTs in non-thyroidal illness. He suggests that plasma thyroid concentrations can be very misleading. He confirms that low T4, low T3, and normal TSH are the usual findings in physically ill patients without thyroid disease. He feels the central issues are:

(i) Are the TFT changes physiological, e.g. an adaptive procedure response reducing protein catabolism and lipogenic enzyme secretion? Initially protective, true hypothyroidism might develop if these responses are sustained. Research in calorie-deprived animals (presumably corresponding to ill, malnourished humans) suggests that at least some T3 mediated responses are normal, e.g. the formation of x-glycerophosphate dehydrogenase.

(ii) Are the low TFTs, especially low T3, clinically important, and should they be treated?

Oppenheimer (1982) comments that even hyper- and hypothyroidism are complex clinical and chemical states and that the low T3 seen in ill patients does not usually represent homeostatic failure. The possible benefit of thyroid hormones in these circumstances has not been experimentally checked, and such treatment would certainly not usually seem to be indicated if the TSH levels are normal.

(h) A very interesting survey of 645 patients with acute psychiatric disorders showed hyperthyroxinaemia in 33 per cent, elevated FTI in 18 per cent, usually with a low T3, although T3 levels were sometimes normal or even slightly raised (Spratt *et al.*, 1982). TSH–TRH responses were sometimes blunted and varied during the progress of the psychiatric disorder. The elevated T4 levels were usually transient.

Hyper- and hypothyroidism can both cause or aggravate acute and chronic psychiatric disorders, including confusion in the elderly (with or without underlying dementia). Psychotropic drugs could also affect TFTs (see below). It is somewhat surprising that these authors apparently found no sustained thyroid dysfunction, i.e. true thyroid disease, although their concluding comment is very important in the light of the large numbers in the survey and the transience of the hyperthyroxinaemia: 'If screening is to be done, it may be more effective to obtain a serum T4 determination at least one week after admission.'

The raised T4 levels could, of course, have contributed to psychiatric symptoms and signs, albeit transiently.

Thyroid Function Tests

A decision to order further investigations into, or start treatment of, suspected thyroid dysfunction should be based on careful history-taking, thorough examination, and selective tests – repeating tests serially is often useful. High and low thyroid screening tests are often due to non-thyroidal factors and may return to normal fairly quickly, especially if an 'ill' old person gets better. Serial testing is also indicated during treatment in order to monitor and titrate the treatment for both hypo- and hyperthyroidism.

In the case of thyrotoxicosis it is important to see when treatment can be reduced and stopped (if a thyroidal blocker such as carbimazole has been used) and for long-term follow-up to ensure early diagnosis of hypothyroidism after RAI or surgical treatment of hyperthyroidism.

Even when falsely positive tests are excluded it may be reasonable to include appropriate TFTs in the routine screening in ill old people, even if there are no specific clinical features of thyroid dysfunction.

The timing of tests is important. There is an overall circadian rhythm of TSH and hour-to-hour variations in T4, T3, and TSH, depending on such factors as stress, nutrition, fluid balance, exercise, and environmental temperature. If the patient is taking T4 the test results may be influenced by when the last dose was taken, as the peak serum T4 is 4 to 6 hours after an oral dose.

For many years endocrinologists have tried to find an ideal single test, and failing that indices such as the FTI or mathematical discriminant or computer-based analysis of several tests or measurements of free T4 and T3 have been suggested. There is no ideal test, especially as disease, drugs, and changes in target organ responsiveness to T3 and T3 are so common in older patients. Some people have suggested that the TRH test should be used as the baseline screen. This needs an injection and at least 3 blood samples, and is better at identifying hyper- than hypothyroidism and can be affected by disease and medication.

Figure 6 shows a rather complex flow chart of diagnostic tests used in elucidating and following treatment. Essentially:

(a) Serum T4, $\pm$ T3 (i.e. the total levels), and/or FTI, and serum proteins should be measured.
(b) TSH is indicated if hypothyroidism is suspected.
(c) Low T4 results should be checked with a TSH. A raised TSH supports the diagnosis of hypothyroidism.
(d) Conflicting tests, especially where thyrotoxicosis is suggested clinically or by initial high test results, should be checked by a TRH test. Glandular autonomy suggests thyrotoxicosis.

Some cautionary points are:

(a) It has been suggested that *calculated* free thyroid hormones compare well with *measurement* of free T4 and T3 in hypo- and hyperthyroid and in sick euthyroid subjects (Fresco *et al.*, 1982). The concentrations of FT4 and FT3 are low and more 'difficult' to measure than calculating the FT4I or FT3I. However, there is evidence that the correlation of indirect indices of FT4 and measured values of FT4 is uncertain and that FT4 assays are particularly useful in diagnosing 'covert' thyroid disease (Symons, Walichnowski, and Murphy, 1982), which is the norm in old age.
(b) Corticosteroids, oestrogens, and L-dopa as well as thyroid hormone or antithyroid treatment can affect TRH tests.
(c) TRH may cause serious symptoms. Dolva, Riddervold, and Thorsen (1983) suggest that the test dose should be 200 rather than 400 to 500 μg. They question the need for this test!

Despite the many problems of choosing and interpreting TFTs in the elderly, Caird's comments made more than 10 years ago are just

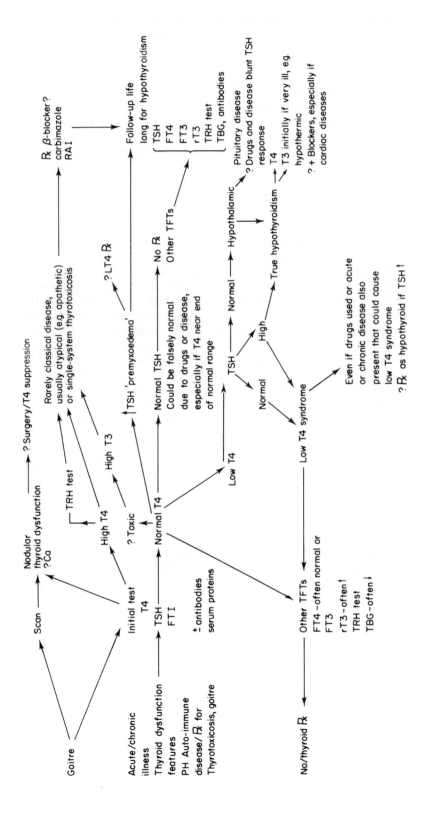

Figure 6   Diagnosis and treatment of thyroid disease in ill elderly people

as valid today (Caird, 1973): 'Laboratory investigations are essential for the accurate diagnosis of many treatment conditions common in the elderly. The proper interpretation of the results of such investigations demands a knowledge both of the normal values encountered in old age and of the numerous factors which may produce misleading results.'

Drugs, Thyroid Function, and Thyroid Function Tests

Older people often take prescribed and/or bought medicines. These can distort TFTs, often by affecting protein-binding, but they can affect virtually any part of the thyroid axis (see Chapter 7.1). Sometimes they can precipitate or cause actual thyroid disease. Obviously, altered TFT and thyroid function due to diseases for which the drugs have been taken may also be present.

An important example of how drugs can affect thyroid function tests – but not clinical status – is the reduction of the circulating total, and to a lesser extent the free, T4, and T3 hormones by fenclofenac. This effect is seen in thyrotoxic and euthyroid subjects. Fenclofenac is a non-steroidal anti-inflammatory drug that can actually reduce toxic levels of total T4 to normal, and also reduces free T4, total T3, and rT3 levels (Pearson *et al.*, 1982). The total T4 and T3 in euthyroid subjects taking fenclofenac may fall to 30 to 40 per cent. of the initial concentration and could therefore cause diagnostic confusion, especially if too much significance is placed on screening tests.

There is no change in clinical thyroid status in thyrotoxic or euthyroid subjects so this drug is of no therapeutic benefit in treating hyperthyroidism; nor will it cause iatrogenic hypothyroidism.

The effect is mediated by competitive inhibition of T4 and T3 binding to TBG (Kurtz *et al.*, 1981). Although no clinical disturbance has been measured the effects of thyroid function tests are so striking that it is possible that thyroidal or even pituitary function could be altered, albeit transiently, by the changes in free T4 and T3 that have been recorded.

The antiarrhythmic iodine-containing drug, amiodarone, can affect TFTs and also thyroid function, which is clearly important if used in elderly patients with cardiac arrhythmia and unsuspected thyroid dysfunction.

Patients taking amiodarone may remain euthyroid, although altered peripheral T4 metabolism may increase the T4/T3 ratio (Pritchard, Singh, and Hurley, 1975) and more rT3 may be produced. A low T3 level is usual; the FTI may be raised (in normal limits). Thyroid dysfunction can occur, usually hypothyroidism probably due to 'iodine overload'. The drug's main effect is on the peripheral conversion of thyroxine that obviously affects the interpretation of TFTs, but as well as occasionally producing thyroid dysfunction the drug's β- and α-blocking actions may also modify the clinical features of cardiac and thyrocardiac disease. A history of thyroid disease may be a contraindication to amiodarone therapy (Jonckheer, 1981). Underdiagnosis as well as false positive overdiagnosis could be a consequence of amiodarone therapy. It may interfere with radioiodine therapy and should usually be used with a specific blocking agent such as carbimazole (Sheldon, 1983).

Bromocriptine is a third interesting example of how drugs affect thyroid function. The drug appears to affect circadian TSH secretion and lowers TSH levels (Sowers, Catania, and Hoshman, 1982), and suppresses the TSH response to i.v. TRH (Yap *et al.*, 1978). This drug could be used in thyrotoxicosis (Connell *et al.*, 1982). The time of administration of the drug may be critical in evaluating effects on TSH and other TFTs, in view of the circadian rhythm of TSH and many other neurotransmitters. Tarquini and coworkers (1981) investigated the effect of bromocriptine in elderly men with prostatic hypertrophy and found a reduction in TSH and prolactin and commented that the time of drug administration and taking of samples radically affected the findings.

Krulich (1982) has reviewed the neurotransmitter control of thyrotropin secretion. He suggests that dopamine, bromocriptine (a dopamine receptor agonist), and L-dopa (a dopamine precursor) decrease circulating TSH and may inhibit the secretion of TSH in response to TRH, especially in hypothyroid subjects (Simonim, 1972; Spaulding, 1972). This would obviously affect the interpretation of TRH tests in Parkinsonian patients treated with these drugs. A single dose of L-dopa lowers raised TSH levels in hypothyroid patients without modifying TRH responses (Refetoff, 1974), but repeated doses are required

Table 2 ↑ TT4 possible drug causes/effects

Drug	Other TFTs, possible explanation	Clinical comment
GH	↑ T3, ↑ T4 ÷ T3 conversion	Goitre, thyroid dysfunction
Androgen	Normal/low FT4I, TT3 ↓ carrier proteins, ↓ binding capacity	
ACTH	↓ TBG, ↓ T4 synthesis	
Salicylates	↑ FT4, ↓ TT3 and FT3I Competition for binding sites on carrier proteins	Hypothyroid patients may have 'rheumatism'
Fenclofenac	↓ FT4, ↓ FT4I, ↓ TT3, ↓ FT3 Displaces hormone from TBC ?Also pituitary effect	
Ranitidine	↓ TRH response ?Histamine involvement in thyroxine regulation	
Heparin	↑ FT4, ↑ FT4I Probably competitive binding	Iodine containing contrast media used to investigate DVTs may precipitate thyrotoxicosis
Diazepam	↓ FT4 ?Protein binding effect	
Diphenyl-hydantoin	↓ FT4, ↓ FT4I, ↓ FT3I normal or 1 TT3, FT3	
Phenobarbitone	↓ FT4, ↓ or ↑ FT4I normal or ↓ TT3	
Primidone	↓ FT4I	
Carbamazepine	↓ All other serum indices All anticonvulsants induce liver enzymes May also competitively bind	
Ethionamide	↓ all indices	May be antithyroid effect
Sulphonylureas chlorpropamide	Displace T4 from TBG	(Insulin ↑ TT4)
Phenothiazine	Hepatic microsomal effect	Abnormal psychiatric state may be caused by hypo- or hyperthyroidism. Also psychiatric disorders tend T4
Cholestyramine, thiazides	↓ intestinal T4 absorption Change distribution volume?	
Iodine compounds		
Oestrogens HRT in women Stilboestrol in men	↑ FT4I Normal/Low FT4I, T3	Altered binding capacity of transport problems
Diamorphine (in myocardial infarction, 'terminal pain')	Normal FT4I, mormal ↑ TT3	Heart disease may be caused by thyroid diseases or aggravated by thyroid treatment
Propranolol, e.g. in hypertensin, thyrotoxicosis, LT4 R of hypothyroidism	↓ TT3 Inhibitin peripheral converision T4–T3	?Cardiac failure, also FTI ?Effect on thyroid function
Digoxin	↑ FTI	
Amiodarone	↑ FT4 Inhibition of peripheral conversion of T4– ↓ TT3 T3. Preferential T4–T3 conversion. ?Anti ↑ rTE T4 effect. Increased TSH response to TRH	
Insulin	Liver release T4	
Orphenadrine in Parkinsonism, especially phenothiazine[1] induced	↑ FT4I ↓ TT3	
L-dopa and bromocriptine normally decrease TSH, inhibit cold-induced TSH. Decrease TSH response to TRH Piribedil – depresses or inhibits cold-induced release of TSH	CNS hypothalmic pituitary dopamine effect	Misleading TFTs in euthyroid and hypothyroid states ?could actually cause thyroid abnormality
Cotrimoxazole	Sulphonamides are potential goitrogens	

[1]Phenothiazine may decrease T4.

to abolish the TRH–TSH response in euthyroid subjects. Bromocriptine decreases TSH levels and blunts the TRH–TSH response in hypothyroid patients (Miyai, 1974). There is conflicting evidence as to whether this drug affects TRH response or not in euthyroid subjects. These drugs decrease TRH-stimulated release TRH and therefore presumably work via the pituitary.

Conversely, dopamine receptor blockers such as metoclopramide have an opposite effect to dopaminergic agonists. TSH levels are elevated when metoclopramide (Scanlon, 1977), sulpiride (Zanoboni, Zanoboni-Muciaccia, and Zanussi, 1979), or domperidone (Delitala, Devilla, and Lotti, 1980) are given. The effect is more marked in women and more marked in hypothyroid subjects (Kamijo *et al.*, 1981), the TSH response being inversely related to the severity of the thyroid deficiency. The response is greater in the middle of the night when TSH responses is at its zenith and less at the nadir in the middle of the day. Haloperidol and pimozide are also dopamine receptor blockers that elevate TSH levels (Delitala *et al.*, 1981). Clearly these groups of drugs can actually influence thyroid function rather than just effect TFTs.

Presumably the dopaminergic system has a tonic inhibitory effect buffering the normal negative feedback mechanism on TSH levels and may help set the diurnal rhythm of TSH. The complex and somewhat variable results of animal investigations of norepinephrine and serotonin (5HT) effects on the hypothalamus and pituitary have not been repeated and confirmed satisfactorily in man. Krulich (1982) has shown that TSH in rats can be stimulated or inhibited depending on which alphanergic blocker is involved, and the level of adrenergic blockade may be critical in determining response. Therapeutic adrenergic blockades is widely used in medicine, including the treatment of thyrotoxicosis and sometimes during the early stage of treating hypothyroidism. Adrenergic blockade could produce a variety of effects on thyroid function.

Conclusion

T4 and other TFTs are more often lowered than raised as a result of drug effects and/or the diseases the drugs are treating. False positive high or low tests may obscure the diagnosis of true thyroid disease, e.g. by producing a high normal range result when toxicosis is present. Measurement of free levels of T4 and T3, TSH levels and the TRH–TSH test, the use of serial measurements, and always combining test results with clinical assessment are all necessary.

THYROID DISEASE

Introduction

Thyroid dysfunction is a potent cause of disabling clinical morbidity and can be lethal. The classical clinical features, e.g. of Graves' disease or Hashimoto's thyroiditis, are rarely seen in older patients, who usually show modified or frankly atypical presentations. Goitres are usually nodular rather than diffuse. The clinical effects of thyroid disease are not only complicated by a tendency to modified or atypical presentation but by the frequent coexistence of other diseases. Thyroid dysfunction can affect any tissue but the heart and the CNS are most often affected in older people.

While thyroid disease is fairly common as a cause of illness in old people there is no evidence that ageing generally is caused by thyroidal ageing or thyroid disease.

The interpretation of laboratory tests in older people is often complicated by age-related changes, e.g. in serum proteins, and by disease or drug effects. The complexities of thyroid physiology and pathology in the older age group highlight many fascinating aspects of geriatric medicine. Understanding them will help the clinician come to an accurate thyroidal diagnosis in ill old people in whom thyroid disease may be a cause of illness and disability.

Even though the various changes in thyroid function and thyroid function tests in old age are increasingly well understood it is still not 'possible to rationalize the age-related deviations found into an integrated, internally consistent pattern of function' (Ingbar, 1978), the main difficulty being the elusiveness of a reproducible, convenient, and reliable measure of 'thyroid function state at the peripheral tissue level' (Ross, 1981).

Anatomy

Most authorities have observed that the thyroid gland shows characteristic age-related changes of atrophy (Pitman, 1962), fibrosis, and nodularity (McKeown, 1965) with advancing age. Increasing nodularity may be associated with a higher rather than a lower gland weight, but if nodularity is excluded there is no age relationship with gland weight (Denham, 1977). One series found that 70 per cent. of women over 60 had multinodular goitres at post-mortem (Mortensen, Woolner, and Bennett, 1955) compared with 50 per cent. of routine autopsies on subjects of all ages showing thyroid nodules (Ibbertson, 1964). Clinical and histological nodularity may of course be a response to dietary iodide insufficiency in goitrogenic areas, but also seems to be a common sporadic finding in the elderly. Most nodules in the elderly are involutional rather than inflammatory or neoplastic. A 2 per cent. incidence of symptomless carcinoma *in situ* has been recorded (Mortensen, Woolner, and Bennett, 1955). Like all thyroid disease nodularity is commoner in women.

Denham and Will's (1980) post-mortem study in a non-goitrogenic area showed that nodularity may be pathological, i.e. associated with increased risk of disease, usually hyperthyroidism. Even macroscopically normal glands tended to show fibrosis and colloidal nodules. Nodules were found in 27 per cent. of post-mortem cases and focal and lymphocytic infiltration was observed in one-fifth of these elderly patients at post-mortem. No clear link was established between lymphocytic infiltration, implying auto-immune thyroiditis, and thyroid dysfunction. There is, however, evidence that circulating thyroid antibodies are correlated with histological thyroiditis in the elderly (Chomette *et al.*, 1966).

Prevalence

Thyroid disease and abnormal thyroid function tests are common in the elderly. Sometimes the clinical features are obvious but two important clinical points are a frequent source of confusion:

(a) Thyroid symptomatology and objective signs are frequently modified or frankly atypical in the elderly.
(b) Suspicious clinical features are not necessarily diagnostic in mild hypothyroidism at any age and in the elderly, particularly, constipation, obesity, dislike of cold weather, deafness, and depression could all be due to myxoedema, but any one or all could be caused by many different pathologies.

The relatively high prevalence of clinically significant, i.e. morbid and potentially mortal, thyroid dysfunction and the frequently blurred clinical picture justify routine laboratory screening of all ill old people. At the same time all results – low, normal, or high – should be analysed critically to see if coexistent disease or drug effects might be altering the interpretation of the results.

The precise incidence of thyroid disease in old age is somewhat uncertain. Of more than 300 acute admissions to the Northwick Park Geriatric Department 3.8 per cent. had hypothyroidism, with an overall prevalence of hyper- and hypothyroidism of 5.7 per cent. (Jeffreys, 1972). Later the same department published a lower figure of 2.3 per cent. of admissions being hypothyroid (Bahemuka and Hodkinson, 1975). Somewhat surprisingly a similar percentage was discovered in long-stay patients (Kind and Ghosh, 1976). Martin (1981) gives a total figure of 3 per cent. of the over sixty-fives as having thyroid disease and some five-sixths as being myxoedematous. The substantial differences between their surveys could be due to local demographic factors such as the long-recognized frequency of thyroid problems in iodine-deficient areas such as Derbyshire or to different selection factors in the research survey, e.g. age (Northwick Park patients had an average age of 80) or local differences in admission policies. Some geriatric departments admit unselectively all people over a certain age; others 'compete' with general medical firms by taking whatever admissions GPs and accident and emergency departments refer to them.

In the latter case it seems likely that admissions to a geriatric department would be more likely to have modified to atypical presentations. It is interesting to note that 2½ per cent. of the unselected Northwick Park admissions were not suspected clinically of having thyroid dysfunction. Conversely, a recent review of biochemical screening for thyroid disease in elderly patients in a general medical ward suggested that TFTs were often abnormal when suspicious clinical features were present

(3 out of 6) but no abnormal TFTs were found in 44 other ill patients with no suggestion of thyroid dysfunction (Sewell *et al.*, 1981). This in itself was surprising as low T4s usually due to low proteins are often found in ill elderly people, as are other thyroid function test abnormalities.

Melmed and Hershman (1982) in Korenman's excellent review of endocrine aspects of ageing highlight another aspect of this interesting matter of the prevalence of thyroid disease and abnormal tests. Titres of circulating antithyroglobulin and antithyroid microsomal antibodies increase with age. Almost 20 per cent. of women over 70 have antithyroglobulin antibodies (Howel *et al.*, 1967). Of postmenopausal women in a large community survey 10 per cent. were shown to have antibodies to thyrocytoplasm and raised circulating TSH levels; 17.4 per cent. of women and 3.5 per cent. of men over 75 had TSH levels above 6 international units. Only 0.5 per cent. of this group had obvious hypothyroidism (Tunbridge *et al.*, 1977).

Another survey of healthy subjects over 60 years of age showed a slightly lower percentage of raised TSH; as before, more women showed this abnormality than men (Sawim, 1979). There is, of course, considerable uncertainty about the significance of raised TSH levels in the absence of definite clinical or laboratory evidence of functional thyroid deficiency, but the findings certainly imply an increased risk of hypothyroidism developing subsequently. There is also argument about how high is the upper limit of 'normal' TSH but 10 μU/ml is often taken as the upper limit. Incipient thyroid failure stimulating the raised TSH to maintain euthyroidism may become decompensated at any time, but one could arbitrarily argue that TSHs well above 10 μU/ml suggest imminent if not actual thyroidal hypofunction.

These observations are important for two reasons. Firstly, the significance of raised TSHs and the natural history of the 'pre-hypothyroid' state and thyroiditis, as suggested by raised circulating antibody levels, are not clear. Secondly, the very low prevalence of actual thyroid dysfunction in the well elderly in the community, as distinct from those who are unwell and attending or admitted to hospital, and a relatively low (but definite) level of auto-immune abnormalities and raised TSH levels

suggest that thyroid disease will be more prevalent with an ageing population.

The results of some of the various hospital and community surveys are summarized in Table 3. The test(s) used and the population studied will obviously influence the prevelnce figures. A much higher yield is likely in surveys of ill old people admitted to hospital. Surveys of 'geriatric' admissions may include more atypical presentations than general medical or endocrine admissions.

TYPES OF THYROID DISEASE

After allowing for false positive tests hypothyroidism is found in 3 to 4 per cent. of ill old people admitted to hospital, which is some 5 to 6 times more common than hyperthyroidism. Thyroid disease is 4 to 5 times more likely to develop in women. Thyroid disease in the elderly is often described as occult or masked. The clinical features are often modified or atypical and other diseases may distort the clinician from the correct diagnosis. The main effects may fall on one system, e.g. cardiac, GI, or CNS.

Thyrotoxicosis

This is very much a disease of late middle and old age. The so-called classical presentation with a large goitre, exophthalmos, and symptoms and signs of virtually every system – Graves' disease – seen in younger people hardly ever occurs in old age.

Causes of hyperthyroidism

(a) *Auto-immune disease, nearly always without classical features of Graves' disease.* The presence of circulating antithyroid antibodies and/or a history of auto-immune disease in the patient or relatives (e.g. PA) do not in themselves confirm a diagnosis of thyroid dysfunction, merely an increased risk of developing thyroid disease at some time. High titres are more significant than low titres which are common in the general population, and antithyroid cell (i.e. mitochondrial) antibodies are more significant than antithyroglobulin antibodies. Thyroglobulin antibodies which are often present in thyroid disease including hyperthyroidism and thyroid cancer may bind with thyroglobulin and lower otherwise abnormally raised titres (Ratcliffe, Ayoub, and Pearson, 1981).

There is often no goitre and eye signs are rarely seen (Davis and Davis, 1974). A single or multinodular goitre may be present but is often not very obvious clinically (Bartels, 1965). Nodular goitre is not usually an auto-immune induced change. This is probably the reason why the exophthalmos and pre-tibial myxoedema associated with Graves' disease are rarely seen in the elderly.

Table 3   Reported prevalance of thyroid disease

Hospital

Background	Results	Reference
Over sixties	37% of cases of thyrotoxicosis in this age group	Lamberg (1960)
Over sixties	30% of cases of thyrotoxicosis in this age group	Thommesen (1971)
Unselected geriatric admissions	3.8% with thyroid disease	Jeffreys (1972)
Over sixties attending endocrine outpatients	Yearly incidences of thyrotoxicosis 7 times greater than in the under sixties	Ronnov-Jenssen and Kirkegaard (1973)
64 inpatients 24 outpatients Over sixties	2 hypothyroid 37% thyrotoxics had no palpable gland	Davis and Davis (1974)
Acute geriatric admissions	2.3% hypothyroid	Bahemuka and Hodkinson (1975)
Long-stay wards	2% hypothyroid	Kind and Ghosh (1976)
Geriatric admissions	2.6% hypothyroid	Palmer (1977)
Psychogeriatric admissions	1.2% hypothyroid	Henschke and Pain (1977)
1,200 psychiatric admissions	0.7% thyrotoxic	McLarty *et al.* (1978)
Geriatric patients	3.0% thyroid disease	Martin (1981)
Acute medical admissions	3 of 6 suspected were hypothyroid; none of 44 without clinical features	Sewell *et al.* (1981)
Acute geriatric admissions (serial measurements to allow illness effects to abate)	6 of 120 hypothyroid (4 clinically suggestive), 1 thyrotoxic	Rai (1982)

Community

Background	Results	Reference
Living at home	4%	Taylor *et al.* (1974)
Residential homes	None of 100	Kind and Ghosh (1976)
Living at home	2 of 114 subjects	Hodkinson (1977)
Community	0.5% overt hypothyroidism	Tunbridge *et al.* (1977)

Mixed community/residential home/hospital

Background	Results	Reference
559 subjects over 65	Prevalence in over 80 group 0.94% hypothyroid 0.47% hyperthyroid 5 of 7 subjects with thyroid disease were suspected	Campbell *et al.* (1981)

(b) *A functioning thyroid cancer can cause thyrotoxicosis*. Ectopic hormone production could produce hyperthyroidism, e.g. in association with calcium of the bronchus, probably from increased TSH secretion rather than excess T4 production.

(c) *Excess intake of T4 or increased responsiveness due to 'normal' doses of T4*. The clinical observation that older people often need less T4 (i.e. up to a daily maximum of 0.2 mg) than younger people to restore euthyroidism in the hypothyroid state could indicate increased cellular/intracellular sensitivity to T4 and T3. It can also indicate increased peripheral T4 to T3 conversion, but what evidence there is suggests a slight decrease in this conversion with ageing and an increased proportion of rT3 being produced. It could also be due to a variety of changes affecting the thyroid pool, e.g. in protein-binding, hepatic and renal clearance, body size, and lowered metabolic demand, even in active elderly people, i.e. it is compensatory.

The important clinical point is that unnecessary T4 supplementation up to the maximum saturation level merely shuts off endogenous intrinsic T4/T3 production through feedback adjustment. Above saturation level the body cannot compensate for excess administered T4 and thyrotoxicosis develops.

(d) It is widely believed that stress can precipitate hyperthyroidism. Psychological stress such as bereavement or depression and many acute physical stresses such as illness, pain, and operations do sometimes seem to act as the provoking factor of thyrotoxicosis.

(e) Radioactive I[125]-labelled fibrinogen used in the investigation of deep venous thrombosis has been shown to precipitate thyrotoxicosis, presumably by blocking thyroidal iodine uptake.

Clinical Features

The presence of other diseases and the modified or atypical presentation of thyrotoxicosis have already been referred to. However, even though cardiac, gastrointestinal, or psychiatric symptoms may predominate, symptoms and signs suggestive of thyroid dysfunction are often present in other systems. For instance, 'apatethic' thyrotoxics have often lost weight and may have cardiovascular abnormalities. Nevertheless, a non-specific presentation – the 'failure-to-thrive' syndrome, or non-specific clinical features – depression, constipation, or deafness may very well be caused by thyroid disease.

Some or all of the classical features may be present, and sometimes the large goitre of Graves' disease (rather than the nodular goitre or autonomous adenomas of Plummer's disease) and exophthalmos and ophthalmoplegia. Thyrocardiac disease is dealt with in Chapter 14.7. In other systems important features are:

(a) *CNS*. Depression, agitation, confusion, or apathy may be present. Apathetic thyrotoxicosis (Lahey, 1932) may be due to T3 as much as T4 toxicosis (Fairclough and Besser, 1973). This is one of the potentially lethal but imminently remediable diseases often mislabelled as 'senility'. An apathetic hyperthyroid presentation may occur in 10 to 15 per cent. of older subjects. Apathy is not the only presentation and agitation, confusion, manic behaviour, and even encephalopathic features may develop. Paranoid delusions may occur. Obviously, psychiatric features may be due to a worsening of preexisting dementia but bizarre, distressing, and even antisocial behaviour can be cured by controlled thyrotoxicosis.

(b) *Gastrointestinal*. Weight loss, anorexia, and diarrhoea (or, interestingly, constipation) that may be regarded as common in old age, possibly caused by an underlying malignancy that cannot be treated, should be investigated. Hepatomegaly is often present in elderly thyrotoxics. The anorexia contrasts with the increased appetite in younger patients.

(c) *Musculoskeletal*. Tremor, muscle wasting, and weakness are common. Characteristically there is severe temporal muscle wasting and a marked proximal myopathy.

(d) *Hypercalcaemia and/or osteoporosis may develop*. Thyroid hormones increase bone turnover and can lead to negative mineral balance. Macfarlane and coworkers (1982) have described altered vitamin D status in hyperthyroidism with a rise in 24, 25-$(OH)_2D_3$ and a fall in 1,25-$(OH)_2D_3$. These changes will tend to affect renal enzymes secondarily, but T3 may also have a direct effect on renal 24-hydroxylase.

(e) *Other.* Dyspnoea is fairly common, even in the absence of cardiac dysfunction (Ayres *et al.*, 1982). Diabetes mellitus may be aggravated and become more difficult to control due to effects on carbohydrate metabolism. Glaucoma may be aggravated or precipitated.

Treatment

Surgery is rarely required for goitre. Medical management is the rule and may be needed urgently. Radioiodine (RAI) is simple and non-toxic but takes time (often several months) to control the toxic state and may be followed by hypothyroidism almost immediately, or years later. The usual explanation is a combination of mitotic damage from the RAI and underlying auto-immune damage.

Thyroid blockade with carbimazole is often necessary. A starting dose of 10 to 25 mg a day is usually all that is needed, followed by a maintenance dose of 5 to 10 mg/d. Hypothyroidism may develop. It is difficult to know how long to continue this treatment as the time before the underlying thyrotoxicosis remits is very variable, but a common practice is to try reducing the dose after 6 to 12 months. Side-effects are rare, but include skin rashes and agranulocytosis. Regular clinical and biochemical monitoring are obligatory during treatment and should be continued for the rest of the patient's life after stopping the carbimazole because of the slight risk of recurrent toxicity and the higher risk of myxoedema.

Despite the risk of cardiac (hypotension and heart failure) and respiratory (bronchospasm) side-effects, peripheral sympathetic effects of thyrotoxicosis are often treated with beta-blockers. Propranolol can produce great sympathetic relief, even after one dose. However, this is not a definitive treatment and has a minimal effect on the levels of thyroid hormones (O'Malley *et al.*, 1982). Higher plasma propranolol levels found in elderly hyperthyroid subjects are effectively counterbalanced by decreased sensitivity of propranolol receptors (Feehy and Stevenson, 1979).

Hypothyroidism

Hypothyroidism in the elderly is caused by:

(a) Auto-immune disease.
(b) The effects of treatment of thyrotoxicosis (e.g. partial thyroidectomy, radioactive iodine, or blocking agents) and often combined with continuing auto-immune damage.
(c) Hypothalamic–pituitary disease. Hypothyroidism is nearly always primary in old age, i.e. due to thyroid disease, but hypopituitarism has been reported (Exton-Smith, 1972).

The age distribution of auto-immune diseases varies, e.g. active rheumatoid arthritis is uncommon in the elderly, whereas polymyalgia rheumatica and temporal arteritis are very much diseases of old age. It is interesting that a decline in T-suppressor cells has been noted in auto-immune thyroiditis (Thielemans *et al.*, 1981) as an age-related decline in immunological competence may be an important factor in the increased risk of developing infections, and various malignancies.

Symptomatic auto-immune thyroiditis may lead to subsequent clinical hypothyroidism. An elevated TSH is a strong predictor of subsequent hypothyroidism and these subjects should be carefully followed (Gordin and Lamberg, 1981). Doniach and Bottazzo (1983) comment that 10 to 20 per cent. of the 20 per cent. of middle aged women who show thyroid antibodies eventually show evidence of thyroid deficiency. They advise permanent replacement therapy to those with raised basal TSH levels in the belief that these subjects have progressive thyroiditis. They also give a 6 months trial of T4 to those whose normal basal level rises steeply after i.v. TRH, and check TFTs including TRH response after this trial.

A raised TSH after thyroidectomy is a much less reliable predictor of hypothyroidism (Hennemann *et al.*, 1975). This has also been found after RAI (radioiodine) (Tunbridge *et al.*, 1977), although the widespread unselective mitotic effect of RAI throughout the gland might be expected to summate with any progressive auto-immune thyroiditis, however careful the dose schedule. Many of these subjects with raised TSHs have normal T4s and are clinically euthyroid. Patients have been seen by the author with even slightly low T4s, whose euthyroidism was maintained by modestly elevated T3 levels with nominal TSHs, after surgery for toxic and non-toxic goitres.

Clinical Features

This tends to be insidious at any age and is a potent cause of the geriatric presentations of 'gone off her feet', 'failure-to-thrive', and senility. It may cause many of the common problems of old age, such as immobility and instability (leading to falls), constipation, deafness, confusion, and depression. Patients with myxoedema may present acutely or chronically to virtually any hospital department, e.g.:

(a) Endocrine – the diagnosis is suspected!
(b) General or special medical – cardiovascular (bradycardia, angina, heart failure, myocardial infarction, pericardial effusion, cardiomyopathy, claudication)
    Gastroenterology (constipation, ascites)
    Haematology (stiffness and weakness, arthralgia and vague rheumatism, falls)
    Dermatology (dry skin, vitiligo, and alopecia – loss of eyebrow hair is a poor diagnostic sign as it is common in the elderly and may not be present in those who are hypothyroid)
    Thoracic (dyspnoea, pleural effusion)
    Haematological (normochromic normocytic marrow 'depression'/chronic illness effect or macrocytosis/PA) and
    Neurological (cerebellar ataxia, coma, cramps and paraesthesiae, carpal tunnel syndrome and peripheral neuropathy, myopathy, deafness, psychiatric disorder)
(c) Accident and emergency (falls, hypothermia)
(d) Orthopaedic surgeons (falls and fractures)
(e) Surgeons (goitre, deafness)
(f) Psychiatric (depression, agitation, paranoia, 'dementia')
(g) Geriatric (any of the above problems, especially if blunted/modified clinical features and/or social problems)

As with thyrotoxicosis, the usual presence of other pathology often confuses the picture. More than one pathology may be present in the same system, e.g. anaemia (hypothyroidism + iron deficiency), confusion (myxoedema + dementia, arthritis and myopathy).

The elderly tend to grossly under-report illness and under-demand medical help. This may be because of excessive stoicism, reduced symptoms (e.g. pain or fever), or because of a misconceived low expectation of what they deserve at their age. The clinical features of myxoedema often mimic the archetype of a 'senile' old person – often obese, deaf, confused, constipated, immobile most of the time, but ataxic if they get up, huddling up to the fire.

The symptoms and signs may be non-specific but a history of thyroid disease or thyroid medication, a scar in the neck, a goitre, vitiligo, and a person or family history of auto-immune disorders (e.g. PA) are all pointers to the diagnosis. Bradycardia is not always present but there are relatively few other causes of a slow pulse in old people (conduction defects such as heart block due to IHD rather than myxoedema; obstructive jaundice, excessive digoxin, or beta-blockade) who are unlikely to have a significant sinus bradycardia because of athletic fitness. The 'myotonic' tendon reflex is a poor sign unless the myxoedema is grossly obvious and in any case many older people have absent ankle jerks – the place where it is best tested.

Hypothyroidism is nearly always due to primary thyroid disease, but hypopituitarism can occur. Whether or not a suggestive history, symptoms, and signs are elicited, unwellness *per se* merits checking TFTs for hypothyroidism.

Management

It is better to be euthyroid than hypothyroid, which is a morbid and mortal condition. Except in the special circumstances of hypothermia (q.v.) where rapid-acting LT3 is indicated, LT4 is the drug of choice. A once-a-day dosage is all that is needed as the half-life is 7 to 8 days, and titration relies on clinical and biochemical monitoring. T4 is preferable to T3 and to biologically derived thyroid hormone such as desiccated thyroid or thyroglobulin (Leboff *et al.*, 1982).

The need for caution in the presence of cardiac disease, and of cardiac decompensation even without coexistent IHD, has already been mentioned. Doses of the order of 25 to 50 mcg incrementally increased by the same amount every 2 to 3 weeks, with or without beta-blockade, are indicated in this situation. Complications due to excessive stimulation of other tissues may develop, such as thyroid-induced mania (Josephson and Mackenzie, 1980), while myxoedema madness, apparent dementia, and depression may be cured by restoring euthyroidism, or transient neural thyrotoxicosis may develop due to the abnormal modulation of catechol receptor sensitivity.

Older people often seem to need less LT4 to restore and maintain euthyroidism. The difference is most marked between old and young men, as many older women seem to need similar dosages to younger patients (Sawin *et al.*, 1983). Nevertheless, caution should be exercised when increasing the dose to more than 200 μg of thyroxine a day. These observations tally with the finding that thyroid hormone secretion tends to fall with advancing age, presumably because a variety of metabolic changes maintain a normal level of free T4 acting on receptors. Treatment should be maintained lifelong.

Hypothermia

This is rarely due to thyroid deficiency although hypothermic victims often look myxoedematous and may have abnormal TFTs. Hypothyroidism can directly cause a reduced deep body temperature via central pathways and lowered basal metabolism. Obviously coexistent cardiorespiratory, infective, musculoskeletal, and cerebral disease coupled with falls and/or inadequate heating or bad weather may summate with even mild hypothyroidism to precipitate hypothermia. A case has been reported of reversible myxoedema coma being induced in a 65 year old woman by a beta-blocker; the patient's core temperature had fallen to the 'prehypothermic' level of 35.5 °C (Murakami *et al.*, 1982).

TFTs may be truly abnormal in hypothermic victims but obviously a decision on treatment is needed before even the best laboratory can supply results. Specific treatment with LT3 can successfully revive even comatose myxoedematous patients (Graham and Harding, 1977). A clear history, e.g. of myxoedematous features, of stopping thyroid tablets, or possibly of just finding a thyroidectomy scar, might jus-

tify LT3 treatment. This should be given i.v. in small doses, e.g. 10 μg 6 to 8 hourly, and of course other non-specific resuscitative measures will be needed. LT4 in very small doses can then be introduced into the regime to replace the LT3 as the patient recovers.

ADRENAL FUNCTION

Adrenocortical Function

Ageing

Adenomatous and nodular hyperplastic changes have been reported in the cortex of adrenal glands from elderly subjects (Dobie, 1969). These changes are often multifocal and in both glands, and may be due to hyperplasia reactive to a reduced blood supply. Hyper- and hypoadrenalism can occur in the elderly and Cushings' syndrome can also develop secondary to pituitary dysfunction. Kernohan and Sayre (1956) reported a chromophobe adenoma in an 85 year old. Small adenomata are fairly often found at post-mortem in pituitaries from the elderly, but as with the adrenal changes they rarely seem to reflect any clinical abnormality.

The main age-related changes in adrenal function are summarized in Fig. 7. They include a tendency to reduced production and utilization and clearance (metabolism plus excretion) of cortisol and its metabolites. Romanoff and coworkers (1961) showed a 25 per cent. drop in daily cortisol production in relatively young old men compared to 21 to 35 year olds. Although most surveys have confirmed these changes, Murray and coworkers (1981) did not find any age-related differences in cortisol production or urinary excretion.

There is also a tendency to a blunting or abolition of the nocturnal drop in cortisol levels compared with the daytime levels – the circadian or nyctohemeral rhythm. The daytime levels may be raised somewhat above normal basal levels but still remain within the normal range. These changes are thought to be partly due to increased physical, psychological, or environmental stress, e.g. any acute or chronic physical illness, surgery, anxiety, or cold. It has been suggested that depressive illness may blunt CNS–adrenal sensitivity (Carroll, 1969).

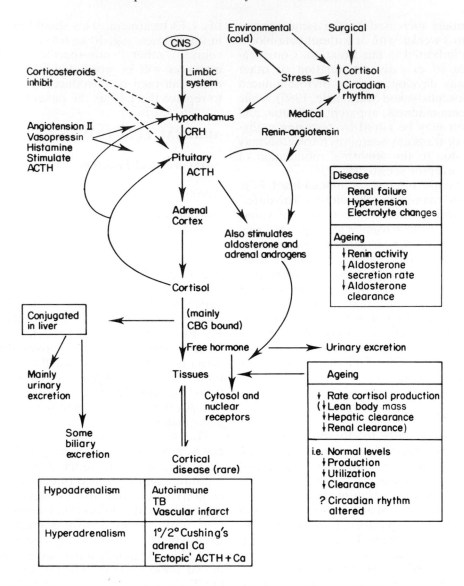

Figure 7   Adrenal function

As with the basic observation of reduced glucocorticoid turnover, not all surveys have confirmed a blunted or abolished circadian rhythm of cortisol in the elderly. Murray and coworkers (1981) only found significantly increased night-time cortisol levels in elderly men, but as already mentioned they had shown 'normal' values for mean cortisol production and urinary excretion of free cortisol. Colucci and coworkers (1975) found a normal circadian rhythm in 'healthy' and hemiplegic elderly subjects, the rhythm being abolished in blind eld-

erly subjects. Dean and Felton (1979) found no evidence of altered periodicity and suggested that the method of assaying cortisol was particularly important as it might be affected by disease or drugs.

Reduced turnover and sustained night-time cortisol levels is possibly due to reduced utilization and clearance of cortisol in the elderly. Renal impairment would obviously reduce renal clearance and altered cyclic AMP/adenyl cyclase/cell receptor systems, particularly in the liver, could reduce cortisol conjugation and metabolism. Reduced muscle mass which is a common finding in old age and generally reduced basal metabolism could also diminish cortisol 'needs'. The intact negative feedback system through the CNS would down-regulate cortisol secretion to ensure normal circulating levels, unless more is required to response to stress. Even the relatively well elderly with apparently normal feedback mechanisms may have sustained nocturnal cortisol levels because they are being stressed.

Insomnia from whatever cause, or waking to empty the bladder, could, presumably, contribute to sustained nocturnal cortisol levels. We did not study the sleep patterns of our subjects in detail but they were asleep during the night-time investigations and blood samples were taken gently from an indwelling catheter (Friedman, Green, and Sharland, 1969; Green and Friedman, 1968).

All the surveys of old subjects seem to agree that the hypothalamic–pituitary–adrenal response and levels of circulating ACTH are normal in the elderly. Our own work that had shown evidence of reduced circadian rhythm showed normal responses to hypoglycaemia and dexamethasone suppression. Synthetic ACTH produced a normal response but ACTH injections caused a higher-than-expected cortisol response, presumably due to reduced adrenal responsiveness and/or clearance. A variety of tests such as insulin hypoglycaemia measuring the cortisol and growth hormone response, the Metyraprone test of the hypothalamic–pituitary–adrenal access (best done by i.v. testing), and ACTH and dexamethasone suppression have confirmed the normal functioning of the CNS–adrenal access in the elderly (Cartlidge *et al.*, 1970; Laron, Doron, and Amilkan, 1970; West *et al.*, 1961).

Clinical Features

Happily, there seems to be little evidence that hyper- or hypoadrenalism are common occurrences in the elderly. However, rarities do occur, and the presentation of disease is so often modified in the elderly that a potentially treatable endocrine rarity can be missed. The clinical features of hypoadrenalism are particularly insidious and hypotension and/or abnormal electrolytes may be assumed to be due to di-

uretics or to severe illness from some other cause. Subnutrition could lead to cortisol depletion or abnormal adrenocortical tests. Vitamin C deficiency might lead to adrenocortical inadequacy because this vitamin is involved in the synthesis of steroids. Dubin, MacLennan, and Hamilton (1978) did not find any evidence of adrenal insufficiency associated with low leucocyte ascorbic acid levels that are thought to reflect poor nutrition.

The elderly are particularly susceptible to the many side-effects of corticosteroids which may cause or aggravate preexisting osteoporosis, diabetes mellitus, gastrointestinal ulceration, hypertension, and psychological disturbance. Prednisolone in a dose of 5 to 7.5 mg a day is roughly equivalent to the normal intrinsic cortisol production, and dosages of this level are unlikely to lead to Cushingoid problems in younger subjects and in some elderly subjects. In elderly people with reduced cortisol clearance, especially those with small body masses, even this modest dose might be potentially harmful. Obviously, the dose of corticosteroids used will be indicated by the clinical condition requiring them. For instance, high doses of corticosteroids are usually used, at least initially, in the treatment of temporal arteritis, polymyalgia rheumatica, and pemphigus.

In every case the dose of corticosteroid should be reviewed regularly, particularly with a view to reducing the dose to the 'physiological' range and if possible stopping it. Abrupt withdrawal of corticosteroids may be followed by a period of adrenal suppression which is potentially serious if the patient is subjected to stress. Normal basal cortisol levels return very quickly after stopping corticosteroids but it may take weeks or even months for full responsiveness of the access to return. This problem can arise even after using modest doses of corticosteroids.

Topical steroids can be absorbed sufficiently to affect adrenocortical function, especially if used over large areas of skin or for a long time. They may also damage skin causing atrophy (especially the fluorinated compounds), or heighten the risk of bacterial or fungal infection of the skin, eye, or mucous membranes. Ageing skin is obviously particularly vulnerable.

There is no evidence that 'shocked' or very

ill old people are likely to have adrenal failure. Blichert-Toft (1975) confirmed this in elderly surgical patients. Mills (1976) found no evidence of hypoadrenalism in hypothermic victims. Corticosteroids have been used to minimize shock. There is no evidence that they are non-specifically beneficial in very ill elderly people.

The use of the corticosteroid dexamethasone as an antioedema agent in treating acute shock is now debatable.

Conclusion

Corticosteroids should be used with care in the elderly, especially on a long-term basis. There is no indication for their use in 'shock' or hypothermia. Screening tests for adrenal dysfunction should be considered in very ill patients, especially those with septicaemia, tuberculosis, disordered electrolytes, or hypotension (that may be caused by or reflect hypoadrenalism).

OESTROGENS AND OVARIAN FUNCTION

The primary event in human female gonadal ageing is a failure, usually relatively abrupt, of ovulation in the face of normal continuing hypothalamic–pituitary gonadotrophin stimulation. The cyclical hormonal pattern initiated at the menarche ceases at the menopause as ovarian follicles fail to mature and menstruation stops. The ovarian stroma becomes fibrotic and collagen is deposited.

Circulating oestrogen levels fall which is thought to be the cause of the characteristic short-term physical (e.g. hot flushes) and psychological (e.g. anxiety) effects known overall as the climacteric, and longer-term pathology including skin and vulvo–vaginal atrophy, increased risk of the syndrome of 'bone loss of ageing', and an increased risk of cardiovascular disease.

In most mammals studied ovarian involution is much slower and menstrual cycles may continue into old age, sometimes even with normal ovulation. Functional follicles may be found in most aged mammals, e.g. the rat and the monkey (Norris and Taylor, 1968). In most cases in animals, ovarian involution seems to be secondary to primary hypothalamic–pituitary fail-

ure and the ovaries tend to remain sensitive to gonadal stimulation.

The Menopause

The perimenopause is the pattern of hormonal and clinical changes occurring before, during, and after the menopause which is marked by the permanent cessation of menstrual cycles. Although the number of oocytes in the ovary falls between pubity and the menopause, some ovarian follicles can be found in the ovary after menstrual cycles cease. However, the number of oocytes has decreased from more than 700,000 at birth and 400,000 at puberty to only about 10,000 by the menopause (Block, 1952). In many women anovular cycles occur with increasing frequency before the menopause in the premenopause. Some ovarian oestrogenic function may continue, albeit declining, for 10 to 15 years after the menopause – the postmenopause.

The length of the menstrual cycle tends to decrease with increasing age but the follicular phase shortens. The central event in the perimenopause is a primary failure of ovarian follicles despite continued and rising stimulation by the pituitary gonadotrophins)GDH); the cessation of menstrual cycles between 40 and 57 with a median age of about 50 years does not seem to have changed for centuries (Jones, 1975). Of course, only the minority of women in the past reached this age. Probably 95 per cent. of women in Western society now reach the menopause and well over half of them live to 75 years.

Further tangential evidence confirming the continuing responsiveness of the pituitary in the face of ovarian failure comes from measurement of drug-induced changes in GDH. For instance, dopamine treatment decreases LH levels mainly by effects on neurones in the median eminence (Pehrson, Jaffee, and Vaitukaitis, 1983) and digoxin suppresses urinary FSH secretion in older women (Burckhardt *et al.*, 1968). This may be because digitalis has a central oestrogen-like effect or because there is some peripheral effect on renal function.

The implications of possibly pathological consequences and deficiency replacement treatment are enormous and tantalizing. Pregnancy is virtually the only condition that cannot occur in old age, and women with climacteric symptoms (most?) may benefit from treatment while appropriate hormonal therapy (HRT) might prevent serious morbidity due to bone or cardiovascular pathology.

Why should the cyclical ovarian–pituitary axis fail? It is not clear whether the failure is simply a consequence of the relative and gross decline in functioning follicles after many years of cyclical ovulation so that normal complete follicular maturation can no longer occur and inadequate levels of progesterone and then oestrogen increasingly fail to prime the necessary pendular and cyclical hormonal changes. There may be a much more intrinsic time and age-related senescent failure of ovarian function.

Less and less progesterone is secreted in the perimenopause but the pituitary continues to produce GDH. In the premenopause LH is grossly elevated, especially at the start of and during the luteal phase of cycles, then FSH rises, cyclical variations in FSH and LH disappear, and postmenopausally FSH rises well above LH levels.

In some women with regular menstrual cycles FSH rises even before the age of 40 (Reyes *et al.*, 1976). It has been suggested that it is the lack of ovarian production of a non-oestrogenic hormonal factor that normally exerts a negative feedback on GDH that prompts the rise in GDH postmenopausally. High levels of GDH are sustained into extreme old age and may still be raised in centenarians, but do tend to drop towards premenopausal levels in most very old women.

It is remarkable that, although the pituitary GDH-producing cells may become hyperplastic postmenopausally in trying to stimulate the non-responsive ovary, there are no records of autonomous nodularity occurring despite the long sustained overactivity of these cells due to the increased feedback stimulation caused by the failure of the target organ.

The rising levels of GDH and falling levels of progesterone are associated with a clear fall in oestradiol but a lesser fall in oestrone and androstenedione because of a sustained or increased peripheral conversion of adrenal hormones, mainly androgens. Oestradiol can be made from testosterone that in itself can be made from adrenal androstenedione. Oestrone can also be made from androstenedione.

The general decline of all ovarian hormones is probably responsible for the physical and psychological clinical features of the perimenopause, but the variability of adrenal androgen conversion is thought to be central to the contribution that ovarian lack makes to postmenopausal/senile osteoporosis (bone loss of ageing). Oestradiol is considerably more potent than oestrone and is the main premenopausal oestrogen, with levels ranging from 100 to 1,000 pmol/l during the menstrual cycle and falling to less than 60 pmol/l postmenopausally. Oestrone levels of 150 to 600 pmol/l with a mean of 320 fall comparatively much less to 50 to 250 pmol/l with a mean of 140 (Crilly, Francis, and Nordin, 1981). This is because relatively more oestrone is derived premenopausally from adrenal androstenedione.

Androstenedione secretion and therefore oestrone production tend to fall with increasing age – the adrenopause. The hormonal conversion of androgen precursors of oestrone and to a lesser extent of oestradiol postmenopausally is mainly in the liver and peripherally, the latter being influenced mainly by body size and fat distribution.

The postmenopausal decline in oestrogens seems to play an important part in the bone loss of ageing because bone is more sensitive to parathormone (PTH).

The general postmenopausal oestrogen drop is obviously a factor in osteoporosis but it has also been suggested by Crilly, Francis, and Nordin (1981) that women with osteoporotic fractures, especially cortical rather than tubecular, have particularly low levels of oestrogen, i.e. they have minimal adrenal production and/or conversion of hormones which in other women may be sufficient to maintain bone mass despite the loss of ovarian oestrone and oestradiol. Whether or not this group have a specific enzyme defect in the adrenal without evidence of other adrenal insufficiency has not yet been established. Early and/or severe and multiple osteoporotic fracture in ageing women reflecting accelerated bone loss obviously does suggest that some other factors are operating in them over and above the general decline in oestrogens, and the increasing likelihood of a poor diet and reduced mobility.

The main suggestion that has been made to account for this, especially in terms of trabecular osteoporosis, is a malabsorption of calcium, but whether this is due to dietary insufficiency or some specific malabsorptive defect possibly caused by lack of small intestinal responsiveness to vitamin D is not clear.

Slight rises in plasma calcium and phosphate and urinary calcium excretion as well as urinary hydroxyproline and alkaline phosphatase are thought to be due to oestrogen lack. Despite a readjustment of PTH secretion there is a net negative balance of calcium associated with slightly increased bone absorption. This loss affects trabecular more than cortical bone, especially in the first few postmenopausal years, although effects on cortical loss may continue much longer. Obviously osteoporosis/bone loss of ageing is complex and hormonal factors may only be pathologically significant if superimposed on previously poor bone mass or associated with other aetiological factors such as inadequate diet or immobility.

However, it is generally agreed that an early and/or severe adrenopause and also of course an early menopause (especially due to oophorectomy) predisposes to earlier and more severe osteoporosis. As so often happens in preventive medicine, it is difficult to translate possible/probable explanations of disease aetiology into effective prophylaxis. Should one look among all menopausal women for those most severely oestrogen deficient, i.e. with little or no adrenal androgen production or conversion of adrenal androgens to oestrogens? This would of course be a vast screening programme involving difficult and expensive blood and urinary assays. Those identified would be presumed to be the most at risk of developing bone, cardiovascular, and skin problems (see below). Even if the benefit of giving HRT to this group can only be detected for 5 to 10 years postmenopausally, as some authorities believe, it would still be theoretically valuable for these individuals to have HRT. If this group could be identified how should they and older women with established fractures be treated? Should hormones be oestrogens or oestrogen/progestagen or hormones with dietary supplements, e.g. calcium, vitamin D, fluoride, or some combination? (See Chapter 25.2.)

The details of hormonal treatment of the climacteric and the pros and cons of which drug(s) and at what dose, and whether HRT should be given cyclically and for how long are obviously not usually a problem for doctors dealing with the elderly. Even if a satisfactory and effective HRT regime could be devised in terms of relieving the very real climacteric symptoms experienced by many women, with minimal thromboembolic, carcinogenic (to breast and endometrium), or hyperlipidaemic risk would this regime be applicable to use in older women prophylactically? In other words, are conclusions about women in the immediate postmenopausal period of their lives relevant to older women? Somewhat surprisingly a significant proportion of geriatric physicians as well as orthopaedic surgeons, urologists, and others interested in the treatment of urinary incontinence do use HRT in very elderly women. Boyle (1981) reported a survey among 650 specialists, with rather more than one-third of geriatricians using oestrogens for postmenopausal osteoporosis, while about one-quarter of orthopaedic surgeons used oestrogen treatment and almost 100 per cent. of gynaecologists used oestrogens in elderly women. The gynaecologists almost always combined oestrogen with a progestagen while geriatricians and rheumatologists usually did not. He also commented that vitamin D was widely used with or without calcium as a treatment for osteoporosis.

It has also been suggested that anabolic steroids are a more effective way of reducing fracture rates in elderly women than oestrogens, calcium, and vitamin D supplements maintaining mobility, fluoride or calcitonin, or any combination of these treatments (Clements and Hamilton, 1983).

The increasing risk of ischaemic heart disease in older women and the preponderance of older women suggest that it would be worth looking for possible factors such as the hormonal decline in older women if one wanted to try and prevent heart disease in the elderly, although of course men are more likely to develop ischaemic heart disease, at least in middle age. There does not seem to be very strong evidence that early menopause or artificial delay of the menopause or HRT at the menopause or in old age will have a preventive effect on ischaemic heart disease (Leader, 1977). The counterproductive thromboembolic effect of hormonal replacement therapy must be taken into account.

Rakoff and Nowroozi (1978), in reviewing

the female climacteric, discuss the pros and cons of oestrogen therapy in postmenopausal women. Although they clearly recognize the untoward effects of oestrogens, including the possible absorption of topical oestrogens used as vaginal creams or suppositories, they believe that HRT can help atrophic vulvo-vaginitis, osteoporosis, and vague psychological feelings of malaise. As with so many experts in this field, they refer to the problem of 'breakthrough bleeding' whether or not the patient is on cyclical or continuous therapy. Such bleeding not only calls for pelvic examination, cytological smears, temporary stopping of therapy, but may also require diagnostic curettage. The bleeding may be caused by benign polyps or myomas or hyperplasia rather than carcinoma.

North American gynaecologists appear to be more prepared to take on the follow-up of large numbers of oestrogen-treated elderly women than in other parts of the world. Ross and coworkers (1980) do not feel that all women at the menopause subsequently should be given oestrogens but that:

> . . . until enough substantiated data are available to resolve these points of controversy, many clinicians, including ourselves, follow an intermediary course centered on the potential benefits and hazards for the individual patient. Oestrogen therapy is recommended for the treatment of the menopausal syndrome and is given cyclically in the smallest effective dose. Risk factors are evaluated on an individual basis. . . . Oestrogen therapy is initiated or continued in postmenopausal patients who develop clinical or radiologic evidence of osteoporosis. The possible benefits and risks are discussed with the patient not only to obtain informed consent but to provide information which will help her make a decision.

Ross and coworkers (1980) concluded that:

> . . . a woman undergoing natural menopause at age 50 years who receives 1.25 mg of replacement oestrogen therapy daily for approximately 3 years would increase her lifetime probability of getting breast cancer by age 75 from 6–12 per cent. if no latency is required to almost 10 per cent. if a 5 year latency is required, and to 9 per cent. allowing for a 10 year latency.

They felt that the sizeable increases in predicted mortality meant that the benefits of oestrogen therapy at this dosage would have to be great to warrant such a risk. At lower doses the risk-to-benefit ratio would be more favourable, but they also estimated that breast cancer risk was likely to be raised if a total cumulative dose of 1,500 mg of oestrogen had been ingested.

Whedon (1981) believes that low-dose oestrogen therapy, e.g. 0.625 mg of conjugated oestrogen per day, which definitely slows the rate of bone resorption is a justifiable prophylactic treatment. He states that even the possible induction of endometrial carcinoma is acceptable and that this form of cancer is often easily detected and has a high cure rate. He states that cyclic administration of oestrogen with an added progestin during the final 5 days of the cycle can reduce the risk of endometrial carcinoma. Jensen *et al.* (1982) also inclined to this view.

Studd and Thom (1981) are protagonists of HRT treatment of the climacteric and the menopause. They 'have one of the largest menopause clinics in Europe . . . and have collected data from over 1,000 patients who have received oestrogen preparations for up to 30 years' and do not feel that gloomy predications about thromboembolic complications, diabetes mellitus, hypertension, strokes, heart attacks, and breast and endometrial carcinoma are justified. If anything they believe that oestrogen therapy not only reduces osteoporosis but may also reduce the incidence of hypertension, strokes, and heart attacks.

Crilly, Francis, and Nordin (1981), in reviewing steroid hormones, ageing, and bone, discuss the menopause and adrenopause. They state that postmenopausal 'hormonal' status is perhaps more closely related to cortical than trabecular bone loss, but these two types of bone are of course interrelated and hormonal deficiency and calcium malabsorption should both be regarded as risk factors in most types of osteoporosis.

Clements and Hamilton (1983) state dogmatically that oestrogens in any form will prevent rapid bone loss following oophorectomy and that the effect persists for 5 to 10 years. Then, however, age-related loss supervenes. They remind the reader that corticosteroids reduce bone formation and reduce calcium absorption from the gut by an effect on vitamin D. It may also directly affect adrenal oestrone production. Thyrotoxicosis directly affects bone by increasing resorption and in diabetes insulin deficiency impairs bone formation so that osteoporosis is more likely in patients with these endocrine disorders, especially if they have other adverse risk factors or a low bone mass to start with. They review the evidence for the use of oestrogens and suggest that a major reason for the protection from fracture is by decrease in bone resorption caused by a rise in plasma calcitonin. Once again they remind us that oestrogens are most effective in the rapid phase of bone loss immediately post-menopausally, but that their longer term use has not been established. They give some guidelines to selecting the subgroup of the population most likely to be at risk of fracture, e.g. small, fairskinned, nulliparous women with little body hair and particularly of Scottish, Irish, or Anglo-Saxon extraction, as well as obviously those who have had a premature menopause resulting from oophorectomy. They list a variety of contraindications to oestrogens including a history of carcinoma or various uterine conditions, hypertension, cardiovascular disease, varicose veins, gallstones, and liver disease and they dogmatically state that women over 65 should not receive oestrogens.

The need to try and organize a more rational and national approach for the community treatment of the menopause was reviewed recently by Cooke in a *British Medical Journal* Leader (1983), and Craig, 1983 (Cooke, 1983; Craig, 1983). The main objectives are to give advice to women at the menopause, to help relieve unpleasant menopausal symptoms, and prophylactically to reduce later life complications, particularly bone problems. Cooke, in the *British Medical Journal* Leader, suggests that an attempt should be made to treat all perimenopausal women even though only half have symptoms. He believes that as much as 15 years of treatment is needed to reduce the impact of osteoporosis in older women who will therefore need to take it from at least 50 to the age of 65. He reminds us that one-quarter of all women over 60 will develop vertebral collapse and one-fifth will have had a fractured hip by the age of 90. Eighty per cent. of elderly women with fractured hips have osteoporosis and one in seven will be dead within 3 months. While Cooke does not seem too concerned about the neoplastic complica-

tions of oestrogens, especially when combined with a sequential progestagen for 10 days, he suggests that a non-hormonal alternative might be preferable. Craig's guidelines for community and menopausal clinics is a helpful and well-thought-out summary of how to help menopausal women, but understandably does not really tackle the major problem of what to do in much older women.

HRT Treatment

If it is decided to give oestrogens to a menopausal or elderly woman despite the possible thromboembolic, arterial, hepatic, gall-bladder, and neoplastic risks the following guidelines would seem to be the most acceptable:

(a) Use the lowest effective dose to control symptoms. This criteria could not be applied, of course, in the prophylactic treatment of osteoporosis.

(b) Use an oestrogen/progestagen combination.

(c) Most authorities seem to recommend cyclical treatment for perimenopausal women but are more inclined to use sequential therapy in the elderly (e.g. the progestagen is given for 10 days in every 28), the oestrogen being given continuously.

(d) If the diagnosis and management of bleeding is likely to be a particular problem, e.g. in the older woman, oral oestradiol is probably preferable to conjugated oestrogens. It is suggested that problems, particularly endometrial proliferation, are minimized by using daily doses of less than 1 mg of oestradiol and less than 0.625 mg of conjugated oestrogens.

(e) The patient should be examined regularly, e.g. at least 6-monthly, and curettage should be considered yearly as a precaution as well as curettage in case of breakthrough bleeding in people taking continuous therapy and abnormal bleeding in those on cyclical therapy.

(f) Repeat prescriptions should only be issued after review of the patient, in particular in respect of the development of complications and contraindications.

(g) Most authorities believe that HRT should not be given for periods of more than 5 years, even where there are clinical symptoms rather than just the use of prophylactic hormone.

(h) Topical oestrogen therapy particularly for vulvo-vaginitis and urinary incontinence thought to be due to local dermal, subdermal, and muscular atrophy should also be given at the lowest possible dose to control symptoms and again only for relatively short periods.

(i) There appears to be no justification for the use of stilboestrol in women.

(j) As already pointed out, corticosteroids accentuate the bone loss of ageing and should be avoided if possible. If required, e.g. to treat temporal arteritis, polymyalgia, rheumatica, or pemphigus, the dose should be reduced to below 5 to 7.5 mg/d as soon as possible.

Although women may get considerable physical and psychological benefit from oestrogens in the perimenopause and oestrogens may be justified prophylactically and therapeutically in older women there is certainly no justification on the evidence at present for giving HRT to all women to prevent 'ageing'. There is no evidence that a hormonal elixir of life, including oestrogens, can prevent senescence or increase life expectation.

Hormonal Tumours in Women

Virtually any hormone or hormone analogue or hormone stimulating or inhibiting hormone can be produced by tumours, especially bronchogenic carcinoma which may occur in the elderly. Although ACTH-like substances are probably the commonest hormones produced by tumours, hypercalcaemia, hypernatraemia, and other hormone/electrolyte changes may be due to underlying neoplasia. Ovarian and other specific hormonal tumours may occur in the elderly. An interesting example was described by De Lange, Pratt, and Doorenbos (1980). They reported an adrenal cortical adenoma producing testosterone. The tumour was gonadotrophin responsive.

Ovarian tumours may occur in the menopause and may secrete hormones. The commonest is a granulosa-theca cell tumour. As already mentioned, tumours may produce hormones other than their own primary secretion (in this case oestrogens and progesterone), and

may produce ACTH parathormone, thyroxine, androgens, gonadotrophins, and corticosteroids.

Granulosa-theca cell tumours account for more than two-thirds of oestrogen-secreting tumours and about 60 per cent. occur in postmenopausal women. Most of these tumours are small and the prognosis after surgery is good, although they tend to recur – even up to 15 years after the original surgical removal. These tumours tend to present with the secondary effects of increased oestrogens including uterine bleeding (which may also be due to endometrial carcinoma which may be associated with these tumours), uterine enlargement, and breast enlargement. Ash and Greenblatt (1978) have reviewed these and other endocrine tumours including virilizing ovarian and adrenal tumours in elderly women.

Breast cancer is of course the commonest cancer in women and occurs in older women. Although the traditional view has been that premenopausal women with advanced breast cancer may respond to oestrogen ablation and postmenopausal women with advanced/metastatic breast cancer are relatively oestrogen responsive, individuals do not always conform to these guidelines. Androgens as well as oestrogens may cause tumour aggression in elderly women, and sometimes multiply therapy may be effective including the use of androgens after oestrogens. The drug Tamoxifen, which in simple terms is an antioestrogen, seems to be very effective in most elderly women, which appears to contradict the guideline that these patients should respond to oestrogen supplementation. Tamoxifen acts by blocking the entry of oestrogen into target organs by binding onto cytocell oestrogen receptors.

TESTICULAR FUNCTION

The physical, psychological, and biochemical changes of the menopause may vary in the acuteness of their onset and severity, but inevitable irreversible ovarian involution is a relatively abrupt event. It is usually completed in 1 to 2 years and at about 50 years of age or soon after all women show no ovarian function, i.e. no ovulation and no ovarian oestrogen production. As already discussed, menopausal ovarian failure is not yet explained but the most likely reason is a primary reduction in ovarian sensitivity to gonadotrophins – cause unknown.

Testicular function and androgen production decline with advancing age in men, but gradually and starting at a later age, i.e. over 60. Some men retain fertility – not the only but an important aspect of normal testicular function – well into old age and sexual activity *per se* does not seem to be related to testosterone levels. There is some disagreement about the gonadotrophin levels in older men which, on logical grounds and by a comparison with postmenopausal women, one would expect to rise. Most researchers have suggested that there is an elevation of serum gonadotrophins (Kley, 1976; Sterns *et al.*, 1974), but not to the levels seen in postmenopausal women.

The andropause, if it exists at all, therefore seems to differ endocrinologically speaking from the menopause. Furthermore, the mechanism of seminiferous failure actually seems to be more clearly worked out, resulting from a decrease in Leydig cell mass and responsiveness due to a reduced blood supply (Albeaux-Fernet *et al.*, 1972). The reduced blood supply is presumably due to arteriosclerosis. It has been suggested that the central hormone lesion is a reduced level of steroid precursors in mitochondria, rather than a failure of steroid formation by the mitochondria (Takahashi *et al.*, 1983).

The Andropause

In general terms the pathophysiological changes in men as they age are:

(a) A decreased Leydig cell mass and cell number. It has, however, been suggested that Leydig cell volume has actually increased. The testicles in older men are usually normal in size (Hudson, Coghlan, and Dulmanis, 1976).

(b) Testosterone and some of its normal immediate precursors, e.g. dihydroepiandrosterone, tend to decrease in testicular and spermatic vein plasma after the age of 60 (Pirke, Sintermann, and Vogt, 1980). Elderly men may have normal adult testosterone levels, albeit at the lower end of the normal range.

(c) These somewhat conflicting observations may be explained by a general but not individually inevitable negative imbalance of total testosterone production. This tendency results from the mixture of reduced total testosterone secretion, increased testosterone binding globulin (TeBG), and a consequent reduction in free active hormone and of reduced metabolic clearance. The average serum testosterone in men aged from 60 to 90 is 3 ng/ml, normal being 4 to 12 ng/ml (Nieschlag *et al.*, 1973).

(d) Pituitary gonadotrophin (FSH and LH) levels do not seem to rise in all older men, as they do in women postmenopausally. Gonadotrophin levels are generally elevated (Baker *et al.*, 1976), but not to levels one may expect to result from target organ failure, even allowing for the later and slower decline in seminiferous tubular function compared with the ovaries. Some elderly male individuals may have low gonadotrophin levels. Leydig cell failure seems to provoke a rise in LH as testosterone falls. Sertoli cell dysfunction causes faulty spermatogenesis and a rise in FSH. The rise in FSH is usually more than that in LH.

(e) The current explanation is that the Sertoli cells secrete a hormone, known as inhibin or factor X, that inhibits the production of gonadotrophin.

This low molecular weight non-steroidal peptide hormone is produced as long as spermatogenesis is continued or Sertoli cells are still functioning, even if plasma testosterone levels are very low (see also (h) below). Inhibin is apparently presenting the pituitary gonadotrophin response to low plasma testosterone levels (Leonard *et al.*, 1972; Peek and Watkins, 1980). The Leydig cells in older men do not seem to respond properly to stimulation with HCG.

(f) Some testosterone precursors such as progesterone and cell 17-alpha hydroxyprogesterone show a relative and sometimes absolute increase in free and protein bound levels in testicular tissue and spermatic vein plasma levels in older men (Pirke, Sintermann, and Vogt, 1980). The postulated explanation is that hypoxia presumably due to atherosclerosis favours testosterone production via progesterone and 17-alpha hydroxyprogesterone precursors rather than via 17-alpha hydroxypregnenolone. This has been supported by *in vitro* testicular tissue incubation experiments. This explanation is preferred to an idiopathic, i.e. unexplained, primary failure of Leydig cell function, possibly due to deficiencies of enzymes needed for normal testosterone synthesis, e.g. C-17, 20-lyase, or 17-beta hydroxylase. The hypoxic/atheromatous explanation is further supported by the finding of atherosclerotic changes in testicular blood vessels and of degenerative tubular changes in old men.

(g) Similarly, 5-alpha metabolites of testosterone and dehydrotesterone such as 5-alpha androstane/3-alpha, 17-beta diol tend to decrease markedly with advancing age, especially compared to 5-beta metabolites (Ghanadian and Puah, 1981).

(h) Plasma oestrogens are clearly raised in older men (Kley *et al.*, 1976). This seems to be due to:

   (i) Increased peripheral androgen conversion, e.g. testosterone to oestrodiol and androstenedione to oestrone.

   (ii) A greater protein binding affinity of TeBG for androgens than oestrogens, especially if TeBG is increased, as it often seems to be in older men, rather than an increased Leydig cell oestrogen production. The relative and sometimes absolute rise in oestrogens, especially in the free form, may be a factor in blocking the expected pituitary gonadotrophin response to declining testosterone levels.

Clinical Implications

The implications of these chemicopathological observations is not clear. The more gradual and later effects of defective testicular function compared with the menopause makes it difficult to establish that psychological, physomatic, and physical symptoms in older men are due to testicular deterioration. Even specific sex-related problems such as impotence are rarely due to easily remediable sex hormone deficiency at any age.

Albeaux-Fernet, Bohler, and Karpas (1978) strongly support the idea, based on their clinical and research observations, that symptoms such as impotence, depression, fatigue, 'cluster' headaches, various forms of arthritis, a variety of so-called psychoneurotic symptoms of lassitude and anxiety, possible scrotalpruritis, and bladder tone problems 'not due to prostatism' may be caused by testosterone deficiency and respond to replacement therapy. They believe that the diagnosis is supported by finding low plasma testosterone levels, especially if LH and/or FSH are related and the free plasma oestrogen ratio is particularly abnormal.

These hormonal parameters are rarely tested for in older men; perhaps they should be. Certainly it is perfectly proper to try and diagnose and treat even the most specific and apparently psychosomatic/neurotic symptoms. Older men and their spouses/consorts do not often ask for advice about their physical or emotional relationships, but if they do then a full history and examination are justified, possibly followed by suitable endocrine investigations.

The proof of a correct diagnosis is, of course, successful treatment. Greenblatt and the other protagonists of androgen replacement therapy in selected elderly men with low hormone levels, i.e. those correctly diagnosed, believe that the andropause is an endocrinopathy sometimes requiring replacement therapy.

The data of Davidson and coworkers (1983) support the conclusion that hormonal changes in older men are related to sexual activity and to a lesser extent to libido. The hormone relationship changes were not caused by drugs or disease.

The protagonists believe that the advantages of male sex hormone replacement are:

(a) Amelioration (cure) of the physical and psychological andropausal symptoms as described above.

(b) A decrease in cholesterol when used in modest doses and then, therefore, a possible decrease in cardiovascular disease.

(c) Improvement in 'arthritic' symptoms. A possible explanation is that testosterone displaces protein-bound cortisol and increases the free active levels of cortisol, or that some testosterone is converted to oestrogens which also increase unbound cortisol levels.

(d) An anti-ageing effect due to a reduction in transcription errors in the RNA synthesis.

(e) A possible reduction in the risk of metabolic bone disease. Androgens might reduce the risk of oesteoporosis (osteopenia) by an anabolic effect or by contributing to the pool of androgens available for conversion to oestrogens. However, oesteoporosis seems to be much less common in older men. This is thought to be due to greater bone mass in men, more likelihood of sustained periosteal stimulation because of greater physical activity in men, and adequately maintained levels of oestrogen in older men (derived from testicular and adrenal androgens).

Against these possible advantages testosterone and its esters may cause:

(a) Cholestatic liver damage
(b) Gynaecomastia
(c) Prostatic hypertrophy and even malignant change
(d) An increase in atheroclerotic complications, especially cardiac
(e) An increased haemoglobin due to an increased red cell number (androgens having been used in the treatment of aplastic anaemia)

If it is decided to use androgens in older men oral preparations are usually preferred to regular injections of long-acting steroids (which have to be given at weekly or fortnightly intervals) or parenteral pellet implants (renewed 4 to 6 monthly). Fluoxymesterone is more potent and less toxic than methyltestosterone. A starting dose of 10 to 25 mg a day is titrated downwards or upwards depending on the clinical responses and side-effects, and then continued for 3 to 6 months. This is repeated once or twice a year. Absolute contraindications to this form of therapy would be a history or finding of benign hypertrophy or malignant change of the prostate. An elevated haemaglobin or abnormalities of liver function tests occurring during treatment would indicate a need to reduce and probably stop the androgen.

Prostatic Disease

The general observation that testicular failure occurs without any gross rise in gonadotrophins in ageing men may be an important factor in the low incidence of testicular hyperplasia and frank malignancy in old men, in contrast to the situation described for women (Hughes and Caron, 1975). At the same time, a sustained production of extratesticular oestrogens in old age and a continuing conversion of some of the testicular testosterone which is still being produced, and possibly a proportionate increase in the oestrogen/androgen ratio, could all be important hormonal factors in the aetiology of benign prostatic hypertrophy (BPH) and possibly malignant prostatic disease. Perhaps 80 per cent. of 65 year old men have nodular hyperplasia (which is BPH) and 20 to 25 per cent. of older men will have significant outflow obstruction. Carcinoma of the prostate has been said to be found on microscopic examinations in a very large proportion of glands studied at post-mortem, although it is clinically manifest in a relatively small number of elderly men.

Whatever the hormonal links and similarities, BPH and prostatic cancer are not the same disease and will not necessarily have the same aetiology. BPH develops as a nodular hyperplasia in the proximal periurethral pelvic urethra. Prostatic cancer usually seems to start in the capsule and spreads through and out of the normal prostatic tissue.

There has been considerable interest in the possible hormonal aetiology of cancers which are 'sex-linked', such as malignancies of the breast, uterus, and prostate. It is often difficult to decide whether abnormal levels of sex hormones and metabolites might be primarily contributing to the pathology or simply a consequence of disorders of tissues involved in the production or metabolism of sex hormones. Prostatic hypertrophy and tumours do not occur in early hypophysectomized or castrated men or animals. Prostatic nodularity in castrated dogs can be induced using androgen and oestrogen (Jacobi, Moore, and Wilson, 1978).

It has been found that:

(a) 5-Alpha dihyroxytesterone (DHT) accumulates in benign prostatic hypertrophy (BPH) tissues. These tissues show a relative reduction in metabolites of this hormone. These findings are perhaps due to reduced levels of 5-reductase.

(b) Patients with BPH tend to have higher serum levels of DHT, presumably secreted by the BPH tissues. They also tend to have slightly higher than normal free and active serum levels of testosterone.

Hammond and coworkers (1978) recorded significantly higher serum levels of DHT and 17-alpha OH progesterone in elderly men with BPH than normal elderly and younger men. Those with BPH also showed somewhat elevated plasma concentrations of progesterone and testosterone. High normal levels of DHT and 17-alpha OH progesterone occur in patients with carcinoma of the prostate. The serum levels of other sex hormones and metabolites studied (pregnanolone, androstenedione, andosterone, and oestradiol) were not altered in the BPH and carcinoma groups. Geller and Albert (1982), in reviewing several surveys of plasma steroids and ageing in patients with BPH, feel that there is no difference in testosterone, but probably an increase in DHT in BPH. All these findings should be considered against the general background of a down-trend in the levels of testosterone with advancing age.

Somewhat higher total levels of oestrogens (e.g. oestradiol) in older men may not be significant as there is a parallel increase of binding globulin, i.e. there is no significant increase in free (active) oestrogen. The evidence on whether oestrogen receptors are present in normal or BPH prostate tissue is conflicting.

The generally raised hormone levels do not, however, appear to be sufficiently abnormal to be used as simple screening/diagnostic tests to confirm BPH or Ca.

It is suggested that testosterone and DHT stimulate the growth of prostatic tissue, thus contributing to benign and nodular hyperplasia and possibly to malignant change. It has also been suggested that stimulating circulating steroids does not necessarily reflect the intraprostate hormonal climate. It is often difficult to be sure whether carcinoma of the prostate is coexistently present with BPH, and the endocrinological abnormalities described do not help further in deciding whether these two prostatic pathologies have a common hormonal aetiology. In particular they do not resolve the problem already raised of hormonal abnormalities being a primary cause or merely due to secondary metabolic consequences of hyperplasia or malignancy. At least half the men with cancer of the prostate have coincidental BPH.

Patients with prostatic disease may have altered androgen receptors. This could be an aetiological factor. It could also affect the response to treatment.

Cancer of the Prostate

The most striking thing about the present treatment for cancer of the prostate is that there is no universally agreed treatment. This is a disease of old age, being 200 times commoner in 60 to 80 year old men compared with 20 to 29 year olds.

This is worrying because it is a common disease. There are 8,000 new cases a year in the United Kingdom. Cancer of the lung, bowel, and skin in both sexes, of the breast in women, and prostate in men are the commonest malignancies in older people. Cancer of the prostate is the commonest genitourinary neoplasm and accounts for 10 per cent. of cancer deaths in men. It is very much a disease of older men – both the clinical disease and the *in situ* growths of uncertain significance so often noted during careful histological examination of the gland. Ninety-five per cent. of victims are over the age of 60. It has been estimated that more than 50 per cent. of 80 year old men have *in situ* neoplasia when serial sections of the prostate are examined (Franks, 1976; Swyer, 1944).

The majority have disseminated, often advanced, malignancies at the first presentation – 75 to 80 per cent. in some series. Untreated, the average life expectation is about 2 years, but a life expectation of several years is still possible in treated patients, who may live for as long as 10 years. The commonest metastatic site is bone, causing pain, fracture, and hypercalcaemia, so specific antiprostatic treatment would be preferable to just relying on a nonspecific palliative approach, however skilled (e.g. pain relief, terminal care, nursing, and so on). Ideally, the two should go side by side.

Aetiology

Cancer is common in old age, probably because of several carcinogenic factors, e.g.:

(a) long exposure to carcinogens (this might well apply to genitourinary neoplasia where dietary or tobacco chemicals or metabolites might be excreted over a long period),

(b) an increased chance of mitosis throwing up neoplastic clone during a long life, especially in damaged cells, which might be combined with

(c) decreased immunological surveillance/competence.

The relative frequency of the disease in Caucasians and American negroes, and rarely in Orientals, is unexplained. Men living in rural areas have a slightly higher risk of developing prostatic cancer.

As far as specific factors are concerned, the most striking finding is evidence of relatively increased testosterone and testosterone metabolite levels, including oestrogens, which may also be derived from conversion of adrenal steroids. The combination of raised testosterone and oestrogen is thought to be a cause rather than just a marker of the disease. Prostatic cancer does not occur in men who have had an 'early' hypophysectomy or castration. The disease can be prevented in dogs by castration and potentially malignant nodularity can then be induced in these experimental animals by giving them testosterone and oestrogen.

Similar hormonal abnormalities have been found in benign prostatic hypertrophy (BPH), particularly raised levels of dihydrotestosterone (DHT) and diol. This confuses the issue because some 80 per cent. of 75 year old men are thought to have histological BPH, two-thirds of older men have symptoms due to BPH, and about 15 to 20 per cent. of them may need definitive treatment for resulting urinary tract outflow obstruction (Flocks, 1964). The frequent coexistence of benign and malignant prostatic disease is probably coincidental as there does not appear to be any specific link between the two despite the apparent common hormonal factors. The malignant prostate usually retains hormonal responsiveness to DHT, i.e. the success of endocrine therapy often seems to depend on reducing cell growth by antiandrogen treatment.

Research into androgen cytosol receptors and cellular extracts suggests that there may be some difference in the level of these receptors in the two conditions and that both have levels differing from the normal. There is, however, disagreement about the best method of measuring these receptors and interpretation of the results (Shain *et al.*, 1979). Measurement of androgen receptors might not only indicate a possible cause but might also be relevant to selecting patients most likely to respond to androgen blockade (Bruchovsky *et al.*, 1980).

Cancer of the prostate is not a homogeneous disease. There is a spectrum of histological types ranging from a fast-growing small cell type with few cellular androgen receptors which would be likely to be hormone resistant to a well-differentiated slow-growing indolent hormone-sensitive cancer. Androgen receptor assay might be able to indicate the degree of cancer cell differentiation (Krieg *et al.*, 1979).

Diagnosis

Rectal examination is obligatory in patients with prostatism, urinary retention, bone pain, and fracture. It is not always easy to distinguish BPH from prostatic cancer, or cancer from chronic prostatitis.

Enzyme tests. The significance of raised formol stable acid phosphatase levels is still uncertain. Multiple infarcts in prostatitis may also release this enzyme. A very high level probably reflects an underlying neoplasm. Rising or clearly raised levels are useful in confirming recurrence and spread in proven cases (Gittes, 1983).

Calcium. The frequency of bone involvement and sometimes of the marrow justify bone biochemistry: calcium, inorganic phosphate, and alkaline phosphatase with appropriate protein correction. Hypercalcaemia is usually due to bone invasion, but can also be caused by non-metastic hormonal effects.

A full blood count and ESR. Anaemia may be normocytic, normochromic, especially if uraemia is present, or is sometimes leukoerythroblastic.

Urea and electrolytes. Outflow obstruction may cause renal impairment.

Appropriate skeletal X-rays of symptomatically affected bones may be indicated, i.e. those that hurt and those that break. Prostatic cancer causes osteosclerotic secondaries. An i.v. pyelogram may be needed.

Bone scans may show 'hot spots'. These are usually indicative of malignancy but suggestive areas can sometimes be demonstrated in osteoporosis.

Abdominal ultrasound is not very helpful but rectal probe ultrasound can be very useful in delineating the prostate and indicating the extent of extraprostatic pelvic spread.

Lymphangiography may be useful as pelvic, periaortic, and hepatic spread is common.

Biopsy. Many surgeons regard this as a useful diagnostic tool. Transrectal biopsy may cause urinary tract infection and transperineal biopsy is therefore preferable. Any biopsy may miss cancerous foci. The diagnosis may only be discovered or confirmed during histological examination of prostatic tissue removed at transurethral resection prostatectomy (TURP).

Radiotherapists and oncologists like to know how anaplastic and invasive or well differentiated the cancer is when advising on treatment.

Urinary cytology is of no use.

Treatment
Relief of outflow obstruction. About two-thirds of patients have significant 'prostatism' and one-fifth present in retention.

A few enthusiasts sometimes carry out total prostatectomy and do achieve a cure of early localized disease.

However, TURP is the standard procedure on the basis that it is simple and only needs a short anaesthetic. It can be repeated if symptoms recur. The well-known complications are postoperative infection and bleeding, and urinary incontinence. This may be due to infection, to anatomical damage to outflow mechanisms, or because removal of an obstruction has revealed unsuspected detrusor instability. There is also a possibility that the more extensive the TURP resection is in an attempt

to remove as much neoplastic tissue as possible, the more likely it is that malignant cells are spilled into pelvic veins and lymphatics. If this argument is valid, it would support those who prefer to catheterize for a short period while one of the following antioestrogen treatments is started, in order to avoid surgery.

Endocrine manipulation. As men with prostatic cancer tend to have higher levels of testosterone and/or sex steroid metabolites than age-matched controls this logical approach has been widely used. Measurement of testosterone levels might reflect the response to treatment. As with any antimalignancy treatment one would want a high rate of control, no or low toxicity, and satisfactory compliance. Several of the treatments currently used do cause worrying levels of toxicity.

(a) Stilboestrol has been successfully used for many years, despite other oestrogenic 'challengers'. The doses used have gradually been reduced but, even when given in the range of 0.5 to 1 mg once to three times a day, side-effects are common. Gynaecomastia and even breast cancer (in men), fluid retention, and the precipitation of heart failure are common, but the most worrying problem is a generally increased risk of thromboembolism. It has been suggested that the morbidity and mortality of this drug are worse than the grim toll of prostatic cancer itself, especially in older men who so often have widespread vascular disease.

Although cytotoxic drugs are unrewarding in treating cancer of the prostate and are likely to have a high level of toxicity, a combination of Normustine and Oestradiol (Estramustine phosphate) is said to have a specific affinity to prostatic tissue with relatively low cytotoxic toxicity. It is suggested the beneficial action is considerably stronger than might be expected from the separate effects of oestrogen and cytotoxic agent. It has been recommended for primary treatment (Nilsson and Jonsson, 1978), for long-term control, and particularly for use in recurrent (relapsing) oestrogen-resistant disease (Andersson *et al.*, 1977). Disappearance of soft tissue and bony metastases has been reported (Nilsson and Jonsson, 1978).

(b) Androgen blockade. Whether or not androgen receptors are increased in prostatic cancer, drugs which block these receptors could slow down or arrest the malignant process in secondary as well as primary growth. Cyproterone is an antiandrogen which has been available for almost 20 years. Its role is still not fully established, probably more because of the surprising lack of large-scale controlled longitudinal trials of treatment than through any fault of the drug. Combination treatments also make trials difficult to carry out, e.g. the use of Cyproterone with or without orchidectomy. Cyproterone has a good effectiveness/toxicity ratio.

It has been used to good effect on metastases (in combination with orchidectomy) (Pescatore *et al.*, 1980), to reduce tumour size (Varenhorst *et al.*, 1981), and to palliatively reduce pain in refractory advanced metastatic bone disease (Fox and Hammonds, 1980).

(c) LHRH analogues/agonists. These act somewhat paradoxically by opposing and therefore effectively reducing testicular androgen production. Small numbers of patients with advanced prostatic cancer have responded to Buserelin (a gonadotrophin-releasing hormone analogue) (Waxman *et al.*, 1983) and to ICI 118630 (an LHRH agonist) (Allen *et al.*, 1983; Leader, 1983; Walker *et al.*, 1983). Unfortunately, Buserelin has to be taken as a snuff and ICI 118630 has to be given by subcutaneous injection. Nevertheless, these do appear to be effective treatments as symptomatic relief is obtained and gonadotrophin and testosterone levels were significantly suppressed to levels comparable with those following castration. They do not seem to cause the fluid retention and thromboembolic complications seen with oestrogen treatment. Depot preparations are being developed. Their greatest use may be in combination with an antiandrogen. They may also be useful to test for hormone dependency/responsiveness.

(d) Subcapsular orchidectomy. This is a simple operation but still leaves the man with some apparent testicular tissue. Inert material can be inserted. It is widely believed that this is a very effective way of slowing or arresting prostatic cancer, often for a long time. It would certainly seem to be preferable to the use of stilboestrol. Many surgeons use it in association with TURP but, as already suggested, it could also be used in a temporarily catheterized patient to avoid vesico-urethral instrumentation.

Some specialists feel that the castration approach is undertaken too lightly in an unproven or exaggerated belief in its success.

Radiotherapy. Hemi-body irradiation using modern equipment, e.g. linear accelerators, of the lower half of the body can be as successful as some of the treatments already discussed. Enthusiasts believe it is the treatment of choice, if necessary using temporary catheterization in the presence of outflow obstruction. Radiation proctocolitis, sometimes permanent, is the major problem.

Pituitary or adrenal ablation does not seem to be worth while.

Other treatments. Appropriate treatment may also be needed for hypercalcaemia, pain, fracture, anaemia, postprostatectomy incontinence, etc.

There does not seem to be a consensus of opinion as to which treatment or combination should be used for different stages, i.e. at first diagnosis or at recurrence, or for disease localized to the prostate or spread into the pelvis, or distantly into bone. There does not seem to be agreement on what subsequent treatment should be used if and when disease recurs after a period of remission.

The normal criteria of cure and 5 year survival rate are often inappropriate in reviewing this disease. Control and time to relapse are more useful terms. There is insufficient evidence to indicate the treatment of choice at first diagnosis and relapse, and the decision may very well depend on local facilities and enthusiasms.

The current view would usually be that orchidectomy or oestrogen or cyproterone blockade of androgen secretion and androgen receptors would be appropriate hormonal treatment as a primary or secondary measure. Failure of primary hormonal treatment might be followed by the use of an LHRH analogue/agonist. These could not be expected to work in orchidectomized patients and might not be effective in 'hormone-relapsed' subjects.

The treatment at relapse will obviously depend on a particular permutation of urinary obstruction, local spread, bony and other metastasis, marrow invasion, hypercalcaemia, etc.

Concern over the long-term side-effects of oestrogen therapy has encouraged many centres to adopt a programme which broadly advocates:

(a) If localized disease at first presentation with no significant outflow obstruction – orchidectomy. Confirmation of localized disease would depend on IVP and rectal ultrasound.
(b) If localized but some outflow obstruction – catheterization rather than TURP.
(c) Pelvic or distant spread at first presentation, no outflow obstruction – orchidectomy plus radiotherapy.
(d) Pelvic or distant spread with outflow obstruction – orchidectomy plus radiotherapy. TURP may be required rather than catheterization as some outflow obstruction may persist, even after orchidectomy plus radiotherapy.

CALCIUM ABNORMALITIES

'Normal' Levels and Ageing

Normal values for many laboratory tests in the elderly should probably be taken as the same as in younger people, but the 'normal' range for serum calcium is rather higher in old age (Reed *et al.*, 1972). Some elderly women may have levels of calcium as high as 2.70 mmol/l (Caird and Judge, 1979). Average levels of 2.43 ± 0.13 mmol/l were noted by Leask, Andrews, and Caird (1973) and of 2.44 ± 0.09 mmol/l by Hodkinson (1977) in fit elderly women. The figures for men are a little lower.

The semantics of normal, physiological, and pathological are difficult if one is trying to be dogmatic about laboratory tests in the elderly.

Calcium is a good example of this problem. Borderline high calcium levels, especially after correction of any protein abnormalities (see below), should be regarded as suspicious, i.e. pathological rather than acceptably physiological. This is obviously more important and critical in an unwell old person, but biochemical screening may suggest hyperparathyroidism at an early stage in an asymptomatic well old person. It is generally accepted that this slight age-related rise in calcium levels and the somewhat higher level in women is due to the lower levels of sex hormones in postmenopausal women allowing a somewhat greater effect of parathomone (PTH) on bone absorption by osteoclasts (Riggs *et al.*, 1969).

Investigation of calcium biochemistry, i.e. serum calcium, inorganic phosphate, and alkaline phosphatase, should be included in the basic biochemical screening of ill old people. The many factors that could affect calcium levels in the elderly mean that every result from this basic screening – whether high, normal, or low – should be examined critically, especially in the ill patient. The problems of diagnosing bone disease (osteomalacia, osteoporosis, and Paget's) are dealt with in Chapter 25.2, but the same general principles apply to interpreting high and low levels of calcium and normal levels when calcium abnormalities are clinically suspected:

(a) Blood should be taken without a cuff.
(b) Inorganic phosphate and alkaline phosphatase levels should be measured concurrently with the calcium levels, along with liver function tests (LFTs). These may indicate whether a raised phosphatase is likely to be bony or hepatic, although isoenzyme separation is the only definite way to be sure of this.
(c) Serum proteins, particularly albumin, should be measured concurrently. Calcium levels may be corrected for protein abnormalities by a correction factor (e.g. by 0.02 mmol for every deviation of 1 gm/l serum albumin from 40 g/l) or by using a nomogram (Hodkinson, 1977). It is difficult to measure ionized/free calcium accurately.
(d) Concurrent renal function tests are obligatory. Creatinine levels are not always a good guide to renal function in the elderly because of changes in muscle/lean body mass. Renal failure may cause or be

caused by hypo- or hypercalcaemia. Dehydration is frequently associated with renal disease and with hypercalcaemia.

(e) A drug history is obligatory, e.g. asking specifically about diuretics and vitamins, including those self-administered.

(f) Transient disturbances of calcium biochemistry are common and should be monitored by serial estimation. Drugs such as thiazides, and disturbances of serum proteins, fluid balance, electrolyte, and renal function are the usual reasons.

(g) Assays of vitamin D or its various metabolites may be useful but do not, of course, correlate directly with calcium levels, especially if renal impairment is present. 25-Hydroxycholecalciferol (25-HCC) is the most widely measured vitamin D analogue and (1,25-DHCC) is the most active metabolite. Vitamin D assays may help in the distinction of osteomalacia from other causes of hypocalcaemia.

Although low circulating vitamin D levels associated with low calcium and inorganic phosphate and raised bone enzyme levels are the hallmarks of osteomalacia, Kafetz and Hodkinson (1981) have reported osteomalacia in the presence of normal 25-OH vitamin D levels.

(h) PTH assays may be useful, especially if hyperparathyroidism is suspected. Hypercalcaemia usually suppresses PTH and a normal PTH level virtually rules out a diagnosis of hyperparathyroidism. In hypercalcaemia associated with malignancy, assay may or may not identify raised levels of PTH or PTH-like hormones secreted by the tumour (Posen *et al.*, 1976).

Immunoassay of PTH may be helpful (iPTH), but assayed iPTH is not automatically equatable with biologically active PTH. Unless sophisticated radioimmunoassays are used that only measure the fully active hormone molecule, circulating inactive PTH metabolites may give falsely high results, especially if renal failure is present, because it reduces renal excretion of these metabolites. The many hormonal influences on calcium, including malignancy and diseases such as renal failure that are likely to be present in older subjects, may exert a powerful effect on PTH effectiveness as well as on circulating levels. iPTH falls in men after middle age (Roof and Gordan, 1978). Black menopausal women have much lower levels of iPTH and higher calcium levels, which appear to correlate with a much lower prevalence of osteoporosis. Oriental women have similar findings.

Most researchers have reported raised levels of PTH in older women (Gallagher *et al.*, 1980; Joffe *et al.*, 1975; Roof and Gordan, 1978; Wiske *et al.*, 1979). The usual explanation is that reduced intestinal calcium absorption and lowered circulating calcium levels stimulate an age-related secondary hyperparathyroidism, albeit usually very mild. Reduced exposure to sunlight in the immobile and house-bound will also impair dermal manufacture of vitamin D and accentuate any dietary defiencies. The consequence hyperparathyroidism will explain the tendency for serum phosphate to fall with advancing age. Reduced renal degradation and excretion of PTH might be another important factor. However, Petersen and coworkers (1983) recently reported that ill old people tend to have raised iPTH levels thought to be due to vitamin D deficiency rather than renal failure, but that normal old people tend to have low PTH concentrations. Hodkinson's (1977) elderly patients had lower calcium values, related to lower serum proteins rather than the result of primary PTH changes.

A small but treatable group of elderly people with osteoporosis have normacalcaemic hyperparathyroidism (Gallagher *et al.*, 1980). They have clearly raised PTH levels but normal or only borderline raised serum calcium levels. Parathyroidectomy is indicated in this group.

(i) There is, as yet, no consistently reliable scanning procedure to visualize the parathyroids. CT scanning and/or parathyroid scintigraphy using radioactive pertechnetate and thallium imaging may demonstrate non-thyroidal functioning nodules in the thyroid or elsewhere, very suggestive of parathyroid adenoma (ta).

(j) Skeletal X-rays and bone scanning may be indicated in suspected cases of hyperparathyroidism, solid malignancies, and haematological malignancies such as myeloma.

Patients with hyperparathyroidism do not always have radiologically obvious bony lesions. Malignant metastatis lesions may be lytic or sclerotic. Lack of new bone formation, e.g. in myeloma, may give a negative bone scan despite bony erosion. Vertebral collapse and other bony involvement in osteoporosis may given rise to hot spots and be difficult to distinguish from malignant secondaries.

(k) The well-known corticosteroid suppression test is still sometimes used. Patients with hypercalcaemia due to primary hyperparathyroidism usually show no change in the serum calcium, e.g. after 30 mg of Prednisolone a day for 10 days. Patients with increased intestinal calcium absorption and some patients with malignancy hypercalcaemia will suppress when given corticosteroids. This approach has also been used in the treatment of symptomatic hypercalcaemia.

(l) Obviously, many of these tests are difficult to perform, not easily automated, and are expensive. The use of biochemical laboratory-based discriminant to differentially diagnose hyperparathyroidism has been suggested. Johnson and coworkers (1982) consider that it is possible to negatively discriminate some non-hyperparathyroid causes of hypercalcaemia and sometimes possible to identify positively some cases of primary hyperparathyroidism by mathematical maximization of normally available laboratory data.

Calcium Homeostasis

The main normal influences affecting circulating calcium levels are dietary vitamin D and calcium, gastrointestinal absorption, protein binding, and renal excretion. These can be abnormal if disease states are also affected by drug effects, but imbalance of the normal bone turnover equation is also a potent cause of calcium abnormalities in disease states (see Fig. 8).

The main causes of hypo- and hypercalcaemia are summarized in Table 4. As so often happens in older patients, several different diseases/pathological processes may be present in the same person. It is important to screen for hypo- and hypercalcaemia in mentally as well as physically ill old people as control of calcium abnormalities may cure or alleviate morbid and even potentially mortal illness.

Hypocalcaemia

Although bone disease (osteomalacia) is a frequent cause of hypocalcaemia there are several important non-bony disorders that may be the cause of lowered calcium:

(a) Serum proteins are often lowered in ill elderly people, due to dietary inadequacy or to a variety of acute or chronic diseases. The hypocalcaemia is usually due to a lowered albumin and is 'benign' as the free ionized calcium levels are normal. This can also be due to a specific deficiency of vitamin D binding globulin, e.g. in liver disease (Barragry *et al.*, 1978).

(b) Renal disease may cause hypocalcaemia due to a reciprocal effect to phosphate retention and/or to acidosis. Hydrogen ion retention tends to protect from tetany due to hypocalcaemia. Chronic hypocalcaemia and chronic renal failure eventually provoke hyperparathyroidism secondarily so that there are many possible permutations of calcium biochemistry in an aged subject with chronic renal failure. They may develop vitamin D resistant osteomalacia, i.e. requiring a higher than normal dose of vitamin D to correct the bone lesions.

(c) Drugs given for a variety of diseases may cause a lowered calcium level, e.g. sex hormones, stilboestrol, anabolic steroids, carbenoxolone, i.v. glucose, and aminoglycosides.

Hypoparathyroidism is a rare disease, usually arising after surgery for parathyroid disease. Idiopathic primary disease has been described in the elderly associated with fits (Graham, Williams, and Rowe, 1979) and incontinence (Baker, 1982). Baker suggests that 'all patients with urinary or faecal incontinence of recent onset should be investigated for calcium abnormalities'.

Hypocalcaemia and Hypomagnesaemia

It has been suggested that the aminoglycosides may cause hypocalcaemia because of hypomagnesaemia due to excessive renal loss. Hypomagnesaemia from various causes may often be associated with hypocalcaemia and the clinical features may mimic hypocalcaemia, e.g. weakness, anorexia, nausea, tremors and cramps, ataxia, convulsions or tetany, and depression (Massry and Seelig, 1977). PTH inhibits intestinal magnesium and increases renal magnesium reabsorption.

The causes of hypomagnesaemia include decreased intake and reduced intestinal absorption, and/or excessive loss in the urine seen in alcoholics, diabetics, and due to diuretics and excessive loss of body fluids, e.g. from diarrhoea (Heath, 1980).

Hypomagnesaemia may itself cause hypo-calcaemia which will not improve until the low magnesium level is corrected, if necessary by i.m. or i.v. magnesium sulphate.

Magnesium is an important trace element involved in many enzymatic processes, in protein synthesis, and in neuromuscular transmission. The non-specific symptomatology of hypermagnesaemia especially causing neuromuscular disturbance suggests that estimates of serum magnesium should sometimes be added to the biochemical screening of ill old people. McConway and coworkers (1980), however, have reported that minor degrees of hypomagnesaemia are common in the elderly admitted to hospital, are not obviously related to hypoalbuminaemia or diuretics, and should

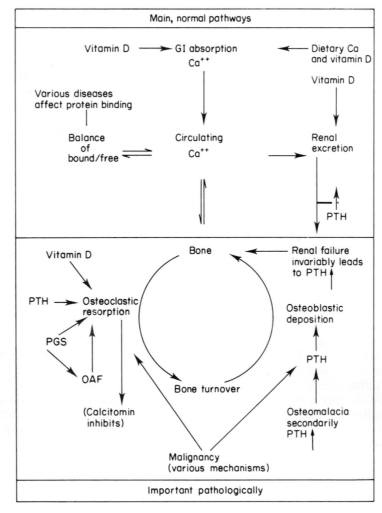

Figure 8   Calcium homeostasis

be interpreted with caution. As with calcium, magnesium disturbance may often be secondary to disease and drugs and may only be transient.

Hypocalcaemia and Cardiovascular Disease

The many diseases and age-related pathological processes that may cause hypocalcaemia have recently acquired another possible important significance.

Raised blood pressure is a relatively common finding in old age. Although the aetiology of hypertension is usually not clearly identifiable it may often be multifactorial and calcium abnormalities may play an important, possibly central, role.

Although hypertension associated with hypercalcaemia due to hyperparathyroidism is usually cured by parathyroidectomy, hypocalcaemia seems to play a much more important role in hypertension. Apparently, hypertensive patients often have a lowered serum ionized calcium, thought to be due mainly to a reduced dietary intake of calcium. A low dietary calcium is associated with sodium retention.

The entry of calcium into cells through so-called channels 'trans membraneous calcium influx' releases vasopressin amines and prostaglandins and stimulates aldosterone release.

Calcium influx stimulates sodium retention in the body and increases the level of ionized intracellular sodium. This is known to aggravate or cause hypertension. Hypernatraemia also tends to affect calcium influx and further aggravate the hypertension.

Increasing dietary intake of calcium may therefore reduce the risk of hypertension in old age, as well as reducing osteomalacia and even osteoporotic bone damage. In established hypotensives, calcium channel blockers/calcium antagonists are being increasingly used.

Drugs such as Nifedipine and Verapamil seem to act directly on the contractile mechanism of the vascular musculature. They may cause fluid retention and are probably used with a diuretic in the treatment of hypertension (Murphy, 1983).

Calcium abnormalities may also directly affect the response of the heart to hypertension and to circulating pressor amines. Though levels of serum calcium tend to reduce the therapeutic effectiveness of digitalis glycosides, hypercalcaemia may cause digoxin toxicity at therapeutic and even subtherapeutic dosage levels. Calcium and other important electrolytes affecting cardiac functions such as sodium and potassium are particularly likely to be affected by nutrition and diuretic use.

Table 4   Causes of hyper- and hypocalcaemia

Hypocalcaemia	
↓ + ↑ age in men	↓ PTH, ↓ serum proteins (cancel out slow ↓ of sex hormones)
Ill elderly	1. ↓ Serum proteins (dietary insufficiency)
	2. Renal disease
	3. Bone disease (e.g. osteomalacia)
	4. Drug effects
Hypoparathyroidism	Usually postoperative
Hypomagnesaemia	↓ Intake/absorption: ↑ loss in urine or body fluids
Acute pancreatitis	
Hypercalcaemia	
↑ + ↑ age in women	↓ Sex hormone effect; ? ↑ PTH
Hyperparathyroidism (1°, 2°, 3°)	May be asymptomatic or a variety of clinical features, including psychiatric
Malignancy	Various mechanisms, often ↑ osteolysis ± ↓ renal clearance, e.g. cancer of lung, prostate; myeloma
Renal failure	May be caused by or cause hypercalcaemia; causes deficiency of active vitamin D metabolites
Bone disease	Especially + immobilization or treatment, e.g. Paget's, malignancy
Thyroid disease	Hyperthyroidism (causing ↑ osteolysis); commoner cause than hypothyroidism (causing ↓ deposition)
Dehydration	↑ Ca due to ↓ GFR excretion may be aggravated by ↑ Ca or aggravate renal failure
GI absorption	Excess vitamin D, milk alkali syndrome
Drugs	e.g. thiazides, excess vitamin D

Hypercalcaemia

Primary hyperparathyroidism with an annual incidence rate of 250 new patients per million per year is a commoner cause of raised calcium than the hypercalcaemia of malignancy (150 new patients per million per year) (Mundy and Martin, 1982). The prevalence of hyperparathyroidism and malignancy hypercalcaemia in older people is not clear, but cancers associated with abnormal calcium levels are relatively common in old age. Certainly, primary hyperparathyroidism does occur in older people and has been found by biochemical screening in ambulant, asymptomatic old people (Heath, Hodgson, and Kennedar, 1980; Mundy, Cove and Fisken, 1980).

Two surveys carried out before biochemical screening was established suggested that hyperparathyroidism was rare in old age. Norris (1947) reported that the condition was about twice as common in late childhood and early old age compared with the seventh and eighth decades, and Mcgeown (1964) found only two patients over 70 in 102 clinical cases. However, Biswas, *et al.* (1982) recently described 3 cases of primary hyperparathyroidism presenting to their geriatric department, each with very different clinical features.

Grero and Hodkinson (1971) found hypercalcaemia in more than 1 per cent. of geriatric admissions, due mainly to osteolytic bone secondaries, primary hyperparathyroidism, carcinoma of the bronchus without secondaries, and lymphoma without bony involvement. The frequency of malignant disease in their survey confirms other studies showing a preponderance of malignancy-associated hypercalcaemia over parathyroid disease in hospital patients.

For some reason most elderly patients with primary hyperparathyroidism are women. The characteristics and biochemical profile of these patients is of a very low phosphate and potassium. The associated biochemistry in solid tumours and haematological neoplasms such as myelomas and lymphomas is variable and phosphate levels are not usually as low as in primary hyperparathyroidism; when bony involvement is extensive, the alkaline phosphatase is likely to be raised.

Primary hyperparathyroidism can coexist with malignant disease. Hypercalcaemia from whatever cause is a potent and potentially re-

medial/reversible cause of acute and chronic physical and mental symptoms and signs.

The complex interrelationships of renal disease in calcium abnormalities have already been mentioned. Renal failure which is common in the elderly virtually leads automatically to eventual secondary hyperparathyroidism (Ross, 1981). This is because of a failure of synthesis of active vitamin D metabolites, especially 1,25-DHCC.

Elucidation of the two main causes of elevated calcium in the elderly, i.e. parathyroid disease and malignant disease, is an example of the need for considerable clinical skill and understanding of laboratory results in the management of elderly patients. Hypercalcaemia from whatever cause can be associated with serious morbidity and mortality and should be treated, if possible, even if as in the case of hypercalcaemia associated with malignancies the primary cause cannot always be removed.

Hypercalcaemia and Malignant Disease

Several pathways lead to hypercalcaemia in malignant disease. Sometimes there is a clearly raised level of iPTH and presumably of biologically active PTH. Bockman (1980) and Mundy and Martin (1982) highlight the many possible reasons for hypercalcaemia and emphasize that if the cause(s) can be sorted out it may lead to a more symptomatically effective treatment. The elderly may develop malignant-associated hypercalcaemia from one or more of the three main mechanisms so far identified (Fig. 9). They may suffer from haematological or solid tumours with or without metastases, the latter possibly secreting PTH or PTH-like chemicals ectopically, e.g. carcinomas of the lung, breast, or pancreas. Solid tumours with metastasis are by far the commonest cause of hypercalcaemia of malignancy, probably representing about 70 to 80 per cent. of the total. The hypercalcaemia is usually a function of the total tumour mass, especially bony metastases. The patients have suppression of intrinsic PTH secretion and may or may not have raised iPTH. They have normal renal function, at least initially, with normal renal cAMP and no disturbance of renal phosphate handling.

Clinical Features of Hypercalcaemia

Obviously, symptoms of primary or associated diseases such as malignancy ('debility', anorexia, or bone pain) or hyperparathyroidism (bone pain) or renal failure will often be present. The clinical presentation of symptomatic hypercalcaemia is usually non-specific with a wide spectrum of possible symptoms and signs. These include:

(a) GI disturbance	Anorexia, nausea, vomiting
	Abdominal pain
	Ileus
	Constipation
(b) Renal	Polyuria, nocturia
	Thirst, polydipsia
	Dehydration
	Nephrocalcinosis, renal stones
(c) CNS	Weakness
	Sleepiness
	Confusion
(d) Musculoskeletal	Myopathy
	Bone pain, tenderness
	Fracture
(e) Other	Band keratopathy

Management of Hypercalcaemia

This is usually determined mainly by the level of the serum calcium and the stability of the hypercalcaemia (Hosking, 1983). The need for treatment may outweigh the need for investigation. Dysequilibrium, with a rising calcium, is likely to occur if bone destruction outweighs bone formation and urinary calcium excretion.

Renal failure, which may be preexisting or caused by the hypercalcaemia, further impairs the body's ability to excrete calcium. Hypercalcaemia reduces the distal tubular ability to conserve salt and water and the effect on sodium further aggravates the renal ability to excrete calcium. A vicious spiral of an unstable and rising calcium level is likely to be accelerated by the reduction in extracellular fluid caused by the sodium changes and by the anorexia and vomiting and may be caused by malignancy or hyperparathyroidism, by other diseases, or by a variety of drugs as well as by the hypercalcaemia itself. Immobilization, e.g. in Paget's disease, the treatment of malignant bone disease, and the use of diuretics may pre-

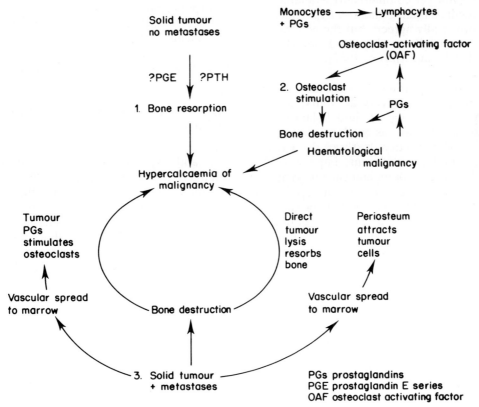

Figure 9   Causes of hypercalcaemia in malignancy

cipitate dysequilibrium in a previously stable hypercalcaemia state. Elderly people with asymptomatic hypercalcaemia or who are discovered during screening of renal calculi or of confusion and appear to have static hypercalcaemia may go subsequently into dysequilibrium. It is therefore important to try and elucidate the underlying cause and regularly check on renal and electrolyte status in case emergency treatment is required.

Obviously, it is best to try and treat any underlying primary condition. Removal of a solitary parathyroid adenoma may effect a complete cure, especially if there is no significant renal damge. Treatment of myeloma, cancer of the prostate, or other malignancy may produce a very satisfactory remission and a restoration of normocalcaemia. Specific drugs such as oral diphosphonates are being investigated to control hypercalcaemia and would obviously be useful in old people with the 'benign' condition of hyperparathyroidism who are considered unfit for surgery or have multiple or inaccessible adenomata, but these drugs are not yet commercially available.

The medical management of hypercalcaemia is not universally agreed, but the general principles are as follows (Heath, 1980; Hosking, 1983; Mundy and Martin, 1982):

(a) Rehydrate, using intravenous normal saline up to 6 l every 24 hours, with frequent monitoring of fluid balance, urea, and electrolytes as well as the calcium level. Rehydration restores the extracellular fluid compartment, improves GFR, and reduces sodium and calcium reabsorption in the kidneys. Potassium supplements are usually needed to avoid hypokalaemia. No other treatment may be required to restore normocalcaemia, even in severe dysequilibrium states due to disseminated carcinoma.

(b) Loop diuretics: frusemide increasing urinary calcium output and can be given in addition to the forced saline diuresis, e.g. up to 100 to 200 mg 2 hourly. Again, great care must be taken to monitor fluids and electrolyte balance.

(c) Intravenous phosphate is an effective therapy but is hazardous. Patients may collapse and die during treatment. This therapy is virtually guaranteed to reduce the calcium

so if other methods fail it might still be used in the last resort.

(d) Dialysis. Peritoneal rather than renal dialysis is probably preferable for what is usually only short-term treatment.

(e) Inhibition of bone absorption. Calcium and diphosphonates may be useful. Inhibitors of prostaglandin synthetase such as indomethacine may help alleviate bone pain of malignancy, but despite the central involvement of prostaglandin metabolism in many cases of malignancy hypercalcaemia the NSAIs do not seem to be very effective in lowering hypercalcaemia.

(f) Corticosteroids rarely influence hypercalcaemia due to hyperparathyroidism. They can be useful in malignancy hypercalcaemia but the response is unpredictable and often too slow to deal with severe dysequilibrium.

The above measures are more likely to be needed in severe or dysequilibrium hypercalcaemia. In mild and stable hypercalcaemia, particularly where a primary cause such as hyperparathyroidism cannot be dealt with, e.g. in a very elderly ill person, no treatment may be indicated. As already indicated, a rise in the serum calcium may merit starting a treatment aimed at reducing the serum calcium.

ELECTROLYTES AND HORMONAL INFLUENCES

Altered sodium levels, especially hyponatraemia, and hypokalaemia and dehydration are relatively common problems in the elderly and are important causes of ill-health. Hypernatraemia, hyperkalaemia, and overhydration are also potent causes of clinical illness.

Potassium, sodium, and fluid volume disturbances are often symptomatologically nonspecific and there are no characteristic clinical signs. Even when 'screening' biochemistry reveals electrolyte abnormalities they may not be blamed for physical or psychological illness. In many cases drugs, especially diuretics, often given inappropriately or continued when the original reason for their prescription has resolved (Burr *et al.*, 1977) and i.v. fluids are the cause rather than a primary disease. Pituitary–hormonal changes may result from electrolyte imbalance or be caused by primary endocrine disturbance or hormonal changes secondary to disease or drugs.

As sodium is the main extracellular ion and determinant of plasma osmolality, abnormal sodium levels revealed on screening are likely to be clinically significant. High or low potassium levels less accurately reflect cerebral, cardiac, and skeletal muscle tissue levels.

When interpreting biochemical screening results the simple rule should be remembered that 'however important it may be to look for unsuspected occult disease in ill older patients, an abnormal result may be due to a non-pathological reason'. It is well known that false hyperkalaemia may be caused by the release of potassium from lysed red cells which may occur because of a delay in separating and assaying blood samples taken from, for example, patients in long-stay hospitals, old people's homes, or at home. While flame photometry accurately measures plasma sodium concentration, sodium ion activity as measured by direct ion selective electrode instruments more accurately reflects biological activity. This does not usually matter but the clinician should be aware of the possibility of 'pseudo-hyponatraemia' suggested by flame photometry. This method measures the electrolyte in the total plasma volume while the selective ion method measures the electrolyte in the plasma water. A significant difference is likely to occur in patients with hyperlipidaemia and hyperproteinaemia, e.g. diabetes or myeloma, or those receiving i.v. nutrition (Worth, 1983).

Abnormal electrolyte levels are particularly likely to occur in older people with renal impairment or as a result of drugs, particularly diuretics. In addition, however, older patients may have unsuspected alterations in the levels of, or abnormal responses to, hormones involved in salt and water homeostasis – of aldosterone, renin, and antidiuretic hormone (ADH), which is also known as arginine vasopressin (AVP).

Sunderam and Mankikar (1983) have shown how important diuretics are as a cause of hyponatraemia and Brooks and Ritch (1983) have emphasized that potassium-conserving/sparing diuretics such as amiloride may cause a significant fall in plasma sodium levels. It is obviously important to distinguish diuretic-induced hyponatraemia from the primary dilutional hyponatraemia of heart failure caused by fluid 'overload' with or without secondary hormonal influences. The treatment of the two causes will be diametrically opposite (Roskovec and Marshall, 1983).

Although diuretics are the commonest cause of hyponatraemia – in itself a common finding (more than 11 per cent. of Sunderam and Mankikar's admissions had hyponatraemia) – about a quarter of their group had a non-diuretic explanation for the low sodium level, mainly abnormal ADH levels secondary to other diseases, or diabetes mellitus.

Ageing and Aldosterone

The renin–angiotensin and aldosterone systems may become more active with increasing age as a result of disease such as renal damage from a variety of causes, from liver disease, especially cirrhosis, or from drugs. A decreased effective circulating blood volume and/or decreased renal blood flow associated with diseases, with 'arteriosclerotic' (ageing?) narrowing of renal arteries, or altered intake or loss of salt and water may be responsible. Excessive sodium reabsorption may aggravate hypersecretion of aldosterone by decreasing renal blood flow.

Secondary hyperaldosteronism may particularly occur in heart failure and/or be caused by diuretics and aggravate and perpetuate the oedematous state. This counterproductive response can be explained as a normal renin–angiotensin reaction to a decrease in effective ECG. Drugs other than diuretics may affect salt and water, e.g. carbenoxolone is thought to have a mineralocorticoid-like effect on the distal renal tubules.

In liver disease, especially cirrhotic liver damage, aldosterone secretion is increased mainly as a result of changes in the renin–angiotensin system. The plasma sodium concentration also probably has an important effect on aldosterone secretion. The situation may also be complicated both in terms of clinical effect and laboratory measurement of hormone levels by abnormalities in the conjugation and excretion of circulating hormones (Wilkinson *et al.*, 1981).

The secretion rate of aldosterone, which is the main mineralocorticoid, tends to fall significantly with advancing age. The elderly show a reduced aldosterone response to a low sodium diet, and have somewhat lower levels of aldosterone in the upright position before as well as after sodium restriction compared with samples taken when lying down. There is no such postural difference in younger people (Weidmann *et al.*, 1975). Although the basal aldosterone level is lower and there is this postural difference in elderly subjects, there is no difference in the aldosterone response of older people to ACTH. This suggests that the age-related change is a consequence of altered renin–angiotensin pathways.

Although a low sodium diet tends to cause less of an increased aldosterone response in elderly subjects compared with younger people (Flood *et al.*, 1967), altered dietary intake of sodium and postural changes in the elderly do not seem to be the prime cause of the altered aldosterone secretion and clearance rates.

Possible age-related changes in aldosterone secretion must be taken into account when investigating elderly hypertensives for possible primary aldosteronism, i.e. low renin hypertension may be overdiagnosed. The concomitant finding of a low potassium level will tend to support the diagnosis of hyperaldosteronism, both primary and secondary.

Studies by Hegstad and coworkers (1983) confirmed that aldosterone secretion decreases in 'young' older subjects. They suggest that the decrease in secretion of aldosterone with ageing is greater than the decline in aldosterone clearance. They found that 'older' subjects had lowered urinary aldosterone secretion before and after sodium depletion and had lower plasma aldosterone levels before and after sodium depletion when studied in the upright position. They confirmed that plasma renin activity declined with advancing age in normo- and hypertensive subjects.

Their findings highlight the need:

(a) to investigate elderly hypertensives for primary aldosteronism in the upright position and on an unrestricted sodium diet and
(b) to correct for age when interpreting aldosterone excretion rates in elderly subjects being investigated for aldosterone-secreting adenomata.

Sonkodi and coworkers (1981) have confirmed that serum and plasma sodium levels fall significantly from the supine to the upright position.

Is there any point in looking for primary aldosterone abnormalities in older people? Annat and coworkers (1981) did not conclude that the renin–angiotensin–aldosterone system plays an important part in hypertension in the elderly. It is certainly rare to find a primary cause for hypertension at any age. Various degrees of renal failure are commonly found but are thought to be due to hypertension or to other diseases rather than being the prime cause of the hypertension. Primary hyperaldosteronism, characterized by hypertension, hypokalaemia, and low plasma renin may be due to an andrenocrotical adenoma or more rarely to adrenal hyperplasia. These conditions are almost certainly excessively rare in old age, but could occur. The hallmark of primary hyperaldosteronism is persistent and severe hypokalaemia in both untreated and treated hypertensives, but use of diuretics to treat hypertensive subjects will obviously confuse the issue. The serum potassium may also be normal. If a raised blood pressure or low potassium cannot be controlled medically, more specialized investigation should be initiated (Swales, 1983).

The plasma renin activity (PRA) in hypertensives decreases with age and is particularly low in black patients, with low renin essential hypertension being present in 50 per cent. of hypertensive black subjects (Mroczek, Finnerty, and Catt, 1973). The frequency with which aldosterone is not increased in elderly hypertensives may be related in some way to the aetiology of the hypertension (Nowaczynski *et al.*, 1977).

There are also, of course, many other variables in the maintenance of blood pressure that may be abnormal in the elderly and may secondarily affect hormonal systems. Ageing seems to be associated with increased peripheral alpha-adrenergic sympathetic nerve activity without any parallel increase in the sympathetic adrenal medullary beta-adrenergic activity (Tuck and Sowers, 1982). Plasma epinephrine and dopamine levels do not increase with ageing (Franco-Morselli *et al.*, 1977), although plasma and urinary norepinephrine levels do increase (Ziegler, Lake, and Kopin, 1976), probably because of increased conversion of dopamine to norepinephrine by the enzyme dopamine beta-hydroxylase (Freedman *et al.*, 1972).

Tuck and Sowers (1982) remind us that other variables may be operating, including increased vascular resistance and reduced vascular elasticity, variable postural blood pressure responses ranging from slow to accelerated, changes in left ventricular filling and myocardial relaxation, impaired baroreceptor arcs, and even abnormalities of the complex hypothalamic and other central baroreceptor blood pressure control reflex arcs. This latter may explain the common hypotensive side-effect of bromocriptine and L-dopa, often most marked in getting up from the lying or sitting position.

As long ago as 1971 Finlay and coworkers demonstrated that L-dopa significantly increased the glomerular filtration rate, renal plasma flow, and renal excretion of sodium and potassium in Parkinsonian patients. The sodium loss is probably an important factor in the orthostatic hypotension so often seen in patients taking anti-Parkinsonian drugs.

In essence, the assessment of aldosterone status, plasma renin activity, and catecholamine levels in elderly hypertensives may reveal abnormalities due to cardiovascular adaptations to high blood pressure and ageing changes, but rarely to primary aldosterone abnormalities (Messerli *et al.*, 1983). Essential hypertension in the elderly tends to be associated with a low cardiac output, raised peripheral and renal vascular resistance, reduced renal blood flow, and low plasma renin activity.

The renin-angiotensin-aldosterone system may be activated in congestive cardiac failure. This may aggravate and perpetrate the heart failure because secondary hyperaldosteronism leads to fluid retention and vasodilators are less effective.

Successful diuresis is associated with a very substantial drop in aldosterone levels associated with natriuresis, but subsequently aldosterone levels increase again. This is thought to be due to activation of the renin–angiotensin system (Nicholls *et al.*, 1974).

The important clinical point is that secretion of the sodium-retaining hormone aldosterone is a response to urinary sodium loss induced by diuretics and this may then perpetuate, aggravate, or cause a recurrence of oedema. Patients with oedema associated with heart failure, cirrhosis (Wilkinson *et al.*, 1981), or nephrosis may have hyperaldosteronism on presentation and this can only be aggravated by 'successful' diuretic therapy.

Spironolactone, usually at a dose of 100 mg a day, has been used for a long time as an adjuvant to diuretic therapy in resistant congestive cardiac failure and in the oedema of hepatic failure. Its success, sometimes dramatic, has been ascribed to control of secondary hyperaldosteronism. It is a so-called potassium-sparing diuretic and is probably less likely to cause hyperkalaemia than other so-called potassium-conserving diuretics such as Amiloride or Triamterene.

The problem of hyponatraemia in the elderly, particularly due to diuretics, has already been mentioned. It is suggested that the elderly are particularly at risk of sodium loss from the distal nephron (Macías Núnez *et al.*, 1980). They suggest that this is not due to hypoaldosteronism but to a deficit of Na–K–ATPase and/or interstitial fibrosis in the renal medulla.

The oral angiotensin II converting inhibitor Captopril has been introduced as a quasiphysiological way of inactivating the renin–angiotensin system in disease states associated with hypertension, heart failure, and oedema. It is effective in normotensive as well as hypertensive heart failure and reduces pre- and afterload as well as affecting sodium retention.

Arginine Vasopressin (AVP)/Antidiuretic Hormone (ADH)

This hormone, along with aldosterone, is the main hormonal influence on salt and water, basically causing water retention and sodium loss. Like aldosterone it is mainly controlled by changes in salt and water and these changes secondarily influence aldosterone levels. Figure 10 summarizes the main relationships of aldosterone and ADH secretion.

AVP/ADH is mainly synthesized in the supraoptic nucleus, but is also made in the paraventricular nucleus and adjoining non-nuclear CNS cells. The hormone is then carried by the transporter peptide neurophysin in axonal extensions from the manufacturing cells to be stored in the posterior pituitary. Its release then depends on hypothalamic stimulation.

Somewhat surprisingly the hypothalamic posterior pituitary tracts do not seem to share in the tendency for most ageing organs to become somewhat fibrotic or arteriosclerotic, or develop specific changes such as the lipofuchsin pigment accumulation seen in other parts of the CNS (Buttlar-Brentano, 1954; Christ, 1951). Helderman (1982) comments from the lack of published data about ageing and AVP/ADH and his own group's work that there is no evidence of any primary, i.e. intrinsic, CNS abnormality of secretion or clearance of this important hormone.

The most important AVP/ADH changes in older subjects are listed in Table 5; they are usually secondary to other pathologies.

Table 5 Causes of AVP/ADH abnormalities in the elderly

---

1. Increased hypothalamic osmostat sensitivity.
2. Abnormal salt and water intake or loss, i.e. changes in extracellular ion and blood volume. Effects are central and peripheral.
3. Non-central or non-osmotic effects
   (a) Age-related decline in response of stretch and pressure receptors to postural change. Receptors are in arteries, aorta, and carotid sinus.
   (b) Age-related decline in response of these receptors to catecholamines and vasoactive drugs.
   (c) Drugs such as opiates and alcohol stimulate AVP/ADH secretion centrally, as does Chlorpropamide.
   (d) Decreased GFR and chronic renal failure affect ADH responsiveness only secondarily.
   (e) Various diseases may be associated with SIADH via peripheral, central, or renal pathways.
   (f) Ectopic AVP/ADH secretion by tumours and with pneumonic lesions.

The increased sensitivity of the hypothalamic osmostat to osmolar stimuli seems to be a primary defect rather than a response to the frequent alterations in salt and water balance or in volumes of the hormonal distribution or its clearance. The osmostat set-point is the same as in younger people but more ADH is secreted for a given stimulus, e.g. a water load (Helderman, 1982). Frolkis and coworkers (1982) have confirmed a general rise in the level of circulating AVP/ADH with age.

The main osmotic plasma ion is sodium. Hypo- and hyperkalaemic states remain important causes of ill-health in the elderly but increased awareness of the need to biochemically screen ill old people has increasingly shown the frequency of sodium abnormalities. These may be important markers of potentially reversible morbidity and even mortality, especially due to hyponatraemia. Altered hydration effects AVP/ADH mainly by affecting sodium balance. As already stated, this is substantially an extracellular ion and levels clearly outside the normal/reference range should be regarded with respect as they are likely to reflect a true alteration in total body sodium. Dehydration and hypotension will also secondarily affect the osmostat and renal clearance of salt and water by reduced perfusion.

Neurogenic non-osmotic factors also affect AVP/ADH secretion and release. Intrathoracic stretch (low pressure) and baroreceptor (high pressure) receptors in the left atrium and arterial walls transmit messages to the central neuroendocrine centres via the parasympathetic fibres in the vagus. Defects in this pathway may account for the tendency to a blunting of the usual rise in hormone produced by the upright posture. Catecholamines, vasoactive drugs, and other drugs such as opiates may alter AVP/ADH secretion by central or peripheral effects. SIADH due to chlorpropamide rarely causes hypernatraemia in younger people but in older diabetics it may cause hyponatraemia because of the increased hypothalamic osmostat sensitivity. Altered central or renal AVP/ADH responsiveness has also been described with tricyclic antidepressants, carbenoxolone, carbamazepine, and intravenous dextrose. The diuretic effect of ethanol is thought to be due to central suppression of AVP/ADH secretion.

Altered/reduced ADH responsiveness in chronic renal failure (often seen in the elderly) because of a reduced glomerular filtration rate (GFR) may be secondary effects, but there is no evidence of primary renal ADH unresponsiveness in the elderly. Indeed, the increased central osmostat sensitivity and the tendency for higher than average circulating levels of AVP/ADH may very well be a normal reaction to maintain blood flow and urine output, if necessary by relatively increased function of the remaining nephrons.

Other clinically significant abnormalities of AVP/ADH – SIADH – occur in association with primary and secondary cerebral and cerebellar tumours, head injuries including subdurals, encephalitis and CVAs, cardiac failure and chest infections, diabetes mellitus, hypothryoidism, and hypoadrenalism.

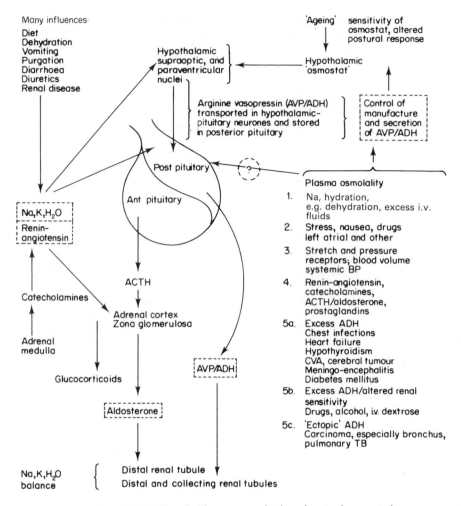

Figure 10   AVP/ADH and aldosterone and salt and water homeostasis

Ectopic, i.e. non-centrally secreted AVP/ADH hormone or analogue, may be produced by carcinomata, especially bronchogenic, and sometimes apparently in association with pulmonary tuberculosis.

Investigation and Treatment of AVP/ADH Abnormalities

In practice the usual diagnostic problem is hyponatraemia. The rate of fall in sodium levels may be as important as the actual level, but even apparently modest chronic hyponatraemia may be symptomatically significant. Weakness and lethargy, hypotension, confusion, restlessness, encephalopathy, focal CNS signs, fits, and coma are possible consequences of hyponatraemia and mental damage may be irreversible.

The history of coexistent diseases such as cirrhosis or renal failure and what drugs are being taken are obviously important to know. Estimation of plasma and urine osmolality will help elucidate the cause. Diuretics are by far the commonest cause of hyponatraemia rather than cranial or nephrogenic diabetes insipidus/SIADH. Renal dysfunction is an important cause of excessive natriuresis.

Treatment of hyponatraemia due to AVP/ADH abnormalities is by removal of the primary cause if possible. Water restriction even to 500 ml per day and/or diuretic administration with extra sodium and/or administration

of the sodium-retaining mineralocorticoid fludrocortisone at a dose of 0.5 to 1 mg/d may
help disabling symptoms even if the primary
cause cannot be removed, e.g. in association
with a bronchogenic carcinoma. Lithium has
also been used but doxycycline seems a less
toxic alternative and can sometimes dramatically reverse the hyponatraemia for a while.

REFERENCES

Albeaux-Fernet, M., Bellot, L., Duribruxj, J., and
Gelinet, M. (1972). 'Appreciation de l'androgen-
cite chez homme', *Ann. Endocrinol. (Paris)*, **24**,
105.

Albeaux-Fernet, M., Bohler, C. S-S., and Karpas,
A. E. (1978). 'Testicular function in the ageing
male'. In *Geriatric Endocrinology* (Ed. R. B.
Greenblatt), *Aging*, Vol. 5, pp. 201–216, Raven
Press, New York.

Allen, J. M., O'Shea, J. P., Mashiter, K., Williams,
G., and Bloom, S. R. (1983). 'Advanced carcinoma of the prostate: Treatment with a gonadotrophin releasing hormone agonist. Papers and
short reports', *Br. Med. J.*, **286**, 1607–1609.

Andersson, L., Edsmyr, F., Jonsson, G., and
Konvves, I. (1977). 'Estramustine phosphate
therapy in carcinoma of the prostate', *Recent Results in Cancer Reserach*, **60**, 73–77.

Annat, G., Vincent, M., Tourniaire, A., and Sas-
sard, J. (1981). 'Relationships between blood
pressure and plasma renin, aldosterone and dopamine–β-hydroxylase in the elderly. Studies in
patients over 70 years of age. *Clinical Section,
Gerontology*, **27**, 266–270.

Ash, R. H., and Greenblatt, R. (1978). 'The aging
ovary: Morphologic and endocrine correlations',
in *Geriatric Endocrinology* (Ed. R. B. Greenblatt), *Aging*, Vol. 5, pp. 141–164, Raven Press,
New York.

Ayres, J., Rees, J., Clark, T. J. H., and Maisey,
M. N. (1982). 'Thyrotoxicosis and dyspnoea',
Clin. Endocrinol., **16**, 65–71.

Bahemuka, M., and Hodkinson, H. M. (1975).
'Screening for hypothyroidism in the elderly patient', *Br. Med. J.*, **2**, 601–603.

Baker, H. W. G., Burger, H. G., de Kretser, D.
M., Hudson, B., O'Connor, S., Wang, C., Mi-
rovics, A., Court, J., Dunlop, M., and Rennie,
G. C. (1976). 'Changes in the pituitary–testicular
system with age', *Clin. Endocrinol.*, **5**, 349–372.

Baker, S. (1982). 'Idiopathic hypoparathyroidism
presenting as urinary and faecal incontinence',
Br. Med. J., **2**, 963–964.

Barragry, J. M., Corless, D., Anton, D., Carter,
N. D., Long, R. G., Maxwell, J. D., and Switala,
S. (1978). 'Plasma vitamin D-binding globulin in

vitamin D deficiency, pregnancy and chronic liver
disease', *Clinica Chim. Acta*, **87**, 359–365.

Bartels, E. C. (1965). 'Hyperthyroidism in patients
over 65', *Geriatrics*, **20**, 459–462.

Biswas, C. K., Bhattacharya, B. K., Datta, S. R.,
and Horrocks, P. (1982). 'Asymptomatic primary
hyperparathyroidism', *Geriatr. Med.*, **12**, 39–41.

Blichert-Toft, M. (1975). 'Secretion of corticotrophin and somatotrophin by the senescent adenohypophysis in man', Thesis, *Acta Endocrinol.
(Kbh.)* (Suppl.), **195**.

Blichert-Toft, M., Christensen, V., Engquist, A.,
Fog-Moller, F., Kehlet, H., Nistrup Madsen,
S., Skovsted, L., Thode, J., and Olgaard, K.
(1979). 'Influence of age on the endocrine-
metabolic response to surgery', *Ann. Surg.*, **190**,
761–770.

Block, E. (1952). 'Quantitative morphological investigations of the follicular system in newborn
female infants', *Acta Anat.*, **17**, 201.

Bockman, R. S. (1980). *Hypercalcaemia in Malignancy in Endocrinology and Cancer* (Ed. K.
Abe), Vol. 9, No. 2, pp. 317–333, Sanders CVB.

Boyle, I. T. (1981). 'Treatment for postmenopausal
osteoporosis', *Lancet*, **1**, 1376.

British Medical Journal (1977). **1**, 598.

Brooks, R. W. S., and Ritch, A. E. S. (1983). 'New
drugs: modern diuretic treatment', *Br. Med. J.*,
296, 1971–1972.

Bruchovsky, N., Callaway, T., Lieskovsky, G., and
Rennie, P. S. (1980). 'Markets of androgen action
in human prostate: Potential use in clinical assessment of prostatic carcinoma', in *Steroid Receptors, and Hormone Dependent Neoplasia* (Eds J.
L. Wittliff and D. Dapunt), pp. 121–131, Masson,
New York.

Burckhardt, D., Cesar, A. Vera, and LaDue, J. S.
(Sloan-Kettering Inst.) (1968). 'Effect of digitalis
on urinary pituitary gonadotrophin excretion: A
study in postmenopausal women', *Ann. Int.
Med.*, **68**, 1069–1071.

Burr, M. L., King, S., Davies, H. E. S., and Pathy,
M. S. (1977). 'The effect of discontinuing long
term diuretic therapy in the elderly', *Age Ageing*,
6, 38.

Burrows, A. W., Shakespear, R. A., Hesch, R. D.,
Cooper, E., Aickin, C. M., and Burke, C. W.
(1975). 'Thyroid hormones in the elderly sick: T4
euthyroidism', *Br. Med. J.*, **4**, 437–439.

Buttlar-Brentano, von K. (1954). 'Zur Lebensges-
ichte des Nucleus basalis, tuberomammllaris, su-
praopticus and paraventricularis unter normalen
und pathogenen', *Bedingungen. J. Hirnforsch.*, **1**,
337.

Caird, F. I. (1973). 'Problems of interpretation of
laboratory findings in the old', *Br. Med. J.*, **4**,
348–351.

Caird, F. I., and Judge, T. G. (1979). *Assessment*

of the Elderly Patient, Pitman Medical.

Campbell, A. J., Reinken, J., and Allan, B. C. (1981). 'Thyroid disease in the elderly in the community', *Age Ageing*, **10**, 47–52.

Carroll, B. J. (1969). 'Hypothalamic–pituitary function in depressive illness, insensitivity to hypoglycaemia', *Br. Med. J.*, **3**, 27–28.

Cartlidge, N. E. F., Black, M. M., Hall, M. R. P., and Hall, P. (1970). 'Pituitary function in the elderly', *Gerontol. Clin.*, **12**, 65.

Christ, J. (1951). 'Zur Anatomie des Tuber cinerum beim erwachsenen Menschen', *Deutsche Zeitschrift für Nervenheilkunde*, **165**, 340.

Chomette, G., Pinandean, Y., Brocherion, C., Auriol, M., and Pfister, A. (1966). 'La thyroide du lieillarde, caracteres anatomiques et essai d'interpretation physiopathologique', *Arch. Anat. Path.*, **14**, 233–245.

Clements, M. R., and Hamilton, D. V. (1983). 'Management of osteoporosis', Special article, *Hospital Update*, **1983**, 607–620.

Colucci, C. F., D'Alessandro, B., Bellastella, A., and Montalbetti, N. (1975). 'Circadian rhythm of plasma cortisol in the aged (Cosinor method)', *Gerontol. Clin.*, **17**, 89–95.

Comfort, A. (1979). *The Biology of Senescence*, p. 226, Churchill Livingstone.

Connell, J. M. C., McGruden, D. C., Davies, D. L., and Alexander, W. D. (1982). 'Bromocriptine for inappropriate thyrotrophin secretion', *Ann. Int. Med.*, **96**, 251–252.

Cooke, I. D. (1983). 'Treating the menopause'. *Br. Med. J.*, **286**, 2001.

Craig, G. M. (1983). 'Guidelines for community menopausal clinics', *Br. Med. J.*, **286**, 2033–2035.

Crilly, R. G., Francis, R. M., and Nordin, B. E. C. (1981). 'Steroid hormones, ageing and bone', in *Clinics in Endocrinology and Metabolism: Endocrinology and Ageing*, Vol. 6, pp. 115–139, W. B. Saunders.

Davidson, J. M., Chen, J. J., Crapo, L., Gray, G. D., Greenleaf, W. J., and Catania, J. A. (1983). 'Hormonal changes and sexual function in aging men', *J. Clin. Endocrinol. Metabl*, **57**(1), 71–72.

Davidson, M. D. (1979). 'Ageing and carbohydrate metabolism', *Clin. Exp. Metabol.*, **28**, 693.

Davis, P. J., and Davis, F. B. (1974). 'Hyperthyroidism in patients over the age of 60 years', *Medicine (Baltimore)*, **53**, 161.

Dean, Sandra, and Felton, S. P. (1979). 'Circadian rhythm in the elderly: A study using a cortisol-specific radio-immuno-assay' *Age Ageing* **8**, 243.

De Lange, W. E., Pratt, J. J., and Dorrenbos, H. (1980). 'A gonadotrophin responsive testosterone producing adrenocortical adenoma and high gonadotrophin levels in the elderly woman', *Clin. Endocrinol.*, **12**, 21–28.

Delitala, G., Devilla, L., Canessa, A., and D'Asta,

F. (1981). 'On the role of dopamine receptors in the central regulation of human TSH', *Acta Endocrinol.*, **98**, 521–527.

Delitala, G., Devilla, L., and Lotti, G. (1980). 'Domperidone, an extracerebral inhibitor of dopamine receptors, stimulates thyrotropin and prolactin release in man', *J. Clin. Endocrinol. Metab.*, **50**, 427–1130.

Denham, M. J. (1977). 'An autopsy study of the thyroid in elderly patients', Personal communication.

Denham, M. J., and Wills, E. J. (1980). 'A clinico-pathological survey of thyroid gland in old age', *Gerontology*, **26**, 160–166.

Dobbie, J. W. (1969). 'Adrenocortical nodular hyperplasia; the aging adrenal', *J. Path. Bact.*, **99**, 1–18.

Dolva, L. O., Riddervold, F., and Thorsen, R. K. (1983). 'Side effects of thyrotrophin releasing hormone', *Br. Med. J.*, **287**, 532.

Doniach, D., and Bottazzo, G. F. (1983). 'Autoimmune endocrine disorders', *Hospital Update*, **1983**, 1145–1159.

Dubin, B., MacLennan, W. J., and Hamilton, Judith C. (1978). 'Adrenal function and ascorbic acid concentrations in elderly women', *Gerontology*, **24**, 473–476.

Exton-Smith, A. N. (1972). Personal communication.

Fairclough, P. D., and Besser, G. M. (1973). 'Apathetic T-3 toxicosis', *Br. Med. J.*, **1**, 364–365.

Feehy, J., and Stevenson, I. H. (1979). 'The influence of ageing on propranolol concentration, binding and efficacy in hyperthyroid patients', *J. Clin. Exp. Gerontol.*, **1**, 173–184.

Finlay, G. D., Whitsett, T. L., Cucinell, E. A., and Goldberg, L. I. (1971). 'Augmentation of sodium and potassium excretion, glomerular filtration rate and renal plasma flow by Levodopa', *New Engl. J. Med.*, **284**(16), 865–870.

Fisher, D. A., and Odell, W. D. (1971). 'Effect of cold on TSH secretion in man', *J. Clin. Endocrinol. Metab.*, **33**, 859–862.

Flocks. R. H. (1964). 'Benign prostatic hypertrophy: Its diagnosis and management', *Med. Times*, **92**, 519–530.

Flood, C., Gherondache, C., Pincus, G., Tait, J. F., Tait, S. A. S., and Willoughby, S. (1967). 'The metabolism and secretion of aldosterone in elderly subjects', *J. Clin. Invest.*, **46**, 960.

Fox, M., and Hammonds, J. C. (1980). 'Palliative effect of cyproterone acetate in carcinoma of the prostate with widespread metastatic bone disease', *Br. J. Urol.*, **52**, 402.

Franco-Morselli, R., Elghozi, J. L., Joly, E., Di Gruilco, S., and Meyer, P. (1977). 'Increased plasma adrenalin in benign essential hypertension', *Br. Med. J.*, **2**, 1251–1254.

Franks, L. M. (1976). 'The natural history of prostatic cancer', in *Prostatic Disease* (Eds H. Marberger, H. Haschek, H. K. A., Schirmer, J. A. C., Colston, E. Witkin), Vol. 6, p. 103, Liss, New York.

Freedman, L. S., Ohuchi, T., Goldstein, M., Axelrod, F., Fish, I., and Dancis, J. (1972). 'Changes in human serum dopamine-β-hydroxylase activity with age', *Nature (Lond.)*, **236**, 310–311.

Fresco, G., Curti, G., Biggi, A., and Fontana, B. (1982). 'Comparison of calculated and measured free thyroid hormones in serum in health and in abnormal states', *Clin. Chem.*, **28**, 1325–1329.

Friedman, M., Green, M. F., and Sharland, D. E. (1969). 'Assessment of hypothalamic–pituitary–adrenal function in the geriatric age group', *J. Gerontol.*, **24**, 292.

Friedman, R. B., Anderson, R. E., Entine, S. M., and Hirshberg, S. B. (1980). 'Effects of diseases on clinical laboratory tests', *Clin. Chem.*, **26**(4), 1D–4D.

Frolkis, V. V., Golovchenko, S. F., Medved, V. I., and Frolkis, R. A. (1982). 'Vasopressin and cardiovascular system in aging', *Gerontology*, **28**, 290–302.

Gallagher, J. C., Riggs, B. L., Jerpbak, C. M., and Arnaud, C. D. (1980). 'The effect of age on serum immunoreactive parathyroid hormone in normal and osteoporotic women', *J. Lab. Clin. Med.*, **95**, 373–385.

Geller, J., and Albert, J. (1982). 'The effect of aging on the prostate', in *Endocrine Aspects of Aging* (Ed. S. G. Korenman), pp. 137–162, Elsevier Biomedical.

Ghanadian, R., and Puah, C. M. (1981). 'Age related changes of serum 5 alpha. Androstane-3 alpha 17 beta diol in hormonal men', *Gerontology*, **27**, 281–285.

Gittes, R. F. (1983). 'Editorial retrospective. Serum acid phosphatase and screening for carcinoma of the prostate', *New Engl. J. Med.*, **309**(14), 852–853.

Gordin, A., and Lamberg, B.-A. (1981). 'Spontaneous hypothyroidism in symptomless autoimmune thyroiditis. A long-term follow-up study', *Clin. Endocrinol.*, **15**, 537–543.

Graf, R. J., Halter, J. B., and Porter, D., Jr (1978). 'Glycosylated haemoglobin in normal subjects with maturity onset diabetes. Evidence for a saturable system in man', *Diabetes*, **27**(A), 834–839.

Graham, J. J., and Harding, P. E. (1977). 'Case of myxoedema coma successfully treated by low dose oral tri-iodothyronine', *Aust. NZ J. Med.*, **7**, 163.

Graham, K., Williams, B. O., and Rowe, M. S. (1979). 'Idiopathic hypoparathyroidism; a cause

of fits in the elderly', *Br. Med. J.*, **1**, 1460–1461.

Green, M. F., and Friedman, M. (1968). 'Hypothalamic–pituitary–adrenal function in the elderly', *Gerontol. Clin.*, **10**, 334–339.

Greenblatt, R. B. (Ed.) (1978). *Geriatric Endocrinology: Aging*, Vol. 5, Raven Press, New York.

Hammond, G. L., Kontturi, M., Vihko, P., and Vihko, R. (1978). 'Serum steroids in normal males and patients with prostatic diseases', *Clin. Endocrinol.*, **9**, 113–121.

Heath, D. A. (1980). *Disorders of Calcium and Magnesium in Endocrine and Metabolic Emergencies* (Eds P. H. Sönksen and C. Lowry), Vol. 9, No. 3, pp. 499–500, W. B. Saunders.

Heath, H. W., III, Hodgson, S. F., and Kennedar, M. A. (1980). 'Primary hyperparathyroidism. Incidence, morbidity and potential economic impact on the community', *New Engl. J. Med.*, **302**, 189–193.

Hegstad, Rebecca, Brown, R. D., Jiang, N-S, Kao, P., Weinshilboum, R. M., Strong, C., and Wisgerhof, M. (1983). 'Aging and aldosterone', *Am. J. Med.*, **74**, 442–448.

Helderman, J. H. (1982). 'The impact of normal aging on the hypothalamic–neurohypophyseal–renal axis', in *Endocrine Aspects of Aging* (Ed. S. G. Korenman), Elsevier Biomedical.

Helderman, J. H., Vestal, R. E., Rowe, J. W., Tobin, S. D., Andres, R., and Robertson, G. L. (1978). 'The response of arginine vasopressin to intravenous ethanol and hypertonic saline in man: The impact of aging', *J. Gerontol.*, **33**, 39–47.

Hennemann, G., Van Welsum, M., Bernard, B., Docter, R., and Visser, T. J. (1975). 'Serum thyrotrophin concentration: An unreliable test for detection of early hypothyroidism after thyroidectomy', *Br. Med. J.*, **2**, 129–130.

Henschke, P. J., and Pain, R. W. (1977). 'Thyroid disease in a psychogeriatric population', *Age Ageing*, **6**, 151–155.

Hodkinson, H. M. (1973). 'Serum calcium in a geriatric inpatient population', *Age Ageing*, **2**, 157–162.

Hodkinson, H. M. (1977). *Biochemical Diagnosis of the Elderly*, Chapman and Hall.

Hodkinson, H. M., and McPherson, C. K. (1973). 'Alkaline phosphatase in a geriatric in-patient population', *Age Ageing*, **2**, 28.

Holmegaard, S. N. (1982). 'Measurement of cyclic AMP in clinical investigations (i p. 6 ii). Variations in cAMP under physiological conditions', *Acta Endocrinologica*, Suppl. **249**, 20–22.

Hosking, D. J. (1983). 'Dysequilibrium hypercalcaemia', *Br. Med. J.*, **286**, 326–327.

Howel, E. A. W., Woodrow, J. C., McDougall, C. D., Chew, A. R., and Evans, R. W. (1967). 'Antibodies in families of thyrotoxic patients', *Lancet*, **1**, 636–639.

Hudson, B., Coghlan, J. P., and Dulmanis, A. (1976). 'Testicular function in man', in *Ciba Foundation Colloquia on Endocrinology* (Section in the text is edited by C. E. Woolstenholme and M. O'Connor), pp. 149–152, Little, Brown & Co., Boston.

Hughes, F. S., and Caron, M. (1975). 'Les tumeurs leydigiennes. Etude générale a propos d'une observation', *Sem. Hop. Paris*, **52**, 1157.

Ibbertson, H. K. (1964). 'The thyroid. Normal physiology and biochemistry'. In *Recent Advances in Medicine* (Eds D. N. Baron, N. Compston, and A. M. Dawson), 14th ed., p. 353, Churchill Livingstone, London.

Ingbar, S. H. (1978). 'The influence of aging on the human thyroid hormone economy', in *Geriatric Endocrinology* (Ed. R. B. Greenblatt), *Aging*, Vol. 5, p. 13, Raven Press, New York.

Jacobi, H., Moore, R. J., and Wilson, J. D. (1978). 'Studies on the mechanism of 3α-androstonediol-induced growth of the dog prostate', *Endocrinology*, **102**, 1748–1755.

Jeffreys, P. M. (1972). 'The prevalence of thyroid disease in patients admitted to a geriatric department', *Age Ageing*, **1**, 33–37.

Jensen, F. G., Christiansen, C., and Transbøl, J. (1982). 'Treatment with post-menopausal oestrogens. A controlled therapeutic trial comparing oestrogen/progestagen 1,25–dihydroxyvitamin D and calcium. Osteoporosis; a multi-disciplinary problem: The Royal Society of Medicine, International Congress and Symposium No. 55', *J. Clin. Endocrinol.*, **16**, 515.

Joffe, B. I., Seftel, H. C., Goldberg, R. C., Bersham, I., and Hacking, W. H. L. (1975). 'Metabolic bone disease with the elderly. Biochemical studies in three different racial groups living in South Africa', *S. Afr. Med. J.*, **49**, 965–966.

Johnson, K., Howarth, A. T., Hamilton, M., and Mascall, G. C. (1982). *Clin. Chem.*, **28/2**, 333–338.

Jonckheer, M. (1981). 'Amiodarone and the thyroid gland. A review', *Acta Cardiologica*, **3**, 199–205.

Jones, E. C. (1975). 'The post-reproductive phase in mammals. Estrogens in the postmenopause', *Front. Horm. Res.*, **3**, 1–19.

Josephson, A. M., and Mackenzie, T. B. (1980). 'Thyroid-induced mania in hypothyroid patients', *Br. J. Psychiatry*, **137**, 222–228.

Kafetz, K., and Hodkinson, H. M. (1981). 'Osteomalacia in presence of "normal" serum 25-hydroxy cholecalciferol concentration'. *Br. Med. J.*, **283**, 1437.

Kahana, L., Keidar, S., Sheinfeld, M., and Palant, A. (1983). 'Endogenous cortisol and thyroid hormone levels in patients with acute myocardial infarction', *Clin. Endocrinol.*, **19**, 131–139.

Kamijo, K., Kato, T., Saito, A., Suzuki, M., and

Yachi, A. (1981). 'Evidence of sex differences in dopaminergic modulation of serum TSH secretion in primary hypothyroidism', *Endocrinol. Jpn*, **28**, 127–131.

Kanungo, M. S. (1980). *Biochemistry of Ageing*, pp. 165–168, Academic Press.

Kanungo, M. S., Patnaik, S. K., and Koul, O. (1975). 'Decrease in 17 beta-oestradiol receptor in brain of ageing rats', *Nature*, **253**, 366–367.

Kaplan, M. M., Larsen, P. R., Crantz, F. R., Dzau, V. J., Rossing, T. H., and Haddow, J. E. (1982). 'Prevalence of abnormal thyroid function test results in patients with acute medical illnesses', *Am. J. Med.*, **72**, 9–16.

Kapstein, E. M., Weiner, J. M., Robinson, W. J., Wheeler, W. S., and Nicoloff, J. T. (1982). 'Relationship of altered thyroid hormone indices to survival in nonthyroidal illnesses', *Clin. Endocrinol.*, **16**, 565–574.

Keating, F. R., Jones, J. D., Elveback, L. R., and Randal, R. V. (1969). 'The relation of age and sex to distribution of values in healthy adults, serum calcium, inorganic phosphorus, magnesium, alkaline phosphatase, total proteins, albumin and blood urea', *J. Lab. Clin. Med.*, **73**, 825.

Kernohan, J. W., and Sayre, G. P. (1956). 'Tumors of the pituitary gland and Infundibulum'. In Section 10, Fascille 36, *Atlas of Tumors of Pathology*. pp. 1–81. United States. Ward Department. Surgeon General's Office. Army Institute of Pathology.

Kind, P. R. N., Ghosh, S. (1976). 'Observations on thyroid function tests in the elderly', *Age Ageing*, **5**, 141–148.

Kley, H. K., Nieschlage, D., Wiegelmann, W., and Kruskemper, H. K. (1976). 'Sexual hormone', *Bieu alteruden MANN. Aktuel gerontol.*, **6**, 61.

Korenman, S. G. (Ed.) (1982). *Endocrine Aspects of Aging*, Current Endocrinology Series, Elsevier Biomedical.

Krieg, M., Bartsch, W., Janssen, W., and Voigt, K. D. (1979). 'A comparative study of binding, metabolism and endogenous levels of androgens in normal, hyperplastic and carcinomatous human prostate', *J. Steroid Biochem.*, **2**, 615–624.

Krulich, L. (1982). 'Neurotransmitter control of thyrotropin secretion', *Neuroendocrinology*, **35**, 139–147.

Kurtz, A. B., Capper, S. J., Clifford, J., Humphrey, M. J., and Lukinac, L. (1981). 'The effect of fenclofenac on thyroid function', *Clin. Endocrinol.*, **15**, 117–124.

Lahey, F. H. (1932). Management of severe and of atypical hyperthyroidism. *Ann. Int. Med.*, **5**, 1123–1128.

Lamberg, B. A. (1960). 'Present status of disorders of the thyroid gland in Finland'. *Dia. Med.*, **32**, 1890–1894.

Laron, Z., Doron, M., and Amilkan, B. (1970). 'Plasma growth hormone in men and women over 70 years of age', in *Medicine and Sport*, Vol. IV. pp. 126–131, Petah Tigra-Karger, Basel.

Leader (1983). 'New treatment for prostatic cancer', *Lancet*, **2**, 438.

Leask, R. G. S., Andrews, G. R., and Caird, F. I. (1973). 'Normal values of 16 blood constituents in the elderly', *Age Ageing*, **2**, 14–23.

Leboff, M. S., Kaplan, M. M., Silva, J. E., Larsen, P. R. (1982). 'Bioavailability of thyroid hormones from oral replacement preparations', *Metabolism*, **31**(9), 900–905.

Leonard, D. J. M., Leach, R. B., Coutur, E. M., and Paulson, C. H. (1972). 'Plasma and urinary FSH levels in oligo-spermia', *J. Clin. Endocrinol.*, **209**, 24.

McConway, M. G., Martin, B. J., Nugent, M., Lennox, I. M., and Glen, A. C. A. (1981). 'Magnesium status in the elderly on hospital admission', *J. Clin. Exp. Teront.*, **3**(4), 367–379.

Macfarlane, I. A., Mawer, E. B., Berry, J., and Hann, J. (1982). 'Vitamin D metabolism in hyperthyroidism', *Clin. Endocrinol.*, **17**, 51–59.

Mcgeown, M. G. (1964). Personal communication to F. McKeown quoted in *Pathology of the Aged*, 1965, p. 218, Butterworths.

Macías Núñez, J. F., Iglesias, G., Tabernero Romo, J. M., Rodríguez Commes, J. L., Becerra, L. C., and Sanchez Tomero, J. A. (1980). 'Renal management of sodium under indomethacin and aldosterone in the elderly', *Age Ageing*, **9**, 165–172.

McKeown, F. (1965). *Pathology of the Aged*, Butterworths, London.

Martin, A. (1981). *Problems in Geriatric Medicine*, p. 179, MTP Press Ltd.

Massry, S. G., and Seelig, M. S. (1977). 'Hypomagnesaemia and hypermagnesaemia', *Clin. Nephrol.*, **7**, 147–153.

McLarty, D. G., Ratcliffe, W. A., Ratcliffe, J. G., Shimmins, J. G., and Goldberg, A. (1978). 'A study of thyroid function in psychiatric in-patients', *Br. J. Psychiatry*, **133**, 211–218.

Melmed, S., and Hershman, J. M. (1982). 'The thyroid and aging', in *Endocrine Aspects of Aging* (Ed. S. G. Korenman), p. 41, Elsevier Biomedical.

Messerli, F. H., Sundgaard–Riise, K., Ventura, H. O., Dunn, F. G., Glade, L. B., and Frohlich, E. D. (1983). 'Essential hypertension in the elderly: Haemodynamics, intravascular volume, plasma renin activity, and circulating catecholamine levels', *Lancet*, **7**, 983–985.

Mills, G. (1976). Personal communication.

Miyai, K., Onishi, T., Hosokava, M., Ishibashi, K., and Kumahara, Y. (1974). 'Inhibition of thyrotropin and prolactin secretion in primary hypo-thyroidism by 2-Br-alpha-ergocryptine', *J. Clin. Endocrinol. Metab.*, **39**, 391–394.

Mondal, C. K., and Sinha, T. K. (1979). 'How acromegaly can creep up on the elderly', *Ger. Med.*, **4**, 50–53.

Mondal, B. K., and Biswas, R. K. (1979). 'An unusual complication of thyrotoxicosis', *Ger. Med.* **9**, Pt 8, 31–32.

Mortensen, J. D., Woolner, L. B., and Bennett, W. H. (1955). 'Gross and microscopic findings in clinically normal thyroid glands', *J. Clin. Endocrin. Metab.*, **15**, 1270–1280.

Mroczek, W. J., Finnerty, F. A., and Catt, K. J. (1973). 'Lack of association between plasma renin and history of heart attack or stroke in patients with essential hypertension', *Lancet*, **2**, 464–468.

Mundy, G. R., Cove, D. H., and Fisken, R. (1980). 'Primary hyperparathyroidism – changes in the pattern of clinical presentation', *Lancet*, **1**, 1317–1320.

Mundy, G. R., and Martin, T. J. (1982). 'The hypercalcaemia of malignancy; pathogenesis and management', *Metabolism*, **31**(12), 1247–1277.

Murakami, K., Kasama, T., Hayashi, R., Tsushima, M., Nashioheda, Y., Koh, H., Nambu, S., and Ikeda, M. (1982). 'Myxoedema coma induced by beta-adrenoreceptor-blocking agent', *Br. Med. J.*, **2**, 543–544.

Murphy, M. B. (1983). 'Calcium and hypertension', *Hospital Update*, **8**, 1119–1126.

Murray, D., Wood, P. J., Moriarty, J., and Clayton, B. E. (1981). 'Adrenocortical function in old age', *J. Clin. Exp. Gerontol.*, **3**(3), 255–268.

Nicholls, M. G., Espiner, E. A., Donald, R. A., and Hughes, H. (1974). 'Aldosterone and its regulation during diuresis in patients with gross congestive heart failure', *Clin. Sci. Molec. Med.*, **47**, 301–315.

Nieschlag, E., Kley, H. K., Wiegelmann, W., Solbach, H. J., and Kruskemper, H. L. (1973). 'Lebensalter und endikrine funktion der testes der erwachsenen mannes', *Pat, DTSH, M. Med, Wochenschr.*, **98**, 1281.

Nilsson, T., and Jonsson, G. (1978). 'Estramustine phosphate (Estracyt) as a primary treatment of prostatic cancer', in *Current Chemotherapy* (Eds W. Siegenthaler and R. Luthy), Vol. II, pp. 1282–1283, Am. Soc. for Microbiology.

Norris, E. H. (1947). 'Parathyroid adenomas. Study of 322 cases', *Ann. Int. Surg.*, **84**, 1.

Norris, H. J., and Taylor, H. B. (1968). 'The ovaries in endocrine disorders', in *Endocrine Pathology* (Ed. J. M. B. Bloodworth Jr), Williams & Wilkins, Baltimore.

Nowaczynski, W., Genest, J., Kuchel, O., Messerli, F. H., Guthrie, G. P., and Richardson, K. (1977). 'Age- and posture-related changes in plasma protein binding and metabolism of aldosterone in essential and secondary hypertension', *J. Lab. Clin. Med.*, **90**, 475–489.

O'Malley, B. P., Abbott, R. J., Barnett, D. B., Northover, B. J., and Rosenthal, F. D. (1982). 'Propranolol versus carbimazone as the sole treatment for thyrotoxicosis. A consideration of circulating thyroid hormone levels and tissue thyroid function', *Clin. Endocrinol.*, **16**, 545–552.

Oppenheimer, J. H. (1982). 'Thyroid function tests in nonthyroidal disease', *J. Chron. Dis.*, **35**, 697–701.

Palmer, K. T. (1977). 'A prospective study into thyroid disease in a geriatric unit', *NZ Med. J.*, **86**, 323–324.

Pearson, D. W. M., Ratcliffe, W. A., Thomson, J. A., and Ratcliffe, J. G. (1982). 'Biochemical and clinical effects of Fenclofenac in thyrotoxicosis', *Clin. Endocrinol.*, **16**, 369–373.

Peek, J. C., and Watkins, W. B. (1980). 'Synergism between bovine seminal plasma extract and testosterone propionate in suppressing serum concentrations of gonadotrophins in acutely castrated rats: a role for inhibin', *J. Endocrinol.*, **86**, 349–355.

Pehrson, J. J., Jaffee, W. L., and Vaitukaitis, J. L. (1983). 'Effect of dopamine on gonadotropin-releasing hormone-induced gonadotropin secretion in postmenopausal women', *J. Clin. Endocrinol. Metab.*, **56**(5), 889–892.

Pescatore, D., Giberti, C., Martorana, G., Natta, G., and Giuliani, L. (1980). 'The effect of cyproterone acetate and orchidectomy on metastases from prostatic cancer', *Eur. Urol.*, **6**, 149–153.

Petersen, M. M., Briggs, R. S., Ashby, M. A., Reid, R. I., Hall, M. R., Wood, P. J., and Clayton, B. E. (1983). 'Parathyroid hormone and 25-hydroxy vitamin D concentrations in sick and normal elderly people', *Br. Med. J.*, **287**, 521–523.

Pirke, K. M., Sintermann, R., and Vogt, H. J. (1980). 'Testosterone and testosterone precursors in the spermatic vein and in the testicular tissue of old men', *Gerontology*, **26**, 221–230.

Ptiman, J. A. (1962). 'The thyroid and aging', *J. Am. Geriatr. Soc.*, **10**, 10–30.

Posen, S., Kleerekoper, M., Ingham, J. P., and Hirshorn, J. E. (1976). 'Parathyroid hormone assay in clinical decision-making', *Br. Med. J.*, **1**, 16–19.

Pritchard, D. A., Singh, B. N., and Hurley, P. J. (1975). 'Effects of Amiodarone on thyroid function in patients with ischaemic heart disease', *Br. Heart J.*, **37**, 856–860

Grero, P. S., and Hodkinson, H. M. (1977). 'Hypercalcaemia in elderly hospital inpatients; value of discriminant analysis in differential diagnosis', *Age Ageing*, **6**, 14.

Rai, G. S. (1982). 'Cardiac arrhythmias in the elderly', *Age Ageing*, **11**, 113–115.

Rakoff, A. E., and Nowroozi, K. (1978). 'The female climacteric', in *Geriatric Endocrinology* (Ed. R. B. Greenblatt), *Aging*, Vol. 5, pp. 165–190, Raven Press, New York.

Ratcliffe, J. G., Ayoub, L. A. W., and Pearson, D. (1981). 'The measurement of serum thyroglobulin in the presence of thyroglobulin antibody', *Clin. Endocrinol.*, **15**, 507–518.

Reed, A. H., Cannon, D. C., Winkelman, J. W., Bhasin, Y. P., Henry, R. J., and Pileggi, V. J. (1972). 'Estimation of normal ranges from a controlled sample, Survey 1. Sex and age related influence on SMA 12/60. Screening group of test', *Clin. Chem.*, **18**, 57–66.

Refetoff, S., Fang, V. S., Rapoport, B., and Frisen, H. G. (1974). 'Interrelationships in the regulation of TSH and prolactin secretion in man: Effects of L-dopa TRH and thyroid hormone in various combinations', *J. Clin. Endocrinol. Metab.*, **38**, 450–457.

Reyes, F. I., Winter, J. S., and Faiman, C. (1976). 'Pituitary gonadotropin function during human pregnancy: serum FSH and LH levels before and after LHRH administration', *J. Clin. Endocrinol. Metab.*, **42**, 490–592.

Riggs, B. L., Joursey, J., Kelly, P. J., Jones, J. D., and Maher, F. T. (1969). 'Effect of sex hormones on bone in primary osteoporosis', *J. Clin. Invest.*, **48**, 1065–1072.

Romanoff, L. P., Morris, C. W., Welch, P., Rodriguez, R. M., and Pincus, G. (1961). 'The metabolism of cortisol-4-C^{14} in young and elderly men', *J. Clin. Endocrinol.*, **21**, 1413.

Ronnov-Jenssen, A., and Kirkegaard, C. (1973). 'Hyperthyroidism; a disease of old age', *Br. Med. J.*, **1**, 41.

Roof, B. S., and Gordan, G. S. (1978). 'Hyperparathyroid disease in the aged'. In *Geriatric Endocrinology* (Ed. R. B. Greenblatt), *Aging*, Vol. 5, pp. 33–79, Raven Press, New York.

Roskovec, A., and Marshall, A. J. (1983). 'New drugs: Modern diuretic treatment', *Br. Med. J.*, **286**, 1971–1972.

Ross, H. (1981). 'Endocrinology', in *Geriatrics for Everyday Practice* (Ed. J. Andrews), pp. 30–45, Karger, Basel.

Ross, R. K., Paganini–Hill, A., Gerkins, V. R., Mack, T. M., Pfeffer, R., Arthur, M., and Henderson, B. E. (1980). 'A case control study of menopausal estrogen therapy and breast cancer', *J. Am. Med. Assoc.*, **243**, 1635–1639.

Salomon, Y., Elhanan, E., and Amir-Zaltsman, Y. (1981). 'The role of GTP in luetropin-induced desensitization of the GTP regulatory cycle and adenylate cyclase in the rat ovary', in *Advances in Cyclic Nucleotide Research* (Eds J. E. Dumont, P. Greengard, and G. A. Robinson), Vol. 14, pp. 101–109, Raven Press, New York.

Sawin, C. T., Chopra, D., Azizi, F., Mannix, J. E., and Bacharch, P. (1979). 'The aging thyroid: Increased prevalence of elevated serum thyrotropin in the elderly', *J. Am. Med. Assoc.*, **242**, 246–250.

Sawin, C. T., Herman, T., Molitch, M. E., London, M. H., and Kramer, S. M. (1983). 'Aging and the thyroid. Decreased requirement for thyroid hormone in older hypothyroid patients', *Am. J. Med.*, **75**, 206–209.

Scanlon, M. F., Weightman, D. R., Mora, B., Heath, M., Shale, D. J., Snow, M. H., and Hall, R. (1977). 'Evidence of dopaminergic control of thyrotropin secretion in man', *Lancet*, **2**, 421–423.

Sewell, J. M. A., Spooner, L. L. R., Dixon, A. K., and Rubenstein, D. (1981). 'Screening investigations in the elderly', *Age Ageing*, **10**, 165–168.

Shain, S. A., Boesel, R. W., Lamm, D. L., and Radwin, H. M. (1979). 'Androgen receptors of the normal and neoplastic human prostate and lymph node metastases of prostate adenocarcinoma', *Am. Soc. Androl. 4th Annual Meeting, Houston, Texas. Programs and Abstracts*, p. 50 (abstract 32).

Sheldon, J. (1983). 'Effects of amiodarone in thyrotoxicosis', *Br. Med. J.*, **286**, 267–268.

Simonin, R., Roux, H., Oliver, C., Jacquet, P., Argemi, B., and Vague, Ph. (1972). 'Effect d'une prise orale de L-dopa sur les taux plasmatiques de TSH, ACTH et GH chez les sujets normaux', *Ann. Endocrinol.*, **33**, 294–296.

Snyder, P. J., Reitano, J. F., and Utiger, R. D. (1975). 'Serum LH and FSH responses to synthetic gonadotrophin releasing hormone in normal men', *J. Clin. Endocrinol. Metab.*, **41**, 938–945.

Sonkodi, S., Nicholls, M. G., Cumming, A. M. M., and Robertson, J. I. S. (1981). 'Effects of change in body posture on plasma and serum electrolytes in normal subjects and in primary aldosteronism', *Clin. Endocrinol.*, **14**, 613–620.

Sowers, J. R., Catania, R. A., and Hoshman, J. M. (1982). 'Evidence of dopaminergic control of circadian variations in thyrotropin secretion', *Clin. Endocrinol. Metab.*, **54**, 673–675.

Spaulding, S. W., Burrow, G. N., Donabedian, R., and Woert, M. van (1972). 'L-dopa suppression of thyrotropin releasing hormone in man', *J. Clin. Endocrinol. Metab.*, **35**, 182–185.

Spencer, C. A., Lum, S. M. C., Wilber, J. F., Kaptein, E. M., and Nicoloff, J. T. (1983). 'Dynamics of serum thyrotropin and thyroid hormone changes in fasting', *J. Clin. Endocrinol. Metab.*, **156**(5), 883–888.

Spratt, D. I., Pont, A., Miller, M. B., McDougall, I. R., Bayer, M. F., and McLaughlin, W. T. (1982). 'Hyperthyroxinemia in patients with acute psychiatric disorders', *Am. J. Med.*, **73**, 41–48.

Sterns, E. L., MacDonnell, J. A., Kaufman, B. J., Padua, R., Lucman, T. S., Winter, J. S. D., and Faiman, C. (1974). 'Declining testicular function with age', *Am. J. Med.*, **57**, 761–766.

Studd, J. W. W., and Thom, M. H. (1981). 'Ovarian failure and aging', in *Clinics in Endocrinology and Metabolism: Endocrinology and Ageing*, Vol. 5, pp. 89–113, W. B. Saunders.

Sunderam, S., and Mankikar, G. (1983). 'Hyponatraemia in the elderly', *Age Ageing*, **12**, 77–80.

Swales, J. D. (1983). 'Primary aldosteronism: How hard should we look? *Br. Med. J.*, **287**, 702–703.

Swyer, G. I. M. (1944). 'Post-natal growth changes in the human prostate', *J. Anat.*, **78**, 130–145.

Symons, R. G., Walichnowski, C. M., and Murphy, L. J. (1982). 'Effectiveness of analysis of free thyroxin concentration in serum for diagnosis of covert thyroid disease', *Clin. Chem.*, **28/2**, 266–270.

Takahashi, J., Higashi, Y., Lanasa, J. A., Yoshida, K-I., Winters, S. J., Oshima, H., and Troen, P. (1983). 'Studies of the human testis. XVII. Simultaneous measurement of nine intratesticular steroids: Evidence for reduced mitochondrial function in testis of elderly men', *J. Clin. Endocrinol. Metab.*, **56**(6), 1178.

Tarquini, B., Halberg, F., Seal, U. S., Benvenuti, M., and Cagnoni, M. (1981). 'Circadian aspects of serum prolactin and TSH lowering by bromocriptine in patients with prostatic hypertrophy', *Prostate*, **2**, 269–279.

Thielemans, C., Vanhaelst, L., de Waele, M., Jonckheer, M., and Camp, B. van (1981). 'Autoimmune thyroiditis: A condition related to a decrease in T-suppressor cells', *Clin. Endocrinol.*, **15**, 259–263.

Tuck, M., and Sowers, J. (1982). 'Hypertension and aging', in *Endocrine Aspects of Aging* (Ed. S. G. Korenman), p. 97, Elsevier Biomedical.

Tunbridge, W. M. G., Evered, D. C., Hall, R., Appleton, D., Brewis, M., Clark, F., Evans, J. G., Young, E., Bird, T., and Smith, P. A. (1977). 'The spectrum of thyroid disease in a community: The Wickham Survey', *Clin. Endocrinol.*, **7**, 481–493.

Vierhapper, H., Laggner, A., Waldhäusl, W., Grubeck-Loebenstein, B., and Kleinberger, G. (1982). 'Impaired secretion of TSH in critically ill patients with 'low T_4-syndrome', *Acta Endocrinologica*, **101**, 542–549.

Walker, K. J., Nicholson, R. I., Turkes, A. O., Turkes, A., and Griffiths, K. (1983). 'Therapeutic potential of the LHRH agonist, ICI 118630, in the treatment of advanced prostatic carcinoma', *Lancet*, **2, 1983**, 413–415.

Waxman, J. H., Wass, J. A. H., Hendry, W. F., Whitfield, H. N., Besser, G. M., Malpas, J. S., and Oliver, R. T. D. (1983). 'Treatment with gonadotrophin releasing hormone analogue in advanced prostatic cancer', *Br. Med. J.*, **286**, 1309–1312.

Weetman, A. P., Weightman, D. R., and Scanlon, M. F. (1981). 'Impaired dopaminergic control of thyroid stimulating hormone secretion in chronic renal failure', *Clin. Endocrinol.*, **15**, 451–456.

Weidmann, P., Myttenaere-Bursztein, S., Maxwell, M. H., and Lima, J. (1975). 'Effect of aging on plasma renin and aldosterone in normal man', *Kidney Int.*, **8**, 325.

Wenzel, K. W. (1981). 'Progress in endocrinology and metabolism. Pharmocalogical interference with in-vitro tests of thyroid function', *Metabolism (Clinical and Experimental)*, **XXX**(7), 717–732.

West, C. D., Brown, H., Simons, E. L., Carter, D. B., Kumagai, L. F., and Englebert, E. L. (1961). 'Adrenocortical function and cortisol metabolism in old age', *J. Clin. Endocrinol. Metab.*, **21**, 1197–1207.

Whedon, G. D. (1981). 'Osteoporosis', *N. Engl. J. Med.*, **305**(7), 397–398.

Wiersinga, W. M., Lie, K. I., and Touber, J. L. (1981). 'Thyroid hormones in acute myocardial infarction', *Clin. Endocrinol.*, **14**, 367–374.

Wilkin, T. J., Storey, B. E., Isles, T. E., Crooks, J., and Swanson Beck, J. (1977). 'High TSH concentrations in "euthyroidism": Explanation based on control-loop theory', *Br. Med. J.*, **1**, 993–996.

Wilkinson, S. P., Wheeler, P. G., Jowett, T. P., Smith, I. K., Keenan, J., Slater, J. D. H., and Williams, R. (1981). 'Factors relating to aldosterone secretion rate, the excretion of aldosterone 18-glucuronide, and the plasma aldosterone concentration in cirrhosis', *Clin. Endocrinol.*, **14**, 355–362.

Wiske, P. S., Epstein, S., Bell, N. H., Queener, S. F., Edmondson, J., and Johnston, C. C. (1979). 'Increases in immunoreactive parathyroid hormone with age', *N. Engl. J. Med.*, **300**, 1419–1421.

Worth, H. G. J. (On behalf of the Scientific Committee, Association of Clinical Biochemists) (1983). 'Plasma sodium concentration: bearer of false prophecies?' *Br. Med. J.*, **287**, 567–568.

Yap, P. L., Davidson, N. McD., Lidgard, G. P., and Fyffe, J. A. (1978). 'Bromocriptine suppression of the thyrotrophin response to thyrotrophin releasing hormone', *Clin. Endocrinol.*, **9**, 179–183.

Young, D. S., Thomas, D. W., Friedman, R. B., and Pestaner, L. C. (1972). 'Bibliography: Drug interferences with clinical laboratory tests', *Clin. Chem.*, **18**(10), 1041–1303.

Zanoboni, A., Zanoboni-Muciaccia, W., and Zanussi, C. (1979). 'Enhanced TSH stimulating effect of TRH by sulphiride in man', *Acta Endocrinol. (Copenhagen)*, **91**, 257–263.

Ziegler, M. G., Lake, C. R., and Kopin, I. J. (1976). 'Plasma noradrenaline increases with age', *Nature (Lond.)*, **261**, 333–335.

22
Obesity

22.1

Obesity

J. Runcie

INTRODUCTION

Obesity is the most important nutritional disorder in Western or Westernized societies where food is abundant, readily available, and cheap. It is a major health problem in Western Europe, North America, and Australasia. In these communities obesity has attained epidemic proportions – 'the commonest metabolic disorder of the age' (Mérimée, 1971). The susceptibility of the individual (to obesity) is not uniform. The disorder has unusual sex and social characteristics. It is difficult to treat, a feature which it shares with alcoholism, where the emotive term 'carboholic' has been coined to describe a rare form of obesity due to carbohydrate addiction (Bloom and Clarke, 1964). The disease is characteristically one of middle adult life. Since obesity rarely arises *de novo* in the elderly its persistence into this age group reflects the features of chronicity and therapeutic failure and is inevitably attended by the major complications of the disorder.

THE DEFINITION OF OBESITY

Obesity is due to the excessive accumulation of fat in its storage form (neutral triglyceride) in specialized cells (adiopocytes) which become hyperplastic and hypertrophic to form adipose tissue. This results in a variable increase in body weight, the central phenomenon of the disorder. This can be massive, with weight increases 5 to 10 times greater than comparable normal weight subjects. Since specific measurements of body fat content are not yet possible, an empirical approach to the definition of obesity has been adopted whereby weight at death in insured subjects has been compared with the life expectancy of normal weight subjects. Tables of normal or ideal weights and the changes with age have been constructed (Society of Actuaries, 1959). This concept, though valuable to the actuary, has been an unfortunate development. It informs on nor defines the functional deficit in obesity. The data source – young American males between the two world wars – is not relevant to the major problem of obesity, which is that of the ageing disadvantaged parous female (Goldblatt, Moore, and Stunkard, 1965), nor does it take into account the changes in height and weight which have occurred in the young since the 1940s (the potential second-generation obese).

THE MAINTENANCE OF NORMAL BODY WEIGHT

In the normal weight subject physical maturity is attained in early adult life. Thereafter weight remains constant with surprisingly little variation until old age when weight loss commonly occurs. Over this approximate 50 year period a representative subject will, each year, ingest food with an energy equivalent of approximately 1 million calories. In some occupations energy requirements may be much higher – up to 5 million calories. That the body weight remains essentially constant throughout this period is remarkable and represents a matching of food intake (energy provision) to physical activity (energy consumption) of a very high order. The sophisticated control mechanism operating here is unknown but clearly is important to a proper understanding of obesity.

NORMAL BODY COMPOSITION

It is helpful to regard body mass as a potential energy store reflecting food intake and tissue breakdown in which some constituents are readily available for energy transformations and others not. Instantaneous body weight therefore represents a dynamic equilibrium between these opposing effects. In this context the body has three constituents, a fixed skeletal mass and two variable components, lean tissue (muscle) and adipose tissue. The growth of lean tissue is determined by physical activity (exercise) in the presence of an adequate protein and calorie supply. In some circumstances, e.g. athletes, muscle hypertrophy of sufficient degree to increase whole body weight can occur. It is interesting that this form of 'over-weightness' carries none of the metabolic or other hazards of obesity (Kalkoff and Ferrou, 1971). In dietary deficiency the amino acids of muscle may undergo gluconeogenesis to provide energy in the form of glucose. Since muscle is composed of 25 per cent. protein and 75 per cent. water its energy yield is 1 cal/g. Muscle is an inefficient energy source. More importantly, there are severe and ultimately lethal metabolic complications associated with lean tissue breakdown. This is hypercatabolic injury seen most commonly in diabetic ketoacidosis and most characteristically following major trauma, including surgical intervention. Under conditions of chronic food excess, conversion to neutral fat (lipogenesis) and storage in the fat depots occurs with the consequent development of obesity. Since adipose tissue contains 85 per cent. fat it has a calorie yield of 8 cal/g. In functional terms adipose tissue represents a massive energy store. Reduction in this fat mass is difficult, requiring a period of negative calorie balance, either by reducing food intake (reduction dieting) or increasing physical activity without increasing food intake or some combination of these effects.

EPIDEMIOLOGY

The concept of obesity is a familiar one. The condition is difficult to define and arbirtrary weight values (>10 per cent. above ideal weight) have been adopted to indicate its occurence in the individual. On such a basis about 40 per cent. of young and middle aged adults in Great Britain could be considered to be obese. Moderate overweightness is an aesthetic judgement and not a clinical disease. It does not carry the major hazards to health, including premature death, that severe or massive obesity (>25 per cent. above ideal weight) does. The factors which give rise to this severe form of obesity are not known. It is not known why at a certain level of obesity the risk to the individual's well-being becomes so much greater.

AETIOLOGY

Parity and Socioeconomic Status

The important studies of Stunkard and Mclaren-Hume (1959) have defined the liability to obesity more closely. Their findings indicate that the most vulnerable group is the economically and socially disadvantaged parous female (Goldblatt, Moore, and Stunkard, 1965). These findings have been corroborated by Silverstone (1968) and closely parallel the author's clinical experience. When asked, most women relate the onset of obesity to excessive weight gain in pregnancy and failure to regain their prepregnancy weight.

Prolonged Immobility

In males particularly the onset of obesity can be related to a period of immobility, usually following a major bone fracture. This factor can also be traced in some subjects who had previously undergone a sanatorium regimen for the treatment of tuberculosis. In yet other subjects a life threatening illness (meningitis, rheumatic carditis) had occurred in childhood or adolescence following which strenuous physical activity had been discouraged. This may have been compounded by protective or compensatory overfeeding by the mother.

Alcohol Abuse

In obese males a history of excessive alcohol intake can frequently be elicited. It is not clear whether food ingestion parallels the alcohol but certainly such subjects have a limited or little used capacity for effort.

Reduced Levels of Spontaneous Physical Activity

The importance of physical inactivity rather than excessive eating in the pathogenesis of obesity was first demonstrated in adolescent schoolgirls (Johnson, Burke, and Mayer, 1956). These were important observations and underlined the dual nature of the problem of obesity, viz. food ingestion and physical activity. It also meant that the prevailing simplistic concept of obesity being due to overeating or gluttony was inadequate and suggested why the therapeutic extension of this view, reduction dieting, was so ineffective in the management of the obese subject (Stunkard and McLaren-Hume, 1959).

PSYCHOLOGICAL ASPECTS OF OBESITY

The aetiological role of psychological abnormalities in obesity remains a controversial issue. There is general agreement that there is no increase in neuroticism in obese subjects but that they show abnormal levels of anxiety (Silverstone, 1968). This finding is consistent with the earlier view of Simon (1963) who described obesity as a 'depressive equivalent'. The supportive data for this hypothesis is tenuous but does highlight the other major problem in the development of obesity, namely non-physiological eating or the urge to eat which is not generated by hunger. The value of food as a comforter has been recognized for centuries and more recently its role in the relief of anxiety has been formally accepted – solace eating. If all behaviour is goal orientated, a common psychoanalytical view of human behaviour, it means that in some obese subjects at least the psychobiological value of eating at any time outweighs the obvious and well-publicized dangers of obesity. The psychological stresses which generate this response are worthy of intensive study. A related problem which has only recently become apparent is that some women in the face of stress retreat into physical inertia. The value of this to the individual is not clear but it does indicate the existence of important functional links between stress and/or anxiety and physical activity which also merit further study.

DIAGNOSIS

Body Weight

The diagnosis of obesity is most simply and accurately established by weighing the individual. Serial measurements are similarly helpful in monitoring the progression or regression of the disorder. Other indices have been suggested, such as the ponderal index, $weight^3\sqrt{}$, in an effort to relate weight to frame size. The advantage of such manipulations is not obvious to the author and tends to suggest the existence of a scientific precision which is illusory in this field.

Physical and Anthropometric Measurements

Skin Fold Thickness

Measurements of skin fold thickness in prescribed areas (subscapular, biceps, and triceps areas) have been used as an index of body fat content (Durnin and Rahman, 1967). The value of such measurements is limited. They are of little value in the individual subject but may be so in large-scale population surveys, particularly if serial values can be recorded in a population identifiable as being at risk.

Body Density Measurements Derived from Flotation

Estimates of body fat content can be made from body density measurements derived from weighing subjects in air and in water. The technique is cumbersome. It is applicable only to the fit subject and is mainly of historical interest.

Needle Biopsy of Adipose Tissue

This technique was introduced some years ago. It is simple, atraumatic, and can be repeated as often as required in the obese subject. It has generated important data relating fat content in the adipocyte to the insulin resistance which has been known to be present in the obese subject for many years (Hirsch and Gallion, 1968). It is also suitable for use in children. It is likely to prove an important investigative and epidemiological tool, particularly in states of developing or regressing obesity.

Body Composition Measurements

Techniques are now available to measure accurately the body muscle mass (lean tissue). These depend on measuring the radioactivity of whole body concentrations of muscle constituents and converting this into its equivalent of lean tissue. This radioactivity may be naturally present as a whole body potassium measurement of ^{42}K or induced in the nitrogen nuclei of protein molecules by bombardment in a cyclotron (^{15}N).

Whole Body Potassium Measurements

This depends on measuring the body content of the naturally occurring potassium isotope, ^{42}K, by passing the patient through a ring of six sodium iodide counters (Fig. 1). The method is non-invasive, atraumatic, and accurate. It is ideally suited to investigate changes in lean tissue mass in general and is of particular value in groups such as the elderly. In conditions where body weight or composition is changing, since skeletal mass is constant, measurement of one of the two variables (lean and adipose tissue) allows accurate measurement of both. Unfortunately there are limited numbers of such counters available throughout the country. Their wider application would generate much important metabolic data in the obese and other patient groups.

Whole Body Nitrogen Measurements Following Cyclotron Excitation of the Nitrogen Nuclei

This is a more recent technique and an interesting application of high technology to medicine. It provides the same information as whole body potassium measurements except that it measures relative change and does not provide an absolute mass for protein content. This

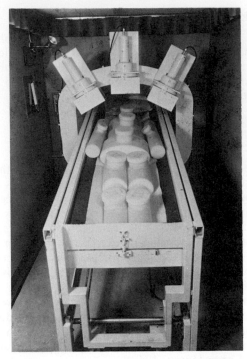

Figure 1   Whole body monitor used to measure total body potassium

technique, though procedurally simple and accurate, is of research interest only.

The Biochemistry of Fat Formation and Breakdown

Fat synthesis (lipogenesis) takes place in adipose tissue predominantly from glucose and fatty acid precursors resulting in the formation of triglyceride (neutral fat). This results from the oxidative phosphorylation of glucose, its subsequent isomerization, and then cleavage to produce the trioses, 3-phosphoglyceraldehyde and dihydroxyacetone. The triose fragment dihydroxyacetone phosphate is reduced to 1-glycerol phosphate which is subsequently esterified with fatty acid resulting in the formation of triglyceride. The sequential reactions are under close enzymatic control, the rate limiting step being the initial phosphorylation controlled by hexokinase(s). The origin of free fatty acid, either in adipose tissue or liver, remains controversial. Irrespective of the site the basic mechanism is probably the same and involves a condensation reaction between acetyl-CoA and units of malonyl-CoA under the control of a cytoplasmic multienzyme complex called fatty acid synthetase.

Lipolysis

In fasting or conditions of nutrient deficiency, fat is released from adipose tissue (lipolysis). This is not a simple reversal of lipogenesis. Under the control of intracellular lipases, stepwise hydrolysis of the glyceride esters occurs, resulting ultimately in the release into the blood of glycerol and long-chain fatty acid (1 mole of glycerol and 3 moles of fatty acid).

Normal Lipogenesis and Lipolysis in Obesity

In human obesity there is no abnormality of lipogenesis such as that which occurs in some genetically obese laboratory animals (mouse, rat). Similarly no abnormality of lipolysis preventing the breakdown or utilization of fat has been observed analogous to those in the different forms of glycogen storage disease in humans. Therefore primary abnormalities of fat formation and dissimilation play no part in the complex metabolic disturbances of obesity.

There are two abnormalities of fat metabolism known to occur in some obese subjects.
(a) The failure of free fatty acid release from adipose tissue in response to adrenaline stimulation in the hypothyroid subject (Galton, 1971). The exhibition of thyroid hormone rapidly restores the response to normal.
(b) Schwartz and Brunzell (1981) have recently reported persistently elevated lipoprotein lipase activity in obese subjects 4 to 28 months following weight loss. Since this enzyme is rate limiting for the uptake of triglyceride by adipose tissue its persistence at this time may perpetuate the obese state. It would be of interest to know whether this effect reflects degree and/or duration of obesity.

A number of hormonal abnormalities have been observed in obesity. The most important include hyperinsulinaemia, both fasting and following a glucose load, impaired growth hormone release affecting basal responses and in response to fasting and insulin stimulation and insulin resistance. The relation of these functional responses to the development or maintenance of the obese state remains an unresolved problem.

SPECIAL FEATURES OF OBESITY IN THE ELDERLY

The assessment and management of the elderly obese subject is made difficult by the paucity of data in this group. There are few large-scale surveys of the changes in energy requirements, physical activity, and food intake in the ageing subject, notable exceptions being the studies of Parizkova and Eiselt (1971) and Milne and Lonergan (1977). Nonetheless, there are a number of distinctive characteristics of obesity in this group.

Sex Difference in Incidence

Severe obesity (>25 per cent. above ideal weight) in the elderly is for practical purposes confined to the female. Severely obese men rarely survive middle adult life due to the poorer prognosis of ischaemic heart disease and idiopathic hypertension in the male, conditions which are both aggravated by obesity.

Pathogenetic Differences

In the complex metabolic disturbance of obesity, physical inactivity can be seen to be a particular problem in the elderly. Social isolation is common. There is little incentive to leave home. The development of major complications, such as osteoarthritis, renders significant physical activity increasingly more difficult. These curtail the potential for expending energy in the group. In the obesity associated with hypothyroidism, physical inactivity is its cardinal feature. The likelihood of effective therapeutic intervention in these circumstances is correspondingly more difficult.

THE CLINICAL FEATURES OF OBESITY IN THE ELDERLY

The obese elderly subject does not present for treatment of her obesity, which she regards as untreatable, but for the complications of the disorder. These include the following.

Osteoarthritis of the Major Weight-Bearing Joints

This is invariably present, the knees and hip joints being most frequently and severely involved. Physical activity is progressively reduced. The long-term use of analgesic drugs exposes such patients to dangers, iron deficiency anaemia from chronic gastrointestinal blood loss, and analgesic nephropathy, which in this form of renal involvement is complicated by secondary renal tubular acidosis.

Diabetes Mellitus (Non-Insulin Dependent)

Diabetes mellitus is an important complication of obesity, being related to both the severity and duration of the disease. Its development in the individual is attended by its major complications, nephropathy, retinopathy, enteropathy, and skin involvement (pruritus), in addition to its ischaemic vascular complications (myocardial infarction, cerebral thrombosis, gangrene). The importance of diabetes mellitus may be gauged from the fact that diabetic eye disease is the commonest cause of new blindness in middle age and beyond in America (American Diabetes Association, 1976).

Panniculitis

Some elderly obese females present with a complaint of pain and tenderness of the skin and subcutaneous tissue, of the legs usually. In the author's experience this has only been observed in women. It is resistant to drugs and to physiotherapy and only responds to significant weight loss.

Paradoxical Subnutrition in the Elderly Obese

It has recently become apparent that the elderly obese subject may develop serious nutritional deficiencies. Impaired mobility makes them excessively reliant on others, restricts shopping and choice of foods, often forcing them on to a diet of easily cooked, convenience foods, carbohydrates mainly – 'the empty calorie syndrome'. Such diets are particularly deficient in the water-soluble vitamins and biochemical testing will frequently reveal significant deficiencies. Obese subjects are perforce restricted to the home. Their opportunity for sunlight exposure is greatly reduced and they can develop severe vitamin D deficiency resulting in painful metabolic bone disease which further restricts physical activity.

THE TREATMENT OF OBESITY IN THE ELDERLY

The treatment of obesity in the elderly is difficult, many would say impossible. Conventional therapy can be listed as follows:
(a) reduction dieting – ineffective and irrelevant (Stunkard and McLaren-Hume, 1959);
(b) anorexiant drugs – effects are short lived; the drugs are addictive and in extended use are psychotomimetic, particularly in the female (Seton *et al.*, 1961).

There are two components to the effective treatment of obesity, weight loss and the subsequent maintenance of this reduced weight. In the severely obese the first can be best achieved by supervised starvation in hospital and by small bowel bypass surgery.

Therapeutic Starvation (The Water Diet)

Starvation is well tolerated by obese subjects, including the elderly. Weight loss is significant, rapid, and predictable (Runcie and Hilditch, 1974). The procedure is safe. There is one established contraindication. No patient should undergo starvation within six months or preferably one year of suffering from an episode of cardiac failure because of the risk of ventricular fibrillation and/or cardiac arrest (Spencer, 1969). Intercurrent disease, including myocardial infarction, is otherwise not a contraindication. Starvation should only be undertaken in hospital. The duration of starvation is related to the patient's prefast weight. In general terms if a patient merits consideration for starvation, a minimum period of 4 weeks is necessary. The impact of fasting on patients aged 60 years is recorded in Table 1.

Small Bowel Bypass Surgery

Surgical, short-circuiting operations on the small bowel are highly effective in promoting weight loss. The procedure is hazardous with a significant primary mortality (5 to 10 per cent.) and a remote mortality due to hepatic

TABLE 1 Weight loss responses in elderly, fasting subjects

Patient	Fast (days)	Weight loss (kg)	Side-effects
S. McB.	48	20.5	None
T. McG.	42	14.5	None
I. H.	58	17.3	Fluid retention
M. F.	44	16.4	None
A. S.	20	11.8	Abdominal pain
M. D.	30	7.3	None
E. McG.	112	38.2	Fluid retention
H. R.	23	10	Nausea
R. McB.	33	17.7	None
M. D.	249	34.1	Fluid retention
R. A.	79	31.8	None
S. McA.	33	11.4	None

necrosis. There are major complications – intractable diarrhoea, renal stone formation. There is little information on the results of such procedures in the elderly but it must be assumed that the mortality and complication rate will be higher, and, in the present state of knowledge, unacceptable in this group.

POST WEIGHT LOSS MANAGEMENT

Once significant weight loss is achieved, usually by fasting, management thereafter should be directed at improving the individual's mobility. This involves careful attention to:

(a) Foot and footwear problems.
(b) Vigorous management of joint dysfunction, including operative intervention (joint replacement).
(c) Overcoming social isolation – geriatric day hospital attendance, organized support in the community.
(d) Psychological assessment and the institution of any necessary therapy, e.g. stress or anxiety management.
(e) Formal dietetic guidance to eliminate faulty eating habits and ensure adequate nutrition.
(f) Frequent follow-up by an interested physician. Obese subjects respond, perhaps abnormally, to the personality of the doctor. Such a structured follow-up, usually in association with a home visiting nursing sister, provides an effective programme of management and one in which the patient can have confidence.

Obesity is a painful and disabling disorder in the elderly. Its treatment is difficult and unsatisfactory. It is an important area for the practice of preventative medicine. Available data indicate that the postnatal clinic is the most important focus for such an exercise. In established obesity in the elderly effective management requires a complete knowledge of the social and psychological status of the individual and the formulation of an individual patient treatment plan. It is only with the adoption of these time-consuming measures that any prospect of alleviation can be held out to the affected subject.

REFERENCES

American Diabetes Association (1976). *Fact Sheet on Diabetes*, American Diabetes Association, New York.

Bloom, W. L., and Clarke, M. B. (1964). 'The obese carboholic', *J. Obesity*, **1**, 10–14.

Durnin, J. V. G. A., and Rahman, M. M. (1967). 'The assessment of the amount of fat in the human body from measurements of skin fold thickness', *Br. J. Nutr.*, **21**, 681–689.

Galton, D. J. (1971). *The Human Adipose Cell*, p. 119, Butterworths, London.

Goldblatt, P. B., Moore, M. E., and Stunkard, A. J. (1965). 'Social factors in obesity', *JAMA*, **192**, 1039–1044.

Hirsch, J., and Gallion, E. (1968). 'Methods for the determination of adipose cell size in man and animals', *J. Lipid. Res.*, **9**, 110–119.

Johnson, M. L., Burke, B. S., and Mayer, J. (1956). 'Relative importance of inactivity and overeating on the energy balance of obese high school girls', *Am. J. Clin. Nutr.*, **4**, 37–42.

Kalkhoff, R., and Ferrou, C. (1971). 'Metabolic differences between obese overweight and muscular overweight men', *N. Engl. J. Med.*, **284**, 1236–1239.

Mérimée, T. J. (1971). 'Editorial', *N. Engl. J. Med.*, **285**, 856–857.

Milne, J. S., and Lonergan, M. E. (1977). 'A five year follow up study of bone mass in older people', *Ann. Hum. Biol.*, **4**, 243–252.

Parizkova, J., and Eiselt, E. (1971). 'A further study in somatic characteristics and body composition of old men followed longitudinally for 8–10 years', *Hum. Biol.*, **43**, 318–325.

Runcie, J., and Hilditch, T. E. (1974). 'Energy provision, tissue utilisation and weight loss in prolonged starvation', *Br. Med. J.*, **2**, 352–356.

Schwartz, R. S., and Brunzell, J. D. (1981). 'Increase of adipose tissue lipoprotein lipase activity with weight loss', *J. Clin. Invest.*, **67**, 1425–1430.

Seton, D. A., Duncan, L. J. P., Rose, K., and Scott, A. M. (1961). 'Diethylpropion in the treatment of refractory obesity', *Br. Med. J.*, **1**, 1009–1011.

Silverstone, J. T. (1968). 'Psychosocial aspects of obesity', *Proc. R. Soc. Med.*, **61**, 371–375.

Simon, R. I. (1963). 'Obesity as a depressive equivalent', *J. Am. Diet Assoc.*, **183**, 208.

Society of Actuaries (1959). *Build and Blood Pressure Study*, Society of Actuaries.

Spencer, I. O. B. (1968). 'Death during therapeutic starvation for obesity', *Lancet*, **1**, 1288–1290.

Stunkard, A., and McLaren-Hume, M. (1959). 'Results of treatment for obesity: Review of literature and report of series', *Arch. Intern. Med.*, **103**, 79–85.

23
Diabetes

23.1

Diabetes

R. A. Jackson

INTRODUCTION

Diabetes mellitus is a universal health problem affecting societies at all stages of development and with the ageing of populations the numbers of reported cases are increasing rapidly. In some countries more than one-third of older adults have diabetes and a majority will eventually develop the disease while in other societies rates of diabetes are as low as 2 per cent. in the elderly (West, 1978). In the United States and Western Europe the disease now affects about 16 per cent. of those aged 65 and over and the size of the diabetic population is likely to double in 15 years.

It is clear, therefore, that the disease has a tremendous impact not only on the health of individuals but also on the health care system of the country. In adult-onset diabetes in Europe and North America, life expectancy averages about 70 per cent. of normal and the leading cause of death is coronary disease, responsible for about half the mortality. Ischaemic heart disease, glomerulosclerosis, retinopathy, gangrene of a lower extremity, neuropathy, stroke, and cataract are major causes of prolonged ill health and while some diabetics live long lives with little indisposition, their rates of disability are in general about 2 to 3 times greater than in non-diabetics. In diabetes blindness is about 10 times and gangrene 20 times more common and some 14 per cent. of diabetics (usually the elderly) are bedridden for an average of six weeks per year.

Fundamental to improved health for the elderly diabetic is a well-organized multidisciplinary approach through the coordination and integration of many social and medical skills for the provision of health care, research, and education. As in all other areas of geriatric care, treatment of the elderly diabetic is essentially a team responsibility, shared on the one hand by the doctor and staff in the hospital and, on the other hand, by those in the community, viz. the general practitioner, the social workers, and, most importantly, the patient's family. The affected person, in particular, should take major responsibility for his or her own health and become as self-sufficient and independent as possible. Patient education is the cornerstone of treatment and countries that have health care systems with the major emphasis on the community lend themselves naturally to the care of the diabetic.

Thus while the same general principles of treatment apply to diabetics of all ages, in the elderly patient the approach and priorities are somewhat changed and total care involves considerations which extend far beyond pure metabolic control. Emphasis should be placed more on the overall welfare of the person and less on the metabolic disorder, and the goal should be to achieve a degree of control through an approach built around the patient's established pattern of living. The principal aim of therapy is the relief of symptoms of hyperglycaemia and the maintenance of a sense of well-being at the expense, if necessary, of achieving absolute normoglycaemia while nevertheless taking adequate precautions to prevent any tendency to develop ketoacidosis. Whether or not complications are preventable 15 years hence by excellent control is of secondary importance in a person who develops diabetes at the age of 65.

Since diabetes is a lifelong disease, continuing medical supervision at regular intervals is essential in order to render patients asymptomatic and to allow them to lead as normal a life as possible within the constraints of their disease. Many clinical judgements required in the treatment of heart disease, renal disease, cerebrovascular disease, etc., are similar in diabetics and non-diabetics and although conditions such as bacterial and fungal infections may have distinctive features in diabetics, the same basic decisions of management apply. On the other hand, several clinical decisions apply only to diabetics, e.g. in the regulation of diet, oral therapy, and insulin. Strict dietary control is almost impossible to enforce and acceptance of this in the elderly will avoid the making of unrealistic demands and thereby promote the development of a good doctor–patient relationship. In any event, it is generally agreed that a less rigid approach should be adopted to blood glucose regulation in the elderly so that due account is taken of all aspects of the patient's physical and mental condition and social circumstances.

PHYSIOLOGICAL CHANGES IN GLUCOSE HOMEOSTASIS WITH AGE

In 1920 Spence was the first to document that glucose metabolism was impaired in subjects over 60 years and since this initial observation numerous reports have appeared (Davidson, 1979) confirming the progressive deterioration of glucose tolerance with age in men (Fig. 1) and women (Fig. 2). This decline begins in the third decade and appears to be continuous throughout the entire adult life span. Blood glucose levels occurring one or two hours after a 50 g oral load rise by about 6 to 13 mg/dl (0.3 to 0.7 mmol/l) per decade and tend to be about 10 mg/dl (0.6 mmol/l) higher for women than men at all ages, whereas the fasting plasma glucose concentration is much less affected and rises by only 1 to 2 mg/dl per decade (O'Sullivan, 1974). In view of the above, three questions arise, viz:

(a) What is the mechanism of the loss of glucose tolerance with age?
(b) How should the results be interpreted according to present criteria?
(c) What is the appropriate therapeutic approach to hyperglycaemia in the elderly?

Answers to these problems will be attempted in this and subsequent sections in this chapter.

With regard to the first question, growing interest in this area has resulted in several recent studies dealing with the mechanisms of age-related glucose intolerance. There is general agreement that changes in glucose absorption are unlikely to play a major role since both oral and intravenous glucose tolerance are similarly affected by age while direct studies of absorption in man have failed to demonstrate any significant age-related influence (Davidson, 1979). There is also now considerable evidence to show that insulin metabolism remains unchanged with ageing and that if abnormalities in insulin secretion exist, either in degree or timing, they are subtle and insufficient to contribute substantially to the observed impairment in glucose tolerance. The excellent review by Davidson (1979) has indicated that neither the insulin responses to glucose nor insulin–glucagon relationships are altered by ageing, and that the higher glucose levels prevailing in the elderly may be associated with higher insulin levels than those observed in younger subjects. Furthermore,

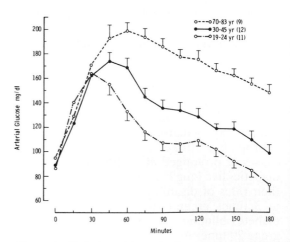

Figure 1 Variation with age in the response to 100 g oral glucose load in healthy men. Figures in parentheses indicate the number in each group. (From Jackson *et al.*, 1982)

recent studies (McGuire *et al.*, 1979) have failed to detect any significant change in insulin secretion, hepatic extraction of insulin, peripheral insulin removal, insulin half-life, or insulin metabolic clearance rate in the elderly. The proportion of proinsulin in total immunoreactive insulin in the basal state is similar in elderly and younger subjects (Jackson *et al.*, 1982), but after glucose loading tends to be somewhat greater in the elderly (Duckworth and Kitabchi, 1976); this increase, however, is small and insufficient to lend any support to the loss of biological activity of circulating immunoreactive insulin as a mechanism of glucose intolerance.

A significant impairment in peripheral glucose uptake with ageing has been strongly suggested by two studies (DeFronzo, 1979; Jackson *et al.*, 1982), one of which employed the human forearm technique to investigate peripheral glucose utilization directly (Jackson *et al.*, 1982). In the latter, the use of a variable intravenous glucose infusion after glucose loading allowed the plasma glucose and insulin levels to be equated in elderly and younger subjects during oral glucose tolerance tests; this manoeuvre revealed that in the presence of similar circulating levels of glucose and insulin, peripheral glucose uptake in the elderly was only one-third that in younger subjects. The failure to find any difference in the numbers and affinity of insulin receptors between

elderly and younger groups in this study suggests that the defect(s) in peripheral uptake is likely to reside at the postreceptor level.

Finally, the possible existence of an age-related loss of hepatic as well as peripheral insulin sensitivity requires further study. The hepatic response to glucose loading comprises at least two components, i.e. a decrease in glucose production and an increase in glucose uptake, and it is likely that these responses do not simply represent a reversal of the same metabolic pathway. Although insulin-induced suppression of hepatic glucose output appears unimpaired by age (DeFronzo, 1979), it may be that a loss of hepatic sensitivity may develop with respect to glucose uptake so that an increase in the latter is delayed in the elderly. This delay, then, would promote a greater rise in arterial glucose concentrations in older subjects by allowing the unrestricted escape of absorbed glucose into the systemic circulation to continue for longer before the increase in hepatic glucose extraction limits this passage.

Hitherto causal roles in the reduction of glucose tolerance with age have been attributed by some to changes in diet, loss of muscle mass, and decreased physical activity. There is now general agreement, however, from both direct and indirect evidence that none of these changes plays any significant role in this regard (Davidson, 1979; DeFronzo, 1981; Jackson *et al.*, 1982). In elderly subjects in whom glucose intolerance has been demonstrated, dietary intake of carbohydrate was adequate and all were fully ambulant while no correlation could be found between peripheral glucose uptake and muscle mass.

In the current state of knowledge, therefore, the glucose intolerance of ageing would appear to reflect a major reduction in peripheral tissue responsiveness to glucose and insulin due to a postreceptor defect and possibly, also, a decrease in hepatic responsiveness with respect to glucose uptake.

DEFINITION OF DIABETES IN THE ELDERLY

While diagnostic difficulty will not arise in classifying obviously severe metabolic disturbances or glucose tolerance test data which are unequivocally normal by any criteria, considerable uncertainty remains concerning the large

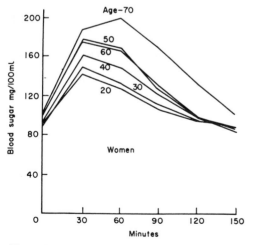

Figure 2 Variation with age in the response to 50 g oral glucose load in healthy women. (From Butterfield, 1964)

intermediate group falling between these extremes since there is no universal agreement on the definition of diabetes. A recent textbook (Davidson, 1981) defines diabetes as 'a disorder in which the level of blood glucose is persistently raised above the normal range' – but in older subjects, what is the normal range?

If it is accepted that the changes observed in the elderly are physiological rather than pathological concomitants of age, any criteria describing the normal response to glucose loading will need to take account of two fundamental considerations: (a) the true magnitude of the age-associated change in glucose tolerance and (b) the technique used for blood sampling. Unfortunately, neither of these points were considered by the National Diabetes Data Group (1979) in their recent determination of normal criteria for glucose tolerance. The extent of the age-related rise in glucose levels based on available literature has been indicated above. In studies in the author's laboratory the mean rise in fasting glucose concentrations per decade in men aged from 19 to 24 years to 70 to 83 years was 2 mg/dl in arterial or venous plasma, in agreement with previous estimates noted above. After a 100-g oral glucose load a similar difference was noted at 30 min but from 60 to 180 min the mean rise per decade was 14 to 16 mg/dl (Fig. 1).

The glucose concentration of a particular plasma sample will be influenced significantly by the site of venepuncture. Large arterio-venous glucose differences develop across the deep muscle compartment of the forearm after glucose loading in both young and elderly subjects. In antecubital veins draining predominantly muscle, glucose levels may be 40 to 45 mg/dl (2.1 to 2.5 mmol/l) less than those in arterial plasma, and intermediate concentrations are found in superficial venous plasma; indeed, the latter may approach arterial concentrations, especially with elevations in the forearm blood flow. The results of the same test therefore may differ substantially depending on the site(s) chosen for venous sampling and the level of local blood flow. Thus in some elderly subjects, glucose levels in arterial or superficial venous blood may exceed the 'normal' criteria, whereas levels in antecubital venous blood draining mainly muscle may fall within the 'normal' range. Thus in the absence of a sampling procedure similar to that em-

ployed in the forearm technique (Jackson *et al.*, 1973), the misinterpretation of a glucose tolerance curve will be best avoided by adopting criteria based on arterial or capillary glucose concentrations. Accordingly, the upper limits of normality in elderly subjects should be raised to avoid the erroneous diagnosis of mild diabetes or impaired glucose tolerance.

Recommendations for Normal Criteria in the Elderly

The fasting plasma glucose concentration remains the most stable and reproducible in elderly as well as younger subjects and should form the principal index of assessment. Using the glucose oxidase method the upper limit of the normal fasting plasma glucose level for the elderly should not exceed 115 mg/dl. The National Diabetes Data Group (1979) suggested (Table 1) that fasting plasma glucose concentrations between 125 and 139 mg/dl are probably abnormal but in the opinion of the present author these levels are unequivocally abnormal, even in the elderly, though clearly they do not reflect a major disturbance in glucose homeostasis.

Table 1 Venous glucose concentrations (mg/dl) after 75-g oral glucose load. (From National Diabetes Data Group, 1979)

	Time (minutes)				
	0	30	60	90	120
Normal	< 115 (100)[a]	←	< 200 (180)	→	< 140 (120)
Impaired glucose tolerance	< 140 (120)	←	> 200[b] (180)	→	140–200 (120–180)
Diabetes	<140 or >140	←	> 200[a]	→	> 200

[a] Quoted values refer to plasma, with levels for whole blood in parentheses. Criteria for capillary blood are the same as those for venous whole blood in the fasting state and those for venous plasma from 30 to 120 minutes.
[b] Levels need exceed 200 mg/dl only once during this period.

With regard to the results of the oral glucose tolerance test, it is the author's view that greater latitude should be allowed than indicated in Table 1 in order to avoid the erroneous diagnosis of impaired glucose tolerance or mild diabetes in a normal elderly subject. It is suggested therefore that the more appropriate upper limits of the normal response to oral glucose loading in the aged are the following: 240 mg/dl (13.3 mmol/l) from 30 to 90 min, 220 mg/dl (12.2 mmol/l) at 120 min, 200 mg/dl (11.1 mmol/l) at 150 min, and 190 mg/dl (10.6 mmol/l) at 180 min. Because 120 min is a relatively short period within which to determine the trend at high levels, it seems desirable to continue observations for 180 min to clarify the direction and rate of change in plasma glucose concentrations. These criteria also imply a fall in glucose levels of 50 mg/dl (2.8 mmol/l) or more from 60 to 180 min, and this index may be used in addition to the above whether or not intermediate blood samples are taken.

A 100-g load was used in the authors' studies whereas 75 g is the load specified by the National Diabetes Data Group (1979). This seems unlikely to invalidate the above as very little difference exists between the responses to 75 or 100 g. Some may view the suggested new criteria for the elderly as being 'too high', but they are likely to be only marginally so and this is more than outweighed by the advantage that healthy elderly individuals will not be misdiagnosed as having impaired glucose tolerance. In his extensive review of the glucose tolerance test, Siperstein (1975) proposed even greater latitude in the elderly in concluding that the response may become statistically abnormal only when blood glucose levels exceed 260 mg/dl (14.4 mmol/1) at one hour, although the recommendation at two hours was similar to that suggested above.

CLINICAL FEATURES

Clinical Presentation

Clinically there are two fairly distinct types of diabetics (Table 2). The previous classification which referred to types 1 and 2 as juvenile-onset and maturity-onset was unsatisfactory because insulin-dependent diabetes may develop in the seventh and eighth decades while non-insulin dependent diabetes may develop in the young. Furthermore,a irrespective of age of onset, insulin-requiring diabetics have the same HLA-determined susceptibility to insulin deficiency which emphasizes environmen-

tal factors (such as viruses) and autoimmunity in its pathogenesis. In contrast, maturity-onset diabetes is not associated with any particular HLA haplotype but has a strong familial inheritance. Thus Cudworth (1976) proposed the term 'type 1' diabetes to include all insulin-dependent patients regardless of age and 'type 2' diabetes to include those insulin-independent patients previously classified as 'maturity-onset' and which includes the vast majority of elderly diabetics. At least two-thirds of all diabetics are non-insulin-dependent.

Table 2   Clinical types of diabetes

	Type 1 (juvenile onset)	Type 2 (maturity onset)
Age	Children and young adults	Middle-aged and elderly
Sex	Male = female	Male < female
Onset	Acute or subacute	Gradual
Symptoms	Present	Present or absent
Obesity	Absent	Often present
Weight loss	Marked	Often absent
Ketosis	Common	Slight or absent
Response to oral agents	Absent	Present
Response to insulin	Sensitive	Relatively insensitive
Serum insulin	Low or absent	Normal or raised

Patients with insulin-dependent diabetes usually present with the classical symptoms of marked hyperglycaemia and glycosuria, i.e. thirst, polyuria, tiredness, and weight loss with or without ketoacidosis (see below). In contrast, in non-insulin-dependent diabetes constitutional symptoms may be absent or mild, and weight loss is seldom a marked feature. Nevertheless, thirst, polyuria, pruritus vulvae, and undue tiredness may occur, and in elderly men frequency and nocturia may be wrongly attributed to prostatic enlargement. In long-undiagnosed cases, the patient may present with features of the late complications, the commonest being deterioration in vision due to retinopathy, lesions of the feet due to neuropathy or ischaemia, or claudication or angina resulting from occlusive vascular disease. Some cases are asymptomatic and diabetes is discovered as a result of a routine urine examination, but even in such cases direct questioning may reveal that diabetic symptoms have been present for some time but disregarded. On the other hand, the severe untreated diabetic may look wasted and ill, loss of weight being due to a combination of dehydration and loss of subcutaneous fat. Heavy glycosuria and hyperglycaemia often produce vulvitis or, less commonly, balanitis and extension of monilial infection from the vulva may cause pruritus ani. Other physical signs will reflect the complications of diabetes discussed below.

Complications

Ketoacidosis

Ketoacidosis may be precipitated in known diabetics for various reasons, such as failure to take drugs or undue stress such as infections or surgical procedures, but a small but important group of elderly diabetics may present with this complication. Loss of consciousness in this condition should be distinguished from other causes of coma (Table 3). Patients with ketoacidosis should be given intensive care yet in spite of advances in the latter, a mortality of 50 per cent. or more is not uncommon in the elderly.

The clinical presentation of ketoacidosis has been well described (Alberti and Hockaday, 1977; Davidson, 1981) and is characterized by hyperglycaemia, glycosuria, ketosis, acidosis, and dehydration. The prime considerations in treatment are correction of acidosis, fluid and electrolyte repletion, insulin administration, and treatment of the underlying cause where

possible. Traditionally, insulin was given in comparatively large doses (80 to 200 units) by simultaneous intravenous and intramuscular injections at intervals of about 2 hours, but it is now recognized that such doses are far in excess of those which are physiologically appropriate. Furthermore, this approach carries the risk of inducing late hypoglycaemia, osmotic disequilibrium, and hypokalaemia, and it has been replaced by safer, alternative approaches. Accordingly, simplified regimes of low-dose insulin administration by continuous infusion or intermittent intramuscular injections have been introduced successfully in the past few years (Davidson, 1981).

In the infusion method, insulin in normal saline is infused at a rate of 4 to 10 units/hour and adjustment of the infusion rate is made according to the results of frequent (usually hourly) blood glucose estimations; an initial small bolus of 10 units may be given intravenously at the beginning of the infusion.

When the blood glucose level falls to 180 to 288 mg/100 ml (10 to 16 mmol/l) the rate of infusion is slowed and glucose may be added to the infusion to prevent hypoglycaemia. Because of the short half-life of insulin given intravenously, changing the infusion rate will result in the establishment of a new steady-state insulin concentration within 10 to 15 min. This method of insulin administration is simple and flexible and is also applicable to the treatment of hyperosmolar non-ketotic coma (see below). The second method employs the intramuscular injection of 5 to 10 units/hour insulin after an initial dose of 10 to 20 units, and may be particularly useful outside specialized units.

Table 3   Coma in the elderly diabetic. (From Jackson, 1980. Reproduced by permission of MTP Press Ltd, Lancaster, England.

Clinical and biochemical features	Ketoacidotic hyperglycaemia	Non-ketotic hyperosmolar hyperglycaemia	Lactic acidosis	Hypoglycaemia	Cerebrovascular disease
Kussmaul breathing	++	0	++	0	0
Dehydration	+++	+++	0 or +	0 or +	0 or +
Neurological signs focal deficit	0	0 or +	0	0 or +	0 or +++
Blood glucose	+++	+++	N or +	−	N or +
Ketosis	+++	0	0 or +	0 or +	0 or +
Acidosis	+++	0	+++	0	0

The use of both these methods produces a steady fall in blood levels of glucose, ketones, free fatty acids, and glycerol while the likelihood of hypokalaemia is reduced and the maintenance of normokalaemia requires less potassium than with high-dose insulin regimes. In general there is probably little to choose between these two methods of low-dose insulin treatment though in severely ill patients with significant peripheral circulatory insufficiency, the infusion method is preferable. The protagonists of the intramuscular method have suggested that in such patients an initial intravenous pulse of insulin may be advisable.

Recently, attention has been drawn to the association between diabetic ketoacidosis and hypothermia in the elderly (Gale and Tattersall, 1978). In one series of patients hospitalized for hypothermia, ketoacidosis was more common than hypothyroidism, and it may be that the occurrence of hypothermia in the course of diabetic ketoacidosis is more frequent than has been recognized hitherto, although the mechanisms of this association are complex. Conversely, hypothermia may aggravate uncontrolled diabetes. At low temperatures insulin secretion is impaired, glucose utilization is reduced, resistance to exogeneous insulin develops, and the secretion of insulin antagonists in the form of cortisol and catecholamines is increased. Thus although loss of diabetic control is not inevitable in severe hypothermia, the metabolic disturbance, when it occurs, is characteristically severe and the mortality high.

Hyperosmolar Non-ketotic Coma

Hyperosmolar non-ketotic coma tends to be found more commonly in the elderly and is about one-sixth as common as diabetic ketoacidosis (Davidson, 1981). The affected patients are almost always mild maturity-onset diabetics or previously undiagnosed diabetics who do not require insulin once the disturbance has been corrected. A minority of patients are insulin-requiring diabetics while patients who are actually non-diabetic may be precipitated into hyperosmolar coma by the administration of excessive amounts of carbohydrate. Precipitating factors, particularly infection or drugs including diuretics and steroids can be implicated in many patients (Table 4).

Table 4 Conditions associated with the onset of hyperosmolar nonketotic coma. (From Davidson, 1981. Reproduced by permission of Garland Publishing Co., John Wiley & Sons, Inc.)

Diseases	Drugs	Miscellaneous
Diabetes mellitus[a]	Diuretic (potassium-depleting)	Burns
Infections	Diazoxide	Hemodialysis
Acute pancreatitis	Diphenylhydantoin	Peritoneal dialysis
Pancreatic carcinoma	Propanolol	Hypothermia
Acromegaly	Glucocorticoids	Heat stroke
Cushing's syndrome	Hypertonic NaHCO$_3$	
Thyrotoxicosis		
Subdural hamatoma		
Uraemia (with vomiting)		

[a] Initial manifestation without known precipitating cause.

The condition resembles severe ketoacidosis in presenting with marked hyperglycaemia, increasing weakness, polyuria, polydipsia, dehydration, clinical shock, and deepening stupor, but differs from ketoacidosis in that both acidosis and severe ketosis are absent. Most patients manifest profound alterations in their state of consciousness but occasionally may be alert and well-orientated. The mechanisms of the disturbance in cerebral function are poorly understood but may be due to reduced cerebral perfusion consequent on shock, and this may be especially important in the elderly who might already have areas of compromised circulation. The hyperosmolarity is predominantly a consequence of the hyperglycaemia, but uraemia, and in some cases hypernatraemia, may contribute. Dehydration is the most striking finding on examination and is due to the osmotic diuresis resulting from glycosuria, vomiting, and an inadequate intake of glucose-free water appropriate to the dehydration. Despite the absence of ketoacidosis, many patients have significant reductions in plasma pH as a result of lactic acidosis, uraemia, or unknown factors. The average blood glucose is usually greater than 1,000 mg (55.6 mmol/l) and the plasma osmolality exceeds 350 mosmol/l while the serum sodium has varied from 118 meq/l to as high as 188 meq/l. The development of shock has been an important factor in the high mortality of this condition which in most series has been about 50 per cent. but has fallen to 15 to 25 per cent. in more recent studies. Of the 34 fatal cases of hyperosmolar coma analysed by McCurdy (1970) about half the deaths were due to the preexisting or precipitating illness while the other half reflected the severe dehydration of the patients.

The pathogenesis of the syndrome remains poorly understood. One of the main unsolved aspects of this disorder is the absence of ketosis. In the present state of knowledge it seems likely that decreased mobilization of free fatty acids from adipose tissue may be an important factor contributing to the absence of ketosis and this could be due to the antilipolytic action of insulin which, though deficient, may be present in significantly higher concentrations than the very low levels which characterize ketoacidosis.

Treatment of this condition should be carried out in an intensive care unit where the most important aspects of therapy are rapid fluid replacement with hypotonic saline (0.45 per cent.) at the rate of 1 to 2 l/hour and treatment of the precipitating condition. Insulin should be used in doses half those recommended in ketoacidosis as these patients are often sensitive to insulin and too rapid a reduction in the blood glucose level and plasma osmolality might result in osmotic disequilibrium and cerebral oedema. Occasional patients, however, have demonstrated insulin resistance. A reasonable regimen, therefore, is the initial administration of 10 units intravenously followed by a constant infusion of 3 to 4 units/hour (or 5 units/hour by intramuscular injection) with hourly monitoring of blood glucose levels for 2 to 3 hours before deciding the level of further insulin dosage.

The Diabetic Foot

Care of the feet is of particular importance in the elderly since, with the advances in metabolic control and the increase in their life expectancy, longer-term diabetic complications are presenting with growing frequency. This is seen in the diabetic foot where the pathology is characterized by occlusive vascular disease, neuropathy, and sepsis, either separately or in combination.

The most important aspect of management is prevention and it cannot be overemphasized that even the most severe lesions in the foot may be painless – so that normal sensation cannot be relied upon to warn of extending disease. All diabetics should have a clear programme of conscious inspection and prophylactic care with foot hygiene in order to reduce the possibility of amputation. Smoking should be actively discouraged at all times and in other respects treatment of vascular disease and sepsis should follow conventional principles. Cramp in the calf muscles at night is a common complaint of the diabetic and may not be associated with neuropathy or ischaemic disease. It can usually be prevented, as in the non-diabetic, by taking a tablet (200 mg) of quinine sulphate before retiring.

Disorders of the Eye

Older people with diabetes are potentially subject to the same complications as younger diabetics but in as much as the appearance of complications is related to the duration of diabetes, their prevalence is not high among persons with onset of diabetes late in life.

Diabetic retinopathy is a major cause of blindness affecting 5 to 10 per cent. of diabetics surviving 20 years from diagnosis, and is classified as either non-proliferative (background) or proliferative. The former is characterized by retinal venous dilatation and microaneurysmal formation which, together with the associated leakage of plasma (exudates) or whole blood (dot and blot haemorrhages), comprises the well-described fundal appearances. Loss of vision is minimal or absent with the rare exception of a haemorrhage at the fovea and the most important duty of the physician at this stage is to ensure adequate follow-up so that treatment will not be delayed should deterioration supervene. Visual loss is, however, associated with maculopathy, i.e. involvement of the macula by a hard exudate or the local oedema associated with the presence in this region of exudates, microaneurysms, and haemorrhages. Proliferative retinopathy is characterized by the growth of new vessels from the optic disc or retinal periphery and is more serious because of the liability of vitreous haemorrhage or retinal detachment to cause serious visual loss.

In the elderly exudates in the macular area

are the commonest cause of defective vision resulting from diabetic retinopathy. Photocoagulation using xenon arc or argon laser treatment has significantly improved the prognosis for vision and is now the therapy of choice for maculopathy and new vessel formation. Good diabetic control offers the best hope of avoiding retinopathy and, indeed, considerable amelioration of changes already present can occur with improved control (Kohner, 1977). In many diabetics, however, good control cannot be achieved and, in others, retinopathy develops even when control is apparently satisfactory. In the last few years vitrectomy has been widely used in the treatment of vitreous haemorrhage and vitreous membranes. In general the results in diabetes are not as good as in other conditions leading to vitreous haemorrhage as the retina behind the haemorrhage may be too badly damaged to have any function.

Diabetic lens opacities are often associated with senile opacities and the combined effect gives rise to more visual difficulty than either alone so that senile cataract is said to occur at an earlier age in diabetics. This combined effect probably causes operation for senile cataract to be about 5 times more common in diabetics than in non-diabetics (Caird, Hutchinson, and Pirie, 1965), and indeed a number of elderly diabetics come to diagnosis because of cataract.

Urinary Tract Disease

Standard principles govern the management of urinary tract infections which in diabetics are common and sometimes difficult to eradicate. Chronic or recurrent infections are indications for urological examination to rule out an obstructive lesion, and this is of particular importance in relation to prostatic hypertrophy in elderly men. The neurogenic and atonic bladder is another occasional predisposing factor that requires attention; a far more common problem may be the presence of an indwelling catheter, for which antibiotic treatment is useful in the shortterm, but has no place in long-term therapy, and indeed a recent study has demonstrated the failure of bladder irrigation with antibiotics to reduce the incidence of urinary tract infection (Warren *et al.*, 1978).

Therapy of the nephropathy is limited to maintaining good diabetic control in the hope that this will either prevent or retard the progression of renal disease. No specific treatment is available since renal transplant has no place in the management of the elderly diabetic.

Neuropathy

Diabetic neuropathy is principally peripheral and autonomic and the former may be a subacute, mixed or a chronic, sensory variety.

The subacute, mixed variety is often called motor neuropathy but the evidence of some sensory involvement in most cases makes the term 'mixed' more appropriate. This variety tends to improve rapidly with good metabolic control although symptoms may increase initially. Mononeuropathy may occur acutely in the elderly with involvement of the oculomotor and abducent nerve, and reassurance regarding the likelihood of spontaneous recovery is the only 'therapy' available. In chronic sensory neuropathy symptoms are unlikely to disappear and the treatment is confined to general measures and symptomatic relief associated with maintenance of optimal diabetic control. Symptoms consist of burning sensations, tingling, numbness, and pain in the lower extremities, especially starting in the feet. The pain may become severe but may be relieved by walking and is often worse at night. Numbness is a particular hazard as the patient cannot then appreciate trauma and take appropriate protective measures. Neuropathic ulcers are important in this regard as is the arthropathy characterized by the Charcot joint.

Pain relief may require simple analgesics such as aspirin, but in more severe cases methadone, dihydrocodeine, or mefenamic acid are indicated, and if pain is very severe in the acute stages even pethidine may be given; carbamazepine or phenytoin is occasionally helpful in severe cases. Because adequate sleep is important, the inclusion of a hypnotic in the treatment is usually necessary. Alcohol may aggravate the condition and should be forbidden or at least restricted. In more severe cases, admission to hospital may be the most useful approach to reviewing overall management. If weakness is present, muscle wasting may be diminished by electrical stimulation and intensive physiotherapy should be employed to maintain and improve mobility of the patient.

Other measures, such as correction of foot drop, may be required. Because of the sensory loss in the legs, care of the feet is vital. Vitamins may be given if there is any doubt regarding the patient's nutritional state.

Elderly men with mild diabetes particularly may be affected by diabetic amyotrophy. The condition is usually self-limiting if the diabetes is carefully controlled but symptomatically the most important factor is the severe pain which it may cause in affected muscle groups, sometimes resistant to treatment and severe enough to prevent sleep. The condition, often unilateral, typically involves proximal muscles of the limbs, especially the quadriceps and pelvic girdle, and is often accompanied by wasting and fasciculation with loss of knee reflexes but with little distal involvement.

Autonomic neuropathy is usually associated with diabetes of long duration and the commonest manifestations involve the genitourinary and gastrointestinal tracts. Impotence and an atonic bladder are the usual clinical features relating to the genitourinary tract. The latter may be present with chronic retention without evidence of obstruction and is more often seen in elderly patients, especially men, in whom it may mimic prostatic obstruction and where catheterization will occasionally be required. Symptoms referable to the gut take the form either of intermittent or persistent diarrhoea which is often worse at night, or of delayed gastric emptying termed 'gastroparesis diabeticorum'. Treatment of the diarrhoea is symptomatic, codeine being the most effective drug, but antibiotics may produce striking relief. Gastroparesis may lead to unpredictable absorption of food and affect metabolic control. Symptoms include a sensation of fullness, nausea, and vomiting after small meals, and it is common for the vomitus to contain food eaten many hours before. Treatment is confined to advising small frequent feedings.

Other disorders that may occur secondary to autonomic neuropathy include orthostatic hypotension and unexplained tachycardia.

TREATMENT—GENERAL CONSIDERATIONS

Broadly, diabetics are treated in one or more of the following situations: (a) as a hospital inpatient where initial stabilization or restabilization is achieved or where control is maintained during admission for unrelated factors; (b) as a hospital outpatient attending the geriatric clinic and/or diabetic clinic; (c) as an outpatient attending the interested general practitioner in the community; and (d) as an outpatient who is seen at home on a domiciliary visit.

Education of the Patient

The Report of the National Commission on Diabetes to the Congress of the United States (10 December, 1975) contained the unqualified statement that 'the cornerstone of good medical treatment . . . is the acceptance by the health professionals, patients and their families that, for diabetes, *patient education is treatment*'. The italics are those of the Commission. The diabetic clinic should provide educational facilities for the patient dealing with all aspects of their disease. Often a short discussion using illustrative slides with 10 or 12 patients in a group can be the most useful of all approaches. All patients should receive instruction regarding dietary modifications, methods of urine testing and recording results, care of the feet, and the influence of intercurrent infections on diabetic control. Where appropriate, patients should be informed about the dosage, administration, and side-effects of oral hypoglycaemic agents (OHA) and/or insulin with special reference to hypoglycaemia and drug interactions.

Since diabetes remains a lifelong problem it is of fundamental importance that patients become as expert as possible in the day-to-day management of their own disease. Ideally, education of the patient must be the shared responsibility of the hospital and/or diabetic clinic on the one hand and the general practitioner or district nurse on the other, and should begin, at least, at the first encounter or clinic visit. Other members of the family or close friends should be encouraged to become a member of the care 'team' at an early stage when reassuring the patient of support in living with their disease is crucial. The repeated instruction which will be needed with some patients should always be undertaken with patience and understanding and this alone will allay fears of being able to cope with a new disease.

In the United Kingdom an educational programme is available as a slide/tape package from the British Diabetic Association and an active local branch of the Association can also contribute fully to the education of diabetic patients. Detailed booklets of all the implications of being a diabetic are available and should be supplied to every patient.

The Hospital Diabetic Clinic

The diabetic clinic provides a centre for clinical assessment of new patients, follow-up of old patients, regulation of therapy, and the opportunity for discussions with the general practitioner and relatives. In addition, the patient has the opportunity to consult other members of staff with special interests in aspects of diabetic care, e.g. the dietitian, chiropodist, ophthalmologist, the dental or general surgeons, neurologist, and social workers. Traditionally patients with diabetes have been managed almost exclusively in a hospital diabetic clinic and this is particularly so in the elderly, where the majority do not require insulin. Diabetic clinic facilities have not increased at a rate commensurate with the expanding diabetic population; many patients wait unduly long and are often seen by a different doctor each visit. The latter should be avoided if at all possible and the importance of not hurrying consultations cannot be overestimated.

Specific aspects of follow-up care are considered elsewhere in this chapter. In general, however, the patient should be asked about symptoms and particularly about hypoglycaemic attacks and, most important of all, confirmation must be obtained that the prescribed treatment is indeed being taken. Finally, it is vital that all missed appointments be investigated immediately and a further consultation arranged.

Care in the Community

A major development in the management of diabetes has been the shift of patient care from the hospital to community. The developments to accommodate this need have included the general practitioner based miniclinic, community care schemes, and the use of specially trained diabetic health visitors and district nurses liaising between the hospital clinic, the general practitioner, and the various community services (social, medical, dietetic, chiropodial, etc.) (Editorial, 1982; Judd *et al.*, 1976; Ruben, 1976; Thorn and Russell, 1973). Thus, debilitated patients can be seen in the home by the district nurse, and the interested practitioner or specialist nurse can measure blood glucose levels on the spot and recommend changes in treatment in order to improve control without requiring the patient to reattend the hospital. Alternatively, a domiciliary visit by the hospital doctor may be required to give advice when difficulties arise in housebound patients or those who cannot easily visit the hospital. A further aid to assist patients with poor vision are preset 'blocked' syringes to eliminate the burden of drawing up the correct dose; in addition, premixed solutions of soluble and isophane insulin may be provided in more severe cases where twice daily injections are required.

The passage of time will establish the merits of these various schemes but such developments are of particular importance in relation to the elderly. With relief of some of the pressure on the hospital diabetic clinic, more time can be given to those patients who do need to attend while those seeing their general practitioner will be spared the journey and have their contact with their doctor reinforced. The full potential for diabetic care in the community, however, depends on good communication and an efficiently functioning team, and therefore patients must be encouraged to seek help whenever necessary.

Role of the General Practitioner

A family doctor who is interested in diabetes and who is familiar with the emotional and personal background of his patient is best placed to provide continuity of care for his diabetic patients once the initial clinical and biochemical assessment is completed.

To undertake this responsibility the family doctor must have adequate facilities for arranging blood sugar estimations, and in some practices a specific time can be set aside for this purpose in the form of a diabetic miniclinic. These miniclinics are less inhibiting to most patients than hospital clinics and reduce both travelling time and expense, so important to the elderly (Thorn and Russell, 1973). The vast majority of maturity-onset diabetics can be supervised in this way, perhaps with an occasional visit to the hospital when a particular problem arises requiring a second opinion or further investigation.

Emotional Impact of Illness on the Patient

The diagnosis of an illness, however mild, can be a threatening and frightening experience for a patient at any age but particularly so in the elderly in whom the awareness of age and the possibility of death is that much greater and intensified. The emotional reaction of the patient is central to management and may take several forms. The patient may see the illness as a challenge to be met and the necessary adjustments will be made without undue disruption of daily life. For some patients, however, the discovery of illness is a devastating blow and, however mild, may represent a misfortune too great to be coped with. The patient may either deny the existence of the disorder altogether or regress to a more helpless form of behaviour. Undue depression, introversion, and withdrawal from the reality of the situation may follow. On the other hand, the illness may be exploited and used as a means of attracting attention in a manipulative way where purely medical indications are not correspondingly pressing. It may be difficult to distinguish organic factors from psychosomatic aspects of the case, yet a judgement has to be made and is an essential prerequisite to optimal care.

Skill and experience is required from doctors, nurses, and social workers in supporting and advising the patient as well as family and friends in a balanced approach to the illness. Of the various complications to which the diabetic is susceptible, perhaps blindness and amputation carry the most serious social implications in terms of overdependence and disability. Where poor vision or blindness is present or where amputation is indicated and major physical disability and rehabilitation are added challenges, management may become even more complex, and from time to time the help of an experienced psychotherapist or psychiatrist may prove essential.

TREATMENT – SPECIFIC CONSIDERATIONS

Diet

Diet is the key element in treatment of the elderly diabetic. Dietary advice should always be based on the patient's habitual food patterns in order to maximize the chance of compliance. The prescribed diet should achieve, where appropriate, adequate weight reduction, avoidance of refined sugar, adequate intake of vitamins, minerals, and protein, and a reasonable distribution of meals. Exchange lists for meal planning prepared by the American and British Diabetic Associations are a valuable guide to patients for alternative food choices and emphasize the potential for individualization of meal planning rather than a fixed diet schedule.

The majority of elderly diabetics are obese and do not require insulin; calorie restriction is the overriding consideration. The elderly often lack motivation which is not infrequently due to loneliness, depression, and lack of interest after death of the spouse. Since many elderly patients will not adhere to dietary restriction, optimum control is unlikely to be achieved. In one respect this does not present too serious a problem because older patients with a milder and more stable variety of diabetes can be allowed a little more latitude than younger diabetics. Cost may be a factor in non-compliance and keeping up a rigorous regime which requires the weighing of foodstuffs is usually beyond the patient's competence. The patient may have difficulty in obtaining the correct food, as is the case with those having meals-on-wheels and while residential care may solve some problems it may also create others related to incorrect feeding.

The major step in ordering diet is deciding the dietary composition. Until recently, low-carbohydrate (about 30 to 35 per cent. of calories) diets were routinely prescribed which necessitated a high-fat content (about 40 to 45 per cent. of calories). The rationale was the assumption that diabetics would have difficulty metabolizing dietary carbohydrates, although it was shown over 45 years ago and has been demonstrated repeatedly since that this is not the case (Committee on Food and Nutrition of the American Diabetes Association, 1979;

West, 1973). Because of the lack of evidence that high-carbohydrate diets are detrimental to diabetics and because a higher fat intake may adversely affect the vascular system, recent recommendations emphasize the inclusion of more liberal amounts of carbohydrate in the diabetic diet. The form of carbohydrate, however, is critically important. Simple sugars such as the disaccharides sucrose, lactose and maltose and the monosaccharides glucose and fructose, appear rapidly in the bloodstream causing marked hyperglycaemia. In contrast, the complex carbohydrates, the majority of which are starches, are broken down relatively slowly in the gut to di- and monosaccharides and their more gradual absorption results in lower glucose concentrations, putting less demand on the β-cell. Thus the intake of simple sugars should be sharply curtailed. In fruit and milk about 10 to 15 per cent. of the total number of calories will be in the form of simple carbohydrates, and the remaining carbohydrate intake (about 35 to 40 per cent. of total calories) should be mainly in the form of starches.

The most recent recommended daily allowance for protein intake is 0.8 g/kg of ideal body weight (National Academy of Sciences, 1980) but from a practical point of view, the protein content of the diet should make up 17 per cent. of the calories ingested. It is probably wise to reduce cholesterol and saturated fat intake in diabetics. Limiting cholesterol intake and increasing the ratio of unsaturated to saturated fat will lower serum cholesterol concentrations in diabetics if the total fat intake is decreased or even kept constant (Kaufmann, Assal, and Soeldner, 1975; Stone and Connor, 1963). An acceptable fat intake is one in which the latter constitutes 33 per cent. of calories, cholesterol intake is less than 300 mg/day, and the ratio of saturated to unsaturated fat is 1.2, the latter containing equal proportions of monounsaturated and polyunsaturated fat.

There is growing interest in the effect of the fibre content of the diet on diabetes mellitus. Dietary fibres are constituents of plants that are not absorbed or metabolized by the small intestine and therefore reach the large intestine unchanged in form. Whatever mechanism(s) are involved, the addition of fibre to a meal decreases postprandial glucose and insulin concentration in both normal subjects and non-insulin-requiring diabetics (Anderson and Chen, 1979). Chronic ingestion of a high-carbohydrate (60 per cent. of the total calories), high-fibre (about 25 g of plant fibre/1,000 calories) diet may also profoundly affect patients whose diabetes is severe enough to require insulin or OHA (oral hypoglycaemic agents). In due course OHA may be discontinued and insulin dosages reduced considerably or discontinued altogether (Andersen and Chen, 1979; Andersen, Midgley, and Wedman, 1979). There is also some evidence that on a chronic basis, glucose tolerance improves following long-term consumption of diets containing large amounts of insoluble fibres (e.g. wheat, bran), but little change was noted with diets rich in soluble fibres (e.g. pectins).

The current approach, therefore, is to impose calorie restriction when indicated and to encourage the intake of high-carbohydrate, high-fibre diets without radically changing the eating habits of the patient.

Exercise

Sustained, regular physical activity is of major importance in the management of diabetes and part of the plan for every older diabetic, where possible, should include programmes of physical activity. An increased amount of exercise of even a modest degree, if maintained, will facilitate both weight reduction and metabolic control by increasing glucose utilization in insulin-sensitive tissues.

Oral Hypoglycaemic Agents

General Approach

Oral hypoglycaemic agents (OHA) now have an established place in treatment and are used by 30 to 50 per cent. of all diabetics and a higher proportion of elderly diabetics. The drugs which fall broadly into two categories, the sulphonylureas and the biguanides (Fig. 3), have an excellent record of safety with a minimum of side-effects.

The sulphonylureas appear to act by both pancreatic and extrapancreatic effects but there is no doubt that some endogenous insulin must be present for these drugs to be effective. An acute action of sulphonylureas is to stimulate insulin release from the β-cell and in animals the newer preparations have been reported to stimulate β-cell replication as well (Sonksen and West, 1978). However, the main hypoglycaemic action of these drugs in long-term therapy may be extrapancreatic due possibly to reduced hepatic glucose output or increased effectiveness of endogenous insulin (Perkins *et al.*, 1975).

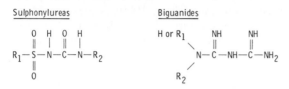

Figure 3   General chemical structures of oral hypoglycaemic agents

The mode of action of the biguanides, however, is uncertain. These drugs do not stimulate insulin secretion and do not lower the blood glucose of non-diabetics but they may reduce appetite and intestinal absorption, inhibit hepatic gluconeogenesis, or increase glucose uptake by muscle. Their hypoglycaemic action is less powerful than that of the sulphonylureas, but when the drugs are given together, their effects are additive.

OHA should be prescribed when dietary modification alone has failed to restore control and in many diabetics they obviate the need for insulin administration. In practice most patients who respond to simple dietary restriction do so within about two weeks and this period should be allowed to assess the response before introducing OHA. The latter, however, are absolutely contraindicated in situations where the immediate institution of insulin therapy is imperative; these are (a) the presence of or liability to ketoacidosis, (b) uncontrolled diabetes in emergencies, (c) acute onset of diabetes with severe hyperglycaemic symptoms and weight loss, and (d) after total pancreatectomy. Nevertheless, a single episode of ketosis or even coma in the past is not necessarily a contraindication to OHA and occasionally such patients may subsequently remain well controlled on drugs and diet alone.

Figure 4 illustrates the general approach to treatment. There are no absolute rules regarding the type of drug to be used and this depends entirely on the preferences of the

physicians concerned. In many clinics the choice of agent in the initial treatment of maturity-onset diabetes is determined by the body weight of the patient. The sulphonylureas tend to increase body weight whereas the biguanides, by causing anorexia, tend to cause weight loss. Thus the sulphonylureas should be used as primary treatment in non-obese patients, reserving the biguanides for those who are overweight. If primary failure occurs, i.e. that control remains poor after 3 to 6 weeks despite satisfactory dietary adherence and the administration in maximum doses of either a sulphonylurea or biguanide alone, the second type of drug should be added and the dosage increased as required to maximum levels (Table 5). Since the biguanides and sulphonylureas have different modes of action, their hypoglycaemic effects are additive. Thus, if, for example, 15 mg/day glibenclamide does not restore control, the addition of 1 to 3 g/day of metformin may prove effective. If at this stage control still remains poor with or without the tendency to develop ketoacidosis, the use of insulin becomes mandatory.

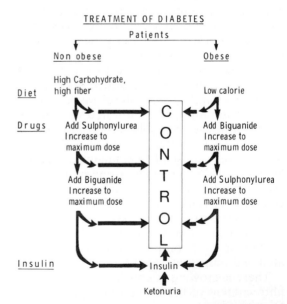

Figure 4   Suggested approach to the treatment of type 2 (maturity-onset, non-insulin dependent) diabetes

In general there is no 'best' choice as far as sulphonylureas are concerned. Experience should be gained with the responses of two or three agents and, if necessary, changes can

Table 5   Oral hypoglycaemic agents

Drug	Proprietary name	Tablet size (mg)	Dose range (mg/day)
Sulphonylureas			
Tolbutamide	Rastinon, Orinase	500	500–2,000
Chlorpropamide	Diabinese	100, 250	100–500
Acetohexamide	Dimelor	500	500–1,500
Tolazamide	Tolanase	100, 500	100–750
Glibenclamide	Daonil, Euglucon	2.5, 5	2.5–20
Biguanide			
Metformin	Glucophage	500, 850	1,000–3,000

then be made in the light of the patient's idiosyncrasy.

The 'second-generation' sulphonylureas, such as glibenclamide which, weight for weight, are 100 times more potent than the older drugs, are not necessarily more effective in the management of diabetes. Indeed, differences between preparations in terms of hypoglycaemic potency are marginal, and there is nothing to be gained by using more than one sulphonylurea preparation at a time and no evidence that if one has failed after maximum doses have been used, another will be more successful. Most authorities will agree that some 60 to 70 per cent. of adult-onset diabetics benefit from the sulphonylureas.

Continuing management on OHA may develop in one of three ways. Firstly, a patient who has initially needed OHA to establish control may be later found able to maintain normal blood glucose levels without drug therapy. Thus, after good diabetic control has been sustained with OHA for at least some months, reduction of dosage and/or drug withdrawal becomes possible; indeed, about one-third of patients requiring OHA for stabilization will subsequently remain well after their withdrawal. Secondly, control may remain stable on OHA but it will be always apparent that uninterrupted drug administration is essential and that therapy will need to continue indefinitely with minor modifications from time to time. Thirdly, late or secondary failure may occur, i.e. patients who respond well initially to sulphonylureas subsequently become uncontrolled despite continuing treatment, and this is an indication for either the addition of metformin or the introduction of insulin. The need

to change to insulin occurs most frequently during the first few months, but secondary failure can occur even after years of successful treatment. Biguanides have been used in the past in conjunction with insulin in order to obtain smoother control but such a regimen offers no advantage and is not to be encouraged.

Although it is generally accepted that patients are less liable to suffer complications the more normal the blood glucose levels, the evidence that OHA delay or prevent cardiovascular complications is conflicting. In the American University Group Diabetes Program Trial (University Group Diabetes Program, 1975) newly diagnosed maturity-onset diabetics had a higher cardiovascular mortality when treated with tolbutamide or phenformin than when treated with a placebo. The results are controversial and the chief merit of the study is that it has caused a more cautious use of OHA. While not altering practice in the United Kingdom the study has emphasized that oral agents are potentially dangerous and should be used only in patients likely to benefit from them and then only in the minimum doses necessary to maintain control.

The Sulphonylureas

Glibenclamide and tolbutamide have a short–intermediate duration of action and are the drugs of choice in the elderly. Chlorporpamide has a prolonged action with a half-life of pharmacological activity of 35 hours and is *best avoided in the elderly because of the risk of hypoglycaemia*. Tolbutamide is given in divided doses and while glibenclamide may also be given divided doses it is best given as a single daily dose. The initial dose should be low, e.g. 500 mg of tolbutamide twice or thrice daily or 2.5 to 5.0 mg of glibenclamide daily, until the effect in each individual patient can be assessed. Doses may be increased every 4 to 7 days and in the case of tolbutamide should be by 500 mg/day and with glibenclamide by 5 mg/day. Unless glycosuria persists responses should be confirmed by fasting blood sugar estimations before a further dose increase is recommended. Where renal failure is present, these drugs must be used with caution.

The sulphonylureas are well tolerated and remarkably safe and although many toxic effects have been reported including rashes, jaundice, leucopenia, and antithyroid activity, these are infrequent. The symptoms of flushing, headache, and nausea induced by alcohol in some patients taking chlorpropamide are far less common with tolbutamide and avoided if glibenclamide is used. The most serious side-effect is that of hypoglycaemia, which, broadly, can occur in three situations. Firstly, the prescribed dose may be too large. Secondly, the patient may fail to take an adequate diet, particularly with regard to the evening meal, rendering nocturnal hypoglycaemia more probable, even when the dose is satisfactory. Thirdly, drug interactions (Table 6) can dangerously enhance the hypoglycaemic action of the sulphonylureas – a factor of particular importance in the elderly because of the prevalence of polypharmacy in this age group.

Hypoglycaemia due to sulphonylureas develops more insidiously than with insulin and may present with confusion and drowsiness – features which are common in the elderly, even in non-diabetics. Typical symptoms and signs may be masked by autonomic neuropathy: the possibility of hypoglycaemia, therefore, must be constantly borne in mind by the entire care team and patients should receive specific instruction in its recognition and management. Accordingly, the aim in treatment should be to err, if anything, in keeping the patient slightly hyperglycaemic.

The Biguanides

Metformin and phenformin are the two commonly available drugs in this group and each have a duration of action of 8 to 12 hours. However, because phenformin predisposes to the development of lactic acidosis, this drug is no longer recommended. The use of biguanides, therefore, is confined to taking metformin, which, in a dose of 850 mg twice daily will help to reduce blood glucose levels satisfactorily in the majority of maturity-onset diabetics. Since biguanides are short-acting drugs, the response to a change in dosage may be assessed within a few days, and, as with the sulphonylureas, the problem of drug interactions must be borne in mind (Table 6). Gastrointestinal discomfort is more troublesome than with the sulphonylureas and the drugs should be taken with food to reduce these effects. The symptoms are often transient and include nausea, an unpleasant metallic taste in the mouth, indigestion, and diarrhoea. Some patients develop an insidious malaise and some taking large doses of metformin have been reported to develop vitamin B_{12} malabsorption (Tomkin *et al.*, 1971), but this does not appear to be a serious clinical problem.

The most serious side-effect of the biguanides is lactic acidosis which has been well reviewed recently (Assan *et al.*, 1977; Cohen, 1978; Cohen and Woods, 1976). Lactic acidosis is probably precipitated by excessive accumu-

Table 6* Principal drug interactions with OHA and insulin.

Drug group	Interacting drug	Hypoglycaemic effect
Sulphonylureas, biguanides and insulin	Drugs influencing glucose metabolism, such as salicylates, adrenoceptor blocking drugs, monoamine oxidase inhibitors	potential
	Thiazide diuretic, glucocorticoids, oestrogens, sympathomimetics, barbiturates, diazoxide, epanutin	antagonized
Sulphonylureas only	Drugs metabolizing microsomal enzyme inhibitor agents: such as coumarin anticoagulants, monoamine oxidase inhibitors	potentiated
	Displacement from plasma protein drug-binding sites, such as clofibrate, phenylbutazone, sulphonamides, ergotamines	potentiated

* From Jackson (1980), reproduced by permission of MTP Press Ltd.

lation of the drug in blood and/or tissues. Most cases have occurred in patients on phenformin and buformin (used in Europe), and while some cases have been associated with metformin, the incidence is far less than with phenformin. The diagnosis may be confirmed by finding a large anion gap not accounted for by ketoacidosis, salicylate ingestion, or uraemia and by a blood lactate concentration greater than 7 mmol/l. The mortality in phenformin-associated lactic acidosis is 50 per cent. (and may be as high in patients not taking phenformin) and rises even further when shock supervenes. Poor renal function and even minor degrees of hepatic failure predispose to the complication and cardiovascular insufficiency is frequently an associated finding. Excessive alcohol intake may precipitate lactic acidosis and in the elderly, where nutrition may be poor, it is important to avoid the use of fructose or sorbitol since the latter are rapidly metabolized to lactate. For the present, then, it seems reasonable to prescribe metformin in the elderly provided that the patient is watched carefully and that the serum creatinine is normal. Where the latter is elevated, however, or where cardiovascular or hepatic insufficiency is present, metformin is contraindicated.

Insulin

General Approach

The administration of insulin in elderly patients is governed broadly by the same principles which apply in younger patients. The emphasis is on simplifying treatment by the administration of only one injection daily whenever possible. As with OHA, it is wise to err on the side of underprescribing, in order to minimize the risk of hypoglycaemia. In general, patients can be satisfactorily managed with a single daily injection of intermediate-acting isophane or long-acting lente insulin when the total daily requirement is less than 20 to 30 units. Patients with larger requirements (i.e. 30 to 80 units/day) can also be maintained on single daily injections of lente insulin when their diabetes is fairly stable. In the minority of elderly insulin-dependent patients with unstable diabetes, the use of short-acting soluble insulin in combination

with the intemediate-acting isophane insulin given twice daily is indicated. The relative proportions and doses of short- and intermediate-acting insulin at each injection will vary from patient to patient and can only be decided on the basis of serial glucose estimations in blood and urine at appropriate times during the day (fasting, pre-lunch, pre-supper, and before retiring), while the patient is following the prescribed diet. Conversion to a twice or thrice daily regimen using soluble insulin only may become necessary during periods of unusual stress such as those relating to surgery and intercurrent infections. This may apply both to patients previously controlled on longer-acting preparations as well as some patients who are not normally insulin-dependent.

The administration of insulin by continuous subcutaneous infusion has received considerable attention recently (Pickup and Keen, 1980) but serious problems attend this method of treatment which has not been applied in the elderly as yet.

Highly Purified Insulins

Until recently, most commercial insulin preparations have consisted of mixtures of porcine and bovine insulin, but interest in the purification of insulin has been stimulated by the finding that even with apparently pure preparations, almost all insulin-treated diabetics have insulin-binding antibodies in their blood. For any patients requiring insulin for the first time, highly purified preparations should be used and transfer to the latter is indicated in the presence of insulin allergy, lipoatrophy, and insulin resistance, i.e. when the daily requirement is 100 units or more in the absence of any recognizable cause.

Insulin requirements usually fall when patients are changed to highly purified insulin but the fall, associated with a reduction in the titre of insulin antibodies, is unpredictable both in magnitude and timing and can only be determined by trial and error. If the daily requirement exceeds 100 units, the transfer to highly purified insulin should be made in hospital. For outpatients the daily dose should be reduced by about 20 per cent. and the patient instructed about the need for subsequent alterations. Some patients have complained that their warning symptoms of hypoglycaemia are reduced or lost after starting on highly purified insulin. The latter may be due to the rapidity with which blood glucose levels fall and this can be corrected by reducing the dose prescribed.

Assessment and Regulation of Diabetic Control

As already noted, the fasting blood glucose concentration is the best and most stable index of metabolic control. Postprandial glucose levels are more variable and, therefore, less reliable. Reasonable goals for therapeutic control are fasting plasma glucose values under 140 mg/dl (7.8 mmol/l) and 2- to 3- hour postprandial concentrations less than 160 to 180 mg/dl (8.9 to 10.0 mmol/l) and to give added confidence to the assessment these levels should represent the average of at least two or three estimations.

When the fasting blood glucose concentration exceeds 115 mg/dl (6.4 mmol/l) but remains consistently below 140 mg/dl (7.8 mmol/l) no specific therapy is indicated and the patients may be simply kept under observation with the fasting blood glucose level being checked at 6-monthly intervals. When fasting blood glucose levels exceed 140 mg/dl, treatment should be instituted and according to the severity of the diabetes a decision taken as to whether OHA or insulin administration is required. As noted above, insulin will be indicated immediately in only a small minority of elderly diabetic patients and in the vast majority of patients a programme of dietary modification with or without OHA will be appropriate. When fasting glucose levels range between 140 and 180 mg/dl (7.8 and 10.0 mmol/l) at presentation, dietary modification alone may suffice, but when levels exceed 180 mg/dl, the addition of OHA is likely to become necessary, particularly in non-obese patients. Satisfactory metabolic control can be achieved in the majority of diabetics with diet alone or in combination with OHA, even when initial fasting glucose levels are markedly elevated (Fig. 5). There will be, however, a number of patients in whom fasting blood glucose levels will remain between 140 and 200 mg/dl (7.8 and 11.1 mmol/l) despite strict dietary adherence and taking maximum doses of OHA. In

these diabetics it will be reasonable to persist with OHA provided that ketonuria is not present and that regular testing of blood and urine samples can be ensured. Insulin administration, however, will become unavoidable should any further loss in control take place.

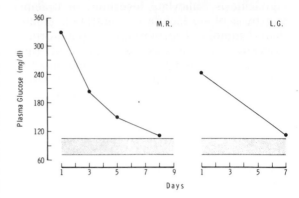

Figure 5 Initial response of fasting blood glucose concentrations to treatment in two type 2 diabetics (M. R. and L. G.). In each patient therapy began on day 1 and comprised dietary modification, glibenclamide 15 mg daily, and metfromin 850 mg twice daily in combination. The shaded area indicates the normal range for fasting blood glucose concentrations

Routine testing of fasting urine samples provides a useful but far less accurate guide to the degree of stabilization. When diabetic control is satisfactory, the absence of fasting glycosuria provides reassurance that all is well while persistent glycosuria will warn of the need to revise therapy. In order to validate the significance of urine testing, however, it is essential to determine the renal threshold whenever possible. If the latter is normal, i.e. 180 mg/dl (10 mmol/l), the morning fasting urine test will provide an acceptable index of overall control. A high renal threshold, as may occur in the elderly, will render urine testing a poor reflection of control, and treatment should then be regulated according to the fasting blood glucose level. A low renal threshold is less common in the elderly but again estimating fasting blood glucose concentrations offers the safest means of avoiding overtreatment and the risk of precipitating hypoglycaemia. If blood sampling presents practical difficulties, then clearly total reliance on urine testing may be unavoidable.

Patients whose values for glucose tolerance

fall in the borderline range should be followed up with regular fasting blood glucose estimations, preferably at 6-monthly intervals. The only specific advice recommended to such patients in the present state of knowledge should refer to weight loss for those who are obese.

Until recently it has not been possible to assess the accuracy of control without frequent blood glucose estimations, but the estimation of glycosylated haemoglobin, i.e. haemoglobin Alc (HbAlc), now provides a solution to this problem (Gonen *et al.*, 1977). It is known that the presence of circulating glucose in high concentrations results in the continuous formation and accumulation of HbAlc within the red cells, which correlates closely with the degree of control as assessed either by fasting plasma glucose levels or mean daily glucose levels observed over the previous few weeks. Thus HbAlc measurements serve as both a screening test for uncontrolled diabetes and as an indicator of the efficiency of various therapeutic regimens while serial estimations allow an objective assessment of control over much longer periods.

Home blood glucose monitoring can also be used to assess long-term control (Schade *et al.*, 1981) and has the advantage of enabling diabetic control to be substantially improved by modification of treatment in the community. In this regard, the special and important place of nurses in the management of diabetes has been recently emphasized (Editorial, 1982). Far fewer elderly diabetics will be involved in self-monitoring than is the case with younger patients since the incidence of insulin-requiring diabetes, where self-monitoring is particularly applicable, is so much less in the older patients. Nevertheless, there are a small selected group of patients, possibly those insulin-requiring diabetics presenting only late in life or those in whom the renal threshold for glucose may be increased, in whom extra efforts are desirable to improve metabolic control. Where such patients have the desire and capability to participate more intensively in their own management, this should receive every encouragement.

ACKNOWLEDGEMENTS

I am grateful to Sir John Nabarro for helpful criticisms of the manuscript and to Miss Marietta de Souza and Miss Fiona Whichelow for their secretarial expertise during its preparation.

REFERENCES

Alberti, K. G. M. M., and Hockaday, T. D. R. (1977). 'Diabetic coma: a reappraisal after five years', *Clin. Endocrinol. Metab.*, **6**, 421–455.

Anderson, J. W., and Chen, W. L. (1979). 'Plant fiber, carbohydrate and lipid metabolism', *Am. J. Clin. Nutr.*, **32**, 346–363.

Anderson, J. W., Midgley, W. R., and Wedman, B. (1979). 'Fiber and diabetes', *Diabetes Care*, **2**, 369–379.

Assan, R., Heuclin, C., Ganeval, D., Bismuth, C., George, J., and Girard, J. R. (1977). 'Metformin-induced lactic acidosis in the presence of acute renal failure', *Diabetologia*, **13**, 211–217.

Butterfield, W. J. H. (1964). 'The Bedford Diabetes Survey', *Proc. Roy. Soc. Med.*, **57**, 196–200.

Caird, F. I., Hutchinson, M., and Pirie, A. (1965). 'Cataract extraction in an English population', *Br. J. Prev. Soc. Med.*, **19**, 80–84.

Cohen, R. D. (1978). 'Prevention and treatment of lactic acidosis', in *Topics in Therapeutics* (Ed. D. W. Vere), pp. 191–197, Pitman, London.

Cohen, R. D., and Woods, H. F. (1976). *Clinical and Biochemical Aspects of Lactic Acidosis*, Blackwell, Oxford.

Committee on Food and Nutrition of the American Diabetes Association (1979). 'Principles of nutrition and dietary recommendations for individuals with diabetes melitus', *Diabetes Care*, **2**, 520–523.

Cudworth, A. G. (1976). 'The aetiology of diabetes', *Br. J. Hosp. Med.*, **16**, 207–216.

Davidson, M. B. (1979). 'The effect of aging on carbohydrate metabolism. A review of the English literature and a practical approach to the diagnosis of diabetes mellitus in the elderly', *Metabolism*, **28**, 688–705.

Davidson, M. B. (1981). *Diabetes Mellitus, Diagnosis and Treatment*, Wiley, New York.

DeFronzo, R. A. (1979). 'Glucose intolerance and ageing. Evidence for tissue insensitivity to insulin', *Diabetes*, **28**, 1095–1101.

DeFronzo, R. A. (1981). 'Glucose intolerance and ageing', *Diabetes Care*, **4**, 493–501.

Duckworth, W. C., and Kitabchi, A. E. (1976). 'The effect of age on plasma proinsulin-like material after oral glucose', *J. Lab. Clin. Med.*, **88**, 359–367.

Editorial (1982). 'The place of nurses in management of diabetes', *Lancet*, **1**, 145–146.

Gale, E. A. M., and Tattersall, R. B. (1978). 'Hypothermia: a complication of diabetic ketoacidosis', *Br. Med. J.*, **2**, 1387–1389.

Gonen, B., Rubenstein, A., Rochman, H., Tanega, S. P., and Horwitz, D. L. (1977). 'Haemoglobin A1: An indicator of the metabolic control of diabetic patients', *Lancet*, **2**, 734–737.

Jackson, R. A. (1980). 'Treatment of the elderly diabetic', in *The Treatment of Medical Problems in the Elderly*, (Ed. M. J. Denham), pp. 159–213, MTP Press, Lancaster.

Jackson, R. A., Blix, P. M., Matthews, J. A., Hamling, J. B., Din, B. M., Brown, J. C., Belin, J., Rubenstein, A. H., and Nabarro, J. D. N. (1982). 'Influence of ageing on glucose homeostasis', *J. Clin. Endocrinol. Metab.*, **55**, 840–848.

Jackson, R. A., Peters, N., Advani, W., Perry, G., Rogers, J., Brough, W. H., and Pilkington, T. R. E. (1973). 'Forearm glucose uptake during the oral glucose tolerance tests in normal subjects', *Diabetes*, **22**, 442–458.

Judd, S. L., O'Leary, E., Read, P., and Fox, C. (1976). 'The changing role of nurses in the management of diabetes', *Br. J. Hosp. Med.*, **16**, 251–255.

Kaufmann, R. L., Assal, J. P., and Soeldner, J. S. (1975). 'Plasma lipid levels in diabetic children', *Diabetes*, **24**, 672–679.

Kohner, E. M. (1977). 'Diabetic retinopathy', *Clin. Endocrinol. Metab.*, **6**, 345–375.

McCurdy, D. K. (1970). 'Hyperosmolar hyperglycaemic nonketotic diabetic coma', *Med. Clin. North Am.*, **54**, 683–699.

McGuire, E. A., Tobin, J., Berman, M., and Andrres, R. (1979). 'Kinetics of native insulin in diabetic, obese and aged men', *Diabetes*, **28**, 110–120.

National Academy of Sciences (1980). *Recommended Dietary Allowances*, 9th ed. National Academy of Sciences, Washington, D.C.

National Diabetes Data Group (1979). 'Classification and diagnosis of diabetes mellitus and other categories of glucose intolerance', *Diabetes*, **28**, 1039–1057.

O'Sullivan, J. B. (1974). 'Age gradient in blood glucose levels. Magnitude and clinical implications', *Diabetes*, **23**, 713–715.

Perkins, J. R., Hay, B. J., Judd, S. L., Quine, K. H., West, T. E. T., and Sonksen, P. H. (1975). 'Effect of diet, sulphonylurea and placebo therapies on glucose tolerance, blood metabolites and insulin secretion in diabetes', *Diabetoligia*, **11**, 369.

Pickup, J. C., and Keen, H. (1980). 'Continuous subcutaneous insulin infusion: a developing tool in diabetes research', *Diabetologia*, **18**, 1–4.

Report of the National Commission on Diabetes to the Congress of the United States, 10 December, 1975 (1975). 'Long range plan to combat diabetes', *Diabetes Forecast*, **28**, Suppl. 1, 1.

Ruben, L. A. (1976). 'Diabetes and the general practitioner', *Br. J. Hosp. Med.*, **16**, 241–246.

Schade, D. S., Eaton, R. P., Mitchell, W. J., and Friedman, N. M. (1981). 'Intravenous home blood glucose monitoring', *Diabetes Care*, **4**, 420–423.

Siperstein, M. D. (1975). 'The glucose tolerance test: A pitfall in the diagnosis of diabetes mellitus', *Adv. Intern. Med.*, **20**, 297–373.

Sonksen, P. H. and West, T. E. T. (1978). 'Carbohydrate metabolism and diabetes mellitus', in *Recent Advances in Endocrinology and Metabolism* (Ed. J. L. H. O'Riordan), pp. 161–186, Churchill Livingstone, Edinburgh.

Spence, J. W. (1920–21). 'Some observations on sugar tolerance with special reference to variations found at different ages', *Quart. J. Med.*, **14**, 314–326.

Stone, D. B., and Connor, W. E. (1963). 'The prolonged effects of a low cholesterol, high carbohydrate diet upon the serum lipids in diabetic patients', *Diabetes*, **12**, 127–132.

Thorn, P. A., and Russell, R. G. (1973) 'Diabetic clinics today and tomorrow, mini-clinics in general practice', *Br. Med. J.*, **ii**, 534–536.

Tomkin, G. H., Hadden, D. R., Weaver, J. A., and Montgomery, D. A. D. (1971). 'Vitamin – B₁₂ status of patients on long term metformin therapy', *Br. Med. J.*, **ii**, 685–687.

University Group Diabetes Program (1975). 'A study of the effects of hypoglycaemic agents on vascular complications in patients with adult-onset diabetes V. Evaluation of phenformin therapy', *Diabetes*, **24**, Suppl. 1, 65–184.

Warren, J. W., Platt, R., Thomas, R. J., Rosner, B., and Kass, E. H. (1978). 'Antibiotic irrigation and catheter-associated urinary tract infections', *New Engl. J. Med.*, **299**, 570–573.

West, K. M. (1973) 'Diet therapy of diabetes: An analysis of failure', *Ann. Intern. Med.*, **79**, 425–434.

West, K. M. (1978). *Epidemiology of Diabetes and Its Vascular Complications*, Elsevier, New York.

24

Cancer in the Elderly Patient

Principles and Practice of Geriatric Medicine
Edited by M. S. J. Pathy
© 1985 John Wiley & Sons Ltd

24.1

Cancer in the Elderly Patient

T. J. Deeley

INTRODUCTION

It is a reflection of present-day medical philosophy that an oncologist should be asked to contribute to a textbook of geriatric medicine. Regrettably many, including the health professions, have accepted malignancy as a hopeless disease for which little if anything could be done. In elderly patients malignancy was considered a merciful release from a long life. The study of geriatric medicine has brought about a greater realization of the scope for treatment of elderly subjects. As a consequence the oncologist's advice is sought more frequently, not merely to palliate but to achieve cure or control. Technical advances in radiotherapy have resulted in improved results of treatment with considerably less damage and effect on normal tissues. Surgical procedures are very carefully controlled and it is possible to carry out surgical removal in older patients with relatively little upset. More radical treatment is now given to the elderly and more patients are treated with the hope of a cure. Early diagnosis before metastases have occurred is perhaps the most important factor affecting the prognosis. The danger that elderly people may fail to recognize or ignore suspicious symptoms requires vigilance.

This chapter will look at cancer in the elderly, will briefly describe the incidence, diagnosis, treatment, and after-care, and will look at special factors which may be relevant because of the patient's age.

THE SPECIAL PROBLEMS OF CANCER IN THE ELDERLY

There are particular problems which may need to be considered when dealing with the elderly patient.

Diagnosis

Cancer is usually diagnosed when a patient presents with suspicious symptoms. A few cancers are detected before symptoms develop, either because the patient has attended with some other disease or has had a special detection test, such as a cervical smear. Diagnosis may be delayed in the elderly because they fail to recognize suspicious symptoms and may present with advanced lesions. There may be some reluctance to subject a frail patient to the necessary distressing or prolonged examinations needed to substantiate the diagnosis.

Choice of Treatment

Age may be an important factor in selecting the method of treatment. Modern surgical and anaesthetic techniques are considerably less upsetting than they were some years ago and may be undergone by even the very elderly. Radiotherapy has made tremendous advances and there is usually little or no upset to the patient while on treatment and slow healing 'radium burns' are no longer seen. However, the tissues of the elderly do not heal as well as young tissues. While little can be done in the surgical field to reduce the damage that has to be repaired, in radiotherapy the dose of radiation given can be adjusted to take account of the response of the normal tissues to irradiation. While it is not always possible to limit the scope of surgery, especially that needed to provide access to the site, the radiation may be limited to the site of the primary tumour and the immediately surrounding potentially involved normal tissues.

Other Diseases

The presence of other serious diseases, especially those which are likely to have a fatal outcome, may well restrict the attack made on the malignant lesions. A fatal outcome must not be assumed because the patient has cancer. A reassessment of the whole clinical picture may result in a positive attack being made on both conditions, both of which may be successful. Even if radical treatment for the cancer is not possible, distressing symptoms may still be palliated to make the last few days of the patient's life more endurable.

The General Condition of the Patient

Before embarking on any treatment the general condition of the patient has to be considered and if possible improved to reduce possible sequelae and complications. Factors to be considered are:

(a) *Nutrition*. Many elderly patients have an inadequate diet, dictated usually by convenience or economy; protein and vitamin C may be particularly lacking. Some malignant diseases especially of the throat and digestive tract may cause deficiencies in diet or in eating and the patient may be malnourished or dehydrated. High protein food supplements or intravenous nutrients may be required before starting treatment.

(b) *Anaemia*. Chronic bleeding from a malignancy may result in anaemia. The efficacy of radiation treatment is related to the degree of oxygenation of the tissues; well-oxygenated tissues show a good response to irradiation while relatively anoxic tissues show little response and the tumour may well be protected (Gray *et al.*, 1953).

It is usual to improve the blood count by blood transfusion before treatment.

(c) *Electrolytes*. Electrolyte depletion may result from fluid loss or malabsorption due to malignancy and quite marked changes may need to be corrected.

(d) *Infection*. With infection anywhere in the body the patient's general condition is worsened. Secondary infection of the primary site may be superimposed on the trauma from surgery or radiation. Sources of infection, e.g. in the bowel or mouth, require treatment with appropriate antibiotics before the cancer therapy.

After-Care

Readjustment after treatment may produce problems for the elderly. Follow-up clinics are essential to monitor progress of the disease and to treat possible recurrences or distressing symptoms. Placement of a patient may produce problems depending on the degree of care required. Pain, needing medication, may necessitate admission because of the difficulty of supervision; terminal care brings its own problems.

Psychological Factor

Particular psychological factors may be more pronounced in the elderly. These patients are reluctant to have new experiences, to leave their home, spouse or animals. While the patient may accept the urgency of the condition and its possible outcome, he may well request that he be left alone at his age. The elderly sick, especially those with cancer, may accept the situation with equanimity. The uncertainty of their future, certainty of their own mortality, and reluctance to make the increasing effort necessary to go on living all colour their attitude to treatment. Perhaps more than death itself they fear the process of dying: the loss of dignity, possibility of pain, likelihood that they will lose control of themselves and the situation.

Many of the public's attitudes to cancer stem from a lack of knowledge and a fear of the disease which has been present for many years, and these patients cannot be expected to think as rationally as we would like.

THE INCIDENCE OF CANCER

The considerable successes in medicine in this century have meant that many causes of death have been eliminated or controlled. Cancer is an acute disease which can occur at any age but which is found increasingly as life continues. Figure 1 shows the percentage of patients dying with cancer for each 5-year age group.

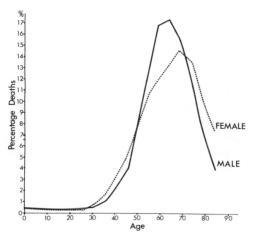

Figure 1   Percentage deaths from cancer for male and females according to age

'Cancer' is a generic term covering a range of malignancies extending from very acute lesions which may terminate life in a matter of days or weeks to the slow-growing lesions that may take many years to develop and produce symptoms. There is a preponderance of slow-growing lesion in old age. This may be because it takes years for such tumours to develop. The blood supply may be impaired in old age and this may affect the rate of growth, or patients with rapidly growing tumours, which often have a poor prognosis, will have died earlier in life.

PATHOLOGY

The pathology of malignant lesions is well covered in the literature and only certain details which are preponderant in the elderly patient will be mentioned here.

The incidence of differing cancers is related to the age and sex of the patient. In early years the common lesions are leukaemia, the reticuloses, and the cancers arising from embryonic tissues. In middle age cancers of the breast in females and bronchus in males predominate while in old age the alimentary tract is more involved. (see Table 1).

Table 1   The three commonest cancers for the 10-year age groups

Age	Male	Female
0–10	Leukaemia, CNS, kidney	Leukaemia, CNS, kidney
10–20	Leukaemia, Hodgkin's disease, CNS	Leukaemia, Hodgkin's disease, CNS
20–30	Leukaemia, Hodgkin's disease, testes	Leukaemia, Hodgkin's disease, ovary
30–40	Leukaemia, colon, rectum	Uterus, colon, rectum
40–50	Bronchus, colon, rectum	Breast, uterus, colon
50–60	Bronchus, stomach, colon	Breast, uterus, colon
60–70	Bronchus, stomach, colon	Breast, uterus, stomach
70–80	Prostate, colon, rectum	Breast, stomach, uterus
80+	Colon, rectum, prostate	Breast, colon, rectum

The higher incidence of gastrointestinal disease in the elderly creates problems of diagnosis requiring a high index of suspicion in the presence of vague ill-health. It also dictates to a large extent the treatment to be given. While rectal and oesophageal lesions can be dealt with by radiation, the intestines are more suited to surgery.

There is some evidence to suggest that tumours in the elderly are more slowly growing, e.g. a common breast tumour in the elderly is the scirrhous carcinoma which has a high proportion of fibrous tissue. In cancer of the lung well-differentiated lesions were found in 76 per cent. of patients aged 60 years or over while only 50 per cent. were found in patients under 60 years.

The relatively poor blood supply of the ageing tissues may result in a less vascular tumour and this may become necrotic when it reaches a certain size, presumably when it outgrows its blood supply or obstructs the feeding blood vessels. Thus, a cancer of the breast may be present as a slowly growing lump for some time, then the overlying skin breaks down, and growth continues at the periphery, the centre being necrotic and eventually infected.

Biopsy

A diagnosis of malignant disease can only be confirmed on histological examination of tissue removed at biopsy. Clinical examination and investigations only provide increasing degrees of probability that a lesion is malignant. Every effort should be made to obtain tissue with as little upset and trauma to the patient as is possible. This is reasonably easy in relatively accessible lesions and needle or drill biopsy may be used. The patient's poor general condition will sometimes preclude histological confirmation of the diagnosis and the clinician then has to rely on the clinical picture and progression of the disease. Treatment must not be delayed unduly because metastatic spread greatly reduces the prognosis and may produce greater and more distressing problems.

Metastases

Metastasis from a malignancy may be by direct extension, which includes transcoelomic spread, seeding along natural lines such as the central nervous system and ureters; lymphatic system; and circulatory system. Some tumours have a predilection for one or other method, some for combinations. It is a clinical impression that metastases are less frequent in the elderly and there is some experimental work in animals to support this. Possible reasons why spread may be less likely in old age than it is in younger patients include:

(a) The tumour is slower growing.
(b) There is more impairment of the blood supply.
(c) The lymphatics and the lymphatic nodes may be fibrosed from previous infections.
(d) The normal tissues may be relatively avascular or fibrotic and incapable of supporting growth.

It has been shown that the breast is an unlikely site of mestastases in old age because much of the tissue is replaced by fibrous tissue and fat (Deeley, 1965).

Solitary metastases may be found with some tumours. In cancer of the lung cerebral metastases were found to be solitary in 20 per cent. of necropsies (Deeley and Rice-Edwards, 1968). If there is no clinical evidence of other metastatic lesions it is possible to give radical treatment to both primary and secondary sites.

TREATMENT

Policy

Once a diagnosis of malignancy is established, a decision on appropriate treatment methods will be influenced by many factors. There are four possible lines of treatment: radical, control, palliative, and none; each is an important medical decision.

Radical

This implies that the lesion is curable and an attempt is made to achieve cure. This is possible only if the lesion is localized, so that it can be removed by surgical operation or can be covered by fields of radiotherapy. Metastases away from the primary site reduce the chances of cure and multiple metastases mean that these two methods of treatment are not applicable and cure can be achieved only if the lesion is very sensitive to cytotoxic drugs in the concentrations it is possible to obtain within the body. Radical implies also that the patient has no other serious lesion which is likely to curtail life. To achieve a cure there is likely to be a proportion of patients who have serious sequelae or complications from the therapy. Surgically, this may involve the loss of a limb, or severe radiation damage from radiotherapy. These possible sequelae must be considered before subjecting the patient to treatment.

Control

It may not be possible to cure, but the lesion may be controlled for a long period of time extending up to the normal life expectancy. This may occur with the irradiation of relatively slow-growing tumours. Therapy aimed at control may be suggested when there is no hope of cure because the dose of irradiation necessary could not be tolerated by the normal tissues.

Palliation

If cure is not possible and the patient has symptoms causing distress, an attempt may be made to palliate. For example, intestinal obstruction may be relieved by a bypass operation, a fungating offensive breast tumour may be excised even though there are secondary deposits.

Cerebral metastases or bone metastases, troublesome bleeding, or fungating growths may be irradiated. Complications must not develop as a result of palliative treatment and the minimal treatment is given to ease distress, e.g. radiotherapy is stopped when bone pain is relieved.

None

If there is no chance of cure or control and no distressing symptoms then a positive decision of no active treatment is made. This decision is of equal importance to the others. General supportive care and nursing care and analgesics are given as required.

Treatment Techniques

There are three main treatment techniques which must be considered: surgical removal, radiotherapy, and chemotherapy singly or in combination. The treatment adopted for a particular patient is dictated by various factors: the primary site, the presence of metastatic spread, the stage of the disease, the histology, the known response to that treatment, and the age of the patient. On the whole radical treatment is possible in localized slowly growing lesions, i.e. the early stages. Broadly, stage I lesions are localized and have no nodes, stage II have mobile nodes which often can be removed, stage III have a tumour fixed to deep structures or with fixed nodes, and stage IV have spread beyond the original confines. Well-differentiated tumours where the histological appearances show cells similar to the parent tissue are usually more slowly growing than poorly differentiated or anaplastic tumours, where the cells are bizarre, show a large number of metastases, and where is it impossible to determine the cell of origin. The feasibility of operation depends on the anatomical site and the patients suitability for the trauma of surgery. Radiotherapy has a much wider application and can be used for inaccessible lesions where surgery is impossible or would produce crippling sequelae. Chemotherapy is used to augment the other two techniques, to ablate small foci of growth remaining after operations, to deal with occult metastases, or may be used as the primary method of treatment in some widespread sensitive lesions, such as leukaemia or the reticuloses.

Treatments may be combined., e.g. in cancer of the breast a radical operation may remove the primary lesion and the axillary lymph nodes, and the lymphatic nodes in the supraclavicular fossa and internal mammary chains are treated with radiation. In a simple mastectomy the axilla is not dissected but is irradiated. A simple mastectomy may be considered more appropriate in the elderly patient. There is a move towards even less trauma in the treatment of breast cancer. Minimal removal of the primary mass is followed by radiation to the primary and node areas; even less traumatic may be a drill or needle biopsy to obtain tissue for histology, followed by radiation to primary and node areas. Such methods of treatment may be particularly suitable for the elderly because there is not the disturbance, physical and psychological, of admission to hospital and operation; radiation may be given as an outpatient and with very little upset to the patient.

Cooperation

Perhaps the greatest advance in oncology that has been made in recent years is the considerable cooperation between all medical workers in the field. Surgery or radiotherapy is no longer the treatment given because the patient was first seen by the surgeon or the radiotherapist. Combined clinics, often with a pathologist, have helped us to consider each patient individually and to give the best treatment for that individual.

Surgery

Surgical removal of a tumour implies that the visible and palpable tumour is removed, together with a surrounding zone of tissue where cancer cells may have infiltrated into surrounding tissues and a clear zone of apparently uninvolved normal tissues. This may be removed in continuity with the local lymph nodes, but this is not always possible. If technically possible, lymph nodes will be removed if they are involved or there is a high probability of involvement. Such operations leave a defect and this must be repaired, or continuity of an organ reestablished or some artificial appliance provided. The procedures may be spread over a period of time and more than one operation be required.

Some lesions are best treated surgically. These include (a) lesions which are known to be relatively radio-resistant – the adenocarcinomas, (b) lesions which are difficult or impossible to localize for a radical course of radiotherapy – mobile gut tumours. At other sites both surgery and radiotherapy may give good results. In early cancer of the larynx the 5-year survival rates are over 90 per cent. by both surgery and radiotherapy, but the former leaves an aphonic patient while the latter causes little or no effect on the voice; surgery can be resorted to should radiotherapy treatment fail.

The disadvantages are that elderly patients need to be relatively fit for an operation and anaesthetic, and need hospital admission. There may be marked psychological problems with operations for diseases at some sites. The advantage is that often everything is done in one operation.

Radiotherapy

The armamentarium of the radiotherapy department includes X-ray machines varying in energy from about 50,000 to 10,000,000 volts with facilities for electron therapy up to 20 or 30 million volts. Much of the routine work is carried out by radioactive cobalt machines which give gamma radiation. Essentially the deeper the tissue to be irradiated lies beneath the skin, the greater will be the energy of the radiation. For very superficial skin lesions a voltage of 50,000 may be adequate: for thicker skin lesions, such as the typical rodent ulcer, 100,000 volts may be required; for deep-seated tumours, e.g. of the bladder, supervoltage therapy at about 5 million volts is used and three of four fields may be applied from different angles around the pelvis crossfiring on the bladder. The planning of treatment is complex and may take some days; in recent years the use of computers has helped to speed up the process and also to produce several alternative plans from which the radiotherapist can accept the most suitable. The aim of radiotherapy is to give an ablating dose of radiation to the selected tumour volume but to cause as little damage as possible to the surrounding normal tissues. The position of the entrance and exit of the fields are marked on the patient's skin and he is advised not to remove these marks. Usually the skin is kept dry during treatment and the patient is advised not to wet the treated area. The application of heavy metals to the skin actually increases the dose to this structure because secondary electrons are produced which have only a short penetration; thus zinc oxide must be avoided both in strapping and in talcum powders. Untoward effects, e.g. reddening of the skin with desquamation, should be watched for and reported to the radiotherapist. Diarrhoea can be alarming and if treatment persists can lead to profound fluid loss and dehydration. Irradiation of the liver or upper abdomen often produces nausea. Nausea and vomiting may occur from breakdown tissue products in the blood and can often be eased by increasing the fluid intake. Dysphagia affecting the epithelial layer may result from irradiation of the oesophagus; it will often resolve if treatment is stopped, but if continued may take a considerable time to resolve.

Radioactive sources may be inserted directly into a tumour using specially made applicators, or wire or needles. The patient needs an anaesthetic for insertion and may need sedation for the time the implant is in position; this method of treatment is not used as frequently as it once was.

The results of treatment, especially the cosmetic results, are better if treatment is fractionated over a period of time, but with very elderly patients whose expectation of life is limited, we are less concerned with the possible late effects of treatment occurring years later and it is expedient to cut down the number of visits. Many skin lesions in the elderly are treated by a single application as outpatients with the treatment producing minimal trauma.

Chemotherapy

The chemotherapeutic agents available fall into two groups: cytotoxic drugs which kill tumour cells or inhibit their growth, and hormones acting on hormone-dependent tumours.

Cytotoxic Drugs

These drugs may destroy the malignant cell at any stage of the cell cycle or may specifically produce damage at one part of the cycle. There are now many compounds, but only a relatively small number have proved to be successful in the treatment of malignancies, and their application is confined to a small number of tumours. Initially, a single drug was given but the effect of the drug on normal tissues restricted the dose and limited success. Recently drug combinations are chosen so that the effect on the malignant lesion is summated or even accentuated, and the effects on normal tissues are spread over a number of organs so that the final toxic effect to the patient is reduced.

The success of cytotoxic drugs depends on the relative sensitivity of the tumour cells compared with those of the normal tissues; the drugs are diluted in the circulation and in body tissues and will only be effective in sensitive tumours such as leukaemia and the reticuloses. They may be used to augment other methods of treatment or to palliate. However, the side-effects must be carefully considered in the elderly and the benefits of palliation must clearly outweigh the distress. The considerable upset which may be caused by these drugs is not justified in elderly patients whose tumour is clearly not responding and in whom there is no hope of cure.

Hormones

Some tumours are known to be hormone dependent and the rationale is to reduce the amount of this hormone by giving opposing ones; thus, in cancer of the prostate, stilboestrol may be given and in the elderly female patient who is more than 10 years past the menopause, the same hormone may be given. When using this drug a watch should be made for bleeding or thromboembolic phenomena. Hormones may be useful in cancer of the breast in elderly females and may keep the lesion under control for long periods. The corticosteroids may also play a role, either on the tumour itself or on certain complications of malignant disease, e.g. hypercalcaemia or cerebral oedema or on general well-being and appetite.

Immunotherapy

This method aims at developing the body's own defence mechanism against the cancer cells which are in effect foreign bodies. There is little indication, at present, that there is an application to the clinical therapeutic field.

COMPLICATIONS

The complications of treatment may come on during or immediately after treatment or may be later.

Immediate Complications of Treatment

In radiotherapy any tissue irradiated may produce an untoward effect, and some tissues are particularly prone to damage. Early reactions on the skin and mucous membranes are shown by erythema. This may proceed to at first patchy and then confluent desquamation of the skin, or a patchy and confluent membrane reaction of mucous membrane composed of discharge and desquamated cells – both may go on to necrosis if treatment continues.

Moist skin at natural folds, the axilla, groins, inframammary regions, and the perineum together with the skin of the dorsum of the foot, does not stand radiation well. The treated skin may need to be protected from the scratching of elderly patients. Irradiation of the lungs may produce the reaction of pneumonitis which is a non-specific response to an irritant similar to that produced after inhalation of toxic gases such as chlorine and phosgene; if this does not produce actual tissue death the reaction will clear. The irradiated lung is very prone to infection. Dysphagia results from reaction of the oesophagus; a similar reaction in the intestine stimulates fluid output in the lumen and quite profuse diarrhoea results. Nausea and vomiting, lethargy, anorexia, and being 'off-colour' may result from circulating breakdown tissue products. Alopecia may occur but may recover after treatment, the hair sometimes growing in its original colour.

Cytotoxic drugs affect varying tissues and may produce nausea and vomiting, stomatitis, alopecia, diarrhoea, bone marrow depression, effects on the heart, and so on. Manoeuvres such as the phasing of the drugs and the use of folinic acid with methotrexate may reduce these effects. A full blood count has to be taken before treatment and frequently throughout. Usually patients are admitted for short courses of therapy.

Surgery has its own particular catalogue of complications to which the elderly are prone.

The acute reactions after radiotherapy may heal without permanent damage, but if tissues have been destroyed they can only be replaced by fibrosis. In the lung pneumonitis may resolve, but if the elastic tissue around the alveoli is destroyed, there is permanent fibrosis. This may be quite extensive and pull the mediastinum to the affected side, the chest wall inwards, cause tenting of the diaphragm, emphysema of the opposite lung, and even scoliosis. Damage leading to scarring may be from the cancer and/or treatment, but often this represents a successful outcome to the disease. Damage from radiation may occur to any organ. Some organs are more susceptible than others and the effects disabling. e.g. in the lens producing a cataract, in the kidneys causing hypertension, in the spinal cord producing radiation myelitis. These reactions take some time to fully develop and such long-term effects are not a contraindication to treatment in the elderly.

There are a few late effects of chemotherapy which are applicable to the elderly, the most upsetting effects being the immediate ones caused by the drugs.

FOLLOW-UP

Patients who have received treatment for a malignant disease are seen regularly at follow-up:

(a) Further treatment may be given for a recurrent lesion.
(b) Distressing sequelae or complications may be relieved.
(c) Minor adjustments or procedures may be carried out, e.g. trimming of a colostomy, changing a tracheostomy tube, correcting anaemia, and so on.
(d) The patient builds up a relationship with the oncologist and is encouraged to report untoward effects.
(e) A careful analysis of the results of treatment helps the oncologist to improve the results of treatment.

There is a tendency to waive follow-up examination in the elderly patient, presuming that the effort of coming for examination may be too demanding. However, if there is a possibility of recurrence and possibly further treat-

ment, patients should be encouraged to attend. Patients receive a psychological boost when told that the disease is under control, or the comfort of knowing that they can come back if they are concerned.

REHABILITATION

It is desirable to rehabilitate the elderly cancer patient as quickly as possible to normal life. It is necessary to overcome a natural reluctance to subject an elderly cancer patient to the organization that may be necessary. Many relatives and health care workers acting out of sympathy will try to disturb him as little as possible. Return to normal requires an active role from the patient.

The elderly patient may well have a suspicion of the nature of the disease. Some will not be interested, some will withdraw from the reality of the diagnosis and prefer not to discuss it, some will assume the worse, a few may ask for clarification. Old age often brings acceptance of circumstances, and it is inevitable that the patient accepts the worst possible diagnosis, resigning himself to the hopelessness of the situation – whatever the prognosis may be. Whenever possible, the patient should be told the facts, simply and as unembellished as possible, and be given some indication of what treatment will entail, what possible complications there are, and what will be done for him after treatment. If the prognosis is fairly good, the patient will be told what is expected of him after he has had treatment and what efforts will be made to rehabilitate him. Any scheme of rehabilitation must be discussed with his relatives and their full cooperation sought. It is important that he is led to understand that life can go on and will go on but that he will need to make a special effort. This psychological approach to rehabilitation must start as quickly as possible.

The toxic effects of cancer and of radiotherapy impair normal vigour and appetite. Radiotherapy, especially to the upper abdomen, and cytotoxic drugs may induce nausea and vomiting and further compromise a fragile nutritional state. Small frequent meals, even hourly, with appropriate vitamin supplements are often necessary. An alcoholic apéritif often aids the appetite.

Age does not deny the appropriateness of a

prosthesis. Hair loss may be particularly upsetting and a wig should be provided. Some elderly women welcome an artificial breast after mastectomy. Skin scars may cause embarrassment and require cosmetic disguises.

RECURRENCE AND RETREATMENT

The popular belief that once treatment has been given nothing more can be done is often incorrect. Should the initial treatment fail, other treatments may be given, sometimes with a chance of cure. For example, if surgical removal fails to cure, a course of radiotherapy or cytotoxic therapy may be given; regular follow-up irrespective of age is therefore important.

Failure to cure by radical treatment may lead to a recurrence of distressing symptoms, these may be palliated and the patient have relief of symptoms for the rest of his life. For example, if radical treatment to a carcinoma of the bladder is unsuccessful and haematuria develops, it can often be stopped with a relatively short course of radiation, only sufficient treatment being given to stop bleeding. Cerebral metastases may show quite dramatic relief with only two treatments of radiation to the brain. Comatosed patients may recover and use return to paralysed limbs, this makes nursing much easier and, is better for the patient and for his relatives. Bone secondaries can be relieved with a single treatment of radiation, obviating the need for sedation and analgesics with upsetting side-effects. Further recurrence may be treated with further radiation.

CARE OF THE PATIENT AFTER TREATMENT

We must now consider the continuing care of the cancer patient.

Care at Home

The elderly patient with malignant disease often returns from hospital to inadequate home or support facilities. Problems of general and nursing care must be discussed before the patient is discharged. There may be an offensive discharge requiring home nursing. In terminal patients incontinence and pain have to be catered for by the family doctor, district nurse, and social services, but they are not always brought to light sufficiently early to be anticipated.

After-Care Homes

In recent years after-care or continuing care facilities have become more available. Ideally these should be sited in a small hostel dedicated to this particular work. Such a home would provide:
(a) convalescent care bridging the gap between the acute ward and the conventional convalescent home;
(b) facilities for admission for minor procedures, blood transfusion, changing tracheostomy tubes, and so on;
(c) for some, rehabilitative instructions and demonstration;
(d) facilities to take in the chronically sick patients for a few days so that they and their relatives may get a rest;
(e) the terminally ill cancer patients.

All these patients would be admitted for a relatively short period only. An important aspect of the work of such homes is the domiciliary service provided; patients would be visited at their homes and help given to the community team; admission would be arranged quickly if necessary.

These homes also have an important role in the tuition of all involved in the care of the malignant patient. Too often oncologists are mainly concerned with radical treatment aimed at a cure; if this is not achieved, it is considered a failure. There is a tendency to pay less attention to the patient whose treatment has been unsuccessful, but it is just these patients who need so much after-care.

Terminal Care

For the patient whose treatment has been unsuccessful and who is steadily declining, there comes the phase of terminal care. At this time there is often realization of impending death and the patient, even the elderly, may react in several ways: resignation and acceptance may occur; in many there is disbelief and lingering hope; some are actively resentful; and some will resist. Contrary to popular belief the terminal stages of cancer are not accompanied by excruciating pain. While about one-half of patients may experience some pain, this may not be severe, may be chronic in nature, and may be controlled by simple drugs such as aspirin or paracetamol. In only about 12 per cent. of patients is powerful narcotic medication with perhaps admission to hospital required. Analgesics should be given regularly to prevent pain (see Chapter 31).

Nausea and vomiting, apprehension, secondary deposits, or fungating offensive discharges or ulceration require appropriate management. Even in the terminal stages an adequate diet should be given and attention taken of the bowels to ensure the patient's comfort.

The final terminal stage may last for a few weeks only and a decision must be made about where the patient is to die. The choice must lie between a special terminal home – dedicated to the care of the terminal cancer patients— and the patient's own home. So much will depend on the individual, his desires and those of his relatives, and the facilities available.

Bereavement

All careworkers are familiar with bereavement and this is an important aspect of oncological care. While every effort is being made to help the patient, the relatives must not be forgotten. The bereaved elderly spouse often has little incentive to carry on or want to live; the dread of cancer adds a further bitterness which may be accentuated if there has been suffering, pain, or distress. In relatively recent years the process of prebereavement has been recognized. This is a time of considerable stress, especially to the elderly, and accentuated by the knowledge that the disease is hopeless, that there is no cure, that death will occur. It is sharpened by a lack of knowledge of when death will occur and how it will happen. The expectant spouse naturally is worried by the thought that the patient may be in pain, may be unprepared, or may lose dignity, but worried also by a fear of their own reaction. Will they cope? What should they do? Is there a danger that they may fail to notice some important symptom? These people need considerable help well before the patient is terminal to prepare them for what is to come.

CANCER INFORMATION

There is need for a greater awareness of the incidence and presenting features of malignancy in old age. Successful treatment usually depends on early detection and elderly persons in long-term residential care may profit by regular surveillance. The old themselves should be encouraged to appreciate that unusual symptoms are due to disease and not to old age.

CONCLUSION

Age by itself is not a contraindication to the treatment of malignant diseases. Early lesions are much easier to deal with and have a better prognosis; therefore all those responsible for the care of the elderly must be alert to the possibility of these diseases developing.

BIBLIOGRAPHY

Alper, T. (1979). *Cellular Radiobiology*, Cambridge University Press.
Bagshawe, K. D. (Ed.) (1975) *Medical Oncology, Medical Aspects of Malignant Disease*, Blackwell, Oxford.
Barnes, P. A., and Rees, D. J. (1972). *A Concise Textbook of Radiotherapy*, Faber and Faber, London.
Calman, K. C., Smyth, S. F., and Tattersall, M. H. N. (Eds) (1980). *Basic Principles of Cancer Chemotherapy*, Macmillan.
Deeley, T. J. (1976) *Principles of Radiation Therapy*, Butterworths, London.
Deeley, T. J. (1979). *A Guide to the Radiotherapy and Oncology Department*, John Wright, Bristol.
Deeley, T. J. (1980). *Attitudes to Cancer*, SPCK, London.
Hall, E. J. (1978). *Radiobiology for the Radiologist*, Harper and Row, Hagerstown, Maryland.
Haskell, C. M. (Ed.) (1980). *Cancer Treatment*, W. B. Saunders, Philadelphia.
Holland, J. P., and Frei, E. III (1973). *Cancer Medicine*, Lea and Febiger, Philadelphia.
Louis, C. J. (1978). *Tumours, Basic Principles and Clinical Aspects*, Churchill Livingstone, Edinburgh.
Lowry, S. (1974). *Fundamentals of Radiation Therapy and Cancer Chemotherapy*, EUP, London.
Price, C. A., Will, B. T., and Ghilchick, M. W. (1980). *Safer Cancer Chemotherapy*, Baillière Tindall, London.
Priestman, T. J. (1980). *Cancer Chemotherapy, An Introduction*, Montedison Pharmaceuticals.

Raven, R. W. (Ed.) (1978) *Principles of Surgical Oncology*, Plenum, New York.

Saunders, C., Summers, D. H., and Tellurn, N. (1981). *Hospice the Living Idea*, Edward Arnold, London.

Scott, R. B. (1979). *Cancer, The Facts*, Oxford University Press.

Thompson, I. (Ed.) (1979). *Dilemmas of Dying*, Edinburgh University Press.

Walter, J. (1971). *Cancer and Radiotherapy, a Short Guide for Nurses and Medical Students*, Churchill Livingstone, Edinburgh.

Waterhouse, J. A. H. (1974). *Cancer Handbook of Epidemiology and Prognosis*, Churchill Livingstone, Edinburgh.

Willis, R. A. (1973). *The Spread of Tumours in the Human Body*, Butterworths, London.

REFERENCES

Deeley, T. J. (1965). 'Secondary deposits in the breast', *Br. J. Cancer*, **19**, 738–743.

Deeley, T. J., and Rice-Edwards, P. (1968). 'Radiotherapy in the management of cerebral secondaries for bronchial carcinoma', *Lancet*, **1**, 1209–1211.

Deeley, T. J. (1982). *Cancer*. Tenovus Cancer Information Centre. Cardiff.

Deeley, T. J. (1984). *After care of the cancer patient*. Tenovus Cancer Information Centre. Cardiff.

Gray, L. H., Conger, A. D., Ebert, M., Hornsey, S., and Scott, O. C. A. (1953). 'The concentration of oxygen dissolved in tissues at the time of irradiation as a factor in radiotherapy', *Br. J. Radiol.*, **26**, 638–648.

25

The Musculoskeletal System

Principles and Practice of Geriatric Medicine
Edited by M. S. J. Pathy
© 1985 John Wiley & Sons Ltd

25.1

Diseases of Muscle and Connective Tissue

M. Denham

DISEASES OF CONNECTIVE TISSUE

Ageing Changes

Connective tissue contains collagen, lipids, and sometimes elastin, in a matrix of ground substance and fibrous protein, while elderly tissue also contains pseudo-elastin and cellulose fibres.

Collagen

The basic macromolecule of collagen consists of three separate protein chains, each arranged in a helix, and all are twisted about each other in one large helix. Increasing age is associated with an increase in the crosslinkages between the protein chains and a slowing of collagen synthesis. Many attempts have been made to apply physical laws of load and extension to connective tissues, but with limited success. Tendon has been studied since it contains collagen as a major component. Viidik (1967), for example, has shown that there is a linear relationship between load and extension, but only over short ranges of the latter. The slope of the line is a measure of the 'stiffness' of the tendon and this changes with age, which is in keeping with Ridge and Wright's (1966) finding that tendon stiffens with age.

Collagen is degraded by collagenases, resulting in the excretion of hydroxyproline in the urine, amounts of which decrease with increasing age. Bacterial enzyme studies suggest that collagen is less susceptible to enzyme attack with increasing age of the human subject (Hall and Reed, 1973) which may be due to the increased crosslinks found in 'elderly' collagen.

Elastin

Elastin fibres are mainly found in skin, the walls of the major blood vessels, the heart, lungs, and ligaments. They are arranged in different ways according to their site – thus, fibres found in the aorta are arranged in a circumferential manner. The elastin content of the aorta increases up to the age of about 20 years, but decreases thereafter. This change may be physiological or related to atherosclerosis. As the elastin content falls, there is an increase in pseudo-elastin (Hall, 1964) which stains similarly to elastin, but is insoluble in the usual collagen solvents. The amounts of elastin vary from tissue to tissue, and from one pathological state to another.

Elastase

The elastin content of connective tissue is controlled by the exocrine secretion of elastase by the pancreas. The concentration of this enzyme in plasma and pancreas falls with age – in men the fall occurs after the age of about 40 years, while in women it falls from about the age of 10 years, with a temporary rise during the menopause (Tesal and Hall, 1972). The increase in the amount of elastolysis which occurs with increasing age, even in the presence of a fall in the concentration of elastase, may be due to a simultaneous fall in the level of plasma es-tastase inhibitor (Hall, 1968). The elastase content of serum can be used as a prognostic sign after a 'stroke' since in those who survive there is a rise followed by a slow fall to normal levels, while there is a dramatic rise in those who die (Hall *et al*, 1980).

Cellulose Fibres

Hall and Saxl (1960) have shown the presence of anisotropic fibres which consist of a central protein core, similar to pseudo-elastin, sur-rounded by cellulose. These fibres appear in subjects over the age of 20 years, and increase with age and disease.

Polymyalgia Rheumatica and Giant Cell Arteritis

Polymyalgia rheumatica (PMR) is a condition of older people, characterized by aching, pain, and stiffness of the proximal muscles (neck, back, shoulder, buttocks, and thighs) without weakness or atrophy, persisting for at least one month. The ESR is greater than 50 mm per hour and there is dramatic relief with steroids (Healey, Parker, and Wilske, 1971). Giant cell arteritis (GCA) is a granulamatous inflamma-tory disease of large and medium sized arter-ies, particularly involving the temporal and ophthalmic arteries. The relationship between PMR and GCA is illustrated by the findings of Fauchald, Rygold, and Lystese, (1972) who studied 94 patients with PMR or GCA. In 61 cases positive temporal biopsies were ob-tained, while 33 patients with clinical PMR had negative results. Of 49 patients with myalgia, but with no clinical abnormality of the cranial arteries, 20 had positive temporal artery biop-sies. Jones and Hazleman (1981) found clinical evidence of GCA in 55 per cent. of all patients with PMR and considered temporal artery bi-opsy to be of little value in predicting patients likely to develop GCA.

Pathology

Pathological investigations in PMR are unhelp-ful. Muscle biopsy, muscle enzyme, and EMG studies are normal, although some patients may have a positive temporal artery biopsy.

The histological picture of active temporal arteritis is characteristic. The lumen is reduced and in the late stage the intima is thickened by fibrosis. The inflammatory cell infiltrate mainly involves the media and adventitia. In the ad-ventitia there may be fibrosis, with mono-nuclear cellular infiltration. The media contains lymphocytes, giant cells, neutrophils, plasma cells, eosinophils, and macrophages. The internal elastic lamina is often destroyed. Skip lesions occur and consequently changes can vary in different sections taken from the same artery. Usually both temporal arteries are affected, even when only one is clinically involved (Cohen and Smith, 1974). Larger ar-teries, such as the aorta, may show arteritic changes (Klein *et al.*, 1975).

Aetiology

The cause of PMR and GCA remains unclear, but immunological factors may be involved. Immunoglobulin has been found in the media of affected arteries. There is an increase in the transformation response of peripheral blood lymphocytes to human muscle antigen in vitro and to arterial antigen in vitro (Esiri, McLen-nan, and Hazelman, 1973). In addition, there is evidence of an association with the immune gene HLA-B8 (Hazleman, Goldstone, and Voak, 1977). However, infective causes are possible in view of the apparent association with upper respiratory tract infections (Bell and Klinefelter, 1967).

Incidence

The majority of cases of PMR occur in those over the age of 60 years – women are more commonly affected than men. The incidence of cases seen at a rheumatology clinic varies from 1.3 to 4.5 per cent. of all referred patients (Dixon *et al.*, 1966; Mowat and Hazleman, 1974). The incidence in the general population is calculated to be 3 per 1,000 population (Dixon, 1970).

The majority of cases of GCA occur in those over the age of 60 years and women are more commonly affected (Hauser *et al.*, 1971). The calculated incidence rate of cases is about 2.2 to 2.9 per 100,000 of the population (Hauser *et al.*, 1971; Ostberg, 1971). However, a post-mortem study, not surprisingly, gave a higher incidence of 1 per cent. (Ostberg, 1971).

CLINICAL FEATURES

The onset of PMR may be acute or gradual over a few days, sometimes commencing with a 'flu-like illness, associated with fever, weight loss, and synovitis. Typically, there is a history of muscle stiffness and aching pains in the muscles of the shoulder and pelvic girdles to such an extent that the patient may have difficulty in getting out of bed or a chair. The symptoms are usually worse after a period of inactivity, hence the characteristic morning stiffness. True synovitis may occur.

GCA may present in a similar non-specific manner with general malaise, anorexia and weight loss, and mild fever. In addition, the patient complains of sudden or gradual onset of a throbbing or aching headache, which is usually unilateral. The temporal arteries may be red, swollen, and tender. The scalp may be tender when the hair is combed. Severe arteritis can lead to infarction of the scalp (Fig. 1). Some patients experience pain over the jaw on eating – jaw claudication – which suggests involvement of other cranial arteries.

The feared complication of GCA is involvement of the eye, leading to blindness; indeed, about 40 per cent. of patients with GCA develop ocular symptoms (Hauser *et al.*, 1971). Visual loss, due to involvement of the ophthalmic artery, may be sudden or gradual over a few days, with warning episodes of blurring of vision. If treatment is commenced early enough, it is possible to prevent permanent blindness, but fully established blindness responds poorly to treatment. The height of the ESR does not correlate with the risk of developing visual loss (Ellis and Ralston, 1983).

Involvement of other arteries causes symptoms appropriate to the organ concerned. Mental changes, such as confusion and depression, are considered to be due to intracranial involvement, which may also result in acute cerebral infarction or brain stem ischaemia. GCA involvement of the aorta, coronary arteries, common iliacs, and the visceral arteries can cause angina or myocardial infarction, while peripheral arterial insufficiency can cause, with intermittent claudication, paraesthesia and Raynaud's phenomenon.

Diagnosis

Patients with PMR typically have an ESR over 50 mm per hour and usually nearer 100 mm per hour. Unfortunately a significant number of patients with PMR/GCA may have an ESR less than 50 mm per hour (Ellis and Ralston, 1983). Other non-specific changes include a mild normo- or hypochromic anaemia and a leucocytosis. Tests for rheumatoid factor are usually negative, while the serum alkaline

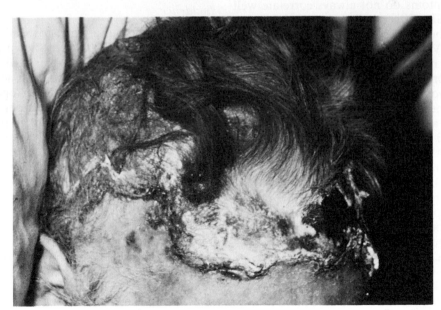

Figure 1   Infarcation of the scalp resulting from severe arteritis

phosphatase and 5-nucleotidase may be elevated. Protein electrophoresis may show a non-specific rise in alpha-2 globulin. The serum albumin level may be raised and serum fibrinogen elevated. Serum complement is normal, while the SCAT is negative and LE cells are not found. Tests of muscle disease, such as the muscle enzyme and EMG are normal. Muscle biopsy may show only mild atrophic changes.

Patients with GCA are likely to show the same features, but with a positive temporal artery biopsy. The results from arterial arteriography may be used to help localize the best site for biopsy. The presence of giant cells in biopsy material has no apparent influence on the clinical course (Huston *et al.*, 1978).

PMR and GCA can be differentiated from cervical and lumbar spondylosis by the ESR and x-rays of the vertebrae. The ESR may or may not be helpful.

Treatment

Although the side-effects of steroids in the elderly are well recognized, prednisolone is essential in the treatment of GCA in order to prevent blindness. The initial starting dose is 60 mg per day with subsequent doses being titrated against the patient's clinical condition and ESR. The aim is to get this below 20 mm per hour. Unfortunately , however the patient's symptoms do not always correlate well with the ESR (Ellis and Ralston, 1983). Treatment may be required for 2 years before being tailed off. Vertebral compression and myopathy are the most serious complications of therapy (Huston *et al.*, 1978). Early mortality is low and most commonly is due to vertebral arteritis. The need for high-maintenance doses of steroids and visual loss are associated with a shortened life span (Graham *et al.*, 1981).

PMR in the absence of classical features of GCA and in the presence of a normal arterial biopsy can be treated with non-steroidal anti-inflammatory drugs. However, such treatment leaves the patients open to the risk of developing temporal arteritis later and therefore they must be carefully watched. Consequently, many physicians prefer to treat with high doses of steroids, even if the biopsy is normal. The disease tends to remit between 6 months to 2 years after onset, but a few cases persist for as long as 5 years.

Polymyositis and Dermatomyositis

Polymyositis (PM) is a diffuse, non-hereditary inflammatory condition of striated muscle. When it is associated with an erythematous skin rash it is known as dermatomyositis (DM).

Pathology

The muscle fibres show widespread degeneration with or without evidence of phagocytosis and regeneration. Inflammatory cells are found around blood vessels and between muscle fibres. As the disease progresses there may be evidence of fibrosis and muscle atrophy. Skin changes include dermal infiltration with lymphocytes, plasma cells, and histiocytes, while the epidermis may show signs of atrophy. Calcification may be seen.

Aetiology

The exact cause of the condition is not known. However, the histological changes, serological findings, lymphocytic studies, and the association with connective tissues known to have an immune basis suggest that polymyositis may have a similar causation. However, genetic factors are involved, since cases can occur in the same family.

Incidence

PM–DM can occur at any age. Medsger, Dawson, and Masi, (1970) have shown a bimodal distribution of incidence against age, with most cases occurring in childhood or in adults in the fifth or sixth decade, giving an age-adjusted incidence of 5 cases per million per year. The condition is more common in men, particularly when there is an association with malignancy (De Vere and Bradley, 1975). This association with malignancy occurs in the adult population rather than in childhood, and is more marked in those with DM.

Diagnostic Criteria of PM–DM

Bohan and Peter (1976) consider that 5 major criteria are required to diagnose PM or DM. These are:
(a) proximal symmetrical muscle weakness of upper and lower extremities;

(b) characteristic muscle biopsy findings;

(c) elevation of serum enzymes: including, in particular, creatine phosphokinase (CPK), as well as the transaminases (SGOT and SGPT), aldolase (ALD), and lactic dehydrogenase (LDH);

(d) characteristic EMG findings;

(e) dermatological manifestations of DM.

Bohan and Peter suggest that the diagnosis of definite DM requires 3 or 4 criteria, plus the rash, while definite PM requires 4 criteria. Possible and probable diagnoses require fewer criteria.

Clinical Features

'Pure' Polymyositis. Usually there is progressive, symmetrical muscle weakness of upper and lower extremities, as well as the neck, abdominal, and paraspinal muscles, with or without dysphagia or respiratory muscle weakness. The weakness advances fairly rapidly over weeks or months, unlike muscle dystrophies, which progress over the years. Distal strength is characteristically good. Facial muscles are usually not involved. There is relatively good retention of tendon reflexes and no sensory loss.

The muscle weakness results initially in difficulties in getting out of bed, climbing stairs, or combing hair. As the disease advances, the muscles of respiration may be involved, as well as those of speech or swallowing. The muscles may be tender. To start with, there is little muscle wasting, but in the later phases contractures can develop. The speed with which the disease advances varies considerably. Progress may be rapid with death within a few weeks, or it may last several months or even years, and show relapses and remissions.

Sometimes the disease involves the viscera, resulting in pulmonary fibrosis and oesophageal smooth muscle hypomotility, which may be associated with oesophageal diverticulae. Rarely the heart may be affected, producing dysrhythmias.

'Pure' dermatomyositis. In DM the symptoms and signs of polymyositis are associated with skin rash. This classically consists of a purplish discolouration of the periorbital region. In addition, there may be an erythematous rash over the cheek, neck, upper chest, the extensor surface of the knees, the elbows, and the knuckles. Sometimes telangiectasia and splinter haemorrhages may be seen.

Polymyositis with features of other connective tissue disorders. These patients have the features of polymyositis together with signs and symptoms of systemic lupus erythematosis, progressive sclerosis, rheumatoid arthritis, Sjögren's syndrome, or Raynaud's phenomenon.

DM (PM) with malignancy. This association is more marked with dermatomyositis. The most frequent sites for tumour are the lungs, ovaries, prostate, breast, gastrointestinal tract, and reticuloses (Bohan *et al.*, 1977; De Vere and Bradley, 1975). Although malignancy may precede or coincide with the development of polymyositis, more commonly it follows some months later.

Investigations and Diagnosis

As indicated earlier, three investigations can give useful diagnostic information:

1. Muscle enzyme levels. The most useful of these is creatine phosphokinase (CPK), but others used include ALD, LDH, SGOT, SGPT. Since not all enzymes may be raised in one particular patient, it is usual to measure two or three at one time. Elevated values indicate active disease and can warn of a relapse, while low values indicate remission or a chronic stage.

2. EMG studies. The three classical features are: firstly, spontaneous fibrillation; secondly, short-duration, low-amplitude polyphonic motor unit potential; and thirdly, salvoes of high-frequency, bizarre repetitive discharge (Bohan *et al.*, 1977). These changes help to differentiate lower motor neurone lesions and muscular dystrophy. Nerve conduction studies are of little diagnostic help.

3. Muscle biopsy. In order to reduce the risks of a negative biopsy, the muscle chosen should not be excessively weak, atrophic, or appear clinically normal.

Other investigations give little specific help. The ESR and serum globulins may be normal or raised, while the SCAT and ANF may or may not be positive. Urinary investigations may show creatinuria and albuminuria. X-rays may show calcification of the skin.

PM–DM can be distinguished from hereditary neuromuscular disorders by the duration of the disease and family history; from motor neurone disease by the distribution of the muscle weakness, muscle fasciculation, and the muscle histology; from PMR by the absence of true muscle weakness and the high ESR; and from inflammatory myopathies by the general clinical condition, while the proximal muscle weakness is less prominent.

Treatment and Progress

The basic treatment for patients without malignancy is steroid therapy. An initial dose of 60 mg prednisolone daily can result in dramatic relief of symptoms and improvement in long-term prognosis. The dose is titrated against clinical state and serum enzyme levels. Steroids are likely to be required indefinitely. Sometimes response is slow, and therefore no change of treatment should be made until about 2 months has elapsed. Alternative treatments include methotrexate, azathioprine, and cyclophosphamide (Pirofsky and Bardana, 1977). Some patients have responded well to thymectomy. In addition to these treatments, all patients are likely to benefit from physiotherapy.

Patients with DM (PM) associated malignancy should have the tumour treated if possible. Successful treatment is usually followed by improvement.

The overall mortality rate is 28 per cent. (De Vere and Bradley, 1975). In general, the earlier the disease is treated, the better the outcome, but the prognosis in the elderly is often not good, due to the association with malignancy and cardiorespiratory problems. The extension of malignancy, the appearance of sepsis, or the development of an aspiration pneumonia are all bad prognostic signs.

Amyloid

Amyloid is an homogenous eosinophilic, protein-like material laid down extracellularly in one or more sites. Its pathogenesis remains unknown, but immune mechanisms are probably involved.

Classification

Various classifications have been proposed, which depend on the presence or absence of predisposing disease or on the distribution of the amyloid. None are entirely successful due to overlap between the suggested groups. At present, a classification based on clinical features is probably most helpful (see Table 1).

Table 1   Classification of amyloidosis

1.	Primary amyloidosis – no recognized predisposing conditions
2.	Secondary amyloidosis – associated with predisposing causes
3.	Amyloidosis—associated with multiple myeloma
4.	Heredofamilial amyloidosis
5.	Local amyloidosis
6.	Amyloidosis of ageing

Primary amyloidosis differs from secondary in the distribution and nature of the amyloid material. Primary amyloid is typically distributed in heart, tongue, skeletal and visceral muscle, nerves, and gastrointestinal tract, and is laid down in relation to the collagen fibres of the adventitia of blood vessels. Patients with primary amyloidosis often show evidence of an abnormal production of an immunoglobulin light chain and some are later found to have an occult plasma cell dyscrasia. In addition, the amyloid fibrils of primary and myeloma-associated amyloidosis appear to have similar N-terminal amino acid sequence, which strengthens further the connection between these two types of amyloidosis (Glenner *et al.*, 1971).

Secondary amyloidosis may be found in a number of conditions, including chronic sepsis such as osteomyelitis, tuberculosis, rheumatoid arthritis, ulcerative colitis, Crohn's disease, malignant lymphoma, and carcinoma. Amyloid in this situation is usually found in the liver, kidney, spleen, and suprarenal glands, and is laid down in association with the endothelial basement membrane of blood vessels. Secondary amyloid does not appear to have an immunological origin and the terminal

N amino acid sequence is different from that in the primary variety (Benditt *et al.*, 1971).

Amyloid may be found in small focal amounts, particularly in the lung, skin, larynx, eye, and bladder. There is usually no evidence of systemic disease. Amyloid may also be found in small amounts particularly in the brain, heart, pancreas, and spleen of the elderly. The cause is unknown. Hereditary amyloidosis is due to autosomal dominant or recessive transmission, and is seen in familial Mediterranean fever.

Pathology

Amyloid, when laid down in large amounts, gives an organ a waxy, greasy appearance and is usually associated with enlargement of that organ. Deposits may be localized or diffuse. Amyloid material can be identified by various staining techniques, including congo red viewed with polarization, thioflavine T staining viewed with ultraviolet light, and sulphonated alcein-blue staining. Unfortunately, not all techniques are specific, which partly accounts for the variation in the reported incidence of the disease. Electron microscopy studies show that amyloid consists of fibrils which are usually arranged in a random fashion, unless they are near cells when there is a degree of parallelism.

Clinical Features

The clinical features depend on the site and the amount of the amyloid deposit. Renal involvement is potentially the most serious, although it may have been present for some years before symptoms appear. Initially, there is proteinuria, which is usually non-selective. The glomerular filtration rate is more impaired than tubular function. The nephrotic syndrome may occur in as many as half the cases. However, patients can retain quite reasonable renal function for long periods, in spite of the amyloid infiltration (Triger and Joekes, 1973).

Cardiac amyloidosis increases in incidence with age and is commoner in women. It is associated with an increased incidence of both cardiac failure and atrial fibrillation. However, an association with ischaemia and ECG changes other than atrial fibrillation is disputed (Hodkinson and Pomerance, 1977). Cardiac amyloidosis is not associated with increased sensitivity to digoxin. It is difficult to prove the existence of cardiac amyloid in life, since rectal biopsies are usually negative, although a raised alkaline phosphatase may be a diagnostic pointer, when other causes of elevation are eliminated.

Symptoms of amyloidosis of the gastro-intestinal tract may be due to direct involvement of the gut or the autonomic nervous system. Clinical features, which are commoner in the primary form, include macroglossia, obstruction, ulceration, malabsorption, haemorrhage, protein loss, and diarrhoea. Liver amyloidosis is not uncommon, but when present is not usually associated with severe dysfunction. The serum alkaline phosphatase may be raised and brom-sulphthaline (BSP) retention present.

Neurological involvement occurs more commonly in the primary amyloidosis and can lead to sensory or motor neuropathies. Deposition of amyloid in the autonomic nervous system can lead to diarrhoea and postural hypotension.

Other organs involved include the lungs, joints, and skin. The former can cause hoarseness of the voice, haemoptysis, and epistaxis. Large joint involvement can mimic rheumatoid arthritis, but microscopic deposits are asymptomatic and are not associated with any pathological condition (Goffin, Thoua, and Patvliege, 1981). Small deposits may also be found in large osteoarthritic joints (Egan *et al.*, 1982). Amyloidosis of the skin produces waxy plaque formation, usually in the axilla, inguinal region, face, or neck. Purpuric areas and alopecia may be seen.

Diagnosis

Diagnosis depends mainly on biopsy, usually from the rectum or from the kidney or liver if involvement of these organs is suspected. The congo red test can be used to assist diagnosis, but false negative results are not uncommon. Routine laboratory investigations are of little diagnostic value.

Treatment

There is no certain curative treatment, but clearly when secondary amyloidosis develops, the precipitating disease should be treated. Reabsorption of amyloid material may occur, but is more likely to persist. The longer the precipitating cause has been present, the less the chance of improvement. Kyle and Bayrd (1975) found that mean survival times for secondary amyloidosis was just over 1 year from the time of diagnosis, and just under 1 year for primary type, but some much longer individual cases of survival times have been found (Hobbs, 1973; Missen and Taylor, 1956). Ravid and coworkers (1982) report some benefit with prolonged demethylsylphoxide treatment in patients with secondary amyloidosis.

DISEASES OF MUSCLE

Ageing Changes in Muscles

It is well known that muscle strength declines with increasing age. Burke and coworkers (1953) have shown that maximum grip strength falls to almost half between the ages of 25 and 79 years. Anderson and Cowan (1966), in their study of larger numbers of elderly people, confirmed steady deterioration in grip strength with age, but also demonstrated a correlation with body weight and sex. However, physical training, even in the elderly, can increase muscle power (Ariansson *et al.*, 1980).

Pathological studies show that as muscles age, they become atrophic and lose the usual red-brown colour of normal muscle. Instead, they may become yellow due to the deposition of lipochrome pigment or grey due to increased amounts of fibrous tissue. Microscopically, muscle fibres are reduced in number and usually show an increased variation in size. There may also be perinuclear lipoprotein pigmentation and nuclear clumping. There is a concomittant increase in fat cells and interstitial connective tissue. Little inflammatory reaction or acute necrosis of muscle cells is seen. Jennekens, Tomlinson and Walton (1971) consider that the muscular atrophy of old age is a complex phenomena due to many causes, including disuse, inadequate nutrition, myopathic changes of undetermined cause, as well as slow progressive denervation and reinnervation. Tomonaga (1977) considered that the changes were due to neuropathic and myopathic causes.

Physiological studies show that muscle wasting and weakness in muscles such as the extensor digitorium brevis result from loss of functioning motor units. The surviving motor units are often enlarged and tend to be of the slow twitch type (Campbell, McComas, and Petito, 1973). Motor nerve conduction velocity is reduced, while muscle and nerve fibres show increased refractoriness with increasing age (Delbeke, Kopec, and McComas, 1978; Farmer, Buchthal, and Rosenfalck, 1960). Campbell, McComas, and Petito (1973) consider senile muscle atrophy to be due to motor neurone dysfunction, but, since motor nerve conduction velocity is reduced in dements (Levy, Isaacs, and Hawks, 1970) and grip strength is related to mental impairment (Denham, Hodkinson, and Qureshi, 1973), loss of muscle power may also be a manifestation of generalized central nervous system involvement.

Loss of muscle power has been related to loss of fat-free mass (FFM). Forbes and Reina (1970) showed a decline in FFM with increasing age, but few of their patients were elderly. However, MacLennan and coworkers (1980) found that the effect of age on grip strength was independent of FFM and thought this might be due to the replacement of muscle by fibrous tissue, thus producing only a marginal reduction in FFM.

Muscle power is also related to dietary potassium. Judge and Cowan (1971) found that grip strength declined as dietary intake of potassium fell. It is interesting to note that Frolkis, Martynenko, and Zamostynan (1976) found that intracellular potassium fell with age.

Myopathies

Although congenital myopathies are important, few patients with these conditions survive into old age. Consequently, acquired causes, such as those due to drugs, non-metastatic carcinomas, endocrine, or metabolic diseases, are more important in the elderly.

Drug-Induced Myopathies

Lane and Mastaglia (1978) have reviewed and classified the cause of drug-induced myopathies. A number are found in the elderly.

Focal myopathies. These can follow injections of drugs such as pethidine (Mastaglia, Gardner-Medwin, and Hudgson, 1971), pentacozine (Steiner, Winkelman, and De Jesus, 1973), antibiotics (Saunders, Hoefnagel, and Staples, 1965), chlorpromazine (Cohen, 1972), digoxin, diazepam, and paraldehyde. Evidence of acute muscle damage is shown by a rise in CPK enzyme levels (Steiness *et al.*, 1978). Repeated injections may result in fibrosis and contractures.

Acute or subacute painful proximal myopathy. This can follow the use of vincristine (Bradley *et al.*, 1970), lithium carbonate (Ghose, 1977), bumetamide, salbutamol (Palmer, 1978), levodopa (Wolff, Goldberg, and Verity, 1976), cimetidine (Blackwood *et al.*, 1976), and can cause pain and weakness in proximal limb muscles. The CPK level may be elevated.

Localized or generalized weakness, with depressed tendon reflexes, may follow hypokalaemia due to diuretics, carbenoxolone, liquorice, or purgative abuse. Symptoms tend to occur when the serum potassium is less than 3 mmol/l.

Chronic painless symmetrical proximal myopathy. This can follow the prolonged use of high doses of steroids, particularly of the fluorinated type. Reflexes and CPK levels are usually normal. Where possible, the drug should be stopped or the dose reduced. Chloroquine can cause the same features.

Myasthenic syndrome. D. penicillamine and aminoglycosides (Wright and McQuillen, 1971) can cause a myasthenic syndrome, while beta blocker drugs (Herishanu and Rosenberg, 1975), chlorpromazine (McQuillen, Gross, and Johns, 1963), and phenytoin (Yaari, Pincus, and Argov, 1977) can exacerbate existing myasthenia gravis.

Chronic alcoholics. Such people can develop acute or subacute myopathies. In the acute condition, the muscles may become painful and the serum potassium raised. In the subacute disease there is symmetrical proximal muscle weakness with elevation of CPK.

Malignant hyperpyrexia. This is characterized by muscle rigidity, hyperpyrexia, disseminated intravascular coagulation, metabolic acidosis, and myoglobinuria, which can be caused by anaesthetic drugs or tricyclic antidepressants (Denborough and Lovell, 1960; Newson, 1972). Susceptibility is thought to be transmitted by autosomal dominant inheritance with variable penetrance. Dantrolene is the treatment of choice (Austin and Denborough, 1977).

Non-metastatic Carcinomatous Myopathies

Non-metastatic carcinoma may cause a number of muscle disorders.

Cachexia. The cachexia of carcinoma is due to loss of fat and diffuse symmetrical muscle wasting. However, muscle power is reasonably well retained, considering the degree of wasting. Histological examination shows a variation in muscle fibre size with little cellular reaction. The exact cause is uncertain, but may be myogenic or neurogenic in origin.

Proximal muscle wasting and weakness. This may occur with carcinoma of the lung, breast, prostate, and gastrointestinal tract. It may be myogenic or neurogenic in origin. Prognosis depends on the ability to treat the carcinoma.

Myasthenic syndrome. Patients with this syndrome have muscular fatiguability which is most marked proximally, especially the pelvic muscles. It is exacerbated by exertion, but not always improved by rest. Ptosis, diplopia, and some muscle wasting may be seen. Tendon reflexes are usually depressed. The response to neostigmine is variable and there is marked sensitivity to muscle relaxants. Symptoms of weakness and fatiguability are improved by guanidine hydrochloride (Oh and Kim, 1973). The carcinoma most likely to produce this syndrome is the oat cell bronchial carcinoma – less commonly carcinomas of the breast, prostate, stomach, and rectum are implicated.

Acute necrotizing myopathy. This uncommon condition is characterized by widespread muscle necrosis with little inflammatory reaction. It occurs with carcinoma of the lung, breast, bladder, and gastrointestinal tract.

Dermatomyositis (See Chapter 20.1) *and poly-myositis*. This syndrome may occur in association with carcinoma.

Endocrine Myopathies

Two main types of endocrine myopathies, steroid and thyroid, can affect the elderly; others are less common.

Steroid myopathy. Steroids, particularly the fluorinated types, may cause gradual or sudden onset of myalgia and/or proximal muscle weakness (Askari, Vignos, and Moskowitz, 1976). Women are more affected than men. The EMG shows no consistent changes and the CPK levels are usually normal. Histologically there is evidence of atrophy of type II muscle fibres. Treatment is to reduce or stop the steroid.

Thyroid myopathies. A number of myopathies are associated with abnormal thyroid function (Millikan and Haines, 1953). Thyrotoxic myopathies occur predominantly in men who develop proximal limb muscle weakness, although in some the weakness is both distal and proximal. The thyrotoxicosis may be mild and long standing. The CPK levels are usually not increased but the EMG shows a decrease in the mean duration of motor unit potential and an increase in polyphasic potentials. Symptoms improve on treatment of the thyrotoxicosis.

Exophthalmic ophthalmoplegia is associated with painful exophthalmos and diplopia. Corneal ulceration, papilloedema, and optic atrophy may occur. Patients may be euthyroid or mildly thyrotoxic. The condition is usually self-limiting – some cases improve spontaneously – but severe cases may need treatment with prednisolone, irradiation, or surgical decompression. The cause is uncertain, but may be due to a delayed hypersensitivity response against the orbital contents (Mullins *et al.*, 1977).

Other thyroid myopathies include myasthenia gravis, periodic paralysis associated with thyrotoxicosis (see below), and weak, painful muscles with depression of tendon reflexes, which is found in hypothyroidism.

Metabolic Myopathies

Hyperparathyroidism and osteomalacia may be associated with symmetrical proximal muscle weakness, pain on movement and pressure over bones, and brisk tendon reflexes. The serum alkaline phosphatase is raised, while the serum calcium level is typically raised in hyperparathyroidism and lowered in osteomalacia. Treatment is the treatment of the primary condition, where this is possible.

Hypokalaemia, particularly when due to gastrointestinal or renal loss, can occur in the elderly, causing a periodic muscular weakness, as detailed earlier. Hypokalaemia periodic paralysis can also occur in thyrotoxicosis. Serum potassium levels are lowered in attacks and tend to be depressed between them. Oral glucose and subcutaneous insulin can precipitate periods of paralysis. Short-term improvement occurs with oral potassium chloride, but longer-term treatment requires correction of the thyroid state. Periodic paralysis may also occur in hyperkalaemia due to renal failure, particularly when the serum potassium is greater than 7 mmol/l.

Miscellaneous Muscle Conditions

Other conditions can affect muscles in the elderly. They include contractures, the stiff man syndrome, acute compression syndrome, menopausal myopathy, and tumours.

Contractures

Contractures develop when drugs, neurological or muscular diseases cause non-active contraction and shortening of muscles. Initially, the situation is reversible, but after fibrosis occurs it may become irreversible. Since contractures present major rehabilitation problems, much emphasis is placed on prevention. However, established contractures may be treated with serial plasters or by tenotomy. Muscle spasms, which can predispose to contractures, can be treated with Baclofen (Lioresal), diazepam (Librium), or orphenadrine (Norflex) but results are not very encouraging.

The Stiff Man Syndrome

Examples of this condition have been described in older people. Characteristically, there is progressive, fluctuating, symmetrical rigidity and muscle spasm which can be precipitated by stimuli such as noise or passive stretching of the muscles (Gordon, Januszko, and Kaufman, 1967). The spasm may be so severe as to cause spontaneous fracture of bones or prostheses (Asher, 1958). The condition disappears in sleep and is abolished by diazepam or muscle relaxants. The main finding on clinical examination is board-like muscles. EMG shows evidence of persistent contraction. Muscle biopsy shows no characteristic change. CPK levels may be normal. The cause is unknown. The disease progresses over several years.

Acute Muscle Compartment Compression Syndrome

Severe pain can develop in the anterior crural muscles (anterior tibial syndrome) when the muscles are subjected to unaccustomed exercise or as the result of arterial thrombosis or embolism. The muscles are enclosed in a tight fibrous sheath which therefore limits the ability of the muscles to expand when there is increased vascularity following exercise or oedema following ischaemic necrosis. Pain produced by exercise is usually relieved by rest, but for persistent pain decompression of the compartment may be necessary. A similar syndrome occurs in Volkmann's ischaemic contracture when postischaemic fibrosis involves the long flexors of the fingers.

Late Onset of Limb Girdle Myopathy

A 'menopausal' proximal myopathy has been described (Corsi, Gentili, and Todesco, 1965) which occurs mostly in women in their forties but can occur in older men and women. Serum enzymes are normal and EMG gives non-specific results. Histological examination shows muscle atrophy and an increase in the number of sarcolemmal nuclei. Though fibrosis is seen, there is little inflammatory response. Progress of the disease is variable – in most patients there is steady progression.

Myositis

Pain in muscles can follow viral infections, such as influenza, coxsackie, and echoviruses, as well as protozoeal and worm infections. The origin is thought to be due to a myositis.

Tumours

Primary tumours of muscle, such as rhabdomyomas and rhabdomyosarcomas, are uncommon. Stout (1946) reviewed 121 cases of rhabdomyosarcoma and found the peak incidence in middle age, but some cases did occur in the elderly. It is an extremely malignant tumour, presenting as a swelling, usually of muscles in the legs. Prognosis after surgical treatment is variable.

Secondary tumours are clinically rare, although histological studies (Pearson, 1959) suggest that tumour embolization to muscle is more common than previously thought. Tumours most likely to embolize are the carcinomas and lymphomas. Muscles may also be involved by direct extension of carcinomas.

REFERENCES

Anderson, W. F., and Cowan, N. R. (1966). 'Hand grip pressure in older people', *Brit. J. Prev. Soc. Med.*, **20**, 141–147.

Ariansson, A., Granby, G., Rundgren, A., Svanborg, A., and Orlander, J. (1980). 'Physical training in old men', *Age Ageing*, **9**, 186–187.

Asher, R. (1958). 'A woman with the stiff man syndrome', *Br. Med. J.*, **1**, 265–266.

Askari, A., Vignos, P. J., and Moskowitz, R. W. (1976). 'Steroid myopathy in connective tissue disease', *Am. J. Med.*, **61**, 485–492.

Austin, K. L., and Denborough, M. A. (1977). 'Drug therapy of malignant hyperpyrexia', *Anaesth. Intensive Care*, **5**, 207–213.

Bell, W. R., and Klinefelter, H. F. (1967). 'Polymyalgia rheumatica', *Johns Hopkins Med. J.*, **121**, 175–187.

Benditt, E. P., Erikson, N., Hermodsen, M. A., and Ericson, L. H. (1971). 'The major proteins of human and monkey amyloid substance: Common properties including unusual N-terminal amino acid sequences'. *FEBS Lett.*, **19**, 169–173.

Blackwood, W. S., Mandgal, D. P., Pickard, R. G., Laurence, D., and Northfield, T. C. (1976). 'Cimetidine in duodenal ulcer', *Lancet*, **2**, 174–176.

Bohan, A., and Peter, J. B. (1976) 'Dermatomyositis and polymyositis. A review of basic concepts', in *Recent Advances in Rheumatology* (Eds W. W. Buchanan and W. C. Dick), pp. 39–66, Churchill Livingstone, Edinburgh and London.

Bohan, A., Peter, J. B., Bowman, R. L., and Pearson, C. M. (1977). 'A computer assisted analysis

of 153 patients with polymyositis and dermatomyositis', *Medicine*, **56**, 255–286.

Bradley, W. G., Lassman, L. P., Pearce, G. W.,
and Walton J. N. (1970). 'The neuromyopathy of
vincristine in man. Clinical, electrophysiological
and pathological studies'. *J. Neurol. Sci.*, **10**, 107–
131.

Burke, W. E., Tuttle, W. W., Thompson, C. W.,
Janney, C. D., and Weber, R. J. (1953). 'The
relation of grip strength and grip-strength endurance to age'. *J. Appl. Physiol.*, **5**, 628–630.

Campbell, M. J., McComas, A. J., and Petito, F.
(1973). 'Physiological changes in ageing muscles',
J. Neurol. Neurosurg. Psychiatry, **36**, 174–182.

Cohen, D. N., and Smith, T. R. (1974). 'Skip lesions in temporal arteritis: Myth versus fact',
Trans. Am. Acad. Opthalmol. Otolaryngol., **78**,
772.

Cohen, L. (1972). CPK test – effect of intramuscular
injection in myocardial infarction', JAMA, **219**,
625–626.

Corsi, A., Gentili, C., and Todesco C. V. (1965).
'The relationship of menopausal muscular dystrophy to other diseases of muscle. A study of 17
cases', *J. Neurol. Sci.*, **2**, 397–418.

Delbeke, J., Kopec, J., and McComas, A. J. (1978).
'Effect of age, temperature and disease on the
refractoriness of human nerve and muscle', *J.
Neurol. Neurosurg. Psychiatry*, **41**, 65–71.

Denborough, M. A., and Lovell, R. R. H. (1960).
'Anaesthetic deaths in a family', *Lancet*, **2**, 45.

Denham, M. J., Hodkinson, H. M., and Qureshi,
K. N. (1973). 'Loss of grip in the elderly', *Gerontol. Clin. (Basel)*, **15**, 268–271.

De Vere, R., and Bradley, W. G. (1975). 'Polymyositis; Its presentation, morbidity and mortality', *Brain*, **98**, 637–666.

Dixon, A. St. J. (1970). 'Polymyalgia rheymatica
and giant cell arteritis', *Br. Med. J.*, **4**, 235–236.

Dixon, A. St. J., Beardwell, C., Kay, A., Wanka,
J., and Wong, Y. T. (1966). 'Polymyalgia rheumatica and temporal arteritis', *Ann. Rheum. Dis.*,
25, 203–208.

Egan, M. S., Goldenberg, D. L., Cohen, A. S., and
Segal, D. (1982). 'The association of amyloid deposits and osteoarthritis', *Arth. Rheum.*, **25**, 204–
208.

Ellis, M. E., and Ralston, S. (1983). 'The ESR in
the diagnosis and management of the polymyalgia
rheumatica/giant cell arteritis syndrome', *Ann.
Rheum. Dis.*, **42**, 168–170.

Esiri, M. M., MacLennan, I. C. M., and Hazleman,
B. C. (1973). 'Lymphocyte sensitivity to skeletal
muscle in patients with polymyositis and other
diseases', *Clin. Exper. Immunol.*, **14**, 25–35.

Farmer, T. W., Buchthal, F., and Rosenfalck, P.
(1960). 'Refractory period of human muscle after
the passage of a propagated action potential',
Electroencephalogr. Clin. Neurophysiol., **12**, 455–
466.

Fauchald, P., Rygvold, O., and Lystese, B. (1972).
'Temporal arteritis and polymyalgia rheumatica.
Clinical and biopsy findings', *Ann. Intern. Med.*,
77, 845–852.

Forbes, C. B., and Reina, J. C. (1970). 'Adult lean
body mass declining with age: Some longitudinal
observations', *Metabolism*, **19**, 653–663.

Frolkis, V. V., Martynenko, O. A., and Zamostynan, V. P. (1976). 'Ageing of the neuromuscular apparatus', *Gerontology*, **22**, 244–279.

Ghose, K. (1977). 'Lithium salts: Therapeutic and
unwanted effects', *Br. J. Hosp. Med.*, **19**, 578–
583.

Glenner, G. G., Terry, W., Harada, M., Isersky,
C., and Page, D. (1971). 'Amyloid fibril protein;
proof of homology with immunoglobulin light
chain by sequence analyses', *Science*, **172**, 1150–
1151.

Goffin, Y. A., Thoua, Y., and Potvliege, P. R.
(1981). 'Microdeposition of amyloid in the joints',
Ann. Rheum. Dis., **40**, 27–33.

Gordon, E. E., Januszko, D. M., and Kaufman, L.
(1967). 'A critical survey of stiff man syndrome',
Am. J. Med., **42**, 582–599.

Graham, E., Holland, A., Avery, A., Ross Russell,
R. W. (1981). Prognosis in giant cell arteritis. *Br.
Med. J.* **282,** 269–271.

Hall, D. A. (1964). In *Elastolysis and Ageing*, C.
C. Thomas, Springfield.

Hall, D. A. (1968). 'Age changes in the levels in
elastase and its inhibitor in human plasma', *Gerontology*, **14**, 97–108.

Hall, D. A., Middleton, R. S. W., El-Ridi, S. S.,
and Zajac, A. (1980). 'Serum elastase levels following a stroke in elderly subjects', *Gerontology*,
26, 167–173.

Hall, D. A., and Reed, F. B. (1973). 'Protein/po-
lysaccharide relationships in tissues subjected to
repeated stress throughout life. II. The intervertebral disc', *Age Ageing*, **2**, 218–224.

Hall, D. A., and Saxl, H. (1960). 'Human and other
animal cellulose', *Nature*, **187**, 547–550.

Hauser, W. A., Ferguson, R. H., Holley, K. E.,
and Kurland, L. T. (1971). 'Temporal arteritis in
Rochester, Minnesota, 1951 to 1967', *Mayo Clin.
Proc.*, **46**, 597–602.

Hazleman, B., Goldstone, A., and Voak, D.
(1977). 'Association of polymyalgia and giant cell
arteritis with HLA-B8', *Br. Med. J.*, **2**, 989–991.

Healey, L. A., Parker, F., and Wilske, K. R.
(1971). 'Polymyalgia and giant cell arteritis', *Arthritis Rheum.*, **14**, 138–141.

Herishanu, Y., and Rosenberg, P. (1975). 'β blockers and myasthenia gravis', *Ann. Intern. Med.*,
83, 834–835.

Hobbs, J. R. (1973). 'An ABC of amyloid', *Proc.
Roy. Soc. Med.*, **66**, 705–710.

Hodkinson, H. M., and Pomerance, A. (1977). 'The clinical significance of senile cardiac amyloidosis; a prospective clinico-pathological study', *Quart J. Med.*, **46**, 381–387.

Huston, K. A., Hunder, G. G., Lie, J. T., Kennedy, R. H., and Elveback, L. R. (1978). 'Temporal arteritis. A 25 year epidemiologic, clinical and pathologic study', *Ann. Int. Med.*, **88**, 162–167.

Jennekens, F. G. I., Tomlinson, B. E., and Walton, J. N. (1971). 'Histo chemical aspects of five limb muscles in old age. An autopsy study', *J. Neurol. Sci.*, **14**, 259–276.

Jones, J. G., and Hazleman, B. C. (1981). 'Prognosis and management of polymyalgia rheumatica'. *Ann. Rheum. Dis.*, **40**, 1–5.

Judge, T. G., and Cowan, N. R. (1971). 'Dietary potassium intake and grip strength in older people', *Geront. Clin. (Basel)*, **13**, 221–226.

Klein, R. G., Handler, G. G., Stanson, A. W., and Sheps, S. G. (1975). 'Large artery involvement in giant cell (temporal) arteritis', *Ann. Int. Med.*, **83**, 806–812.

Kyle, R. A., and Bayrd, E. D. (1975). 'Amyloidosis; review of 236 cases', *Medicine*, **54**, 271–299.

Lane, R. J. M., and Mastaglia, F. L. (1978). 'Drug induced myopathics in man', *Lancet*, **2**, 562–566.

Levy, R., Isaacs, A., and Hawks, G. (1970). 'Neurophysiological correlates of senile dementia', *Psychol. Med.*, **1**, 40–47.

MacLennan, W. J., Hall, M. R. P., Timothy, J. I., and Robinson, M. (1980). 'Is weakness in old age due to muscle wasting?', *Age Ageing*, **9**, 188–192.

McQuillen, M. P., Gross, M., and Johns, R. J. (1963). 'Chlorpromazine induced weakness in myasthenia gravis', *Arch. Neurol.*, **8**, 286–290.

Mastaglia, F. L., Gardner-Medwin, D., and Hudgson, P. (1971). 'Muscle fibrosis and contractures in a pethidin addict', *Br. Med. J.*, **4**, 532–533.

Medsger, T. A., Dawson, W. N., and Masi, A. T. (1970). 'The epidemiology of polymyositis'. *Am. J. Med.*, **48**, 715–723.

Millikan, C. H., and Haines, G. F. (1953). 'The thyroid gland in relation to neuromuscular disease', *Arch. Intern. Med.*, **92**, 5–39.

Missen, G. A. K., and Taylor, J. D. (1956). 'Amyloidosis in rheumatoid arthritis', *J. Path. and Bact.*, **71**, 179–192.

Mowat, A. G., and Hazleman, B. L. (1974). 'Polymyalgia rheumatica – a clinical study with particular reference to arteral disease', *J. Rheumatol.*, **1**, 190–192.

Mullins, B. R., Levinson, R. E., Friedman, A., Henson, D. R., Winand, R. J., and Kohn, L. D. (1977). 'Delayed hypersensitivity in Graves disease and exophthalmos. Identification of thyroglobulins in normal human orbital muscle', *Endocrinology*, **100**, 351–366.

Newson, A. J. (1972). 'Malignant hyperthermia; three case reports', *N.Z. Med. J.*, **75**, 138–143.

Oh, S. J., and Kim, K. W. (1973). 'Guanidine hydrochloride in the Eaton–Lambert syndrome', *Neurology (Minneap.)*, **23**, 1084–1090.

Ostberg, G. (1971). 'Temporal arteritis in a large necropsy series', *Ann. Rheum. Dis.*, **30**, 224–235.

Palmer, K. N. V. (1978). 'Muscle cramp and oral salbutamol', *Br. Med. J.*, **3**, 833.

Pearson, C. M. (1959). 'The incidence and type of pathologic alterations observed in muscles in a routine autopsy survey', *Neurology (Minneap.)*, **9**, 757–766.

Pirofsky, B., and Bardana, E. J. (1977). 'Immunosuppressive therapy in rheumatic disease', *Med. Clin. North Am.*, **61**, 419–437.

Ravid, M., Shapira, J., Lang, R., and Kedar, I. (1982). 'Prolonged dimethylsulphoxide treatment in 13 patients with systemic amyloid', *Ann. Rheum. Dis.*, **41**, 587–592.

Ridge, M. D., and Wright, V. (1966). 'The ageing of skin'. *Gerontology*, **12**, 174–192.

Saunders, F. P., Hoefnagel, D., and Staples, O. S. (1965). 'Progressive fibrosis of the quadriceps muscles', *J. Bone Joint Surg.*, **47A**, 380–384.

Steiner, J. C., Winkelman, A. C., and De Jesus, P. V. (1973). 'Pentazocine-induced myopathy', *Arch. Neurol.*, **28**, 408–409.

Steiness, E., Rasmussen, F., Svendsen, O., and Nielsen, P. (1978). 'A comparative study of serum creatine phosphokinase (CPK) activity in rabbits, pigs and humans after intra-muscular injection of local damaging drugs', *Acta. Pharmacol. Toxicol. (Copenh.)*, **42**, 357–364.

Stout, A. P. (1946). 'Rhabdomyosarcoma of the skeletal muscles', *Ann. Surg.*, **123**, 447–472.

Tesal, S., and Hall, D. A. (1972). 'The hormonal control of enzymes involved in the age mediated degradation of connective tissue. Report of 9th Internat. Assoc', *Gerontol. Kiev.*, **2**, 58–60.

Tomonaga, M. (1977). 'Histochemical and ultrastructural changes in senile human skeletal muscle', *J. Am. Geriat. Soc.*, **25**, 125–131.

Triger, D. R., and Joekes, A. M. (1973). 'Renal amyloidosis – a fourteen year follow up', *Quart J. Med.*, **165**, 15–40.

Viidik, A. (1967). 'Experimental evaluation of the tensile strength of isolated rabbit tendons', *Biomed. Eng. (NY)*, **2**, 64–67.

Wolff, S., Goldberg, L. S., and Verity, A. (1976). 'Neuromyopathy and periarteriolitis in a patient receiving levadopa', *Arch. Intern. Med.*, **136**, 1055–1057.

Wright, E. A., and McQuillan, M. P. (1971). 'Antibiotic induced neuromuscular blockade', *Ann. N.Y. Acad. Sci.*, **183**, 358–368.

Yaari, Y., Pincus, J. H., and Argov, A. (1977). 'Depression of synaptic transmission by diphenylhydantoin', *Ann. Neurol.*, **1**, 334–338.

25.2

Bone Disorders

P. Courpron, M. Druguet

INTRODUCTION

Bone disorders constitute a heterogeneous group of diseases among which primary osteoporosis and Paget's disease are the most frequently encountered in the elderly. Heterogeneity is illustrated by the fact that these diseases can be clinically silent or dramatic, localized or generalized, malignant or benign, responsible for hyper- or hypocalcaemia, rapid or slow in their evolution, secondary to a well-established aetiology or still considered as idiopathic. Four circumstances lead to the discovery of metabolic bone diseases in clinical practice: pain, fracture, bone deformity and occasional radiography. While some symptoms are very suggestive of precise disease, none is really pathognomonic, so diagnosis will take into account not only clinical information and radiological features but also laboratory findings and very often bone histological data.

Radiological findings roughly allow metabolic bone diseases to be classified into fragilizing bone diseases on the one hand (primary and secondary osteoporoses, lytic metastasis, multiple myeloma, osteomalacia, hyperparathyroidism) and osteosclerotic bone diseases (Paget's disease of bone, sclerotic bone metastasis, fluorosis, renal osteodystrophy) on the other hand. This radiological classification of bone disorders is useful in practice because it anatomically correlates with a localized or generalized decrease of mineralized bone tissue in fragilizing bone diseases and an increase of the amount of bone tissue in osteosclerotic

bone diseases. This chapter will particularly emphasize osteoporosis and Paget's disease, being the most common metabolic disorders of the skeleton in ageing.

PHYSIOLOGICAL OSTEOPENIA AND BONE TISSUE MECHANISMS UNDERLYING BONE LOSS

The skeleton of young people progressively increases its bone mass, whereas that of the adult progressively decreases the capital of bone tissue acquired during growth. 'The term osteopenia is used to designate a loss of absolute bone volume without fracture, whereas osteoporosis will imply the presence of osteopenia in addition to mechanical failure of the skeleton' (Thomson and Frame, 1976). Physiological osteopenia corresponds to a progressive loss of compact and spongy bone tissue with ageing. It is clinically silent. Its radiological appearance includes an increased transparency of the skeleton, no deformation of vertebral bodies, and a progressive cortical thinning (Courpron, 1972; Giroux, Courpron, and Meunier, 1975).

It has been suggested that bone loss begins at 40 or 45 years of age in women (Morgan, 1973a; Morgan and Newton-John, 1969) and between 50 and 60 years of age in men (Beck and Nordin, 1960; Caldwell and Collins, 1961; Morgan et al., 1967; Mueller, Trias, and Ray, 1966) for compact and spongy bone. Arnold et al. (1966) and Courpron (1972) consider that bone loss begins at the end of the growth period. All workers in this field agree that bone loss is more pronounced in females than in males. However, it is difficult to quantify precisely its magnitude because of the variety of techniques used and the many bone sampling sites concerned. The mean percentage of cortical bone loss seems to be 10 per cent. per decade in females and 5 per cent. in males (Morgan, 1973). The major studies indicate a trabecular bone loss of 10 per cent. per decade in females and in males, but some authors found an earlier and a more rapid loss in females (Bartley and Arnold, 1967; Doyle, 1972). Others did not find any loss of spongy bone in males (Dequeker, 1972; Mazess and Cameron, 1973). If histomorphometric studies give the most reliable data (calcified tissue plus osteoid tissue) (Bordier and Tun Chot, 1972; Giroux, Courpron, and Meunier, 1975; Melsen, 1978; and Schenk and Merz, 1969) then males between 20 and 80 years of age have lost approximately 30 per cent. of the iliac spongy bone in an essentially linear fashion. In females, a break occurs in this curve between 50 and 70 years of age because of a more rapid bone loss during this period. At 80 years of age females have lost approximately 40 per cent. of the iliac spongy bone tissue they had at age 20 (Courpron *et al.*, 1973).

The relation between menopause and the accelerated bone loss in females remains unclear. As most studies dealing with bone ageing are cross-sectional, we do not know precisely whether bone loss occurs in every individual or not (it does seem probable), whether the magnitude of osteopenia is the same in absolute value for each individual or not (whatever may be the bone capital acquired during growth), or whether or not the rate of bone loss is constant during life (which is not true in

females, at least after the menopause). Some authors (Courpron, 1972; Newton-John and Morgan, 1968, 1970) claim that bone loss is a universal phenomenon occurring in all individuals. Longitudinal studies have, however, noted differences among individuals (Johnston, 1979). In spite of this persisting lack of precise information, we can accept the fact that human ageing is accompanied by a progressive global loss of compact and spongy bone tissue.

Bone Structure

Compact and spongy bone tissue are composed of elementary morphological units called basic structural units (BSU), which are clearly visible under polarized light (Fig. 1). They look like ellipses or circles in compact bone, according to the plane of section, and correspond to secondary osteons or haversian systems. They appear as arch-like structures in trabecular bone (Fig. 2). In both compact and cancellous bone, BSU represent the final product of the continuous adult bone remodelling by functional bone units (basic multicellular units). Each of these BMU combines in time and space a sequential and stereotyped activity, characterized by the following sequence of events: activation (A), resorption (R), and formation (F). Each BMU cycle is characterized by a certain amount of bone resorbed by osteoclasts and a certain amount of bone newly formed by osteoblasts (Jaworski, 1981).

Bone Formation and Resorption

In adults, the gain or loss of bone tissue is the direct consequence of the cumulative bone balance occurring at the individual BMU level. The direction (positive or negative) and the

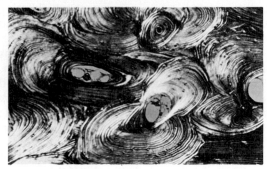

Figure 1   Bone structure units of the cortex

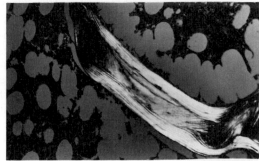

Figure 2   Bone structure units of the spongiosa.

magnitude of changes in the amount of bone tissue will depend on two variables of the BMU system, namely (a) the nature and the value of the imbalance between bone resorption and bone formation at the BMU level and (b) the generation rate of BMU per unit volume of bone tissue. The bone tissue balance at the BMU level differs from one skeletal envelope to another, as follows:

(a) The external diameter of bone increases progressively with age, depending upon the bone sampled. This means that each periosteal BMU is characterized by a lesser quantity of bone resorbed (qR) than formed (qF). Thus, the tissue balance of the periosteal BMU is positive.

(b) Intracortical porosity does not vary much with age (Courpron *et al.*, 1973). This means that in each haversian BMU the quantity of bone resorbed essentially equals the quantity of bone formed. Thus, the tissue balance of the haversian BMU is in equilibrium.

(c) In spongy bone, ageing is characterized by a progressive atrophy and a decrease in the number of trabeculae (Courpron *et al.*, 1973). This means that in the cortico-endosteal and the trabecular endosteal BMU more bone is resorbed than formed. Thus, the tissue balance of the endosteal BMU is negative.

A progressive cortical thinning occurs during ageing because the positive tissue balance on the periosteal envelope does not compensate the negative tissue balance on the endosteal envelope.

In adults, variations in the amount of cortical bone tissue depend upon bone remodelling activity occurring on periosteal, haversian, and subcortical endosteal envelopes; whereas variations in spongy bone mass depend on endosteal BMU activity. By postulating that 'pathological factors' will modify only the birth-rate of BMU by increasing or decreasing it without inducing any modification in the tissue BMU balance that characterizes each skeletal envelope, one can define three possible tissue consequences of such variation of the BMU birth-rate as follows:

(a) A normal generation rate on the three skeletal envelopes is responsible for so-called 'physiological osteopenia'.

(b) An increased BMU generation rate should induce a high bone remodelling state and so accelerate the onset of the physiological osteopenia.

(c) A decreased generation rate should create a low bone remodelling situation and so slow down the physiological osteopenic process. However, other 'pathological factors' may also act independently on the different skeletal envelopes and on other BMU variables (Courpron, 1981).

FRAGILIZING BONE DISEASES – OSTEOPOROSIS

Quantitatively osteoporosis represents a reduced amount of bone tissue as compared with controls of the same age and sex. This quantitative fact leads to mechanical failure of the skeleton that results in the occurrence of fracture with minimal trauma.

Fracture Threshold

Measurements of iliac trabecular bone volume in osteoporotic patients having at least one vertebral collapse have shown that the mean trabecular bone volume is the same in both sexes whatever the aetiology of the osteoporosis (secondary or primary osteoporosis). The mean value was 11 ± 3 per cent (SD). There is a critical amount of iliac spongy bone tissue below which a high risk of vertebral collapse exists, the 'vertebral fracture threshold' (Meunier *et al.*, 1973). It corresponds approximately to a loss of 50 per cent. of the spongy bone observed in controls at 20 years of age. This suggests that a diagnosis of osteoporosis based only on quantitative histologic measurement may be possible even in the absence of vertebral deformation. A comfortable margin separates the physiological osteopenia curve from the fracture threshold in young adults but then decreases progressively with age (Fig. 3) (Courpron *et al.*, 1976). However, there is a wide overlap between trabecular bone values in controls and in osteoporotic women after the age of 50.

Cortical loss can be monitored at the mid-point of the second metacarpal of the right hand on good quality radiographs; medullary and total width are measured with needle calipers and cortical and total cross-sectional areas calculated on the assumption that the bone is tubular. The mean cortical area / total area ratio (CA/TA) in premenopausal women is 0.86 and this falls to 0.60 by the age of 85. The male value falls much less, from 0.82 to 0.74. Here, too, a fracture threshold can be defined corresponding to the lower limit observed in young normal women, and below this the femoral neck fracture incidence rises steeply (Nordin, 1979). After the age of 60, the number of femoral neck fractures double every 5 years in women and every 7 years in men (Alfram, 1964) and are a significant cause of death in the elderly.

The Clinicoradiological Syndrome

Clinical Features

The most frequent symptom is back pain. This may begin suddenly with great intensity and may occur with almost no trauma (bending to tie a shoe or turning over in bed). It is sharp in character, is aggravated by movement and weight bearing, and is improved by bed rest. It reflects an underlying compression fracture of a vertebral body. The twelfth thoracic and first lumbar vertebrae are most often affected.

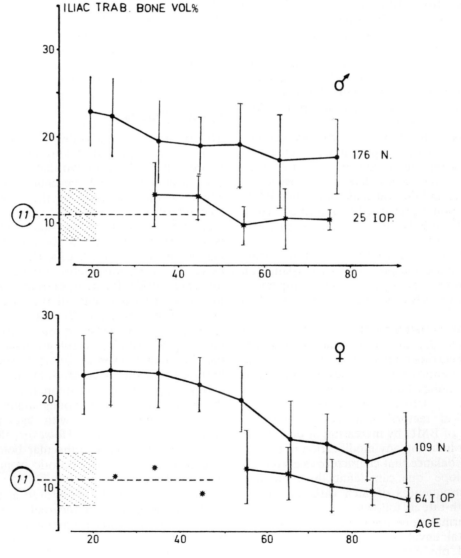

Figure 3   The vertebral fracture threshold (11 per cent.)

The pain usually persists for four to eight weeks and gradually subsides. Residual pain may reflect spasm of the paravertebral muscles. Deformity of the spine may slowly evolve in the absence of back pain, and osteoporosis is frequently discovered as an incidental finding during the examination of a patient for an unrelated complaint. A progressive loss in height occurs as a result of compression of the vertebral bodies. The loss generally ranges from 2 to 20 cm. With progression, recurrent fractures of vertebral bodies result in kyphosis of the dorsal spine, reduction of the lumbar lordosis, and protuberance of the abdomen, producing the typical Dowager's hump deformity (Urist, Gurvey, and Fareed, 1970). Deformity may cause the lower ribs to touch the iliac crests.

Fractures of the femoral neck, distal radius, ribs, and proximal humerus are usually associated with the disease. As for vertebral collapse, they are prone to develop after apparently trivial trauma (a fall from ground level being the most common).

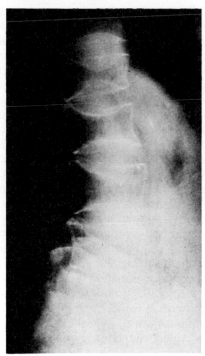

Figure 4   The osteoporotic spine

Radiographic Findings

Several means of quantitating trabecular and cortical bone density, using non-invasive methods, have been proposed to assess osteoporosis. Lateral thoracic and lumbar spine radiographs show typically a loss of transverse trabeculation and an accentuation of the density of the cortex and vertical trabeculae. More characteristic are ballooning of the nuclei pulposi into the vertebral bodies, producing the classical biconcave or so-called 'cod-fish deformity' of British literature, and vertebral collapse which may appear as anterior wedging of the vertebrae or as complete compression. Marked thinning of the cortex is observed on peripheral long bone X-ray. Barzel (1978), points out that the 'practitioner of geriatric medicine should be alert to the fact that there is generally nothing specific and pathognomonic in radiographs in early osteoporosis. The relative decrease in bone or the lesser density of bone should be best described as 'osteopenia'. The loose manner in which the term 'osteoporosis' is used by some radiologists should not mislead the physician to accept it as an accurate diagnosis until the differential diagnosis is fully satisfied. Morphometric measurements of vertebral biconcavity or the degree of anterior wedging of vertebral bodies are of limited value because of difficulty in reproducing the appropriate views of the spine. For the same reason, X-ray densitometric measurements of the spine have been described but not widely used. The most common means of quantitating trabecular bone density is by photon beam absorptiometry of the distal radius (Cameron and Sorenson, 1963). Assessment of cortical bone density has also been made by photon beam absorptiometry of the midshaft of the radius and measurements of cortical thickness of the second metacarpal (Morgan, 1973b). None of these non invasive techniques can be shown to be effective in detecting the early stage of osteoporosis (before the occurrence of vertebral body deformities) in individuals.

Primary Osteoporosis

Primary osteoporosis is also described by such terms as 'senile', 'involutional', 'postmenopausal' (Albright, Smith, and Richardson, 1941), or 'idiopathic' osteoporosis.

Incidence

Clinically, osteoporosis is encountered more frequently in women than in men. It is four times more prevalent in women (Lender *et al.*, 1976). In women the incidence has been reported to be between 3 per cent. at 60 and 20 per cent. at 80 years of age (Gerson-Cohen *et al.*, 1953; Smith and Rizek, 1966; Urist, 1973). It is more frequent in Caucasians and Northern Europeans than in Negroes and peoples from warmer climates.

Laboratory Findings

Serum calcium, serum phosphorus levels, and serum alkaline phosphatase are typically normal. However, the alkaline phosphatase activity may be slightly elevated in patients with acute fractures. Generally the urinary calcium and the urinary hydroxyproline excretion are in the normal range according to age. The urinary phosphorus excretion varies greatly with the dietary phosphorus intake and is therefore not useful. Blood sedimentation rate and plasma electrophoresis are normal. In fact, the diagnosis of primary osteoporosis is basically one of exclusion and more specific laboratory investigations must be done each time that clinical associated symptoms make a particular aetiology possible.

Bone Histology

It is possible to perform a routine iliac bone biopsy under local anaesthesia by using a Bordier trephine without any discomfort to the patient. The classic microscopic examination of such a bone sample shows a thin cortex and atrophy of trabeculae which are less numerous and decreased in their width than in controls. No specific anatomical finding other than a diminished amount of normally mineralized bone tissue seems to exist. However, a histomorphometric analysis of 154 undecalcified transiliac bone samples by Meunier and his coworkers (1972b) has shown an obvious histologic heterogeneity of primary osteoporosis. This osteoporotic population included 106 postmenopausal women and 48 men. Results showed that in 33 per cent. of the cases osteoclastic resorption surfaces were greater (2 SD) than control values; in 21 per cent osteoid sur-

faces were greater (2 SD) than normal; and of 109 cases doubly labelled with tetracycline (Frost, 1969) 21 per cent. showed an abnormally low calcification rate.

In an analysis of these different histological variables, roughly three groups emerge:

(a) The first group includes 30 per cent. of the osteoporotics and is characterized by increased osteoclastic resorption surfaces, increased osteoid surfaces, and normal calcification rates.

(b) The second group includes 20 per cent. of the cases characterized by a normal extent of osteoclastic resorption surfaces, a normal extent of osteoid surfaces, and a decreased calcification rate.

(c) The third group includes approximately 50 per cent. of the cases and does not differ from the control group. It may correspond to the lower fringe of senile physiological osteopenia and may represent only a consequence of bone ageing.

Pathogenesis

Several theories have been proposed to explain the pathogenesis of involutional osteoporosis: mainly hormonal imbalance, dietary factors, and the direct consequence of bone ageing. None is actually proven but one must remember the histological heterogeneity of the disease – one or a combination of causes will eventually explain the disease. A viewpoint is that the amount of bone present at skeletal maturity, before the onset of age-related bone loss, governs the risk of developing clinical osteoporosis (Thomson and Frame, 1976). The universal bone loss which inevitably occurs during and after the menopause may then cause symptomatic osteoporosis in those women who had a reduced bone mass prior to the menopause. Failure to develop a normal skeletal mass during the growth period might result from poor nutrition, severe illness, prolonged immobilization, or genetic influences (Kleerekoper, Talia, and Parfitt, 1981). According to this hypothesis osteoporosis appears to be the clinical expression (pain, fracture, spinal deformity) of age-related bone loss and it recognizes the same bone tissue mechanisms as physiological osteopenia (Courpron, 1981). Other explanations are more biological and not necessarily in disagreement with the one above. The calcium deficiency hypothesis (Nordin, 1961) postulates that a reduced calcium absorption, a diminished calcium intake, or an increased urinary calcium loss will induce a state of secondary hyperparathyroidism (Lutwak, Singer, and Wrist, 1974) to enable the body to maintain serum calcium levels within a normal range, the subsequent elevated parathyroid hormone then, in turn, producing a loss of bone tissue by increasing bone resorption. Tetracycline labelling techniques have shown a decrease in bone remodelling with formation more depressed than resorption in most of the cases (Courpron, 1981; Wu and Frost, 1969). Iliac trabecular bone volume measurements in primary hyperparathyroidism do not demonstrate an associated bone loss in elderly patients (Courpron *et al.*, 1976). The prevalent hormonal factor usually implicated in causing postmenopausal osteoporosis is oestrogen deficiency (Gallagher *et al.*, 1978). Four general observations have suggested the relationship between lack of oestrogens and osteoporosis: the temporal association of osteoporosis and the menopause (Garn, 1970; Johnston *et al.*, 1968); age-related bone loss is greater in women than in men (Garn, 1970); oestrogen deficiency whether abrupt in onset as after bilateral oophorectomy or more gradual in onset as with natural menopause is followed by at least a twofold increase in bone turnover (Heaney *et al.*, 1978b), and osteoporosis is more common in women than in men (Garn, 1970). The mechanism whereby oestrogen deficiency initiates rapid bone loss remains unknown and several theories have been proposed concerning indirect effects of oestrogen deficiency on bone (Kleerekoper, Tolia, and Parfitt, 1981), including an interaction with parathormone, 1–25-dihydroxycholecalciferol, calcitonin, and cortisol secretion.

Treatment

The goals in treating osteoporotic patients are the following: treat fracture and subsequent pains, prevent rapid bone loss following the menopause, induce a positive bone tissue balance in order to add new bone to a higher level than the fracture level.

Colles' fractures are treated with a cast allowing callus formation and bone healing until union is complete. Femoral neck and intertrochanteric fractures are treated with prothesis or nailing followed by early mobilization and adequate physiotherapy. An acute vertebral compression fracture requires complete bed rest until the acute pain subsides and the use of effective analgesics. During this phase of treatment most patients will need stool softeners and laxatives daily and high fluid intake should be encouraged to avoid faecal impaction associated with bed rest. After this period a corset with expanding front and steel ribs is fitted to the patient. Once the patient is able to sit comfortably, walking begins progressively. The corset will serve the patient for approximately 8 weeks, during which time increased activity will be encouraged, and it needs to be worn only when the patient is up. Of available modes of activity swimming in heated pools is probably the best. Lordotic low back pain increased by activity may occur some two months or so post fracture. An intermittent horizontal rest during the day will provide considerable relief in such cases (Frost, 1981). The patient should be taught that recurrent episodes of fractures are the rule and that they are unpredictable but that several years may pass between episodes. The problem of calcium intake and its relationship with bone mass and interaction with sex hormones remains complex and partly understood. It seems that high calcium intake, about 1 to 1.5 g per day, is effective to preserve the skeleton in postmenopausal women. However, calcium supplements alone have not been shown to increase bone mass. Adequate intake of calcium associated or not with oestrogens seems more important as prophylaxis of bone loss than as a treatment for overt osteoporosis (Recker, 1981). Although the present therapeutic programmes proposed to treat osteoporosis may be classified into those that have been shown to inhibit bone resorption (oestrogens, calcium, anabolic steroids, calcitonin) and those that stimulate bone formation (combination of fluoride, vitamin D, calcium) we will discuss here only oestrogens and fluoride because there is no firm evidence for a long-term effect for calcium supplements alone, there is no evidence that androgens are beneficial, and the results obtained with calcitonin have not been encouraging (Thomson and Frame, 1976).

There is wide agreement that age-related bone loss can be inhibited in healthy postmenopausal women by the administration of oestrogens (Aitken, Hart, and Lindsay, 1973; Lindsay *et al.*, 1980; Meema, Bunker, and Meema, 1975; Recker, Saville, and Heaney, 1977). There is some evidence that oestrogen treatment reduces the incidence of lower forearm and hip fractures (Hutchinson, Polansky, and Feinstein, 1979) and the risk of vertebral compression fractures (Lindsay *et al.*, 1980), but the protective effect lasts only as long as the treatment is maintained (Lindsay *et al.*, 1978) and there is no reliable method of screening the healthy population for detection of those at risk of osteoporosis (Recker, 1981). The usefulness of oestrogen treatment for symptomatic osteoporosis is not so obvious. Oestrogen risks include that of endometrial carcinoma which seems however to be low at the doses known to be effective in preserving bone (Smith *et al.*, 1975; Weiss and Sayvetz, 1980). Cases where oestrogens are contraindicated are those with ischaemic heart disease, hypertension, history of thromboembolism or breast cancer (Exton-Smith, Hodkinson, and Stanton, 1966). The lowest dose known to be effective in preventing bone loss in post-menopausal women is 0.625 m per day of conjugated equine oestrogens or its equivalent (Recker, Saville, and Heaney, 1977) given 3 weeks each month, possibly combined with a progestagen in the third week to ensure adequate shedding of the endometrial mucosa (Nordin, 1979). The type of oestrogen used does not seem to matter (Heaney, Recker, and Saville, 1978a; Nordin *et al.*, 1980; Recker, Saville, and Heaney, 1977). Nordin and coworkers (1980) have used 1αOHD$_3$ in conjunction with oestrogens in patients with post menopausal osteoporosis and have demonstrated inhibition of bone loss, decrease in fractures, and, perhaps, a small gain in bone mass.

Introduced 20 years ago (Rich and Ensink, 1961) fluoride therapy has been shown to be effective in osteoporosis by inducing new bone formation. In his most recent report, Meunier and his colleague (Briançon and Meunier, 1981) have shown a positive response with increased trabecular bone volume in 66 per cent. of the treated patients and restored bone mass in 35 per cent. by thickening the trabeculae after 2 years of therapy. The histological changes were very similar to those observed previously in osteoporotic patients following long-term treatment with sodium fluoride. The dose administered was 50 mg per day of sodium fluoride (25 mg twice a day), given orally 1 hour before meals to improve drug absorption, in the form of a gastric acid resistant capsule to minimize gastric irritation – it was taken alone for 1 month and subsequently associated with 800 IU per day of vitamin D$_2$ and 1 gm of elemental calcium. To prevent any malabsorption resulting from CaF$_2$ formation, calcium was given at least 3 hours before or after sodium fluoride. Side effects may occur in patients treated, including gastric discomfort and articular pains.

Secondary Osteoporosis

Corticosteroid-Induced Osteoporosis

Prolonged corticosteroid therapy (as well as Cushing's disease) very often induces osteoporosis (Bressot *et al.*, 1976). Morphologically, the periosteal diameter of such bones remains normal, the marrow cavity enlarges (that is a marked cortical thinning is observed), the cortex exhibits essentially normal intracortical porosity, and spongy bone mass decreases, often dramatically. The bone loss that characterizes this condition occurs primarily on the endosteal envelope. Biologically, the serum calcium level is moderately decreased, serum phosphorus and alkaline phosphatase levels are generally normal, calciuria is often normal and sometimes increased, and urinary excretion of hydroxyproline is in the normal range. Histologically, an increase in the bone resorption surface has been observed (Frost, 1973), contrasting with a decrease in the appositional rate (Bressot *et al.*, 1976). The mean level of serum immunoreactive parathyroid hormone has been found elevated, in direct relationship with the daily steroid dose (Bressot *et al.*, 1979). Thus, hyperparathyroidism seems to exist, possibly secondary to a decreased intestinal calcium absorption, itself secondary to the chronic corticosteroid therapy. Furthermore, a direct antianabolic effect of the steroid glucocorticoids on bone formation would enhance the endosteal BMU bone balance deficit. If steroid therapy cannot be stopped, vitamin D$_2$ or one of its metabolites have been proposed in order to increase intestinal calcium absorption and so to prevent secondary hyperparathyroidism (Klein *et al.*, 1977).

Osteoporosis Associated with Hyperthyroidism

This is not very frequent. Hyperthyroidism can generally be easily diagnosed from clinical features and with the use of appropriate laboratory studies. However, asymptomatic hyperthyroidism is more common in the ageing population and must be systematically suspected. Vertebral signs are very similar to those observed in idiopathic osteoporosis. The metacarpal index (combined cortical thickness/ total metacarpal width) is decreased among older hyperthyroid patients and more frequently in women than in men (Smith, Fraser, and Alilson, 1973). Microradioscopic examination of the fine structures of metacarpal bones has disclosed an abnormal intracortical striation in hyperthyroid patients (Meema and Meema, 1972; Meema and Schatz, 1970). Serum calcium and phosphorus are usually normal, but a mild hypercalcaemia and an increased calciuria are not rare. The serum concentration of alkaline phosphatase and the urinary excretion of hydroxyproline are generally increased. Bone histology shows a high level of bone remodelling embracing increased cortical porosity, an increase of resorption of osteoid surfaces, a normal or accelerated calcification rate, and a decreased trabecular bone volume in the iliac crest (Melsen and Mosekilde, 1977; Meunier *et al.*, 1972a; Mosekilde, 1979). The severity of thyrotoxicosis does not seem to correlate with the decrease of trabecular bone volume, but there does seem to be a correlation with its duration.

Static and dynamic histomorphometric studies suggest that the causative bone tissue mechanisms include an increased generation-rate of BMU on the haversian and endosteal envelopes and a uniform decrease of the formative and resorptive phase of remodelling units (Courpron, 1981).

Osteoporosis Secondary to Immobilization

Osteoporosis secondary to immobilization or so-called disuse osteoporosis may be localized to a single part of the skeleton as in plaster casting or more generalized as seen in the para-

plegic or the quadriplegic patient. Localized osteoporosis is often associated with hemiplegia, fractures, and severe arthritis and prolonged bed-rest may lead to generalized osteoporosis. The radiographic appearance of this osteoporosis has been described as diffuse osteoporosis, spotty osteoporsis, and linear radiolucent cortical bands (Louis, 1976). The excessive release of calcium from bones leads to increased urinary calcium and hydroxyproline excretion and frequently to stone formation. While numerous radiodensitometric and biological studies have been made about disuse osteoporosis, histological studies are scarce. Bone biopsies reveal an increase in osteoclastic bone resorption and reduced osteoblastic bone formation (Minaire *et al.*, 1974). The lack of muscular activity in an unknown manner produces the localized bone loss. Therefore, mobilizing the immobilized patient as soon as possible is the only logical treatment.

Miscellaneous

Osteoporosis has been reported in many other pathological conditions such as: diabetes mellitus, chronic heparin therapy, systemic mastocytosis, rheumatoid arthritis, liver disease and prolonged intake of aluminium containing antacids, use of loop diuretics, and cigarette smoking.

OTHER FRAGILIZING BONE DISEASES

Osteomalacia

Aetiology

One of the most important conditions to be differentiated from osteoporosis is osteomalacia. It is characterized by an excess of unmineralized bone resulting from an impairment of bone mineralization. Vitamin D deficiency is responsible for the lack of mineralization of bone collagen elaborated by osteoblasts in most cases. Systematic use of bone biopsy has shown unsuspected osteomalacia in many patients with femoral neck fractures (Aaron, Gallagher, and Anderson, 1974). A pronounced and prolonged vitamin D deficiency is necessary to develop clinical and radiological osteomalacia. In most cases subclinical evidence of hypovitaminaemia is demonstrated by blood vitamin assays, biochemical changes in calcium and phosphorus metabolism, or bone histology. A variety of causes and mechanisms is responsible for this lack of vitamin D. Inadequate ultraviolet light exposure resulting in defective photosynthesis secondary to confinement indoors, dietary vitamin D lack, and malabsorption predominate in the elderly (Frame and Parfitt, 1978). Malabsorption of cholecalciferol may occur in many digestive tract diseases, particularly adult coeliac disease; it is also a sequela of gastrectomy, exocrine pancreatic insufficiency, chronic biliary obstruction, and indeed all other causes of steathorrhea. Disorders in hepatic 25-hydroxylation may be due to hepatic cirrhosis or to drug enzymatic induction, as seen in anticonvulsant osteomalacia. Osteomalacia is found in renal osteodystrophy as a consequence of disorders in renal 1–25-hydroxylation due to reduced renal tissue, impaired stimulation, or inhibition of l-α-hydroxylase. Patients on long-term anticonvulsant therapy may develop osteomalacia (Hahn, 1975).

Metabolism of Vitamin D

Vitamin D_3 can be produced in the skin from 7-dehydrocholesterol under the influence of ultraviolet light or ingested in the diet. It accumulates very rapidly in the liver where it undergoes 25-hydroxylation, yielding 25-OH-D_3 (the major circulating metabolite of the vitamin). This proceeds to the kidney where it undergoes one of two hydroxylations. If there is a biological need for calcium or for phosphate the kidney is stimulated to convert 25-OH-D_3 to the 1,25-$(OH)_2$-D_3, a calcium-phosphate-mobilizing hormone. If, however, supplies of calcium and phosphate are sufficient, the l-hydroxylase is shut down and instead the 25-OH-D_3 is converted to a 24,25-$(OH)_2$-D_3, the role of which remains unknown; it may be an intermediate in the inactivation–excretion mechanism. 1,25-$(OH)_2$-D_3 proceeds to the intestine where it stimulates intestinal calcium and phosphate transport (DeLuca, 1976).

Vitamin D_2, irradiated ergosterol, a synthetic form of vitamin D, appears to be metabolized in the same manner as the natural vitamin D_3 and has the same biological effects.

Clinical Manifestations

Bone pain is the most common symptom of osteomalacia. It is made worse by muscle strain, weight bearing, or pressure. A limp may result from pains in the pelvis and lower extremities. However, skeletal pains are often vague and ill defined. In patients with severe osteomalacia of long duration, abnormal spinal curvature, a bell-shaped thorax, or pelvic deformity may develop due to softening of the bones. Occasionally spinal deformity with kyphosis and decreased height may occur with relatively little skeletal pain. Proximal muscle weakness in the lower extremities may lead to a waddling gait similar to that seen in muscular dystrophy or a proximal myopathy (Schott and Wills, 1976). Occasionally, hypocalcaemia is present in such a degree that paraesthesias, muscle cramps, and frank tetany may occur.

Radiographic Features

The radiological features of osteomalacia to a great extent mimic those of osteoporosis (Mankin, 1974). A decrease in radiodensity with thinning of the cortex is indistinguishable from that found in osteoporosis. In some cases the trabecular pattern is coarsened, whereas in others it is replaced by a homogeneous ground-glass appearance. Paradoxically, osteosclerosis (especially of the spine) may occur, but is more often manifest during the healing phase of the disease. In some patients radiographic evidence of secondary hyperparathyroidism, due to hypocalcaemia, may be manifested by subperiosteal resorption of the phalanges or bone cysts. The most distinctive radiographic feature of osteomalacia is the occurrence of symmetrical radiolucent bands, adjacent and usually perpendicular to the periosteal surface in ribs, pubic rami, outer borders of the scapulae, in the shafts of long bones, in clavicles, and bones of feet and hands (Parfitt and Duncan, 1975). They are known as Looser's zones or Milkman fractures (Fig. 5) and represent stress fractures in which the normal process of healing is impaired by the mineralization defect. Looser's zones may progress to complete fractures. The fractures and pseudo-fractures of osteomalacia usually show increased uptake of bone-seeking isotopes with external scanning (McFarlane, Lutkin, and Burwood, 1977).

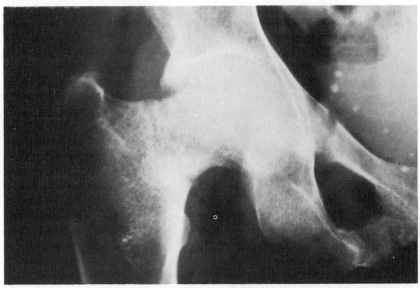

Figure 5   Milkman fractures of the hip

Clinical Biochemistry

The biochemical changes may depend on the cause of osteomalacia. In conditions leading to vitamin D deficiency alkaline phosphatase is usually increased, sometimes to a high level, but occasionally is normal; urinary calcium excretion is low; and in severe cases blood phosphorus and blood calcium levels may fall. 25-Hydroxyvitamin D_3 serum levels can be obtained using a variety of methods, but establishing normal ranges is difficult because of seasonal variations (Stryd, Gilbertson, and Brunden, 1979).

Bone Histology

The criteria used to confirm the diagnosis of osteomalacia on an undecalcified bone sample are both an excess of unmineralized osteoid and a decrease in the rate of bone mineralization, as determined by double labelling of bone tissue with tetracycline – the increase in osteoid is reflected by the greater extent of osteoid seams, the increase of osteoid volume, and an increased width of the seams.

Treatment

Prevention of vitamin D deficiency can be accomplished through dietary means by providing a recommended intake of 100 IU (2.5 μg) daily. In patients with established bone disease, these doses would be adequate to produce full healing. However, to hasten the clinical course towards more rapid recovery, two-to tenfold higher doses have been given. Adequate dietary calcium and phosphorus intake must also be maintained to optimize the healing process. The treatment of vitamin D malabsorption is dependent upon the ability of the physician to correct the underlying disease and in some patients parenteral vitamin D administration may be necessary. Prophylactic administration of vitamin D_2 has been reported to prevent or reduce the severity of anticonvulsant-induced bone disease – doses of 3,000 units or greater per week have been used.

Primary Hyperparathyroidism

The disease is prominent in postmenopausal women (Muller, 1969) and is not rare in the elderly. Signs and symptoms associated with hyperparathyroidism are the following: systemic (fatigue, weakness, malaise), musculoskeletal (bone pain, arthralgia, joint effusion, myalgia, muscle weakness), genitourinary (polyuria, nocturia, renal colic), neuropsychiatric (impaired concentration, lethargy, confusion, depression, coma), gastrointestinal (anorexia, nausea, vomiting, polydipsia). Chondrocalcinosis is found in 50 per cent. of the cases (Menkes *et al.*, 1980). The biochemical findings include hypercalcaemia, decreased serum phosphate concentration, hypercalciuria, and elevated clearance of phosphorus. The radioimmunoassay of parathyroid hormone has significantly simplified the diagnosis. Radiological features are those of subperiosteal bone resorption, a loss of bone density of the skull which gives a 'salt and

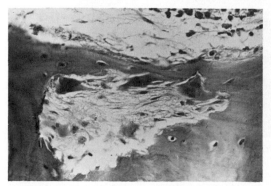

Figure 6   Osteoclasts and fibrovascular marrow in primary hyperparathyroidism

pepper' appearance, and occasionally a generalized osteopenia or solitary lesions of variable size corresponding to brown tumours or cysts. Bone histology shows characteristically an increased number of osteoclasts, a dense fibrovascular marrow with numerous fibroblasts, and an osteocytic osteolysis (Meunier *et al.*, 1972a) (Fig. 6). Even in the elderly treatment of primary hyperparathyroidism is surgical.

Multiple Myeloma

Multiple myeloma (synonyms = plasma cell myeloma, myelomatosis, Kahler's disease) represents the commonest primary malignant disorder affecting the skeleton in the elderly. In its classic and advanced stage, myelomatosis is often accompanied by severe and persistent bone pains, anorexia, weight loss, anaemia, and less often by a pathological fracture or even paraplegia. While punched-out radiolucent skull lesions are considered characteristic of the disease (Fig. 7), osteoporosis may be the only radiological manifestation. Multiple

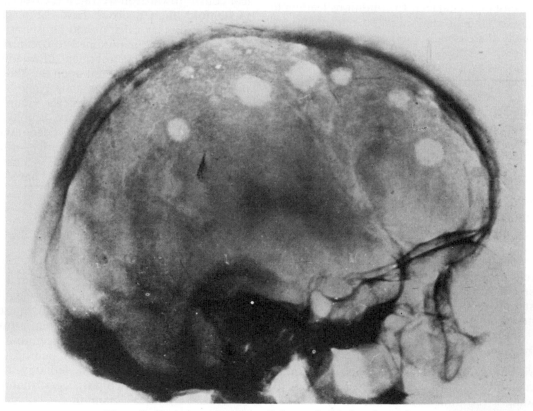

Figure 7   Typical punched-out radiolucent skull lesions in myeloma

myeloma must be ruled out in every case of osteoporosis. Diagnosis and treatment are discussed in Chapter 12.

Neoplastic Bone Disease (Fig. 8)

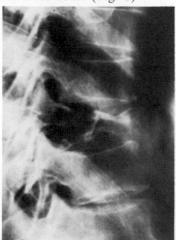

Figure 8   Metastatic osteolytic bone lesion secondary to a carcinoma of the kidney

Osteoporosis must be differentiated from metastatic osteolytic bone diseases, a common finding in the elderly, because the only objective manifestation in such cases may be radiographic evidence of osteoporosis. However, the discovery of osteolytic bone lesion is very suggestive of malignancy. A search for a primary neoplastic lesion, such as a carcinoma of the breast, kidney, lung, thyroid, female genitalia, and less often of the intestinal tract, should be made. In such cases hypercalcaemia may be indicative of a neoplastic process associated with permanent pains and weight loss – tumour cells in bone marrow aspirates or bone biopsy may reveal the correct diagnosis.

OSTEOSCLEROTIC BONE DISEASES

Even in the elderly, cortical and cancellous bone tissue is subjected to permanent remodelling due to the destructive activity of osteoclasts followed by the constructive activity of osteoblasts. Physiological bone tissue balance resulting from these two antagonistic activities is negative and leads to senile osteopenia. Contrariwise, when bone tissue balance is positive because of bone formation exceeding osteoclastic resorption, thickening of cortices may appear and trabecular bone volume may in-

crease, leading to an osteosclerotic condition. We will consider only diffuse bone sclerosis and we will not discuss here localized change. Paget's disease of bone and metastatic prostatic carcinoma is the main diagnosis to be discussed for the elderly.

Paget's Disease of Bone (osteitis deformans)

The disease was first described by Sir James Paget in 1877 (Paget, 1877). It is characterized by pain, deformity, and sometimes fracture of involved bones. The characteristic radiological findings include enlargement and sclerosis of pathological bones. Serum alkaline phosphatase level and urinary level of hydroxyproline are increased, both attesting a high bone remodelling state clearly visible on bone biopsies. This disease is rare before the age of 30. Its prevalence was found to be 3 to 3.7 per cent. over the age of 40 years (Pygott, 1957), but as high as 11 per cent. in women over the age of 85 years. The mean age of affected patients varies from 65 to 70 years of age. Men are more commonly found to have Paget's disease than women, the ratio being 4:3 Ultrastructural studies have revealed nuclear inclusions in osteoclasts very similar to those in various viral diseases and, therefore, a viral aetiology has been considered (Rebel *et al.*, 1976).

Symptomatology

Symptoms and complications in Paget's disease may arise from bone pain, deformity or fracture of involved bones, a change in the temperature of skin overlying the involved bones, compression of neural structures, alteration of joint structure and function, and as a consequence of increased vascularity or shunting (Krane, 1977). However, a significant proportion of patients are diagnosed because of an incidental radiological examination or blood chemistry screening.

Pain is the most common presenting complaint. It is, however, absent in approximately 50 per cent. of the patients. Bone pain is usually of mild to moderate degree but permanent. It is localized to the involved bone and may be worsened by weight-bearing. Joint pains are mainly localized to hip and knee joints. Nerve compression may produce excruciating pain in the lower extremities. The skeletal deformities are characterized by both abnormal shape and increase in size of the affected bones. In the lower extremities the force of weight-bearing leads to progressive lateral bowing of long bones. The skull may be enlarged but the face is usually not involved. The spine may sink and seems to be shorter with greatly increased dorsal and lumbar curves. The pelvis may become wide. The disease may involve a single bone (monostotic) or many bones (polyostotic).

There is a characteristic increase in skin temperature over affected extremity bones in many patients due to an increase in blood flow (Heistad *et al.*, 1975).

Radiological and Scintigraphic Findings

The earliest manifestation of Paget's disease is a localized osteolytic lesion. When the osteolytic phase involves the skull, it is termed osteoporosis circumscripta. It usually begins in the frontal or occipital areas and may spread to involve the entire calvarium. Pagetic involvement of a long bone is usually initially manifest radiographically as a V-shaped resorption front beginning at one end of the bone. The speed of this process has been considered to be 8 to 20 mm per year and the evolution of osteolytic lesions to the late osteosclerotic phase may take many years. In the skull, a patchy increase in bone density is frequent (Fig. 9) and has been termed a 'cotton

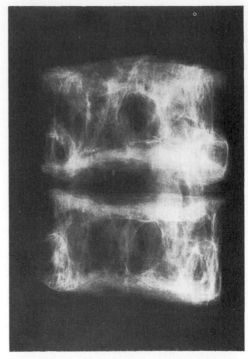

Figure 10 Paget's disease of the vertebral bodies – the 'picture frame' appearance

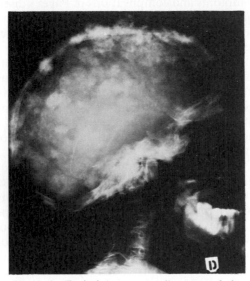

Figure 9   Typical 'cotton wool' aspect of the skull in Paget's disease

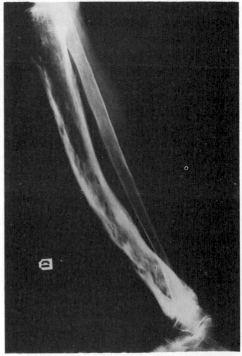

Figure 11   Paget's disease of the tibia

wool' shadowing. This appearance is quite unique for this disease. In far-advanced disease platybasia or basilar invagination may occur. Paget's disease may produce enlargement of the body of a single involved vertebra (Corcoran and Reeder, 1977), and osteosclerotic lesions may result in a 'picture frame' appearance (Fig. 10). A thickening of the pelvic brim is very characteristic. Involvement of the bones adjacent to the hip joint may result in protrusio acetabuli. In long bones thickening of the cortex and a coarsened trabecular pattern of the epiphysis are typical features (Fig. 11). Incomplete fractures, also termed fissure fractures, may occur at areas of tension, characteristically on the convex border of the bone. Bone scans employing a variety of radiotracers, such as technetium diphosphonate, have proved to be useful in the early diagnosis of the disease and in the evaluation of its extent and of its activity (Waxman *et al.*, 1977) (Fig. 12). The most recent scintigraphic study (Salson, 1981) has demonstrated that the decreasing frequency with which various bones are involved by the pagetic process is the following – pelvis, lumbar spine, femur, dorsal spine, sacrum, skull, tibia, humerus, scapula, ribs, sternum, facial bones, calcaneus, metacarpal bones, foot. The disease is never seen to affect the entire skeleton and usually affects a segment of the bone.

Clinical Biochemistry

The hyperactivity of bone remodelling is reflected by the elevation of the serum alkaline phosphatase and of the urinary hydroxyproline. Alkaline phosphatase is considered as an index of osteoblastic activity. It is usually considerably elevated in patients with Paget's dis-

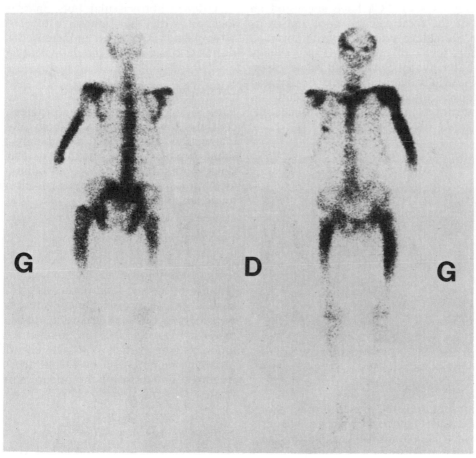

Figure 12 Bone scintigraphy in a polyostotic Paget's disease

ease. It tends to increase with time but often shows fluctuation with a periodicity of months to years. Osteoclastic activity is conventionally monitored utilizing urinary levels of hydroxyproline, a non-essential amino acid found in the body almost exclusively in collagen. While the urinary excretion of hydroxyproline on a low gelatin diet is less than 50 mg per day, daily excretion in Paget's disease may be elevated to more than 2,000 mg. The level correlates with the extent of the disease and its activity. Serum alkaline phosphatase and urinary hydroxyproline levels tend to be closely correlated. In monostotic disease involving a small bone such as a clavicle or in the burned-out phase of the disease, the level of these parameters may be normal. The serum calcium concentration and urinary calcium excretion are almost always normal (Nagant de Deuxchaisnes and Krane, 1964); calciuria is variable. Calcium kinetics studies utilizing the radiotracers ^{45}Ca or ^{47}Ca have suggested an increase of the total calcium pool and of its turnover. Serial levels of parathyroid hormone and urinary levels of cyclic AMP are usually normal but may be elevated in some cases. Serum uric acid concentration may be elevated with extensive disease, perhaps reflecting increased turnover in the numerous bone cells (Franck *et al.*, 1974).

Bone Histology (Fig. 13)

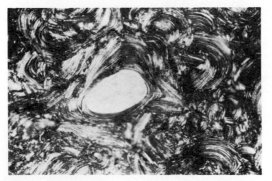

Figure 13   The mosaic aspect of bone histology in Paget's disease

One major feature is the presence of an excessive bone tissue balance with increased remodelling which is responsible for the abnormal architecture and pattern of bone tissue. A net accretion of bone occurs on both the periosteal and endosteal surfaces, leading to an increase in both the transverse diameter and cortical thickness of bone and to a loss of corticomedullary differentiation. The lamellar bone which is characteristically deposited in a 'mosaic' pattern nevertheless appears to undergo mineralization normally, and double labelling of the calcification front with tetracycline often reveals an increased rate of bone formation. The trabecular bone volume is largely increased. Under polarized light the anarchic orientation of collagen fibres leads to an appearance of 'woven bone'. These abnormalities denote that the Pagetic bone, although densified, has lost a part of its elastic properties.

The number of osteoclasts per square millimetre of bone surface is greater than normal. These cells are large and multinucleated and they may contain up to 100 nuclei per cell. The number of osteoblasts is also increased.

A dense fibrovascular bone marrow is associated with the intense osteoclastic and osteoblastic activity and an increased vascularization is observed on the periosteal envelope.

Evolution and Complications

Paget's disease is very slow in progress. It may continue for many years without any consequence on general health and may give no other trouble than those due to changes in shape and size of the involved bones. It may lead, however, to a variety of local and systemic complications.

Pathological Fractures

Pathological fractures of the vertebral bodies, femur, and tibia are not uncommon. Complete fracture of a long bone occurs as a transverse chalk-stick fracture. Healing of these fractures is usually good, but according to the study made by Dove (1980) the incidence of non-union may be as high as 40 per cent. the main problems being posed by the subtrochanteric fractures and those of the upper shaft of the femur.

Sarcomatous Degeneration

A variety of osseous neoplasms have been recognized as complications of Paget's disease.

They have been classified as osteosarcomas, chondrosarcomas, fibrosarcomas, and benign or malignant giant cell tumours. The bones most commonly affected by sarcomatous degeneration are the femur, humerus, skull, pelvis, and tibia (Singer, 1977a). Sarcoma has been estimated to develop in 0.9 to 2 per cent. of larger series of patients. Presenting symptoms of degeneration include localized intense and permanent pain, rapid swelling, pathological fracture associated with fever, and a marked acceleration of the ESR. X-rays may show an osteolytic zone with rupture of the cortex and involvement of soft tissues. Diagnosis is usually confirmed by local bone biopsy. Sarcomas are notoriously resistant to therapy, with only transient palliation from radiotherapy. Metastatic development is usual and death occurs in a few months.

Neurological Complications

Neurological complications may arise by several mechanisms such as pressure exerted by pathological bones along the neuroaxis, changes in the weight-bearing ability of bones, local invasion by areas of neoplastic degeneration, and vascular insufficiency of neural structures (Schmidek, 1977). Compressive phenomena may result in cranial nerve dysfunction. Weakening of bone at the base of the skull permits the skull to sag on the vertebrae, the odontoid process projects through the foramen magnum, producing pressure at the cervicomedullary junction as well as compression of posterior fossa structures. Obstructive hydrocephalus as well as brain stem and cerebellar dysfunction may result. Pagetic involvement of the vertebral column may result in spinal cord compression by bone enlargement. Involvement of the thoracic spine most often produces symptoms as the vertebral canal is narrowest in that portion. Spinal involvement may also produce nerve root compression by encroachment on intervertebral foramina.

Hearing Loss

In approximately 30 to 50 per cent. of patients with Paget's disease involving the skull, loss of auditory acuity is present. This hearing loss is most often mixed in nature with both sensorineural and conductive deficit.

High-Output Congestive Heart Failure

High cardiac output states may occur when 35 per cent. or more of the skeleton is involved. Haemodynamic studies suggest that this results from functional arteriovenous communications (Howarth, 1953). This could contribute to the development of congestive heart failure and myocardial infarction, particularly in the elderly. Blood flow through the external carotid system was found to be much greater than normal in patients with involvement of the skull. This may shunt blood away from the brain – a so-called Pagetic steal syndrome.

Treatment

It is important for the treating physician to keep in mind that in most patients with Paget's disease no treatment is indicated and that some pains are due to osteoarthritis of a joint of an involved extremity. Large doses of aspirin, 4 to 5 g per day, have been suggested as a therapeutic measure. During the past decade two drugs of choice in long-term therapy have been proposed – calcitonin and diphosphonates.

Calcitonin. This is a hormone elaborated by the medullary cells of the thyroid, and has been found empirically to be useful in the treatment of Paget's disease (Bijvoet and Jansen, 1967). Porcine salmon and human calcitonins have been administered in a wide variety of dosage regimens (Singer, 1977b) – the immediate effect is a decrease in bone resorption (Singer, Melvin, and Mills, 1976), followed on long-term administration by a decrease in bone formation. Calcitonin is generally administered subcutaneously at a dose of 50 to 100 MRC units daily for 3 to 5 weeks during the initial phase of the treatment and 3 times a week during the following months. Chronic treatment results in an average reduction of 50 per cent. of both serum alkaline phosphatase and urinary hydroxyproline within the first 3 to 6 months of therapy. Cessation of therapy is followed by reactivation of the Pagetic process in a few weeks or months. Symptomatic relief of bone pain attributable to direct Pagetic involvement has been achieved in most treated patients. Improvement in congestive heart failure may result in part from decreased skeletal blood flow and in part from a natriuretic effect of calcitonin. A variety of neurologic deficits along the neuraxis may decrease with therapy. However, the leading indication for treatment with calcitonin is bone pain – it has not been determined what the optimal duration of treatment should be. Side-effects include transient nausea and vomiting, flushing of the hands and face – they are generally not severe enough to cause discontinuation of the therapy.

Diphosphonates. The diphosphonates are analogues of pyrophosphate (POP) and constitute a class of compounds that inhibits both bone resorption and formation (Russell and Fleisch, 1975). Disodium etidronate (disodium salt of (1-hydroxyethylidene) diphosphonic acid) referred to in the literature as EHDP has been approved for the treatment of Paget's disease. It acts primarily on bone – it can modify the crystal growth of calcium hydroxyapatite by chemisorption onto the crystal surface. Histological examination of bone from Pagetic patients on EHDP therapy shows a reduction in the excessive cellular activity accompanied by a suppression of bone resorption and accretion and a return towards normal histological patterns. Unfortunately, high doses induce a mineralization defect which may lead to pathological fractures (Khairi *et al.*, 1977). For this reason the recommended dose of EHDP is 5 mg/kg body weight per day given orally for a period of 6 months. In the treated patients, the elevated urinary hydroxyproline and serum alkaline phosphatase decrease by 30 per cent. or more in about 4 out of 5 patients. These actions usually occur after 1 to 3 months of medication and a prolonged suppression of biochemical parameters is common after stopping treatment. In controlled studies, approximately 3 out of 5 patients experienced decreased pain and improved mobility. Retreatment should be undertaken only after a drug-free period of at least 3 months and after it is evident that reactivation of the disease has occurred.

Mithramycin. This drug has been administered intravenously at a dose of 15 to 50 μg/kg body weight, utilizing a variety of treatment schedules (Lebbin, Ryan, and Schwartz, 1974). Marked suppression of the activity of the disease as well as relief of bone pain has been reported. However, side-effects and toxicity are frequent, particularly nausea and vomiting, platelet abnormality leading to haemorrhage, malaise, elevation of liver enzymes. The availability of calcitonin and disodium etidronate make it unlikely that mithramycin will be a commonly used drug in the future.

Other Osteosclerotic Bone Diseases

Metastatic Bone Diseases

Metastatic bone diseases, frequently encountered in the elderly, may lead to sclerotic bone lesions. The radiological densification of involved bones is secondary to a stimulation of osteoblast synthesis by malignant cells, leading to a positive bone tissue balance and consequently to an increase in the amount of bone. In such cases pains are usually permanent and more severe during the night. They are ill improved by bed-rest or by usual analgesics. Anorexia, weight loss, anaemia, and neurological symptoms such as neuralgia or progressive paraplegia are commonly associated with pain. The most frequent primary neoplastic lesion is prostatic carcinoma, whereas carcinoma of the breast, intestinal tract, lung, kidney, thyroid, or ovary usually cause osteolytic or mixed lesions.

Radiologically, the initial picture is characterized by nodular opacities. Then a whole bone, such as a vertebral body, may be involved, leading to the typical 'ivory' vertebrae (Fig. 14). The shape and size of involved bones are not modified and this is an important radiological feature in discussing the differential diagnosis with Paget's disease of bone in which involved bones are enlarged. A biological profile similar to the one observed in typical osteomalacia is sometimes observed. Commonly calcium and phosphorus serum levels are normal and serum level of alkaline phosphatase is increased. Discovery of tumour cells in iliac bone biopsy or bone marrow aspirate may confirm the diagnosis.

Diseases of the Haemopoietic Tissue

These disorders may be associated with bone sclerosis. An example is primitive myelofibrosis in which osteosclerosis is due to secondary ossification of the medullary fibrosis. This osteopathy is usually asymptomatic. Radi-

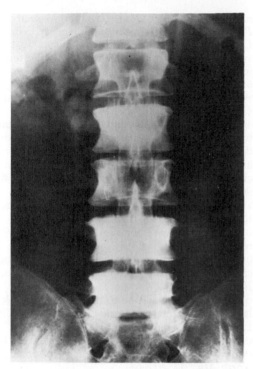

Figure 14   Sclerotic bone metastasis secondary to prostatic carcinoma – the 'ivory vertebrae'

ographic findings are characterized by the prevalence of sclerotic lesions in haemopoietic bones. Bone morphology is not modified but in some cases periostosis is observed at the internal edge of the femoral diaphysis and at the external and proximal part of the tibia. Bone sclerosis has rarely been described associated with Hodgkin's disease and myeloma.

Endocrine and Metabolic Diseases

These may lead to osteosclerosis.

Chronic Renal Failure

Chronic renal failure is a classical aetiological factor in osteosclerosis (Avioli, 1978). Its pathogenesis includes osteomalacia and secondary hyperparathyroidism. Bone pain and muscle weakness are prominent clinical features. Serum calcium concentration may be low, serum phosphorus is amost always elevated, and alkaline phosphatase activity is often elevated. Radiologically, osteosclerosis is a common finding, most often seen in the spine.

The 'rugger jersey' spine is characterized by sclerosis of the inferior and superior portions of the vertebral bodies. Sclerosis may also be found in the skull and long bones.

Primary Hyperparathyroidism and Osteomalacia

These disorders may sometimes be responsible for osteosclerotic lesions.

Fluorosis

Fluorosis is typically a generalized sclerotic bone disease. While rare in the elderly it is described here because of the present tendency to treat osteoporosis with sodium fluoride. This disease is most often asymptomatic and appears on X-ray of the skeleton as a generalized sclerosis without any bone deformity. It is secondary to a thickening of bone trabeculae. Ossification of ligaments, tendons and interosseous membranes, clearly visible on radiographs, constitute an important sign for diagnosis. Serum calcium and phosphorus are normal and alkaline phosphatase activity is usually markedly increased. Fluoride is elevated in serum, urine, and bone tissue.

REFERENCES

Aaron, J. E., Gallagher, J. C., and Anderson, J. (1974). 'Frequency of osteomalacia and osteoporosis in fractures of the proximal femure', *Lancet*, **1**, 229–233.

Aitken, J. M., Hart, D. M., and Lindsay, R. (1973). 'Oestrogen replacement therapy for prevention of osteoporosis after oophorectomy', *Br. Med. J.*, **3**, 515–518.

Albright, F., Smith, P. H., and Richardson, A. M. (1941). 'Post menopausal osteoporosis', *JAMA*, **116**, 2465–2474.

Alexanian, R., Salmon, S., Bonnet, J., Gehan, J., Haut, A., and Weich, J. (1977). 'Combination therapy for multiple myeloma', *Cancer*, **40**, 2765–2771.

Alfram, P. A. (1964). 'An epidemiologic study of cervical and trochanteric fractures of the femur in an urban population', *Acta Orthop. Scand. (Suppl.)*, **65**, 1–109.

Arnold, J. S., Bartley, M. H., Tont, S. A., and Jenkins, D. P. (1966). 'Skeletal changes in aging and disease', *Clin. Orthop.*, **49**, 17–38.

Avioli, L. V. (1978). 'Renal osteodystrophy', in *Metabolic Bone Disease*, (Eds L. V. Avioli and

S. M. Krane). Vol. II, Academic Press, New York.

Bartley, M. H. and Arnold, J. S. (1967). 'Sex differences in human skeletal involution', *Nature*, **214**, 908–909.

Barzel, U. S. (1978). 'Common metabolic disorders of the skeleton in aging', in *Clinical Aspects of Aging* (Ed. W. Reichel), pp. 277–287, Williams and Wilkins, Baltimore, Maryland.

Beck, J. S., and Nordin, B. E. C. (1960). 'Histological assessment of osteoporosis by iliac crest biopsy', *J. Pathol. Bact.*, **80**, 391–397.

Bijvoet, O. L. M., and Jansen, A. P. (1967). 'Thyrocalcitonin in Paget's disease', *Lancet*, **2**, 471–472.

Bordier, P., and Tun Chot, S. (1972). 'Quantitative histology of metabolic bone disease', *Clin. Endocrinol. Metab.*, **1**, 197–215.

Bressot, C., Courpron, P., Edouard, C., and Meunier, P. J. (1976). 'Histomorphometrie des osteopathies endocriniennes', Monographie du Laboratoire de Recherches sur l'Histodynamique osseuse, Lyon.

Bressot, C., Meunier, P. J., Chapuy, M. C., Lejeune, E., Edouard, C. and Darby, A. (1979). 'Histomorphometric profile, pathophysiology and reversibility of corticosteroid-induced osteoporosis', *Metab. Bone Dis. Relat. Res.*, **1**, 303–311.

Briançon, D. and Meunier, P. J. (1981). 'Treatment of osteoporosis with fluoride, calcium and vitamin D', *Orthop. Clin. North Am.*, **12**, 629–648.

Caldwell, R. A., and Collins, D. H. (1961). 'Assessment of vertebral osteoporosis by radiographic and chemical methods post mortem', *J. Bone Joint Surg.*, **43B**, 346–361.

Cameron, J. R., and Sorenson, J. (1963). 'Measurement of bone mineral in vivo: an improved method', *Science*, **142**, 230–232.

Corcoran, R. J., and Reeder, M. M. (1977). 'Enlargement of one or more vertebrae', *JAMA*, **238**, 1555–1556.

Courpron, P. (1972). 'Données histologiques quantitatives sur le vieillissement osseux humain', Thesis, Lyon.

Courpron, P. (1981). 'Bone tissue mechanisms underlying osteoporoses', *Orthop. Clin. North Am.*, **12**, 513–545.

Courpron, P., Meunier, P. J., Bressot, C., and Giroux, J. M. (1976). 'Amount of bone in iliac crest biopsy', in *Bone Histomorphometry* (Ed. P. J. Meunier), pp. 39–53, Lyon.

Courpron, P., Meunier, P. J., Edouard, C., Bernard, J., Bringuier, J. P., and Vignon, G. (1973). 'Données histologiques quantitatives sur le vieillissement osseux humain', *Rev. Rhum. Mal. Osteoartic.*, **40**, 469–483.

DeLuca, H. F. (1976). 'Vitamin D endocrinology', *Ann. Intern. Med.*, **85**, 367–377.

Dequeker, J. (1972). *Bone Loss in Normal and Pathological Conditions*, University Press, Louvain.

Dove, J. (1980). 'Complete fractures of the femur in Paget's disease of bone', *J. Bone Joint Surg.*, **62B**, 12–17.

Doyle, F. H. (1972). 'Involutional osteoporosis', *Clin. Endocrinol. Metab.*, **1**, 143–167.

Exton-Smith, A. N., Hodkinson, H. M., and Stanton, B. R. (1966). 'Nutrition and metabolic bone disease in old age', *Lancet*, **1**, 999.

Frame, B., and Parfitt, A. M. (1978). 'Osteomalacia: current concepts', *Ann. Intern. Med.*, **89**, 966–982.

Franck, W. A., Bress, N. M., Singer, F. R., and Krane, S. M. (1974). 'Rheumatic manifestations of Paget's disease of bone', *Am. J. Med.*, **56**, 592–603.

Frost, H. M. (1969). 'Tetracycline-based histological analysis of bone remodeling', *Calcif. Tissue Res.*, **3**, 211–237.

Frost, H. M. (1973). Bone Remodeling and its Relationship to Metabolic Bone Diseases, pp. 1–210, Ed. C. C. Thomas. Springfield, Illinois.

Frost, H. M. (1981). 'Clinical management of the symptomatic osteoporotic patient', *Orthop. Clin. North Am.*, **12**, 671–681.

Gallagher, J. C., Riggs, B. L., Hamtra, A., and DeLuca, H. F. (1978). 'Effect of estrogen therapy on calcium absorption and vitamin D metabolism in postmenopausal osteoporosis', *J. Clin. Res.*, **26**, 415A.

Garn, S. M. (1970). The Earlier Gain and the Later Loss of Cortical Bone, C. C. Thomas, Springfield, Illinois.

Gerson-Cohen, J., Rechtman, A. M., Schraer, H., and Blumberg, N. (1953). 'Asymptomatic fractures in osteoporotic spines of the aged', *JAMA*, **153**, 625.

Giroux, J. M., Courpron, P., and Meunier, P. J. (1975). 'Histomorphometrie de l'osteopénie physiologique sénile', Monographie due Laboratoire de Recherches sur l'Histodynamique Osseuse, Lyon.

Hahn, T. J. (1975). 'Anticonvulsant osteomalacia', *Arch. Intern. Med.*, **135**, 997–1000.

Heaney, R. P., Recker, R. R., and Saville, P. D. (1978a). 'Menopausal changes in calcium balance performance', *J. Lab. Clin. Med.*, **92**, 953.

Heaney, R. P., Recker, R. R., and Saville, P. D. (1978b). 'Menopausal changes in bone remodeling', *J. Lab. Clin. Med.*, **92**, 964.

Heistad, D. D., Abboud, F. M., Schmid, P. G., Mark, A. L., and Wilson, W. R. (1975). 'Regulation of blood flow in Paget's disease of bone', *J. Clin. Invest.*, **55**, 69.

Howarth, S. (1953). 'Cardiac output in osteitis deformans', *Clin. Sci.*, **12**, 271.

Hutchinson, T. A., Polansky, S. M., and Feinstein, A. R. (1979). 'Post menopausal oestrogens protect against fractures of hip and distal radius', *Lancet*, **2**, 705.

Jaworski, Z. F. G. (1981). 'Physiology and pathology of bone remodelling', *Orthop. Clin. North Am.*, **12**, 485–512.

Johnston, C. C. (1979). 'Age-related bone loss', in *Osteoporosis II* (Ed. U. S. Barzel), p. 91–100, Grune and Stratton, New York.

Johnston, C. C., Smith, D. M., Yu, P. L., and Deiss, W. P. (1968). 'In vivo measurement of bone in the radius', *Metabolism*, **17**, 1140–1153.

Khairi, M. R. A., Altman, R. D., DeRosa, G. P., Zimmermann, J., Schenk, R. K., and Johnston, C. C. (1977). 'Sodium etidronate in the treatment of Paget's disease of bone. A study of long-term results', *Ann. Intern. Med.*, **87**, 656.

Kleerekoper, M., Tolia, K., and Parfitt, A. M. (1981). 'Nutritional, endocrine, and demographic aspects of osteoporosis', *Orthop. Clin. North Am.*, **12**, 547–558.

Klein, R. G., Arnaud, S. B., Gallagher, J. D., DeLuca, H. F., and Riggs, B. L. (1977). 'Intestinal absorption in exogenous hypercortisonism', *J. Clin. Invest.*, **60**, 253.

Krane, S. M. (1977). 'Paget's disease of bone', *Clin. Orthop.*, **127**, 24–36.

Lebbin, D., Ryan, W. G., and Schwartz, T. B. (1974). 'Outpatient treatment of Paget's disease of bone with mithramycin', *Ann. Intern. Med.*, **81**, 635.

Lender, M., Makin, M., Robin, G., Steinberg, R., and Menczel, J. (1976). 'Osteoporosis and fractures of the neck of the femur. Some epidemiologic considerations', *Isr. J. Med. Sci.*, **12**, 596.

Lindsay, R., Hart, D. M., Forrest, C., and Baird, C. (1980). 'Prevention of spinal osteoporosis in oophorectomised women', *Lancet*, **2**, 1151.

Lindsay, R., Hart, M. D., MacLean, A., Clark, A. C., Kraszewski, A., and Garwood, J. (1978). 'Bone response to termination of oestrogen treatment', *Lancet*, **1**, 1325.

Louis, J. M. (1976). 'The radiographic appearance of osteoporosis secondary to immobilization', *J. Amer. Pediatric. Ass.*, **66**, 242–251.

Lutwak, L., Singer, F. R., and Urist, M. R. (1974). 'Current concepts of bone metabolism', *Ann. Intern. Med.*, **80**, 630–644.

McFarlane, J. D., Lutkin, J. E., and Burwood, M. A. (1977). 'The demonstration by scintigraphy of fractures in osteomalacia', *Br. J. Radiol.*, **50**, 369–371.

Mankin, H. J. (1974). 'Rickets, osteomalacia and renal osteodystrophy', *J. Bone Joint Surg.*, **56A**, 101.

Mazess, R. B., and Cameron, J. R. (1973). 'Bone mineral content in normal U.S. whites', International Conference on Bone Mineral Measurement, University of Wisconsin, Chicago, Illinois.

Meema, H. E., and Meema, S. (1972). 'Comparison of microradioscopic and morphometric findings in the hand bones with densitometric findings in the proximal radius in thyrotoxicosis and renal osteodystrophy', *Invest. Radiol.*, **7**, 88–96.

Meema, H. E., and Schatz, D. L. (1970) 'Simple radiologic demonstration of cortical bone loss in thyrotoxicosis', *Radiology*, **97**, 9–15.

Meema, S., Bunker, M. L., and Meema, H. E. (1975). 'Preventive effect of estrogen on postmenopausal bone loss', *Arch. Intern. Med.*, **135**, 1436–1440.

Melsen, F. (1978). 'Histomorphometric analysis of iliac bone in normal and pathological conditions', Thesis, University Institute of Pathology, Aarhus, Denmark.

Meema, H. E., and Schatz, D. L. (1970) 'Simple radiologic demonstration of cortical bone loss in thyrotoxicosis', *Radiology*, **97**, 9–15.

Menkes, C. J., Simon, F., Duveau, J., Chapuis, Y., and Delbarre, F. (1980). 'L'hyperparathyroidisme primitif du sujet âgé. A propos de 16 adenomes opérés', *Ann. Med. Intern.*, **131**, 393.

Meunier, P. J., Bianchi, G. G. S., Edouard, C., Bernard, J., Courpron, P., and Vignon, G. (1972a). 'Bony manifestations of thyrotoxicosis', *Orthop. Clin. North Am.*, **3**, 745–774.

Meunier, P. J., Courpron, P., Edouard, C., Bernard, J., Bringuier, J. P., and Vignon, G. (1973). 'Physiological senile involution and pathological rarefaction of bone', *Clin. Endocrinol. Metab.*, **2**, 239–256.

Meunier, P. J., Vignon, G., Bernard, J., Edouard, C., and Courpron, P. (1972b). 'Quantitative bone histology as applied to the diagnosis of hyperparathyroid states', in *Clinical Aspects of Metabolic bone Disease* (Eds B. Frame, A. M. Parfitt, and H. Duncan), p. 215, Excerpta Medica, Amsterdam.

Minaire, P., Meunier, P. J., Edouard, C., Bernard, J., Courpron, P., and Bourret, J. (1974). 'Quantitative histological data on disuse osteoporosis', *Calcif. Tissue Res.*, **17**, 57–73.

Morgan, D. B. (1973a). 'Aging and osteoporosis, in particular spinal osteoporosis', *Clin. Endocrinol. Metab.*, **2**, 187–201.

Morgan, D. B. (1973b). 'Osteomalacia, renal osteodystrophy and osteoporosis', C. C. Thomas, Springfield, Illinois.

Morgan, D. B., and Newton-John, H. F. (1969). 'Bone loss and senescence', *Gerontologia*, **15**, 140–154.

Morgan, D. B., Spiers, F. W., Pulvertaft, C. N., and Fourman, P. (1967). 'The amount of bone in metacarpal and the phalanx according to age and sex', *J. Clin. Radiol.*, **18**, 101–108.

Mosekilde, L. (1979). 'Effects of thyroid hormone(s) on bone remodeling bone mass and calcium-phosphorus homeostasis in man', Thesis, University Institute of Pathology, Aarhus, Denmark.

Mueller, K. H., Trias, A., and Ray, R. D. (1966). 'Bone density and composition age-related and pathological changes in water and mineral content', *J. Bone Joint Surg.*, **48A**, 140–148.

Muller, H. (1969). 'Sex, age and hyperparathyroidism', *Lancet*, **1**, 449.

Nagant de Deuxchaisnes, C., and Krane, S. M. (1964). 'Paget's disease of bone: clinical and metabolic observations', *Medicine*, **43**, 233–266.

Newton-John, H. F., and Morgan, D. B. (1968). 'Osteoporosis: disease or senescence?', *Lancet*, **1**, 232–233.

Newton-John, H. F., and Morgan, D. B. (1970). 'The loss of bone with age, osteoporosis and fractures', *Clin. Orthop.*, **71**, 229–252.

Nordin, B. E. C. (1961). 'The pathogenesis of osteoporosis', *Lancet*, **1**, 1011–1014.

Nordin, B. E. C. (1979). 'Treatment of postmenopausal osteoporosis', *Drugs*, **18**, 484–492.

Nordin, B. E. C., Horsman, A., Grilly, R. G., Marshall, D. H., and Simpson, M. (1980). 'Treatment of spinal osteoporosis in postmenopausal women', *Br. Med. J.*, **280**, 451.

Paget Sir, J. (1877). 'On a form of chronic inflammation of bones (osteitis deformans)', *Med. Chirg. Trans.*, **60**, 37–64.

Parfitt, A. M., and Duncan, H. (1975). 'Metabolic bone disease affecting the spine', in *The Spine* (Eds R. Rothman and F. Simeone), pp. 599–720, Saunders, Philadelphia.

Pygott, F. (1957). 'Paget's disease of bone – The radiological incidence', *Lancet*, **1**, 1170–1171.

Rebel, A., Malkani, D., Basle, M., and Bregeon, C. (1976). 'Osteoclast ultra-structure in Paget's disease', *Calcif. Tissue Res.*, **20**, 187.

Recker, R. R. (1981). 'Continuous treatment of osteoporosis: current status', *Orthop. Clin. North Am.*, **12**, 611–627.

Recker, R. R., Saville, P. D., and Heaney, R. P. (1977). 'Effect of estrogens and calcium carbonate on bone loss in postmenopausal women', *Ann. Intern. Med.*, **87**, 649–655.

Rich, C., and Ensink, F. (1961). 'Effect of sodium fluoride on calcium metabolism of human beings', *Nature*, **191**, 184.

Russell, R. G. G., and Fleisch, H. (1975). 'Pyrophosphate and diphosphonates in skeletal metabolism', *Clin. Orthop.*, **108**, 241.

Salson, C. (1981). 'Distribution squelettique de la maladie de Paget evaluée par la scintigraphie osseuse quantitative dans 170 cas', Thesis, Lyon.

Schenk, R. K., and Merz, W. A. (1969). 'Histologic-morphometric studies of old age strophy and senile osteoporosis in the crest of ilium', *Dtsch. Med. Wochenschr.*, **31**, 206–208.

Schmidek, H. H. (1977). 'Neurologic and neurosurgical sequelae of Paget's disease of bone', *Clin. Orthop.*, **127**, 70–77.

Schott, G. D., and Wills, M. R. (1976). 'Muscle weakness in osteomalacia', *Lancet*, **1**, 626–629.

Singer, F. R. (1977a). 'Human calcitonin treatment of Paget's disease of bone', *Clin. Orthop.*, **127**, 86–93.

Singer, F. R. (1977b). 'Paget's disease of bone', Plenum Medical, London.

Singer, F. R., Melvin, K. E. W., and Mills, B. G. (1976). 'Acute effects of calcitonin on osteoclasts in man', *Clin. Endocrinol. (Oxf.)*, 5–333.

Smith, D. A., Fraser, S. A., and Wilson, G. M. (1973). 'Hyperthyroidism and calcium metabolism', *Clin. Endocrinol. Metab.*, **2**, 333–354.

Smith, D. C., Prentice, R., Thompson, D. J., and Herrmann, W. L. (1975). 'Association of exogenous estrogen and endometrial carcinoma', *N. Engl. J. Med.*, **293**, 1164–1167.

Smith, R. W., and Rizek, J. (1966). 'Epidemiologic studies of osteoporosis in women of Puerto Rico and South Eastern Michigan with special reference to age, race, national origin and to other related or associated findings', *Clin. Orthop.*, **45**, 31–48.

Stryd, R. P., Gilbertson, T. J., and Brunden, M. N. (1979). 'A seasonal variation study of 25-hydroxyvitamin D3 serum levels in normal humans', *J. Clin. Endocrinol. Metab.*, **48**, 771–775.

Thomson, D. L., and Frame, B. (1976). 'Involutional osteopenia: current concepts', *Ann. Intern. Med.*, **85**, 789–803.

Urist, M. R. (1973). 'Orthopedic management of osteoporosis in post menopausal women', *Clin. Endocrinol. Metab.*, **2**, 159–176.

Urist, M. R., Gurvey, M. S., and Fareed, D. O. (1970). 'Long-term observations on aged women with pathologic osteoporosis', in *Osteoporosis* (Ed. U. S. Barzel), pp. 3–37, Grune and Stratton, New York.

Waxman, A. D., Ducker, S., McKee, D., Siemsen, J. K., and Singer, F. R. (1977). 'Evaluation of 99m Tc diphosphonate kinetics and bone scans in patients with Paget's disease before and after calcitonin treatment', *Radiology*, **125**, 761.

Weiss, N. S., and Sayvetz, T. A. (1980). 'Incidence of endometrial cancer in relation to the use of oral contraceptives', *N. Engl. J. Med.*, **302**, 551.

Wu, K., and Frost, H. M. (1969). 'Bone formation in osteoporosis', *Arch. Pathol.*, **88**, 508–510.

Principles and Practice of Geriatric Medicine
Edited by M. S. J. Pathy
© 1985 John Wiley & Sons Ltd

25.3

Disease of Joints

T. Gibson

DISEASES OF JOINTS

The pattern and prevalence of rheumatic diseases in the elderly reflect two things. Firstly, certain disorders arise more frequently with increasing age and are relatively uncommon in middle life. Secondly, since many joint diseases are chronic, there is a steady cumulative effect on their prevalence with age. Thus, by the time of retirement, 80 per cent. of the population has some rheumatological disorder (Kolodny and Klipper, 1976) and one-third of those with a rheumatic complaint are aged between 65 and 74 (Harris, 1971). For those still at work, and taking all diseases into consideration, there is a tendency for the rate of incapacity to decline with increasing age. In contrast to this general trend, incapacity due to rheumatic complaints increases with age, and is maximal in the years preceding retirement (Wood and McLeish, 1974). Beyond this period it is the problems of added illness, frailty, diminished motivation, and social isolation which increasingly affect the management and outcome of the rheumatological disorders (Gibson and Grahame, 1981).

Two diseases whose onset is characteristically seen in the ageing population are polymyalgia rheumatica and pseudo-gout. Two examples of chronic diseases whose high frequency in old age are the result of a continual addition of new cases from middle age onwards are rheumatoid arthritis and osteoarthritis. The latter condition is so common among the elderly that it is often assumed to be physiological rather than pathological. Kellgren (1961) observed that radiological changes of osteoarthritis were universal in the later decades of life but also noted that most of such changes were not associated with significant pain or disability. The dividing line between disease and what is a normal ageing phenomenon in this context is moot. If the clinical and radiological features of osteoarthritis are so common, are they manifestations of age related degeneration of the cartilage?

THE EFFECT OF AGE ON JOINT CARTILAGE

At autopsy, limited osteophytes of the femoral head occur in 33 per cent. of those beyond 49 years of age but this appears to be non-progressive and a purely age-related phenomenon (Byers, Contempomi, and Farkas, 1970). Using Indian ink staining to define areas of cartilage roughening, changes occur in all joints and are often seen as early as the second decade, spreading from the periphery of the joint with age (Meachim and Emery, 1973). Interference and scanning electron microscopy reveal that cartilage surfaces, which appear smooth to the naked eye, are covered with undulations and small hollows. The latter increase in both depth and diameter with advancing age and other surface irregularities become more common (Longmore and Gardner, 1975). It is doubtful whether these consistent surface changes are relevant to the development of osteoarthritis which, although common, is not invariable. Osteoarthritis is associated with cartilage thinning and it is often presumed that its loss precedes other changes. It is therefore puzzling to note that, in general, cartilage actually becomes thicker with increasing age, even in the presence of slight surface fibrillation (Armstrong and Gardner, 1977; Meachim, 1971). Patellar cartilage appears to be an exception to this rule, and thins progressively with age, especially in females (Meachim, Bentley, and Baker, 1977).

As cartilage ages, its mechanical properties alter, becoming increasingly compliant and less elastic (Armstrong, Barhzani, and Gardner, 1977). It has been suggested that this permits easier fatigue and greater susceptibility to osteoarthritis but some difficulty has been experienced in explaining this phenomenon in precise biochemical terms (Freeman, 1975).

Joint cartilage is an extracellular matrix of proteolglycans and collagen, both of which are synthesized by chondrocytes. The proteoglycans are proteins with several attached glycosaminoglycans (Chondroitin sulphate and keratan sulphate). Each proteoglycan is linked to hyaluronic acid to form a high molecular weight aggregate (Moskowitz, 1977). Many studies of cartilage have been conducted on costal cartilage but it is now quite clear that age-related changes at this site are not mirrored by articular cartilage. After the third decade, progressive pigmentation of costal cartilage occurs, probably due to the deposition of amino acid derivatives. These changes are much less obvious in joint cartilage (Van der Korst, Sokoloff, and Miller, 1968). A gradual reduction of collagen also takes place in rib cartilage but not in articular cartilage (Miller, Van der Korst, and Sokoloff, 1969). Similarly, a linear reduction of chondroitin sulphate occurs with age in costal cartilage (Kaplan and Meyer, 1959) but not in joint cartilage (Bollet, Handy, and Sturgill, 1963). Furthermore, no change of cartilage water content occurs as subjects grow older (Linn and Sokoloff, 1965). This feature invariably accompanies the early stages of osteoarthritis. Thus, the lack of any demonstrable biochemical hallmark of ageing has prompted Ball and Sharp (1978) to argue that there is no generalized time-dependent deterioration of chondrocyte function in articular cartilage.

THE PATTERN OF RHEUMATIC DISEASE IN THE ELDERLY

The explanation for the very high prevalence of osteoarthritis and rheumatoid disease in the ageing population has already been discussed. Symptomatic osteoarthritis, although most often manifest for the first time beyond the age of 60, usually represents a disease process which begins at a much younger age. In this sense, it is misleading to refer to the frequent onset of osteoarthritis in the elderly. By constrast rheumatoid disease is clinically evident more or less from the time of its development and it is quite clear that while the incidence of new cases declines beyond the peak seen between the ages of 30 and 50, the prevalence continues to increase up to the age of 70 (Mikkelsen et al., 1967).

Painful syndromes affecting the neck and lower back are very common in all age groups and, overall, represent the most common rheumatic complaints. The prevalence of symptomatic disease of the spine, unlike that of peripheral osteoarthritis, does not continue to increase with age. This may reflect declining physical activity, especially among those in whom occupational factors are paramount. For example, back pain due to lumbar disc protrusion is approximately 9 times more common in the fourth decade compared with ages beyond 60 (Kelsey, 1975). The prevalence of soft tissue rheumatism also shows no increase with age and this, too, probably reflects a decrease of vigorous physical activities.

Acute arthritis affecting one or more joints is common among the elderly and the distribution of causes differs from that of the young and middle aged. The declining incidence of rheumatoid arthritis and other causes of chronic polyarthritis make these rather less likely to present in late life as an acute illness. However, rheumatoid arthritis remains the most common cause of acute arthritis while crystal-induced synovitis is as likely to be due to pseudo-gout as gout and septic arthritis is a more important consideration than Reiter's syndrome or ankylosing spondylitis (Gibson and Grahame, 1973).

DIAGNOSTIC DIFFICULTIES IN THE ELDERLY

Establishing the diagnosis of an arthritis, especially when it is acute, tends to be more problematic in the elderly, especially if synovial fluid is unavailable for examination. Despite intensive investigation there may remain instances where it is not possible to attribute the cause. The common concurrence of X-ray evidence of chondrocalcinosis and diuretic induced hyperuricaemia may introduce the possibility of either pseudo-gout or gout and there may be occasions when no diagnostic clues are available (Gibson and Grahame, 1973). It has been suggested that some cases represent an entity termed 'senile monarticular arthritis' (Benians, 1969) but the existence of such a disease has not been substantiated. The precision of diagnosis may be further compounded by some resemblance between polymyalgia rheumatica (see Chapter 25.1) and rheumatoid arthritis. The former, a disease almost exclusively confined to those of more than 60 years of age, may exhibit the clinical features of a polyarthritis (Henderson, Tribe and Dixon, 1975), and radionuclear scanning has suggested that joint involvement is common (O'Duffy, Wahner, and Hander, 1976). On the other hand, rheumatoid arthritis may present in the elderly with prominent shoulder pain and stiffness resembling polymyalgia rheumatica (Dimant, 1979). Furthermore, the natural increase of the erythrocyte sedimentation rate with age (Boyd and Hoffbrand, 1966; Kulvin, 1972) may suggest an inflammatory basis for joint pain where none exists. The presence of a positive test for rheumatoid factor may erroneously indicate the presence of rheumatoid arthritis. The prevalence of rheumatoid factor in the serum increases with age (Heimer, Levin, and Ludd, 1963) and 35 per cent. of all individuals over the age of 70 may exhibit a positive latex slide test for rheumatoid factor (Dequecker, Layer, and VandePitte, 1969).

AUTOANTIBODY PRODUCTION IN RELATION TO RHEUMATIC DISEASES AND AGEING

In parallel with the increase of rheumatoid factor, autoantibodies to nuclear and tissue specific antigens are found with greater frequency in the elderly (Goidl *et al.*, 1981; Mackay, 1972). The connective tissue diseases associated with positive tests for antinuclear antibodies are with the exception of rheumatoid arthritis, rare in this age group.

Paradoxically, the heightened immunological activity which results in the increased prevalence of antibodies is associated with decreased cellular immunity. Lymphocytes from old persons have a decreased mitogenic response to plant mitogens (Weksler and Hutteroth, 1974). It has been suggested that the two phenomena may be directly related and may be the result of a diminution of T-cell activity. Thus, generalized T-cell hyporeactivity may result in the observed impairment of cellular immunity and the increase of antibody production may reflect the specific disappearance of suppressor T cells and their controlling influence on B-cell function (Stobo and Tomasi, 1975). A relative deficiency of suppressor T cells has been observed in rheumatoid arthritis and presented as an hypothesis to explain many of the immune mediated aspects of the disease (Janossy *et al.*, 1981). If this were true and relevant to the aetiology of rheumatoid disease and perhaps other connective tissue diseases, one might anticipate an increase in the incidence of these illnesses in the elderly in view of the evidence for T-cell deficiency in this age group. This is not the case.

OSTEOARTHRITIS

Epidemiology

There is always a semantic problem to be overcome when discussing the epidemiology of osteoarthritis. Most population surveys have emphasized the radiological evidence of osteoarthritis, especially in the hands. Such features are so widespread in the elderly and so often unassociated with symptoms that they may hardly warrant consideration as a disease process. In a study of 380 people aged 55 to 64, 60 per cent. of the females and 40 per cent. of the males had radiological evidence of osteoarthritis involving the distal interphalangeal joints (Kellgren and Lawrence, 1958). Other joints commonly involved on X-ray are proximal interphalangeal, first carpometacarpal, knees, and first metatarsophalangeal (Kellgren, 1961). The frequency of radiological abnormalities increases with age and several studies have confirmed that finger involvement, especially of the distal interphalangeal joints, occurs much more often in females (Acheson and Collart, 1975; Caird, Webb, and Lie, 1973).

The principal radiological features of osteoarthritis are loss of joint space and osteophyte formation. These are the characteristics sought in epidemiological studies but osteophytes may be a purely age-related phenomenon, unassociated with cartilage pathology (Byers, Contempomi, and Farkas, 1970). Osteophytes of the knees tend to increase in size up to the age of 70 and are not invariably associated with other evidence of osteoarthritis (Hernborg and Nilsson, 1973). In people aged more than 60, radiological evidence of osteophytes or joint space narrowing may occur in as many as 70 per cent. of knees, of which less than half will be sites of pain, stiffness, or deformity (Gresham and Rathey, 1975). Estimates of prevalence of osteoarthritis of the hip have been more realistically linked to the presence of symptoms. In a Swedish population of more than 65 years old, this figure was 6 per cent. (Danielsson, 1966). This is very similar to the 5.6 per cent. prevalence determined in a British population aged more than 66 (Wilcock, 1979).

Aetiology

The frequency of X-ray features of osteoarthritis in the distal interphalangeal joints and of the associated deformities (Heberden's nodes) with osteoarthritis at other sites implies an inherited susceptibility which is expressed most strongly in females (Acheson and Collart, 1975; Kellgren, Lawrence, and Bier, 1963). If this predisposition is related to a biochemical or metabolic deficiency of cartilage it has yet to be defined. However, the familial association of Heberden nodes is beyond dispute and these occur in 45 per cent. of female relatives of those with nodes and in only 13 per cent. of those without nodes (Kellgren, Lawrence, and Bier, 1963). Osteoarthritis at other sites appears to be more severe when associated with Heberden nodes. Further evidence of a familial trait derives from the association of generalized osteoarthritis in the absence of Heberden nodes, with inflammatory polyarthritis (Kellgren, Lawrence, and Bier, 1963). These latter observations pertain to women and imply that some cases of primary generalized osteoarthritis may be preceded by mild or unrecognized inflammatory joint disease. This points to the heterogeneity of aetiological factors in osteoarthritis. Epidemiological surveys have suggested that in men trauma may be a more important factor (Kellgren and Lawrence, 1958). There are prolific data which clearly illustrate how repetitive minor occupational damage or more dramatic injuries, such as torn menisci or fractures, may result in mechanical dysfunction or joint surface incongruity and, in time, the development of osteoarthritis at the site of injury. Other factors such as preexisting arthritis due to recurrent crystal synovitis, acute sepsis, chronic polyarthritis, such as rheumatoid disease, or abnormal subchondral bone, as in Paget's disease, may all result in the common clinical picture of osteoarthritis. To these may be added osteoarthritis of the knee secondary to disparities of leg length; congenital or hereditary defects such as epiphyseal dysplasia or congenital dislocation of the hip; and endocrine and metabolic diseases such as acromegaly or ochronosis. There is some evidence that obesity may be a predisposing factor, affecting joints other than those which bear weight (Acheson and Collart, 1975), although this has been disputed (Goldin *et al.*, 1976). Diabetes may be an additional endocrine disorder which predisposes to osteoarthritis, although this association requires confirmation (Waine *et al.*, 1961). The radiological features of osteoarthritis may occasionally be associated with such severe juxta-articular bone destruction that cause and effect may be difficult to determine. This picture occurs most often in the hip joint (Fig. 1). The appearance is often attributed to avascular necrosis which has been followed by osteoarthritis as a secondary event. In the elderly it is probable that bone necrosis is more usually a sequel to osteoarthritis. True avascular necrosis is not rare and most often occurs in the elderly after subcapital femoral neck fractures. Other clinical associations need to be considered where avascular necrosis is suspected, and these include alcohol abuse and corticosteroid administration (Herndon and Aufranc, 1972).

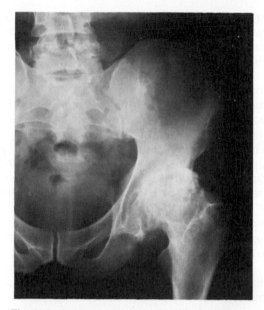

Figure 1 Severe osteoarthritis of the hip with loss of joint space, osteophytes, and sclerosis. The femoral head is disintegrating and the picture resembles that of avascular necrosis

However, not infrequently, avascular necrosis occurs in the hip without a recognizable cause. Analogous spontaneous osteonecrosis of the femoral condyle has been documented in the elderly, leading to severe osteoarthritis of the knee (Smith, Zaphiropoulos, and Polyzoides, 1981).

A classification of causes of osteoarthritis has been proposed on the basis of whether (a) abnormal forces operate on normal cartilage, e.g. injury, (b) normal forces on abnormal cartilage, e.g. preexisting arthritis, or (c) normal forces act on abnormal subchondral bone, e.g. Paget's disease and avascular necrosis (Mitchell and Cruess, 1977). Many instances defy such a ready classification. For example, in the majority of patients with hip disease, there is neither evidence of generalized osteoarthritis nor any other cause. That does not preclude some unrecognized event or circumstance which may have preceded the development of osteoarthritis.

The role of inflammation in the pathogenesis of osteoarthritis is readily appreciated among those patients who exhibit features of a classical disease such as rheumatoid arthritis. In other cases it is rather more difficult. Acute inflammation may appear to precede the de-velopment of Heberden nodes and the analogous osteophytic deformities of the proximal interphalangeal joints (Bouchard nodes), and may give rise to simultaneous articular erosions reminiscent of the purely inflammatory joint diseases (Ehrlich, 1972a; Peter, Pearson, and Marmor, 1966). Whether such cases represent an entity is not clear. In such instances the synovium may be indistinguishable from the chronically inflamed picture seen in rheumatoid arthritis and a proportion of patients so described may subsequently develop typical rheumatoid arthritis (Ehrlich, 1972b).

A modest degree of joint inflammation may be clinically obvious in a very large number of osteoarthritis joints. To what extend this may accentuate cartilage damage is uncertain.

Further evidence for an inflammatory aetiology has been speculated on the basis of the identification of calcium hydroxyapatite crystals in the synovial fluid of patients with generalized osteoarthritis (Dieppe *et al.*, 1976). These may be recognized only by using electron microscopy techniques but their presence in synovial fluid obtained from patients with other joint diseases makes it less plausible that they have an important primary role in the pathogenesis of osteoarthritis (Schumacher *et al.*, 1977). It is possible that such crystals are a secondary phenomenon and since their phlogistic properties have been well demonstrated, some of the inflammatory features of osteoarthritis could be due to their presence. Similar claims have been made for cholesterol crystals which have also been demonstrated in osteoarthritic synovial fluid (Fam *et al.*, 1981) and shown to induce synovitis in animals (Pritzker *et al.*, 1981).

Pathology

It is thus clear that a wide range of miscellaneous insults may precede the pathological picture of osteoarthritis. The initial changes in the cartilage tend to be focal (Mankin *et al.*, 1971). To the naked eye, the cartilage loses its healthy gloss, becoming dull and roughened. Under the light microscope, surface fibrillation proceeds vertically and horizontally, eventually producing deep clefts extending to the subchondral bone. It has been argued that the diminishing strength and stiffness of cartilage with age reduces its fatigue resistance and that breaches of the articular surface represent stress fractures, an important primary event (Freeman, 1975). Alterations in the cartilage are paralleled by increased bone metabolism in the subchondral region, especially in areas which bear weight (Reimann, Mankin, and Trahan, 1977). This results in hardening of the subchondral bone, the increased density of which is a characteristic X-ray feature of osteoarthritis. According to Radin (1976), hardening of the bone increases the stress on the cartilage and provides an alternative mechanical explanation for the development of the clefts. Light microscopy also reveals that, in the early stages, chondrocytes appear larger and tend to clump together instead of being evenly distributed. There is evidence that the metabolic activity of the chondrocytes increases in an attempt at repair (Mitrovic *et al.*, 1981), although this has been disputed (Moskowitz, Goldberg, and Malemud, 1981). Histochemical staining suggests that, in the early stages, the ratio of chondroitin sulphate to keratan sulphate is increased, resembling immature cartilage. This is consistent with an increase of chondrocyte activity during which chondroitin sulphate synthesis is accentuated (Thompson and Oegema, 1979). Similar alterations of glycosaminoglycan production have been demonstrated in experimental osteoarthritis where there is also an initial increase of cartilage thickness and water content (McDevitt and Muir, 1976). These biochemical events in animals precede evidence of fibrillation and cleft formation. The sequence in man is less certain but there is a correlation between the severity of the histological changes and the increase of glycosaminoglycan synthesis (Mankin *et al.*, 1971). However, at a certain stage of severity, the chondrocytes decrease in number and total glycosaminoglycan content declines despite increased synthesis. Cellular depletion and loss of proteoglycans, most severe where there is fibrillation, may extend into nonfibrillated areas, providing further evidence to suggest that cellular and biochemical events may precede the fissuring of the cartilage (Meachim, Ghadially, and Collino, 1965). At an early stage of osteoarthritis, the increase of subchondral bone synthesis is associated with bone remodelling and the formation of osteophytes. This is probably another reparative

process and even in advanced osteoarthritis the cartilage covering of bone osteophytes is biochemically almost normal (Mankin *et al.*, 1971).

Where osteoarthritis progresses to its extreme, the cartilage disintegrates and the bone surface may become totally denuded so that bone articulates with bone. Cysts may develop within the subchondral bone at various stages. These may represent extensions of cartilage clefts along which synovial fluid may flow and help to expand the cysts or they may result from multiple small fractures which coalesce. When large they may collapse, especially in weight-bearing joints. This is one explanation for the radiological picture which resembles avascular necrosis of the hip joint.

Although the aetiopathogenesis of osteoarthritis is conventionally, and correctly, discussed with reference to the cartilage, changes also occur in the synovium and joint capsule. The joint capsule becomes thickened as does the synovium which may also be infiltrated to a greater or lesser extent by chronic inflammatory cells. Not infrequently, the inflammatory changes of the synovium may be florid and indistinguishable from those of rheumatoid arthritis (Soren, Klein, and Huth, 1976). The synovial fluid may occasionally contain large numbers of granulocytes, reflecting the inflammatory component of the disease (Dieppe *et al.*, 1976). It is possible that inflammation, perhaps in some instances induced by crystals of hydroxyapatite or cholesterol, may accelerate the degradation of cartilage by releasing proteinases such as collagenase from granulocytes, synovium, or even the chondrocytes themselves (Bayliss and Ali, 1978; Ehrlich *et al.*, 1977; Jubb and Fell, 1980).

Clinical Features

Pain is the presenting complaint. This is usually confined to the involved joint but may be diffuse and poorly localized. The pain is described as a continuous ache, accentuated during or soon after activity, but which is paradoxically worse after rest and often disturbs sleep. It may be intermittent in mild to moderately severe disease. Trauma or overuse may be clearly related to each recurrence or to episodes of worsening. Stiffness is a usual accompaniment but tends to be less severe than in rheumatoid arthritis. It may be especially prominent after periods of inactivity. Bearing in mind the increased prevalence of asymptomatic radiological abnormalities in the elderly, pain and stiffness arising from joints which exhibit X-ray evidence of osteoarthritis may have some alternative explanation. Functional impairment may be insidious and relegated in the list of symptoms, but incapacity which intrudes on day to day activities such as dressing or walking may be foremost. Difficulty coping with a lavatory is very common but rarely volunteered by patients.

In general, the signs are those of (a) deformity caused by joint swelling; subluxation; loss of cartilage ligament and joint capsule laxity; (b) muscle wasting; (c) joint tenderness; (d) warmth; (e) synovial effusion; (f) restriction of passive and active movement; (g) crepitus. None of these findings is specific and all may be found to a variable extent in other joint diseases.

Generalized Osteoarthritis

The work of Kellgren, Lawrence, and Bier, (1963) not only illustrated how a susceptibility to osteoarthritis may be inherited but also im-plied that there were two patterns of inherited disease. In one, characterized by Heberden nodes and called nodular primary generalized osteoarthritis, radiological involvement of the distal interphalangeal joints was more likely to be associated with similar changes of other sites but especially the small joints of the hands (Figs. 2). In the other, a generalized pattern occurred in the absence of Heberden nodes. In both cases, the pattern did not appear to follow simple Mendelian inheritance and showed a predeliction for females. Heberden nodes may be asymptomatic and are not always associated with more generalized arthritis. Occasionally, they may become intermittently painful, red, and swollen or expand into cysts which contain a mucus material (Fig. 3). Heberden nodes may also be features of those patterns of generalized osteoarthritis which have been termed inflammatory (Peter, Pierson, and Marmor, 1966) and erosive osteoarthritis (Ehrlich, 1972b). Osteoarthritis of the fingers, with or without Heberden nodes, may be associated with intermittent soft tissue swelling, redness, and increased tenderness.

Involvement of the proximal interphalangeal joints, giving rise to the bone swelling of Bouchard nodes, is most often seen as part of the

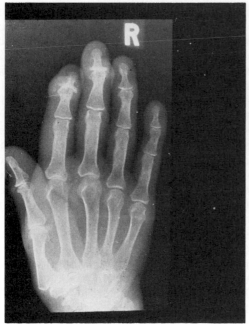 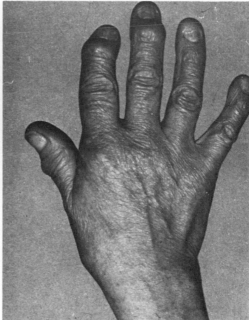

Figure 2   Osteoarthritis of the distal interphalangeal joints (Heberden nodes) in a patient with generalized osteoarthritis

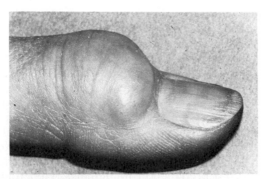

Figure 3   Cystic changes in a Heberden node. This is warm and tender and contains mucus

picture of so-called primary generalized osteoarthritis. The metacarpophalangeal joints are less frequently affected.

Osteoarthritis of the carpometacarpal joint of the thumb may be seen in association with generalized involvement of the hands, but is just as likely to occur in isolation (Fig. 4). It is exceedingly common in the aged and is the most common cause of thenar eminence wasting. The muscle wasting and pain are often mistakenly attributed to carpal tunnel syndrome. The presence of adduction deformity of the thumb, causing a rectangular appearance to the hand, together with pronounced local tenderness, crepitus, and pain on movement help to distinguish it. Osteoarthritis of the fingers, and particularly of the carpometacarpal joints of the thumbs, may cause considerable disability by interfering with the fine movements necessary for such activities as doing up buttons or sewing.

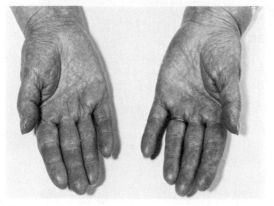

Figure 4   Osteoarthritis of the carpometacarpal joints of the thumbs preventing abduction. There is associated wasting of the thenar eminence on both sides

Other Upper Limb Involvement

Osteoarthritis of the wrists occurs less often than that of fingers, even in the presence of a generalized pattern of involvement. Radiological evidence of osteoarthritis of the elbow is more common in elderly men than women and occupational factors may be important. Such changes are often asymptomatic but are usually associated with restriction of elbow extension. Symptoms may only arise when osteophyte encroachment impinges on the ulnar nerve giving rise to pain, paraesthesiae, or weakness of the hand. Osteoarthritis of the shoulder is sufficiently unusual to be mistaken for frozen shoulder when pain and stiffness at this site are associated with restricted movement. Bilateral involvement with radiological evidence of osteoarthritis may occasionally be the result of hydroxyapatite crystal deposition in the shoulder joint cavity, a condition recently described and termed 'Milwaukee shoulder' (McCarty *et al.*, 1981).

Hip Involvement

This affects women more than men and is usually unilateral. Pain and stiffness are situated in the groin and less commonly around the buttock. Referral of pain to the knee is characteristic and it is axiomatic that patients with knee pain should receive a careful examination of the hip since pain may be confined entirely to the knee. Pain may impair walking to a variable degree. Nocturnal pain may be severe and is by itself a recommendation for surgical treatment. The signs are (a) an abnormal gait due to weakness of the hip abductors on the involved side, allowing the pelvis to tilt to the contralateral side (Trendelenberg gait); (b) shortening of the leg due to loss of joint cartilage, collapse of the femoral head, or flexion deformity; (c) wasting of the quadriceps; (d) painful restriction of hip movement, initially affecting internal rotation; (e) loss of hip extension progressing to flexion deformity. Pain in the buttock needs to be distinguished from that arising in the spine. The two may coexist, especially where leg shortening causes tilting of the pelvis and a compensatory scoliosis of the lumbar spine.

Knee Involvement

Pain is usually confined to the knee and worsened by walking. Osteoarthritis of the patellofemoral compartment causes pain which is characteristically worse on walking up an incline. Nocturnal pain may be a feature. The signs are (a) a limp; (b) wasting of the quadriceps; (c) swelling due to thickness of the joint capsule and synovium or formation of a joint effusion; (d) valgus or, less commonly, varus deformity with collateral and cruciate ligamentous laxity; (e) warmth; (f) painful restriction of movement with loss of full extension; (g) crepitus arising from the patellofemoral compartment. Osteoarthritis of the knee with valgus deformity (Fig. 5) not uncommonly occurs in the contralateral limb where there is shortening of one leg due to hip disease or other causes (long leg arthropathy).

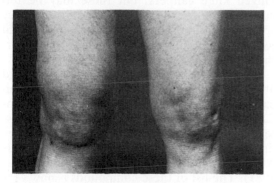

Figure 5 Osteoarthritis of the knees giving rise to a large effusion on the right side

With the exception of the ubiquitous osteoarthritis of the first metatarsophalangeal joint (hallux rigidus) which commonly follows long-standing deformity of the big toe (hallux valgus), involvement of the feet is uncommon. Osteoarthritis of the ankles, subtalar or midtarsal joints may supersede severe trauma but is otherwise rare.

Investigation

The symptoms and signs of osteoarthritis are not specific and even in the presence of radiological features, the diagnosis may rest on the exclusion of other possibilities. The radiological hallmarks are loss of joint space due to cartilage destruction (sometimes apparent in the knee only on weight-bearing X-ray films),

osteophytes, subchondral bone sclerosis, and cysts. Painful finger joints, even in the presence of Heberden nodes and X-ray changes of osteoarthritis, may be due to the later onset of rheumatoid arthritis. Elevation of sedimentation rate and the presence of circulating rheumatoid factor may be useful discriminating investigations but need to be interpreted with caution in view of the natural increase of ESR and positive rheumatoid latex tests in the elderly. However, an ESR in excess of 40 mm/h and a positive sheep cell agglutinating test (as opposed to the latex test) for rheumatoid factor, especially if the test is positive in high titre, may help to differentiate. Examination of synovial fluid is a much neglected diagnostic aid in this context. It should always be aspirated where possible and is most readily obtainable from the knee. Where osteoarthritis is the sole cause of symptoms the synovial fluid is likely to be clear, relatively viscous, and to contain less than 2,000 white cells/ml. Samples should be examined routinely by compensated polarizing microscopy to exclude the presence of monosodium urate or calcium pyrophospate crystals. Culture of synovial fluid for tuberculosis is also mandatory since, unlike infection with pyogenic microorganisms, the clinical picture may be insidious and the synovial fluid may be clear and exhibit the other characteristics of osteoarthritis. A high sedimentation rate, clinical and radiological evidence of osteoarthritis affecting a single large joint, and a history of tuberculosis at some other site should heighten suspicion. In the United Kingdom this possibility should always be excluded when the patient is an Asian immigrant, even in the absence of previous infection (Halsey, 1982). Where the index of suspicion is strong, synovial biopsy is warranted since isolation of acid fast bacilli from synovial fluid is not always possible. The synovium may reveal evidence of typical tuberculous granuloma.

Treatment

General

Osteoarthritis is not always relentlessly progressive and involvement of a single joint does not imply that more widespread arthritis will ensue. Furthermore, symptoms may fluctuate for reasons which are not always apparent or may be accentuated by minor trauma or over-use. When these facts are made known to patients, the dread of unremitting pain or total disability may be mitigated. At the same time, unrealistic expectations must not be encouraged since conservative treatment is at best palliative. The aims are essentially to reduce pain and stiffness, eradication of excessive joint strain and stress, and the preservation of function.

Specific

Rest is an important but neglected component of treatment. Patients may benefit from simply relaxing in a chair for an hour each day, elevating the legs if hip or knees are involved. Activities may need to be modified if these clearly impose unusual strain on affected joints. For example, patients with lower limb disease should be discouraged from frequent use of stairs and should be advised to sit while performing tasks about the house. Such simple advice makes it easier for a patient to alter life-long habits even when the suggestions are obvious.

Stresses on the joints can be relieved in other ways. Reduction of body weight in the obese may have a profound effect on hip or knee pain. The provision of a stick and, equally important, instruction in its proper use may redistribute body weight from the involved limb as well as aiding confidence in walking. Disparities in leg length should be corrected with a heel or shoe raise, thus relieving the strains of the contralateral knee in long leg arthropathy and lessening the risk of low back pain. A shoe raise should not attempt to correct the disparity precisely since this will create a sense of imbalance. A useful rule is to raise the shoe by half the length of the shortening.

Exercise should not be neglected but patients often need to be disabused of the notion that an affected joint will cease moving if not exercised rigorously. Furthermore, there is no justification for trying to increase the range of joint movement by exercises, supervised or otherwise. This invariably worsens pain. The only muscle group which requires regular attention is the quadriceps. These waste rapidly in osteoarthritis of the hip and knee. Non-weight-bearing exercises can rebuild muscle mass which is so important for retention of an efficient gait and knee joint stability. Physical treatments other than exercise may play an important role in alleviating symptoms. Heat applied at home with a hot water bottle or a radiant heat lamp may lack the psychological impact of hospital-based therapy but may be equally effective. Short-wave diathermy in osteoarthritis of knee or hip is of proven value although the effects may be short lived (Wright, 1964). Exercises in a heated pool offer the dual benefits of warmth and muscle strengthening exercises made easier by the buoyant effect of water.

Splints are of limited value. Inpatient treatment of knee flexion deformities may be attempted by serial plaster splints employing a diminishing angle of flexion. This usually produces only a temporary improvement. Severe ligamentous laxity of the knee associated with valgus or varus deformities may be braced by hinged knee calipers, but these may be too cumbersome for the aged. A plastic or plaster splint which immobilizes the carpometacarpal joint of the thumb may be helpful when arthritis involves this joint.

Drug treatment is ostensibly straightforward and is usually necessary at some time in all cases. Presumably because of the modest inflammatory component so often seen in osteoarthritis, non-steroidal anti-inflammatory drugs are more effective than those medicines which are purely analgesic (Kale and Jones, 1981). The list of these compounds is now very long and the choice is wide. None has been shown to be more effective than salicylates but many compounds confer the benefit of once or twice daily dosage and better gastrointestinal tolerance. These are substantial benefits for the elderly. Anti-inflammatory agents are, with few exceptions, inhibitors of prostaglandin synthetase. This implies that they will invariably have some effect on the gastric mucosa, even when given as a pro-drug. It also implies that glomerular filtration may be impaired and this is an important point to recognize in those elderly persons who already exhibit more renal dysfunction than can be attributed to ageing. The latter effect is usually temporary and previous renal function can be restored by withdrawal of the drug. The following list is not exhaustive but illustrates those categories of drugs which may be tried with the expectation of some benefit:

(a) salicylates: diflunisal, aloxiprin, benory-late;
(b) propionic acids: ibuprofen, ketoprofen, naproxen;
(c) anthranilic acids: flufenamic acid;
(d) arylacetic acids: diclofenac;
(e) heteroaryl acetic acids: tolmetin;
(f) indole and indene acetic acids: indometh-acin, sulindac;
(g) enolic acids: azapropazone.

It needs to be emphasized that all of these compounds may have undesirable effects but an idiosyncratic response does not preclude substituting one for another. There are no acknowledged advantages in prescribing com-binations of anti-inflammatory drugs and the habit is to be deprecated because while their combined therapeutic effect is less than their sum, the potential for toxicity is increased doublefold. Indomethacin has an effect on the central nervous system which causes muzziness and occasional confusion. It should not there-fore be used in the elderly person already exhibiting such symptoms. There is no role for phenylbutazone and oxyphenbutazone in the elderly. Their potent fluid-retaining properties precipitate heart failure all too readily in this vulnerable group.

Intra-articular corticosteroid preparations may occasionally be of benefit in patients who have acute worsening of symptoms, especially following trauma. For practical purposes, this measure is performed mainly on the knee. Where an increased effusion and signs of in-flammation occur after a fall, joint aspiration is a necessary prerequisite since the effusion may represent an haemarthrosis, removal of which should suffice. In general, the effects of intra-articular injections last less than four weeks in osteoarthritis (Friedman and Moore, 1980). For this reason, patients may anticipate and demand regular injections. Even though the risks of corticosteroid injections on carti-lage metabolism have probably been exagger-ated (Gibson *et al.*, 1977) it is imprudent to repeat this procedure more frequently than two or three times each year in a single joint.

Less conventional treatments may include irradiation of large joints but it is doubtful whether this is more beneficial than placebo (Gibson, Winter, and Grahame, 1973). The use-fulness of acupuncture has yet to be meas-ured but may have a role. The management of osteoarthritis of the hip and knee has been transformed by prosthetic replacement. All pa-tients with severe pain should be considered for this procedure. The extent of the demand is illustrated by a survey of 838 people over the age of 66 of whom 5.6 per cent. had symp-toms of hip osteoarthritis and 1.2 per cent. had or would have benefited from hip replacement (Wilcock, 1979). Resources cannot meet this challenge in the United Kingdom and there are many patients who wait inordinate periods in severe discomfort. Delays among the elderly carry the risk that other illnesses may super-vene and thus increase the risks of surgery. These are not inconsiderable and the incidence of post-operative complications is high in this age group (Feinstein and Habermann, 1977).

RHEUMATOID ARTHRITIS

Epidemiology

The prevalence of rheumatoid arthritis has been determined in many populations and with surprisingly little variance. Unfortunately, most surveys have applied the loose set of cri-teria defined by the American Rheumatism Association (Ropes *et al.*, 1958). These em-body criteria for classical, definite, and prob-able examples of the disease. Taking into consideration only those patients with a clas-sical or definite clinical picture, the prevalence in adult United States populations is approxi-mately 1 per cent. (Engel, Roberts, and Burch, 1966; Mikkelsen *et al.*, 1967) and in the United Kingdom 1.8 per cent. (Lawrence, 1961).

Little of aetiological significance has derived from these studies except that rheumatoid ar-thritis has a worldwide distribution. One inter-esting observation has been that whereas 3 per cent. of an urban African population had rheu-matoid disease, the prevalence among the same people living in a rural environment was less than 1 per cent., implicating some envi-ronmental precipitating factor associated with life in a township (Solomon *et al.*, 1975).

The prevalence among females is in excess of that of males, in the ratio of approximately 2:1. The overall prevalence increases with age up to the seventh decade. Between 35 and 44 years of age the prevalence has been estimated as 0.5 per cent. in an English population, rising to 8 per cent. in the age range 65 to 74 (Lawrence, 1961). In another study of an urban population aged 55 to 64 the prevalence of those with X-ray or serological evidence of rheumatoid arthritis was 4 per cent. (Kellgren and Lawrence, 1956). There is some evidence that in the elderly there is a relatively increased involvement of males (Mikkelsen *et al.*, 1967) and a more equitable sex distribution (Adler, 1966; Brown and Sones, 1967).

Aetiology

Whereas epidemiological surveys have provided no firm clues as to the causes of rheumatoid arthritis, a genetic association has now become firmly established. Antigens on two loci of the major histocompatibility complex have been implicated, namely HLA D4 and HLA DR4. It has been noted that whereas HLA D4 was found in only 16 per cent. of healthy subjects, the antigen occurred in 59 per cent. of rheumatoid patients (Stastny and Fink, 1977). The HLA DR4 antigen is more easily determined than HLA D4 but their relationship is as yet unclear. The former antigen has been found in 50 per cent. of rheumatoid patients compared with 33 per cent. in a control population (Panayi, Wooley, and Batchelor, 1978). There is some evidence that the presence of this antigen is more likely to be associated with severe disease and the presence of rheumatoid factor (Roitt *et al.*, 1978). Others have found that high titres of rheumatoid factor are more likely to be linked to the antigen HLA DR3 (Panayi, Wooley, and Batchelor, 1979).

These findings have provided fresh impetus for the quest for environmental factors. There may be a telling analogy with Reiter's syndrome and reactive arthritis, where genetic susceptibility is increased by the presence of the histocompatibility antigen HLA B27 and arthritis is induced by recognizable infectious agents. The suspicion that microorganisms may cause rheumatoid arthritis has existed for many decades. There are no convincing data to support the involvement of one particular agent and the evidence for an infectious aetiology is at best controversial.

The search for organisms which might be implicated has been wide-ranging. Much interest has been aroused by the observation that patients with rheumatoid disease may produce an antibody which reacts with nuclear antigens of B lymphocytes transformed by Epstein–Barr virus (Alspaugh *et al.*, 1978). However, rheumatoid patients do not exhibit more direct evidence of Epstein–Barr virus infection. Another virus which is known to cause a usually self-limiting arthritis is rubella. This has been isolated from a group of patients with a miscellaneous pattern of chronic joint diseases including a seronegative polyarthritis resembling rheumatoid disease (Grahame *et al.*, 1981). It is known that viral genomes may modify the antigenic surface of a host cell and it is possible that such a mechanism may induce 'autoimmune disease' states such as in rheumatoid arthritis (August and Strand, 1977).

The fact that mycoplasma strains may cause chronic arthritis in a large number of animals has not unnaturally made these a prime target of study. Organisms with the characteristics of mycoplasmas have been isolated from human joint tissue (Markham and Myers, 1976). Many attempts have failed to confirm this finding. Another organism which has been incriminated is *Clostridium perfringens*, a bacteria which has been found more commonly in the faeces of rheumatoid patients (Olhagen and Mansson, 1968). It is also possible that in a genetically susceptible individual, there could be several infectious agents which may be capable of initiating the disease.

Pathology

A lot is now known about the mechanisms of joint inflammation and there is a plethora of information about the immunological phenomena which accompany these changes. These have led in turn to many speculative proposals about the cause and chronicity of the disease. A central role for the lymphocyte in the perpetuation of joint inflammation derives from the clinical improvement seen after their artificial depletion by thoracic duct drainage (Paulus *et al.*, 1973). One of many paradoxes is that in active rheumatoid disease there is a spontaneous lymphopenia (Basch *et al.*, 1977). Although somewhat controversial, it is likely that the relative proportions of circulating T and B lymphocytes are unaltered whereas in the inflamed synovium there is a predominance of T lymphocytes. Suppression of skin reactivity to injected antigens and decreased in vitro transformation of blood lymphocytes to plant mitogens indicate a qualitative deficiency of lymphocytes. It is not clear whether this is due to humoral factors which suppress lymphocyte function or to some disorder of lymphocyte regulation or merely reflects the preoccupation of rheumatoid lymphocytes which have been committed to the disease process.

Levels of immunoglobulins are increased in the blood and in the joint where they are produced locally by the inflamed synovium. They may exhibit the features of rheumatoid factors and act as antibodies against antigenic determinants of IgG. In both the blood and joint cavity, rheumatoid factors may be IgM, IgG, or IgA immunoglobulin but it is the IgM rheumatoid factor which is most readily detectable and which produces the positive Rose Waaler test. The importance of rheumatoid factors in the pathogenesis of rheumatoid arthritis is not clear but it is known that IgM rheumatoid factor may fix complement and the presence of low complement levels in synovial fluid, together with immune complexes containing rheumatoid factors, may denote that they are an important component of the mechanism which perpetuates the synovitis. In the circulation, high titres of IgM rheumatoid factor are associated with worse disease and an increased likelihood of extra-articular manifestations. IgM rheumatoid factor may also be found in health and in a number of other connective tissue diseases as well as other chronic inflammatory or infectious illnesses. In rheumatoid arthritis it is found by conventional tests in about 70 per cent. of patients.

In the synovial fluid, the most common leukocytes are polymorphs and these may be present in large numbers. They enter the joint cavity rapidly and few can be detected in the synovium. It is presumed that complement activation or other mechanisms of chemotaxis attract the polymorphs to the site of injury. They phagocytose immune complexes but also contribute to enhancement of the inflammation by release of prostaglandins, superoxide radicals, and chemotactic factors, some of which operate through complement activation. They also release proteinases such as collagenase, cathepsin D and G, and elastase. All of these are potentially destructive to the cartilage but whether they are liberated in excess of their natural inhibitors is unclear. In the joint and, to a lesser extent, the blood, the polymorphs of rheumatoid disease show evidence of impaired phagocytosis, possibly due to prior ingestion of immune complexes (Wilton, Gibson, and Chuck, 1978). This may partly explain the susceptibility of rheumatoid patients to infections and to septic arthritis in particular.

The synovial lining, normally one or two cells thick, becomes hypertrophied and the cells hyperplastic. In the early stages, the subsynovial layer becomes more vascular and infiltrated with mononuclear cells, most of which are T lymphocytes (see Fig. 6). These changes are by no means specific and are characteristic of chronic inflammatory joint disorders. Later, mononuclear cells consisting of lymphocytes and plasma cells aggregate around vessels. These synthesize immunoglobulins including rheumatoid factors. The hypertrophy of the synovium progresses with the chronicity of the arthritis, forming finger-like villi. These become layered with a deposit of fibrin. The synovium encroaches on the joint cavity spreading over the articular cartilage to form a pannus. At the margins of the pannus, cartilage and subchondral bone is destroyed by an obscure process, producing the characteristic erosions. The joint capsule becomes thickened and chronic inflammatory changes may occur in overlying joint tendons. Subchondral cysts occur as in osteoarthritis and these may be partly the effect of raised intra-articular pressure.

Rheumatoid nodules (Fig. 7) occur over subcutaneous areas subjected to trauma and almost invariably are confined to patients with circulating IgM rheumatoid factor. Each nodule has a typical appearance with a central necrotic area surrounded by densely layered fibroblasts and other mononuclear cells arranged in palisades.

Clinical Features

The onset of rheumatoid arthritis is usually insidious and may be preceded by a history of malaise, fever, or weight loss extending over a period of weeks or months. Characteristically, joint inflammation occurs symmetrically, affecting the hands and feet at an early stage.

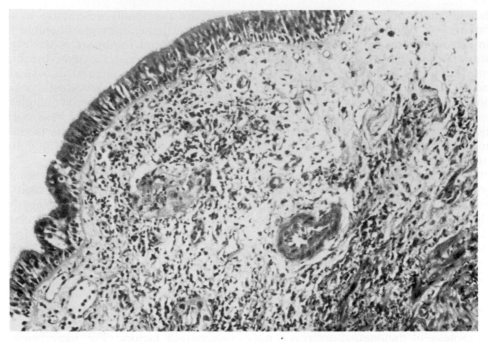

Figure 6 Synovium from the knee of a patient with rheumatoid arthritis. There is thickening of the synovial lining which is normally one or two cells thick. The subsynovium is infiltrated with chronic inflammatory cells

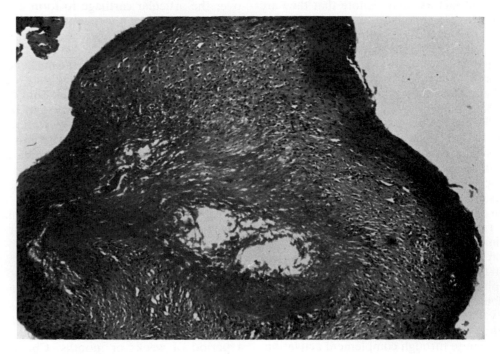

Figure 7   A Subcutaneous rheumatoid nodule. There is a central necrotic surrounded by layers of histiocytes, fibrocytes, and chronic inflammatory cells

However, in the elderly, an explosive onset is common (Brown and Sones, 1967) and initial shoulder involvement is often a feature (Ehrlich, Katz, and Cohen, 1970). This form of presentation creates confusion and is easily mistaken for polymyalgia rheumatica (Dimant, 1979; Weinberger, 1980), or shoulder–hand syndrome (Ehrlich, Katz, and Cohen, 1970). Involvement of a single large joint before obvious polyarticular disease is less characteristic but has also been described as more common in the elderly (Oka and Kytila, 1957). Recurrent acute and transient arthritis is sometimes referred to as palindromic rheumatism, but 25 per cent. of such cases evolve into rheumatoid arthritis.

No synovial joint is immune from involvement, including those of the cervical spine. Symmetrical joint swelling due to synovial thickening and effusions precede deformities due to contractures or subluxation. The small joints of the extremities often bear the brunt with typical ulnar deviation of the hands, subluxation of the metacarpophalangeal joints, or boutonnière and swan-neck finger deformities. Subluxation of the metatarsal heads are associated with callus formation and patients complain that foot pain is like walking barefoot on pebbles. Juxtarticular muscle wasting may proceed rapidly leading to profound weakness.

The course of rheumatoid disease is highly variable. Some are chronic and either benign or aggressive while others remit spontaneously after a short history. In the elderly, it has been claimed that the disease is milder (Erhlich, Katz, and Cohen, 1970) but this is not predictable. Disease to which a patient has accommodated over many years may become intolerable when added to the frailty and illnesses associated with advancing age.

Large joint involvement may be particularly disabling. Restriction of shoulder movement has a disproportionate effect on upper limb function. Hip, knee, and ankle disease may impair mobility. Chronic distension of the knee joint capsule and ligaments together with cartilage loss may result in severe instability with valgus or varus deformities. Flexion deformities of the elbow and knee are common.

Complications of Articular Disease

Involvement of the cervical spine may cause subluxations at any level but particularly of the atlantoaxial joint (Fig. 8). This occurs in 25 per cent. of patients (Conlon, Isdale, and Rose, 1966) and carries the risk of cervical cord compression in a small percentage (Mathews, 1974). This complication is related to the severity and duration of the arthritis and must always be sought in patients undergoing anaesthesia because cord damage may follow manipulation of the head or neck. The altas may be partly destroyed allowing upward luxation of the axis into the base of the skull. This may cause medullary compression and bulbar palsy. Dysphagia may be the first indication of this problem and has been described almost exclusively in the elderly (Gow and Gibson, 1977).

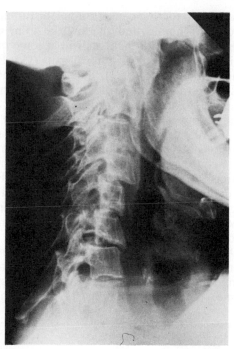

Figure 8 Rheumatoid arthritis affecting the cervical spine and causing anterior subluxation at several levels

Ankylosis of involved joints, including the cervical spine, may be a tendency displayed by patients who have been bedridden for long periods. This finding is also a feature of older patients and has been termed ankylosing rheumatoid arthritis (Grahame *et al.*, 1975).

Popliteal extension of joint effusions (Baker's cysts) may extend into the calf or rupture, causing painful swelling of the calf which simulates deep vein thrombosis. This has been described in other joint diseases but is more commonly a feature of rheumatoid arthritis.

Septic arthritis is a feared yet frequently overlooked complication. It must be suspected whenever a single joint is disproportionately inflamed and especially if there is a focus of infection such as leg or foot ulceration (Morris and Eade, 1978). There is a high mortality rate from this complication.

Involvement of cricoarytenoid and cricothyroid joints may cause hoarseness and in the elderly deafness may be the result of inflammation of the ossicles in the middle ear.

Extra-Articular Complications

In addition to the constitutional disturbance which may herald and shadow the joint disease, 76 per cent. of patients will at some time exhibit involvement of other organs (Gordon, Stein, and Broder, 1973). Subcutaneous nodules over the ulnar border of the forearms, occiputs, Achilles tendons, and buttocks are common but may be more widespread and affect internal organs. Other common skin manifestations are palmar and nail fold erythema. Cutaneous vasculitis may be manifest by small infarcts around the margins of the nails (Fig. 9), digital infarction, and leg ulceration (Fig. 10). Digital vessels may be narrowed by intimal hyperplasia, a picture which is distinct from vasculitis.

Ocular involvement may take different forms. Episcleritis and scleritis are more common in those with associated Sjogren's syndrome (McGavin *et al.*, 1976). Corneal

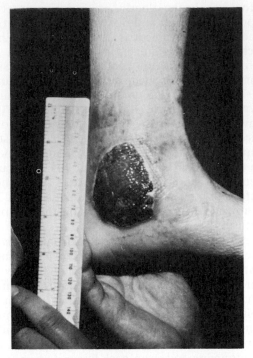

Figure 10   A large ulcer over the medial malleolus. This was caused by rheumatoid vasculitis

ulceration, keratolysis, and perforation may also occur.

Lymph node enlargement is common and may raise the suspicion of lymphoma. Splenomegaly may be a concomitant feature and when associated with neutropenia constitutes the picture of Felty's syndrome. This usually occurs in patients with severe joint disease but may become manifest when the arthritis is quiescent. It is associated with leg ulceration, positive tests for antinuclear factor, and increased susceptibility to infection (Barnes, Turnbull, and Vernon-Roberts, 1971).

The most common neurological complication is carpal tunnel syndrome. A mild sensory peripheral neuropathy is common and of no great consequence. A more severe mixed neuropathy or mononeuritis multiplex are also features and are associated with a poor prognosis. Peripheral neuropathies tend to occur in association with evidence of cutaneous vasculitis, nodules, and high titres of IgM rheumatoid factor (Chamberlain and Bruckner, 1970).

Sjögren's syndrome may be associated with all connective tissue diseases or may exist as an entity (sicca syndrome). Chronic inflam-

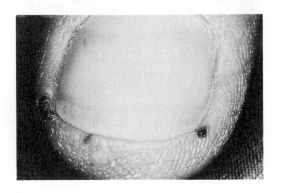

Figure 9   Nail-fold infarcts as a manifestation of cutaneous vasculitis in a patient with rheumatoid arthritis

matory cell infiltration and fibrosis of the salivary, mucosal, and lachrymal glands have the expected result of dry eyes and mouth. Elderly subjects in general and 50 per cent. of women over the age of 80 have keratoconjunctivitis sicca, so dry eyes and a positive Schirmer test in this age group does not necessarily denote the presence of Sjögren's syndrome (Whaley *et al.*, 1972).

Osteoporosis is usual in bone adjacent to inflamed joints but may be a generalized phenomenon. It is not clear whether this reflects disuse or is a more direct manifestation of the disease. The natural thinning of the skeleton with age may thus be accelerated and spontaneous fractures of long bones (Fig. 11) and wedging of vertebrae are frequent.

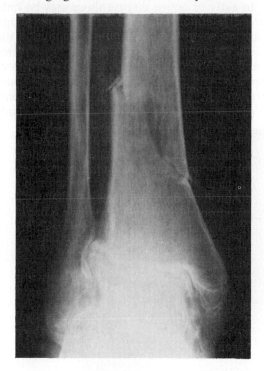

Figure 11 Fracture of the tibia in a patient with osteoporosis and rheumatoid arthritis. Note the severe arthritis of the ankle joint

Internal organ involvement only rarely causes symptoms but may be detected frequently when sought. The lungs may be affected by exudative pleural effusions (Fig. 12), the most striking characteristic of which is their low glucose content. The lung parenchyma may be involved by fibrosis of the lower zones. Rheumatoid nodules may occur as isolated lesions when they need to be distinguished from tumours. When multiple, they may coalesce and cavitation occurs occasionally. Multiple nodules are more common among men with a history of exposure to industrial dusts (Caplan's syndrome). Smokers may be more prone to pulmonary complications but airways obstruction occurs more frequently than can be attributed to smoking alone (Geddes, Webley, and Emerson, 1979).

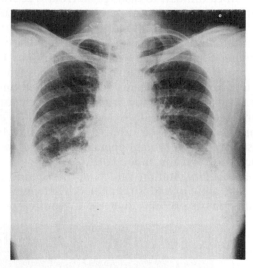

Figure 12 Pleural effusions and lower zone pulmonary fibrosis in a patient with rheumatoid arthritis

The heart may rarely be affected in a clinical sense. Pericarditis occurs in a third of patients at some time but only rarely gives rise to symptoms. Constrictive pericarditis is exceedingly rare, occurs more often in men, and is often wrongly attributed to right heart failure (Burney *et al*, 1979). Valvular dysfunction and conduction defects due to endocardial and myocardial granulomata are equally rare causes of symptoms.

Renal dysfunction may be apparent in a large number of patients but this may be partly the effect of drugs causing reversible impairment or an interstitial nephritis. Heavy proteinuria, if not attributable to drug treatment, may imply amyloid nephropathy. The presence of amyloid deposition on rectal biopsy is highly indicative of this disorder but a negative result does not preclude the diagnosis which may be established only by renal biopsy (Hajzok, Tomik, and Hajzokova, 1976).

Investigation

There are a wide number of investigations which are helpful in determining the severity of the disease and monitoring its progress. Few are of diagnostic value.

Anaemia is usual in active disease and responds promptly to effective control of the disease process. The red cells are hypochromic and associated with a low serum iron. It is therefore difficult to distinguish from true iron deficiency which may also be present as a result of gastrointestinal blood loss secondary to anti-inflammatory drugs. An elevated iron-binding capacity or low serum ferritin may be helpful discriminating investigations but, when equivocal, iron deficiency may be gauged only be determining marrow iron stores. In the anaemia of rheumatoid disease these tend to be normal or increased. Active disease may be associated with lymphopenia, polymorph leucocytosis, and thrombocytosis.

The sedimentation rate is a good guide to disease activity and is paralleled by changes of acute phase proteins such as C-reactive pro-tein. The latter has been claimed to represent a better indicator of joint damage (Amos *et al.*, 1977).

Serum protein electrophoresis usually reveals elevation of all immunoglobulin levels. A positive rheumatoid latex test for IgM rheumatoid factor is by no means diagnostic. The sheep cell agglutination test (Rose Waaler test) is marginally more specific and high titres are very suggestive of rheumatoid arthritis. Tests for antinuclear antibodies are positive in 10 per cent. but DNA binding and the Crithidia test for antibodies against double stranded DNA are negative. Serum complement levels are normal except where there is much extra-articular vasculitis and prima facie evidence of immune complex deposition.

In early or active disease there may be mild liver enzyme abnormalities and serum albumin tends to be lowered. Radiology provides the best available information about disease progression and response to treatment. X-rays of hands and feet in early disease may reveal unexpected loss of joint cartilage and erosions, even at sites devoid of pain. The small joints

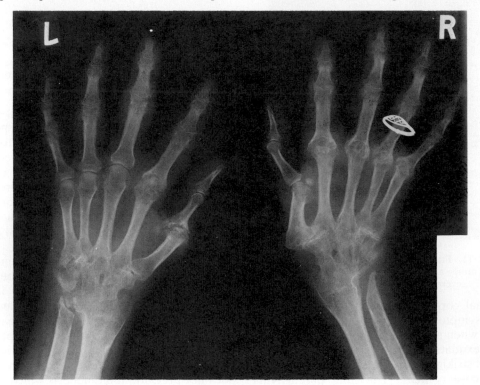

Figure 13　Rheumatoid arthritis. Erosive changes have caused extensive damage to the metacarpophalangeal joints and ulnar styloids. The carpi have been resorbed and ankylosed

of the extremities and the ulnar styloids are common sites of early damage. Loss of joint space, erosions, osteoporosis, and subluxations may be seen at any involved joint. Loss of bone may be extreme, especially at the wrists where whole carpi may disappear (Fig. 13). Ankylosis may be a feature but clinically stiff joints are not usually the result of bony anky-losis. At the hips, concentric loss of cartilage is characteristic of inflammatory joint disease in general and contrasts with the more common picture in osteoarthritis where the loss is most evident on the superior, weight-bearing aspect. Views of the cervical spine must be taken in flexion so that subluxations may be more easily demonstrable. Cord compression does not correlate with the severity of atlan-toaxial subluxation.

Treatment

General

Many elderly patients with rheumatoid disease cope with their illness throughout middle age but then find that declining reserve, concomi-tant diseases and changing social factors such as the loss of an active spouse, force them to seek help.

As in osteoarthritis, rest is an important component of treatment. This may be achieved at home by ensuring patients spend some time each day either lying flat or at least in a com-fortable chair. When warranted, complete bed-rest can lessen disease activity dramati-cally. For those who lack help at home, and this applies to large numbers of the elderly, hospital admission is the only way of achieving this.

Rest of specific joints may be obtained by splinting and when this is combined with bed-rest, disease activity may be contained by such measures alone (Partridge and Duthie, 1963). A week in bed is usually adequate and in the elderly should not exceed this because of the risks of accelerated muscle wasting, osteopo-rosis and bed sores. Muscle strengthening exercises, especially of the quadriceps, are im-portant during periods of enforced rest. In hos-pital, these can be easily encouraged by a physiotherapist but it is useful for patients to be familiarized with exercises they can perform at home. These need to be simple and the

objectives carefully explained. Balancing the respective roles of exercise and rest may be difficult, but in the elderly patient the import-ance of physical treatment and an aggressive approach to rehabilitation have been emphas-ized (Nastro, 1969; Steele, 1970).

Specific

All patients with rheumatoid disease require drug treatment at some time. Non-steroidal anti-inflammatory drugs are the sheet-anchor. Some of the choices have been summarized in the section on osteoarthritis. It is worth em-phasizing that those preparations which have a long half life and which need to be given only once or twice daily have an obvious advantage for the elderly (Mowat, 1979). Suppositories used at night may lessen early morning symp-toms but the aged patient is often unable to insert these. Patients with xerostomia due to Sjögren's syndrome may experience great dif-ficulty in swallowing tablets and so liquid prep-arations such as benorylate should be considered. There is evidence that patients with Sjögren's syndrome are more prone to drug toxicity. It is also possible that adverse effects are in general more common in the elderly (Hurwitz, 1969). Non-steroidal anti-in-flammatory drugs may produce a large number of side-effects, the most common of which are gastrointestinal intolerance, gastric bleeding, peptic ulceration, and rashes. Intolerance or lack of efficacy with one preparation does not preclude the use of others and it is fortunate that the choice is wide. These drugs lessen joint inflammation but do not have a more fundamental effect on the disease process as manifest by reductions of ESR or rheumatoid factor. Such claims have been made but the evidence is not wholly convincing.

So called second-line drugs such as sodium aurothiomalate, D-penicillamine, the antima-larials (chloroquine and hydroxychlorine), im-munosuppressives, and levamisole do exhibit a different mode of action. Their delayed res-ponse together with improvements of labora-tory indices of disease activity suggest that they are capable of altering the course of the ar-thritis (Highton *et al.*, 1981).

Complete remissions may be achieved with some of these drugs and radiological deterio-ration may be halted (Gibson *et al.*, 1976).

This belief has prompted their earlier use before permanent joint damage has occurred. The risks of serious toxicity have in the past deterred their use but increased experience and careful monitoring have lessened the chances of life-threatening side-effects. These treatments should not be denied to elderly patients whose response may be excellent (Ehrlich, Katz, and Cohen, 1970).

Sodium aurothiomalate and D-penicillamine are equally efficacious. Gold injections lessen the chances of poor patient compliance which may be a problem among the elderly. The conventional approach involves a test dose of 10 mg followed by weekly injections of 50 mg until substantial improvement or a total of 1.0 g has been achieved. Maintenance injections of the same dose at monthly or more frequent intervals may help to sustain improvements. Unfortunately, the incidence of toxicity is high in the first 6 months of treatment and up to half may be withdrawn for this reason. Lack of effect is often encountered and relapse may occur despite maintenance therapy. Various permutations of dose and frequency of injection have been attempted to overcome these problems but without obvious benefit (Griffin *et al.*, 1981; McKenzie, 1981). A flexible regime does not necessarily confer a better chance of uninterrupted treatment.

Side-effects are, in order of frequency, skin rashes, proteinuria, mouth ulcers, thrombocytopenia, and bone marrow suppression. Tests of urine and blood counts are mandatory precautions to be performed before or at the time of each injection. Reintroduction of sodium aurothiomalate at a smaller dose may be attempted when side-effects have resolved. Recurrence of toxicity demands that the treatment be abandoned. D-penicillamine has a similar range of major side-effects but rashes tend to be less common and less severe. Loss of taste is frequent but is usually restored despite continued treatment. The incidence of side-effects is reduced by starting treatment with 125 mg daily and increasing the dose by 125 mg increments at monthly intervals. Response is often achieved with a total daily dose of 750 mg or less but doses up to 1.0 g may be necessary. The precautions advised for gold therapy are equally important for D-penicillamine. Some authorities have advocated continuance of treatment when proteinuria occurs but this policy is imprudent because nephrotic syndrome may be a severe, debilitating complication.

The antimalarials are of certain benefit but somewhat less effective than gold. Side-effects include gastrointestinal intolerance, headaches, and ocular toxicity. Corneal and retinal deposition occur and the latter constitutes a serious risk of blindness. All patients receiving antimalarials must therefore have an ophthalmic examination every 4 to 6 months. Evidence of retinal change demands withdrawal of treatment. This complication has discouraged wider use of antimalarials. It occurs in approximately 10 per cent., is related to the dose and duration of treatment, and may be an increased risk in the elderly (Marks and Power, 1979).

A number of immunosuppressive agents have been used to treat rheumatoid disease. Azathioprine is the most popular and is probably as effective as gold and penicillamine but is more toxic (Berry *et al.*, 1976; Dwosh *et al.*, 1977). Cyclophosphamide and chlorambucil have also been employed but are limited to a greater extent by adverse effects. All of these drugs are potentially oncogenic. Levamisole is also much limited by its toxicity which includes bone marrow suppression. The place of this drug, if any, has not yet been defined.

Corticosteroids are deprecated in chronic rheumatic diseases. Intra-articular injections of long-acting preparations are useful adjuncts to treatments when a small number of joints is active. They may also be used to inject inflamed tendon sheaths. Their effect tends to last no longer than several weeks. In cases where all other therapeutic avenues have been reasonably explored, systemic corticosteroids in small doses have a role. In elderly patients who would be otherwise immobile their use may be fully justified.

Severe skin ulcers or life-threatening complications of vasculitis are refractory to treatment with oral corticosteroids. When given as a series of intravenous pulses of 1.0 g methylprednisolone they may be effective. Some advocate the concurrent intravenous administration of cyclophosphamide. In general, leg ulcers are resistant to treatment and skin grafting may effect only temporary improvement.

The rehabilitation of elderly patients with rheumatic diseases, and especially rheumatoid

arthritis, demands a disproportionate investment of time and skills so it is essential to know
what a patient wants and what is practicable
(Ditunno and Ehrlich, 1970). In the United
States, 33 per cent. of females aged between
65 and 74 live alone and this illustrates how
elderly people with joint diseases are disadvantaged in terms of help from a spouse (Rivlin,
1981). Deafness, impaired sight, loss of taste,
inadequate nutrition, and poor housing may
add to social isolation and make attempts at
rehabilitation more difficult. The presence of
other diseases such as strokes, Parkinsonism,
and heart failure may impede attempts to
achieve independence (Schutt, 1977). Hospital
admission and assessment by occupational
therapists and physiotherapists with appropriate instruction and practice are desirable for
those whose disabilities are severe. It must be
remembered that hospital admission may itself
precipitate fresh problems such as falls, untoward drug reactions, and infections in as many
as 30 per cent. of elderly inpatients (Rosin and
Boyd, 1966). Infection in particular must be
rigorously sought and treated since this is the
major single cause of death in rheumatoid arthritis (Rasker and Cosh, 1981). The provision
of aids for walking, toilet, and household tasks
are an important aspect of rehabilitation (see
Fig. 14). A wheelchair may be necessary and
electric models should not be considered impracticable in the elderly (Winyard, Luker,
and Nichols, 1976).

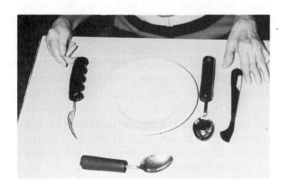

Figure 14   Varieties of eating utensils used by a patient
with rheumatoid arthritis. These are a few of many
available cutlery modifications which allow patients a
better grip

NON-INFLAMMATORY SPINAL DISORDERS

Epidemiology

Pain in the neck or back is the most common
rheumatic complaint and few people escape at
least one episode in a lifetime. In one large
survey, neck and arm pain was present in 21
per cent. and back or sciatic pain in 30 per
cent. of all subjects (Lawrence, 1969). The
self-limiting nature of spinal pain makes it difficult to determine exact prevalence but there
is no convincing evidence that symptoms are
more common in the elderly.

Radiological evidence of lumbar and cervical
disc degeneration increases with age (Kellgren,
1961). Among men, these changes are more
frequent and occur earlier. Between the ages
of 65 to 74, 87 per cent. of males and 74 per
cent. of females have cervical disc degeneration (Lawrence, De Graffe, and Laine, 1963).
A lesser prevalence of 72 per cent. in males
and 65 per cent. in females has been determined in an American population of similar
age (Mikkelsen, Duff, and Dodge, 1970). Disc
degeneration of the lumbar and cervical spine
is more frequent and occurs earlier among men
who have engaged in occupations which involve strenuous physical activity (Lawrence,
1969). There is a broad correlation between
severe X-ray changes and pain, but many subjects with radiological disc disease are asymptomatic. The converse is also true, especially
in young subjects where neck and low back
pain may occur in the absence of X-ray
abnormalities.

Pathology

An appreciation of the anatomy of the spine
makes it clear why radiological abnormalities
may be irrelevant. Pain may derive from soft
tissues such as ligaments, muscles, and nerve
roots as well as from facetal and intervertebral
joints. In the neck, the joints of Luschka,
which are contiguous with the intervertebral
discs, are lined with synovium and may
undergo inflammatory changes in rheumatoid
disease. Osteophytes on vertebral bodies may
be apparent as early as the age of 20 and increase with age thereafter. Over the age of 40

all skeletons exhibit spinal osteophytes which occur mainly on the anterior aspect and are more frequent in males (Nathan, 1962). In the cervical spine these occur predominently on the lower vertebrae where they are often but not invariably associated with disc degeneration. Osteoarthritis of the apophyseal joints tends to affect the upper segment of the cervical spine (Holt and Yates, 1966). In the lumbar spine, osteophytes and disc degeneration predominently affect the lower vertebrae.

The nucleus pulposus of discs undergo qualitative changes with age. The water content and the molecular size of their proteoglycans decrease while keratan sulphate content increases (Adams and Muir, 1976). The gelatinous nucleus becomes more fibrous with age and is eventually indistinguishable from the surrounding annulus. These changes make the disc less able to absorb energy. Stresses are transmitted more readily to the vertebral bodies and the facetal joints. The vertebral end plate cartilage becomes thinned and fibrillated and osteoarthritic changes take place at the facets.

In the elderly, spinal pain is more likely to denote serious pathology although disc degeneration, osteoarthritis of the facets, and soft tissue sprains remain the most common causes. Osteoporosis, osteomalacia, and Paget's disease of vertebral bodies, infection of discs and vertebral osteomyelitis, myelomatosis, and secondary malignant deposits are all more common in this age group and need to be excluded with care (Bandilla, 1977; Davison, 1980; Sarkin, 1977).

NECK PAIN

Clinical Features

Symptoms arising from the neck are often difficult to attribute to precise pathology. Their classification into acute stiff neck, cervical radiculopathy, cervical myelopathy, and vertebro-basilar insufficiency (Jeffreys, 1980) are four acceptable clinical categories which are not mutually exclusive and do not invoke a pathological mechanism.

An acute stiff neck may occur after periods of unaccustomed activity, sleep in awkward positions or prolonged abnormal posture. The pain may be very severe and associated with gross limitation of head rotation. Muscle spasm may be accompanied by slight tilting of the head. Tenderness may be localized or diffuse, extending to the dorsal vertebrae and trapezius muscles. Usually, the pain and stiffness settle spontaneously within a week. When such abrupt symptoms are associated with pain or paraesthesiae referred into the arm or hand, it may be presumed that the cause is an acute cervical disc prolapse. The frequency with which disc prolapse occurs in the absence of radicular symptoms or signs is unknown. Objective evidence of nerve root compression substantiates the diagnosis. Weakness of deltoid or biceps with diminution of the biceps reflex indicates involvement of the C5 root, weakness of wrist extension and diminution of the brachoradialis reflex; that of the C7 root and weakness of grip or finger abduction denote T1 root involvement. Sensory impairment of light touch or pin prick may be found in the distribution of C5, 6, 7 and T1 dermatomes. The natural history is one of spontaneous resolution over a period of 1 to 2 months.

A story of chronic or intermittent neck pain with or without radicular symptoms is more likely to be caused by degenerative changes of the intervertebral or facetal joints (cervical spondylosis). Headache is not uncommon and may be occipital or frontal in distribution. Pain or paraesthesiae may be experienced in the arm, hand, or scapular region. The signs are similar to those described above with a similar pattern of neurological deficit. Diminished reflexes may occur in 16 per cent. and sensory impairment in a similar proportion (Brooker and Barter, 1965). In one study of 50 unselected inpatients of more than 50 years of age it was claimed that 60 per cent. had some neurological abnormality consistent with cervical spondylosis, many in the absence of symptoms (Pallis, Jones, and Spillane, 1954). Head flexion associated with an electric shock sensation in arms or legs (Lermitz's sign) is strongly suggestive of cervical cord compression. Accentuated reflexes, clonus, and an extensor plantar response are certain signs of cervical myelopathy.

Pain or paraesthesiae in the upper arm or hand need to be distinguished from periarthritis of the shoulder, medial and lateral epicondylitis, ulnar nerve lesions, and carpal tunnel syndrome. Painful restriction of the shoulder may be secondary to cervical spondylosis and there is some evidence that carpal tunnel syndrome is more common in patients with narrow spinal canals. Nerve conduction studies may be necessary to differentiate peripheral nerve lesions.

Vertebrobasilar artery narrowing due to atheroma may be accentuated by osteophytic pressure. Symptoms and signs of brain stem ischaemia may be related to head movements (Brain, 1963).

Investigations

Cervical spine X-rays are mandatory. The presence of disc space narrowing and osteophytes are not necessarily related to neck pain but neurological symptoms occur in 0.3 per cent. of subjects with mild and 1.7 per cent. of those with severe radiological changes (Lawrence, 1969). Oblique views may reveal foraminal narrowing due to osteophytes arising from vertebral bodies or facetal joints, and 40 per cent. of such patients may exhibit signs of nerve root compression (Pallis, Jones, and Spillane, 1954). Subluxation may be associated with the risk of myelopathy. In general, cord compression is more likely where there is constitutional or acquired narrowing of the sagittal diameters of the cervical canal and subluxation is associated with the most severe cases of cord compression (Nurick, 1972).

A major purpose of cervical spine X-rays is to rule out serious pathology. Infection will produce loss of disc space and bone destruction with soft tissue shadowing due to abscess formation. Malignant disease or myelomatosis may produce vertebral collapse with little alteration of adjacent disc spaces. Collapse due to metabolic bone disease is unusual in the cervical spine. A chest X-ray is of equal importance and may reveal evidence of past or active tuberculosis, bronchial carcinoma, or secondary deposits. Haemoglobin, ESR, white cell count, serum protein electrophoresis, detection of Bence Jones proteinuria, and bone biochemistry may provide additional evidence of serious disease. Pancoast tumours must not be overlooked as a cause of neck and arm pain. The concurrence of Horner's syndrome is a helpful clue to this diagnosis but ESR estimations may be normal (Wilson, 1979). Where

there is evidence of cord compression, cervical myelography will delineate the level of the lesion. In suspected infection of the cervical spine, blood culture, antistaphylolysin titres, and a Mantoux test may help to determine the organism. Where serious disease is suspected and X-rays are normal, [99]technetium bone scanning may define the site of abnormality. Areas of the spine defined either by X-ray or bone scan may be biopsied under X-ray control, thereby yielding tissue for histology and culture.

Treatment

In acute, self limiting neck pain with or without root symptoms, the principal aim is pain relief. This may be partially achieved by analgesics and non-steroidal anti-inflammatory drugs. The provision of a soft collar for use at night and a firmer collar for the day may be helpful. Some patients may prefer to provide head support at night by making a deep hollow in a pillow. More than one pillow increases the chance of stretching painful tissue during sleep and should be discouraged. Manual traction, heat applications, and vertebral 'mobilization' by anteroposterior manipulation of the vertebral bodies may help to relieve muscle spasm. Vigorous rotational manipulations may relieve acute neck pain in a dramatic fashion but should not be attempted in the presence of neurological symptoms or signs. Physical treatments such as traction, short-wave diathermy, collars, and exercises do not appreciably influence the natural history of acute neck pain (BAPM, 1966; Goldie and Landquist, 1970). Sleep should be ensured by prescription of an hypnotic if necessary.

The chronic or intermittent discomfort of cervical spondylosis may be managed in an identical fashion. Fortunately, most patients do not have persistent, severe pain. Even so, frequent exacerbations of symptoms and the interruptions of sleep which may ensue create tiredness and depression. It is often tempting for doctors to ascribe intractable neck pain to depression but this merely reflects the inadequacy of available treatments. Antidepressant drugs may be useful in lightening a patient's mood and making symptoms more tolerable.

Spinal decompression and spinal fusion may be warranted in the face of cord compression.

Serious pathology warrants treatment of the underlying disease process.

BACK PAIN

Clinical Features

Many of the considerations discussed in relation to the source of neck pain apply to back pain. The ubiquitous presence of lumbar disc degeneration and vertebral osteophytosis may be unrelated to symptoms. Nevertheless, as in cervical spondylosis, nerve root compression is slightly more likely to occur in those with severe X-ray changes (Lawrence, 1969).

Acute back pain and stiffness may arise from the structures outlined for neck pain but pain or paraesthesiae referred into the buttock or leg are very likely to imply nerve root compression. When such symptoms are acute it is reasonable to assume that the cause is a lumbar disc prolapse, although it is possible that pain arising from ligaments, facetal joints, or muscle may be distributed in a similar fashion (Kellgren, 1977). In the elderly, such acute symptoms are less common than in younger subjects. This may partly be due to an absence of occupational factors such as lifting heavy loads and partly to the less gelatinous structure of the nucleus pulposus. Pain may extend in a sciatic (sciatica) or femoral nerve (cruralgia) distribution and the latter may be a more common feature of back pain in the elderly. Referred pain accentuated by coughing or straining suggest nerve root irritation.

Back pain is invariably associated with restriction of lumbosacral movement. A scoliosis is usually functional and when associated with nerve root compression is often accentuated by forward flexion. Alternatively, it may be due to disparities of leg length which cause tilting of the pelvis to the short side. Measurement of leg length is therefore an important aspect of spinal examination and shortening of one limb may be constitutional or secondary to hip disease. Long-standing scoliosis leads to disc degeneration, osteophytosis on the concave aspect of the curvature, and to backache. Spinal tenderness is often diffuse and may be experienced over the sacroiliac joints and buttocks, some distance from the site of the problem. Unilateral restriction of straight leg raising and increased pain on dorsiflexion of the foot are good indicators of sciatic nerve root irritation. Pain in the thigh or back on flexing the knee with the patient lying prone may denote femoral nerve root involvement (femoral nerve stretch test). Wasting or weakness of the quadriceps and reduction of the knee jerk implicate L3, 4 nerve root compression, while wasting or weakness of the calf and a diminished ankle jerk suggest S1 root compression. Weakness of foot eversion and of extensor hallucis longus indicate L5 involvement. Sensory impairment usually conforms to one or more dermatomes but when pain is severe, sensory changes may affect the whole limb.

Pain which is worse on lying down and relieved by sitting or walking should suggest the possibility of an intraspinal tumour. Pain in the back, buttock, or leg which is induced by walking and relieved by rest may be mistaken for peripheral vascular disease. So-called intermittent claudication of the cauda equina is usually a feature of lumbar spinal stenosis. This clinical picture is most often seen in the elderly and is due to large osteophytes or bulging discs encroaching on the spinal canal. It may also be seen in Paget's disease, spondylolisthesis, or any condition which occludes the canal. Back pain and stiffness which is worse at night or in the morning suggest sacroiliitis but the diseases which cause inflammatory spinal disease almost always begin in youth or middle age.

Investigation

Plain X-rays of the lumbosacral spine, pelvis, and chest are the minimal investigations for severe or persistent back pain. These may reveal any of the serious pathologies outlined for neck pain. Spondylolisthesis may be associated with disc degeneration or defects of the pars interarticularis which are best visualized by oblique views of the spine. A view of the pelvis is often neglected but is important because it may be the site of infectious or neoplastic disease causing back pain. Sacroiliitis may be manifest by sclerosis and irregularity of the sacroiliac joint margins and hip disease may be demonstrated. Where the clinical picture or the additional investigations referred to in the discussion of neck pain suggest serious disease, a bone scan and needle biopsy may help to establish the diagnosis. In those rare instances where recent back pain of the elderly has the characteristic features of sacroiliitis, a quantified scintiscan of the sacroiliac joints may confirm the suspicion of inflammation. Osteoporosis in the elderly may make it difficult to define the margins of the sacroiliac joints on X-ray.

When there is diagnostic uncertainty or surgical intervention is contemplated, the level and nature of any lesion causing nerve root compression may be defined by injection of X-ray contrast material into the subarachnoid space. Radiculography using a water soluble material has largely replaced myelography with oil-based media. The advantages include rapid clearance and better definition of nerve root pouches. One disadvantage is the risk of convulsions. Lumbar puncture headaches are a common side-effect. Other techniques using contrast material for outlining the nerve roots include spinal venography and epidurography (McCormick, 1978). A clearer picture of the status of intervertebral discs may be obtained by discography but this procedure is painful and only rarely demanded.

Nerve conduction studies are advocated by some as a means of defining the distribution of nerve root involvement. This approach may be useful in distinguishing root pain due to diabetic radiculopathy when radiculography is normal (Child and Yates, 1978). Ultrasound has been used to measure the dimensions of the spinal canal and provides a potential non-invasive assessment for suspected spinal stenosis. Computerized axial tomography scans – also have a role in this context as well as in the investigation of root compression.

Treatment

The vast majority of episodes of back pain resolve spontaneously within days and most patients do not consult their practitioners. For those with persistent discomfort, modified activities, simple analgesics, and local applications of heat at home suffice for the majority. Some patients are susceptible to recurrent episodes which may be induced by physical activities such as gardening or lengthy car journeys. For these, prevention may be achieved by advising that such activities be interspersed with frequent rest periods. Patients with pro-

longed backache are often referred to hospital. For this minority, the investigations outlined above are essential.

The treatment of persistent back pain in the absence of radicular symptoms and signs is empirical. Hospital experience suggests that even including those with root symptoms, less than 10 per cent. will require· surgery or become regular attenders (Currey *et al.*, 1979). A survey of physiotherapy departments in the United Kingdom revealed that back extension exercises and short wave diathermy were the most popular treatments (Anderson, 1978). Other therapies commonly employed are lumbar traction, manipulation, corsets, hydrotherapy, and isometric flexion exercises. All of these may induce some symptomatic improvement but there is no evidence that any alters the natural history of the condition (Mathews and Hickling, 1975; Sims-Williams *et al.*, 1978) nor that one treatment is more effective than another (Doran and Newell, 1975). The difficulty of assessing the comparative value of available treatments is compounded by the heterogeneous pathology of back pain and its natural history (Grahame, 1980). In practice, those few patients with chronic pain who do not have a surgically remediable lesion are offered successive treatments. The whole range of 'remedies' may be exhausted in these unfortunate individuals.

Patients with acute pain and symptoms or objective evidence of nerve root compression are most likely to have a lumbar disc protrusion. Such symptoms may be preceded by less specific back pain and, in a sense, the advent of root symptoms makes management easier because the pathology can be surmised. Rest in bed is the most effective means of inducing improvement. For those who insist upon remaining ambulant, a surgical corset may provide partial relief. If facilities permit, bed-rest in hospital is desirable for those who cannot be nursed at home. Epidural injections of corticosteroid preparations can speed resolution of pain and encourage an earlier return to normal activities (Dilke, Burry, and Grahame, 1973; Yates, 1978). Intermittent claudication of the cauda equina may also be helped by this measure, but long-term relief usually requires surgical decompression of the narrow spinal canal. For patients with proven disc protrusions who fail to respond to rest, a corset, epidural injection, or the physical treatments which are often prescribed for lumbar disc protrusions, discectomy with or without laminectomy, is warranted. Injection of chymopapain into the lumbar discs (chemonucleolysis) is an alternative conservative approach which is practised in a few centres and has been claimed to offer benefits over laminectomy (Nordby and Lucas, 1973). Spondylolisthesis with nerve root compression may respond temporarily to an epidural injection but a corset is the best long-term treatment. In the elderly, this condition is usually associated with marked disc degeneration and osteoarthritis of the facetal joints. Surgical fusion of the subluxing vertebra therefore carries a diminished chance of relieving pain and is not readily contemplated by orthopaedic surgeons.

DISSEMINATED SKELETAL HYPEROSTOSIS

Disseminated skeletal hyperostosis is essentially a radiological entity since many patients with this finding are free of symptoms. Large osteophytes bridge the intervertebral space, superficially resembling the syndesmophytes of ankylosing spondylitis (Fig. 15). The frequency of the finding increases with age and was detected in 12 per cent. of one series of autopsy subjects (Vernon Roberts, Pirie, and Trenwith, 1974). The dorsal spine is predominently affected but the cervical and lumbar regions may also be involved. The osteophytes occur mainly on the anterolateral margins of the vertebrae. Characteristically, the disc spaces are preserved and although the bone outgrowths appear to be ankylosed with each other on X-ray, they rarely are (Vernon Roberts, Pirie, and Trenwith, 1974). Pain or stiffness of the spine tends to be absent or mild. Limitation of spinal movement may be moderate to severe (Harris *et al*, 1974). Haematological and biochemical investigations are normal although the prevalence may be increased among diabetics (Julkunen, Heinmann, and Pyorola, 1971). X-rays of other areas of the skeleton may reveal fluffy new bone formation at the insertion of muscles and tendons (Utsinger and Shapiro, 1976). The osteophytes may on occasion be sufficiently large to cause dysphagia (Meeks and Renshaw, 1973) and when they occur to any extent on the posterior aspect of

the cervical spine, there is a risk of cord compression (Gibson and Schumacher, 1976). Specific treatment is not usually necessary.

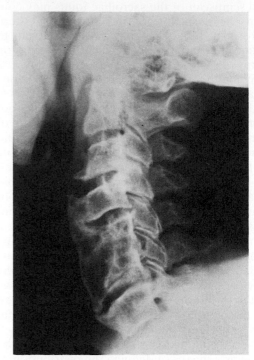

Figure 15 Ankylosing hyperostosis of the cervical spine showing large anterior osteophytes which bridge the disc spaces

ANKYLOSING SPONDYLITIS

Epidemiology

The prevalence of ankylosing spondylitis in two separate surveys has been estimated to be 0.4 per cent. in males and 0.05 per cent. for females (Lawrence, 1963; Mikkelsen *et al*., 1967). The maximal prevalence occurs between the ages of 40 and 59, beyond which it is of the order of 0.3 per cent. (Mikkelsen *et al*., 1967). This frequency and the male predominance has been challenged by reference to all subjects who carry the HLA B27 antigen. Assessment of genetically susceptible populations has suggested that the frequency of ankylosing spondylitis has been underestimated and many less than florid examples remain unrecognized (Calin and Fries, 1975). Most patients develop the disease in their second and third decades but since it does not materially affect life expectancy, a number of elderly patients experience the sequelae of this inflammatory spinal disorder.

The prevalence among non-Caucasian populations is less than the figures quoted above. This reflects the racial distribution of the antigen HLA B27 which is found less frequently among populations where ankylosing spondylitis is uncommon.

Pathology

Approximately 95 per cent. of Caucasian patients with ankylosing spondylitis carry the antigen HLA B27. This is but one of several hundred genes on the major histocompatibility complex segment of the sixth chromosome. Relatively few of these have so far been identified. Those which have been designated to the three series HLA, A, B and C are found on the surface of most cells. By contrast, the HLA DR series (see the section on rheumatoid arthritis) has a more restricted distribution.

Although peripheral arthritis with synovial inflammatory changes similar to those seen in rheumatoid arthritis occurs, it is the axial skeleton which is principally involved. The essential pathological changes are currently considered to be distinct from rheumatoid disease and occur not in synovium but at the insertion of ligaments and muscles. This concept is embodied in the term 'enthesopathy'. A low-grade inflammatory process is followed by a striking tendency to ossification. Bilateral sacroiliitis leading to bony ankylosis is the pathological hallmark. Ossification of the outer margins of the discs often begins at the dorsilumbar junction, but the cervical spine or other areas may be strikingly involved in the early stages. Spinal ligaments and facetal joints become involved in the process of ossification which may be limited or extend throughout the spine.

It has been long recognized that some patients with inflammatory bowel disease, Reiter's syndrome, and psoriatic arthropathy may develop sacroiliitis and a clinical picture which is indistinguishable from idiopathic ankylosing spondylitis. In these instances there remains a strong association with HLA B27. It is reasonable to assume that since recognizable diseases and infections seem to initiate the spondylitis in these related disorders, there must be some initiating event in those cases where the disease appears in isolation. An association between active disease and the isolation of faecal *Klebsiella aerogenes* has been claimed (Eastmond *et al.*, 1982; Ebringer *et al.*, 1978).

Clinical Manifestations

Although the disease usually begins in youth, it may go unrecognized until late life. In one series, less than 2 per cent. of cases developed symptoms for the first time beyond the age of 50 (Wilkinson and Bywaters, 1958). Spinal pain, especially low back pain, begins insidiously and is associated with stiffness. Both symptoms are characteristically worse in the morning or may awaken the patient at night. Elderly patients with the clinical and radiological features of ankylosing spondylitis may have inactive disease with little pain and indeed may recall no such history. Examination reveals limited movement of the spine and usually little else.

Peripheral arthritis, most commonly of knees and ankles, occurs in about 20 per cent. of patients at some time and may be the initial complaint. Involvement of other peripheral joints occurs and joint deformities may be a feature.

Anterior uveitis occurs in 25 per cent. of patients. Aortic regurgitation, other heart valve involvement, and conduction defects are rare and related to chronic severe disease, usually accompanied by peripheral joint involvement. Such extra-articular complications may become manifest in those with disease which remains active in late life. Apical pulmonary fibrosis is another rare extra-articular manifestation but is of little consequence.

In general, the activity of the disease lessens after a period of several years. Onset of eye inflammation or peripheral arthritis is exceptional in the elderly (Wilkinson and Bywaters, 1958). Despite a disease of more than 20 years' duration, severe deformities are uncommon and functional capacity tends to be little impaired.

With the advance of osteoporosis related to ageing, spines which are severely involved by ankylosis are susceptible to fracture after trauma. Cord compression may result from this dramatic sequel. Intermittent claudication of the cauda equina may also occur as a late complication (Young *et al.*, 1981).

Investigation

The clinical suspicion of ankylosing spondylitis can best be confirmed radiologically. Back pain and stiffness due to non-inflammatory causes may sometimes be difficult to distinguish on a clinical basis. In the elderly modest elevation of ESR is not a reliable guide to the existence of spondylitis but values in excess of 40 mm/hr may point the clinician in the right direction.

The X-ray appearance may be confused with ankylosing hyperostosis because in the elderly the syndesmophytes of ankylosing spondylitis are thicker than in younger subjects (Lawrence, 1977). The presence of unequivocal sacroiliitis on pelvic X-ray is confirmatory. Unfortunately, the sacroiliac joints may be poorly visualized in elderly patients because of adjacent osteoporosis. Furthermore, degenerative changes at this site may simulate sacroiliitis causing loss of joint space, subchondral sclerosis, and occasional ankylosis (Resnick, Hiwayama, and Goergen, 1977). The cervical spine is less likely to be involved when the disease begins late in life and erosions of the margins of the vertebral bodies (Romanus lesions) are less common (Riley, Ansel, and Bywaters, 1971). The vertebral bodies may acquire a square shape but, by itself, this is not a helpful radiological sign. X-rays of peripheral joints, especially the hips, may reveal loss of cartilage. Joint erosions are uncommon but do occur. New bone formation may occur at sites of muscle and tendon insertion.

Quantified scintiscans of the sacroiliac joints after withdrawal of anti-inflammatory drugs may indicate active inflammation if X-rays are unhelpful. Tissue typing may weight the evidence in favour of spondylitis if HLA B27 is present, but this finding is in no sense diagnostic.

Treatment

General

The majority of elderly patients with spondylitis have relatively quiescent disease but are likely to be troubled by spinal stiffness. Daily exercise of the spine is recommended. Marginal increases of movements may thus be achieved and there is reason to believe that regular exercise, preferably after instruction by a physiotherapist, can retard the process of stiffening.

Specific

Pain and stiffness often respond dramatically to indomethacin or phenylbutazone. The latter should not be used in elderly patients. Gastric intolerance, headaches, or other central nervous system side-effects demand replacement of indomethacin with other non-steroidal anti-inflammatory drugs. These tend to be less effective than indomethacin.

Irradiation of the sacroiliac joints and spine is no longer employed on a regular basis because of the risks of leukaemia and other malignant diseases. These do not apply so readily to elderly patients and in the rare instances where symptoms cannot be contained by anti-inflammatory drugs, or where these are contraindicated, it is a justifiable remedy.

OTHER SPONDYLARTHROPATHIES

These represent a group of clinical by clinically related disorders in which sacroiliitis and ankylosing spondylitis are variable features. Their prevalence is uncertain. The pathology of the peripheral joints is indistinguishable from that of rheumatoid arthritis and that of the spine is the same as idiopathic ankylosing spondylitis. The granulomata associated with rheumatoid arthritis do not occur.

Psoriatic Arthropathy

Clinical Features

Approximately 10 per cent. of patients with psoriasis will develop joint inflammation. The age of onset is similar to that of rheumatoid arthritis with a peak between 36 and 45 years. However, 10 per cent. begin beyond the age of 66 and unlike rheumatoid arthritis the sex distribution is equal (Roberts *et al.*, 1976). There are no special characteristics of the disease when it begins in the elderly. In 70 per cent. of patients there is an asymmetrical peripheral arthritis affecting a few joints. Large and small joints may be involved. Inflammation of the distal interphalangeal joints is characteristic but is rarely the sole feature (Moll and Wright, 1973). Involved digits may assume a sausage shape. Psoriatic nail changes are more common in psoriatic arthritis than in psoriasis without arthritis and there is some relationship between nail dystrophy and distal interphalangeal arthritis (Green *et al.*, 1981). The pattern of joint involvement may resemble rheumatoid arthritis in 5 per cent. of cases and this is sometimes severely destructive (arthritis mutilans).

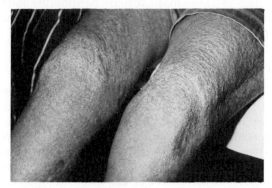

Figure 16 Severe psoriasis with arthritis of both knees

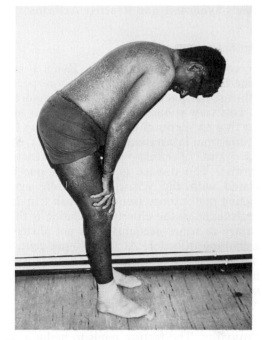

Figure 17 Psoriatic arthritis with clinical evidence of spondylitis. The patient is attempting forward flexion but his spine is rigid and movement is occuring mainly at the hips

Patients with severe psoriasis (Fig. 16) are probably more likely to develop joint disease but the arthritis may precede skin lesions. In some cases, the rash is restricted to obscure areas such as the scalp, umbilicus, or anal cleft and the diagnosis may be established only after a careful examination of these sites. Radiological evidence of sacroiliitis and spondylitis occurs in 20 to 40 per cent. of patients but clinical features of spinal disease occur in only a quarter of these (Fig. 17).

Extra-articular complications are much less frequent than in rheumatoid disease. Conjunctivitis and anterior uveitis occur rarely. Plantar fasciitis and tenosynovitis are common.

Investigation

There are no specific laboratory tests. Sedimentation rates are usually elevated and a mild anaemia may be a feature of severe disease. Tests for IgM rheumatoid factor are positive no more frequently than in the healthy population. The tissue antigen HLA B27 is found in 30 to 50 per cent. of those with sacroiliitis but is not a feature of those with peripheral arthritis alone.

X-rays of peripheral joints may resemble those of rheumatoid arthritis. Bone lysis may be extreme and may involve the terminal tufts. Changes of sacroiliitis, spondylitis, and fluffy new bone at sites of tendon or muscle insertion are similar to those of idiopathic ankylosing spondylitis, but syndesmophytes tend to arise from the main body of the vertebrae rather than the margins.

Treatment

General management is similar to that of rheumatoid arthritis. Sodium aurothiomalate is effective even in the presence of sacroiliitis. D-penicillamine has not been properly assessed. Antimalarials are contraindicated because they may worsen the rash. The immunosuppressive drugs azathioprine and methotrexate have been shown to be beneficial but their use is confined to those patients in whom severe disease is unresponsive to gold. The frequency of severe disability is much less than that of rheumatoid arthritis and the majority of patients with psoriatic arthropathy have an excellent prognosis.

Reiter's Syndrome and Reactive Arthritis

Clinical Features

The conventional concept of Reiter's syndrome is of an illness comprising non-specific urethritis, peripheral arthritis, and conjunctivitis. This view is hardly tenable since it is now clear that an identical clinical picture may follow intestinal infestation with *Salmonella*, *Shigella*, and *Yersinia* organisms (reactive arthritis). The disease is very much one associated with the young and middle aged, affecting males more frequently than females. Its relevance to the elderly population is that, contrary to some accounts, it is not always a self-limiting disorder. At least 40 per cent. of those affected develop chronic or intermittent joint symptoms (Sairanen, Paronen, and Mahonen, 1969).

When the arthritis is persistent, it follows patterns which are similar to those of psoriatic arthropathy. The picture tends to be intermittent or one of chronic low-grade joint inflammation punctuated by episodic acute arthritis. Conjunctivitis, iritis, plantar fasciitis, tendonitis, or a circinate balanitis may accompany flares of the arthritis. An exfoliative rash (Fig. 18), indistinguishable from pustular psoriasis, may occur on the soles and palms (keratodermia blenorrhagica). Nail changes identical with those of psoriasis may be a feature.

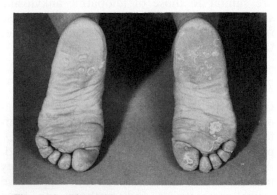

Figure 18   The rash of keratodermia blenorrhagica in a patient with Reiter's syndrome

Sacroiliitis occurs in 20 per cent. of patients and may be associated with the clinical picture of ankylosing spondylitis. Some cases of spondylitis presenting in later life without other symptoms may be examples of Reiter's syndrome in whom a precipitating infection has been overlooked or forgotten.

Investigation

There are no diagnostic tests. There is a strong relationship with the tissue antigen HLA B27 which has been reported in approximately 80 per cent. of patients and unlike psoriatic arthropathy is not confined to those with sacroiliitis. X-rays may reveal peripheral joint erosions and the changes of ankylosing spondylitis.

Treatment

The peripheral arthritis is notoriously resistant to treatment but non-steroidal anti-inflammatory drugs, splints, and intra-articular corticosteroids may ameliorate acute episodes. There is no evidence that the so-called second-line drugs employed in rheumatoid arthritis are helpful. Involvement of the axial skeleton demands the measures outlined for idiopathic ankylosing spondylitis. Profound disability is unusual.

Arthritis of Inflammatory Bowel Disease

A peripheral arthritis occurs in 10 to 20 per cent. of young and middle aged patients with Crohn's disease and ulcerative colitis. This tends to be a problem in the first few years of the illness and to fluctuate with the activity of the bowel disease. A similar pattern of arthritis, perhaps mediated by the same mechanism, has been described in subjects who have undergone intestinal bypass surgery for obesity.

Radiological or bone scan evidence of sacroiliitis occurs in almost half of patients with inflammatory bowel disease. This is asymptomatic in the majority but 4 per cent. of those with Crohn's or ulcerative colitis develop clinical and radiological evidence of ankylosing spondylitis. The tissue antigen HLA B27 occurs in 70 per cent. of these but is not found in association with asymptomatic sacroiliitis. When spondylitis occurs it pursues a course which is independent of the bowel disease and progression may continue into old age. The principles of investigation and management are those of ankylosing spondylitis.

Behcet's Disease

This is a multisystem disorder which shares some of the characteristics of the spondylarthropathies. It is rare in the United States and Europe, occurring more commonly in Japan and the Mediterranean countries. The peak age of onset is similar to that of rheumatoid arthritis. The major clinical features are peripheral arthritis, iritis, aphthous and genital ulceration, erythema nodosum, and central nervous system involvement. It is distinguished from the diseases discussed above by the absence of spondylitis and any clear association with HLA B27. Anti-inflammatory drugs including systemic corticosteroids are the treatments of choice. The activity of the disease tends to regress with age but sequelae such as hemiplegia and blindness may be causes of severe disability in the elderly.

CRYSTAL INDUCED ARTHRITIS

Gout

Epidemiology

The overall prevalence rate for gout is 0.5 per cent. for males and 0.3 per cent. for females with a peak in the fifth and sixth decades (Mikkelsen *et al.*, 1967). The prevalence of gout in females rises after the menopause and more closely approximates that of males. This reflects the distribution curves of blood uric acid levels which peak at an older age in females. The prevalence of hyperuricaemia is approximately 18 per cent. (O'Sullivan, 1972).

Pathology

Acute gout is due to the precipitation of monosodium urate crystals within the joint cavity. It is unlikely that these develop abruptly and under favourable circumstances are released from small tophaceous deposits within the synovium. The slow accumulation of urate crystals in the synovium is invariably the consequence of sustained hyperuricaemia. Tophi are deposited preferentially in the synovial lining of joints and bursae as well as in the cartilage of joints and the pinnae of the ears. When large,

these deposits may replace joint cartilage and excavate subchondral bone.

The causes of hyperuricaemia are many. There is a good correlation of blood uric acid with indices of obesity and alcohol consumption (Gibson and Grahame, 1974). A family history of gout occurs in almost 40 per cent. of cases (Grahame and Scott, 1970) and the majority of gouty subjects exhibit impaired renal clearance of uric acid, a mechanism which probably accounts for their natural susceptibility to hyperuricaemia (Gibson *et al.*, 1980). Diuretics reduce uric acid excretion and are a major cause of hyperuricaemia and gout in the elderly.

Clinical Features

Gout usually presents as an acute monoarthritis. The first metatarsophalangeal joint is the most frequently affected, followed by the ankles, knees, wrists, and other small joints of the extremities. A polyarticular onset is less common but recurrent attacks are more likely to involve several joints simultaneously. Pain is extreme and the taut skin overlying the swollen joint may be hot, shiny, and red. It tends to exfoliate as the arthritis regresses. Each episode is self-limiting, lasting for several days or a few weeks. Attacks may be precipitated by other acute illness or surgical procedures. Some elderly patients present with deforming arthritis and large intra-articular tophi but little pain and no history of acute gout (See Fig. 19). The evident lack of an inflammatory response in these cases is poorly understood (Arnold and Simmons, 1980). Visible tophi on the ears or at other sites are of great diagnostic value.

Hypertension may be a feature in as many as 18 per cent. of gout patients (Gibson *et al.*, 1979). There is disputed evidence that the risks of coronary artery disease are increased, possibly by virtue of the increased prevalence of obesity in gout (Klein *et al.*, 1973). Hypertriglyceridaemia is a frequent finding and mediated by obesity and alcohol abuse (Gibson and Grahame, 1974). Renal calculi are more common but severe renal insufficiency is rare. Renal impairment does occur but tends to be mild and slowly progressive (Fig. 20) (Gibson *et al.*, 1980). Evidence now exists to suggest that hypouricaemic treatment may retard the progression of renal dysfunction, implying that

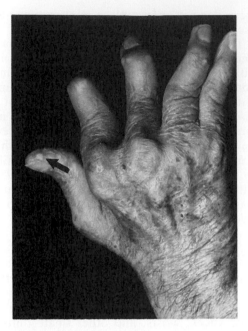

Figure 19 Chronic tophaceous gout in an elderly patient with no history of acute arthritis. There are multiple-joint deformities and tophi are visible beneath the skin on the thumb (arrow)

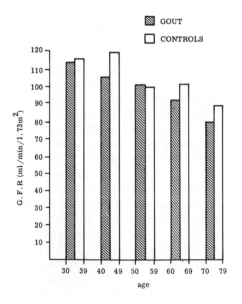

Figure 20 Glomerular filtration rates in gout and age-matched controls. Renal function declines with age in both groups but at a somewhat faster rate in the gouty population. (From Gibson *et al.*, 1980. Reproduced with the kind permission of the Editor of the *Annals of Rheumatic Diseases)*

urate crystal deposition within the renal parenchyma may be implicated (Gibson *et al.*, 1982).

Investigation

The difficulties of establishing a cause of acute arthritis in the elderly have been discussed. Gout may account for 8 per cent. of such cases (Gibson and Grahame, 1973). When only one joint is inflamed the most likely possibilities are pseudo-gout, gout, or sepsis. Aspiration of synovial fluid is the single most important diagnostic step.

In some elderly patients the duration of a joint effusion is often difficult to judge historically and an apparent acute monoarthritis may have been present for some time. Naked eye examination of the fluid may be helpful (see Table 1). A haemarthrosis will become self-evident. Turbid fluid denotes an inflammatory disease process but purulent material does not always imply sepsis. Crystal synovitis may produce a dense effusion which may be distinguished from infection by the identification of crystals. An ordinary light microscope may be adequate to view crystals but a polarizing microscope with a first-order red compensator will allow distinction of monosodium urate from the calcium pyrophosphate crystals of pseudo-gout. Crystals have birefringent properties and a compensator which excludes green will provide a pink background against which urate and pyrophosphate crystals are yellow or blue depending on the direction of their long axes. When aligned with the slow ray of the compensator, urate crystals are brightly yellow (negatively birefringent) and pyrophosphate are blue (positively birefringent). When the crystals are aligned at right angles to the compensator they change to the opposite colour. The colours of pyrophosphate crystals are less brilliant and the transition from blue to yellow on realigning their axes is less striking than with those of urate. Calcium pyrophosphate crystals tend to be chunky and rhomboid whereas those of urate are thin and needle shaped (Fig. 21). However, distinction on a morphological basis is less reliable than on the optical properties. Many of the crystals will be seen residing within white cells. A synovial fluid white cell count, Gram stain, and culture are of inestimable value in discriminating infectious causes of acute arthritis (Table 1). In purulent samples where crystals are not visualized it is best to presume infection. The incidence of septic arthritis is increased in the elderly, especially where there is preexisting joint disease, malignancy, diabetes or other debilitating illness (Newman, 1976; Willkins, Healey, and Decker, 1960). Septic arthritis affects the knee, hip, ankle and sacroiliac joints in that order of frequency (Kelly, Martin, and Coventry, 1970). Where there is a suspicion of infection and Gram's stain reveals no organisms, synovial fluid lactate levels are a rapid and reliable guide to the presence or absence of infection (Behn, Mathews, and Phillips, 1981). Rarely, crystals of both urate and pyrophosphate are found simultaneously. Crystal-induced synovitis has also been described in the presence of septic arthritis (Smith and Phelps, 1972).

Blood uric acid estimation is of obvious importance in the diagnosis of gout when synovial fluid cannot be obtained. However, hyperuricaemia by itself is not diagnostic proof. Diuretic-induced retention of uric acid is so common in the elderly that the concurrence of an acute arthritis cannot be presumed to represent gout unless the clinical picture is unequivocal. Elevation of ESR and a leucocytosis may be present.

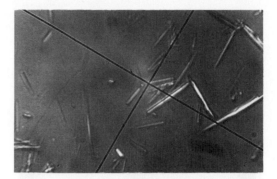

Figure 21 The needle-shaped crystals of monosodium urate. These were obtained from a tophus and there are no surrounding white cells

Radiological examination of involved joints and of the feet may reveal erosions due to tophaceous deposits (Fig. 22).

Treatment

Acute gout demands prompt diagnosis and treatment with anti-inflammatory drugs. Aspirin is contraindicated because in low doses it will accentuate hyperuricaemia. The best choice in the elderly is indomethacin but, when contraindicated, other non-steroidal anti-inflammatory drugs such as naproxen may be used. Colchicine has been superseded because, although very effective, the doses required to

TABLE 1   Characteristics of synovial fluid in different joint disorders

	Appearance	Viscosity	WBC (10^9l)	Polymorphs (%)	Crystals
Haemarthrosis	Blood	—	—	—	—
Sepsis	Turbid — purulent	High or low	>30	>90	None
Osteoarthritis	Clear	High	<2.0	<25	None
Trauma and mechanical joint disease	Clear	High	<2.0	<25	None
Inflammatory joint disease e.g. rheumatoid arthritis	Turbid	Low	>2.0	>90	None
Gout	Turbid — purulent	Low	>2.0	>90	Needle shaped; negative birefringence
Pseudo-gout	Turbid — purulent	Low	>2.0	>90	Rhomboid; weakly positive birefringence

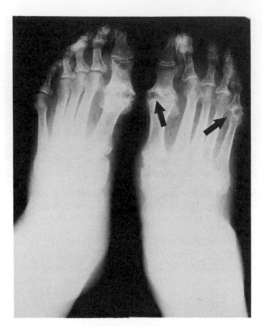

Figure 22   X-rays showing joint erosions (arrows)
caused by chronic tophaceous gout

alleviate an acute episode invariably cause
diarrhoea, nausea, or abdominal cramps. In
low doses, however, it is a useful drug for
preventing recurrences during the early stages
of hypouricaemic treatment. Only when the
arthritis has resolved should attempts be made
to tackle persistent hyperuricaemia. Rapid
fluctuations of blood uric acid levels will increase the risk of further gout. Withdrawal of
diuretics, limitation of alcohol intake, and
weight reduction may suffice. A single attack
of gout does not necessarily demand sustained
hypouricaemic therapy unless blood uric acid
levels remain very high. Probenecid is the
cheapest drug but allopurinol is the choice if
there is evidence of renal dysfunction or renal
calculi. In the first three months of hypouricaemic treatment, it is prudent to continue
either colchicine or a non-steroidal anti-inflammatory drug.

Pseudo-Gout and Calcium Pyrophosphate Deposition Disease

Epidemiology

Calcification of hyaline and fibrocartilage is an
age-related phenomenon. Whenever it occurs

within a joint there is a risk of acute or chronic
pseudo-gout. The menisci and articular cartilage of the knee are the most commonly affected sites (Fig. 23) and this has been described
in 7 to 28 per cent. of two elderly populations
(Bocher *et al.*, 1965, Ellman and Levin, 1975).
Many subjects are asymptomatic and others
have pain due to concomitant osteoarthritis.
Other sites of chondrocalcinosis are the wrist,
symphysis pubis, hips, and small joints of the
fingers. The prevalence of wrist joint calcification has been estimated to be 2.5 per cent.
in a population aged more than 60 (Dodds and
Steinbach, 1969).

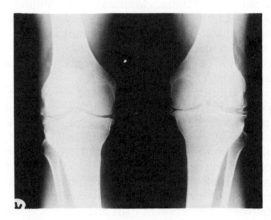

Figure 23   X-rays showing chondrocalcinosis of the
knees. Menisci and articular cartilage are both
involved

Pathology

Unlike calcification at other sites, which tends
to be principally the result of calcium hydroxyapatite deposition, the major salt in calcified
cartilage is calcium pyrophosphate dihydrate.
In the majority of instances it may simply reflect an ageing process but in rare cases it has
a familial association. Widespread chondrocalcinosis may be a feature of hyperparathyroidism, occurring in as many as 40 per cent. (Glass
and Grahame, 1976).

There are also associations with haemochromatosis, hypothyroidism, and diabetes
mellitus.

Crystals may also be deposited within the
synovium. No inflammatory cells are seen
around crystals either at this site or in cartilage.
It seems that acute inflammation is provoked
only by crystals within the joint cavity. In both
gout and pseudo-gout sparse crystals may be

seen without inflammation and it seems likely that an inflammatory response only occurs when crystals of a critical, but undetermined, number and size are present (Bjelle, 1979).

Clinical Features

The typical episode of pseudo-gout is a mono-arthritis, most often affecting the knee. The inflamed joint resembles that of gout and like gout is often associated with fever. A mistaken diagnosis of septic arthritis is not infrequent, especially if purulent synovial fluid is aspirated and not examined for crystals (Angevine and Jacox, 1973; Bong and Bennett, 1981). Attacks may be precipitated by surgery or intercurrent illness.

Less well known is a picture of chronic pyrophosphate synovitis with moderate joint swelling (Bjelle, 1979). This is usually associated with X-ray evidence of osteoarthritis so it is often difficult to determine cause and effect.

Investigation

There are no biochemical hallmarks. The presence of hypercalcaemia should raise the suspicion of hyperparathyroidism. During acute attacks, ESR and white cell counts are elevated.

Chondrocalcinosis is a radiological diagnosis. The presence of cartilage calcification and acute arthritis do not necessarily denote pseudo-gout. Examination of synovial fluid is of paramount importance in excluding other causes of acute arthritis (see the section on gout). Occasionally, X-rays reveal a destructive joint lesion associated with the chondrocalcinosis. This more resembles avascular necrosis rather than an erosive arthropathy (Richards and Hamilton, 1974).

Treatment

The tenets of treatment are joint aspiration, rest, non-steroidal anti-inflammatory drugs, and, if necessary, intra-articular corticosteroids. The usefulness of colchicine is uncertain. There are no specific prophylactic measures analogous to the hypouricaemic therapy of gout. Recurrent episodes of pseudo-gout occur but tend not to be frequent.

ADHESIVE CAPSULITIS OF THE SHOULDER

Epidemiology

Painful restriction of the shoulder may have several local causes. Lesions of specific tendons which make up the rotator cuff are sometimes identifiable, especially during the early stages. Usually there is evidence of painful dysfunction of several tendons by the time of presentation. The painful abduction of supraspinatus tendonitis or subacromial bursitis is one example of single-tendon involvement.

Painful and concentric restriction of shoulder movement implies adhesive capsulitis. The condition has several synonyms including frozen shoulder and periarthritis. The peak age of onset is 54 to 60 but 40 per cent. of patients are more than 60. Females are more likely to be affected in a ratio of 3:2. In the elderly, trauma and hemiplegia are common causes and an association with conditions producing referred pain to the shoulder region is well known. Thus, a history of angina, myocardial infarction, gall bladder disease, and cervical nerve root pain are frequent findings. Other factors which are related include diabetes mellitus, epilepsy and its treatments, pulmonary tuberculosis, and thyroid disease (Wright and Haq, 1976). A premorbid personality showing increased anxiety has been claimed (Fleming *et al.*, 1976).

Pathology

The condition is associated with varying degrees of inflammation of the bursae surrounding the shoulder. The shoulder capsule becomes thickened and contracted, adhering to the humeral head. Fibrosis with minor inflammatory changes characterize the changes in the subsynovium (Neviaser, 1945).

An association with the tissue antigen HLA B27 has been reported (Bulgen, Hazleman, and Voak, 1976) but this claim has not be substantiated. Decreased levels of serum IgA and an impaired in vitro lymphocyte response to phaetohaemagglutinin provide further unconfirmed evidence that immune mediated factors may be somehow involved in the pathogenesis (Bulgen *et al.*, 1978).

Clinical Features

The onset is usually insidious. Patients note pain and difficulty in elevating the arm. Dressing becomes a problem and sleep is disturbed by lying on the involved side. There are no clinical findings other than painful restriction of movement in several directions. Additional findings such as evidence of cervical spondylosis may denote the initiating cause.

Investigation

An X-ray of the chest and shoulder are important to exclude serious disease. Pancoast tumour may present as pain in the shoulder and malignant skeletal deposits need to be ruled out. Views of the shoulder may show roughening at the site of rotator cuff insertion or calcification of the supraspinatus tendon. The history and clinical findings are quite distinct from polymyalgia rheumatica, but an elevated ESR should force reconsideration of this possibility.

Treatment

The condition is preventable in many instances. Patients with a history of trauma or hemiplegia should receive regular passive or active movement to prevent stiffening (Jayson, 1981). Local corticosteroid injections either into the joint cavity or shoulder capsule usually induce some improvement but may not be curative. Any measure which limits pain is appreciated by patients. Physical treatments which provide heat in one form or another may achieve this and allow exercises. There is some evidence that ice applications are more helpful in lessening pain temporarily (Benson and Copp, 1974). Injections of steroid or heat treatment combined with exercises are more effective than analgesics alone (Lee *et al.*, 1974). Manipulation of the shoulder is favoured by some and it has been claimed that when manipulation is combined with a corticosteroid injection the effect is better than an injection alone (Thomas, Williams, and Smith, 1980). Usually the shoulder returns to normal within 18 months although treatment can accelerate improvement and, more importantly, reduce pain. Nevertheless, 40 per cent. of patients do have minor limitation of movement which persists for as long as 6 years (Clarke *et al.*, 1975).

SYSTEMIC LUPUS ERYTHEMATOSUS (SLE)

Epidemiology

In the United Kingdom this is a rare disease but in the United States the prevalence among Caucasian females is roughly 0.1 per cent. The disease is more common among blacks and is unusual in males. The peak age of onset is in the third decade of life but the illness can occur in elderly subjects.

Pathology

In the majority of patients there is evidence of multiple-organ involvement. This may occur over a long period of time in a sporadic pattern which affects only one or a few systems at a time. It is now thought that the various manifestations are the consequence of soluble immune complex deposition. Antigen–antibody complexes containing immunoglobulin and complement can be demonstrated in the skin, blood vessels, and kidneys. A low serum total haemolytic complement in active SLE provides indirect evidence for the role of immune complexes. Serological abnormalities abound but their pathogenetic significance is uncertain. Antibodies against single- and double stranded DNA, nucleolar and cytoplasmic antigens may all occur. Those directed against double-stranded DNA are the most specific for SLE. Other immunoglobulin mediated phenomena may include a positive Coomb's test and a biological false positive test for syphilis. Antibody against nuclear ribonucleoprotein (n-RNP) has been associated in high titres with a variant of SLE. This is considered by some to be an entity and called mixed connective tissue disease because it combines features of SLE and scleroderma with little major organ disease.

Despite the occasional seriousness of SLE, ordinary light microscopy reveals very little histopathological change except in the kidneys. True vasculitis can be rarely demonstrated.

The cause of SLE is obscure. In the elderly, drug induced disease is common. Several preparations have been incriminated and these include hydralazine, procainamide, isoniazid, methyldopa, D-penicillamine, beta blockers, and lithium.

Clinical Features

The disease may produce a wide range of features. These usually evolve over months or years, involvement of one system resolving while that of another becomes evident. Long periods of remission are common. The most common clinical manifestations is a non-deforming polyarthritis affecting small and large joints. Facial erythema, alopecia, photosensitivity, pleurisy or pericarditis, Raynaud's phenomenon, oral or nasal ulceration, discoid lupus, psychoses, convulsions, and renal disease are the most common additional features.

In the elderly, rash, arthritis, lymph node enlargement, and pleurisy or pericarditis are more common than in younger patients (Foad, Sheon, and Kironer, 1972; Wilson *et al.*, 1981). Pneumonitis is also thought to be a characteristic of this age group (Baker *et al.*, 1979; Urowitz, Stevens, and Shulman, 1967). Neuropsychiatric features are thought to be less common (Baker *et al.*, 1979) and in one study of nervous system involvement there were no patients older than 60 (Gibson and Myers, 1976). There is uncertainty about whether glomerulonephritis is less frequent (Wilson *et al.*, 1981) or the same as in younger subjects (Baker *et al.*, 1979). In those cases which are drug related, neurological and renal involvement are unusual (Hess, 1981).

Investigation

The diagnosis of SLE may be supported by routine laboratory findings such as leucopenia and thrombocytopenia. Biological false positive tests for syphilis and a positive Coomb's test are additional features which if present may help substantiate a diagnosis. The possibility of SLE is difficult to countenance in the absence of antibodies against DNA. These can be detected by the LE cell test, although few laboratories still favour this in preference to the immunofluorescent tests for antinuclear antibodies. Tests for antibodies against double-stranded DNA are generally considered to be more specific for SLE.

Screening tests for antibodies against DNA

may also detect those directed against single-stranded DNA. These may be found in a small percentage of healthy elderly subjects as well as in rheumatoid arthritis and other connective tissue diseases. Antibodies against double-stranded DNA are rare in drug-induced SLE and it seems probable that they may be absent in some elderly subjects with otherwise classical disease (Wilson *et al.*, 1981). They are measured by the immunofluorescent *Crithidia luciliae* test or by the DNA-binding test. The titre of such antibodies is not a predictable guide to disease activity. Serum complement levels, on the other hand, tend to be reduced when SLE is active, especially when there is renal involvement.

Examination of urine for cells, casts, and protein, together with tests of glomerular filtration, are mandatory investigations. Renal biopsy may be indicated if there are abnormal urinary findings. Some prognostic indication may be gleaned from renal histopathology.

Radiological examination of the chest may reveal pneumonitis or pleurisy. Views of the joints are usually normal although joint space narrowing and small erosions have been described. The presence of prominent articular destruction probably denotes a mistaken diagnosis.

Skin biopsy with immunofluorescent staining may reveal immunoglobulin deposition at the dermal–epidermal junction, even in uninvolved skin. This is referred to as the lupus band test.

Treatment

The course of SLE in the elderly is usually benign (Foad, Sheon, and Kirsner, 1972) and treatment should therefore be conservative. Arthritis may be improved by non-steroidal anti-inflammatory drugs and antimalarials such as chloroquine may reduce both joint symptoms and rashes. Avoidance of bright sunlight will aid those with photosensitivity. Corticosteroids in small or modest doses, given for limited periods if possible, may be required for pleurisy, pericarditis, and other non-fatal manifestations. Severe clinical renal disease and neuropsychiatric involvement demand larger doses of corticosteroids supplemented by immunosuppressive agents. There is no convincing evidence that one regime is better than another or perhaps better than no treatment at all (Steinberg, 1981). Plasmapheresis and intravenous pulse therapy with methylprednisolone may be helpful adjuncts. A constant awareness of infection must be maintained, particularly among those receiving corticosteroids. This is the commonest cause of mortality.

SCLERODERMA

Epidemiology

This disease is rare but in the initial stages may be confused with rheumatoid arthritis. About 10 per cent. of cases begin after the age of 60 and the incidence increases with age, reaching a peak of 7.6 per million population per year for persons older than 65 (Medsger and Masi, 1971). This is distinct from SLE which has its highest incidence in the child-bearing years. Females are affected twice as commonly as men.

Pathology

The cause is unknown. Involvement of skin, joints, and internal organs such as heart, lungs, and bowel is characterized by the deposition of dense collagen fibres with little inflammation. Morphological abnormalities of skin capillaries may precede cutaneous changes. When the kidneys are affected, intimal hyperplasia and fibrinoid necrosis occur in the small arteries. Calcium hydroxyapatite deposits occur at sites of involvement, particularly in the skin.

Clinical Manifestations

The illness may be preceded by fatigue and peripheral oedema. Raynaud's phenomenon is usual and may antedate other features by years. The most evident manifestation is skin disease. This may become thickened, pigmented, and immobile over the face, trunk, and upper aspects of the limbs. The skin of the hands becomes tight and shiny (sclerodactyly) (Fig. 24) and the face may be similarly affected. Telangiectasia may occur on the trunk and extremities and subcutaneous calcification may be painful and ulcerate. Joint pain is common but severe destructive arthritis is unusual. Ten-

don fibrosis and contractures may combine with taut skin to produce flexion deformities of the skin. Muscle weakness and wasting may denote myositis.

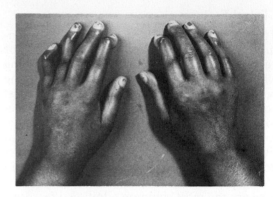

Figure 24   Sclerodactyly in a patient with severe scleroderma

In some patients the disease may be mild and non-progressive. Others have a fulminant illness. The constellation of calcinosis, Raynaud's phenomenon, and sclerodactyly is often referred to as the CRST syndrome. The majority of patients with this picture do not develop proximal cutaneous changes or serious internal organ disease. This mild variant is often overlooked in elderly patients (Dalziel and Wilcock, 1979; Hodkinson, 1971).

Serious disease manifestations include pericarditis, conduction defects of the heart, pleurisy, and pulmonary fibrosis. These may cause chest pain, dyspnoea, heart failure, and arrythmias. Involvement of the oesophagus leads to disordered motility and, at a later stage, dilatation. Indigestion, heartburn, and, less commonly, dysphagia result. Dilatation and hypomotility of the small bowel may be associated with intestinal bacterial overgrowth and malabsorption. Hypertension is a grave complication and is usually accompanied by rapidly progressive renal impairment.

Investigation

Anaemia is common. Urinalysis and tests of renal function are usually normal except in those cases associated with hypertension. Antibodies against single-stranded DNA occur in 75 per cent. Elevated creatine phosphokinase and electromyography should be requested where myositis is suspected. Investigation of internal organs may reveal evidence of early, subclinical disease. Chest X-ray and respiratory function tests, faecal fat estimation, barium swallow, and small bowel examination may all reveal unsuspected evidence of involvement. An electrocardiogram may indicate conduction defects. X-rays of the extremities will often show extensive soft tissue calcification and there may be resorption of the terminal tufts of the fingers.

Treatment

There is no really effective treatment. Malabsorption due to bacterial overgrowth may respond to a broad-spectrum antibiotic and dietary supplements. Hypertension demands aggressive treatment with vasodilators and other appropriate hypotensive drugs. Nonsteroidal anti-inflammatory drugs may alleviate joint pain and corticosteroids in small dosage may be necessary for myositis, pleurisy, and pericarditis. D-penicillamine may reduce the relentless progression of skin involvement but an effect may be apparent only after treatment for a year or longer.

REFERENCES

Acheson, R. M., and Collart, A. B. (1975). 'New Haven survey of joint diseases. XVII. Relationship between some systemic characteristics and osteoarthrosis in a general population', *Ann. Rheum. Dis.*, **34**, 379–387.

Adams, P., and Muir, H. (1976). 'Qualitative changes with age of proteoglycans of human lumbar discs', *Ann. Rheum. Dis.*, **35**, 289–296.

Adler, E. (1966). 'Rheumatoid arthritis in old age'. *Isr. J. Med. Sci.*, **2**, 607–613.

Alspaugh, M., Jensen, F., Rabin, H., and Tan, E. M. (1978). 'Lymphocytes transformed by Epstein–Barr virus: Induction of nuclear antigen reactive with antibody in rheumatoid arthritis', *J. Exp. Med.*, **147**, 1018–1027.

Amos, R. S., Constable, T. J., Crockson, R. A., Crockson, A. P., and McConkey, B. (1977). 'Rheumatoid arthritis: Relation of C-reactive protein and erythrocyte sedimentation rates to radiographic changes', *Br. Med. J.*, **1**, 195–197.

Anderson, J. A. D. (1978). 'Working group on back pain', *Facuity Comm. Med., R. Coll. Physicians Newsletter*, **5**, 72–79.

Angevine, C. D., and Jacox, R. F. (1973). 'Pseudogout in the elderly', *Arch. Intern. Med.*, **131**, 693–696.

Armstrong, C. G., Barhrani, A. S., and Gardner, D. L. (1977). 'Changes with age in the compliance of human femoral head articular cartilage', *Lancet*, **1**, 1103–1104.

Armstrong, C. G., and Gardner, D. L. (1977). 'The thickness and distribution of human femoral head articular cartilage changes with age', *Ann. Rheum. Dis.*, **36**, 407–412.

Arnold, W. J., and Simmons, R. A. (1980). 'Clinical variability of the gouty diathesis', *Adv. Exp. Med. Biol.*, **122A**, 39–46.

August, J. T., and Strand, M. (1977). 'Type C oncornoviruses and autoimmunity', *Arthritis Rheum.*, **20** (Suppl.), 64–73.

Baker, S. B., Rovira, J. R., Campion, E. W., and Mills, J. A. (1979). 'Late onset systemic lupus erythematosus', *Am. J. Med.*, **66**, 727–732.

Ball, J., and Sharp, J. (1978). 'Osteoarthrosis', in *Copeman's Textbook of the Rheumatic Diseases* (Ed. J. T. Scott), 5th ed., pp. 595–644, Churchill Livingstone, Edinburgh, London, New York.

Bandilla, K. K. (1977). 'Back pain: osteoarthritis', *J. Am. Geriatr. Soc.*, **25**, 62–66.

Barnes, C. G., Turnbull, A. L., and Vernon-Roberts, B. (1971). 'Felty's syndrome. A clinical and pathological survey of 21 patients and their response to treatment', *Ann. Rheum. Dis.*, **30**, 359–374.

Basch, C. M., Spitler, L. E., Engleman, E. L., and Engleman, E. P. (1977). 'Cellular immune reactivity in patients with rheumatoid arthritis and effects of levamisole', *J. Rheumatol.*, **4**, 377–378.

Bayliss, M. T., and Ali, S. Y. (1978). 'Studies on cathepsin B in human articular cartilage', *Biochem. J.*, **171**, 149–154.

Behn, A. R., Mathews, J. A., and Phillips, I. (1981). 'Lactate UV-system: a rapid method for diagnosis of septic arthritis', *Ann. Rheum. Dis.*, **40**, 489–492.

Benians, R. G. (1969). 'Senile monoarticular arthritis', *Geront. Clin.*, **11**, 109–114.

Benson, T. B., and Copp, E. P. (1974). 'The effects of therapeutic forms of heat and ice on the pain threshold of the normal shoulder', *Rheumatol. Rehabil.*, **13**, 101–104.

Berry, H., Liyange, S. P., Durance, R. A., Barnes, C., Berger, L., and Evans, S. (1976). 'Azathioprine and penicillamine in treatment of rheumatoid arthritis: A controlled trial', *Br. Med. J.*, **1**, 1052–1054.

Bjelle, A. (1979). 'Pyrophosphate arthropathy', *Scand. J. Rheumatol.*, **8**, 145–153.

Bocher, J., Mankin, H. J., Berk, R. N., and Rodnan, G. P. (1965). 'Prevalence of calcified meniscal cartilage in elderly persons'. *N. Engl. J. Med.*, **272**, 1093–1097.

Bollet, A. J., Handy, J. R., and Sturgill, B. C. (1963). 'Chondroitin sulphate concentration and protein–polysaccharide composition of articular cartilage in osteoarthritis', *J. Clin. Invest.*, **42**, 853–859.

Bong, D., and Bennett, R. (1981). 'Pseudogout mimicking systemic disease', *JAMA*, **246**, 1438–1440.

Boyd, R. V., and Hoffbrand, B. I. (1966). 'Erythrocyte sedimentation rate in elderly hospital inpatients', *Br. Med. J.*, **1**, 901–902.

Brain, R. (1963). 'Some unsolved problems of cervical spondylosis', *Br. Med. J.*, **1**, 771–777.

British Association of Physical Medicine (1966). 'Pain in the neck and arm: A multicentre trial of the effects of physiotherapy', *Br. Med. J.*, **1**, 253–258.

Brooker, A. E., and Barter, R. W. (1965). 'Cervical spondylosis. A clinical study with comparative radiology', *Brain*, **88**, 925–936.

Brown, J. W., and Sones, D. A. (1967). 'The onset of rheumatoid arthritis in the aged', *J. Am. Geriatr. Soc.*, **15**, 873–880.

Bulgen, D. Y., Hazleman, B. L., and Voak, D. (1976). 'HLA B27 and frozen shoulder', *Lancet*, **1**, 1042–1044.

Bulgen, D., Hazleman, B., Ward, M., and McCallum, M. (1978). 'Immunological studies in frozen shoulder', *Ann. Rheum. Dis.*, **37**, 135–138.

Burney, D. P., Martin, C. E., Thomas, C. S., Fisher, R. D., and Bender, H. W. (1979). 'Rheumatoid pericarditis. Clinical significance and operative management', *J. Thorac. Cardiovasc. Surg.*, **77**, 511–515.

Byers, P. D., Contempomi, C. A., and Farkas, T. A. (1970). 'A post mortem study of the hip joint including the prevalence of features on the right side', *Ann. Rheum. Dis.*, **29**, 15–31.

Caird, F. I., Webb, J., and Lee, P. (1973). 'Osteoarthrosis of the hands in the elderly', *Age Ageing*, **2**, 150–156.

Calin, A., and Fries, J. F. (1975). 'The striking prevalence of ankylosing spondylitis in healthy W27 positive males and females. A controlled study', *N. Engl. J. Med.*, **293**, 835–839.

Chamberlain, M. A., and Bruckner, F. E. (1970). 'Rheumatoid neuropathy: Clinical and electrophysiological features', *Ann. Rheum. Dis.*, **29**, 609–616.

Child, D. L., and Yates, D. A. (1978). 'Radicular pain in diabetes', *Rheumatol. Rehabil.*, **17**, 195–196.

Clarke, G. R., Willis, L. A., Fish, W. W., and Nichols, P. J. R. (1975). 'Preliminary studies in measuring range of motion in normal and painful stiff shoulder', *Rheumatol. Rehabil.*, **14**, 39–46.

Conlon, P. W., Isdale, I. C., and Rose, B. G. (1966). 'Rheumatoid arthritis of the cervical spine'. *Ann. Rheum. Dis.*, **25**, 120–126.

Currey, H. L., Greenwood, R. M., Lloyd, G. G., and Murray, R. S. (1979). 'A prospective study of low back pain', *Rheumatol. Rehabil.*, **18**, 94–104.

Dalziel, J. A., and Wilcock, G. K. (1979). 'Progressive systemic sclerosis in the elderly', *Postgrad. Med. J.*, **55**, 192–193.

Danielsson, L. (1966). 'Incidence of osteoarthritis of the hip', *Clin. Orthop.*, **45**, 67–72.

Davison, S. (1980). 'Rheumatic disease in the elderly', *Mt Sinai J. Med (NY)*, **47**, 175–180.

Dequeker, J. V., Noyen, R. van, and VandePitte, J. (1969). 'Age-related rheumatoid factors – instance and characteristics', *Ann. Rheum. Dis.*, **28**, 431–436.

Dieppe, P. A., Huskisson, E. C., Crocker, P., and Willoughby, M. D. (1976). 'Apatite deposition disease', *Lancet*, **1**, 266–268.

Dilke, T. F. W., Burry, H. C., and Grahame, R. (1973). 'Extradural corticosteroid injection in the management of lumbar nerve root compression', *Br. Med. J.*, **2**, 635–637.

Dimant, J. (1979). 'Rheumatoid arthritis in the elderly, presenting as polymyalgia rheumatica', *J. Am. Geriatr. Soc.*, **37**, 183–185.

Ditunno, J., and Ehrlich, G. E. (1970). 'Care and training of elderly patients with rheumatoid arthritis', *Geriatrics*, **25**, 164–172.

Dodds, W. J., and Steinbach, H. L. (1969). 'Triangular cartilage calcification in the wrists: Its incidence in elderly persons', *Am. J. Roentgen.*, **105**, 850–852.

Doran, D. M., and Newell, D. T. (1975). 'Manipulation in the treatment of low back pain: A multi-centre study', *Br. Med. J.*, **2**, 161–164.

Dwosh, I. L., Stein, H. B., Urowitz, M. B., Smythe, H. A., Hunter, T., and Ogryzlo, M. A. (1977). 'Azathioprine in early rheumatoid arthritis. Comparison with gold and chloroquine', *Arthritis Rheum.*, **20**, 685–692.

Eastmond, C. J., Calguneri, M., Shinebaum, R., Cooke, E. M., and Wright, V. (1982). 'A sequential study of the relationship between faecal *Klebsiella aerogenes* and the common clinical manifestations of ankylosing spondylitis', *Ann. Rheum. Dis.*, **41**, 15–20.

Ebringer, R. W., Cawdell, D. R., Cowling, P., Ebringer, A. (1978). 'Sequential studies in ankylosing spondylitis. Association of *Klebsiella pneumoniae* with active disease', *Ann. Rheum. Dis.*, **37**, 146–151.

Ehrlich, G. E. (1972a). 'Inflammatory osteoarthritis 1. The clinical syndrome', *J. Chronic. Dis.*, **25**, 317–328.

Ehrlich, G. E. (1972b). 'Inflammatory osteoarthritis. 2. The superimposition of rheumatoid arthritis', *J. Chronic. Dis.*, **25**, 635–643.

Ehrlich, G. E., Katz, W. A., and Cohen, S. H. (1970). 'Rheumatoid arthritis in the aged', *Geriatrics*, **25**, 103–113.

Ehrlich, M. G., Mankin, H. J., Jones, H., Wright, R., Crispen, C., and Vigliani, C. (1977). 'Collagenase and collagenase inhibitors in osteoarthritis and normal human cartilage', *J. Clin. Invest.*, **59**, 226–233.

Ellman, M. H., and Levin, B. (1975). 'Chondrocalcinosis in elderly persons', *Arthritis Rheum.*, **18**, 43–47.

Engel, A., Roberts, J., and Burch, T. (1966). *Rheumatoid Arthritis in Adults. United States 1960–62*, Vital and Health Statistics, Public Health Service, Government Printing Office, Washington.

Fam, A. G., Pritzker, K. P. H., Cheng, P. T., and Little, A. H. (1981). 'Cholesterol crystals in osteoarthritic joint effusions', *J. Rheumatol.*, **8**, 273–280.

Feinstein, P. A., and Habermann, E. T. (1977). 'Selecting and preparing patients for total hip replacement', *Geriatrics*, **32**, 91–96.

Fleming, A., Dodman, S., Beer, T. C., and Crown, S. (1976). 'Personality in frozen shoulder', *Ann. Rheum. Dis.*, **35**, 456–457.

Foad, B. S. I., Sheon, R. P., and Kirsner, A. B. (1972). 'Systemic lupus erythematosus in the elderly', *Arch. Intern. Med.*, **130**, 743–746.

Freeman, M. A. R. (1975). 'The fatigue of cartilage in the pathogenesis of osteoarthrosis', *Acta Orthop. Scand.*, **46**, 323–328.

Friedman, D. M., and Moore, M. E. (1980). 'The efficacy of intra-articular steroids in osteoarthritis', *J. Rheumatol*, **7**, 850–856.

Geddes, D. M., Webley, M., and Emerson, P. A. (1979). 'Airways obstruction in rheumatoid arthritis', *Ann. Rheum. Dis.*, **38**, 222–225.

Gibson, T., Burry, H. C., Poswillo, D., and Glass, J. (1977). 'Effect of intra-articular corticosteroid injections on primate cartilage', *Ann. Rheum. Dis.*, **36**, 74–79.

Gibson, T., and Grahame, R. (1973). 'Acute arthritis in the elderly', *Age Ageing*, **2**, 3–13.

Gibson, T., and Grahame, R. (1974). 'Gout and hyperlipidaemia', *Ann. Rheum. Dis.*, **33**, 298–303.

Gibson, T., and Grahame, R. (1981). 'Rehabilitation of the elderly arthritic patient', *Clinics Rheum. Dis.*, **7**, 485–495.

Gibson, T., Highton, J., Potter, C., and Simmonds, H. A. (1980). 'Renal impairment and gout', *Ann. Rheum. Dis.*, **39**, 417–423.

Gibson, T., Highton, J., Simmonds, H. A., and Potter, C. (1979). 'Hypertension, renal function and gout', *Postgrad. Med. J. Suppl.*, **3**, 21–25.

Gibson, T., Huskisson, E. C., Wojtulewski, J. A., Scott, P. J., Balme, H. W., Burry, H. C., Grahame, R., and Hart, F. D. (1976). 'Evidence that D-penicillamine alters the course of rheumatoid arthritis', *Rheumatol. Rehabil.*, **15**, 211–215.

Gibson, T., and Myers, A. R. (1976). 'Nervous system involvement in systemic lupus erythematosus', *Ann. Rheum. Dis.*, **35**, 398–406.

Gibson, T., Rodgers, V., Potter, C., and Simmonds, H. A. (1982). 'Allopurinol treatment and its effect on renal function in gout: A controlled study', *Ann. Rheum. Dis.*, **41**, 59–65.

Gibson, T., and Schumacher, H. R. (1976). 'Ankylosing hyperostosis with cervical spinal cord compression', *Rheumatol. Rehabil.*, **15**, 67–70.

Gibson, T., Winter, P. J., and Grahame, R. (1973). 'Radiotherapy in the treatment of osteoarthrosis of the knee', *Rheumatol. Rehabil.*, **12**, 42–46.

Glass, J. S., and Grahame, R. (1976). 'Chondrocalcinosis after parathyroidectomy', *Ann. Rheum. Dis.*, **35**, 521–525.

Goidl, E. A., Michelis, M. A., Siskind, G. W., and Weksler, M. E. (1981). 'Effect of age on the induction of autoantibodies', *Clin. Exp. Immunol.*, **44**, 24–30.

Goldie, I., and Landquist, A. (1970). 'Evaluation of the effects of different forms of physiotherapy in cervical pain', *Scand. J. Rehabil. Med.*, **2**, 117–121.

Goldin, R. H., McAdam, L., Louie, J. S., Gold, R., and Bluestone, R. (1976). 'Clinical and radiological survey of the incidence of osteoarthrosis among obese patients', *Ann. Rheum. Dis.*, **35**, 349–353.

Gordon, D. A., Stein, J. L., and Broder, I. (1973). 'The extra-articular manifestations of rheumatoid arthritis. A systematic analysis of 127 cases', *Am. J. Med.*, **54**, 445–452.

Gow, P. J., and Gibson, T. (1977). 'Dysphagia due to vertical subluxation of the axis in rheumatoid arthritis', *Rheumatol. Rehabil.*, **16**, 155–157.

Grahame, R. (1980). 'Clinical trials in low back pain', *Clinics Rheum. Dis.*, **6**, 143–157.

Grahame, R., Armstrong, R., Simmons, N. A., Mims, C. A., Wilton, J. M. A., and Laurent, R. (1981). 'Isolation of rubella virus from synovial fluid in five cases of seronegative arthritis', *Lancet*, **2**, 649–651.

Grahame, R., Calin, A., Tudor, M., Kennedy, L., and Perrin, A. (1975). 'Ankylosing rheumatoid arthritis', *Rheumatol. Rehabil.*, **14**, 25–30.

Grahame, R., and Scott, J. T. (1970). 'Clinical survey of 354 patients with gout', *Ann. Rheum. Dis.*, **29**, 461–468.

Green, L., Meyers, O. L., Gordon, W., and Briggs, B. (1981). 'Arthritis in psoriasis', *Ann. Rheum. Dis.*, **40**, 366–369.

Gresham, G. E., and Rathey, U.K. (1975). 'Osteoarthritis in knees of aged persons. Relationship between roentgenographic and clinical manifestations', *JAMA*, **233**, 168–170.

Griffin, A. J., Gibson, T., Huston, G., and Taylor, A. (1981). 'Maintenance chrysotherapy in rheumatoid arthritis. A comparison of two dose schedules', *Ann. Rheum. Dis.*, **40**, 250–253.

Hajzok, O., Tomik, F., and Hajzokova, M. (1976). 'Amyloidosis in RA. A study of 48 histologically confirmed cases', *Z. Rheumatol.*, **35**, 356–362.

Halsey, J. P., Reeback, J. S., and Barnes, C. G. (1982). 'A decade of skeletal tuberculosis', *Ann. Rheum. Dis.*, **41**, 7–10.

Harris, A. I. (1971). *Handicapped and Impaired in Great Britain*, Part 1, Social Survey Division, Office of Population Censuses and Surveys, HMSO, London.

Harris, J., Carter, A. R., Glick, E. N., and Storey, G. O. (1974). 'Ankylosing hyperostosis 1. Clinical and radiological features', *Ann. Rheum. Dis.*, **33**, 210–215.

Heimer, R., Levin, F. M., and Rudd, E. (1963). 'Globulins resembling rheumatoid factor in serum of the aged', *Am. J. Med.*, **35**, 175–181.

Henderson, D. R. F., Tribe, C. R., and Dixon, A. S. (1975). 'Synovitis in polymyalgia rheumatica', *Rheumatol. Rehabil.*, **14**, 244–249.

Hernborg, J., and Nilsson, B. E. (1973). 'The relationship between osteophytes in the knee joint, osteoarthritis and ageing', *Acta Orthop. Scand.*, **44**, 69–74.

Herndon, J. H., and Aufranc, O. E. (1972). 'Avascular necrosis of the femoral head in the adult', *Clin. Orthop.*, **86**, 43–62.

Hess, E. V. (1981). 'Introduction to drug-related lupus. Proceedings of the Kroc Foundation Conference on drug induced lupus', *Arthritis Rheum.*, **24**, 6–9.

Highton, J., Panayi, G. S., Shepherd, P., Faith, A., Griffin, J., and Gibson, T. (1981). 'Fall in immune complex levels during gold treatment of rheumatoid arthritis', *Ann. Rheum. Dis.*, **40**, 575–579.

Hodkinson, H. M. (1971). 'Scleroderma in the elderly, with special reference to the CRST syndrome', *J. Am. Geriatr. Soc.*, **19**, 225–228.

Holt, S., and Yates, P. O. (1966). 'Cervical spondylosis and nerve root lesions', *J. Bone Joint Surg.*, **48B**, 407–423.

Hurwitz, N. (1969). 'Predisposing factors in adverse reactions to drugs', *Br. Med. J.*, **1**, 536–539.

Janossy, G., Panayi, G., Duke, O., Bofill, M., Poulter, L., and Goldstein, G. (1981). 'Rheumatoid arthritis: A disease of T-lymphocyte/macrophage immunoregulation', *Lancet*, **2**, 839–842.

Jayson, M. I. V. (1981). 'Frozen shoulder: Adhesive capsulitis', *Br. Med. J.*, **283**, 1005–1006.

Jeffreys, E. (1980). *Disorders of the Cervical Spine*, p. 95, Butterworths, London, Boston, Sydney.

Jubb, R. W., and Fell, H. B. (1980). 'Changes resembling osteoarthrosis induced by the used culture medium of synovium in organ culture', in *The Aetiopathogenesis of Osteoarthrosis* (Ed. G. Nuki), pp. 139–143, Pitman Medical, Tunbridge Wells.

Julkunen, H., Heinonen, O. P., and Pyorala, K. (1971). 'Hyperostosis of the spine in an adult population: Its relation to hyperglycaemia and obesity', *Ann. Rheum. Dis.*, **30**, 605–612.

Kale, S. A., and Jones, J. V. (1981). 'Rehabilitating the elderly arthritic', *Geriatrics*, **36**, 101–105.

Kaplan, D., and Meyer, K. (1959). 'Ageing of human cartilage', *Nature*, **183**, 1267–1268.

Kellgren, J. H. (1961). 'Osteoarthrosis in patients and populations', *Br. Med. J.*, **2**, 1–6.

Kellgren, J. H. (1977). 'The anatomical source of back pain', *Rheumatol. Rehabil.*, **16**, 3–12.

Kellgren, J. H., and Lawrence, J. S. (1956). 'Rheumatoid arthritis in a population sample', *Ann. Rheum. Dis.*, **15**, 1–11.

Kellgren, J. H., and Lawrence, J. S. (1958). 'Osteoarthrosis and disc degeneration in an urban population', *Ann. Rheum. Dis.*, **17**, 388–397.

Kellgren, J. H., Lawrence, J. S., and Bier, F. (1963). 'Genetic factors in generalised osteoarthritis', *Ann. Rheum. Dis.*, **22**, 237–255.

Kelly, P. J., Martin, W. J., and Coventry, M. B. (1970). 'Bacterial arthritis in the adult', *J. Bone Joint Surg.*, **52A**, 1595–1602.

Kelsey, J. L. (1975). 'An epidemiological study of acute herniated lumbar intervertebral discs', *Rheumatol. Rehabil.*, **14**, 144–159.

Klein, R., Klein, B. E., Cornoni, J. C., Maready, J., Cassel, J. C., and Tyroler, H. A. (1973). 'Serum uric acid. Its relationship to coronary heart disease risk factors and cardiovascular disease. Evans County, Georgia', *Arch. Int. Med.*, **132**, 401–410.

Kolodny, A. L., and Klipper, A. R. (1976). 'Bone and joint diseases in the elderly', *Hosp. Pract.*, **11**, 91–101.

Kulvin, S. M. (1972). 'Erythrocyte sedimentation rates in the elderly', *Arch. Ophthalmol.*, **88**, 617–618.

Lawrence, J. S. (1961). 'Prevalence of rheumatoid arthritis', *Ann. Rheum. Dis.*, **20**, 11–17.

Lawrence, J. S. (1963). 'The prevalence of arthritis', *Br. J. Clin. Pract.*, **17**, 699–705.

Lawrence, J. S. (1969). 'Disc degeneration. Its frequency and relationship to symptoms', *Ann. Rheum. Dis.*, **28**, 121–137.

Lawrence, J. S. (1977). *Rheumatism in Populations*, p. 70, William Heinemann, London.

Lawrence, J. S., De Graff, R., and Laine, V. A. (1963). 'Degenerative joint disease in random samples and occupational groups', in *The Epidemiology of Chronic Rheumatism*, (Ed. J. H. Kellgren, M. R. Jeffrey and J. Ball), Vol. 1, p. 98, Blackwell Scientific Publications, Oxford.

Lee, P. N., Lee, M., Haq, A. M., Longton, E. B., and Wright, V. (1974). 'Periarthritis of the shoulder. Trial of treatments investigated by multivariate analysis', *Ann. Rheum. Dis.*, **33**, 116–119.

Linn, F. C., and Sokoloff, L. (1965). 'Movement and composition of interstitial fluid of cartilage', *Arthritis Rheum.*, **8**, 481–494.

Longmore, R. B., and Gardner, D. L. (1975). 'Development with age of human articular surface structure', *Ann. Rheum. Dis.*, **34**, 26–37.

McCarty, D. J., Halverson, P. B., Carrera, G. F., Brewer, B. J., and Kozin, F. (1981). 'Milwaukee shoulder – association of micro-spheroids containing hydroxyapatite crystals, active collagenase and neutral protease with rotator cuff defects 1. clinical aspects', *Arthritis Rheum.*, **24**, 464–473.

McCormick, C. E. (1978). 'Radiology in low back pain and sciatica. An analysis of the relative efficacy of spinal venography discography and epidurography in patients with a negative or equivocal myelogram', *Clin. Radiol.*, **29**, 393–406.

McDevitt, C. A., and Muir, H. (1976). 'Biochemical changes in the cartilage of the knee in experimental and natural osteoarthritis in the dog', *J. Bone Joint Surg.*, **58-B**, 94–101.

McGavin, D. D., Williamson, H., Forrester, J. V., Foulds, W. S., Buchanan, W. W., Dick, W. C., Lee, P., MacSween, R. N. M., and Whaley, K. (1976). 'Episcleritis and sleritis. A study of their clinical manifestations and association with rheumatoid arthritis', *Br. J. Ophthalmol.*, **60**, 192–226.

Mackay, I. (1972). 'Aging and immunological function in man', *Gerontologia*, **18**, 285–304.

McKenzie, J. M. (1981). 'Report on a double-blind trial comparing small and large doses of gold in the treatment of rheumatoid disease', *Rheumatol. Rehabil.*, **20**, 198–202.

Mankin, H. J., Dorfman, H., Lippiello, L., and Zarins, A. (1971). 'Biochemical and metabolic abnormalities in articular cartilage from osteoarthritis human hips', *J. Bone Joint Surg.*, **53-A**, 523–537.

Markham, J. G., and Myers, D. B. (1976). 'Preliminary observations on an isolate from synovial fluid of patients with rheumatoid arthritis', *Ann. Rheum. Dis.*, **35**, 1–7.

Marks, J. S., and Power, B. J. (1979). 'Is chloroquine obsolete in treatment of rheumatic disease?', *Lancet*, **1**, 371–373.

Mathews, J. A. (1974). 'Atlanto-axial subluxation in rheumatoid arthritis. A five year follow up study', *Ann. Rheum. Dis.*, **33**, 526–531.

Mathews, J. A., and Hickling, J. (1975). 'Lumbar traction: A double blind controlled study for sciatica', *Rheumatol. Rehabil.*, **14**, 222–225.

Meachim, G., Bentley, G., and Baker, R. (1977). 'Effect of age on thickness of adult patellar articular cartilage', *Ann. Rheum. Dis.*, **36**, 563–568.

Meachim, G., and Emery, I. H. (1973). 'Cartilage fibrillation in shoulder and hip joints in Liverpool necropsies', *J. Anat.*, **116**, 161–179.

Meachim, G., and Emery, I. H. (1973). 'Cartilage fibrillation in shoulder and hip joints in Liverpool necropsies', *J. Anat.*, **116**, 161–179.

Meachim, G., Ghadially, F. N., and Collins, D. H. (1965). 'Regressive changes in the superficial layer of human articular cartilage', *Ann. Rheum. Dis.*, **24**, 23–30.

Medsger, T. A., and Masi, A. T. (1971). 'Epidemiology of systemic sclerosis (Scleroderma)', *Ann. Int. Med.*, **74**, 714–721.

Meeks, L. W., and Renshaw, T. S. (1973). 'Vertebral osteophytosis and dysphagia', *J. Bone Joint Surg.*, **55-A**, 197–201.

Mikkelsen, W. M., Dodge, H. J., Duff, I. F., and Kato, I. H. (1967). 'Estimates of the prevalence of rheumatic disease in the population of Tecumseh, Michigan, 1959–60', *J. Chronic. Dis.*, **20**, 351–369.

Mikkelsen, W. M., Duff, I. F., and Dodge, H. F. (1970). 'Age-specific prevalence of radiographic abnormalities of the joints of the hands, wrists and cervical spine of adult residents of Tecumseh', *J. Chronic. Dis.*, **23**, 151–159.

Miller, E. J., Van der Korst, J. K., Sokoloff, L. (1969). 'Collagen of human articular and costal cartilage', *Arthritis Rheum.*, **12**, 21–29.

Mitchell, N. S., and Cruess, R. L. (1977). 'Classification of degenerative arthritis', *Can. Med. Assoc. J.*, **117**, 763–765.

Mitrovic, D., Gruson, M., Demignon, J., Mercier, P., Aprile, F., and De Seze, S. (1981). 'Metabolism of human femoral head cartilage in osteoarthrosis and subcapital fracture', *Ann. Rheum. Dis.*, **40**, 18–26.

Moll, J. M. H., and Wright, V. (1973). 'Psoriatic arthritis', *Semin. Arthritis Rheum.*, **3**, 55–78.

Morris, I. M., and Eade, A. W. T. (1978). 'Pyogenic arthritis and rheumatoid disease: The importance of the infected foot', *Rheumatol. Rehabil.*, **17**, 222–226.

Moskowitz, R. W. (1977). 'Cartilage and osteoarthritis, current concepts'. *J. Rheumatol.*, **4**, 329–331.

Moskowitz, R. W., Goldberg, V. M., and Malemud, C. J. (1981). 'Metabolic responses of cartilage in experimentally induced osteoarthritis', *Ann. Rheum. Dis.*, **40**, 584–592.

Mowat, A. G. (1979). 'Drug treatment of arthritis in the elderly', *Age Ageing*, **8** (Suppl.), 14–25.

Nastro, L. J. (1970). 'Aggressive management of rheumatoid arthritis in the elderly', *J. Am. Geriatr. Soc.*, **18**, 63–66.

Nathan, H. (1962). 'Osteophytes of the vertebral column. An anatomical study of their development according to age, race and sex', *J. Bone Joint Surg.*, **44-A**, 243–268.

Neviaser, J. S. (1945). 'Adhesive capsulitis of the shoulder; a study of the pathological findings in periarthritis of the shoulder', *J. Bone Joint Surg.*, **27-A**, 211–222.

Newman, J. H. (1976). 'Review of septic arthritis throughout the antibiotic era', *Ann. Rheum. Dis.*, **35**, 198–205.

Nordby, E. J., and Lucas, G. L. (1973). 'A comparative analysis of lumbar disk disease treated by laminectomy or chemonucleolysis', *Clin. Orthop.*, **90**, 119–129.

Nurick, S. (1972). 'The pathogenesis of the spinal cord disorder associated with cervical spondylosis', *Brain*, **95**, 87–100.

O'Duffy, J. D., Wahner, H., and Hander, G. G. (1976). 'Joint imaging in polymyalgia rheumatica', *Arthritis Rheum.*, **19**, 815.

Oka, M., and Kytila, J. (1957). 'Rheumatoid arthritis with the onset in old age', *Acta Rheum. Scand.*, **3**, 249–258.

Olhagen, B., and Mansson, I. (1968). 'Intestinal *Clostridium perfringens* in rheumatoid arthritis and other collagen diseases', *Acta Med. Scand.*, **184**, 395–402.

O'Sullivan, J. B. (1972). 'Gout in a New England Town. A prevalence study in Sudbury, Massachusetts', *Ann. Rheum. Dis.*, **31**, 166–169.

Pallis, C., Jones, A. M., and Spillane, J. D. (1954). 'Cervical spondylosis, incidence and implications', *Brain*, **77**, 274–289.

Panayi, G., Wooley, P., and Batchelor, J. (1978). 'Genetic basis of rheumatoid disease: HLA antigens, disease manifestations and toxic reactions to drugs', *Br. Med. J.*, **2**, 1326–1328.

Panayi, G., Wooley, P., and Batchelor, J. (1979). 'HLA-DRw4 and rheumatoid arthritis', *Lancet*, **1**, 730.

Partridge, R. E., and Duthie, J. J. (1963). 'Controlled trial of the effect of complete immobilisation of the joints in rheumatoid arthritis', *Ann. Rheum. Dis.*, **22**, 91–99.

Paulus, H. E., Machleder, H. I., Peter, J. B., Goldberg, L., Levy, J., and Pearson, C. M. (1973). 'Clinical improvement of rheumatoid arthritis during prolonged thoracic duct lymphocyte drainage', *Arthritis Rheum.*, **16**, 562.

Peter, J. B., Pearson, C. M., and Marmor, L. (1966). 'Erosive osteoarthritis of the hands', *Arthritis Rheum.*, **9**, 365–388.

Pritzker, J. P. H., Fam, A. G., Omar, S. A., and Gertzbein, S. D. (1981). 'Experimental choles-terol crystal arthropathy', *J. Rheumatol.*, **8**, 281–290.

Radin, E. L. (1976). 'Mechanical aspects of osteoarthrosis', *Bull. Rheum. Dis.*, **26**, 862–865.

Rasker, J. J., and Cosh, J. A. (1981). 'Cause and age at death in a prospective study of 100 patients with rheumatoid arthritis', *Ann. Rheum. Dis.*, **40**, 115–120.

Reimann, I., Mankin, H. J., and Trahan, C. (1977). 'Quantitative histologic analyses of articular cartilage and subchondral bone from osteoarthritis and normal human hips', *Acta. Orthop. Scand.*, **48**, 63–73.

Resnick, D., Niwayama, G., and Goergen, T. G. (1977). 'Comparison of radiographic abnormalities of the sacroiliac joint in degenerative disease and ankylosing spondylitis', *Am. J. Roentgen.*, **128**, 189–196.

Richards, A. J., and Hamilton, E. B. (1974). 'Destructive arthropathy in chondrocalcinosis articularis', *Ann. Rheum. Dis.*, **33**, 196–203.

Riley, M. J., Ansel, B. M., and Bywaters, E. G. (1971). 'Radiological manifestations of ankylosing spondylitis according to age of onset', *Ann. Rheum. Dis.*, **30**, 138–148.

Rivlin, R. S. (1981). 'Nutrition and aging: Some unanswered questions', *Am. J. Med.*, **71**, 337–340.

Roberts, M. E. T., Wright, V., Hill, A. G. S., and Mehra, A. C. (1976). 'Psoriatic arthritis: Follow up study', *Ann. Rheum. Dis.*, **35**, 206–212.

Roitt, I. M., Corbett, M., Festenstein, H., Jarequemada, D., Papasteriadis, C., Hay, F. C., and Nineham, L. J. (1978). 'HLA Drw4 and prognosis in rheumatoid arthritis', *Lancet*, **1**, 990.

Ropes, M., Bennett, G., Cobb, S., Jacox, R., and Jessar, R. (1958). 'Revision of diagnostic criteria for rheumatoid arthritis', *Bull. Rheum. Dis.*, **9**, 175–176.

Rosin, A. J., and Boyd, R. V. (1966). 'Complications of illness in geriatric hospital patients', *J. Chronic. Dis.*, **19**, 307–313.

Sairanen, E., Paronen, I., and Mahonen, H. (1969). 'Reiters syndrome: A follow up study', *Acta. Med. Scand.*, **185**, 57–63.

Sarkin, T. L. (1977). 'Backache in the aged', *South Afr. Med. J.*, **51**, 418–420.

Schumacher, H. R., Somlyo, A. P., Tse, R. L., and Maurer, K. (1977). 'Arthritis associated with apatite crystals', *Ann. Intern. Med.*, **87**, 411–416.

Schutt, A. H. (1977). 'Physical medicine and rehabilitation in the elderly arthritic patient', *J. Am. Geriatr. Soc.*, **25**, 68–75.

Sims-Williams, H., Jayson, M. I., Young, S. M., Baddeley, H., and Collins, E. (1978). 'Controlled trial of mobilisation and manipulation for patients with low back pain in general practice', *Br. Med. J.*, **2**, 1338–1340.

Smith, D. A., Zaphiropoulos, G. C., and Polyzoides, A. J. (1981). 'Spontaneous osteonecrosis of the femoral condyle', *Rheumatol. Rehabil.*, **20**, 136–142.

Smith, J. R., and Phelps, P. (1972). 'Septic arthritis, gout, pseudogout and osteoarthritis in the knee of a patient with multiple myeloma', *Arthritis Rheum.*, **15**, 89–96.

Solomon, L., Beighton, P., Valkenburg, H. A., Robin, G., and Soskolne, G. (1975). 'Rheumatic disorders in the South African Negro. 1. Rheumatoid arthritis and ankylosing spondylitis'. *South Afr. Med. J.*, **49**, 1292–1296.

Soren, A., Klein, W., and Huth, F. (1976). 'Microscopic comparison of the synovial changes in rheumatoid arthritis and osteoarthritis', *Z. Rheumatol.*, **35**, 249–263.

Stastny, P., and Fink, C. W. (1977). 'HLA-DW4 in adult and juvenile rheumatoid arthritis', *Transplant Proc.*, **9**, 1863–1866.

Steele, A. D. (1969). 'Arthritis in the aged. Medical aspects', *Postgrad. Med.*, **46**, 168–171.

Steinberg, A. D. (1981). 'Management of systemic lupus erythematosus', in *Textbook of Rheumatology*, (Eds W. N. Kelly, E. D. Harris, S. Ruddy, and C. B. Sledge), pp. 1133–1150, W. B. Saunders, Philadelphia.

Stobo, J. D., and Tomasi, T. B. (1975). 'Aging and the regulation of immune reactivity', *J. Chronic. Dis.*, **28**, 437–440.

Thomas, D., Williams, R. A., and Smith, D. S. (1980). 'The frozen shoulder: A review of manipulative treatment', *Rheumatol. Rehabil.*, **19**, 173–179.

Thompson, R. C., and Oegema, T. R. (1979). 'Metabolic activity of articular cartilage in osteoarthritis', *J. Bone Joint Surg.*, **61-A**, 407–416.

Urowitz, M. B., Stevens, M. B., and Shulman, L. E. (1967). 'The influence of age on the clinical pattern of systemic lupus erythematosus', *Arthritis Rheum.*, **10**, 319–320.

Utsinger, P. O., and Shapiro, R. (1976). 'Diffuse skeletal abnormalities in Forestier's disease'. *Arch. Int. Med.*, **136**, 763–768.

Van der Korst, J. K., Sokoloff, L., and Miller, E. J. (1968). 'Senescent pigmentation of cartilage and degenerative joint disease', *Arch. Path.*, **84**, 40–46.

Vernon Roberts, B., Pirie, C. J., and Trenwith, V. (1974). 'Pathology of the dorsal spine in ankylosing hyperostosis', *Ann. Rheum. Dis.*, **33**, 281–288.

Waine, H., Nevinny, D., Rosenthal, J., and Joffe, I. (1961). 'Association of osteoarthritis and diabetes mellitus', *Tufts Folia Med.*, **7**, 13–19.

Weinberger, K. A. (1980). 'Rheumatoid arthritis masquerading as polymyalgia rheumatica: Report of two cases', *J. Am. Geriatr. Soc.*, **7**, 13–17.

Weksler, M. E., and Hutteroth, T. H. (1974). 'Impaired lymphocyte function in aged humans', *J. Clin. Invest.*, **53**, 99–104.

Whaley, K., Williamson, J., Wilson, T., McGavin, D., Hughes, G. R. V., Hughes, H., Schmulian, L. R., MacSween, R. N. M., and Buchanan, W. W. (1972). 'Sjogrens syndrome and autoimmunity in a geriatric population', *Age Ageing*, **1**, 197–206.

Wilcock, G. K. (1979). 'The prevalence of osteoarthrosis of the hip requiring total hip replacement in the elderly', *Int. J. Epidemiol.*, **8**, 247–250.

Wilkinson, M., and Bywaters, E. G. (1958). 'Clinical features and course of ankylosing spondylitis as seen in a follow up of 222 hospital referred cases', *Ann. Rheum. Dis.*, **17**, 209–228.

Willkens, R. F., Healey, L. A., and Decker, J. L. (1960). 'Acute infectious arthritis in the aged and chronically ill', *Arch. Int. Med.*, **106**, 354–364.

Wilson, D. S. (1979). 'Pain in the neck and arm', *Rheumatol. Rehabil.*, **18**, 177–180.

Wilson, H. A., Hamilton, M. E., Spyker, D. A., Brunner, C. M., O'Brien, W. M., Davis, J. S., and Winfield, J. B. (1981). 'Age influences the clinical and serologic expression of systemic lupus erythematosus', *Arthritis Rheum.*, **24**, 1230–1235.

Wilton, J. M., Gibson, T., and Chuck, C. M. (1978). 'Defective phagocytosis by synovial fluid and blood polymorphonuclear leucocytes in patients with rheumatoid arthritis. 1. The nature of the defect', *Rheumatol. Rehabil. Suppl.*, **17**, 25–36.

Winyard, G. P. A., Luker, C., and Nichols, P. J. R. (1976). 'The uses and usefulness of electrically powered indoor wheelchairs', *Rheumatol. Rehabil.*, **15**, 254–263.

Wood, P. H., and McLeish, C. L. (1974). 'Statistical appendix. Digest of data on the rheumatic diseases', *Ann. Rheum. Dis.*, **33**, 93–105.

Wright, V. (1964). 'Treatment of osteoarthritis of the knees', *Ann. Rheum. Dis.*, **23**, 389–391.

Wright, V., and Haq, A. M. (1976). 'Periarthritis of the shoulder. 1. Aetiological considerations with particular reference to personality factors', *Ann. Rheum. Dis.*, **35**, 213–219.

Yates, D. W. (1978). 'A comparison of the types of epidural injections commonly used in the treatment of low back pain and sciatica', *Rheumatol. Rehabil.*, **17**, 181–186.

Young, A., Dixon, A., Getty, J., Renton, P., Vacher, H. (1981). 'Cauda equina syndrome complicating ankylosing spondylitis: Use of electromyography and computerized tomography in diagnosis', *Ann. Rheum. Dis.*, **40**, 317–322.

26

The Genitourinary System

Principles and Practice of Geriatric Medicine
Edited by M. S. J. Pathy
© 1985 John Wiley & Sons Ltd

26.1

Gynaecology of the Elderly

Joan Andrews

The elderly female patient presents to the gynaecologist by referral from the general practitioner or geriatrician and only rarely because of clinical findings at a well woman's clinic. These older patients differ in several significant ways from the younger. Many women, particularly those referred by geriatricians, will have little in the way of symptoms referrable to the pelvis, but during the course of investigations for concurrent disease have been suspected of having some pelvic abnormality. Sometimes the diagnosis is clinically obvious as with carcinoma vulva or procidentia but the ideal management may be less clear. Once the diagnosis of malignant disease has been made then treatment can proceed on standard lines modified only by the physical and mental fitness of the patient to tolerate surgery, radiotherapy, or cytotoxic drugs. In contrast, where a benign condition such as procidentia is found during the course of the routine general medical examination it is essential that treatment is not an unnecessary intrusion into the woman's way of life.

A decision to proceed with surgery must be based on the wishes of the patient and family taken after full medical consultation. The medical advice depends on the presence of concurrent disease in relation to anaesthetic, life expectancy, and any technical difficulties anticipated with surgery because of arthritic hips and knees preventing adequate surgical access. These must be balanced against the prognosis of the gynaecological condition and the problems likely to occur if the disease is untreated.

A decision that treatment is justified needs to be made with especial care where the pelvic abnormality has been found during the course of radiological or ultrasonic examination for non-gynaecological symptoms. A common referral is the patient in whom a pelvic mass is seen pressing on the bladder (Fig. 1) at intravenous pyelogram or distorting the bowel at barium enema. While it is obviously important to diagnose and treat malignant disease of uterus or ovary it is unusual for either of these conditions to occur in the absence of postmen-

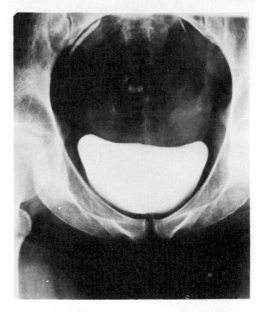

Figure 1 Intravenous pyelogram. Bladder shown compressed by dermoid cyst containing teeth

opausal bleeding or pelvic pain. A good ultransonic scan (Figs 2 to 4) associated with
careful history and examination should distinguish the occasional mass requiring treatment
from the more common benign fibroid uterus
(Fig. 5) which in the postmenopausal patient
will always be asymptomatic and require no
treatment.

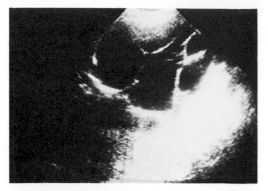

Figure 2   Ultrasonic scan (sector). Multilocular
ovarian cyst

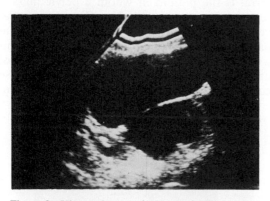

Figure 3   Ultrasonic scan (transverse). Simple cyst
– larger translucent area is bladder

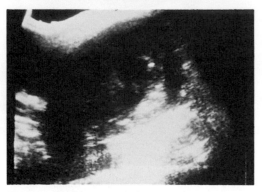

Figure 4   Ultrasonic scan (longitudinal). Fibroids

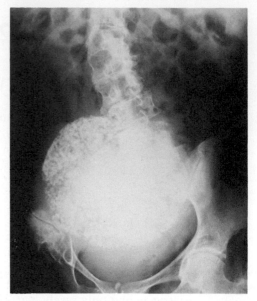

Figure 5   Plain X-ray. Calcified fibroid

It should be superfluous to say that the elderly patient's symptoms may not always be easily understood by the doctor. There is still a
diffidence among some older women in describing symptoms referrable to the pelvis, and
postmenopausal bleeding, pruritis vulvae, vaginal discharge, incontinence, and in particular
any sexual difficulties may not be volunteered
(see Chapter 3.5). Difficulties also arise as
memory becomes poor and the length of symptoms is usually underestimated. A relative may
be able to help but where an old lady lives
alone then it is unwise to rely solely on the
short time scale to which she relates her
symptoms.

It is particularly important to have privacy
for any patient with gynaecological problems
during history taking and examination. When
deafness and some mental confusion are also
present then it is both more difficult to achieve
and even more important. On the ward there
should always be a single room which can be
used for history taking, undressing, and examination as well as subsequent discussion. It
is also a real advantage if, when the patient is
from a home or hospital ward, the accompanying person is someone the elderly lady knows
and trusts and who can help clarify any doubt
about her symptoms.

For the examination a firm couch or bed at reasonable height is essential, as is a good light. An accurate assessment can never be made in a soft, low, ward bed with a wavering torch as the only illumination. Arthritis of hips or knees may make examination difficult and here the left lateral position may be helpful. Where an old lady is very dyspnoeic, the upper chest and head can be lifted on pillows, but still allow abdomen and pelvis to be flat on the couch, something which is impossible if the usual hospital bed rest is not removed.

Examination will not only be easier for the patient but also for the doctor if the patient is clear first as to what is intended. Many of todays older patients may have had babies, but been delivered in their own homes by midwives and never before been subjected to pelvic examination. The single, nulliparous patient will invariably have an intact hymen, having lived through years when extramarital sex was rare and tampons unavailable.

Examination should include a brief general examination with emphasis on clinical anaemia, presence of enlarged lymph glands, breasts, varicose veins, and oedema. Assessment of the cardiorespiratory state will be necessary in conjunction with geriatrician and anaesthetist where surgery is contemplated. In abdominal examination it may at times be difficult for the woman to relax her rather tense or obese abdomen and where there is doubt in regard to the presence of an abdominal mass percussion is a valuable addition to palpation. It should be unnecessary to remind oneself that the bladder must be empty. Vaginal examination is usually possible providing the hymen is not intact and gentleness is used. Speculum examination should follow and it is important to have available the small size Cusco and Sims speculae as ageing inevitably narrows the introitus. A rectal examination should no more be forgotten by the gynaecologist than vaginal examination by the general surgeon, particularly where the diagnosis is obscure.

At the completion of examination some explanation must be offered. This should not be thrust at the half-dressed woman on the couch, but given when the patient is sitting down fully dressed. Whatever is said often needs to be reinforced later and ideally where the patient is confused or liable to forget relatives should be seen.

EFFECTS OF AGEING ON GENITAL TRACT

Symptoms referrable to the pelvic organs are dependent in part on the changes that the pelvic organs undergo at the menopause and into old age.

The vulva and vagina, and indeed the urethra, all change during the years of oestrogen withdrawal with thinning and atrophy of mucosa and loss of pubic hair. Glycogen disappears from the vaginal epithelium with the reaction becoming neutral or alkaline. In some women a non-infective vaginitis of so-called senile or atrophic type occurs (Fig. 6). This may lead to scanty postmenopausal bleeding, dryness at coitus, and the urethral syndrome of frequency and urgency of micturition. Rarely, especially if coitus occurs after an interval of time, there may be a vaginal tear with frank bleeding.

The vaginal smear of the postmenopausal woman shows fewer cells, a fall in the proportion of superficial to intermediate cells and a lower cornification index (CI) of 5 or 10 unless the woman is receiving oestrogen therapy. In very old age there is a preponderance of parabasal cells with large deeply staining nuclei (Figs 7 and 8).

The cervix becomes shorter and the ectocervix becomes flush with vaginal vault. The squamo-columnar junction withdraws into the cervical canal.

The uterus itself undergoes atrophy of myometrium and concomitant diminution in size of any benign fibromyoma. The endometrium is no longer influenced by ovarian hormones, since the ovary becomes unresponsive to increasingly high levels of pituitary gonadotrophin produced as the pituitary is released from the inhibitary effect of oestrogen. The endometrium no longer undergoes cyclical change and becomes a thin epithelium over dense stroma with occasional inactive gland.

Characteristic levels of postmenopausal female sex hormones are shown in Table 1. Subsequent to the initial rise of gonadotrophins to a peak some 3 years after the menopause the level gradually declines and in 30 per cent. of women 20 to 30 years after the menopause the mean concentrations of luteinizing and follicle-stimulating hormones are lower than the levels in reproductive life (Chakravarti *et*

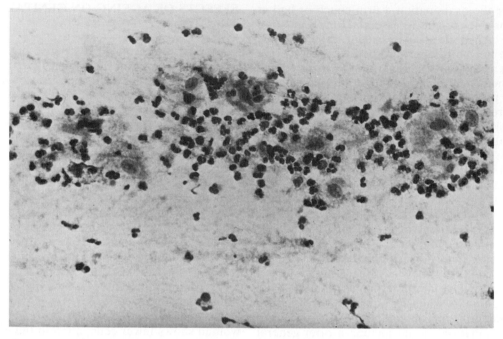

Figure 6   Vaginal smear (Papanicolaou). Leucocytes of atrophic vaginitis. (From Schnell and Meinrenken, 1975. Reproduced by permission of Dr Johannes D. Schnell)

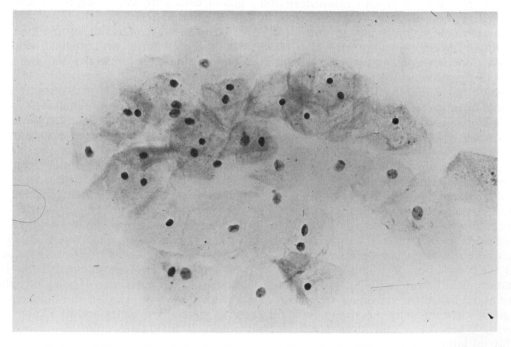

Figure 7   Vaginal Smear (Papanicolaou). Women aged 22 on day 8 of 28-day cycle – superficial old
intermediate cells. (From Schnell and Meinrenken, 1975. Reproduced by permission of Dr Johannes D.
Schnell)

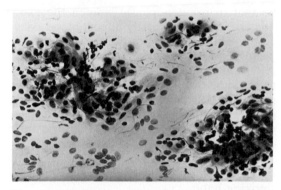

Figure 8　Vaginal smear (Papanicolaou). Women aged 78, postmenopausal – parabasal cells, many becoming autolysed. (From Schnell and Meinrenken, 1975. Reproduced by permission of Dr Johannes D. Schnell)

al., 1976). The sources and concentration of steroids have been reviewed (Hutton, Jacobs, and James, 1979). Subsequent to the menopause there is a shift of oestrogen production from oestradiol 17B of ovarian origin to oestrone synthesized in body fat from precursors such as androstenedione in adrenal and ovarian stroma (Monroe and Menon, 1977). The ovary becomes smaller and sclerotic with progressive depletion of ova, failure of ovulation and decreased output of ovarian hormones. This gradual process may take up to 20 years from the onset of decreased fertility, through this menopause and into old age.

The Fallopian tubes become shorter with muscle replaced by fibrous tissue. The endopelvic fascia sheathing the genital and urinary tract and the bowel below the pelvic peritoneum of Pouch and Douglas and uterovesical pouch atrophies as do the fascial condensations of cardinal and uterosacral ligaments. The muscle tone of the pelvic floor diminishes.

HORMONE REPLACEMENT THERAPY
(see also Chapter 21)

In addition to the changes in genital organs associated with oestrogen withdrawal other systems are affected. Whether such changes are part of normal ageing or should be considered as disease is arguable.

Psychiatric symptoms especially depression have been ascribed to oestrogen withdrawal possibly associated with changes in plasma tryptophan.

Symptoms of vasomotor instability are experienced by about 75 per cent. of women and untreated will last from 1 to 5 years.

Atrophy of skin, hair, and breasts occur with loss of fatty tissue.

Probably the most important effects are osteoporosis and cardiovascular change. Osteoporosis continues progressively over the years with fractures being 5 times as common in women than men by the seventh decade (Knowelden, Buhr, and Dunbar, 1964). It seems probable that the extent of postmenopausal loss of bone is governed by the conversion of adrenal and possibly ovarian stroma androgen to oestrogen and such conversion is dependent on the bulk of fat present.

There is no doubt that at surgery in the absence of malignant disease ovarian function should be preserved as prophylaxis against early development of menopausal symptoms. Even in the postmenopausal woman when

TABLE 1　Hormone levels in postmenopausal women. (From Chakravarti *et al.*, 1976. Reproduced by permission of J. Studd)

	Premenopausal Days 1–10 of menstrual cycle	Ten years after menopause	Conversion SI to traditional units
	Mean and range	Mean and range	
Plasma FSH U/L	3.6 (1.5–7.0)	42.1 (25.5–79.0)	
Plasma LH U/L	17.8 (4.1–41.7)	55.3 (32.2–63.8)	
Testosterone nmol/l	1.42 (0.6–2.24)	1.49 (0.59–2.98)	1 nmol/l = 28.8 ng/100 ml
Oestrone pmol/l	439.1 (158.7–664.2)	34.3 (9.2–101.4)	1 pmol/l = 0.0270 ng/100 ml
Oestradiol 17B pmol/l	250.3 (90.4–600.8)	43.4 (18.4–91.9)	1 pmol/l = 0.270 ng/100 ml

ovarian oestrogen production falls the stroma does continue to produce androstenedione and testosterone – both precursors of oestrogen (Asch and Greenblatt, 1977). Forty per cent. of women maintain a well-oestrogenized vaginal smear until over the age of 70.

Similarly there is agreement that short term oestrogen replacement therapy is justified in the treatment of vasomotor symptoms, dyspareunia, and the urethral syndrome. There is more room for argument as to the place of hormone replacement therapy in the long term to minimize osteoporosis (Aitken, Hart, and Lindsay, 1973), fractures (Hutchinson, Polansky, and Feinstein, 1979), and coronary artery disease (Parrish *et al.*, 1967; Robinson, Higano, and Cohen, 1959). Oestrogen can be given as natural or synthetic hormone by oral route, injection, or implant. Arguments against use include expense, some coagulation changes, withdrawal bleeding, an increased incidence of endometrial hyperplasia, and possibly carcinoma of the body of the uterus where unopposed oestrogen therapy is given. A recent survey from the United States showed some 24 per cent. of women over 70 to be receiving oestrogen (Barrett-Connor *et al.*, 1979) although the incidence in Britain is almost certainly much lower.

Cholesterol levels can be shown to be higher in postmenopausal women than the premenopausal and to exhibit an inverse relationship with oestrogen level (Magnani and Moore, 1976). Triglyceride levels show less clear trends increasing with age and also showing an increase at the menopause independent of the age at which menstruation ceases. There are apparently less marked coagulation changes where so-called natural conjugated oestrogen is used as compared with the synthetic compounds in oral contraception therapy but factor VII and X levels are increased (Bonnar *et al.*, 1976; Notelovitz, 1977). There is some evidence that long-term oestrogen replacement may be effective in preventing atherosclerosis or myocardial infarction (Higano, Robinson and Cohen, 1963; Ross *et al.*, 1981).

It seems paradoxical that the use of oral contraception in premenopausal women appears to predispose to thromboembolism and arterial disease whereas in the postmenopausal it is apparently lack of oestrogen which predisposes to myocardial infarction. It may

be that in premenopausal women the exogenous oestrogen primarily affects blood coagulation while in the postmenopausal the low oestrogen levels predispose to atherosclerosis. Alternatively these differences may be related to the type of oestrogen used or their relative potency and to date there are no clinical reports of cardiovascular disease as a result of oestrogen replacement therapy in the postmenopausal woman (Adam, Williams, and Vessey, 1981). Any hazard there is may well be greater in those with prior thromboembolism or heavy smoking habit.

There is a possible association between exogenous oestrogen prescribed for menopausal symptoms and the development of endometrial carcinoma (Smith *et al.*, 1975). Such induced carcinomas appear to be very localized and the preceding hyperplastic change may be reversed by cessation of treatment or addition of progesterone. Uterine bleeding is certainly a practical problem for the older woman receiving hormone replacement therapy. Withdrawal bleeding after cessation of oestrogen is an indication for curettage as is breakthrough irregular loss while still on therapy. Some would advise that an endometrial biopsy be performed on all women after two years on oestrogen therapy. The use of progesterone with low-dose oestrogen replacement therapy has been shown to reduce the incidence of hyperplasia and such therapy is to be preferred to oestrogen alone (Paterson *et al.*, 1980). Obesity is a relative contraindication to oestrogen use because of association with increased risk of endometrial cancer.

SYMPTOMS

These are modified by increasing age.

Postmenopausal Bleeding

(Differentiate from haematuria or rectal bleeding.)
(a) Carcinoma body – frank loss, may not be heavy.
(b) Atrophic vaginitis – not common in the very old. May follow examination or coitus.
(c) Trophic ulceration from prolapse or foreign body.
(d) Cervical polyp – usually benign.

(e) Carcinoma cervix – often associated with offensive vaginal discharge.

(f) Oestrogen withdrawal after medication.

(g) Pyometra.

Vaginal Discharge

(a) Atrophic vaginitis — brown.

(b) Pyometra with or without underlying carcinoma – may be episodic, usually offensive.

(c) Pessary or foreign body.

Pruritis Vulvae

It is important that the symptom is irritation and not soreness or pain. It is made worse by local heat from clothing, oily local applications, and lack of hygiene.

(a) Vulval dystrophy.

(b) Chronic irritation – scratching leading to lichenification presenting as thick rigid skin often extending on to thighs.

(c) Exclude anal irritation – worm infestation, liquid paraffin, haemorrhoids.

(d) Fungus infection – not common unless precipitating cause such as antibiotics.

(e) Diabetes mellitus – undiagnosed or badly controlled.

(f) Local allergic reaction to toilet preparations.

Urinary Incontinence

(a) Urgency – may follow infection/illness.

(b) Stress incontinence – as on coughing.

(c) True – fistula or neurogenic

(d) Retention with overflow.

Dyspareunia

(a) Atrophic vaginitis/oestrogen withdrawal.

(b) Urethral caruncle.

(c) Vaginal stenosis – post-operative, kraurosis, or radiotherapy.

Faecal Incontinence

(a) Old third-degree tear.

(b) Faecal impaction with spurious diarrhoea – confused by attendants as coming from vagina.

PROLAPSE

Many elderly women tolerate a large prolapse for years. This may be partly because of diffidence in seeking medical aid but also because they have made a conscious decision that therapy by either pessary or surgery is not justified. In contrast, other women may present with a very short history of sudden development of prolapse subsequent to problems with lifting a heavy invalid relative.

The two principle factors responsible for the development of prolapse are damage occurring during childbirth and subsequent weakening of fascia and muscle support following the menopause. Raised intra-abdominal pressure from an abdominal mass or chronic cough is a contributory factor in some women as is congenital or postoperative weakness.

Most commonly the presenting symptom is a feeling of a lump coming down in the vulval region. This may be constantly present, may disappear on lying down and may need to be replaced before initiating micturition. A minor prolapse may become symptomatic in the presence of marked atrophic vaginitis. Trophic ulceration may occur with discharge and bleeding. Rarely a woman presents with an irreducible mass at the vulva needing reduction of oedema before replacement is possible. The symptoms of prolapse depend very much on the anatomical relationships of the wall or walls of vagina which prolapse (Fig. 9).

A common mistake is to blame the development of urinary symptoms in the elderly upon a prolapse which may well have been present since soon after the menopause and has pre-dated the problems of micturition by many years. Farrar (Chapter 26.3) describes the limited number of symptoms by which disordered micturition is manifest and any of these may be associated with, or less frequently caused by, gynaecological conditions.

The commonest cause of urge incontinence in the elderly is detrusor instability. This may be associated with a defective urethral closure mechanism so that even relatively weak detrusor contractions overcome the sphincteric action and cause incontinence.

Defective control of urethral closure is often a result of pelvic floor damage and in these cases stress incontinence occurs with any in-

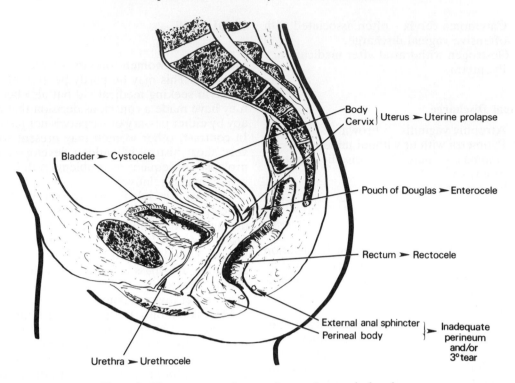

Figure 9 The anatomy and nomenclature of utervaginal prolapse

crease of intra-abdominal pressure caused by coughing, sneezing, or laughing.

A common difficulty is the patient with only a small cystourethrocele whose symptoms include both urge (unstable) and stress incontinence. Differentiation is aided by careful history taking, clinical examination of the patient with a full bladder, and, at times, by urodynamic investigation. The more specialized examination can be justified where the history is confusing, where simple empirical treatment has failed, and especially prior to consideration of surgery for urinary symptoms associated with minimal prolapse. The investigations and management of urinary symptoms in the elderly may be improved by a standard scheme (Hilton and Stanton, 1981).

Dysuria and frequency caused by frank infection are more common with prolapse, especially with a marked cystocele where stagnation of urine occurs.

True incontinence from fistula formation may present in the postoperative period after major gynaecological surgery, but should be both very rare and easily recognized.

Rectal function is very tolerant even of ma-

jor rectal prolapse and bowel symptoms are uncommon. Rectocele should not be confused with faecal impaction presenting as urinary retention and overflow incontinence.

Where the perineum related normally to the lower third of the vagina has been completely torn at the time of childbirth (and no primary repair of the third degree tear has been effected) faecal incontinence does not usually occur while levator muscle activity remains good and faeces normal. With ageing and general muscle weakness, however, especially if diarrhoea develops due to other conditions such as diverticulitis, then incontinence occurs.

Operative treatment by repair of prolapse with or without vaginal hysterectomy is usually better tolerated than abdominal surgery. All pelvic surgery carries a risk of thromboembolism (Jeffcoate and Tindall, 1965) of the order of 3 per cent. Prophylaxis in the form of anticoagulation or embolism stockings should reduce this figure. Obesity, heavy smoking habit, and chronic constipation require improvement before surgery.

Where surgery is contraindicated or refused by the patient then pessary therapy is an alternative. A soft ring pessary of the Portex type will be successful providing there is adequate perineum to retain the pessary. Some patients, particularly those with large prolapse and very little perineum, may do better with a Simpson shelf pessary (Fig. 10). This type is not well tolerated by the active woman but is useful for the bedridden patient. Either type requires changing at approximately 3-monthly intervals and the vagina should be regularly inspected by speculum to ensure no ulceration has occurred. To achieve this not all pessary changes should be delegated to a nurse. Once a pessary is fitted there must be careful oversight of the patient with regular follow-up appointments as a pessary neglected can ulcerate even into the bladder.

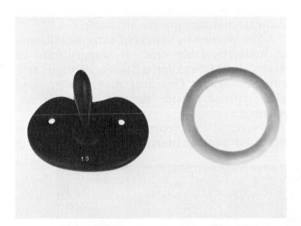

Figure 10   Simpson shelf and plastic ring pessaries

VULVAL DYSTROPHY

Vulval dystrophy is a generic term used to include leukoplakia, lichen sclerosis of the vulva, and kraurosis. The latter is considered by some to be a final atrophic stage of lichen sclerosis (Jeffcoate and Woodcock, 1961), and lichen sclerosis itself to be similar to the atrophic phase of leukoplakia. Leukoplakia has come to mean to some any disease causing white patches on the vulva, but others use it only to apply to vulval dysplasia with a histological picture of keratinization and hyperplasia of epidemis on a thinning dermis with loss of collagen and elastic fibres. At a later stage the epidemis atrophies and the dermis undergoes fibrosis.

Chronic epithelial vulval dystrophy is considered to be premalignant, although there is little evidence to prove this contention and it is possible that dystrophic change and carcinoma of vulva may develop together. Ulceration or extensive fissuring is an indication for biopsy. In the absence of such signs of premalignancy, treatment is conservative with limited local application of corticosteroid in a water-miscible base. Adjuvent therapy includes cool cotton clothing, avoidance of oily local preparations, and the antihistamine Promethazine may be helpful in obtaining sleep and avoiding the irritation which is so often worse at night. Intractable pruritis requires local vulvectomy but, unfortunately, symptoms tend to recur in surrounding skin.

Bowen's disease or carcinoma in situ presents as one or more elevated reddened areas and is treated by wide excision or local vulvectomy.

INFECTION

Infection of the genital tract is unusual in the postmenopausal woman. Sexually transmitted disease is rare but does occur and gonorrhoea or trichomonal infection may spread to Fallopian tubes. Monilia vaginitis occurs but irritation is more often due to vulval pruritis from other causes.

Vaginal infection may occur, especially with neglected pessaries or other foreign bodies. Neglected late carcinoma cervix or vulva will become secondarily infected with associated offensive discharge.

The atrophic vaginitis of the postmenopausal is associated with the decrease of acidity. Organisms other than Doderlein's will colonize the vagina giving a low-grade pyogenic infection which responds to local or systemic oestrogen therapy. A similar condition in the uterus, endometritis, may result in pus being retained in the uterus if the cervix is fibrosed, as after previous surgery or radiotherapy. Pyometra presents as offensive vaginal discharge and occasionally as pelvic peritonitis. An underlying carcinoma of the body of the uterus must be excluded by curettage when the pyometra is drained by cervical dilatation.

A tubo-ovarian abscess can occur either due to rare ascending infection or secondary to cancer of the bowel.

CARCINOMA OF THE UTERINE BODY

The presenting symptom of this neoplasm in the elderly is almost always postmenopausal bleeding and if ignored late symptoms include pain, heavy discharge especially from pyometra or symptoms from peritoneal spread and liver and chest involvement. Postmenopausal bleeding is recognized even by the elderly as abnormal and is usually reported.

An incidence rate of 30 to 45 per 100,000 female population is reported for women in the 60 to 94 age range (Waterhouse, 1974; see Table 2). Obesity is associated with increased risk possible because of higher oestrogen levels found in overweight women.

Clinical examination and cytology (Fig. 11) may suggest the diagnosis but do not adequately exclude intrauterine neoplasia and a diagnostic curettage is essential.

Surgery for the elderly is dependent largely on the ability of the patient to cope with anaesthesia and a skilled anaesthetist is essential. With preoperative assessment even the very elderly can usually withstand surgery. When the diagnosis is obvious it may be possible to proceed with abdominal hysterectomy and bilateral salpingo-oophorectomy under the same

TABLE 2 Gynaecological cancer — incidence. (From Waterhouse, 1974. Reproduced by permission of J. A. H. Waterhouse)

	Mean age (Years)	95% Between ages	Proportion of all cancers in women
Carcinoma endometrium	60.9	41–83	4.9
Carcinoma ovary (including Fallopian tube)	57.9	31–83	4.7
Carcinoma vulva	67.2	36–89	1.0
Carcinoma cervix			
– in situ	42.0	25–66	—
– invasive	55.0	33–84	6.2

anaesthetic. If the disease is subsequently shown to extend into the myometrium, then radiotherapy with radium to vaginal vault and also external therapy are advisable.

A few women by reason of extreme infirmity or understandable fear of surgery can be treated by Medroxyprogesterone acetate as a cytotoxic agent. This drug may also be used where spread outside the pelvis has already occurred.

A survival rate (corrected to allow for the increased general mortality with age) of 77.5

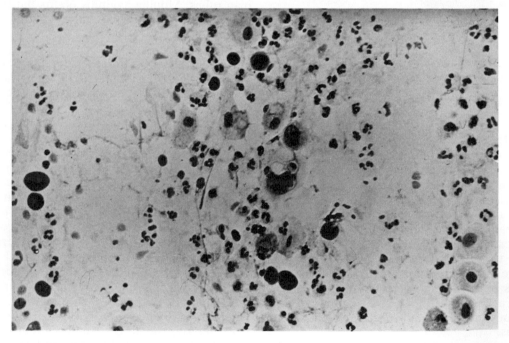

Figure 11   Cervical smear (Papanicolaou). Adenocarcinoma tumour cells. (From Schnell and Meinreken, 1975. Reproduced by permission of Dr Johannes D. Schnell)

per cent. after radical treatment has been reported from the Birmingham region (Waterhouse, 1974; see Table 3).

TABLE 3 Gynaecological cancer corrected five year survival rate. (From Waterhouse, 1974. Reproduced by permission of J. A. H. Waterhouse)

	All Cases %	Following radical treatment
Carcinoma endometrium	69.6	77.5
Carcinoma ovary (including Fallopian tube)	25.6	46.8
Carcinoma vulva	52.2	59.1
Carcinoma cervix		
– in situ	90.7	91.3
– invasive	43.5	51.7

Sarcoma of the uterus is a rare tumour but incidence increases with age. Treatment is essentially the same as for carcinoma but the prognosis is worse.

CARCINOMA OF THE OVARY

This tumour can occur at any age but, sadly, tends to present late, only causing symptoms after the tumour has spread outside the ovary.

The incidence rises during young adult life with a sharp increase during the decade 40 to 49 but subsequently remains steady at about 40 per 100,000 women until the age of 80. Carcinoma of the ovary is now the commonest cause of death from gynaecological malignancy in the United Kingdom but at the present time many attempts are being made to improve this poor prognosis. There is no effective screening programme possible at the early curable stage and efforts are aimed at improving the treatment of patients with advanced disease.

A corrected 5-year survival rate of 46.8 per cent. after radical treatment is reported by Waterhouse (1974). Once the tumour has breached the ovarian capsule spread is direct, transcoelomic, lymphatic, and blood borne. The transcoelomic route is particularly emphasized as cells shed from the tumour surface may seed throughout the peritoneal cavity and up the paracolic gutters and drain by the lymphatics on the under surface of the diaphragm to subpleural lymph nodes.

The histological type of tumour is probably of less prognostic significance than the extent of spread, although in general the poorly differentiated tumour has the worse prognosis.

Age inevitably worsens the prognosis and in the Medical Research Council Study (1981) on chemotherapy in advanced ovarian cancer women aged 70 or over had a mortality approximately double that of those aged under 50.

Diagnosis may at times be made at an early stage when an otherwise symptomless mass is found on examination of the abdomen. Later symptoms include abdominal pain, nerve root pain, symptoms of deep vein thrombosis or symptoms referrable to bowel involvement, the development of ascites or pleural effusion.

A certain number of ovarian tumours will be secondary to primary tumour of stomach or bowel and the presenting symptom may be of the primary tumour. It is unusual for a patient with ovarian tumour to present with postmenopausal bleeding, although the rare functional granulosa cell tumours may do so and even less often the stroma of other malignant ovarian tumours may be hormonally active. A masculinizing tumour of ovary such as arrhenoblastoma is again rare.

The provisional diagnosis can be reviewed in the light of ultrasonic scan, paracentesis, and intravenous pyelogram and barium studies but the final diagnosis can only be confirmed by laparotomy. In the symptomatic elderly patient this is almost always justified as the prognosis is improved and the patient made more comfortable by the removal of the main tumour mass. Where at all possible surgery will include both bilateral oophorectomy and usually hysterectomy. Omentectomy has also been recommended as an opportunity to remove occult metastases. At laparotomy search is made for spread not only in liver and pelvic lymph nodes but also for subdiaphragmatic nodules and para-aortic nodes.

Subsequent to surgery cytotoxic therapy is usually preferred to abdominal radiotherapy although trials are in progress comparing the two courses of action.

The main drugs used to treat ovarian cancer are the alkylating agents – in particular cyclophosphamide, Melphalan, and Chlorambucil. Between 35 and 65 per cent. of patients have been reported as showing initial response with 5 to 15 per cent. still responding after 2 years (Young, 1975).

These poor results have prompted a number

of current trials. Drugs used include the anti-metabolites such as 5-fluorouracil and anti-tumour antibiotics such as Doxorubicin. Recently Cisplatin (*cis*-dichlorodiammine platinum) has been used both as initial chemotherapy and when other drug therapy has been associated with a lack of response. Initially response was measured by clinical findings alone, but both laparoscopy and repeat laparotomy are being increasingly used (Lambert, 1981).

All the cytotoxic drugs are toxic and may cause serious side-effects and in the elderly more than in any other patient the quality of remaining life has to be weighed against the possibility of response.

My own practice at present is to reserve cytotoxic therapy for those women where disease has spread outside the ovary, but who are otherwise medically and physically fit. Even the regular hospital attendance for blood tests and particularly for intravenous therapy puts an added strain on the elderly patient and her often elderly relatives.

In the absence of a caring family or hospice facility, the woman with terminal gynaecological cancer appreciates readmission to a ward where she knows the auxillaries, nurses, and doctors and can obtain maximum relief for her symptoms from people already familiar to her.

CARCINOMA OF THE VULVA

Carcinoma of the vulva is particularly a disease of the elderly (Table 2). The histology is usually squamous but basal cell tumour (rodent ulcer) and adenocarcinoma of Bartholin's gland may occur as can the rare melanoma. Presenting symptoms are of soreness, irritation, ulceration, nodularity, or actual bleeding or discharge. At times the history may be prolonged due either to the patient failing to report symptoms or to coexistant vulval dystrophy. Diagnosis can only be confirmed by biopsy or biopsy excision of a small lesion.

The basal cell tumour can be treated by wide local excision but squamous and adenocarcinoma require radical surgery. Response to radiation is poor and experience with cytotoxic therapy limited. Radical surgery includes local vulvectomy with bilateral inguinal and femoral lymphadenopathy. The extent of skin excision may be more limited than that originally described by Way (1982) and primary skin closure is usually achieved. Despite the apparent extensive nature of the surgery, pain is not great and postoperative care is aimed at maintaining fluid balance and avoiding infection. Where prolonged general anaesthetic is better avoided epidural anaesthesia gives good conditions for surgery. Radical vulvectomy is justified in any but the most frail as the results are good unless disease has already spread outside the primary lymphatic drainage area. Untreated carcinoma of vulva will slowly spread as a large necrotic ulcer with secondary infection and lead to death from cachexia or renal failure.

CARCINOMA OF THE CERVIX

The Asymptomatic Patient

Well women's clinics have developed in recent years and examination of the asymptomatic patient has been aimed particularly at the early diagnosis of carcinoma of the cervix and also other pelvic pathology.

Reporting from British Columbia (Fidler, Boyce, and Worth, 1968) found a prevalence rate of 4.31 per 1,000 of carcinoma in situ among women screened for the first time. The prevalence was highest for women in the 40 to 44 years age group, falling to 3.85 for women aged 60 to 64, down to 1.29 for those aged 80 or over.

The Cardiff Cervical Cytology Study (Sweetnan *et al.*, 1981) aimed primarily at screening married women between the ages of 25 and 69 resident in the Cardiff City area. Of the defined population of 80,869, 65 per cent. had one or more tests but the initial acceptance rate fell from 91.7 per cent. in the age group 25 to 29 to 33.5 per cent. in those women aged 60 to 64 and to 25.8 per cent. in those of 65 to 69. The very low acceptance rate among older women influences the estimates of prevalence and incidence in these groups. The prevalence of suspicious or positive smears increased with age to a maximum of 11.2 per 1,000 in the age group 45 to 49 and then decreased slightly to 8.1 per 1,000 in the age group 60 to 64 and 8.8 among those aged 65 to 69. These cytological findings are regarded as an indication for operation to ascertain a histological diagnosis and

97 per cent. were subjected to surgery. The resultant histological diagnosis correlated well with the cytological findings with 93 per cent. showing carcinoma in situ or invasive carcinoma and only 7 per cent. dysplasia or lesser abnormality.

In the Cardiff study the prevalence of previously unrecognized clinically invasive cervical cancer increased with age, reaching 6.6 per 1000 in the age group 65 to 69.

A woman may be assumed to be no longer at risk for the development of squamous carcinoma of the cervix when having previously had normal cytological findings she reaches the age of 60 (Walton Report, 1976).

At present Ministry policy recommends that women up to the age of 65 should have regular cervical screening but that no further tests be taken for women over 65 who have had two recent negative smears and no prior abnormality.

The management of the asymptomatic older woman with an abnormal smear differs from that of her younger sister in several ways. Investigation by colposcopy often has to exclude study of the squamo-columnar junction which is frequently within the external cervical os and in that this is the primary site of neoplastic change normal colposcopic findings do not exclude in situ or invasive disease within the canal and surgical biopsy is indicated. Similarly the recent technique of laser therapy for in situ disease is less applicable in the older woman as the disease more commonly extends up the canal and only lesions visible to colposcopic examination are amenable to laser therapy. When surgical biopsy excision is indicated hysterectomy is more often resorted to in the older woman in contrast to simple cone biopsy, not only because she is more likely to have other uterine pathology but also because there is no concern regarding subsequent childbearing.

Patients previously treated for carcinoma in situ of the cervix should continue to have cytological follow-up for life as they remain at greater risk of developing disease than the population at large (Bevan *et al.*, 1981).

Invasive Carcinoma of the Cervix

Invasive carcinoma of the cervix can occur at any age but the mean age for diagnosis is 55.5 compared with 42.0 for in situ disease with a rate of 30+ per 100,000 for women aged 60 and over (Waterhouse, 1974).

Presenting symptoms include postmenopausal bleeding and discharge and spread outside the cervix to involve parametrium, vagina, lymphatic glands, or distant organs. Severe nerve root pain and uraemia may develop when spread reaches the pelvic wall and rarely a rectovaginal or vesicovaginal fistula occurs.

Treatment is primarily by radiotherapy and results depend on the original extent of disease and degree of tumour differentiation. The advantage of presymptomatic diagnosis is shown in the contrasting survival rates (Table 3).

REFERENCES

Adam, S., Williams, V., and Vessey, M. P. (1981). 'Cardiovascular disease and hormone replacement treatment', *Br. Med. J.*, **282**, 1277–1278.

Aitken, J. M., Hart, D. M., and Lindsay, R. (1973). 'Oestrogen replacement therapy for prevention oesteoporosis after oophorectomy', *Br. Med. J.*, **3**, 515–518.

Asch, R. H., and Greenblatt, R. B. (1977). 'Steroidogenesis in the post-menopausal ovary'. The climacteric, *Clin. Obstet. Gynecol.*, **4**, 55–106.

Barrett-Connor, E., Brown, W. V., Turner, J., Austin, N., and Criquit, M. H. (1979). 'Heart disease risk factors and hormone use in post-menopausal women', *JAMA*, **241**, 2167–2169.

Bevan, J. R., Attwood, M. E., Jordan, J. A., Lucan, A., and Newton, J. R. (1981). 'Treatment of preinvasive disease of the cervix by cone biopsy', *Br. J. Obstet. Gynaecol.*, **88**, 1140–1144.

Bonnar, J., Haddon, M., Hunter, D. M., Richards, D. H., and Thornton, C. (1976). 'Coagulation system changes in postmenopausal women receiving oestrogen therapy', *Postgrad. Med.*, **52** (Suppl. 6), 30–34.

Chakravarti, S., Collins, W. P., Forecast, J. D., Newton, J. R., Oram, D. H., and Studd, J. W. W. (1976). 'Hormonal profiles after the menopause', *Br. Med. J.*, **2**, 784–786.

Fidler, H. K., Boyce, D. A., and Worth, A. J. (1968). 'Cervical cancer detection in British Columbia', *J. Obstet. Gynaec. Brit. Comm.*, **75**, 392–404.

Higano, N., Robinson, R. W., and Cohen, W. D. (1963). 'Increased incidence of cardiovascular disease in castrated women', *New Engl. J. Med.*, **268**, 1123.

Hilton, P., and Stanton, S. L. (1981). 'Algorithric method for assessing urinary incontinence in elderly women', *Br. Med. J.*, **282**, 940–942.

Hutchinson, T., Polansky, S., and Feinstein, A. R. (1979). 'Postmenopausal oestrogens protect against fractures of hip and distal radius', *Lancet*, **705**, 709.

Hutton, J. D., Jacobs, H. S., and James, V. H. T. (1979). 'Steroid endocrinology after the menopause', *J. R. Soc. Med.*, **72**, 835–841.

Jeffcoate, T. N. A., and Tindall, V. R. (1965). 'Venous thrombosis and embolism in obstetrics and gynaecology', *Aust. N.Z. J. Obstet. Gynaecol.*, **5**, 119–130.

Jeffcoate, T. N., and Woodcock, A. S. (1961). 'Premalignant conditions of the vulva', *Br. Med. J.*, **11**, 127–134.

Knowelden, J., Buhr, A., and Dunbar, O. (1964). 'Incidence of fractures in persons over 35 years of age', *Br. J. Prev. Soc. Med.*, **18**, 130–141.

Lambert, H. (1981). 'Treatment of epithelial ovarian cancer', *J. Obstet. Gynaec. Brit. Comm.*, **88**, 1169–1173.

Magnani, H. N., and Moore, B. (1976). 'The effect of sequential mestranol/norethisterone on the circulating lipid levels of pre- and postmenopausal women', *Postgrad. Med.*, **52** (Suppl. 6), 55–58.

Medical Research Council Study (1981). 'Chemotherapy in advanced ovarian cancer', *Br. J. Obstet. Gynaecol.*, **88**, 1174–1185.

Monroe, S. E., and Menon, K. M. J. (1977). 'Changes in reproductive hormone secretion during the climacteric and postmenopausal periods', *Clin. Obstet. Gynecol.*, **20**, 113–122.

Notelovitz, M. (1977). 'Coagulation, oestrogen and the menopause. The climacteric', *Clin. Obstet. Gynecol.*, **4**, 119–125.

Parrish, H. M., Carr, C., Hall, D., and King, T. M. (1967). 'Time interval from castration in premenopausal women to development of excessive coronary atherosclerosis', *Am. J. Obstet. Gynecol.*, **99**, 155–162.

Paterson, M. E., Wade Evans, T., Sturdee, D., Thom, M. H., and Studd, J. W. (1980). 'Endometrial disease after treatment with oestrogens and progestogens in the climacteric', *Br. Med. J.*, **280**, 822–824.

Robinson, R. W., Higano, N., and Cohen, W. D. (1959). 'Incidence of coronary artery disease after castration', *Arch. Intern. Med.*, **104**, 908.

Ross, R. K., Hill, A. P., Mack, T., Arthur, M., and Henderson, B. (1981). 'Menopausal oestrogen therapy and protection from death from ischaemic heart disease', *Lancet*, **1**, 858–860.

Schnell, J. D., and Meinrenken, H. (1975). *Cytology and Microbiology of the Vagina*, S. Karger, Basel.

Smith, D. C., Prentice, R., Thompson, D. J., and Herrman, W. L. (1975). 'Association of exogenous oestrogen and endometrial cancer', *New Engl. J. Med.*, **293**, 23, 2164–2167.

Studd, J., Chakravarti, S., and Oram, D. (1977). 'The climacteric', *Clin. Obstet. cynecol.*, **4**, 1, 3–29.

Sweetnan, P., Evans, D., Hibbard, B. M., and Jones, J. M. (1981). The Cardiff Cervical Cytology Study', *J. Epidemiol. Community Health*, **35**, 83–90.

Walton Report (1976). 'Cervical cancer screening program', *Can. Med. Assoc. J.*, **114**, 1003–1012.

Waterhouse, J. A. H. (1974). *Cancer Handbook of Epidemiology and Prognosis*, Churchill Livingstone, Edinburgh and London.

Way, S. (1982). *Malignant Disease of the Vulva*, Churchill Livingstone, Edinburgh and London.

Young, R. C. (1975). 'Chemotherapy of ovarian cancer', *Semin. Oncol.*, **2**, 267–276.

26.2

Renal Disease

J. R. Cox, W. A. Shalaby

PHYSIOLOGY AND RENAL FUNCTION TESTS

Function of the Kidney

(a) Excrete waste products of metabolism.
(b) Adjust the amount of water and electrolytes excreted to keep the body fluid relatively constant in volume and composition.
(c) Help in keeping the pH of the blood constant through secretion of hydrogen ions, a buffer system converting monohydrogen phosphate to dihydrogen phosphate and formation of ammonia.

All this is achieved through urine formation.

Endocrine Function of the Kidney

(a) Regulate the blood pressure through the renin – aldosterone mechanism.
(b) A role in calcium metabolism through the conversion of 25-hydroxycholecalciferol to active vitamin D 1–25-dihydroxycholecalciferol.
(c) Help in keeping Hb constant under certain circumstances by formation of erythropoeitin.

Function of the Bladder

Acts as a reservoir for urine until the proper amount has been collected and the time is suitable to void it.

Tests of Renal Function

Urine Tests

(a) 24-hour urine volume
(b) Urine analysis: specific gravity, urinary pH, microscopic examination, detection of proteinuria, haematuria, glycosuria, culture and sensitivity and 24-hour solute excretion
(c) Urine concentration tests
(d) Urine dilution tests

(a) Blood urea. The normal concentration of blood urea is 4 to 7 mmol/l. Low values are found in children, during pregnancy, and in liver failure. As urea is mainly cleared by the glomeruli through the glomerular filtrate, one anticipates an increase in the plasma urea by reduction of the glomerular filtration rate. Unfortunately there are a lot of factors interfering with this and make its use less valuable. The plasma concentration depends on the rate of urea production and elimination. It is affected by the amount of ingested protein, the state of protein metabolism, as well as the glomerular filtration rate. Plasma urea rises disproportionately for a given glomerular filtration rate (GFR) or if a patient has a high protein intake, protein is catabolized following surgery, trauma, infection, or under the influence of corticosteroids or tetracyclines. Urea concentration falls out of proportion to GFR during sodium depletion, anabolism of pregnancy, and liver disease. A common cause of a high

blood urea is dehydration due to excessive diuretic therapy. However, increased plasma urea should generally reflect the state of the glomerular filteration rate.

(b) Creatinine. This is a more accurate measure of GFR as it is not affected by protein metabolism. Normal plasma creatinine is 60 to 120 mmol/l. However, the rate of production of creatinine will affect its blood level.

(c) Serum electrolytes. These are not usually diagnostic of renal disease, but may reflect excessive loss by the kidneys due to renal disorder. For example, low potassium might be due to potassium-losing nephritis or possibly chronic pyelonephritis. A high concentration of electrolytes may reflect a state of dehydration.

Clearance Tests

The clearance of a substance is the volume of plasma cleared completely of this substance through passage in the kidney in one minute. It is calculated from the following equation:

Volume of plasma cleared

$$= \frac{\begin{array}{c}\text{Volume of}\\\text{urine/min}\end{array} \times \begin{array}{c}\text{Concentration in}\\\text{urine}\end{array}}{\text{Concentration of substance in plasma}}$$

The clearance is used in the following measurements:

(a) Measurement of glomerular filtration rate. Ideally we should use a substance which passes freely through the glomeruli, travelling downwards without being subtracted or added to by the tubular cells. The amount that is excreted in the urine in 1 minute is therefore the same as that which is filtered.

Inulin clearance. This is the ideal substance as it is neither excreted nor reabsorbed by the renal tubule. In practice it is a difficult procedure. Inulin has to be injected i.v. either as a bolus or a drip, and many blood samples should be taken to make the average concentration. Urine should be collected by a catheter to avoid incomplete bladder emptying. It is only used for research purposes. EDTA (ethylene diamine tetracetic acid) is handled the

same way as inulin by the kidneys. ^{51}Cr EDTA makes the calculation easier. Concentration is calculated using a gamma counter.

Creatinine clearance. It is slightly greater than inulin indicating that some creatinine is actively secreted by the tubules. It is a much more convenient method than that of inulin, for creatinine is already present in body fluids and its plasma concentration is fairly steady through 24 hours. Only one blood sample is needed plus a 24-hour urine collection which minimizes the effect of bladder emptying and emotional reactions.

Urea clearance. Urea is a small highly diffusable molecule; a great deal is reabsorbed as it passes down the tubules. Urea clearance is about 35 per cent. of the glomerular filtration rate at maximum urinary concentration and rises to about 70 per cent. with water diuresis over 2 ml/min. It is inferior to creatinine clearance.

(b) Measurement of renal blood flow. Renal plasma flow can theoretically be calculated by the Fick principle using any substance excreted in urine provided renal arterial and venous concentrations are known:

Renal plasma flow

$$= \frac{\text{amount of substance excreted in urine/min}}{\text{arteriovenous difference}}$$

This laborious procedure is not necessary as renal plasma flow can be measured using a substance which is completely cleared in one passage through the kidneys, e.g. para-aminohippuric acid (PAH). It would mean under such circumstances that the volume of plasma which would supply the amount of substances excreted in the urine is equal to renal plasma flow. Para-aminohippuric acid is infused intravenously until a steady plasma concentration is achieved and the renal plasma flow is calculated using the following equation:

Renal plasma flow

$$= \frac{\begin{array}{c}\text{volume}\\\text{of urine}\end{array} \times \begin{array}{c}\text{concentration of PAH}\\\text{in the urine}\end{array}}{\text{concentration of PAH in plasma}}$$

In other words, para-aminohippuric acid clearance is equal to renal plasma flow. The simplest way to perform a PAH clearance now is to use ^{125}Hippuran and the concentration is calculated by a gamma counter.

Radiological Examination

(a) Plain X-ray. Give information about the size, shape, and position of the kidneys, nephrocalcinosis, stones, calcification of the arteries, tumours, and cysts along with prostatic calcification.

(b) Excretion urography. It is now the backbone of radiological examinations of the urinary tract. The kidneys, calyces, ureters, and bladder are visualized.

(c) Retrograde urography. Retrograde pyelography is useful in non-excreting kidneys to exclude urinary tract obstruction. It defines the calyceal details or shows the site of obstruction if present.

(d) Cystourethrography. Abnormalities of the bladder neck and urethra are demonstrated by this method. The micturating cystogram is the most useful single radiological investigation of the lower urinary tract and it is the only reliable method for demonstration of vesicoureteric reflux.

(e) Retroperitoneal air insufflation. Injection of gas into the fat-containing layer will improve radiological contrast around the structure within that layer. If air is injected through the parasacral fat, it will spread continually to the perirenal fat.

(f) Renal angiography. Its main use is to diagnose localized disease of renal arteries, and the peripheral arterial and capillary system, arterial distortion due to tumours or hydronephrosis, abnormal vessels, areas of ischaemia or infarction, arteriovenous malformation, ectopic or absent renal tissue.

Instrumentation

Catheterization is rarely used to measure the residual urine. Urethroscopy, cystoscopy, and ureteric catheterization are done under anaesthesia. They give direct magnified vision to the inside of the urethra, bladder, and ureters. Ureteric catheterization is also important in assessment of split renal function tests in suspected unilateral disease.

Isotope Study

(a) Renography. The renal accretion and release of intravenously injected radioactive substance has been used to assess renal function. It includes serial images using a gamma camera which add regional assessment to previous measurements. Some curve patterns have been correlated with specific disease processes.

(b) Renal scanning. This is useful to identify parenchymal function when the kidneys are not visualized by intravenous pyelography to detect renal masses and to distinguish between disease and anatomic variations and areas of regional abnormalities.

Ultrasonic Study

As ultrasound does not depend on the function of an organ, it is very valuable when other techniques such as urography are unsatisfactory. A classical example of its use is to demonstrate the nature of a non-visualized kidney. It is not invasive so is of particular importance in frail patients. The most important uses are in a differential diagnosis of renal masses and polycystic disease.

Renal Biopsy

This is indicated in cases of unexplained proteinuria, haematuria, expected renal involvement in systemic disease, and renal homograft failure. Exact diagnoses may be revealed in difficult cases.

Other Tests

Percutaneous renal puncture Antegrade Pyelography Renal pressure flow study

EFFECT OF AGE ON URINARY FUNCTION AND RENAL FUNCTION TESTS

Ageing is known to be associated with a decrease in functional capacity of a number of organs and systems (Szilard, 1959). This occurs particularly in tissues of adult animals where cellular division is absent, e.g. muscles, heart, and kidney, but not in those where mitosis still occurs – liver. There is a wide variation of opinion as to why age effects performance.

After the age of 30 there is a gradual reduction in renal functional capacity. By the age of 60 these functions decrease to half their value at the age of 30. There are two hypotheses regarding this clinical decline in renal function:

(a) There is a progressive physiological change due to gradual loss of nephron population and inability of the aged kidney to regenerate – an ageing phenomenon.

(b) Renal function remains fairly steady until a pathological process, particularly vascular insufficiency, causes it to suddenly deteriorate.

Though there is no doubt that pathological changes which occur and cause rapid deterioration of function at any age do occur more frequently and produce more sinister results in the elderly, gradual deterioration of function without any obvious pathological cause are now documented. Data collected from a normal ageing population (Davies and Shock, 1950; Shock, 1946) show that there is a decrease in the mean renal function with age in each decade. Moreover the process is accelerated with advancing age'. Phillips and Leong (1967) measured the proliferative activity in the kidneys after unilateral nephrectomy using tritiated thymidine autoradiography, and found the activity was three times as great in young rats, i.e. weaning rats, compared to adult animals. However, although the proliferative activity was much lower in adult animals, a similar response qualitatively was obtained in both groups, i.e. elderly rats respond in the same way as young rats but to a lesser degree. A similar finding by Barrows, Falzone and Shock (1960) showed that the rate of oxidative phosphorylation and accumulation of succinoxidase is significantly decreased in homogenate prepared from kidney cortex of older animals.

Beauchene, Fanastil and Barrows (1965) also noted that there is a decrease in PAH accumulation by aged rat kidney slices as well as a decrease of sodium and potassium activated ATPase activity of renal tissue. It seems that gradual deterioration of renal function occurs with age either due to decreased nephron population or diminished enzyme activity in the kidney. On the other hand, the increase in incidence of pathological changes, especially ischaemic lesions, does occur with advancing age. Friedman and coworkers, (1972) found abnormal kidney scarring in 25 out of 35 elderly patients; 46 per cent. showed focal areas of diminished uptake representing an ischaemic lesion. In all patients the intravenous pyelogram (IVP) was normal and there was no proteinuria. On the other hand Howell and Piggot, (1948) reported that in a series of 300 postmortem examinations of patients above the age of 65 no gross renal change appeared in 47 per cent.; a fifth of the cases showed finely granular structures and diminution of the cortex. Grossly scarred kidneys were found in a seventh of the cases examined. Microscopic examination showed degenerative changes in the tubules, especially the proximal convoluted tubules, with cloudy swelling and atrophy of the tubular wall and tubular collapse. Other tubules were dilated. Fibrotic change was seen in the glomeruli with areas of hyalinization. (Rosen, 1976). These changes are presumably due to structural changes in renal vasculature. Arteriolar hyalinization and intimal thickening in small arteries usually associated with essential hypertension are seen in normotensive elderly people. To summarize, lesions due to pathological abnormality occur more in the elderly; however, decrease in renal activity with increasing age takes place without evidence of pathological changes.

It is well recognized that water and electrolyte metabolism are more critical in aged people with no gross signs or laboratory tests indicating renal dysfunction.

The ability to concentrate or dilute urine is gradually lost, with the result that the elderly person is unable to cope maximally with either dehydration or water load. Elderly persons are more prone to develop hypokalaemia and hyponatraemia during diuretic therapy or due to an inadequate diet. On the other hand, excess salt intake may result in heart failure. Elderly subjects show a high renal sodium loss and this loss is exclusively through the distal nephron (Nunez *et al.*, 1978). This would explain why aged individuals easily become dehydrated and develop acute renal failure. Body potassium content of the elderly has been shown to be less than in the young (Cox and Shalaby, 1981). There is a linear correlation between potassium content and age, even when the potassium content is related to lean body weight and fat-free body weight. This might be partly due to excessive loss of potassium by renal tissue, as well as poor intake.

Specific gravity of 1.040 during water deprivation tests are rarely seen in individuals above the age of 20 years. The maximum attainable specific gravity in Chelsea pensioners over the age of 65 was 1.030. (Howell and Piggot, 1948). The ability of the distal renal tubules of older individuals to perform osmotic work when provided with a standardized amount of antidiuretic hormone is impaired (Miller and Shock, 1953).

Lindeman and coworkers (1966) suggested that the ability of cellular membranes in the distal nephron to become more water permeable in response to ADH was possibly diminished only in patients with chronic pyelonephritis and severe hypertension. Recently the problem has been further investigated by Bengele and coworkers (1981) who studied the water metabolism in aged rats and concluded that the decrease in responsiveness of collecting duct tubular epithelium to circulatory ADH is the most likely explanation for the impairment of urine concentrating ability. Reduced hypophyseal function seems to play no role in this defect.

In response to the same osmotic challenge old subjects increase the circulatory antidiuretic hormone to a concentration higher than young subjects (Helderman *et al.*, 1978). Whatever the cause of this abnormality there is no doubt about the inability of the aged kidney to concentrate urine and the ease with which the elderly person may develop acute renal failure as a consequence. As long as the water intake is adequate (2.51 to 3.01 per day) the condition will remain under control. Crises will arise when water intake diminishes because the patient becomes either disinterested, lonely, immobile, depressed, confused, or frightened of incontinence. This may also be induced by the unnecessary use of diuretics. Dehydration and electrolyte imbalance are important factors in the development of acute renal failure in elderly patients (Kumar, Hill, and McGeown, 1973). Although it might be partly the inability of the kidney to handle water load, other factors such as a marginal cardiac decompensation could be responsible. Acid excretion is decreased in advanced age, probably due to decreased renal tubular mass rather than specific tubular defect (Adler *et al.*, 1968).

Proteinuria is not generally accepted as a result of ageing. Alt and coworkers (1980) demonstrated greatly increased renal excretion of albumin in rats with increased age. However, the total protein excretion stays the same or even decreases slightly as the rats age, due to loss of molecular sex dependent proteins excreted by the young ones. A comparable state of affairs might occur in human beings.

Bacteriuria used to be accepted in the elderly as harmless if asymptomatic. However, Dontas and coworkers (1966) found that the glomerular filtration rate, renal plasma flow, and tubular function are significantly reduced in elderly patients with bacteriuria as compared with people of the same age group who had no bacteriauria. This point will be discussed further later on.

Blood urea and blood creatinine are usually normal in aged healthy individuals. This does not necessarily mean that the glomerular filtration rate is normal. Blood urea may be reduced due to diminished protein intake which is common in the elderly, and very rarely is due to liver disease and inefficient production of urea. Normal serum creatinine may reflect low production. Reduced muscle mass is common in aged individuals and may account for the normal plasma creatinine.

The average inulin and diodrast clearance decrease linearly beyond the age of 30 years (Davies and Shock, 1950). Olbrich and coworkers (1950) agreed that both inulin and diodrast clearance decreased with age reflecting a diminution in the glomerular filtration rate and renal plasma flow. They suggested that these results do not signify impairment of glomerular filtration capacity but that due to decreased renal plasma flow associated with vascular changes. Brod (1968) showed that in both men and women renal blood flow, renal plasma flow, and the glomerular filtration rate were significantly lower in a group of people aged 41 to 60 years as compared to another group aged 21 to 40 years. Moreover, McDonald, Solomon, and Shook (1951) concluded by administration of pyrogen that the reduced renal blood flow observed in the aged is partly reversible and therefore is not a result of structural damage in the renal vessels. The glomerular filtration rate and renal tubular absorption of glucose decrease with advancing age (Miller 1952).

In a longitudinal study of 844 patients Rowe and coworkers (1976) showed a decrease in creatinine clearance with age, which they regarded as representing true renal ageing and not secondary to disease. They constructed a nomogram providing a normative age-corrected standard for creatinine clearance.

It is therefore clear that GFR and RPF are significantly reduced in the elderly. This might be of crucial importance, particularly in view of multiple drug therapy, so common in this age group. Drugs excreted by the kidneys may accumulate in the body and exert their toxic effect. Although routine techniques to measure the glomerular filtration rate are available, the patient may be incontinent, confused, or uncooperative, and making 24-hour urine collections may not only be difficult but sometimes impossible without successful catheterization. Clinical conditions such as this are not uncommonly due to infection and a delay of 24 hours before initiation of a drug is not ideal. Gral and Young (1980) compared an endogenous creatinine clearance (24-hour urine collection) with estimated (calculated) creatinine in 26 elderly subjects. The calculated creatinine clearance was obtained by a formula suggested by Lott and Hayton (1978), namely:

Creatinine clearance
$$= \frac{(140 - \text{age}) \times \text{lean body weight}}{72 \times \text{serum creatinine}}$$

This formula is a modification of the formula designed by Cockcroft and Gault in 1976:

Creatinine clearance
$$= \frac{(140 - \text{age}) \times \text{body weight}}{72 \times \text{serum creatinine}}$$

All subjects studied were fairly stable and on adequate food and fluid. In all subjects creatinine clearance was reduced in spite of the normal serum creatinine level and the result of endogenous creatinine clearance was compared with the estimated (calculated) one. The correlation coefficient was highly significant in all instances. It was concluded that a fairly accurate assessment of renal function can be obtained based on the patient's age, weight, and serum creatinine level.

The original formula designed by Cockcroft and Gault is simple and reasonably accurate and provides a rapid bedside estimation of the renal status in the acute situation. The modified formula needs the estimation of lean body weight, although tables are available for this estimation.

The abnormality of renal function could be explained by a recent study by Smalley (1980). Human glomerular basement membrane (HGBM) was isolated in highly purified form from the kidney cortex of a number of individuals ranging from 27 to 90 years after routine biopsy. An increase of HGBM per unit with age was found and a progressive decrease in the quantities of amino acids: threonine, methionine, isoleucine, leucine, tyrosine, phenylalanine, hydroxylysine, and histidine (3.7 per cent. reduction per decade). It was concluded from this that there was a diminution of the collagenous component present in the HGBM with increasing age.

An electron microscopy study on mice kidney glomeruli shows that there is a significant age-related increase in glomerular diameter and number of microvilli on the podocyte surface (Johnson and Barrows, 1980). Feeding the rats with a diet containing 4 per cent. protein resulted in a smaller diameter of the glomeruli and decreased numbers of podocytes, as compared to those fed on a control diet containing 24 per cent. protein. Dietary restriction has been shown to increase the life of the laboratory animals. The relationships between diet and ageing, particularly dietary deficiencies, is important but the above findings seem to suggest that a very high protein intake may result in renal ageing.

In summary, there is good evidence that renal function deteriorates with age. The aged kidney is unable to concentrate urine as much as the young kidney and because of this the elderly are more easily dehydrated and therefore more liable to develop acute renal failure. The ageing kidney is unable to handle large amounts of solute or hydrogen ions and cannot conserve maximally potassium and sodium like the young healthy kidney. Urea and creatinine are generally normal in the elderly individual but this may reflect a state of reduced production rather than normal elimination. The glomerular filtration rate as well as renal plasma flow show a linear reduction with increased age. Undoubtedly this decline in function is accentuated in the elderly who are more prone to renal damage, particularly by pyelonephritis and ischaemic changes.

Endocrine Function of the Kidney and Ageing

Serum 1–25-dihydroxy vitamin D_3 decreases with age, while 25-hydroxy vitamin D_3 remains constant (Gallagher *et al.*, 1979). Calcium absorption is decreased with age (Bullamore *et al.*, 1970). There is a marked decrease in the capacity of the vitamin D deficient adult rat as compared to younger rats to convert 25-hydroxy vitamin D_3 to 1–25-dihydroxy vitamin D_3, probably due to a decreased capacity of the adult kidney to 1–25-hydroxylate and 25-hydroxylate vitamin D_3 (Armbrecht, Zensen, and Davis, 1980). This change with age of the endocrine function may be one of the reasons for the increased incidence of osteomalacia in the aged and why it is difficult to treat with simple vitamin D supplementation. This is supported by the findings of Kafetz and Hodkinson (1981) who reported two cases of osteomalacia in patients aged 74 years and 87 years diagnosed histologically in whom the serum 25-hydroxycholecalciferol concentration was close to mean in elderly patients.

Radiography of the Aged Kidney

The intravenous pyelogram is usually normal in patients with a moderate reduction in the glomerular filtration rate. It is only when the glomerular filtration rate is reduced below 10 ml/min that visulization of the kidneys is greatly reduced. It is important to rehydrate the patient before the procedure. Renal scan shows significant abnormalities in 70 per cent. of the elderly, including asymmetric areas of decreased uptake, frequent inequality of the

two kidneys, and considerable reduction of the active kidney area. These might represent areas of ischaemia. In general it is expected in elderly individuals and should not cause alarm in asymptomatic patients.

Ultrasound examination is one of the most valuable non-invasive techniques for the non-functional kidney. It can usually differentiate tumours from staghorn stones. This could be invaluable in a frail elderly person.

RENAL DISEASES IN THE AGED

Renal disorders as they occur in the young and middle aged, e.g. acute nephritis, collagen disorders, and malignant hypertension, are uncommon in old age. If they occur they do not show a basic difference in mode of presentation. Essentially the same investigations and treatment are carried out. Acute and chronic renal failure are essentially similar to the same conditions in younger age groups. Apart from a more critical water and electrolyte balance and a greater tendency to develop cardiac failure, causes, symptomatology, and investigation are principally the same as in the young.

The common renal problems affecting the aged population are:
(a) bacteriuria, urinary tract infection, acute and chronic pyelonephritis;
(b) drugs and the aged kidney;
(c) kidney and hypertension;
(d) renal failure;
(e) miscellaneous disorders.

Bacteriuria and the Urinary Tract Infection in Old Age

Bacteriuria is one of the most common human infections. It is present in a relatively asymptomatic population. It is commonly agreed that the presence of bacteriuria will proceed to the development of acute infection in the urinary tract with probable renal invasion. People at risk are pregnant women, people who undergo urinary tract instrumentation, and the elderly. Partial obstruction by an enlarged prostate is one of the most common causes of bacteriuria and of actual urinary tract infection (Kass, Savage, and Santamario, 1964).

The incidence of bacteriuria increases with advancing age. It is more common in females, both young and old, but is markedly more common in elderly males when compared to young males (Rosen, 1976).

Possible causes of increased incidence of bacteriuria in old people are:

(a) urinary stasis and obstruction;
(b) vascular insufficiency;
(c) diminished immunity;
(d) instrumentation, especially catheterization.

Ascending infection is often seen in the presence of stasis or catheterization, but haematogenous infection is not uncommon. In addition in vascular insufficiency due to nephrosclerosis and diminished power of immunity, vescicourethral reflux has been implicated.

Causes of urinary tract obstruction in the elderly are:

(a) prostatic hypertrophy, benign or malignant;
(b) uterine prolapse, and preurethral gland hypertrophy in females;
(c) stones;
(d) strictures;
(e) tumours of the urinary tract and pelvis;
(f) sloughed papillae due to diabetes mellitus or drugs.

Neurogenic bladder due to diabetes mellitus, posterior roots, and posterior column dysfunction results in retention of urine with similar results to that of mechanical obstruction.

Bacteriuria has been extensively studied in the elderly. Sourander (1966) found asymptomatic bacteriuria in 30 per cent. of women and 7 per cent. of men in a random sample of the population above the age of 65 years. In chronically ill patients Mou, Siroty, and Ventry (1962) found a high bacterial count in 20 per cent. of men and 61 per cent. of women, all of geriatric age. Similar findings were reported by Wolfson (1965). They found an increase in incidence of asymptomatic bacteriuria with age. They also suggested that impaired resistance could be a factor in patients in whom urinary tract obstruction is not found. Brocklehurst and coworkers (1968) noted that in males aged 65 to 70 the incidence of bacteriuria was only 3 per cent. Above this age and in all women over 65 the average was 20 per cent. It is obviously markedly less than in institutionalized patients which means that aged populations taking regular exercise have a lower incidence of urinary tract infections. Brocklehurst also found that there is no correlation between bac-

teriuria and symptoms such as precipitancy. The possibility remains that in men and some women these symptoms are the result of the disease which causes the bacteriuria in the first place, e.g. obstruction or neurogenic bladder. The increased incidence of predisposing factors might be used to explain the greater frequency of bacteriuria in old age, but there is a significant number of patients where definite predisposing factors cannot be found. It can be assumed in these cases that they either have diminished immunity or a deficient blood supply.

More recently Kasviki-Charwati and coworkers (1982) have shown in a study of 352 residents in a home for the elderly that significant susceptibility to infection does exist in old age coupled with a lesser trend towards a spontaneous cure. Thus the prevalence rises steadily in old age. Secondly, a previous history of bacteriuria in a subject with currently sterile urine increases his chances of reinfection or recurrence 2 to 7 times compared to those of subjects without past infection.

The significance of asymptomatic bacteriuria is unknown. It is possible that the bacteriuria noted represents just a urine infection without tissue involvement. Dontas and coworkers (1966) investigated 53 ambulant aged patients who had no clinical evidence of renal disease. He found that 25 per cent. had bacterial counts exceeding 10.000/ml. Renal function tests revealed a significant impairment of tubular capacity in a group with bacteriuria as compared with the group of non-bacteriurias. Glomerular and circulatory deficits were also found to be pronounced in the first group. The same problems were further studied by the same authors in 1968. They supported their previous findings of prevalence of bacteriuria in the elderly and its deleterious effect on the glomerular filtration rate, renal plasma flow, and tubular function. All showed significant impairment as compared to the group with no bacteriuria. They concluded that bacteriuria in old age is a contributary factor in accelerating the pre-existing renovascular disease and suggested that the non-bacteriuria group display renal function homogeneity at progressive levels of nephrosclerosis, but in the presence of bacteriuria this pattern is modified by superimposed qualitative functional abnormalities.

Investigation by Miall and coworkers (1962)

showed that in the Jamaican as well as in the Welsh population the bacteriuric woman has somewhat higher blood pressure than do aged matched non-bacteriuric women. There is as yet no clear indication that bacteriuria leads to the development of chronic pyelonephritis; the association of bacteriuria and hypertension is not clear. Hypertension is familial while bacteriuria is not. There may be a reason to question just how much of the chronic pyelonephritis is due to infection.

There is thus evidence to suggest that treatment of bacteriuria and certainly urinary tract infections is worth while. Classification and line of treatment is not different from that applied in young people. Brown (1980) has proposed the following classification for urinary tract infections:

(a) Bacteriuria: when there are laboratory findings of bacteriuria in the urine. It is mostly asymptomatic.

(b) Urinary tract infection: bacteriuria with signs and symptoms involving the tissue of the tract including kidney, ureter, prostate, bladder, or urethra.

(c) Acute pyelonephritis: bacteriuria with or without lower urinary tract symptoms but including chills, fever, flank pain, and tenderness.

(d) Chronic pyelonephritis: renal disease believed but not proved to be due to previous intermittent or chronic infection. It can be caused by other factors like analgesics, X-ray irradiation, and accompanied by renal scarring.

(e) Urethral syndrome in women: symptoms of urgency, frequency, and dysuria in the absence of an easily identifiable microorganism in the culture.

The most common cause of a urinary tract infection (UTI) is *Escherichia coli* (85 per cent.). In cases of complicated urinary tract infection, if treatment is carried out efficiently and the cause is removed 50 per cent. full recovery is expected. Where chronic or persistent infection is established with evidence of chronic pyelonephritis, poor urinary concentration, hypertension, inability to conserve electrolytes, and rising blood urea, even the relief of urinary tract obstruction, may not help the patient. In such cases 90 per cent. may be expected to continue with slowly progressive renal failure.

Usually patients are treated for at least 5 days with the appropriate antibiotic, but it is interesting that Harbord and Gruneberg (1981) have shown 95, 87.5, and 90 per cent. cure rates in three different groups of patients after a single dose of amoxycillin, cotrimoxazole and trimethoprim, respectively. Furthermore Rapoport and coworkers (1981) stated that the conventional dose of cotrimoxazole repeated on 2 successive nights (total of 6 tablets) was as effective as conventional treatment (14 or more tablets) in eliminating acute uncomplicated urinary infection in patients treated at home. The use of such short-term antibiotic therapy could be of great advantage in elderly in whom compliance is difficult and drugs often more toxic.

Drugs and the Ageing Kidneys

The very elderly, i.e. those aged 75 years and over, constitute an increasing percentage of the population. The increased standards of living, better housing, better diet, and the elimination of infectious diseases in the Western world have increased the number of people reaching old age.

Lengthy exposure to the hazards of life makes them more likely to be suffering from chronic conditions needing multiple-drug therapy as well as the inevitable effects of age itself. Many are receiving or have received prolonged courses of treatment by one or more drugs (Lyle, 1977).

In a survey of a Canadian town Skoll, August, and Johnson (1979) found that during 1976, 77.3 per cent. of the population above the age of 65 received at least one prescription, in comparison with the age group 35 to 54 years. Prescriptions issued and drugs used per person was higher than average among the elderly. Altered and unexpected responses to treatment can be caused by physiological changes that occur with ageing. These changes can affect the absorption, distribution, metabolism, and elimination of drugs. Changes in renal function, body composition, and gastrointestinal tract are variables influencing a drug's mechanism of action (Vancura, 1979) and an understanding of these variables is essential to avoid therapeutic problems. Although basic absorption is unchanged, many elderly patients are prone to chronic diarrhoea or constipation, either of which may alter intestinal contact time and thus absorption (Ward and Blatman, 1979). The problems of drug interaction are also important, as elderly patients commonly receive multiple-drug therapy. One of the major routes of drug elimination is the kidneys. Before prescribing drugs in elderly patients the following questions should be proposed:

(a) Is the drug mainly excreted by the kidneys?
(b) Does it especially affect the kidney's which are the subject of previous damage?
(c) What is the side-effect of such a drug?

The effects of drugs and their relationship to the kidney may be considered in two ways.

(a) The problems posed by the potentially toxic effect of certain drugs on the kidneys.
(b) Toxicity of drugs that are prescribed for patients with diminished renal function.

Toxic Effects of Drugs on the Kidneys

The kidneys are particularly susceptible to the toxic effect of drugs and other chemical agents (Evans, 1980) for the following reasons:
(a) rich blood supply;
(b) drugs are concentrated in the hypertonic medulla;
(c) drug accumulation associated with impaired renal function;
(d) hypersensitivity reaction with vasculitis is common in the kidney;
(e) concomitant inhibition of hepatic enzymes increases drug toxicity.

There are many different mechanisms involved in drug-induced renal disorders (Curtis, 1980). There is evidence that metabolic activation of some drugs within the kidneys is responsible for nephrotoxicity while other drug reactions seem to be immunologically mediated. Certain drugs produce their side effects as a result of fluid and electrolyte disturbances, calculus formation, or crystalluria. Some of these occur only in genetically predisposed individuals.

Drug Toxicity

This can cause:
(a) acute nephrotoxicity: secondary hypovolaemia, acute tubular necrosis, acute interstitial nephritis, acute vasculitis, arteriolar damage, tubular block, osmotic nephrosis, ureteric obstruction, or acute urinary retention;
(b) drug-induced syndromes such as systemic lupus erythematosis and nephrotic syndrome;
(c) chronic renal failure.

Mechanisms Producing Renal Damage

The mechanisms by which drugs produce renal damage (Cove-Smith, 1980) are as follows:
(a) prerenal uraemia;
(b) obstructive uropathy;
(c) vascular lesions;
(d) glomerular damage;
(e) interstitial and tubular damage;
(f) papillary necrosis.

(a) Prerenal uraemia. Diuretics and laxatives cause dehydration. The effect is accentuated by concomitant potassium loss. Glucocorticoids and tetracyclines raise blood urea by increasing catabolism.

(b) Obstructive uropathy. Retroperitoneal haemorrhage and ureteric obstruction caused by blood clot due to anticoagulants or fibrinolytic therapy. Retroperitoneal fibrosis occurs with methysergide and methyldopa. Ureteric fibrosis and sloughed papillae can be caused by the chronic use of analgesics. Crystalluria can be caused by increased uric acid levels, acetazolamide, mercaptopurine, or methotrexate. Tubular blockage can be caused by material used in intravenous pyelography in tubules already partially blocked by Bence Jones' proteins in myeloma. Haemolysis and blockage of tubules can be caused by sulphonamides and antimalarials in cases of glucose-6-phosphate dehydrogenase deficiency or by rifampicin. Excessive use of vitamin D can result in tubular blockage by calcium. The elderly are perhaps more prone to vitamin D deficiency and thus not uncommonly may undergo treatment with vitamin D.

(c) Vascular lesions. Vascular occlusion occurs with oestrogen therapy. Hypersensitivity angiitis may be caused by thiazides. Vascular damage plays a part in drug-induced systemic lupus erythematosis.

(d) Glomerular damage. This might present as a nephrotic syndrome due to ampicillin, gold, mercurials, penicillin, probenecid, sulphonamide, and tolbutamide.

Systemic lupus erythematosis-like syndrome may be caused by hydrallazine, isoniazid, procainamide, tetracycline, penicillin, carbamazepine, phenytoin, methyldopa, penicillamine, and phenylbutazone. It usually occurs in genetically predisposed individuals.

(e) Interstitial and tubular damage. Acute interstitial nephritis usually occurs as part of generalized hypersensitivity reaction, due to penicillins, sulphonamides, rifampicin, thiazides, and frusemide.

Acute tubular necrosis occurs with heavy metals, aminoglycosides, colistin, polymyxin B, cephalosporins, and may be potentiated with frusemide. Other drugs which may cause this are amphotericin B, analgesic overdose, and radiological contrast media.

(f) Papillary necrosis. Chronic ingestion of analgesics may cause necrosis of the renal papillae and interstitial nephritis resulting in chronic renal failure due to obstruction caused by the detached papillae.

There is little doubt that the elderly are more likely to be affected by the use of drugs than the young. The elderly kidneys are basically as susceptible as the young, but two facts should always be remembered:

(1) The elderly are more susceptible to dehydration and electrolyte imbalance which potentiates the toxicity of drugs. This is caused by their deteriorating renal function and poor fluid and electrolyte intake.

(2) In view of the present prescribing habits and multiple pathology associated with old age, the elderly are more exposed to prolonged and multiple drug therapy.

Toxicity of the Drugs when Administered to Patients with Diminished Renal Function

This depends on multiple factors, e.g. the proportion of the drug normally excreted by the kidneys and the likely toxic effect of drugs. As previously noted, renal function diminishes with age.

The reduction in renal clearance of a drug caused by renal impairment is proportional to reduction in renal clearance of creatinine (Levy, 1977). If a standard dose of a drug cleared through the kidney was given to an elderly patient, accumulation is likely to occur in blood and tissue far higher than that necessary for therapeutic benefit and may certainly result in serious side-effects with iatrogenic disease. The elderly patients are more susceptible to ototoxicity and nephrotoxicity with aminoglycosides, neuropathy with nitrofurantoin, hypoglycaemia with chlorpropamide, lactic acidosis with biguanides, and intoxication with digoxin (Castleden, 1978). Penicillin half-life increases in the elderly corresponding to the decrease in creatinine clearance (Hansen, Kampmann, and Laursen, 1970).

Equidoses of digoxin produce higher blood levels and a longer blood half-life in old subjects when compared with young subjects (Ewy *et al.*, 1969).

Ideally doctors should be prepared to treat the individual elderly patient with the appropriately reduced dose as there is a great variability of absorption, distribution, metabolism, and excretion (Stevenson, 1978). Dose adjustment may be achieved by reducing the amount given at the same intervals or by giving the same dose at longer intervals. Both methods are acceptable and each is recommended by a number of authors. In case of doubt, measuring the creatinine clearance would be a safe method to judge the dangers of drug dosage. The formula created by Cockcroft and Gault (1976):

Creatinine clearance

$$= \frac{(140 - \text{age}) \times \text{body weight}}{72 \times \text{serum creatinine}}$$

seems to be quite satisfactory, especially in cases where 24-hour urine collection is impossible or in urgent cases where treatment cannot be delayed.

Some drugs are of particular interest as regards the elderly. Digoxin is often prescribed for a very prolonged period. As it is excreted mainly by the kidney it is very unlikely that the elderly will need normal digitalization as given to the young. The dose 0.25 to 0.5 mg is nearly always sufficient and the maintenance dose is usually 0.0625 to 0.125 mg. Its cardiac toxicity is enhanced by hypokalaemia, a very common association due to the concomitant use of diuretics and the known tendency of the elderly to take a diet deficient in potassium. The serum potassium may be little guide to total body potassium content, though low serum levels are nearly always associated with low total body levels (Cox Pearson, and Speight, 1971). It might be wise to review regularly the need and dosage of digitalis as well as renal function in patients who are on a maintenance regime of digoxin. Another group of drugs commonly used in the elderly are diuretics. Thiazides are ineffective at a low glomerular filtration rate. Frusemide, bumetanide, and ethacrynic acid can still be effective at a glomerular filtration rate of only 3 ml/min. Ethacrynic acid and frusemide can be ototoxic and bumetanide may cause myopathy. All these drugs can cause severe hypokalaemia in the elderly and may result in dehydration if given in large doses over a prolonged period. Hypokalaemia itself may produce renal damage. In cases of acute renal failure potassium-conserving diuretics can cause serious hyperkalaemia.

Hypokalaemia has been reported following the treatment with a combination of thiazide and beta blockers. Skehan and coworkers (1982) reported profound hypokalaemia following the use of hydrochlorothiazide sotazide and 25 mg of hydrochlorothiazide Thus the combination of beta blocker and diuretic does not necessarily protect against potassium deficiency.

Anti-inflammatory non-steroidal drugs can affect renal function in various conditions including nephrotic syndrome (Dunn and Zambraski, 1980).

Baumelou and Legrain (1982) used indomethacin to produce a medical nephrectomy in order to prevent protein leakage in a patient with nephrotic syndrome having regular dialysis. These drugs can affect the elderly kidney in the same way as it is universally agreed that as people age the renal function deteriorates. Paracetamol can induce renal failure in the absence of signs of fulminant liver damage (Cobden *et al.*, 1982).

Hypotensive agents can accumulate in the body due to their poor excretion by the elderly kidney. They can cause devastating postural hypotension, a condition which may result in confusion, falls, and immobility. Adjustment of the dose is necessary and review of the condition at intervals is important.

Anticholinergic drugs and drugs with anticholinergic effects may accumulate with severe side-effects. They may be prescribed in large doses which cannot be handled by the elderly kidney and also sometimes in combination. A common example of this iatrogenic condition occurs in the prescribing of anticholinergic drugs for Parkinsonism, antidepressants, and drugs to control the bladder; all may have a strong anticholinergic effect on an elderly person whose kidneys may be unable to deal with even normal doses of drugs and whose brain is highly susceptible to confusional states (see Chapter 5).

Kidney and Hypertension

Renal diseases have long been associated with hypertension. Some renal disorders as well as acute and chronic failure may cause hypertension. On the other hand, hypertension itself can result in renal damage.

The role of the kidney in essential hypertension has always been a subject of great interest and debate. Guyton and coworkers (1972) maintain what is called resetting of pressure natriuresis as a feature of all hypertensive states. It is known that a rise in arterial blood pressure increases urinary sodium excretion. Reduction in the ability of the kidney to excrete sodium at a given arterial blood pressure leads to sodium retention, which raises blood pressure to the point where sodium balance can be restored. Another theory suggested by Parfrey and coworkers (1981a) is that in patients with essential hypertension, the blood pressure is sensitive to sodium intake. This may partly be due to changes either produced by or associated directly with hypertension. A decreased responsiveness of the renin-angiotensin-aldosterone system may account for the result. Parfrey and coworkers (1981b) further suggested that a genetically determined susceptibility to the pressor effect of low dietary potassium is important in the early stages of hypertension, followed later by increased susceptibility to dietary sodium. The potassium effect is mediated through the autonomic nervous system. A rise in arterial pressure with age in Western society may result from increase in dietary sodium or decreased dietary potassium or both. It was proposed by Lever and coworkers (1981) that the two mechanisms, the so-called resetting of pressure natriuresis as well as dietary sensitivity, may operate together in essential hypertension. They suggested that in the early stages of the disease, blood pressure is raised by abnormal processes related to potassium and sodium intake, perhaps more closely to potassium than sodium. A renal lesion develops later, possibly as a consequence of this primary increase in blood pressure. This is associated by resetting of pressure natriuresis so that higher blood pressure is needed to maintain a given sodium excretion.

Reubi and Weidman (1980) concluded that in essential hypertension disturbances of renal function are related to the severity and duration of the disease and that this disturbance can be arrested by antihypertensive therapy. They suggested that there is little to suggest the hypothesis that sodium retention contributes to the developments of essential hypertension. Sodium clearance, plasma aldosterone, and their interrelationship are similar in patients with essential hypertension and normal subjects.

Serious renal damage resulting in renal failure cannot be expected to be caused by benign or essential hypertension. Ljugman and coworkers (1980) found that with increasing blood pressure there was a decrease in renal blood flow and an increase in renovascular resistance and filtration fraction. The glomerular filtration rate was unchanged as was the renal concentrating capacity. These changes in renal haemodynamics occurred gradually from low to high blood pressure and did not start at any particular blood pressure level. It seems that renal haemodynamics in essential hypertension are adjusted mainly to ensure a consistent glomerular filtration rate.

On the other hand, malignant or accelerated hypertension can result in serious renal damage. Diastolic blood pressure above 140 mmHg damages the renal arterioles causing fibrinoid

necrosis, areas of endothelial cell rupture, dilation of muscular wall, and entering of plasma into the media. Clinically it results in renal failure. Sometimes renal function deteriorates suddenly and unexpectedly in hypertensive patients. This condition is commonly due to obstruction of main renal arteries by atheroma, either on both sides or on one side where there is a previously damaged kidney on the other. This is one of the causes of so-called renovascular renal failure. Reconstructive surgery might restore the blood pressure.

Hypertension is a common complication of renal diseases. Parenchymal renal disease such as glomerulonephritis, pyelonephritis, interstitial nephritis, and polycystic disease are all associated with hypertension. In these cases control of hypertension is an essential part of controlling the patient's condition. A potentially reversible renal hypertension occurs in obstructive uropathies, renovascular hypertension due to atheroma, fibromuscular hyperplasia, and renal artery stenosis. Medically treated renal diseases which can cause hypertension are: pyelonephritis, tuberculosis, and diabetes mellitus. Hypertension is commonly associated with acute and chronic renal failure regardless of aetiology. Pathogenesis of renal hypertension (Ledingham, 1975) is as follows

(a)   overactivity of renin-angiotensin system;
(b)   salt and water retention;
(c)   central neurogenic mechanism;
(d)   changes in cardiac output and vascular reactivity.

How they react and the individual importance of each is not clear.

Renal Failure

This can clinically be classified into:
(a)   acute renal failure;
(b)   chronic renal failure.

Acute Renal Failure

Acute renal failure is a condition which occurs, when there is a sudden loss of the kidneys contribution to the body metabolism (Clarkson, 1980). Regardless of the cause, urea, creatinine, and waste products of metabolism accumulate in the body. There is ineffective salt and water homeostasis and hydrogen ion excretion. Oliguria defined as less than 400 ml of urine per 24 hours and hyperkalaemia are very common.

Established acute renal damage is an uncommon medical emergency occurring every 1 to 2 per 1,000 hospital admissions. Mortality is 90 per cent. if not treated early and efficiently.

Aetiology of acute renal failure. Commonly it is divided into prerenal, renal, and postrenal uraemia.

(a) Prerenal causes are:
   (1) loss of fluids, e.g. vomiting and diarrhoea;
   (2) inadequate fluid, intake associated with the overuse of diuretics and laxatives (a very important cause in the elderly);
   (3) loss of plasma, e.g. burns;
   (4) loss of blood in haemorrhage;
   (5) shock, e.g. cardiogenic and septicaemic shock.

(b) Renal causes are:
   (1) acute tubular necrosis due to the persistance of the state of prerenal uraemia and to nephrotoxins such as sulphonamides;
   (2) rapidly progressive damage due to poststreptococcal nephritis, collagen disorders, Goodpasture's syndrome, Henoch-Schoenlein purpura, etc;
   (3) arterial or venous thrombosis;
   (4) acute interstitial nephritis usually due to toxicity with drugs;
   (5) bilateral cortical necrosis associated with pregnancy.

(c) Postrenal causes are due to urinary tract obstruction (Beck, Francis, and Scuhami, 1977):
   (1) obstruction at the level of renal pelvis and ureters: stones, blood clot, carcinoma, papilloma, retroperitoneal fibrosis, aortic aneurysm, and tuberculosis;
   (2) obstruction at the level of bladder and urethra by benign prostatic hypertrophy, carcinoma of prostate, median bar hypertrophy (Marion's syndrome), urethral stricture, carcinoma of the urethra, and rarely urethral stone.

Acute renal failure in the elderly was studied by Kumar, Hill, and McGeown (1973). Dehydration and electrolyte imbalance were present in 50 per cent. of the cases studied. Only in 10 out of 122 patients was a primary renal disease responsible. The rest of the patients conditions were due to urinary tract obstruction. Among the last group prostatic enlargement was the main predisposing factor. Primary renal disorders are slightly higher in young people (20 per cent.) (Clarkson, 1980). It was found that among all age groups the most common cause of acute tubular necrosis occurs as a result of prolonged prerenal uraemia. A major contribution to development of prerenal uraemia in the elderly is deficient fluid and electrolyte intake associated with the common use of diuretics and prolonged use of laxatives. The inevitable loss of water, sodium, and potassium lead to acute renal failure.

The establishment of the cause of renal failure is important. It is critical to differentiate between prerenal uraemia and established acute renal failure, whatever its cause. It is summarized by Kleinknecht (1975).

	Pre-renal	Established renal failure
Urine osmolarity (mosmol/kg m)	>500	<400
Urine/plasma osmolarity ratio	>1.5	<1.1
Urine Na (meq/litre)	<20	>40
Urine/plasma urea ratio	>10	<10
Response to Mannitol	Yes	No
Response to IV Lasix	Yes	No

In short, the usual renal response to poor perfusion is the excretion of small volumes of highly concentrated urine of (osmolarity 600 mosmol) which is low in sodium content (20 mmol/l) because of maximum reabsorption. Also there is a higher urine-to-plasma ratio of both urea and creatinine. This condition is characteristically reversible but acute renal failure inevitably occurs if the factors predisposing to renal ischaemia are not corrected. Once acute renal failure is established, restoration of blood volume will not result in recovery of renal function. In those circumstances the small volume of urine excreted is isoosmotic with plasma (approximately 300 mosmol/kg m) and contains a high concentration of sodium. There is also a low urine-to-plasma ratio of urea and creatinine.

Obstruction must be considered in any patient with acute renal failure. It is one of the commonest causes of renal failure in the elderly frequently caused by prostatic enlargement. Difficulty in micturition, loin pain, oliguria alternating with polyuria, or complete anuria are all suggestive. Pre-renal tests should be performed routinely and residual urine should always be measured.

Clinical features of acute renal failure

(a) *Gastrointestinal*: anorexia, nausea, vomiting, diarrhoea, ulceration of the mouth, adynamic ileus, gastrointestinal bleeding, stress ulcers.
(b) *Respiratory*: dyspnoea due to metabolic acidosis, infection, or pulmonary oedema.
(c) *Circulatory*: usually normal blood pressure. Hypertension may occur with acute glomerulonephritis, renal infarction, cortical necrosis, and thrombotic microangiopathy. Pericarditis may occur and ECG changes as a result of metabolic abnormalities.

Infection and haemorrhage is common.

Management

(a) Differentiate between prerenal and established renal failure.
(b) Exclude obstruction.

Treatment

(a) Intravenous replacement of fluid and electrolytes.
(b) Manitol 100 to 150 ml of 10% to be repeated in 3 or 4 hours if response occurs.
(c) Frusemide 100 to 250 mg i.v. to be repeated every 3 or 4 hours if diuresis started.
(d) Fluid depletion should be replaced by 5% glucose containing 4.6 gm of Na/l + 1 to 1.6 gm of K/l.
(e) Specific treatment of any treatable cause, e.g. chelating agents in heavy metal poisoning. Hypertension should be treated simultaneously.

Management of established acute renal failure

(a) General measure: care of skin, mouth, bladder catheter, fluid charts, blood pressure charts.
(b) Replace fluid output plus 500 ml/day (adjusted according to presence of fever, excessive sweating, etc.).
(c) Treat hyperkalaemia, acidosis, infection, hypertension according to the standard method.
(d) Dialysis whether peritoneal or haemodialysis. During the diuretic phase, fluid and electrolyte replacement should be carried out carefully.
(e) Obstructive lesions should be relieved surgically whenever possible.
(f) Immediate commencement of treatment of reversable conditions such as diabetes, tuberculosis, renal infection, collagen disorders, etc.

Chronic Renal Failure

Chronic renal failure results from gradual progressive failure of the kidney to maintain the internal environment of the body. It is a disease that affects mainly young and middle aged individuals. The commonest cause in the elderly is progressive renal sclerosis and chronic pyelonephritis.

The causes of chronic renal failure among 772 patients on regular dialysis (Linton, 1980) were found to be as follows:

Glomerulonephritis	37.2%	Hypertensive nephrosclerosis	7.5%
Pyelonephritis	10.9%	Analgesic nephropathy	2.1%
Polycystic disease	9.3%	Hereditary nephropathy	1.5%
Diabetic nephropathy	9.0%	Others	22.4%

Other patients with these problems do not survive into old age.

The mechanisms by which the failing kidney may produce specific clinical features are (Jones and Ledingham, 1975):
(a) Uraemic toxins: diminishes the GFR and may result in accumulation of toxic material which affects the body enzymatic activity.

(b) Electrolyte and water disturbances which may result in circulatory failure, dehydration, or hyper-or hypokalaemia.

(c) Erythropoeitin and 1–25 di-hydroxycholecalciferol deficiency result in anaemia and low calcium, respectively.

(d) Derangement of the renin-aldosterone mechanism results in hypertension.

(e) Phosphate retention results in secondary hyperparathyroidism and renal osteodystrophy.

Management

(a) Establish the cause and treat accordingly.

(b) Correct water and electrolyte disturbances.

(c) Treat infection, whether renal or extrarenal.

(d) Treat hypertension and circulatory abnormalities.

(e) Perform renal dialysis either in the form of regular haemodialysis or chronic ambulatory peritoneal dialysis.

(f) Consider renal transplant.

Miscellaneous Disorders

Renal Tuberculosis

It is an uncommon disease at the present time. The diagnosis depends on the isolation of myobacterium tuberculosis from the urine; 3 to 6 urine samples should be examined. Intravenous pyelogram using a high dose of the radioopaque dye, retrograde pyelogram, or percutaneous translumbar pyelogram can be performed to investigate the extent of the disease. The classic way of treatment was to use a combination of three of the standard drugs such as streptomycin, isoniazid, PAS for 2 years or even longer. After the discovery of rifampicin a shorter course of treatment can now be successful. At present rifampicin and pyrazinamide are the most potent drugs (being bacteriocidal) followed by isoniazid. Ethambutol may have less effect as it is bacteriostatic.

Hepatorenal Syndrome

The classical definition of hepatorenal syndrome is unexplained renal failure that complicates hepatic cirrhosis. A pseudo-hepatorenal syndrome is a condition in which renal and hepatic function are simultaneously affected, e.g. leptospirosis, heart failure, eclampsia, and renal diseases with hepatic complications such as hypernephroma with liver secondaries.

Hepatic disease can affect the kidney. An example is obstructive jaundice which may lead to renal failure.

Chronic Interstitial Nephritis Due to Nephrotoxic Agents

The insidious development of renal fibrosis due to chemical agents is being increasingly recognized. The essential features are focal or diffuse interstitial nephritis leading to fibrosis in the later stages. Commonest agents are phenacetin, chronic lead poisoning, uric acid in gout, and irradiation. The history is one of slowly developing renal failure in patients with a specific past history.

Renal Lesions in Diabetes Mellitus

Renal disease is now one of the commonest fatal complications of diabetes. It is due to the fact that hyperglycaemia and ketosis are now well controlled; thus patients live longer to develop vascular complications. The condition first described by Kimmelstiel and Wilson and known by that name is intercapillary glomerulosclerosis. Clinically long-standing proteinuria with gradual decline in renal function leads to development of nephrotic syndrome, hypertension, and heart failure. Other types of renal involvement in diabetes are ischaemic atrophy due to atherosclerosis, which tends to be more common in diabetics, and ascending pyelonephritis may occur in a particularly intense form leading to papillary necrosis.

Renal Amyloidosis

Amyloid disease of the kidney is always secondary to long-standing disease such as bronchiectasis, rheumatoid arthritis, pulmonary tuberculosis, and myelomatosis. It is not uncommon in the elderly. Primary renal amyloidosis is a rare disease. Amyloidosis presents with proteinuria and gradual renal impairment, leading to nephrotic syndrome and renal failure. Hypertension is uncommon. Treatment is that of the primary disorder.

Collagen Disorders

Collagen disorders are chronic progressive inflammatory diseases commonly involving the kidneys. The lesion is always some form of vasculitis. In systemic lupus erythematosis, necrosis and thrombosis of small vessels lead to ischaemic changes. In polyarteritis nodosa it is a focal panarteritis starting in the media with neutrophil infiltration and fibrinoid necrosis leading to thrombosis. In progressive systemic sclerosis there is obliterative thickening of the intima of the small arteries and thickening of basement membrane due to fibroblastic proliferation and deposition of collagen. Rheumatoid arthritis commonly affects the kidney; the common feature is proteinuria with renal impairment. Nephritic and nephrotic syndrome, renal hypertension, a fulminating picture of acute renal failure, or chronic renal failure may occur. Hypertension is unusual in progressive systemic sclerosis and rheumatoid disease, while it is very common in polyarteritis nodosa. Renal failure is not uncommonly the cause of death in these disorders.

BIBLIOGRAPHY AND REFERENCES

Adler, S., Lindeman, R. D., Yiengst, M. J., Beard, E., and Shock, N. W. (1968). 'Effect of acute acid loading on urinary acid excretion by ageing human kidney', *J. Lab. Clin. Med.*, **72**, 278–289

Alt, J. M., Hackbarth, F., Deerberg, F., and Stolte, H. (1980). 'Proteinuria in rats in relation to age-dependent renal changes', *Laboratory Animals*, **14**, Part 2, 95–101.

Armbrecht, H. J., Zenser, T. V., and Davis, B. B. (1980). 'Effect of age on the conversion of 25 hydroxy Vit D$_3$ to 1, 25 hydroxy vitamin D$_3$ by the kidney of rat', *J. Clin. Invest.*, **66**, 1118–1123.

Barrows, C. H., Falzone, J. A. and Shock, N. W. (1960). 'Age difference in the succinoxidase activity of homogenates and mitochondria from the livers and kidneys of rats', *J. Gerontol.*, **15**, 130–133.

Bates, C. P., and Corney, C. E. (1971). 'Synchronous cine/press/flow cystography. A method of routine urodynamic investigation', *Br. J. Radiol.*, **44**, 44–50.

Baumelou, A., and Legrain, M. (1982). 'Medical nephrectomy with anti-inflammatory non-steroidal drugs', *Br. Med. J.*, **284**, 234.

Beauchene, R. E., Fanestil, D. D., and Barrows, C. H. (1965). 'The effect of age on active transport and sodium – potassium-activated ATPase activity in renal tissue of rats', *J. Gerontol.*, **20**, 306–310.

Beck, E. R., Francis, J. L., and Souhami, R. L. (1977). 'Practice problems in clinical medicine', *Hospital Update*, **3**(3), 133.

Bengele, H. H., Mathias, R. S., Perkins, J. H., and Alexander, E. A. (1981). 'Urinary concentrating defect in the aged rat', *Clin. J. Physiol.*, **240** (2), 147–150.

Brocklehurst, J. C., Dillane, J. B., Griffiths, L., and Fry, J. (1968). 'The prevalence and symptomatology of urinary infection in an aged population', *Gerontol. Clin.*, **10**, 242–253.

Brocklehurst, J. C., and Hanley, T. (1976). *Geriatric Medicine for Students*, pp. 70–89, Churchill Livingstone.

Brod, J. (1968). 'Changes of renal function with age', *Scripta Medica*, **1968**, 223–229.

Brown, C. B. (1980). 'Urinary tract infection', *Medicine*, **26**, 1341–1346.

Bullamore, J. R., Wilkinson, R., Gallagher, J. C., Nordin, B. E., and Marshall, D. H. (1970). 'The effect of age on Ca absorption', *Lancet*, **2**, 535–537.

Castleden, C. M. (1978). 'Prescribing for the elderly', *Prescriber's J.*, **18**(4), 90.

Clarkson, A. R. (1980). 'Acute renal failure', *Medicine*, **3** 25, 1279.

Cobden, I., Record, C. O., Ward, M. K., and Kerr, D. N. S. (1982). 'Paracetamol induced acute renal failure in the absence of fulminating liver damage', *Br. Med. J.*, **284**, 21–22.

Cockcroft, D. W., and Gault, M. H. (1976). 'Prediction of creatinine clearance for serum creatinine', *Nephron*, **16**, 31–41.

Cove-Smith, R. (1980). 'Drugs causing renal disease', *Medicine*, **1980**, 3rd series. 1361–1364.

Cox, J. R., Pearson, R. E., and Speight, C. J. (1971). (Changes in potassium and body fluid spaces in depression and dementia', *Gerontol. Clin.*, **13**, 233–245.

Cox, J. R., and Shalaby, W. A. (1981). 'Potassium changes with age', *Gerontol.*, **27**, 340–344.

Curtis, J. R. (1980). 'Drug induced disorder of the urinary tract', *Br. J. Hosp. Med.*, **1980**, 29–33.

Davies, D. R., and Shock, N. W. (1950). 'Age changes in glomerular filtration rate, effective renal plasma flow and tubular excretory capacity in adult males', *J. Clin. Invest.*, **29**, 496–507.

Dontas, A. S., Papanayiotou, P., Marketos, S. G., Papanicolaou, N., and Economou, P. (1966). 'The effect of bacteriuria on renal function pattern in old age', *Clin. Sci.*, **34**, 73–81.

Dontas, A. S., Papanayiotou, P., Marketos, S. G., and Papanicolaou, N. T. (1968). 'Bacteriuria in old age', *Lancet*, **2**, 305.

Dunn, M. J., and Zambraski, E. J. (1980). 'Renal effects of drugs that inhibit prostaglandin synthesis', *Kidney Int.*, **18**, 609–622.

Evans, D. B. (1980). 'Drugs and the kidney', *Br. J. Hosp. Med.*, **24**, 244–251.

Ewy, A., Kapadia, G. G., Yao, L., Lullin, M. and Marcus, F. I. (1969). 'Digoxin metabolism in the elderly', *Circulation*, **39**, 449–453.

Friedman, S. A. Raizner, A. E., Rosen, H., Solomon, N. H., and Wilferdo, S. Y. (1972). 'Functional defects in the ageing kidney', *Ann. Intern. Med.*, **76**, 41–45.

Gallagher, J. C., Riggs, B. L., Eisman, J., Hamstra, A., Arnaud, S. B., and Deluca, H. F. (1979). 'Intestinal Ca absorption and serum vitamin D metabolites in normal subjects and osteoporotic patients', *J. Clin. Invest.*, **64**(3), 729–736.

Ganong, W. F. (1975). *Review of Medical Physiology*, Vol. 3, p. 536, Lange Medical Publication.

Garland, M. H., and James, M. (1978). 'Incontinence in the elderly', *Hospital Update*, **4** (12), 819.

Gral, T., and Young, M. (1980). 'Measured versus estimated creatinine clearance in the elderly as an index of renal function', *J. Am. Geriatr. Soc.*, **28**(2), 492–496.

Guyton, A. C., Coleman, T. G., Cowley, A. W., Scheel, K. W., Manning, R. D., and Normar, R. A. (1972). 'Arterial pressure regulation, over-riding dominance of the kidneys in long-term regulation and hypertension', *Am. J. Med.*, **52**, 584–594.

Hansen, J. M., Kampmann, J., and Laursen, H. (1970). 'Renal excretion of drugs in the elderly', *Lancet*, **1**, 1170.

Harbord, R. B., and Gruneberg, R. N. (1981). 'Treatment of urinary tract infection with a single dose of amoxycillin, co-trimoxazole or trimethoprim respectively', *Br. Med. J.*, **283**, 1301.

Helderman, J. H., Vestal, R. E., Rowe, J. W., Tobin, J. D., Andres, R., and Robertson, G. L. (1978). 'The response of arginine vaso-pressin to intravenous ethanol and hypertonic saline in man', *J. Gerontol.*, **33**, 39–47.

Howell, T., and Piggot, A. P. (1948). 'Kidney in old age', *J. Gerontol.*, **3**, 124–128.

Hutch, J. A. (1965). 'A new theory of the internal sphincter and the physiology of micturition', *Invest. Urol.*, **3**, 36–58.

Isaacs, B. (1973). 'Treatment of the irremedial elderly patient', *Br. Med. J.*, **3**, 566–568.

Jeffcoate, T. N. A., and Roberts, H. (1952). 'Stress incontinence of urine', *J. Obstet. Gynaecol.*, **59**, 685–720.

Johnson, J. H., and Barrows, C. H. (1980). 'Effects of age and dietary restriction on the kidney glomeruli of mice', *Anat. Rec.*, **196**, 145–151.

Jones, N., and Ledingham, J. G. G. (1975). *Chronic Renal Failure.* Part 1, 2nd series, p. 1502.

Kafetz, K., and Hodkinson, H. M. (1981). 'Osteomalacia in the presence of "normal" serum 25-hydroxycholecalciferol concentration', *Br. Med. J.*, **283**, 1437.

Kass, E. H., Savage, W., and Santamario, B. (1964). *International Symposium on Pyelonephritis, Boston*, Vol. 3, S. A. Davis, Philadelphia.

Kasviki-Charvati, P., Droletti-Kafakis, B., Papanayiotou, P. C., and Dontas, A. S. (1982). 'Turn over of bacteriuria in old age', *Age Ageing*, **11**, 169–174.

Kerr, D. N. S. (1980). 'The assessment of renal function and detection of urinary abnormalities', *Medicine*, **25**(1), 1269–1274.

Kleinknecht, D. (1975). 'Acute renal failure', *Medicine*, **28**(1), 1488.

Kumar, C., Hill, M., and McGeown, G. (1973). 'Acute renal failure in the elderly', *Lancet*, **13**, 90–91.

Lapides, J. (1958). 'Further observation on pharmacologic reaction of the bladder', *J. Urol.*, **80**, 34.

Ledingham, J. G. (1975). 'Hypertension and the kidney', *Medicine*, **(2)**, 2nd Series, Part 2, 1611–1617.

Lever, A. F., Beretta-Piccoli, C., Brown, J. J., Fraser, D. L., and Robertson, J. I. S. (1981). 'Sodium and potassium in essential hypertension', *Br. Med. J.*, **283**, 463–468.

Levy, G. (1977). 'Pharmacokinetics in renal disease', *Clin. J. Med.*, **63**(4), 461–465.

Lindeman, R. D., Lee, T. D., Yiengst, M. J., and Shock, N. W. (1966). 'Influence of age, renal diseases, hypertension, diuretics and calcium on antidiuretic responses to suboptimal infusion of vasopressin', *J. Lab. Clin. Med.*, **68**, 206–223.

Linton, A. (1980). 'Chronic renal failure', *Medicine*, **3**, 1285–1288.

Ljugman, S., Aurell, M., Hartford, M., Wikstrand, J., Wilhelmsen, L., and Berglund, G. (1980). 'Blood pressure and renal function', *Acta Med. Scand.*, **208**, 17–25.

Lott, R. S., and Hayton, W. C. (1978). 'Estimation of creatinine clearance for serum creatinine concentration. A review', *Drug Intelligence and Clinical Pharmacy*, **12**, 140.

Lyle, W. M. (1977). 'Drugs prescribed for the elderly', *J. Am. Optom. Assoc.*, **48**(8).

McDonald, R. K., Solomon, D. H., and Shock, N. W. (1951). 'Ageing as factor in renal hemodynamic changes induced by standardized pyrogen', *J. Clin. Invest.*, **30**, 457–462.

McNaught, A. B., and Callander, R. (1975). *Illustrated Physiology*, Vol. 1, Churchill Livingstone.

Malvern, J. (1981). 'Incontinence of urine in women', *Br. J. Hosp. Med.*, **25**, 224–231.

Miall, W. L., Kass, E. H., Ling, J., and Stuart, K. L. (1962). 'Factors influencing arterial pressure in general population in Jamaica', *Br. Med. J.*, **2**, 497.

Miller, J. H. (1952). 'Age changes in maximal rate of renal tubular re-absorption of glucose', *J. Gerontol.*, **7**, 196–200.

Miller, J. H., and Shock, N. W. (1953). 'Age differences in renal tubular response to antidiuretic hormone', *J. Gerontol.*, **8**, 446–450.

Mou, T. L., Siroty, R., and Ventry, P. (1962). 'Bacteriuria in elderly chronically ill patients', *J. Am. Geriatr. Soc.*, **10**, 170–178.

Nunez, M., Iglesias, C. G., Roman, A. B., Commes, J. L. K., Becerra, L. C., Rome, J. M. T., and Del Pozo, S. D. (1978). 'Renal handling of sodium in old people. A functional study', *Age Ageing*, **7**, 178–181.

Olbrich, O., Ferguson, M. H., Robson, J. S., and Stewart, C. P. (1950). 'Renal function in aged subjects', *Edinburgh M. J.*, **57**, 117–127.

Parfrey, P. S., Condou, K., Wright, P., *et al.* (1981a). 'Blood pressure and hormonal changes following alteration in dietary sodium and potassium in young men with and without familiar predisposition to hypertension', *Lancet*, **1**, 113–117.

Parfrey, P. S., Markandu, N. D., Roulston, J. E., Jones, B. E., and MacGregor, G. A. (1981b). 'Relation between arterial blood pressure, dietary sodium intake and renin system in essential hypertension', *Br. Med. J.*, **283**, 94.

Phillips, T. L., and Leong, G. F. (1967). 'Kidney cell proliferation after unilateral nephrectomy as related to age', *Cancer Res.*, **27**, 286–292.

Potchen, E. J., Koehler, P. R., and Davis, D. O. (1971). *Principles of Diagnostic Radiology*, pp. 245–288, McGraw Hill.

Rapoport, J., Rees, G. A., Willmott, N. J., Slack, R. C. B., and O'Grady, F. W. (1981). 'Treatment of acute urinary tract infection with three doses of co-trimoxazole'. *Br. Med. J.*, **283**, 1301–1302.

Reubi, F. C., and Weidman, P. (1980). 'Relationships between sodium clearance, plasma renin activity, plasma aldosterone, renal haemodynamics and blood pressure in essential hypertension', *Clin. Exp. Hypertension*, **2**(3&4), 593–612.

Rosen, H. (1976). 'Renal disease of the elderly', *Med. Clin. North Am.*, **60**(6), 1105.

Rowe, W., Andres, R., Tobin, J. D., Norris, A. H., and Shock, N. W. (1976). 'The effect of age on creatinine clearance in man', *J. Gerontol.*, **31**, 155–163.

Shanks, S. C., and Kerley, P. (Eds) and Hodson, C. J., and Edwards, D. (authors) (1970). *Textbook of X-ray Diagnosis*, Vol. 5 (4), H. K. Lewis and Co. Ltd.

Shock, N. W. (1946). 'Kidney function tests in aged males', *Geriatrics*, **1**, 232–239.

Shock, N. W. *Surgery of the Aged and Debilitated Patients*, p. 10, Saunders, New York, London.

Skehan, J. D., Barnes, J. N., Drew, P. J., and Wright, P. (1982). 'Hypokalaemia induced by a combination of beta blocker and thiazide', *Br. Med. J.*, **284**, 83.

Skoll, S. L., August, R. J., and Johnson, G. E. (1979). 'Drug prescribing for the elderly in Saskatchewan during 1976', *Can. Med. Assoc. J.*, **121** (8), 1074–1081.

Smalley, J. W. (1980). 'Age related changes in the amino acid composition of human glomerular basement membrane', *Exp. Gerontol.*, **15**(1), 43–52.

Sourander, L. B. (1966). 'Urinary tract infection in the aged', Aura print of *Turku and Ann. Med. Intern. Fenn.*, **55**, Suppl. 45.

Stanton, S. L. (1980). 'Gynaecological aspect of incontinence', in *Incontinence and Its Management* (Ed. D. Mandelstam), p. 55, Croom Helm, London.

Stevenson, I. H. (1978). 'Drug metabolism in the elderly', *Age Ageing*, **7** (Suppl.), 131–133.

Szilard, C. K. (1959). 'On the nature of the ageing process', *Proc. Natl. Acad. Sci. USA*, **45**, 30–45.

Tanagho, E. A., and Smith, R. D. (1966). 'The anatomy and function of the bladder neck', *Br. J. Urol.*, **38**, 54–71.

Vancura, E. J. (1979). 'Guard against unpredictable drug responses in the ageing', *Geriatrics*, **34**(4), 63–65, 69–70.

Ward, M., and Blatman, M. (1979). 'Drug therapy in the elderly', *Am. Fam. Physician*, **19**(2), 143–152.

Wardner, H. E. de (1973). *The Kidney*, 4th ed., Churchill Livingstone.

Warrell, D. W. (1969). 'Urinary incontinence', in *Modern Trends in Gynaecology* (Ed. R.J. Kellar), Vol. 4, pp. 186–214, Butterworth, Sevenoaks.

Wolfson, S. (1965). 'Epidemiology of bacteriuria in predominantly geriatric male population', *Am. J. Med. Sci.*, **250**, 168–173.

26.3

The Bladder and Urethra

D. J. Farrar

Normal control of bladder and urethral function is taken for granted by the majority of the population. Disorders of the lower urinary tract which interfere with this control are increasingly common in old age. They affect a population whose ability to cope with the resulting problems are often compromised by disorders of locomotion or by degrees of brain failure. The disturbances may be such that they dictate the patient's whole pattern of life.

Urinary incontinence is the main threat to the elderly. It conjures up fears (often real) of rejection by relatives, friends, and not infrequently by medical and nursing personnel. As a result many patients are unwilling to admit to their incontinence or to seek advice. Others consider incontinence to be a normal facet of ageing. A recent survey in the United Kingdom showed that incontinence occurred regularly in 11.6 per cent. of females and 6.9 per cent. of males over the age of 65 and this was more than 4 times greater than the incidence of incontinence presenting to the local health and social services (Thomas *et al.*, 1980).

Prostatic hyperplasia is the principal cause of disordered micturition in the ageing male although there is a wide variation, both in the degree of obstruction to the urinary flow this causes and the severity of the resulting symptoms. Patients' tolerance to obstructive symptoms is also variable. It has been estimated that 1 in 10 males will require prostatectomy at some time (Lytton, Emery, and Harvard, 1968) and many of these patients will present initially to geriatric units. More than 50 per cent. of patients undergoing prostatectomy are over the age of 70 (Singh, Tressidder, and Blandy, 1973).

As the elderly population continues to increase, so naturally will the incidence of urinary tract problems. An understanding of the complexities of normal bladder and urethral function is important if these problems are to be managed effectively.

BLADDER AND URETHRAL FUNCTION

Continence and Voiding

The bladder is essentially an organ of storage which under control of the higher centres discharges its contents at convenient intervals. Between voidings, continence is maintained by the ability of the bladder to accommodate increasing volumes of fluid without significant intravesical pressure rise and by a competent urethral closure mechanism.

Continence

The muscular wall of the bladder is composed of a complex meshwork of interlacing bundles of smooth muscle with longitudinally orientated bundles predominating on the inner and outer aspects of the muscle coat (Gosling and Dixon, 1975; Hunter 1954). During filling the bladder's ability to accommodate fluid without significant pressure rise is in part dependent upon the inherent physical properties of this muscular wall and in part upon an intact nervous system. As fluid enters the bladder impulses pass along the afferent limb of the reflex arc to the spinal cord. In the cord itself above the micturition centre are areas extending up to the level of the hypothalamus which act either to facilitate or inhibit micturition (Tang and Ruch, 1955).

As bladder filling continues the facilitatary impulses become more frequent, overcome the inhibitory mechanism, and impinge on consciousness as a desire to micturate. Micturition can indeed be facilitated or inhibited at any time voluntarily from the highest centres of the cerebral cortex. The part of the cortex which is thought to be responsible lies in the frontal lobes between the superior frontal gyrus and the anterior end of the cingulate gyrus (Andrew and Nathan, 1965; Pool, 1954). These

areas control the septal and hypothalamic nuclei which are in turn responsible for the organization of the total act of micturition. Interference with any part of this mechanism above the sacral micturition centre may result in uninhibited detrusor contractions.

It is clear from combined cystometric and radiological studies that the primary defence mechanism against incontinence is the bladder neck (Fig. 1). This mechanism is usually both cough-proof and strain-proof (Turner-Warwick *et al.*, 1973) and only opened in association with a detrusor contraction. The anatomical configuration of the bladder neck has been the subject of much debate and has led to the advancement of a number of concepts (Denny-Brown and Robertson. 1933; Hutch, 1965; Tanagho and Smith, 1966), often conflicting.

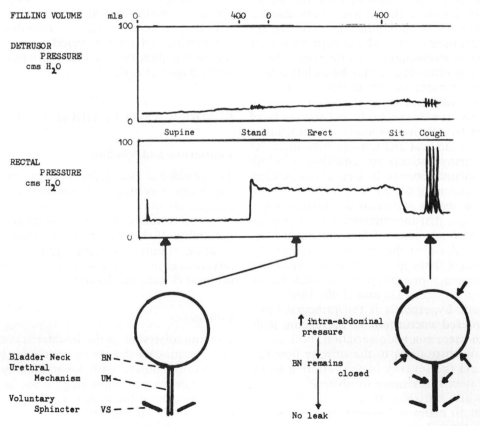

Figure 1 Diagramatic representation of bladder and urethral function with normal filling cystometrogram. Detrusor pressure is derived by subtracting rectal (intra-abdominal) pressure from intravesical pressure

Recent work has clarified the situation and shown that there are basic differences in bladder neck and urethral anatomy between the sexes (Gosling and Dixon, 1975). There exists in the male a well-defined collar of smooth muscle around the bladder neck which is not continuous with the detrusor muscle but extends distally to surround the preprostatic urethra. This collar of muscle is thought to be genitally orientated and prevent reflux ejaculation. Its presence, however, would fit with the clinical observation that bladder neck incompetence in the male in the absence of surgical intervention is uncommon.

The bladder neck closure mechanism in the female, on the other hand, is less well defined. The smooth muscle, which has no distinct circular component at the bladder neck but runs an oblique or longitudinal course in the urethral wall fading out in the distal part of the urethra, would seem illsuited to maintain bladder neck competence. It is presumed that other components present at the bladder neck, such as elastic tissue, striated muscle, and even vascular tissue, must play a significant part. The anatomical differences in bladder neck anatomy between the sexes is reflected clinically in that bladder neck incompetence is much commoner in the female than the male.

When the bladder neck mechanism is incompetent continence is then dependent on the urethral mechanism. This is mainly an involuntary mechanism composed of specialized striated muscle, morphologically different from the striated muscle of the pelvic floor and external sphincter, which is capable of maintaining tone. This muscle which in the male lies in the distal part of the prostatic urethra and in the female surrounds the middle third of the urethra is supplied by pelvic splanchnic nerves running with the pudendal nerve (Gosling *et al.*, 1981). The position of the muscle correlates well with the site of the maximal closure pressure recorded on urethral pressure profile measurements.

The voluntary striated sphincter, innervated by the pudendal nerve, plays little part in day-to-day continence except in times of emergency or at the termination of micturition. Continence can be maintained following paralysis of the pudenal nerves (Lapides, Gray, and Rawling, 1955).

The presence of an intra-abdominal segment of urethra would also seem to be necessary for continence, allowing for changes in intra-abdominal pressure to be transmitted equally to this segment and to the bladder, hence maintaining the pressure differential between the bladder and urethra (see Fig. 1) (Enhorning, Miller, and Hinman, 1964). The male urethra is well supported and rarely displaced. The female urethra, however, is prone to displacement as a result of weakening of the supporting ligaments by childbirth and ageing with a resulting loss of the intra-abdominal segment of uretha, and when this is combined with bladder neck incompetence continence is inevitably compromised.

Voiding

Voiding results from an active contraction of the detrusor muscle with opening of the bladder neck and urethra and relaxation of the pelvic floor. The actual mechanism of the bladder neck opening is uncertain. The view that it is actively pulled open by a detrusor contraction (Lapides, 1958) would seem to be difficult to correlate with the anatomical findings which show the detrusor and bladder neck musculature to be separate (Gosling and Dixon, 1975). An active role for the trigonal musculature has been advanced (Tanagho *et al.*, 1966) but its role is doubtful (Homsey, 1967). The cystometric observation that in females efficient voiding may occur without a significant detrusor contraction supports the view that active urethral relaxation plays a part in voiding.

At the end of micturition the voluntary sphincter contracts and urine remaining in the posterior urethra is 'milked back' into the bladder by the urethral mechanism. The bladder neck closes and the voluntary sphincter relaxes.

The detrusor receives its motor supply through parasympathetic fibres originating from the lateral horns of S2-4.

Age Changes

Bladder and urethral function in the elderly are influenced by the physiological ageing processes of a number of different systems. In the nervous system, cerebral control of micturition may be affected by the progressive atrophy of the cerebral cortex and by the loss of neurones, the latter being more marked in patients with senile dementia (Bowen and Davison, 1978). Autonomic function also steadily declines with age, leading to impairment of autonomic reflexes. Marked impairment of autonomic function as a result of age has been demonstrated in cases of atonic bladder (Collins *et al.*, 1980).

Ageing of striated muscle involves a diminution in the number of cells and their replacement by fat and fibrous connective tissue. Muscle bulk may be reduced by half by the eighth decade of life. The reduction in muscle strength as a result of these changes is relevant when considering voluntary sphincteric and pelvic floor activity in the elderly.

There is little information on age changes in detrusor smooth muscle. A general reduction in the number of autonomic nerves has been noted (Gosling and Dixon, 1981) and Brocklehurst (1972) observed that marked trabeculation was present in the majority of post-mortem specimens of bladders in elderly females. This trabeculation may result from obstruction uninhibited detrusor activity or be due merely to prominence of the muscle bundles in a thin-walled bladder.

There is a gradual decline in oestrogen activity in the female after the menopause, although the rate of decline is variable. The distal urethra, which with the vagina has a common embrylogical origin from the urogenital sinus and is lined by oestrogen-sensitive squamous epithelium, is affected by this decline, resulting in decreased cellularity and subsequent atrophy of the epithelial lining (Smith, 1972).

The prostate is also affected by ageing. Hyperplasia proceeds at a variable rate but its aetiology is unknown. Carcinoma is rare before the age of 50 but then the incidence increases rapidly up till the age of 80 when the rate slows. Many of these carcinomas, however, are inactive and latent (Franks, 1973).

BLADDER AND URETHRAL DYSFUNCTION IN OLD AGE

A basic understanding of the disorders which can affect the lower urinary tract is an essential requirement for the effective management of bladder and urethral dysfunction in the elderly. It is as illogical, for example, to believe that all cases of incontinence can be treated in the same way as to attempt to apply a single treatment to all cases of indigestion. Not all cases of urinary dysfunction in the elderly present to the geriatric service, and some that do will require referral for urological or gynaecological treatment, and vice versa. A multidisciplinary approach, especially to a problem such as incontinence, has much to commend it.

Clinical Presentation

The bladder on the whole is an unreliable witness. There are only a limited number of symptoms by which disordered micturition is manifest, and hence there is considerable overlap in the clinical presentation of disorders of bladder and urethral function.

Inflammatory Disorders

Bacterial urinary tract infections are a common problem in the elderly. They have been shown to occur in 20 per cent. of patients over the age of 65 compared with an incidence of only 3.2 per cent. in the 45 to 65 age group (Brocklehurst *et al.*, 1972). This increased incidence is in part due to the presence of residual urine, which results from less efficient bladder emptying. The presentation of bacterial infection in the elderly is not always as cystitis; it may manifest as incontinence or may be asymptomatic. Where infection persists, despite treatment, or relapses frequently after treatment, other underlying pathology such as urinary stones, neoplasia, or vesicointestinal fistula should be considered. In the male, recurrent infections are most frequently the result of prostatic outflow obstruction and its sequelae.

Dysuria and frequency in the absence of bacterial infection in the aged female is often described as the urethral syndrome. It is thought to be due primarily to changes in the hormone-sensitive squamous epithelium of the distal urethra resulting in an atrophic urethritis. Secondary bacterial infection may occur and in some cases the urethritis may progress to cause a degree of urethral stenosis (Smith, 1979).

Persistent symptoms of frequency and dysuria without bacterial infection should raise in both sexes the possibility of carcinoma *in situ* of the bladder or tuberculous cystitis, especially if cells are present in the urine; in the female, chronic interstitial cystitis (Hunner's ulcer) should also be considered. These conditions, however, are relatively uncommon.

Incontinence

Incontinence should be considered as a symptom resulting from a number of different disorders of micturition. It should be distinguished from urinary leakage as a result of a vesicovaginal fistula.

Genuine stress incontinence. This results when the bladder neck mechanism is incompetent and the distal urethral mechanism is unable to cope with the passive rise in intravesical pressure resulting from a rise in intra-abdominal pressure on coughing or sudden movement (Fig. 2). The dynamic behaviour of the bladder

is normal, and bladder neck incompetence results from a congenital weakness, bladder neck surgery, or in the female from childbirth, age, or hormone deficiency. This type of incontinence occurs almost exclusively in the female but would appear to be relatively uncommon in the elderly, accounting for less than 4 per cent. of cases presenting to two geriatric units (Eastwood, 1979; Overstall, Rounce, and Palmer, 1980).

Unstable incontinence. Uninhibited detrusor contractions will also render the bladder neck incompetent; incontinence will occur if the distal urethral mechanism is unable to cope with the resulting active rise in intravesical pressure (Fig. 3). This is the commonest type of incontinence in the elderly, the incidence ranging

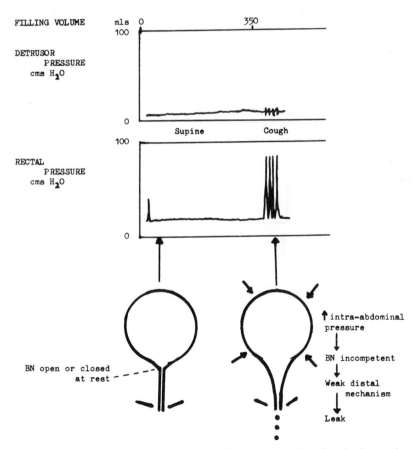

Figure 2   Diagramatic representatipon of bladder and urethral function in genuine stress incontinence. Normal filling cystometrogram. Detrusor pressure is derived by subtracting rectal (intra-abdominal) pressure from intravesical pressure

from 57 to 68 per cent. in reported series (Castleden, Duffing, and Asher, 1981; Overstall, Rounce, and Palmer, 1980). The effect of these contractions is to cause both diurnal and nocturnal frequency of micturition, and urgency. The degree of incontinence depends upon the severity of the uninhibited contractions and the efficiency of the urethral sphincter mechanism.

Bladders presumed clinically to have uninhibited activity are commonly referred to as being unstable, but the term detrusor instability should strictly only be applied to those cases where the diagnosis has been confirmed cystometrically.

Overflow incontinence. This results from an excessive volume of residual urine. There may be true organic obstruction as in prostatic disease, with a subsequent failure of the detrusor over a prolonged period to sustain an adequate contraction, or the failure may be primarily of detrusor contractility. The latter occurs in about 10 per cent. of cases in the elderly (Castledon *et al.*, 1981; Overstall, Rounce, and Palmer, 1980) although a detectable neurological cause is not always apparent.

This type of incontinence may present as enuresis or a persistent daytime dribble; a distended bladder can usually be palpated or percussed.

Others. Postprostatectomy incontinence is most commonly a result of bladder instability which persists following relief of the obstruction. Incontinence from sphincter damage with a stable detrusor is uncommon although overflow incontinence from residual obstruction (prostatic or a urethral stricture) may occur.

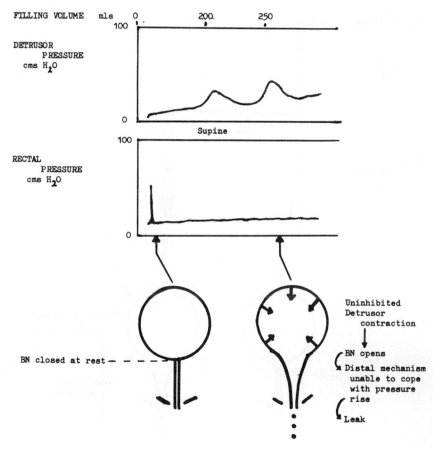

Figure 3 Diagramatic representation of bladder and urethral function in unstable incontinence. Detrusor pressure is derived by subtracting rectal (intra-abdominal) pressure from intravesical pressure

A prolonged postmicturition dribble in the male may be a source of embarrassment. It results from failure of the bulbocavernosus muscle to expel urine remaining in the bulb of the urethra at the end of voiding (Claridge, 1966). It may or may not be associated with outlet obstruction (Stephenson and Farrar, 1977).

Outlet obstruction. The classical symptoms of prostatic outflow tract obstruction – delay, poor stream and terminal dribbling – result from the encroachment of the prostate on the urethral lumen. The degree of encroachment, however, is not necessarily reflected in the prostatic size found on rectal examination, the importance of which lies more in deciding the type of prostatectomy required, i.e. transurethral or suprapubic.

Incontinence as a symptom of prostatic disease in the elderly is of three types: urge incontinence which is a manifestation of the detrusor instability demonstrated to be present in 75 per cent. of cases of prostatic outflow tract obstruction (Farrar, 1979) and usually associated with frequency and nocturia; overflow incontinence which is a result of chronic urinary retention; and incontinence from a prolonged postmicturition dribble.

Outflow obstruction in the male may also result from prostatic carcinoma which is increasingly common in the elderly or from urethral stricture.

Outlet obstruction in the female is more ill defined in terms of clinical presentation (Farrar et al., 1976). It may present as frequency, as recurrent urinary tract infections, or as incontinence either of an urge type or as retention with overflow. Obstruction occurs either in the distal urethra or at the bladder neck, the latter more frequently being associated with an acontractile or poorly functioning detrusor. Urethral obstruction in the female may also result from a large prolapse causing urethral distortion, voiding efficiency being restored by digital reduction of the prolapse. Rarely a urethral neoplasm may cause obstruction.

Neuropathic Bladder

Bladder dysfunction resulting from demonstrable neurological disease is more accurately described as neuropathic; the term neurogenic which is in common use merely assumes the presence of a neurological disorder.

Many classifications of neuropathic bladder dysfunction have been proposed. The most commonly used describes uninhibited bladder, autonomous bladder, automatic bladder, and atonic bladder and is based on the site and degree of neurologic damage (Band, 1945). The advent of urodynamic investigation has meant that more emphasis is being placed on the detrusor and sphincter, and a description of neuromuscular dysfunction is defined in terms of detrusor and sphincter activity based on urodynamic investigation (International Continence Society, 1981).

Disorders of the highest centre of the cerebral cortex with resulting uninhibited detrusor activity are the commonest lesions in the elderly. They include senile dementia and ageing itself. The sensory pathway is normal in this group but the ability to suppress the micturition reflex is diminished and urgency and urge incontinence result. If the frontal lobes are involved micturition may be precipitant with no warning. The effect of a cerebral vascular accident on bladder function is dependent upon the site of the lesion: where the micturition pathway is involved retention may occur in the early stages, but later as activity returns the detrusor becomes uninhibited.

Lesions involving the spinal cord above the sacral micturition centre such as disseminated sclerosis usually result in an uninhibited bladder. The development of residual urine in these cases is dependent upon the degree of detrusor/sphincter dyssynergia present. Complete spinal transection with an automatic bladder is uncommon in the elderly.

Lesions of the cord involving the sacral micturition centre, e.g. tumour or vascular accident, interfere with the efferent side of the reflex arc and result in an atonic bladder. The motor supply of the bladder may also be compromised by damage to the pelvic nerves during surgical mobilization of the rectum (Fowler, 1973). Overflow incontinence may occur if the bladder is allowed to become overdistended.

Loss of bladder sensation as a result of degenerative changes in the posterior roots, posterior root ganglia, and posterior column of the cord may occur in diabetes and in tabes dorsalis. Progressive distention of the bladder occurs and eventually results in atonicity. Cystometric studies have shown that in diabetes the degree of bladder dysfunction is related to the severity of the disease rather than the duration (Buck, McRae, and Chisholm, 1974). eighty per cent. of Buck's series of 40 diabetic patients had abnormal bladder function, i.e. increased bladder capacity and diminished sensation; only 15 per cent. were atonic.

Bladder dysfunction may also occur in Parkinson's disease, the type of dysfunction depending on the site of the lesion in the extrapyramidal system. The bladder may be uninhibited or a significant residual urine may develop because of diminished detrusor activity.

Others

Nocturnal frequency of micturition is increasingly common in old age (Milne *et al.*, 1972; Osborne, 1976). It is important to differentiate true nocturia, i.e. the arousal from sleep to void, which usually implies underlying bladder pathology, e.g. unstable bladder or urinary tract infection, from the poor sleeper who voids when awake (and often makes a cup of tea which exacerbates the nocturia!).

Neoplasms affecting the lower urinary tract are most commonly transitional cell carcinomas of the bladder. They classically present as painless haematuria, but in the elderly presentation may be as incontinence or persistent urinary tract infection. Urethral neoplasms are an uncommon cause of outlet obstruction in the female.

INVESTIGATION OF BLADDER AND URETHRAL FUNCTION

Advances in technology over the last decade have improved the diagnostic techniques which are available to investigate bladder and urethral function. While some of the techniques will remain confined to the larger centres because of cost, the ability to measure bladder pressure or access to such a system should be available to all geriatric units.

The mainstay of any investigation, however, is an accurate history and relevant physical examination.

History and Examination

An accurate micturition history should involve direct questioning about individual urinary symptoms. The all-embracing question 'Do you have any trouble with your waterworks?' may evoke a negative response when subsequent questioning reveals this is not the case, incontinence in particular often being considered by the elderly to be a normal facet of ageing.

Inquiry should be made into the patient's medication. Diuretics are a potent cause of urinary problems and tranquillizers or sedatives may depress the awareness of bladder sensation.

Relevant examination includes assessment of the patient's mental state, degree of mobility, and any neurological deficit present. Abdominal examination should exclude a chronically distended bladder, although this may be difficult in the obese without careful percussion and palpation. The use of a diagnostic catheter to detect chronic retention should be a last resort because of the danger of introducing infection. In the male, the size and consistency of the prostate is important. In the female, examination of the external genitalia should include an assessment of the degree of incontinence, if any, on coughing, leakage on the first cough being more suggestive of pure sphincter weakness than detrusor instability. Prolapse of the urethral mucosa at the external meatus is common in the elderly female and should not be confused with the uncommon urethral caruncle. Atrophic changes should also be noted. In both sexes a rectal examination will exclude faecal impaction as a cause of overflow incontinence of urine.

The value of charting either in a ward situation or in the home cannot be overemphasized. It frequently allows a more accurate assessment of the urinary problem to be made than can be ascertained from a history, and may give a guide to possible treatment, e.g. more frequent voiding to preempt incontinence. It is preferable that the patient should be required to keep the chart if possible as this may serve as a form of bladder training.

Some assessment of the degree of incontinence is required if incontinence aids are to be supplied. Clinical observation is often all that is necessary but objective methods of measuring urine loss are available as the Urilos electronic nappy and the more simple technique of weighing pads before and after use (Walsh and Mills, 1981).

Culture of a midstream urine specimen should be a routine part of the examination of any patient with bladder dysfunction, as should the testing of the urine for sugar.

Intravenous Urogram

Radiological assessment of the urinary tract is essential for haematuria (painless or painful), persistent urinary tract infections, and symptoms related directly to the upper urinary tract. The significance of residual urine on the post-micturition film of the urogram should be interpreted with caution, the circumstances of the examination not always being conducive to efficient voiding.

Cystometry

The measurement of bladder pressure is an essential requirement for the study of bladder function. The classical single-channel technique measuring intravesical pressure only, fails to differentiate accurately pressure changes resulting from either of the two components of intravesical pressure, i.e. detrusor muscle pressure and intra-abdominal pressure. While in the supine posture with the patient lying at rest the intra-abdominal pressure component is negligible and therefore the intravesical pressure can roughly be equated with detrusor pressure, any attempt at either postural change or movement by the patient makes the interpretation of the intravesical pressure recording very difficult.

The minimum requirement for meaningful filling cystometry is a two-channel system measuring intravesical pressure (most commonly via a small diameter tube per urethram) and intra-abdominal pressure (via a similar small diameter tube per rectum). Subtraction of the latter from the intravesical pressure either electronically or visually gives a measure of the detrusor muscle pressure. During voiding a third channel is required to record the flow rate.

The actual technique of cystometry has been well documented (Arnold, 1974; Bates, 1971;

Whiteside, 1972) including its use in geriatric practice (Castleden *et al.*, 1981). Attempts to standardize both the techniques used and the interpretation of the recordings has been made by the International Continence Society (1976).

Cystometry investigates two phases of bladder function: filling and voiding. During filling an assessment is made of bladder sensation but basically the cystometrogram aims to detect the presence or absence of uninhibited detrusor contractions. While in the younger age group up to 55 per cent. of the uninhibited contractions will be missed if postural cystometry, i.e. standing and erect filling is omitted (Arnold, 1974), in the elderly this percentage falls to 4 per cent. (Hilton and Stanton, 1981). Nevertheless, if supine cystometry only is used the absence of uninhibited contractions does not exclude the presence of an unstable bladder.

The voiding phase of the cystometrogram gives information about detrusor contractility and when combined with a measured flow rate provides an assessment of the degree of outlet resistance. It is desirable that separate catheters are used for bladder filling and pressure recording so that the former can be removed prior to voiding.

The role of cystometry in geriatric practice has yet to be fully defined. It is both impracticable and unnecessary to submit all patients with disorders of bladder function to cystometry and this includes patients with incontinence. Nevertheless, the main role of cystometry in the elderly is to investigate incontinence and some selection of cases for investigation is therefore required. Cystometry is not usually required where a diagnosis can be established clinically, i.e. overflow incontinence as a result of prostatic obstruction, where there is a treatable predisposing cause for the symptoms, e.g. infection, or where the symptoms respond to simple bladder training. Failures of simple empirical treatment do require investigation, as do cases where the clinical diagnosis is uncertain and there is a need to establish accurately the type of bladder dysfunction before treatment can be planned intelligently. A simple flow chart as advanced by Hilton and Stanton (1981) as a guide to the need for investigation has much to commend it.

Gas Cystometry

This technique using CO_2 has the advantage of being quick and clean. It is, however, basically a one-channel system and detects only grossly uninhibited detrusor contractions. The carbon dioxide is more irritant to the urothelium than water and the system also suffers from gas leakage. Nevertheless, it may be valuable as a screening test to detect or eliminate grossly uninhibited detrusor contractions.

Cystography

Micturating Cystography

The use of this investigation without reference to cystometric function has a limited place in assessing bladder dysfunction. There are basic difficulties in interpreting function from changes in anatomical configuration and this is compounded if static films only are studied.

The examination of micturating cystography is enhanced if both filling and voiding phases are screened and the relevant information recorded on video tape for more detailed study later. The findings should be evaluated in the light of a recent cystometric examination.

Micturating cystography is of value to determine the site of a proven outlet obstruction in patients with voiding dysfunction.

Combined Synchronous Pressure Flow Cystography

The limitations of both pressure flow measurement and cystography individually are overcome if the two investigations are combined and viewed simultaneously (Bates and Corney, 1971). The observed changes in the bladder and urethral configuration can be interpreted in conjunction with the synchronous pressure record, and this is particularly valuable in assessing urethral closure mechanisms and the severity and site of outflow obstruction. There is no doubt that the simultaneous study provides valuable information which in some cases, especially of voiding dysfunction, can be obtained in no other way.

The radiological apparatus required is standard in most X-ray departments and is readily combined with the pressure recorders. Recording of the information on video tape is preferable to allow for subsequent review.

Uroflowmetry

The measurement of the peak urinary flow rate is the simplest screening test to exclude outflow obstruction and is applicable, particularly in the male, when the diagnosis of prostatic obstruction is uncertain clinically. A flow rate of less than 15 ml/s on an adequate voided volume (preferably greater than 200 ml) can be considered to indicate obstruction (Farrar *et al.*, 1976; Holm, 1962).

Uroflowmetry independent of any instrumentation is also indicated when the voiding pattern during pressure flow cystometry is abnormal, to determine whether the usual flow pattern has been affected by the presence of the urethral pressure catheter.

Urethral Pressure Profile

This investigation measures urethral closure pressure and functional urethral length. The actual technique has been well documented (Harrison and Constable, 1970). A low urethral closure pressure is found in cases of incontinence with poor sphincter activity and a high pressure is equated with spasm of the external sphincter. The range of values recorded for urethral closure pressure in normal individuals, however, shows a wide variation and in the female the values decline with age (Edwards and Malvern, 1974). Individual recordings are therefore often of little diagnostic significance and many clinicians feel they get a better return from other investigations.

The use of microtip transducers to measure urethral pressure changes would seem to offer considerable advantages, although further evaluation is still required.

Electromyography

The measurement of striated muscle EMGs of the voluntary sphincter and pelvic floor are now well established, but have little place in the routine investigation of urethral dysfunction in the elderly. EMG recordings of detrusor smooth muscle have been attempted but the results are not satisfactory (Stanton, Hill, and Williams, 1973).

Cystoscopy

This is an essential investigation if intra-vesical pathology is suspected. It can conveniently be performed in the female under local anaesthesia if necessary.

MANAGEMENT OF BLADDER AND URETHRAL DYSFUNCTION

The principals of treatment which apply to the younger age group are also applicable to the elderly, although cure may be more difficult to achieve in the latter because of the effects of tissue ageing or from poor patient cooperation. Nevertheless, the aim in these patients should still be to achieve effective management of their urinary problem.

Inflammatory Disorders

The treatment of urinary tract infection should be based on the result of a culture of a midstream urine specimen and the effect of treatment checked by a further specimen; regular voiding and a high fluid intake should also be advised. In the male, infections associated with outflow obstruction require relief of the obstruction: in the female with frequent recurrent infections in the absence of intravesical pathology, the results of urethrotomy are very satisfactory (Farrar, Green, and Ashken, 1973).

Bacterial infection associated with the presence of an indwelling urethral catheter is difficult to eradicate, either with antibiotics or urinary antiseptics administered orally, or with bladder washouts, although the latter do reduce the episodes of catheter blockage (Brocklehurst and Brocklehurst, 1978). Antibiotics are best reserved for symptomatic infections.

Symptoms of frequency and dysuria in the female associated with atrophic changes of the external genitalia may respond to the administration of oestrogens either orally or vaginally; the latter is less prone to complications but may be unacceptable or impracticable with some patients. Urethral dilatation is of value in those cases which do not respond to oestrogen therapy and those with symptoms and no obvious atrophic changes (Roberts and Smith, 1968).

Incontinence

Genuine Stress Incontinence

The treatment of this type of incontinence is aimed at improving the efficiency of the distal urethral sphincter mechanism. Urethral sphincter and pelvic floor exercises (Kegel, 1951) are valuable in this respect and can readily be practised by the patient: a perineometer is useful to assess progress. Electrical stimulation (faradism or interferential therapy) used to increase striated muscle tone can also help reeducate the patients in the use of their pelvic floor.

An already weak sphincter may be compromised further by obesity or a chronic cough associated with bronchitis and smoking, and advice should therefore be given. Oestrogen therapy (oral or vaginal) may have a beneficial effect where oestrogen deficiency has been demonstrated.

Surgical treatment should be considered for major degrees of genuine stress incontinence; the age of the patient should not necessarily be a contraindication.

The use of mechanical intravaginal devices which compress the urethra against the symphysis pubis are applicable to this type of incontinence but are not well tolerated by the elderly and because of vaginal laxity are poorly retained. The same applies to intravaginal electronic stimulators.

Pads and pants may be required on a temporary or permanent basis for this group. The choice of system should be determined by the degree of incontinence—the more inobtrusive the better.

Unstable Incontinence

Drugs are the most widely used treatment for this type of incontinence. Unfortunately there is no single preparation which significantly influences detrusor activity without affecting other aspects of the autonomic nervous system. Anticholinergic agents, particularly Emepronium and Flavoxate, are the most commonly used, and while they have a clinical effect, the response to treatment in individual patients is very variable. This is not unexpected, for while Emepronium is effective when given by injection the drug is poorly absorbed from the gut and therapeutic levels are not always obtained (Rich *et al.*, 1977); similarly there are no consistent cystometric changes following the administration of Flavoxate (Briggs, Castleden, and Asher, 1980). Propantheline and Imipramine, which are less commonly used, also have anticholinergic properties, but again the therapeutic response to these agents is variable. As all these drugs have to be used in high doses to gain maximum clinical benefit, side-effects are common. A combination of drugs may be more effective than single agents alone.

A large number of different types of drugs has been advanced for the treatment of detrusor instability but few have stood the test of time. Recently prostaglandin inhibitors (Cardoza *et al.*, 1980) and calcium antagonists (Palmer, Worth, and Exton-Smith, 1981) have been tried with beneficial effects, but further evaluation is required.

Bladder retraining with or without the addition of drugs is an important part of the treatment of detrusor instability. Its efficacy in younger patients has been adequately demonstrated (Frewen, 1978) and its adaptation for elderly patients has also produced satisfactory results (Overstall, Rounce, and Palmer, 1980). A form of bladder training which uses intermittent bladder distension has been shown to be of value (Willington, 1978) but has the disadvantage that it may require repeated catheterization. Bladder training aims to increase functional bladder capacity and decrease the frequency of voiding and should be distinguished from regular toileting which aims to preempt leakage in those whose mental state or mobility makes bladder training difficult.

Attention should be paid to factors which precipitate incontinence such as the timing of administration and usage of diuretics, patient mobility, the accessability of toilet facilities, and the treatment of urinary tract infections. General and specific measures to improve the efficiency of the urethral sphincter mechanism as previously discussed are also valuable. Intravaginal compression devices and electrical stimulators are of limited value, however, because the degree of urethral obstruction they cause is frequently overcome by the force of the uninhibited detrusor contraction.

Pads, pants, and appliances are widely used in the management of incontinence, unfortunately often without medical or nursing supervision, having been obtained by the patient from mail order firms through the columns of newspapers. The selection of suitable aids, however, is important and depends upon the degree of incontinence with which they are required to cope and the patient's ability to understand their use; a specialized nurse advisor in incontinence can be very valuable in this respect. It behoves the clinician, however, to be aware of the available products and their correct use; publications by the Disabled Living Foundation are very helpful on this aspect.

The use of indwelling catheters should be the last resort in the management of incontinence. With unstable incontinence, leakage around the catheter is a major problem resulting from either blockage of the catheter by debris or more commonly from uninhibited detrusor activity exacerbated by infection or the presence of the catheter. Repeated changing of the catheter merely compounds the latter problem and attention should be directed to treating the infection and suppressing detrusor activity. Silicone catheters are preferable to latex for long-term catheterization as they require less frequent changing and on the whole are less likely to encrust.

Overflow Incontinence

Chronic urinary retention resulting from prostatic enlargement requires prostatectomy. Preliminary catheterization is required where there is biochemical evidence of significant renal impairment to allow renal function to recover or where intensive medical treatment is required prior to surgery.

Treatment of retention with overflow in the female depends upon the cause. Faecal impaction and gynaecological pathology should be excluded. Urological treatment by urethral dilatation or bladder neck incision depends upon the site of the obstruction (Farrar *et al.*, 1976).

The use of cholinergic drugs in this group should be restricted to cases where the need for surgical treatment to relieve obstruction has been excluded. Regular voiding should also be advised.

The technique of intermittent self-catheterization (Lapides *et al.*, 1972) is rarely applicable to the elderly. Permanent catheterization may be required where surgical treatment is contraindicated or medical management fails.

Careful management of the catheter is important if complications are to be minimized (Ferrie, Glen, and Hunter, 1979).

Outlet Obstruction

Outlet obstruction as a result of benign prostatic disease is best managed by prostatectomy. Improved techniques have meant that mortality rates are now as low as 1.4 per cent. (Singh, Tressidder, and Blandy, 1973) and the only contraindications are brain failure and gross immobility.

The treatment of outlet obstruction in the female is dependent upon the site of obstruction (Farrar *et al.*, 1976).

Neuropathic Bladder

Treatment of this group should be based upon the symptoms and the type of detrusor and/or sphincter dysfunction present.

Uninhibited bladder activity is less amenable to bladder training or pharmacological manipulation than those with no overt neurological disease, but the same principles apply.

Where bladder sensation is diminished regular toileting is required to prevent overdistension. Bladder neck surgery may be required for hypo- or acontactile detrusors if obstruction is present because of a failure of bladder neck opening.

Others

Where nocturia is the main symptom in the absence of outlet obstruction large doses of Emepronium (Brocklehurst *et al.*, 1969) and Imipramine (Castleden *et al.*, 1981) have been found to be of value, although the latter would seem to be more effective.

CONCLUSION

Advances in diagnostic techniques, in endoscopy and anaesthesia, and an increasing awareness of the needs of the elderly incontinent patient have led to a great improvement in the potential for managing lower urinary tract disorders in the elderly. The application of these advances to routine clinical practice is necessary, however, if patients are to benefit.

REFERENCES

Andrew, J., and Nathan, P. W. (1965). 'The cerebral control of micturition', *Proc. Roy. Soc. Med.*, **58**, 553–555.

Arnold, E. P. (1974). 'Cystometry: Postural effects in incontinent women', *Urol. Int.*, **29**, 185–186.

Band, D. (1945). 'Cystometry', *Br. J. Urol.*, **17**, 1–25.

Bates, C. P. (1971). 'Continence and incontinence', *Ann. R. Coll. Surg. Engl.*, **49**, 18–35.

Bates, C. P., and Corney, C. E. (1971). 'Synchronous cine pressure flow cystography: A method of routine urodynamic investigation', *Br. J. Radiol.*, **44**, 44–50.

Bowen, D. M., and Davison, A. N. (1978). 'Biochemical changes in the normal ageing brain and in dementia', in *Recent Advances in Geriatric Medicine* (Ed. B. Issacs), pp. 41–59, Churchill Livingstone.

Briggs, R. S., Castleden, C. M., and Asher, M. J. (1980). 'The effect of Flavoxate on uninhibited detrusor contractions and urinary incontinence in the elderly', *J. Urol.*, **123**, 665–666.

Brocklehurst, J. C. (1972). 'Bladder outlet obstruction in elderly women', *Mod. Geriat.*, **2**, 108–113.

Brocklehurst, J. C., and Brocklehurst, S. (1978). 'The management of indwelling catheters', *Br. J. Urol.*, **50**, 102–105.

Brocklehurst, J. C., Fry, J., Griffiths, L. L., and Kalton, C. (1972). 'Urinary infection and symptoms of dysuria in women aged 45–64 years: Their relevance to similar findings in the elderly', *Age Ageing*, **1**, 41–47.

Brocklehurst, J. C., Dillane, J. B., Fry, J., and Armitage, P. (1969). 'Clinical trial of emepronium bromide in nocturnal frequency', *Br. Med. J.*, **2**, 216–218.

Buck, A. C., McRae, C. U., and Chisholm, G. D. (1974). 'The diabetic bladder', *Proc. Roy. Soc. Med.*, **67**, 81–83.

Cardoza, L. A., Stanton, S. L., Robinson, H., and Hole, D. (1980). 'Evaluation of flurbiprofen in detrusor instability', *Br. Med. J.*, **280**, 281–282.

Castleden, C. M., Duffin, H. M., and Asher, M. J. (1981). 'Clinical and urodynamic studies in 100 elderly incontinent patients', *Br. Med. J.*, **282**, 1103–1105.

Castleden, C. M., George, C. F., Renwick, A. G., and Asher, M. J. (1981). 'Imipramine. A possible alternative to current therapy for urinary incontinence in the elderly', *J. Urol.*, **125**, 318–320.

Claridge, M. (1966). 'Analysis of obstructed micturition', *Ann. R. Coll. Surg. Engl.*, **39**, 30–52.

Collins, K. J., Exton-Smith, A. N., James, M. H., and Oliver, D. J. (1980). 'Functional changes in autonomic nervous responses with ageing', *Age Ageing*, **9**, 17–24.

Denny-Brown, D., and Robertson, E. G. (1933). 'On the physiology of micturition', *Brain*, **56**, 149–190.

Eastwood, H. D. H. (1979). 'Urodynamic studies in the management of urinary incontinence in the elderly', *Age Ageing*, **8**, 41–48.

Edwards, L., and Malvern, J. (1974). 'The urethral pressure profile: theoretical considerations and clinical application', *Br. J. Urol.*, **46**, 325–336.

Enhorning, G., Miller, E. R., and Hinman, F., Jr (1964). 'Urethral closure studied with cineroentgenography and simultaneous bladder/urethra pressure recording', *Surg. Gynaecol. Obstet.*, **118**, 507–516.

Farrar, D. J. (1979). *Detrusor Instability: Its Significance in Bladder Outlet Obstruction*, M.S. Thesis, University of London.

Farrar, D. J., Green, N. A., and Ashken, M. H. (1973). 'An evaluation of otis urethrotomy in female patients with recurrent urinary tract infections', *Br. J. Urol.*, **45**, 610–615.

Farrar, D. J., Osborne, J. L., Stephenson, T. P., Whiteside, C. G., Weir, J., Berry, J., Milroy, E. J. G., and Turner-Warwick, R. T. (1976). 'A urodynamic view of bladder outlet obstruction in the female: Factors influencing the results of treatment', *Br. J. Urol.*, **47**, 815–822.

Ferrie, B. G., Glen, E. S., and Hunter, B. (1979). 'Long-term urethral catheter drainage', *Br. Med. J.*, **2**, 1046–1047.

Fowler, J. W. (1973). 'Bladder function following abdominoperineal excision of the rectum for carcinoma', *Br. J. Surg.*, **60**, 574–576.

Franks, L. M. (1973). 'Etiology, epidimiology and pathology of prostatic cancer', *Cancer*, **32**, 1092–1094.

Frewen, W. K. (1978). 'An objective assessment of the unstable bladder of psycho-somatic origin', *Br. J. Urol.*, **50**, 246–249.

Gosling, J. A., and Dixon, J. S. (1975). 'The structure and innervation of smooth muscle in the wall of the bladder neck and proximal urethra', *Br. J. Urol.*, **47**, 549–558.

Gosling, J. A., and Dixon, J. S. (1981). Personal communication.

Gosling, J. A., Dixon, J. S., Critchley, H. O. D., and Thompson, S. A. (1981). 'A comparative study of the human external sphincter and periurethral levator ani muscles', *Br. J. Urol.*, **53**, 35–41.

Harrison, N. W., and Constable, A. R. (1970). 'Urethral pressure measurement: A modified technique', *Br. J. Urol.*, **42**, 229–233.

Hilton, P., and Stanton, S. L. (1981). 'Algorithmic method of assessing urinary incontinence in elderly women', *Br. Med. J.*, **282**, 940–942.

Holm, H. H. (1962). 'A uroflowmeter and a method for combined pressure and flow measurement', *J. Urol.*, **88**, 318–321.

Homsey, G. E. (1967). 'The dynamics of the ureterovesical and vesico-urethral junctions', *Invest. Urol.*, **4**, 399–407.

Hunter, D. W. T., Jr (1954). 'A new concept of urinary bladder musculature', *J. Urol.*, **71**, 695–704.

Hutch, J. A. (1965). 'A new theory of the anatomy of the internal urinary sphincter and the physiology of micturition', *Invest. Urol.*, **3**, 36–58.

International Continence Society (1976). 'First report on the standardisation of terminology of lower urinary tract function', *Br. J. Urol.*, **48**, 39–42.

International Continence Society (1981). 'Fourth report on the standardisation of terminology of lower urinary tract function', *Br. J. Urol.*, **53**, 333–335.

Kegel, A. H. (1951). 'Physiologic therapy for urinary stress incontinence', *JAMA*, **146**, 915–917.

Lapides, J. (1958). 'Structure and function of the internal vesical sphincter', *J. Urol.*, **80**, 341–353.

Lapides, J., Diokno, A. C., Silber, S. J., and Lowe, B. S. (1972). 'Clean, intermittent self catheterisation in the treatment of urinary tract disease', *J. Urol.*, **107**, 458–461.

Lapides, J., Gray, H. O., and Rawling, J. C. (1955). 'Function of striated muscles in control of urination. (1) Effect of pudendal block', *Surg. Forum.*, **6**, 611–612.

Lytton, B., Emery, J. M., and Harvard, B. M. (1968). 'The incidence of benign prostatic obstruction', *J. Urol.*, **99**, 639–645.

Milne, J. S., Williamson, J., Maule, M. M., and Wallace, E. T. (1972). 'Urinary symptoms in older people', *Mod. Geriat.*, **2**, 198–213.

Osborne, J. L. (1976). 'The management of the menopause and post-menopause years', in *Proceedings of an International Symposium* (Ed. S. Campbell), p. 285, MTP Press, Lancaster, England.

Overstall, P. W., Rounce, K., and Palmer, J. H. (1980). 'Experience with an incontinence clinic', *J. Am. Geriatr. Soc.*, **28**, 535–538.

Palmer, J. H., Worth, P. H. L., and Exton-Smith, A. N. (1981). 'Flunarizine: A once-daily therapy for urinary incontinence', *Lancet*, **2**, 279–281.

Pool, J. L. (1954). 'The visceral brain of man', *J. Neurosurg.*, **11**, 45–59.

Rich, A. E. S., Castleden, C. M., George, C. F., and Hall, M. R. P. (1977). 'A second look at emepronium bromide in urinary incontinence', *Lancet*, **1**, 504–506.

Roberts, M., and Smith, P. (1968). 'Non-malignant obstruction of the female urethra', *Br. J. Urol.*, **40**, 694–702.

Singh, M., Tressidder, G. C., and Blandy, J. P.

(1973). 'The evaluation of transurethral resection for benign enlargement of the prostate', *Br. J. Urol.*, **45**, 93–102.

Smith, P. (1972). 'Age changes in the female urethra', *Br. J. Urol.*, **44**, 667–676.

Smith, P. (1979). 'The management of the urethral syndrome', *Br. J. Hosp. Med.*, **22**, 578–587.

Stanton, S. L., Hill, D. W., and Williams, J. P. (1973). 'Electromyography of the detrusor muscle', *Br. J. Urol.*, **45**, 289–298.

Stephenson, T. P., and Farrar, D. J. (1977). 'Urodynamic study of 15 patients with post micturition dribble', *Urology*, **9**, 404–406.

Tanagho, E. A., Miller, E. R., Meyers, F. H. L., and Corbett, R. K. (1966). 'Observations on the dynamics of the bladder neck', *Br. J. Urol.*, **38**, 72–84.

Tanagho, E. A., and Smith, D. R. (1966). 'The anatomy and function of the bladder neck', *Br. J. Urol.*, **38**, 54–71.

Tang, P. C., and Ruch, T. C. (1955). 'Non-neurogenic basis of bladder tonus', *Am. J. Physiol.*, **181**, 249–257.

Thomas, T. M., Plymat, K. R., Blannin, J., and Meade, T. W. (1980). 'Prevalance of urinary incontinence', *Br. Med. J.*, **281**, 1243–1245.

Turner-Warwick, R. T., Whiteside, C. G., Worth, P. H. L., Milroy, E. J. G., and Bates, C. P. (1973). 'A urodynamic view of the clinical problems associated with bladder neck dysfunction and its treatment by endoscopic incision and trans trigonal posterior prostatectomy', *Br. J. Urol.*, **45**, 44–59.

Walsh, J. B., and Mills, G. L. (1981). 'Measurement of urinary loss in elderly incontinent patients', *Lancet*, **1**, 1130–1131.

Whiteside, C. G. (1972). 'Video-cystographic studies with simultaneous pressures and flow recordings', *Br. Med. Bull.*, **28**, 214–219.

Willington, F. L. (1978). 'Therapeutic distension for detrusor instability in the elderly', in *Proceedings of International Continence Society, 1978 Meeting*, Pergamon Press.

Principles and Practice of Geriatric Medicine
Edited by M. S. J. Pathy
© 1985 John Wiley & Sons Ltd

26.4

Incontinence in the Community

J. A. Muir Gray

Because the term incontinence is interpreted differently by different people its precise incidence and prevalence is difficult to determine. The range of values for the prevalence of incontinence found by different research workers is from 2 to 42 per cent., and for men the prevalence ranges from 2 to 26 per cent. However, one well-conducted study found that incontinence occurred regularly in 6.9 per cent. of men aged over 65 and 11.6 per cent. of females of the same age (Thomas *et al.*, 1980).

BELIEFS AND ATTITUDES ABOUT INCONTINENCE

Even though incontinence is a distressing problem it is not uncommon for the affected person to suffer without seeking help. There are two common reasons for this failure to seek help: a pessimistic belief that nothing can be done, and a feeling of shame.

Pessimistic Beliefs

Many elderly people are both fatalistic and pessimistic about their problems (see page 48), and incontinence is often accepted as inevitable and untreatable. Some elderly people believe that incontinence is a normal concomitant of ageing and because they know that there is no treatment for ageing they assume that their incontinence is untreatable. This is particularly the case with stress incontinence.

Pessimism about the efficacy of the treatment of disease in old age may be so profound that the old person may not refer the problem to the general practitioner or may refuse his offer of referral to a specialist unit for investigation and treatment (see chapter 26.3).

Shame

Many old people are ashamed or embarrassed by their incontinence but fortunately this usually motivates them to seek help. For a small number, however, such feelings induce the affected old person to try to conceal the problem from friends, neighbours, and professional helpers, and sometimes even from the general practitioner.

Practical Implications

Because of these beliefs and attitudes it is necessary to:
(a) make specific enquiry about difficulty with micturition and defaecation;
(b) repeat the enquiry on each occasion an old person is seen, as the old person may become more willing to reveal her problem as her confidence grows;
(c) emphasize to the old person who is suffering from incontinence that her problems are not due to 'old age' but to a disease which can be treated (see page 1160);
(d) take every opportunity when speaking to old people, their relatives, or groups of voluntary or professional helpers that incontinence is not a normal manifestation of the ageing process and that it should be referred to a doctor if it develops.

ENVIRONMENTAL INCONTINENCE

Whether or not a person who suffers from urgency will be incontinent depends upon three factors:

(a) her degree of urgency, i.e. the time between the sensation of need and moment when an irresistable urge to evacuate occurs (T);

(b) the distance she has to travel to the lavatory (D);

(c) the speed at which she can travel (S).

When $T < D/S$ the person will be incontinent. This type of incontinence may be called environmental incontinence and occurs when there is urgency, although the time taken to reach the lavatory is also of importance in stress incontinence.

To prevent and treat incontinence when the person is suffering from urgency it is obviously necessary to try to achieve two objectives:

(a) to cure or alleviate the urgency (see page 1160);

(b) to reduce the time taken to reach the lavatory by increasing the person's speed of walking (i.e. by increasing S) or by making the journey to the lavatory easier or shorter by decreasing D.

It is the second of these approaches which is of particular relevance in the community, both in the treatment and in the prevention of environmental incontinence, although in this section I wish to emphasize one aspect of the management of incontinence which is frequently ignored but which is of vital importance in the community – education of the patient's relatives (Table 1).

Table 1 Advice for relatives in coping with urgency

1. Encourage your elderly relative to keep as mobile as possible: do not do too much for him and inform the doctor if he becomes less mobile.
2. Remember that an old person with urgency may become very tense and anxious. If an 'accident' occurs it is better not to say simply 'don't worry', but to accept that it is very distressing and to give comfort and support while showing that you do not mind the mess.
3. Inform the doctor or nurse if 'accidents' become more common or if the old person becomes more distressed by them.
4. Try to keep the old person's bowels regular by a high fibre diet.

The excellent study of *The Elderly at Home* conducted by Audrey Hunt for the Social Survey Division of the Office of Population Censuses and Surveys found that over 5 per cent. of people over the age of 80 are either totally unable to reach the lavatory or are only able to do so with help (Table 2). The survey did not record those for whom the journey to the lavatory was difficult or for whom 'incontinence' occurred regularly or occasionally because of environmental problems, but there is no doubt that many people have difficulty of this sort because the survey also revealed that 'about one elderly person in nine has an outside lavatory only, and a further one in ten has no lavatory on the same floor as either bedroom or living room'. Furthermore, about 40 per cent. of people aged over 80 live alone so that many people over the age of 80 who need help to go to the lavatory are unable to receive it, because, as Audrey Hunt emphasizes, 'bathing or washing can be, at a pinch, postponed until help is available, but obviously the need to use a lavatory cannot'.

Table 2 Survey of those unable to get to the lavatory. (From Hunt, 1978))

Age range	Percentage totally unable to get to toilet or unable without help
65–69	0.4
70–74	1.3
75–79	2.8
80–84	5.1
85 and over	6.2

The emotional reaction of someone who has to wait for someone else so that they can use the lavatory has been eloquently described by Alexander Solzhenitsyn:

But there's not that much to laugh at. We are dealing with that crude necessity which it is considered unsuitable to refer to in literature (although there, too, it has been said, with immortal adroitness: 'Blessed is he who early in the morning . . .'). This allegedly natural start of the prison day set a trap for the prisoner that would grip him all day, a trap for his spirit – which was what hurt. Given the lack of physical activity in prison, and the meagre food and the muscular relaxation of sleep, a person was just not able to square accounts with nature immediately after rising. Then they quickly returned you to the cell and locked you up – until 6 p.m., or, in some prisons, until morning. At that point, you would start to get worried and worked up by the approach of the daytime interrogation period and the events of the day itself, and you would be loading yourself up with your bread ration and water and gruel, but no one was going to let you visit that glorious accommodation again, easy access to which free people are incapable of appreciating. This debilitating, banal need could make itself felt day after day shortly after the morning toilet trip and would then torment you the whole day long, oppress you, rob you of the inclination to talk, read, think, and even of any desire to eat the meagre food (Solzhenitsyn, 1973).

Practical Implications

When a person suffers from urgency and is regularly or occasionally incontinent it is important not only to try to cure or alleviate the urgency but also to consider the problems faced by the old person in reaching the lavatory 'in time'. The approach to this can be set out in an algorithm:

House Adaptation

Because the only lavatory is so frequently on the first floor in British houses the stairs present problems to many people with urgency. The first approach is to try to improve the mobility of the affected person to see whether or not she can be helped to regain the strength, skill, and confidence to climb the stairs quickly enough. It is often possible for a physiotherapist to help a disabled person climb the stairs which were once an insurmountable obstacle, but for someone with urgency it may prove impossible for her to climb them quickly enough to reach the lavatory in time.

A stair rail, along the wall, will often help the disabled person and should be tried if her own powers are insufficient for her to go up stairs quickly and safely, but even a stair rail will not increase the speed of ascent significantly for someone who has severe impairment of mobility and urgency. If the staircase is straight a stair lift may provide the solution to the problem and the advice of a domiciliary occupational therapist should be sought. However, the time taken to reach the bottom of the lift and to reach the lavatory from the top of the lift may still make the total length of time needed to reach the lavatory greater than

the time the person can hold her water, and if the occupational therapist's assessment is that a stair lift would not solve the problem she will recommend the installation of a lavatory downstairs. In some houses it is possible to install a toilet under the stairs, in others an extension is required, with grants and loans for people who are private tenants or who own their own houses.

Commodes

The choice of the most appropriate commode is very important. The domicilliary occupational therapist or nurse is able to advise the disabled person and her relatives, bearing the following points in mind:

(a) The height should be the same as the chair or bed in which the old person is sitting, but care should be taken that the old person can sit with her feet on the ground when on the commode.

(b) The best type of commode has both arms and a back, but if lateral transfer is necessary one arm must be movable.

(c) Care should be taken to teach the old person how to transfer.

Chemical closets have the advantage that they require emptying less frequently than commodes, but a chemical closet is more obtrusive than the commode, which looks more like normal furniture and is usually preferable to the affected person. For some people the 'Sani-chair', a toilet seat set on wheels, is appropriate because it allows the disabled person to be wheeled, or to push herself over to a lavatory or commode.

Urinals

The many different sorts of urinal may be grouped into two main types.

The objective of the first is to allow the person who has difficulty in reaching the lavatory or commode to urinate cleanly and easily. The male 'bottle' is well known and widely used, but the female urinals which can be equally effective are not so widely used as they could be. The St Peter's boat is a pointed plastic urinal with a handle which can be slipped between the legs while sitting or standing. Easier to use is the Suba-seal female urinal which is

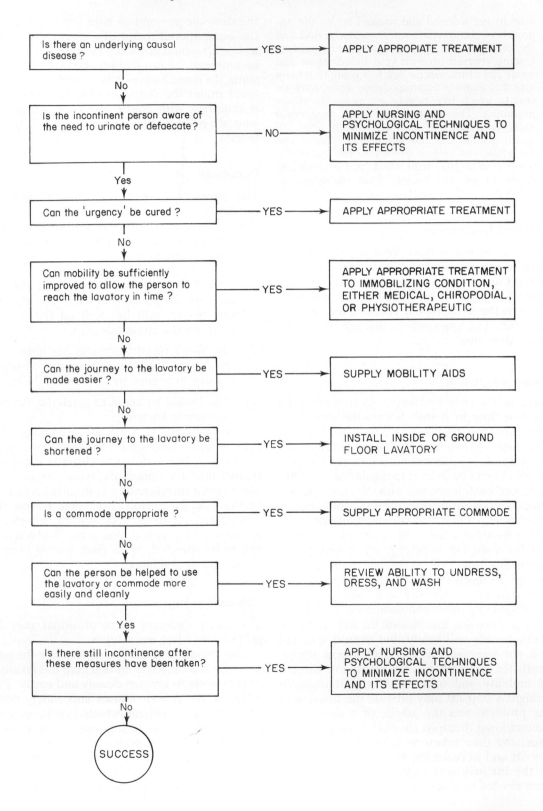

shallower and cannot be spilled (Mendelstam, 1980).

For travelling, both men and women can use the Reddy-Bottle, which is a disposable urinal with a one-way valve.

The second type of urinal is for the person who is continuously incontinent: it is similar to the catheter. The only type in common use is the condom type of urinal, which is, of course, only suitable for men. Although there are advantages over catheterization the use of a permanent urinal gives rise to many problems, particularly if the old person is confused.

Skin Protection

If incontinence cannot be prevented by the approaches which have been described it is essential to protect the skin. This can be done in two ways:

(a) by absorbing any urine which is passed if the person cannot change their clothing or bedding immediately;
(b) by careful washing and drying of the skin which is soaked by urine.

For many years incontinent people have sat on incontinent pads but this is an unsatisfactory and unhealthy life style. In recent years, however, a number of different types of pants which allow the person to walk about with an absorbent pad held in the perineum have been developed. The ordinary sanitary towel is the simplest form of pad and is suitable for people who lose small amounts of urine when coughing or laughing. The Gelulose Pad looks like an ordinary sanitary towel but it contains not only a deodorant but also a chemical substance which forms a gel when wet, allowing the pad to hold more urine than an ordinary pad. Larger pads can be held in adult diapers, such as the Molnycke Adult Inco Diaper, or in the pouch of a pair of Kanga Pants. The latter are simple but ingenious because they are made of a fabric which allows urine to pass only from the inside to the outside of the pants where it is absorbed in a pad held in a plastic pouch.

The domiciliary nurse should have a range of different designs and sizes, to allow the old person and her relatives to choose the most appropriate, and is also the best person to advise on skin care. Every person who is continuously or intermittently incontinent should have a nursing assessment to work out a care plan for her skin.

PROBLEMS AT THE LAVATORY

For many people with urgency or stress incontinence the last few seconds are the most difficult. They have reached the lavatory, they can see it, their need for evacuation is at its height, yet they still have to undress and, in the case of women, sit down. In addition, even people who do not have either stress incontinence or urgency but who have disabilities may have difficulty in using the lavatory cleanly and safely. Careful enquiry about this should be included in a comprehensive assessment of a person who has a disorder of balance, co-ordination, or immobility.

The problems which can occur when using the lavatory and the steps which can be taken to alleviate them can also be summarized in an algorithm.

Undressing quickly and safely

A zip-fly is easier than buttons for most people although the small tab may present difficulties to the person whose ability to see or grasp is impaired. For some people, therefore, a Velcro fly and waist fastening are easier than a zip and clip at the waist band. For men who have difficulty in using a bottle a pair of trousers with a fly which is longer than usual will be helpful. Braces present problems if they are under layers of clothing, but it is often difficult for a person who is overweight to keep his trousers up by any other method. Women who have difficulty in undressing can often be helped if they are given a wraparound skirt or dress, although pants can then still cause difficulty.

The domiciliary occupational therapist or incontinence adviser at the local hospital will be able to advise the old person or her relatives about the adaptation of her clothes or, if necessary, the purchase of new clothes.

Sitting Down Quickly and Safely

A firmly attached handrail on the wall beside the lavatory is useful for almost every disabled person, although some will need rails on both sides of the lavatory.

For the person whose hips are stiff a raised lavatory seat will be helpful.

Once the person has urinated or defaecated

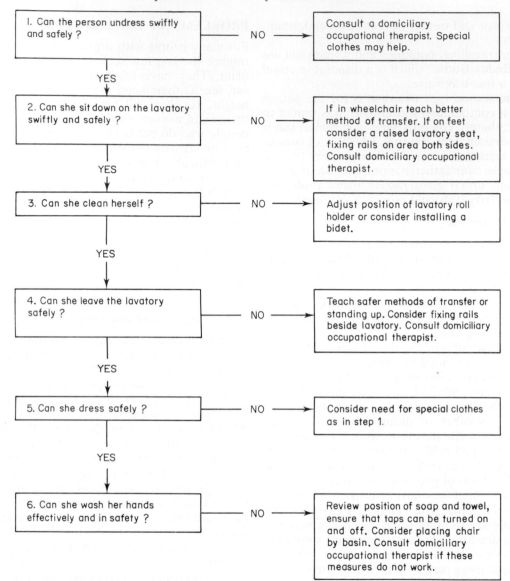

the need for speed is over, although the need for safety is just as great. A comprehensive home assessment should include a review of the person's ability to clean herself, stand up, dress, and wash her hands.

PROBLEMS AT NIGHT

When supporting an incontinent old person at home it is essential to pay detailed attention to the night time for two reasons:
(a) Sleep disturbance is a common problem for the relatives of old people and incontinence at night or a trip to the toilet is one of the causes of sleep disturbance.
(b) A fall may occur while the person is going to the toilet due to one or more of the following factors: postural hypotension, the effect of hypnotics, and micturition syncope.

To prevent incontinence at night the following measures are helpful:
(a) Moderate fluid restriction: the old person should not be forced to go to bed thirsty but excessive intake of fluid, alcohol, or caffeine should be avoided in the evening.
(b) Hypnotics and tranquillizers should be avoided if possible.

(c) A bedside light whose switch can easily be reached should be provided.

(d) A urinal or commode should be provided in the bedroom.

(e) The mattress should be protected by a plastic cover and drawsheet which protect the bed. The use of an undersheet of a 'one-way' material which allows the urine to drain through leaving a dry surface in contact with the skin helps to protect the skin. The Kylie Absorbent Bedsheet is the best of these drawsheets.

The domiciliary nurse can help the old person and her relatives plan a series of measures which will preclude nocturnal incontinence and relatives should be told to seek help if the incontinence increases in frequency.

RELATIVES' PROBLEMS

The mainstay of the system of support for elderly people at home is still their relatives and frequently it is the relatives who bear most of the burden of coping with incontinence. The problems faced by relatives are:

(a) laundry,

(b) smell, and

(c) embarrassment and disgust.

Laundry

The best way to tackle the problem of incontinent laundry is obviously to prevent it by curing the incontinence or by the provision of an adequate supply of effective pads and pants. However, no matter how much care is taken with the provision of pads and pants, sheets and clothes will occasionally be soaked in urine or soiled with faeces. Often, unfortunately, they are soaked and soiled regularly.

To deal with laundry in the most effective way relatives should be given a simple set of instructions (Table 3).

Table 3   Useful advice for relatives in coping with incontinent laundry

1. Sluice soaked and soiled clothes as soon as possible: a rubber hose attached to the bath taps is often helpful.
2. Soak the clothes and sheets in a bucket of cold water; buy a bucket with a tight-fitting lid to reduce the smell.
3. Wash the clothes and sheets with a biological powder.
4. Ask for help if the incontinence becomes more frequent or if you find the laundry particularly irksome or trying.

Relatives should be relieved of the burden if it is proving very tiring by the provision of an incontinent laundry service or, if this does not exist, the services of a home help.

Smell

Careful attention to dirty laundry should minimize the smell but there are other causes of an unpleasant smell and relatives need to be given careful advice.

Table 4   Useful advice for relatives on how to prevent smells

1. Deal with soiled or soaked clothes or bedding quickly.
2. Burn incontinent pads quickly, or if you do nor have an open fire, wrap them in newspaper and put them in a polythene bag as quickly as possible.
3. Encourage and help the old person to wash regularly.
4. Keep the room and house adequately ventilated.
5. Dispose of carpets, rugs, and chairs which have been soiled.
6. Remember that the old person's sense of smell may not be as acute as it was and if she refuses to admit that there is a problem seek the help of the health visitor and district nurse.

Embarrassment and Disgust

Because of the taboos associated with faeces and urine in developed societies and the significance given to the attainment of continence in childhood incontinence is a problem which causes embarrassment and sometimes disgust in the minds of relatives. For example, relatives may be unable to tell an old person that she is smelling or that she is soiling an expensive chair. Relatives, therefore, often need not only practical help but psychological support when caring for someone who is incontinent.

REFERENCES

Hunt, A. (1978). *The Elderly at Home*, (Ed.) HMSO, London.

Mendelstam, B. (1980). *Incontinence and Its Management*, pp. 218–224, Croom Helm, London.

Solzhenitsyn, A. (1973). *The Gulag Archipelago*, Vol. 1, pp. 204–205, Fontana.

Thomas, T. M., Plymat, K. R., Blannin, J., and Meade, T. W. (1980). 'Prevalence of urinary incontinence', *Br. Med. J.*, **281**, 1243–1245.

27
Anaesthesia and Surgery in the Elderly

27.1

Anaesthesia and Surgery in the Elderly

D. Crosby, G. Rees

INTRODUCTION

A substantial proportion of the work in most surgical specialties is now concerned with patients over 65 years of age and it seems inevitable that this proportion will continue to increase in the coming decades.

The problems associated with such surgery are widely known: the elderly patient frequently has multiple-system diseases, while the signs and symptoms of disease may be altered by the ageing process itself. Much of the increased postoperative mortality occurring in such patients may well be due to delayed diagnosis, and correspondingly more advanced pathology. This in turn may be due to the difficulties of history-taking because of impaired mental acuity or emotional disturbances. Also, elderly patients are often willing to accept symptoms as part of the ageing process, rather than attribute them to disease.

Modern techniques of anaesthesia and the comprehensive supportive care now available to critically ill patients make it possible to undertake major surgical procedures in patients of advanced age, which would scarcely have been considered possible or appropriate 30 years ago. Thus, it is no longer exceptional for octogenarians to undergo major joint replacement, resection of aortic aneurysms, and major gastrointestinal resections.

Though the technical aspects of surgery differ very little in elderly patients, its practice poses greater demands in regard to diagnosis, clinical judgement, anaesthesia, and post-operative care than that required in younger patients. Consequently, the achievement of good results demands great vigilance in the exercise of clinical skills and can therefore be highly rewarding to both surgeon and patient. While other chapters have dealt with special aspects of surgery, it is the purpose of this contribution to outline certain general principles of management, with particular reference to major abdominal surgery.

OBJECTIVES

In elderly patients, the objectives of surgical treatment are frequently more limited than those in younger age groups. While the prolongation of active, enjoyable, and worthwhile life is the prime objective, the successful return to gainful employment or to vigorous leisure pursuits is seldom necessary. Though it is important not to deny any patient the possible surgical cure or palliation of a particular disease, it is also important to avoid operations from which the patient can derive no benefit.

FACILITIES

Though surgical techniques differ very little in elderly patients, certain additional facilities and services are particularly valuable in their postoperative care. The familiar hazards of immobility and mental confusion must be anticipated, and, with few exceptions, early ambulation pursued vigorously with the assistance of both nurses and physiotherapists.

Perhaps what is needed most by the clinical team is the attitude of mind that recognizes and accepts the increased demands that elderly patients are bound to make on acute hospital resources. As in so many difficult clinical situations, teamwork is an essential prerequisite to good management, and in this context must usually involve surgeon, anaesthetist, geriatrician, rehabilitation services, patient's family and the general practitioner, if the best possible results are to be achieved.

The organization and delivery of the care needed by such patients following major surgery must be considered carefully by any unit undertaking this work on a regular basis. The heavy demands on nursing services alone, which on some wards may be difficult to provide continuously, are best satisfied by the provision of high-dependency nursing areas (Fig. 1) (Crosby and Rees, 1983). In such areas, the detailed monitoring of critically ill patients can be much more readily undertaken. This in turn implies acceptance of the concept of progressive patient care so that available resources can be allocated most effectively and efficiently.

PATHOPHYSIOLOGICAL AND PHARMACOLOGICAL ASPECTS OF AGEING

Age is associated with profound changes at the cellular level. The tissues of the elderly show a decrease in the number of functional cells but the loss of these cells is compensated for by an increase in the interstitial substances so that there is no net loss of weight. Although many cells in the body can regenerate, other cells – particularly nerve cells – cannot be replaced.

These changes at the cellular level are obviously of fundamental importance but it is the overall performance of organ systems, particularly under stress, that determines whether the patient survives. Thus, it is common to observe a decline in cardiac function and renal function, muscle weakness (including the respiratory muscles), and mental acuity in the elderly.

The elderly patient is likely to present with deviations from the normal. It is often difficult to determine whether these changes are the result of biological ageing or due to degenerative disease. In practice, such differentiation is irrelevant as long as the clinical implications of these changes are appreciated.

The efficiency of many physiological functions diminish in the elderly, which in the main are due to degenerative processes. Although all systems in the body are involved, the cardiorespiratory system is predominantly affected.

It is essential for the successful management of surgery in the elderly that the anaesthetist and surgeon are aware of these profound physiological, pharmacological, and pathological disturbances in organ systems that may accompany old age. Failure to recognize these changes will result in an increased morbidity and mortality.

Respiratory Function

Pulmonary function is markedly reduced with increasing age. The degenerative changes involving the lung structure and the chest wall result in substantial changes in respiratory parameters.

The total lung capacity is not significantly affected by advancing years. There is, however, a marked fall in vital capacity but an increase in residual volume and functional residual capacity (FRC) (Turner, Mead, and Wohl, 1968). The vital capacity at the age of 70 is approximately 70 per cent. of that of a 20-year old and there is a 50 per cent. increase in residual volume over the same period of time (Zamost and Benumof, 1981).

A change in lung volumes of even greater import is the increased closing capacity with age which becomes equal to the FRC in the supine position at about 44 years and the upright position at 66 years (Leblanc, Ruff, and Milic-Emili, 1970). Although the FRC is increased with age, the closing capacity increases at an even faster rate (Holland *et al.*, 1968).

A result of the increase in closing capacity is that in the elderly some airways will be closed in all positions during normal tidal breathing. This will lead to an imbalance between pulmonary ventilation and perfusion, the end result being a reduction in arterial oxygen tension (PaO_2).

The anatomical and physiological dead spaces increase with age. The increase in anatomical dead space is mainly due to associated chronic bronchitis with enlargement of the

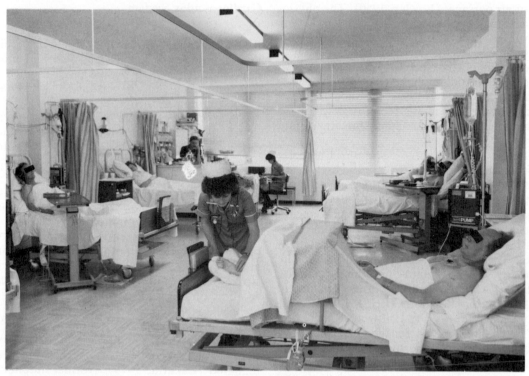

Figure 1   (a) General view of the high-dependency unit ward area. (b) Facilities at the bedside in the high dependency unit

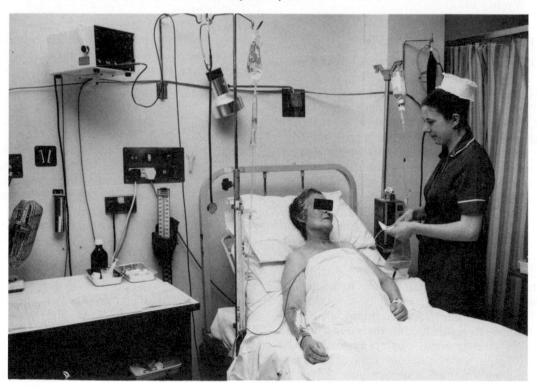

major air passages (Fowler, 1950). The physiological dead space increases by slightly less than 1 ml per year (Harris *et al.*, 1973). A consequence of the increase in physiological dead space is that the ratio of physiological dead space to tidal volume (VD/VT) increases with age. Although the physiological dead space rises, the $PaCO_2$ remains constant as there is a concomitant fall in metabolic rate (White, 1980).

There is a progressive decrease in alveolar surface area so that at 80 years the area available for gas exchange is reduced by 30 per cent. (Zamost and Benumof, 1981). At the same time there is a fall in diffusion capacity. Also, the muscles of respiration become progressively weaker and there is a fall in compliance. These effects are responsible for the decrease in maximum breathing capacity (MBC), forced expiratory volume (FEV), and peak expiratory flow rates (PEFR) that accompany ageing.

The changes in lung mechanics, lung volumes and ventilation/perfusion imbalance lead to a reduction in arterial oxygen tension that is progressive. The reduction is predictable and can be calculated from the formula (Marshall and Wyche, 1972).

$$PaO_2 = 102 - \frac{Age}{3} \text{ mmHg}$$
$$\text{or } PaO_2 = 13 \cdot 6 - 0.044 \text{ (years of age) KPa}$$

However, the findings of Phillips and Tomlin (1977) indicate that the rate of decrease of PaO_2 is increased over the age of 80 years.

In addition to the biological process of ageing, the elderly are subjected to specific disease entities. There is a higher incidence of chronic obstructive lung disease as a result of chronic bronchitis and emphysema, carcinoma of the lung, and even tuberculosis. In addition, they are very susceptible to pneumonia and pulmonary embolism, particularly postoperatively.

Pulmonary function is therefore diminished not only by the biological process of ageing but also by the specific pulmonary diseases that are associated with the older age group. Therefore additional 'stress', which in the young may be of little consequence, can easily lead to the development of respiratory failure and postoperative pulmonary complications.

Cardiovascular System

The changes in the cardiovascular system in the elderly are caused, not only by the biological process of ageing but also and more importantly by degenerative diseases such as atherosclerosis and hypertension which are more common in this group.

These changes commonly manifest themselves as myocardial infarction, conduction defects, cerebral vascular disorders, renal impairment, vascular insufficiency, and cardiac failure.

As well as the gross pathological effects attributable to the pathological changes of age, there are profound physiological changes in the cardiovascular system. The cardiac output falls from 5 to 6 l/min in the young to 3.8 l/min at the age of 80 as a result of the decline in stroke volume and heart rate. Similarly, circulation time is prolonged by 33 per cent. at the age of 80 and myocardial contractility is diminished (Zamost and Benumof, 1981).

The influence of the autonomic nervous system on reflex compensatory mechanisms is attenuated (Lakatta, 1979). Normal autonomic reactivity is altered and is characterized by increase in vagal tone and a decrease in sympathetic activity.

These major physiological and pathological changes limit the ability of the cardiovascular system to respond to stress so that cardiac decompensation is readily precipitated in the elderly.

Nervous System

Biological ageing together with cerebral vascular disease often leads to diminished mental alertness or organic dementia, the latter being characterized by memory deficits, emotional lability, restlessness, and confusion, which in themselves cause serious communication difficulties. The problem of communication is often compounded by a loss of hearing and poor eyesight.

Compensatory reflexes such as those associated with cardiovascular stability and protection of the respiratory tract are depressed. As already mentioned, autonomic nervous tone is greatly diminished.

Temperature regulation is less effective and this is partly due to a fall in the number of skin capillaries with a consequent reduced capacity for vasodilation and vasoconstriction and to a decreased facility for sweating due to atrophy of the sweat glands. The elderly are therefore less able to adapt to ambient temperature changes, especially cold. Elderly patients living alone during the winter months often develop accidental hypothermia which is life-threatening and requires treatment prior to anaesthesia and surgery.

Renal Function

The kidney undergoes age-related changes in structure and function (Shock, 1979). Renal blood flow, renal glomerular flow, and the glomerular filtration rate decrease with age and there is an increasing elevation in the blood urea. Specific organ diseases common in the elderly, such as prostatism, cause urinary tract obstruction, which not only exacerbates the deterioration in renal function but is frequently associated with urinary tract infection. Other diseases such as atherosclerosis, hypertension, and diabetes cause structural renal damage and further renal impairment. Finally, extra renal problems such as hypovolaemia, electrolyte problems, and cardiac failure may further diminish renal reserve. The kidney is thus a vital organ particularly vulnerable in the elderly and impairment of renal function has important implications in management.

Hepatic Function

Although the liver does not show structural changes with advancing age, there is a deterioration in function, presumably related to a fall in hepatic blood flow as a consequence of the decline in cardiac output. This has pharmacological implications in that metabolism will be substantially altered, particularly if associated with superimposed liver disease (*vide infra*).

Structural Changes in Skin, Muscular Skeletal System, and Dentition

With advancing age, the skin loses its elasticity and vascularity which makes it vulnerable to trauma. The hands in particular bruise easily. Orofacial structures, including the muscles, show a loss of elasticity and tone. In addition, many elderly patients are edentulous which,

with the other changes, causes the cheeks to have a concave appearance. Finally, mobility of the neck and jaw can be limited due to osteoarthritic changes in the cervical spine and mandibular joints.

Osteoarthritic changes occur at other sites, especially the lumbar spine, hips, and knees. The result is fixation and immobility of the joints and in the spine there is a reduction in the size of the intervertebral spaces and a narrowing of the intervertebral foramina.

The bones show a progressive decalcification with age so that they become increasingly osteoporotic, and this process is accentuated by bed rest and immobilization. These changes predispose to fractures, particularly of the hip and the femur.

The posture of the elderly is typically one of flexion, especially of the head and neck, together with kyphosis of the dorsal spine.

Pharmacological Aspects

Changes in hepatic and renal functions have a profound influence on pharmacological behaviour. Impaired hepatic function diminishes drug metabolism and this with impaired renal function leads to an increased blood level of the drug and prolongation of its half-life. In addition, due to change in the plasma proteins, there is an elevation in the blood level of the active component of the drug. Finally, drugs administered on a weight basis will produce more powerful effects because there is a loss of cellular structures which are replaced by interstitial connective tissue and fat.

There is also a change in pharmacodynamic activity with age because for a given tissue there is a fall in the number of receptors.

The practical implications of these alterations in pharmacological activity is that the amount of drug required for a given effect is substantially reduced in the elderly. Also, because of lack of receptors, the response is delayed. In addition, the physiological effects of ageing, particularly on the cardiovascular system, diminish the ability of the aged to compensate for a drug effect.

Although anaesthetic drugs have not been fully investigated in the elderly, some drugs which are of considerable interest to anaesthetists have been the subject of particular study (Table 1).

Table 1   Effect of ageing on pharmacology of drugs commonly used in anesthesia

Drugs	Type	Name	References

Drugs commonly prescribed in the elderly	Cardiac glycosides
	Diuretics
	β-blockers
	
	Tricyclic antidepressants
		Digoxin
		Frusemide
		Propranolol
		Practolol
			Editorial, 1978
			Castleden, Kaye, and
			  Parsons, 1975
			Edwards *et al.*, 1979;
			  Glisson, Fajardo, and
			  El-Etr, 1975

Drugs used for premedication	Benzodiazepines
	Anticholinergics
	Narcotic analgesics
		Diazepam
		Atropine
		Morphia
		Pethidine
			Klotz *et al.*, 1975;
			  Reidenberg *et al.*, 1978
			Virtanen *et al.*, 1982
			Kaiko, 1980
			Chan *et al.*, 1975; Mather
			  et al., 1975

Anaesthetic drugs and agents	Induction agents
	Inhalation agents
	
	Muscle relaxants
	Regional anaesthesia
		Thiopentone
		Halothane/isoflurane
		Enflurane
		Pancuronium
		Lignocaine/mepivacaine/
		  bupivacaine
			Christensen, Anderson,
			  and Jansen, 1981
			Gregory, Eger, and
			  Munson, 1969;
			Stefansson, Wicksrom,
			  and Haljamae, 1982a,
			  1982b; Stevens *et al.*,
			  1975
			McLeod, Hull, and
			  Watson, 1979
			Anderson and Cold, 1981;
			  Bromage, 1969;
			  Nightingale and
			  Marstand, 1981;
			  Rosenberg, Saramies,
			  and Alila, 1981

To conclude, drugs used in the elderly should be administered in smaller doses, particularly if given intravenously. Also, the increased half-life of all drugs should be borne in mind when determining the time interval between drug administrations.

Finally, counter measures should be available to deal with any deleterious drug effect due to the failure of compensatory mechanisms.

PREOPERATIVE CLINICAL ASSESSMENT

The discovery of a disease which may be amenable to surgical treatment is no more than an indication for a full and detailed assessment of the patient concerned. Only when this has been done can a responsible opinion be given as to whether an operation is appropriate. Though not separated in practice, there are two principal aims.

To Obtain a Precise Preoperative Diagnosis

This is necessary so that the requirements of the relevant operation can be assessed and properly planned. For example, in obstructive jaundice, a knowledge of the exact cause of the obstruction will usually facilitate the speed and ease with which the operation can be done, thereby improving its safety. Accurate diagnosis of the extent of the disease is also of the greatest importance since, in this way, operations which are unlikely to help the patient can be avoided: e.g. the discovery of extensive metastatic disease or the spread of disease to such an extent that the patient would be unable to withstand the magnitude of operation required. At the same time, it is important not to advise unpleasant, invasive, costly, and sometimes hazardous investigations unless the information they can provide will affect the clinical decision which needs to be made.

To Discover Concomitant Disorders

Only when these are known can the risks of surgery be properly assessed. Thus, cardiorespiratory, renal, and metabolic disorders must be sought, and the nutritional status of the patient assessed. To this end all patients should have a chest X-ray, ECG, full blood count, serum electrolyte and urea estimations, and examination of urine, especially for glucose. Also, sputum culture and pulmonary function tests including blood gas levels may be appropriate. As far as possible, all deviations from normal should be corrected preoperatively, particularly cardiac failure, chest infection, hypovolaemia and electrolyte imbalance.

Preoperative evaluation of the mental state and psychological attitude of the patient is also important when advising major surgery, since it clearly has a bearing on the difficulties of postoperative management. Anxiety, agitation, and confusion may be due to correctable organic causes such as metabolic disturbance, drug therapy, and hypoxia. It is self-evident that the active and willing cooperation of the patient who accepts and understands the need and nature of an operation must result in an improved chance of recovering from it.

SURGICAL DECISION

The timing of surgery has to be a balance between the possible improvement in the patient's condition that can be obtained by preoperative measures and the progressive nature of the condition for which surgery is indicated. The final decision is a matter of clinical judgement by the surgeon in consultation with other colleagues, and this must depend on balancing the chances of success, the risks of failure, and the likely course if surgery is not performed.

These factors can only be assessed against the background of knowledge and expertise of the surgical team concerned. Thus, it is the obligation of any clinician active in geriatric surgery to audit the mortality and morbidity rates engendered in the surgical treatment of various disorders in relation to advancing age. The course of the untreated disease is less easy to determine since, in many instances, properly controlled clinical trials are ethically difficult to justify; e.g. those involving the treatment of non-obstructive intra-abdominal malignancy. Therefore, for various reasons, a surgeon often has to make a decision about whether or not an operation is indicated on evidence which is inevitably incomplete.

CONSENT TO OPERATION

Only when a patient has been fully assessed is it legitimate to offer an opinion concerning the need for surgical treatment. In offering this opinion, the surgeon should allow time and opportunity for the patient and the patient's family to comprehend the risks of having, or not having, the operation which is recommended. Often it is preferable for the surgeon to return after sufficient time has been allowed for the patient to assimilate the advice which has been given. While many patients will readily accept what is offered, and even prefer not to discuss any details, there are those who will wish to crossexamine the surgeon about the risks, the nature of the operation, and the chances of success. When the offer of surgery is declined, the surgeon should ensure that the possible effects of refusal or delay are fully explained. At the same time, it must be openly acknowledged that refusal to agree to surgery is the patient's privilege, as is the freedom to alter the decision at a later date. In some cases it may be appropriate to encourage the patient to take a second opinion. On no account should patients ever be persuaded or seduced to agree to surgical treatment.

The question of consent in the demented or confused patient obviously poses special difficulties. Normally, this will need the signed agreement of available relatives. In this situation, major surgery will usually be restricted to those procedures which will either relieve pain or distress, or which will make the situation easier for those caring for the patient to manage. Thus, for example, excision of an ulcerating tumour, amputation of a gangrenous limb, or relief of intestinal obstruction are operations which will relieve suffering. On the other hand, elective surgery for extensive non-obstructive malignant disease is less easy to recommend in a severely demented patient. Hard and fast rules cannot and should not be laid down, and all patients must be considered individually.

SPECIFIC PREOPERATIVE MEASURES

Anticoagulants

The prevention of postoperative deep vein thrombosis by perioperative administration of anticoagulants such as low-dose heparin or high-molecular-weight dextran has been the subject of many clinical trials (Anonymous, 1979; Klein *et al.*, 1975). Graduated compression stockings have also been claimed to be effective (Scurr, Ibrahim, and Faber, 1977). Though these measures reduce the incidence of deep vein thrombosis and pulmonary embolism as detected by I^{125} radioisotope scanning and lung perfusion studies, respectively, the statistical proof that there is a reduction in postoperative mortality has been difficult to obtain (International Multicentre Trial, 1975; Kiil *et al.*, 1978). Nevertheless, there is considered to be sufficient supportive evidence to justify the routine use of anticoagulant measures during major surgery, particularly in those with increased risk of thromboembolic disease. The risk factors are agreed to include advancing age, obesity, malignant disease, post or family history of thrombosis, and certain operations, such as those on the hip (Anonymous, 1979). Such prophylactic measures are associated with some bleeding problems such as wound bruising and haematomata but not with major haemorrhage requiring transfusion (Gallus, Hirsh, and O'Brien, 1976; Kelton and Hirsh, 1980).

There have been a number of reports over the past 5 years which suggest that the substitution of regional anaesthesia for general anaesthesia is protective against deep vein thrombosis (Davis, Quince, and Laurenson, 1980; Hendolin, Mattila, and Poikolainen, 1981; Modig, Malmberg, and Saldeen, 1980 Thorburn, Louden, and Vallance, 1980) and is associated with a decrease in the number of deaths from pulmonary embolism in surgical patients (McKenzie *et al.*, 1980; McLaren, Stockwell, and Reid, 1978).

It is postulated that the changes in blood flow and coagulability that occur with spinal and epidural anaesthesia are responsible for the apparent protective effects (Davis, Quince, and Laurenson, 1980; Modig, Malmberg, and Saldeen, 1980).

Prophylactic Antibiotics

The severity and incidence of postsurgical wound infections, and other infective complications, have been greatly reduced in recent years by the administration of prophylactic antibiotics (Keighley and Burdon, 1979). Patients undergoing gastrointestinal and biliary tract surgery have been shown to benefit in a number of clinical trials; in particular there has been a marked reduction in wound infections following colorectal surgery (Chodak and Plaut, 1977; Keighley, 1977).

Nutrition

Problems of malnutrition are more common in the elderly. They may result from a combination of long-standing inadequate dietary intake, for social or habitual reasons, and the effects of a pathological process such as gastro-intestinal malignancy. As well as the catabolic effects of major surgery there may be further depletion of nutritional status, due to feeding difficulties in the postoperative period. There have been many reports of both enteral and parenteral feeding before and after major surgery and beneficial effects are claimed in regard to both postoperative mortality and morbidity (Heatley, Harris, and Lewis, 1979; Hill, 1981; Souchon *et al.*, 1979). However, it must be stressed that parenteral feeding itself carries risks if there is not detailed attention to the techniques of administration (Mitchell *et al.*, 1982).

Diabetes

Diabetes is a common disorder in the aged, being 10 times more common in people over 45. It is a condition associated with an increase in atherosclerosis, particularly of the coronary and cerebral arteries and vessels of the lower limbs, microangiopathy of retinal and renal vessels, infection, and, especially in the elderly, obesity. It is for these reasons that they often require surgery, particularly in the latter part of life, and it has been estimated that 50 per cent. of all diabetics will require operative treatment at some time of their life (Root, 1966).

Elderly diabetic patients undergoing surgery are a high-risk group. Mortality rates for diabetics undergoing surgery have been reported as being between 3 and 4 per cent. (Alberti and Thomas, 1979). The major causes of mortality and morbidity are myocardial infarction and infection. Myocardial infarction postoperatively presages an ominous outcome in the diabetic.

Another factor increasing postoperative morbidity and mortality is the finding that diabetics present *de novo* on the surgical wards. It has been estimated that 25 per cent. of diabetic patients on surgical wards are newly diagnosed cases often requiring emergency treatment (Beaser, 1970).

There is increasing evidence (Goodson and Hunt, 1977; Nolan, Beaty, and Bagdale, 1978; Toker, 1974) that maintaining a normal blood glucose intraoperatively and in the postoperative period is associated with a more favourable surgical outcome than would otherwise be achieved. However, this can only be achieved by 'tight metabolic control' during and following surgery since it has been shown that the popular convenient arbitrary regimes recommended in the management of diabetic surgical patients are associated with wide fluctuations of blood glucose levels (Bowen *et al.*, 1982; Walts *et al.*, 1981).

Tight metabolic control requires that control of the blood sugar is carried out on an individual basis. This is best achieved by the use of controlled insulin and glucose intravenous infusions and best managed in a high-dependency unit (Fig. 2).

ANAESTHETIC MANAGEMENT

General Considerations

The principles when providing anaesthesia for the elderly are no different from those that apply to the general population. Nevertheless, there are certain considerations which commonly apply to the aged and these must be borne in mind when deciding which anaesthetic technique is most appropriate in an individual case.

Premedication

The elderly, unlike the young, usually do not exhibit anxiety when faced with the prospect of anaesthesia and surgery. Therefore, the need for preoperative medication is lessened and in many patients can be omitted. A preoperative visit by the anaesthetist during which he elicits any anxieties the patient may have and specifically deals with them will usually suffice. Unfortunately, in some patients communication is difficult due to confusion, deafness, or blindness.

Since the elderly are sensitive to drugs (*vide supra*) the fact that premedication may not be required simplifies the anaesthetic management and promotes safety. However, in certain circumstances of gross anxiety and agitation, preoperative medication will be necessary. The need to use antisialogogues, such as atropine, is less in the elderly since all oropharyngeal secretions decrease with age (Zamost and Benumof, 1981).

Anatomical

The degenerative changes in orofacial structures, cervical spine, mandibular joints, and dentition can cause problems of airway management. Firstly, due to a loss of orofacial supporting structures there are difficulties in maintaining a tight fit with the anaesthetic face mask. Secondly, loose teeth can be dislodged with consequent pulmonary aspiration, particularly following endotracheal intubation. In order to obviate any medicolegal problems, an explanation should be given concerning the necessity to remove loose or carious teeth during anaesthesia. Thirdly, osteoarthritic changes involving the cervical spine and temporomandibular joints can reduce neck and jaw mobility and can make endotracheal intubation difficult because of the inability to visualize the vocal cords. The preoperative anaesthetic evaluation must involve assessment of neck and jaw movements. Finally, vigorous manipulations, especially overextension of the head and neck, must be avoided, since such movements can further compromise the circulation through the vertebral arteries, which may be already impaired because of osteo-arthritic changes involving the vertebral canal.

The techniques of spinal and epidural anaesthesia are made more difficult not only because the spine becomes fixed and rigid but also because the intervertebral spaces become nar-

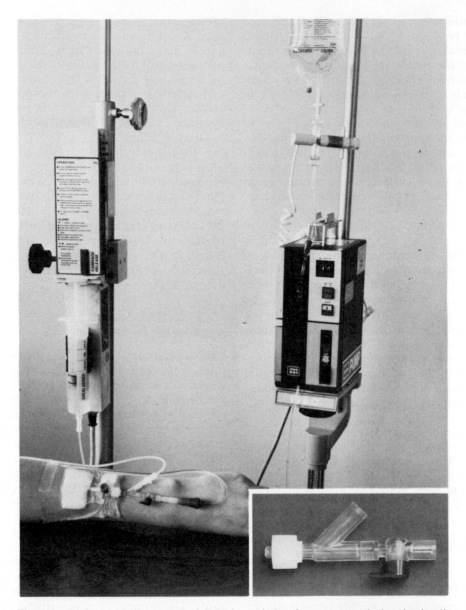

Figure 2   'Tight metabolic control' of diabetic surgical patient postoperatively using insulin
pump, controlled infusion of dextrose solution, and Cardiff valve (inset)

row, and calcification of ligaments is common. The patient showing anatomical deformities should have a preoperative X-ray of the lumbar spine. The inability to flex the vertebral column plus widespread calcification often makes the midline approach impossible. In such cases a paramedian approach is often successful. In addition, blocking of the intervertebral foramina by osteoarthritic changes leads to a high spread of local anaesthetic solution

with epidural anaesthesia (Mostert, 1960). Therefore, the volume and concentration of the local anaesthetic solution should be reduced accordingly (Bromage, 1969).

Posture on the operating table needs careful consideration. Degenerative changes in bones can easily lead to fractures if the patient is clumsily handled.

The degenerative and atrophic changes in the skin and mucosa make them susceptible to trauma. Cannulation of the veins is more difficult because they are fragile and haematomas are common unless particular care is taken. Techniques of intravenous cannulation should be used which allow the intravenous sites to be visible. Also bleeding can occur from the nasal and oral mucosa from roughly placed nasal tubes and oral airways.

Physiological

The limited cardiac reserve together with impaired reflex compensatory mechanisms affect the anaesthetic management in many important ways.

The prolonged circulation time suggests that time should be allowed to assess the effects of intravenous anaesthetic drugs during induction of general anaesthesia. These drugs, particularly the thiobarbiturates such as thiopentone, can produce severe hypotension. At the same time, laryngoscopy and intubation can cause arrhythmias and hypertension (Prys-Roberts *et al.*, 1971).

The combined effect of hypotension and/or hypertension during induction of general anaesthesia can be of limited importance in the young. However, in the elderly either effect may cause severe myocardial ischaemia.

Induction of general anaesthesia should therefore be carried out by the use of small doses of barbiturates or even by the substitution of drugs such as diazepam or ketamine or, in special circumstances, by the use of inhalation agents. The use of beta blockers to attenuate the circulatory responses to upper airway stimulation should be considered and a means of measuring blood pressure at 1 minute intervals during induction should be utilized (Dynamap).

Although laryngeal reflexes can cause reflex hypertension during induction of anaesthesia, the major problem in the elderly is that these reflexes are imparied and so facilitate pulmonary aspiration whether it be gastrointestinal contents, blood, or carious or loose teeth. Priority should be given to ensure that the respiratory tract is fully protected. It is vital at all times when aspiration is a problem that the respiratory tract is protected either by the use of a cuffed endotracheal tube or, alternatively, by the use of local anaesthetic techniques.

Pharmacology

All anaesthetics cause depression of the cardiovascular system and this is even more pronounced in the elderly because of the limited cardiac reserve and impaired reflex compensatory mechanisms.

The effect of all inhalation agents is further compounded if changes in minimal alveolar concentration (MAC) are not appreciated (Eger, 1974). The quantitative aspects of the relationship of MAC to age of some inhalation agents have been determined. For example, at the age of 80 years the MAC for halothane and isoflurane are 0.64 and 1.95, respectively.

In the aged there is a decrease in muscle tissue power so that the dose of muscle relaxant required to produce satisfactory operating conditions is reduced. Residual postoperative muscle paresis is a problem in that the capacity of the residual muscle fibres to increase power is diminished. This effect can on occasion lead to postoperative respiratory failure.

Finally, other pharmacological effects of muscle relaxants may be deleterious in the elderly: for example, the tachycardia associated with gallamine, the hypotension caused by curare, and hyperkalaemic and dual-block response to suxamethonium are not tolerated to the same extent as they are in the young. Age is an important factor when regional techniques are used. The increase in spread and duration of epidural anaesthesia with age is probably related to anatomical changes in the spinal canal rather than to reduced vascular perfusion, as the increase in spread is not associated with lower plasma levels of the local anaesthetic drugs (Scott *et al.*, 1972).

Another factor may be the increased half-life of local anaesthetic agents with age. The half-life of lignocaine is increased by 70 per cent. in the seventh decade (Nation, Triggs, and Selig, 1977). Finally, the decline in neuronal population and the deterioration in neural connective tissue probably plays an important part. The combination of adrenaline with local anaesthetic solutions for epidural anaesthesia should probably be avoided as the blood supply to the spinal cord may be compromised in the elderly. This is particularly so if generalized arterial disease exists.

The problem that is clinically important with both epidural and spinal anaesthesia is arterial hypotension following the block. This is important in the elderly who are unable to compensate, and this can lead to severe myocardial ischaemia or even cardiac arrest. It is therefore essential that drugs and intravenous fluids required to elevate the blood pressure, together with all forms of resuscitation, are immediately to hand.

Monitoring

The safety of the aged during anaesthesia and surgery is enhanced when moment-to-moment observation is carried out. Thus, full and adequate monitoring is a priority during the intraoperative period so that adverse trends can be detected and corrected. The cardiorespiratory status should be assessed by non-invasive techniques. Where indicated, direct intra-arterial and central venous pressure measurements together with blood gas studies should be made. The measurement of body temperature with a digital thermometer should be carried out routinely in major operative procedures and in this context consideration should be given to warming of all intravenous fluids such as blood, colloid, or crystalloid solutions.

ANAESTHETIC TECHNIQUES

Local Anaesthesia

The operative procedures that are well suited to local anaesthetic techniques in the elderly are operations on the extremities, cataract surgery, and dental extractions. Infiltration, intravenous regional blockade, or peripheral neural blockade are techniques that when properly performed cause little systemic effect, which is of considerable advantage.

Regional blockade, however, is associated with profound physiological changes and the choice between it and general anaesthesia in an individual case is a matter of fine judgement. The major haemodynamic changes that are characteristic of spinal and epidural anaesthesia must be balanced against the problems inherent to general anaesthesia.

Operative procedures where regional anaesthesia is widely used, often in preference to general anaesthesia, are operations on the lower extremities, particularly hip replacement and fracture of the femur, perineal procedures such as haemorrhoidectomy, vaginal hysterectomy, transurethral resection of the prostate, and some procedures in the lower abdomen and inguinal region. This is particularly so if patients scheduled for such procedures have either severe pulmonary disease and/or evidence of disturbed respiratory function. It is essential, however, that when regional anaesthesia is used in the elderly, the anaesthetist is cognizant of the altered response of the aged to the physiological and pharmacological effects of these techniques.

An advantage of regional anaesthesia that is becoming increasingly appreciated in contemporary practice is its value in the relief of post-operative pain. The analgesic effect of spinal anaesthesia extends well into the post-operative period. However, when epidural anaesthesia is used, this time can be extended further, even indefinitely, by the use of epidural catheter.

Two contraindications for the use of regional anaesthesia are local sepsis and the use of anticoagulants (Bromage, 1969). The latter is an important consideration as many patients are given miniheparin prophylactically so as to diminish the incidence of deep vein thrombosis and pulmonary embolism.

General Anaesthesia

Although certain operative procedures are better performed under local anaesthesia, there are circumstances when general anaesthesia is preferable and safer. Examples of the latter are when control of the airway's is a problem or when the patient has poor respiratory function due to severe pulmonary disease and requires assisted respiration and tracheobronchial toilet. The advantage of general anaesthesia vis-à-vis regional anaesthesia is that the former, despite all its problems, provides the anaesthetist with moment-to-moment control of the patient's vital functions which, in the situations referred to above, promotes safety. There is little doubt that upper abdominal, intrathoracic, and intracranial operations in the elderly are better carried out under general anaesthesia.

The problem of cardiovascular stability during general anaesthesia, particularly during induction, is always a matter of some concern in the elderly (*vide supra*). It is for this reason that ketamine with its sympathomimetic effects has been advocated in selected cases. Also, during induction of anaesthesia, the effects on the uptake and distribution of inhalation agents, low cardiac output and diminished ventilation that accompany ageing should be taken into account.

In contemporary practice, general anaesthesia is usually maintained either by the use of nitrous oxide with a narcotic analgesic such as fentanyl or phenoperidine or by the combination of nitrous oxide with another inhalation agent such as halothane, enflurane, methoxyflurane, or even trichlorethylene. Occasionally the two techniques are combined. Either of these techniques when properly managed lead to minimal depression of the cardiovascular or respiratory systems.

Many of the operative procedures requiring general anaesthesia also require intermittent positive pressure ventilation either with or without muscle relaxation. The pharmacokinetic studies that have been carried out on the muscle relaxants in current use demonstrate that dose for dose their effects on the elderly are more intense and prolonged (McLeod, Hull, and Watson, 1979). This should counsel caution, particularly if they are used in patients with pulmonary disease when not infrequently there is difficulty in reestablishing spontaneous respiration at the end of the operation.

Adverse cerebral effects following what is often apparently uneventful general anaesthesia and surgery are most distressing to both the patient and his relatives. The effects can range from extreme dementia to diminished intellectual ability and memory deficits (Bedford, 1955). The aetiology is obscure, but two factors that should be considered when the cause is not obvious are unrecognized hypoxia and hypocarbia. Hypocarbia leads to a reduction in cerebral blood flow which may have serious implications in elderly patients, particularly those with cerebrovascular disease. This reinforces the need to closely monitor the geriatric surgical patient so as to detect and correct hypoxia and/or hypocarbia.

The most common cause of death following general anaesthesia in the elderly is due to pulmonary aspiration of gastrointestinal contents. They are especially vulnerable to this complication because the protective laryngeal reflexes are impaired and there is an increased incidence of hiatus hernia with gastrooesophageal reflux. This hazard can be completely averted by sealing off the respiratory tract from the gastrointestinal tract with a cuffed endotracheal tube. There are many techniques available to accomplish this but they all require expertise.

Finally, the anaesthetic requirements for all drugs is reduced, which necessitates additional caution when anaesthetizing elderly patients – somewhat trite, but sound advice.

SPECIFIC SURGICAL CONDITIONS AND PROBLEMS

Carcinoma of Stomach

As with a number of intra-abdominal malignancies, the incidence of carinoma of the stomach rises with age, and it carries a gloomy prognosis (Office of Population Censuses and Surveys, 1976; Thompson, 1982). Its insidious onset, and initially vague symptoms, make early diagnosis the exception rather than the rule. Barium studies and endoscopic biopsy are the usual methods of diagnosis, and liver isotope imaging is sometimes useful to identify metastases. However, the latter is obviously unnecessary if a clinical decision to advise operation has already been made, for example, because of evidence of gastric outlet obstruction.

At laparotomy, extensive macroscopic evidence of tumour spread may be found, both to adjacent lymph nodes as well as to other viscera and the peritoneum. However, palliative excision of the primary tumour may be feasible, thus ridding the patient of an ulcerated and bleeding lesion. Occasionally, a bypass procedure such as gastrojejunostomy or exclusion gastrectomy may provide useful palliation by relieving gastric outlet obstruction. If no macroscopic evidence of extra gastric tumour spread is discovered at laparotomy, a wide resection of the gastric tumour is justified. If the primary lesion is in the antrum or body of the stomach, a subtotal gastrectomy is usually possible. If a more extensive lesion is present, or if the gastric fundus is involved, total gastrectomy with resection of the lower oesophagus may be necessary if the patient is sufficiently fit to withstand such a major procedure. For such extensive operations, a 20 per cent. mortality rate may be expected, while a 5-year survival rate of 15 per cent. is seldom exceeded (Paulino, 1973). The morbidity of the procedure is also considerable (Bradley *et al.*, 1975; Longmire, 1980).

Dysphagia

Two of the more common causes of dysphagia of recent onset in an elderly patient are malignant disease of the oesophagus and benign oesophageal stricture secondary to gastrooesophageal reflux. The differential diagnosis, which is sometimes difficult despite barium studies, must normally be confirmed by endoscopic biopsy. Achalasia (cardiospasm), neurological disorders such as bulbar palsy, and pharyngeal pouch are also sometimes the underlying causes in elderly patients presenting with dysphagia.

Carcinoma of Oesophagus

This disease carries a grim prognosis with 5-year survival rates following treatment seldom exceeding 20 per cent. (Orel, Erzen, and Hrabar, 1981; Roberts, 1980). Though some patients may be cured, in many the main aim of treatment must be to relieve the distressing effects of dysphagia. There are no experimental data to prove that either surgery or radiotherapy is preferable in the management of various categories of oesophageal cancer. However, where both radiotherapy and surgical services are highly developed, optimal benefit is likely to be achieved if patients with squamous carcinoma of the middle and upper thirds of the oesophagus are treated initially by radiotherapy, and patients with squamous carcinoma of the lower third and all adenocarcinomas are treated surgically unless medically unfit (Pearson, 1981). Thus, in patients in whom extensive or metastatic disease has been excluded, successful surgical excision is often the most effective means of alleviating dysphagia, though many patients will be found insufficiently fit for the extensive thoracoabdominal procedure which is usually necessary. If surgical excision of the tumour is not considered possible, some form of palliative

surgical bypass procedure may be feasible (Ong, 1975). Palliative intubation of inoperable tumours may also be possible, even in very frail patients. However, it is important to realize that even when this is successfully achieved, only a liquidized diet can usually be tolerated. Consequently, intubation should only be considered when patients have reached the stage when they are unable to swallow fluids. Palliative intubation can be successfully performed non-operatively using fibre-optic endoscopy (Atkinson, Ferguson, and Parker, 1978; Pfleiderer, Goodall, and Holmes, 1982).

Achalasia (Cardiospasm)

This remains a rare and interesting neuromuscular cause of dysphagia. Until recent years Heller's operation, viz. oesophagomyotomy, was the treatment of choice. However, forcible endoscopic dilation of the oesophagogastric junction under radiographic control has now been shown to be a relatively safe and effective alternative method of treatment (Okike *et al.*, 1979; Orringer, 1979).

Hiatus Hernia and Gastrooesophageal Reflux

Hiatus hernia with associated reflux oesophagitis is a common condition in the elderly, and its management does not differ significantly from that in other age groups. Fortunately, symptoms are usually mild and intermittent, and satisfactorily controlled with conservative measures including postural advice and antacid medications. Perhaps the main hazard of this condition is that it may be blamed for symptoms which are actually due to more serious intra-abdominal disorders, such as early gastrointestinal neoplasms. Also, though peptic oesophagitis is sometimes associated with iron deficiency anaemia due to occult blood loss, it is most important to exclude other possible causes such as colonic tumours.

In those patients where symptoms have become intractable, and who are confirmed by endoscopy to have persistent and severe oesophagitis, surgical reduction of the hernia and repair of the hiatus may become necessary. Transabdominal repair usually entails fundoplication as described by Nissen (1956). Alternatively, transthoracic repair, such as the Belsey operation, may be preferred by some surgeons (Singh, 1980).

When reflux oesophagitis is complicated by stricture formation, with associated dysphagia, in an older patient, the magnitude of the surgery required to correct the situation is such that endoscopic dilatation, together with strict medical treatment, is usually the first line of treatment. When this fails to provide relief, surgical control of gastrooesophageal reflux may be necessary by one of the procedures mentioned above. Resection of the stricture may sometimes also prove necessary if it is confirmed to be mainly fibrous, rather than due to associated spasm.

Gastric Ulceration

This may present, persist, or recur in the aged. Assuming malignant change has been excluded by adequate endoscopic biopsy, initial treatment may be conservative with particular regard to nutritional problems, and the exclusion of ulcerogenic medications which the patient may be receiving for other disorders. Carbenoxalone, which is certainly efficacious in this condition, must however be used with caution because of its fluid-retaining and hypokalaemic side-effects. Failure to obtain healing of a gastric ulcer, doubt about its histological nature, and evidence of bleeding are all indications for partial gastrectomy. The Billroth I operation with anastomosis of the gastric remnant to the duodenum is the most favoured surgical technique.

Gastric ulcers which perforate or bleed are particularly dangerous, and are usually dealt with by resection rather than simple suture, since the latter is often complicated by reperforation or recurrent bleeding. If simple suture of the ulcer has to be performed because the patient's state is too poor to withstand partial gastrectomy, it is important to biopsy the edge of the ulcer in order to exclude malignant change.

Duodenal Ulceration

Uncomplicated duodenal ulceration seldom needs surgical treatment in the aged, and can usually be controlled by medical treatment. This may be due to natural regression of the disease, which has a peak age incidence of onset in the third and fourth decades. Also, perhaps those requiring surgical treatment have already been dealt with earlier in life. Nevertheless, older patients with bleeding, perforating, or stenosing chronic duodenal ulcers are not infrequently seen as surgical emergencies, and pose particular difficulties.

Perforation of Peptic Ulcer

This diagnosis is not always obvious in the older patient. As with other intra-abdominal catastrophies, the initial symptoms and signs may be insidious rather than dramatic. Once the diagnosis has been made, usually by the radiological demonstration of free gas in the peritoneal cavity, laparotomy is normally undertaken, with simple suture of the perforation. If the patient is sufficiently fit, and if the ulcer is evidently chronic in nature, some surgeons consider it appropriate to proceed to definitive surgical treatment of the ulcer by some form of vagotomy at the same procedure. In those patients believed to have perforated their ulcers more than 48 hours prior to diagnosis, and whose general condition remains reasonably good and without clinical evidence of peritonitis, there is a case for conservative treatment which will usually include continuous nasogastric suction, intravenous fluids, and antibiotics (Rossoff, Puig-La-Calle and Luder, 1980).

Haematemesis and Melaena

The risk of life of this dangerous condition is well known to increase with advancing age, and the reasons for this are well recognized (Dronfield and Langman, 1978; Thomas *et al.*, 1980). Apart from the presence of other disorders which may prejudice survival, the primary cause of bleeding is itself more likely to be chronic and advanced, and associated with arteriosclerosis which impedes physiological haemostatic mechanisms. It is important, therefore, that investigative procedures such as barium studies, endoscopy, and arteriography designed to establish the exact diagnosis in such patients are performed with urgency. As a general principle, surgery for bleeding peptic ulcers will need earlier consideration in older patients since bleeding is less likely to stop spontaneously; also, the hazards of massive blood transfusion are greater.

Gall-Bladder Disease

The incidence of gall-bladder disease rises steadily with advancing years, as does the mortality of surgical treatment (Bateson and Bouchier, 1975; Editorial, 1981; Glenn, 1981). Not infrequently, gallstones are an incidental discovery during the course of investigations for other disorders, and close questioning of the patient may fail to elicit symptoms attributable to the biliary tract. While there is little controversy about the need for cholecystectomy in patients with recurrent cholecystitis, biliary colic, or associated pancreatitis, there is less conviction of the need for cholecystectomy in those who are asymptomatic (Bates, 1981).

The increased risk of gall-bladder surgery in older patients is in some measure probably due to more advanced disease and the increased incidence of common bile duct exploration for the removal of ductal calculi shown by operative choledochography. The need for emergency laparotomy because of spontaneous perforation of the gall-bladder is certainly more common in older patients.

In patients shown to have radiolucent calculi in a functioning gall-bladder, and in whom there are increased hazards of cholecystectomy, because of other medical disorders, dissolution of calculi by chenodeoxycholic acid may be considered. However, the long-term success of this method remains unproven (Anonymous, Polli *et al.*, 1981; Schoenfield and Lachin, 1981; Summerfield, 1979). Surgery may also be avoided in some patients discovered to have stones in the common bile duct, since such stones can often be removed by duodenoscopic sphincterotomy (Mee *et al.*, 1981).

Gallstone intestinal obstruction is a rare and interesting complication of biliary tract disease. It is most commonly seen in elderly women and is usually due to ulceration of a large cholesterol stone from the gall-bladder into the duodenum, thus forming a biliary enteric fistula. The obstruction is often intermittent, and diagnosis is frequently delayed due to the gradual onset of the obstruction. It is a dangerous condition and early, correct, preoperative diagnosis usually rests on a high index of suspicion, together with the radiological identification of gas in the biliary tract (Day and Marks, 1975; Heuman, Sjodahl and Wet-

terfors, 1980). Removal of the obstructing gallstone, which is usually found to be impacted in the terminal ileum, is best performed by milking it proximally before removing it by enterotomy. The associated gall-bladder disease may need surgical treatment at a later date, since patients are usually quite ill by the time intestinal obstruction has been diagnosed and relieved. Recurrent obstruction due to the passage of further stones may occasionally occur.

Obstructive Jaundice

In elderly patients, the most likely causes of obstructive jaundice are malignant disease and biliary calculi. The differential diagnosis between these and other causes of jaundice has been made considerably easier in recent years by advances in investigative techniques including ultrasonic scanning, transhepatic fine-needle cholangiography, arteriography, and endoscopic cannulation of the sphincter of Oddi (Blumgart, 1978; Bouchier, 1981).

It is thus possible to have accurate knowledge of the requirements of any proposed operation to relieve jaundice before it is undertaken. This in turn makes it possible to undertake appropriate preoperative preparations, including adequate blood transfusion, if there is a possibility of major surgery such as pancreatic resection. All jaundiced patients undergoing surgery should normally be checked for coagulation defects and vitamin K given in order to correct reduced prothrombin levels. During operation it is customary to administer an osmotic diuretic such as mannitol, since this is believed to reduce the risk of renal failure, to which such patients are more vulnerable. When this is done, a urethral catheter should be inserted so that urine output can be monitored. In deeply jaundiced patients, it may sometimes be advantageous to decompress the biliary tree by preoperative transhepatic cannulation of the bile ducts, leaving a catheter *in situ* for a number of days, during which time other measures may be undertaken aimed at improving the patient's preoperative state (McPherson *et al.*, 1982).

In many elderly patients with obstructive jaundice due to a malignant cause, only palliative surgical measures will be possible. This will usually be due to the discovery of malignant disease beyond the scope of surgical resection, while some of those with a small tumour (e.g. periampullary carcinoma) may be too frail to withstand a Whipple's type pancreaticoduodenal resection. Nevertheless, worthwhile palliation with relief of jaundice can often be achieved with surgical bypass procedures of various kinds. In those cases where the obstruction lies below the origin of a patent cystic duct, as in carcinoma of the head of the pancreas, it is customary to anastomose the fundus of the distended gall-bladder to the proximal jejunum. A Roux en Y type of reconstruction is often performed in this situation, since this reduces the likelihood of recurrent ascending cholangitis. Alternatively, the distended common bile duct, or common hepatic duct, may be anastomosed to the duodenum or proximal jejunum. In recent years, it has been shown that patients with tumours or strictures of the bile ducts causing obstructive jaundice can also be successfully palliated by percutaneous transhepatic or transduodenoscopic intubation using stents of various kinds (Cotton, 1982; Irving, 1981).

Appendicitis

There is some evidence to suggest that the incidence of appendicitis is falling (Donnan and Lambert, 1976; Raguveer-Saran and Keddie, 1980). Nevertheless, it remains a dangerous disease, particularly in the elderly. A recently reported survey (Peltokallio and Tykka, 1981) showed a mortality rate of 4 per cent. in patients over 60, while the average age of all patients who died was 70. Perforation of the appendix is much more common in the elderly and occurs in over 40 per cent. of those with appendicitis, compared with about 18 per cent. in younger patients. Also, perforation occurs earlier in the disease, and this has been attributed to loss of appendicular lymphoid tissue and ischaemia, or previous weakening of the appendix. It seems certain that the mortality and morbidity rates for acute appendicitis in the aged would be improved by earlier diagnosis, and appendicectomy prior to perforation.

Colorectal Cancer

More than half of all cases of carcinoma of the large intestine occur over the age of 60. The peak incidence for carcinoma of the rectum is between 60 and 69 years, and there appears to be an increasing tendency to develop rectal cancer with advancing age (Goligher, 1980, p. 378; Office of Population Censuses and Surveys, 1976). The diagnosis should not be difficult provided there is a high index of suspicion in regard to the discovery of iron deficiency anaemia, changes in bowel habit, and rectal bleeding. Approximately half of all large bowel cancers are within easy range of biopsy by sigmoidoscopy, while the remainder can usually be identified by barium enema examination. Colonoscopy is a useful investigation for colonic lesions which are of a doubtful nature following radiography.

Surgical excision of such tumours remains the mainstay of treatment, since they are relatively resistant to other therapeutic methods such as radiotherapy or chemotherapy. The majority of patients can be dealt with on an elective basis, and cancer-specific survival rates of around 50 per cent. at 5 years can be obtained in operable patients. Between 5 and 40 per cent. of patients present as emergencies with intestinal obstruction, depending on the site of the primary tumour (Goligher, 1980, p. 419; Irvin and Greaney, 1977). When the latter occurs due to a tumour in the right colon, primary resection with restoration of intestinal continuity by ileo-colic anastomosis is usually possible. If the primary obstructing tumour is unresectable a palliative ileocolic anastomosis will provide relief of obstruction. However, when obstruction is due to a tumour in the left side of the colon, it is usual to perform a proximal colostomy as an emergency procedure, with a view to later definitive resection of the obstructing tumour and closure of the colostomy.

Extensive tumours in the lower third of the rectum are still usually dealt with by abdominoperineal resection and the construction of a permanent colostomy in the left iliac fossa. However, in recent years the increasing use of various stapling devices has facilitated the performance of anastomoses deeper in the pelvis, thus reducing the number of patients requiring permanent colostomies (Goligher, 1979). While there have been apprehensions that this might result in incomplete tumour excision, there is evidence to support the view that an adequate margin of tumour removal is still obtained (Heald, 1979).

In frail patients considered insufficiently fit to withstand total removal of the rectum by abdominoperineal excision, the Hartmann's procedure, which leaves the rectal stump distal to the tumour *in situ*, has much to recommend it, particularly in tumours causing some degree of obstruction. Also, it retains the possibility of colostomy closure at a later date by colorectal anastomosis, when the patient's general condition has improved, provided no evidence of tumour recurrence has subsequently appeared. The reported 5-year survival rates for all patients undergoing colorectal cancer resection are between 50 and 60 per cent. in most series. There is close correlation between survival rates and the extent of tumour spread at the time of operation, as classified by Dukes (McDermott *et al.*, 1981).

Severe Rectal Bleeding

Sudden profuse bright red rectal bleeding of life-threatening severity is an indication for the emergency admission to hospital of elderly patients. There are a number of possible causes for such bleeding including ulcerative colitis, mesenteric infarction, colonic tumours, and diverticular disease. In recent years, with the advent of more detailed investigation by mesenteric arteriography, many such patients have been discovered to have angiodysplastic lesions in the submucosa of both the large and small bowels or, more frequently, in the ileocaecal region (Baum *et al.*, 1977; Boley *et al.*, 1979; Broor *et al.*, 1978). In those patients with recurrent severe bleeding, resection of the involved segment of bowel may become necessary. There have been some reports of therapeutic embolization of such lesions, with variable success (Allison, 1980). When the origin of recurrent bleeding cannot be identified, total colectomy with ileorectal anastomosis may sometimes prove necessary (Goligher, 1980, p. 906).

Complete Rectal Prolapse

This is a not uncommon reason for the surgical referral of elderly patients. It is clearly a distressing disorder and commonly associated with faecal incontinence. Females are preponderant by at least 4:1 and, interestingly, the condition appears to be relatively more common in nulliparous women (Henry, 1980). Sometimes it is also associated with complete uterine prolapse. In many cases, the underlying cause of the condition is believed to be an intussusception of the rectum, which in turn may be due to a disorder of the neuromuscular control of defaecation. The pelvic floor musculature and anal sphincter mechanism become lax and stretched, probably as a result of the prolapse. A deep rectovaginal or recto-vesical peritoneal pouch is a commonly associated finding.

Though many of the older patients suffering from this condition are very frail, many can be made sufficiently fit to withstand transabdominal repair and fixation of the prolapse. Many ingenious abdominopelvic surgical manoeuvres have been devised with variable success. Currently, the most favoured method is the Ivalon sponge rectopexy. This involves transabdominal mobilization of the rectum, followed by a simple and incomplete wrapping of the rectum in a sheet of polyvinyl sponge, which itself is sutured to the hollow of the sacrum. A high success rate has been reported in regard to control of the prolapse, though complete recovery of the associated faecal incontinence is not always obtained (Penfold and Hawley, 1972). The insertion of a Thiersch wire or nylon purse string suture in the perianal region is a very simple procedure and is still used for complete rectal prolapse in those patients who remain unfit for major abdominal surgery. However, it is not always satisfactory, since when the suture is sufficiently tight to prevent rectal prolapse, it often results in faecal impaction, which can only be prevented by frequent enemata.

Colonic Diverticular Disease

This is increasingly common with advancing age, mainly affecting the sigmoid colon, and a troublesome cause of lower abdominal pain and bowel disturbance. Fortunately, in most patients, it pursues a relatively benign course and symptoms are often improved with high roughage diets (Hyland and Taylor, 1979, 1980). However, a small proportion of patients suffer dangerous complications, including pericolic abscess, peritonitis, and fistula formation with adjacent viscera.

Minor inflammatory episodes may be treated successfully with antibiotics, intravenous fluids, and nasogastric suction. Evidence of spreading peritonitis is an indication for laparotomy; if a localized pericolic abscess is discovered, this can be drained and peritoneal lavage with antibiotics performed in addition to systemic chemotherapy. Evidence of intestinal obstruction is an indication for proximal colostomy, with resection of the diseased segment of bowel at a later stage when the patient's condition has improved. However, the staged operations necessary for proximal colostomy, bowel resection, and closure of colostomy, all carry their own morbidity and mortality rates.

Sigmoid Volvulus

This is an occasional, but well-recognized, cause for emergency admission of elderly patients. The clinical features of complete intestinal obstruction, drum-like abdominal distension, and characteristic radiological appearances, are well known. There is often a long past history of intractable constipation with institutionalized patients seeming to be more prone to this condition. Deflation of the distended sigmoid colon by passage of a sigmoidoscope and flatus tube is usually effective as an emergency procedure. However, abdominal tenderness or other evidence of peritonitis, which may be due to non-viability of the twisted bowel, is an indication for laparotomy. Elective surgical intervention may also be necessary for recurrent sigmoid volvulus, and sigmoid colectomy is sometimes required. If circumstances are unfavourable for a primary anastomosis, staged procedures involving resection and temporary colostomy are relatively safe alternatives (Goligher, 1980, pp. 927–929).

Colostomy

At any age, colostomy is an undesirable alternative to normal defaecation. In the elderly, the difficulties of colostomy care are often aggravated by poor vision, loss of dexterity, social problems, and general debility. It is well known that some patients who never 'accept' their colostomies become depressed and socially reclusive. Nevertheless, many patients of advanced years do cope remarkably well and suffer minimal social or physical inconvenience.

The difficulties of colostomy life may be reduced by the following measures:

(a) Patient preparation. When the operation leading to colostomy is elective, the fullest possible explanations should be given to the patient and family concerning its implications. Personal counselling by the surgical team should be supported by information booklets and, if available, a stomatherapist can demonstrate the various appliances in current use. In addition, there are many patient organizations which are helpful in this way. A useful step is to fit the patient with a colostomy device which can be worn for several days prior to surgery. In this way, the optimum siting of the colostomy stoma can be identified; also, the patient can begin to learn its acceptance.

(b) In those circumstances where colostomy has been performed at an emergency operation, and where there has consequently been insufficient time to prepare the patient for its necessity, it is important that more time is allowed in the postoperative period for instruction and supervision. Ideally, patients should not leave hospital until they have demonstrated some degree of independence in coping with the stoma. Whenever possible, close relatives should also be instructed in colostomy care so that they are able to provide whatever support may be necessary.

(c) Patients with a colostomy generally find a constipated stool easier to cope with and learn to adjust their diets accordingly. Additional assistance in this direction can sometimes be obtained with preparations containing codeine phosphate or methylcellulose. Regular self administered colostomy irrigation has not, thus far, proved generally successful (Doran and Hardcastle, 1981).

Herniae

Inguinal

The surgical repair of inguinal herniae can usually be safely achieved in even the most frail and elderly patients. However, before undertaking this operation, it is particularly important to exclude any underlying causes for raised intra-abdominal pressure, such as prostatism, subacute intestinal obstruction, or ascites. Similarly, it is important to remember that elderly patients are sometimes apt to attribute various abdominal symptoms to a long-standing groin hernia which may be irrelevant to their real cause. With these provisos, indirect inguinal herniae, particularly if causing discomfort, and especially if difficult to reduce, should normally be dealt with surgically. Certainly, the risks of elective surgery for this condition are much less than those when an emergency operation for strangulation is necessary (Vowles, 1979). The repair of long-standing large and sometimes huge scotal herniae pose special risks. They are more often found in patients with severe obstructive airways disease, and the reduction of bulky viscera to the abdomen can cause further respiratory embarrassment. The surgical repair of recurrent inguinal herniae is often technically difficult, and in elderly males the operation can sometimes be made easier by division of the spermatic cord and orchidectomy. Clearly if this is contemplated, the patient should be advised of this possibility and his consent sought. Not infrequently, bilateral inguinal herniae exist and it is sometimes necessary to operate on them simultaneously. Small direct and easily reducible inguinal herniae are often evident in elderly men, who are frequently quite unaware of their presence. These do not normally require surgical treatment and are best left alone.

Femoral

The diagnosis of femoral hernia is not always easy, particularly in obese patients. The sac is often small and easy to miss on a cursory clinical examination of the abdomen. Also, even when strangulated, it is not always acutely tender – hence the frequent advice to clinical students that the groins should be carefully examined in any patient with abdominal – and particularly obstructive – symptoms. Once diagnosed, at any age, and with few exceptions, surgical treatment should be advised for femoral hernia. Obviously, if strangulation is suspected, the operation will need to be an emergency procedure. In this situation, the McEvedy surgical approach is especially useful since it allows easier access to the abdomen should bowel resection prove necessary (McEvedy, 1966).

Umbilical

Paraumbilical herniae are more common in multiparous, obese, elderly women in whom they sometimes become enormous. In general, they are considered to carry a high risk of strangulation, though this impression may be partly due to the fact that it is mostly those who are symptomatic who present themselves for treatment. Certainly, those patients describing pain or discomfort in relation to such herniae should normally be advised to undergo surgical repair. This is often a taxing technical procedure, since the sac may be multilocular and the abdominal parietes tenuous, making a satisfactory repair difficult to achieve.

Abdominal Incisional Herniae

These may sometimes become quite massive and pose a daunting challenge to surgical care. Nevertheless, when pain and irreducibility coexist, there is no option to surgical intervention. However, many are large and easily reducible, with a wide underlying defect in the abdominal wall; these are sometimes best controlled with an abdominal support.

Hydrocele and Epididymal Cysts

In elderly patients these often attain an enormous size before medical attention is sought because of social embarrassment. In these circumstances, simple tapping will usually solve the diagnosis, as well as the immediate problem, provided elementary clinical competence has excluded the presence of a scrotal hernia. However, recurrence of the hydrocele or epididymal cyst will usually occur within a few weeks or months, though some cures have been described for idiopathic hydrocele using a sclerosant following aspiration. The surgical alternatives involve excision, obliteration, or eversion of the hydrocele sac, though all these procedures are not devoid of morbidity, particularly scrotal haematomata. Epididymal cysts usually require excision. Occasionally, orchidectomy may be necessary in order to effect a permanent cure should recurrence occur.

POSTOPERATIVE CARE

An important contribution to the reduction of mortality and morbidity following major surgery in the elderly is obtained by the avoidance of postoperative complications (Szauer and Zukaukas, 1975). Preoperative measures designed to prevent postoperative morbidity, such as the administration of antibiotics or anticoagulants, have already been mentioned. The anticipation, identification, and early treatment of complications is also of the greatest importance. Thus, a short period of mild postoperative confusion resulting in a minor fall can lead to the most disastrous sequelae in an aged patient recovering from abdominal surgery. This 'cascade effect' whereby complications pave the way for increasingly dangerous complications is, unfortunately, an all too common experience in caring for the elderly.

MORBIDITY AND MORTALITY

Many retrospective studies of surgical procedures in the elderly indicate an increased morbidity and mortality (Palmberg and Hirsjarvi, 1979; Soper and McPeek, 1980; Ziffren and Hartford, 1972). There is no doubt that there is an increased mortality postoperatively in elderly surgical patients with coexisting medical conditions such as a recent myocardial infarction (Knapp, Topkins, and Artusio, 1962; Tarhan *et al.*, 1972) and cardiac failure from any cause. The life-threatening complications associated with cardiovascular disease usually occur in the early postoperative period and they emphasize the need for adequate preoperative assessment and treatment (Foëx, 1980). There is some evidence that a reduction in postoperative morbidity and mortality can be achieved by better medical and anaesthetic management (Djokovic and Hedley-White, 1979; Rao and El-Etr, 1981; Steen, Tinker, and Tarhan, 1978).

The Cardiff Anaesthetic Records System provides detailed information on patients subjected to anaesthesia and surgery over the past 20 years (Lunn *et al.*, 1982). Table 2 compares the mortality rates for the general population during two 6-year periods, namely 1958–63 and 1972–77. It can be seen that the mortality rates fell from 2.9 in the first period to 2.2 per hundred patients in the second period (Farrow *et al.*, 1982).

Table 2 Mortality rate of surgical patients of all ages 1958–1963 and 1972–1977

Year	Number	Number of deaths	Percentage
1958–63	53,541	1,532	2.9
1972–77	108,878	2,391	2.2

Tables 3 and 4 show that the mortality rates for males and females over 75 is nearly twice that for those over 65, and over 85 it is trebled. This approximates to the findings reported in the Wisconsin series (Sikes and Detmer, 1979).

Table 3 Mortality rate of male surgical patients 1972–77

Age	Number	Number of deaths	Percentage
65+	6,701	333	4.97
75+	2,683	189	7.04
85+	365	56	15.34
Total	9,749	578	5.90

Table 4 Mortality rate of female surgical patients 1972–77

Age	Number	Number of deaths	Percentage
65+	5,551	235	4.23
75+	2,908	264	9.08
85+	652	113	17.3
Total	9,111	612	6.7

Table 5 breaks down the mortality rate for 5 common but different operative procedures performed in the elderly. The high mortality rates for abdominal aneurysm reflect the number of emergency operations performed for ruptured aneurysms. The overall rate for cholecystectomy was 0.8 per cent. as against 1.8 and 3.18 per cent. for males and females over 65, respectively. Emergency procedures are undoubtedly associated with a far greater risk, particularly in gastrointestinal surgery (Gerson-Greenburg *et al.*, 1981).

Table 5   Mortality rates for surgical operations on patients aged more than 65 years 1972–1977

Operation	Male	Female
Fractured femur	18.9%	13.9%
Inguinal hernia	1.61%	0.88%
Cataract	0.16%	
Gall-bladder	1.8%	3.18%
Aneurysm	28.3%	40%

Reduction of mortality and morbidity rates at any age must depend on the continuing refinement of pre-and postoperative managements, along the lines already referred to in this chapter.

A certain number of deaths following surgery in the elderly is virtually inevitable, when the underlying condition proves terminal; e.g. advanced mesenteric infarction and carcinomatosis. Such deaths can only be avoided by improvements in diagnostic techniques so that surgery can be avoided in such situations.

Finally, attitudes to mortality rates in frail elderly patients must be based to some extent on a philosophical attitude to the risks involved. Thus, a simple and effective means of reducing the mortality rates for some major surgical procedures lies in the avoidance of surgery in high risk situations. However, the implication of this approach would be that some patients with potentially recoverable conditions would be denied the possible benefits of surgical treatment. The continuing reappraisal of the results of surgery in elderly patients remains the principal way in which a satisfactory balance between its risks and benefits can be maintained.

REFERENCES

Alberti, K. G. M. M., and Thomas, D. J. B. (1979). 'The management of diabetes during surgery', *Br. J. Anaesth.*, **51**, 693–710.

Allison, D. J. (1980). 'Therapeutic embolisation and venous sampling', in Recent Advances in Surgery (Ed. Selwyn Taylor). Vol. X, Chap. 2, Churchill-Livingstone, Edinburgh.

Anderson, S., and Cold, G. E. (1981). 'Dose-response studies in elderly patients subjected to epidural analgesia', *Acta. Anaesth. Scand.*, **25**, 279–281.

Anonymous (1972). 'Prevention and treatment of deep-vein thrombosis', *Drug Ther. Bull.*, **10**, 21–24.

Anonymous. (1979). 'Low dose heparin preparations for prophylactic use', *Drug Ther. Bull.*, **15**, 21–22.

Anonymous (1981). 'Dissolving hopes for gallstone dissolution?' *Lancet*, **2**, 905–906.

Atkinson, M., Ferguson, R., and Parker, G. C. (1978). 'Tube introducer and modified Celestin tube for use in palliative intubation of oesophago-gastric neoplasms at fibre-optic endoscopy', *Gut*, **19**, 667–671.

Bates, T. (1981). 'One man's view: Gallstones – to cut or not to cut?', *Surgery Today*, **2**, 49–50.

Bateson, M. C., and Bouchier, I. A. D. (1975). 'Prevalence of gallstones in Dundee, a necropsy study', *Br. Med. J.*, **4**, 427–430.

Baum, S., Athanasoulis, C. A., Waltman, A. C., Galdabini, J., Schapiro, R. H., Warshaw, A. L., and Ottinger, L. W. (1977). 'Angiodysplasia of the right colon: A cause of gastrointestinal bleeding', *Am. J. Roentgenol.*, **129**, 789–794.

Beaser, S. B. (1970). 'Surgical management', in *Diabetes Mellitus: Theory and Practice.* (Eds M. Ellenberg and H. Rifkin), pp. 746–757, McGraw Hill, New York.

Bedford, P. D. (1955). 'Adverse cerebral effects of anaesthesia on old people', *Lancet*, **2**, 259–263.

Blumgart, L. H. (1978). 'Biliary tract obstruction: New approaches to an old problem', *Am. J. Surg.*, **135**, 19–31.

Boley, S. J., DiBlase, A., Brandt, L. J., and Sammartano, R. J. (1979). 'Lower intestinal bleeding in the elderly', *Am. J. Surg.*, **137**, 57–64.

Bouchier, I. A. D. (1981). 'Diagnosis of jaundice', *Br. Med. J.*, **2**, 1282–1284.

Bowen, D. J., Nancekeivill, M. L., Proctor, E. A., and Norman, J. (1982). 'Perioperative management of insulin-dependent diabetic patients. Use of continuous intravenous infusion of insulin-glucose-potassium solution', *Anaesthesia*, **37**, 825–855.

Bradley, E. L. III, Isaacs, J., Hersh, T., Davidson, E. D., and Millikan, W. (1975). 'Nutritional consequences of total gastrectomy', *Ann. Surg.*, **182**, 415–429.

Bromage, P. R. (1969). 'Ageing and epidural dose requirements: Segmental spread and predictability of epidural analgesia in youth and extreme age', *Br. J. Anaesth.*, **41**, 1061–1022.

Broor, S. L., Parker, H. W., Ganeshappa, K. P., Komaki, S., and Dodds, W. J. (1978). 'Vascular dysplasia of the right colon. An important cause of unexplained gastrointestinal bleeding', *Am. J. Dig. Dis.*, **23**, 89–92.

Castleden, C. M., Kaye, C. M., and Parsons, R. L. (1975). 'The effects of age on plasma levels of propanol and practolol in man', *Br. J. Clin. Pharmacol.*, **2**, 303–306.

Chan, K., Kendall, M. J., Mitchard, M., Wells, W. D. E., and Vickers, M. D. (1975). 'The effect of ageing on plasma pethidine concentration', *Br. J. Clin. Pharmacol.*, **2**, 297–302.

Chodak, G. W., and Plaut, M. E. (1977). 'Use of systemic antibiotics for prophylaxis in surgery: A critical review', *Arch. Surg.*, **122**, 326–334.

Christensen, J. H., Andreason, F., and Jansen, J. A. (1981). 'Influence of age and sex on the pharmacokinetics of thiopentone', *Br. J. Anaesth.*, **53**, 1189–1195.

Cotton, P. B. (1982). 'Duodeoscopic placement of bilary prostheses to relieve malignant obstructive jaundices', *Br. J. Surg.*, **69**, 501–503.

Crosby, D. L., and Rees, G. A. D. (1983). 'Postoperative care: The role of the High Dependency Unit', *Ann. R. Coll. Surg. Engl.*, **65**, 391–393.

Davis, F. M., Quince, M., and Laurenson, V. G. (1980). 'Deep vein thrombosis and anaesthetic technique in emergency hip surgery', *Br. Med. J.*, **2**, 1528–1529.

Day, E. A., and Marks, C. (1975). 'Gallstone ileus. Review of the literature and presentation of thirty-four new cases', *Am. J. Surg.*, **129**, 552–558.

Djokovic, J. L., and Hedley-White, J. (1979). 'Prediction of outcome of surgery and anesthesia in patients over 80'. *JAMA*, **242**, 2301–2306.

Donnan, S. P. B., and Lambert, P. M. (1976). 'Appendicitis: Incidence and mortality', *Pop. Trends*, **5**, 26–28.

Doran, J., and Hardcastle, J. D. (1981). 'A controlled trial of colostomy management by natural evacuation, irrigation and foam enema', *Br. J. Surg.*, **68**, 731–733.

Dronfield, M. W. and Langman, M. J. S. (1978). 'Acute upper gastro-intestinal bleeding'. *Br. J. Hosp. Med.*, **19**, 97–108.

Editorial (1978). 'Diuretics in the elderly', *Br. Med. J.*, **1**, 1092–1093.

Editorial (1980). 'Facts and fallacies about gallstones', *Br. Med. J.*, **2**, 171.

Edwards, R. P., Miller, R. D., Roizen, M. F., Ham, J., Way, W. L., Lake, C. R., and Roderick, L. (1979). 'Cardiac responses to imimpramine and pancuronium during anesthesia with halothane or enflurane', *Anesthesiol.*, **50**, 421–425.

Eger, E. I. II (1974). *Anesthetic Uptake and Actions*, Williams & Wilkins Company, Baltimore, Maryland.

Farrow, S. C., Fowkes, F. G. R., Lunn, J. N., Robertson, I. B., and Samuel, P. (1982). 'Epidemiology in anaesthesia. II. Factors affecting mortality in hospital', *Br. J. Anaesth.*, **54**, 811–817.

Foëx, P. (1980). 'Preoperative assessment of patients with cardiac disease', in *Hypertension; Ichaemic Heart Disease and Anesthesia*, (Ed. C. Prys-Roberts), pp. 81–110, International Anesthesiology Clinics, Little Brown and Co., Boston.

Fowler, W. S. (1950). 'Lung function studies. V. Respiratory dead space in old age and in pulmonary emphysema', *J. Clin. Invest.*, **29**, 1439–1444.

Gallus, A. S., Hirsh, J., and O'Brien, S. E. (1976). 'Prevention of venous thrombosis with small subcutaneous doses of heparin', *JAMA*, **235**, 1980–1982.

Gerson-Greenburg, A., Sail, R. P., Coyle, J. J., and Peskin, G. W. (1981). 'Mortality and gastrointestinal surgery in the aged. Elective vs. emergency procedures', *Arch. Surg.*, **116**, 788–791.

Glenn, F. (1981). 'Surgical management of acute cholecystitis in patients 65 years of age and older', *Ann. Surg.*, **193**, 56–59.

Glisson, S. N., Fajardo, L., and El-Etr, A. A. (1978). 'Amitriptyline therapy increases electrocardiographic changes during reversal of neuromuscular blockade', *Anesth. Analg.*, **57**, 77–83.

Goligher, J. C. (1979). 'Use of circular stapling gun with peripheral insertion of anorectal purse-string suture for construction of very low colorectal or colo-anal anastomoses', *Br. J. Surg.*, **66**, 501–504.

Goligher, J. C. (1980). *Surgery of the Anus, Rectum and Colon*, 4th ed., Balliere-Tindall, London.

Goodson, W. H. III, and Hunt, T. K. (1977). 'Studies of wound healing in experimental diabetes mellitus'. *J. Surg. Res.*, **22**, 221–227.

Gregory, G. A., Eger, E. I. III, and Munson, E. S. (1969). 'The relationship between age and halothane requirement in man', *Anesthesiol.*, **30**, 488–491.

Harris, E. A., Hunder, M. E., Seelye, E. R., Vedder, M., and Whitelock, R. M. L. (1973). 'Prediction of the physiological dead-space in resting normal subjects', *Clin. Sci.*, **45**, 375–386.

Heald, R. J. (1979). 'A new approach to rectal cancer', *Br. J. Hosp. Med.*, **22**, 277–281.

Heatley, R. V., Harris, A., and Lewis, M. H. (1979). 'Pre-operative intravenous feeding – a controlled trial', *Postgrad. Med. J.*, **55**, 541–545.

Hendolin, H., Mattila, M. A. K., and Poikolainen, E. (1981). 'The effect of lumbar epidural analgesia on the development of deep vein thrombosis of the legs after open prostatectomy', *Acta. Chir. Scand.*, **147**, 425–429.

Henry, M. M. (1980). 'Rectal prolapse', *Br. J. Hosp. Med.*, **24**, 302–307.

Heuman, R., Sjodahl, R., and Wetterfors, J. (1980). 'Gallstone ileus: An analysis of 20 patients', *World J. Surg.*, **4**, 595–598.

Hill, G. L. (Ed.) (1981). 'Nutrition and the surgical patient', *Clinical Surgery International*, Vol. 2, Churchill Livingstone, Edinburgh.

Holland, J., Milic-Emili, J., Macklem, P. T., and Bates, D. V. (1968). 'Regional distribution of pulmonary ventilation and perfusion in elderly subjects', *J. Clin. Invest.*, **47**, 81–92.

Hyland, J. M. P., and Taylor, I. (1979). 'Diverticular disease – has natural history altered?', *Gut*, **20**, A441.

Hyland, J. M. P., and Taylor, I. (1980). 'Does a high fibre diet prevent the complications of diverticular disease?', *Br. J. Surg.*, **67**, 77–79.

International Multicentre Trial (1975). 'Prevention of fatal postoperative pulmonary embolism by low doses of heparin', *Lancet*, **2**, 45–51.

Irvin, T. T., and Greaney, M. G. (1977). 'The treatment of colonic cancer presenting with intestinal obstruction', *Br. J. Surg.*, **64**, 741–744.

Irving, J. D. (1981). 'Relief of bilary obstruction', *Br. J. Hosp. Med.*, **26**, 329–338.

Kaiko, R. F. (1980). 'Age and morphine analgesia in cancer patients with postoperative pain', *Clin. Pharmacol. Ther.*, **28**, 823–826.

Keighley, M. R. B. (1977). 'Prevention of wound sepsis in gastrointestinal surgery', *Brit. J. Surg.*, **64**, 315–321.

Keighley, M. R. B., and Burdon, D. W. (1979). *Antimicrobial Prophylaxis in Surgery*, Pitman Medical, Tunbridge Wells.

Kelton, J. G., and Hirsh, J. (1980). 'Bleeding associated with antithrombotic therapy', *Semin. Hematol.*, **17**, 259–291.

Kiil, J., Kiil, J., Axelsen, F., and Anderson, D. (1978). 'Prophylaxis against postoperative pulmonary embolism and deep vein thrombosis by low-dose heparin', *Lancet*, **2**, 1115–1116.

Klein, A., Hughes, L. E., Campbell, H., Williams, A., Zlosnick, J., and Leach, K. G. (1975). 'Dextran 70 in prophylaxis of thromboembolic disease after surgery: A clinically oriented, randomized, double-blind trial', *Br. Med. J.*, **2**, 109–112.

Klotz, H., Avant, G. R., Hoyumpa, A., Schenker, S. and Wilkinson, G. R. (1975). 'The effects of age and liver disease on the disposition and elimination of diazepam in adult man', *J. Clin. Invest.*, **55**, 347–359.

Lakatta, E. G. (1979). 'Alterations in the cardiovascular systems that occur in advanced age', *Fed. Proc.*, **38**, 163–167.

Leblanc, P., Ruff, F., and Milic-Emili, J. (1970). 'Effects of age and body position on airway closure in man', *J. Appl. Physiol.*, **28**, 448–451.

Longmire, W. R. (1980). 'Gastric carcinoma: Is radical gastrectomy worthwhile?', *Ann. R. Coll. Surg. Engl.*, **62**, 25–30.

Lunn, J. N., Farrow, S. C., Fowkes, F. G. R., Robertson, I. B., and Samuel, P. (1982) 'Epidemiology in Anaesthesia. I: Anaesthetic practice over 20 years', *Br. J. Anaesth.*, **54**, 803–809.

Knapp, R. B., Topkins, M. J., and Artusio, J. F. (1962). 'The cerebrovascular accident and coronary occlusion in anesthesia', *JAMA*, **182**, 332–334.

McDermott, F. T., Hughes, E. S. R., Pihl, E., Milne, B. J., and Price, A. B. (1981). 'Comparative results of surgical management of single carcinomas of the colon and rectum: A series of 1939 patients managed by one surgeon', *Br. J. Surg.*, **68**, 850–855.

McEvedy, P. G. (1966). 'The internal approach for inguinal herniae', *Post-grad. Med. J.*, **42**, 548–550.

McKenzie, P. J., Wishard, H. Y., Dewar, K. M. S., Gray, I., and Smith, G. (1980). 'Comparison of the effects of spinal anaesthesia on postoperative oxygenation and perioperative mortality', *Br. J. Anaesth.*, **52**, 49–54.

McLaren, A. D., Stockwell, M. C., and Reid, V. T. (1978). 'Anaesthetic technique for surgical correction of fractured neck of femur. A comparative study of spinal and general anaesthesia in the elderly', *Anaesthesia*, **33**, 10–14.

McLeod, K., Hull, C. J., and Watson, M. J. (1979). 'Effects of ageing on the pharmacokinetics of pancuronium', *Br. J. Anaesth.*, **51**, 435–438.

McPherson, G. A. D., Bejamin, I. S., Habib, N. A., Bowley, N. B., and Blumgart, L. H. (1982). 'Percutaneous transhepatic drainage in obstructive jaundice: advantages and problems', *Br. J. Surg.*, **69**, 261–264.

Marshall, B. E., and Wyche, M. Q. (1972). 'Hypoxaemia during and after anaesthesia', *Anesthesiol.*, **37**, 178–209.

Mather, L. E., Tucker, G. E., Pflug, A. E., Lindop, M. J., and Wilkerson, C. (1975). 'Meperidine kinetics in man', *Clin. Pharmacol. Ther.*, **17**, 21–30.

Mee, A. S., Vallon, A. G., Croker, J. R., and Cotton, P. B. (1981). 'Non-operative removal of bile-duct stones by duodenoscopic sphincterotomy in the elderly', *Br. Med. J.*, **1**, 521–523.

Mitchell, A., Atkins, S., Royle, G. T., and Kettlewell, M. G. W. (1982). 'Reduced catheter sepsis and prolonged catheter life using tunnelled silicone rubber catheter for total parental nutrition', *Br. J. Surg.*, **69**, 420–422.

Modig, J., Malmberg, P., and Saldeen, T. (1980). 'Comparative effects of epidural and general anesthesia on fibrinolysis function, lower limb rheology and thromboembolism after total hip replacement', *Anesthesiol.*, **53**, S 34.

Mostert, J. W. (1960). 'Risk of epidural block in old people', *Br. J. Anaesth.*, **32**, 613–615.

Nation, R. L., Triggs, E. J., and Selig, M. (1977). 'Lignocaine kinetics in cardiac patients and aged subjects', *Br. J. Clin. Pharmacol.*, **4**, 439–448.

Nightingale, P. J., and Marstrand, T. (1981). 'Subarachnoid anaesthesia with bupivacaine for orthopaedic procedures in the elderly', *Br. J. Anaesth.*, **53**, 369–371.

Nissen, R. (1956). 'Eine einfach Operation zur Beeinflussung der Refluxoesophagitis', *Schweig. Med. Wochenschr.*, **86**, 590.

Nolan, C. M., Beaty, H. N., and Bagdale, J. D. (1978). 'Further characterisation of the impaired bactericidal function of granulocytes in patients with poorly controlled diabetes', *Diabetes*, **27**, 889–894.

Office of Population Censuses and Surveys (1976). *Cancer Statistics; Registrations*, HMSO, London.

Okike, N., Payne, W. S., Neufeld, D. M., Bernata, P. E., Pairolero, P. C., and Sanderson, D. R. (1979). 'Esophagomyotomy versus forceful dilation for achalasia of the esophagus: Results in 899 patients', *Ann. Thorac. Surg.*, **28**, 119–125.

Ong, G. B. (1975). 'Unresectable carcinoma of the oesophagus', *Ann. R. Coll. Surg.Engl.*, **56**, 3–14.

Orel, J. J., Erzen, J. J., and Hrabar, B. A. (1981). 'Results of resection of carcinoma of the oesophagus and cardia in 196 patients', *World J. Surg.*, **5**, 259–267.

Orringer, M. B. (1979). 'The treatment of achalasia: Controversy resolved?', *Ann. Thorac. Surg.*, **28**, 100–102.

Palmberg, S., and Hirsjarvi (1979). 'Mortality in geriatric surgery, with special reference to the type of surgery, anaesthesia, complicating diseases and prophylaxis of thrombosis', *Gerontology*, **25**, 103–112.

Paulino, F. M. (1973). 'Carcinoma of the stomach with special reference to total gastrectomy', *Curr. Prob. Surg.*, **7**, 32–72.

Pearson, J. G. (1981). 'Radiotherapy for oesophageal carcinoma', *World J. Surg.*, **5**, 489–497.

Peltokallio, P., and Tykka, H. (1981). 'Evolution of the age distribution and mortality of acute appendicitis', *Arch. Surg.*, **116**, 153–156.

Penfold, J. C. B., and Hawley, P. R. (1972). 'Experiences of Ivalon-sponge implant for complete rectal prolapse at St. Mark's Hospital, *1960–70*', *Br. J. Surg.*, **59**, 846–848.

Pfleiderer, A. G., Goodall, P., and Holmes, G. K. T. (1982). 'The consequences and effectiveness of intubation in the palliation of dysphagia due to benign and malignant strictures affecting the oesophagus', *Br. J. Surg.*, **69**, 356–358.

Phillips, G., and Tomlin, P. J. (1977). 'Arterial oxygen tensions in elderly and injured elderly patients', *Br. J. Anaesth.*, **49**, 514–515.

Polli, E. E., Bianchi, P. A., Conti, D., and Sironi, L. (1981). 'Treatment of radiolucent gallstones with CDCA or UDCA: A multicentre trial', *Digestion*, **22**, 185–191.

Prys-Roberts, C., Green, L. T., Meloche, R., and Foëx, P. (1971). 'Studies of anaesthesia in relation to hypertension II: Haemodynamic consequences of induction and endotracheal intubation', *Br. J. Anaest.*, **43**, 531–547.

Raguveer-Saran, M. K., and Keddie, N. C. (1980). 'The falling incidence of appendicitis', *Br. J. Surg.*, **67**, 681.

Rao, T. L. K., and El-Etr, A. A. (1981). 'Myocardial reinfarction following anesthesia in patients with recent infarction'. *Anesth. Analg.*, **60**, 271–272.

Reidenberg, M. M., Levy, M., Warner, H., Coutinho, C. B., Schwartz, M. A., Yu, G., and Cheripko, J. (1978). 'Relationship between diazepam dose, plasma level, age and central nervous system depression', *Clin. Pharmacol. Ther.*, **23**, 371–374.

Roberts, J. G. (1980). 'Cancer of the oesophagus – how should tumour biology affect treatment?', *Br. J. Surg.*, **67**, 791–797.

Root, H. F. (1966). 'Preoperative care of the diabetic patient', *Postgrad. Med.*, **40**, 439–445.

Rosenberg, P. H., Saramies, L., and Alila, A. (1981). 'Lumbar epidural anaesthesia with bupivicaine in old patients; effect of speed and direction of infection', *Acta Anaesth. Scand.*, **25**, 270–274.

Rossoff, L., Puig-La-Calle, R., and Luder, M. (1980). 'Dealing with the perforated gastroduodenal ulcer', in *State of the Art of Surgery* (Eds M. Allgower and F. Harder), Summaries of the Breakfast and Lunchtime Panels of the 28th Congress of the Societe Internationale de la Chirugie, San Francisco.

Schoenfield, L. J., and Lachin, J. M. (1981). 'Chenodiol (chenodeoxycholic acid) for the dissolution of gallstones: The National Cooperative Gallstone Study', *Ann. Int. Med.*, **95**, 257–289.

Scott, D. B., Jebson, P. J. R., Braid, D. P., Ortengren, B., and Frisch, P. (1972). Factors affecting plasma levels of lignocaine and prilocaine', *Br. J. Anaesth.*, **44**, 1040–1049.

Scurr, J. H., Ibrahim, S. Z., and Faber, R. G. (1977). 'The efficacy of graduated compression stockings in the prevention of deep vein thrombosis'. *Br. J. Surg.*, **64**, 371–373.

Shock, N. W. (1979). 'Systems physiology and ageing: Introduction', *Fed. Proc.*, **38**, 161–162.

Sikes, E. D., and Detmer, D. E. (1979). 'Ageing and surgical risk in older citizens of Wisconsin', *Wis. Med. J.*, **78**, 27–30.

Singh, S. V. (1980). 'Present concept of the Belsey Mark IV procedure in gastro-oesophageal reflux and hiatus hernia', *Br. J. Surg.*, **67**, 26–28.

Soper, K., and McPeek, B. (1980). 'Predicting mortality for high risk surgery', in *Health Care Delivery in Anaesthesia* (Eds R. A. Hirsch, W. H. Forrest, F. K. Orkin, and H. Wollman, pp. 99–103), G. F. Strickley Co.

Souchon, E. A., Englert, D., Duke, J. H., Jr., and

Dudnick, S. J. (1979). 'Intravenous hyperalimentation in 342 surgical patients', *Rev. Surg.*, **33**, 297–299.

Steen, P. A., Tinker, J. H., and Tarhan, S. (1978). 'Myocardial reinfarction after anesthesia and surgery', *JAMA*, **239**, 2566–2570.

Stefansson, T., Wicksrom, I., and Haljamae, H. (1982b). 'Cardiovascular and metabolic effects of halothane and enflurane anaesthesia in the geriatric patient', *Acta. Anaesth. Scand.*, **26**, 378–385.

Stefansson, T., Wickstrom, I. and Haljamae, H. (1982a). 'Halothane and enflurane in the geriatric patient', *Acta. Anaesth. Scand.*, **26**, 371–377.

Stevens, W. C., Dolan, W. M., Gibbons, R. T., White, A., Eger, E. I., II, Miller, R. T., de Jong, R. H., and Elashoff, R. M. (1975). 'Minimum alveolar concentrations (MAC) of isoflurane with and without nitrous oxide in patients of various ages', *Anesthesiol.*, **42**, 192–205.

Summerfield, J. A. (1979). 'Medical treatment of gallstones', *Br. J. Hosp. Med.*, **21**, 482–489.

Szauer, J., and Zukaukas, C. (1975). 'The problems of abdominal operations in elderly patients', *Geriatrics*, **30**, 57–64.

Tarhan, S., Moffat, E. A., Taylor, W. F., and Guilliani, E. R. (1972). 'Myocardial infarction after general anesthesia', *JAMA*, **220**, 1451–1454.

Thomas, G., Venables, C. W., Hoare, A. M., and Allison, D. J. (1980). 'Gastro-intestinal bleeding', *Br. J. Hosp. Med.*, **23**, 333–366.

Thompson, H. (1982). 'Gastric cancer', *Brit. J. Hosp. Med.*, **284**, 684–685.

Thorburn, J., Louden, J. R., and Vallance, R. (1980). 'Spinal and general anaesthesia in total hip replacement: Frequency of deep vein thrombosis', *Br. J. Anaesth.*, **52**, 1117–1121.

Toker, P. (1974). 'Hyperosmolar hyperglycemic, non-ketotic coma: A cause of delayed recovery from anaesthesia', *Anesthesiol.*, **41**, 284–285.

Tomebrandt, K., and Fletcher, R. (1982). 'Pre-operative chest X-rays in elderly patients', *Anaesthesia*, **37**, 901–902.

Turner, J. M., Mead, J., and Wohl, M. E. (1968). 'Elasticity of human lungs in relation to age', *J. Appl. Physiol.*, **25**, 664–671.

Vaughan, M. S., Vaughan, R. M., and Cork, R. C. (1981). 'Postoperative hypothermia in adults: Relationship of age, anesthesia and shivering to rewarming', *Anesth. Analg.*, **60**, 746–751.

Virtanen, R., Kanto, J., Iisalo, E., Iisalo, E. U. M., Salo, M., and Sjovall, S. (1982). 'Pharmacokinetic studies on atropine with special reference to age', *Acta. Anaesth. Scand.*, **26**, 297–300.

Vowles, K. D. J. (1979). *Surgical Problems in the Aged*, pp. 98–108, John Wright & Sons Limited, Bristol.

Walts, L. F., Miller, J., Davidson, M. B., and Brown, J. (1981). 'Perioperative management of diabetes mellitus', *Anesthesiol.*, **55**, 104–109.

White, D. G. (1980). 'Anaesthesia in old age', *Br. J. Hosp. Med.*, **24**, 145–150.

Zamost, B., and Benumof, J. L. (1981). 'Anaesthesia in geriatric patients', in *Anaesthesia and Uncommon Diseases* (Eds J. Katz, J. Benumof, and L. B. Kadis), pp. 98–118, W. B. Saunders, Philadelphia.

Ziffren, S. E., and Hartford, C. E. (1972). 'Comparisons of mortality rates for various surgical operations according to age groups', *J. Am. Geriatr. Soc.*, **20**, 485–489.

28
Orthopaedic Management of the Elderly

28.1

Orthopaedic Management of the Elderly

M. B. Devas

INTRODUCTION

Geriatric orthopaedics is the practice of combined care of the elderly by an orthopaedic surgeon and a physician in geriatric medicine. The highest standards of medical and surgical skills are required if the patient is to obtain the greatest benefit. It is a stimulating discipline and faces an increasing demand in both its acute and elective branches because there is a real increase in the numbers of elderly patients presenting with fractured necks of femur (Lewis, 1981) and the demand for arthroplasty is also increasing (OHE, 1982). Good management and consideration of the patient as a whole is essential in order to achieve a return home, thus realizing the full benefit of the treatment received.

It must be emphasized that the surgical operation itself is only an incident in, and a small part of, the whole treatment. It must be considered in relation to rehabilitation of the whole patient, particularly in emergency cases. This philosophy of management underlies successful treatment of all geriatric orthopaedic problems.

THE ORGANIZATION

The Team

In order to treat an old person quickly, efficiently, and properly the surgeon and geriatric physician must give combined care from the moment of admission. Old age is in itself an indication for internal fixation of fractures so most acute admissions will require operation and early involvement of the anaesthetist is essential. Resuscitation of the shocked or hypothermic patient so that there is minimal delay before operation is his responsibility. Later the patient may require care from the endocrinologist for diabetes, the urologist for bladder problems, and the psychogeriatrician for brain failure. Geriatric Orthopaedic Units combining such skills are rare but the need for them is becoming apparent.

The Ward

Since repeated moves from ward to ward after admission are likely to exacerbate confusion in elderly patients it is a major benefit if one ward can be earmarked for geriatric orthopaedic admissions. Preoperative assessment and immediate postoperative care should be shared between the disciplines and after a few days the true accident in an otherwise fit old person is very clearly distinguishable from the case in which an underlying condition or conditions require further geriatric care.

The geriatric physician will be competent in the management of medical rehabilitation of the patients, calling occasionally on specialist colleagues as mentioned previously. The rest of the geriatric orthopaedic team will consist of nurses, physiotherapists, social workers, occupational therapists, and a secretary.

A grand round attended by all members of the team, including the medical and surgical consultants, should be held weekly to correlate treatment. Every detail of each patient should be considered and the future programme outlined for as far ahead as is practical so that objectives and time scale are known and understood by all members. By sharing information, care, and responsibility of the elderly patients all aspects of their condition can be dealt with quickly and thoroughly.

Day to day care of elderly patients postoperatively by medical staff of a geriatric unit will ensure that no unsolved orthopaedic problems are missed. A satisfactory choice and technique of operation are essential to ensure complete repair of a fracture so that further surgical consideration, other than removal of stitches in due time, is unnecessary.

The management of a patient with a fracture near the hip is an ideal example of the benefits of management in a Geriatric Orthopaedic Unit.

FRACTURES NEAR THE HIP

The management of an old lady (9 out of 10 such patients in Britain are female) with a fracture near the hip must include effective early stabilization of the fracture, proper medical rehabilitation by the geriatrician, and careful consideration of a precipitating condition which may also need treatment. Thirty per cent. of patients admitted with such fractures will have such a precipitating condition.

This latter group of patients will not achieve full independence unless treatment is correct and prompt. Even in the best circumstances they may require a higher standard of care at home than before the accident, but it should always be possible to avoid a very lengthy stay in hospital or so-called 'bed blocking' by such patients.

The distinction between the true accident and that precipitated by underlying disease is difficult to make on admission when patients will be shocked, mentally distressed, and apparently gravely ill. Even an apparently clear history of a fall in the street may conceal the first occurrence of a drop attack or minor stroke. A few days postoperatively, however, the patient with the true accident will be up and about, getting ready for discharge, while the progress of the other will be noticeably slower.

Delay in operating for treatment of heart failure or diabetes should not exceed 24 hours. Medical treatment is easier when the fracture has been cured since proper assessment of the patient is then possible.

A satisfactory operation will control the fracture so completely that the patient can walk forthwith so that function is restored immediately. Loss of function and thus loss of independence are thereby eliminated. To achieve a satisfactory outcome all fractures of the neck of femur must be treated by replacement hemiarthroplasty. Other techniques cause greater difficulties in rehabilitation and the results are poor, especially when avascular necrosis is considered (Barnes *et al.*, 1976).

The late results of replacement arthroplasty can also give problems. Acetabular erosion (Figs 1 to 3) occurs most frequently in younger and more active patients and is not a consequence of osteoporosis or even of osteomalacia. Erosion of the head of the prosthesis upwards into the bone of the acetabulum with pain and loss of function can occur at various times after operation. The incidence is about 11 per cent. (D'Arcy and Devas, 1976). The probable cause is point-bearing of too small a head in the acetabulum (Figs. 4 to 8). The newly introduced Hastings hip prosthesis with a double head appears to overcome this problem (Figs 9 to 12).

All trochanteric fractures must be fixed, usually with a pin and plate (Figs 13 and 14).

No operation should be considered and no routine ever instituted that does not allow elderly patients to have their operation within 24 hours of admission and to walk the following day. This is the most important of all criteria in geriatric orthopaedics.

THE GERIATRIC ORTHOPAEDIC UNIT

Any hospital can have a unit for the rehabilitation of the elderly after orthopaedic problems have been dealt with. This requires only the mutual regard of the orthopaedic surgeon and the geriatric physician, and a determination on the part of both to improve the treatment of the elderly patient who has usually had a fracture. If no separate ward is available part of an existing orthopaedic or geriatric ward can be used.

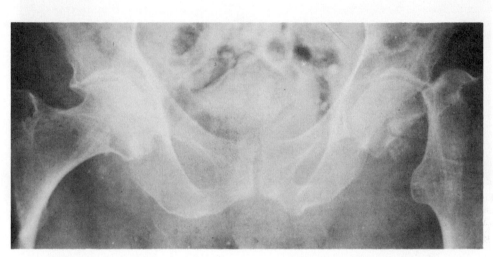

Figure 1   A man in his eighties, much given to cycling, fell and broke his left hip

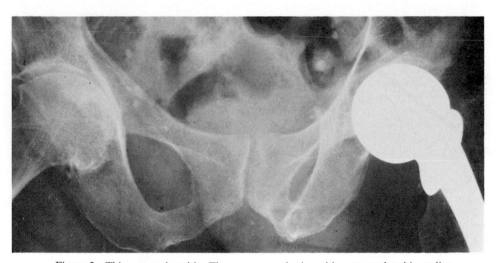

Figure 2   This was replaced by Thompson prosthesis and he returned to his cycling

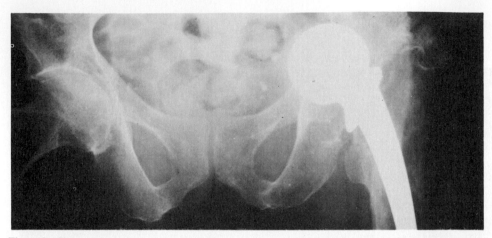

Figure 3   Six months later he returned with pain in the hip. The prosthesis has eroded the acetabulum and is now in the pelvis. This occurs in some 11 per cent. of patients, varying according to age and activity

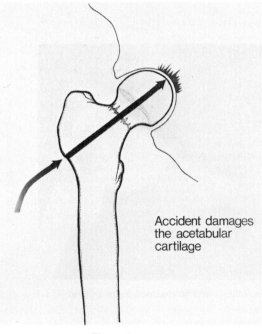

Accident damages
the acetabular
cartilage

Figure 4

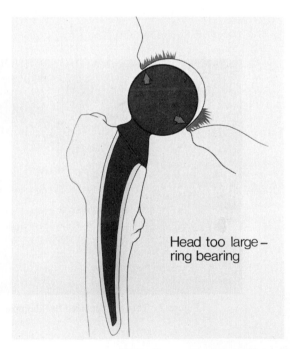

Head too large –
ring bearing

Figure 5

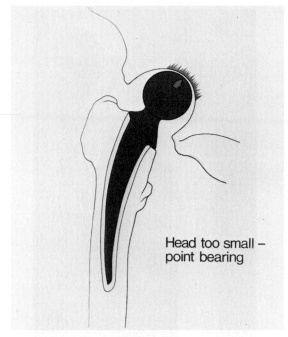

Figure 6

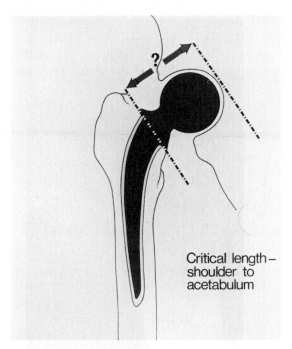

Figure 7

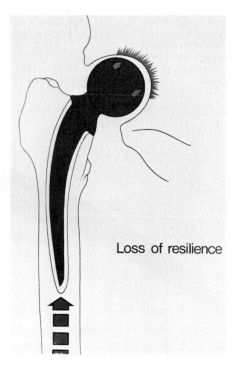

Figure 8

Figures 4 to 8   These figures illustrate the possible causes of acetabular erosion. First, it is possible that the accident damages the acetabulum (Fig. 4). Second, the prosthetic head may be too large (Fig. 5) or too small (Fig. 6), the latter cause being thought to be the most important of all. Finally, a variable neck length or loss of resilience because of the firmly cemented prosthesis in the uppermost third the femur have to be considered (Figs 7 and 8)

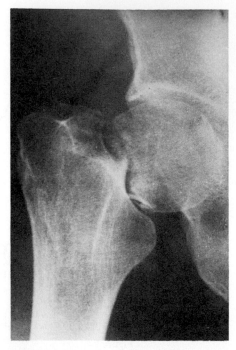

Figure 9   The fractured neck of femur can still be the 'unsolved fracture', but only of it being wrongly treated. This is the radiograph of the fracture of a women of 64. It was not replaced with a cemented Thompson, because she would have had a 50 per cent. chance of erosion at her age with that treatment

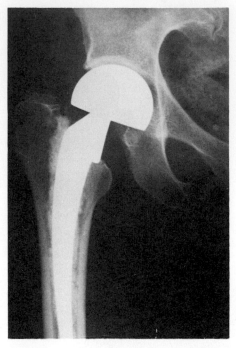

Figure 10   Instead, the patient ws treated by replacement with a Hasting hip. It has shown no erosion over 4 years. She has a normal gait, a full range of movement, a no pain

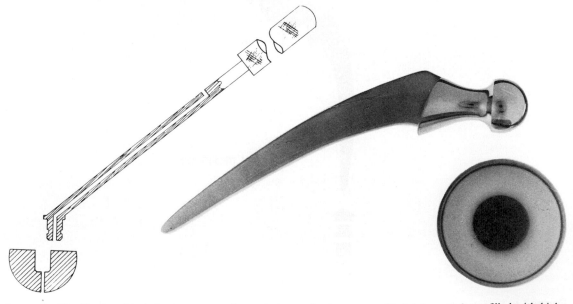

Figure 11   The Hastings hip is in two parts, a femoral stem and a loose, snap-fit stainless steel cup filled with high-density polythene. The design ensures the movement of the cup in the acetabulum as well as on the femoral stem head. The sizer is also in two parts, the hollow handle and the millimetre-variable acetabular hemispheres. Suction, by blocking the hole in the handle, gives a very accurate method of sizing the head

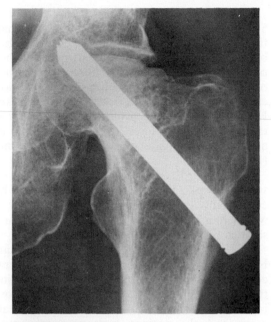

Figure 12   The Smith–Peterson nail did more for patients with fractured femoral necks than any other surgical advance. It saved the patient's life, but not always did it save the hip. Here avasular necrosis is seen to have occured. This happens in a great number of patients if it is looked for. Two cross-screws or pins are now more commonly used by those who pin, but even so there is a 25 per cent. failure rate

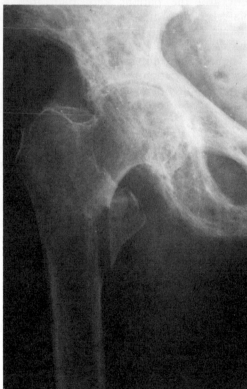

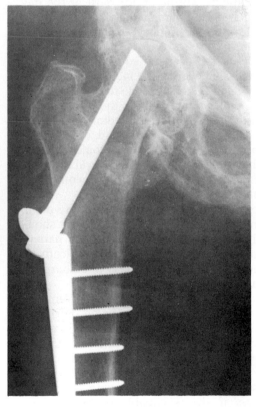

Figures 13 and 14   Radiographs of the pertrochanteric fracture of a septuagenarian before (Fig. 13) and after (Fig. 14) a McLaughlin pin and plate was applied. At first glance this seems to have secured the fractured well; nevertheless the pin is much too high in the neck and enters the lateral aspect of the head. Also it is placed at too acute an angle; it should lie more horizontally. These defects and others similar lead to a 10 per cent. failure rate of this method. Unfortunately there is no better procedure available at the moment

At least one-third of the patients have had the fracture because of one or more of the conditions that beset the elderly. These have been well documented and all need urgent treatment. Wild, Nayak, and Isaacs (1981) found that out of every 100 old people who had falls, some 30 per cent. were dead within one year. Only 3 per cent. had fractures near the hip but the same outcome, i.e. 30 per cent. mortality within one year, can be presumed to occur. This correlates well the findings of D'Arcy and Devas (1976). Thus the patients presenting to the Geriatric Orthopaedic Unit are very acute and can be most rewarding in their response to the investigations and treatment that is available in the Unit.

The Unit is not a convalescent unit but one designed to give a high level of geriatric care. The patient must be seen as soon as she arrives, an immediate medical and social assessment done, and any treatment started at once. Patients will be up for most of the day, walking and dressing is a daily routine, and in general the whole emphasis will be on progress homewards.

The Unit must be staffed as an acute geriatric admission ward; the medical staff under the physician are responsible for the day to day care of the patients and for the intensive and thorough investigation on admission to the Unit. The physiotherapists and occupational therapists who staff the Unit should also deal with the other geriatric wards, as will the social worker. The secretary should also come from the geriatric department office.

No special equipment is needed. By definition, no patient transferred to the Unit should be still suffering from a fracture. All patients should be up and dressed, unless physically too ill, but there must be no surgical embargo on such activity.

Once a week there is the ward round, as previously described in the section on organization. Decisions on discharge will be made at that time. For example, if it is uncertain whether a certain patient could manage at home a domiciliary visit is arranged with the occupational therapist going with the patient to assess if she is capable of living alone. Alternatively, a provisional discharge can be made with the patient's bed in the ward being kept available for a short period in case the patient cannot manage on her own.

Most patients will stay in the Unit for about 5 weeks. Patients requiring a longer stay than this should be transferred to a geriatric rehabilitation ward provided no untreated orthopaedic problem remains. These patients are often those in which the underlying condition causing the fall and the fracture was a stroke. However, with more prolonged rehabilitation these patients also have a very good chance of achieving independence and discharge home (Irvine, 1981).

At the ward round every patient should be seen to walk. It is vital that this should be continually emphasized. The ordering of a wheelchair should be strenuously avoided and seen as the failure of the team.

Where a fracture is recognized to be a harbinger of dissolution and the patient's general condition is clearly terminal, overenthusiastic treatment should not be instituted. Tender loving care should be continued as the only treatment and the patient kept pain free with opiates given as necessary. Occasionally such patients, free of all drugs, make an almost miraculous recovery.

The high mortality consequent on operating on all elderly patients who have a fracture near the hip should not daunt the surgeon, since the aim is to restore life to a satisfactory quality rather than solely to preserve it. Once this is understood surgeon and anaesthetist will willingly accept the risks since operation is the only hope for the patient of a life worth living. Even severely osteoporitic bone unites and will support a replacement prosthesis.

Visiting should be encouraged in the Unit, both to comfort the patient and to assist the staff in assessment by obtaining the observations of family and neighbours.

ARTHROPLASTY

The very old will often accept a painful hip for a long time consoling themselves with the ever-present thought that they have not long to go and that it will last them out. Sometimes, a spouse needs to be looked after and help is not sought until later. It is often anxiety, about the ability to remain independent and to continue to live alone, that brings the patient for advice. Sometimes, however, the pain itself is so distressing that the patient will tell the surgeon that life is not worth living and thereby instruct the surgeon in the indication for surgery. No patient is ever too old or decrepit; once life is no longer acceptable in its present state then not to operate is to deny the patient hope. The increased risk of an operation in the aged and feeble patient is small compared to the normal adult, but nevertheless is present. Some of the risk is that of old age only; actuarily about 10 per cent. of octogenarians die before the next birthday. Anaesthetic mortality is not a problem in the hands of a competent anaesthetist in the operating theatre. Wound healing is excellent and osteoporosis need not cause technical anxiety but only precautions. The slight overall higher mortality can usually be discounted against the increased risk of falls, accidents, or of being knocked over in the street through lack of agility.

The elderly are fully occupied with the activities of daily living. With age, movements become slower and quite simple tasks are more difficult; living alone, often without a spouse, is a problem and the added disability of an arthritic joint compounds these difficulties. Age is no bar to an operation. Nevertheless, the patient does not always know this and at the first consultation it is important to achieve confidence and understanding so that questions may be asked and reassurance given. The old person does not fear death. It is inevitable, sooner or later. It is to achieve the best quality of life that is so important. Even if the patient has some other condition which will limit the expectation of life there is no reason why the remaining months should not be enjoyed.

Replacement of the hip and knee are very satisfactory procedures in the elderly and are rightly popular with patient and surgeon as a means of restoring an enjoyable life. However, in many places the demand exceeds supply and in some hospitals there are long waiting lists for these operations. Despite the recommendation of a working party (DHSS Orthopaedic Services, 1981), delays in emptying beds still remain with consequent delays in admission. An adequate management system is required to overcome delays by maintaining a rapid throughput in the wards and also for the benefit of the patient. To organize a satisfactory system a clinical manager is necessary. This should be a person with a sound experience of orthopaedics and organization and may be promoted from the nursing or secretarial staff.

The prime duty of the manager is to supervise the well-being of the patient; she is directly responsible to the consultant orthopaedic surgeon in charge.

Assessment is an important part of treatment of the elderly. Whereas the surgeon will obtain some details of how life is led, and where, he will not have time to go into minutiae. The assessment is designed to be the beginning of a total care system. In the orthopaedic outpatient clinic, the time available is limited and misunderstandings may occur. The patient may leave the clinic knowing only that she is to have an operation but very often she knows little more. Assessment by the team 2 or 3 weeks after the outpatient appointment should allow 2 to 3 hours so that the patient is unhurried, the tempo is slow, and she can be asked questions. Communication is important at any age of life, but it is much more so to the elderly, and at this assessment session the ability to communicate will be explored by all members of the team. The clinical manager will assess the social circumstances of the patient, including family or other support, and find out a suitable time for admission. The occupational therapist will assess the activities of daily living and will determine what may be needed preoperatively, postoperatively, and what achievements will be necessary to allow the patient to return to living alone after the operation. The physiotherapist will be interested in housing details, e.g. whether there are stairs or if there are lifts, so that a record can be made of the level of muscular achievement that will be necessary before the patient returns home. The nursing assessment will explore the medical background of the patient and present any therapy and current medical conditions. Finally, there will be a discussion on the best dates for operation with the patient and the whole team, and a case discussion to make sure all are fully informed. The reassured patient is sent home but her doctor is asked to send her back if she deteriorates. The patient is next sent about 6 weeks before admission and a further assessment done. Up-to-date information on the general condition and on drugs being taken (which is so important in the elderly and especially so before surgery) is obtained from the doctor. Enquiries are made about help at home after discharge, about staying with relatives, or the financial possibility of a short holiday in a hotel or other suitable place. The patient is told about drips and drains so that, on recovery from the anaesthetic, the coils of tubing around her do not cause alarm. The necessary investigations are repeated, blood is kept for crossmatching later, and the blood bank warned of the impending admission so that suitable blood may be available. The patient is then referred to the anaesthetic clinic.

All these measures prevent delay in the ward because there is now no reason for it to occur: the patient is not found to have diabetes or heart failure at the last moment; the chest radiograph will not show an unexpected lesion; nor, when it is time to go home, will the family have gone away for a month.

The patient is admitted, operated upon the next day, and is walked the day after. Early walking is highly beneficial in preventing deep vein thrombosis and is also a remarkable tonic to the elderly who, despite the discomfort, appear anxious to do this when they have been told about it at assessment. The first day the patient is stood with a walking frame, takes a step to a chair, and sits there for a while before returning to bed. The next day many of the tubes will have been removed, with the exception of the vacuum drains, and proper walking is encouraged. Each day this continues in greater amount; the patient will dress once the drains are out.

From 5 days after operation, the patient may be considered for discharge. There is no necessity to keep the patient in hospital merely to take out the sutures. According to the assessment before admission and its continuation by the clinical manager during the time in hospital, most patients will go home, or to a low dependancy unit, within 8 days. The latter, previously known as a convalescent home, is useful for those who live alone or with a debilitated spouse who could not manage for two. Before discharge, the primary health care team is alerted to make sure all is well and to visit the patient at home on the day of discharge.

While the patient with an arthroplasty is in hospital the assessment continues and any lapse from the planned schedule is noted so that this will not disrupt the general ward programme.

With rapid progress patients never remain as convalescents. Thus a ward with efficient throughput, such as has been described, needs a nursing staff at the same level as an intensive care unit. A further problem is that operation time is much longer if the proper precautions are taken, such as the use of a clean air theatre. However, a low or non-existent morbidity from sepsis amply pays for the extra care and effort.

Clinical Monitoring

In the same way that the clinical manager organizes the continuing care of the arthroplasty patients, so will she continue assessment of those patients admitted as emergencies and who were not assessed as outpatients. It is usually several days after the fracture has been dealt with, if such was the diagnosis, before a final progress report and future plans are formulated.

Once the management of the two conditions, the acute fracture near the hip and the replacement of the arthritic hip, are understood then all other orthopaedic problems in the elderly will be managed just as readily with the same approach.

THE SPINE

The spine attracts attention because of the osteoporotic deformity that occurs in most old ladies and some old men. The surgeon will note this as an indication of the severity of the osteoporosis he will find when he is doing a knee replacement or treating a fracture near the hip.

Osteoporosis in the spine gives rise to pain. This is secondary to the weakness which occurs with the loss of bone. The vertebrae concerned are being stressed to such an extent that they will in a short while collapse. The pain is present in just the same way as a stress fracture can produce pain in the otherwise normal healthy bone of the young adult. In osteoporosis the bone is normal but there is less of it and so it is weak and there is insufficient strength to withstand the stress of everyday use and so collapse occurs with the classic wedge deformity. Often a trivial injury such as a simple jolt will allow the compression to occur with a sudden increase in pain. The unwary clinician may tell the patient that she has broken her back and that this is the cause of her pain. The alarm and despondency is intense in both patient and relatives alike; it is then difficult to persuade the patient that the injury is in fact trivial in itself but needs urgent activity for rehabilitation. It is far better to tell the patient that the slight injury has caused heavy bruising of the bone, which is painful but not at all serious, and that after resting for a little in bed, she may get up again and start walking. The latter is achieved by giving the patient as many pillows as possible for comfort on admission and soon she is sitting upright, usually within a day or two. Then she may be seated upright in a chair. Having achieved this, it should be explained to the patient that although she will get pain if she stands and walks she will not become stiff and immobile: she will then walk, often without recourse to analgesics. It is the knowledge that the doctor knows there is pain and the assurance that the pain is not important that allows the patient to do this in her own interest.

With this regimen there is very rarely any necessity for the patient to stay in hospital longer than 3 or 4 days; some form of back support may be applied which may or may not be necessary to support the spine but is helpful in reassuring the patient.

Spinal Stenosis

Computerised-Axial Tomography

The Computerised-Axial Tomography (CAT) scan is of most help to the orthopaedic surgeon in diagnosing the size and shape of the lumbar spine when it has become stenosed, or for rheumatoid arthritis in the upper cervical spine. As a diagnostic tool other than for these sites it does not normally lend itself to orthopaedic, as opposed to neurosurgical, problems in the elderly. Problems with the rheumatoid patient occur especially at the occipito-cervical complex, sometimes with subluxation. Although this can be measured by careful radiology, it is not actually possible to see the amount of space left for the cord or conus medullaris in that region. The CAT scan will show this clearly.

However, the CAT scan is not quite as simple as scintigraphy and is not so comfortable for the patient; it is costly in time and money and gives a moderately high X-ray dosage so it should not be used without proper consideration for its indications.

Lumbar stenosis causes bizarre symptoms in an old person that have been, and still are, attributed to ageing. Old age may be associated with factors increasing the effect of the stenosis, but it is not old age itself that causes the patient gradually to sink into a chair, and from the chair into the grave. It is the inability to support themselves on their own legs that causes them to sit. This is due to the inability to walk for more than a few yards without the feeling of being unable to stand any longer, with odd, peculiar, and unpleasant sensations in the legs.

The activities of daily living are lost, nutrition may fail, and friends, relations, and neighbours will consider the patient is failing – and indeed she is.

A fatal outcome may occur if treatment is not given to enable the patient to look after herself and to remain independent. The patient with lumbar stenosis who is seen in a clinic has usually been sitting for some while awaiting her turn and, when examined, there will be no physical signs. However, if the diagnosis is considered and if the history is taken fully and carefully, it will suggest the diagnosis. It may be possible to watch the patient at exercise and see the gradual failure of walking, the increasing unsteadiness, and the increased distress as walking continues. Plantar reflexes will probably be flexor throughout unless the patient has an associated cervical spondylosis causing pyramidal tract compression. The only way to prove or disprove that the patient has a lumbar stenosis is by a lumbar scan or by radiculogram. Either of these will show the stenosis but the CAT scan will show the actual compression of the nerve roots as they pass laterally to the foramena better than will the radiculogram. Myelography, while not giving the same detail as radiculography, is quite sufficient to give the main levels of stenosis and to be used as a diagnostic aid before operation.

The treatment of lumbar stenosis is by decompression of the affected spine, usually at the third or fourth lumbar level but often involving several levels. The stenosis is caused by encroachment on the spinal canal by osteophytes from the facet articulations and from protruding discs, often ossified, with narrowing of the foramena through which the nerves pass. A congenitally narrow lumbar canal may predispose to the condition.

Operation is the only treatment; without it the condition progresses. Decompression is neither dangerous nor difficult but it may be tedious if many nerve roots have to be decompressed. Fusion after operation is rarely necessary. The aftercare is important; micturition may be affected for the first few days and care must be taken to ensure the bladder is not overflowing and giving rise to false incontinence. It is wise to catheterize men and women before operation, removing it at 2 days after operation when the patient is able to stand or sit on a commode. Long bed-rest is not indicated after operation but a spinal support, measured and made before operation, helps considerably.

FRACTURES IN GENERAL

There are two reasons for the old person being admitted to hospital after an injury. The first is social, because it is not possible for the patient to continue to live at home, as, for example, the patient with bilateral Colles's fractures with both wrists in plaster. The other indication is the severity of the fracture or its pain; internal fixation is then indicated when it is feasible. The technique, with one or two exceptions, is the same as at any other age.

Plating osteoporotic bones has its problems but these are largely overcome by the use of proper methods and it need cause no anxiety as to the quality of fixation. It is imperative to use the proper size of drills followed by the correct tap and then the correct length of non-self-tapping screws (most orthopaedic screws are self-tapping). Finally, if the bone is still not gripped satisfactorily, a high-density polythene plate is put on the opposite side of the bone with a small hole drilled where the screw will come, and the latter is then driven home until it grips the polythene plate and pulls it firmly against the bone. This will give a very firm fixation even in the most osteoporotic bone.

In the very decrepit patient, often bedridden, the femoral shaft may break without any injury of note – even during simple nursing care, as in lifting the patient. Such a patient may well be unable to stand a long operation of internal fixation and open reduction and for these patients a very simple technique has been developed. Under the anaesthetic of choice, the patient is placed on the operation table with the knees bent over the end. It is then easy to open the knee, make a hole into the femur between the two condyles and then insert the guide wire up the femoral shaft. Often, by simple traction, the fracture will reduce sufficiently to allow the guide wire to enter the upper fragment. X-ray control, or the image intensifier, will confirm this. If the reduction is not good enough a small incision, anteriorly and over the fracture site, will allow sufficient room for the bone ends to be aligned. An intramedullary nail is then inserted and the hole in the femur plugged with cement. The patient may walk forthwith (Devas, 1977).

Another fracture that used to cause problems in the elderly is that of the lower end of the femur, often 'T' shaped into the knee. However, by the use of the special pin and plate with a compression screw medially the fracture can be held as securely as that of the trochanteric region, thus allowing the patient to walk at once.

Fractures of the Tibia

In the same way that the femur can have an intramedullary nail put up the shaft, so can one be put down the tibia in order to fix it quickly, easily, and firmly. Few fractures in old people are caused by high-velocity injuries, which are so common in the tibia in youth, and as a consequence union of the bone occurs quite readily and without undue delay, even if the internal fixation seems a little loose.

The approach is through an incision on one or other side of the patellar tendon; the front of the tibial plateau outside and anterior to the capsule of the knee is cleared. This part of the plateau lies over the centre of the tibial shaft owing to the backward bend of the uppermost third of the tibia. A hole is made in the plateau and a straight rod can be dropped down with the greatest ease. If there is displacement of the fracture then the position of the leg with the knee flexed at the end of the table is usually sufficient to reduce the fragments, but if not it is easily achieved by extra traction and manipulation. A firm dressing with or without an eggshell plaster is sufficient to preserve comfort and stability and the patient may get up and walk with a frame.

Eggshell Plasters

Many orthopaedic procedures use a firm pressure dressing after operation. In one way or another these are based on the Robert Jones bandage which was alternate layers of Gamgee and unbleached calico bandages. Nowadays cotton wool is wrapped round the part and crepe bandages applied over it. If one, or occasionally two, plaster bandages are applied outside this pressure dressing it adds some stiffening without much weight and is excellent for ankles, knee, or arms in the elderly, for whom heavy plaster casts are not indicated as a routine.

Intramedullary Fixation of Osteoporotic Bone

The osteoporotic bone has a very large medullary cavity and it may be that a large intramedullary nail is insufficient in itself to hold the bone. In these circumstances it is possible to 'stack' the Kuntschner nail. Because the nails are of clover-leaf design one nail can be interlocked with another thereby increasing the overall size. The 'stacked' nail need not, of course, be the same length as the first nail. This technique is especially suitable to stabilize the lowermost third of the femoral shaft when the fracture is at the junction of the middle and lowermost thirds.

Potts' fractures, even if not severe, can often immobilize the elderly because they find it very difficult to manage a walking plaster, however light and skilfully applied. Open reduction and screw fixation is then indicated, using strong implants so that the patient, supported only by firm crepe bandages, can walk.

The very painful fracture of the neck of the humerus that can occur in the osteoporotic old lady sometimes necessitates admission. If this is so, then at operation it is quite simple to put a Rush pin through the head of the humerus and down the shaft to control the movement at the fracture site and thereby eliminate the pain and allow the patient to be up and about again. Early movements are instituted.

The Treatment of Fractures in Outpatients

Old bone unites as readily as does younger bone and age by itself is no indication for admission if the patient can walk; indeed age is a contraindication because being in hospital is harmful. This also means that the fracture clinic must be properly organized. It is important to make quite certain that the elderly, who perhaps are less inclined to participate in the exercises they are told to do than would a young man, have a proper organization of rehabilitation from the moment that they arrive to final discharge. One method of treating such patients has been found to be eminently satisfactory; a Colles fracture will be used as an example. The patient has a manipulation under general anaesthetic (when the displacement warrants it) and application of a plaster backslab, and is then referred to the physiotherapy department for individual exercises to make sure that the immediate swelling after the accident and manipulation is dispersed by activity. When seen at the next fracture clinic, the swelling should be controlled and movement should be starting in the fingers. If the check radiograph is satisfactory the patient can have the plaster completed and is then referred to the occupational therapy workshop for further assessment and treatment. Here the patient is seen and the activities of the injured limb are noted. The range of movement of shoulder, elbow, and fingers is recorded and the patient is given activities suitable to her injury. Often these are preceded by a period of exercises in the 'hot box', an apparatus with hot air circulating in it. The limb, in plaster, is held in the box and some simple activity given for a few minutes until the hand is warm. The patient then continues with the activities ordered which may be anything from making a jigsaw puzzle to placing pegs in holes or even setting type and printing. As activity proceeds, assessment continues and finally the occupational therapist will decide that the patient needs no further treatment and can be discharged from the workshop. At the end of 5 weeks the fracture will have united and the plaster is removed, and it will be found that the patient has excellent movements of shoulder, elbow, and fingers and good movements of the wrist which, although not full, soon becomes so with normal use.

A similar regime can be applied to practically every fracture that is treated as an outpatient. Because it is group treatment, it is more economical than individual treatment by the physiotherapist, or the dull wrist and foot classes in which the elderly patient appears to achieve nothing more than boredom.

Pathological Fractures

Scintigraphy

This procedure is now well established and needs no special description but the technique as applied to the elderly does need some attention.

Firstly, it is a quick, easy, and comfortable investigation which, although invasive, is not harmful in any way. Normally it is the first choice to determine if metastatic deposits in bone have occurred. The Technitium 99^M scan will show secondaries in bone well before normal radiological methods. Secondly, because it is a total body scan, no part is missed but no extra time is taken doing this, unlike the ordinary radiological skeletal survey.

It is also very useful in certain hip or knee problems which have had prosthetic replacements because, if there is loosening of either one or other part of the prosthesis, this will show as a 'hot spot' (provided the replacement is at least 1 year old).

Sometimes the increased physical activity after a very painful hip or knee has been replaced causes a stress fracture. This will also produce a 'hot spot' long before it can be seen in the normal radiograph.

Almost invariably a metastatic deposit from a primary growth elsewhere or multiple myelomatosis causes the fracture. All such fractures should be treated by internal fixation at the earliest possible moment. If the fracture is in the femoral head or neck, a cemented replacement is the best treatment.

No pathological fracture which is causing distress should be left unoperated upon because the patient is going to die; this is medicine at its worst. It is a surgeon's privilege to be able to operate, cure, or ameliorate a painful fracture which will destroy any pleasure in the last few days or weeks of life.

All such patients must have skeletal surveys because often other bones may be affected. This may be radiological or by means of scintigraphy with Technietum 99^M. When an important long bone appears to be about to fracture through a deposit it should be treated by an intramedullary rod, which is easy to do before the fracture occurs but can be very difficult afterwards.

It must also be remembered that any bony deposit treated by radiotherapy will not begin to respond in strength until at least 6 weeks have elapsed, and this gives another reason for pinning a bone of doubtful strength.

PARAPLEGIA FROM METASTASES

Any patient who develops paraparesis must be considered to be developing a paraplegia and once bladder function has been lost for 2 or 3 hours, it is very difficult to regain it. Never wait until the next day. A radiculogram must be done at once and the theatre prepared for operation. Only by treating this condition with the utmost alacrity can the patient make a full recovery. There is often no indication of where the primary is and no time should be wasted searching for it; no other specialist advice is needed other than that of the anaesthetist, who should never refuse an anaesthetic to such a patient, knowing that without decompression the patient will spend a few miserable weeks or months doubly incontinent, in pain, and with no hope of recovery.

The radiculogram is all important. The straight radiograph may well show the vertebra affected, eroded and perhaps partially destroyed. However, until the block is clearly defined it is not possible to eliminate a vascular lesion that has obliterated the arterial supply to cause the paraplegia. Also, the soft tissue block may extend some distance from the level of the bone destruction, and only the radiculogram will show this.

Once the block is demonstrated, that part of the spine is decompressed. Starting either above or below the lesion the laminae are nibbled away until the spinal cord is seen free and pulsating. Usually this is all that needs to be done, especially in the thoracic spine. Sometimes the growth may have so damaged the stability of the lumbar spine that it may be necessary to stabilize it with two spinal plates.

CONCLUSION

Geriatric orthopaedics demands a very active approach to the problems that arise. It is only by taking time by the forelock and treating the emergencies with the outmost celerity that success will be apparent; it is only by insisting on shared responsibility that the proper methods of rehabilitation will be used; and finally it must always be remembered that without the trained and enthusiastic team of nurses, therapists, and social workers the erudition of the doctors would be of no avail.

REFERENCES

Barnes, R., Brown, J. T., Garden, R. S., and Nicholl, E. A. (1976). 'Subcapital fractures of the femur', *J. Bone Joint Surg.*, **58B**, 2–24.

D'Arcy, J., and Devas, M. (1976). 'Treatment of fractures of the femoral neck by replacement with the Thompson prosthesis', *J. Bone Joint Surg.*, **58B**, 279.

Department of Health and Social Security Orthopaedic Services (1981). *Waiting Time for Outpatient Appointments and Inpatient Treatment*, HMSO, London.

Devas, M. (1977). *Geriatric Orthopaedics*, Academic Press, London.

Irvine, R. E. (1981). Personal communication.

Lewis, A. F. (1981). 'Fracture neck of femur; changing incidence', *Br. Med. J.*, **283**, 1217–1220.

Office of Health Economics (1982). *Hip Replacement*, London.

Wild, W., Nayak, U. S. L., and Isaacs, B. (1981). 'How dangerous are falls in old people at home?', *Br. Med. J.*, **282**, 266–268.

29
Rehabilitation of the Elderly

Principles and Practice of Geriatric Medicine
Edited by M. S. J. Pathy
© 1985 John Wiley & Sons Ltd

29.1

Rehabilitation of the Elderly

K. Andrews

Rehabilitation has been defined as 'the restoration of a patient to his fullest physical, mental and social capability' (Mair, 1972) and this is the basis of geriatric medicine. In practice it is usually more appropriate to aim for optimal recovery of abilities which allow the patient to adjust to his own environment, not only within the limitations of his capabilities but also within the limits of his determination and desires.

This chapter aims to describe the rehabilitation possibilities of conditions which commonly present in geriatric rehabilitation units without attempting to cover all those disorders which are managed in such units.

THE ELDERLY REHABILITEE

The elderly person requiring rehabilitation presents with additional problems to those found in the younger disabled. Apart from being generally more frail, the elderly have a greater tendency to multiple pathology, especially of a degenerative vascular nature. This is a particular problem when it involves the cerebral circulation predisposing to falls, confusion, and poor concentration.

The energy requirements of even young non-disabled people using crutches is double that of normal walking (Fisher and Patterson, 1981). When additional disabilities, due for instance to brain damage (Richerson and Richerson, 1981) or amputation (Gonzalez, Concoran, and Reyes, 1974), are added they result in greatly increased energy expenditure

for even simple tasks. In the elderly the energy requirement to overcome disability is complicated by cardio-respiratory conditions or anaemia. In addition, muscle wasting and increased tendency to degenerative joint disease make mobilization more difficult to achieve and prolongs the rehabilitation programme.

Elderly people are socially vulnerable, being more likely to live alone or be dependent on an equally elderly spouse, sibling, or neighbour. Social service departments, although very supportive, are often reluctant to supply expensive aids or modifications to the home and some grants, such as mobility allowances, are not available to the elderly.

The aim is for the elderly patient to live independently, although this is often only achieved by extensive support of family and neighbours as well as social and nursing services rather than by the provision of complex equipment, aids, and adaptations.

GENERAL APPROACH TO REHABILITATION OF THE ELDERLY

The aim of rehabilitation is to obtain the maximum degree of social independence for the individual patient. This requires a wide range of professional skills (Table 1) aimed at correcting, or adapting to, a disability together with the psychological support of the patient and family. The rehabilitation process also includes the planning of a safe return home and good communications with those providing community support.

Table 1   The rehabilitation team

PATIENT AND FAMILY	
Geriatric Unit	*Community*
Geriatrician	Family Doctor
Nurse	District Nurse
Physiotherapist	Health Visitor
Occupational Therapist	Home Help
Speech Therapist	Meals-on-Wheels
Social Worker	Social Worker
Chiropodist	Neighbourhood Visitor
Dietician	Rehabilitation Officer
	Therapists
Hospital	Volunteers
Surgeon	Day Centres
Prosthetist	Clubs for Disabled
Technicians	
Artificial Limb and	
Appliance Centre	

There are several basic concepts in the rehabilitation of the elderly. At the start of the rehabilitation programme it is necessary to determine the 'goals' for the patient and the rehabilitation team since the expectations and hopes of the patient, relatives, and staff can differ widely (New, Ruscio, and George, 1969). It is not unusual for considerable effort to be put into making the patient independent in activities which neither the patient nor his relative want or utilize when the patient returns home.

Many elderly people have difficulty in adapting to new ideas and it is usually more helpful to modify existing equipment than to provide complex aids. Some patients, especially those with confusion, anxiety, depression, loss of confidence, or perceptual disorders, do not benefit from intensive complex therapeutic activity and seem to progress better when treated on the ward than in remedial therapy departments. Some patients will even progress better when treated by gentle nursing encouragement than by active 'rehabilitation'.

Activities assessed in hospital are often unrelated to what happens at home. This may be due to lack of involvement of the family in the rehabilitation programme. The space available in the rehabilitation unit is usually much greater than that at home; thus the walking frame which enabled safe mobilization in hospital becomes a hazard in the confines of the patient's home. Positioning of furniture and carpets at home present obstacles which were not a problem in hospital. A home visit with

the patient and his family prior to discharge permits assessment of potential problems that are likely to arise and provides advice on avoiding dangers or on provision of appropriate aids.

SPECIFIC MEASURES

Many of the conditions requiring similar treatment are found in several disorders and therefore it is appropriate to discuss management of the clinical features rather than list them separately under specific diagnoses.

Prevention

Much can be done to prevent disabilities. The value of correct positioning to prevent pressure sores, spasticity, painful shoulders, and contractures is a particularly good illustration of prevention.

The painful shoulder following a stroke is not only distressing to the patient but inhibits the recovery of function in that limb. Placing the patient in the correct antispastic position along with passive mobilization and muscle strengthening actively prevents shoulder problems (Caillet, 1980; Johnstone, 1983).

The shoulder should be moved through external rotation and flexion and this is not achieved by the pulleys normally used in rehabilitation units. Passive mobilization in inexperienced hands can also produce trauma to the shoulder capsule, especially when abduction is carried out beyond 90 degrees.

The use of a sling to prevent the painful shoulder is debatable. Hurd, Farrell, and Waylonis (1974) were unable to show any benefit though Miglietta, Lewitan, and Rogoff (1959) found it useful. The sling does not necessarily prevent subluxation of the shoulder, though the additional support of an axillary pad may help. When the arm is flaccid the provision of a flail arm splint will support the shoulder blade as well as the arm while allowing movement to take place.

Appropriate measures may avoid exaggerating the deformity of rheumatoid joints. Immobilization by splinting and avoidance of active exercise is important in the acutely inflamed joint. As the inflammation settles this is followed by passive then active mobilization. Function is helped by the provision of aids and the use of the correct techniques of carrying out activities (Brattström, 1973). It is, for instance, useful to advise the removal of jar tops and turning on of taps with the left hand and replacing with the right hand to avoid exacerbation of the ulnar deformity of rheumatoid fingers.

Pain

The treatment of pain obviously depends on accurate diagnosis of its cause. In addition to analgesic drugs several physical measures symptomatically relieve pain. Heat can be provided superficially (hot-water bottles, electric pads, paraffin wax, and infrared radiation) or to deep tissues with ultrasound or electromagnetic radiations of various wavelengths. In general heat should be used with caution where there is acute inflammation, venous obstruction, ischaemia, or problems with coagulation; ultrasound is contraindicated in vascular disease, malignancy, pulmonary tuberculosis, and near the eye (Stewart, Abzug, and Harris, 1980) as well as over metal prostheses. The potential temperature rise in metal prostheses has caused some concern, though Lehmann (1965) found that the heat is quickly conducted away and does not produce clinical problems; he does not, however, say whether there is any loosening of the fixing cement surrounding the prostheseis due to the microvibration.

Pain can also be relieved by ice packs (Grant, 1964; Hayden, 1964; Lane, 1971; Lorenze Caratonis, and De Rosa, 1960) though this is also contraindicated in ischaemia, anaesthetic areas, and vasculitis.

Transcutaneous electrical stimulation relieves pain in a proportion of cases (Ebersold *et al.*, 1975; Loeser, Black, and Christman, 1975; Long and Hagfors, 1975) and modern equipment can achieve significant pain relief in up to half of those with peripheral neuropathy, arthropathy, phantom limb, and stump pain and in nearly three-quarters of those with hemiplegic shoulder – hand syndrome (Birkhan *et al.*, 1980). Prolonged electrical stimulation has also been reported to improve postherpetic neuralgia in about one-third of cases (Nathan and Wall, 1974).

Although backache responds to bed-rest in 60 per cent. of cases (Wiesel *et al.*, 1980) rehabilitation to increase the range of move-

ment, strengthen the support muscles, and correct postural deformities is also effective (Kendall and Jenkins, 1968) while avoiding the dangers of bed-rest.

Splinting of painful joints is useful in the acutely inflamed phase though it should be discouraged, except during rest periods, in chronic arthroses since it tends to produce osteoporosis and makes the patient dependent.

The rest pain and walking distance in intermittent claudication can be improved by exercise (Ekroth *et al.*, 1978 Hayne, 1980; Jonason *et al.*, 1979; Zetterquist, 1970) and early experience with pneumatic intermittent compression of the legs is showing promising results.

Tissue Healing

Each clinician has his preferred potion for the treatment of ulceration but the physiotherapist can aid with certain techniques. Ultrasound has been shown to stimulate new tissue growth in the laboratory (Dyson and Pond, 1970) and clinically significantly improves the rate of healing of varicose ulceration (Dyson and Suckling, 1978). Other physical methods include the use of dry air currents (Davis and Chu, 1974), ultraviolet light, and pneumatic intermittent compression.

An increased rate of healing of bone fractures has also been reported using electrical stimulation across the fracture site (Brighton *et al.*, 1981; Jorgensen, 1977) or pulsing electromagnetic induction (Bassett, Mitchell, and Gaston, 1981; Heckman *et al.*, 1981; Sutcliffe, Sharrard, and MacEarchern, 1980) .

Balance

Balance problems are probably responsible for the major workload of a geriatric rehabilitation unit. Management depends on the cause of the unsteadiness and therefore the appropriate treatment is required for weak muscles, Parkinson's disease, flaccidity, spasticity, visual problems, and lack of confidence.

Proprioceptive feedback is diminished in the elderly (Levin and Benton, 1973) and therefore stimulation needs to be at a higher level than in younger individuals. The patient should not be expected to stand until he has achieved sitting balance, nor should he be expected to walk until standing balance is satisfactory.

Backward leaning presents particular difficulties. Helping the patient to stand by supporting under the arm at the shoulder exacerbates the backward lean and therefore the patient should be encouraged to push up from a chair or pull against the hands of the attendant. Once on his feet the patient walks better when pushing a wheelchair (with a nurse sitting on it!) or a weighted frame with wheels. Chairs which encourage the patient to sit leaning backwards and prolonged rest should be avoided. Some patients benefit from standing leaning forward over a support for 15 minutes three or four times a day while others benefit from wearing shoes with raised heels.

The patient who lacks strength and is apprehensive of standing, such as after fracture of the femur, often responds to gradually taking the weight through the feet using a tilting table.

Wright (1979) has described the technique for mobilizing those patients where the feet seem to stick to the ground when beginning to walk or on changing direction (stammering gait). He suggests that once the first step is made, for instance by stepping over a flexible band attached to the back legs of the walking frame, then a good walking pattern can be established.

Ataxia can be stabilized by providing the patient with a smock weighted with lead or sand-bags. Correction of ataxic muscle imbalance using resistive exercise to improve proprioception and increase strength endurance are also beneficial (Kabat, 1965) while Morgan (1980) has suggested simple aids such as the use of non-slip mats, weighted dishes and pans, wheeled walking frames, and limb restraint by weighted leather wristbands.

STROKE

More has been written about stroke rehabilitation than the rehabilitation of almost any other physical disability. Many techniques have been described but most therapists on geriatric units adapt these for the particular problems of individual patients. The complexity of stroke has made it doubtful whether satisfactory randomly controlled trials can be carried out.

Techniques fall into two major groups: (a) the compensation approach, training the patient to compensate using the non-affected side, and (b) the neurophysiological approach which uses neurological reflexes to encourage recovery of the affected side.

The best-known neurophysiological approach is that advocated by Bobath (Bobath, 1978; Semans, 1967) which concentrates on inhibiting abnormal synergic patterns. The Brunnstrom approach (Brunnstrom, 1970; Perry, 1967), on the other hand, uses synergic reflex patterns to produce improvement in movement. Both of these techniques, along with others such as the Rood approach (Stockmeyer, 1967) and proprioceptive neuromuscular facilitation (Knott and Voss, 1968; Voss, 1967), have something to offer individual patients.

There are three phases in the rehabilitation process of the stroke patient: (a) the acute phase; (b) the rapid recovery phase; (c) the slow recovery phase. Patients pass through these phases at varying rates.

Acute Phase

Emphasis in the acute phase is on prevention – of deformities, spasticity, pressure sores, pulmonary stasis, and depression. Prevention of spasticity and pressure sores depends on the correct positioning of the patient. Supporting the seated patient in a chair prevents the development of orthostatic pneumonia, increases the proprioception necessary for maintaining the balance mechanism, and prevents the development of abnormal postures. Passive movement of the affected joints prevents spasticity and maintains a good range of joint movement, especially at the shoulder.

During the acute phase both the patient and his family are vulnerable to pessimism and depression about the future. Explanations and planning of rehabilitation goals at this stage can go a long way to preventing these psychological problems.

Rapid Recovery Phase

This is the phase where spontaneous recovery is most marked and gives the greatest opportunity for modifying the recovery process. The rehabilitation programme aims to correct:
(a) muscle weakness and patterns of movement,
(b) postural imbalance,

(c) abnormal tone,
(d) sensory loss,
(e) visual disturbances,
(f) gait and mobility difficulties,
(g) activities of daily living,
(h) speech problems.

Muscle Power

Improving motor power is classically achieved by resistive exercises but it is so limited by disturbance of muscle tone, proprioceptive, sensory, or perceptual problems that if these can be overcome then improvement in muscle power usually follows. It is important to recognize that recovery depends on control of the central mechanism of movement rather than building up strength of individual muscle groups.

Balance

Patients cannot be expected to stand until they have sitting balance; nor should they be expected to walk until they have standing balance.

Sitting balance is achieved either passively (supported in the upright position when seated rather than leaning to one side, and the avoidance of tip-back chairs) or actively. Rocking the patient from side to side increases proprioception. This can further be increased by encouraging the patient to grip the affected hand with the normal hand and moving both from side to side and up and down while sitting unsupported.

Similarly, standing balance can be achieved by rocking while standing and using a full-length mirror to provide visual feedback of the patient's position.

Abnormal Tone

Classically initial flaccidity is followed by spasticity. However, flaccidity may be a persistent problem in about one-fifth of patients. This may result in subluxation of the shoulder or hyperextension of the knee. Gentle handling, good positioning, and support of the affected joints is therefore essential. Passive movement requires support above and below the joint. Inflatable splints (Johnstone, 1983) (Fig. 1) or lightweight plastic splints are both supportive and protective.

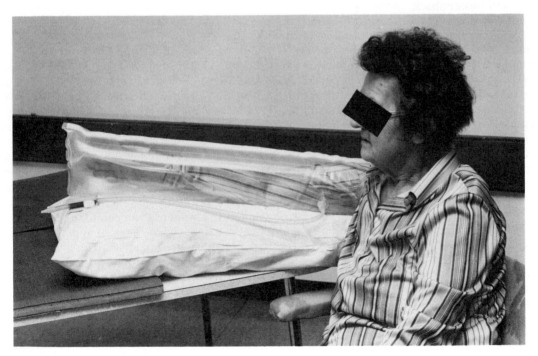

Figure 1   Inflatable arm splint

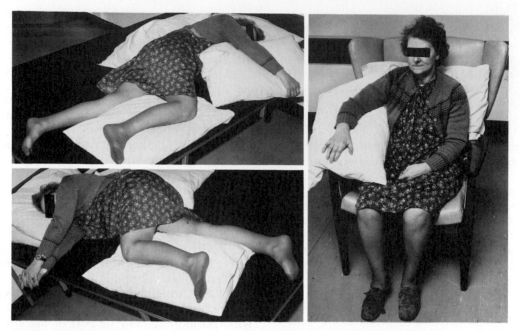

Figure 2   Positioning the stroke patient to prevent spasticity, pressure sores, and subluxation of the shoulder. Right hemiplegic patient in the lateral and siting positions

Techniques which help to increase tone are weight-bearing (Bobath, 1978), vibration (Carr and Shepherd, 1980), ice (Lee and Warren, 1978), and biofeedback.

Spasticity presents a different problem. Uncorrected, contractures and deformities of the affected limb occur. These can be prevented to a large extent by correct positioning in the early stages (Fig. 2). It is also important to avoid exercises which increase the abnormal tonic reflexes – squeezing a ball comes into this category. Other methods include weight-bearing in the normal position and the use of ice (Knutsson, 1970; Miglietta, 1973).

Prolonged spasticity results in contractures which are severely disabling and difficult to treat. Although surgery may be required, serial splinting using a skin-tight plaster of Paris weight-bearing inhibitory support has been used successfully (Ada and Scott, 1980; Hayes and Burns, 1970); however, high pressure pneumatic intermittent compression over the joint along with night-splinting is often more easily tolerated by the patient. The passive stretching should be supported by strengthening of the weak agonist muscle along with local inhibition of spasticity (Cherry, 1980). Rizk and Park (1981) have also described the ben-

eficial effect of transcutaneous electrical nerve stimulation with an extensor splint in treating contracture of the knee.

Sensory Loss

This occurs in about one-third of strokes (Anderson, 1971; Gresham *et al.*, 1975; Marquardsen, 1969). Sensory awareness has been improved by increased stimulation (Fox, 1964; Weinberg *et al.*, 1979), whilst sensation of movement has been improved by EMG biofeedback techniques (Inglis *et al.*, 1976).

Sensory loss may be due to internal capsule or cortical hemisphere damage. The main difference is that in internal capsule damage there is recognition of the hemisensory loss and therefore compensation can take place. In cortical damage a wide range of agnosias is found, all of which are major barriers to recovery, even when they are found in association with very little muscle weakness.

The most obvious tactile agnosia is that of unilateral neglect of the affected side. This may range from 'forgetting' the limb when the attention is distracted, to complete inability to recognize the affected side. Increased sensory input can improve awareness of the affected side (Anderson and Choy, 1970; O'Brien and Pallett, 1978; Siev and Freishtat, 1976), and this can be achieved by massaging the limb with ice or warm packs, using high-pressure pneumatic intermittent (fast-cycle) compression, drawing the patient's attention to the affected side, encouraging bilateral use of the limbs, and constant handling of the affected side. It is essential that all staff and relatives are aware of the problem so that a constant flow of stimulation can be achieved.

Visual Problems

These are also common. Homonymous hemianopia is found in 20 to 40 per cent. of stroke patients (Gresham *et al.*, 1975; Waylonis, Keith, and Aseff, 1973) and some degree of perceptual abnormality is present in 90 per cent. of those with hemianopia (Andrews *et al.*, 1980). Patients with hemianopia bump into objects on the affected side but they can compensate by scanning. On the other hand, the patient with unilateral visual neglect, due to parieto-occipital cortical damage, is unaware that the hemianopic visual field exists and therefore scanning does not take place. These patients do not recognize an object in the affected visual field even if it has been slowly moved from the normal field. When asked to draw a picture only one half of the object will be drawn. Food is eaten from only one half of the plate and the time can only be seen when the pointers are in the normal visual field. It is important for nurses and relatives to recognize these problems to avoid placing the bedside container on the affected side and to prevent the environment from becoming unnecessarily limited, e.g. by putting the patient in bed whilst all the activity is taking place in the agnostic visual field. Management is by persistent encouragement and training the patient to scan (Weinberg *et al.*, 1977).

Another form of disturbance of visual memory results in difficulty in remembering the relationship of one part of an object when visual attention moves to another part. This makes activities such as dressing and feeding very difficult. Management is to break down activities into as few basic processes as possible and carry them out in a set order, giving as many auditory and tactile clues as possible. More complex tasks cannot be performed until the patient has mastered the basic steps of each activity. It is sometimes helpful to do activities by numbers – i.e. each action is given a number and then each activity is carried out in a set sequence.

Difficulty in judging distances results in an inability to find the way around even familiar surroundings (atopographagnosia). Since the patient cannot cope with more than a very limited environment, the bed should remain in the same position and all activities, including therapy, should be carried out at the bedside. As the patient adapts to his immediate environment he can then gradually extend his area of activity. In mild cases the patient may be unable to judge the relationship of one object to another and therefore appears clumsy.

It is important in all these forms of agnosia to simplify the activity to basic actions and provide as little distraction as possible.

Gait

A good walking gait is one of the main goals of the rehabilitation programme. Disturbance of gait may be due to a combination of muscle weakness, flaccidity, spasticity, proprioceptive loss, unilateral tactile neglect, postural instability, apraxia, or contracture. Previous disabilities such as Parkinson's disease, arthritis, or amputation obviously complicate the picture.

Gait-training is a complex process but a few points may be made:

(a) Sitting and then standing balance should be achieved before walking is attempted.

(b) Although support by two persons may be required in the early stages the use of a gutter frame (Fig. 3) may give a greater sensation of independence to the patient.

(c) A frame is preferable to a stick in the preindependent stage since this allows the centre of gravity to fall between the feet, therefore producing a more normal walking pattern. A stick encourages the centre of gravity to fall to one side and produces a rolling gait.

(d) Foot drop requires a wedge support while sitting. This enables the foot to remain near to a right angle – a preferable alternative is for the patient to sit with the lower part of the legs vertical but this is tiring for long periods. When walking the ankle can

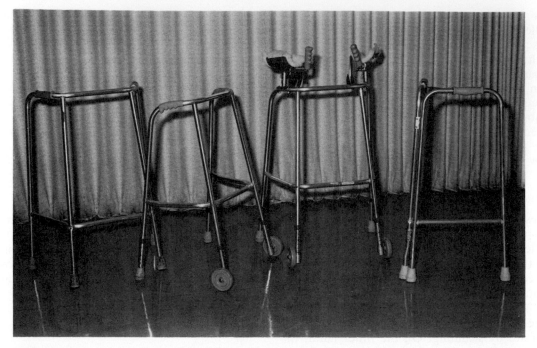

Figure 3   Types of frame (from left to right): lightweight frame (Zimmer), wheeled frame, gutter wheeled frame, triangular folding frame

be supported by a lightweight splint which fits into the shoe. A caliper with a toe spring increases spasticity in the calf muscles and is often too heavy for the already weak leg.

(e) Walking between parallel bars gives the patient confidence while allowing unimpeded walking. A mirror at the end of the bars aids the patient to correct the tendency to lean to one side; it also makes him look ahead instead of at his feet.

(f) Sitting in a rocking chair can help proprioception while increasing muscle strength, even during rest periods.

(g) Walking in the gym gives no indication of the ability to manage irregular surfaces such as curbs, steps, or stairs.

(h) Patients should know how to fall safely and to get up again. This realistic approach seems to add to the patient's confidence.

Activities of Daily Living

The aim of rehabilitation is to obtain independence in activities of daily living, even where there is poor neurological recovery. This can be achieved by training in compensatory techniques or the provision of aids and appliances.

In general, the elderly stroke patient does not adapt to complex aids. Nevertheless, simple aids such as non-slip mats and food buffers on plates are useful (Fig. 4). Multipurpose cutlery is of limited use but the rocker knife (Fig. 4) which enables food to be cut by rocking the cutting surface against food is particularly helpful where the food cannot be steadied with the hemiplegic hand.

Aids are available for just about every activity. Bath and toilet aids and appliances are required for all but a few patients.

Speech Therapy

Few patients manage to receive an adequate amount of speech therapy. Since dysphasia results in learning defects (Katz, 1958; Rosenberg and Edwards, 1964; Tikofsky and Reynolds, 1962) it is not surprising that it is associated with poor functional recovery (Baker, Schwartz, and Ramseyer, 1968; Marquardsen, 1969). However, Pesczczynski (1961) found that receptive, and sometimes global, dysphasia did not necessarily interfere

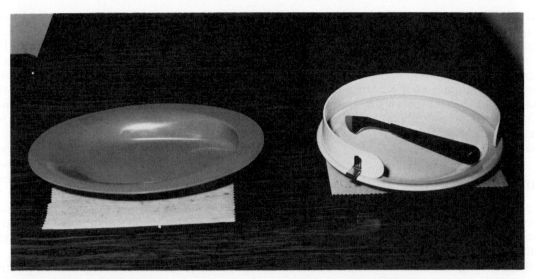

Figure 4   Plates for hemiplegic patients. Left – plate with one vertical side. Right – ordinary plate with buffer, containing a 'rocker' knife. Both plates on non-slip mats

with the patient's ability to walk, dress, or feed independently.

The value of speech therapy is as yet undecided. Attempts at controlled trials (Sarno *et al.*, Silverman, and Sands 1970; Vignolo, 1964) have been unable to show the benefit of speech therapy.

Even in the absence of evidence of the benefit of speech therapy in dysphasia the speech therapist does help the other members of the rehabilitation team to understand the patient's problems, and this is of major importance in the rehabilitation programme (see Chapter 19.1).

Slow Recovery Phase

Most studies (Carroll, 1962; Cassvan *et al.*, 1976; Katz *et al.*, 1966; Stern *et al.*, 1971) have found that the maximal recovery occurs within the first few months, with little recovery taking place after the first 6 months. There are, however, some reports (Adams and Hurwitz, 1975; Adams and McComb, 1953) of improvement continuing beyond 6 months. Certainly many patients tell of improvement up to several years. In our own study (Andrews *et al.*, 1981), 29 per cent. of patients with severe disability 3 months following the stroke continued to improve during the following 3 months. We also found that recovery continued between 6 months and one year in 21 per cent. for mo-

bility, and 14 per cent. for activities of daily living.

These figures are important since rehabilitation resources are scarce and it seems logical to concentrate effort where it is likely to be the most successful.

Experience shows that many patients who have responded to a rehabilitation programme do not persist with the activities when they return home. We found (Andrews and Stewart, 1979) that patients attending the day hospital were carrying out fewer activities at home than they were capable of at their rehabilitation assessment. Much of this was due to lack of appreciation by relatives of what the patient could do or impatience or reluctance on their behalf to allow the activities to be carried out at home. This emphasizes the importance of training the relative as well as the patient. Domiciliary rehabilitation may be more effective in achieving this.

The role of volunteers in the long term management of stroke should not be ignored. There are at least two excellent schemes. Stroke clubs are organized by local volunteers (often patients or relatives themselves) to provide a social outlet for the stroke family. In addition the clubs act as an education forum for the discussion of problems about stroke and disability.

The second scheme is for dysphasic patients (Griffiths, 1975, 1980; Griffiths and Miller,

1980). A local organizer supervises several groups of volunteers, each group attaching themselves to one dysphasic patient. They do not replace the speech therapist but act as informed 'friends' who have access to a large amount of training material. Since they work closely with the local speech therapist they are an important method of helping the patient to practice speech away from the speech therapy department.

AMPUTATION OF THE LOWER LIMB

Amputation is too often regarded as a surgical failure and delay in rehabilitation is common, though this is often due to concomitant disease (Hamilton and Nichols, 1972). The poor prognosis and long rehabilitation time has led Harris and coworkers (1974) to urge the development of residential units for the rehabilitation of the elderly amputee.

The first aim of rehabilitation is to prevent the need for surgery. Rest pain and walking distance in intermittent claudication can be improved by exercise (Ekroth *et al.*, 1978; Hayne, 1980; Jonason *et al.*, 1979; Zetterquist, 1970) and early experience with pneumatic intermittent compression of the limbs is showing promising results in delaying the need for surgery (Fig. 5).

Amputation is traumatic emotionally as well as physically and it is important that the patient is prepared psychologically for the future. Patient and family should have the opportunity preoperatively of discussing with the rehabilitation doctor a positive programme for the postoperative period. This is important since many patients have prolonged mourning for lost limb and feel that they have no future. It is equally important that unrealistic promises are not made since the patient's progress may be inhibited if high expectations do not come to fruition. It is also helpful at this stage to introduce the patient to someone who has successfully adapted to amputation since this usually has more impact than anything the professional team can say.

Physical preparation is important. Control of concomitant heart failure, anaemia, diabetes and general disability of poor nutrition results in optimal success for operation and rehabilitation. Pre-operative exercises prevent joint contracture, improve balance, and increase muscle strength in preparation for postoperative rehabilitation. Vitali and Redhead (1967) describe the use of a prosthesis on which the patient kneels prior to operation (Fig. 6). This provides some preparation for the future prosthesis while improving balance and strength.

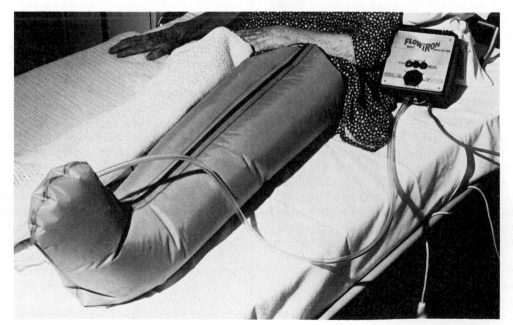

Figure 5   Pneumatic intermittent compression

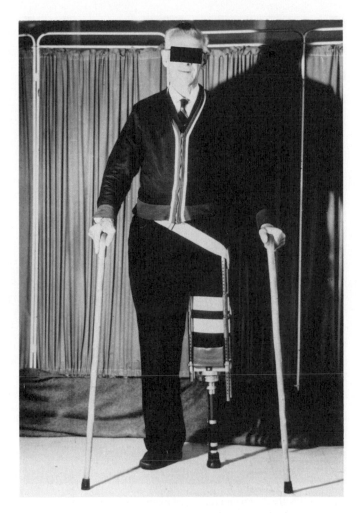

Figure 6   Preamputation training prosthesis

Correct positioning in the early postoperative period prevents contractures and the development of pressure sores. The heel of the so called 'good leg' is particularly vulnerable and must be protected at all costs. Skilled pressure gradient bandaging (Callen, 1981) helps to reduce oedema and results in a good shaped stump.

The occupational therapist is meanwhile training the patient to dress and carry out the activities of daily living. The physiotherapist supervises the exercises to strengthen muscles while maintaining a good range of joint movement and training the patient in balance techniques. Therapists and nurses, including night staff, should all be using the same techniques for transferring and all general activities.

Early mobilization on a temporary prosthesis improves the morale of the patient, lowers the postoperative mortality and morbidity, and results in a higher rate of patients walking at the time of discharge (Hutton and Rothnie, 1977). Mooney and coworkers (1971) have suggested that immediate use of the temporary prosthesis inhibits wound healing and recommended that mobilization is delayed until the wound has healed. However, if an ischial weight-bearing prosthesis is used, where there is no pressure on the stump, the increased circulation due to activity seems to improve the rate of healing.

The difficulty of getting frail elderly patients to limb-fitting centres for a temporary prosthesis has been overcome by the availability of

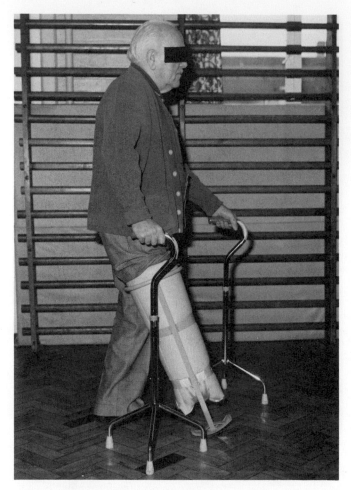

Figure 7   Pneumatic postamputation mobility aid

modular devices or the use of a pneumatic postamputation mobility aid, (Fig. 7). This is a metal cage with a rocker foot into which the stump is placed surrounded by an inflatable cuff. The patient can then use this as a pylon prior to receiving a definitive pylon (Fig. 8) and eventual cosmetic prosthesis (Fig. 9).

The use of wheelchairs in the early stage of rehabilitation is controversial. Some believe that wheelchairs deter the patient from trying to walk but there is a great psychological value in being able to get about the ward independently. Some elderly amputees do not achieve walking ability and therefore early wheelchair training prevents prolonged stay in hospital.

To prevent the patient toppling backwards a wheelchair with wheels set farther back than normal is required to counteract the change in the centre of gravity due to loss of the weight of the legs.

Assessment for the appropriate prosthesis requires the skilled teamwork of the artificial limb and appliance centre. Unfortunately these centres are often far from the patient's home and follow-up rehabilitation may be required from the local geriatric unit.

Much of the excellent work of limb-fitting centres is wasted if a comprehensive rehabilitation programme is not available. Van de Ven (1981) found that many problems exist because home visits were not made or were made after discharge with little planning for the future. She also found that many patients provided with a prosthesis did not use them after discharge from hospital. This emphasizes the need for careful planning at regular case con-

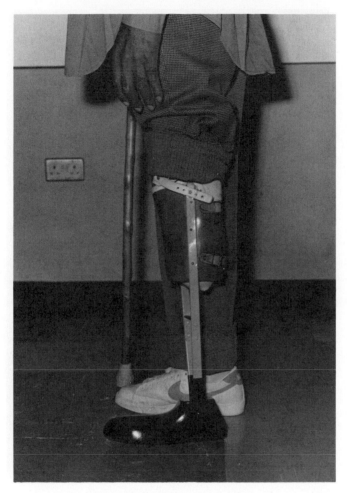

Figure 8   Below knee pylon

ferences with appropriate goal-setting. It is important at an early stage to have an assessment by therapists and social workers of the type of accommodation the patient will return to, the preamputation ability, and the expectations and hopes of the patient and his family.

There are three criteria for a prosthesis to be used: (a) it must be easy to fit – the patient who has difficulty will not wear it; (b) it must be practical – the patient who is frightened of falling or who has to cope with steps or uneven ground will discard the prosthesis; (c) it must be acceptable – many patients, especially women, demand a cosmetic limb that looks as much like the normal limb as possible. All of these facts must be considered when the team plans the rehabilitation programme.

The double amputee presents further prob-

lems. Sakuma *et al* (1974) and Weaver and Marshall (1973) found that about half of bilateral amputees were discharged walking. However, the older the patient the greater the problems with balance, cardiovascular disease, and basic strength. Even those patients who learn to balance on short rocker pylons may have difficulty managing at home since furniture is the wrong height and only a few, usually young below-knee amputees, progress onto full-length pylons.

Discharge needs careful planning. A predischarge home visit with the patient will allow any unexpected difficulties in the home to become known and resolved, increasing the patient's confidence of success. Discussion with the other professional staff who will be involved, viz. district nurse, health visitor, social

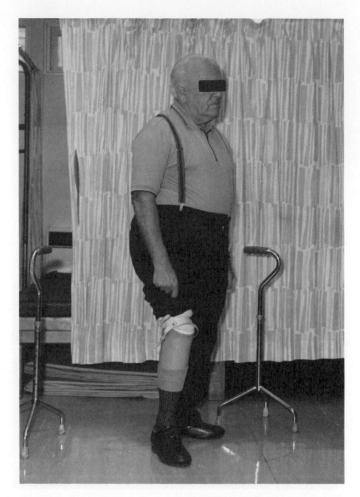

Figure 9   Patela tendon bearing prosthesis

worker, and community rehabilitation officer, should ensure that appropriate aids, adaptations, and services are available and that there is a coordinated programme of care. Weekend discharge should be avoided in order to allow optimum availability of necessary services.

Follow-up by the domiciliary physiotherapist will encourage achievement and maintenance of independent living and thus a resumption of previous social activities.

Social adaptation is often difficult and requires full discussion and understanding by the rehabilitation team, including the patient and his family. The counselling role of the social worker plays a vital part in the process of restoring the patient to a satisfactory place in his community.

AIDS AND APPLIANCES

There are numerous aids and appliances available for the disabled but a few principles can be indicated.

Elderly patients often have difficulty in adapting to new ideas and therefore it is wise to keep aids as simple as possible. For instance, few patients can cope with multipurpose equipment and therefore simple adaptation of their own cutlery is often more acceptable physically and emotionally.

Walking aids need careful selection. It is important for stability that the centre of gravity falls between the feet and therefore in the early stage of rehabilitation a frame is more useful than a stick because the latter encourages the balance to be shifted to one side. It must, however, be recognized that a frame is a prop and does not allow normal gait, the patient having to stop at each step to move the frame on. In this case a frame with wheels is more practical (Fig. 3).

Limb prostheses and wheelchairs require specialist assessment if inappropriate devices are to be avoided. Even so, Harris and coworkers (1974) found that only two-thirds of amputee survivors were using the prescribed artificial limb to any extent. Hollings and Haworth (1978) and Thornely, Chamberlain, and Wright (1977) have shown that up to one-third of aids provided are not used and Haworth and Hopkins (1980) found 46 per cent. of aids were not being used 3 months after operation for fractured femur. This suggests that careful selection and follow-up of the use of appliances is important.

THE REHABILITATION TEAM

The success of rehabilitation depends on the close liaison between all members of the rehabilitation team and this includes the patient and relative. Many so-called 'teams' are nothing more than a group of professionals who individually provide their specific skills in the management of the patient. Ideally the team must meet frequently, each aware of the progress being made by the others and using all the same techniques. Unless this happens the patient becomes confused by the different advice being given by each professional. It is also important that goals are planned and constantly reviewed with the patient and his relative.

Lubbock and Wright (1979) have suggested that updating in the case conference can be improved by recording progress on videotape which can then be shown to other members of the team, including night staff and the community liaison officers.

The role of the family cannot be overemphasized. Anderson, Anderson, and Kottke (1977) have shown that functional levels are maintained as much through the education of the patient's family as through the use of professional resources.

We have found (Andrews and Stewart, 1979) that about half of the stroke patients could carry out many more activities in the day hospital than they were attempting at home. In nearly every case this was because the relative had either not understood what the patient could do or insisted on carrying out the activities because of impatience or unnecessary concern.

A predischarge home visit can be useful in assessing those problems likely to occur in the home because of the physical environment and in the assessment of the psychosocial adjustment, not only of the patient but also of relatives and, just as important, neighbours.

ORGANIZATION

There are several potential methods of organizing rehabilitation for the elderly. Day hospitals were developed to separate the therapeutic from the hotel aspects of care (Brocklehurst, 1973) and to enable earlier discharge from hospital (Brocklehurst, 1964; Woodford-Williams et al., 1962). The role of day hospitals varies from providing social relief to those with a major emphasis on rehabilitation (Brocklehurst and Tucker, 1980).

Apart from the economic advantages to the hospital of not having to provide 24 hour staff and beds, the patient gains by being able to practice the relearned skills at home while still receiving treatment. Day hospitals are not without disadvantages. Ambulance delays and travelling to hospital can be demanding for the elderly (Beer et al., 1974). Frazer (1979) found that an ambulance was cancelled on at least one occasion for 20 per cent. of patients attending the day hospital and Prinsley (1971) has shown the deleterious effect of interrupted ambulance service on patients attending for rehabilitation. As many as eleven per cent. of patients cancel the appointment (Peach and Pathy, 1981), suggesting that day hospitals are not necessarily efficient in providing rehabilitation for all patients.

Home rehabilitation has been assessed by several workers (Frazer, 1979; Holgate, 1977; Partridge and Warren, 1977) and has been shown to be less expensive and required less treatment time than day hospital rehabilitation (Frazer, 1979) while relatives can be more easily involved in the rehabilitation programme.

SPECIALIZED REHABILITATION UNITS

There have been few studies on the value of inpatient rehabilitation therapy, but there is a great interest in the development of specialized units. The value of stroke units is as yet undecided. Some workers (Cooper, Olivet, and Woolsey, 1972; Drake *et al.*, 1973; Taylor, 1970; Truscott, 1972) have found that stroke units result in a fall in mortality, others (Kennedy *et al.*, 1970; Pitner and Mance, 1973) have been unable to find any associated reduction in death rate. In Britain the Royal College of Physicians (1974) felt that there was no need to duplicate the intensive care facilities already available, but that there were advantages in grouping stroke patients together to make the best use of the limited number of remedial therapists with a special experience and expertise in stroke rehabilitation.

Rehabilitation stroke units may increase the discharge rate (Dow, Dick, and Crowell, 1974), especially for severe strokes (Blower and Ali, 1979). McCann and coworkers (1976) found that although the stroke unit was no more successful than a general unit in rehabilitating patients with moderate or profound strokes, it was significantly better for treating those patients with severe strokes.

A stroke unit has been shown to improve the level of independence at the time of discharge (Garraway *et al.*, 1980a) though by the end of the first year there was no difference from the levels of independence from those discharged from a general medical ward (Garraway *et al.*, 1980b).

The incidence of fracture of the femur rises dramatically with increasing age (Donaldson, Stoyle, and Clarke, 1979) and as many as 17 per cent. of those patients admitted from home require long-stay care (Jensen, Tønderold, and Sørensen, 1979) while those who do return home often require markedly increased domestic support (Ceder *et al.*, 1979). In view of these difficulties orthopaedic – geriatric units have been set up (Clarke and Wainwright, 1966; Devas, 1964, 1974, 1976) to combine the specific skills of the orthopaedic surgeon and the geriatrician in the management of these patients.

It cannot be overemphasized that rehabilitation is more than specialist techniques. Rehabilitation at its best involves a large team of professionals working with a patient and his relative towards the goal of a happy, confident, and independent family. This can only be achieved when the team works together, each member knowing what the others are doing and with an agreed programme of techniques and goals.

REFERENCES

Ada, L., and Scott, D. (1980). 'Use of inhibitory, weight-bearing plasters to increase movement in the presence of spasticity', *Aust. J. Physiother.*, **26**)2), 57–61.

Adams, G. F., and Hurwitz, L. J. (1975). 'Rehabilitation of hemiplegia: Indices of assessment and prognosis', *Br. Med. J.*, **1**, 94–98.

Adams, G. F., and McComb, S. G. (1953). 'Assessment and prognosis in hemiplegia', *Lancet*, **2**, 266–269.

Anderson, E. K. (1971). 'Sensory impairment in hemiplegia', *Arch. Phys. Med. Rehabil.*, **52**, 293–297.

Anderson, E., Anderson, T. P., and Kottke, F. J. (1977). 'Stroke rehabilitation: Maintenance of achieved gains', *Arch. Phys. Med. Rehabil.*, **58**, 345–352.

Anderson, E. K., and Choy, E. (1970). 'Parietal lobe syndrome in hemiplegia', *Am. J. Occup. Ther.*, **24**, 13–18.

Andrews, K., Brocklehurst, J. C., Richards, B., and Laycock, P. J. (1980). 'The prognostic value of picture drawings by stroke patients', *Rheumatol. Rehabil.*, **19**, 180–188.

Andrews, K., Brocklehurst, J. C., Richards, B., and Laycock, P. J. (1981). 'The rate of recovery from stroke – and its measurement', *Int. Rehabil. Med.*, **3**, 155–161.

Andrews, K., and Stewart, J. (1979). 'Stroke recovery: He can but does he?', *Rheumatol. Rehabil.*, **18**, 43–48.

Baker, R. N., Schwartz, W. S., and Ramseyer, J. C. (1968). 'Prognosis among survivors of ischaemic stroke', *Neurology (NY)*, **18**, 933–941.

Bassett C. A. L., Mitchell S. N., and Gaston S. R. (1981). 'Treatment of ununited tibial diaphyseal fracture with pulsing electromagnetic fields', *J. Bone Joint Surg.*, **63A**, 511–523.

Beer, T. C., Goldberg, E., Smith, D. S., and Mason, A. S. (1974). 'Can I have an ambulance doctor?', *Br. Med. J.*, **1**, 226–228.

Birkhan, J., Carmon, A., Meretsky, P., and Zinder, H. (1980). 'Clinical effects of a new TENS using multiple electrodes and constant energy', *Acta. Anaesthesiol. Belg.*, **31** (Suppl.), 239–245.

Blower, P., and Ali, S. (1979). 'A stroke unit in a district general hospital: The Greenwich experience', *Br. Med. J.*, **2**, 644–646.

Bobath, B. (1978). 'Adult hemiplegia: Evaluation and treatment', 2nd ed., William Heineman, London.

Brattström, M. (1973). *Principle of Joint Protection in Chronic Rheumatic Disease*, Wolfe Medical Books, London.

Brighton, C. T., Black, J., Friedenberg, Z. B., Esterhai, J. L., Day, L. J., and Connolly, J. F. (1981). 'Multicentre study of treatment of non-union with constant direct current', *J. Bone Joint Surg.*, **63A** (1), 2–13.

Brocklehurst, J. C. (1964). 'The work of the geriatric day hospital', *Gerontol. Clin.*, **6**, 151–166.

Brocklehurst, J. C. (1973). In *Textbook of Geriatric Medicine and Gerontology*, (Ed. J. C. Brocklehurst), pp. 683–686, Churchill Livingstone.

Brocklehurst, J. C., and Tucker, J. S. (1980). *Progress in Geriatric Day Care*, King Edward's Hospital Fund.

Brunnstrom, S. (1970). *Movement Therapy in Hemiplegia*, Harper and Row.

Caillet, R. (1980). *The Shoulder in Hemiplegia*, F. A. Davis, Philadelphia.

Callen, S. (1981). A modern method of stump bandaging', *Physiotherapy*, **67** (5), 137–138.

Carr, J. H., and Shepherd, R. (1980). In *Physiotherapy in Disorders of the Brain*, pp. 378–382, Heinmann Medical.

Carroll, D. (1962). 'The disability in hemiplegia caused by cerebrovascular disease', *J. Chronic Dis.*, **15**, 179–189.

Cassvan, A., Ross, A. L., Dyer, P. R., and Zane, L. (1976). 'Lateralisation in stroke syndrome. A factor in ambulation', *Arch. Phys. Med. Rehabil.*, **57** (12), 583–587.

Ceder, L., Ekelund, L., Inerot, S., Lindberg, L., Odberg, E., and Sjölin, C. (1979). 'Rehabilitation after hip fracture in the elderly', *Acta. Orthop. Scand.*, **50**, 681–688.

Cherry, D. B. (1980). 'Review of physical therapy alternative for reducing muscle contractures', *Phys. Ther.*, **60** (7), 877–881.

Clarke, A. N. G., and Wainwright, D. (1966). 'Management of the fractured neck of femur in the elderly female: A joint approach of orthopaedic surgery and geriatric medicine', *Gerontol. Clin.*, **8**, 321–326.

Cooper, S. W., Olivet, J. A., and Woolsey, F. M. (1972). 'Establishment and operation of Combined Intensive Care Units', *NY J. Med.*, **72**, 2215–2220.

Davis, S. W., and Chu, D. S. (1974). 'Air current treatment for decubitus ulcers', *Arch. Phys. Med. Rehabil.*, **55**, 138–139.

Devas, M. B. (1964). 'Fracture in the elderly', *Gerontol. Clin.*, **6**, 347–359.

Devas, M. B. (1974). 'Geriatric orthopaedics', *Br. Med. J.*, **1**, 190–192.

Devas, M. B. (1976). 'Geriatric orthopaedics', *Ann. Roy. Coll. Surg. Engl.*, **58** (1), 16–21.

Donaldson, L. J., Stoyle, T. F., and Clarke, M. (1979). 'Fractured neck of femur in Leicestershire', *Public Health*, **93**, 285–289.

Dow, R. S., Dick, H. L., and Crowell, F. A. (1974). 'Failures and successes in a stroke programme', *Stroke*, **5**, 40–47.

Drake, W. E., Hamilton, M. J., Carlsson, M., and Blumenkrantz, J. (1973). 'Acute stroke management and patient outcome: The value of neurovascular care unit', *Stroke*, **4**, 933–945.

Dyson, M., and Pond, J. M. (1970). 'Effect of pulsed ultrasound on tissue regeneration', *Physiotherapy*, **56**, 136–142.

Dyson, M., and Suckling, J. (1978). 'Stimulation of tissue repair by ultrasound: A survey of the mechanisms involved', *Physiotherapy*, **64** (4), 105–108.

Ebersold, M. J., Laws, E. R., Stonnington, H. H., and Stillwell, G. K. (1975). 'Transcutaneous electrical stimulation for treatment of chronic pain: A preliminary study', *Surg. Neurol.*, **4**, 96–98.

Ekroth, R., Dahllöf, A., Gunderall, B., and Holm, J. (1978). 'Physical training of patients with intermittent claudication: Indications, methods and results', *Surgery*, **84**, 640–643.

Fisher, S. V., and Patterson, R. P. (1981). 'Energy cost of ambulation with crutches', *Arch. Phys. Med. Rehabil.*, **62**, 250–256.

Fox, J. V. D. (1964). 'Cutaneous stimulation effects on selected tests of perception', *Am. J. Occup. Ther.*, **18**, 53–55.

Frazer, W. F. (1979). *Evaluation of a Domiciliary Physiotherapy Source to the Elderly*, M. Phil. Thesis, University of Aston and Birmingham.

Garraway, W. M., Akhtar, A. J., Prescott, R. J., and Hockey, L. (1980a). 'Management of acute stroke in the elderly: Preliminary results of a controlled trial', *Br. Med. J.*, **1**, 1040–1043.

Garraway, W. M., Akhtar, A. J., Hockey, L., and Prescott, R. J. (1980b). 'Management of acute stroke in the elderly: Follow up of a controlled trial', *Br. Med. J.*, **2**, 826–829.

Gonzalez, E. G., Corcoran, P. J., and Reyes, R. L. (1974). 'Energy expenditure in below knee amputees: Correlation with stump length', *Arch. Phys. Med. Rehabi.*, **55**, 111–119.

Grant, A. E. (1964). 'Massage with ice in the treatment of painful conditions of the musculoskeletal system', *Arch. Phys. Med. Rehabil.*, **45**, 233–238.

Gresham, G. E., Fitzpatrick, T. E., Wolf, P. A., McNamara, P. M., Kannel, W. B., and Dawbert, T. R. (1975). 'Residual disability in survivors of stroke – The Framinham Study', *New Engl. J. Med.*, **293**, 954–956.

Griffiths, V. E. (1975). 'Volunteer scheme for dysphasia and allied problems in stroke patients', *Br. Med. J.*, **3**, 633–635.

Griffiths, V. E. (1980). 'Observation on patients dysphasic after a stroke', *Br. Med. J.*, **2**, 1608–1609.

Griffiths, V. E., and Miller, C. L. (1980). 'Volunteer stroke scheme for dysphasic patients with stroke', *Br. Med. J.*, **2**, 1605–1607.

Hamilton, E. A., and Nichols, P. J. R. (1972). 'Rehabilitation of the elderly lower limb amputee', *Br. Med. J.*, **2**, 95–99.

Harris, P. L., Read, F., Eardley, A., Charlesworth, D., Wakefield, J., and Sellwood, R. A. (1974). 'The fate of elderly amputees', *Br. J. Surg.*, **61**, 665–668.

Haworth, R. J., and Hopkins, J. (1980). 'Use of aids following total hip replacement', *Brit. J. Occ. Therap.*, **43**, 398–400.

Hayden, C. A. (1964). 'Cryokinetics in early treatment programme', *Phys. Ther.*, **44**, 990–993.

Hayes, N. K., and Burns, Y. R. (1970). 'Discussion on the use of weight bearing plasters in the reduction of hypertonicity', *Aust. J. Physiother.*, **16** (3), 108–117.

Hayne, J. A. (1980). 'The effect of exercise with early claudication'. *Physiotherapy*, **66** (8), 260–261.

Heckman, J. D., Ingram, A. J., Lloyd, R. O., Luck, J. V., and Mayer, P. W. (1981). 'Non-union treatment with pulsed electromagnetic field', *Clin. Orthopaed.*, **161**, 58–66.

Holgate, B. (1977). 'Report of a pilot scheme for a domiciliary physiotherapy service', *J. Chest Heart and Stroke Assoc.*, **2**, 38–42.

Hollings, E. M., and Haworth, R. J. (1978). 'Supply and use of aids and appliances – a study of 119 patients with rheumatoid arthritis', *Brit. J. Occ. Therap.*, **41**, 336–337.

Hurd, M. M., Farrell, K. H., and Waylonis, G. W. (1974). 'Shoulder sling for hemiplegia, friend or foe?', *Arch. Phys. Med. Rehabil.*, **55**, 519–522.

Hutton, I. M., and Rothnie, M. G. (1977). 'The early mobilization of the elderly amputee', *Br. J. Surg.*, **64** (4), 267–270.

Inglis, J., Sproule, M., Leicht, M., Donald, M. W., and Campbell, D. (1976). 'Electromyographic biofeedback treatment of residual neuromuscular disabilities after cerebrovascular accident', *J. Can. Physiother. Assoc.*, **28** (5), 260–264.

Jensen, J. S., Tønderold, E., and Sørensen, P. H. (1979). 'Social rehabilitation following hip fracture', *Acta. Orthop. Scand.*, **50**, 777–785.

Johnstone, M. (1983). *Restoration of Motor Function in the Stroke Patient*, 2nd ed., Churchill Livingstone.

Jonason, T., Jonzon, B., Ringqvist, I., and Oman-Rydberg, A. (1979). Effect of physical training on different categories of patients with intermittent claudication', *Acta. Med. Scand.*, **206**, 253–258.

Jorgensen, T. E. (1977). 'Electrical stimulation of human fracture healing by means of a slow pulsating, asymmetrical direct current', *Clin. Orthop.*, **143**, 124–127.

Kabat, J. (1965). 'Analysis and therapy of cerebellar ataxia and asynergia', *AMA Arch. Neurol.*, **4**, 375–382.

Katz, L. (1958). 'Learning in aphasic patients', *J. Consult. Clin. Psychol.*, **22**, 143–146.

Katz, S., Ford, A. B., Chinn, A. B., and Newill, V. (1966). 'A prognosis after stroke. Part II. Long term course of 159 patients', *Medicine (Balt.)*, **45**, 236–246.

Kendal, P. H., and Jenkins, J. M. (1968). 'Exercises for backache: A double blind controlled trial', *Physiotherapy*, **54**, 154–157.

Kennedy, F. B., Pozen, T. J., Gabelman, E. H., Tuthill, J. E., and Zaentz, S. D. (1970). 'Stroke intensive care – an approval', *Am. Heart J.*, **80** (2), 188–196.

Knott, M., and Voss, D. E. (1968). *Proprioceptive Neuromuscular Facilitation*, Harper and Row, New York.

Knutsson, E. (1970). 'Topical cryotherapy in spasticity', *Scan. J. Rehab. Med.*, **2**, 159–163.

Lane, L. E. (1971). 'Localised hypothermia for relief of pain in musculoskeletal injuries', *Phys. Ther.*, **51**, 182–183.

Lee, J. M., and Warren, M. P. (1978). In *Cold Therapy in Rehabilitation*, pp. 51–53, Bell and Hyman.

Lehmann, J. F. (1965). 'Ultrasonic Therapy', in *Therapeutic Heat* (Ed. S. Licht), pp. 326–386, Waverley Press, Baltimore, Maryland.

Levin, H. S., and Benton, A. L. (1973). 'Age effects in proprioceptive feedback performance', *Gerontol Clin. (Basel)*, **15**, 161–169.

Loeser, J., Black, and R., Christman, A. (1975). 'Relief of pain by transcutaneous stimulation', *J. Neurosurg.*, **42**, 308–314.

Long, D. M., and Hagfors, N. (1975). 'Electrical stimulation in the nervous system', *Pain*, **1**, 109–123.

Lorenze, E. J., Carantonis, G., and De Rosa, A. J. (1960). 'Effect on coronary circulation of cold packs to hemiplegic shoulder', *Arch. Phys. Med. Rehabil.*, **41**, 394–399.

Lubbock, G., and Wright, W. B. (1979). 'How video tape has improved the case conference', *Ger. Med.*, **9** (11), 3.

McCann, R. C., and Culbertson, R. A. (1976). 'Comparison of two systems for stroke rehabilitation in a general hospital', *J. Am. Geriatr. Soc.*, **24** (5), 211–216.

Mair, A. (1972). *Report of Subcommittee of the Standing Medical Advisory Committee*, Scottish Health Service Council on Medical Rehabilitation, HMSO, Edinburgh.

Marquardsen, J. (1969). 'The natural history of acute cerebrovascular disease', *Acta. Neurol. Scand.*, **45** (Suppl., 38).

Miglietta, O. (1973). 'Action of cold on spasticity', *Am. J. Phys. Med.*, **52** (4), 198–205.

Miglietta, O., Lewitan, A., and Rogoff, J. B. (1959). 'Subluxation of the shoulder in hemiplegic patients', *NY State J. Med.*, **59**, 457–460.

Mooney, V., Harvey, J. P., Jr, McBride, E., and Snelson, R. (1971). 'Comparison of post operative stump management: Plaster vs soft dressing', *J. Bone Joint Surg.*, **53A** (2), 241–249.

Morgan, M. H. (1980). 'Ataxia – its causes, measurement and management', *Int. Rehabil. Med.*, **2**, 126–132.

Nathan, P. W., and Wall, P. D. (1974). 'Treatment of post herpetic neuralgia by prolonged electrical stimulation', *Br. Med. J.*, **3**, 645–647.

New, P. K., Ruscio, A. T., and George, L. A. (1969). 'Toward an understanding of the rehabilitation system', *Rehabil. Ltd.*, **30**, 130–139.

O'Brien, M. T., and Pallet, P. J. (1978). In *Total Care of the Stroke Patient*, Little, Brown and Co., Boston.

Partridge, C. J., and Warren, M. D. (1977). *Physiotherapy in the Community*, Health Services Research Unit, University of Kent at Canterbury.

Peach, H., and Pathy, M. S. (1981). 'Role of non-attendance statistics in assessing the efficiency of geriatric day hospitals', *Community Med.*, **3**, 123–130.

Perry, C. E. (1967). 'Principles and techniques of Brunnstrom approach to the treatment of hemiplegia', *Am. J. Phys. Med.*, **46**, 789–815.

Pesczczynski, M. (1961). 'Prognosis for rehabilitation of the older adult and the aged hemiplegic patient', *Am. J. Cardiol.*, **7**, 365–369.

Pitner, S. E., and Mance, C. J. (1973). 'An evaluation of Stroke intensive care: Results in a municipal hospital', *Stroke*, **4**, 737–741.

Prinsley, D. M. (1971). 'Effects of industrial action by the ambulance service on the day hospital patient', *Br. Med. J.*, **3**, 170–171.

Richerson, R. L., and Richerson, M. E. (1981). 'Energy expenditure in simulated tasks: Comparison between subjects with brain injury and able-bodied persons', *Arch. Phys. Med. Rehabil.*, **62**, 212–214.

Rizk, T. E., and Park, S. J. (1981). 'Transcutaneous nerve electrical stimulation and extensor splint in knee scleroderma knee contracture'. *Arch. Phys. Med. Rehabil.*, **62**, (2) 86–88.

Rosenberg, B., Edwards, A. (1964) 'The performance of aphasia in three automated perceptual discrimination programs', *J. Speech Hear Res.*, **7**, 295–298.

Royal College of Physicians, London (1974). *Report on the Geriatrics Committee Working Group on Strokes*.

Sakuma, J., Hinterbuchner, C., Green, R. F., and Silber, M. (1974). 'Rehabilitation of geriatric patients having bilateral lower extremity amputations', *Arch. Phys. Med. Rehabil.*, **55**, 101–111.

Sarno, M. T., Silverman, M., and Sands, E. (1970). 'Speech therapy and language recovery in severe aphasia', *J. Speech Hear Res.*, **13**, 607–623.

Semans, S. (1967). 'The Bobath concept in the treatment of neuromuscular disorders', *Am. J. Phys. Med.*, **46**, 732–788.

Siev, E. and Freishtat, B. (1976). In *Perceptual Dysfunction in the Adult Stroke Patient*, Charles B. Slack.

Stern, P. H., McDowell, F., Miller, J. M., and Robinson, M. (1971). 'Factors influencing rehabilitation', *Stroke*, **2**, 213–215.

Stewart, H. F., and Abzug, J. L., and Harris, G. R. (1980). 'Consideration in ultrasound therapy and equipment performance', *Phys. Ther.*, **60** (4), 424–428.

Stockmeyer, S. A. (1967). 'An interpretation of the approach of Rood to the treatment of neuromuscular dysfunction', *Am. J. Phys. Med.*, **46**, 900–961.

Sutcliffe, M. L., Sharrard, W. J. W., and MacEarchern, A. G. (1980). 'The treatment of fracture non-union by electromagnetic induction', *J. Bone Joint Surg.*, **63B**, 123–127.

Taylor, R. R. (1970). 'Acute stroke demonstration project in a community hospital', *J. SC Med. Assoc.*, **66**, 225–227.

Thornely, G., Chamberlain, M. A., and Wright, V. (1977). 'Evaluation of aids and equipment for the bath and toilet', *Br. J. Occup. Ther.*, **40**, 243–244.

Tikofsky, R. S., and Reynolds, G. (1962). 'Preliminary study: Non-verbal learning and aphasia', *J. Speech Hear Res.*, **5**, 133–143.

Truscott, B. L. (1972). 'Health care delivery in the community: Use of available resources', *JAMA*, **221**, 289–291.

Van de Ven, C. M. C. (1981) 'An investigation into the management of bilateral amputees', *Br. Med. J.*, **283**, 707–710.

Vignolo, L. A. (1964). 'Evolution of aphasia and language rehabilitation', *Cortex*, **1**, 344–367.

Vitali, M., and Redhead, R. G. (1967). 'The modern concept of the general management of amputee rehabilitation'. *Ann. Roy. Coll. Surg. Engl.*, **40**, 251–260.

Voss, D. E. (1967). 'Proprioceptive neuromuscular facilitation'. *Am. J. Phys. Med.*, **46**, 838–899.

Waylonis, G. W., Keith, M. W., and Aseff, J. N. (1973). 'Stroke rehabilitation in a Midwestern county', *Arch. Phys. Med. Rehabil.*, **54**, 151–155.

Weaver, P. C., and Marshall, S. A. (1973). 'A functional and social review of lower-limb amputees', *Br. J. Surg.*, **60** (9), 732–737.

Weinberg, J., Diller, L., Gordon, W. A., Gerstman, L. J., Lieberman, A., Lakin, P., Hodges, G., and Ezzrachi, O. (1977). 'Visual scanning training effect on reading, related tasks in acquired right brain damage', *Arch. Phys. Med. Rehabil.*, **58**, 479–486.

Weinberg, J., Diller, L., Gordon, W. A., Gerstman, L. J., Lieberman, A., Lakin, M. A., Hodges, G. and Ezrachi, O. (1979). 'Training sensory awareness and spatial organisation in people with right brain damage', *Arch. Phys. Med. Rehabil.*, **60**, 491–496.

Wiesel, S. W., Cuckler, J. M., Deluca, F., Jones, F., Zeide, M. S., and Rothman, R. H. (1980). 'Acute low back ache: An objective analysis of conservative therapy'. *Spine*, **5** (4), 324–330.

Woodford-Williams, E., McKeon, J. A., Trotter, I. S., Watson, D., and Bushby, C. (1962). 'The day hospital in the community care of the elderly', *Gerontol. Clin.*, **4**, 241–256.

Wright, W. B. (1979). 'Stammering gait', *Age Ageing*, **8** (1), 8–12.

Zetterquist, S. (1970). 'Effect of daily training on the nutritive blood flow in exercising ischaemic legs', *Scand. J. Clin. Lab. Invest.*, **25**, 101–111.

30
Delivery of Health Care

Principles and Practice of Geriatric Medicine
Edited by M. S. J. Pathy
© 1985 John Wiley & Sons Ltd

30.1

Delivery of Health Care in the United Kingdom

M. R. P. Hall

HISTORICAL DEVELOPMENTS

The delivery of health care to the elderly has evolved gradually in the United Kingdom over the course of the last hundred years. Following the introduction of the Poor Law, poor houses developed and it was to these that the destitute elderly went. As a result of improved living standards, following the industrial revolution, more people began to reach old age and the need to care for the elderly sick, who were also poor, led to the development of the poorhouse infirmaries so that, by the 1930s, every poor house had its own infirmary. While the nursing care in these infirmaries was usually excellent, the medical care was rudimentary until in 1935 the West Middlesex hospital took over the adjacent poor law infirmary. The task of looking after the large numbers of aged chronic sick which this institution contained was given to Dr Marjory Warren. It is as a direct result of her work and that of other pioneers like her that the specialty of geriatric medicine has developed.

The evolution of geriatric medical services in the United Kingdom has recently been reviewed by Anderson (1981) who has emphasized the important part that many disciplines have to play in the geriatric team. The doctor and the nurse need help to deal with the special problems of old people and they may be assisted by the physiotherapist, occupational therapist, speech therapist, chiropodist, and the social worker, who in their turn can call upon many social services as well as enlist the support of voluntary agencies and helpers.

GERIATRIC MEDICINE

Geriatric medicine has been defined as that branch of medicine which is concerned with the clinical, rehabilitative, preventive and social aspects of health and illness in the elderly. Like any short definition, this one has its drawbacks. Nevertheless, it can be made to cover all aspects of the care of the elderly if the word clinical is used to cover both physical and mental illness, and prevention is understood to include the maintenance of health as well as the prevention of illness. Any total health care programme which is going to maintain health and prevent illness as well as treat and rehabilitate those who are ill, will inevitably involve many disciplines and an enormous spread of resources. The potential resources needed to provide a comprehensive health care service are listed in Table 1. Most of these resources, if not all, will be available in every health district.

There seems to be little doubt that the delivery of health care to the elderly is a growth industry. Indeed, a recent working party has published the results of its findings under the title *The Impending Crisis of Old Age, a Challenge to Ingenuity*. The reasons for this are many. Better living standards and public health, for instance, have meant that more people are surviving into old age. Families are smaller and consequently contain fewer young people to care for the old who survive. Changes in society and in employment opportunities mean that families may need to move away from their home towns in search of jobs.

Table 1   Potential resources needed to provide a comprehensive service to the elderly

1. Geriatric hospital beds
2. Hospital services of other specialities (general medicine, surgery, orthopaedics, etc.)
3. Psychogeriatric beds
4. Geriatric day hospitals
5. EMI or psychogeriatric day hospitals
6. Geriatric outpatient clinics
7. Psychogeriatric outpatient clinics
8. General practitioners
9. Domiciliary nurses
10. Psychogeriatric domiciliary nurses
11. Health visitors
12. 'Hospital at home' service
13. Occupational therapists and aides
14. Physiotherapists and aides
15. Speech therapists and aides
16. Hearing therapists
17. Clinical psychologists
18. Chiropodists
19. Pharmacists and pharmacies
20. Social Workers
21. Local Authority residential homes for the elderly
22. Day centres and luncheon clubs for the elderly
23. Home helps (including a 'heavy duty' squad)
24. Meals-on-wheels
25. Loans/aids/adaptors
26. Telephone installation
27. Sheltered housing (warden-assisted)
28. Private nursing homes and rest homes
29. Care attendant service
30. Evening and night nursing services
31. Home sitting service
32. Tucking-in service
33. Voluntary services, visiting schemes, clubs, etc.
34. Transport (e.g. concessionary bus fares, OAP rail concession)
35. Telephone service
36. Education
37. Leisure activities, 'sport for all'
38. Money

The old are left behind, frequently in inappropriate housing, in decaying city centres. They become therefore more dependent on health and social services than previous generations.

In the United Kingdom, the development of the National Health Service has meant that the old poor law infirmaries have been taken under the wing of district general hospitals. The medical work-load necessary to provide appropriate care for these supposedly 'chronic sick' has been recognized and general physicians trained in modern medical technology have used their skill and ingenuity to ameliorate degenerative diseases so that many elderly patients have been rehabilitated to lead relatively independent lives in their own homes. More-

over, advances in medical technology mean that potentially better care becomes available as a result of more accurate diagnosis. Methods of organ imaging have become less invasive and more accurate, so that ethical problems which might previously have caused one to baulk at further investigations are no longer applicable. Consequently, Charcot's dream of a better understanding of senile pathology is now attainable (Charcot, 1881).

This means that geriatric medicine or clinical gerontology has a 'respectable' base in scientific technological medicine. Undergraduate medical students and others can see it as a satisfying branch of medicine from which the rewards of cure have not been banished. As a result of this development Chairs of Geriatric Medicine, the Health Care of the Elderly, and even Gerontology have been created and research into various aspects of ageing and its problems is developing. This is obviously most important. Nevertheless, while it may be possible to reduce the total amount of morbidity which occurs in old age, some will remain and the irremediable frail patient will continue to exist (Isaacs, Livingstone, and Neville, 1972). The need to cater for these people must remain part of the care of the elderly. It is important that geriatric medicine itself does not become so specialized that it forgets the needs of those whom it cannot cure or rehabilitate.

We are, however, a long way from this stage. As yet, the attitudes of a great many professionals and most of the general public need to be altered with regard to the old and the subject of ageing. There is still a great necessity to research the needs of individuals and what happens to them when they are old. Ingenuity is necessary to provide the appropriate services and above all there is need to educate the young and middle aged about ageing. Pre-retirement education and preparation for retirement is of vital importance.

THE INFLUENCE OF GOVERNMENTAL AND NATIONAL BODIES ON THE HEALTH CARE OF THE ELDERLY

The provision of an efficient health care service for the elderly depends on many people, resources and organizations. While the actual delivery of health care to the individual depends on the arrangement and provision of local services the influence that governmental or national bodies and institutions have on this is substantial but often unrecognized.

Department of Health and Social Security

The Department of Health and Social Security (DHSS) is the central government agency which ensures that parliamentary legislation enacted with regard to the health and social care of the elderly is put into effect. From time to time it issues guidelines in the form of health memoranda and circulars as well as letters to the Regional Health Authorities (DHSS, 1971a, 1971b, 1972a). These have laid down guidelines for the number of hospital beds and day places for geriatric and psycho-geriatric patients (DS329/71 and HM72/71); and for social services provision (HM35/72) consultative documents such as *Priorities for Health and Personal Social Services in England* (DHSS, 1976) have been issued and more recently, a discussion document 'A Happier Old Age' has appeared (DHSS, 1978). Within the DHSS some medical officers and administrators are given special responsibility to oversee the health care needs of the elderly. They are advised by clinicians practising in the field of geriatric medicine and psychiatry and initiate research into aspects of health care so that appropriate advice may be given to the Secretary of State and Minister of Health. The DHSS has also encouraged the establishment of Chairs of Geriatric Medicine throughout the United Kingdom and it has also been responsible for setting up the Health Advisory Service.

There is no doubt that the DHSS and its officers have done a very great deal in the past 15 to 20 years to improve the health care service for the elderly.

Health Advisory Services (HAS)

This service was set up in 1969 to look at the psychiatric service after a series of 'scandals' had been reported in the press. Since some of these involved the care of the elderly people, the service was expanded to monitor both the Psychogeriatric and Geriatric Medical Services. The role of the HAS is to create and stimulate change by the creation of good practice. Its multidisciplinary team comprising doc-

tor, nurse, administrator, therapist, and perhaps social worker, visits a district service and discusses its operational policy and performance with the district's own team of doctors, nurses, therapists, administrators, and social workers. In its reports it praises what is good and criticizes what is poor in the district's service for the health care of the elderly. It also issues advice and makes recommendations. Unfortunately, it is not always possible for districts to implement the recommendations as rapidly as they are needed. While the HAS has no direct power to force local health authorities to improve services there is no doubt that its presence has increased standards of care throughout England and Wales. A district receiving an adverse report may be asked for its comments and further visits from an HAS team may be made to monitor progress and help the district with further suggestions.

General Medical Council, Royal Colleges, and the British Medical Association (BMA)

Recently the education committee of the General Medical Council (1980) has issued new recommendations concerning the medical undergraduate curriculum. This now emphasizes that 'principles of demography should also be taught, including the effects upon society, and upon medical practice, of the increasing number of elderly people in the population . . .'. Also that during his or her clinical studies the 'attention of the student should be constantly directed to the importance of the inter-relationship of the physical, psychological and social aspects of disease and the growing importance of the problems posed by disability and disease in an increasing elderly population.' Moreover, 'students should be introduced to the care of the chronic elderly psychiatric sick . . .' and 'should receive instruction in the special problems of diagnosis and treatment of illness in the elderly and in maintaining mental and physical health in old age. He should be introduced to the range of domiciliary and institutional services available for the care of the elderly.'

This means that geriatric medicine and psychiatry must be included in undergraduate medical curricula. This should mean that all doctors will, on qualification, have some knowledge of the health care of the elderly.

The Royal Colleges, particularly the Royal Colleges of Physicians of London and Edinburgh, have been at the forefront of looking at the problems relating to the care of the elderly. The Joint Committee on Higher Medical Training of the Royal Colleges has a specialist advisory committee in geriatric medicine which is responsible for the inspection and approval of training posts in the specialty of geriatric medicine as well as the accreditation of specialists who have carried out appropriate training. The London College has a geriatric medical sub-committee, and has recently published a report on the *Medical Care for the Elderly* (1977), while the Edinburgh College published a similar report on the *Care of the Elderly in Scotland* in 1963, and a follow-up report in 1970. These reports have done much to establish the specialty of geriatric medicine throughout the United Kingdom and have had considerable influence on the delivery of health care to the elderly.

Similarly, the British Medical Association published its first report on the care and treatment of the elderly and infirm in 1949 and up-dated this report in 1976.

The British Geriatrics Society and Other Professional Bodies

In 1947 a small group of interested doctors practising in the field of the care of the elderly decided to meet together in order to discuss their experience. They elected a Chairman, Lord Amulree, and formed a society for the medical care of the elderly. Over the years, this society has blossomed and become the British Geriatrics Society. Its influence on the medical care of the elderly has been profound. A medical officer from the Department of Health attends its Council meetings as an observer, it nominates members to the Geriatric Medical Subcommittee of the Council of the Royal College of Physicians in London, and it nominates the members of the specialist advisory committee to the Joint Committee for Higher Medical Training of the Royal Colleges. Its opinion is sought by government whenever matters which may relate to the medical care of the elderly are being promulgated or discussed. Its main objective is to promote and improve the health care of the elderly and to achieve this it has promoted research, initiated working parties, organized multidisciplinary conferences, as well as holding biannual meetings of its members.

Examples of some of its work has been a paper on the training of general practitioners in geriatric medicine, issued jointly with the Royal College of General Practitioners (British Geriatrics Society and RCGP, 1978); a paper in collaboration with the Royal College of Psychiatry's section for the psychiatry of old age on the care of the elderly mentally infirm; a booklet entitled *Improving Geriatric Care in Hospitals* published as a result of a joint working party with the Royal College of Nursing. The Society's journal is *Age and Ageing*.

The Nursing Profession

In addition to publishing the above report the Royal College of Nursing has established its own group of nurses interested in geriatric nursing. This group meets regularly and has held joint conferences with the British Geriatrics Society and its members.

In addition, the Joint Board of Clinical Nursing Studies has approved post basic courses in the care of the elderly. One of these courses lasts for about 6 months and is designed to train nurses in all aspects of the specialty including the clinical, social, psychological, and psychiatric aspects of care. Another course is of much shorter duration, being of approximately 10 to 15 days in length and is run on a day-release basis. Both courses are certificated on completion.

Professions Supplementary to Medicine

Recent reports on rehabilitation (Tunbridge Report: DHSS, 1972b) and speech therapy (Quirk Report: Dept. Ed. & Sci., 1972) have both emphasized the important role which members of these professions have to play in the care of the elderly. Study days and conferences on this topic have been organized on a local or regional basis, and in Wessex the Association of Occupational Therapists have formed a special interest group with regard to the care of the elderly which holds a biannual day conference.

Social Work

The Central Council for Education and Training in Social Work has recognized the important part that social work has to play in the care of the elderly by ensuring that the Certificate of Social Work has an option on the elderly which can be taken by students during this course. It has also approved a postqualification course in social work for the elderly which is held yearly at the University of Southampton, who grant a Diploma to those who participate successfully.

The British Society for Behavioural and Social Gerontology which was formed in 1970 has recently changed its title to the British Society of Gerontology. It holds regular meetings and has initiated an excellent journal entitled *Ageing and Society*.

British Society for Research into Ageing (BSRA) and the British Foundation for Age Research (BFAR)

The British Society for Research into Ageing was founded by the late Dr Vladimir Korenchevesky and has formed a focal point for those scientists and biologists who have developed an interest in the ageing process in living cells and tissues. The Society is a small one but has fulfilled the important function of keeping alive an interest in experimental gerontology. This has recently reached a climax with the foundation of the Wolfson Institute of Gerontology in the University of Hull which has given a big boost to interest and development in the sphere of ageing research.

The British Foundation for Age Research was born as a result of Age Action Year (1976). This is a charitable fund-raising body whose objectives are to stimulate research into all aspects of ageing as well as encouraging educational activities in this field. At present the Foundation acts purely as a fund-raising organization but it has already promoted research into incontinence, senile dementia, and other topics.

Voluntary Organizations

Age Concern

Age Concern is an organization of voluntary workers who have a special interest in the care and support of elderly people in the United Kingdom. England, Scotland, Wales, and Northern Ireland each have their national Age Concern organization. Age Concern is a registered charity, whose main objective is to promote the welfare of elderly people. It brings together all the major national voluntary and professional groups throughout Britain who provide support services to the elderly. These include visiting schemes for the lonely, day centres, lunch clubs, transport schemes, promotion of leisure activities, craft exhibitions, and many other services. Age Concern (England) produces an excellent journal, *New Age*, a monthly information circular, and many other publications of importance to the elderly.

It has stimulated much research through its own research committee as well as a number of action studies (e.g. *Going Home*: Age Concern, Liverpool, 1975), and its national conferences have produced a series of excellent publications on various aspects of the care of the elderly (*The Manifesto*: Age Concern, England, 1974).

Help the Aged

Help the Aged has done much to promote better care of the elderly through its fund-raising activities. It has helped to develop day centres, improve hospital resources with the National Health Service, provide minibuses for the elderly, and many other facilities. It has also promoted various publications and has recently entered the educational field and shown itself willing to help with the promotion of research.

Centre for Policy for Ageing

Until recently this body has been known as the National Corporation for the Care of Old People. It was set up with a grant from the Nuffield Foundation and has remained under the umbrella of that particular organization. It has promoted a considerable amount of research into the social aspects of ageing and has maintained a register of social research.

Preretirement Association

This is another charitable body founded in 1958, whose main objective is to promote education so that when people retire they will be able to enjoy their retirement. Through its local branches it organizes preretirement courses either by encouraging local organizations or large firms to put on their own courses or through educational bodies such as the Workers' Education Association (WEA) or local colleges of further education.

King Edward's Hospital Fund for London

Better known by its abbreviated title, The King's Fund, the King Edward's Hospital Fund for London has done much to promote a better delivery of health care for the elderly, not only in London but throughout the whole of Great Britain. It has achieved this either by promoting working groups whose reports have resulted in such excellent books as *Living in Hospital* (Elliott, 1975) or *The Geriatric Day Hospitals* (Brocklehurst, 1970) or by holding conferences at the Hospital Centre. In addition, in conjunction with the British Geriatrics Society, it holds a yearly management course for senior registrars in geriatric medicine.

British Red Cross Society (BRCS)

In many places the BRCS provides a variety of services for the elderly and, in particular, aids to facilitate the nursing of the elderly sick.

Womens Royal Voluntary Services (WRVS)

The WRVS often play an important part in providing meal services, particularly meals-on-wheels in rural areas.

Other Voluntary Bodies

Many other voluntary bodies exist which may play an important part in providing care or funds which may help the elderly: examples are the Distressed Gentlefolks Association, The Association of Carers, the Crossroads Care Attendant Scheme, and community care groups often formed as a result of action by Councils of Community Service.

The Crossroads Care Attendant Scheme

These schemes began as a result of a fictional story on the popular television programme and an initial grant of £10,000 from ATV. The first pilot scheme began in 1974 and by 1981, 31 schemes were operative in various parts of the United Kingdom with a further 20 being planned. Each scheme has a management committee who employs a coordinator who recruits care attendants for training. The coordinator visits referrals, assesses needs, and allocates care attendants to the client. Care attendants are paid an hourly wage with extra pay for unsocial hours. The types of care given are shown in Table 2. Schemes are funded by grants from Social Service Departments, Health Authorities jointly, or other means such as Urban Aid or local fund raising activities (Phillips, 1982).

Table 2 Type of care provided by Crossroad scheme

1. Getting disabled person up or put to bed
2. Visiting when carer out
3. Staying overnight to allow carer rest
4. Helping with specific tasks, e.g. bathing
5. Provide regular relief break for carer
6. Provide occasional longer relief for carer, e.g. weekend
7. Provide emergency help

THE ORGANIZATION OF SERVICES AT THE LOCAL LEVEL

General Considerations

Needs and Wants

'Wants' may be defined as a need which is perceived by individuals themselves whereas 'needs' are shortcomings which have been perceived by another person who may be either a professional or a non-professional. The balance of the equation between 'wants' and 'needs' would depend on a variety of factors. Stoicism or lack of stoicism in the individual may lead to either an apparent absence of need or excessive demand. Similarly, the professional assessment of 'need' may vary considerably from that of the non-professional whose assessment may be influenced by their relationship to the individual. Studies comparing the 'wants' of an individual with their perceived 'need' as assessed by a layperson and professional workers are rare.

It is, moreover, difficult to assess their value since the professional workers may be biased by the lack of resources available to them so that on the one hand they may underestimate need as they know they cannot meet it, while on the other hand they may overestimate need in order to emphasize the lack of resources to the providers of services.

Recently, attempts have been made to try to look at needs in the context of resources. Balance of care studies have been performed by the DHSS operational research unit in Wiltshire and by Exeter University's biometry team in Devon (Wright and Canvin, 1982), and most District Health Authorities perform some sort of stock-taking exercise relating this to demand as part of their health care planning for the elderly.

A recent study in a London borough (Chapman, 1979) looked specifically at unmet needs and the delivery of care. Earlier, surveys in the 1960s had shown (Townsend and Wedderburn, 1965) that a wide range of health, social, and economic needs were unmet and it was estimated that perhaps four times as many people qualified for a need than those for whom the need was met. If this was true, it is hardly surprising that the needs are not always expressed by the elderly.

With increasing numbers of elderly, particularly in the age groups of over 75 and over 85, the amount of perceived need is likely to increase. This, linked to limitation of services by inflation and reduction in proportional budget, means potentially reducing resources while needs are actually increasing. In order to meet 'needs' it will be essential to look carefully at resource utilization. Can one afford to spend, for instance, a large proportion of the money available to provide residential and hospital accommodation for the long term care of the elderly frail and sick, when perhaps a more appropriate disposition of that money might provide support for a much greater number, thereby keeping more out of hospital or residential care? It would seem that to provide complete comprehensive care for the elderly and to meet all their perceived needs is beyond the capability of the economy of any Western country (Grimley Evans, 1981). Moreover, intensive domiciliary care may prove more expensive than residential or hospital care (Opit, 1977). It would appear, therefore, that a variety of services are necessary in an appropriate proportion and even then their use will need to be rationed and monitored.

Perhaps the most important 'want' of the elderly person, as suggested by Chapman's (1979) study, is to be able to express that want to a sympathetic person who will do something to relieve the need expressed. In a recent text-book on caring for the elderly sick, Chalmers (1980) recounts that when telling a group of students that old people did not complain he received the instant reply: 'You should hear my granny.' Old people do complain. However, they and their relatives often do not know to whom they should complain and when they do they frequently complain to the wrong people at the wrong time about the wrong things.

Figure 1 shows the organization of services and the interaction which may exist between them, while Table 1 lists the potential resources upon which the elderly may call. This formidable list excludes private resources which the elderly may provide for themselves or which they may have earned during the course of their working lives, such as an occupational pension, their own house, or other accommodation. For the old person, therefore, to discover his entitlement and how to meet his needs may represent a considerable problem. The voluntary organization Age Concern (England) has done a great deal to ease this position for the elderly in the publication annually of its booklet *Your Rights* (see Age Concern, 1982).

Housing

Good housing is probably one of the best measures available to ensure good health, yet as far as the elderly are concerned they are often badly housed in old accommodation in a run-down area with few amenities. However, they are often unwilling to move. A good housing policy is therefore essential and the position in Scotland has been reviewed by Thorn (1981).

In England and Wales each local district council has its housing department which is responsible for the provision of council hous-

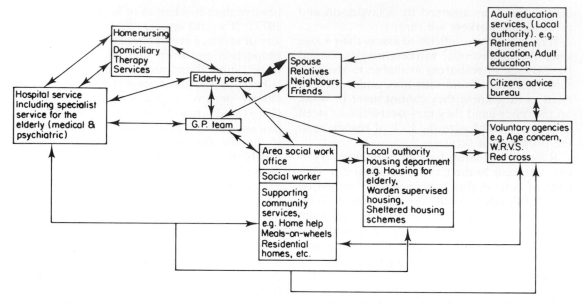

Figure 1   Diagram to show organization of and interaction between services available at local district level for the care of the elderly

ing. Within this provision will be special provision for the elderly. Most elderly people, though, will be housed within the ordinary housing stock and the better the design of this ordinary 'mainstream' housing the less likely will be the need for the elderly to move if they become disabled. However, in addition to this main stock the local housing department provides special housing designed specifically for old people, sometimes known as 'amenity housing'. If this is then connected by some form of communication system to a warden, then it becomes known as sheltered housing.

Sheltered Housing

While norms exist for hospital beds and residential home places, the government has never issued guidelines with regard to sheltered housing provision. Yet some authorities consider that the provision of sheltered housing has done much to prevent deterioration and keep these tenants out of residential and hospital care. There is no doubt that sheltered housing places have increased enormously in numbers in recent years, rising from about 36,000 in 1963 to 300,000 in 1976 and nearly ½ million in 1979, or sufficient to accommodate 7 per cent. of the over-65 population. The subject

has been well reviewed by Peckham (1981) and there is no doubt that the increasing frailty of tenants has meant increasing demands on wardens who are often asked to perform duties for which they are untrained. The need for closer collaboration between housing and social services departments has also increased. This is leading to interesting experiments in care which will need to be monitored and published. One such has been described by Holt (1981) and the monitoring report published (Hampshire County Council Social Services Department, 1981). In this study additional resident warden support was provided to give 24-hour cover to tenants in a 32-place sheltered housing block (Kinloss Court) and a further 2 blocks of 58 places had communication links. The 90 tenants were compared to residents in a 40-place residential home for the elderly. It was found that there was little difference between the frailty of residents in the home and tenants living in Kinloss Court, though the residents in the other two blocks were fitter. The conclusion was that such provision enabled very frail elderly to be cared for in an independent living situation. However, additional community support services were necessary to enable them to achieve this and no cost comparisons were made.

In addition to such statutory provision, many 'private' or housing association schemes (e.g. Anchor Housing Association, Abbeyfield Homes) exist in which the elderly may participate. These provide various levels of care. Some of these may be purchased (if the individual has the money), while others are provided by voluntary agencies at relatively low costs.

Citizens Advice Bureau

While the Citizens Advice Bureau is not usually considered as having an important part to play in the delivery of health care for the elderly, it nevertheless represents a most important information source. The Bureau will have a central office and perhaps subsidiary offices in larger towns. These offices will provide advice and information on all types of problems which may relate to the elderly and will advise them where to go for help in case of trouble. The role played by Citizens Advice Bureaux is often underestimated.

Social Services Departments

Many of the services necessary to meet the needs of elderly people in their own homes are provided by the social services departments of the local civic authorities in the United Kingdom. The members of these local authorities are elected by the general public at local council elections and form part of the party political organization. Each local authority will have as a sub-committee of its council a Social Services Committee on which there will be appropriate party representation. This Social Services Committee will be served by a paid Director of Social Services and the staff which will be allocated to him by the Social Service Committee as part of the budget of the local authority. While the Director of Social Services and his team can advise the Social Services Committee on the most appropriate use of resources to provide services for the care of the elderly, this advice may often be tempered by political considerations necessary to fulfil the promises made by the political party which has been most successful at the local elections.

Fortunately the basic pattern of social services for the elderly is mandatory, i.e. councils are required to provide them. Hence, major changes are not possible and only minor variations within the permissive powers of councils are possible. The services provided by these local authority social service departments are shown in Table 3.

Table 3   Services provided by local authority social services departments to the elderly

Social work
Residential care
Home help
Meals-on-wheels service and luncheon clubs
Day care
Aids and adaptions
Laundry service for incontinent clients (sometimes provided by the Health Authority)
Support and encouragement of voluntary agencies
Community care schemes
Telephone installation and rental services

Social Work

The role of the social worker in support of the elderly is a most important one. The old often require advice about the resources which are available to them, and the social worker, by enabling the elderly to use those resources, will enable the elderly client to lead a happier and fuller life. In addition to seeing that elderly clients avail themselves of the resources which are available to them, the social worker must ensure their best possible use. Social workers will often need to use considerable judgement, and experience and training is essential. The easy solution to the care of a disabled, lonely 85 year old woman, unable to do her own shopping or get out of her own house, may be to place her in a local authority residential home. However, placement in such a home may be an expensive option and not necessarily the right one for the individual concerned. The client might be happier in a smaller, more intimate home run privately. While she herself may not have the financial resources to pay for this, a combination of her old age pension, supplementary benefit, and the attendance allowance, all of which she may be able to claim, may make this solution possible. Organization of such a place will obviously place greater demands on social work time and skills while a more complex solution to the old lady's predicament, such as providing day care, arranging a good neighbour scheme, or support by a neighbourhood care group, or other community care scheme if available, combined with the continuing monitoring of the client's welfare when the arrangements have been made, can involve the social worker in even more work, yet be the most acceptable solution to the client. Social workers and social work assistants who have been specially trained in the needs of the elderly or who can work under the direction of trained social workers, are therefore necessary if the easiest options, which may not always be in the best interests of the client, are not to be adopted. On the other hand, the pressure of work which these more difficult options engender must be recognized.

The Department of Health (HM35/72) suggests that 50 to 60 social workers are needed to cater for a standard population of 100,000 people (DHSS, 1972a). However, in some British coastal resorts where the proportion of elderly may approach 33 per cent. of the total population, considerably more social workers may be necessary. Obviously, the more resources which are available to the client, the greater will be the client's choice and the more difficult the work of the social worker in enabling the client to make that choice. Social workers therefore need to have in their training a considerable knowledge of how age affects human beings and they need to be able to recognize the hazards and risks to which their clients may be subjected by disease and the ageing process (Brearley, 1982).

The social worker may have a most important role to play in relation to bereavement in the elderly. Resettlement of the elderly client within the family may prove difficult and sons, daughters, and even grandchildren may require the social worker's services as much as the elderly client themselves.

Close collaboration and consultation between medical and social services with regard to the elderly is most important. This can be made much easier if the geographical area served by health and social services as well as the housing and education departments is the same – making general planning of services and husbanding of resources much easier. Collaboration can lead towards a single service partnership such as that which has been described between hospital and social services in the Halton district of Cheshire (Shegog, 1981).

Residential Care

HM35/72 suggested (DHSS, 1972a) that the local authority should provide 25 places in residential homes per thousand elderly aged 65 years or more. Charges are made according to the resident's income and wealth for these places unless the individual has less than £1,200 capital and no income with the exception of supplementary benefit and the old age pension. However, the old age pension in these cases is lost but the individual is allowed a basic allowance of £7.15 for personal expenses.

The 25 places per thousand aged 65 years or more are intended to cater not only for the elderly infirm but also for the elderly mentally infirm. Policy on placement of clients in residential care varies from authority to authority and several experiments in management and design of residential care have been attempted. Many residential homes, however, have not been built for the purpose of housing the elderly infirm but are adaptations of large houses so that the elderly often have to share a bedroom with four or five others. This is obviously an unsatisfactory state of affairs which is recognized by local authorities who have long-term plans to replace unsatisfactory accommodation with accommodation which has been designed for the purpose. Some authorities allocate special functions to some of their residential homes, e.g. some homes have been reserved specifically for the elderly blind or for the elderly mentally infirm. In the case of the latter, links have been developed with health services so that consultant psychiatrists with a special interest in the elderly may have contractural sessions relating to these homes. On the other hand, some authorities have designed homes so that residential accommodation is grouped to allow people of similar ability to be accommodated together.

The type and design of home limits the type of care that can be given within the home and consequently the type of client that can be accommodated. Moreover, it often means that clients are unable to bring their own possessions or furniture with them when they move into residential care. While considerable lip service is paid to the desirability of allowing clients to bring their own furniture and possessions into residential accommodation, the ultimate decision is often left to the officer in charge of the home and clients are often limited to small personal possessions such as pictures or photographs and larger items of furniture are not accepted.

The selection and allocation of people for residential places varies depending on the policy laid down by the local authority's social services departments. The type of accommodation available may also influence placement since some homes may not be suitable for wheelchair-fast clients. Most authorities operate some form of panel system with representatives from social work areas, the residential homes themselves, and health services. Once a person has been allocated a place then they are usually taken to view the home by the social worker and the ultimate decision as to whether or not the place is accepted is that of the client. Usually, there is some lapse of time between the panel's decision that a person is suitable for residential care and the allocation of a place in a residential home. Some places in homes may be reserved for intermittent care of clients so that appropriate relief of client's carers may be given.

The degree of urgency for admission to residential care is also usually assessed by the panel, and vacancies given to those clients who seem in most urgent need. Criteria with regard to assessment of need will depend on the policy of the admission panel if this exists. These policies vary considerably from district to district and decisions as to whether to take somebody who is living in their own home, as against somebody who is in hospital, and thereby blocking a hospital bed, can sometimes be very difficult. Usually such priorities are decided as the result of a pragmatic decision such as every second, third, or fourth vacancy being allocated to 'hospital patients'. A recent study on decision making with regard to placement in residential care (Spackman, 1982) suggests that greater priority should perhaps be given to the 'hospital patient' as opposed to the client who is living in the community. As Brearley (1975) points out, a multidisciplinary approach to the delivery of health care of the elderly is essential if appropriate decisions are to be taken in order to enable individuals to lead healthy and happy lives.

Private Rest Homes

In addition to providing residential homes for the elderly which are under their own direction, the local authority has responsibility for the licensing of private rest homes which can also provide residential care for the elderly. All homes which cater for more than 4 people must be registered with the local authority. In order to obtain registration, the proprietors of such rest homes must fulfil criteria which will enable them to comply with fire regulations and also with appropriate standards of care. In this way, all such licensed homes should be above an appropriate standard. In addition to this, many private homes have for their own sakes banded together to form their own professional associations (e.g. the Hampshire Rest Homes Association), thereby creating their own standards which they must fulfil and meet. This means that the standard of rest home care has been steadily rising in recent years and the public has been, to a certain extent, safeguarded against homes of poor quality whose proprietors have the sole objective of making a large profit.

Day Care

Many elderly are lonely and isolated. Their lot may be eased if they are involved in activities which alleviate the tedium of life. The provision of day centres and day clubs may do much to achieve this objective. HM35/72 suggests (DHSS, 1972a) that local authorities should provide 50 places per 100,000 total population in day centres for the elderly. Such day centres would aim to provide day care for the frail elderly, thereby combating loneliness, providing them with a good substantial meal, and engaging them in activities which might relieve their boredom. While it is recognized that it is important to provide day centres for the frail elderly, very few local authorities have been able to find capital resources to build the centres. Where greater provision exists, it has often been provided by voluntary organizations who have developed day centres in collaboration with social services departments. There is no doubt that day centres are essential as supporting elements to day hospitals and where they do not exist, the day hospital is often forced to take over 'a social role'.

Meals-on-Wheels and Luncheon Clubs

Nutrition of the elderly is important and though surveys (DHSS, 1979) have shown the incidence of subnutrition to be only 7 per cent. overall, its incidence doubles in the over 80s and is particularly associated with medical and social 'risk' factors. Without a meals-on-wheels service there is no doubt that subnutrition would be greater. HM35/72 suggests (DHSS, 1972a) that mobile meals should be provided for approximately 20 per cent. of the elderly population. While there is no doubt that some elderly need meals taken to them in their own homes, it can be argued that there are others who would benefit more if they were stimulated to go out for a meal. Consequently, the provision of luncheon clubs or senior citizens' clubs which, in addition to providing a social function, also provide food form an important element in the overall provision of services for the elderly. Moreover, some authorities have experimented with extending neighbourhood schemes to provide food to those who need it as well as company and help in the home (Bytheway, 1980).

Home Help

A good home help service is essential if reasonable standards of cleanliness and tidiness are to be maintained in the homes of disabled or aged elderly people. In 1975 there were 6.5 home helps per thousand elderly in the United Kingdom (Bytheway, 1980). HM35/72 suggests (DHSS, 1972a) that the norm should be 12 per thousand.

The home help service can, however, be supplemented by good neighbour schemes and neighbourhood care schemes. An examination of the role of home helps and district nurses has shown that there is considerable overlap in their roles (Barsoum, 1982). The local authority has an important role to play in stimulating voluntary agencies to provide this type of service for the elderly. Moreover, some local authorities (Kent Community Care Project) have evolved schemes whereby local volunteers have been paid relatively small amounts to perform tasks for clients. These tasks might range from basic personal care such as toileting, dressing, etc., through to companionship such as social visits with the objective of raising

morale, or simply 'one off' tasks such as accompanying an elderly person to the out-patient department of a hospital, etc. (Challis, 1982).

Aids and Adaptions

Home adaptions and aids to enable infirm elderly people to maintain their independence may often be vitally important. Local authorities may undertake or financially assist the adaptions. Many local authorities employ occupational therapists to advise them and the elderly client and their families with regard to what particular aid or adaption is necessary. Adaptations may include heat insulation and improved heating, the provision of handrails on stairs or near the bath or lavatory, ramps on steps, alterations to kitchens, and even major alterations such as widening doorways for a wheelchair. In special cases adding a downstairs lavatory or shower may be agreed.

There are a great many aids available for the elderly disabled. However, one of the problems in providing aids is that responsibility for provision may be divided between the local authority, the health authority, or even a voluntary association. Voluntary associations such as the British Red Cross Society may often act as agents for the local authority with regard to the provision of aids. Consequently, the elderly person or the relative or chief carer in search of an aid may have to seek it from different people. There is much to be said for a single combined agency which would provide all aids and adaptions. Experiments along these lines have been successful (Robertson and Hains, 1978) and should be encouraged (Hall, 1980). The Central Council for the Disabled, the Scottish Information Service for the Disabled, the Disabled Living Foundation, and the British Red Cross Society publish books and pamphlets which give details of many of the aids and appliances which are available.

Provision of Telephones

Local authorities also have a duty to provide a telephone for any elderly or handicapped person who may require assistance in an emergency because of a serious medical condition, but who are themselves unable to afford this. The level of provision of this also varies between authorities, but most provide installation costs and pay the basic rental charge for a number of old people who fulfil the local criteria for such provision.

Laundry Service

Local authorities, or in many districts health authorities, provide a special laundry service to old people who may suffer from urinary incontinence and some local authorities will also supply additional bed linen. Some experiments have also linked laundry services with the services of an incontinence advisory nurse who is available to advise relatives and patients.

DISTRICT HEALTH SERVICES

The prime responsibility for the delivery of health care to the elderly person rests with the general practitioner and his primary health Care team. In order to receive health care under the provision of the National Health Service, individuals need to be registered with a doctor of their choice. While such registration is not compulsory, people who do not register are not able to receive free care from a family doctor. They could, however, employ a doctor through a private agreement and pay his fees as the need arose. They would, however, need to pay for their medicine, though if they required the services of the district nursing service or admission to an NHS hospital, these would be available to them free as of right. While it is possible to take out private health insurance which could cover most of the charges which are likely to be incurred by private medical care at home or in a private hospital bed, it is very unlikely that any private health insurance company would be prepared to pay institutional fees for an indefinite period to support the individual with irremediable disease. Moreover, the cost of providing round the clock nursing to keep somebody in their own home would prove prohibitive to all but the very wealthy (a recent example was a £20,000 per year bill for agency nursing provided on a 24-hour, 7-day per week basis). Consequently, it behoves the general practitioner and his team to provide an appropriate service to his elderly patient. General practitioners usually form themselves into partnerships of two or more doctors who agree to provide a service to the patients who register with them. A few general practitioners still work in single-handed practice but this is gradually becoming less common and there is a tendency for groups to work together from health centres or fairly large group practice premises. Various experiments of organization have been tried and some practices have attempted to specialize, individuals catering for various age groups. This has led to the GP paediatrician, the GP mediatrician, and the GP geriatrician. While this system may have certain advantages, particularly for the elderly, the idea has not proved popular with doctors who have preferred to cover the whole span of life.

Screening and Prevention

One of the most important needs of the elderly is to be encouraged to seek advice early from their general practitioner before loss of function becomes detrimental. The elderly, however, are often unwilling to trouble their general practitioners unnecessarily, consequently the general practitioner needs to guide and educate the patient with regard to the early detection and prevention of disease. This topic has been excellently reviewed by Anderson (1978). That a large amount of 'unreported' illness exists among old people was highlighted by Williamson and Stokoe (1964) and has been confirmed by many others (Akhtar *et al.*, 1973; Andrews, Cowan, and Anderson, 1971). The problem remains, how to persuade the elderly to report their disability. The GP and his attached nurse and health visitor form a team who through their practice record system should be in a position to know which of their elderly patients are particularly at risk. It is, moreover, possible for them to make contact with all their elderly patients so that some form of intermittent regular contact can be maintained. In order to achieve this, however, a good general practice record system must be organized. Computerization of medical records is one possibility but the use of a specially designed coloured card may be just as successful in spot-lighting those who are at risk (Munday and Rowe, 1979).

The most essential element, however, to any general practice screening programme is an age/sex register. General practitioners in the United Kingdom can form age/sex registers for the elderly with the help of their Family Practitioner Committees. These age/sex registers can take many forms from a simple register book to a card index system on which simple details of the patient's age, sex, address, occupation, etc., may be recorded. Such age/sex registers can be linked to computers, especially for research purposes. Age/sex registers, however, are not mandatory and Family Practitioner Committees may be reluctant or even refuse to provide them.

In order for screening to be successful the general practice team has to be committed to the programme. All have to be in agreement that it is necessary and of importance. Many general practitioners are, however, unconvinced of the value of the screening, feeling that those in need are brought to their notice anyway and those who are not do not need attention. This may well apply in the case of practitioners whose standard of everyday practice is high, for some general practitioners will see 95 per cent. of their clientele over a period of 12 to 18 months. In order to aid screening some general practitioners have developed special clinics for the elderly. These are often run on days and times when the practice is comparatively slack. At them the elderly can be seen at greater leisure and consequently more attention paid to their needs.

Perhaps the most famous of such clinics was that run on a voluntary basis not by general practitioners but by a Medical Officer of Health and a Professor of Geriatric Medicine – the Rutherglen clinic (Anderson and Cowan, 1955).

While their value today may be questioned, such clinics initially served the most important function of focusing the attention of doctors, nurses, and the elderly themselves on the physical illness which is a concomitant of old age and its amelioration. They have done much to change the attitudes of all towards better standards of medical care and treatment for the elderly.

The Primary Health Care Team

Medical treatment and advice with regard to the physical and mental problems which are associated with ageing form the major part of the work of the general practitioner and the nurses attached to his team. A good family practitioner service is the foundation on which a good geriatric service can be built, for unless there is good medical and nursing care in the home, no geriatric service will be able to fulfil its aim. Fortunately, in the British National Health Service, it is possible to integrate family medical and nursing services based in the community with those that are based in the hospital.

The GP will be supported by a nurse either employed by him or attached to him from the Health Authority District Nursing Service and will also be able to call on the services of a health visitor. In addition, general practitioners must provide their own secretarial support and practice receptionist who has a vital role to play in communications between doctor and patients as well as the maintenance of a record system and communications with various hospital services. The general practice team will be able to call upon the various resources provided by the local authority social services department and voluntary organizations which have already been described. In addition, the District Health Authority will provide additional resources through its community medical and nursing services. For instance, a night nursing or attendant service may be an integral part of the district's home nursing service.

Liaison with the hospital geriatric or psychogeriatric team will usually be on an *ad hoc* consultative basis. The patients are seen by a member of the appropriate hospital team in their own home (domiciliary consultation or home assessment visit) or else are referred to the hospital geriatric outpatient clinic. Alternatively, a senior member of the hospital team may hold regular consultation clinics in the family doctor's premises. This can be justified when family doctors work in large groups or from a health centre which services a defined geographical area (MacLennan and Hall, 1980). Similarly the psychiatrist with a special interest in the elderly, together with his team of doctors and nurses, will often develop a special liaison with the general practitioner teams in the area in which he works. In this way, patients with mental illness who are over 65 years of age may be assessed and a programme of long-term care worked out with the general practitioners concerned.

In addition, the general practitioner's team will be supported by remedial therapists who work in the community treating patients in their own homes and in some cases developing treatment groups which may be formed into clubs such as 'stroke' clubs.

Community Medicine

Each health district has a specialist in community medicine as a member of the district medical team. This doctor is the direct descendent of the Medical Officer of Health and is the medical coordinator of a team of doctors, nurses, and administrators who are responsible for organizing supporting health services in the community as well as developing collaboration with social services and monitoring the delivery of health care to all groups including the elderly. One task is to organize and administer a health care planning team for the elderly. This team has a multidisciplinary representation and will contain representatives from those people who are particularly concerned with the care of the elderly.

The composition of such a team is shown in Table 4. The principal objective of such a team is to plan health services in relation to social services and a well organized team can do much to promote good care of the elderly.

Table 4 Example of membership of Health Care Planning Team for the elderly

District Medical Officer, or
Specialist in Community Medicine (Elderly/Social Services),
Consultant Physician in Geriatric Medicine,
Consultant Psychiatrist with special interest in the elderly,
A General Practitioner,
A senior hospital nurse,
A senior community nurse,
District Occupational Therapist,
District Physiotherapist,
A representative from Social Services Department,
A representative from Local Housing Authority,
A member of the District Health Authority,
A member of the Community Health Council,
Voluntary services Liaison Officer,
A member of District Administrators' Team

Since the District Medical Officer has responsibility for the whole range of health services, he will often detail one of the medical members of his team to take a special responsibility for establishing good services for the elderly and liaisoning with social services. This coincides with the recommendations of the BMA's report of 1976.

In addition, it is the responsibility of the community physician and his team to develop health education programmes and some of these need to be directed towards the elderly. The hospital geriatric team can also play a major part in these educational activities, taking part in the training programmes of all who are involved with the care of the elderly, whether they be professionals or lay persons. They also have an important role in promoting preretirement education.

The Hospital Service

In Great Britain this service is provided by the National Health Service though a small proportion of people who are over the age of 65 years may be treated on a short-term basis by private medicine. Usually, however, such individuals belong only to social class 1 and the majority of the population over the age of 65 years get their hospital services from the National Health Hospitals.

All the services available within the hospital are available to patients who are over the age of 65. The decision as to which service the patient is referred is in the hands of the general practitioner. He decides whether his patient is best treated by a general physician with a special interest such as gastroenterology, by a surgeon, or an audiologist or an opththalmologist, or an orthopaedic surgeon or other specialist. Most districts, however, now have an organized geriatric medical service and a psychogeriatric service. If these services are to be successful they must concentrate on supporting the community element already described. They must try and stimulate early referral of patients by general practitioners and by appropriate treatment maintain the function of the individuals at a high level. They must also educate all their colleagues working in the hospital service with regard to the role that geriatric medicine and psychiatry can play in the role of the treatment of their patients.

Nursing Homes

Homes which provide continuous nursing care for patients exist within the boundaries of most Health Districts. They may be run by voluntary organizations (often religious nursing orders) or by private individuals. They are licenced and inspected by the Health Authority and are required to have at least one fully qualified nurse (SRN or SRMN) on duty at all times, thus distinguishing them from private residential homes. They can make a substantial contribution to the overall service.

Geriatric Medical Services

In 1972 a Working Party commissioned by the Wessex Regional Hospital Board defined the needs of the elderly that the hospital geriatric services should meet (Table 5). In order to do this, the geriatric service will require resources and the DHSS (1971a) has suggested the norms, which are shown in Table 6. These norms, however, can be queried and the bed norm in particular has been criticized as being deficient. Indeed, the Scottish Home and Health Department has suggested a figure of 15 beds as being more appropriate than 10. However, the trends which have taken place in geriatric medicine in the United Kingdom in the past 20 years suggest that these norms may be more than sufficient if the length of patient stay continues to fall and the discharge rates rise. Indeed, Slattery and Bourne (1979) have argued for a lower bed norm. In assessing norms it is necessary to take into account the success of community services available, in which case the norms suggested by Slattery and Bourne may be more appropriate. Moreover, the goal of 50 per cent. of the geriatric beds being placed in the district general hospital is often unattainable and the more recently proposed figure of 30 per cent. by the DHSS (1976) is probably more realistic.

Even more recently, the DHSS has suggested that long-term care of the elderly irremediable patient should be undertaken not in large long-stay hospitals but in smaller nursing units for the elderly. Currently, three such experimental units have been commissioned and their development will be watched with interest.

Table 5   Needs of the elderly which the hospital geriatric service should meet

1. At the outset of the incapacity, to receive an expert opinion at an early stage and to receive treatment for that incapacity without or with admission to hospital.
2. If admission to hospital is appropriate, then the patient will need access to all diagnostic facilities and specialist services.
3. If urgent admission is required then this must be available.
4. Since recovery from illness in old age is often slow, continuing treatment will need to be in active rehabilitation wards which are geared to meet the needs of the elderly.
5. Some patients will prove irremediable and require longer rehabilitation programmes or even permanent long-term care in accommodation which is suited to their needs.
6. Where relatives bear a heavy nursing or caring load at home, intermittent admissions may be necessary to relieve the burden of care.
7. Some patients will need admission for the terminal period of their illness.

Table 6   Health services provision

Hospital beds
  Medical: 10 per 1,000 aged 65 years or more
  Psychiatric: 2.5–3 per 1,000 aged 65 years or more
  Medical/psychiatric assessment: 10–20 per 250,000 total population
Day hospital places
  Medical: 2 per 1,000 aged 65 years or more
  Psychiatric: 2–3 per 1,000 aged 65 years or more

GERIATRIC MEDICAL SERVICES

In addition to their need for beds in the District General Hospital, Geriatric Hospitals or DHSS Nursing Homes, Geriatric Services also need other facilities.

Day Hospitals

The day hospital movement began in Britain before World War II as a way of treating patients with mental illness on an outpatient or daily basis. The geriatric day hospital has developed from the psychiatric day hospital and the first major study of geriatric day hospitals was published by Brocklehurst in 1970. The geriatric day hospital may be defined as a hospital ward from which the patient returns to his own home to sleep each night. However, while the main accent is on medical treatment and rehabilitation, many day hospitals have had, in the absence of day centres, to fulfil also a social side in preventing loneliness and keeping the elderly active in the community. This is an inappropriate use of an expensively staffed resource, and can be avoided only by constant and careful audit of the operations of the day hospital. Individual assessment to formulate a management plan, followed by repeated views of progress and discharge as soon as optimal recovery has been achieved, is essential to ensure that the day hospital remains cost-effective.

The most appropriate size for a day hospital is in considerable dispute, but it would seem likely that the large 50 place day hospital which was once thought to be the most appropriate is not the most suitable. One of the major problems with regard to day hospital care is the provision of appropriate transport facilities. If severely disabled patients are brought to the day hospital for treatment then obviously ambulances will be necessary for their transport.

The priorities and time-tabling of this transport is often so delayed that the day hospital becomes little more than a 'lunch hospital'. The fewer the number of places, the easier it is to get patients there and the more are the staff able to concentrate on their treatment. This has led Martin and Millard (1978) to suggest that day hospitals should not exceed 18 places and they have argued the case for good therapist staffing on the grounds that this increases the throughput of the unit. Irvine (1980), however, has made the point that the average number of visits to the day hospital per patient is approximately 20 and this is spread over the average period of 3 months. This length of time coincides with the natural period of recovery following many causes of disabilities such as arthritis or stroke and it may be that to take the therapist to the patient would be a more effective form of management of their disability than to bring the patient to a central therapeutic unit. Much more research into the use of day hospitals needs to be done, but at the present time it would certainly seem that they form a useful and essential part of any geriatric service. A good review of the day hospital in its present form has recently been written by Tucker (1982).

Outpatient Clinics

The facility to hold outpatient clinics in geriatric medicine is one of the requirements laid down by the Royal College of Physicians in its approval of the job description of Consultants in Geriatric Medicine in England and Wales. Most physicians in geriatric medicine hold at least one outpatient clinic per week and this is usually held in the District General Hospital. Additional outpatient clinics may, however, be held in group practice surgeries or health centres, as has already been described, or else in smaller peripheral hospitals or even in day hospitals.

In addition to holding outpatient clinics, the Consultant Physician in Geriatric Medicine is available to the general practitioner for consultation, and domiciliary consultations, for which a fee can be paid, will often be done jointly with the general practitioner. Equally, if resources are short, patients may sometimes have their need assessed by the Consultant or a member of his team making a home assessment visit.

Psychiatric Services for the Elderly

Considerable overlap exists between geriatric medicine and psychiatry. As a result, a certain amount of conflict has existed between physicians in geriatric medicine and psychiatrists with a special interest in the elderly. This has been well described and reviewed by Godber (1978).

The specialty of 'psychogeriatrics' has developed only recently. The impetus for setting up this specialty has come from the epidemiological studies performed in Newcastle-upon-Tyne in the early 1960s (Kay, Beamish, and Roth, 1964). These drew attention to the enormous amount of mental ill-health which existed among the elderly, and the need to provide not only a service for patients with senile dementia but also for those suffering from affective disorders. Close collaboration between medical and psychiatric services is essential and although the provision of a complete 'geriatrician' would probably not be an appropriate answer to all the needs of the elderly, both physicians in geriatric medicine and psychiatrists with a special interest in the elderly need training in each other's specialties.

They also need appropriate resources and if these can be provided along the lines shown in Table 6, then collaboration between the two health services for the elderly, as well as the Primary Medical Care Service, can be much closer. Good examples of such close collaboration exists (Arie and Dunn, 1973; Donovan, Williams, and Wilson, 1971; Robinson, 1981). Moreover, in Nottingham, an attempt has been made to formally link psychiatrists and physicians together within a single department headed by a Professor for the Health Care of the Elderly, who is a psychiatrist.

REFERENCES

Age Concern (England) (1974). *The Manifesto.*

Age Concern (England) (1984). *Your Rights.*

Age Concern (Liverpool) (1975). *Going Home.*

Akhtar, A. J., Broe, G. A., Crombie, A., McLean, W. M. R., Andrews, G. R., and Caird, F. I. (1973). 'Disability and dependence in the elderly at home', *Age Ageing*, **2**, 102–111.

Anderson, W. F. (1978). 'The early detection and prevention of disease in the elderly', in *Recent Advances in Geriatric Medicine* (Ed. B. Isaacs), Chap. 11, p. 143, Churchill Livingstone, Edinburgh.

Anderson, W. F. (1981). 'The evolution of services in the United Kingdom'. in *The Provision of Care for the Elderly* (Eds J. Kinnaird, J. Brotherston, and J. Williamson), p. 117, Churchill Livingstone, Edinburgh.

Anderson, W. F., and Cowan, N. R. (1955) 'A consultative health centre for older people; Rutherglen experiment', *Lancet*, **2**, 239–240.

Andrews, G. R., Cowan, N. R., and Anderson, W. F. (1971) 'The practice of geriatric medicine in the community: An evaluation of the place of health centres', in G. McLachlan (Ed.) *Problems and Progress in Medical Care, Essays on Current Research*, p. 58, Oxford University Press.

Arie, T., and Dunn, T. (1973). 'A "do it yourself" psychiatric–geriatric joint patient unit', *Lancet*, **2**, 1313–1316.

Barsoum, M. (1982). Personal communication.

Brearley, C. P. (1975). *Social Work, Ageing and Society*, Routledge and Kegan Paul, London.

Brearley, C. P. (1982). *Risks and Ageing*, Routledge and Kegan Paul, London.

British Geriatrics Society and Royal College of General Practitioners (1978). 'Training general practitioners in geriatric medicine', *J. R. Coll. Gen. Pract.*, **28**, 355.

British Medical Association (1949). *The Care and Treatment of the Elderly and Infirm*, BMA House, London.

British Medical Association (1976). *Care of the Elderly*, BMA House, London.

Brocklehurst, J. C. (1970). *The Geriatric Day Hospitals*, King Edward's Hospital Fund, London.

Bytheway, W. R. (1980). 'United Kingdom', in *International Handbook on Ageing* (Ed. E. Palmore), p. 418, Macmillan Press, London.

Challis, D. S. (1982). 'Towards more creative social work with the elderly: The community care project', in *Care in the Community: Recent Research and Current Projects* (Ed. F. Glendening), p. 43–60, Beth Johnson Foundation.

Chalmers, G. L. (1980). *Care of the Elderly Sick*, Pitman Medical, Tunbridge Wells.

Chapman, P. (1979). 'Unmet needs and the delivery of care', Occasional Papers in Social Administration no. 61, Bedford Square Press, London.

Charcot, J. M. (1881). *Clinical Lectures on Senile Diseases*, The New Sydenham Society, London.

Department of Education and Science (1972). *Speech Therapy Services*, HMSO, London.

Department of Health and Social Security (1971a). *Hospital Geriatric Services*, HMSO, London. DS329/71.

Department of Health and Social Security (1971b). *Services for Mental Illness Related to Old Age*, HMSO, London. HM72/71.

Department of Health and Social Security (1972a). *Local Authority Services 10 Years Development Plan, 1973–1983*, HMSO, London. HM35/72.

Department of Health and Social Security (1972b). *Rehabilitation – Report of the Sub-committee of the standing Medical Advisory Committee*, HMSO, London.

Department of Health and Social Security (1976). *Priorities for Health and Personal Social Services in England*, HMSO, London.

Department of Health and Social Security (1978). *A Happier Old Age*, HMSO, London.

Department of Health and Social Security (1979). *Nutrition and Health in Old Age*, HMSO, London.

Donovan, J. F., Williams, I. E. I., and Wilson, T. D. (1971). 'A fully integrated psychogeriatric service', in *Recent Developments in Psychogeriatrics* (Eds D. W. K. Kay and A. Walk), Chap. 10, p. 113–125, RMPA, London.

Elliott, J. R. (1975). *Living in Hospital*, King Edward's Hospital Fund, London.

General Medical Council (1980). *Recommendations on Basic Medical Education*, General Medical Council, London.

Godber, C. (1978). 'Conflict and collaboration between geriatric medicine and psychiatry', in *Recent Advances in Geriatric Medicine* (Ed. B. Isaacs), p. 131, Churchill Livingstone, Edinburgh.

Grimley Evans, J. (1981). 'Demographic implications for the planning of services in the United

Kingdom', in *The Provision of Care for the Elderly* (Eds J. Kinnaird, Sir J. Brotherston, and J. Williamson), Chap. 1, iii, p. 8, Churchill Livingstone, Edinburgh.

Hall, M. R. P. (1980). 'Supplying the demand', *Health and Social Sciences J.*, **90**, 47.

Hampshire County Council Social Services Department (1981). Kinloss Court Sheltered Housing Scheme. 'A report on three years monitoring', Research Report No. 29.

Holt, J. (1981). 'Kinloss Court sheltered housing scheme, Southampton', in *Care in the Community: Recent Research and Current Projects* (Ed. F. J. Glendening), p. 120, Beth Johnson Foundation.

Irvine, R. E. (1980). 'Geriatric day hospitals: Present trends', *Health Trends*, **12**, 68.

Isaacs, B., Livingstone, M., and Neville, Y. (1972). *Survival of the Unfittest*, Routledge and Kegan Paul, London.

Kay, D. W. K., Beamish P., and Roth, M. (1964). 'Old age mental disorders in Newcastle upon Tyne. A study of prevalence', *Br. J. Psychiat.*, **110**, 146–158.

MacLennan, W. J., and Hall, M. R. P. (1980). 'Geriatric clinics in general practitioner surgeries', *The Practitioner*, **224**, 687–689.

Martin, A., and Millard, P. H. (1978). *Day Hospitals for the Elderly: Therapeutic or Social*', St. George's Hospital, London.

Munday, M., and Rowe, J. (1979). *Care of the Elderly in Devon*, King's Fund Publication, London.

Opit, L. J. (1977). 'Domiciliary care for the elderly: Economy or neglect?', *Br. Med. J.*, **1**, 30.

Peckham, D. (1981). 'Sheltered housing', in *The Impending Crisis of Old Age* (Ed. R. F. A. Shegog), p. 91, Oxford University Press.

Phillips, D. (1982). 'The Crossroads care attendant scheme', in *Care in the Community* (Ed. F. Glendening), p. 91, Beth Johnson Foundation, University of Keele, and Age Concern (England).

Robertson, J., and Hains, J. R. (1978). 'A community hospital home aids loan scheme based on a rehabilitation demonstration centre', *Health* Trends, **10**, 15.

Robinson, R. (1981). 'Psychiatric care of the elderly', in *The Provision of Care for the Elderly* (Eds J. Kinnaird, Sir J. Brotherston, and J. Williamson), Chap. 11, p. 159, Churchill Livingstone, Edinburgh.

Royal College of Physicians (Edinburgh) (1963). *The Care of the Elderly in Scotland*, no. 22, Royal College of Physicians, Edinburgh.

Royal College of Physicians (Edinburgh) (1970). *The Care of the Elderly in Scotland: A Follow Up Report*, Royal College of Physicians, Edinburgh, HMSO.

Royal College of Physicians (London) (1977). *Report of the Working Party on Medical Care for the Elderly*, Royal College of Physicians, London.

Shegog, R. F. A. (1981). *The Impending Crisis of Old Age – A Challenge to Ingenuity*, Nuffield Provincial Hospitals Trust, Oxford University.

Slattery, M., and Bourne, A. (1979). 'Norms and recent trends in geriatrics', *J. Clin. Exp. Gerontol.*, **1**, 79.

Spackman, A. (1982). 'Decision making and residential home placement of the elderly', Ph.D. Thesis, University of Southampton.

Thorn, W. T. (1981). 'Housing policies', in *The Provision of Care for the Elderly* (Eds J. Kinnaird, Sir J. Brotherston, and J. Williamson), Chap. 2, iii, p. 31, Churchill Livingstone, Edinburgh.

Townsend, P., and Wedderburn, D. (1965). *The Aged in the Welfare State*, Bell, London.

Tucker, J. S. (1982). 'The day hospital', in *Establishing a Geriatric Service* (Ed. D. Coakley), Chap. 4, p. 58, Croom Helm Publishers, London.

Wessex Regional Hospital Board (1972). *Report of a Working Party on the Care of the Elderly*, Wessex Regional Hospital Board.

Williamson, J., and Stokoe, I. H. (1964). 'Old people at home: their unreported needs', *Lancet*, **1**, 1117.

Wright, W. B., and Canvin, R. W. (1982). 'Geriatric medicine and the computer', in *Establishing a Geriatric Service* (Ed. D. Coakley), Chap. 12, p. 181, Croom Helm Publishers, London.

Principles and Practice of Geriatric Medicine
Edited by M. S. J. Pathy
© 1985 John Wiley & Sons Ltd

30.2

Delivery of Health Care in the United States

R. W. Lindsay

DEMOGRAPHY

The following quotation is from Dr Robert N. Butler's Pulitzer Prize winning book, *Why Survive? Being Old in America:*

What are an individual's chances for a 'good old age' in America, with satisfying final years and a dignified death? Unfortunately, none too good. For many elderly Americans, old age is a tragedy, a period of quiet despair, deprivation, desolation and muted rage. This can be a consequence of the kind of life a person has led in younger years and the problems in his/her relationships with others. There are also inevitable personal and physical losses to be sustained, some of which can be overwhelming and unbearable. All of this is the individual factor, the existential element. But old age is frequently a tragedy, even when the early years have been fulfilling and people seemingly have everything going for them. Herein lies what I consider to be a genuine tragedy of old age in America. We have shaped a society which is extremely harsh to live in when one is old. The tragedy of old age is not the fact that each of us must grow old and die but that the process of doing so has been made unnecessarily, and at times excruciatingly painful, humiliating, debilitating, and isolating through insensitivity, ignorance and poverty. The potentials for satisfactions and even triumphs in late life are real and vastly under-explored. For the most part, the elderly struggle to exist in an inhospitable world (Butler, 1975).

One of the major forces involved in the struggle of the elderly is the health care delivery system. Butler's book included the challenge for significant changes in the United States' health care delivery system for the elderly. This chapter will assess the status of these changes and will include a discussion of the various types of health care facilities (both institutional and community-based) that are available to the elderly in the United States. The financing of health care in the United States will be examined, and recent developments in geriatric education will be reviewed. The chapter will conclude with a discussion of the possible future for the geriatric health care delivery system in the United States.

The elderly in this chapter are defined as those citizens 65 years of age and older. Health care is defined in its broadest sense and includes areas other than those encompassed by the traditional medical definition – including economic, nutritional, social and mental health components.

One of the major concerns of health planners at various levels of government in the United States is the rapidly changing demography of its population. In 1900, there were some 3 million Americans over the age of 65, nearly 4 per cent. of a population of some 76 million. By 1950, the elderly had increased to approximately 12 million. By 1980, this figure had risen to approximately 25 million Americans, or roughly 12 per cent. of the total population of the United States. The forecast calls for an even more striking increase in our elderly population, brought about as a result of the maturing of the post World War II 'baby boom'. Forecasters estimate that by the year 2030, 55 million Americans will be over the age of 65 (Soldo, 1980, p. 7).

Many factors have been put forward as reasons for this dramatic increase in our elderly population during the past 80 years. One is the high birth-rate that occurred in the early part of this century. Another is the rapid decline in infant and child mortality. Other reasons given include improvements in childhood immunization programmes, medical care, and public health measures. Regardless of the cause, more and more citizens of the United States are surviving the early years of life and are living into their sixth and seventh decades. As a result, we are also seeing much larger numbers of our older population who are suffering from degenerative and chronic diseases, impairing the quality of life and the function of the individual rather than leading directly to death.

It is also important to note that the elderly population of the United States is predominantly female, and as the age level rises, this female predominance becomes more apparent. It is predicted that by 2000 there will be 150 females per 100 males at 65 years of age; and in the 75-year age range the ratio will be 191 females to 100 males (U.S. Department of Health, Education and Welfare, 1978).

Within the expanding elderly population, the segment that will be growing at the most rapid rate will be the so-called 'old/old' or the 'frail' elderly (over 75 years of age) and will include many of our minority group elderly (Fig. 1). Currently, approximately 40 per cent. of elderly Americans are over the age of 75 and this will increase to approximately 45 per cent. by the year 2000 (Soldo, 1980, p. 11). In that same year, 1 of 11 elderly persons in the United States will be aged 85 or over. This is the age group that will manifest the greatest degree of limitation in functional capabilities, and the group that will call for the maximal outlay of resources, financial support, and coordination of all the elements of the health care delivery system. The need for assistance in certain basic daily activities is significantly greater in this older age group (Fig. 2).

The health and social needs for our elderly population may be better appreciated by fo-

Percent change in number of elderly by age groups and race: United States, 1950–2000 and 2000–2050

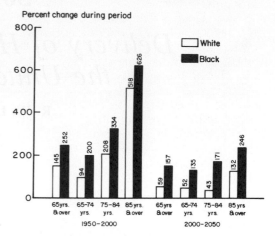

Figure 1 Percentage change in the number of elderly by age groups and race: United States, 1950–2000 and 2000–2050. (From US Department of Health and Human Services, 1981)

Percent of elderly needing assistance in four activities of daily living by age groups: United States, 1978.

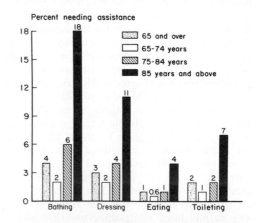

Figure 2 Percentage of elderly needing assistance in four activities of daily living by age groups: United States, 1978. (Note: This excludes elderly in institutions.) (From US Department of Health and Human Services, 1981)

cusing briefly on the functional status of the elderly and their use of the current health care delivery system.

Approximately 5 per cent. of the elderly population in the United States is institutionalized at any one time, and furthermore an elderly individual living in the community stands a one in five chance of being institutionalized for some period of time before they die (Technical Committee on Health Services, 1981, p. 2). For every institutionalized elderly individual it is estimated that there are two more in the community setting with an equal degree of infirmity or impairment (Shanas, 1980). In addition, 46 per cent. of the persons over the age of 65 report some chronic limitation of functional activity (Fig. 3). Cardiovascular and arthritic conditions account for approximately one-half of those with limitations (Technical Committee on Health Services, 1981, p. 4).

The elderly have approximately one more physician visit per year than the population as a whole (Fig. 4). Those above 85 show a decrease in frequency of visits, perhaps because more are institutionalized.

The use of short-stay hospitals increases dra-

Visits to physicians by the elderly by age groups: United States

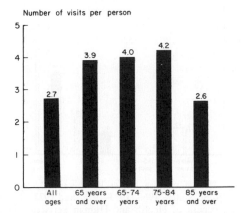

Figure 4   Visits to physicians by the elderly by age groups: United States, (Note: This excludes telephone contacts and visits to clinics and emergency rooms.) (From US Department of Health and Human Services, 1981)

Percent of elderly with limitation of activity due to chronic condition by age groups and type of limitation: United States, 1978

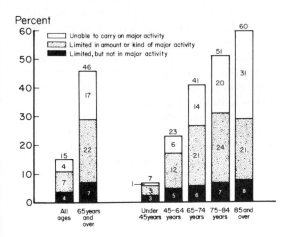

Figure 3   Percentage of elderly with limitation of activity due to chronic condition by age groups and type of limitation: United States, 1978. (Note: This includes only those persons with an activity limitation due to a chronic condition and excludes elderly in insitutions.) (From US Department of Health and Human Services, 1981)

matically with age, as is reflected in the number of discharges per 1,000 patients. Between 1965 and 1978 there was a 46 per cent. increase in the number of discharges per 1,000 patients of 65 years of age and over, while all other age groups showed only an 8 per cent. increase during the same period (U.S. Department of Health and Human Services, 1981, p. 40).

The special needs for the elderly over the age of 85 are reflected in a hospital discharge rate 70 per cent. greater than that for people in the 65 to 74 age range.

The most striking difference in utilization of facilities occurs in the nursing home (Fig. 5). Elderly individuals over the age of 75 are approximately 30 times more likely to be in a nursing home than those in the 45 to 64 age range, and 8 times more likely than those aged 65 to 74 (Technical Committee on Health Services, 1981, p. 7).

The maximum demands on the health care delivery system in the United States are posed by that segment of the population who are 65 years of age and older. In addition, the rapid increase in total numbers of elderly will pose an even greater burden on a system which has not proven itself adequate in dealing with the present needs.

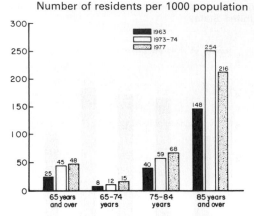

Figure 5 Use of nursing homes by the elderly by age groups: United States, 1963, 1973–1974, and 1977. (From US Depaertment of Health and Human Services, 1981)

FINANCING OF GERIATRIC CARE

During the 1960s, the costs of health care escalated rapidly, and many elderly were unable to meet them. The total health care expenditures in the United States were 4.0 billion dollars in 1940, but by 1965 this figure had climbed to 41.7 billion, and it was at this time that the Medicare programme was enacted in the United States (Gibson and Waldo, 1981, p. 19). This programme was a form of National Health Insurance, but unlike the British system and that found in some other Western European nations, this programme was directed largely at the elderly. Its goal was to protect the elderly from the high costs of health care. Those persons eligible included anyone over the age of 65 who met the requirements for social security or railroad benefits. The coverage has since been expanded to include patients with chronic renal disease and totally disabled patients. Currently some 27 million citizens are covered by the programme; in 1977, Medicare covered most short-term acute hospital expenses.

The Medicare programme was not designed to cover all health care costs. It excluded such items as long-term nursing home care and out-of-hospital prescription medications. The programme is a complex one, and an explanation of it may provide some idea of the problems involved in determining a person's eligibility.

Part A of the Medicare programme is hospital insurance, which is financed through payroll taxes. There are no premiums required but there is a deductible of approximately $307 before benefits begin. In addition, there are payments of approximately $76 a day for a hospital stay beyond 60 days. It is, therefore, still possible for the elderly to have a significant hospital bill even though they are covered by Medicare.

Part B of the Medicare programme was designed to assist in payments for physicians' services and some outpatient hospital services. Part B is a voluntary plan that requires payment of premiums to supplement general revenue funds. Reimbursement for physicians under this programme is dependent upon whether or not the physician accepts the 'assignment of benefits'. For those physicians who do accept assignment of benefits, direct billing is then carried out through the third party Medicare carrier, and payments are received by the physician directly from that firm. On the other hand, if the physician does not accept assignment of benefits, the patient is billed and is responsible for forwarding the bill to the medical insurance carrier, and also for reimbursing the physician. In both instances, Medicare only reimburses the patient for 80 per cent. of that portion of the bill defined as a 'reasonable charge'. This reasonable charge is based upon current regional physicians' fees, or the customary fees charged by that individual physician during a period of time. However, if the physician does not accept the assignment of benefits, then he/she can charge fees considerably over what the Medicare programme considers 'reasonable charges' and the patient is liable for the difference. The number of physicians accepting assignment of benefits has decreased over the duration of the programme, and some physicians are refusing to accept the assignment of benefits at all because of low fee schedules, payment delays, and increased paper work.

The Medicare programme has done a good job in the area of acute hospital-related expenses. In 1977, Medicare covered 88 per cent. of the cost of acute community hospital care for the elderly. The problems with Medicare relate to the areas of non-coverage, in that it does not cover 'custodial' care such as personal care which includes eating, dressing, assistance in walking and bathing, or activities that could be provided by a non-skilled or untrained person. This exclusion, probably more than any other, seems contradictory to one of the major goals of long-term care; i.e. assisting in the maintenance of the elderly individual at the highest level of function possible.

The Medicare programme also excludes payment for preventive services such as routine physical examinations, immunizations, routine foot care, eye and hearing examinations, and many home services. Some recent changes in the programme have liberalized the number of allowable home visits under Medicare and have eliminated a particularly vexing problem which requires a three-day hospitalization period prior to coverage for home health care benefits under Part A (Technical Committee on Health Services, 1981, p. 32).

The associated programme that was to provide an additional 'safety net' for the elderly is called Medicaid. It is a joint federal and state programme originally targeted as medical assistance to families of dependent children, as well as the aged, blind, permanently and totally disabled individuals whose incomes were insufficient to meet the costs of necessary medical services.

This programme uses a means test to define an indigent person. Rather than serving solely as a backup to Medicare, Medicaid has come to represent a major source of support for the long-term care of the chronically impaired elderly, particularly nursing home residents. In 1978, Medicaid financed 46 per cent. of the total national nursing home bill. Medicaid covers the cost of skilled nursing facility services. Those services are defined as any requiring skilled nursing personnel or other skilled rehabilitation services.

The costs for this programme have also escalated tremendously, and since a significant portion of the fiscal responsibility falls upon the states, further nursing home bed construction has been halted in some states. Since 1976, 27 per cent. of Medicaid costs went directly to nursing home care, compared to only 3 per cent. of Medicare. In 1980, the total Medicaid benefit cost to the states and the federal government was 25.3 billion dollars (Gibson and Waldo, 1981, p. 14).

It is important to note that the Medicaid payments are substantially lower than those provided under Medicare or private health insurance (Somers and Fabian, 1980, p. 7). As a result, some proprietors of nursing homes, and others, have sought to limit their clientele to those persons who possess either private insurance, private funding, or Medicare.

A problem occurs with Medicaid when individuals who are financially independent on admission to the nursing home wish to become eligible for coverage under Medicaid. At that time they must liquidate almost all their assets, including their homes. This process is called 'spending down'. After having spent one's life savings for care in the nursing home up to that point, this liquidation of assets precludes an opportunity to return home after rehabilitation.

Another criticism that has been leveled at the Medicaid programme is that payment is not contingent upon patient outcomes, thus supporting the status quo of the patient. Kane has suggested that reimbursement for nursing homes should be tied in with actual patient outcome. Under his proposal, each patient would be periodically assessed, compared with an expected course, and if the patient did as well as, or better than expected, the nursing home would be paid an amount greater than the estimated cost of the patient's care. On the other hand, if the outcome was less than optimal, or the patient's level of function deteriorated, then the reimbursement would be less than cost (Kane and Kane, 1978, p. 918).

In the case of both Medicare and Medicaid, the number of gaps in covered services and the widely varying state eligibility requirements, and the maze of rules regarding copayments and deductibles, present such a bewildering obstacle that the elderly individuals or their families find it almost impossible to obtain optimal patient coverage. In many instances, this leads to denial of benefits for those who are in fact eligible.

PRIVATE INSURANCE

In 1979, 76 per cent. of the population of the United States was covered by private health insurance for hospital care (Gibson and Waldo, 1981, p. 11). In 1975, 62.7 per cent. of the elderly were reported to have insurance for hospital care (Feder and Holahan, 1979). Private insurance, however, still covers less than 6 per cent. of the expenditures for the care of the elderly (Ball, 1981, p. 22). Currently, the major use of private health insurance is to supplement Medicare, and to reimburse by paying the co-payments and deductibles that arise for covered services. For the most part, private insurance does not provide payments for services that are not covered by Medicare or Medicaid, such as long-term nursing home care.

SOCIAL SECURITY

Somers has stated that the number one health programme in the United States is social security, her point being that an adequate income which sustains an individual above the poverty level is in fact one of the major contributors to good health (Somers and Fabian, 1980, p. 9). The social security programme is a federally operated programme based upon payroll deductions from workers and their employers. It provides monthly benefits to the retired and disabled, their dependents, widows, widowers, and children of deceased workers (Ball, 1978). In 1976, the Congressional Budget Office indicated that 60 per cent. of the families headed by persons over the age of 65 would be 'poor' (according to the rock-bottom definition of poverty), without social security benefits (Ball, 1981, p. 24).

Because some individuals have had only minimal participation in the payroll deduction system, there are still individuals whose benefits would be inadequate to maintain them above the poverty level. The United States has a programme to aid these individuals, entitled 'Supplemental Security Income'. This programme is not funded through payroll deductions, and it is means-tested to determine the needs of the individual. This programme guarantees a monthly income, albeit a small one. In 1983, the amount was $304.30 for single individuals and $456.40 for couples.

HEALTH CARE DELIVERY SYSTEM FOR THE ELDERLY

Before looking at the health care delivery system for the elderly, it is important to review briefly the development of the overall health care system in the United States.

The practice of medicine in the United States prior to World War II could be charac-

terized as being oriented to the non-specialist/general practitioner. Many of the health care needs, as well as the social needs, were met by personal family physicians who were available to make house calls and whose practices were carried on outside of hospitals. During this era, many families had three generations living under the same roof, and the elderly often lived out their later years surrounded by loved ones. The intimate experiences with death and dying were part of each family's life, and frequently occurred in the home.

Following World War II, a tremendous explosion of new biomedical research and information occurred. During these same years, the American family became more mobile and many families lived in physically separate dwellings, and frequently in widely separate geographic areas. Many elderly lived alone by choice although families with initially strong ties retained them, and their children continued to be responsible for many parents' needs in their later years.

During the 1950s and early 1960s, a continuous decline in the number of general practitioners occurred. Concomitant with this decline, the availability of home health care decreased markedly. Health care delivery became focused on hospitals and hospital emergency rooms. The initial work-up frequently occurred in doctors' offices, but then the patient was referred to the hospital, a site where there was more sophisticated equipment for diagnostic testing. Medical education and medical training programmes of this era produced increasing numbers of specialists, a fact which plays a major role in the fragmentation of health care for the elderly today. Because the elderly frequently suffer multiple chronic disorders and are also under a wide variety of significant social and economic pressures, the effect of a poorly coordinated fragmented health care system frequently exerts maximal impact upon this group.

During the 1960s and 1970s, the growth in the number of nursing homes in the United States was phenomenal. Two years before Medicare and Medicaid, there were slightly more than 8,100 nursing homes; today there are 18,300 (Pearson and Wetle, 1981, p. 224). With that background, this section will examine some of the significant parts of the health care delivery system for the elderly.

Ambulatory Care

The overwhelming majority (95 per cent.) of the elderly do not live in institutions. For these individuals, ambulatory care is of great importance. Kovar has reported that about three-quarters of all visits made by the elderly are to office-based physicians. The family practitioners and the general internists are responsible for 66 per cent. of these visits (Kovar, 1977, p. 14).

Acute Hospitals

There are several types of hospitals in the United States but the most common one is the voluntary (not for profit) general (non-special) short-term hospital. The acute hospitals in the United States were changing dramatically in the 1970s, with more and more acute specialty care units being established within each institution. With the growth of these specialty units, patients were able to receive more sophisticated high technology critical care. In the case of the elderly, chronic problems might be overlooked and sensitive personal care often diminishes.

The acute care hospitals also added key services such as rehabilitation, social, psychiatric, and family care services to those already existing in medicine and nursing. Therefore, within the acute hospital, several levels of care were available. The hospital became a model of coordinated services which the rest of the nonhospital care system was unable to provide.

The acute care hospital was also the point at which many elderly individuals began their formal contact with the established health care system. Unfortunately, the links between the acute care hospital and the services in the community (both of a social and medical nature) were frequently lacking. Currently, more acute hospitals in the United States are establishing associations with chronic care facilities.

Long-Term Care Facilities

Long-term care institutions include nursing homes, homes for the aged, rest and convalescent homes. A nursing home is defined by the Long-Term Care Minimum Data Set Report of the National Committee on Vital and Health Statistics as, 'an establishment with three or more beds whose primary function is to serve unrelated persons who do not need hospitalization but require nursing services and other health related services. It includes facilities that are certified or licensed as skilled nursing facilities and/or intermediate care facilities and uncertified facilities that provide the equivalent levels of skilled or limited nursing services' (Monahan and Greene, 1981).

In 1973, the United States had 1,327,704 nursing home beds. At the same time, there were a total of 1,030,432 hospital beds, directing attention to the fact that there were now more nursing home beds than acute hospital care beds (Kane and Kane, 1978, p. 914). These nursing home beds were mostly in institutions with capacities of between 25 to 200 beds. During this time, 76.6 per cent. of nursing homes were proprietary (being operated for profit); 17.3 per cent. were non-profit, and 6.1 per cent. were government operated (Scanlon, Difederico, and Stassen, 1979, p. 60).

In 1973, 83 per cent. of nursing home residents were 75 years of age and over, and almost 75 per cent. of them were women. Out of these, one-third to one-half were incontinent, two-thirds were estimated to be senile, and one-third were either bed- or chair-fast (Kovar, 1977, p. 18).

Nursing homes are classified into two categories: skilled and intermediate care facilities. A skilled facility must provide complete care and have a registered nurse on duty 24 hours a day. Although not a required part of the staff, a physician must supervise the health care of each patient and must be available for emergencies. Such a facility must offer a regular programme of independent medical review of patients in order to assess their progress and appropriateness of their placement.

Intermediate care facilities deliver less intensive care than the skilled institutions, and are not required to have a registered nurse on duty 24 hours a day. Rather, a registered nurse or licensed practical nurse must supervise the provision of services only during the day shift.

Although many nursing homes provide good care, there are deficiencies in terms of the availability of many vital services such as rehabilitation, occupational therapy, and mental health services. These are the services so vital in maintaining the activities of daily living of the elderly at their highest level.

Another problem with the nursing home industry has been the tremendously high turnover rate among personnel who have had very little geriatric training. Some authors suggest that the annual turnover rate of staff in nursing homes approaches 75 per cent. (Pearson and Wetle, 1981, p. 225). The industry has also been plagued by scandals in the form of Medicare/Medicaid fraud, poor enforcement of regulations, patient abuse, and tragic fires.

Personal Care Homes and Domiciliary Care Facilities

Other facilities in which nursing home care is not provided include personal care and domiciliary care units. In 1973, a report stated there were a total of 11,107 beds in these facilities. Most of these facilities contained less than 25 beds (Scanlon, Difederico, and Stasson, 1979, p. 65).

In a personal care home, therapy can be given following a physician's order. The main function of the units is to assist with activities of daily living – bathing, toileting, eating, transferring, and ambulation. In a personal care home, three or more of these services are provided to each resident.

In the domiciliary care facility, no medical services are provided, and only one or two activities of daily living services are provided for each resident. Neither of these facilities is eligible for Medicare.

Foster Care Homes

The foster care home is a private dwelling in which the owner becomes the careprovider responsible for housekeeping services, meals, personal care, minimal observation, and the provision of a room for the elderly patient. Information on the number of foster care homes is difficult to obtain, as evidenced by the Congressional Budget Office which estimates that between 75,000 and 635,000 units exist in foster care homes and congregate care centres. This estimate was made in 1977 (Scanlon, Difederico, and Stasson, 1979, p. 68). Both of these units are important parts of the community health care system.

Eighty per cent. of the home care to the elderly people in the United States is delivered by their own families (Brody, 1977). The costs of maintaining an elderly person at home are borne largely by the family with assistance from the elderly individual's various pension or supplemental social security income plans. Paradoxically, governmental benefits are reduced when the eligible elderly person resides with the family.

Congregate Facilities

Congregate housing facilities include both government-supported facilities and private retirement villages, sectarian elderly housing developments, and other non-profit institutions. Common to these facilities is the sharing of such functions as housekeeping, meals, health, and transportation.

Non-Institutional Housing

Many American elderly rent individual apartments, or in the case of those with restricted incomes, community housing has been especially designed for older residents and offers the convenience of emergency call system or the availability of social services. For those with adequate incomes, the United States has popularized the concept of retirement villages. Individual lots and homes may be purchased – some with combined medical facilities and common social centres such as golf courses, etc. Of significance is the fact that the cost of many retirement communities is beyond the means of great numbers of elderly individuals.

More recently, the development of facilities with several levels of care and types of living quarters in one location have become available. These may include apartments, single-unit dwellings, a nursing home (including a skilled care capability), and congregate living facilities. Certain facilities allow individual clients to pay an initial fee that entitles them to a lifetime use of the facility. There is usually a monthly charge for maintenance services and operating costs, and at the end of the individual's lifespan, the facilities revert to the property of the sponsor.

Community Services

From its outset, the British National Health System included a community-based programme whose goal was to meet the needs of the population outside the hospital. There was, and is, no similar programme in effect in the United States. Instead, the specific needs were frequently approached by the development of a separate programme under the auspices of either the federal, state, or local government or volunteer groups. Programmes for the blind and deaf, those in need of additional fuel for heating their homes, nutritional programmes, social programmes, etc., were instituted by various governmental bodies. Each of these programmes had specific eligibility criteria for a specific target population. Each programme frequently had financial support from both the federal and state government, and existed in a separate geographic location. No attempts were made to coordinate many of these programmes, and very frequently the elderly individuals or their families were required to seek out the services rather than be contacted by the agency. The varied eligibility requirements and locations of these agencies often represented an insoluble puzzle for the elderly and their families. Again, because they frequently are victims of multiple chronic disorders, the elderly would have to visit multiple locations to receive appropriate services and coverage. More important, no single site or facility existed in which the actual needs of the patient could be determined and from which the social and medical services could be coordinated to meet those needs.

The availability of community-based services in the United States, such as day care, provision of meals, homemaker services, etc., varies widely from community to community. Many of these targeted services are more readily available in the urban areas then in the rural areas where transportation is a much more significant problem. The rural situation is also complicated by the lack of large numbers of skilled personnel.

Many of these services are provided by government agencies but volunteer community groups and other organizations, such as churches, also plan an important role. Personal care services such as assistance in the activities of daily living are being provided by home health aides. Each home health aide must be supervised by a registered nurse if the service is to be reimbursed by Medicare. This is a cumbersome aspect of the programme.

Homemakers and home health aides are re-quired by Medicare to complete a formal geriatric instruction programme during the first 6 months of their work. The funding for these home services available under Medicare is almost solely for skilled services, i.e. the patient must be home-bound and under the care of a physician. The need for homemaker home health aides far exceeds the supply in the United States. Silverstone has estimated that there are 30,000 homemaker home health aides to meet a need of 300,000 clients (Silverstone, and Hyman, 1976).

Originally, proprietary home health agencies were not reimbursed by Medicare, but this has recently been changed to allow them to qualify for payment. Some funding is also available under Medicaid but this remains a small proportion of the overall programme which is oriented towards institutional care. Both Medicare and Medicaid have remained relatively small contributors to home health care and there is considerable fear that if home care benefits were expanded, the huge cost of these programmes would be prohibitive. The Congressional Budget Office estimates that less than 10 per cent. of public expenditures goes into non-institutional care settings (Scanlon, Difederico, and Stassen, 1979, p. 96).

Homemaker services such as laundry, grocery shopping, home repairs, groundskeeping, home alterations, etc., receive minimal allocations of public or voluntary funds. Some funding is available under the Social Security Act but the elderly must compete with all other age groups for this money.

Meals-on-Wheels and Congregate Meals

The two major programmes currently available in the United States to provide adequate nutrition for the elderly are 'meals-on-wheels' and the congregate meals programme. 'Meals-on-wheels' is a voluntary programme and is frequently operated by civic or religious groups. The programme delivers meals to the home and utilizes a sliding scale of payments for their recipients based upon their income; it is important to note that they operate in several rural areas in the United States. Funding is largely from private sources.

The congregate meals programme is a federally funded nutrition programme. In 1977, 225 billion dollars in federal funds were appropriated for this programme which served an estimated 2.8 million elderly persons in congregate settings. Under this programme, citizens were served one hot meal per day, and approximately 15 per cent. of these meals were delivered to the home. The need for both of these programmes exceeds current delivery capability.

Day Care Programmes

Day care programmes for the elderly are still underdeveloped and relatively unavailable in the United States. The programmes vary in the amount of medical services versus social services that they offer. The day care hospital concept which has been developed in Great Britain exists in only a handful of locations in the United States. One facility, located at the Burke Rehabilitation Center in White Plains, New York, was established for research into this concept (Brocklehurst and Tucker, 1980). The major problem facing these institutions is reimbursement, since most services are not covered under existing legislation.

Another important problem inhibiting the day hospital concept has been the lack of an integrated and coordinated transportation network in most communities. Figures from a 1980 directory indicate 600 day care programmes serving 13,500 persons (Robins, 1981). Medicaid coverage is only offered by some states.

Hospice Care

It has been estimated today that some 70 per cent. of deaths in the United States take place in hospitals or other institutions which could be characterized by impersonal surroundings and lack of humanistic concern (Technical Committee on Health Services, 1981, p. 25). In 1979, a survey revealed more than 57 active, planned, and community support hospices in the United States and Canada (Cohen, 1979). This number has continued to grow and the concept seems firmly rooted in America's health care scheme. Reimbursement for hospice service is only slowly becoming available, but is included in the new Medicare legislation.

Mental Health Services

Fifteen per cent. of all older people within the community and up to 70 per cent. of those who are institutionalized manifest significant mental and/or emotional problems. The striking fact is that only 1.5 per cent. of all mental health resources in the United States are expended on elderly patients (Technical Committee on Health Services, 1981, p. 10). This lack of mental health service for the elderly is particularly acute in the institutional setting where the problems are so prevalent. When the large mental hospitals were being decompressed by placing the patients in the community, a community mental health programme was established in the United States. Its purpose was to assist the integration of those elderly individuals with mental problems into the community. Unfortunately, many of these patients ultimately were placed in nursing homes, and currently only 4 per cent. of the caseloads of community mental health centres and outpatient services are comprised of elderly clients (Fig. 6).

Use of mental health services by the elderly
United States, 1971 and 1975

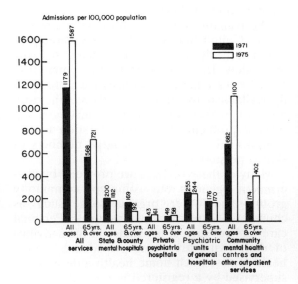

Figure 6   Use of mental health services by the elderly: United States, 1971 and 1975. (From US Department of Health and Human Services, 1981)

Dental Care

In 1971, over 50 per cent. of elderly white males in the United States were found to be edentulous. Although this figure has been declining recently, the elderly continue to have a very high incidence of periodontal problems. Of those elderly fortunate enough to have dentures, 27 per cent. report their dentures need refitting or replacement (Kovar, 1977, p. 15). A 1978 survey indicated that 60 per cent. of the total population over the age of 65 has not visited a dentist in two or more years (U.S. Department of Health and Human Services, 1980). These statistics indicate there is a large population of elderly who need dental care, some of whom do not receive it because of a lack of financial resources. Medicare offers essentially no dental benefits.

GERIATRIC EDUCATION AND MANPOWER NEEDS

This section will review the current situation in the United States in regard to the geriatric educational and training programmes in medicine and nursing, as well as the projected manpower needs.

A 1977 survey of the American Medical Association, seeking to determine physicians' professional activities, generated an 88 per cent. response rate from 363,619 active practitioners. Of this group, geriatrics was listed as a primary specialty only by 371; as a secondary specialty by 187; and as a tertiary specialty by 71, making a grand total of 629 physicians (roughly 0.2 per cent.) of the practising physician community (Kane *et al.*, 1980a). These figures indicate a severe shortage of physicians in the geriatric field.

A report in 1977 by the American Geriatrics Society indicates that the creation of a new geriatrics specialty would lead not only to friction and confusion about the medical specialty organizations and their training programmes, but would also lead to confusion for the lay public (Reichel, 1977). The Society felt that another specialty would only confuse the elderly patient in terms of further fragmentation of the responsibility for their care.

A second report in September 1978 from the prestigious Institute of Medicine of the National Academy of Sciences recommended against the establishment of a formal practice specialty in geriatrics but favoured the recognition of gerontology and geriatrics as academic disciplines within the relevant medical specialties (Committee of the Institute of Medicine, 1978).

Others have felt that geriatrics does represent a specific body of knowledge and should become a separate specialty. The discussion continues as to whether certificates of special geriatric competence will be issued within the current specialties, i.e. family practice, internal medicine, and psychiatry; or whether in fact there will be a separate specialty Board.

Geriatrics in Medical Schools

In 1976, there were only a few programmes in geriatrics in medical schools in the United States. By 1979, 81 medical schools were in the process of developing such programmes at this level – a substantial increase over 1976. In Robins' survey of 108 medical school programmes, 82.4 per cent. remain elective and are in various stages of development (Robbins, Vivell, and Beck, 1982, p. 85). A great deal of this new interest in geriatric education has been stimulated through federal grant support. In addition, some states, such as Ohio, have actually legislated geriatric programmes into the medical school curriculum.

The recent White House Conference on Aging produced many recommendations to expand the amount of geriatric training that is offered not only to physicians but to nurses and other health professionals.

Geriatric Fellowship Programmes

A survey reporting on the 1980–81 academic year found 36 geriatric fellowship training programmes in the United States, most of which were started in the last two years (Robbins, Vivell, and Beck, 1982, p. 82). Prerequisites for these programmes included Board eligibility in either internal medicine, psychiatry, and/ or family practice. The number of actual training positions for the academic year 1981 was 87.

The geriatric fellowship programmes vary a great deal in composition but most offer experience in long-term care facilities and emphasize working with other health professionals, including nurse practitioners, social workers, rehabilitation specialists, community health workers, and volunteers. Training is also offered in geropsychiatry, rehabilitation, neurology, and community health, as well as other electives.

There is a critical shortage of faculty to staff both undergraduate and graduate geriatric training programmes in the United States. As a result, the major thrust of many of the currently operational programmes is to provide an educational experience that will allow the fellow in the future to train more geriatric physicians and allied health personnel in the geriatric area.

In 1980, Kane and coworkus (1980b) estimated the needs for geriatric manpower in the United States for the next 50 years. The calculations were done using four different models of care. The first model utilized the status quo with little delegation of responsibility to nurse practitioners and social workers. The second model provided a cadre of geriatricians who would function solely in an academic setting. The third model extended the clinical role of the geriatrician outside of the academic settling, but limited his function to that of a consultant who would see elderly patients on a 'referral basis' only. This use of the geriatrician is similar to the British geriatric specialist. In the fourth model, the geriatrician would provide some of the primary care to the elderly as well as function as a specialist. Each model was then analysed using varying delegation of care responsibility to social workers, nurse practitioners, and physicians' assistants. The delegation of responsibility was characterized as minimal, moderate, and maximal, with minimal corresponding to the situation as it exists today.

The authors concluded that by 1990 the United States will require approximately 8,000 geriatricians, based on the following assumptions: (a) most specialized geriatric care would be given to patients who were at least 75 years of age, (b) there would be a moderate degree of delegation of care to social workers and nurse practitioners, and (c) there would be an increase in the depth of care (Kane *et al.* 1980b).

The study indicated that the results did not call for an absolute increase in the number of physicians but would depend upon some re-allocation of current training programme positions. Whether one agrees with the calculations or not, most experts in the field agree there is an absolute shortage of adequately trained manpower to deal with the rapidly expanding geriatric population in the United States.

In addition, if the system requires the delegation of responsibility to other health professionals, such as geriatric nurse practitioners, social workers, or physicians' assistants, there will have to be a concomitant increase in faculty, as well as students, enrolled in these programmes to meet the projected needs.

Geriatric Education in Nursing

The situation in nursing education is similar to that found in medical education. An extremely small fraction of the United States' nursing school graduates seek employment in nursing homes. In 1976, only 5 per cent. of approximately 700,000 registered nurses in the United States were employed in nursing homes (Heller and Walsh, 1976).

In an article in 1975, the authors commented on the fact that nursing curricula include in their clinical theory courses experience in obstetrics and maternity, paediatrics, surgery, and psychiatry. Few include theoretical content or clinical practice in geriatrics (Kayser and Minnigerode, 1975). Currently a small but increasing number of nursing schools, including the University of Rochester, Duke University, and Case Western Reserve, are offering graduate level training programmes for geriatric nurse practitioners (Lindsay, 1979). The total production of these programmes is minuscule. Required geriatric course material at the nursing undergraduate level is still scarce.

Recent Developments in Geriatric Education

In 1978, the National Institute on Aging, under the leadership of Dr Robert Butler, established a programme entitled, 'The Geriatric Medicine Academic Award'. This programme is designed to stimulate faculty and curriculum development in geriatric medicine and research in geriatrics and gerontology. This programme has become the nucleus for the development of geriatric medicine in the medical schools across the United States. The National Institute on Aging has been instrumental in fostering research and teaching in the long-term carre field. The Institute is sponsoring a programme entitled 'Teaching Nursing Homes'. This has as its goal the development of teaching in the long-term care setting and research into all aspects of nursing homes.

CHALLENGES OF THE FUTURE

The problems facing the United States in caring for its elderly population are being identified. The next 40 years will see these problems increase in magnitude (Fig. 7). The increase in the size of the elderly population will impact directly on the future use of health services.

Projections of the use of health services by the elderly United States, 1978 and 2000

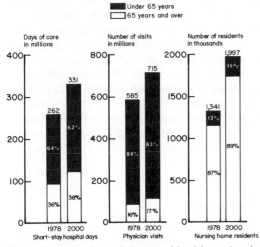

Figure 7 Projections of the use of health services by the elderly: United States, 1978 and 2000. (Note: Physician visits exclude contacts and visits to clinics and emergency rooms.) (From US Department of Health and Human Services, 1981)

The United States faces the problems of the elderly with a patchwork system of expensive medical services. The total projected health care expenditures for 1990 will be 758 billion dollars (U.S. Department of Health and Human Services, 1981, p. 52). Significantly, at a time when health care costs are rising exponentially, many elderly individuals are living on relatively fixed incomes of below $6,000/year (Fig. 8).

Percent distribution of families and unrelated individuals by income levels: United States, 1978

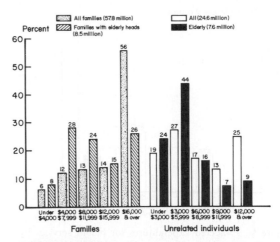

Figure 8 Percentage of distribution of families and unrelated individuals by income levels: United States, 1978. (Note: Income categories are smaller for unrelated individuals due to lower poverty thresholds and excludes unrelated individuals under 14 years.) (From US Department of Health and Human Services, 1981)

The United States' acute care hospital system is a superb one, capable of delivering the finest in high technology intensive care. However, as stated previously, this does not always meet the needs of the elderly.

The long-term care and chronic care system is also expensive. The current costs of nursing homes in the United States is $16 billion annually, with projected increases to $76 billion by 1990 (Fig. 9). This is paying for a system which fails to provide many of the essentials necessary to optimize a patient's functional capability, and which favours an institutional setting for patient care over a home setting.

The community-based, non-institutional services of the United States are seriously underdeveloped and underfinanced. These include both social and medical services. This lack of institutional alternatives often forces institutional care on individuals who do not need it, and contributes to the tremendous costs of nursing home care. Currently, many of these non-institutional services are undergoing substantial cuts in federal funding while the demand increases. The future must see greater efforts by volunteer organizations if progress is to be made.

Projected expenditures for health services by type of service: United States, 1978 and 1990

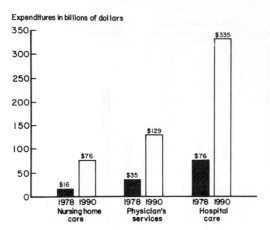

Figure 9   Projected expenditures for health services by type of service: United States, 1978 and 1990. (Note: This assumes that historical trends and relationships from 1965 to 1978 will continue into the future.) (From US Department of Health and Human Services, 1981)

The family which is the primary care giver in the United States' system will in the future have to receive a greater level of support if home care is to increase and needless institutionalization is to decrease. Suggestions of direct payments and other services to families are now being made in both national and state forums. Currently, programmes of respite care for families are rare and this type of care is not reimbursable.

In the future, community-based systems of coordinated care will be essential. Several pilot programmes have been operating with a goal of providing cost–benefit information and operational research. One such programme, The Wisconsin Community Care Organization, allows elderly individuals to contact one organization when they need assistance to remain in or return to the community. This single organization can provide eligibility information, needs assessment, service planning, service delivery, and manage payments (American College of Physicians, 1980). The information provided by such programmes will allow sensible design of future non-institutional care systems.

The health planners of the future must also address the problems of health care delivery for the rural elderly. The current lack of skilled personnel and services in the rural setting must

be overcome. The transportation situation, a major problem for all elderly in the United States, is a particular challenge in the rural area. Some rural areas have tackled the problem of rural health care by moving the service to the elderly in mobile vans containing laboratory facilities and health care personnel.

The future must see more legislation directed towards assisting the elderly. The recent White House Conference on Aging indicated the growing political strength of the elderly. It is hoped that this strength will lead to increased resource allocation to programmes for the elderly.

The future must see a critical examination of the reimbursement mechanism for non-institutional care and services. Until these services can be covered by either governmental or private insurance, developments in this sphere of health care will be slow.

Finally, the integration of the social and medical parts of geriatric health care delivery systems will continue to evolve and grow. The model community care projects are now providing experience in multidisciplinary care and coordination of services. The new efforts in geriatric medical education at the undergraduate and graduate levels are a major step in preparing physicians and nurses to be important parts of the future health care delivery system for the elderly.

REFERENCES

American College of Physicians (1980). *Proceedings of the Conference on the Changing Needs of Nursing Home Care*, American College of Physicians, Washington, D. C.

Ball, R. M. (1978). Social Security: Today and Tomorrow. Columbia University Press, p. 1.

Ball, R. M. (1981). 'Rethinking national policy on health care for the elderly: An introduction to gerontology and clinical geriatrics', in *The Geriatric Imperative* (Eds A. R. Somers and D. R. Fabian), Appleton-Century Crofts.

Brocklehurst, J. D. and Tucker, J. S. (1980). *Progress in Geriatric Day Care*, King Edward's Hospital Fund, London.

Brody, E. M. (1977). *Long-Term Care of Older People: A Geriatric Guide*, p. 65, Human Sciences Press, New York.

Butler, R. N. (1975). *Why Survive? Being Old in America*, p. 2, Harper and Row, New York.

Cohen, K. P. (1979). *Hospice: Prescription to Terminal Care*, p. 155, Aspen Systems Corporation. Rockville, USA.

Committee of the Institute of Medicine (1978). *Report of a Study on Aging and Medical Education*, Publication No. 10M–78–04, p. xiii, Washington, D.C.

Feder, J., and Holahan, J. (1979). *Financing Health Care for the Elderly. Medicare, Medicaid and Private Health Insurance*, p. 43, Health Policy and Elderly Series, The Urban Institute.

Gibson, R. M., and Waldo, D. R. (1981). 'National health expenditures, 1980', *Health Care Financing Review*, **1981**, 11–19.

Heller, R. R., and Walsh, F. J. (1976). 'Changing nursing students' attitudes toward the aging: An experimental study', *J. Nurs. Ed.*, **15** (1), 9–17.

Kane, R. W., and Kane, R. A. (1978). 'Care of the aged: Old problems in need of new solutions', *Science*, **200**, 914–918.

Kane, R. L., Solomon, D. H., Beck, J. C., Keeler, E., and Kane, R. A. (1980a). *Geriatrics in the United States. Manpower Protection and Training Considerations*, p. 14, Publication No. R 2543–HJK, Rand Corporation, Santa Monica, California.

Kane, R. L., Solomon, D. H., Beck, J. C., Keeler, E., and Kane, R. A. (1980b). 'The future need for geriatric manpower in the U.S.: A special article', *N Engl. J. Med.*, **302**, 1332.

Kayser, J. S., and Minnigerode, F. A. (1975). Increasing nursing students' interest on working with aged patients', *Nursing Res.* **24** (1), 23–26.

Kovar, M. D. (1977). 'Health of the elderly and use of health services', in *Health of the Elderly. Public Health Reports*, **92**, No. 1, 14–18.

Lindsay, R. W. (1979). 'A survey of geriatric medicine and nursing education in the United States'. Monograph. Virginia Centre on Aging at Virginia Commonwealth University, Richmond, Virginia, p. 27.

Monahan, D. J., and Greene, V. L. (1981). 'Long term care: Concepts and definitions, Generations', *Quart J. Western Gerontol. Soc.*, **5** (3), 8.

Pearson, D. A., and Wetle, T. T. (1981). *Long-Term Care in Health Delivery in the U.S.*, Springer Publishing Co., Inc., New York.

Reichel, W. (1977). 'Graduate education: Rejection of C model', *J. Am. Geriat. Soc.*, **XXV**, No. 11, 489.

Robbins, A. S., Vivell, and S., Beck, J. C. (1982). 'A study of geriatric training programs in the United States', *J. Med. Ed.*, **57**, No. 2, 82–85.

Robins, E. G. (1981). 'Adult day care: Growing fast but still for lucky few', *Generations*, **V**, No. 3, 22–23.

Scanlon, W., Difederico, E. and Stassen, M. (1979). *Long-Term Care. Current Experience and a Framework for Analysis*, Health Policy and the Elderly Series. The Urban Institute, Washington, D.C.

Shanas, E. (1980). The status of health care for the elderly', in *Health Care of the Elderly* (Ed. Gari Lesnoff-Caravaglia), pp. 167–176, Human Sciences Press, New York.

Silverstone, B., and Hyman, H. K. (1976). 'You and your aging parent', in *The Modern Family's Guide to Emotional, Physical and Financial Problems*, Pantheon Books, New York.

Soldo, B. J. (1980). 'Americas' elderly in the 1980s', *Population Bulletin*, **35**, No. 4, 7–11.

Somers, A., and Fabian, D. (1980). 'Rethinking health policy for the elderly: A six-point program', *Inquiry*, **17**, 7–9.

Technical Committee on Health Services (1981). *Report of the 1981 White House Conference on Aging*, pp. 2–25, U.S. Government Printing Office, Washington D.C.

United States Department of Health, Education and Welfare (1978). *Public Policy and the Frail Elderly: A Staff Report*, DHEW Publication No. (OHDS) 79–20959, Office of Human Developments Services, Federal Council on Aging, Washington, D.C.

United States Department of Health and Human Services (1980). *Health, United States*, p. 47, DDHS Publication No. (PHS) 81–1232, Hyattsville, Maryland.

United States Department of Health and Human Services (1981). *The Need for Long-Term Care*, A Chartbook of the Federal Council on Aging, DHHS Publication No. (OHDS) 81–20704, Office of Human Development Services, Washington, D.C.

Principles and Practice of Geriatric Medicine
Edited by M. S. J. Pathy
© 1985 John Wiley & Sons Ltd

30.3

Delivery of Health Care in Japan

J. Ohmura

ILL-HEALTH IN THE ELDERLY

Ill-health in the elderly increases with senescence. Even when there is no sickness the physical and mental reserve decline. However, human functions do not decline uniformly with ageing. Vision and hearing are the first to show the symptoms of ageing, followed by the simple locomotor functions, and finally by complicated integrated functions like muscle coordination. Maintenance of homeostasis enables the elderly to continue to lead a normal healthy life despite reduced physiological functions. The particular characteristic of the elderly is that their ability to cope with stress is significantly less than that of younger adults and their physiological reserves decline.

Socioeconomic Background

Upon retirement from his main occupation the elderly person can retreat or possibly take on a second job which is comparatively dull. Along with this there is a narrowing of personal relationships.

At home the parent–child relationships change, the elderly person may be bereaved of spouse and close friends, and the children establish separate households. His income is reduced, he has to live on a pension, or he loses his economic independence and has to rely on others. As a consequence the standard of living of the elderly person declines.

In the European and North American countries the family is centred on the husband and wife. When the children grow up and marry it is common practice for them to live apart from their parents. In Japan, although there is a trend towards nuclear families, 74.2 per cent. of the 65 year olds and over still live with their children (*Fact-Finding Survey on the Elderly*, Social Welfare Bureau, Ministry of Health and Welfare, 1973). This is extremely high compared with Europe and America.

From a period of high birth and death rates in the 1940s, Japan has experienced a very rapid change to a period of low birth and death rates since the 1960s.

Before World War II, the rate of increase in the population aged 65 and over was low and was 4.1 per cent. for the 10 year period from 1920 to 1930, but 12.7 per cent. for the 10 years from 1930 to 1940. After the War this demographic change continued and the rate of increase of the Japanese population over 65 rose 30.3 per cent. from 1950 to 1960, to 37.0 per cent. from 1960 to 1970, and to 48.3 per cent. from 1970 to 1980. The percentage of the total population aged 65 and over was stable before the War, but increased rapidly after the War to 9.05 per cent. in 1980, which was still less than that of other advanced countries. However, it is expected to grow rapidly, according to estimates published in November 1981 by the Institute of Population Problems, Ministry of Health and Welfare. The population projection, based on the medium variant for TFR, (Total Specific Fertility Rate) is shown in Table 1. The percentage of persons 65 and over in the population is estimated at 11.65 in 1990, 15.57 in the year 2000, and 21.29

Table 1   Trends of ageing of the Japanese population

	Total[a]	Age 0 to 14	Age 15 to 64	Age 65 and over	Age 75 and over	Ratio, age 65 and over (%)	Crude birth rate (per 1,000)	Crude death rate (per 1,000)
Actual								
1920	55,963	20,417	32,606	2,941	732	5.26	36.20	25.41
1930	64,540	23,579	37,808	3,063				
1940[b]	71,933	26,383	42,097	3,454	903	4.80	29.40	16.50
1950[b]	83,199	29,428	49,659	4,109	1,057	4.93	28.10	10.88
1960[b]	93,419	28,067	60,002	5,350	1,626	5.72	17.19	7.56
1970	103,119	24,645	71,164	7,311	2,209	7.09	18.76	6.91
1980	116,916	27,547	78,791	10,578	3,645	9.05	13.57	6.22
Estimated[c]								
1990	122,834							
		22,512	86,032	14,290	5,553	11.65	11.42	7.47
2000	128,119	22,561	85,615	19,943	7,473	15.57	13.34	9.31
2025	127,184	21,929	78,176	27,079	13,840	21.29	12.86	14.13
2050	120,790	21,909	73,375	25,506	13,291	21.12	13.01	14.31
2075	118,395	22,141	73,000	23,253	11,126	19.69	12.90	12.95

[a] Population figures are in thousands.
[b] Okinawa prefecture is excluded.
[c] Estimation from *The New Estimate of Future Population of Japan* by the Institute of Population Problems, Ministry of Health and Welfare, November 1981. The figures are calculated based on the medium variant.

in 2025. This last estimate is higher than the estimated ratio for all other countries except Luxembourg and Switzerland, according to the United Nations projections.

Within the aged population, the proportions of higher age groups are markedly increasing. The percentage of persons 75 and over, within the aged population, decreased slightly before the War. However, it increased from 25.7 per cent. in 1950 to 34.5 per cent. in 1980. The percentage is expected to be up to 38.9 per cent. in 1990.

A significant characteristic of the ageing of the Japanese population is its speed. It will have taken Japan only 67 years to bring the percentage of persons 65 and over from the 4.76 of 1930 to 14.43 in 1997. The United Kingdom, on the other hand, took 129 years to raise it from 4.65 in 1851, to 14.14 in 1980. The speed of ageing of the Japanese population is twice as fast as that of the United Kingdom.

The population distribution according to age groups for the years 1980 to 2000 is shown in Figure 1. The form can be seen to be changing from a bell- to a jar-type outline.

In Japan, households with persons aged 60 and over can be broken down as follows: single households – 10.3 per cent., nuclear family households – 30.6 per cent., three-generation households – 46.9 per cent., and others – 12.3

per cent.. (*Health and Welfare Administrations Basic Survey*, Statistics and Information De-

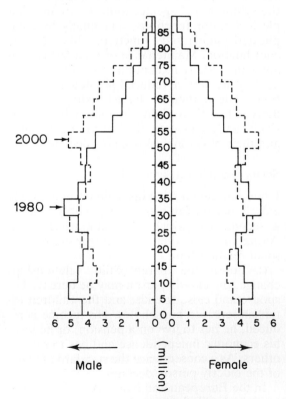

Figure 1   Japanese population distribution according to age groups for the years 1980 and 2000

partment, Minister's Secretariat, Ministry of Health and Welfare, 1976). The proportion of nuclear families decreases with age because of the loss of the spouse. Because of the difference in age between husband and wife and the fact that women on average live longer than men, there are more women who are in single households or being looked after by their children.

In Japan 30 per cent. of the bedridden old people are accommodated in hospitals or nursing homes, while the remainder are cared for at home. Over half of the men requiring care received it from their wives or, in many cases, from their daughters-in-law. In the case of women, over half are cared for by their daughters-in-law or, secondly, by their daughters (*Fact-Finding Survey on Care for the Elderly*, Interim Report, Japan Social Welfare Council, 1977).

MENTAL DISORDERS OF THE ELDERLY

Within the planning for a health system for the elderly, it is necessary to consider their particular mental characteristics. Like other internal organs the brain cannot escape from senescence. In addition to the effects of the biological ageing of the brain, the mental and psychological condition of elderly people is also often affected when they cannot adapt to social and economic changes.

There are several reasons (physical, psychological, and social) for the occurence of mental disorders in old age. The introduction of preventative measures and the use of early intervention resources may stem the development or advance of mental disorders in the elderly.

PRIMARY CARE FOR THE ELDERLY

While the elderly population is small there is no necessity to consider the particular medical systems for them. However with the increase in the number of elderly people there is a growing necessity for special planning.

The health care system for each country has developed historically its own particular structure, and the medical care system for the aged can hardly be regarded as separated from the system as a whole. For primary health care to be complete, provision must be made for the aged and as they frequently suffer from chronic

diseases comprehensiveness and continuity of the care is especially important. Home medical care is mainly provided by the family doctor and the visiting nurse. If hospital admission is necessary it is appropriate that accommodation at a general or special hospital be available for the elderly patient. However, because of their particular characteristics, it is desirable that a geriatric department be provided to meet the special health needs of elderly people.

PREVENTION OF DISEASE AND DISABILITY

Genetic enviromental, and occupational factors can cause diseases in old age. The overt manifestations of sickness may be long delayed and subsequent treatment may need to be prolonged and is often incomplete. For preventing adult illnesses it is imperative that healthy living habits are followed when young and precautions are taken against chronic diseases. For example, the number of bedridden elderly persons in Japan is estimated to be 400,000. The reasons for this are: stroke – 35.3 per cent., hypertension – 18.1 per cent., rheumatism and neuralgia – 9.5 per cent., senility – 9.5 per cent. and others – 27.6 per cent. (*Fact-Finding Survey on the Elderly*, Social Welfare Bureau, Ministry of Health and Welfare, 1980). About half of these cases of bedfastness could be prevented by control of hypertension.

There are no standard methods for adult health screening but for certain high-risk groups it is important that enforcement plans be established after consideration of cost-benefit analyses. In Japan urine, blood pressure, and electrocardiogram check-ups are carried out together with various blood tests. As a result of subsequent health guidance given to control blood pressure, the corrected death rate due to cerebrovascular diseases fell by 36.4 per cent. in the 10 years from 1968 to 1978. Over recent years the smear test for uterine cancer screening has become more popular by self-collection methods.

More important than expensive medical examinations, is to teach elderly people to regulate their lives and become conscious of protecting their own health by maintaining good health habits. A health facility called Promotorium (health promotion sanatorium) has been established experimentally in Japan. Elderly people live there for a period to learn and practice good health habits.

INTEGRATION OF SERVICES

Health maintenance and its related needs pose various problems in old age. There are also many problems concerning the home and other living environments. Consequently, it is necessary that a comprehensive health service incorporating health promotion, prevention, cure and rehabilitation, and a welfare service including support for everyday life and recreation be fully integrated. It is now desirable that this integrated service, based on the community, be planned to make efficient use of social resources in accordance with the needs of the elderly.

PROMOTION OF HOME CARE

Apart from elderly people living alone, it is preferable that those living with their families remain at home provided that the condition of their ill health allows it. Accommodation in an institution means separation from the family, and prolonged institutionalization may occur and the costs become high.

Some of the obstacles against the trend for home care are: cramped and inferior living conditions, children moving away from home, the increase in the number of elderly living alone, and the ageing and fatigue of family members undertaking the care of elderly relatives. To contain these problems requires comprehensive community health and welfare services. These include government assistance for home improvements, a visiting health team service involving doctors, nurses, rehabilitation technicians, and social workers, together with guidance for the family members, the development of day care health facilities, the provision of meals-on-wheels and domestic helps, and the encouragement of assistance by volunteers. The short-stay programme is a health facility for the elderly when family members nursing them are themselves taken ill or suffer from accidents, or so that the latter can have a brief respite from the task, is also valuable.

NEEDS OF MULTIPURPOSE FACILITIES

The types of facilities in which elderly people in Japan are accommodated are various. Hitherto the system has been to classify those accommodated according to their physical condition and social situation, and to place them in a facility in accordance with these factors. However, while the health, social, and economic surroundings of the elderly are quite changeable, it is often difficult to transfer inmates after changes of condition have occurred. With this in mind multipurpose facilities and mutually complementary facilities on the same site or in close proximity to each other have been encouraged in recent years.

TYPES OF HEALTH SERVICE FOR THE ELDERLY

Hospital Medical Care (Fig. 2)

The so-called geriatric hospital is a form of chronic hospital and accommodates many of the elderly. However, few of the hospitals are specialized in treatment and research of the diseases of the elderly.

The importance of geriatric medicine is accepted and in many countries universities have established chairs in this field. It is desirable that there be geriatric departments in general hospitals, but there are still countries where there is no official recognition of geriatrics, as in the cases of the Netherlands and Japan.

In Japan there are only a few general hospitals having adequate rehabilitation facilities, and when this stage is reached the patient is usually moved to a chronic hospital. General hospital beds occupied by the elderly are increasing year by year and the needs of specialized long-term wards or long-term care hospitals is increasing.

In the United States, Japan, and Denmark there are many nursing homes providing day care. In the United States and Europe the contents of day care services are various, be they independent centres or attached to other facilities, but many of them emphasize community service. In the United States, also, other names are in use such as recreation and education centres, drop-in centres, and information and referral centres.

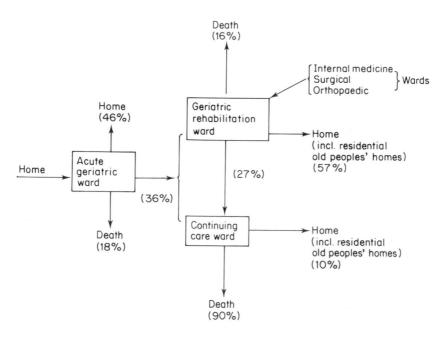

Figure 2   Hospital medical care

Nursing Homes

Nursing homes comprise a wide range of institutions other than hospitals which provide various levels of maintenance and personal or nursing care to people who are unable to care for themselves and who may have health problems which range from minimal to the very serious. While there are differences in the types of patients admitted, facility, equipment, and staff provision, they are quite widespread in the United States and Europe.

In Japan nursing homes have not been developed as medical care institutions but as welfare facilities for the elderly. Known as Tokuyo (special homes for the care of the elderly), they are mostly operated at public expense and medical care insurance is not applicable to them. The Act for the Welfare of the Elderly designates the Tokuyo as 'facilities for those 65 years old and over in need of regular nursing due to marked physical or mental inpairment, and for whom it is difficult to receive such at home'. The staff ratios for Tokuyo are fixed at one nursing aid per 5 elderly persons, one doctor per 300 persons, and 3 nurses per 100 persons. Moreover, for those elderly needing medical treatment, it is stipulated that a Tokuyo must ensure agreement with a hospital for its cooperation for medical care in advance.

In 1979 there were 907 Tokuyo accommodating 71,307 elderly people. Within a period of 10 years the number of facilities has increased 6 times and the number of those accommodated 6.2 times (*Report of Social Welfare Facilities Survey*, Statistics Information Department, Minister's Secretariat, Ministry of Health and Welfare, 1979).

According to a survey in Metropolitan Tokyo, elderly people were admitted to Tokuyo thus: from hospitals – 37.4 per cent., from homes for the elderly – 33.5 per cent., and from their own homes – 25.3 per cent. Reasons for discharge were classified as: death after hospitalization (while registered at a Tokuyo) – 58.1 per cent., death at the Tokuyo facility – 23.4 per cent., transfer to a general hospital – 12.6 per cent., transfer to a mental hospital – 1.8 per cent., discharge home – 2.3 per cent. (*Investigative Report on Tokuyo and Those Who Use Them*, Tokyo Metropolitan Institute of Gerontology, 1981).

Home-Health Care

For the severely ill people of advanced age and elderly people with no close relations, admission into a residential facility is necessary at the time of sickness or disablement. However, in cases where it is possible to treat the patient at home (and assuming he is satisfied with this arrangement), it is more economical.

The visiting nurse system allows for a degree of home nursing which had hitherto only been thought possible where the patient was admitted to hospital; with guidance in nursing methods the level of proficiency of the family members involved can be improved. With regard to rehabilitation also it was considered that this had to be done at a residential facility and that there were certain difficulties in conducting such training at home. It is now seen that the effects can be more permanent if it is carried out in the home environment.

In order to promote home medical care, assistance for families providing nursing care must be reinforced and social services made available to support them. That is to say, the provision of home helps and services for bathing, meals-on-wheels, and changing bed-linen should be community responsibilities, to be planned and operated continuously. With the cooperation of volunteers a comprehensive community service should be developed. For home medical care to be effective it is essential that there be close liaison with hospitals and other facilities. It is not unusual that the elderly require emergency hospitalization and the necessity for short-term hospitalization for health check-ups and special treatment also arises. Where medical care is home-based and short-term hospitalization is repeated according to necessity, this is referred to as intermittent hospitalization. Also beneficial are link-ups with day care and short-stay facilities, participation in group work devoted to functional rehabilitation, and the promotion of arrangements for respite from their duties of those in charge of care.

The nuclei for implementation of the home nursing service are the local health departments, hospitals, private agencies, and so on. In the United Kingdom they provide for the care of the elderly living at home. In Japan and the United States, in addition to local health department's visiting nurses, there are many cases where the hospitals themselves have established visiting nurse departments and run extended nursing services.

Terminal Care and Hospice

Although the percentage of those who die purely from mental and physical senescence and not as a result of sickness is small, senescence is more or less a factor in the deaths of elderly people.

Terminal care is concerned with assisting the elderly person to live through his latter days in a mode worthy of a human being. On the physical side it attempts to ensure that he is comfortable and applies his remaining abilities effectively, and on the psychological side it is concerned to reduce anxiety and fear to the minimum so that he can accept death naturally. Moreover, it is essential that the elderly person has contact with close acquaintances until the end, and that community assistance through the work of doctors, nurses, and others involved, together with cooperation of the family, be encouraged, so that death can be approached with dignity.

In recent years this service to assist people in meeting death in a dignified and peaceful manner has been popularized as the Hospice Movement. Hospice is a programme which provides palliative and supportive care for terminally ill patients and their families, either directly or on a consulting basis with the patient's physician or another community agency such as a visiting nurse association.

A hospice programme can be a free-standing hospice, operated independently, a home-care-based hospice, offering assistance for home care, or a hospital based hospice.

BIBLIOGRAPHY

Birchenall, J. M., and Streight, M. E. (1982). *Care of the Older Adult*, 2nd. ed., pp. 15–131 and 242–260. J. B. Lippincott, New York.

Brocklehurst, J. C. (1975). *Geriatric Care in Advanced Societies*, MTP Press.

Brocklehurst, J. C. (Ed.) (1978). *Geriatric Medicine and Gerontology*, Part III. *Medical and Community Care*, 2nd ed., pp. 747–806, Churchill Livingstone.

Brocklehurst, J. C., and Tucker, J. S. (1980). *Progress in Geriatric Day Care*, King Edward's Hospital Fund.

Cohen, K. P. (1979). *Hospice, Prescription for Terminal Care*, Aspen Systems Corp.

Davidson, G. W. (1979). *The Hospice, Development and Administration*, Hemisphere Pub.

Dunlop, B. D. (1979) *'The Growth of Nursing Home Care'*, Lexington Books. Lexington, USA.

Fact Finding Survey on Care for the Elderly. Interim Report, Japan Social Welfare Council (1977).

Fact Finding Survey on the Elderly, Social Welfare Bureau, Japanese Ministry of Health and Welfare (1973).

Furukawa, C., and Shomaker, D. (1982). *Community Health Service for the Aged*, Aspen Systems Corp, Maryland.

Gilmore, A. J. J., Svanborg, A., Moris, M., Beattie, W. M., and Pitrowski, J. (Eds) (1981). *Aging: A Challenge to Science and Society*, Vol. 2, *Medicine and Social Science*, Chap. V, pp. 165–242, Oxford University Press.

Health and Welfare Administrations, Japan Basic Survey (1976). Statistics and Information Department, Ministers Secretariat, Ministry of Health and Welfare.

Hodkinson, H. M. (1981). *An Outline of Geriatrics*, 2nd ed., pp. 1–9 and 26–69, Academic Press, London.

Investigative Report on Tokyo Metropolitan Institute of Gerontology (1981).

The new estimate of the future population of Japan, Institute of Population Problems. Ministry of Health and Welfare (1981).

Kart, C. S., Metress, E. S., and Metress, J. S. (1978). *Aging and Health*, Chaps. 12, 13, 14, 15, pp. 196–269, Adison-Wesley, Reading, USA.

Weiler, P. G. (1978). *Adult Day Care, Community Work with the Elderly*, Philip G. Weiler Springer Pub, New York.

Wells, T. (1982). *Aging and Health Promotion*, Aspen Systems Corp, Maryland.

WHO (1974). *Planning and Organization of Geriatric Services*, Technical Report no. 548 of the WHO Expert Committee.

Principles and Practice of Geriatric Medicine
Edited by M. S. J. Pathy
© 1985 John Wiley & Sons Ltd

30.4

Health Problems of Older People in the Developing World

A. Kalache , J. A. Muir Gray

The usual picture of the demographic conditions in the developing world is of a high birth rate and a large proportion of the population under the age of 15. This is certainly the case in some developing countries, although in many the infant mortality rate is falling and in fewer the birth rate is falling. However, the numbers of elderly people are also increasing and by the year 2000 there will be many more old people in developing countries than in the developed world. Although still a small proportion of the total population (see Fig. 1), the absolute numbers, and that is what counts, represent many people needing help and support.

Just as the health problems of an old person cannot be considered in isolation from his social and economic situation, so the health problems of elderly people as a whole have to be considered in their social and economic context and this is of particular importance when discussing the problems of older people in the developing world.

THE ECONOMIC CONTEXT

Older people in the developing world live in countries whose economies are under severe and increasing pressure as a result of oil price rises, reduced trade consequent on the world recession, and the necessity of maintaining capital and interest repayments on large loans negotiated in more optimistic times. Protectionism which is becoming increasingly apparent in the developed countries accentuates these difficulties.

THE DEMOGRAPHIC CONTEXT

The problem of population ageing in the developing world has been largely overlooked for two reasons. The first is preoccupation with its high birth rate and population growth; the second, the common tendency to speak of population ageing in proportionate terms, thus masking the fact that the absolute increase in numbers is very great.

Concern has been voiced in the developed world about the rate of increase of the elderly population, particularly the rate of increase of the very elderly population, but this rate of increase is small compared to that in many developing countries (Table 1).

THE SOCIAL CONTEXT

The developing countries are not simply repeating the pattern of development which was experienced in Europe and North America in the last hundred years. They are not simply one hundred years behind the developed countries because their rate of development is very much greater than that which we have experienced. Urbanization and industrialization have taken place and are continuing at a tremendous pace with consequent social turbulence. Furthermore, the change does not necessarily affect the whole of the society but may affect only part of it, so that in many developing countries a peasant culture coexists with a society in which jet travel and computers are familiar components. The phenomenon of ur-

Table 1 Changes in the population of countries that will have more than 15 million people aged 60 and over in 2025

	Rank in 1950	Population aged over 60				Rank in 2025	Magnitude of the increase (1950 to 2025)
		1950	1975	2000	2025		
China	1	42.5	73.7	134.5	284.1	1	6.8 China
India	2	31.9	29.7	65.6	146.2	2	4.6 India
U.S.S.R.	4	16.2	33.9	54.3	71.3	3	4.4 U.S.S.R.
United States	3	18.5	31.6	40.1	67.3	4	3.6 United States
Japan	8	6.4	13.0	26.4	33.1	5	5.2 Japan
Brazil	16	2.1	6.2	13.9	31.8	6	15.1 Brazil
Indonesia	10	3.8	6.8	14.9	31.2	7	8.2 Indonesia
Pakistan	11	3.3	3.6	6.9	18.1	8	5.5 Pakistan
Mexico	25	1.3	3.1	6.6	17.5	9	13.4 Mexico
Bangladesh	14	2.6	3.3	6.5	16.8	10	6.4 Bangladesh
Nigeria	27	1.3	2.6	6.3	16.0	11	12.3 Nigeria
Italy	9	5.7	9.7	13.5	15.9	12	2.8 Italy
West Germany	6	7.0	12.3	13.3	15.1	13	2.2 West Germany

banization merits special attention because of the problems that are developing in the rapidly growing cities of the Third World and in the countryside which the migrants have left.

Accustomed as we are to think of cities such as London or Toronto or Chicago as being large cities, they will be small in comparison with the huge conurbations of Third World countries such as Sao Paulo, Mexico City, Calcutta, and Manila; these will be huge by the end of the century and will present health planners with major challenges.

In the countryside that has been left behind problems are also developing and this is where many elderly people live. In the early days of urban migration the young people who went to the cities were often able to send money back to support elderly relatives at home, but with the recession and inflation they have found it much more difficult to support their elderly relatives and thus many elderly people now live in rural areas without the social support offered by the extended family and without the financial support which they had formerly. However, the problems of elderly people in the country are in general less than those of elderly people in the cities, particularly those who live in the makeshift dwellings in the unstable crowded communities that have grown up round most cities.

Furthermore, the difficulties of delivering services to old people are often immense, even when the resources are available and there is willingness to help. We take for granted a literate society in which the telephone works, the post arrives, and roads reach every village.

These conditions are not universal and neither is the existence of an efficient and uncorrupt bureaucracy. These are significant factors which affect the well-being of elderly people.

THE HEALTH CONTEXT

Just as developing countries have seen a social revolution which has taken place at such a rate that the technology that we associate with nineteenth or even eighteenth century life exists alongside twentieth century technology, so the evolution of the health care of these countries has also been telescoped in time. The health ministers, health planners, and the public health doctors still struggle with the diseases which were defeated in the developed countries by public health measures in the nineteenth century, namely tuberculosis, cholera, typhoid, typhus, malaria, and, in childhood, gastroenteritis and respiratory infections associated with malnutrition. However, they also have to tackle many twentieth century health problems. Road traffic accidents are now epidemic in many developing countries, alcohol consumption has increased in some, and, the most serious epidemic which now constitutes a pandemic, cigarette smoking, has become widely prevalent due to aggressive marketing. The effects of this social change on mortality and morbidity figures are starting to become evident.

Furthermore, these health problems are having to be tackled in countries in which food supplies are often limited, in which the climate is often harsh, in which parasites abound, and in which the infrastructure on which health planning and health service delivery depends has never been developed to a degree which would allow the sort of health service planning that we take for granted.

This is not to say that nothing is happening. On the contrary, there are many experiments based on the principles of primary health care planning adopted by the World Health Assembly and disseminated by the World Health Organisation as a means of reaching the goal of health for all by the year 2000 (WHO, 1981).

Primary health care is care that is:

(a) universally accessible,
(b) acceptable,
(c) at a cost that the community and country can afford, i.e. it uses appropriate technology,
(d) planned to meet the needs of the whole population.

Primary health care planning has two other important principles which, like those listed above, are particularly relevant to the developing world. One is that health service planning must be integrated with the planning and delivery of other services such as education and housing. The second, which poses an equal challenge to those working in basing countries, is that elderly people should participate both individually and collectively in the planning and management of their services. Some developing countries are developing their services on these principles and there is much that doctors, nurses, and health planners in the developed world can learn from developing countries (King, 1966).

THE PREVALENCE OF DISABILITY

The main threat to life and health in the developing world occurs in the early years of life (see Fig. 2). Some of the great killers in middle and old age in the developed world are relatively uncommon in most Third World countries, e.g. ischaemic heart disease, stroke, and cancer. The life style in the developed world is healthy for children but not so healthy for adults.

However, this does not mean that the adults and old people in developing countries are healthier and less disabled than old people in the developed countries. On the contrary, there is a high prevalence of disability in mid-

dle and old age with the result that people who are sixty in developing countries are, in general, a group which has a higher prevalence of disability than those of the same age in the developed world. In part this is due to the long-term effects of diseases that occurred in childhood and early adult life (see Table 2).

Table 2   Third World health problems causing permanent disability

Tuberculosis
Poliomyelitis
Leprosy
Trachoma
Accidents
Infections associated with malnutrition occurring in people who do not have easy access to antibiotics, leading to disorders such as empyema and osteomyelitis

New causes of disability are experienced, notably those experienced at work, for the working environment is less well protected by the type of legislation that we take for granted in the developed world.

The health of women declines at an earlier age than in developed countries because of the demands and risks of pregnancy, childbirth, and lactation. The health of men also declines more quickly because of adverse working and living conditions, with the result that the prevalence of disability and therefore the need for assistance increases at much earlier ages than in the developed world. The population over the age of 75 is usually taken to be that which will require large amounts of resources in the developed world. Detailed data on the needs of people in developing countries are not available but it seems probable that the age at which the prevalence of problems increases significantly is 10 or 20 years earlier than the age of 75 (King, 1983).

THE CONTRIBUTION OF DEVELOPED COUNTRIES

One way in which developed countries can help is by providing training opportunities. The view that a Western type of medical training is appropriate for people from developing countries is dying fast, although it is not yet extinct. The contrary view, namely that the developed world has nothing to offer developing countries, which is held by some people, has not gained universal acceptance by either developed or developing countries. The truth is somewhere in the middle. People from developing countries can learn much that is helpful to them provided those trying to teach them bear in mind the technology on which they will be able to call when they return and the infrastructure of the country, namely its level of administration, the presence or absence of corruption, and the effectiveness of communications, for these have a very important influence on the delivery of health services.

In part a trainee from the developing world benefits simply by being away from the pressure of work in his home country with the opportunity to read and discuss ideas in receptive environments.

Official bodies such as the World Health Organisation which has an important Global Programme for the Aged and the British Council sustain links with many developing countries. However, help for the developing world requires a bigger sacrifice than has been available hitherto.

Support for Charities

Two United Kingdom charities have been particularly active in providing support for elderly people in the developing world, namely Oxfam and Help the Aged, which were both founded by one man, Cecil Jackson-Cole. The United Nations has suggested that each developed country should give 0.7 per cent. of its GNP to underdeveloped countries as aid and that is perhaps a target for an individual to consider as the basis for deciding on his personal contribution to foreign aid. Charitable aid has been criticized and while it is true that some money does not reach those in need many more poor people would suffer and die if it were not for charitable aid.

Statutory Aid

The whole subject of foreign aid is politically controversial. The World Bank has shifted its policy in recent years away from massive projects, which benefitted the countries from the developed world who won the contracts as much as the developing countries, towards much smaller scale projects employing appropriate technology and building on the self-reliance of the individuals in small communities.

THE NATURE OF THE CHALLENGE

The ageing of populations in developing countries will lead to a heavy demand of social and health services in these countries in the near future. That is easily predictable considering the very nature of the problems commonly associated with old age: chronic, long-term diseases which often cause diabilities and the supportive services for the remainder of the patient's life. In the meantime societies in these countries will continue to experience drastic changes. In Brazil, for example, the total population has more than doubled (from 45 to 50 million to over 120 million) during the last 30 years. In 1950 only one-third of the population lived in urban areas while now it is over 70 per cent. This rapid process of urbanization simultaneouly with industrialization has changed Brazilian society immensely, with an important impact on family life. There are now far more women in the working force and the trend towards nuclear families is marked, particularly in the big cities. Houses are smaller and it is more difficult to accommodate an extra adult person. Social as well as geographical mobility have created visible gaps. Finally, the introduction of advanced technology in many sectors of the economy has made the knowledge and experience accumulated throughout life by older people seem of rather less practical use; that combined with the changes in family life have, and will, alter old people's preceptions and attitudes, which are particularly important in respect to social roles that may be left for them to play. Looking at these aspects in perspective, the situation in a country like Brazil will pose many challenges to health planners and administrators. From 1980 to the year 2000 the elderly population in that country will increase by around 140 per cent., while the increase in the total population will be about 70 per cent. due to a decline in the birth rate (see Table 3). However, in the meantime other problems which are clearly of great relevance will not have been solved, such as high infant mortality, lack of basic sanitation for large segments of the population, high morbidity and mortality rates for infectious diseases, etc. The classical problems of a developing country will coexist with the new challenges created by the ageing of the population.

It is now imperative to pay more attention to the problems of the elderly in developing countries. Without proper plans following careful studies we may be heading for very serious difficulties in the near future – a future when most of us will be elderly ourselves.

REFERENCES

World Health Organization (1981). *Global Strategy for Health for All by the Year 2000*, WHO, Geneva.

King, M. H. (1966). *Medical Care in Developing Countries*, Oxford University Press.

King, M. H. (1983). 'Medicine in an unjust world', in *Oxford Textbook of Medicine* (Eds D. J. Weatherall, J. G. G. Ledingham and D. A. Warrell), pp. 3.3–3.11, Oxford University Press.

Siegal, J. S. (1982). *Demographic Aspects of the Health of the Elderly to the Year 2000 and Beyond*, Vol. 1982.3, WHO/Age.

United Nations (1980). Population Division Working Paper ESA/P/WP 65, 2 Jan. 1980.

Table 3   Percentage increases in the population of countries from 1980 to 2000. (From UN, 1980)

	Total population			Population 60+			Population 70+		
	1980	2000	Increase (%)	1980	2000	Increase (%)	1980	2000	Increase (%)
Argentina	27.1	32.8	21	3.39	4.72	39	1.44	2.30	59
Australia	14.5	17.8	23	1.93	2.67	39	0.83	1.32	58
Brazil	126.0	212	68	6.97	14.3	105	2.39	5.68	138
Egypt	42.0	64.7	54	2.38	4.64	94	0.82	1.73	110
Federal Republic of Germany	60.0	60.0	2.2	11.5	13.4	17	6.04	6.19	2
France	53.4	57.3	7.2	9.07	10.7	18	5.04	5.51	9
India	694	1,037	49	33.6	61.5	83	11.7	21.8	87
Israel	3.95	5.62	42	0.45	0.62	38	0.20	0.30	50
Italy	57.0	61.0	7.1	10.0	13.5	35	4.97	6.87	38
Japan	116	129	11	14.7	25.5	74	6.38	11.3	77
Kenya	16	33.6	105	0.65	1.32	103	0.23	0.50	118
Nigeria	77.1	149	93	3.12	6.36	104	1.02	2.24	120
Phillipines	51.0	84.4	64	2.47	4.67	89	0.89	1.65	86
Poland	35.8	41.2	15	4.69	6.83	46	2.29	3.20	40
Sweden	8.3	8.5	3.0	1.81	1.77	2.2	0.89	0.98	10
United Kingdom	55.9	56.7	1.4	11.1	11.3	1.3	5.45	5.96	9
United States	222	260	17	34.7	42.0	21	16.2	22.6	38
North America	246	290	18	37.8	46.4	23	17.6	24.8	41
South America	245	392	60	15.7	28.8	83	5.91	12.0	103
Europe (excl. Israel, Turkey, U.S.S.R.)	484	520	7.6	81.6	101	24	41.2	50.1	21
Africa	469	828	76	22.8	42.7	87	7.86	15.6	98
Middle East, SW Asia (incl. Israel & Turkey)	98.2	164	67	5.72	10.9	91	2.31	4.25	84
Asia (excl. SW Asia)	2,459	3,447	40	164	279	70	61.9	109.3	76
Oceania	22.8	29.6	30	2.61	3.70	41	1.11	1.77	59
World	4,415	6,199	40	372	580	56	157	248	58

REFERENCES

World Health Organization (1984). Global Strategy for Health for All by the Year 2000, WHO, Geneva.

King, M. H. (1966). Medical Care in Developing Countries, Oxford University Press.

Muir, M. H. (1984). Medicine in an urban society, in Oxford Textbook of Medicine (eds D. A. Weatherall, J. G. G. Ledingham and D. A. Warrell), vol. 1, pp. 3.11–3.12, Oxford University Press.

Strehl, J. S. (1985). Demographic Aspects of the Population and Literacy in the Year 2000 and Beyond, Vol. 1982, WHO, Rome.

United Nations (1982). Population Division, Working Paper No. ESA/WP/43, p. 9.

31

The Management of
the Dying Patient

Principles and Practice of Geriatric Medicine
Edited by M. S. J. Pathy
© 1985 John Wiley & Sons Ltd

31.1

The Management of the Dying Patient

Brian Livesley

'"Would you like me to have left that in her stomach?" said N aggressively, showing me the jar full of a yellowish substance. I did not reply. In the corridor he said, "At dawn she had scarcely four hours left. I have brought her back to life." I did not venture to ask him "For what?".'

(De Beauvoir, 1980)

'While we must adhere to medicine's traditional role of life prolongation, we now have to decide in each case when this becomes an appropriate goal. Perhaps we should ask ourselves: "What would I wish if the patient were my own Mother?", or, even more pertinently: "What if I were the patient?".'

(Williamson, 1981)

THE DIAGNOSIS OF THE DYING PATIENT

While all doctors have occasion to certify death, dying is the diagnosis commonly overlooked or evaded. This curious paradox is the result of at least two factors: firstly, the virtual absence today of those life-threatening epidemic diseases that previously provided almost daily experience with dying patients of all ages; secondly, the easy availability of persistent diagnostic and therapeutic endeavour associated with high-technology medicine.

Unfortunately, the scientific basis of medical practice can lift clinical thoughts far from the real problems patients are having with their diseases. All too often an observer may be left asking the question, 'Are you doing this for the patient, doctor, or is he doing it for you?'. Contrariwise, once a diagnosis of chronic disability or 'untreatable' illness has been made, patients can be rejected even by those whose job it is to care. This overlooking of the needs of affected patients has given rise to the Hospice Movement for the Care of the Dying and the continued need for geriatric medicine as a distinct speciality for the care of the ageing patient.

Since about one third of patients admitted to a modern geriatric medical unit die there, how is the diagnosis of dying made and what management is required for this large group of patients? It will be realized, of course, that the principles of management are the same whether the patient is in hospital or at home.

There are 500,000 deaths each year in the United Kingdom and, while 50 per cent. occur in those aged over 74 years and 20 per cent. in those aged over 84 years, no one dies merely of old age. At least one specific factor, among the plethora of multiple pathology common to the old, ends intellectual and brainstem function. This can occur after an abrupt syncope or a more prolonged period of exhaustion and coma. The nature and severity of sudden illness can point out dramatically that death is inevitable. It is important to ensure that inappropriate resuscitative measures are not instituted.

On the ward round, as in the home, many elderly and aged patients can appear initially to be recovering from an acute illness or making satisfactory progress with chronic disability. A stealthy deterioration in their condition is then not immediately apparent and, in the absence of depression, it can result from the inexorable progress of the presenting illness; the masked development of added cardiovascular complications; or the onset of hypostatic pneumonia. The patient's failure to thrive is clearly shown by a passive unwillingness and inability to respond to otherwise practical rehabilitative and therapeutic efforts. This may be the primary result of unexpected complications of drug therapy that can be overlooked by the unwary. The appropriate withdrawal of tranquillizers and hypnotics can allow affected patients to become active again. Similarly, correction of an unsuspected dehydration can produce dramatic improvement, especially when aggravating diuretic therapy is stopped. For no obvious reason, the patient's general condition may improve for a brief period only to deteriorate as unexpectedly. This can be followed by further cycles of apparent improvement and obvious deterioration. This yo-yo effect can be very disturbing for inexperienced carestaff – especially if initial directions for terminal care are then reversed by the false expectation of recovery. During this period inappropriate rehabilitation exercises may be instituted and then withdrawn on a go-stop-go-stop policy that varies with the yo-yo phases of the patient's condition. When patients are failing to thrive and deterioration has occurred the real diagnosis may be that the patient has begun to die.

This is the time to review the problems and needs of the patient, and also to consider the effects the now-terminal illness is having on others. In some circumstances, particularly when anxious relatives are present at the bedside, this can be a complex business at a very emotional time. A compassionate, unhurried, and professional approach goes a long way to instilling confidence, restoring calm, and assisting others to come to terms with their dilemma. If death is not imminent, and with the patient's consent, the visiting relatives and friends (on ward rounds this also includes all team members except the senior nurse and one student) should be asked to withdraw for a short time. This creates a more dignified and private opportunity for the patient to express any problems and enables the doctor quietly to decide what is required to ensure the patient's personal comfort; it also allows the relatives and other team members time to compose their thoughts and prepare their questions.

This is the time for the doctor also to consider the ways in which the religious/cultural attitudes and beliefs of the patient may affect the treatment and care required. Although the caring professions are expected to meet all the needs of the sick and dying in our increasingly multiethnic society, the general and ethical problems affecting the many religions and cultures of patients being nursed in our hospitals have only recently received special attention (Sampson, 1982).

INAPPROPRIATE TREATMENT OF THE DYING: THE 'NOT ALLOWED TO DIE' SYNDROME

'A doctor aged 68 . . . had . . . a large carcinoma of the stomach . . . . On the tenth day after gastrectomy the patient collapsed with . . . massive pulmonary embolism. Pulmonary embolectomy was successfully performed in the ward by a Registrar . . . The patient collapsed again, two weeks after . . . with acute myocardial infarction and cardiac arrest – he was revived . . . . His heart stopped on four further occasions . . . and each time was restarted artificially. The body then recovered sufficiently to linger for three more weeks . . . Intravenous nourishment was carefully combined with blood transfusion . . . to maintain electrolyte and fluid balance . . . preparations were being made for . . . an artificial respirator, but the heart finally stopped . . . .'

(Symmers, 1968)

Doctors and nurses need to know when to move from the 'diagnostic–investigative–attempting-to-cure' mode to the as complex and equally important 'diagnosis-of-dying-with-its-implications-for-care' mode. Medical and nursing staff of all grades should be made aware that, with the high technology now available, an initial, ill-judged decision can set in motion an inappropriate, but in the correct context, completely logical sequence of events. The performance of this can overlook the patient's real needs for care while it satisfies the real needs of the professional staff to offer attempted cure. Although the circumstances of individual patients obviously differs, each unit should develop a mutually agreed policy that is led by competent medical advice and communicated to all concerned – who then have the opportunity to ask questions and obtain answers to their eventual satisfaction – especially as staff change. The constant introduction of students, nursing, and others to the wards provides senior staff with the repeated educational obligation tactfully to seek out any questions about the management of dying patients and to use for discussion the practical problems that present themselves as part of the daily work.

Once the diagnosis of dying has been made the patient's treatment should be reviewed and, by active decision-making, inappropriate therapy not given. The nursing–medical team should know that resuscitation is not indicated and if attempted could unnecessarily, indeed cruelly, add to the patient's distress. Other positive decisions are also required. This is not the time to provide pretentious medicine (e.g diuretics can disturb the bladder and leave the dying patient in an uncomfortably wet bed); not the time to give undue injections; and not the time to perform unwarranted investigations. Neither is this the time for nasogastric tubes, oxygen masks, intravenous fluids, nor artificial life-support systems. As both the patient and the team move into the final-care mode remember to stop active physiotherapy; do not insist patients sit-out in a chair – with gentle nursing care allow patients to die comfortably in bed. Finally, remember this is not the time to force food or drinks; if dying patients do not want them, do not press them, but ensure that nursing staff do not feel this as a failure on their part.

APPROPRIATE TREATMENT

Assisting the Patient

'Care of the dying patient is best learnt by practice, a film or lecture can be stimulating, but it is no substitute for personal experience.'
(Lamerton, 1973)

It is important first to confirm the patient is dying; then to consider what palliative measures, if any, are required. Clinical and, whenever possible, pathological evidence should be collected to determine the actual diagnoses present without subjecting the patient to unnecessary investigations and anxiety. This requires an objective but compassionate and careful review of the symptoms and physical signs in a patient who is usually already apprehensive if not mentally confused and physically distressed. It is essential to demonstrate willingness to kindly seek out needs and patiently listen to problems. It is as important to show an appreciative awareness of the communication difficulties of those who are dysphasic, deaf, blind, and muddled in thought. Particular attention should be directed to identifying and relieving all conditions producing obvious concern. These commonly include pain, dyspnoea, nausea, vomiting, constipation, urinary incontinence, and impaired mental state.

Pain Relief

As a result of the excellent work already published from St Christopher's Hospice (Baines, 1981, Saunders, 1978); a great deal is known about effective pain control. No patient need now suffer recurrently when pain has once been relieved. It should be stressed that analgesia is being used as a supplement to, and not a replacement for, good basic nursing care. Skilful positioning of a patient can relieve the aches and strains of prolonged lying. This is especially true when the limbs are paralysed or affected by muscle atrophy and have carried the unaccustomed burden of bedclothes. As the patient and the nurse share the problems, lessened tensions and anxieties can reduce the need for tranquillizers which otherwise may be required to augment the effect of analgesics. When adequate pain control has been obtained the observer can sometimes be misled into recommending the dosage be increased. This is most likely to occur in those patients who can have an 'alarm response' to being disturbed – particularly when they are blind, deaf, confused, or have been asleep. Sometimes these patients may call out when they are unattended not because they are in obvious pain but because they need to be reassured they are not alone. Since rest on its own can relieve pain, movement of patients to reposition them can aggravate severe pain and analgesics may need adjusting to anticipate this problem. Tranquillizers can aid pain relief by reducing the patient's restlessness as well as by raising their anxiety threshold. It can be difficult to differentiate the severe pain response to positional change from the sometimes considerable discomfort that patients can experience when they are moved from a settled position. If a patient's symptoms are immediately relieved once they have been repositioned this 'disturbance reaction' does not require a further prescription for analgesics. Medical and nursing staff will become aware of the particularly gentle handling required by this group of patients.

Other specific pain-relieving measures should not be overlooked. While painful aphthous ulceration in the mouth can respond to hydrocortisone lozenges BPC (2.5 mg, 4 times daily), monilial infection is the most common and frequently unconsidered cause of a painful mouth and dysphagia in the dying patient. This infection does not mean necessarily that nursing attention to oral hygiene has been overlooked but that more attention needs to be helped by prompt administration of nystatin oral suspension (100,000 units, four hourly). Pain elsewhere can be relieved by other valuable specific measures including expertly performed selective nerve blocks for irremedially ischaemic limbs or malignant conditions, as well as radiotherapy to isolated bony metastasis.

Choosing the Analgesic Drug

It is important to become familiar with a few drugs to use them well and, therefore, only a small range will be described. As a guide to treatment, it should be remembered that simple pains require simple drugs. Aspirin and paracetamol are the most useful mild analgesics providing they are given in adequate dosage. Two aspirin tablets (600 mg) four-hourly may not be enough, whereas 3 or 4 tablets (900 to 1200 mg) four-hourly may provide satisfactory symptom relief.

Aspirin and the many other non-steroidal anti-inflammatory drugs now available form the first-line treatment of choice for the relief of bone pain due to metastases. (Remember, in the elderly, bone pain may be due to osteomalacia, and this can be quickly and totally relieved by oral treatment with calcium and vitamin D.) For the early treatment of pain due to lesions only in soft tissues, paracetamol (1g) four-hourly is the drug of choice and does not produce the perspiration that can follow aspirin. When pain arises in both bone and soft tissues it is convenient to use a compound tablet containing 500 mg of aspirin and 8 mg of codeine phosphate or 300 mg of aspirin and 250 mg of paracetamol.

Analgesics may be introduced gradually beginning with aspirin or paracetamol in appropriate doses and then introducing major analgesics if more effective pain control is required. Alternatively, in very apprehensive patients and those who have become severely distressed by uncontrolled pain, it may be necessary to give major analgesics immediately to demonstrate that pain can be controlled effectively. When apprehension was previously a major factor, and once the pain and the patient have been relieved and with the patient's understanding and agreement, it may be possible to reduce the dose or substitute a milder analgesic, particularly when anxious fears have been calmed or pain relieved by other measures including nerve blocks and radiotherapy. These are important considerations since the patient can then have the dignity of feeling more in control of the situation.

Alert patients can gain excellent relief from moderate to severe pain by using oxycodone pectinate suppositories (30 mg). These are convenient for use in the home and when inserted at eight-hourly intervals have a morphine-equivalent dosage of 15 mg four-hourly.

A large number of aged patients experiencing pain also have mental impairment during their final illness. Clouding of consciousness leading to coma relieves the anxiety of the patient and often too that of the observer. Mental function, however, can cause problems not only due to the constant demand for considerate attention but also because confusion in susceptible patients may actually be precipitated by peaks of pain. Effective management here requires an increase in the continuing analgesic therapy and the addition of a sedative, as discussed later.

Some patients with more severe pain of non-bony origin are helped by morphine sulphate twelve-hourly in a time-released tablet. Eight-hourly dosage may be required despite the manufacturer's recommended twelve-hourly regime.

Unlike morphine, diamorphine is completely absorbed from the gastrointestinal tract, and, perhaps because of this, rarely produces the disturbing gastrointestinal symptoms that can be such a troublesome problem when morphine is used. If allowance is made for this there is no difference in analgesic effect between morphine and diamorphine which have an equianalgesic ratio of 1.5:1 respectively (Twycross, 1977). When injections are necessary, however, the greater solubility of diamorphine hydrochloride (1g in 1.6 ml) gives it a further important practical advantage over morphine sulphate or hydrochloride (1g in more than 20 ml). Indeed, injections of diamorphine only rarely need to exceed 0.1 ml.

When major analgesics are required they should not be withheld from the dying patient because of the unfounded nursing or medical anxiety that dependence is likely to occur. It is unethical to withhold effective analgesic therapy from a dying patient. The effectiveness of an initial oral dose of 2.5 to 5 mg of diamorphine (5 to 10 mg of morphine) should be charted and subsequent doses adjusted if necessary, given on a regular, recorded, four-hourly basis. This regime is based on the known half-life of the drugs. If oral medication is not appropriate because of uncontrolled vomiting or inability to swallow then diamorphine by injection has an already stated advantage over morphine. Indeed, diamorphine hydrochloride is so soluble that only 0.04 ml of fluid need be used to inject 20 mg of the drug subcutaneously. This has an obvious advantage for the patient requiring repeated injections for maintenance therapy, since both diamorphine and morphine have to be given four-hourly. These drugs are more potent when given by injection and it is usual to begin by injecting half of the oral dose.

Note:
Diamorphine is available on prescription only in the United Kingdom and Belgium. In the United States of America and elsewhere in the world, morphine is the most suitable alternative.

Practical Points

The dose of analgesic should be the lowest compatible with adequate pain control during the whole day, and for this both diamorphine and morphine need to be given four-hourly. If they induce nausea and vomiting, prochlorphenazine (5 mg orally) or chlorpromazine (25 to 50 mg orally) can be given concurrently in elixir or tablet form. If vomiting is troublesome either of these drugs can be given as suppositories or by injection. Both drugs have anti-emetic and tranquillizer actions, potentiate the analgesic effect of morphine and diamorphine, and unless used in overdosage do not contribute to respiratory depression. Mixtures of prochlorphenazine or chlorpromazine with diamorphine or morphine are reported as not being stable for storage but are usually active for up to 3 weeks. Certainly, the big disadvantage of such mixtures is that simply doubling the dose for greater analgesic effect can be associated with unwanted sedation.

Solutions for Oral Administration
Diamorphine hydrochloride, 5 mg in 5 ml of chloroform water (10, 15, or 20 mg of diamorphine can be substituted or 60 to 90 mg if a higher dose is required). The mixture is to be given four-hourly. For use at home, a volume of 500 ml can be provided. This is stable at room temperature for 1 month.

Morphine sulphate or hydrochloride, 10 mg in 5 ml of chloroform water (20, 30, or 60 mg of morphine can be substituted and rarely is 120 mg required). The mixture is to be given four-hourly.

Simple elixirs of morphine or diamorphine should be prescribed by writing the formula in full, for example:

Diamorphine hydrochloride, 5 mg
Chloroform water to 5 ml
To take 5 ml four-hourly

The total quantity to be supplied should be added in both words and figures, together with other details required for controlled drug prescription (British National Formulary, 1981).

Solutions for Injection
Diamorphine is prepared for injection by adding sterile water to ampoules containing 5, 10, or 30 mg of the powered hydrochloride.

As stated above, and unlike morphine, diamorphine can be dissolved in a minimal quantity of water (up to 20 mg in 0.04 ml), making it particularly suitable for repeating subcutaneous injections.

Morphine for injection is provided in ampoules containing 1 ml solution of 10, 15, 20, or 30 mg of morphine sulphate.

Dyspnoea

In resting elderly and aged patients dyspnoea is most commonly due to obstructive airways disease or left ventricular failure. Difficulty with breathing can be a very distressing symptom and should be relieved by specific treatment with a bronchodilator (salbutamol, syrup or tablets, 2 to 4 mg, eight-hourly); a diuretic in patients alerted by heart failure; and an opiate as necessary. Airways obstruction in dying patients is not a contraindication to the use of opiates for the relief of pain or distressing breathlessness. Breathlessness can be aggravated by an anaemia that may be due to dietary factors; associated with gastrointestinal haemorrhage; or secondary to advanced malignant disease. Relief of the immediate precipitating condition (whether obstructive airways disease or left ventricular failure) is invariably all that is required in the treatment of such dyspnoea. Concurrent anaemia, although an aggravating factor, rarely if ever requires specific treatment with transfusion. Tapping a large, malignant pleural effusion, however, can make a simple but significant contribution to relieving breathlessness.

Bronchopneumonia as a new event in a dying patient, and in the absence of previously untreated respiratory tract infection, is invariably due to hypostasis. Its effects become particularly obvious as unconsciousness supervenes. Antibiotic therapy is never indicated under these circumstances. Stertorous breathing can be controlled by correct positioning of the patient and the removal of dentures. Secretion retention in the large bronchi and trachea, augmented by saliva pooling at the back of the throat, can produce wheezing and a 'death-rattle' that is particularly distressing to observers. It can be alleviated by atropine (0.6 to 1.2 mg) given by intramuscular injection.

Gastrointestinal Symptoms

In dying patients nausea and vomiting are commonly side-effects of digoxin and morphine. The former should be withdrawn and potassium deficiency sought and corrected to provide early symptomatic relief. Prochlorphenazine or chlorpromazine should be given with the required dose of morphine, and may need to be given by suppository or injection until nausea and vomiting are relieved, but oversedation is to be avoided. Vomiting unresponsive to the usual antiemetics may be associated with hypercalcaemia resulting from widespread bony metastases. This can be relieved by prednisolone (10 mg, twice daily). 'Steroid responsive vomiting' has also been described in the presence of metastases but the absence of hypercalcaemia (Baines, 1978).

Severe constipation in the elderly can also precipitate nausea and vomiting. Repeated enemata should be prescribed to clear the loaded large bowel before aperients are given. Indeed, in dying patients, bulk-producing agents not only add to distress by causing abdominal colic, especially if codeine or morphine is also being given, but also produce unnecessary repeated calls to stool. A low residue diet with a disposable phosphate enema on alternate days is usually all that is required. Diarrhoea is commonly spuriously associated with constipation; may be drug-induced; is occasionally due to subacute obstruction; and is associated with pancreatic carcinoma. This last, although rare, has a peak incidence in those aged over 80. Constipation with faecal overflow requires clearance of the lower bowel. Careful review of drug therapy can allow withdrawal of the offending agent – many drugs, including of course laxatives, antibiotics, and digoxin, can produce diarrhoea in the elderly. Diarrhoea due to subacute obstruction can be relieved by diphenyloxylate hydrochloride. The bulky and offensive stools of malabsorption from pancreatic insufficiency can be reduced by pancreatic replacement therapy.

In all patients a gently performed rectal examination at the time of the patient's first assessment, repeated after 3 to 4 days, can do much to alleviate anxiety about the state of the bowel when the results are communicated to both the patient and the nursing staff, and the appropriate treatment recommended.

Urinary Incontinence

For the dying patient the most satisfactory method of controlling the difficult problem of urinary incontinence is by sustained bladder catheterization. It is important, however, to ensure that incontinence is not being aggravated by: unnecessary diuretic therapy; an osmotic diuresis due to uncontrolled diabetes mellitus or hypercalcaemia; or even excessive fluid intake. Inappropriate diuretics should be withdrawn and diabetes corrected by oral hypoglycaemic agents (insulin is rarely required at this stage). Occasionally urinary incontinence is a feature of retention with overflow due to remediable constipation and, in men, this may be aggravated by the effects of prostatism. For the majority of affected patients, however, incontinence is a complication of irreversible cerebral damage with uninhibited bladder activity. A self-retaining catheter positioned using an aseptic technique is quite painless and prevents the discomfort of wet clothing and the hazards of skin maceration. Urinary tract infections following catheterization are not usually a problem. If suprapubic pain does occur or the confused patient becomes more restless, suggesting that acute bladder infection has developed, examination of the urine will confirm the diagnosis. The bladder should be treated with washouts of chlorhexidine solution (1 in 5,000) or irrigation with the more expensive 1 to 2.5% noxythiolin solution. Routine systemic antibiotic therapy is not indicated.

Mental Impairment

Acquired impairment of intellect and memory is age-related and affects 1 in 20 aged between 65 and 79 years, but 1 in 5 aged over 80. These deficiencies are not usually a problem when afflicted patients are dying of specific physical diseases. If, however, dying is heralded by progressive mental impairment this can be a worrying experience full of practical problems.

Relatives, friends, and nursing staff need to be reassured that when the patient has been calmed it will be possible then to manage more

effectively both urinary and faecal incontinence. Sedation is, however, but a part of management. It is important to attend to the patient's general condition including the adequate relief of other physical symptoms.

Relief of Agitated Confusion Occurring in the Dying

Thioridazine can be presented as syrup or tablets, the latter in 10, 25, and 50 mg doses. It is important to adjust the dose to achieve optimum effects. Treatment should begin with 10 mg three times daily and the dose increased as necessary, up to 200 mg three times daily.

Promazine is presented as the embonate in suspension and the hydrochloride in 25, 50, and 100 mg tablets. A dose of 12.5 to 50 mg up to three times daily is usually sufficient.

When patients are at risk because of their persistent, agitated confused state and refuse to take oral medication, fluphenazine decanoate in a single (depot) injection can have a sustained calming effect, for as long as a month. The response to an initial intramuscular injection of 12.5 mg is best observed in hospital. After 5 to 7 days the dose can be repeated and then given at 2 to 4 weekly intervals, increasing to 25 mg if required.

Sedation for Severely Disturbed Patients

An acutely disturbed and aggressive patient, who is a risk to himself and unwilling or unable to take oral medication, can be calmed by chlorpromazine, (50–100) mg given in a single, deep intramuscular injection.

SPEAKING OF DEATH

'The frequently debated question, "Should the doctor tell?", tends to carry a false implication that the doctor knows all about the patient's approaching death and the patient knows nothing; the resultant discussion and controversy is therefore often irrelevant . . .'

(Hinton, 1979)

The doctor may be unaware that the patient is dying but the patient may already know. If at this stage his questions are summarily dismissed as an unnecessary morbid preoccupation it denies his hope for help, understanding, and reassurance. More than this, it prevents the doctor from recognizing that the dying patient now has a new series of needs. In more acute illness, or after the confirmed diagnosis of neoplastic disease, the doctor is usually the first to know the seriousness of the patient's condition. What then does he say? There are at least two considerations here. Firstly, to respond immediately to the patient's expressed need to know or not to know. Secondly, simply to ask the patient what he thinks about his condition and what questions he wishes to ask. This presents the patient with the opportunity to be told or not, according to his own desire and at his own pace. The patient who is seeking to come to terms with his dilemma can be eased into a gradual grasping of the truth in three simple stages by leading him from awareness through understanding to realization. This involves his awareness that full recovery is not possible; his understanding that deterioration may be expected; and his realization that the illness may end fatally. Whatever the patient's response a close and responsible relative should be made aware of the seriousness of the patient's condition. The doctor and his supporting team then have the important task of offering advice and providing help to both the patient and the family. This commonly includes going over the problems again and listening sympathetically as people proffer their life's difficulties, while with disbelief they deny and then bargain with the future, prior to accepting the inevitable.

THE DYING PATIENT

Apart from the presence of mental impairment associated with confusional states, the patient's perception of the environment and his dilemma may be impaired by the effects of both necessary and unnecessary drug therapy; a masked sensory stroke associated with cerebral ischaemia/infarction; and secondary cerebral deposits. It can be very difficult to calm the fears and anxieties of such affected patients. They have a bruised perception of their present problem, their lost past, and their impending, inevitable future. They require particularly sympathetic handling and should not be oversedated merely to relieve the anxieties of relatives or caring staff. Such patients, like many others when they are dying, can have an over-

whelming distortion of their self-image and a desperate need to be listened to – even when they have to struggle with, for example, dysphasia, to discuss apparent trivia. Listening carefully to these patients can go a long way to providing essential reassurance. This can be reinforced by tactfully drawing attention to their immediate personal comfort and in a positive but unpatronizing way, gently and kindly touching them. Regular contact with the patient in the form of turning them in bed; attending to pressure areas; adjusting their posture and pillows; ensuring appropriate comfortable action of bladder and bowels; and preventing and relieving physical symptoms – all offer the reassuring warmth of personal contact, and ease an otherwise frightening loneliness. A busy ward does not necessarily offer security and it is often important that someone sits with the patient just to hold their hand if necessary. The dying patient and their relatives may not have gone through the phases of disbelief, denial, anger, and resentment (Kübler-Ross, 1977), and the caring staff may be unaware of the attitudes and beliefs towards dying and grief of the major ethnic groups now in the United Kingdom (Speck, 1978); but kindness with an obvious concern to help are universal in dispersing emotional barriers providing there is a willingness to be helped.

The mutual acceptance with equanimity of the eventual death by the patient, the relatives, and the carers can only be achieved by a constant readiness on the part of the carers to identify and deal with the provoking physical, emotional, and social factors that otherwise produce disharmony, distrust, and despair. Failure to anticipate and deal with these problems effectively can precipitate resentment and misinterpretation. Medicolegal complications may then become an inevitable part of a pathological bereavement. The determinants of grief and how to help the bereaved have been well described elsewhere (Parkes, 1980).

CARING FOR THE CARERS

As dying patients become weaker many prefer to be propped up in bed. To prevent undue anxiety it is important to ensure visiting relatives and friends are aware of the practical significance of any perceptual problems experienced by the patient including hemianopia, memory impairment, and confusion. Even when the patient is unconscious, relatives, friends, and team members too (particularly students) may need to be reminded that while every reasonable effort has been made to provide a good quality to the patient's life despite the final illness, a continuing positive effort is being made to ensure a comfortable end. Many relatives need someone to listen as their early grieving highlights some personal anxiety, a sense of guilt, or a feeling of frustration. The well-tuned ear of a nurse, doctor, social worker, and always the clerk who handles the details of death certificates and returns the deceased's belongings, can assist the relatives to come to terms with their loss.

The patient's general practitioner should be contacted by telephone or a reliable message left at his surgery as soon after the patient's death as is practicable.

The ward staff (especially student nurses) and other team members also have constant needs requiring careful attention. It should not be forgotten that caring for the elderly and particularly for many dying patients is a constant drain on the emotional resources of staff. This is especially true for those who have to work isolated in low-status institutions, with the chronic problems of overwork, poor staffing, and underfunding. Progressive disillusionment can lead to staff 'burn-out' (Edelwick and Brodsky, 1980), adding a further burden to the other team members. A mutual caring relationship – constantly supported by the team leader's reassurance and his constructive criticism when necessary – fosters the self-esteem and growth needs of the individual team members. It allows staff working for and caring for the elderly to develop confidence and job satisfaction. This positive team approach is reflected as much in the numbers of patients who die in comfort as the numbers of patients who are discharged home. Every individual within the team has to be encouraged to make their own effort to supply their own needs – or to seek help from more experienced staff as necessary. It is important that all staff are aware that this attitude of 'caring for the carers' is quietly surrounding the team at work.

REFERENCES

Baines, M. (1978). 'Control of other symptoms', in *The Management of Terminal Disease*, (Ed. C. M. Saunders), p. 101, Arnold, London.

Baines, M. (1981). 'Drug control of common symptoms', *World Med.*, **17**, No. 4, 47–60.

British National Formulary (1981). *Prescriptions for Controlled Drugs,* No. 1, p. 15, British Medical Association and the Pharmaceutical Society of Great Britain, London.

De Beauvoir, S. (1980). *A Very Easy Death*, p. 25, Penguin, Middlesex.

Edelwich, J., and Brodsky, A. (1980). *Burn-out: Stages of Disillusionment in the Helping Professions*, Human Sciences Press, London.

Hinton, J. (1979). *Dying*, p. 126, Penguin, Middlesex.

Kübler-Ross, E. (1977). *On Death and Dying*, Tavistock Publications, London.

Lamerton, R. (1973). *Care of the Dying*, p. 45, Priory Press, London.

Parkes, C. M. (1980). *Bereavement: Studies of Grief in Adult Life*, Penguin, Middlesex.

Saunders, C. M. (1978). *The Management of Terminal Disease*, Arnold, London.

Sampson, C. (1982). *The Neglected Religious and Cultural Factors in the Care of Patients*, McGraw-Hill, Maidenhead.

Speck, P. W. (1978). 'Cultural factors and grief', in *Loss and Grief in Medicine*, pp. 113–148, Baillière Tindall, London.

Symmers, W. St C. (1968). 'Not allowed to die', *Br. Med. J.*, **1**, 442.

Twycross, R. G. (1977). 'Choice of strong analgesic in terminal cancer: diamorphine or morphine?', *Pain*, **3**, 93–104.

Williamson, J. (1981). 'Doctors and the elderly dying patient', *Geriat. Med.*, **11**, Part 8, 6–8.

Index